Current Pediatric Diagnosis & Treatment 1987

Ninth Edition

Current Pediatric Diagnosis & Treatment 1987

Edited By

C. HENRY KEMPE, MD
Professor of Pediatrics and Microbiology
University of Colorado School of Medicine (Denver)

HENRY K. SILVER, MD
Professor of Pediatrics
University of Colorado School of Medicine (Denver)

DONOUGH O'BRIEN, MD
Professor of Pediatrics
University of Colorado School of Medicine (Denver)

VINCENT A. FULGINITI, MD
Professor of Pediatrics and Vice Dean
University of Arizona College of Medicine (Tucson)

and Associate Authors

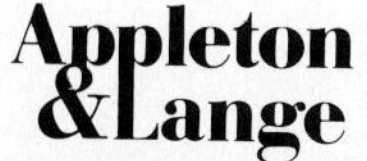

Norwalk, Connecticut/Los Altos, California

0-8385-1414-6

Notice: Our knowledge in clinical sciences is constantly changing. As new information becomes available, changes in treatment and in the use of drugs become necessary. The authors and the publisher of this volume have taken care to make certain that the doses of drugs and schedules of treatment are correct and compatible with the standards generally accepted at the time of publication. The reader is advised to consult carefully the instruction and information material included in the package insert of each drug or therapeutic agent before administration. This advice is especially important when using new or infrequently used drugs.

88 89 90 / 5 4 3

Prentice-Hall of Australia, Pty. Ltd., Sydney
Prentice-Hall Canada, Inc.
Prentice-Hall Hispanoamericana, S.A., Mexico
Prentice-Hall of India Private Limited, New Delhi
Prentice-Hall International (UK) Limited, London
Prentice-Hall of Japan, Inc., Tokyo
Prentice-Hall of Southeast Asia (Pte.) Ltd., Singapore
Whitehall Books Ltd., Wellington, New Zealand
Editora Prentice-Hall do Brasil Ltda., Rio de Janeiro

Spanish Edition: Editorial El Manual Moderno, S.A. de C.V., Av. Sonora 206, Col. Hipodromo, 06100-Mexico, D.F.
Serbo-Croatian Edition: Savremena Administracija, Crnotravska 7–9, 11100 Belgrade, Yugoslavia
Polish Edition: Panstwowy Zaklad Wydawnictw Lekarskich, P.O. Box 379, 00–950 Warsaw 1, Poland
Italian Edition: Piccin Nuova Libraria, S.p.A., Via Altinate, 107, 35121 Padua, Italy
Portuguese Edition: Editora Guanabara Koogan S.A., Travessa do Ouvidor, 11, 20,040 Rio de Janeiro—RJ, Brazil

ISBN: 0-8385-1414-6

PRINTED IN THE UNITED STATES OF AMERICA

Table of Contents

Authors

Roger M. Barkin, MD, MPH
Emergencies & Accidents
Associate Professor of Pediatrics and Surgery, University of Colorado School of Medicine.

Frederick C. Battaglia, MD
The Newborn Infant
Professor and Chairman of Department of Pediatrics, University of Colorado School of Medicine.

Gary K. Belanger, DDS
Teeth
Associate Professor and Chairman, Division of Pediatric Dentistry, University of Colorado School of Dentistry.

Stephen Berman, MD
Ear, Nose, & Throat
Associate Professor of Pediatrics and Director of Ambulatory Care Center, University of Colorado School of Medicine.

Florence B. Blager, PhD
Development of Speech & Language
Associate Professor of Otolaryngology and Psychiatry, University of Colorado School of Medicine.

John G. Brooks, MD
Respiratory Tract & Mediastinum
Associate Professor of Pediatrics, Director of Pediatric Pulmonary Division, and Director of Pediatric Intensive Care Unit, University of Rochester School of Medicine and Dentistry.

John D. Burrington, MD
Emergencies & Accidents
Clinical Professor of Surgery, University of Colorado School of Medicine; Attending Pediatric Surgeon, The Children's Hospital, Denver.

Bonnie W. Camp, MD, PhD
Developmental Disorders
Professor of Pediatrics and Psychiatry, University of Colorado School of Medicine.

Paul S. Casamassimo, DDS, MS
Teeth
Associate Professor and Chairman, Department of Growth and Development, University of Colorado School of Dentistry.

Robert E. Eilert, MD
Orthopedics
Chairman, Department of Orthopedic Surgery, The Children's Hospital, Denver; and Assistant Clinical Professor of Orthopedic Surgery, University of Colorado School of Medicine.

Philip P. Ellis, MD
Eye
Professor and Chairman, Department of Ophthalmology, University of Colorado School of Medicine.

William K. Frankenburg, MD
Development; Developmental Screening
Professor of Pediatrics and Preventive Medicine, University of Colorado School of Medicine.

Vincent A. Fulginiti, MD
Immunization; Infections: Viral & Rickettsial; Infections: Mycotic
Professor of Pediatrics and Vice Dean, University of Arizona College of Medicine, Tucson.

John H. Githens, MD
Hematologic Disorders
Professor Emeritus of Pediatrics and Director of Sickle Cell Treatment and Research Center, University of Colorado School of Medicine.

Benjamin A. Gitterman, MD
History & Physical Examination
Assistant Professor of Pediatrics, University of Colorado School of Medicine.

Stephen I. Goodman, MD
Genetic & Chromosomal Disorders, Including Inborn Errors of Metabolism
Professor of Pediatrics, University of Colorado School of Medicine.

Ronald W. Gotlin, MD
Endocrine Disorders; Diagnostic & Therapeutic Procedures
Associate Professor of Pediatrics and Section Head of Pediatric Endocrinology, University of Colorado School of Medicine.

Donald E. Greydanus, MD
Adolescence
Director of Adolescent Medical Program, Raymond Blank Memorial Hospital for Children, Iowa Methodist Center, Des Moines.

K. Michael Hambidge, MD, FRCP
Normal Childhood Nutrition & Its Disorders
Professor of Pediatrics and Director of Pediatric Clinical Research Center, University of Colorado School of Medicine.

Keith B. Hammond, MS, FIMLS
Normal & Therapeutic Biochemical & Hematologic Values
Senior Instructor of Pediatrics and Director of Pediatric Microchemistry Laboratories, University of Colorado School of Medicine.

William E. Hathaway, MD
Hematologic Disorders
Professor of Pediatrics, University of Colorado School of Medicine.

Anthony R. Hayward, MD, PhD
Immunodeficiency
Professor of Pediatrics and Medicine, University of Colorado School of Medicine.

J. Roger Hollister, MD
Rheumatic Diseases
Associate Professor of Pediatrics and Medicine, University of Colorado School of Medicine; Senior Staff Physician, Department of Pediatrics, National Jewish Hospital and Research Center, Denver.

Richard B. Johnston, Jr., MD
Immunodeficiency
Professor and Chairman of Pediatrics, University of Pennsylvania School of Medicine; Physician-in-Chief, The Children's Hospital of Philadelphia.

C. Henry Kempe, MD*
Anti-infective Chemotherapeutic Agents & Antibiotic Drugs
Professor of Pediatrics and Microbiology, University of Colorado School of Medicine.

Ruth S. Kempe, MD
Personality Development; Child Abuse & Neglect
Associate Professor of Psychiatry and Pediatrics, University of Colorado School of Medicine.

Anthony J. Kisley, MD
Psychosocial Aspects of Pediatrics & Psychiatric Disorders
Assistant Clinical Professor of Psychiatry, University of Colorado School of Medicine.

Georgeanna J. Klingensmith, MD
Endocrine Disorders
Associate Professor of Pediatrics, University of Colorado School of Medicine; Chief of Department of Endocrinology and Metabolism, The Children's Hospital, Denver.

Beverly L. Koops, MD
The Newborn Infant
Professor and Chairman of Pediatrics, Texas A&M School of Medicine; Neonatologist, Scott and White Memorial Hospital, Temple, Texas.

Brian A. Lauer, MD
Infections: Bacterial & Spirochetal
Associate Professor of Pediatrics and Medicine (Infectious Diseases), Assistant Director of Diagnostic Virology Laboratory, and Assistant Director of Clinical Microbiology Laboratory, University of Colorado School of Medicine.

Gary M. Lum, MD
Kidney & Urinary Tract
Associate Professor of Pediatrics and Medicine (Nephrology) and Director of Pediatric Dialysis, University of Colorado School of Medicine.

David K. Manchester, MD
The Dysmorphic Infant
Associate Professor of Pediatrics and Pharmacology, University of Colorado School of Medicine.

Elizabeth R. McAnarney, MD
Adolescence
Associate Professor of Pediatrics and Director, Division of Biosocial Pediatrics and Adolescent Medicine, University of Rochester, New York.

Edward R. B. McCabe, MD, PhD
Genetic & Chromosomal Disorders, Including Inborn Errors of Metabolism
Associate Professor of Molecular Genetics and Pediatrics and Director of the Robert J. Kleberg, Jr., Clinical Center in the Institute for Molecular Genetics, Baylor College of Medicine, Houston.

Kenneth McIntosh, MD
Infections: Bacterial & Spirochetal
Professor of Pediatrics and Chief of Clinical Infectious Diseases, Children's Hospital, Boston.

Paul G. Moe, MD
Neurologic & Muscular Disorders
Associate Professor of Pediatrics and Neurology, University of Colorado School of Medicine; Director of Neurology and EEG Laboratory, The Children's Hospital, Denver.

Gerhard Nellhaus, MD
Neurologic & Muscular Disorders
Associate Clinical Professor of Pediatrics and Neurology, University of California, Davis, Sacramento Medical Center; Neurologist, Napa State Hospital, Napa, California.

Donough O'Brien, MD, FRCP
Normal Childhood Nutrition & Its Disorders; Kidney & Urinary Tract; Diabetes Medicine; Fluid & Electrolyte Therapy; Normal & Therapeutic Biochemical & Hematologic Values
Professor of Pediatrics and Director of Barbara Davis Center for Childhood Diabetes, University of Colorado School of Medicine.

David S. Pearlman, MD
Allergic Disorders
Clinical Professor of Pediatrics, University of Colorado School of Medicine; Attending Allergist, Division of Pediatrics, National Jewish Center for Immunology and Respiratory Medicine, Denver.

* Deceased.

Robert G. Peterson, MD, PhD
Drug Therapy
Associate Professor of Pediatrics and Pharmacology, University of Ottawa; Medical Director, Poison Information Centre, Children's Hospital of Eastern Ontario, Canada.

Dane G. Prugh, MD
Psychosocial Aspects of Pediatrics & Psychiatric Disorders
Professor Emeritus of Psychiatry and Pediatrics, University of Colorado School of Medicine.

C. George Ray, MD
Anti-infective Chemotherapeutic Agents & Antibiotic Drugs
Professor of Pathology and Pediatrics, University of Arizona College of Medicine, Tucson.

L. Barth Reller, MD, DTM&H
Infections: Parasitic
Professor of Medicine and Director of Clinical Microbiology, University of Colorado School of Medicine.

Arthur Robinson, MD
Genetic & Chromosomal Disorders, Including Inborn Errors of Metabolism
Professor of Biochemistry, Biophysics, and Genetics and Professor of Pediatrics, University of Colorado School of Medicine; Director of Cytogenetics, National Jewish Hospital and Research Center, Denver.

Claude C. Roy, MD
Gastrointestinal Tract
Chief, Gastroenterology Unit, Hôpital Ste-Justine, University of Montreal.

Barry H. Rumack, MD
Poisoning; Drug Therapy
Professor of Pediatrics, University of Colorado School of Medicine; Director of Rocky Mountain Poison Center, Denver General Hospital.

Barton D. Schmitt, MD
Ambulatory Pediatrics; Ear, Nose, & Throat
Associate Professor of Pediatrics, University of Colorado School of Medicine; and Director of Consultative Services, The Children's Hospital, Denver.

Craig Schramm, MD
Diagnostic & Therapeutic Procedures
Pediatric Pulmonary Fellow, University of Colorado School of Medicine.

Ziad M. Shehab, MD
Anti-infective Chemotherapeutic Agents & Antibiotic Drugs
Assistant Professor of Pediatrics, University of Arizona College of Medicine, Tucson.

Henry K. Silver, MD
History & Physical Examination; Growth & Development; Endocrine Disorders; Diagnostic & Therapeutic Procedures; Drug Therapy
Professor of Pediatrics & Associate Dean, University of Colorado School of Medicine.

Arnold Silverman, MD
Gastrointestinal Tract; Liver & Pancreas
Professor of Pediatrics, University of Colorado School of Medicine; Director of Pediatrics, Denver General Hospital.

David A. Stumpf, MD, PhD
Neurologic & Muscular Disorders
Children's Memorial Hospital, Chicago.

James K. Todd, MD
Kidney & Urinary Tract
Professor of Pediatrics and Microbiology-Immunology, University of Colorado School of Medicine; Director of Infectious Diseases, The Children's Hospital, Denver.

David G. Tubergen, MD
Neoplastic Diseases
Professor of Pediatrics, University of Colorado School of Medicine; Medical Director, The Children's Hospital, Denver.

William L. Weston, MD
Skin
Professor of Dermatology and Pediatrics and Chairman of the Department of Dermatology, University of Colorado School of Medicine.

James W. Wiggins, Jr., MD
Cardiovascular Diseases
Assistant Professor of Pediatrics and Cardiology, University of Colorado School of Medicine.

Robert R. Wolfe, MD
Cardiovascular Diseases
Associate Professor of Pediatrics and Director of Pediatric Cardiology, University of Colorado School of Medicine.

Anne S. Yeager, MD*
Anti-infective Chemotherapeutic Agents & Antibiotic Drugs
Associate Professor of Pediatrics, Division of Pediatric Infectious Diseases, Stanford University Medical Center.

Preface

The ninth edition of *Current Pediatric Diagnosis & Treatment* features practical, up-to-date information on the care of children from infancy through adolescence. *CPDT* emphasizes the clinical aspects of pediatric care while also covering the important underlying principles.

Students will find that *CPDT* serves as an authoritative introduction to pediatrics and as an excellent source for reference and review. Interns and residents will appreciate the concise descriptions of diseases and diagnostic procedures. Pediatricians, family practitioners, nurses, and other health care providers will find *CPDT* a useful reference work on all aspects of pediatric care.

Coverage

Thirty-nine chapters cover a wide range of topics, including growth and development of the healthy child, preventive medicine, and diagnosis and treatment of specific pediatric disorders. Tables and figures offer ready access to important information such as anti-infective agents, drug dosages, immunization schedules, and developmental screening tests. The last chapter serves as a handy guide to normal and therapeutic laboratory values.

New Features

The ninth edition of *Current Pediatric Diagnosis & Treatment* includes the following new features:

1. Treatment sections revised to reflect the latest medical advances and recommendations.
2. Revised chapters on anti-infective and other pharmacologic agents.
3. Revised chapter on immunizations, including current recommendations for use of *Haemophilus influenzae* type b vaccine.
4. Updated emergency procedures and management of poisoning.
5. Practical information on dental problems, including the current status of orthodontia and prevention of dental caries.
6. Revised sections on acute and serous otitis media, child abuse and neglect, pharmacologic management of asthma and other allergic disorders, and diagnostic uses of recombinant DNA technology.

Acknowledgments

We wish to thank the authors who contributed to this edition and to reaffirm our debt of gratitude to all whose work on previous editions has carried over into this one. Dr C. Henry Kempe's many contributions to this book will be an integral part of it for as long as it continues to be published. Succeeding him as one of the editors is Dr Vincent A. Fulginiti, editor-in-chief of *American Journal of Diseases of Children* and former chairman of the "Red Book" Committee (Committee on Infectious Diseases) of the American Academy of Pediatrics.

We wish to express our thanks to our readers throughout the world who have supplied us with useful suggestions. Comments and recommendations for future editions can be sent directly to us or in care of Lange Medical Publications, Drawer L, Los Altos, CA 94023.

CPDT has been translated into Spanish, Italian, Polish, Serbo-Croatian, and Portuguese.

C. Henry Kempe, MD
Henry Silver, MD
Donough O'Brien, MD
Vincent A. Fulginiti, MD

NOTICE

Not all of the drugs mentioned in this book have been approved by the FDA for use in infants or in children under age 6 or age 12. Such drugs should not be used if effective alternatives are available; they may be used if no effective alternatives are available or if the known risk of toxicity of alternative drugs or the risk of nontreatment is outweighed by the probable advantages of treatment.

Because of the possibility of an error in the article or book from which a particular drug dosage is obtained, or an error appearing in the text of this book, our readers are urged to consult appropriate references, including the manufacturer's package insert, especially when prescribing new drugs or those with which they are not adequately familiar.

—The Editors

History & Physical Examination 1

Henry K. Silver, MD, & Benjamin A. Gitterman, MD

HISTORY

General Considerations in Taking the History

For many pediatric problems, the history is the most important single factor in making a proper assessment.

A. Interpretation of History: The presenting complaint as given by the informant may be a minor part of the problem. One should be prepared to go on, if necessary, to a subsequent phase of the interview, which may have little apparent relationship to the complaint as initially presented.

B. Source of History: The history should be obtained from the mother or from whoever is responsible for the care of the child. Much valuable information can be obtained also from the child, and for this reason the child should be encouraged to contribute. Adolescents should be interviewed, and part of the interview should be without the parents present, since important information is often deliberately withheld in the presence of parents.

C. Direction of Questioning: Allow the informant to present the problem as he or she sees it; then fill in with necessary past and family history and pertinent information. (See also Chapter 24.) The record should include whatever may be disclosed concerning the parents' temperaments, attitudes, and methods of rearing children.

Questions should not be prying, especially about subjects likely to be associated with feelings of guilt or shame; however, the informant should be allowed to volunteer information of this nature when prepared to do so.

D. Recorded History: The history should be a detailed, clear, and chronologic record of significant information. It should include the parents' interpretation of the present difficulty and should indicate the results they expect from consultation.

E. Psychotherapeutic Effects: In many cases, the interview and history taking is the first stage in the psychotherapeutic management of the patient and the parents. The physician should introduce himself or herself and should refer often to the parents and patient by name. Avoid being hurried or perfunctory. Avoid technical or ambiguous language without being condescending. Recognize that socioeconomic and cultural background, education, and knowledge influence physician-patient communication.

During or after the interview, it is useful and frequently desirable for the patient and parents to have some idea of the health provider's impressions. Some idea of the reasoning behind diagnostic and therapeutic considerations and of the possible course of the child's condition should be conveyed. This can decrease anxiety and improve the interactions between family and provider.

HISTORY OUTLINE: GENERAL

The following outline should be modified and adapted as appropriate for the age and sex of the child and the reason for the visit to the physician:

(1) Name, address, and telephone number; sex; date and place of birth; race, religion, and nationality; referred by whom; father's and mother's names, occupations, and business telephone numbers.

(2) Date of this visit.

(3) Hospital or case number.

(4) Previous entries: Dates, diagnoses, therapy, other data.

(5) Summary of correspondence or other information from physicians, schools, etc.

Chief Complaint (CC)

Patient's or informant's own brief account of the complaint and its duration.

Present Illness (PI) (or Interval History)

(1) When was the patient last entirely well?

(2) How and when did the disturbance start?

(3) Health immediately before the illness.

(4) Progress of disease; order and date of onset of new symptoms.

(5) Specific symptoms and physical signs that may have developed.

(6) Pertinent negative data obtained by direct questioning.

(7) Aggravating and alleviating factors.

(8) Significant medical attention and medications given and over what period.

(9) Use of "home remedies," if any.

(10) In acute infections, statement of type and degree of exposure and interval since exposure.

(11) For the well child, determine factors of significance and general condition since last visit.

(12) Examiner's opinion about the reliability of the informant.

Previous Health

A. Antenatal: Health of mother during pregnancy. Medical supervision; diet; infections (eg, rubella) and other illnesses; vomiting, preeclampsia-eclampsia, and other complications; Rh typing and serology; pelvimetry, medications, x-ray procedures, amniocentesis.

B. Natal: Duration of pregnancy, birth weight, kind and duration of labor, type of delivery, sedation and anesthesia (if known), state of infant at birth, resuscitation required, onset of respiration, first cry.

C. Neonatal: Apgar score, color (cyanosis, pallor, jaundice), cry, twitchings, excessive mucus, paralysis, convulsions, fever, hemorrhage, congenital abnormalities, birth injury. Difficulty in sucking, rashes, excessive weight loss, feeding difficulties. Length of hospital stay.

Development

(1) First raised head, rolled over, sat alone, pulled up, walked with help, walked alone, talked (meaningful words; sentences).

(2) Urinary continence during night; during day.

(3) Control of feces.

(4) Comparison of development with that of siblings and parents.

(5) Any period of failure to grow or unusual growth.

(6) School grade, quality of work.

Nutrition

A. Breast or Formula: Type, duration, major formula changes, time of weaning, difficulties.

B. Vitamin Supplements: Type, when started, amount, duration.

C. "Solid" Foods: When introduced, how taken, types, family dietary habits (eg, vegetarian).

D. Appetite: Food likes and dislikes, idiosyncrasies or allergies, reaction of child to eating.

Illnesses

A. Infections: Age, types, number, severity.

B. Contagious Diseases: Age, complications following measles, rubella, chickenpox, mumps, pertussis, diphtheria, scarlet fever.

C. Others.

Immunizations & Tests

Indicate type, number, reactions, age of child.

A. Inoculations: Diphtheria, tetanus, pertussis, measles, poliomyelitis, typhoid, mumps, others.

B. Oral Immunizations: Poliomyelitis.

C. Recall Immunizations: "Boosters."

D. Serum Injections: Passive immunizations.

E. Tests: Tuberculin, Schick, serology, others.

Operations

Type, age, complications; reasons for operations; apparent response of child.

Accidents & Injuries

Nature, severity, sequelae.

Medications

Allergies to medications. Chronic use of medications.

Family History

(1) Father and mother (age and condition of health). What sort of people do the parents characterize themselves as being?

(2) Marital relationships. Little information should be sought at first interview; most information will be obtained indirectly.

(3) Siblings. Age, condition of health, significant previous illnesses and problems.

(4) Stillbirths, miscarriages, abortions; age at death and cause of death of immediate members of family.

(5) Tuberculosis, allergy, blood dyscrasias, mental health impairment, neurologic disease, diabetes, cardiovascular diseases, kidney disease, rheumatic fever, neoplastic diseases, congenital abnormalities, cancer,convulsive disorders, others.

(6) Health of contacts.

Personality History

A. Relations With Other Children: Independent or clinging to mother; negativistic, shy, submissive; separation from parents; hobbies; easy or difficult to get along with. How does child relate to others? Physical deformities affecting personality.

B. School Progress: Class, grades, nursery school, special aptitudes, reaction to school.

Social History

A. Family: Income; home (size, number of rooms, living conditions, sleeping facilities), type of neighborhood, access to playground. Localities in which patient has lived. Who cares for patient if both parents work outside the home? Who else lives in the home besides immediate family?

B. Family Support Systems: Relatives or nearby close friends who provide support and give parents free time away from child.

C. School: Public or private, overcrowded, type of students.

D. Insurance: Private or public health insurance?

Habits

A. Eating: Appetite, food dislikes, how fed, attitudes of child and parents toward eating.

B. Sleeping: Hours, disturbances, snoring, restlessness, dreaming, nightmares.

C. Recreation: Exercise and play.

D. Elimination: Urinary, bowel.

E. Disturbances: Excessive bed-wetting, masturbation, thumb-sucking, nail-biting, breath-holding, temper tantrums, tics, nervousness, undue thirst, others. Similar disturbances among members of family.

F. Adolescent Habits: Adolescents should be asked about smoking, alcohol or substance abuse, sexual activity, and use of birth control measures. These questions should be asked routinely when appropriate to age.

G. Dental Hygiene: Self-care habits (brushing, flossing), most recent preventive examination.

H. Safety Habits of Family: Use of auto restraint for infant or child, carefully stored medicines and toxic substances, covered electrical outlets, other age-appropriate safety measures.

System Review

A. Ears, Nose, and Throat: Frequent colds, sore throat, sneezing, stuffy nose, epistaxis, discharge, postnasal drip, mouth breathing, snoring, adenitis, otitis, hearing problems. When was the last hearing test?

B. Teeth: Age of eruption of deciduous and permanent; number at 1 year; comparison with siblings.

C. Cardiorespiratory System: Frequency and nature of disturbances. Dyspnea, chest pain, cough, sputum, wheeze, expectoration, cyanosis, edema, syncope, tachycardia.

D. Gastrointestinal System: Vomiting, diarrhea, constipation, type of stools, abdominal pain or discomfort, jaundice.

E. Genitourinary System: Enuresis, dysuria, frequency, polyuria, pyuria, hematuria, character of stream, vaginal discharge, menstrual history, bladder control, abnormalities of penis or testes.

F. Neuromuscular System: Headache, nervousness, dizziness, tingling, convulsions, habit spasms, ataxia, muscle or joint pains, postural deformities, exercise tolerance, gait.

G. Endocrine System: Disturbances of growth, excessive fluid intake, polyphagia, goiter, thyroid disease.

H. Special Senses.

I. General Review: Unusual weight gain or loss, fatigue, skin color and texture, abnormalities of skin, temperature sensitivity, mentality. Pattern of growth (record previous heights and weights on appropriate graphs). Time and pattern of pubescence.

The Health Record

Every patient should have a comprehensive medical and health record containing all pertinent information. The parents should be given a summary of this record (including data regarding illnesses, operations, idiosyncrasies, sensitivities, heights, weights, special medications, and immunizations).

PHYSICAL EXAMINATION

Every child should receive a complete systematic examination at regular intervals. One should not restrict the examination to those portions of the body considered to be involved on the basis of the presenting complaint.

Approaching the Child

Adequate time should be spent in allowing the child and the examiner to become acquainted. The child should be treated as an individual whose feelings and sensibilities are well developed, and the examiner's conduct should be appropriate to the age of the child. A friendly manner, quiet voice, and a slow and easy approach will help to facilitate the examination. If the examiner is not able to establish a friendly relationship but feels that it is important to proceed with the examination, it should be done in an orderly, systematic manner in the hope that the child will then accept the inevitable.

The examiner's hands should be washed in warm water before the examination begins.

Observing the Child

Although the very young child may not be able to talk, much information can be gained by being observant and receptive. The total evaluation of the child should include impressions obtained from the time the child first enters the room—ie, not just while on the examining table. This is also the best time to assess parent-child interaction, which should be recorded. In general, more information is obtained by careful inspection than by any other method of examination.

Holding the Child for Examination

A. Before Age 6 Months: The examining table is usually well tolerated.

B. Age 6 Months to 3–4 Years: Most of the examination can be performed while the child is held in the parent's lap or over the shoulder. Certain parts of the examination can sometimes be done more easily with the child prone or held against the parent so that the child does not see the examiner.

Removal of Clothing

Clothes should be removed gradually to prevent chilling and to avoid resistance from a shy child. It saves time and avoids creating unpleasant associations with the doctor in the child's mind if the parent undresses the child and takes the temperature. The child's feelings of modesty should be respected to the extent possible.

Sequence of Examination

It is usually best to begin examination of a young child with an area unlikely to be associated with pain or discomfort. The ears and throat should usually be examined last. The examiner should develop a regular sequence of examination that can be adapted to special circumstances as required.

Painful Procedures

Before performing a disagreeable, painful, or upsetting examination, the examiner should tell the child (1) what is likely to happen and how the child can assist, (2) that the examination is necessary, and (3) that it will be performed as rapidly and as painlessly as possible.

GENERAL PHYSICAL EXAMINATION

Record the temperature, pulse rate, and respiratory rate (TPR); blood pressure; and weight and height. Weight should be measured at each visit, height at monthly intervals during the first year, quarterly intervals in the second year, and twice a year thereafter. Height, weight, and head circumference should be compared with standard charts and the approximate percentiles recorded. The blood pressure should also be compared with standard percentiles. Multiple measurements at intervals are of much greater value than single ones, since they give information regarding pattern of growth. (See also Chapter 2.)

Rectal Temperatures

After the first month of life, the temperature should be taken by rectum (except for routine temperatures in premature infants, in whom axillary temperatures are sufficiently accurate). The child should be laid face down across the parent's lap and held firmly with the parent's left forearm placed flat across the child's back; the parent can separate the buttocks with the left thumb and index finger and insert the lubricated thermometer with the right hand.

Rectal temperature may be 1 °F higher than oral temperature. A rectal temperature up to 37.8 °C (100 °F) may be considered normal in a child.

Apprehension and activity may cause slight fever.

General Appearance

Does the child appear well or ill? Degree of prostration; degree of cooperation; state of comfort, nutrition, and consciousness; abnormalities; gait, posture, and coordination; estimate of intelligence; reaction to parents, physician, and examination; nature of cry and degree of activity; facies and facial expression.

Skin

Color (cyanosis, jaundice, pallor, erythema), texture, eruptions, hydration, edema, hemorrhagic manifestations, scars, dilated vessels and direction of blood flow, hemangiomas, café au lait areas and nevi, mongolian (blue-black) spots, pigmentation, turgor, elasticity, subcutaneous nodules, sensitivity, hair distribution and character, and desquamation.

Practical notes:

(1) Loss of turgor, especially of the calf muscles and skin over the abdomen, is evidence of dehydration.

(2) The soles and palms are often bluish and cold in early infancy; this is of no significance.

(3) The degree of anemia cannot be determined reliably by inspection, since pallor (even in the newborn) may be normal and not due to anemia.

(4) To demonstrate pitting edema in a child, it may be necessary to exert prolonged pressure.

(5) A few small pigmented nevi are commonly found, particularly in older children.

(6) Spider nevi occur in about one-sixth of children under 5 years of age and almost half of older children.

(7) Mongolian spots (large, flat black or blue-black areas) are frequently present over the lower back and buttocks; they have no pathologic significance.

(8) Cyanosis will not be evident unless at least 5 g of reduced hemoglobin is present; therefore, it develops less easily in an anemic child.

(9) Carotenemic pigmentation is usually most prominent over the palms and soles and around the nose and spares the conjunctiva.

(10) Striae and wrinkling may indicate rapid weight gain or loss.

Lymph Nodes

Location, size, sensitivity, mobility, consistency. One should routinely attempt to palpate suboccipital, preauricular, anterior cervical, posterior cervical, submaxillary, sublingual, axillary, epitrochlear, and inguinal lymph nodes.

Practical notes:

(1) Enlargement of the lymph nodes occurs much more readily in children than in adults.

(2) Small inguinal lymph nodes are palpable in almost all healthy young children. Small, mobile, nontender shotty nodes are commonly found as residua of previous infection.

Head

Size, shape, circumference, asymmetry, cephalhematoma, bosses, craniotabes, control, molding, bruit, fontanelles (size, tension, number, abnormally late or early closure), sutures, dilated veins, scalp, hair (texture, distribution, parasites), face, transillumination.

Practical notes:

(1) The head is measured at its greatest circumference; this is usually at the mid forehead anteriorly and around to the most prominent portion of the occiput posteriorly. The ratio of head circumference to circumference of the chest or abdomen is usually of little value.

(2) Fontanelle tension is best determined with the quiet child in the sitting position.

(3) Slight pulsations over the anterior fontanelle may occur in normal infants.

(4) Although bruits may be heard over the temporal areas in normal children, the possibility of an existing abnormality should not be overlooked.

(5) Craniotabes may be found in the normal newborn infant (especially the premature) and for the first 2–4 months.

(6) A positive Macewen sign ("cracked pot" sound when skull is percussed with one finger) may be present normally as long as the fontanelles are open.

(7) Transillumination of the skull can be performed using a flashlight with a sponge rubber collar so that it forms a tight fit when held against the head.

Face

Symmetry, paralysis, distance between nose and mouth, depth of nasolabial folds, bridge of nose, distribution of hair, size of mandible, swellings, hypertelorism, Chvostek's sign, tenderness over sinuses.

Eyes

Photophobia, visual acuity, muscular control and conjugate gaze, nystagmus, mongolian slant, Brushfield's spots, epicanthic folds, lacrimation, discharge, lids, exophthalmos or enophthalmos, conjunctiva, pupils (size, shape, and reaction to light and accommodation), iris (color), media (corneal opacities, cataracts), fundi, visual fields (in older children).

Practical notes:

(1) Newborn infants usually will open their eyes if placed prone, supported with one hand on the abdomen, and lifted over the examiner's head.

(2) Not infrequently, one pupil is normally larger than the other. This sometimes occurs only in bright or in subdued light.

(3) The fundi should be examined with every complete physical examination.

(4) Dilation of pupils may be necessary for adequate visualization of the eyes.

(5) A mild degree of strabismus may be present during the first 6 months of life but should be considered abnormal after that time.

(6) To test for strabismus in the very young or uncooperative child, note where a distant source of light is reflected from the surface of the eyes; the reflection should appear on corresponding portions of the 2 eyes (see Fig 11–2).

(7) Small areas of capillary dilatation are commonly present on the eyelids of normal newborns.

(8) Most infants produce visible tears during the first few days of life.

Nose

Exterior, shape, mucosa, patency, discharge, bleeding, pressure over sinuses, flaring of nostrils, septum.

Mouth

Lips (thinness, downturning, fissures, color, cleft), teeth (number, position, caries, mottling, discoloration, notching, malocclusion or malalignment), mucosa (color, redness of Stensen's duct, enanthems, Bohn's nodules, Epstein's pearls), gums, palate, tongue, uvula, mouth breathing, geographic tongue (usually normal).

Practical note: If the tongue can be extended as far as the alveolar ridge, there will be no interference with nursing or speaking. Frenectomy is not a preventive measure for being "tongue-tied."

Throat

Tonsils (size, inflammation, exudate, crypts, inflamed anterior pillars), epiglottis, mucosa, hypertrophic lymphoid tissue, postnasal drip, voice (hoarseness, stridor, grunting, type of cry, speech).

Practical notes:

(1) It is advisable to examine the mouth before the throat. Permit the child to handle the tongue blade, nasal speculum, and flashlight in order to overcome fear of the instruments. Then ask the child to stick out the tongue and say "Ah," louder and louder. In some cases, this may allow an adequate examination. In others, a cooperative child may be asked to "pant like a puppy"; during this time, the tongue blade is applied firmly to the rear of the tongue. Gagging need not be elicited in order to obtain a satisfactory examination. In still other cases, it may be expedient to examine one side of the tongue at a time, pushing the base of the tongue to one side and then to the other. This may be less unpleasant and is less apt to cause gagging.

(2) Young children may have to be restrained to obtain an adequate throat examination. Eliciting a gag reflex may be necessary if the oral pharynx is to be adequately seen.

(3) The small child's head may be restrained satisfactorily by the parent's hands placed at the level of the child's elbows while the arms are held firmly against the sides of the child's head.

(4) A child old enough to sit up can be held erect in the parent's lap with the child's back against the parent's chest. Holding the child's hands against his or her groin or lower thighs will prevent slipping down. If the throat is to be examined in natural light, the parent faces the light. If artificial light and a head mirror are used, the light should be behind the parent's chair. In either case, the physician uses one hand to hold the patient's head in position and the other to manipulate the tongue blade.

(5) Young children seldom complain of sore throat even in the presence of significant infection of the pharynx and tonsils.

Ears

Pinnas (position, size), canals, tympanic membranes (landmarks, mobility, perforation, inflammation, discharge), mastoid tenderness and swelling, hearing.

Practical notes:

(1) A test for hearing is an important part of the physical examination of every infant and child. If a parent says that the infant is not hearing well, this

must be accepted and investigated until disproved.

(2) Examine the ears of all sick children.

(3) Before actually examining the ears, it is often helpful to place the speculum just within the canal, remove it and place it lightly in the other ear, remove it again, and proceed in this way from one ear to the other, gradually going farther and farther, until a satisfactory examination is completed.

(4) In examining the ears, as large a speculum as possible should be used and should be inserted no farther than necessary, both to avoid discomfort and to avoid pushing wax in front of the speculum so that it obscures the field. The otoscope should be held balanced in the hand by holding the handle at the end nearest the speculum. One finger should rest against the head to prevent injury resulting from sudden movement by the child.

(5) Pneumatic insufflation to test mobility of the tympanic membrane should be part of the examination.

(6) The child may be restrained most easily while lying on the abdomen.

(7) Low-set ears are present in a number of congenital syndromes, including several that are associated with mental retardation. The ears may be considered low-set if they are below a line drawn from the lateral angle of the eye to the external occipital protuberance.

(8) Congenital anomalies of the urinary tract are frequently associated with abnormalities of the pinnas.

(9) To examine the ears of an infant, it is usually necessary to pull the auricle backward and downward; in the older child, the external ear is pulled backward and upward.

Neck

Position (torticollis, opisthotonos, inability to support head, mobility), swelling, thyroid (size, contour, bruit, isthmus, nodules, tenderness), lymph nodes, veins, position of trachea, sternocleidomastoid (swelling, shortening), webbing, edema, auscultation, movement, tonic neck reflex.

Practical note: In the older child, the size and shape of the thyroid gland may be more clearly defined if the gland is palpated from behind.

Thorax

Shape and symmetry, veins, retractions and pulsations, beading, Harrison's groove, flaring of ribs, pigeon breast, funnel shape, size and position of nipples, breasts, length of sternum, intercostal and substernal retraction, asymmetry, scapulas, clavicles.

Practical notes:

(1) At puberty in normal children, one breast usually begins to develop before the other.

(2) In both sexes, tenderness of the breasts is relatively common.

(3) Gynecomastia is not uncommon in boys.

(4) Breast examination of the adolescent female should be routine. This is also a logical time to begin the promotion of self-examination of breasts.

Lungs

Type of breathing, dyspnea, prolongation of expiration, cough, expansion, fremitus, flatness or dullness to percussion, resonance, breath and voice sounds, rales, wheezing.

Practical notes:

(1) Breath sounds in infants and children normally are more intense and more bronchial, and expiration is more prolonged, than in adults.

(2) Most of the young child's respiratory excursion is produced by abdominal movement; there is very little intercostal motion.

(3) If one places the stethoscope over the mouth and subtracts the sounds heard by this route from the sounds heard through the chest wall, the difference usually represents the amount produced intrathoracically.

Heart

Location and intensity of apex beat, precordial bulging, pulsation of vessels, thrills, size, shape, auscultation (rate, rhythm, force, quality of sounds—compare with pulse as to rate and rhythm; friction rub—variation with pressure), murmurs (location, position in cycle, intensity, pitch, effect of change of position, transmission, effect of exercise).

Practical notes:

(1) Many children normally have sinus dysrhythmia. The child should be asked to take a deep breath to determine its effect on the rhythm.

(2) Extrasystoles are not uncommon in childhood.

(3) The heart should be examined with the child erect, recumbent, and turned to the left.

Abdomen

Size and contour, visible peristalsis, respiratory movements, veins (distention, direction of flow), umbilicus, hernia, musculature, tenderness and rigidity, tympany, shifting dullness, tenderness, rebound tenderness, pulsation, palpable organs or masses (size, shape, position, mobility), fluid wave, reflexes, femoral pulsations, bowel sounds.

Practical notes:

(1) The abdomen may be examined while the child is lying prone in the parent's lap, held over the shoulder, or seated on the examining table with the child's back to the physician. These positions may be particularly helpful where tenderness, rigidity, or a mass must be palpated. Examination of an infant may be easier if the child sucks at a "sugar tip" or nurses at a bottle.

(2) Light palpation, especially for the spleen, often will give more information than deep palpation.

(3) Umbilical hernias are common during the first 2 years of life. They usually disappear spontaneously.

Male Genitalia

Circumcision, meatal opening, hypospadias, phimosis, adherent foreskin, size of testes, cryptorchidism, scrotum, hydrocele, hernia, pubertal changes.

Practical notes:

(1) In examining a suspected case of cryptorchidism, palpation for the testicles should be done before the child has fully undressed or become chilled or had the cremasteric reflex stimulated. In some cases, examination while the child is in a hot bath may be helpful. The boy should also be examined while sitting in a chair holding his knees with his heels on the seat; the increased intra-abdominal pressure may push the testes into the scrotum.

(2) To examine for cryptorchidism, start above the inguinal canal and work downward to prevent pushing the testes up into the canal or abdomen.

(3) In the obese boy, the penis may be so obscured by fat as to appear abnormally small. If this fat is pushed back, a penis of normal size is usually found.

Female Genitalia

Vagina (imperforate, discharge, adhesions), hypertrophy of clitoris, pubertal changes.

Practical note: Digital or speculum examination is rarely done until after puberty.

Rectum & Anus

Irritation, fissures, prolapse, imperforate anus, muscle tone, character of stool, masses, tenderness, sensation.

Practical note: The rectal examination should be performed with the little finger (inserted slowly). Examine the stool on glove finger. Perform gross and microscopic examination, culture, and guaiac test as indicated.

Extremities

A. General: Deformity, hemiatrophy, bowleg (common in infancy), knock-knee (common after age 2 years), paralysis, edema, coldness, posture, gait, stance, asymmetry.

B. Joints: Swelling, redness, pain, limitation, tenderness, motion, rheumatic nodules, carrying angle of elbows, tibial torsion.

C. Hands and Feet: Extra digits, clubbing, simian lines, curvature of little finger, deformity of nails, splinter hemorrhages, flatfeet (feet commonly appear flat during first 2 years), abnormalities of feet, dermatoglyphics, width of thumbs and big toes, syndactyly, length of various segments, dimpling of dorsa, temperature.

D. Peripheral Vessels: Presence, absence, or diminution of arterial pulses.

Spine & Back

Posture, curvatures, rigidity, webbed neck, spina bifida, pilonidal dimple or cyst, tufts of hair, mobility, mongolian spot, tenderness over spine, pelvis, or kidneys.

Neurologic Examination (After Vazuka)

A. Cerebral Function: General behavior, level of consciousness, intelligence, emotional status, memory, orientation, illusions, hallucinations, cortical sensory interpretation, cortical motor integration, ability to understand and communicate, auditory-verbal and visual-verbal comprehension, recognition of visual object, speech, ability to write, performance of skilled motor acts.

B. Cranial Nerves:

1. I (olfactory)—Identification of odors, disorders of smell.

2. II (optic)—Distant and near visual acuity, retina, visual fields, ophthalmoscopic examination.

3. III (oculomotor), IV (trochlear), and VI (abducens)—Ocular movements, strabismus, ptosis, dilatation of pupil, nystagmus, pupillary accommodation, pupillary light reflexes.

4. V (trigeminal)—Sensation of face, corneal reflex, masseter and temporal muscles, maxillary reflex (jaw jerk).

5. VII (facial)—Wrinkle forehead, frown, smile, raise eyebrows, asymmetry of face, strength of eyelid muscles, taste on anterior portion of tongue.

6. VIII (acoustic)—

a. Cochlear—Hearing, lateralization, air and bone conduction, tinnitus.

b. Vestibular—Caloric tests.

7. IX (glossopharyngeal) and X (vagus)—Pharyngeal gag reflex; ability to swallow and speak clearly; sensation of mucosa of pharynx, soft palate, and tonsils; movement of pharynx, larynx, and soft palate; autonomic functions.

8. XI (accessory)—Strength of trapezius and sternocleidomastoid muscles.

9. XII (hypoglossal)—Protrusion of tongue, tremor, strength of tongue.

C. Cerebellar Function: Finger to nose; finger to examiner's finger; rapidly alternating pronation and supination of hands; ability to run heel down other shin and to make a requested motion with foot; ability to stand with eyes closed; walk; heel-to-toe walk; tremor; ataxia; posture; arm swing when walking; nystagmus; abnormalities of muscle tone or speech.

D. Motor System: Muscle size, consistency, and tone; muscle contours and outlines; muscle strength; myotonic contraction; slow relaxation; symmetry of posture; fasciculations; tremor; resistance to passive movement; involuntary movement.

E. Reflexes:

1. Deep—Bicep, brachioradialis, tricep, patellar, and Achilles reflexes; rapidity and strength of contraction and relaxation.

2. Superficial—Abdominal, cremasteric, plantar, and gluteal reflexes.

3. Pathologic—Babinski's, Chaddock's, Oppenheim's, and Gordon's reflexes.

Development

Both a history of developmental progress (''milestones'') and formal developmental screening tests are part of the routine physical evaluation.

Practical note: Screening devices may not be diagnostic of a particular problem but may merely indicate a need for further developmental evaluation.

SELECTED REFERENCES

Barness LA: *Manual of Pediatric Physical Diagnosis,* 5th ed. Year Book, 1981.

Bates B: *A Guide to Physical Examination,* 3rd ed. Lippincott, 1983.

DeGowin EL, DeGowin RL: *Bedside Diagnostic Examination,* 4th ed. Macmillan, 1981.

Frankenburg W et al: *Denver Developmental Screening Test Reference Manual,* revised 1975 ed. LADOCA Project & Publishing Foundation, 1975.

Green M, Richmond JB: *Pediatric Diagnosis,* 3rd ed. Saunders, 1980.

Judge RD, Zuidema GD (editors): *Physical Diagnosis: A Physiologic Approach to the Clinical Examination,* 2nd ed. Little, Brown, 1968.

Morgan WL, Engel GL: *The Clinical Approach to the Patient,* Saunders, 1969.

Growth & Development* 2

Henry K. Silver, MD

Body measurements and developmental landmarks provide the best and most practical means of evaluating the health of the individual child, because physical growth and developmental sequence follow a relatively smooth and clearly defined pattern. Growth and development generally progress along expected lines only when the functions of the individual are successfully integrated into a working whole. Failure of the individual to conform to the expected human pattern is completely nonspecific in etiologic terms, since it may equally well result from malnutrition, genetic deficiency, psychologic maladaptation, protracted illness, or a number of other causes. The physician, alerted by disturbances in growth, needs to seek out the specific causes.

Physical or psychologic growth and development generally have a smooth pattern of progression, but some deviation from this pattern is to be expected. The variation between racial groups can be great because of unfavorable factors in some cultures. The reference data given here apply to the USA and other Western countries. The reference "norms" are derived from the measurement of many individuals and may not be entirely applicable to an individual child.

There is no demonstrated advantage for the relatively large child over the relatively small child, although children falling outside the fifth and 95th percentiles are more likely to contract particular diseases or be prone to contract them. Gradual and relatively minor change over a period of months or years from one percentile level within the group to another need not be considered as evidence of disease, but marked deviations should be regarded with suspicion. The physician must constantly bear in mind that integration of function occurs within the individual and that disruption of the child's own pattern of growth and development is of greater significance than a deviation from the total population of any one set of measurements.

A knowledge of growth and development is of practical importance in relation to the sick child. Diseases tend to have more impact and to lead to greater permanent impairment when they occur during periods of rapid growth and development than when they occur during intervals of slower growth. For example, loss of growth in the long bones of one leg over a period of several months because of osteomyelitis or prolonged casting in the preadolescent child is of lesser ultimate significance to alignment of the spine than if the loss occurred at the peak of adolescent growth.

Development and growth are continuous dynamic processes occurring from conception to maturity and take place in an orderly sequence that is approximately the same for all individuals. At any particular age, however, wide variations among normal children reflect the responses of growing individuals to numberless hereditary and environmental factors.

GROWTH

The body as a whole and its various tissues and organs have characteristic growth patterns that are essentially the same in all individuals (Fig 2–1). *Development* signifies maturation of organs and systems, acquisition of skills, ability to adapt more readily to stress and assume maximum responsibility, and the capacity to achieve freedom in creative expression. *Growth* denotes change in size resulting from increase in the number or size of the cells of the body.

Rate of growth is generally more important than actual size, and height and weight data must be considered in relation to the variability within a certain age. For more accurate comparisons, data should be recorded both as absolute figures and as percentiles for a particular age.

A number of extrinsic and intrinsic factors influence the rate of total growth and growth of various organ systems. Some of the more important extrinsic factors are nutritional status, climate, season, illness, and activity.

Serial measurements of growth are the best indicators of health. Pertinent measurements should be plotted to determine the pattern of growth and to compare them with normal standards. Graphs designating percentile distribution are particularly useful.

Fetal Growth

See Figs 2–2 and 2–3 and also Tables 2–1 and 2–2.

A. Placental Transport:

1. Substances that pass through the placenta by

* See also Index and other pertinent chapters.

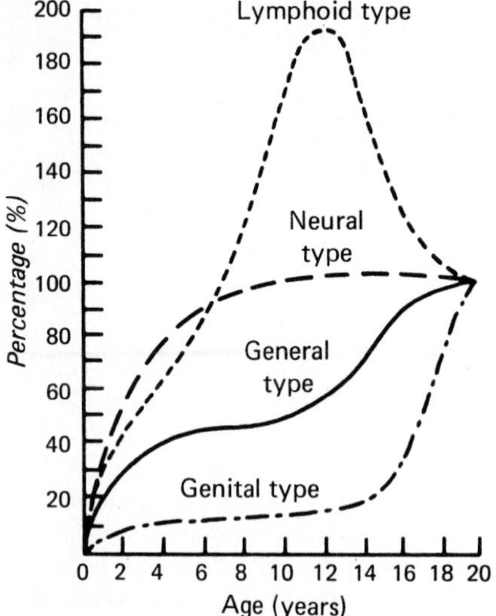

Figure 2–1. Graph showing major types of postnatal growth of various parts and organs of the body. *Lymphoid type:* thymus, lymph nodes, intestinal lymphoid masses. *Neural type:* brain and its parts, dura, spinal cord, optic apparatus, many head dimensions. *General type:* body as a whole, external dimensions (with exception of head and neck), respiratory and digestive organs, kidneys, aorta and pulmonary trunks, spleen, musculature as a whole, skeleton as a whole, blood volume. *Genital type:* testis, ovary, epididymis, uterine tube, prostate, prostatic urethra, seminal vesicles. (From RE Scammon. Redrawn and reproduced, with permission, from Holt LE Jr, McIntosh R, Barnett HL: *Pediatrics,* 13th ed. Appleton-Century-Crofts, 1962, as redrawn from Harris JA et al: *Measurement of Man.* University of Minnesota Press, 1930.)

simple diffusion are oxygen, carbon dioxide, water, and urea. Some that diffuse are present in lower concentration in the fetus (thyroxine, cholesterol, bilirubin, insulin, progesterone, estrogen), whereas still others are transported actively across the placenta and appear in fetal blood in higher concentration than in maternal blood (amino acids, glucose, glycerol, fatty acids, minerals).

2. Phosphorus, iodine, and iron are relatively more concentrated on the fetal side of the placenta. Total calcium is present in higher concentration in the blood of the fetus than in the maternal blood, but ionizable calcium is present in equal concentrations in both.

3. Water-soluble vitamins are found in higher concentrations in fetal blood, but fat-soluble vitamins are present in lower concentrations in the fetus.

4. Lipids cross the placenta poorly.

5. The placenta acts as a barrier against thyroid-stimulating hormone, growth hormone, nucleic acids, neutral fats, and many bacteria and viruses.

6. The placenta produces estrogens, progestins, and gonadotropins.

B. Etiology of Fetal Abnormalities: Dietary deficiencies, infections, and numerous other factors in the pregnant woman may cause no manifest symptoms in her while producing significant abnormalities in the offspring; the pregnant woman may fare better than her offspring. Major malformations are present in 1–3.6% of newborn and stillborn infants; minor anomalies have been noted in as many as 15% of newborns.

C. Metabolic Factors:

1. The main source of energy for the growing fetus is carbohydrate.

2. Oxygen saturation in the fetus is lower than that found after birth.

Length & Height

Data are presented in Figs 2–2 to 2–5, 2–8 to 2–11, and 2–14 and in Tables 2–1, 2–3, and 2–4.

A. In Utero:

1. Maximal growth in length occurs during the sixth and seventh months of pregnancy.

2. During fetal life, the rate of growth is extremely rapid. During the early months, the fetal rate of gain in length is greater than the rate of gain in weight when expressed as percentage of value at birth. By the eighth month, the fetus has achieved 80% of birth length and only 50% of birth weight. After the second fetal month, the greatest relative increase in length is due to an increase in the growth of the extremities.

B. Neonatal:

1. Firstborn infants are usually smaller than later-born ones.

2. At birth, males are slightly taller and heavier than females.

3. At birth, the ratio of the lower to the upper segment of the body (as measured from the pubis) is approximately 1:1.7. Subsequently, the legs grow more rapidly than the trunk (Fig 2–6).

C. Childhood: (Figs 2–4, 2–5; Table 2–3.) Height increases at a slowly declining rate until the onset of puberty, when a great spurt in growth occurs. Changes in height are slower in responding to factors detrimental to growth than are changes in weight.

1. Birth length is doubled by approximately age 4 and tripled by age 13.

2. The average child grows approximately 20 inches (50.8 cm) in the 9 months prior to birth, 10 inches (25.4 cm) in the first year of life, 5 inches (12.7 cm) in the second, 3–4 inches (7.6–10.2 cm) in the third, and approximately 2–3 inches (5.1–7.6 cm) per year until the growth spurt of puberty appears.

3. At 2 years of age, the midpoint in height is the umbilicus, whereas at adulthood the midpoint is slightly below the symphysis pubica.

4. At *3* years of age, the average child is *3* feet (91.4 cm) tall, and at *4* years, *40* inches (101.6 cm) tall. At *3.5* years the average child weighs *35* pounds (15.9 kg).

5. The legs and feet grow more rapidly than the trunk during childhood. During the first 2–3 years, the feet are flat, and there is an inward bowing of the legs from the knees to the ankles. The feet are

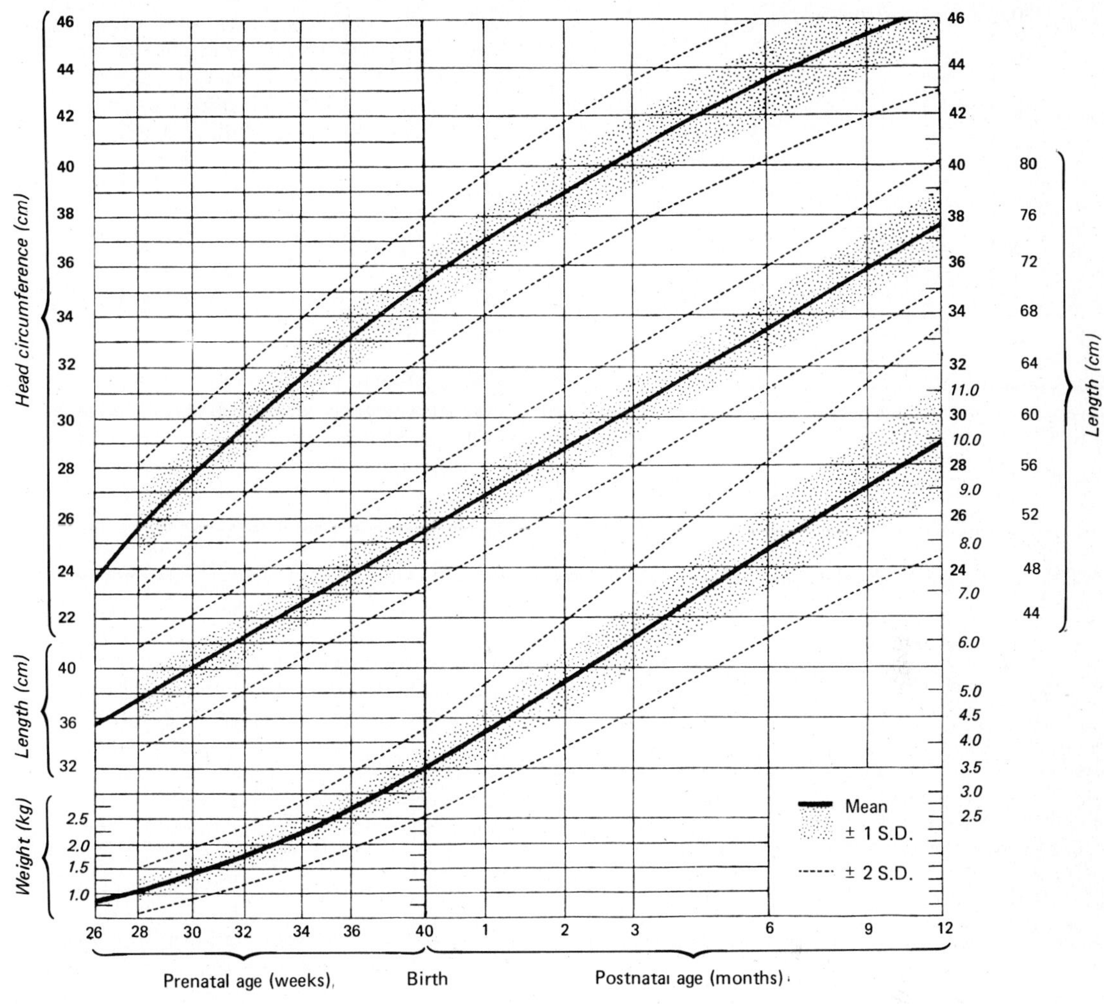

Figure 2–2. Growth record for infants in relation to gestational age and fetal and infant norms (combined sexes). (Modified and reproduced, with permission, from University of Oregon Health Sciences Center form 3.20-2-Rev. 2–3/75.)

often internally rotated (''pigeon-toed'') as a result of internal torsion of the tibia or varus deformity of the medial aspect of the forefoot.

6. During the first year of life, boys grow slightly faster than girls.

7. Between the ages of 1 and 9 years, both boys and girls grow at approximately the same rate.

D. Pubescence:

1. Although children pass through the phase of accelerated growth associated with pubescence at different chronologic ages, the pattern or sequence of pubescent growth tends to be similar in all children.

2. Adolescents undergoing early puberty are taller during early pubescence but have an earlier cessation of growth than adolescents undergoing late puberty.

3. In the period following the menarche, the median growth for girls is approximately 3 inches (7.6 cm), but the range is from less than 1 inch (2.5 cm) up to 7 inches (17.8 cm).

4. Boys whose height is at the median at age 2 are likely to be twice as tall as adults as they were at age 2.

E. Environmental Factors:

1. Children of middle and low socioeconomic groups in this generation are appreciably taller than children in previous generations.

2. Children from high socioeconomic groups are taller and heavier than those from lower socioeconomic groups in the same area.

3. Height gains are maximal in the spring and minimal in the fall. The growth of well-nourished children is less affected by seasons than is the growth of poorly nourished children. The mechanism in seasonal factors affecting growth is not known.

Weight

Body weight is probably the best index of nutrition and growth. Growth responses are noted in changes

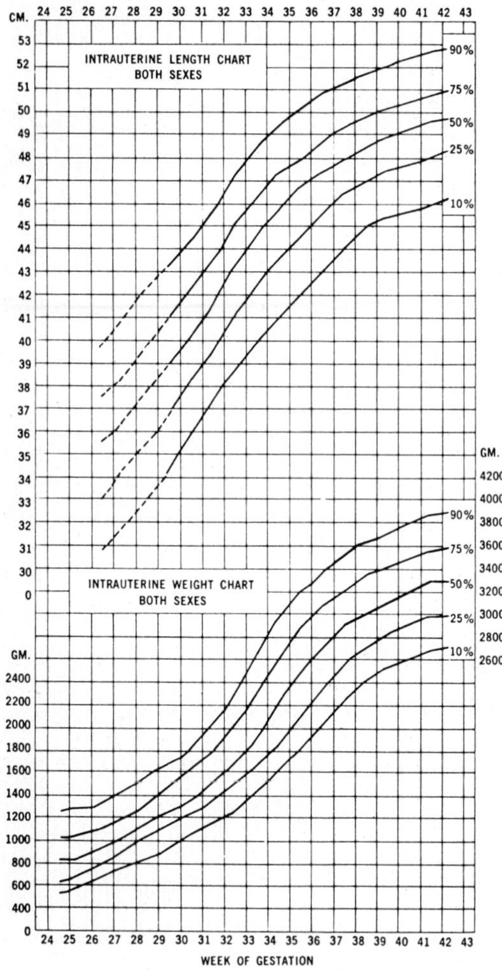

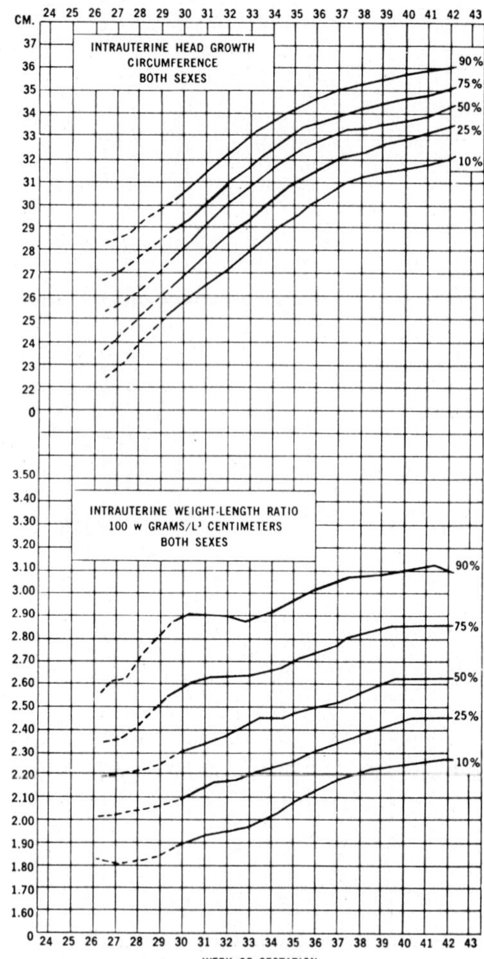

Figure 2–3. Colorado intrauterine growth charts. (Reproduced, with permission, from Lubchenco LO et al: *Pediatrics* 1966;37:403.) These values are lower than those reported by others.

in weight before they are noted in other aspects of growth. The greatest weight gain occurs in the fall and the least gain in the spring. Obese children are usually taller and have advanced bone ages. (See Figs 2–2, 2–3, and 2–7 to 2–11 and also Table 2–4.)

A. Neonatal:

1. The average infant weighs approximately 7 lb 5 oz (3333 g) at birth.

2. Within the first few days of life, the newborn may lose up to 10% of birth weight. This loss is attributable to loss of meconium and urine, physiologic edema, and less intake. Birth weight is usually regained by 10 days of age.

B. Childhood: (Fig 2–7.)

1. The increment in weight is approximately 1 oz (30 g)/d during the early months of life.

2. Between the ages of 3 and 12 months, weight in pounds is equal to age in months plus 11.

3. Birth weight is doubled between the fourth and fifth months of age, tripled by the end of the first year, and quadrupled by the end of the second year. Between the ages of 2 and 9 years, the annual increment in weight averages about 5 lb per year.

4. At 7 years, the average child weighs 7 times his or her birth weight.

C. Adolescence: During adolescence in girls, the most rapid gain in weight usually occurs in the year before menarche.

Head & Skull

Measurements of the head serve as an estimate of brain growth. Growth of the skull as determined by increasing head circumference is a much more accurate index of brain growth than is the presence or size of the fontanelle. (See Figs 2–6, 2–8, 2–9, and 2–12.)

A. In Utero: During pregnancy, the cranium increases in size much more rapidly than the rest of the body.

Table 2–1. Fetal and newborn dimensions and weights of the body and its organs.*

Age (Fetal) in Weeks†	Crown-heel (cm)	Crown-rump (cm)	Head Circ. (cm)	Body Wt (g)	Adrenal (g)	Brain (g)	Heart (g)	Kidney (g)	Liver (g)	Lungs (g)	Pancreas (g)	Pituitary (g)	Spleen (g)	Thymus (g)	Thyroid (g)
Prenatal and Newborn															
12	9.0	7.5	7.4	18.6	.087	2.32	.098	.163	.097	.69	.013		.006	.010	.026
16	16.7	12.8	12.6	100	.417	14.4	.662	.962	5.94	3.23	.095	.011	.086	.122	.133
20	24.2	17.7	17.6	310	1.07	43.0	2.08	2.77	16.8	8.18	.314	.024	.410	.553	.352
24	31.1	21.9	22.3	670	2.02	91.0	4.47	5.69	34.5	15.2	.695	.040	1.16	1.53	.684
28	37.1	25.5	26.3	1150	3.16	153	7.70	9.43	57.4	23.7	1.22	.058	2.43	3.14	1.08
30	39.8	27.1	28.1	1400	3.78	189	9.78	11.5	70.3	28.2	1.53	.067	3.26	4.18	1.33
32	42.4	28.5	29.9	1700	4.44	228	11.6	13.8	84.3	33.0	1.88	.076	4.25	5.41	1.54
34	44.8	29.9	31.5	2000	5.11	268	13.7	16.2	100.0	37.8	2.24	.085	5.36	6.77	1.78
36	47.0	31.2	33.1	2450	5.77	309	15.9	18.6	113.0	42.7	2.61	.094	6.55	8.22	2.01
38	49.1	32.4	34.4	2900	6.45	352	18.2	21.0	129.0	47.5	3.01	.103	7.86	9.82	2.26
40	51.0	33.5	35.7	3150	7.10	394	20.6	23.5	143.5	52.5	3.40	.111	9.22	11.5	2.50
Postnatal															
Age (Years)															
1					4	875	43	62	350	160		0.15	30	23	
5					5	1250	90	110	575	305		0.23	55	28	
10					6	1325	145	150	825	450		0.33	77	31	
15					8	1340	245	220	1275	675		0.48	125	27	
Adult‡															
Male					6	1375	300	320	1600	1000			165	14	
Female					6	1280	250	280	1500	750			150	14	

* Adapted from Edith Boyd.
† Time from first day of last menstrual period.
‡ Adapted from several sources.

Table 2–2. Human fetal development.*

		Fetal Age in Lunar Months
Integument	Three-layered epidermis	3
	Body hair begins	4
	Skin glands form, sweat and sebaceous	4
Mouth	Lip fusion complete	2
	Palate fused completely	3
	Enamel and dentin depositing	5
	Primordia of permanent teeth	6–8
Gastrointestinal	Bile secreted	3
	Rectum patent	3
	Pancreatic islands appear	3
	Fixation of duodenum and colon	4
Respiratory	Definitive shape of lungs	3
	Maxillary sinuses developing	4
	Elastic fibers appear in lung	4
Urogenital	Kidney able to secrete	2½
	Vagina regains lumen	5
	Testes descend into scrotum	7–9
Vascular	Definitive shape of heart	1½
	Heart becomes 4-chambered	3½
	Blood formation in marrow begins	3
	Spleen acquires typical structure	7
Nervous	Commissures of brain complete	5
	Myelinization of cord begins	5
	Typical layers of cortex	6
Special senses	Nasal septum complete	3
	Retinal layers complete, light-perceptive	7
	Vascular tunic of lens pronounced	7
	Eyelids open	7–8

* Reproduced, with permission, from Arey LB: *Developmental Anatomy: A Textbook and Laboratory Manual of Embryology,* 5th ed. Saunders, 1947.

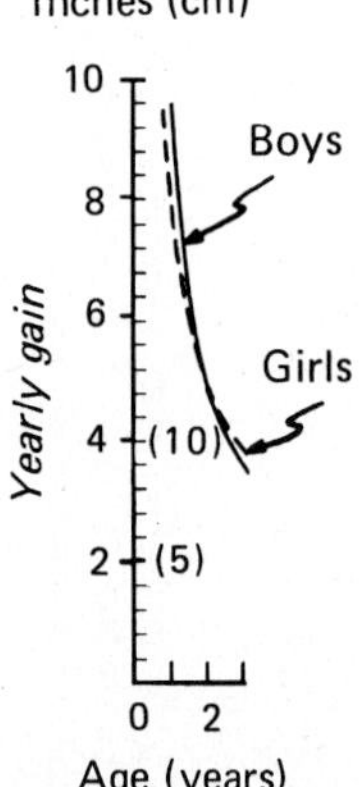

Figure 2–4. Growth rate from birth to age 3 (both sexes).

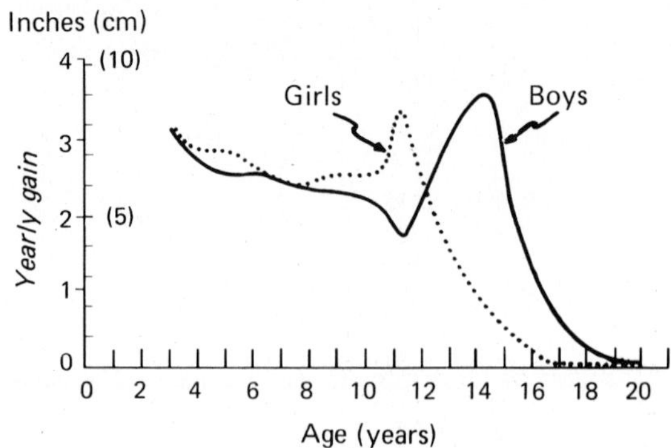

Figure 2–5. Growth rate from age 3 to 20 (both sexes).

Table 2–3. Approximate percentage of mature height achieved at each age.

	Boys			Girls		
Age in Years	**Average**	**Accelerated**	**Retarded**	**Average**	**Accelerated**	**Retarded**
Birth	29			31		
1	42	45	40	45	48	42
2	50	51	47	53	55	50
3	54	56	52	57	60	55
4	58	60	56	62	65	60
5	62	64	60	66	69	64
6	65	68	64	69	73	68
7	69	71	67	74	76	72
8	72	74	70	78	80	75
9	75	77	73	81	84	78
10	78	80	76	84	88	81
11	81	83	80	88	93	85
12	84	87	82	93	97	88
13	87	91	85	97	98	91
14	92	96	88	98	99	95
15	96	98	92	99	99	98
16	98	99	96	99	99	99
16½	98	99	97	99	100	99
17	99	100	98	100		99
18	100		99			100
19			100			

B. Newborn: At birth, the head is approximately three-fourths of its total mature size, whereas the rest of the body is only one-fourth its adult size.

C. Childhood:

1. The brain grows very rapidly during infancy and then less rapidly. At birth, the head makes up one-fourth of the infant's length; by 25 years of age, the head measures only one-eighth of body length.

2. Cranial sutures do not ossify completely until early adulthood.

3. Although the *averages* of head and chest circumference in the first 4 years of life are approximately equal, during this period the head circumference may normally be from 5 cm larger to 7 cm smaller than the chest.

Table 2–4. Percentiles for weight and height: Birth to 5 years and 5–18 years.*

Percentiles (Boys)						Percentiles (Girls)				
3	10	50	90	97		3	10	50	90	97
					Birth					
5.8	6.3	7.5	9.1	10.1	Weight in pounds	5.8	6.2	7.4	8.6	9.4
2.63	2.86	3.4	4.13	4.58	Weight in kg	2.63	2.81	3.36	3.9	4.26
18.2	18.9	19.9	21.0	21.5	Length in inches	18.5	18.8	19.8	20.4	21.1
46.3	48.1	50.6	53.3	54.6	Length in cm	47.1	47.8	50.2	51.9	53.6
					3 Months					
10.6	11.1	12.6	14.5	16.4	Weight in pounds	9.8	10.7	12.4	14.0	14.9
4.81	5.03	5.72	6.58	7.44	Weight in kg	4.45	4.85	5.62	6.35	6.76
22.4	22.8	23.8	24.7	25.1	Length in inches	22.0	22.4	23.4	24.3	24.8
56.8	57.8	60.4	62.8	63.7	Length in cm	55.8	56.9	59.5	61.7	63.1
					6 Months					
14.0	14.8	16.7	19.2	20.8	Weight in pounds	12.7	14.1	16.0	18.6	20.0
6.35	6.71	7.58	8.71	9.43	Weight in kg	5.76	6.4	7.26	8.44	9.07
24.8	25.2	26.1	27.3	27.7	Length in inches	24.0	24.6	25.7	26.7	27.1
63.0	63.9	66.4	69.3	70.4	Length in cm	61.1	62.5	65.2	67.8	68.8
					9 Months					
16.6	17.8	20.0	22.9	24.4	Weight in pounds	15.1	16.6	19.2	22.4	24.2
7.53	8.07	9.07	10.39	11.07	Weight in kg	6.85	7.53	8.71	10.16	10.98
26.6	27.0	28.0	29.2	29.9	Length in inches	25.7	26.4	27.6	28.7	29.2
67.7	68.6	71.2	74.2	75.9	Length in cm	65.4	67.0	70.1	72.9	74.1
					12 Months					
18.5	19.6	22.2	25.4	27.3	Weight in pounds	16.8	18.4	21.5	24.8	27.1
8.39	8.89	10.07	11.52	12.38	Weight in kg	7.62	8.35	9.75	11.25	12.29
28.1	28.5	29.6	30.7	31.6	Length in inches	27.1	27.8	29.2	30.3	31.0
71.3	72.4	75.2	78.1	80.3	Length in cm	68.9	70.6	74.2	77.1	78.8
					15 Months					
19.8	21.0	23.7	27.2	29.4	Weight in pounds	18.1	19.8	23.0	26.6	29.0
8.98	9.53	10.75	12.34	13.33	Weight in kg	8.21	8.98	10.43	12.07	13.15
29.3	29.8	30.9	32.1	33.1	Length in inches	28.3	29.0	30.5	31.8	32.6
74.4	75.6	78.5	81.5	84.2	Length in cm	71.9	73.7	77.6	80.8	82.8
					18 Months					
21.1	22.3	25.2	29.0	31.5	Weight in pounds	19.4	21.2	24.5	28.3	30.9
9.57	10.12	11.43	13.15	14.29	Weight in kg	8.8	9.62	11.11	12.84	14.02
30.5	31.0	32.2	33.5	34.7	Length in inches	29.5	30.2	31.8	33.3	34.1
77.5	78.8	81.8	85.0	88.2	Length in cm	74.9	76.8	80.9	84.5	86.7
					2 Years					
23.3	24.7	27.7	31.9	34.9	Weight in pounds	21.6	23.5	27.1	31.7	34.4
10.57	11.2	12.56	14.47	15.83	Weight in kg	9.8	10.66	12.29	14.38	15.6
32.6	33.1	34.4	35.9	37.2	Length in inches	31.5	32.3	34.1	35.8	36.7
82.7	84.2	87.5	91.1	94.6	Length in cm	80.1	82.0	86.6	91.0	93.3
					2½ Years					
25.2	26.6	30.0	34.5	37.0	Weight in pounds	23.6	25.5	29.6	34.6	38.2
11.43	12.07	13.61	15.65	16.78	Weight in kg	10.7	11.57	13.43	15.69	17.33
34.2	34.8	36.3	37.9	39.2	Length in inches	33.3	34.0	36.0	37.9	38.9
86.9	88.5	92.1	96.2	99.5	Length in cm	84.5	86.3	91.4	96.4	98.7
					3 Years					
27.0	28.7	32.2	36.8	39.2	Weight in pounds	25.6	27.6	31.8	37.4	41.8
12.25	13.02	14.61	16.69	17.78	Weight in kg	11.61	12.52	14.42	16.96	18.96
35.7	36.3	37.9	39.6	40.5	Length in inches	34.8	35.6	37.7	39.8	40.7
90.6	92.3	96.2	100.5	102.8	Length in cm	88.4	90.5	95.7	101.1	103.5
					4 Years					
30.1	32.1	36.4	41.4	44.3	Weight in pounds	29.2	31.2	36.2	43.5	48.2
13.65	14.56	16.51	18.78	20.09	Weight in kg	13.25	14.15	16.42	19.73	21.86
38.4	39.1	40.7	42.7	43.5	Length in inches	37.5	38.4	40.6	43.1	44.2
97.5	99.3	103.4	108.5	110.4	Length in cm	95.2	97.6	103.2	109.6	112.3
					5 Years					
33.6	35.5	40.5	46.7	50.4	Weight in pounds	32.1	34.8	40.5	49.2	52.8
15.24	16.1	18.37	21.18	22.86	Weight in kg	14.56	15.79	18.37	22.32	23.95
40.2	40.8	42.8	45.2	46.1	Length in inches	39.4	40.5	42.9	45.4	46.8
102.0	103.7	108.7	114.7	117.1	Length in cm	100.0	103.0	109.1	115.4	118.8

* See footnote on next page.

Table 2–4 (cont'd). Percentiles for weight and height: Birth to 5 years and 5–18 years.*

Percentiles (Boys)						Percentiles (Girls)				
3	10	50	90	97		3	10	50	90	97
					5 Years					
34.5	36.6	42.8	49.7	53.2	Weight in pounds	33.7	36.1	41.4	48.2	51.8
15.65	16.6	19.41	22.54	24.13	Weight in kg	15.29	16.37	18.78	21.86	23.5
40.2	41.5	43.8	45.9	47.0	Height in inches	40.4	41.3	43.2	45.4	46.5
102.1	105.3	111.3	116.7	119.5	Height in cm	102.6	105.0	109.7	115.4	118.0
					6 Years					
38.5	40.9	48.3	56.4	61.1	Weight in pounds	37.2	39.6	46.5	54.2	58.7
17.46	18.55	21.91	25.58	27.71	Weight in kg	16.87	17.96	21.09	24.58	26.63
42.7	43.8	46.3	48.6	49.7	Height in inches	42.5	43.5	45.6	48.1	49.4
108.5	111.2	117.5	123.5	126.2	Height in cm	108.0	110.6	115.9	122.3	125.4
					7 Years					
43.0	45.8	54.1	64.4	69.9	Weight in pounds	41.3	44.5	52.2	61.2	67.3
19.5	20.77	24.54	29.21	31.71	Weight in kg	18.73	20.19	23.68	27.76	30.53
44.9	46.0	48.9	51.4	52.5	Height in inches	44.9	46.0	48.1	50.7	51.9
114.0	116.9	124.1	130.5	133.4	Height in cm	114.0	116.8	122.3	128.9	131.7
					8 Years					
48.0	51.2	60.1	73.0	79.4	Weight in pounds	45.3	48.6	58.1	69.9	78.9
21.77	23.22	27.26	33.11	36.02	Weight in kg	20.55	22.04	26.35	31.71	35.79
47.1	48.5	51.2	54.0	55.2	Height in inches	46.9	48.1	50.4	53.0	54.1
119.6	123.1	130.0	137.3	140.2	Height in cm	119.1	122.1	128.0	134.6	137.4
					9 Years					
52.5	56.3	66.0	81.0	89.8	Weight in pounds	49.1	52.6	63.8	79.1	89.9
23.81	25.54	29.94	36.74	40.73	Weight in kg	22.27	23.86	28.94	35.88	40.78
48.9	50.5	53.3	56.1	57.2	Height in inches	48.7	50.0	52.3	55.3	56.5
124.2	128.3	135.5	142.6	145.3	Height in cm	123.6	127.0	132.9	140.4	143.4
					10 Years					
56.8	61.1	71.9	89.9	100.0	Weight in pounds	53.2	57.1	70.3	89.7	101.9
25.76	27.71	32.61	40.78	45.36	Weight in kg	24.13	25.9	31.89	40.69	46.22
50.7	52.3	55.2	58.1	59.2	Height in inches	50.3	51.8	54.6	57.5	58.8
128.7	132.8	140.3	147.5	150.3	Height in cm	127.7	131.7	138.6	146.0	149.3
					11 Years					
61.8	66.3	77.6	99.3	111.7	Weight in pounds	57.9	62.6	78.8	100.4	112.9
28.03	30.07	35.2	45.04	50.67	Weight in kg	26.26	28.4	35.74	45.54	51.21
52.5	54.0	56.8	59.8	60.8	Height in inches	52.1	53.9	57.0	60.4	62.0
133.4	137.3	144.2	151.8	154.4	Height in cm	132.3	137.0	144.7	153.4	157.4
					12 Years					
67.2	72.0	84.4	109.6	124.2	Weight in pounds	63.6	69.5	87.6	111.5	127.7
30.48	32.66	38.28	49.71	56.34	Weight in kg	28.85	31.52	39.74	50.58	57.92
54.4	56.1	58.9	62.2	63.7	Height in inches	54.3	56.1	59.8	63.2	64.8
138.1	142.4	149.6	157.9	161.9	Height in cm	137.8	142.6	151.9	160.6	164.6
					13 Years					
72.0	77.1	93.0	123.2	138.0	Weight in pounds	72.2	79.9	99.1	124.5	142.3
32.66	34.97	42.18	55.88	62.6	Weight in kg	32.75	36.24	44.95	56.47	64.55
56.0	57.7	61.0	65.1	66.7	Height in inches	56.6	58.7	61.8	64.9	66.3
142.2	146.6	155.0	165.3	169.5	Height in cm	143.7	149.1	157.1	164.8	168.4
					14 Years					
79.8	87.2	107.6	136.9	150.6	Weight in pounds	83.1	91.0	108.4	133.3	150.8
36.2	39.55	48.81	62.1	68.31	Weight in kg	37.69	41.28	49.17	60.46	68.4
57.6	59.9	64.0	67.9	69.7	Height in inches	58.3	60.2	62.8	65.7	67.2
146.4	152.1	162.7	172.4	177.1	Height in cm	148.2	153.0	159.6	167.0	170.7
					15 Years					
91.3	99.4	120.1	147.8	161.6	Weight in pounds	89.0	97.4	113.5	138.1	155.2
41.41	45.09	54.48	67.04	73.3	Weight in kg	40.37	44.18	51.48	62.64	70.4
59.7	62.1	66.1	69.6	71.6	Height in inches	59.1	61.1	63.4	66.2	67.6
151.7	157.8	167.8	176.7	181.8	Height in cm	150.2	155.2	161.1	168.1	171.6

* The figures for the group from 0 to 5 years are from Studies of Child Health & Development, Department of Maternal & Child Health, Harvard School of Public Health; those for the group from 5 to 18 years are from studies by and are reproduced by courtesy of Howard V. Meredith, Iowa Child Welfare Research Station, the State University of Iowa. The figures for 5 years are given twice; their variations are due to the different populations of children used for each group.

Table 2–4 (cont'd). Percentiles for weight and height: Birth to 5 years and 5–18 years.*

Percentiles (Boys)						Percentiles (Girls)				
3	10	50	90	97		3	10	50	90	97
					16 Years					
103.4	111.0	129.7	157.3	170.5	Weight in pounds	91.8	100.9	117.0	141.1	157.7
46.9	50.35	58.83	71.35	77.34	Weight in kg	41.64	45.77	53.07	64.0	71.53
61.6	64.1	67.8	70.7	73.1	Height in inches	59.4	61.5	63.9	66.5	67.7
156.5	162.8	171.6	179.7	185.6	Height in cm	150.8	156.1	162.2	169.0	172.0
					17 Years					
110.5	117.5	136.2	164.6	175.6	Weight in pounds	93.9	102.8	119.1	143.3	159.5
50.12	53.3	61.78	74.66	79.65	Weight in kg	42.59	46.63	54.02	65.0	72.35
62.6	65.2	68.4	71.5	73.5	Height in inches	59.4	61.5	64.0	66.7	67.8
159.0	165.5	173.7	181.6	186.6	Height in cm	151.0	156.3	162.5	169.4	172.2
					18 Years					
113.0	120.0	139.0	169.0	179.0	Weight in pounds	94.5	103.5	119.9	144.5	160.7
51.26	54.43	63.05	76.66	81.19	Weight in kg	42.87	46.95	54.39	65.54	72.89
62.8	65.5	68.7	71.8	73.9	Height in inches	59.4	61.5	64.0	66.7	67.8
159.6	166.3	174.5	182.4	187.6	Height in cm	151.0	156.3	162.5	169.4	172.2

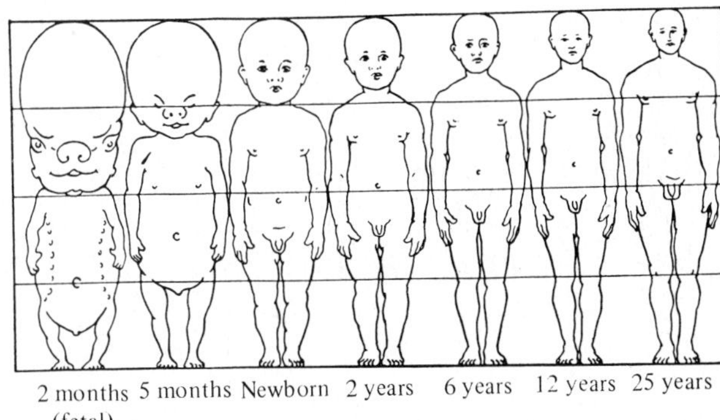

Figure 2–6. Relative proportions of head, trunk, and extremities at different ages. (From Stratz, modified by Robbins WJ et al: *Growth.* Yale Univ Press, 1928.)

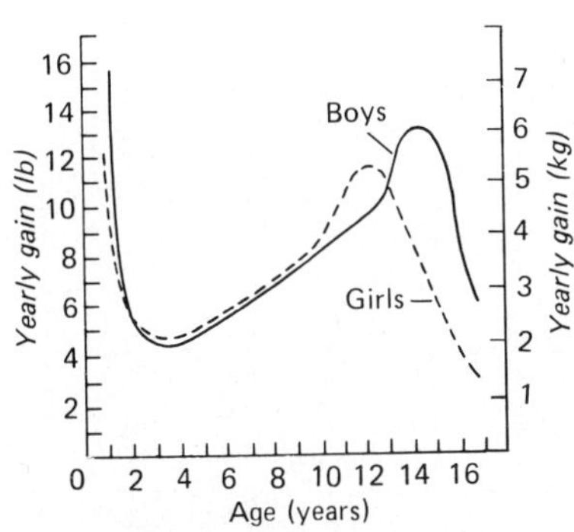

Figure 2–7. Yearly gain in weight. (Redrawn and reproduced, with permission, from Barnett HL: *Pediatrics,* 14th ed. Appleton-Century-Crofts, 1968.)

D. Fontanelles:

1. Six fontanelles (anterior, posterior, 2 sphenoid, and 2 mastoid) are usually present at birth.

2. The anterior fontanelle normally closes between 10 and 14 months of age but may be closed by 3 months or remain open until 18 months.

3. The posterior fontanelle usually closes by 2 months but in some children may not be palpable even at birth.

E. Other:

1. The pineal gland may be seen on x-ray in 10% of children beyond the tenth year and in 80% of elderly adults.

2. The auditory (eustachian) tube is shorter and more horizontal at birth than later.

Nervous System

The central nervous system makes up one-fourth of the total body weight in the second fetal month, one-tenth at birth, one-twentieth at age 5, and only one-fiftieth of the total weight at full maturity.

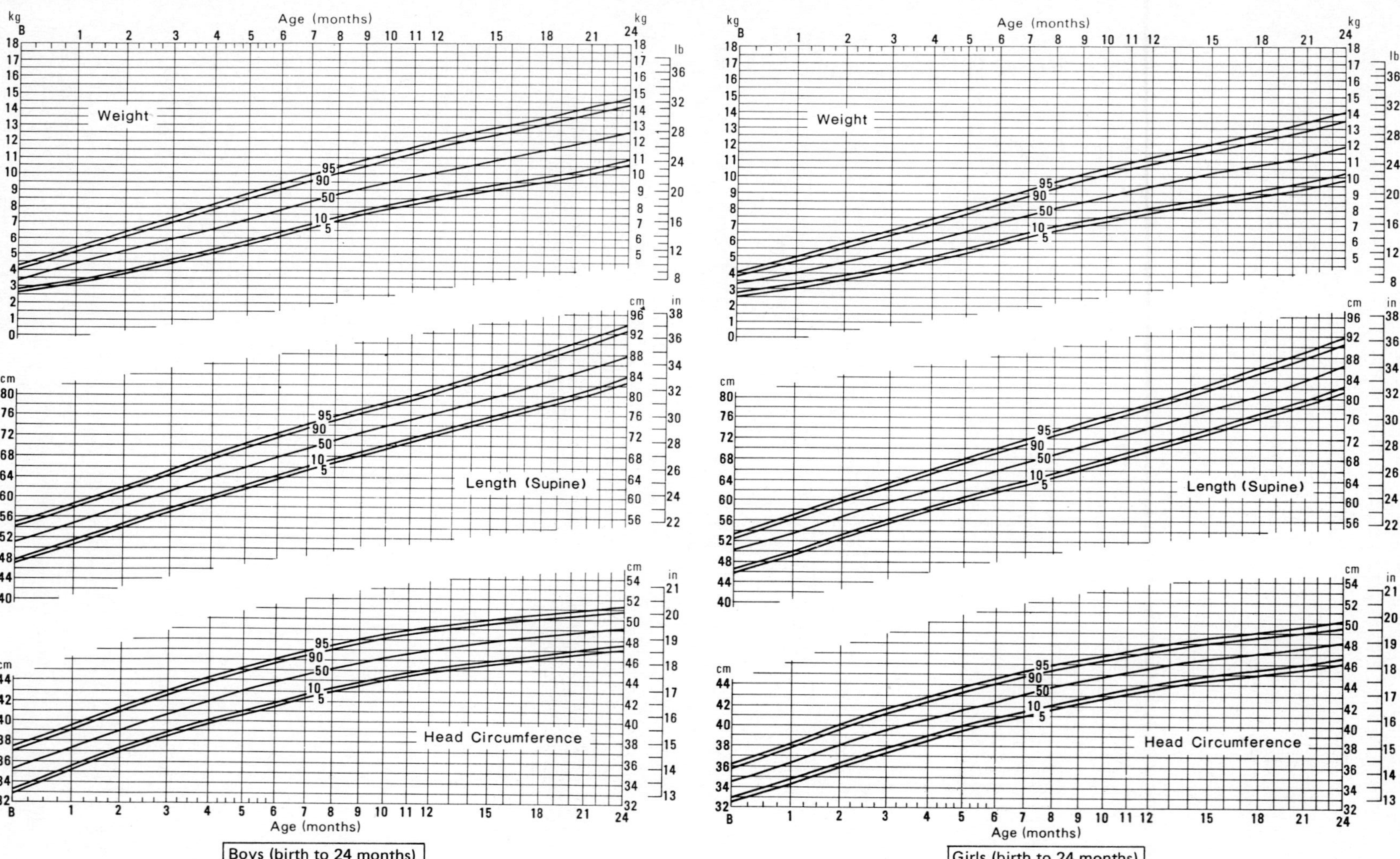

Figure 2–8. Percentile standards for weight, length, and head circumference for boys, birth to 24 months. (University of Colorado Health Sciences Center graph as adapted from NCHS Growth Charts, 1976.)

Figure 2–9. Percentile standards for weight, length, and head circumference for girls, birth to 24 months. (University of Colorado Health Sciences Center graph as adapted from NCHS Growth Charts, 1976.)

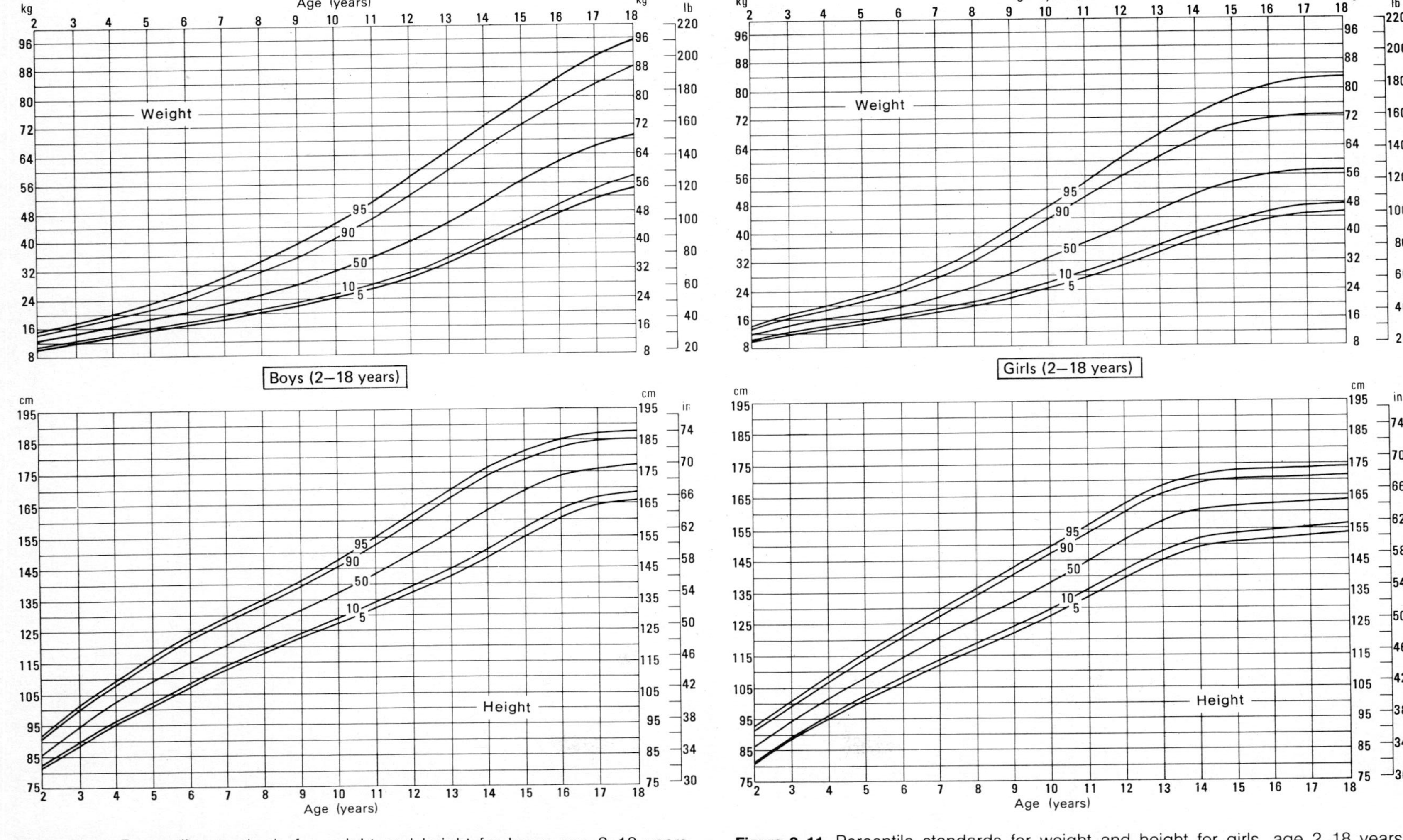

Figure 2–10. Percentile standards for weight and height for boys, age 2–18 years. (University of Colorado Health Sciences Center graph.)

Figure 2–11. Percentile standards for weight and height for girls, age 2–18 years. (University of Colorado Health Sciences Center graph.)

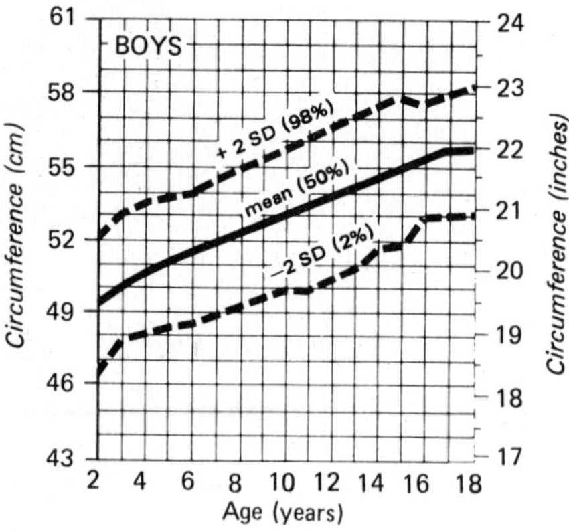

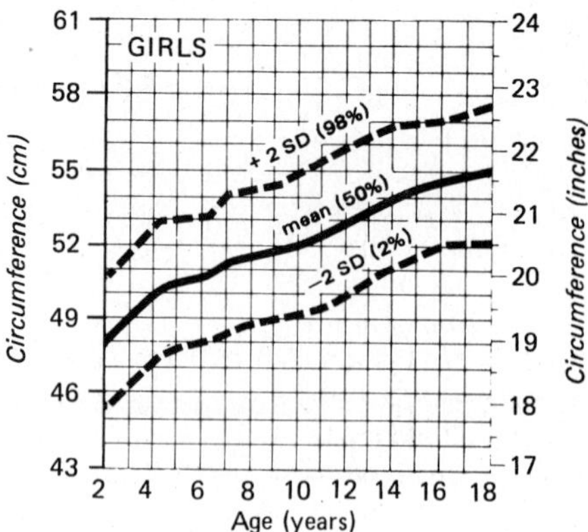

Figure 2–12. Head circumference for boys and girls, 2–18 years. (Modified from Nellhaus G: *Pediatrics* 1968;**41**:106.)

A. Myelinization:

1. Myelinization begins by the fourth fetal month and is evident first in the ventral and dorsal spinal routes. The cerebral cortex and thalamus are the last to be myelinated. Myelinization in the cord proceeds in a cephalocaudal direction. At birth, all the cranial nerves, with the exception of the optic and olfactory nerves, are myelinated. At that time, the autonomic nervous system is mature, and some of the segmented spinal nerves are mature, fully myelinated, and functional.

2. The brain stem, those tracts going to the cortex, and some of the finer configurations of the cortex of the brain, as well as the nerve tracts connecting the cortex with lower centers, are immature and probably incompletely myelinated. Minimal cortical function is present; function is primarily on a subcortical level.

3. Efferent fibers to the voluntary muscles begin to become myelinated soon after birth.

4. Myelinization of the spinal cord, brain stem, and cortex may not be completed for at least 2 years.

B. Reflexes:

1. The cough reflex, Moro reflex, Chvostek's sign, the walking reflex, the patellar reflex, and the grasping reflex are present at birth.

2. The Babinski reflex is seldom elicited in the newborn infant but appears somewhat later and may persist for a year or more.

3. The abdominal and cremasteric reflexes usually cannot be elicited in the neonatal period, nor can the Achilles tendon reflex nor the tonic neck reflex, which is quite inconstant in the newborn but is usually present in the normal 1-month-old infant.

4. By 6 months, superficial reflexes are present.

C. Blood-Brain Barrier: The blood-brain barrier appears to be more permeable during early infancy than later.

The Respiratory System

A. In Utero:

1. Respiratory movements take place in utero; an exchange of amniotic fluid in the alveoli occurs.

2. The first patterns of respiratory movements become manifest at about the 20th week of pregnancy.

3. The fetus and the newborn can withstand anoxia more effectively than can adults.

B. Newborn:

1. The onset of respiration in the newborn infant probably depends on a number of factors, including stimulation of the tactile and thermal receptors on the skin, as well as hypoxia.

2. Respiration in infants is largely diaphragmatic during the first years of life.

C. Childhood:

1. The respiratory rate decreases steadily during childhood, averaging approximately 30/min during the first year, 25/min in the second year, 20/min during the eighth year, and 18/min by the 15th year.

2. As the child becomes older, the amount of oxygen in the expired air decreases and the amount of CO_2 increases.

D. Adult: Men expel more CO_2 with each breath and have a larger alkali reserve in their blood than women.

Sinuses

A. Newborn: At birth, the mastoid process is only a single cell—the mastoid antrum—and has a relatively wide communication with the middle ear. Its cellular structure appears gradually between birth and age 3. Pneumatization of the tip of the mastoid process becomes demonstrable by the fifth year.

B. Childhood:

1. Maxillary and ethmoid sinuses are present at birth but are usually not aerated and usually cannot be seen by x-ray examination for at least 6 months. The sphenoid sinuses are usually not pneumatized (or visible) until after the third year.

2. Frontal sinuses become visible by x-ray between 3 and 9 years of age, usually after age 5.

The Cardiovascular System

A. Heart Rate: The heart rate falls steadily

throughout childhood, averaging about 150 beats/min in utero, 130 beats/min at birth, 105 beats/min in the second year of life, 90 beats/min in the fourth year, 80 beats/min in the sixth year, and 70 beats/min in the tenth year.

B. Blood pressure: (See Table 21–4.)

1. The systolic blood pressure is lower immediately after birth than at any other time.

2. The pulmonary and the systemic pressures are appxoximately equal during the first weeks of life.

C. Heart Sounds:

1. During childhood, the heart sounds have a higher pitch, shorter duration, and greater intensity than later in life. The pulmonary second sound is usually louder than the aortic.

2. Innocent ("functional") murmurs are common during childhood and have been reported to occur in approximately 50% of children at some time during childhood, with a peak incidence between the ages of 6 and 9.

3. Less than 10% of murmurs present at birth are the result of a congenital lesion that will persist.

4. A "venous hum" is commonly noted in childhood. It is continuous, located in the parasternal area, usually accentuated in the upright position, and may be either sub- or supraclavicular in location.

D. Heart Volume: Heart volume decreases an average of 25% from birth to the second day as a result of both the fluid shift from the vascular compartment and a decreasing flow of blood through the ductus arteriosus.

E. Blood Volume: The total blood volume ranges from 80 to 110 mL/kg in the newborn infant; averages 115 mL/kg in the premature infant during the first several weeks of life; and is 75–100 mL/kg in the older infant and child and 70–85 mL/kg in the adult.

F. Electrocardiography: (Table 2–5.) During the first months of life, there is a tendency to right axis deviation on the ECG.

G. Anatomic Changes Occurring at Birth: (Table 2–6.) The ductus arteriosus and the foramen ovale close functionally soon after birth; anatomic obliteration of the ductus is complete by the fourth month of postnatal life, whereas anatomic closure of the foramen ovale does not occur until toward the end of the first year.

Table 2–5. Upper limits of the normal PR interval in children.*

Pulse Rate	Below 70	71–90	91–110	111–130	Above 130
Birth–18 months	0.16	0.15	0.145	0.135	1.125
18 months–6 years	0.17	0.165	0.155	0.145	0.135
6–13 years	0.18	0.17	0.16	0.15	0.14
13–17 years	0.19	0.18	0.17	0.16	0.15

* Reproduced, with permission, from Ashman R, Hull E: *Essentials of Electrocardiography*, 2nd ed. Macmillan, 1941.

H. Other:

1. In early childhood, the axis of the heart is more nearly transverse than in later life.

2. Sinus dysrhythmia is a normal phenomenon during childhood.

The Blood

See Table 16–2 and Fig 2–13.

A. In Utero: The first blood-forming centers in the fetus are found in connective tissue (mesenchyma). This later shifts to the liver (most active), spleen, and mesonephros, and finally to the bone marrow. At birth, production of formed elements in the blood occurs primarily in the bone marrow. The liver and spleen retain the ability to make blood cells until early childhood at times of pathologic stress such as excessive hemorrhage.

B. Newborn:

1. If the umbilical cord is not clamped for 2–3 minutes after delivery of the infant, 75–135 mL of blood will be transferred from the placenta to the infant. Late clamping will produce a red blood cell count that is approximately 1 million/μL higher, a hemoglobin level approximately 2.5 g/dL higher, and a hematocrit 7% higher than if early clamping were carried out.

2. Nucleated red cells and immature lymphocytes may be present in the newborn but disappear within the first week of life.

3. At birth, 5% of all red blood cells may be reticulocytes; they drop to less than 1% after the second week.

4. Up to 5% of nucleated red blood cells (as a percentage of the total number of nucleated cells) may be present normally for several days after birth.

5. Normally, the number of leukocytes and erythrocytes and the amount of hemoglobin are relatively greater immediately after birth than at any other time.

C. Fetal Hemoglobin: Fetal hemoglobin accounts for 80% of total hemoglobin at birth (cord blood), 75% of the total at 2 weeks of age, 55% at 5 weeks, and falls to 5% by 20 weeks.

D. White Cells: (Fig 2–13.)

1. The leukocyte count is high at birth, rises slightly during the first 48 hours, falls for the next 2 or 3 weeks, and then rises again. In some children, it reaches its highest level sometime before the seventh month; the leukocyte count then falls gradually throughout childhood.

2. The lymphocyte count is highest during the first year and then falls progressively throughout childhood.

3. The eosinophil count is higher during early infancy than at any other time.

4. The basophil count remains essentially unchanged during childhood; at puberty, it falls to adult levels.

E. Sedimentation Rate: Children have an elevated sedimentation rate compared to adults.

Table 2–6. Changes in the circulatory mechanism at birth. (Adapted from Scammon.)

Structure	Prenatal Function	Postnatal Function
Umbilical vein	Carries oxygenated blood from placenta to liver and heart.	Obliterated to become ligamentum teres (round ligament of liver).
Ductus venosus	Carries oxygenated blood from umbilical vein to inferior vena cava.	Obliterated to become ligamentum venosum.
Inferior vena cava	Carries oxygenated blood from umbilical vein and ductus venosus and mixed blood from body and liver.	Carries only unoxygenated blood from body.
Foramen ovale	Connects right and left atria.	Functional closure by 3 months, although probe patency without symptoms may be retained by some adults.
Pulmonary arteries	Carry some mixed blood to lungs.	Carry unoxygenated blood to lungs.
Ductus arteriosus	Shunts mixed blood from pulmonary artery to aorta.	Generally occluded by 4 months and becomes ligamentum arteriosum.
Aorta	Receives mixed blood from heart and pulmonary arteries.	Carries oxygenated blood from left ventricle.
Umbilical arteries	Carry oxygenated and unoxygenated blood to the placenta.	Obliterated to become the vesical ligaments on the anterior abdominal wall.

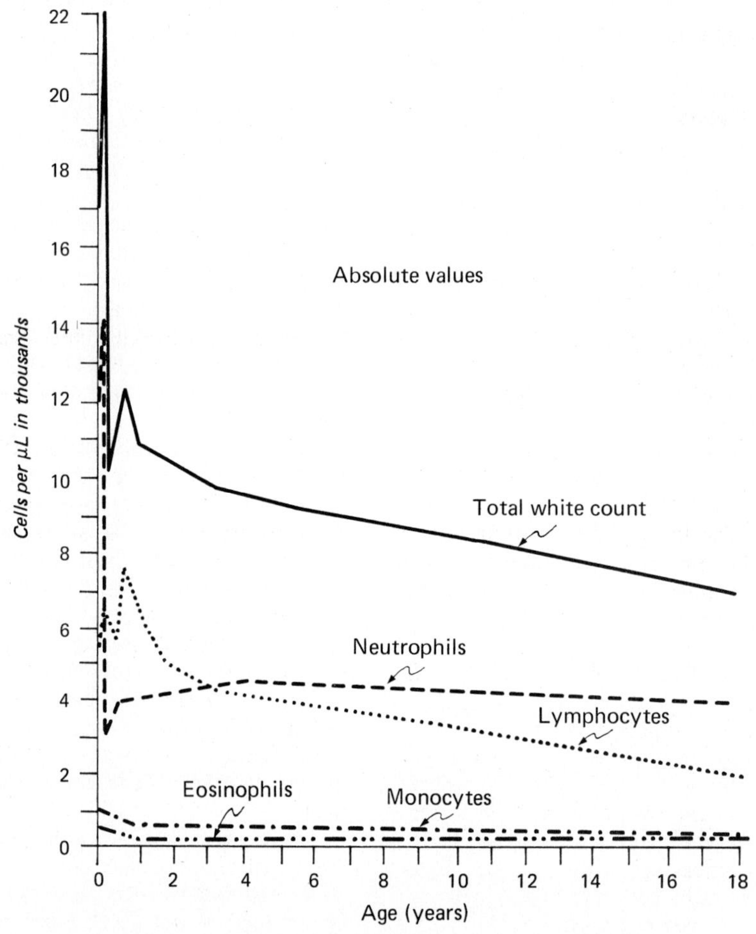

Figure 2–13. Life patterns of leukocytes. (Redrawn and reproduced from Whipple D: *Dynamics of Development: Euthenic Pediatrics*. Copyright © 1966 by McGraw-Hill. Used with permission of McGraw-Hill Book Co.)

The Gastrointestinal Tract

A. Newborn: Gas may be seen on x-ray almost immediately after birth in the stomach, within 2 hours in the ileum, and, on the average, in 3 or 4 hours in the rectum.

B. Enzymes:

1. There is a deficiency of the starch-splitting enzyme amylase during early infancy; this prevents optimal handling of long-chain polysaccharides. Amylase is present in significant amounts in the pancreatic juice by 3 months of age.

2. Lipase activity is low throughout early childhood. In contrast, trypsin activity is adequate from birth except in the premature infant, in whom low levels are often found.

C. Ketone Bodies: Ketone bodies are not formed as readily by the liver of the young infant as by the older child; acetone is seldom found in the urine at any time during the first 6 months of life.

D. Gastric Acidity: Gastric juice acidity is low during infancy and rises during childhood, with a marked increase during adolescence. Acidity is greater in boys than in girls.

E. Transit Time: Food passes through the stomach more rapidly in the infant than in the older child. Protein digestion is less complete in the stomach of the infant than in the older child.

F. Stomach Capacity: The capacity of the stomach is approximately 30–90 mL at birth, 90–150 mL at 1 month, 210–360 mL at 1 year, approximately 500 mL at 2 years, and averages 750–900 mL in later childhood.

G. Other:

1. Some spitting-up is common in early infancy in almost all children.

2. The abdomen tends to be prominent in infants and toddlers. In the infant, the ascending and descending portions of the colon are short compared with the transverse colon, and the sigmoid extends higher into the abdomen than during later life.

The Urinary System

A. In Utero: The kidney functions during fetal life and contributes some urine to the amniotic fluid, but the fetal kidney probably does not participate in the regulation of electrolyte balance.

B. Newborn:

1. In the kidney of the full-term infant at birth, there is a full quota of nephrons, but this may not be the case in the premature infant.

2. The first urine usually has a specific gravity of about 1.015. During the first weeks of life, the urine is scanty and quite dilute, probably as a result of poor response to antidiuretic hormone and immaturity of the renal tubules.

3. During the neonatal period, there is a low clearance of sodium, chloride, and urea, resulting in a hypotonic urine as compared to plasma.

4. The percentage of uric acid is higher in the urine of the newborn than later.

C. Childhood:

1. Renal immaturity probably exists for several months after birth; during the second year of life, the histologic structure of the kidney reaches its mature structure.

2. Glucose and albumin may normally be present in the urine.

D. Urine Volume: The average infant secretes 15–50 mL of urine per 24 hours during the first 2 days of life, 50–300 mL/d during the next week, 250–400 mL/d during the next 2 months, and 400–500 mL/d by the latter half of the first year. There is subsequently a gradual increase in urinary output; 700–1000 mL/d is secreted during ages 5–8 and 700–1500 mL/d between the ages of 8 and 14.

E. Glomerular Filtration: Glomerular filtration rate is low during the first 9 months of life, as are urea clearance, renal plasma flow, and maximal tubular excretory capacity.

F. Creatine and Creatinine:

1. Creatine is excreted in large amounts by the infant and to a lesser degree by children before puberty; men excrete almost no creatine and women very little.

2. Creatinine output increases throughout the growing period, the quantity being directly related to the amount of body musculature.

Fat, Muscle, & Body Water

A. Fat: The body contains equal amounts of fat and protein at or shortly before birth; subsequently, the amount of fat exceeds the amount of protein.

1. Fat is first laid down about the sixth month of pregnancy.

2. The fat of the fetus and newborn infant has a higher degree of saturation, a higher melting point, and contains more palmitic but less stearic and oleic acids than the fat of the older child or adult.

3. There is a gradual decrease in the body stores of fat from the middle of the first year to age 6 or 7 years; girls tend to retain more fat than boys, but the differences are slight during childhood. Fat begins to reaccumulate from age 6–7 up to puberty. At that time, the amount of fat decreases in the male but continues to increase in the female.

B. Muscle:

1. At birth, muscle constitutes a smaller portion (20–25%) of the total body weight than it does in the adult.

2. During the second trimester of pregnancy, skeletal musculature forms about one-sixth of the body weight; at birth, one-fifth to one-fourth; in early adolescence, one-third; and in early maturity, approximately two-fifths. The gain in musculature during childhood equals the growth of all other organs, systems, and tissues combined.

C. Body Water:

1. The water content of the body is approximately 95% by weight in early fetal life; 65–75% at birth; and 55–60% at maturity.

2. The infant ingests and excretes approximately

20% of total body fluid daily, whereas the adult has a water exchange of only 5% of total body fluid. For the infant, this represents nearly 50% of extracellular fluid volume; for the adult, 14% of extracellular fluid volume.

Temperature, Basal Metabolic Rate, & Steroids

A. Body Temperature: (Table 2–7.) Body temperature during childhood is on the average 37.3 °C (99.1 °F) in the first year, 37.5 °C (99.4 °F) in the fourth year, 37 °C (98.6 °F) in the fifth year, and 36.7 °C (98 °F) in the 12th year. During childhood, there is no appreciable difference in the body temperature of boys and girls, but after adolescence, women tend to have a higher temperature than men.

B. Basal Metabolic Rate:

1. Fetal metabolism is lower than that of the newborn.

2. The basal metabolic rate is highest in the young infant and falls continuously throughout life.

3. Boys and girls have comparable basal metabolic rates, but the rate is higher in men than in women.

C. Steroids:

1. Plasma levels of 17-ketosteroids at birth and for a few days thereafter are 2–5 times higher than in the adult; urinary excretion is higher in the neonatal period than later in infancy.

2. The plasma levels and the urinary excretion of 17-hydroxycorticosteroids are decreased in the newborn infant when compared with the mother's levels (which are elevated, particularly during vaginal delivery). Plasma levels remain low for the first 1–2 weeks after birth, gradually rising to adult levels.

Organs of Special Sense

A. Tactile Sensation:

1. At birth, the newborn infant has mature sensory receptors for pressure, pain, and temperature from the entire body surface, from the mouth, and from the external genitalia; the infant also has mature pain receptors in the viscera and proprioceptive receptors in muscles, joints, and tendons.

2. A response to touch is first elicited in the region of the face, particularly the lips.

B. Taste: The ability to taste is present in the newborn infant, and the 4 basic tastes can be distinguished at this time.

C. Smell: The human infant is born with fully mature receptors for olfaction; the infant may have a stronger sense of smell than the older individual, but this is difficult to test.

D. Hearing:

1. Normal infants can hear almost immediately after birth, but because of a lack of myelinization of cortical auditory pathways, they respond to sounds at a subcortical level. Voluntary muscular action in response to sound is present in the average infant by 2 months of age.

2. Although the hearing mechanism in the ear is anatomically mature soon after birth, full maturity of total auditory function may not be present for 5–7 years.

3. The infant can localize a direction of sound by the middle of the first year.

E. Vision: (Table 2–8.) The visual system is relatively immature at birth. The eyeball is less spherical, the cornea is larger, the anterior chamber is more shallow, and the lens more spherical than in the older individual. Because of a lack of myelinization of cerebral neural pathways, the striated muscles that move the eyeballs are not under voluntary control.

1. Anatomic considerations—

a. The macula begins to differentiate during the first month of life, is well organized by 4 months, and is histologically mature by 8 months.

b. Final development of the macula is reached at about 6 years of age.

c. Tears can be produced during the early weeks of life.

d. The newborn infant is hyperopic; the eyeball grows rapidly for the first 8 years of life, becoming even more hyperopic as a result of changes in the cornea and lens. The eyeball reaches adult size at about age 8 and then tends to become comparatively myopic. Thus, hyperopia is to be expected in the preschool and early school years.

e. Some children may have brief episodes of transient strabismus during the first few months of life. These usually clear spontaneously. Irrespective of age, strabismus that is present for prolonged periods needs ophthalmologic consultation and evaluation as soon as recognized. Mature adult function of the eye muscles is usually reached by the end of the first year.

2. Functional considerations—

a. At birth, there is an awareness of light and dark, and an infant is capable of rudimentary fixation on near objects.

b. The newborn is capable of peripheral vision, but other visual functions are deficient.

c. Pupillary response is present in late fetal life.

Table 2–7. Average body temperatures in well children under basal conditions.*

Age	Temperature and Standard Deviation	
	°F	°C
3 months	99.4 (0.8)	37.4 (0.4)
6 months	99.5 (0.6)	37.5 (0.3)
1 year	99.7 (0.5)	37.6 (0.2)
3 years	99.0 (0.5)	37.2 (0.2)
5 years	98.6 (0.5)	37.0 (0.2)
7 years	98.3 (0.5)	36.8 (0.2)
9 years	98.1 (0.5)	36.7 (0.2)
11 years	98.0 (0.5)	36.7 (0.2)
13 years	97.8 (0.5)	36.5 (0.2

* From *Growth and Development of Children,* by Ernest H. Watson, MD. Copyright © 1978. Year Book Medical Publishers, Inc. Used by permission.

Table 2–8. Chronology of visual development.

Age	Level of Development
Birth	Awareness of light and dark. Infant closes eyelids in bright light.
Neonatal	Rudimentary fixation on near objects (3–30 inches).
2 weeks	Transitory fixation, usually monocular at a distance of roughly 3 feet.
4 weeks	Follows large conspicuously moving objects.
6 weeks	Moving objects evoke binocular fixation briefly.
8 weeks	Follows moving objects with jerky eye movements. Convergence beginning to appear.
12 weeks	Visual following now a combination of head and eye movements. Convergence improving. Enjoys light objects and bright colors.
16 weeks	Inspects own hands. Fixates immediately on a 1-inch cube brought within 1–2 feet of eye. Vision 20/300–20/200 (6/100–6/70).
20 weeks	Accommodative convergence reflexes all organizing. Visually pursues lost rattle. Shows interest in stimuli more than 3 feet away.
24 weeks	Retrieves a dropped 1-inch cube. Can maintain voluntary fixation of stationary object even in the presence of competing moving stimulus. Hand-eye coordination appearing.
26 weeks	Will fixate on a string.
28 weeks	Binocular fixation clearly established.
36 weeks	Beginning of depth perception.
40 weeks	Marked interest in tiny objects. Tilts head backward to gaze up. Vision 20/200 (6/70).
52 weeks	Fusion beginning to appear. Discriminates simple geometric forms (squares and circles). Vision 20/180 (6/60).
12–18 months	Looks at pictures with interest.
18 months	Convergence well established. Localization in distance crude—runs into large objects.
2 years	Accommodation well developed. Vision 20/40 (6/12).
3 years	Convergence smooth. Fusion improving. Vision 20/30 (6/9).
4 years	Vision 20/20 (6/6).

d. The ability to fixate well is usually present by 2–3 months of age.

e. Perception of bright colors is probably present at 3–5 months of age.

f. Depth perception develops at about 9 months of age but does not reach a mature level until age 6.

g. Convergence begins to appear at approximately 8 weeks of age. At 4 months, vision is 20/300–20/200 (6/100–6/70). By 7 months of age, binocular fixation is clearly established. Depth perception becomes apparent at 9 months. At 10 months, vision is 20/200 (6/70). At 1 year, fusion is beginning to appear, and at 18 months convergence is well established. At 2 years, accommodation is well developed; vision is 20/40 (6/12). By 3 years, fusion is appearing and vision is 20/30 (6/9). Vision becomes 20/20 (6/6) at age 4.

h. Fusion of images probably occurs by the sixth year.

Immune Mechanisms

See also Chapter 17.

A. In Utero:

1. Antibodies of low molecular weight—7S immunoglobulin G (IgG)—may appear in higher concentration in fetal than in maternal blood. Antibodies of high molecular weight—19S immunoglobulin M (IgM)—are usually found in low concentration in the fetus.

2. The placenta permits the transfer of 7S IgG molecules to the fetus but selectively withholds the IgM and IgA. Transfer of gamma globulin from mother to fetus takes place principally in the last trimester; blood levels of gamma globulin are higher in the full-term infant than in the premature infant.

3. Immunoglobulins are normally not synthesized in utero. Macroglobulins (19S IgM) may be synthesized in response to antigenic stimulation.

B. Newborn Period and Infancy:

1. During the first months of postnatal life, the infant has passive immunity to certain diseases to which the mother was immune, but such immunity is generally limited to those whose antibodies are carried in the 7S IgG fraction. Maternal immunity carried solely in macroglobulins is not passed on.

2. In the newborn period, the blood contains a relatively high level of passively transmitted 7S IgG and no or very little 7S and 19S IgM. The 7S IgG that was passively transferred from the mother gradually disappears from the infant's circulation. The lowest level of gamma globulin is reached about the 15th–80th day.

3. The newborn can manufacture antibody (macroglobulins) as early as the end of the first week of life. By the end of the first year, the child can produce 19S IgM as effectively as the adult. However, the newborn is unable to synthesize 7S IgG.

C. Childhood: In the normal adult, the presence of 19S IgM is followed within 1–2 weeks by the appearance of 7S IgG, but in the infant relatively little 7S IgG appears subsequent to 19S IgM formation.

Adolescent Changes

See Tables 2–9 and 2–10.

A. Both Sexes:

1. The adolescent growth spurt in both sexes is probably due to the production of androgens.

2. Girls mature earlier than boys.

3. Children destined to mature sexually at an early

Table 2–9. Time of appearance of sexual characteristics in North American girls.*

Pelvis	Female contour assumed and fat deposition begins	8–10 years
Breasts	First hypertrophy or budding	9–11 years
	Further enlargement and pigmentation of nipples	12–13 years
	Histologic maturity	16–18 years
Vagina	Secretion begins and glycogen content of epithelium increased with change in cell type	11–14 years
Pubic hair	Initial appearance	10–12 years
	Abundant and curly	11–15 years
Axillary hair	Initial appearance	12–14 years
Acne	Varies considerably	12–16 years

* From *Growth and Development of Children,* by Ernest H. Watson, MD. Copyright © 1978. Year Book Medical Publishers, Inc. Used by permission.

age tend to be tall and have an advanced bone age; late-maturing children are short and show epiphyseal retardation.

4. Sexual maturation is more closely correlated with bone maturation than with chronologic age.

B. Girls: (Table 2–9.)

1. The vaginal mucosa converts from columnar to squamous shortly before menarche. This is associated with an increased glycogen content of the mucosa and a lowering of the pH.

2. The maximal yearly increase in height occurs during the year before menarche in most girls.

3. Climate apparently has little effect on sexual development. Nigerian girls and Eskimo girls have their menarche at approximately the same age.

4. If environmental and nutritional factors are similar, girls of different races tend to have their menarche at the same approximate age.

5. During the first 1–2 years following menarche, the menstrual periods of most girls are anovulatory.

6. The first several menses are often irregular, and the interval between periods may be longer or shorter than is characteristic of later life.

7. Girls with early menarche have a more accelerated growth curve than girls with late menarche, but the duration of their growth is shorter.

8. Girls who mature later are taller (on the average) when final stature is attained.

C. Boys: (Table 2–10.) Some degree of breast hypertrophy (gynecomastia) is relatively common in boys at puberty.

Table 2–10. Time of appearance of sexual characteristics in North American boys.*

Breasts	Some hypertrophy, often assuming a firm nodularity	12–14 years
	Disappearance of hypertrophy	14–17 years
Testes and penis	Increase in size begins	10–12 years
	Rapid growth	12–15 years
Pubic hair	Initial appearance	12–14 years
	Abundant and curly	13–16 years
Axillary hair	Initial appearance	13–16 years
Facial and body hair	Initial appearance	15–17 years
Acne	Varies considerably	14–18 years
Mature sperm	Average range	14–16 years

From *Growth and Development of Children,* by Ernest H. Watson, MD. Copyright © 1978. Year Book Medical Publishers, Inc. Used by permission.

"Bone Age" (Epiphyseal Development)

See Table 2–11 and Fig 2–14.

The ideal method of evaluating bone age would be based upon x-rays of all the bones. However, this is not practical owing to limitations of time, cost, and danger of excessive radiation. At all ages, the most useful areas to evaluate are the wrists and hands; before age 2 years, x-rays of the feet and knees are also valuable.

The time of appearance and union of various epiphyseal centers follows a specific sequential pattern during both intra- and extrauterine life.

At birth, the average full-term infant has 5 ossification centers demonstrable by x-ray; the distal end of the femur, the proximal end of the tibia, the calcaneus, the talus, and the cuboid.

Calcification begins during the fifth fetal week. The clavicle is the first bone to calcify in utero.

Epiphyseal development of girls is consistently ahead of that of boys throughout childhood.

Teeth

See Table 2–12 and Chapter 12.

DEVELOPMENT*

The physician is as responsible for the preservation of health as for the treatment of disease. In order to carry out the former and to identify developmental deviations that may require further assessment, persons responsible for child care must understand the dynamic process involved in what we call development. Development applies to the maturation of organs and systems as well as the acquisition of skills and the ability to adapt to new situations. (See Table 2–15 and Figs 2–15 and 2–16.)

* Edited and revised by William K. Frankenburg, MD.

Table 2–11. Time of appearance of epiphyseal ossification centers.*

Age (Year//Month†) Percentile (Boys)			Epiphyseal Centers	Age (Year//Month†) Percentile (Girls)		
5	50‡	95		5	50‡	95
			Hand and Wrist			
Birth	0 // 2.5	0 // 4	Capitate	< term §	0 // 2.25	0 // 4
Birth	0 // 3.5	0 // 6	Hamate	< term §	0 // 2.5	0 // 5
0 // 8	1 // 0	2 // 0	Distal radius	0 // 6	0 // 10	1 // 6
1 // 0	1 // 6	2 // 0	Proximal third carpal	0 // 9	0 // 11	1 // 3
1 // 0	1 // 6	2 // 0	Proximal second and fourth carpals	0 // 9	0 // 11	1 // 6
1 // 3	1 // 6	2 // 3	Second metacarpal	0 // 9	0 // 11	1 // 6
1 // 0	1 // 6	2 // 3	Distal first carpal	0 // 9	1 // 0	1 // 6
1 // 3	1 // 9	2 // 6	Third metacarpal	0 // 9	1 // 0	1 // 6
1 // 6	2 // 0	2 // 6	Fourth metacarpal	1 // 0	1 // 3	1 // 9
1 // 6	2 // 0	2 // 6	Proximal fifth carpal	1 // 0	1 // 3	2 // 0
1 // 6	2 // 0	2 // 6	Middle third and fourth carpals	1 // 0	1 // 3	2 // 0
1 // 6	2 // 3	3 // 0	Fifth metacarpal	1 // 0	1 // 6	2 // 0
1 // 6	2 // 3	3 // 0	Middle second carpal	1 // 0	1 // 6	2 // 0
1 // 0	2 // 3	4 // 6	Triquetrum	1 // 0	1 // 6	3 // 0
2 // 0	2 // 3	3 // 0	First metacarpal	1 // 6	1 // 6	2 // 6
2 // 6	3 // 0	3 // 6	Proximal first carpal**	1 // 3	1 // 9	2 // 6
2 // 6	3 // 6	5 // 0	Middle fifth carpal**	1 // 6	2 // 0	3 // 3
1 // 6	4 // 0	5 // 6	Lunate**	2 // 6	3 // 0	4 // 0
3 // 6	5 // 3	6 // 6	Greater multangular**	2 // 6	4 // 0	5 // 6
3 // 6	5 // 3	6 // 6	Lesser multangular**	2 // 6	4 // 0	5 // 6
4 // 0	5 // 3	7 // 0	Navicular**	3 // 0	4 // 0	6 // 6
6 // 0	7 // 0	8 // 0	Distal ulna	5 // 0	5 // 6	7 // 0
10 // 0	11 // 0	13 // 0	Pisiform	7 // 6	8 // 0	10 // 6
			Extremities (Excluding Hand and Wrist)			
< term §	< term §	2 weeks	Distal femur	< term §	< term §	1 week
< term §	< term §	2 weeks	Proximal tibia	< term §	< term §	1 week
< term §	2 weeks	6 weeks	Tarsal cuboid	< term §	1 week	2 weeks
Birth	3 weeks	0 // 2	Head of humerus	Birth	2 weeks	0 // 1
0 // 3	0 // 4	0 // 9	Distal tibia	0 // 2	0 // 3	0 // 8
0 // 4	0 // 5	0 // 10	Head of femur	0 // 3	0 // 4	0 // 8
0 // 5	0 // 7	1 // 6	Capitellum of humerus	0 // 3	0 // 5	1 // 0
0 // 7	1 // 0	2 // 0	Greater tuberosity of humerus	0 // 4	0 // 8	1 // 6
0 // 8	1 // 0	2 // 0	Distal fibula	0 // 8	0 // 9	1 // 6
2 // 6	3 // 6	4 // 6	Greater trochanter of femur	2 // 0	2 // 6	4 // 0
3 // 0	4 // 0	5 // 6	Proximal fibula	2 // 0	2 // 6	4 // 6
3 // 6	5 // 0	7 // 6	Proximal radius	3 // 0	4 // 0	6 // 0
4 // 6	6 // 0	8 // 0	Medial epicondyle of humerus	3 // 0	3 // 6	6 // 0
7 // 6	10 // 0	12 // 0	Trochlea of humerus	6 // 0	8 // 0	10 // 0
8 // 0	10 // 6	12 // 0	Proximal ulna	6 // 6	8 // 0	9 // 6
10 // 0	12 // 0	13 // 0	Lateral epicondyle of humerus	8 // 0	9 // 6	11 // 0

* Adapted from Marian Maresh. Compiled from data obtained from the Harvard Growth Study, Fels Institute, Brush Foundation, and the University of Colorado Child Research Council.
† Example of notation: 1 // 3 = 1 year 3 months.
‡ 50th percentile and mean are approximately the same in most studies.
§ < term = before term.
** Centers that are most variable in time and order of appearance.

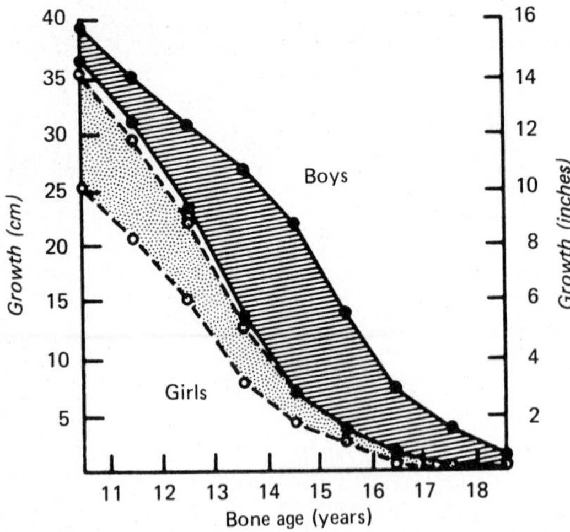

Figure 2–14. Growth expectancy at bone ages indicated. (Redrawn and reproduced, with permission, from Holt LE Jr, McIntosh R, Barnett HL: *Pediatrics*, 13th ed. Appleton-Century-Crofts, 1962, as redrawn from Harris JA et al: *Measurement of Man*. University of Minnesota Press, 1930.)

Progress of Development

Development is a continuous process that starts with conception and follows an orderly sequential course until death. Children sit before they stand, say single words before they speak phrases and sentences, and draw circles before they can draw squares. Development does not proceed at a constant rate but in bursts of rapid progress interrupted by resting plateaus.

The developmental process takes place in a cephalocaudal direction: control of the head precedes control of the arms, and both precede control of the legs.

Development in the extremities progresses in a direction from proximal to distal: control of the arms and legs occurs before control of the wrists and fingers and the feet and toes.

Development proceeds from the massive to the specific. Initially, a young infant responds to seeing a toy by moving the entire body; at a later age, by reaching with one hand to grasp it. The infant who has learned to say "milk" may use the word to mean "Bring me a glass of milk" or "Take the milk"—or the word milk may be used to signify some other drink. Eventually, the word is used to denote what

Table 2–12. Dental growth and development.

Primary (Deciduous) Teeth

	Crown Calcification Begins At	Root Completed At	Maxillary Teeth Erupt At	Mandibular Teeth Erupt At	Maxillary Teeth Exfoliate At	Mandibular Teeth Exfoliate At
Central incisor	14 weeks in utero	18 months	6–10 months	5–8 months	6–7½ years	6–7 years
Lateral incisor	16 weeks in utero	18–24 months	8–12 months	8–13 months	7–8½ years	7–8 years
Cuspid	17 weeks in utero	39 months	16–20 months	16–20 months	10–12 years	9–11 years
First molar	15½ weeks in utero	27–30 months	12–18 months	12–18 months	9–11 years	9–11 years
Second molar	18 weeks in utero	36 months	20–30 months	20–30 months	11–13 years	11–13 years

Secondary (Permanent) Teeth

	Crown Calcification Begins At	Root Completed At	Maxillary Teeth Erupt At	Mandibular Teeth Erupt At
Central incisor	3–4 months	9–10 years	7–8 years	6–7 years
Lateral incisor	Maxilla: 10–12 months Mandible: 3–4 months	10–11 years	8–9 years	7–8 years
Cuspid	4–5 months	12–15 years	11–12 years	9–11 years
First premolar	18–24 months	12–14 years	10–11 years	10–12 years
Second premolar	24–30 months	12–14 years	10–12 years	11–13 years
First molar	Birth	9–10 years	6–7 years	6–7 years
Second molar	2½–3 years	14–16 years	12–14 years	12–14 years
Third molar	7–10 years	18–25 years	17–25 years	17–25 years

we mean by milk and is combined with other words to form phrases and sentences.

Factors Influencing Development

During "critical" growth periods, interference with the normal course of development may result in long-standing developmental deficits. Just as rubella during the first trimester of pregnancy may result in congenital anomalies, so may untreated cretinism, phenylketonuria, galactosemia, or malnutrition during the first few months of life result in developmental problems. When these conditions occur later in life, they are usually not associated with permanent significant developmental deficits.

Emotional and psychologic deprivation early in life may cause personality problems. Lack of appropriate stimulation at critical periods may result in neurologic deficits; eg, persons deprived of light and sound for a prolonged time may develop temporary hallucinations and electroencephalographic changes. The pattern of development can be influenced by genetic determinants, as when several family members have delayed language development. Genetic factors can also cause defective enzyme systems that lead to inborn errors of metabolism.

Whereas biologic factors determine the range of variation, environmental factors may greatly mediate the effect of biologic deficits. For example, an infant genetically destined to develop cretinism can be protected from the associated brain damage by adequate thyroid replacement therapy. Environmental influences can also affect motivation, curiosity, and learning ability.

Several studies have demonstrated that discrepancies in developmental rates due to differing socioeconomic environments may not become apparent until about age 24 months and then will increase with age. The home environment, especially of a child "at risk," must be evaluated by the health care professional. Specific methods of evaluation are available (see references, below).

Coons CE et al: *The Home Screening Questionnaire Reference Manual.* LADOCA Publishing Foundation, 1981.

Sameroff AJ: Early influences in development: Fact or fancy? *Merrill Palmer Quarterly* 1975;**21**:267.

Werner EE, Smith RS: *Kauai's Children Come of Age.* Univ of Hawaii Press, 1977.

DEVELOPMENT OF MOTOR SKILLS

Although practice of motor movements has a slight influence on the rate of development, maturation usually plays a much greater role. The newborn infant can perform a number of motor movements, mainly of a reflex type.

Motor development involving the hands tends to proceed along a definite sequential course. The child first looks from the hand to the object and then attempts to grasp objects with 2 hands. Grasping with the palm of the hand is learned first, using the ulnar side of the hand initially and later the radial side. Eventually, grasping with the thumb and index finger is mastered.

DEVELOPMENT OF SPEECH & LANGUAGE*

The normal development of speech and language requires exposure to language, normal structures of the organs of speech, and the following abilities: normal hearing in the speech frequencies (250–4000 Hz); comprehending what is heard; recalling what has been heard before; formulating a response; and controlling the muscles of speech. On the average, infants manifest speech and language development as shown in Table 2–13.

Normal Variations in Speech & Language Development

A normal 2-year-old child may have a vocabulary varying from a few words to well over 200 words. First children tend to speak earlier than subsequent children; twins later than singletons. In some reported studies, girls develop language earlier than boys. Early development of language is often found in intellectually gifted children. Slow onset of speech may be an indication of a problem in the child's development or environment.

Speech & Language Disorders

Speech and language problems can be detected within the first few years of life, and they should be discovered and treated before school age.

A. Delayed Development of Language: If a child does not produce words by 2 years of age, language may be considered to be retarded. This should be considered a significant delay of language, the principal causes of which are listed below.

1. Hearing loss or hypoacusis—The effect of hearing loss on speech and language development varies with the age at which the loss began (more severe in the younger child), the severity of loss, the configuration of the threshold audiogram, and the efficacy of treatment. (See Chapter 13.) Hypoacusis is frequently associated with incorrect articulation of **b, f,** and **u.** The sounds of **d, y,** and **w** are frequently substituted for **g, l,** and **r,** respectively. The child with a high-frequency hearing loss may react normally to the spoken voice or to sounds of low frequency, clapping of hands, or banging of doors. Hypoacusis, therefore, should only be ruled out by means of a complete audiologic evaluation.

2. Central nervous system dysfunction—The most common type of central nervous system dysfunction associated with delayed language development is mental retardation. Any child with delayed

* Edited by Florence Berman Blager, PhD.

Table 2–13. Normal speech and language development.

Age	Speech	Language	Articulation*
1 month	Throaty sounds		Vowels: /ah/, /uh/, /ee/
2 months	Vowel sounds ("eh"), coos		
2½ months	Squeals		
3 months	Babbles, initial vowels		
4 months	Guttural sounds ("ah," "go")		Consonants: m, p, b
5 months			Vowels: /o/, /u/
7 months	Imitates speech sounds		
8 months			Syllables: da, ba, ka
10 months		"Dada" or "mama" nonspecifically	Approximates names: baba/bottle
12 months	Jargon begins (own language)	One word other than "mama" or "dada"	Understandable: 2–3 words
13 months		Three words	
16 months		Six words	Consonants; t, d, w, n, h
18–24 months		Two-word phrases	Understandable 2-word phrases
24–30 months		Three-word phrases	Understandable 3-word phrases
2 years	Vowels uttered correctly	Approximately 270 words; uses pronouns	Approximately 270 words; uses phrases
3 years	Some degree of hesitancy and uncertainty common	Approximately 900 words; intelligible 4-word phrases	Approximately 900 words; intelligible 4-word phrases
4 years		Approximately 1540 words; intelligible 5-word phrases or sentences	Approximately 1540 words; intelligible 5-word phrases
6 years		Approximately 2560 words; intelligible 6- or 7-word sentences	Approximately 2560 words; intelligible 6- or 7-word sentences
7–8 years	Adult proficiency		

* Data on articulation from Berry MF: *Language Disorders of Children.* Appleton-Century-Crofts, 1969; and from Bzoch K, League R: *Receptive-Expressive Emergent Language Scale.* University Park Press, 1970.

language development should be evaluated intellectually in terms of nonverbal as well as verbal adaptive skills. Neurologic impairments anywhere in the complex speech mechanism may be manifested in delayed speech and language development.

3. Maternal deprivation—Children reared without adequate mothering may have delayed language development. Although other aspects of development may also be delayed, the delay in language is often the most prominent. Inadequate mothering may result in diminished affect, decreased motivation, failure to demonstrate stranger anxiety, inability to communicate nonverbally, and a history of an insatiable appetite.

4. Infantile autism—One of the most common manifestations of autism is a delay in language (see above).

5. Elective mutism—In this condition, children may not talk to certain persons but speak freely at home or elsewhere. Frequently, such children are shy. Birth of a sibling may cause a child to stop talking or to talk less and to regress in development in other ways.

6. Socially disadvantaged background—Since language is learned from other people, deprived environments may fail to provide suitable reinforcement or a sufficient variety of environmental experiences to develop verbal facility. Children from the lower socioeconomic classes may demonstrate significant deficits in vocabulary, in use of adjectives and adverbs, in correct sentence structure, and a general delay in development of articulation. Regional or ethnic dialects can delay acquisition of standard language structures.

7. Familial delay—Occasionally, a delay in language development (possibly resulting from delayed myelinization) affects several members of a family. The child usually comprehends normally. The delay in speech seldom persists beyond 3 years of age.

8. Histidinemia—In this rare familial aminoaciduria, delayed speech development may occur with mental retardation.

9. Twins—Twins are often late talkers.

10. Bilingualism—Bilingual children are usually delayed in early development of speech and language, but with maturity usually show adequate integration of both languages.

B. Voice Defects (Dysphonia): Loss or impairment of vocal quality and volume is due to excessive loudness and pitch. Although it is generally a functional process, it may evolve into an organic condition with the production of vocal cord nodules. It may also be due to structural defects (eg, papilloma of the larynx).

C. Articulation Disorders: Articulation errors may be produced by omissions, distortions, substitutions, additions, or a combination of these.

1. Causes of articulation disorders—

a. Physiologic and anatomic causes—Defects in the cerebrum and cranial nerves that innervate the muscles of the lips, tongue, and palate may produce articulation defects. Inadequate velopharyngeal closure may also cause articulation disorders, since normal articulation involves movement of the velum between the pendant position to closure against the posterior pharyngeal wall. Inappropriate closure removes the nasality from nasal consonants. Inadequate closure results in resonant properties such as "talking through the nose." Causes of inadequate closure are cleft palate, submucous cleft, velar paresis, and disproportion between the soft palate and posterior pharynx. Since the adenoids sometimes form part of the posterior surface against which the soft palate closes, removal of the adenoids may produce inadequate closure. Children with inadequate closure sometimes present with a history of fluids coming out of the nose during drinking. Failure of fusion of the upper lip and hypoplasia of the mandible are other causes of articulation disorders. Hearing loss can also cause articulation problems.

b. Environmental factors—Since a child replicates the speech heard in the home, articulation errors may be due to bilingual, cultural, and regional patterns or to imitation of articulation errors of the parents. The later a child starts to learn a second language, the more difficult it will be to master the necessary articulation skills.

2. Evaluation of articulation disorders—Before age 2½, the child should be producing sounds as shown in the column labeled "articulation" in Table 2–13. After age 2½, the Denver Articulation Screening Exam* is a useful, simple, accurate instrument for determining whether a child's articulation is appropriate for age. The test is designed to detect articulation problems in children age 2½–6 years. To administer the test, one determines the child's ability to correctly articulate each of the 30 italicized sounds found in the following 22 words.

1. *t*able
2. shi*rt*
3. *d*oor
4. tru*nk*
5. *j*umping
6. zi*pp*er
7. *gr*apes
8. *fl*ag
9. *th*umb
10. too*th*brush
11. *s*ock
12. vac*uum*
13. *y*arn
14. *mother*
15. *tw*inkle
16. *w*agon
17. *gum*
18. *h*ouse
19. *p*encil
20. *fish*
21. *leaf*
22. *carrot*

* Amelia F. Drumwright, University of Colorado Medical Center, 1971.

The child's articulation is also evaluated for general intelligibility when words are combined into sentences or phrases (Table 2–14). An abnormal response either in the articulation of single words or in general intelligibility is an indication for diagnostic evaluation by a speech pathologist.

The evaluation should also include a complete neurologic assessment; evaluation of general development or intelligence; assessment of social maturity with a scale such as the Vineland Social Maturity Scale; physical examination of the oropharyngeal cavity; a complete audiologic examination; and a complete pharyngeal assessment for children with severe palatal problems.

D. Dysrhythmia: Three to 4% of children manifest a lack of normal language fluency. There is no current theory that explains dysfluency. Dysrhythmias may be in the form of undue prolongation of word sounds, arrest of speech—mainly at the beginning of a sentence (hesitation)—or repetition of syllables at the beginning of phrases or sentences. Young children 2½–4 years of age normally manifest breaks in the rhythm of speech, with repetitions being most common.

E. Stuttering: Stuttering is a disturbance of rhythm and fluency of speech by an intermittent blocking, convulsive repetition, or prolongation of sounds, syllables, words, or phrases. It is probably caused by many factors. Both organic and psychogenic factors are considered to play a role. Fifty percent of people who stutter begin to do so before age 5, and most begin to stutter before age 11. Between ages 2 and 5, stuttering is usually transient or benign. Stuttering is 2–4 times more frequent in boys. Stuttering causes considerable anxiety in parents, who may then call the child's attention to it. This, in turn, makes the child more anxious and self-conscious and aggravates the problem. The child may avoid words that are difficult to enunciate or may even avoid speaking altogether. Facial and body movements may be associated with stuttering.

F. Cluttering: Cluttering is rapid nervous speech marked by omission of sounds or syllables. The child who clutters may repeat syllables or short words and be unaware that there is any speech disturbance. Clut-

Table 2–14. Evaluation of articulation disorders.*

	Age in Years						
	2½–3	3–3½	4–4½	4½–5	5–5½	5½–6	6 and older
Normal number of sounds articulated correctly	7 or more	15 or more	16 or more	18 or more	22 or more	24 or more	25 or more
Normal intelligibility	Understandable half the time or more	Easy to understand					

* Adapted from Drumwright A et al: The Denver articulation screening exam. *J Speech Hear Disord* 1973;**38**:3.

Table 2–15. Developmental charts for ages 3–15 years.*

Ages 3–4 years

Activities to be observed:

Climbs stairs with alternating feet.
Begins to button and unbutton.
"What do you like to do that's fun?" (Answers using plurals, personal pronoun, and verbs.)
Responds to command to place toy *in, on,* or *under* table.
Draws a circle when asked to draw a man (girl, boy).
Knows own sex. ("Are you a boy or a girl?")
Gives full name.
Copies a circle already drawn. ("Can you make one like this?")

Activities related by parent:

Feeds self at mealtime.
Takes off shoes and jacket.

Ages 4–5 years

Activities to be observed:

Runs and turns without losing balance.
May stand on one leg for at least 10 seconds.
Buttons clothes and laces shoes. (Does not tie.)
Counts to 4 by rote.
"Give me 2 sticks." (Able to do so from pile of 4 tongue depressors.)
Draws a man. (Head, 2 appendages, and possibly 2 eyes. No torso yet.)
Knows the days of the week. ("What day comes after Tuesday?")
Gives appropriate answers to: "What must you do if you are sleepy? Hungry? Cold?"
Copies + in imitation.

Activities related by parent:

Self care at toilet. (May need help with wiping.)
Plays outside for at least 30 minutes.
Dresses self except for tying.

Ages 5–6 Years

Activities to be observed:

Can catch ball.
Skips smoothly.
Copies a + already drawn.
Tells age.
Concept of 10 (eg, counts 10 tongue depressors). May recite to higher number by rote.
Knows right and left hand.
Draws recognizable man with at least 8 details.
Can describe favorite television program in some detail.

Activities related by parent:

Does simple chores at home. (Taking out garbage, drying silverware, etc.)
Goes to school unattended or meets school bus.
Good motor ability but little awareness of dangers.

Ages 6–7 Years

Activities to be observed:

Copies a Δ.
Defines words by use. ("What is an orange?" "To eat.")
Knows if morning or afternoon.
Draws a man with 12 details.
Reads several one-syllable printed words. (My, dog, see, boy.)
Uses pencil for printing name.

Ages 7–8 Years

Activities to be observed:

Counts by 2s and 5s.
Ties shoes.
Copies a ◇.
Knows what day of the week it is. (Not date or year.)
Reads paragraph #1 Durrell:

Reading:

Muff is a little yellow kitten. She drinks milk. She sleeps on a chair. She does not like to get wet.

Corresponding arithmetic:

$$\begin{array}{r}7\\+4\\\hline\end{array}\qquad\begin{array}{r}6\\+7\\\hline\end{array}\qquad\begin{array}{r}6\\-4\\\hline\end{array}\qquad\begin{array}{r}8\\-3\\\hline\end{array}$$

No evidence of sound substitution in speech (eg, *fr* for *thr*).
Adds and subtracts one-digit numbers.
Draws a man with 16 details.

Ages 8–9 Years

Activities to be observed:

Defines words better than by use. ("What is an orange?" "A fruit.")
Can give an appropriate answer to the following: "What is the thing for you to do if . . .
—you've broken something that belongs to someone else?"
—a playmate hits you without meaning to do so?"
Reads paragraph #2 Durrell:

Reading:

A little black dog ran away from home. He played with two big dogs. They ran away from him. It began to rain. He went under a tree. He wanted to go home, but he did not know the way. He saw a boy he knew. The boy took him home.

Corresponding arithmetic:

$$\begin{array}{r}67\\+4\\\hline\end{array}\qquad\begin{array}{r}45\\16\\+27\\\hline\end{array}\qquad\begin{array}{r}14\\-8\\\hline\end{array}\qquad\begin{array}{r}84\\-36\\\hline\end{array}$$

Is learning borrowing and carrying processes in addition and subtraction.

* Modified from Leavitt SR, Goodman H. Harvin D: *Pediatrics* 1963;**31**:499.

[cont'd]

Table 2–15 (cont'd). Developmental charts for ages 3–15 years.*

Ages 9–10 Years

Activities to be observed:

Knows the month, day, and year.

Names the months in order. (Fifteen seconds, one error.)

Makes a sentence with these 3 words in it: (One of 2. Can use words orally in proper context.)

1. work . . . money . . . men
2. boy . . . river . . . ball

Reads paragraph #3 Durrell:

Reading:

Six boys put up a tent by the side of a river. They took things to eat with them. When the sun went down, they went into the tent to sleep. In the night, a cow came and began to eat grass around the tent. The boys were afraid. They thought it was a bear.

Corresponding arithmetic:

$$5204 - 530 \qquad 23 \times 3 \qquad 837 \times 7$$

Should comprehend and answer question: "What was the cow doing?"

Learning simple multiplication.

Ages 10–12 Years

Activities to be observed:

Should read and comprehend paragraph #5 Durrell:

Reading:

In 1807, Robert Fulton took the first long trip in a steamboat. He went one hundred and fifty miles up the Hudson River. The boat went five miles an hour. This was faster than a steamboat had ever gone before. Crowds gathered on both banks of the river to see this new kind of boat. They were afraid that its noise and splashing would drive away all the fish.

Corresponding arithmetic:

$$420 \times 29 \qquad 9\overline{)72} \qquad 31\overline{)62}$$

Answer: "What river was the trip made on?"

Ask to write the sentence: "The fishermen did not like the boat."

Should do multiplication and simple division.

Ages 12–15 Years

Activities to be observed:

Reads paragraph #7 Durrell:

Reading:

Golf originated in Holland as a game played on ice. The game in its present form first appeared in Scotland. It became unusually popular and kings found it so enjoyable that it was known as "the royal game." James IV, however, thought that people neglected their work to indulge in this fascinating sport so that it was forbidden in 1457. James relented when he found how attractive the game was, and it immediately regained its former popularity. Golf spread gradually to other countries, being introduced in America in 1890. It has grown in favor until there is hardly a town that does not boast of a private or public course.

Corresponding arithmetic:

$$536\overline{)4762} \qquad \tfrac{1}{3} + \tfrac{1}{3} \qquad 7\tfrac{1}{6} - \tfrac{3}{4}$$

Reduce fractions to lowest forms.

Ask to write sentence: "Golf originated in Holland as a game played on ice."

Answers questions:

"Why was golf forbidden by James IV?"

"Why did he change his mind?"

Does long division, adds and subtracts fractions.

* Modified from Leavitt SR, Goodman H, Harvin D: *Pediatrics* 1963;**31**:499.

tering is due to a dissociation between thinking and speaking. Thus, a child may "get lost" in the middle of a sentence. Individual sounds may be articulated correctly, but the articulation breaks down when the child speaks in longer sentences. Some children who clutter also manifest dysrhythmic handwriting. There is often a family history of cluttering. Occasionally, cluttering may lead to stuttering.

With a young child, referral for counseling may prevent dysfluencies from becoming habituated. If any secondary facial or body movements are associated with stuttering, the child should be referred to an experienced speech pathologist.

Young children with delays in speech and language should be treated with home stimulation or specific therapy or both to produce maximum development.

Berry M: *Language Disorders in Children.* Appleton-Century-Crofts, 1969.

Blager FB: Speech and language evaluation. In: *Pediatric Developmental Diagnosis.* Frankenburg WK, Thornton GM, Cohrs MG (editors). Thieme-Stratton, 1981.

Drumwright A: *Denver Articulation Screening Exam.* University of Colorado Medical Center, 1971.

Mysak EK: *Pathologies of Speech System.* Williams & Wilkins, 1976.

Pushaw DR: *Teach Your Child to Talk.* Cebco/Standard, 1976.

DEVELOPMENTAL SCREENING*

There is general agreement that the physician and other health care professionals who give routine pediatric care should have some knowledge of child devel-

* Prepared by William K. Frankenburg, MD, and revised by Alma W. Fandal.

opment and be able to identify abnormal delays. The Denver Developmental Screening Test (DDST)† and a newly revised modification (DDST-R) can provide a profile of developmental progress and delays during infancy and the preschool years (Fig 2–15).

The DDST-R consists of a progressive sequence of developmental tasks that test personal-social, fine motor-adaptive, language, and gross motor skills. The order of the items is based on the age at which 90% of children in the original normative study could perform the tasks. Failure to perform an item passed by 90% of the child's age-mates should be considered significant, though not necessarily abnormal. The DDST-R can be easily and quickly administered, and serial evaluations can be scored on the same test sheet.

Test Materials for DDST-R

Skein of red wool, box of raisins, rattle with a narrow handle, small clear bottle with ⅝-inch opening, bell, tennis ball, 8 one-inch cubical colored blocks, pencil.

General Administration Instructions

The parent should be told that this is a developmental screening device to obtain an estimate of the child's level of development and that it is not expected that the child will be able to perform each of the test items. This test relies on observations of what the child can do and on reports by a parent who knows the child. Direct observation should be used whenever possible. Since the test requires active participation by the child, every effort should be made to put the child at ease. The younger child may be tested while sitting on the parent's lap. This should be done in such a way that the child can comfortably reach the test materials on the table. The test should be administered before any frightening or painful procedures. A child will often withdraw if the examiner rushes demands upon the child. One may start by laying out one or 2 test materials in front of the child while asking the parent about the child's mastery of some of the personal-social items. Administer the first few test items well below the child's age level in order to ensure an initial successful experience. To avoid distractions, it is best to remove all test materials from the table except those required for the test.

Steps in Administering the Test

(1) Calculate the exact age of the child in years and months. Place an "X" and the date of the examination next to that age on the scale at the top of the test form.

(2) Use the appropriate vertical line for the age of the child as a point of reference to determine which items should be administered.

(a) Administer the top 3 items in each sector (personal-social, fine motor-adaptive, language, gross motor) that are entirely to the left of the age line. If the child refuses or fails to perform one of these items, continue down the form, testing items to the left of the age line until at least 3 items are passed in each sector.

(b) Administer all items that are intersected by the age line.

(3) Only the items actually performed ("passed") are scored; place a large "P" at the right end of the bar around the item. Since the format of the test resembles that of a growth curve, the Ps will form a curve that makes the developmental progress readily apparent.

(4) If a child refuses to perform an item that must be observed by the examiner and cannot be rated on the basis of a parent's report, ask the parent to administer the item.

(5) Ask the parent if the child's performance is typical of performance at other times.

(6) Note parent and child behavior (how child feels at time of evaluation, relation to examiner, attention span, verbal behavior, self-confidence, etc).

(7) See instructions below for administering footnoted items.

(8) The same form can be used for serial testing by using a different color pencil for dating and scoring.

Interpretation

Each test item is represented by a bar located under the age scale in such a way as to indicate the ages at which 25%, 50%, 75%, and 90% of the standardization population could perform the task. The left end of the bar indicates the age at which 25% could perform the item; the hatch mark along the top line of the bar, 50%; the left end of the shaded area, 75%; and the right end, 90%.

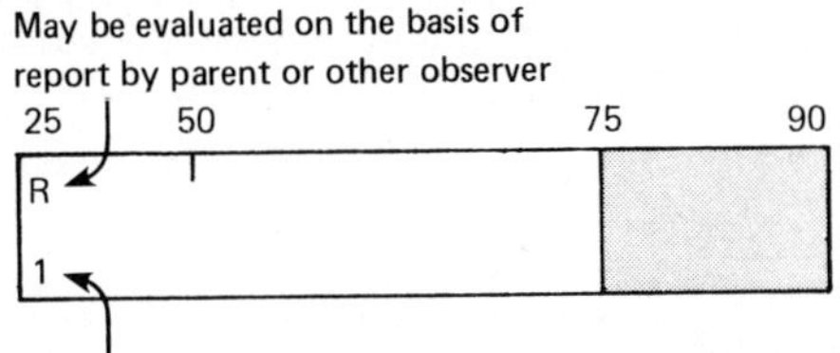

Failure to perform an item passed by 90% of children of the same age should be considered significant. Several delays in one sector are considered an indication of possible delayed developmental progress. These delays may be due to the following factors:

(1) Unwillingness of the child to perform even though capable.

(a) Transient interfering phenomena such as fatigue, fear, illness, hospitalization, or separation from the parent.

† The Denver Developmental Screening Test and Denver Prescreening Developmental Questionnaire can be ordered from LADOCA Project and Publishing Co., a sheltered workshop for retardates, at Lincoln and East 51st Ave., Denver 80216.

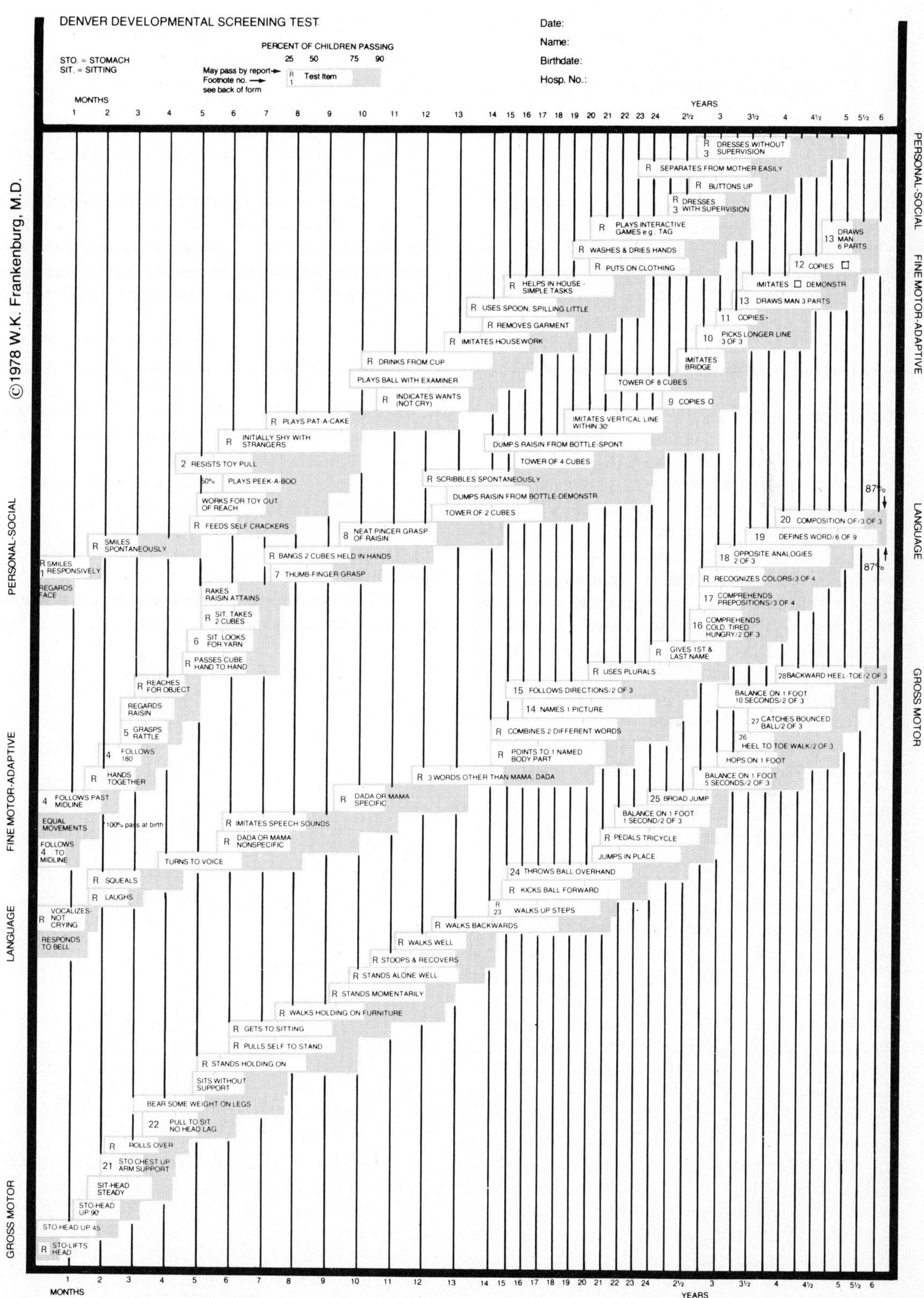

Figure 2–15. Denver Developmental Screening Test, Revised (DDST-R). See text for discussion of footnoted items.

   (b) General unwillingness to do what is asked. (This may be just as detrimental to success socially and in school as inability to perform.)
(2) Inability to perform the item because of—
   (a) General retardation.
   (b) Pathologic factors such as deafness or neurologic impairment.
   (c) Familial pattern of slow development in one or more areas.

If unexplained delays are noted and are a valid reflection of the child's abilities, a second screening examination should be scheduled 1 month later. If the delays persist, further evaluation with more detailed diagnostic studies is indicated.

Caution: The DDST is not an intelligence test. It is intended as a screening instrument for use in a clinical setting to determine whether the development of a particular child is within the normal range.

Abbreviated DDST

For health programs serving children whose parents have less than a high school education and where the schedule prevents administering a complete DDST each time a child is seen for well child care, a 2-stage screening procedure is recommended. First-stage screening with an abbreviated DDST should be followed by second-stage screening with a full DDST or DDST-R when the score of the abbreviated test is suspect. The abbreviated DDST requires the same careful calculation of a child's age as the full test, but only 12 items need be administered. In each of the 4 sectors, the first 3 items immediately to the left of the child's age should be given. If all 12 items are passed, no further testing is needed until the next age on the periodic screening schedule. However, if one or more of the 12 items is refused or failed, the full test should be completed while the child is in the test setting.

Prescreening Developmental Questionnaire (PDQ)

When caring for patients whose parents are likely to have had a high school education or more, developmental screening can be done with an even faster but equally effective parent-answered questionnaire: the Prescreening Developmental Questionnaire (PDQ). The PDQ requires the parent to answer 10 age-appropriate questions formulated from DDST items and related to the child's current developmental status. Scores of 8 or fewer "yes" answers should be considered suspect and require rescreening with the PDQ 2–4 weeks later. A child who receives a score of 6 or fewer "yes" answers on the second PDQ should be referred for diagnostic testing. A score of more than 6 on the second PDQ would indicate that no further testing would be done until that child reaches the next age on the periodic screening schedule.

Note: It should be remembered that nonsuspect screening results are not always a guarantee of problem-free development. If the physician or the parents are concerned about some aspect of a child's development, that child should receive further testing regardless of the screening test score.

Directions for Footnoted Items

(1) Try to get child to smile by smiling or by talking or waving. *Do not touch the child.*

(2) When child is playing with toy, pull it away. Pass if the child resists.

(3) Child does not have to be able to tie shoes or button in the back.

(4) Move yarn slowly in an arc from one side to the other, about 6 inches above child's face. Pass if eyes follow 90 degrees to midline (past midline, 180 degrees).

(5) Pass if child grasps rattle when it is touched to the backs or tips of fingers.

(6) Pass if child continues to look where yarn disappeared or tries to see where it went. Yarn should be dropped quickly from sight from tester's hand without arm movement.

(7) Pass if child picks up raisin with any part of thumb and a finger.

(8) Pass if child picks up raisin with the ends of thumb and index finger using an overhand approach.

(9) Copy. Pass any enclosed form. *Do not name form. Do not demonstrate.*

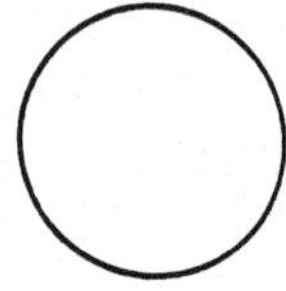

(10) "Which line is *longer?*" (Not *bigger.*) Turn paper upside down and repeat. Pass 3 of 3 or 5 of 6.

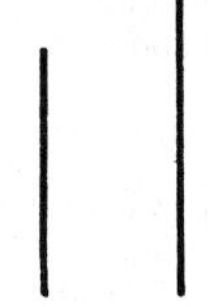

(11) Copy. Pass any crossing lines. *Do not name form. Do not demonstrate.*

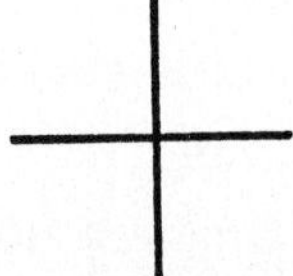

(12) Have child copy first. If the child fails, demonstrate. *Do not name form.*

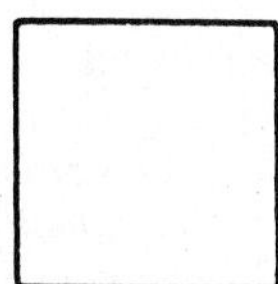

(13) When scoring symmetric forms, each pair (2 arms, 2 legs, etc) counts as one part.

(14) Point to picture and have child name it. (No credit is given for sounds only.)

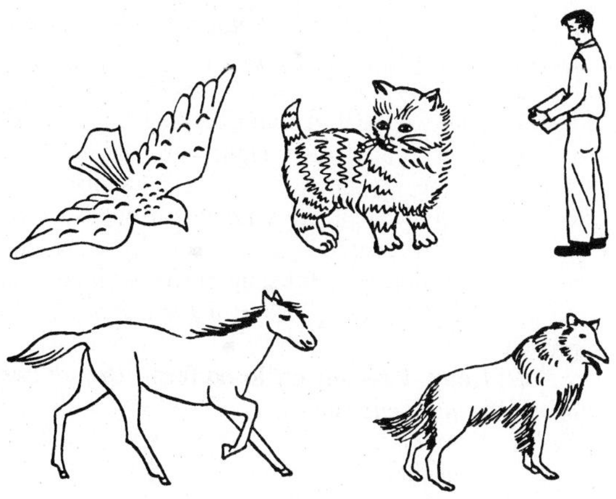

(15) Tell child to: "Give block to Mommy." "Put block on table." "Put block on floor." Pass 2 of 3.

(16) Ask child, "What do you do when you are cold?" "Hungry?" "Tired?" Pass 2 of 3.

(17) Tell child to: "Put block on table." ". . . under table." ". . . in front of chair." ". . . behind chair." Pass 3 of 4. *Do not help child by pointing or by moving head or eyes.*

(18) Ask child, "If fire is hot, ice is —." "Mother is a woman; Dad is a —" (answer must be "man"). "A horse is big; a mouse is —." Pass 2 of 3.

(19) Ask child, "What is a ball?" ". . . a lake?" ". . . a desk?" ". . . a house?" ". . . a banana?" ". . . a curtain?" ". . . a ceiling?" ". . . a hedge?" ". . . a pavement?" Pass if defined in terms of use, shape, what it is made of, or general category (eg, *fruit,* not just *yellow*). Pass 6 of 9.

(20) Ask child, "What is a spoon made of?" ". . . a shoe made of?" ". . . a door made of?" (No other objects may be substituted.) Pass 3 of 3.

(21) When placed on stomach, child lifts chest off table with support of forearms or hands (or both).

(22) When child is on back, grasp by the hands and pull to sitting position. Pass if head does not hang back.

(23) Child may use wall or rail only, not a person. May not crawl.

(24) Child must throw ball overhand 3 feet to within arm's reach of tester.

(25) Child must perform standing broad jump over width of test sheet (8½ inches).

(26) Tell child to walk forward, heel within 1

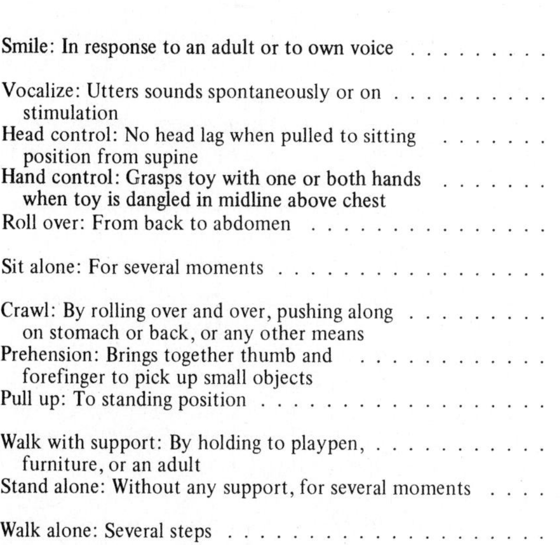

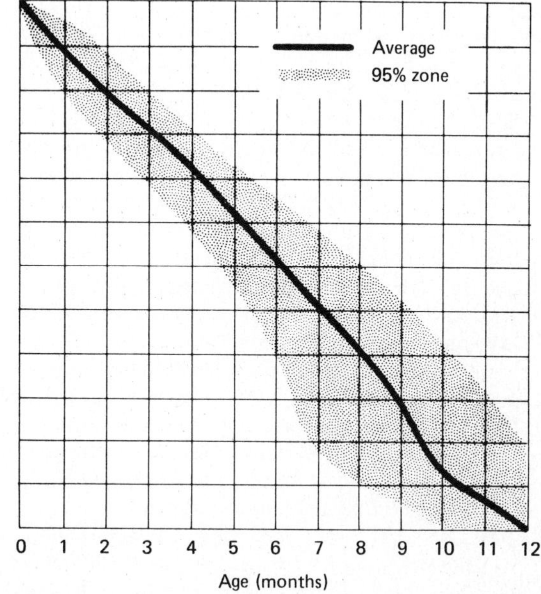

Figure 2–16. Norms of development. (Adapted from Aldrich CA, Norval HA: A developmental graph for the first year of life. *J Pediatr* 1946;**29**:304.)

inch of toe. Tester may demonstrate. Child must walk 4 consecutive steps in 2 out of 3 trials.

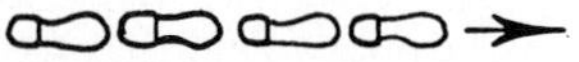

(27) Bounce ball to child, who should stand 3 feet away from tester. Child must catch ball with hands, not arms, in 2 out of 3 tries.

(28) Tell child to walk backward, toe within 1 inch of heel. Tester may demonstrate. Child must walk 4 consecutive steps in 2 out of 3 tries.

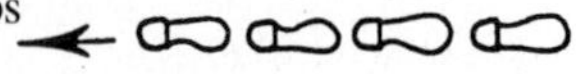

Date and behavioral observations: How child feels at time of test, relation to tester, attention span, verbal behavior, self-confidence, etc.

Frankenburg WK, Dodds JB: The Denver Developmental Test. *J Pediatr* 1967;**71**:181.

Frankenburg WK et al: The newly abbreviated and revised Denver Developmental Screening Test. *J Pediatr* 1981; **99**:995.

PERSONALITY DEVELOPMENT*

Personality development is a dynamic process, and no summary can give a complete picture of what takes place. The goal of the individual, both as a child and as an adult, is to be able to work, to play, to master personal problems, and to love and be loved in a manner that is creative, socially acceptable, and personally gratifying.

The development of personality is a complicated process involving all aspects of the individual and the environment. The process varies from one child to another, but on the whole all children pass through various phases of development of which the broad general outlines are essentially the same.

Each of these successive stages of development is characterized by definite problems the child must solve in order to proceed with confidence to the next. The highest degree of functional harmony will be achieved when the problems of each stage are met and solved at an orderly rate and in a normal sequence. On the other hand, it is well to remember that the successive personality gains the child makes are not rigidly established once and for all but may be reinforced or threatened throughout life. Even in adulthood, a reasonably healthy personality can be achieved in spite of previous misfortunes and defects in the developmental sequence.

In considering psychologic development, it is important to remember that it takes place within a cultural milieu. Not only the form of large social institutions but the framework of family life, the attitudes of parents, and their practices in child rearing will be conditioned by the culture of the period.

Psychologic development in childhood may be roughly divided into 5 stages: infancy (birth to 18 months), early childhood (18 months to 5 years), late childhood (5–12 years), early adolescence (12–16 years), and late adolescence (16 years to maturity).

* Ruth S. Kempe, MD

Infancy

Perhaps the most striking features of the first year are the great physical development that takes place and the infant's growing awareness of *self* as an entity separate from the environment.

Much of the psychologic development of the first year is interrelated with physical development, ie, dependent on the maturation of the body to the extent that the child can discriminate self and nonself. Knowledge of the environment comes with increasing sharpening of the senses (from indiscriminate mouthing to coordinated eye-hand movements). Beginning of mastery over the environment comes with increasingly adept coordination, the development of locomotion, and the beginnings of speech. Perception of the self as an individual in relation to an environment that includes other individuals is the basis on which interpersonal relationships are founded.

The newborn infant is at first aware only of bodily needs—ie, the presence or absence of discomfort (cold, wet, etc). The pleasure of relief from discomfort gradually becomes associated with parenting and later (when perception is sufficient for recognition) with the parents. The child derives a feeling of security when bodily needs are satisfied and from physical contact with the parents. The feeding situation provides the first opportunity for development of this feeling of security, and it is therefore important to make certain that this is a happy event.

The development of the first emotional relationship, then, is derived from close contact with the mother. Meeting the infant's physical needs thus develops into sustained physical contact and emotional interaction with one person. Prolonged deprivation of this relationship is damaging to the personality if no satisfactory substitute is provided. Permanent deprivation leads to restriction of personality development—even to pseudoretardation in all areas. Such behavior may also occur in a home situation, but it is more striking and more common in infants who remain for long periods in hospitals or other institutions where adequate personalized attention is not given to each child. The infant deprived of the security and affection necessary to produce a sense of trust may respond with listlessness, immobility, unresponsiveness, poor appetite, an appearance of unhappiness, and insomnia. In other cases, the continued deprivation of consistent care in infancy may not become apparent until later in life, when the individual feels there is no reason to trust people and thus has no sense of responsibility toward others.

No particular techniques are necessary to develop an infant's feeling of security. The infant is not easily discouraged by an inexperienced mother's mistakes; rather, the child seems to respond to the warmth of her feeling and her eagerness to keep trying. The feeling of security derived from satisfactory relationships during the first year is probably the most important single factor in personality development, making it possible for the child to accept restrictions without fearing that each restriction implies total loss of love.

Toward the end of the first year, other personal relationships are also developing—particularly with the father, who is now recognized as comparable to the mother in importance. During this time, relationships are forming also with siblings.

Early Childhood

In early childhood, the child's horizon continues to widen. Increased body control is followed by the development of many physical skills. The very important development of speech permits extension of the social environment and increasing ability to understand and perfect social relationships.

Perhaps the central problem of early childhood is still, however, the development of control over the instinctive drives, particularly as they arise in relationship to the parents. The acceptance of limitations on the need for bodily love (the realization that complete infantile dependency is not permitted or desirable) and the control of aggressive feelings are prime examples. This control of primitive feelings is largely accomplished through the psychologic process of "identification" with the parents—the desire in the child to be like the parents and to emulate them. With this desire come the beginnings of conscience, as the moral values of the parents are incorporated into the child's own personality.

The child now begins to have a feeling of autonomy—of self-direction and initiative. The child 18 months to 2½ years of age is actively learning to exercise the power of "yes" and "no." The difficulty the 2-year-old has in choosing between the two often leads to misunderstanding; the child may say "no" when "yes" would be better, as if out of some compulsion to exercise this new "will" even when it hurts.

At this period, parental "discipline" becomes very important. Discipline is an educative means by which the parent teaches the child how to become a self-respecting, likeable, and socially responsible adult. Disciplinary measures have value chiefly as they serve this educative function; if used as an end in themselves, to establish the "authority" of the parent irrespective of the issues at hand, they usually lead only to warfare (open or surreptitious) between parent and child.

The goal is to allow the child to develop a feeling of personal responsibility without turning aside from the help and guidance of others in important matters. The favorable result is self-control without loss of self-esteem. Adults must allow children a widening range of choices of experiences they are ready for—teach them also, however, to be able to accept restrictions when necessary.

Discipline must be administered with firmness and consistency to protect the child against the consequences of immature judgment. Perhaps the most constructive rule a parent can follow is to decide which kinds of conformity are really important and then to insist on obedience in these areas. "Discipline" thus seeks the positive goal of making the child a social being who can live comfortably in society without guilt about basic drives, but it must be administered in such a way as not to stifle natural and healthy needs for some expression of independence.

Late Childhood

Late childhood is a period marked by rapid intellectual growth during which the individual actively strives to become a member of society. Psychiatrists call this the latency period because the force of primitive drives has been fairly successfully controlled, expressed in a socially acceptable way, or repressed. The energy derived from instinctive impulses whose direct expression is not permitted by society is diverted into the drive for knowledge—a process of "sublimation." At no time in life does the individual learn more avidly and quickly. Reading and writing (the intellectual skills) and vast bodies of information are quickly assimilated. The preoccupation with fantasy gradually subsides, and the child wants to be engaged in real tasks that can be carried through to completion. Even in play activities, the emphasis is on developing mental and bodily skills through sports and games.

Late childhood is also a period of conformity to the group. The environment enlarges to include the school and, particularly, other children. Much of the emotional satisfaction previously derived from the parents is now derived from relationships with peers. The need to become a member of this larger group tends to encourage cooperation and obedience to the will of the group (elements of democracy). It also paves the way for questioning of the parents' values to the extent that they conflict with those of the group.

Early Adolescence

After the comparative calm of late childhood, early adolescence is a period of upheaval. Along with changes in body size and shape comes a new confusion about the physical self (the "body image"). Sexual maturation brings with it a resurgence of instinctive drives that have been repressed for years. In most modern societies—in contrast to some primitive ones—the sexual drive is not permitted direct expression in adolescence in spite of physical readiness.

The emotional adjustment is disrupted as once again the child must learn to control feelings of love or hate and the impulse to aggression as a response to frustration. Again, the relationship to the parents is disturbed. Docile acceptance of the parents as powerful and wise beings whose domination must be accepted is replaced by rebellious rejection of parental authority. Even so, dependent needs persist as the adolescent continues to reject personal responsibility and rely on parental care.

The emerging young man or woman continues to seek individualization not in the family circle but in the larger society of neighborhood, school, town, and nation. Adolescents are constantly preoccupied with how they appear in the eyes of others as compared with their own conceptions of themselves. They find comfort in conformity with their age-mates, and fads in clothing and manners reach a peak in early adolescence.

Late Adolescence

By the 16th year, most children have again reached comparative equilibrium. Body growth has slowed somewhat, and the adolescent has had time to adapt to the changes. Sufficient mastery over biologic drives has been achieved so that they can be channeled into constructive activities and heterosexual social activity, eventually leading to a choice of companion or marital partner.

The relationship to the parents is now more mature. With the discovery that responsible independence is neither frightening nor overwhelming but a position possible to maintain, the adolescent can cease to rebel and can accept help from the parents in planning constructively for adult responsibilities and rewards.

Again, learning is rapid, particularly for the intelligent young person, who can absorb much more than the conventional school curriculum.

Active preparation for adult life characterizes late adolescence in our culture, although, as in more primitive cultures, some adolescents will have already taken on the responsibilities of job and marriage. Biologically, this is certainly feasible; it is the complexity and competition of our modern culture that so greatly prolong the emergence into adulthood.

SELECTED REFERENCES

Frankenburg WK, Camp W: *Pediatric Screening Tests.* Thomas, 1975.

Kernan KT, Bejab MJ, Edgerton RB: *Environments and Behavior.* University Park Press, 1983.

Levine MD et al: *Developmental-Behavioral Pediatrics.* Saunders, 1983.

Lowrey GH: *Growth and Development of Children,* 7th ed. Year Book, 1978.

The Newborn Infant

3

Beverly L. Koops, MD, & Frederick C. Battaglia, MD

Neonatology is one of several pediatric subspecialties that have blossomed in the last 15 years. These years have been characterized by expanding technology, markedly increased basic and clinical research, and a positive attitude among involved health care professionals about the prognosis of very low birth weight and sick newborns. There has been a dramatic reduction in neonatal deaths in all birth weight and gestational age groups (compare Figs 3–1 and 3–2). The efforts associated with reducing mortality in the very low gestational age and low-birth-weight groups also have had an important impact on the outcome for larger and older infants. The provision of anticipatory care and the increased cooperation between obstetric and pediatric services have markedly lowered the mortality risk for almost all birth weight and gestational age groups.

During the past few years, neonatal services have been divided into 3 levels of infant care (low-risk, level 1; intermediate care, level 2; and intensive care, level 3) and 2 levels of obstetric services (a "regular," or low-risk, service and a high-risk service).

Level 1 nurseries provide primary care to their local communities and are usually for full-term infants. They often function as "rooming-in" units. Level 1 nurseries may also sponsor antepartum classes on birthing and breast feeding. All personnel working in this type of nursery should encourage the development of good parenting skills, should assist and monitor the infant's adjustment to extrauterine life, and should initiate screening tests for various acute and congenital problems such as hypoglycemia, phenylketonuria, and hypothyroidism. Level 1 units should have excellent delivery room and treatment area facili-

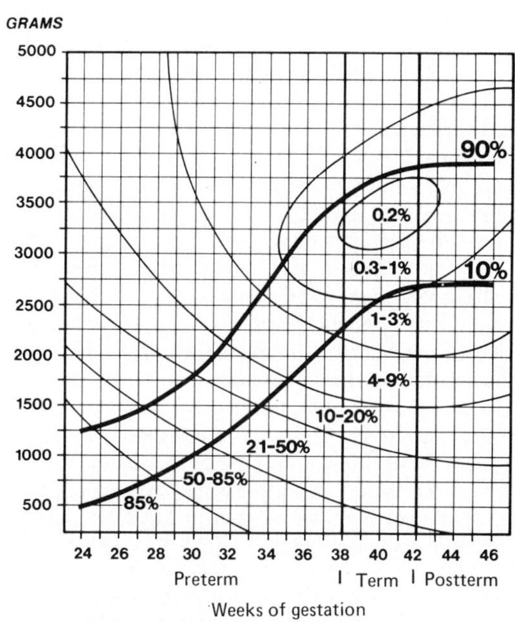

Figure 3–1. Neonatal mortality risk by birth weight and gestational age, 1958–1969, based on 14,436 live births at the University of Colorado Health Sciences Center. (Reproduced, with permission, from Koops BL, Morgan LJ, Battaglia FC: Neonatal mortality risk in relation to birth weight and gestational age: An update. *J Pediatr* 1982;**101**:969.)

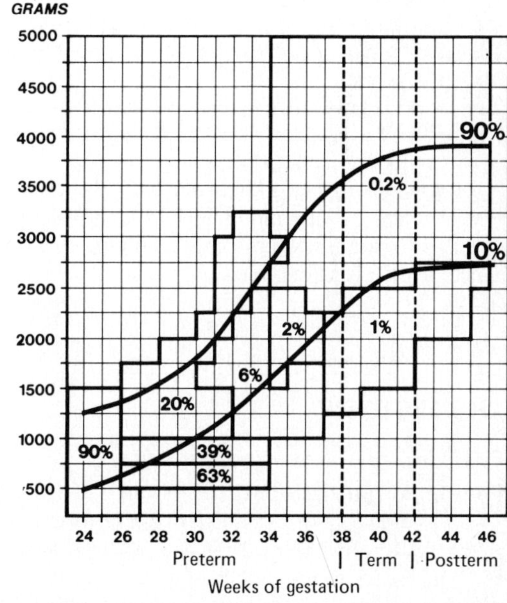

Figure 3–2. Neonatal mortality risk by birth weight and gestational age, 1974–1980, based on 14,413 live births at the University of Colorado Health Sciences Center. (Reproduced, with permission, from Koops BL, Morgan LJ, Battaglia FC: Neonatal mortality risk in relation to birth weight and gestational age: An update. *J Pediatr* 1982;**101**:969.)

ties and personnel capabilities so that infants with unexpected problems in the delivery room or nursery can be cared for briefly and their conditions stabilized in preparation for transport to level 2 or level 3 units.

Level 2 nurseries, in addition to serving the populations seeking level 1 care, also provide care to many newborn infants in whom problems are anticipated, eg, in multiple pregnancy, maternal illnesses such as diabetes, pregnancy complications such as acute hypertension, and fetal problems such as intrauterine growth retardation and premature labor or rupture of membranes. These nurseries also provide care for convalescent and sick newborn infants, including most preterm infants above 32 weeks' gestational age or 1500 g birth weight. These centers attempt to deliver only infants that can be adequately resuscitated and managed there. Facilities must be available for transfer of infants to higher intensity care centers and for care of infants from level 3 nurseries who no longer require intensive nursery care prior to home discharge.

Level 3 centers attempt to care for all infants regardless of gestational age, size, or severity of illness. They deal with the problems of extreme immaturity, major birth defects, and life-threatening illnesses. These centers should have pediatric subspecialty services in anesthesiology, surgery, cardiology, pulmonology, genetics, birth defects, and psychiatry. In addition to acute problems, level 3 nurseries also manage chronic problems that are potentially life-threatening, eg, disorders requiring central alimentation or tracheostomy, bronchopulmonary dysplasia, and blindness in infants who require hospitalization. Transport to nurseries closer to home is appropriate when the infant's condition has stabilized, so that parents can become involved in personal contact and care and bed space can be made available for other infants requiring intensive care.

In addition to being involved with the medical care of infants, health professionals should take part in finding solutions to problems involving finances, ethics, and legislative directives.

THE HISTORY

Past Maternal History

To a considerable extent, the past history of the infant is actually the medical and obstetric history of the mother. A family history of genetically acquired illnesses, unexplained fetal or neonatal deaths, birth defects, or social problems should be noted. Chronic medical illnesses in the mother, such as endocrine abnormalities, heart disease, and immunologic system disorders, are also important.

Previous Obstetric History

The incidence and outcome of previous pregnancies should be reported in detail, including previous therapeutic or spontaneous abortions, miscarriages, premature births, and number of current living children. Intervals between pregnancies and graphs of siblings' birth weights and gestational ages may enable the health care provider to recognize the repetition of a pattern of intrauterine fetal growth or any striking change in growth. A history of infertility in the parents is also pertinent.

Current Obstetric History

Ages, years of education completed, occupations, and the financial circumstances of both parents should be recorded. Information on maternal weight gain or loss, nutritional intake (including adherence to fad diets), and drug use (particularly alcohol and cigarettes) should be obtained. As complete a maternal history as possible, particularly as regards nutrition, should be obtained, since there is convincing evidence that the prepregnancy nutritional status of the mother and her weight gain during the pregnancy are important in determining the infant's birth weight. For example, the incidence of low-birth-weight infants of mothers who are underweight prior to pregnancy and gain less than 9 kg during pregnancy exceeds 50%. Vitamin B_{12} deficiency associated with use of a strict vegetarian diet during pregnancy may result in neurologic problems in the newborn infant. The status of previous medical conditions in the mother and any treatments she is receiving (eg, an asthmatic taking iodides and corticosteroids) are critical data in the assessment of the newborn infant. Acute problems in the mother, such as urinary tract infection, toxemia, or bleeding, must be noted. One should note the fluid and electrolyte management of the mother during labor and delivery, particularly during cesarean section, since both sodium and glucose concentrations and homeostasis in the newborn infant may be disturbed by the administration of large glucose loads to the mother immediately prior to delivery.

Social and work environments have been shown to have important influences on the outcome of pregnancy. Adolescents have no biologic barriers to successful pregnancies, but their own health habits and the positive or negative support of their immediate families alter the risks significantly. Similarly, studies of a large group of women in a socialized medicine system have shown improved pregnancy outcome when risk factors were identified and reduced (eg, by making changes in life-style and reducing physical exertion in the workplace).

American Academy of Pediatrics Committee on Drugs: The transfer of drugs and other chemicals into human breast milk. *Pediatrics* 1983;**72:**375.

Briggs GG et al: *Drugs in Pregnancy and Lactation: A Reference Guide to Fetal and Neonatal Risk.* Williams & Wilkins, 1983.

Milunsky A (editor): Management of the high-risk pregnancy. *Clin Perinatol* 1974;**1:**187.

Papiernik E et al: Prevention of preterm births: A perinatal study in Haguenau, France. *Pediatrics* 1985;**76:**154.

Zuckerman BS et al: Adolescent pregnancy: Biobehavioral determinants of outcome. *J Pediatr* 1984;**105:**857.

INTRAUTERINE GROWTH RATE

The intrauterine growth rate of an infant is affected by many factors, including the mother's general health, the health of the fetus, and the condition of the placenta. During the intrauterine period, virtually any organ system disease can affect the growth rate of the child, sometimes temporarily and in other instances permanently. The weight of the infant reflects the total genetic and environmental status. Thus, maternal toxemia may lead to small-for-gestational-age (SGA) infants; the longer the toxemia has been present during the pregnancy, the more striking the degree of growth retardation. Similarly, congenital viral infection, multiple births, chromosomal aberrations, birth defects, and chronic ingestion of alcohol, nicotine, or heroin often produce some degree of growth retardation. Regardless of the cause of intrauterine growth retardation, these infants tend to be at increased risk of developing fetal distress during labor and delivery, and personnel specially trained in perinatal medicine should be in attendance. Potential problems in the small-for-gestational-age infant include birth asphyxia, meconium aspiration, renal injury leading to oliguria, hyperviscosity syndrome, hypoglycemia, and hypocalcemia.

Conversely, infants of diabetic mothers are large for gestational age (LGA). Excessive size in the infant is associated with an increased incidence of birth trauma, particularly following vaginal delivery. In a vertex delivery, there may be injuries to the head and neck, including stretching or tearing of the cervical or brachial plexus leading to peripheral nerve injuries (eg, Erb's palsy or phrenic nerve paralysis). In addition, these infants are at increased risk of having congenital anomalies, cardiomyopathy, hyperviscosity, hypercoagulability, hyperbilirubinemia, hypocalcemia, and hypoglycemia.

Representative conditions associated with birth weight and gestational age categories are illustrated in Fig 3–3. It can be seen that marked deviations in intrauterine growth rate are often associated with serious problems in the newborn infant.

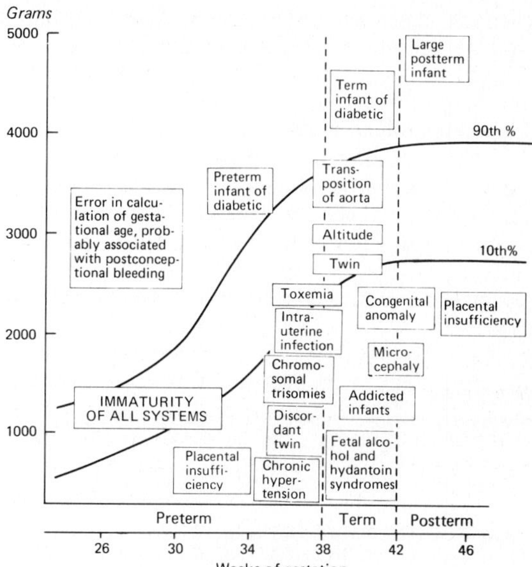

Figure 3–3. Conditions associated with intrauterine growth related to birth weight and gestational age classification. (Reproduced, with permission from Lubchenco LO et al: Factors influencing fetal growth: Aspects of prematurity and dysmaturity. [Second Nutricia Symposium.] HE Stenfert Kroese, NV. Leiden, Holland, 1968.)

Birth Weight

In the past, prematurity was defined as a birth weight of less than 2500 g. Today, the age and the birth weight of an infant are recognized as separate and equally important factors. Birth weight is important because many physiologic and metabolic processes such as temperature regulation and the need for environmental temperature support are a function of size and are relatively independent of the infant's gestational age. Relative surface area increases as weight decreases. For practical purposes, many physicians distinguish a category of "very low birth weight" infants. These are infants with birth weights of less than 1000 g, whose problems of metabolism, thermal regulation, and water and electrolyte balance are exceedingly complex regardless of their gestational age.

Gestational Age

Determination of gestational age must be based on the maternal history correlated with certain findings during the pregnancy, eg, rate of change of uterine height above the symphysis and the time when fetal heart sounds and movement were first noted.

Many additional tests can help to determine gestational age during pregnancy. These include serial ultrasound examinations to determine biparietal diameter and its rate of growth, amniotic fluid examination, and assessment of pulmonary maturity. Correct determination of gestational age is especially important when elective termination of pregnancy is considered.

After delivery, a clinical estimation of gestational age should be based on physical characteristics and the neurologic examination, which change predictably with increasing gestational age (Table 3–2).

Length & Head Size

Most newborn infants who present with intrauterine growth retardation in weight show relatively less deviation from normal in length and head circumference. Length and head growth appear to be protected to some extent under circumstances of intrauterine undernutrition. However, in severe and prolonged intrauterine undernutrition, such as occurs in the discordant twin, all body proportions may be affected.

Weight-Length Ratio

The weight-length ratio aids in identifying fetal growth abnormalities. It increases with fetal age; ie, infants become heavier in relation to their length as they approach full term. In intrauterine growth retardation, the weight-length ratio decreases, since the rate of growth in weight is affected more than length.

Battaglia FC, Lubchenco LO: A practical classification of newborn infants by weight and gestational age. *J Pediatr* 1967;**71:**159.

Jones MD, Battaglia FC: Intrauterine growth retardation. *Am J Obstet Gynecol* 1977;**127:**540.

Lowry GH: *Growth and Development of Children,* 6th ed. Year Book, 1973.

Lubchenco LO, Searls DT, Brazie JV: Neonatal mortality rate: Relationship to birth weight and gestational age. *J Pediatr* 1972;**81:**814.

Lubchenco LO et al: Intrauterine growth in length and head circumference as estimated from live births at gestational ages from 26 to 42 weeks. *Pediatrics* 1966;**37:**403.

PHYSICAL EXAMINATION

The physical examination of the newborn infant should be appropriate for the infant's age. The first examination should be performed immediately after birth, usually in the delivery room, and is aimed at identifying life-threatening abnormalities that require immediate attention and at evaluating the infant's ability to adjust to extrauterine life. A thorough or "complete" examination is not appropriate at this time. The second examination may be done in the "transition" period, which may last 1–4 hours. The infant is observed but not disturbed (unless problems arise) except to be weighed, measured, and classified by birth weight and gestational age. The complete examination and third evaluation are ideally performed after 12–24 hours and should be thorough. The final evaluation is done at the time of hospital discharge. The discharge examination may be brief and is performed in the presence of the mother so that she and the examiner may assess the infant's condition and discuss the findings.

Considerable effort is currently being expended to find ways to evaluate the infant with the least disturbance to the mother-child interaction and with the least disruption of an environment conducive to the development of good parenting patterns.

THE INFANT IMMEDIATELY AFTER BIRTH

Evaluations

A. Apgar Score: Immediate evaluation of the newborn infant at 1 and 5 minutes after birth is a valuable routine procedure (Table 3–1). The infant in the best condition (Apgar score 8–10) is vigorous, pink, and crying. A moderately depressed infant (Apgar score 5–7) appears cyanotic, with slow and irregular respirations, but has good muscle tone and reflexes. The severely depressed infant (Apgar score 4 or less) is limp, pale or blue, apneic, and has a slow heart rate. The 5-minute Apgar score is the more useful indicator of neonatal and long-term prognosis.

One should be cautious, however, in attempting to interpret low Apgar scores in very low birth weight infants. Partly because of their marked immaturity, which militates against normal muscle tone, and partly because of their very small size, which predisposes to more severe shock, very low birth weight infants often have low Apgar scores unassociated with subsequent increased morbidity or mortality rates. The progressive change in the Apgar score of an infant who is born severely depressed is one of the best predictors of the prognosis for the infant. Many very low birth weight infants may have a low initial Apgar score, but if it improves markedly at 5 minutes with adequate resuscitation, the outcome is often good. Serial measurements of the Apgar score can be used as an ongoing bioassay of the degree of damage resulting from in utero or perinatal asphyxia.

B. Chest: Auscultation of the lungs may reveal crackling or wet rales during the first few breaths. In the healthy infant, air exchange is good almost immediately. Respiratory rate ranges from 30 to 60/min for the first few minutes and may be irregular.

Table 3–1. Infant evaluation at birth (Apgar score.)* One minute and 5 minutes after complete birth of infant (disregarding cord and placenta), the following objective signs should be observed and recorded.

Points	0	1	2
1. Heart rate	Absent	Slow (< 100)	> 100
2. Respiratory effort	Absent	Slow, irregular	Good, crying
3. Muscle tone	Limp	Some flexion of extremities	Active motion
4. Response to catheter in nostril (tested after oropharynx is clear)	No response	Grimace	Cough or sneeze
5. Color	Blue or pale	Body pink; extremities blue	Completely pink

* Reproduced, with permission, from Apgar V: *JAMA* 1958;**168:**1985.

The heart rate may be variable but should remain above 100/min and stabilize between 120 and 160/min.

Positive pressure resuscitation is rarely required when the heart rate is consistently above 100/min. Resuscitation and the various stages of physiologic support supplied during resuscitation are discussed later in this chapter.

C. Temperature: The maintenance of body temperature is always important but especially so in the very low birth weight infant and in the infant severely depressed as a result of perinatal asphyxia. The body temperature of a newborn infant must be maintained within a very narrow range of 36.5–37.3 °C (97.7–99.1 °F) in order to minimize the infant's caloric expenditure in responding to heat or cold stress. At birth, the infant's skin must always be toweled dry, because evaporative heat losses are very large and it is difficult to support body temperature if the skin is wet. A radiant heater should be used in the delivery room until the infant is stable and can be given to the mother or taken to the nursery (Fig 3–4).

Body temperature will fall precipitously in a cool environment unless adequate precautions are taken. As a fall in body temperature occurs, the infant becomes cyanotic—first in the hands and feet, then in the face, and finally over the entire body—and may develop grunting respirations and retractions.

A change in cardiac output occurs in infants who are allowed to become hypothermic. This altered state may cause metabolic acidosis, gradually increasing hypoxia, hypoglycemia, and shock. Many of the respiratory and cardiovascular difficulties of the very low birth weight infant in the first few hours of life may be attributable to the fact that these infants often have very low core temperatures, despite attempts to maintain body temperature at an acceptable level. Skin temperatures may be relatively higher than core temperatures because of heaters used for warming.

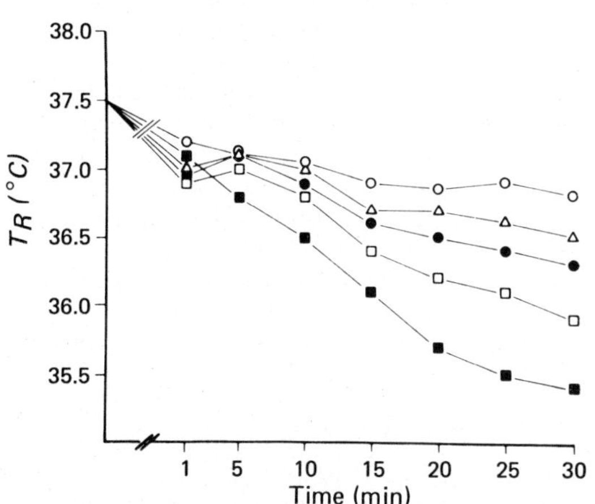

Figure 3–4. Mean deep body temperatures (T_R) of each group during the first 30 minutes of life. T_R is on the ordinate and minutes postdelivery on the abscissa. ■ wet infants in room air; □ dry infants in room air; ● wet infants under the radiant heater; Δ dry infants wrapped in a blanket; ○ dry infants under the radiant heater. (Reproduced, with permission, from Dahm LS, James LS: Newborn temperature and calculated heat loss in the delivery room. *Pediatrics* 1972;**49**:504.)

D. Skin: Cyanosis of the peripheral portions of the extremities is common for a short time after birth. The presence of persistent cyanosis, pallor, petechiae, ecchymoses, or plethora requires further investigation. The amount of vernix should be noted and related to clinical estimation of gestational age. Jaundice at birth is a grave finding and requires immediate evaluation.

Pallor in the newborn infant may indicate possible acute hemorrhage that is draining into the maternal circulation. It may be caused by a tear in a placental vessel. Ecchymoses of the skin, particularly in preterm infants following breech vaginal deliveries, may be a manifestation of extensive hemorrhage into the deep muscles of the back or buttocks and may be severe enough to cause shock. In all cases of suspected hemorrhage, prompt expansion of blood volume should be achieved by means of placental blood, albumin, plasma protein fraction, or some other appropriate colloid solution. Blood volume expansion should be done with care; infusion of blood products and large volumes is not without risk. However, except for infectious or hypoxic shock, there are few conditions occurring in the newborn infant at delivery that are likely to be confused with acute blood loss.

E. Abdomen: The abdomen should be soft and somewhat scaphoid immediately after birth. As the bowel fills with air, the abdomen becomes more full. Abdominal organs are easily palpated during this early period. A marked and persistent scaphoid abdomen suggests diaphragmatic hernia with some abdominal contents within the chest. A distended abdomen suggests such problems as organomegaly, ascites, and bowel obstruction.

F. General Appearance: The infant's sex, size and development in relation to gestational age, and the presence of malformations or deformations should be noted. Any asymmetric movements may suggest an injury to the cervical or the brachial plexus. In such cases, movement of the chest wall should be carefully observed for any suggestion of a phrenic nerve injury producing asymmetric respiration. The examination for possible birth injuries should be especially thorough in infants who are large for gestational age.

Fetal Adnexa

A. Amniotic Fluid: The color, appearance, and estimated volume of amniotic fluid should be noted. Normal amniotic fluid at term is a light straw color. Bright red fresh blood or chocolate-colored old blood pigments may be present.

In normal pregnancy, amniotic fluid volume increases until approximately the 35th week of gestation and then decreases at a rate of approximately 100 mL per week. At term, the volume is about 700 mL. Polyhydramnios is present if the amniotic fluid volume is 3 times the normal value or is greater than 2000 mL. Polyhydramnios occurs in association with those congenital anomalies that prevent normal fetal swallowing or absorption of amniotic fluid, including (1) major central nervous system anomalies such as anencephaly and (2) gastrointestinal tract obstruction. Oligohydramnios occurs in association with lesions that reduce fetal urine production, such as prune-belly syndrome, renal agenesis, or urinary obstruction, which affect a major source of amniotic fluid. When the fluid is meconium-stained, the obstetrician and pediatrician should observe special precautions (see Special Care of the High-Risk Infant, below).

B. Umbilical Cord:

1. Gross appearance—The cord of term infants with small placentas is likely to be thin and stained yellow. Meconium staining of the cord indicates prior fetal distress. The cord is usually inserted concentrically on the placenta. When the insertion is velamentous, arising away from the placental margin and supported only by the amnion, there is increased risk of fetal hemorrhage during delivery. Velamentous insertions of the cord occur more frequently with multiple births.

2. Length—A very short cord is uncommon but can result in abruptio placentae or rupture of the cord. A very long cord ($\geq$ 75 cm) may loop around the body and neck, resulting in a relatively short cord during delivery. Occasionally, a nuchal cord is the cause of fetal distress.

3. Single umbilical artery—The vessels of the umbilical cord are best observed in a freshly cut section at birth. Normally, 2 arteries and one vein are present. A single artery is present in approximately 1% of births. The incidence rises to 5–6% in twins. The twin with a single umbilical artery is often smaller than the twin with 2 arteries. A single umbilical artery is considered a congenital vascular malformation. Associated congenital abnormalities, especially of the cardiovascular, gastrointestinal, or urinary systems, may be present, although the incidence of associated anomalies is not high enough to justify special diagnostic tests in the absence of any specific clinical signs.

4. Prolapsed cord—Prolapsed umbilical cord with compression during labor causes acute fetal distress. This is an obstetric emergency, and prompt treatment is necessary if the life and welfare of the infant are to be preserved. The perinatal mortality rate with prolapsed umbilical cord is about 35%.

C. Placenta: Placental weight and the infant's birth weight are directly related. A small placenta is invariably associated with a small infant. However, large placentas, particularly if they are abnormal (eg, as a result of hydrops fetalis or congenital infections), may occur with infants who are not large. The small placenta with multiple small infarcts is characteristic of the woman with chronic hypertensive vascular disease and is associated with infants who are small for gestational age. Examination of the placenta is particularly helpful in multiple pregnancies. An arteriovenous anastomosis between placentas can be recognized by the injection of a dye or of milk into the placental vessels of one fetus; if one chorion is present, the twins must be monozygotic (identical). When 2 chorions and 2 amnions are present, the twins can be either monozygotic or dizygotic.

THE INFANT DURING THE FIRST FEW HOURS AFTER BIRTH

During the first few hours after birth, the normal infant progresses through a fairly predictable sequence of events in recovering from the stress of delivery and adapting to extrauterine life. The infant neither requires nor easily tolerates the handling involved with a complete physical examination. However, a considerable portion of the physical examination and evaluation of the infant can be based on careful observation. This is especially important during the birth recovery period in order to identify early—but without excessive handling—the infant who is at increased risk of developing problems. Observation of abnormal findings such as hypotension, pallor, cyanosis, plethora, jaundice, birth injury, respiratory distress, abdominal distention, hyperactivity, abnormal birth recovery period, or discrepant clinical estimation of gestational age requires early, more detailed evaluation. The nurses caring for the infant play a vital role in observing and evaluating the infant during this period. (The complete physical examination and routine care of the newborn infant during this period are discussed in subsequent sections.)

Recognition of an abnormal birth recovery period may be an important clue to underlying disease. Significant deviation from the basic sequence of events may result from a variety of influences. The preterm infant's response is prolonged. Infants may have a low Apgar score initially but may then recover rapidly. Drugs administered to the mother, birth trauma, and disease in the newborn may alter the birth recovery events.

Clinical Estimation of Gestational Age

The onset of the mother's last menstrual period is the basic information from which the period of gestation is calculated. During pregnancy, observations of increasing fundal height, onset of fetal movement, detection of fetal heartbeat, and certain laboratory tests aid in determining the degree of fetal maturity.

It is possible to estimate the gestational age of the infant by examination after birth, since fetal physical characteristics and neurologic development progress in a predictable fashion with increasing gestational age. Table 3–2 itemizes the clinical criteria used in determining gestational age and outlines the

Table 3–2. A simplified score for assessment of fetal maturation of newly born infants.*†‡

	0	1	2	3	4	5
Neuromuscular maturity						
Posture	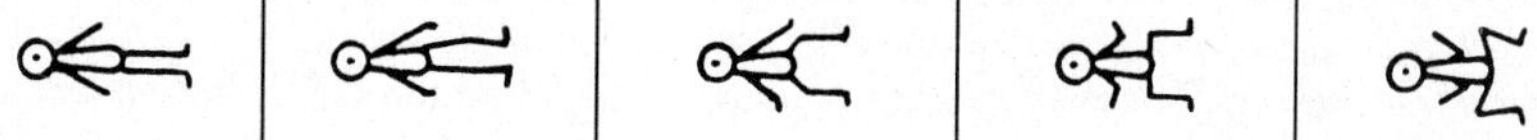					
Square window (wrist)	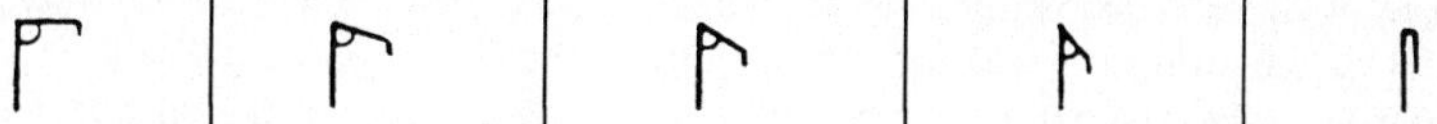 90°	60°	45°	30°	0°	
Arm recoil	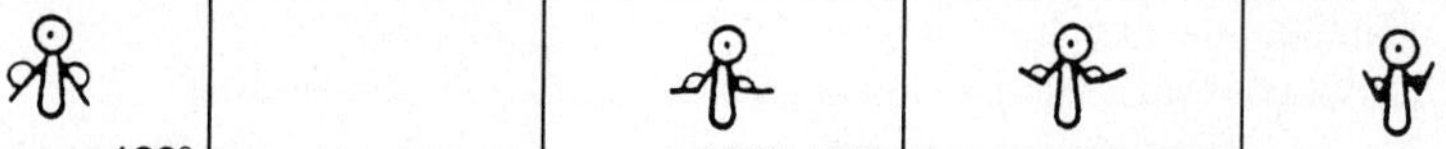 180°		100°–180°	90°–100°	< 90°	
Popliteal angle	180°	160°	130°	110°	90°	< 90°
Scarf sign	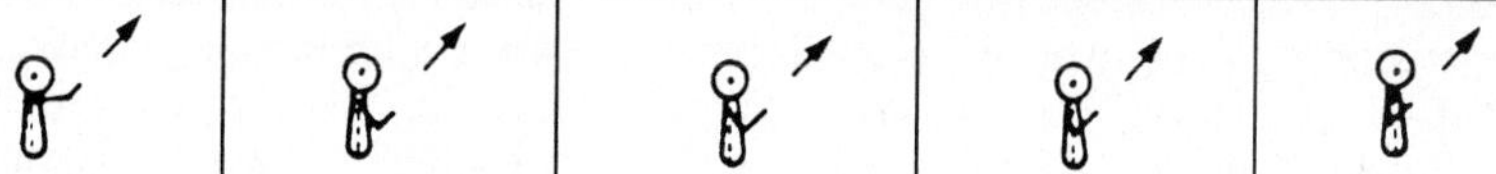					
Heel to ear	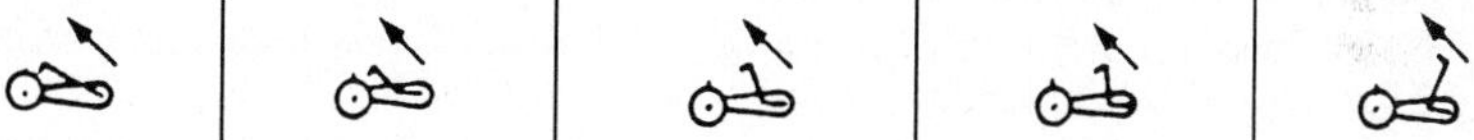					
Physical maturity						
Skin	Gelatinous, red, transparent	Smooth, pink; visible veins	Superficial peeling, rash, or both; few veins	Cracking, pale area; rare veins	Parchment, deep cracking; no vessels	Leathery, cracked, wrinkled
Lanugo	None	Abundant	Thinning	Bald areas	Mostly bald	
Plantar creases	No crease	Faint red marks	Anterior transverse crease only	Creases anterior two-thirds	Creases cover entire sole	
Breast	Barely perceptible	Flat areola; no bud	Stippled areola; bud, 1–2 mm	Raised areola; bud, 3–4 mm	Full areola; bud, 5–10 mm	
Ear	Pinna flat; stays folded	Slightly curved pinna; soft; slow recoil	Well-curved pinna; soft; ready recoil	Formed and firm; instant recoil	Thick cartilage; ear stiff	
Genitalia (male)	Scrotum empty; no rugae		Testes descending; few rugae	Testes down; good rugae	Testes pendulous; deep rugae	
Genitalia (female)	Prominent clitoris and labia minora		Majora and minora equally prominent	Majora large; minora small	Clitoris and minora completely covered	

Score	5	10	15	20	25	30	35	40	45	50
Weeks	26	28	30	32	34	36	38	40	42	44

* Reproduced, with permission, from Ballard JL, Novak KK, Driver M: A simplified score for assessment of fetal maturation of newly born infants. *J Pediatr* 1979;**95:**769.

† Maturity rating.

‡ See text for a description of the clinical gestational age examination.

physical and neurologic findings observed in infants born at various gestational ages.

There are 2 charts presented in Table 3–2 for estimating gestational age. The first is a neuromuscular examination based on items indicating normal neuromuscular development, and the second includes physical characteristics. The examination for gestational age requires very little manipulation of the infant yet gives important data for assessing gestational age. Each physical characteristic is observed and scored from 0 to 5. Similarly, selected neuromuscular characteristics that reflect the infant's muscle tone and strength are examined and scored from 0 to 5. The total score achieved on this "maturity rating" is correlated with the clinical gestational age given in the table. Discrepancies in maturation between the physical and neuromuscular characteristics often indicate a problem in intrauterine growth.

For example, intrauterine growth retardation due to undernutrition—rather than due to fetal malformation—alters the physical more than the neurologic characteristics associated with gestational age as follows:

(1) Diminished growth or absence of breast tissue and, in the female, relatively small labia majora.

(2) Loss of vernix and desquamation of the skin prior to term.

(3) Meconium staining of the skin and nails due to fetal distress with bowel evacuation.

(4) Weight is affected first, followed by decreased growth in length and, in severe undernutrition, head circumference.

(5) Neurologic examination is least affected and is usually appropriate for the actual gestational age.

COMPLETE PHYSICAL EXAMINATION OF THE NEWBORN INFANT

A complete physical examination should be done on each infant within 24 hours after delivery. However, it should be delayed until the infant has stabilized following birth, because of the infant's limited tolerance to handling during the birth recovery period. Careful observation for abnormal findings during this time by the physician and other health care personnel will identify those infants who require earlier, more detailed examination and evaluation.

It may not be possible to complete the entire examination at one time, in which case the balance can (and must) be finished later. One should provide a complete record of the newborn infant that will contain essential information for reference as the infant grows and if later problems develop. If possible, take advantage of quiet periods to perform portions of the examination that require it. The infant can usually be quieted sufficiently by being given a pacifier or by being held by the examiner or the parent.

There are distinct advantages in having the mother present and assisting the examination: (1) Her participation with the examiner in this intimate evaluation of her infant can enhance the development of the normal mother-infant relationship. (2) Her response and involvement with the infant can be observed, allowing early identification of problems in mothering that may exist. (3) She can be reassured immediately about minor variations in normal findings. (4) The meaning and plan for evaluation of significant abnormal findings can be discussed, allowing early involvement with the sick infant.

When abnormal findings are observed, they must be documented and a plan for evaluation developed. In caring for the newborn infant, it is crucial that abnormal findings be reevaluated at frequent intervals. Changes in physical findings such as heart murmurs can occur rapidly.

The basic approach to the newborn physical examination is modified somewhat from that described in Chapter 1 because of the special problems the newborn infant often presents:

(1) Observation: Observation is particularly important in the newborn examination. A major portion of the information gathered will be obtained by patient, careful observation of the infant before the infant is handled and during various stages of activity. The usual order is to observe the infant generally and then to concentrate on specific areas for more detailed observation.

(2) Auscultation: Listen to the heart, lungs, abdomen, and head when the infant is quiet. Be alert for any asymmetry in breath sounds.

(3) Palpation and manipulative procedures: These must be timed in order to obtain reliable information but without disturbing the infant to such a degree that valid observations cannot be made. Adequate palpation of the abdomen and portions of the neurologic examination must be done with the infant quiet; examination of the mouth, throat, and ears can be done adequately even in a crying infant.

General Appearance & Evaluation

A. Vital Signs and Physical Measurements: These may be obtained from the nurse's record or during the course of the examination. It is usually not advisable to make these observations first, since the infant will become fussy. The heart rate for a normal newborn infant ranges from 120 to 160/min. The respiratory rate may be as high as 60/min within the first 1–2 days of extrauterine life but settles to a normal range of 25–40/min. Normal blood pressures are related to the size and postnatal age of the infant (see Fig 3–5 and additional references). Blood pressure should be determined in both upper and lower extremities using the Doppler method (see Chapter 15) and a cuff size that covers two-thirds of the appropriate limb. Length, weight, and head circumference are measured and plotted on the intrauterine growth charts related to gestational age.

B. Appearance: The general appearance, maturity, nutritional status, presence of abnormal facies or body deformities, and state of well-being are noted. Before the infant is disturbed, observe the resting

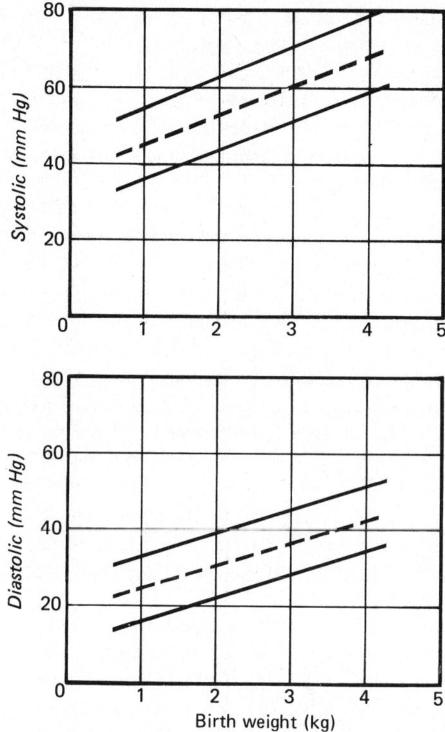

Figure 3–5. Aortic blood pressure during the first 12 hours of life in infants with birth weights of 610–4220 g. (Reproduced, with permission, from Versmold HT et al: Aortic blood pressure during the first 12 hours of life in infants with birth weight 610 to 4,220 g. *Pediatrics* 1981;**67**:607.)

position (which frequently reflects the position assumed in utero), quality of respirations, color, and character of sleep pattern. While the infant is being undressed, observe the response to handling, general muscle tone, and mottling. The usual quieting response upon being picked up and held may be demonstrated after undressing.

Specific Observations

A. Skin:

1. Color and appearance—The skin becomes erythematous for a few hours after birth, then fades to its normal appearance. The presence of **jaundice** and age at onset of jaundice should always be noted. **Peripheral cyanosis** (acrocyanosis) is commonly present, particularly when extremities are cool. **Generalized cyanosis** is an important observation requiring immediate evaluation.

Pallor may be due to acute blood loss at the time of delivery or to gastrointestinal bleeding from a variety of causes or may be iatrogenic, particularly in the preterm infant who has had multiple samples of blood drawn for blood chemistry and blood gas measurements. Even so-called microchemistries can lead to appreciable blood loss in infants weighing less than 1200 g. The amount of blood withdrawn each time for sampling should be recorded. **Plethora** suggests polycythemia, which may lead to hyperviscosity syndrome. It occurs frequently in infants of diabetic mothers, small-for-gestational-age infants, and twins who have received a twin-twin transfusion. **Vernix caseosa,** a whitish, greasy material, normally covers the body of the fetus, decreasing in amount as term approaches. It is usually present in body creases of term infants but may be completely absent on a postterm infant. **Dry skin,** with cracking and peeling of the superficial layers, is common in infants who are postterm or have had intrauterine growth retardation. Normal skin is present underneath. **Edema** may be generalized (usually indicating serious renal, cardiac, or other systemic disease) or localized (dorsum of extremities in Turner's disease, eyelids with acute conjunctivitis). **Meconium staining** of the umbilical cord, vernix, nails, and skin suggests prior fetal distress. The preterm infant's skin is more translucent and may be covered with fine hair **(lanugo).**

2. Skin lesions—Many lesions are present on the skin of normal newborn infants and must be differentiated from significant skin disease. **Mongolian spots**—bluish-black areas of pigmentation over the back and buttocks—are seen frequently in dark-skinned races. **Capillary hemangiomas** are common over the lower occiput, eyelids, forehead, nares, and lips. These lesions tend to decrease in size and intensity as the child grows. A few **petechiae** may be seen over the presenting part. Numerous or fresh petechiae should suggest thrombocytopenia. **Milia** are the small, yellowish-white papular areas over the nose and face. **Erythema toxicum** is characterized by an evanescent rash with lesions in different stages—erythematous macules, papules, or small vesicles containing eosinophils—that spread to a variable extent over the skin, more commonly on the trunk. It occurs with decreasing frequency in preterm infants.

Staphylococcal or streptococcal infection of the skin in preterm infants may resemble erythema toxicum, a diagnosis that should always be made with caution in preterm infants.

B. Head: Note size, shape, symmetry, and general appearance of the head. **Molding** of the presenting part due to pressures during labor and delivery causes transient deformation of the head. **Head circumference** may be affected by molding; therefore, measurement should be repeated at discharge. **Caput succedaneum** is an area of edema over the presenting part that extends across suture lines. This differentiates it from a **cephalhematoma,** bleeding into the subperiosteal space on the surface of a skull bone (most commonly the parietal), which is circumscribed by the borders of the individual skull bone. The quantity of blood draining into a cephalhematoma can be significant in contributing to anemia appearing soon after birth and in causing early hyperbilirubinemia.

Normally, the size of the **anterior fontanelle** varies from 1 to 4 cm in any direction; it is smaller when the sutures are overriding. It is soft, pulsates with the infant's pulse, and becomes slightly depressed when the infant is upright and quiet. The

posterior fontanelle is usually less than 1 cm in diameter. A **third fontanelle,** a bony defect along the sagittal suture in the parietal bones, may be present. The sutures may feel open to a variable degree or may be overriding. These findings are usually of no clinical importance. **Craniosynostosis** may be present as a ridge along one or more sutures and is associated with cranial deformity.

Increased intracranial pressure in the newborn infant is associated with increasing head circumference and a full anterior fontanelle. **Skull fractures** resulting from birth trauma may be linear or depressed and may be associated with a cephalhematoma.

Transillumination—the degree of light transmitted through the head—should be determined in any infant suspected of having neurologic disease. The procedure is done in a completely dark room after the examiner's eyes have become dark-adapted. The circle of light extending beyond the flange of the transillumination flashlight should be no more than 1.5 cm in term or up to 2 cm in preterm infants. Excessive light transmission occurs when diminished brain tissue is present, such as that observed with collection of subdural fluid, hydrocephalus, or brain atrophy.

CT and ultrasound scans in preterm infants may reveal subependymal, intraventricular, or intracerebral hemorrhage during the first 5–10 days of life in the absence of physical signs or symptoms. For this reason, all newborn infants with gestational ages of less than 33 weeks should have a CT or ultrasound scan during the first week of life. If hemorrhage into the ventricles or brain has occurred or if a scan was not done, ultrasonography of the brain is indicated at 10–21 days of age to rule out progressive hydrocephalus. Increasing head circumference is an extremely late sign and cannot be used to determine whether the infant had a hemorrhage. Full-term infants with meningitis or seizures should also have CT scanning and ultrasonography for diagnosis of additional insults to the brain.

C. Face: The general appearance and symmetry of the face are observed. **Odd facies** are often associated with specific syndromes and should alert the examiner to search for other abnormalities. Localized swelling, ecchymoses, or asymmetry of movement may result from birth pressure or the use of forceps during delivery. **Facial nerve palsy** is observed when the infant cries; the unaffected side of the mouth moves normally, giving a distorted facial grimace. When injury is more extensive, the eyelid will remain partially open on the affected side. **Facial edema** can be marked following a face presentation and can be severe enough to cause airway obstruction. A careful evaluation of water intake and output for 24–48 hours is in order for infants with facial edema, because they are prone to dilutional hyponatremia and may need regulation of fluid and electrolyte intake.

D. Eyes: The eyes of every newborn infant should be examined carefully at least once during the nursery stay—preferably before silver nitrate prophylaxis is given, since periorbital edema and conjunctivitis may make examination difficult following the procedure. This is particularly important when eye disease or head trauma is suspected. An ophthalmologist should be available for consultation, since loss of vision may result from delay in proper diagnosis and treatment.

Eye examination should include evaluation of the periorbital structures, nerve function, anterior orbital structures, and light reflex. In infants of less than 38 weeks' gestation, the remnant of the pupillary membrane may be used as an adjunct determination of gestational age. If indicated, an ophthalmoscopic examination through dilated pupils may be done after examination has ruled out the presence of glaucoma or anterior chamber hemorrhage. A weak solution of mydriatic and cycloplegic ophthalmic drops may be instilled to obtain good pupillary dilation. Side effects of the drugs or of the examination include vagal slowing of the heart, cold stress on the infant, acceleration of heart rate to over 180/min, and hypertension.

The eyes are usually open and the infant alert for the first 30 minutes, and the eyes are then closed during sleep for the next few hours. The baby will open its eyes when awake, especially when picked up in a semidark room. The infant will look toward a light and may focus briefly on the examiner's face. The size, shape, and position of the eyes and the presence of epicanthal folds are noted. Eyelid swelling and some conjunctival discharge are frequent within 24 hours after instillation of silver nitrate, but the possibility of infection must always be considered. **Eyelid movement** is observed. Occasional **uncoordinated eye movements** are common, but persistent irregular movements (nystagmus, eye deviation) are abnormal. **Acute dacryocystitis** associated with swelling and redness along the course of the lacrimal duct may become apparent in the newborn period. **Corneal or lens opacities** and **pupil size** can be observed with an ordinary flashlight. **Iris abnormalities,** such as Brushfield's spots and colobomas, are noted. **Anterior chamber hemorrhage** may occur following eye trauma during birth but may not be apparent for several hours. A fluid level of blood will form when the infant is upright. **Congenital glaucoma** must be recognized early to preserve vision. The cornea is larger than 11 mm in diameter and is often cloudy as a result of edema. Photophobia is common. Enlargement of the entire eye is a late finding.

Chorioretinitis may occur as a result of congenital toxoplasmosis, cytomegalic inclusion disease, rubella, or other viral infections. Small **retinal hemorrhages** are commonly observed in normal newborn infants, but more extensive hemorrhage is indicative of trauma or a bleeding disorder. **Tumors** are rare in the newborn infant; retinoblastoma must be considered if the light reflection is grayish-yellow or absent or if strabismus or a dilated pupil is noted. Orbital hemangiomas may displace the eye in the orbit.

E. Nose: The shape and size of the nose are noted. Deformities may be due to in utero pressure, but many congenital syndromes are associated with abnormal nose configuration. Nasal discharge, noisy breathing, or complete obstruction to breathing may be present, suggesting choanal atresia or other nasal abnormality. When nasal obstruction is present, the infant may become cyanotic or apneic, since one-third of term infants are obligatory nasal breathers. Nasal obstruction from mucous discharge can occur in those infants born with an upper respiratory tract infection acquired as a viral infection in utero. Flaring of the alae nasi occurs with increased respiratory effort.

F. Ears: Malformed or malpositioned (low-set or rotated) ears are often associated with other congenital abnormalities, especially of the urinary tract. The amount of cartilage in the pinnas is related to maturity. The **tympanic membranes** may be visualized with careful examination. Fluid may be present behind the drum for the first few hours.

Otitis media occurs fairly frequently in the neonatal period, particularly in preterm infants, in those with deformities of the palate, or in those who have been intubated for long periods of time (particularly with nasotracheal intubations). A careful examination of the eardrums should be made whenever sepsis or other infection is suspected.

Hearing loss may be detected by standardized hearing screening tests in the newborn period (see Chapter 13). It is now practical to test newborn infants for hearing loss. Infants at high risk of hearing loss should be identified in all nurseries. The risk factors of significance include a family history of early hearing loss, congenital infections, structural anomalies of the head and neck, severe birth asphyxia, hyperbilirubinemia requiring exchange transfusion, and birth weight less than 1500 g with a difficult nursery course. Infants with any of these factors should be tested for hearing abnormalities immediately. There are 2 important new tools for accurate auditory testing in the newborn period. One involves electrical monitoring of infant movement in response to a loud stimulus repeated periodically over several hours. A second method is that of brain stem-evoked response audiometry, in which sound stimuli are presented to one or both ears and the electrical responses in the brain stem are monitored from 3 scalp electrodes. Abnormal responses are indicative of conductive or sensorineural hearing loss, and immediate referral and treatment of these infants are indicated.

G. Mouth: Observe the lips and mucous membranes for pallor and cyanosis. The membranes should be moist in a normally hydrated infant. **Epithelial pearls,** or retention cysts, are noted on the gum margins and at the junction of the soft and hard palates. **Natal teeth** may be present—usually soft incisors—and need to be removed if they are loose in order to avoid the risk of aspiration. **High-arched palate** may be present as an isolated finding or may be associated with abnormal facies. **Cleft lip and palate** should be noted. Most newborn infants have relatively small **mandibles** that cause no problem. When the mandibles are very small, as in Pierre Robin syndrome, difficulty in breathing may occur when the tongue blocks the airway as it falls back against the pharynx. In the prone position, the infant usually has less respiratory difficulty. Some **drooling** of mucus is common in the first few hours after birth; excessive drooling occurs with esophageal atresia. The **tonsils** and **adenoids** are quite small in newborn infants.

H. Neck: Position, symmetry, range of motion, and muscle tone are noted. **Webbing** of the neck suggests Turner's syndrome. Enlargement of the **thyroid** may occur in the newborn infant and must be evaluated. **Sinus tracts** may be seen as remnants of branchial clefts. **Torticollis** due to shortening or spasm of one sternocleidomastoid muscle may occur when there is hemorrhage or fibrosis in the body of the muscle. A persistent **tonic neck reflex,** assumed spontaneously and maintained by the infant, may be caused by brain damage. A very **short neck** may be associated with cervical vertebral abnormalities.

I. Vocalization: Note character of the **cry.** A high-pitched cry suggests brain damage. A hoarse cry results from inflammation or edema of the larynx or vocal cord paralysis. A whining "cat's cry" occurs with the syndrome of partial deletion of the short arm of chromosome 5. A weak cry may be a general sign occurring in a sick infant. A delay in vocalizing the cry after the infant appears to be crying is noted in congenital hypothyroidism.

Expiratory grunting occurs with respiratory distress due to many causes—notably the respiratory distress syndrome. **Inspiratory stridor** is associated with partial obstruction of the upper airway during inspiration such as occurs with the soft, collapsible tracheal structures of congenital stridor.

J. Thorax: Note shape, symmetry, position, and development of the thorax, nipples, and breast tissue. Note the respiratory pattern and the character of the respirations.

Absent **clavicles** permit unusual anterior movement of the shoulders. Fracture of the clavicle is detected by tenderness and crepitus at the fracture site and limited movements of that arm. Note movement of arms when the Moro reflex is elicited. After a few days, callus is formed and the deformity can be easily visualized and felt. **"Fullness" of the thorax** due to increased anteroposterior diameter occurs with overexpansion of the lungs. Note asymmetry in expansion of the 2 sides or retractions during inspiration in the subcostal, intercostal, xiphoid, and suprasternal areas. These signs indicate pulmonary disease, airway obstruction, or air leaks.

K. Lungs: Auscultation of lungs in the newborn infant reveals bronchovesicular or bronchial breath sounds. Fine rales may be present during the first few hours. When there is a pneumothorax or pneumomediastinum, the breath sounds and heart sounds may be distant and the percussion sound may be hyperresonant. Decreased air entry and expiratory grunting are noted in respiratory distress syndrome. Because of the limited usefulness of physical findings alone in evaluation of respiratory disease, a chest x-ray must be obtained when abnormal lung findings are suspected.

L. Heart and Vascular System: Physical examination of the heart and vascular system and the physiologic changes of the perinatal period that affect these physical findings are described in detail in Chapter 15. Briefly, perfusion of the skin, strength of the pulses, point of maximal cardiac impulse, and auscultatory findings of the heart sounds and any murmurs, including those heard intermittently, are noted.

M. Abdomen: The abdomen will appear slightly scaphoid at birth but will become more protuberant as the bowel fills with air. The abdominal organs are most easily palpated soon after birth, before the bowel becomes distended. A markedly scaphoid abdomen associated with respiratory distress suggests the presence of a diaphragmatic hernia. These are generally on the left side. An **omphalocele** may be present at birth; sometimes it may be small and may be included in the cord clamp if not recognized. **Umbilical hernias** are common and usually cause no difficulty. **Absence of abdominal musculature** (prune-belly syndrome) may occur in association with severe urinary tract abnormalities.

Abdominal distention may occur with intestinal obstruction or paralytic ileus in an infant with peritonitis or generalized sepsis. Palpation of the abdomen for organs or masses should be done with a light touch. The spleen tip is felt from the patient's right side and is sometimes 2–3 cm below the left costal margin. The liver usually is palpable 1–2 cm below the right costal margin. The lower poles of both kidneys are usually palpable. Abdominal muscle rigidity and apparent abdominal tenderness should be evaluated.

The outline of a distended **bladder** may be seen above the symphysis and may be felt as a ballotable mass in the lower abdomen. Contraction of bladder muscles with voiding often occurs with palpation.

Superficial veins may appear prominent over the abdominal wall with or without pathologic conditions.

The **umbilical cord** begins drying within hours after birth, becomes loose from the underlying skin by 4–5 days, and falls off by 7–10 days. Occasionally, a granulating stump remains that heals faster if treated with silver nitrate cauterization.

N. Genitalia: Male and female genitalia show findings characteristic of gestational age (Table 3–2). In most term male infants, the scrotum is pendulous, with rugae completely covering the sac. The testes have completely descended. The size of the scrotum and the penis varies widely in normal infants. The foreskin is adherent to the glans.

In females, the labia majora at term completely cover the labia minora and clitoris. A hymenal ring may be visible as a protruding tab of tissue. During the first few days after birth, a white mucous discharge that may contain blood issues from the vagina. Occasionally, a thin septum produced by fusion of the labia minora covers the vagina. The fusion is easily disrupted with a blunt probe.

O. Anus and Rectum: Observe anatomy and muscle tone of the anus. **Patency** should be checked if meconium has not been passed; use a soft catheter or little finger—not a rectal thermometer or other rigid object. **Irritation** or **fissures** may occur after the immediate newborn period. A firm **meconium plug** may be present.

Meconium plug syndrome may occur in the newborn infant, with hard meconium producing total intestinal obstruction. These infants generally appear well, despite marked abdominal distention. Once the plug is passed, the distention is rapidly relieved and does not recur. Abnormal meconium, however, which occurs in cystic fibrosis, will cause this syndrome and must be considered.

P. Extremities and Back: The arms and legs should be relatively symmetric in anatomy and function. Obvious **major abnormalities** of the extremities include absence of a bone, clubfoot, fusion or webbing of digits, or missing parts. **Hip dislocation** is suspected when there is limitation of abduction of the hips or when a click can be felt when the femur is pressed downward and then abducted. The legs may be unequal in length and extra skin folds in the affected thigh are seen. **Palsies** involving the extremities are recognized when there are limited movements of the extremities, especially if only one is involved. **Fractures** may present with the same findings, in which case swelling and crepitation may be felt. Note the size and shape of the hands and feet. Deformities are frequent with **chromosomal abnormalities.**

The back is observed for curvature, spinal defects such as meningomyelocele, and dimples or defects overlying the lower lumbar spine.

Q. Neurologic Examination: The neurologic behavior of the newborn infant has become more clearly understood in recent years. Certain test items and observations on muscle tone are useful in assessing gestational age, since normal neurologic development follows a predictable course (Table 3–2).

Other items, described below, are those traditionally associated with abnormal central nervous system function (Prechtl and Beintema), and still others (Brazelton) attempt to test higher centers of central nervous system function. These authors stress the importance of testing the infant during specific awake and asleep states. A guide to the items applicable in each of the neurologic examinations is presented in Table 3–3.

1. Traditional neurologic examination—Examination of head circumference, sutures, and fontanelles and the presence of cephalhematoma have been described. One should note evidence of jaundice, plethora, cyanosis, and sepsis as part of a neurologic examination because of the potential association with central nervous system disorders (eg, kernicterus, meningitis, alteration of central nervous system circu-

Table 3–3. The neurologic examinations of the newborn infant. The first test is evaluation of normal neurologic development; the second is the classic neurologic examination for central nervous system disease; and the third extends the evaluation to study function of higher central nervous system centers and to elucidate individual behavior.

(1) NORMAL NEUROLOGIC DEVELOPMENT
(Estimate of gestational age.)
(From Dubowitz et al.)

Muscle tone
- Resting posture
- Recoil of extremities
- Horizontal suspension
- Vertical suspension
- Heel to ear
- Popliteal angle
- Scarf sign
- Neck extensors } pull to sit
- Neck flexors } pull to sit
- Body extensors
- Standing

Reflexes
- Sucking
- Rooting
- Grasp
- Crossed extension
- Automatic walk
- Moro
- Tonic neck
- Neck righting
- Pupillary
- Glabellar tap
- Babinski
- Magnet

Flexion angles
- Ankle
- Wrist (square window)

(2) ABNORMAL CENTRAL NERVOUS SYSTEM FUNCTION
(From Prechtl & Beintema.)

Muscle tone
- Resting posture and recoil
  - Opisthotonos versus frog position
  - Hypertonic versus hypotonic
  - Flopping hand and foot
    - Unequal tone
  - Pull to sit
  - Spontaneous movements
    - Lack of or excessive
    - Fisting
    - Tremors → seizures
  - Passive movement

Reflexes
- Moro
- Knee jerk
- Ankle clonus
- Biceps
- Suck and root
- Hand grasp
- Plantar grasp
- Tonic neck
- Crawling
- Babinski

Eyes
- Strabismus, nystagmus
- Abnormal movements
- Setting sun
- Doll's eyes
- Corneal reflex
- Ophthalmologic examination

Face
- Expression
- Facial palsies

Cry
- High-pitched

Skull
- Sutures
- Fontanelles
- Cephalhematoma

Other
- Jaundice
- Plethora
- Cyanosis
- Abdominal distention
- Skin turgor

(3) FUNCTION OF HIGHER CENTRAL NERVOUS SYSTEM CENTERS AND BEHAVIOR
(From Brazelton.)

Response decrements
- Visual
- Auditory
- Tactile

Orientation: visual
- Inanimate
- Animate

Orientation: auditory
- Inanimate
- Animate

General behavior (tone, irritability, spontaneous motor behavior, maturity)
- Level of consciousness
  - Initial state
  - Predominant state
  - Alertness
- Lability of state
- Rapidity of buildup

Specific behavior
- Cuddliness
- Consolability
- Hand to mouth
- Self-quieting
- Smiles
- Lability of state
- Lability of skin color
- Rapidity of buildup

Reflexes
- Defensive movements

lation and oxygen supply). Facial palsies and ocular disorders have been described.

Some observations are made while the infant is completely undisturbed; some involve minimal handling; and some can only be made by observing responses to specific stimuli. The infant should not be too hungry or too sleepy. Because a prolonged examination may exhaust the infant or cause irritability, the examination may have to be done in parts.

a. General observations—Paucity of **spontaneous movements** may be as important as abnormal movements. Discordant movements of one limb or of one side, hyperactivity, opisthotonos, athetoid movements, and movements ranging from tremors or jerks to frank convulsions may be seen in the infant with central nervous system damage. Brief seizures may present as momentary cessation of movements in a crying infant. Continuous chewing or sucking movements, protrusion of the tongue, and frequent yawning are other abnormal movements.

Resting position is observed without disturbing the infant. **Asymmetry** of the skull, face, jaw, or extremities may result from intrauterine pressures. The infant may be passively "folded" into the position of comfort assumed in utero.

b. Muscle tone—Test recoil of the extremities. Extend the legs and then release; both legs return promptly to the flexed position in the term infant. Extend arms alongside the body; upon release, there is prompt flexion at the elbows in the term infant. The amount of flexion and extension around joints is further tested at the neck, trunk, shoulders, elbows, wrists, hips, knees, and ankles.

Another means of testing for tone is the so-called passivity test. As the wrist is moved sharply back and forth, the hand flops for a brief period and then the infant resists the movement and holds the hand or wrist firm. In normal term infants, the wrist will be floppy for about as long as it is resistant to this maneuver.

A general impression of hypotonia or hypertonia can be gained from this testing. The **hypertonic** infant is usually jittery and startles easily; the fists are tightly closed, the arms are in tight flexion, and the legs are stiffly extended. The **hypotonic** or **lethargic** infant is "floppy" and has little head control. The extremities fall to the bed loosely when picked up and released. Recoil of arms and legs to the flexed position after being extended helps determine tone as well as gestational age.

c. Rooting reflex—The rooting reflex occurs so early in gestation that its absence in a viable infant should cause concern. However, the rooting reflex is strongest when the infant is hungry and may disappear after feeding. The reflex is elicited in 4 areas: at both corners of the mouth and on the upper and lower lips at the midline. The mouth opens or the head turns toward the side of the stimulus.

d. Sucking reflex—The sucking reflex can be obtained by placing a finger in the infant's mouth and noting the vigor of the movements and the amount of suction produced. A hypertonic or irritable infant makes biting rather than sucking movements.

e. Traction response (head flexion and extension)—The infant is pulled gently to a sitting position, by traction on the hands and wrists. In the term infant, there is at first a head lag and then active flexion of the neck muscles, so that the head and chest are in line when the infant reaches the vertical position. The head is maintained in the upright position for a few seconds and then falls forward. The infant will then raise its head again, either spontaneously or following a slight stimulus such as stroking the upper lip.

f. Grasp reflex—

(1) Fingers—When the palm is stimulated with a finger, the fingers will close on it. A term infant's grasp should be strong enough that it can be lifted from the table by holding onto the examiner's finger.

(2) Toes—Pressing the ball of the foot elicits a definite and prompt toe flexion.

g. Biceps, triceps, knee, and ankle tendon reflexes—These are best elicited with the finger rather than a percussion hammer. The infant must be relaxed.

h. Ankle clonus—This is normally present in newborn infants; sustained clonus is abnormal.

i. Incurvation of the trunk—The infant is lifted up and held over the hand in a prone position. The amount of flexion of the head and body is noted for an additional estimate of tone. The incurvation reflex is obtained by stroking or applying intermittent pressure with the finger parallel to the spine, first on one side and then the other, watching for a movement of the pelvis to the stimulated side.

j. Righting reaction—When the infant is lifted from the table vertically, the legs will usually flex. If the soles of the feet then touch the table, the infant will respond with the righting reflex—ie, first the legs will extend, then the trunk and the head.

k. Placing—The infant is held vertically with its back against the examiner and one leg restrained. The other leg is moved forward so that the dorsum of the foot touches the edge of the examining table. The infant will flex the knee and bring the foot up as though trying to step onto the table.

l. Automatic walking—Following the preceding tests, the ability to perform automatic walking movements is evaluated. The infant is inclined forward to begin automatic walking. When the sole of one foot touches the table, the infant tries to remain upright with that leg and the other foot flexes. As the next foot touches the table, the reverse action occurs. Term infants will walk on the entire sole of the foot, whereas preterm infants often walk on their toes.

m. Moro (startle) reflex—When eliciting the Moro response, observe the arms, hands, and cry. The arms show abduction at the shoulder and extension of the elbow, followed by adduction of the arms in most infants. The hands show a prominent spreading or extension of the fingers. Any abnormality in the movements should be noted, such as jerkiness or tremor, slow response, or asymmetric response. A cry follows the startle and should be vigorous. The nature of the cry is important—absent, weak, high-pitched, or excessive.

The Moro reflex may be elicited in several ways:

(1) While holding the infant's hands, lift the body and neck (but not the head) off the examining table and quickly let go.

(2) While holding the infant with one hand supporting the head and the other the body, allow the head to drop 1–2 cm rather suddenly.

(3) While holding the infant in both hands, lower both hands rapidly a few centimeters so that the infant experiences a sensation of falling.

(4) If the infant is quiet in the bassinet, lift the head of the bassinet a few centimeters and let it drop.

2. The Brazelton examination—This behavioral assessment of the newborn infant is presented as a research tool with an elaborate scoring system, and observer reliability must be established for it. However, items in the examination lend themselves to routine application. The examination includes items from the Prechtl-Beintema examination (Table 3–3).

The various tests and observations are all done in relation to specific states. The infant should pass through 6 states during the examination: quiet sleep, active sleep, drowsy alertness, active alertness, animated alertness, and the irritable or crying awake state.

During the testing, observations on lability of state, skin color, rapidity of buildup, self-quieting activity, startle responses, irritability, and spontaneous movements are noted and recorded.

a. Response decrements—Visual (flashlight), auditory (rattle and bell), and tactile (pinprick) stimuli are presented repetitively to the infants in states 1, 2, or 3. The response to each is noted and the time of the decrement noted.

b. Orientation—The infant's ability to orient to and attend to visual stimuli (animate and inanimate) is tested in state 4, and orientation to auditory stimuli is noted. Again, animate and inanimate sounds are presented.

c. Behavior—Cuddliness is defined as molding of the body of the infant to the examiner and can be elicited in the arms or by placing the infant over the shoulder. Consolability is scored on the number of ways necessary to quiet the infant, ranging from the examiner's face, voice, hand on belly, to holding, rocking, and finally a pacifier. Self-quieting activity is observed when the infant has reached state 6. The infant may not be able to remain quiet at all or may be quiet only for brief periods. The infant may have the capacity to be quiet for sustained periods. Associated with self-quieting is hand-to-mouth facility, which may range from brief swipes to thumb-sucking.

d. Defensive movements—In this part of the examination, the observer tests the infant's ability to remove a cloth placed over the face.

THE DISCHARGE EXAMINATION

Since the complete examination should have been performed earlier, only supplemental observations need be made at discharge, eg, rechecking a heart murmur, vital signs, and growth. The infant should be examined at the mother's bedside, and she should be given ample opportunity to raise questions. The physician should check the late appearance of medical problems such as jaundice, infection, skin rashes, etc, and be aware of maternal behavior that may affect care of the infant. Plans for medical follow-up are made at this time.

American Academy of Pediatrics Joint Committee on Infant Hearing: Position statement 1982. *Pediatrics* 1982;**70:**496.

Aniel-Tison C, Grenier A: *Neurologic Evaluation of the Newborn and the Infant.* Year Book, 1980.

Brazelton TB: *Neonatal Behavioral Assessment Scale.* Spastics International Medical Publications. Heinemann, 1973.

Caputo AR et al: Dilation in neonates: A protocol. *Pediatrics* 1982;**69:**77.

Desmond MM et al: The transitional care nursery: A mechanism for preventive medicine in the newborn. *Pediatr Clin North Am* 1966;**13:**651.

Dubowitz LMS, Dubowitz V: *Gestational Age of the Newborn: A Clinical Manual.* Addison-Wesley, 1977.

Guidelines for Perinatal Care. American Academy of Pediatrics/American College of Obstetrics and Gynecology, 1983.

Hittner HM, Hirsch NJ, Rudolph AJ: Assessment of gestational age by examination of the anterior vascular capsule of the lens. *J Pediatr* 1977;**91:**455.

Illingworth RS: *The Development of the Infant and Young Child: Normal and Abnormal,* 7th ed. Churchill Livingstone, 1982.

Johnson ML, Rumack CM: Ultrasonic evaluation of the neonatal brain. *Radiol Clin North Am* 1980;**18:**117.

Lee BC et al: Neonatal intraventricular hemorrhage: A serial computed tomography study. *J Comput Assist Tomogr* 1979;**3:**483.

Marshall RE et al: Auditory function in newborn intensive care unit patients revealed by auditory brain-stem potentials. *J Pediatr* 1980;**96:**731.

Mizrahi EM, Dorfman LJ: Sensory evoked potentials: Clinical applications in pediatrics. *J Pediatr* 1980;**97:**1.

Smith DW: *Recognizable Patterns of Human Malformation.* Saunders, 1976.

THE NORMAL NEWBORN INFANT

CARE OF THE NORMAL NEWBORN INFANT

Immediately After Delivery

Certain routines must be performed after delivery to make certain that the infant is adapting smoothly to extrauterine life and that there are no immediate life-threatening problems.

A. Nasopharyngeal Suction: Gentle suctioning of the mouth and throat with a bulb syringe is done during or immediately after delivery to remove mucus or blood and to clear the airway of obstructive debris.

B. Breathing: Occasionally, an infant needs help in establishing ventilation. A short period of assistance with bag, mask, and oxygen is often the only therapy necessary. Mild respiratory depression in a full-term infant is most likely the result of anesthetics or analgesics given the mother.

C. Apgar Score: This is determined at 1 and 5 minutes (Table 3–1).

D. Physical Examination: See above.

E. Body Temperature: Every effort should be made to prevent a fall in body temperature. This is especially important in cool, air-conditioned delivery rooms. Evaporative heat loss from wet skin and radiant heat loss into the cool environment can be excessive unless special precautions are taken. The infant should be wiped dry, wrapped in a warm blanket, and placed in a warm environment until stable and able to maintain body temperature well.

F. Stomach Tube: Passing an orogastric tube should *not* be routine. Stimulation of the posterior pharynx and esophagus may cause bradycardia and apnea. Therefore, if the procedure is required, it should be done in the nursery after the infant has stabilized. An exception is a delivery complicated by polyhydramnios, when it is important to rule out the possibility of a tracheoesophageal fistula by passing a soft rubber catheter into the stomach.

G. Umbilical Cord, Membranes, and Placenta: Examine after delivery for abnormalities.

H. Eye Prophylaxis: Routine eye prophylaxis against gonorrheal infection must be done as defined by local health codes. One percent silver nitrate is instilled carefully into each eye so that the conjunctival surface is adequately bathed in the solution. Single-dose vials are preferred. The eyes are not irrigated with water or saline after instillation of silver nitrate.

I. Identification: Bands are placed on the ankle and wrist before the infant is removed from the delivery area.

J. Cord Blood Collection: At least 10–20 mL of clotted cord blood in 2 tubes should be collected. One tube is used for blood typing, Coombs testing, serologic examination, and other tests that may be needed later. The other tube should go to the nursery with the infant and be kept in a refrigerator, where it will be available if other tests are required as the infant is further evaluated. This second tube should be retained for 7 days or should go with the infant if transferred to another nursery for care.

K. Mother-Infant Relationship: Important aspects of developing mother-infant relationships optimally occur in the delivery area. (See Parent-Infant Relationships, below.)

L. Transfer to Nursery: If the nursery is adjacent to the delivery area, the infant may be carried, adequately protected from chilling. For the premature infant, specially designed transport incubators are available for use when the nursery is far removed from the delivery area by time or distance. In addition to heat, these special incubators provide for visibility, easy access to the infant, and oxygen administration.

In the Transitional Nursery Area

An area or room in the nursery should be designated for admission of newborn infants from the delivery room for careful observation during the birth recovery period. All newborn infants should be admitted to this area except sick infants or those at high risk who are admitted directly to the special care nursery. All infants are potentially at risk, and most of those who will become sick during their nursery stay can be identified in the first few hours after birth by careful observation and evaluation. The nursery staff play a vital role during this time in evaluating the infant and identifying those who require special attention.

A. Data Compilation and the Medical Record: Begin the newborn record with the calculated gestational age, birth weight, length, and head circumference. The medical record should be designed to relate to problems that the infant presents as well as to record the data required for the infant's care and for evaluation of the nursery service activities. A nursing checklist of vital signs and observations of the infant's activity and physiologic functioning should be at the bedside during hospitalization and should be made part of the permanent record at discharge.

B. Classification: Based on birth weight and gestational age, each infant may be classified into one of 9 categories: preterm, term, or postterm; and small, appropriate, or large for gestational age. Infants who cannot be categorized as term and appropriate for gestational age must be watched carefully for abnormalities in hematocrit, blood glucose, and temperature regulation.

C. Mortality Risk: Estimate the mortality risk based on birth weight and gestational age (Fig 3–2). In general, infants with a 10% or greater chance of dying, based on these criteria, should be placed in a special care nursery. Other factors that may contribute to the risk of a particular newborn infant must also be considered in determining the level of care that should be given. Examples of these additional factors include maternal hypertension, drug therapy, diabetes, Rh sensitization, bleeding, infection, and previous neonatal deaths.

D. Examination: The appropriate examination at this time includes a review of the maternal and immediate perinatal history, noting whether fetal monitoring was done and, if so, whether results were normal; clinical estimation of gestational age; evaluation of vital signs and pulmonary and cardiac status; and notation of factors that may influence the infant's course. A careful review of potential drug exposure must be made.

E. Birth Recovery Period: The sequence of events related to birth recovery and deviations from normal pattern are noted.

Abnormal symptoms or signs that may suggest developing problems should be noted. Careful reading of the nurse's notes will yield significant information.

F. Temperature Control: After delivery and until the infant has stabilized, the body temperature may be labile. Cooling should be avoided, since it will delay the normal cardiovascular adjustments required of the infant after birth. Radiant heat devices or incubators are ideal for this purpose in the transitional nursery area. For premature or low-birth-weight infants, it is very important to conserve the infant's calorie and oxygen requirements for growth rather than to consume them for temperature maintenance. Therefore, guidelines for starting and adjusting the environmental temperature by birth weight and age of the infant are valuable in the nursery (Table 3–4).

G. Vitamin K: Phytonadione, 1 mg intramuscularly, should be given routinely to every newborn infant as part of the admission procedure to the nursery. Vitamin K is particularly important for the prevention of hemorrhagic disease of the newborn in exclusively breast-fed infants and those born by alternative birthing methods such as home delivery.

H. First Urine and Stool: Time must be noted. If these events have not occurred prior to transfer to the general care nursery, a special note must be made. The normal infant will pass stool and urine within 24–48 hours after birth.

I. Care and Feeding: After the infant stabilizes in good condition, it will usually sleep and then wake

Table 3–4. Neutral thermal environmental temperatures.*

Age and Weight	Starting Temperature† (°C)	Range of Temperature (°C)
0–6 hours		
Under 1200 g	35.0	34.0–35.4
1200–1500 g	34.1	33.9–34.4
1501–2500 g	33.4	32.8–33.8
Over 2500 (and > 36 wk)	32.9	32.0–33.8
6–12 hours		
Under 1200 g	35.0	34.0–35.4
1200–1500 g	34.0	33.5–34.4
1501–2500 g	33.1	32.2–33.8
Over 2500 (and > 36 wk)	32.8	31.4–33.8
12–24 hours		
Under 1200 g	34.0	34.0–35.4
1200–1500 g	33.8	33.3–34.3
1501–2500 g	32.8	31.8–33.8
Over 2500 (and > 36 wk)	32.4	31.0–33.7
24–36 hours		
Under 1200 g	34.0	34.0–35.0
1200–1500 g	33.6	33.1–34.2
1501–2500 g	32.6	31.6–33.6
Over 2500 (and > 36 wk)	32.1	30.7–33.5
36–48 hours		
Under 1200 g	34.0	34.0–35.0
1200–1500 g	33.5	33.0–34.1
1501–2500 g	32.5	31.4–33.5
Over 2500 (and > 36 wk)	31.9	30.5–33.3
48–72 hours		
Under 1200 g	34.0	34.0–35.0
1200–1500 g	33.5	33.0–34.0
1501–2500 g	32.3	31.2–33.4
Over 2500 (and > 36 wk)	31.7	30.1–33.2
72–96 hours		
Under 1200 g	34.0	34.0–35.0
1200–1500 g	33.5	33.0–34.0
1501–2500 g	32.2	31.3–33.2
Over 2500 (and > 36 wk)	31.3	29.8–32.8
4–12 days		
Under 1500 g	33.5	33.0–34.0
1501–2500 g	32.1	32.0–33.2
Over 2500 (and > 36 wk)		
4–5 d	31.0	29.5–32.6
5–6 d	30.9	29.4–32.3
6–8 d	30.6	29.0–32.2
8–10 d	30.3	29.0–31.8
10–12 d	30.1	29.0–31.4
12–14 days		
Under 1500 g	33.5	32.6–34.0
1501–2500 g	32.1	31.0–33.2
Over 2500 (and > 36 wk)	29.8	29.0–30.8
2–3 weeks		
Under 1500 g	33.1	32.2–34.0
1501–2500 g	31.7	30.5–33.0
3–4 weeks		
Under 1500 g	32.6	31.6–33.6
1501–2500 g	31.4	30.0–32.7
4–5 weeks		
Under 1500 g	32.0	31.2–33.0
1501–2500 g	30.9	29.5–32.2
5–6 weeks		
Under 1500 g	31.4	30.6–32.3
1501–2500 g	30.4	29.0–31.8

* Reproduced, with permission, from Klaus M, Fanaroff A: The physical environment. Chap 3, p 68, in: *Care of the High-Risk Neonate.* Saunders, 1973.

† Starting temperature is the first environmental temperature the infant should be placed in.

up hungry and start to cry, usually 2–6 hours after delivery. The infant can be bathed, dressed, and fed at this time. Normal infants tolerate bathing and dressing with little difficulty.

J. Physician Responsibility: The physician responsible for the care of the newborn infant reviews the history and neonatal course and performs a complete physical examination after the infant is stable, preferably before 24 hours of age. The physician should be notified of any significant abnormalities that have been identified before this examination so that problems can be evaluated immediately.

Continued Care in the Level 1 Nursery

Although a registered nurse will supervise the area, the bulk of the day-to-day care in a level 1 nursery may be given by personnel at lower professional levels who are trained in the care of newborn infants. The emphasis is on well infant care, enhancing successful mother-infant relationships, feeding, and teaching care techniques. However, the staff must be continuously alert for any significant evidence of illness that may require evaluation.

A. Admission: The staff should review the infant's history and immediate postnatal events in order to be aware of any problems.

B. Duration of Stay: Following an uncomplicated perinatal course, mother and infant have traditionally stayed in the hospital for 2–3 days. Increased efforts to reduce hospital costs have resulted in a trend toward early discharge, with nearly 50% of mothers and infants being discharged at 12–48 hours. However, cost is only one of the many factors to be taken into account. Infants who have experienced respiratory distress, temperature instability, cyanosis, or other serious problems are not candidates for early discharge. Although medical experience suggests that evidence of such problems is usually apparent in the first 6 hours of life, other neonatal problems such as difficulties in breast feeding or jaundice will not appear until 3–4 days. Another factor for consideration is the level of prenatal care and education of the mother. The teaching of normal newborn care can hardly be accomplished in a few hours with parents who are physically tired and emotionally excited. Therefore, a careful system for following infants in the first few days of life must be established. Physicians and hospital services are currently developing programs for early office visits, home health care involvement, and public health nurse contacts to provide appropriate medical follow-up and teaching.

C. Adapting Nursery Activity to Needs of Mother and Child: The life situation of the mother and the family is important in their acceptance of the newborn infant. Favorable conditions exist when the mother is married, the child is wanted at this time, there is some financial security, and the parents themselves are emotionally mature. Even when these favorable factors are operative, however, there may be adverse factors that interfere with satisfactory adjustment. Problems in pregnancy, a difficult delivery, birth of an abnormal or premature infant, and development of maternal or infant illness are a few such factors. The nursery staff should understand the needs of the mother and child and show their willingness to meet these needs. The following suggestions will help (see also Parent-Infant Relationship, below): (1) Become acquainted with the mother and father—before delivery if possible. (2) Show an interest in the total family unit. (3) Visit the mother daily while she is in the hospital and be attentive to her expressed anxieties. (4) Institute flexible schedules of feeding, especially for mothers who are breast feeding. (5) Institute flexible schedules for the amount of time the infant and mother spend together. (6) Examine the infant in the mother's presence. Above all, it is important that *both* physicians and nurses respect the diversity of life-styles and approaches to parenting. The health care team should *assist* the parents and infant, not *dictate* any particular approach to the family. Parents should not be made to feel guilty if they do not choose to use rooming-in nursery arrangements, natural childbirth, or breast feeding. Criticism is often implied when parents do not choose the same approach to childbirth and infant care that the health care team would, despite the fact that different approaches to parenting and family life are equally compatible with development of a healthy child.

D. Rooming-In: The optimal family-centered program is the rooming-in situation with mother and infant together in the room under the supervision of an understanding and helpful nurse, with unrestricted visiting by the father or other supportive persons. The mother can get instruction in caring for the infant as she watches her infant being examined, and her questions about the significance of findings can be answered as they arise. Continued help and encouragement from well-trained nurses for the mother who is breast feeding are very helpful. Rooming-in may be continuous in a separate unit or modified, using existing postpartum and nursery facilities. Close cooperation between obstetric and pediatric medical and nursing personnel is essential.

1. Continuous rooming-in—A separate unit with separate nursing staff is arranged so that the mothers may have the infants with them as much as they desire. A nursery room located in the unit is available for infants at other times. The nursing staff cares for mothers and infants and plays an essential teaching role, encouraging successful breast feeding when that method is desired and being alert to problems in mother-infant relationships.

2. Modified rooming-in—It is feasible to adapt the routine schedule of activities in the postpartum and nursery units to allow the infants to remain with their mothers for variable periods, depending on the mother's individual desires and needs. Feeding on demand, modification of visiting rules and patient activities, and a helpful, interested attitude on the part of the staff will ensure a successful program of modified rooming-in.

E. Screening for Disease: Since nearly all infants in the USA are born in hospitals, an excellent opportunity exists to screen mother and infant for disease that may not become manifest during their stay in the hospital. Some of these tests can be routine, and some are required by law:

1. Blood type and direct Coombs test to identify potential blood group incompatibilities.
2. Serologic test for syphilis.
3. Elevated serum phenylalanine (causing phenylketonuria); α-keto acids, valine, isoleucine, and leucine (causing maple syrup urine disease); and homocystine (causing homocystinuria).
4. Thyroid function tests, eg, T_4 and TSH, which are more commonly abnormal in premature infants (see Chapter 25).
5. Galactosemia.
6. Sickle cell and other hemoglobinopathies.
7. Other tests have been recommended in some screening programs, eg, G6PD deficiency, IgM, indirect Coombs, histidinemia, adenosine deaminase deficiency.

The major problems in all screening programs consist of the time delay (often 2–6 weeks) between sample collection and reporting of results to health care personnel, who then must locate families and obtain compliance for recall testing, provide follow-up treatment and counseling, and determine the long-term efficacy and cost benefits in alleviating or preventing rare diseases.

Screening programs throughout North America have been very effective in the early identification and treatment of congenital hypothyroidism (1:3500 newborn infants) and phenylketonuria (1:20,000). The effectiveness of massive screening is less clear for the hemoglobinopathies. The levels of fetal hemoglobin are high at birth, and production of adult hemoglobins occurs only gradually over the next 6 months. Thus, the effects of abnormal adult hemoglobins are not immediately apparent. Efforts at early counseling of parents have not been remarkable in terms of preventing sepsis or vascular insults. Additional guidance is needed during the well child visits at 2, 4, and 6 months.

F. Circumcision: The American Academy of Pediatrics has formulated a statement to the effect that there is no longer any medical reason for neonatal circumcision. Parents should be informed of the pros and cons of the procedure in a prenatal visit.

G. Newborn and Infant Safety: Health professionals should emphasize the importance of using the safety precautions available to protect children throughout the first years of life. Safe transport of infants and children begins with the first ride home in a car seat specifically made for the newborn to 4-year-old child. Laws require the use of these safety seats in many states.

H. Preparation for Discharge:

1. Perform a physical examination—preferably with the mother in attendance—and discuss the care of the cord, circumcision, genitalia, etc, as the infant is examined.

2. Make sure the mother has mastered and understood the reasons for procedures for caring for the infant. Give her ample opportunity for questions.

Now that infants are being discharged from the nursery earlier and parents are assuming more of the medical care of the newborn infant at home, it is important to explain to parents the need to observe the infant for jaundice. They should be prepared to bring the infant to their physician as soon as significant signs or symptoms are noted. Parents should be taught to look for poor feeding, lethargy, excessive yawning, and yellow skin extending over the trunk and extremities. Newborn infants with heart murmurs must be watched for poor color, vomiting, poor feeding, and sweating.

3. Give feeding instructions. Careful attention to preparation of the formula is essential, since improperly prepared formula is dangerous to the infant. If coupons or food stamps are used to obtain formula, this—as well as a visit from a public health nurse—should be arranged before discharge.

4. Vitamin and iron supplementation may be required. Most proprietary infant formulas contain adequate vitamins. If breast milk is used exclusively and the mother's diet is inadequate, supplementation with vitamins A, C, and D is recommended. Fluoride supplementation is indicated if there is no fluoride in the local water.

5. Make an appointment for the mother and infant to visit the physician's office or clinic in 2–3 days (for early discharge follow-up) or in 10–14 days (for a well infant care visit).

6. Make sure the parents know whom to call if they have questions or if problems develop.

7. Check identification of the infant and of the person accepting responsibility for the infant at time of discharge.

American Academy of Pediatrics Committee on Fetus and Newborn: Report of fetus and newborn—Report of the ad hoc task force on circumcision. *Pediatrics* 1975;**56:**610.

Barness LA et al: Fluoride supplementation: Revised dosage schedule. *Pediatrics* 1979;**63:**150.

Berger LR et al: Promoting the use of car safety devices for infants: An intensive health education approach. *Pediatrics* 1984;**74:**16.

Britton HL, Britton JR: Efficacy of early newborn discharge in a middle-class population. *Am J Dis Child* 1984;**138:**1041.

Chowdhry P et al: Results of controlled double-blind study of thyroid replacement in very low-birth-weight premature infants with hypothyroxinemia. *Pediatrics* 1984;**73:**301.

Christophersen ER, Sullivan MA: Increasing the protection of newborn infants in cars. *Pediatrics* 1982;**70:**21.

Grossman LK et al: Neonatal screening and genetic counseling for sickle cell trait. *Am J Dis Child* 1985;**139:**241.

Herrera AJ et al: The role of parental information in the incidence of circumcision. *Pediatrics* 1982;**70:**597.

Lane PA, Hathaway WE: Vitamin K in infancy. *J Pediatr* 1985;**106:**351.

Levy HL, Hammersen G: Newborn screening for galactosemia and other galactose metabolic defects. *J Pediatr* 1978;**92:**871.

McCabe ERB et al: Newborn screening for phenylketonuria: Predictive validity as a function of age. *Pediatrics* 1983;**72:**390.

New England Congenital Hypothyroidism Collaborative Study Group: Characteristics of infantile hypothyroidism discovered on neonatal screening. *J Pediatr* 1984;**104:**539.

Nussbaum RL et al: Neonatal screening for sickling hemoglobinopathies. *Am J Dis Child* 1984;**138:**44.

Patel DA, Flaherty EG, Dunn J: Factors affecting the practice of circumcision. *Am J Dis Child* 1982;**136:**634.

Snyderman SE, Sansaricq C: Newborn screening for maple syrup urine disease. *J Pediatr* 1985;**107:**259.

PARENT-INFANT RELATIONSHIP

Mothers' feelings for their newborn infants may vary over a range extending from strong feelings of love and protection to complete rejection. Many factors that affect a woman's capacity for mothering are ingrained, ie, dependent on her genetic endowment, her relationship with her own parents, and cultural practices. Other factors include her marital status, financial situation, and attitudes about the pregnancy. Obstetric and nursery routines and attitudes of hospital personnel also affect the mother's ability to relate to her child. The separation of mother and infant at birth and during much of the postnatal period is probably the most arbitrary and potentially harmful of current postnatal practices.

Development of Maternal Attachment to the Infant

The mother's emotional attachment to the infant begins early in pregnancy. If the fetus or newborn infant dies, she will go through a process of mourning, even following an early abortion. During the early months, she may be preoccupied with a sense of not really being pregnant. Fetal movements are the first concrete evidence that she is truly going to have a baby. These movements are usually pleasant and associated with considerable fantasy. At this time, the parents often decide on a choice of names for the infant.

Behavior After Birth

The mother's initial thoughts at the moment of birth are usually, "Is my baby all right?" and "Is it a boy or a girl?" The answer may provoke profound expressions of joy or, at times, withdrawal and tears. When the mother is given the opportunity in the delivery room to hold her infant, she will regard it with tenderness, tending to concentrate on its eyes. Klaus and Kennell (1982) have observed a pattern of examination and touching that the mother follows when the nude infant is presented to her at about 1 hour of age. She usually begins with fingertip touching of the extremities and proceeds to palm contact of the trunk within a few minutes. There is noticeable attention paid to the infant's eyes.

Both the mother and the infant may go through a stage of wakefulness during the first hour after birth. The infant is wide-eyed, alert, and responsive. The mother's wakefulness may persist until she has held and fed the infant. It is as though the birth process is not finished until she has cared for her child. Following this period of wakefulness, both the mother and the infant fall into a deep sleep lasting several hours.

Implication for Hospital Care of Mother & Infant

Prolonged separation of mother and infant and rigidity of schedules and routine activities in the postnatal areas may be playing a significant negative role in development of normal mother-infant relationships.

Guidelines to Provide Optimal Parent-Infant Relationships

(1) The mother's comfort and access to her infant are of prime importance.

(2) The physician or other health professional responsible for the infant's care should talk with parents—preferably together—at least once a day.

(3) If the infant is ill, it is important to explore the parents' understanding of the infant's illness and its causes. They should be prepared for the infant's appearance and for the equipment used in the special care nursery before visiting the infant. An informed individual must be present to answer questions and give support. Physical contact with the infant should be allowed whenever possible.

(4) The physician and nurse should not overburden the parents with details or concerns of care and prognosis during the early period. Optimism about prognosis is essential whenever possible. The parents are developing an important relationship with the infant during this time that should not be interrupted by needless anxieties.

(5) The teenage mother, especially when unmarried, will need compassionate attention and teaching to help her become attached to her infant and assume the responsibilities of motherhood.

The Sick Infant

Occasionally, an infant has a grave illness or serious congenital anomaly requiring immediate management. If the difficulty has been anticipated, the problems will have been prepared for prior to delivery. If the occurrence is unexpected, the following guidelines will be helpful:

(1) A prompt survey of the seriousness of the condition and decisions about immediate treatment are urgently required. Additional help or immediate transfer to the nursery may be required.

(2) The parents will sense the seriousness of the situation. An absent cry and increased activity around the infant cannot be disguised. A word to the parents that indicates there is a problem and that the infant's welfare is being considered first is vital. Some indication of the type of trouble should be given—eg, "He has a defect of his spine," or "She has difficulty breathing."

(3) If the infant is likely to die or must be removed from the room immediately, the parents should be told these facts and be assured that someone will return soon to report what is happening.

(4) Should the parents see a sick or deformed infant? Yes, for many reasons. Even a glimpse of the infant will prevent a grossly exaggerated imaginary picture from forming in their minds. If possible, they should be allowed to see and touch their infant in order to complete the perinatal experience. If the appearance of the infant is gruesome, the parents will need preparation plus added support and understanding. If the infant dies, it is especially important that they see the infant so that they will be able to accomplish the mourning process. These comments also apply when a stillbirth has occurred.

(5) No emotionally charged comments should be made to the parents. Decisions involving long-term outcome and disposition should be postponed.

(6) The parents of a sick preterm infant will go through a period of shock and disappointment, often associated with feelings of guilt, and will require understanding and emotional support from health professionals during the succeeding days and weeks.

(7) Early separation of infants from their parents, prolonged hospitalization, and socioeconomic problems of parents are common associated problems in extremely premature births. The increased risks of abuse, neglect, and dysfunctional parenting have been well documented for these surviving infants.

Genetic Counseling

The likelihood of genetic defects reappearing in future pregnancies need not be considered or discussed immediately after the birth of an abnormal child. When the parents begin to ask how and why the defects occurred, they will be ready for genetic information and counseling. The information may have to be reviewed over and over again as the parents struggle with the reality of their newborn infant's problems.

Decisions about providing extraordinary life support and aggressive medical care have been intensely debated. Right-to-life advocates demand equal standards for treating every infant with no exceptions. Others feel equally strongly that measures to "prolong life" for infants who have no chance of long-term survival merely serve to prolong the process of dying. A third opinion is that infants and children who have no chance for any intellectual function, and thus no meaningful life, should not be subjected to ventilator care, surgery, and other costly and painful measures. Often, the physician cannot predict exactly how severe a newborn infant's handicaps and retardation will be. These "gray-zone" cases are at the center of this highly charged emotional issue.

Traditionally, decisions were made by the primary physician and immediate family. Subspecialists such as pediatric neurologists and neonatologists were often called upon to give independent medical opinions and predictions of outcome. When this decision-making process was challenged in the USA, the federal government tried to develop laws and regulating agencies attempted to standardize care for all cases. The "Baby Doe" rulings and laws became a national issue. In response, the American Academy of Pediatrics took a public stand supporting the right of involved physicians and family members to continue making decisions, and they recommended that an infant bioethics review committee be established in every hospital or region as a resource for evaluating current cases and addressing issues. These committees have been formed in over 60% of hospitals in the USA.

Grief Counseling

Dealing with death and the dying process in a newborn infant is a major psychologic task for both family and health care professionals. Often these situations must be faced by families with no forewarning. The emotional reactions experienced include shock, denial, sadness, anxiety, anger, and, importantly, resolution. Parents must be assisted in their efforts to work through their grief. Often the 2 parents may not be feeling the same emotion at the same time, and emotional energy may be misdirected against the mate. Psychosomatic symptoms are common and can usually be recognized and resolved. If there is a history of psychiatric illness or if there is no emotional support system, major psychiatric crises may occur. The possible stresses on marriage, family functioning, and siblings should be anticipated and resolved as soon as possible.

Whenever possible, parents should be well informed of the imminence of death and of the medical decisions being made. Religious and ethical issues must be handled sensitively. Parents should be allowed to see the infant before and after death, and, if they wish, they should be allowed to hold the infant during the last moments of life. Dignity, respect, and understanding of the infant and parents need not compromise appropriate medical care.

Decisions regarding autopsy and funeral arrangements are important, and the family should be given adequate time (sometimes several hours) to make such decisions. An autopsy may be beneficial for the parents and may provide a good reason for them to return in 6–12 weeks for counseling with the health care provider. At these times, the health care professional will be able to inform the parents of unexpected findings, refer them for genetic counseling, put to rest their lingering feelings of guilt, and identify any abnormal psychologic patterns of grieving that may be present.

In intensive care units, personnel must also be given assistance in going through the process of grieving. Some nurses and other staff members may be experiencing death for the first time, and they should be allowed to express and helped to deal with their feelings and reactions, which may be quite different from those of the parents.

Mothers have intense emotional reactions to fetal deaths, including stillbirths and very early abortions. Information about the cause of death must be pursued (even if it means performing an autopsy instead of surgical pathologic examination), and the family should be encouraged and supported in viewing the baby. Although this may be a very painful experience, this approach is a more psychologically healthy way of mourning and resolving grief.

Parents experience many of these same emotions when a malformed infant is born. Their task is even more difficult, because they often face living with this child for the rest of their lives. The parents should be helped to learn to live with chronic sorrow and to find joy in life. With time, health care professionals should provide understanding and support for the family's feelings and concurrently encourage them to develop the skills needed to move ahead with caretaking.

Relinquishing an Infant

Although pregnancy in the unmarried does not carry the same social stigma as in the past, there is still much misunderstanding about emotional aspects of the adoption process in such cases. Relinquishment of the infant should be presented as an acceptable alternative to pregnant women carrying an unwanted child. They should be aware of the current favorable adoption statistics showing that infants will almost certainly be placed in appropriate homes. Another popular belief is that "the mother does not want to see or hear about the child"; that "she does not want to become attached to it"; or that "she might change her mind." However, since the mother already has related to the fetus early in pregnancy, special feelings cannot be avoided when she relinquishes the infant for adoption. If she can see and touch the infant, the experience of pregnancy and delivery can be completed rather than be forever shrouded in uncertainty, denial, and fantasy, because the mother can work through her feelings more easily. Predelivery counseling is desirable, including informed discussion of expected emotional reactions after delivery. The process of delivery and immediate handling by the mother may be the same as for the mother who is keeping her infant.

The *earliest possible* placement of the infant in a permanent adoptive home is best for the new parents and for the infant.

American Academy of Pediatrics Committee on Bioethics: Treatment of critically ill newborns. *Pediatrics* 1983;**72:**565.

American Academy of Pediatrics Infant Bioethics Task Force and Consultants: Guidelines for infant bioethics committees. *Pediatrics* 1984;**74:**306.

Brazelton TB: Developmental framework of infants and children: A future for pediatric responsibility. *J Pediatr* 1983;**102:**967.

Helfer RE, Wilson AL: The parent-infant relationship: Promoting a positive beginning through perinatal coaching. *Pediatr Clin North Am* 1982;**29:**249.

Hunter RS et al: Antecedents of child abuse and neglect in premature infants: A prospective study in a newborn intensive care unit. *Pediatrics* 1978;**61:**629.

Klaus M, Kennell J: *Parent-Infant Bonding.* Mosby, 1982.

Lozoff B et al: The mother-newborn relationship: Limits of adaptability. *J Pediatr* 1977;**91:**1.

Nance S: *Premature Babies: A Handbook for Parents.* Priam Books, 1982.

Peppers LG, Knapp RJ: *Motherhood and Mourning: Perinatal Death.* Praeger, 1980.

Schulman JL: Coping with major disease: Child, family, pediatrician. *J Pediatrics* 1983;**102:**988.

Schwiebert P, Kirk P: *When Hello Means Goodbye.* Univ of Oregon Health Sciences Center, 1981.

Strain J: The American Academy of Pediatrics comments on the "Baby Doe II" regulations. *N Engl J Med* 1983;**309:**443.

FEEDING OF THE NEWBORN INFANT*

Feeding schedules in newborn nurseries have tended to be fairly rigid, primarily for the convenience of the staff. The result has been that some infants are awake and hungry for long periods and others must be awakened to be fed, and neither is optimal from the infant's point of view. "Demand feeding"—allowing the infant to eat when awake and hungry—usually leads to optimal intake and eventual establishment of a "schedule" that will be both satisfying to the infant and reasonable for the family. Initiating demand feeding in the nursery is entirely feasible and most easily done with a modified or continuous rooming-in program where the mother can respond to the infant's needs with ease.

* Infant feeding as such is discussed in Chapter 4.

What, When, & How Much to Feed

The first feeding of water should be offered as the birth recovery period is ending and the infant appears hungry, which is normally at 3–6 hours of age. The 3 most important criteria in the decision to begin feedings are that the infant should appear actively hungry, should have normal bowel sounds, and should have no abdominal distention. When these conditions are met, the first feeding of sterile water may be given.

One water feeding is usually sufficient, although in occasional cases several may be required to make certain that feedings are well tolerated. Full-strength milk formula (approximately 20 kcal/oz) or breast feedings can then be given. Ready-to-use formulas rather than concentrates are recommended for use in the nursery, since they provide a maximum of convenience and safety.

The initial feeding may consist of a few swallows or several ounces. As feedings are established, the infant should be allowed to regulate the volume and frequency of feedings so long as fluid and caloric requirements are met. By the third day, the infant should receive a minimum of 100 mL/kg/d and will soon thereafter start taking about 120 kcal and 180 mL/kg/d or more, allowing for hunger satisfaction and optimal growth.

Methods of Feeding

A. Bottle Feeding: Most commercial bottles and nipples are satisfactory. If the nipple hole needs to be enlarged, this can easily be done with a hot needle. For premature or debilitated infants, a soft nipple with easy flow (cross-cut hole) is required.

B. Breast Feeding: (See also Chapter 4.) When a mother wants to nurse her infant, success or failure is related in part to the counseling and emotional support given her by health care personnel. The staff can share the role of listening, giving factual data, and encouraging the mother to continue nursing long enough to overcome problems she may have in establishing lactation. Having a nurse present when the mother first attempts to feed, providing explanation of physiologic processes, and making her physically comfortable will ensure success.

A variable amount of breast engorgement occurs on about the third day after delivery. The engorgement may interfere with nursing because the infant is unable to grasp the nipple. A nipple shield may be used to reduce the areolar engorgement and to draw out the nipple. The infant may then nurse directly from the breast. Prolonged use of the shield interferes with complete emptying of the breasts. Nipple soreness is minimized if the nursing time is kept to approximately 5 minutes during the prelactation period until milk flow is established. Only a bland ointment should be used on the nipples.

The mother should be forewarned that her infant will seem to become more hungry about the fourth or fifth day and will want to nurse more frequently.

This behavior lasts only 1–2 days. The infant will then return to a less frequent feeding schedule.

The mother who wishes to nurse a premature, sick, or debilitated infant may be successful if given some additional suggestions. She must empty her breasts several times a day with a mechanical pump or by manual expression to maintain lactation until her infant is able to nurse from the breast. The healthy premature infant will begin breast feeding at 36–40 weeks' gestation. If the infant does not empty the breast, milk production can be increased if the mother pumps the breast after feedings. She may have insufficient milk for a few days, and a supplement immediately following feeding will be necessary until supply increases.

C. Gavage Feeding: Intermittent gavage feeding should be used when the infant has a weak sucking and swallowing reflex or tires easily. Gavage feeding can be done safely with minimal handling. However, in a sick infant with danger of abdominal distention, regurgitation, and aspiration, gavage feeding has the same risk as nipple feeding.

Indwelling orogastric tubes have been used for long-term feedings of small premature infants. A small polyethylene (rather than rubber) catheter must be used to minimize local irritation. The location of the end of the tube must be checked before each feeding to be sure it has remained in the stomach.

Some centers handling newborn infants prefer nasogastric tubes although these have 2 disadvantages: They tend to obstruct breathing, particularly in preterm infants who are obligate nasal breathers, and since they constitute a foreign body in the nasopharynx, they can predispose to otitis media and blockage of the auditory tube. Occasionally, a preterm infant of less than 32 weeks' gestation may not tolerate gastric feedings. These infants can be fed successfully using oroduodenal tubes or nasojejunal tubes. The use of these tubes may be complicated by bilious reflux or perforation of the viscus with rupture and infection into the peritoneal cavity, the renal pelvis, or the retroperitoneal space. Therefore, the tubes must be taped with clear marking of proper location, must be changed every 5 days, and must never be advanced after initial placement is established.

D. Gastrostomy: This procedure can be done easily and relatively safely in infants in the rare instances when it is indicated. It should be done by an experienced surgeon. The main indications are in surgical conditions such as tracheoesophageal fistula, chest surgery, certain types of bowel surgery to aid in the pre- and postoperative care, and for some children with severe central nervous system dysfunction.

E. Intravenous Fluids: (See Chapter 35.) Intravenous fluids are always required in preterm, very low birth weight, and critically ill infants. The fluids are given primarily to ensure adequate hydration and electrolyte intake. A multivitamin preparation should be added if feedings have not been started. Water and electrolyte intake must be adjusted to the needs of each infant, based on a record of intake and output that should be reviewed at least every 12 hours. The amount administered should maintain normal plasma sodium concentrations, a plasma osmolality of approximately 280 mosm/kg of water, a urine osmolarity between 150 and 250 mosm/kg of water, and a urine flow rate between 1 and 3 mL/kg/h. In general, the amount of water administered in the form of 10% glucose should be in the range of 80–150 mL/kg/d, and sodium intake should be between 2 and 4 meq/kg/d. The higher figures apply to the smaller preterm infants. Potassium, 2 meq/kg/d, should be added to the intravenous fluids after the infant has begun to urinate. If metabolic acidosis is not present, the sodium is given as sodium bicarbonate or chloride and the potassium as potassium chloride. If metabolic acidosis is present, both are given as the salts of metabolizable anions, sodium bicarbonate and potassium acetate.

F. Parenteral Alimentation: The development of effective methods to provide adequate nutrition by the vascular route represents a major advance in meeting nutritional needs in those rare instances where infants cannot take sufficient feedings orally for a prolonged period. Several specific solutions have been devised that consist of water, glucose, amino acids, lipids, electrolytes, and vitamins. The solution is usually delivered through a central venous catheter. Anabolic status can be achieved at 60 kcal/kg/d, and growth may be achieved at 70 kcal/kg/d using parenteral nutrition. However, much greater caloric intake may be necessary for severely ill infants such as those with bronchopulmonary dysplasia or with fresh surgical wounds. Newborns likely to benefit from this technique are primarily those infants with gastrointestinal abnormalities that do not allow adequate oral feedings or infants with associated severe malabsorption.

G. Special Considerations:

1. Termination of intravenous feedings—Intravenous fluids are discontinued gradually to avoid reactive hypoglycemia and to provide supplemental fluids until oral intake is satisfactory. When several oral feedings have been retained, the infusion may be discontinued.

2. Feeding preterm infants—Even in small preterm infants, early feedings are preferred over a period of prolonged starvation and dehydration. For infants who are very small and sick, peripheral alimentation with glucose, maintenance electrolytes, and amino acids provides some calories and nitrogen until oral or gavage feedings can be started safely. The use of intravenous amino acid solutions is not begun until the condition of the infant is stable and the physician is reasonably certain of good liver function, including liver perfusion. Usually this will occur within 24–48 hours after delivery. Infants who are well and who will tolerate oral feedings may be fed by nipple or gavage. The first nipple or gavage feedings should be with sterile water. Formula at standard dilution (20 kcal/oz) is started as soon as water feedings are tolerated. Small infants begin at 1–5 mL per feeding at 2- to 3-hour intervals, gradually increasing to the desired 24-hour volume as tolerated (120 kcal and 180 mL/kg or more). Larger infants begin at 5–15 mL per feeding at 3-hour intervals. With gavage feedings, gastric emptying can be checked by aspirating the stomach before feedings until a regular feeding pattern occurs. Replace aspirated fluid and add milk to the volume desired for that feeding. If the abdomen becomes distended or if bile-stained residuals are aspirated from the stomach, feedings should be withheld and consideration should be given to possible causes such as midgut volvulus, obstruction, infection, or necrotizing enterocolitis.

If mothers wish to breast-feed their premature infants, the use of their milk may be highly advantageous to the infant. Particularly the fresh milk early in gestation seems to have increased calories and may protect against infections, allergies, and later obesity. However, pooled, banked human milk appears to be less advantageous than the special formulas prepared for premature infants.

Nipple feedings can be substituted for gavage feedings gradually at 34 weeks' gestation and when the infant begins sucking on the gavage tube. Transition is made slowly, as infants will tire easily with nipple feedings. Demand feeding of premature infants is desirable. Intake will vary, and each infant will tend to establish an individual pattern. Feeding is satisfactory when optimal weight gain occurs.

3. Discharge formula—A variety of formulas are available for feeding after the infant goes home. Anticipate the confusion that may occur about how to make up the particular formula the infant is given. Clear instructions for preparation of the infant's formula must be written out for the mother's reference.

No prepared formula may be considered ideal to replace mother's milk. However, the standard milk preparations available provide satisfactory nutrition. Proprietary formulas usually come in 3 forms: concentrated liquid, requiring dilution with equal parts of water; ready-to-use, requiring no dilution; and powdered, requiring water dilution according to instructions on the can. An evaporated milk formula is no longer recommended.

American Academy of Pediatrics: Report of the Task Force on the Assessment of the Scientific Evidence Relating to Infant-Feeding Practices and Infant Health. *Pediatrics* 1984;**74 (Suppl)**:579.

Anderson GH: Human milk feeding. *Pediatr Clin North Am* 1985;**32**:332.

Battaglia FC: Umbilical uptake of substrates and their role in fetal metabolism. Pages 83–91 in: *Nutrition and Metabolism of the Fetus and Infant, Fifth Nutricia Symposium*. Visser HKA (editor). Martinus Nijhoff, 1979.

Battaglia FC, Sparks JW: Perinatal nutrition and metabolism. Pages 145–171 in: *Perinatal Medicine*. Boyd RDH, Battaglia FC (editors). Butterworth, 1983.

Butte NF et al: Human milk intake and growth in exclusively breast-fed infants. *J Pediatr* 1984;**104**:187.

Kanareck KS, Williams PR, Curran JS: Total parenteral nutrition in infants and children. Pages 151–181 in: *Advances in Pediatrics*. Vol 29. Barness LA (editor). Year Book, 1982.

Oh W: Fluid and electrolyte therapy and parenteral nutrition in low birth weight infants. *Clin Perinatol* 1982;**9**:637.

Putet G et al: Nutrient balance, energy utilizations, and composition of weight gain in very-low-birth-weight infants fed pooled human milk or a preterm formula. *J Pediatr* 1984;**105**:79.

Sadowitz PD, Oski FA: Iron status and infant feeding practices in an urban ambulatory center. *Pediatrics* 1983;**72**:33.

Workshop on Current Issues in Feeding the Newborn Infant. *Pediatrics* 1985;**75(Suppl)**:135.

SPECIAL CARE OF THE HIGH-RISK INFANT

GENERAL CONCEPTS & PROCEDURES

Each hospital service that delivers infants must be able to respond to the urgent needs of the newborn infant who is acutely ill at birth or develops an acute problem during the newborn stay. In many cases, the danger can be anticipated and appropriate arrangements made for care of the high-risk infant by having needed personnel and equipment available or by transferring the infant to a special care nursery as soon as the need is recognized. Ideally, when the infant's problem is identified during pregnancy, arrangements should be made to deliver at the hospital where special care can be provided. The special care nursery provides specially trained physicians and nurses, related medical subspecialty support (pediatric surgery, birth defects, neurology, etc), service support (x-ray, laboratory), and equipment and facilities geared to the special needs and care of sick newborn infants.

Transport to Special Care Nursery

Referral guidelines should be well established in order to expedite transfer when the need arises. The special care nursery may be in another hospital, perhaps some distance away. Telephone consultation about the infant's problem and management facilitates the transfer and allows the staff to be prepared to provide for the infant's specific needs. Adequate clinical information, a consent for treatment at the referral nursery, a tube of clotted mother's blood, the tube of cord blood, and the placenta should accompany the infant.

Stabilization of the sick newborn infant prior to transport minimizes risk during transport. Temperature maintenance requires special attention. Precautions must be taken to ensure that the skin is dry, to reduce the evaporative losses, and to provide a neutral thermal environment during transportation. Swaddling the infant in specially designed materials that reduce radiant, evaporative, and convective heat loss is very useful as an additional safeguard. A check should be made of the blood glucose and hematocrit. Treatment with 5–10% glucose water at 3–4 mL/kg/h is recommended during transport. Hypoventilation must be recognized and methods of supporting ventilation instituted prior to transport. Evaluation of acid-base status should be made and treatment instituted by means of assisted ventilation or bicarbonate therapy (or both if indicated). Under no conditions should the amount of $NaHCO_3$ exceed 3 meq/kg over a 24-hour period. Hypotension may be detected (Fig 3–5) and may be treated by means of blood volume expanders. Chest x-ray may be indicated.

Certain problems require special attention related to transport, as illustrated by these examples. Any enclosed pocket of air will expand if the infant is transported to a higher altitude. Therefore, pneumothorax, diaphragmatic hernia, and bowel obstruction usually need tube and suction decompression prior to air transport. The blind upper pouch of esophageal atresia needs constant suction to avoid overflow aspiration of saliva. A large omphalocele presents a special problem of temperature control because of the large evaporative surface. This should be covered with gauze packs moistened with warm (37 °C) sterile saline solution and enclosed with plastic wrap during transport in order to prevent evaporative heat loss. Mechanical vibration, high sound levels, compromised lighting, and limited access to the infant during air or ground transport make transport an additional risk for the sick infant, and a degree of stabilization must be achieved for optimal care during transport.

All drugs for use in small infants should be kept in a transport kit and should be appropriately diluted so that the volumes to be administered can be measured accurately. One of the commonest errors made in transport of low-birth-weight infants is the overenthusiastic administration of drugs; vigorous supportive care and thorough evaluation should be used instead.

PERINATAL RESUSCITATION

It is no longer adequate to begin resuscitation of the newborn infant after delivery; instead, the entire sequence of decisions made by obstetricians, pediatricians, and family physicians throughout the course of labor and delivery must be seen as significantly affecting the condition of the infant at birth. Parturition and the many endocrine and cardiovascular changes it induces in the mother and infant begin sometime before uterine contractions actually start. However, attention focuses most closely on the time of labor, when synchronous cervical dilatation and uterine contractions lead to delivery of the infant. Labor constitutes a stress that is perfectly normal and well tolerated by the full-term, healthy infant delivered after an uncomplicated pregnancy. However, the stress of labor and delivery may cause marked fetal distress in pregnancies having one or more complications, eg, intrauterine growth retardation.

For this reason, it is important to emphasize preplanning for delivery by the entire health care team. Careful assessment of perinatal risk factors allows for identification of women whose infants are likely to require resuscitation in the delivery room. Refinements in systems for scoring or ranking risk factors (eg, a history of cesarean sections is less hazardous than fetopelvic disproportion) have improved the process of identifying high-risk situations. On a typical delivery service, one out of every 5–10 infants will require some resuscitation. Therefore, appropriate equipment and trained staff must be ready to respond immediately to an asphyxiated infant. Increasing emphasis is being placed on determining the best setting for delivery before the birth takes place so that the parents can be informed of the option for transporting the mother to a level 3 perinatal center prior to delivery. This contrasts with the past practice of delivery at the local community hospital followed by transport of a critically ill infant to a referral nursery.

Effective preplanning based on multiple assessments of gestational age and maturity can definitely decrease the complication of elective delivery of a preterm infant who subsequently develops iatrogenic hyaline membrane disease.

Intrapartum Resuscitation

In high-risk pregnancies, the obstetrician must continually assess the condition of the fetus through measurements of maternal blood pressure, maternal acid-base status, oxygenation of the mother, intrauterine pressure recordings, instantaneous fetal heart rate recordings, and occasional scalp pH measurements. Any fall in maternal blood pressure is reflected in a fall in uterine blood flow and potential uterine and fetal hypoxia. This is why attempts are made to avoid maternal hypotension by infusing isotonic salt solutions or colloid into the mother or by placing the mother on her side to avoid pressure from the gravid uterus upon the inferior vena cava, which would reduce return of blood to the right side of the heart. Oxygen tension in the most highly oxygenated blood of the fetus, ie, the umbilical venous blood, tends to equilibrate with uterine *venous* P_{O2}, not with maternal arterial P_{O2}. When oxygen in high concentration is given to the mother, her arterial P_{O2} rises to very high levels, but the P_{O2} in the uterine vein increases to a much smaller extent. This increase in uterine vein P_{O2} leads to a small but very important increase in umbilical venous P_{O2}. Since the oxygen affinity of fetal blood is greater than that of adult blood and since the human fetus functions on the steep part of its oxygen dissociation curve, the small change in oxygen tension effects a very large change in oxygen content in the umbilical venous blood. This is why oxygen therapy is used when there is any evidence of fetal distress.

Obstetric Management at Delivery

Because unexpected complications at delivery can develop, it is important—particularly at medical centers where a choice can be made—that the most experienced obstetrician be available for the delivery of high-risk infants. Immediately after delivery of the infant, the obstetrician should draw umbilical artery and umbilical venous blood samples into heparinized 1-mL syringes for blood gas analysis. These data often reflect the degree and longevity of in utero fetal hypoxia.

Whenever meconium-stained amniotic fluid is noticed at delivery, the obstetrician should deliver the head of the infant and then suction the nasopharynx, using a catheter and a DeLee trap before the shoulders are delivered and the thorax expands. This simple procedure has markedly reduced the incidence of severe meconium aspiration pneumonitis. The pediatrician should examine the vocal cords, and if meconium can be seen on them, the infant should be intubated and the trachea suctioned until no meconium returns. Only after suctioning is completed should positive pressure bagging and resuscitation be given.

Resuscitation of the Newborn Infant

The flow chart presented in Fig 3–6 shows the resuscitation procedures for newborn infants according to the severity of the neonatal depression shown at delivery. A few general comments apply to all infants. A physician skilled in the mechanics of resuscitation and in the evaluation of depressed infants of any weight or gestational age should be present for the delivery of every high-risk infant. In multiple pregnancies, there should always be one physician present for each infant. The knowledge of the attending physician should encompass technical skills in airway management and the ability to recognize clinical signs of impending shock. Ideally, a staff nurse from the neonatal intensive care unit should be present at the delivery of a high-risk infant. This enables the high-risk obstetrics nurse to concentrate exclusively upon the care of the mother.

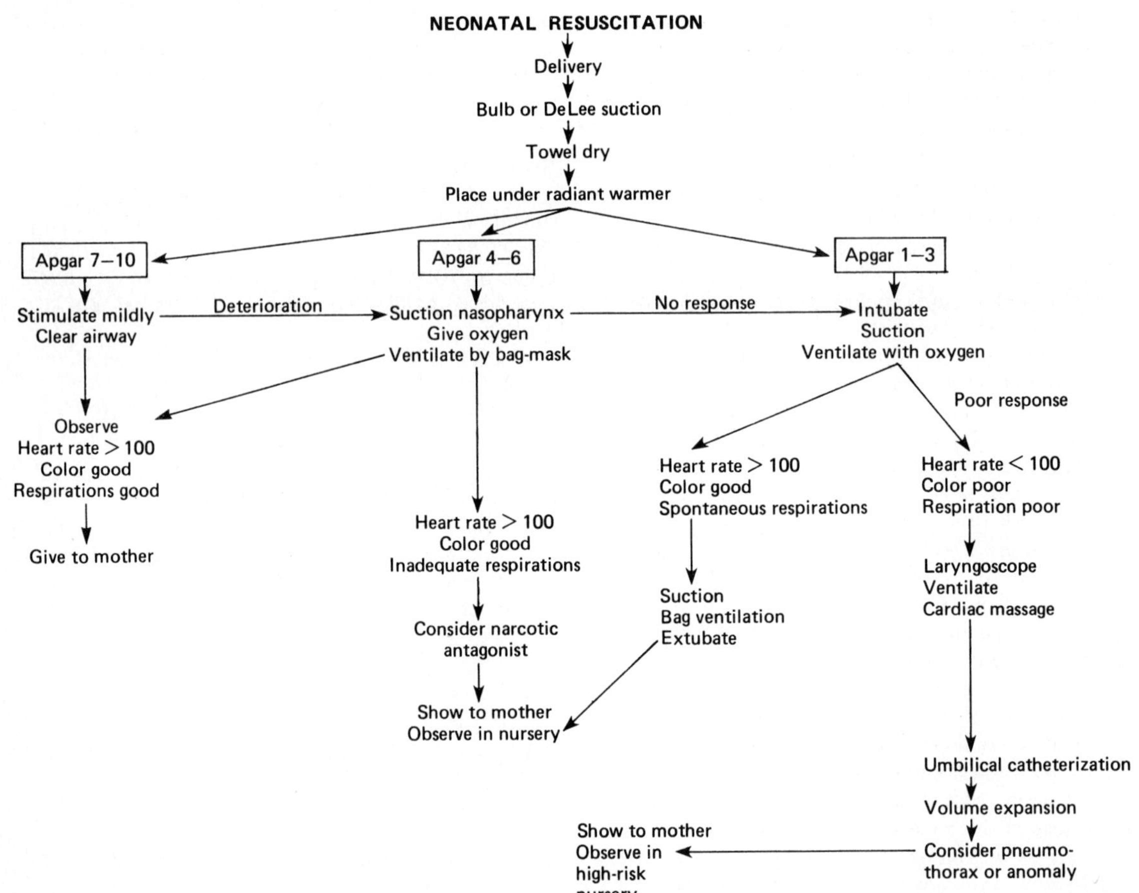

Figure 3–6. Flow diagram for neonatal resuscitation. (Modified and reproduced, with permission, from Lemons JA, Battaglia FC: Resuscitation of the newborn. Pages 811–814 in: *Current Therapy 1977*. Conn HF [editor]. Saunders, 1977.)

The basic approach to resuscitation should center on adequate oxygenation and temperature support of the infant. It should ensure that these needs are met promptly and should de-emphasize pharmacologic management, including sodium bicarbonate. All newborn infants, even the low-risk, full-term newborn infant, require adequate temperature support at delivery. In addition, every delivery suite should have adequate lighting and a gentle suction source for aspiration of the oro- or nasopharynx. There should be a laryngoscope with blades to accommodate premature and term infants, endotracheal tubes with internal diameters ranging from 2.5 to 4 mm, and a bag and mask with a 100% oxygen source readily accessible. Temperature support of the infant requires that a radiant heat source be provided and that the infant's skin be toweled dry.

Very low birth weight infants may have depressed (< 3) initial Apgar scores at 1 minute, even though their subsequent course is uncomplicated and the umbilical venous and arterial pH and base excess were normal at delivery. This suggests that the Apgar score may provide an inadequate assessment of the condition of the very immature infant. *The decision to withhold prompt and effective resuscitative measures should never be made on the basis of the low Apgar score in the very immature infant.* If *prompt* intervention and the establishment of adequate ventilation are carried out in small newborn infants, further steps are rarely required. Closed chest compression is indicated if poor peripheral perfusion, weak or absent pulses, or a heart rate of less than 100/min persists in spite of ventilatory support.

When volume expansion is required, give placental blood, 5% albumin, or plasma protein fraction (Plasmanate), 10 mL/kg. In the rare cases in which sodium bicarbonate may be required for resuscitation of an infant, it should always be diluted to an isotonic solution and should generally be given as 1–2 meq/kg in the 5% albumin solution.

Additional drugs that should be available are 10% dextrose (to be given at a dose of 5 mL/kg); 10% calcium gluconate (100 mg/kg); epinephrine, 1:10,000 solution (0.2 mL via endotracheal tube or intravenously); and naloxone, neonatal injection type (0.1 mg/kg). If the infant makes no respiratory effort or if there is no heartbeat or a very low heartbeat despite adequate ventilation and cardiac massage, drugs may be helpful.

Prognosis

Asphyxiated infants are at high risk for sequelae. The more common sequelae include central nervous system insult with seizures, cerebral edema, and hypoxic ischemic encephalopathy; myocardial dysfunction and dysrhythmias; shock lung; persistent fetal circulation; hypoglycemia; renal insufficiency and acute tubular necrosis; necrotizing entercolitis; and thrombocytopenia. Immediate nursery management for the severely asphyxiated infant (5-minute Apgar score of 3 or less) should include no feedings, intravenous fluids of 10% dextrose at 50–60 mL/kg/d, strict calculation of fluid intake and output, continuous monitoring of vital signs, and observation for abnormal neurologic activity, respiratory distress, and cardiac decompensation. Long-term outcome will depend on events in both the resuscitation room and the transition nursery.

An aggressive approach to the early identification of high-risk pregnancies, transport of mothers prior to delivery to a level 3 center, and presence of high-risk teams at the delivery have markedly reduced mortality rates of very low birth weight infants. Further improvement in outcome of high-risk pregnancies will result from prevention of premature delivery and the development of effective intermediate community-based maternal and neonatal care centers.

Bajo K: Equipment costs. *Clin Perinatol* 1983;**10:**175.

Baum JD, Scopes JW: The silver swaddler. *Lancet* 1978;**1:**672.

Besch NJ et al: The transparent baby bag: A shield against heat loss. *N Engl J Med* 1971;**284:**121.

Bowes WA Jr: Results of the intensive perinatal management of very low birth weight infants (500–1500 grams). Pages 331–355 in: *Preterm Labor.* Anderson A et al (editors). Royal College of Obstetrics and Gynecology, 1978.

Brans YW: Equipment available for nurseries. *Clin Perinatol* 1983;**10:**263.

Buckwald S, Zorn WA, Egan EA: Mortality and follow-up data for neonates weighing 500 to 800 g at birth. *Am J Dis Child* 1984;**138:**779.

Campbell AN et al: Mechanical vibration and sound levels experienced in neonatal transport. *Am J Dis Child* 1984;**138:**967.

Carson BS et al: Combined obstetric and pediatric approach to prevent meconium aspiration syndrome. *Am J Obstet Gynecol* 1976;**126:**712.

Hack M, Fanaroff AA, Merkatz IR: The low-birth-weight infant: Evolution of a changing outlook. *N Engl J Med* 1979;**301:**1162.

Hirata T et al: Survival and outcome of infants 501–750 grams: A six-year experience. *J Pediatr* 1983;**102:**741.

Jung AL, Bose CL: Back transport of neonates: Improved efficiency of tertiary nursery bed utilization. *Pediatrics* 1983;**71:**918.

Koops BL: Extreme immaturity: A frontier in neonatology. (Editorial.) *Am J Dis Child* 1984;**138:**713.

Main DM, Main EK, Maurer MM: Cesarean section versus vaginal delivery for the breech fetus weighing less than 1500 grams. *Am J Obstet Gynecol* 1983;**146:**580.

Pleasure JR, Dhand M, Kaur M: What is the lower limit of viability? Intact survival of a 440-g infant. *Am J Dis Child* 1984;**138:**783.

Press S, Tellechea C, Pregen S: Cesarean delivery of full-term infants: Identification of those at high risk for requiring resuscitation. *J Pediatr* 1985;**106:**477.

Schechner S: For the 1980s: How small is too small? *Clin Perinatol* 1980;**7:**135.

THE PRETERM INFANT

Infants born prematurely make up the major portion of newborns who are at increased risk. (For definitions and classification, see the early sections of this chapter.) Gestational age and birth weight correlate well with mortality risk.

Physiologic Handicaps Due to Prematurity

The increased risk due to prematurity is largely due to the functional and anatomic immaturity of various organs. Some of the more important examples are as follows:

(1) Weak sucking, swallowing, gag, and cough reflexes, leading to difficulty in feeding and danger of aspiration.

(2) Pulmonary immaturity and a pliable thorax, leading to hypoventilation and hypoxia with respiratory and metabolic acidosis.

(3) Decreased ability to maintain body temperature.

(4) Limited ability to excrete solutes in urine.

(5) Increased susceptibility to infection.

(6) Limited iron stores and rapid growth, leading to later anemia.

(7) Tendency to develop rickets due to rapid growth with diminished intake of calcium and vitamin D.

(8) Nutritional disturbances secondary to feeding difficulties and diminished absorption of fat and fat-soluble vitamins.

(9) Immaturity of some metabolic processes, which influences the metabolism of certain nutrients and drugs as well as maintenance of normal homeostasis.

Care of the Preterm Infant

A. Delivery Room: See Perinatal Resuscitation (above) for resuscitation procedures for preterm infants.

B. Care in Nursery: Infants born at 36–38 weeks' gestation may need only routine nursery care, stabilizing uneventfully after birth and going home with the mother. The more premature infant will require special care in either a level 2 or level 3 nursery.

Incubator Care

Small, preterm, or growth-retarded infants should be cared for in incubators set to maintain skin temperature at 36–37 °C (96.8–98.6 °F) with an air temperature of 32–36 °C (89.6–96.8 °F) (see Table 3–4). Incubator care reduces the risk of infection and prevents excessive evaporative water losses.

Satisfactory incubators may be either servocontrolled or manually controlled. The use of manually controlled incubators for temperature regulation encourages observation of the infant's thermal stability and increases the chances that elevations of body temperature will be noted more readily. Humidification of the incubator environment by the addition of water is no longer routine, because the inspired air, supplemented with oxygen, has often already been warmed and humidified. In addition, there is concern that the high humidity within the incubator may encourage the growth of hydrophilic organisms (eg, *Pseudomonas*) on the inner surfaces, thus predisposing to infections with these organisms.

If radiant warmers are used to maintain body temperature in low-birth-weight infants, additional water (20 mL/kg/d) should be provided. Electrolyte needs, however, are not increased. Use of loosely fitting plastic blankets in the radiant warmers may decrease the temperature instability and fluid problems.

Transfer From an Incubator to Bassinet

The premature infant who is swaddled and able to maintain body temperature without added environmental heat is placed in an open bassinet. This usually may be done when the infant reaches 1800–2000 g.

Examination

Evaluation and diagnostic procedures are done gently and carefully. Careful observation will provide much information, diminishing the amount of handling needed for the physical examination. Whenever possible, procedures should be done without removing the infant from the incubator and within the nursery environment.

The advent of relatively noninvasive techniques for physiologic monitoring in infants has greatly reduced the amount of manipulation and handling required. Doppler techniques for measuring arterial blood pressure and transcutaneous electrodes for measuring continuous arterial P_{O2} have reduced the need for long-term umbilical artery catheterization or arteriopuncture (see Chapter 35). Continuous P_{O2} recordings using transcutaneous electrodes are of great help in recognizing specific events that trigger hypoxia in particular infants and in monitoring infants with long-term oxygen dependence.

Growth of Preterm Infant

In order to monitor the growth, hydration, and nutrition of preterm infants, standard postnatal growth curves can be used in conjunction with the infant's own growth curve. Each day the infant's weight, total water intake (in mL/kg/d), and total caloric intake (kcal/kg/d) are plotted on the graph (Fig 3–7).

Nutrition

In feeding premature infants of any size, the goal is not only to achieve adequate caloric intake, but to do so with an appropriately balanced intake of carbohydrates, amino acids, and fats. The general principles—which often require extensive modifications—are as follows:

A. Carbohydrates: Premature infants will require intravenous or intra-arterial infusion of 10% glucose at a rate sufficient to provide approximately 7 mg/kg/min. The rate can then be increased or decreased as required in a particular infant to maintain a blood glucose level greater than 40 mg/dL and under 120 mg/dL. The premature infant should be fed a formula that contains some lactose, since this will be hydrolyzed in the gastrointestinal tract. The galactose released will be rapidly taken up by the liver and converted to glucose and glycogen. The

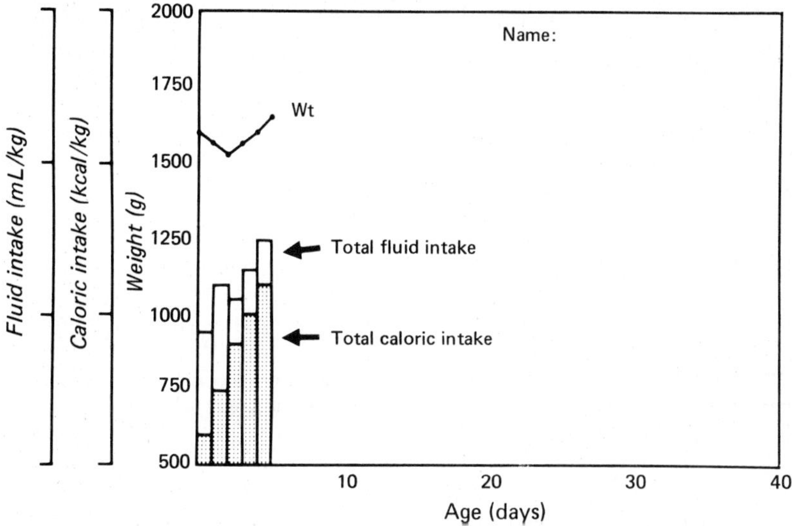

Figure 3–7. A convenient method of presenting a summary of hydration, nutrition, and body weight in newborn infants.

new formulas for premature infants provide some carbohydrate as a glucose polymer and some as lactose. The weaning period from intravenous feeding to milk feeding is a particularly hazardous time for the development of hypoglycemia, since full milk feedings provide a relatively low glucose intake. When full milk feedings are given, gluconeogenesis must provide the additional glucose necessary.

B. Amino Acids: Amino acids can be given intravenously to infants, using any one of several commercially available protein hydrolysates. However, it is preferable whenever possible to provide amino acids as protein contained in milk feedings. Infants will tolerate a wide range of protein intakes, and it is not clear at this time what intake is optimal. The modified cow's milk formulas especially tailored for premature infants contain protein with a high whey/curd ratio and a relatively high protein concentration compared with human breast milk. The use of human milk is discussed in an earlier section of this chapter.

C. Fats: Fat ingestion appears to be important in establishing normal postnatal liver and gastrointestinal function. Formulas with mixtures of medium-chain triglycerides and complex fats should be used. Approximately 3% of total calories should be linoleic acid. When the introduction of milk feedings has been markedly delayed in newborn infants, essential fatty acid intake in other forms must be ensured.

D. Vitamins: For infants receiving adequate amounts of breast milk or a proprietary formula, controversy exists about the need for vitamin supplements. Some recommend vitamin D and intravenous or oral calcium during the first few days to weeks of life to prevent rickets. In addition, for infants of less than 35 weeks' gestation, we recommend 50 mg of vitamin C, 25 IU of vitamin E, and 50 μg of folate daily. Phytonadione (vitamin K_1, AquaMephyton), 1 mg intramuscularly, should be given on admission to the nursery. If oral intake of milk is not adequate, the vitamin K is repeated once weekly.

When infants receive only intravenous or intra-arterial fluids during the first few days of life, a water-soluble multivitamin preparation should be added to the fluids to ensure adequate intake of water-soluble vitamins. This must include vitamin B_{12}.

E. Iron: Infants with birth weights of less than 1800 g need supplemental iron, since their iron stores at birth are limited and there is rapid growth with an increase in red cell mass during the first year of life. Oral iron supplementation is not recommended until 38 weeks' gestation in these infants, because of the hemolysis caused by iron.

F. Calcium and Phosphorus: For very low birth weight infants, both calcium and phosphorus supplements may be necessary to ensure adequate bone mineralization. These additives in premature formulas are frequently changed by the manufacturers, and intake versus need must be watched closely.

G. Trace Metals: Zinc and copper deficiencies have been reported in premature infants and in infants with short bowel or malabsorption syndromes. For diagnosis and treatment, see Chapter 4.

H. Hormones: The availability of circulating thyroxine has been shown to be better in premature infants taking breast milk than in those receiving formula.

Discharge

Discharge from the hospital usually occurs when the infant weighs 2000–2500 g and is eating well and coexistent medical problems have resolved or are under adequate control. In the nursery, the parents are encouraged to visit the infant frequently and help care for and feed their child. A social worker or visiting nurse may be very helpful in aiding the mother to care for the infant and in helping to solve the special problems related to prolonged mother-infant separation, disease, or handicaps.

Follow-Up Care

For infants discharged from level 2 or level 3 nurseries, long-term follow-up care is especially important because of the high incidence of significant handicaps occurring later. In recent follow-up studies, 10–20% of surviving infants who had birth weights of less than 1500 g later had physical problems, neurologic difficulties, visual impairment, deafness, learning and perceptual problems, or mental retardation.

Catch-up growth in premature infants correlates with gestational age, birth weight, severity of neonatal illnesses, and complications. Growth is slower in small-for-gestational-age infants, those of multiple births, and those of low socioeconomic class.

Formal follow-up testing has shown that premature infants usually have lower intelligence scores than their full-term siblings and that they have lower scores on visual-motor and perceptual tests than their full-term classmates. The effects of family characteristics and socioeconomic status on psychomotor achievements of high-risk infants must be taken into consideration during follow-up.

American Academy of Pediatrics Committee on Nutrition: Nutritional needs of low-birth-weight infants. *Pediatrics* 1985;**75**:976.

Battaglia FC, Sparks JW: Perinatal nutrition and metabolism. Pages 145–171 in: *Perinatal Medicine*. Boyd RDH, Battaglia FC (editors). Butterworth, 1983.

Baumgart S: Reduction of oxygen consumption, insensible water loss, and radiant heat demand with use of a plastic blanket for low-birth-weight infants under radiant warmers. *Pediatrics* 1984;**74**:1022.

Beaton GH: Nutritional needs during the first year of life. *Pediatr Clin North Am* 1985;**32**:275.

Drillien CM: Abnormal neurologic signs in the first year of life in low birth weight infants: Possible prognostic significance. *Dev Med Child Neurol* 1972;**14**:575.

Franklin R, O'Grady C, Carpenter L: Neonatal thyroid function: Comparison between breast-fed and bottle-fed infants. *J Pediatr* 1985;**106**:124.

Hack M et al: Catch-up growth in very-low-birth-weight infants. *Am J Dis Child* 1984;**138**:370.

Hillman LS, Hoff N, Salmons S: Mineral homeostasis in very premature infants: Serial evaluation of serum 25-hydroxy vitamin D, serum minerals, and bone mineralization. *J Pediatr* 1985;**106**:970.

Klein N et al: Preschool performance of children with normal intelligence who were very low-birth-weight infants. *Pediatrics* 1985;**75**:531.

Koops BL, Harmon RJ: Studies on long-term outcome in newborns with birth weights under 1500 grams. Pages 1–28 in: *Advances in Behavioral Pediatrics*. Vol 1. Camp BW (editor). JAI Press, 1980.

Kumar SP, Anday EK: Edema, hypoproteinemia, and zinc deficiency in low-birth-weight infants. *Pediatrics* 1984;**73**:327.

Laing IA, Glass EJ, Hendry GMA: Rickets of prematurity: Calcium and phosphorus supplements. *J Pediatr* 1985;**106**:265.

Oberkotter LV et al: Effect of breast-feeding vs. formula-feeding on circulating thyroxine levels in premature infants. *J Pediatr* 1985;**106**:822.

Pape KE et al: The status at two years of low birth weight infants born in 1974 with birth weights of less than 1001 grams. *J Pediatr* 1978;**92**:253.

Sabio H: Anemia in the high-risk infant. *Clin Perinatol* 1984;**11**:59.

Sameroff AJ, Chandler MJ: Reproductive risk and the continuum of caretaking casualty. Pages 187–244 in: *Review of Child Development Research*. Vol 4. Horowitz FD (editor). Chicago Press, 1975.

Sell EJ et al: Early identification of learning problems in neonatal intensive care graduates. *Am J Dis Child* 1985;**139**:460.

MULTIPLE BIRTHS

Twinning occurs in about one out of 90 pregnancies. The incidence of twins increases with the mother's age and parity. There is a familial tendency toward dizygotic twinning.

Dizygotic twinning occurs with increased frequency following the use of drugs, such as clomiphene, which induce ovulation and which may be used in the treatment of infertility. Twins may develop from a single ovum (monozygotic, identical) or from 2 ova (dizygotic, fraternal).

About one-third of twins are of the single ovum type. About one-third of identical twins have a double placenta, amnion, and chorion. However, if the partition between the twins consists of 2 layers of transparent amnion without an intervening chorion, a diagnosis of monozygotic twinning can be made with certainty.

Intrauterine Growth

The fetal growth pattern in multiple pregnancy differs from that of a single fetus. Intrauterine growth retardation occurs at a given total weight of all fetuses regardless of the number. Thus, intrauterine growth retardation appears in each fetus later in gestation in triplets than for quadruplets and still later in twins. In addition, the greater the number of fetuses, the earlier in pregnancy labor will occur—ie, triplets tend to be delivered earlier than twins. Thus, infants in multiple pregnancies are more likely to be affected by problems of preterm delivery and intrauterine growth retardation than are singletons. Discordant twins whose birth weights differ markedly (by at least 20% or more) often are found in association with twin-twin transfusion syndrome and are more common when there is a single chorion, as in monozygotic twins. The larger, plethoric twin tends to be much more ill at birth than the anemic, smaller one when twin-twin transfusion syndrome occurs, perhaps because hypervolemia and hyperviscosity may contribute to the morbidity in the larger twin.

Complications of Multiple Births

(1) Preterm delivery: Pregnancy is usually several weeks shorter with twins.

(2) Polyhydramnios: Ten times more common.

(3) Preeclampsia and eclampsia: Three times more common.

(4) Placenta previa: More frequent, presumably from increased placental mass.

(5) Abruptio placentae: May occur with second twin placenta owing to reduction in size of uterus following delivery of the first twin.

(6) Presentation: Breech and other abnormal presentations are more frequent.

(7) Duration of labor: Usually not much longer, though uterine contractions after delivery may be poor, with subsequent bleeding.

(8) Prolapse of the cord: Seven times more frequent than in single deliveries because of abnormal presentations and rupture of the second twin's membranes when unengaged.

Prognosis

The morbidity and mortality risks in multiple births are greater than with single births. More secondborn twins die than firstborn twins.

Follow-up data on growth and development of twins are conflicting, with some studies supporting a continued discrepancy in size of the 2 twins into adulthood and other studies being unable to demonstrate persistent differences in developmental size from those recorded in single births.

Fujikura T, Froehlich LA: Mental and motor development in monozygotic co-twins with dissimilar birth weights. *Pediatrics* 1974;**53:**884.

Pettersson F, Smedby B, Lindmark G: Outcome of twin birth: Review of 1,636 children born in twin birth. *Acta Paediatr Scand* 1976;**65:**473.

Wilson RS: Twins: Measure of birth size at different gestational ages. *Ann Hum Biol* 1975;**1:**57.

SPECIFIC DISEASES OF THE NEWBORN INFANT

RESPIRATORY DISEASES

1. APNEA

Apnea is defined as cessation of respiration for 20 seconds or longer and is accompanied by cyanosis and bradycardia. It must be distinguished from **periodic breathing** (see below), in which the apnea is brief (usually < 10 seconds) and is not accompanied by cyanosis or bradycardia.

Apnea may be a sign of serious significance in the newborn infant. Apnea can occur at any time during the neonatal period, particularly in very immature infants. Generally, the appearance of severe apneic episodes in a previously well preterm infant signals the onset of some other serious illness (eg, meningitis, sepsis, intracranial hemorrhage, etc), but in some instances apnea apparently unassociated with any metabolic problem or illnesses may occur. Virtually any serious illness may precipitate apneic episodes. For this reason, apneic attacks require a thorough evaluation of the infant's condition, with particular attention directed to any infection or central nervous system disorder as a possible cause of the attacks. Severe apneic attacks in a previously well infant may be an indication for an EEG, because seizures in the newborn infant may present as apnea only. Apneic episodes in infants with neonatal seizures will often stop when seizures are controlled and successfully treated with anticonvulsants. Upper airway obstruction may contribute to apnea in premature infants.

Studies in sleep laboratories and pulmonary function laboratories have supported the hypothesis that premature infants with apnea have a central disturbance in regulation of breathing. Respiratory reflexes are immature, gastroesophageal reflux may precipitate apnea even while the infant is awake, and there is a decreased response to elevated carbon dioxide levels. On the other hand, pulmonary mechanics and oxygenation are normal.

If idiopathic apneic episodes are frequent, an oral loading dose of theophylline, 5 mg/kg, can be given. A blood level reading should be obtained 2 hours after administration of the loading dose, at which time the drug level is likely to be at its peak. A maintenance dose is adjusted on the basis of blood level readings but is generally in the range of 1–2 mg/kg every 12 hours, given orally.

Aranda JV et al: Pharmacokinetic aspects of theophylline in premature newborns. *N Engl J Med* 1976;**295:**413.

Dransfield DA, Spitzer AR, Fox WW: Episodic airway obstruction in premature infants. *Am J Dis Child* 1983;**137:**441.

Durand M et al: Ventilatory control and carbon dioxide response in preterm infants with idiopathic apnea. *Am J Dis Child* 1985;**139:**717.

Gerhardt T, Bancalari E: Apnea of prematurity. (2 parts.) *Pediatrics* 1984;**74:**58, 63.

Spitzer AR et al: Awake apnea associated with gastroesophageal reflux. *J Pediatr* 1984;**104:**200.

2. PERIODIC BREATHING

Periodic breathing is common in newborn and young infants. It is usually not clinically significant, but in some infants, most commonly premature ones, prolonged respiratory pauses may be associated with cyanosis and bradycardia. It then becomes a major problem for diagnosis and management. Reports suggest that irregular respiratory patterns may be due to changes in respiratory drive or effective respiratory timing. Stimulation of laryngeal chemoreceptors may result in slowing or cessation of respiration. Finally, careful monitoring has revealed that active and quiet sleep states may not develop normal cycling and regulation in some premature and term infants.

Follow-up data on these infants have not yet defined the relationship between periodic breathing of prematurity and subsequent risk of sudden infant death syndrome.

Brooks JG: Apnea of infancy and sudden infant death syndrome. *Am J Dis Child* 1982;**136:**1012.

Brooks JG, Grunstein MM: Analysis of the respiratory pattern in newborn and young infants during regular and periodic breathing. *Am Rev Respir Dis* 1978;**117:**288A.

Phillipson EA: Control of breathing during sleep. *Am Rev Respir Dis* 1978;**118:**909.

Sander LW et al: Effects of alcohol intake during pregnancy on newborn state regulation: A progress report. *Alcoholism* 1977;**1:**233.

3. RESPIRATORY DISTRESS

Diagnosis

It is generally useful to divide pulmonary disorders of the newborn infant into 3 categories based upon physical and radiologic findings.

(1) Hyaline membrane disease is characterized by marked hypoexpansion and reduced lung volume and involves all lung fields, so that an inspiratory chest x-ray has thc appcarance of an expiratory film. On physical examination, the findings are consistent with decreased lung volume and include tachypnea, marked intercostal retraction, suprasternal retraction, and grunting. Air entry is uniformly poor throughout all lung fields.

(2) Disorders with increased or normal pulmonary expansion, hilar infiltrates, rales, and rhonchi include congenital bacterial pneumonias, "wet lung" syndrome, transient tachypnea of the newborn infant, and amniotic fluid or meconium aspiration. Wheezing may be present. The chest x-ray shows a slightly enlarged heart and streaky infiltrates radiating from the hilum of the lung and following the general pattern of the lymphatic and venous drainage of the lung. The peripheral lung fields are clear. Areas of infiltrate or atelectasis may be present.

(3) Disorders with normal lung expansion, relatively clear lung fields, and marked hypoxemia are most commonly associated with persistent fetal circulation. Any congenital heart lesion with inadequate pulmonary blood flow will also have these findings. Occasionally, "shock lung" following a severe hypoxic and hypotensive episode will also have these signs. More commonly, shock lung has a clinical spectrum comparable to that of "wet lung" syndrome.

For nasopharyngeal fluid collection, see Chapter 35.

Treatment

Supplemental oxygen administration is needed for infants whose arterial oxygen tensions fall below 50–60 mm Hg. Cyanosis does not provide an accurate indication of arterial oxygen levels and cannot be used as a guide for continued oxygen therapy. Blood gases must be monitored. The use of equipment to maintain an ambient oxygen concentration at less than 40% without monitoring is not recommended, because arterial P_{O2} levels exceeding 100 mm Hg may occur at this concentration and a limit of 40% may be insufficient for an infant with respiratory distress. Oxygen should be warmed, humidified, and given through an air blender, so that the desired concentration may be carefully delivered. The concentration being delivered into the incubator or hood should be monitored by an oxygen analyzer located near the infant's nose. This level of inspired oxygen should be measured and recorded each time a blood gas sample is drawn.

Arterial oxygen should be maintained at 60–70 mm Hg. Arterial oxygen tension determinations may be done from the descending aorta or the temporal, brachial, or radial arteries. Values from blood obtained from a warmed heel are not reliable. Recently, the use of indwelling arterial lines and transcutaneous oxygen analyzers, which give continuous readouts of arterial oxygenation, has shown the rapid and marked swings with handling, suctioning, and simply observing the infant. These methods have the advantages of continuous monitoring and noninvasiveness.

If blood gas measurements are not available, oxygen supplementation may be administered in concentrations just high enough to relieve cyanosis. However, because of the special risk of retrolental fibroplasia and other toxic effects of oxygen administration, the infant should be transferred for care where blood gas measurements are available. Infants with gestational ages of less than 36 weeks who have received oxygen therapy should have a careful eye examination for evidence of retrolental fibroplasia before discharge. The development of retrolental fibroplasia is directly related to increased arterial oxygen tensions in the susceptible premature infant. Prevention of this disease requires careful regulation of arterial P_{O2}. The pathogenesis of retrolental fibroplasia includes retinal vessel dilatation, proliferation into the vitreous, hemorrhage, and fibrosis. This process may spontaneously regress, or it may continue to complete retinal detachment.

A second organ injured by administration of oxygen in high concentrations is the lung. Prolonged exposure to high ambient oxygen concentrations will produce bronchopulmonary dysplasia. Since this condition is caused by exposure of the surface of the respiratory tract to high concentrations of inspired oxygen rather than by a high arterial P_{O2}, it may to some extent be unavoidable in those infants with severe hyaline membrane disease who require high oxygen concentrations to ensure acceptable arterial oxygen tension. Positive pressure ventilation with high oxygen concentrations increases the risk of pulmonary damage.

A. Hyaline Membrane Disease: Treatment includes early administration of continuous positive airway pressure, careful monitoring of inspiratory oxygen concentration, and appropriate supportive care of temperature, hydration, and nutrition. If CO_2 retention is marked or if oxygenation is inadequate, respirator support should be used.

Continuous positive airway pressure (CPAP) is normally begun at pressures of 2–6 cm of water. The concentration of inspired oxygen is adjusted to maintain an arterial P_{O2} greater than 55 mm Hg. If positive pressure ventilation is required, lower pressures can be used to achieve adequate oxygenation if inspiratory-expiratory ratios of 1.0 or greater are used. Peak inspiratory pressures greater than 24–26 cm of water and rates greater than 20–30/min are rarely required. In randomized clinical trials, infants treated with inhalant surfactant were reported to have lower oxygen needs and require reduced ventilator settings in comparison to controls. The clinical severity and risks of hyaline membrane disease, air leaks, and chronic lung disease may also be lessened by use of inhalant surfactant.

General supportive care is crucial in avoiding iatrogenic complications or other problems. Hypothermia should be avoided, since this will increase the infant's oxygen requirements. An infusion of 10% glucose with appropriate sodium intake provided as $NaHCO_3$ should be given, because infants with hyaline membrane disease almost invariably demonstrate combined respiratory and metabolic acidosis. The quantities of water and sodium required will vary depending upon the size and maturity of the infant; general guidelines have been given above. Infants may require circulatory support with intravenous infusion of colloid or crystalloid solutions.

B. Conditions With Infiltrates: In general, infants with diseases in this category will not require respiratory support and can be managed satisfactorily in level 2 nursery units. For infants with respiratory failure, ventilator support and continuous positive airway pressure may be necessary to improve oxygenation while avoiding the risk of excessively high concentrations of inspired oxygen. Since diseases in this category cannot be distinguished early in their courses from congenital bacterial pneumonia, particularly group B streptococcal pneumonia, infants with these diseases should be given antibiotics, and cultures should be performed until infection has been ruled out.

C. Conditions With Clear Lung Fields: In many cases of persistent fetal circulation, CO_2 retention is not marked and respirator care is not required. Therapy consists of frequent adjustments of inspired oxygen concentration. During the first 24–48 hours, pulmonary vascular resistance may increase or decrease at frequent intervals. Hypoxemia and acidemia cause more pulmonary vasoconstriction. For this reason, inspired oxygen concentration must be readjusted often. When transient persistence of the fetal circulation is very severe, ventilator support, muscle relaxation, and pulmonary vascular dilation with tolazoline (Priscoline) in a dose of 1–2 mg/kg intravenously may be required. Tolazoline is a general α-adrenergic blocking agent and has histaminelike activity. As such, it will cause vasodilation in other vascular beds besides that of the lung. Severe and irreversible shock may occur if colloid in the form of plasma or whole blood is not given at the time of tolazoline administration. Mean arterial blood pressure should be carefully monitored during and following tolazoline therapy.

Prognosis

With the advent of ventilators and continuous positive airway pressure devices, the mortality rate from acute respiratory failure in newborn infants has been notably reduced. In hyaline membrane disease, it has decreased from 75 to 25%. Developmental and neurologic evaluations of survivors of hyaline membrane disease have shown that at age 1–2 years, major central nervous system handicaps are not related to the neonatal illness. Infants who develop significant bronchopulmonary dysplasia have up to a 10% risk of death in the first 2 years of life owing to respiratory failure, pulmonary infection, or sudden death. Survivors are at risk of developing systemic hypertension during the first year of life, and developmental follow-up has shown that 40% will have significant delays at 1–2 years. As more infants with extremely low gestational age and severe lung disease have survived and as better tools for evaluating pulmonary function in young infants and children have become available, it appears that high oxygen concentrations may cause long-term sequelae. However, some long-term studies of survivors have shown normal pulmonary function and developmental well-being at 6 years of age.

Abman SH et al: Pulmonary vascular response to oxygen in infants with severe bronchopulmonary dysplasia. *Pediatrics* 1985;**75:**80.

Abman SH et al: Systemic hypertension in infants with bronchopulmonary dysplasia. *J Pediatr* 1984;**104:**929.

An international classification of retinopathy of prematurity. *Pediatrics* 1984;**74:**127.

Enhorning G et al: Prevention of neonatal respiratory distress syndrome by tracheal instillation of surfactant: A randomized clinical trial. *Pediatrics* 1985;**76:**145.

Gidding SS, Rosenthal A, Moorehead C: Transcutaneous oxygen monitoring: Its use in the treatment of outpatients with congenital heart disease. *Am J Dis Child* 1985;**139:**288.

Hallman M, Gluck L: Respiratory distress syndrome: Update 1982. *Pediatr Clin North Am* 1982;**29:**1057.

Hallman M et al: Exogenous human surfactant for treatment of severe respiratory distress syndrome: A randomized prospective clinical trial. *J Pediatr* 1985;**105:**963.

Koops BL, Abman SH, Accurso FJ: Outpatient management and follow-up of bronchopulmonary dysplasia. *Clin Perinatol* 1984;**11:**101.

Krauss AN, Klain DB, Auld PAM: Chronic pulmonary insufficiency of prematurity. *Pediatrics* 1975;**55:**55.

Lucey JF, Dangman B: A reexamination of the role of oxygen in retrolental fibroplasia. *Pediatrics* 1984;**73:**82.

Lyrene RK, Philips JB: Control of pulmonary vascular resistance in the fetus and newborn. *Clin Perinatol* 1984;**11:**551.

Markestad T, Fitzhardinge PM: Growth and development in children recovering from bronchopulmonary dysplasia. *J Pediatr* 1981;**98:**597.

Patz A: New international classification of retinopathy of prematurity. (Editorial.) *Pediatrics* 1984;**74:**160.

Rawlings JS, Smith FR: Transient tachypnea of the newborn: An analysis of neonatal and obstetric risk factors. *Am J Dis Child* 1984;**138:**869.

HEART DISEASE

See Chapter 15 for discussions of physiologic changes in circulation in the perinatal period, specific congenital and acquired heart diseases, and treatment of heart failure in the newborn infant.

Symptoms & Signs of Heart Failure in the Newborn Infant

Heart failure in the newborn infant may be difficult to recognize because the symptoms and signs are not the same as in older infants. The infant in early failure will show only an increased heart and respiratory rate, excessive weight gain, and, perhaps, irritability. As heart failure worsens, sweating, anxiety, and poor feeding occur. Auscultation of the lungs rarely reveals evidence of pulmonary edema. Abnormal heart sounds and murmurs are often not diagnostic. X-ray examination will show the heart to be enlarged.

Increasing liver size is an important finding. An enlarged or enlarging liver, in the absence of other disease, is good evidence of heart failure. Liver size should be followed as a means of evaluating the effectiveness of treatment.

Peripheral edema is frequent in preterm infants but rarely as a sign of heart failure. When it does occur as a result of heart failure, it is a late and ominous sign. In general, peripheral edema reflects excessive sodium and water intake rather than heart failure.

Electrocardiography is important in determining axis and atrial or ventricular dilatation or hypertrophy. Echocardiography, a powerful noninvasive tool requiring little manipulation of the infant, enables physicians to safely perform serial examinations of critically ill infants. It has been useful in assessing the strength of myocardial contractions, facilitating the early diagnosis of various congenital anomalies of the heart, and providing an estimate of left atrial size through measurements of left atrium (LA) and aorta (AO) diameters (LA:AO ratios). However, misinterpretation of the echocardiogram can lead to serious diagnostic errors, and cardiac catheterization is thus indicated for infants with complicated lesions and for those whose clinical condition is worsening.

Patent Ductus Arteriosus

The most common cardiovascular problem in the premature infant, particularly one having very low birth weight or hyaline membrane disease or one receiving prolonged ventilatory and oxygen therapy, is a patent ductus arteriosus causing shunting of blood between the pulmonary artery and aorta, with resultant hypoxemia, fluid retention, pulmonary edema, and heart failure.

The clinical picture may include excessive weight gain and increased respiratory distress, usually on days 3–7 of life, and x-ray findings of an enlarged heart and pulmonary edema or marked opacification of the lung fields. Bounding pulses, widened pulse pressure, and heart murmurs are classic signs but may not always be present.

Treatment

Treatment of congestive heart failure of whatever cause consists of restricting water intake to the amount of evaporative losses and eliminating sodium intake. If water restriction is coupled with complete sodium restriction, hyponatremia will not result even if potent diuretics are used. This regimen can be instituted along with possible use of furosemide and digitalization of the infant. After 12–24 hours, water and sodium intake may then be increased, with the degree of water and sodium administered depending upon the clinical course of the infant.

Specific treatments of the patent ductus arteriosus are surgical ligation and drug treatment with indomethacin. Proper selection of therapy depends on the experience of personnel in neonatology, anesthesiology, and cardiovascular surgery.

Prognosis

Treatment of congestive heart failure depends on the specific lesion. For cyanotic heart disease or persistent congestive heart failure, a palliative procedure or major cardiovascular surgery may be necessary. The mortality rate among infants with congenital heart disease undergoing operative repair now approaches 65%. Deaths are most commonly due to cardiac dysrhythmias and respiratory failure in spite of intensive care support. The long-term morbidity in survivors includes delayed growth and development. The most serious sequela is severe neurologic dysfunction due to hypoxic, ischemic, or embolic insults suffered by the infant in relation to the primary cardiac lesion or major invasive procedures.

Balisteri WF: Neonatal cholestasis. *J Pediatr* 1985;**106:**171.

Bhat R et al: Patent ductus arteriosus: Recent advances in diagnosis and management. *Pediatr Clin North Am* 1982;**29:** 1117.

Gersony WM et al: Effects of indomethacin in premature infants with patent ductus arteriosus: Results of a national collaborative study. *J Pediatr* 1983;**102:**895.

Graham TP: When to operate on the child with congenital heart disease. *Pediatr Clin North Am* 1984;**31:**1275.

Kleinman CS et al: Echocardiographic studies of the human fetus: Prenatal diagnosis of congenital heart disease and cardiac dysrhythmias. *Pediatrics* 1980;**65:**1059.

Lees MH, Sunderland CO: Heart disease in the newborn. Chap 39, pp 619–628, in: *Heart Disease in Infants, Children, and Adolescents,* 2nd ed. Moss AJ et al (editors). Williams & Wilkins, 1977.

Murphy DJ, Meyer RA, Kaplan S: Noninvasive evaluation of newborns with suspected congenital heart disease. *Am J Dis Child* 1985;**139:**589.

Nadas AS: Update on congenital heart disease. *Pediatr Clin North Am* 1984;**31:**153.

Ramsden CA, Oliver RE: Respiratory adaptation. Pages 23–49 in: *Perinatal Medicine*. Boyd RDH, Battaglia FC (editors). Butterworth, 1983.
Sahn DJ, Friedman WF: Difficulties in distinguishing cardiac from pulmonary disease in the neonate. *Pediatr Clin North Am* 1973;**20:**293.
Snider AR: Use and abuse of the echocardiogram. *Pediatr Clin North Am* 1984;**31:**1345.
Stark J: Analysis of factors which might improve the survival rate of infants with congenital heart disease. *Progr Pediatr Surg* 1979;**13:**109.
Teitel D, Heymann MA: Cardiovascular problems of infancy. Pages 50–69 in: *Perinatal Medicine*. Boyd RDH, Battaglia FC (editors). Butterworth, 1983.
Yabek SM: Neonatal cyanosis: Reappraisal of response to 100% oxygen breathing. *Am J Dis Child* 1984;**138:**880.

JAUNDICE IN THE NEWBORN INFANT

Jaundice is the most frequent clinical problem in the neonatal period. The age at onset, the degree of jaundice, and the condition of the infant are important observations in determining the cause and significance of jaundice.

General Considerations

When red blood cells break down, the iron and protein are stored and reused. However, the porphyrin ring is reduced to bilirubin (unconjugated, indirect) in the reticuloendothelial cells and is then transported to the liver, bound to albumin. In the liver, the bilirubin is conjugated mainly to bilirubin diglucuronide (conjugated, direct) and excreted through the biliary ducts to the gut. In the intestine, it would normally be converted to urobilinogen by bacterial action. However, since the newborn infant's intestine is sterile, conjugated bilirubin excreted in the bile can be hydrolyzed back to bilirubin and then reabsorbed if the bowel contents are not evacuated.

The degree of jaundice that develops will depend upon the rate of red cell breakdown (bilirubin load), the rate of conjugation, the rate of excretion, and the amount of bilirubin reabsorbed from the intestine.

Etiology of Jaundice in the Newborn Infant

A. Increased Rate of Hemolysis: All patients in this category have an increased unconjugated bilirubin concentration and an increased reticulocyte count.

1. Patients with positive Coombs test (this category includes all patients with isoimmunization, including ABO incompatibility, Rh incompatibility, etc).
2. Patients with negative Coombs test.
   a. Abnormal red cell shapes (spherocytosis, elliptocytosis, pyknocytosis, stomatocytosis).
   b. Red cell enzyme abnormalities (glucose 6-phosphate dehydrogenase deficiency, pyruvate kinase deficiency).

B. Decreased Rate of Conjugation: Unconjugated bilirubin elevated, reticulocyte count normal.

1. Immaturity of bilirubin conjugation (''physiologic'' jaundice) due to premature birth, maternal diabetes, and male sex.
2. Congenital familial nonhemolytic jaundice (inborn errors of metabolism affecting glucuronyl transferase system and bilirubin transport).
3. Breast milk jaundice.

C. Abnormalities of Excretion or Reabsorption: Conjugated and unconjugated bilirubin elevated, Coombs test negative, reticulocyte count normal.

1. Hepatitis (viral, parasitic, bacterial, toxic).
2. Metabolic abnormalities (galactosemia, glycogen storage diseases, infants of diabetic mothers, cystic fibrosis, hypothyroid ism).
3. Biliary atresia.
4. Choledochal cyst.
5. Obstruction at ampulla of Vater (annular pancreas).
6. Sepsis.
7. Gastrointestinal obstruction (structural or functional).
8. Drugs.

D. Abnormalities of the Blood-Brain Barrier: Autopsy findings of yellow staining of the brain despite low serum bilirubin levels have suggested increased susceptibility in the following clinical situations:

1. Infusion of hypertonic solutions resulting in opening the blood-brain barrier to albumin-bound bilirubin.
2. Prolonged acidosis, hypoxemia, hypothermia, and hypercapnia.
3. Sepsis and meningitis.

Diagnosis of Bilirubin Toxicity

Serum levels of indirect bilirubin should be determined periodically in all jaundiced infants because of the special dangers of sensorineural hearing loss and kernicterus. Guidelines for suggested bilirubin levels for exchange transfusion based on birth weight and clinical course are shown in Table 3–5.

Recent tests that allow determination of unbound bilirubin, albumin-binding capacity, and albumin saturation have not proved to be much better predictors of bilirubin toxicity.

Treatment of Hyperbilirubinemia

Specific recommendations for management are given below in the sections on etiology of jaundice. However, in addition to exchange transfusion (see Chapter 35), the most important therapeutic modality is phototherapy.

Light energy enhances the degradation of unconju-

Table 3–5. Serum levels of indirect bilirubin and exchange transfusion.*†

Birth Weight (g)	Serum Bilirubin Level for Exchange Transfusion (mg/dL)	
	Normal Infants‡	Abnormal Infants§
< 1,000	10.0	10.0**
1,001–1,250	13.0	10.0**
1,251–1,500	15.0	13.0
1,501–2,000	17.0	15.0
2,001–2,500	18.0	17.0
>2,500	20.0	18.0

* Reproduced, with permission, from American Academy of Pediatrics: Page 95 in: *Standards and Recommendations for Hospital Care of Newborn Infants,* 6th ed. American Academy of Pediatrics, 1977. Copyright American Academy of Pediatrics, 1977.

† These guidelines have not been validated.

‡ Normal infants are defined for this purpose as having none of the problems listed below.

§ Abnormal infants have one or more of the following problems: perinatal asphyxia, prolonged hypoxemia, acidemia, persistent hypothermia, hypoalbuminemia, hemolysis, sepsis, hyperglycemia, elevated free fatty acids or presence of drugs that compete for bilirubin binding, signs of clinical or central nervous system deterioration.

** There have been case reports of basal ganglion staining at levels considerably lower than 10 mg.

gated bilirubin in the skin to colorless by-products that are apparently nontoxic. Full-spectrum fluorescent bulbs are preferred to blue lights so that the infant can be observed under normal light. Otherwise, observation of skin color for pallor, cyanosis, or other conditions is virtually impossible. Certain important routines must be followed whenever phototherapy is used:

(1) Phototherapy should be used only when significant unconjugated (indirect) hyperbilirubinemia is present; its use with elevated conjugated (direct) bilirubin levels is contraindicated (''bronze baby syndrome''). It is begun when the bilirubin is approximately 4 mg/dL below the exchange level.

(2) The etiologic basis for jaundice must always be sought.

(3) Bilirubin levels must be determined serially while the infant is receiving phototherapy; skin jaundice is not a reliable indicator of serum bilirubin levels.

(4) The indications for exchange transfusion and other methods of management of neonatal jaundice are not changed by phototherapy.

(5) The eyes should be protected from intense light by appropriate patching. The patch must be applied carefully and should be removed at regular intervals to examine the eyes; conjunctivitis and corneal abrasion are the main hazards. The patch should be removed and phototherapy discontinued when the parents visit, to encourage eye-to-eye contact.

(6) The use of phototherapy or an open radiant heater (or both) produces considerable evaporative water losses in infants. It is customary to increase free water intake during phototherapy by about 25% and to follow urine flow rates and specific gravities carefully in order to readjust fluid intake as required. An increase in the evaporative water loss may be associated with an increase in caloric requirements. This may constitute an additional nutritional problem in certain instances in which nutrition has been inadequate for other reasons. Phototherapy also increases gastrointestinal transit time and may interfere with the absorption of drugs administered orally.

(7) Electrical and mechanical safety of the phototherapy unit must be ensured.

(8) Home phototherapy has been advocated by medical supply companies to reduce hospital costs, shorten hospital stays, and eliminate the adverse effects of parent-child separation. However, clinical experience has shown that onset of treatment is delayed an average of 15 hours and that corneal abrasions and nasal occlusion from inappropriate use of eye patches and temperature derangements are problems. In one study, 10% of ''normal'' children receiving home phototherapy required rehospitalization for dehydration, sepsis, congenital heart disease, or a rapid rise in bilirubin levels. The cost-benefit ratio is not yet clear.

Prognosis

Regardless of etiology, bilirubin causes damage when it passes from the serum into the basal ganglion cells of the brain and the inner ear cells. Sensorineural hearing loss is the most common sequela of excessive bilirubin. Kernicterus is less common, but it refers to the clinical syndrome and pathologic changes in the central nervous system secondary to deposition of unconjugated bilirubin in certain nuclei of the brain. Depending on gestational age, the risk of kernicterus becomes significant at serum bilirubin levels above 10–20 mg/dL. Certain factors predispose to the development of kernicterus at lower serum levels. These factors (acidosis, low albumin levels, sulfonamide administration, elevated free fatty acid, etc) may result in decreased albumin-binding capacity for bilirubin.

The infant with kernicterus initially has severe hyperbilirubinemia, usually secondary to erythroblastosis but in some cases associated with jaundice due to other causes. There is a fairly sudden onset of lethargy and poor feeding; a weak or incomplete Moro reflex; a weak, high-pitched cry; and opisthotonos. In premature infants, slowed respiratory rate and apneic periods may be prominent findings. Apnea, respiratory arrest, and convulsions characterize the terminal episode. Infants who survive have severe motor impairment, including hypotonia, spasticity, and athetosis. Mental retardation is less severe. Fortunately, kernicterus has become extremely rare as techniques for monitoring newborn infants have improved. Kernicterus can be prevented by close monitoring of unconjugated bilirubin concentrations and the initiation of appropriate treatment in jaundiced infants.

1. "PHYSIOLOGIC" JAUNDICE

The diagnosis of "physiologic" jaundice is made by exclusion of specific causes. In normal full-term infants, bilirubin levels peak at 4–5 days; in premature infants, the peak is around 6 days. Exaggerated jaundice (serum bilirubin levels > 12 mg/dL in the full-term infant) occurs in 13% of newborns.

The minimal workup should include a careful maternal and pregnancy history; physical examination of the infant for petechiae, bruising, hepatosplenomegaly, and signs of infection; maternal and neonatal blood typing; direct and indirect Coombs tests; complete blood count, including differential, smear and reticulocyte count; thyroid tests; and examination of urine for reducing substances.

2. ISOIMMUNIZATION DUE TO ABO BLOOD GROUP INCOMPATIBILITY

ABO blood group incompatibility is the most common form of isoimmunization but a less severe clinical problem than Rh-D incompatibility, which is second in frequency.

Diagnosis

There is no satisfactory way to predict which infants with ABO incompatibility will develop significant hyperbilirubinemia. However, the presence of a potential problem can be anticipated by comparing the blood groups of the mother and infant. (Routine blood typing of cord blood should be determined for all infants.) The most common blood group incompatibility is maternal O and infant A or B.

Hemoglobin levels are normal or only slightly low. Mild reticulocytosis may be present. Spherocytes are commonly found on the smear of peripheral blood.

Physical examination is usually normal except for jaundice, which may develop in the first 48 hours. More severe involvement occasionally occurs, usually with B-O incompatibility.

Coombs testing can be done whenever potential incompatibility exists. The direct Coombs test is usually positive if done carefully. The indirect Coombs test will be positive in the presence of antibody if type-specific cells are used, although a strongly positive reaction is uncommon.

Note: Infants who may have both ABO and Rh isoimmunization (eg, mother is type O Rh-negative, and infant is type A Rh-positive) will often be protected from Rh sensitization. However, such an infant with a positive direct Coombs test should have indirect Coombs testing for both antibodies.

Management

Give supportive care and phototherapy as described for Rh sensitization (see below). Exchange transfusion (see Chapter 35) should be used to keep bilirubin levels below the toxic range. Cord values or early rates of bilirubin rise are not indications for transfusion in ABO sensitization, since these do not predict eventual bilirubin levels. Infants should be followed at weekly intervals for up to 6 weeks to be sure serious anemia due to ongoing hemolysis of sensitized red blood cells does not occur.

3. ISOIMMUNIZATION DUE TO Rh & SIMILAR RED CELL ANTIGENS

Isoimmunization due to Rh antigens (D, E, C, d, c, or e), Kell (Kk), Duffy (Fy), Lutheran (Lu), and Kidd (Jk) factors may have a similar clinical picture. The involved red cell antigen is always absent from the mother's red cells; therefore, if fetal red cells containing the antigen cross the placenta, the mother will produce antibodies to the "foreign" antigen. The IgG antibodies cross the placenta and enter the fetal circulation. When antibody forms a complex with fetal red cell antigen, the cells will be removed from the circulation at an increased rate, leading to anemia and increased bilirubin load.

Diagnosis

A. Maternal Past History: There may be a history of an infant who was affected or had unexplained jaundice, anemia, or fetal death.

B. Current Pregnancy: Blood type and antibody screening should be done on all pregnant women as early as possible. Antibody screening is an easy and inexpensive means of demonstrating the presence or absence of red cell antibody. If antibody is absent in an Rh-negative woman early in pregnancy, antibody screening should be repeated frequently throughout the second and third trimesters. Significant sensitization to blood groups other than D is unlikely to occur when no antibody exists in the initial screening. When antibody screening is positive, the specific antibody should be identified and an indirect Coombs titer determined to establish the degree of sensitization.

C. Amniocentesis and Amniotic Fluid Analysis: Amniotic fluid analysis should be done early on all pregnant women with significantly elevated Rh antibody titers to determine if the fetus is affected and to evaluate the severity of the disease. A clinical estimate of severity of disease in the fetus is then made, using the prediction graph based on clinical experience with that method.

D. Infant at Birth: Comparison of the blood type on cord blood with the mother's blood type will indicate potential blood group incompatibility. A direct Coombs test done on cord blood will be positive if the infant's cells are coated with antibody. This is diagnostic of isoimmunization.

Prevention of Rh-D Isoimmunization

The passive administration of human Rh_0(D) immune globulin (RhoGAM) to the Rh-negative, unsensitized mother has proved successful in preventing sensitization when she has delivered an Rh-positive infant.

After delivery, the Rh-negative woman must receive RhoGAM within 72 hours if it is indicated. This is also true after delivery of a stillborn infant or after abortion.

Management

A. During Pregnancy: In severely sensitized women, amniocentesis for testing amniotic fluid bilirubin and intrauterine transfusions may be required for fetal survival. Premature delivery at 34–37 weeks' gestational age may be necessary to prevent in utero fetal hydrops.

B. Infant at Delivery:

1. The first indication for a postnatal exchange transfusion (see Chapter 35) of packed red blood cells immediately after birth is to correct anemia and circulating blood volume, thus helping to alleviate cardiac failure. In such cases, the first exchange transfusion may be done essentially on cardiovascular indications, and the volume should be relatively small—ie, just enough to increase hemoglobin concentration to 13–15 mg/dL and central venous pressure to 8–11 cm of water. An infant with severe disease often requires both paracentesis to reduce the volume of ascitic fluid and positive pressure ventilation on a respirator to ensure adequate oxygenation.

2. A second indication for an immediate exchange transfusion is severe sensitization in an infant who is not hydropic. In this case, an exchange transfusion is done to remove affected red cells, since it is far more efficient to remove potential bilirubin while it is still packaged in red blood cells as hemoglobin rather than when it is free bilirubin distributed in fat depots throughout the body. Sensitization as an indication for exchange transfusion depends on whether or not intrauterine transfusions have been done. When several intrauterine transfusions have been performed, the infant's circulating red blood cells at birth may be virtually all donor red cells. In such a case, an early exchange to remove affected infant cells would be useless. The Kleihauer test and umbilical cord blood typing should be done to determine what percentage of circulating red cells are fetal cells.

3. The third indication for double volume exchange transfusion is to remove the bilirubin that has already formed. This indication for exchange transfusion may develop at any time whether or not intrauterine transfusions have been performed. Guidelines such as those in Table 3–5 should be followed.

Exchange transfusions involve replacement of approximately twice the infant's blood volume. To estimate the volume of donor blood required, the infant's blood volume is usually calculated as constituting 8–10% of body weight. Type O Rh-negative blood may be used, particularly when plans must be made before delivery for an exchange transfusion immediately after birth. ABO type-specific blood may be used if the infant's ABO type is known. Donor blood should always be cross-matched with maternal serum. Fresh heparinized blood may be used safely for exchange transfusion but has little advantage over citrate-phosphate-dextrose (CPD) blood. CPD blood which is less than 48–72 hours old or which can be reconstituted in the blood bank from frozen red cells and fresh frozen plasma is preferable. Blood should not be reconstituted or altered in the nursery, because of the risks of contamination and hemolysis. Attempts to alter blood pH prior to exchange transfusion are not only unnecessary but may be dangerous and lead to an increased risk of cardiac dysrhythmia. Metabolic complications associated with erythroblastosis fetalis include (1) severe hypoglycemia secondary to pancreatic islet cell hyperplasia and occurring most frequently following an exchange transfusion using blood that has a high glucose concentration and (2) cardiac dysrhythmia associated with delayed return of normal calcium activity when citrated blood is used for an exchange transfusion. The fall in calcium activity is not necessarily associated with a fall in total calcium concentration in the plasma. The risk of cardiac dysrhythmia is compounded if calcium activity falls when other factors affecting function may also be changing (temperature of the solution, glucose concentration in the blood, etc). For this reason, all solutions infused into the inferior vena cava should be warmed to body temperature or administered very slowly to avoid any sudden change in temperature within the heart. Because of all the other problems requiring medical management immediately after birth, infants at risk should be delivered if possible at hospitals that can provide optimal obstetric and neonatal care.

All infants with erythroblastosis should be followed closely, particularly for signs of severe anemia or cholestatic syndrome that may develop later in the neonatal period.

The risks of exchange transfusion may be increasing as fewer transfusions are being done. In a recent report, the mortality rate in 190 infants who received transfusions was 14%, and the acute morbidity rate approached 7%. Three deaths occurred within 24 hours of the exchange transfusion. Morbidity included bradycardia, cyanosis, vasospasm, thrombosis, and apnea.

4. OTHER CAUSES OF JAUNDICE

Breast Milk Jaundice

One of the most difficult diagnoses to establish is that of breast milk jaundice in an infant between 3 days and 3 weeks of age who has an indirect bilirubin level of 15–20 mg/dL, with no apparent cause for hemolysis, and who is entirely breast-fed.

The problems of rehospitalization and interruption of breast feeding must be carefully weighed against the uncertain risks of bilirubin toxicity in an otherwise well infant.

Infection

Jaundice secondary to bacterial infection is most commonly due to organisms (*Escherichia coli*, staphylococci, and streptococci) that produce hemolyzing toxins, increasing the rate of red cell breakdown. The bilirubin is mainly conjugated. Jaundice may appear shortly after birth or later in the first week, depending on severity and timing of the infection.

Jaundice due to agents such as viruses (cytomegalic inclusion disease, hepatitis, herpes simplex, rubella, etc), parasites (toxoplasmosis), and *Treponema pallidum* is associated with elevations of both conjugated and unconjugated bilirubin as a result of liver cell injury and obstruction of biliary canaliculi.

Abnormal Red Cell Metabolism

Two inborn errors of metabolism in the red cells may result in an increased rate of hemolysis: glucose 6-phosphate dehydrogenase (G6PD) deficiency and pyruvate kinase deficiency. The first is a very common enzyme defect but usually becomes evident only after coincident exposure of the mother or infant to substances such as naphthalene or primaquine. Hereditary spherocytosis may present with a hemolytic crisis in the newborn period, causing jaundice and anemia. Synthetic vitamin K preparations are oxidants and thus will cause increased hemolysis of red blood cells if administered in excessive amounts to patients with G6PD deficiency.

Extravascular Hemorrhage

Bleeding within the body, as in cephalhematoma, extensive purpura, or central nervous system hemorrhage, may result in elevated levels of unconjugated bilirubin because of the increased load of hemoglobin that is broken down to bilirubin. Recent studies have stressed the tendency to underestimate the degree of bleeding into muscle and soft tissues of preterm infants who have suffered from apparently superficial bruising. In some preterm infants delivered after difficult breech extractions, the bleeding into muscles of the back and buttocks may be extensive enough to cause shock and muscle necrosis in the newborn period.

Immaturity of Glucuronyl Transferase Enzyme System

The cause of jaundice in some newborn infants is a delay in maturation of the glucuronyl transferase enzyme system, which results in decreased conjugated bilirubin, although other factors may also be operative. Serum unconjugated bilirubin is increased, but other laboratory findings are normal.

Treatment consists of adequate hydration and caloric intake. Phototherapy is required occasionally, and exchange transfusions are needed only in premature infants. The prognosis is excellent.

Metabolic Defects in the Liver

Galactosemia and glycogen storage disease may cause jaundice in the newborn infant. In galactosemia, symptoms (which may include hypoglycemia) begin after milk feedings are established. Mild jaundice usually has its onset after the third day and persists into the second week of life.

Obstruction of Biliary Ducts

Bile duct obstruction is manifested principally by an elevation in the level of conjugated bilirubin, but a significant degree of unconjugated bilirubinemia secondary to liver cell injury will also be present. Jaundice may begin on the third day, as with physiologic jaundice, but will persist and become increasingly intense as the conjugated bilirubin levels rise. With persistent jaundice of this type, the skin takes on a greenish-yellow hue.

Gastrointestinal Obstruction

Obstruction of the gastrointestinal tract secondary to structural abnormalities, inability to pass meconium, ileus due to infection, metabolic imbalance, or extreme immaturity will cause excessive gastrointestinal reabsorption of bilirubin. The use of glycerin suppositories may enhance evacuation of meconium from the gastrointestinal tract.

Prolonged & Persistent Jaundice in the Newborn Infant

Most causes of jaundice in the newborn infant are transient. When jaundice persists into the second week of life, consider one of the following conditions:

(1) In small premature infants, jaundice will persist longer due to the delayed maturation of the glucuronyl transferase enzyme system.

(2) Liver disease or anomaly: If there are unabating or increasing levels of conjugated and unconjugated bilirubin, the diagnostic workup is urgent, because irreversible cirrhosis may develop in the presence of a surgically correctable lesion. Therefore, intrahepatic biliary atresia and neonatal hepatitis must be differentiated from extrahepatic atresia, choledochal cysts, or other correctable abnormality. Liver function tests, needle biopsy, and the clinical course may help in differentiation, but open biopsy and operative cholangiogram are usually necessary to identify the cause of the jaundice.

(3) Choledochal cysts cause obstruction by intermittent filling of the cyst with bile, which causes torsion of the duct. The jaundice is usually intermittent and variable and is often associated with a palpable mass in the upper right quadrant of the abdomen.

Bowman JM: Neonatal management. Pages 200–239 in: *Modern Management of the Rh Problem*. Queenan JT (editor). Harper & Row, 1977.

Bratlid D, Cashore WJ, Oh W: Effect of acidosis on bilirubin deposition in rat brain. *Pediatrics* 1984;**73:**431.

Cockington RA: A guide to the use of phototherapy in the management of neonatal hyperbilirubinemia. *J Pediatr* 1979;**95:**281.

Levine RL, Fredericks WR, Rapoport SI: Entry of bilirubin into the brain due to opening of the blood-brain barrier. *Pediatrics* 1982;**69:**255.

Levine RL, Maisels MJ (chairpersons): *Hyperbilirubinemia in the Newborn: Report of the Eighty-Fifth Ross Conference on Pediatric Research.* Ross Laboratories, 1983.

McDonagh AF, Lightner DA: Bilirubin, jaundice and phototherapy. *Pediatrics* 1985;**75:**443.

National Institute of Child Health and Human Development: Randomized, controlled trial of phototherapy for neonatal hyperbilirubinemia. *Pediatrics* 1985;**75(Suppl):**381.

Osborn LM, Reiff MI, Bolus R: Jaundice in the full-term neonate. *Pediatrics* 1984;**73:**520.

Poland RL: Breast-milk jaundice. *J Pediatr* 1981;**99:**86.

Ritter DA et al: A prospective study of free bilirubin and other risk factors in the development of kernicterus in premature infants. *Pediatrics* 1982;**69:**260.

Turkel SB et al: A clinical pathologic reappraisal of kernicterus. *Pediatrics* 1982;**69:**267.

Walker W et al: A follow-up study of survivors of Rh-haemolytic disease. *Dev Med Child Neurol* 1974;**16:**592.

Wennberg RP et al: Abnormal auditory brainstem response in a newborn infant with hyperbilirubinemia: Improvement with exchange transfusion. *J Pediatr* 1982;**100:**624.

INFECTION IN THE NEWBORN

GENERAL APPROACH

The fetus and newborn are especially susceptible to generalized, sometimes overwhelming bacterial, viral, and parasitic infections. Organisms can infect the fetus through hematogenous spread from the placenta or can infect the newborn by colonization during passage through the birth canal or by invasion of fresh wounds, such as the cut surface of the umbilical cord, the circumcision site, or a scalp electrode site. The newborn infant is susceptible because of immature cellular and humoral immune systems. Immunoglobulin G (IgG) is transferred from the mother to the fetus, providing passive protection against some organisms. However, antibodies to gram-negative organisms are contained in the IgM fraction, which is not transferred to the fetus. Toxins may be produced that cause systemic and cellular injury. Symptoms may be deceptively mild until the infection is far-advanced, making early recognition and treatment difficult.

Hospital Precautions

Since newborns are so susceptible to infection, traffic in the nursery must be monitored and controlled. Physicians, nurses, laboratory technicians, parents, students, and anyone else authorized to enter the nursery and handle infants must wash their hands for 3 minutes with a germicidal soap and wear a clean gown. This procedure should be repeated before handling each infant. Herpetic lesions of the lip, infected wounds, etc, must be covered by a mask, gloves, or bandage to prevent spread to the infants. Persons with systemic illnesses such as viral upper respiratory infections or diarrhea must be rigorous about hand washing or be restricted from the nursery. An employee with a diagnosis of bacterial infection based on culture should receive appropriate antibiotic treatment for 24–48 hours before returning to the nursery even if he or she feels well.

If a newborn infant is considered infectious at birth based on clinical signs and symptoms or obstetric history, specific orders must be written for handling the infant, bed linens, waste products, etc. Since these infants are often very sick, they should be placed within immediate reach of monitoring, observation, and treatment. Isolation in a remote place is rarely indicated; if the infant is put in room isolation, appropriate nursing coverage must be arranged. For most infants, the appropriate precautions are careful hand washing, gowning during care, separate disposal of diapers and linens, and, if necessary, gloving while handling. Guidelines for specific infections are outlined in references listed below.

Infants born at home or en route to the hospital and premature infants returning from level 3 units to other medical centers do not need isolation. Breastfeeding mothers of these infants should be allowed to use hospital facilities after they have learned to maintain cleanliness.

Diagnosis

A. History: Maternal and obstetric histories are essential for early diagnosis of congenital neonatal infections. Maternal illnesses that are often associated with neonatal infection include urinary tract infection, amnionitis, prolonged rupture of amniotic membranes, genital herpesvirus infection, gonorrhea, syphilis, vaginal streptococcal infections, tuberculosis, hepatitis, and systemic viral or bacterial illness in the third trimester, especially when they result in premature labor and delivery.

If the mother is ill at the time of delivery, cultures of her blood and the placenta may help diagnose the organism responsible for infections in the infant. Knowledge of previous positive maternal cultures, laboratory reports, and antibiotic treatments is also valuable.

B. Symptoms and Signs: An infected newborn infant does not usually exhibit specific symptoms. The infant may be irritable or lethargic, have difficulty maintaining normal temperature, and feed poorly or regurgitate. Apnea, abdominal distention, hypotension, mottling, and shock are also common symptoms.

C. Laboratory Findings: The white blood cell and differential counts are useful in the early diagnosis of infection, because elevation in number of the band forms of polymorphonuclear cells occurs early in the illness. Extremely low granuloctye counts, particularly in the first 2 hours of life, are an ominous sign and should always be considered an indication of overwhelming infection until proved otherwise. Serial white blood cell counts are often useful, because they may reflect improvement or deterioration in the infant's condition. Platelet counts below 200,000/μL may also indicate infection and correlate with a localized or systemic consumptive coagulopathy.

Treatment

Early diagnosis, supportive care, and specific therapy are essential for effective management of neonatal infection. The infant frequently cannot tolerate oral feedings, and intravenous fluids must be given to maintain normal water, glucose, and electrolyte status. Accurate records of body weight, intake, urine output, and gastrointestinal fluid losses must be kept. Careful attention to these parameters and hourly changes in fluid administration may be necessary in the first few days when infection is not yet controlled. Shock must be treated with blood volume expanders and, rarely, with pharmacologic agents. In the debilitated or neurologically depressed infant, ventilator support may be necessary.

Prognosis

The long-term outcome of neonatal infection is related to the extent and location of the disease and the etiologic organism. The mortality and morbidity rates are very high in neonatal infections, as noted below; therefore, prevention or early recognition and treatment are major goals. In all survivors of congenital or neonatally acquired infection, careful follow-up and early therapy for specific motor, mental, neurologic, visual, and auditory deficiencies are of utmost importance in minimizing sequelae.

SPECIFIC INFECTIONS*

1. BACTERIAL SEPSIS

The most common bacterial organisms infecting newborn infants are group B β-hemolytic streptococci and *Escherichia coli*. However, many other gram-negative and gram-positive bacteria have been proved by positive blood cultures to cause neonatal sepsis. These include *Staphylococcus epidermidis, Staphylococcus aureus,* and *Klebsiella*. Organisms that are usually nonpathogenic in older children may cause clinical disease in a newborn infant. If bacterial infection is suspected, the workup should include 2 blood cultures, suprapubic aspiration or bladder catheterization for urine culture, and lumbar puncture for cerebrospinal fluid culture. The spinal fluid should be analyzed for elevated white blood cell count (especially of neutrophils), elevated protein concentration, and low glucose concentration. Surface cultures and histologic examination of the umbilicial cord, external ear, or stomach contents are not worthwhile unless obtained within 1 hour of birth. Diagnosis is proved if one or more blood cultures are positive. Sepsis may also be diagnosed on the basis of the infant's symptoms even when cultures are negative. Both gram-positive and gram-negative infections should be treated with ampicillin and an aminoglycoside, which have synergistic effects. Specific drug dosages and schedules are given in Chapter 27, but a few principles should be noted here. For infants less than 5–7 days old, adequate antibiotic treatment may be achieved by parenteral dosages at 6- to 8-hour intervals, depending on the drug. Seventy-two hours after cultures are obtained, the diagnosis of infection should be either ruled out or established. Antibiotics are discontinued, changed because of the organism isolated, or continued for 10 days as appropriate. In severe or unresponsive infections, repeat cultures and assays of serum antibiotic levels are indicated. After antibiotics are stopped, hospital observation of the infant must be continued for 2–3 days to watch for recurrence. Negative blood cultures obtained at least 24 hours after discontinuation of antibiotics will confirm the adequacy of treatment. The serious threat of death in neonates with systemic bacterial infections requiring intensive care has led to the addition of white blood cell transfusions for selected infants. In the compromised neonatal host, sepsis with unusual organisms such as coagulase-negative staphylococci and *Candida* should be considered. The mortality rate in neonatal sepsis as reported by several large institutions is 25–50%. The morbidity rate is 30–60% and includes mental retardation, developmental delays, motor handicaps, and hearing loss.

Baumgart S et al: Sepsis with coagulase-negative staphylococci in critically ill newborns. *Am J Dis Child* 1983;**137:**461.

Chin KC, Fitzhardinge PM: Sequelae of early-onset group B hemolytic streptococcal neonatal meningitis. *J Pediatr* 1985;**106:**819.

Christensen RD et al: Granulocyte transfusions in neonates with bacterial infection, neutropenia, and depletion of mature marrow neutrophils. *Pediatrics* 1982;**70:**1.

Edwards MS et al: Long-term sequelae of group B streptococcal meningitis in infants. *J Pediatr* 1985;**106:**717.

Eisenfeld L et al: Systemic bacterial infections in neonatal deaths. *Am J Dis Child* 1983;**137:**645.

Laurenti F et al: Polymorphonuclear leukocyte transfusion for the treatment of sepsis in the newborn infant. *J Pediatr* 1981;**98:**118.

Remington JS, Klein JO (editors): *Infectious Diseases of the Fetus and Newborn Infant,* 2nd ed. Saunders, 1983.

Starr SE: Antimicrobial therapy of bacterial sepsis in the newborn infant. *J Pediatr* 1985;**106:**1043.

Weinstein RA, Boyer KM, Linn ES: Isolation guidelines for obstetric patients and newborn infants. *Am J Obstet Gynecol* 1983;**146:**353.

* Consult the Index for a listing of discussions in other chapters.

2. EPIDEMIC DIARRHEA

Acute diarrhea in infants may be associated with certain types of pathogenic *E coli* and *Klebsiella*. When it occurs in the nursery, it is potentially quite virulent and communicable. Constant surveillance, quick recognition and treatment, and active measures to avoid epidemic spread are required. Spread of infection is chiefly via hand contamination; therefore, hand washing and stool care are the chief measures of control.

The most virulent form of neonatal gastroenteritis is necrotizing enterocolitis. This illness is most common in premature infants and in full-term infants with polycythemia. Infants may present with lethargy, apnea, poor color, or bloody stools. Abdominal distention and x-ray findings of air-fluid levels or distended loops of bowel are consistent with gastroenteritis. Areas of pneumatosis within the bowel wall or peritoneal free air are ominous radiographic signs of bowel necrosis.

Management involves giving prompt fluid and electrolyte replacement by the intravenous route, stopping all oral feedings and medications, performing cultures of stool and blood, and beginning parenteral antibiotics. Treatment of shock with blood volume expanders may be needed. Specific antibiotic therapy may need to be changed, depending upon the organisms isolated and their antibiotic sensitivities.

Immediate prognosis depends on whether organisms are eliminated from the bowel. Infants should be followed closely for recurrence of diarrhea. Long-term outcome depends on whether the infant develops necrotizing enterocolitis, which may lead to immediate death or may necessitate surgical resection of the bowel, leaving the infant with short bowel syndrome.

Abbasi S et al: Long-term assessment of growth, nutritional status and gastrointestinal function in survivors of necrotizing enterocolitis. *J Pediatr* 1984;**104:**550.

Diarrheal disorders. Chap 8, pp 173–204, in: *Pediatric Clinical Gastroenterology,* 2nd ed. Silverman A, Roy CC, Cozetto FJ (editors). Mosby, 1975.

Kosloske AM: Pathogenesis and prevention of necrotizing enterocolitis: Changing hypothesis based on personal observation and a review of the literature. *Pediatrics* 1984;**74:**1087.

LaGamma EF, Ostertag SG, Birenbaum H: Failure of delayed oral feedings to prevent necrotizing enterocolitis. *Am J Dis Child* 1985;**139:**385.

LeBlanc MH, D'Cruz C, Pate K: Necrotizing enterocolitis can be caused by polycythemic hyperviscosity in the newborn dog. *J Pediatr* 1984;**105:**804.

3. PNEUMONIA

The respiratory system of an infant may be infected in utero, during passage through the birth canal, or at any time in the first months of life. The most serious illness is pneumonia. Pneumonia should be suspected in infants with tachypnea, cyanosis, and retractions. Blood gas determinations will show hypoxia. In serious cases, there will be progressive evidence of respiratory failure with hypoxia, hypercapnia, and acidosis. In addition to blood cultures, a deep tracheal aspirate should be performed to obtain fluid for culture and Gram-stain examination. A chest x-ray may reveal infiltrates, atelectasis, and pleural effusion, and films should be repeated to follow the progression and resolution of pneumonia. Treatment includes ventilatory support if respiratory failure occurs, appropriate antibiotics, and percussion, drainage, and suction therapy as frequently as needed to keep the airways clear. Prognosis in group B streptococcal and *Listeria* pneumonia ranges from a fulminating course leading to death within hours in 50% of cases to slow but complete recovery. Other organisms are usually less virulent. In survivors, recovery of normal pulmonary function is anticipated, since the infant can entirely regenerate normal lung tissue.

Boyle RJ et al: Early identification of spesis in infants with respiratory distress. *Pediatrics* 1978;**62:**744.

Klein JO, Marcy SM: Bacterial infections. Chap 17, pp 747–891, in: *Infectious Diseases of the Fetus and Newborn Infant.* Remington JS, Klein JO (editors). Saunders, 1976.

Leonidas JC et al: Radiographic findings in early onset neonatal group-B streptococcal septicemia. *Pediatrics* 1977;**59 (Suppl):**1006.

4. MENINGITIS

The diagnosis of meningitis is suspected in an irritable infant with symptoms of sepsis. Localizing physical findings may include a bulging anterior fontanelle, meningeal irritation with opisthotonos, and convulsions, but more commonly newborn infants respond to central nervous system infection with few if any localizing findings. Laboratory findings include cerebrospinal fluid levels as follows: protein, more than 150 mg/dL; glucose, less than 30 mg/dL; and white blood cells, more than 25/μL. CT and ultrasound scans are important in detecting early cerebral edema and late problems of encephalomalacia, hydrocephalus, or brain abscess.

Treatment should include general supportive care and specific therapy with antibiotics effective against both gram-positive and gram-negative organisms until the etiologic agent is identified. Treatment is continued for a minimum of 3 weeks and until lumbar punctures show completely normal spinal fluid and negative cultures.

The mortality rate for neonatal meningitis remains near 50% in spite of antibiotics and intense supportive care. It is higher with gram-negative organisms and appears to correlate with high cerebrospinal fluid protein levels. Long-term follow-up studies of survivors have suggested that approximately 10% have severe sequelae requiring institutionalization, 30% fall below accepted norms on psychometric assessment, and 60% have electroencephalographic abnormalities with or without seizures. Some children have difficulties with speech and perceptual motor function.

Fitzhardinge PM et al: Long-term sequelae of neonatal meningitis. *Dev Med Child Neurol* 1974;**16:**3.
Overall JC: Neonatal bacterial meningitis. *J Pediatr* 1970; **76:**499.

5. OSTEOMYELITIS

The diagnosis of osteomyelitis is quite rare and is almost always secondary to septicemia in the newborn infant; in rare cases it may be secondary to organisms introduced when a femoral puncture, heel stick, or bone marrow examination is performed. The most common organisms are staphylococci, streptococci, and *E coli.*

Physical examination will reveal localization of the infection to a bone or joint. There will be tenderness, swelling, redness of the area, and limitation of movement of the extremity involved. The diagnosis is confirmed by aspiration of joint or subperiosteal material for smear and culture. X-ray changes (which may not be present for 1–2 weeks) include periosteal elevation and calcification.

Specific antibiotic therapy should be aimed at the organism most likely to cause the disease. Treatment should be continued until the child is completely well, evidence of local inflammation has completely subsided, and x-rays show that healing is well under way. Follow-up examination and x-rays should be done to watch for recurrence. Clinical evaluation, orthopedic consultation, and physical therapy may be needed for several months to ensure good bone growth and joint mobility in the affected area.

Fox L, Sprunt K: Neonatal osteomyelitis. *Pediatrics* 1978; **62:**535.
Kolyvas E et al: Oral antibiotic therapy of skeletal infections in children. *Pediatrics* 1980;**65:**867.

6. URINARY TRACT INFECTION

Newborn infants with symptoms of infection may have a focus of infection in the urinary tract. This is especially true if the infant is suspected of having a urinary tract anomaly or an infection that began 72 hours or more after birth. Septicemia, abnormal fistulous connections between the bowel and the urinary tract, patent urachus, vesicovaginal fistula, or other structural anomaly of the urinary tract associated with obstruction will predispose to urinary tract infection.

A specimen taken by means of suprapubic aspiration (see Chapter 35) is desirable for examination and culture. The presence of organisms in a suprapubic specimen or the presence of colony counts above 10,000 organisms per milliliter of urine in a clean, freshly voided urine specimen should be considered evidence of infection. Jaundice is common in pyelonephritis in the newborn infant. Other diagnostic procedures such as intravenous urography, cystography, renal scanning, and ultrasonography may be needed to demonstrate congenital anomalies or obstruction of the urinary tract.

Treatment with antibiotics should be continued until the urine is normal and cultures negative. An infant with documented urinary tract infection must be followed for a long time with repeated urine cultures to be sure that infection does not recur after therapy is discontinued. Underlying urinary tract anomalies and obstruction make recurrence or continued chronic infection more likely and may necessitate surgical correction.

Visser VE, Hall RT: Urine culture in the evaluation of suspected neonatal sepsis. *J Pediatr* 1979;**94:**635.

7. OMPHALITIS

A normal umbilical cord stump will mummify and separate at the skin level. Saprophytic organisms occasionally cause a small amount of purulent material to form at the base of the cord. Other organisms may colonize and cause infection, especially *E coli,* streptococci, and staphylococci.

Omphalitis is a potential danger when umbilical vessels are catheterized for administration of intravenous fluids or exchange transfusion. Strict aseptic technique and immediate removal of catheters at the first sign of any complication are important.

Signs include redness and edema of the skin around the umbilicus, indicating cellulitis. Serosanguineous or purulent discharge indicates progress of the infection. Systemic reaction occurs as infection becomes more severe. Culture of skin around the cord base and blood cultures should be done.

Treatment with appropriate antibiotics for gram-positive and gram-negative organisms is given until the cause is specifically identified, and antibiotics are continued until all evidence of disease has disappeared and blood cultures are negative.

Local therapeutic measures should also be used and include drying the base of the cord thoroughly with absolute ethanol swabs, swabbing the area with one of the surgical soaps containing an organic iodide, or applying bacitracin.

The extent of infection into omphalic vessels determines the prognosis. Septic thrombophlebitis can lead to hepatic abscess, generalized septicemia, and portal vein thrombosis.

Johnson JD et al: A sequential study of various modes of skin and umbilical care and the incidence of staphylococcal colonization and infection in the neonate. *Pediatrics* 1976;**58:**354.

8. SKIN INFECTIONS

The skin is exposed first to all of the organisms in the birth canal and then to staphylococci upon contact with nursery personnel and the family. Since staphylococcal epidemics in nurseries often begin with an outbreak of several apparently minor infections of the skin in infants, even relatively minor infections should receive aggressive treatment and should stimulate a review of hand-washing techniques among nursery personnel. Treatment of both infants and personnel may be necessary to rid a nursery of a prevailing virulent organism.

Colonization by organisms other than staphylococci—usually *E coli* or *Candida*—may take place in a newborn infant who is debilitated, has received antibiotic therapy, or has been so well isolated that staphylococcal colonization has not taken place.

Symptoms of infection are manifested by skin pustules with an erythematous base. These may rupture, releasing purulent exudate, and become encrusted. The degree of involvement of the skin may be variable, from a few lesions to extensive coalescing lesions spread over most of the body. **Cellulitis** due to streptococci (less often staphylococci) may spread rapidly. **Ritter's disease** is a grave form of cellulitis caused by staphylococci in which invasion of the skin is extremely rapid, with sloughing of the superficial layers, leaving extensive denuded, weeping areas.

Localized infections may occur around the circumcision site or umbilicus. Breast abscess may occur.

Appropriate local cultures and blood cultures should be done. Specific phage typing of staphylococci may be necessary to determine the prevalence of a pathogenic strain in an epidemic.

Systemic antibiotic therapy should always be used for infections that cause more than the most superficial lesions. A clearly localized and superficial infection can be treated by repeated cleansing with a soap containing an organic iodide preparation.

Curran JP, Al-Salihi FL: Neonatal staphylococcal scalded skin syndrome: Massive outbreak due to an unusual phage type. *Pediatrics* 1980;**66**:285.

Hargiss C, Larson E: The epidemiology of *Staphylococcus aureus* in a newborn nursery from 1970 through 1976. *Pediatrics* 1978;**61**:348.

9. OTITIS MEDIA

Otitis media may be present in almost 30% of patients in an intensive care nursery. Otitis may occur concurrently with sepsis or may precede it, and culture of the middle ear fluid is very helpful in determining the causative agent. Follow-up of infants who have had otitis in the nursery is very important for the recognition and, if necessary, treatment of conductive hearing loss.

Berman SA, Balkany TJ, Simmons MA: Otitis media in the neonatal intensive care unit. *Pediatrics* 1978;**62**:198.

10. CYTOMEGALOVIRUS INFECTION

Congenital cytomegalovirus infection usually follows an apparently normal pregnancy and delivery, although the mother may have an infectious mononucleosis-type illness. In severe infection, the infant is acutely ill at birth, with signs of multiple organ involvement. The infant tends to be small for gestational age and to have a disproportionately small head circumference. Central nervous system signs include symptoms of meningoencephalitis and later development of muscle weakness or spasticity. Chorioretinitis has been observed. Mental retardation accompanies the severe form.

In milder infection, the infant may have jaundice, petechiae, feeding difficulties, irritability, muscle weakness, spasticity, and hepatosplenomegaly.

IgM in cord blood is usually elevated. Cerebrospinal fluid is abnormal—with elevated protein and white cell count—and epithelial cells in the urine show inclusion bodies. Cytomegalovirus may be cultured from the urine, saliva, and cerebrospinal fluid. Skull x-rays may show periventricular calcification. Paired sera at birth and at 6 weeks will show rising or persistent cytomegalovirus antibody titer in the infant. Infants may excrete the virus for several years. Therefore, follow-up is indicated to detect late onset of sequelae, and urine cultures should be repeated until the organism is no longer excreted. In the premature sick infant, maternally derived infections and blood transfusion-acquired infections have been documented. Therefore, ongoing surveillance for infection is necessary. Increasing oxygen requirements, neutropenia, lymphocytosis, thrombocytopenia, and hepatosplenomegaly should suggest the possibility of the disease.

Cases have been documented in which no clinical evidence of disease existed and no late sequelae were reported. However, school failures, sensorineural deafness, and lowered performance on standardized mental tests have been reported with asymptomatic congenital infections. Longitudinal studies of infants with congenital disease, both symptomatic and diagnosed by prospective urine culture identification alone, have heightened the concern about late onset of hearing loss and disorders of language and learning.

Alford CA et al: Long-term mental and perceptual defects associated with silent intrauterine infections. Page 377 in: *Intrauterine Asphyxia and the Developing Fetal Brain.* Gluck L (editor). Year Book, 1977.

Hanshaw JB et al: School failure and deafness after "silent" congenital cytomegalovirus infection. *N Engl J Med* 1976;**295**:468.

Pass RF et al: Outcome of symptomatic congenital cytomegalovirus infection: Results of long-term longitudinal follow-up. *Pediatrics* 1980;**66**:758.

Saigal S et al: The outcome in children with congenital cytomegalovirus infection. *Am J Dis Child* 1982;**136**:896.

Williamson WD et al: Symptomatic congenital cytomegalovirus: Disorders of language, learning, and hearing. *Am J Dis Child* 1982;**136**:902.

Yeager AS et al: Prevention of transfusion-acquired cytomegalovirus infections in newborn infants. *J Pediatr* 1981;**98**:281.

Yeager AS et al: Sequelae of maternally derived cytomegalovirus infections in premature infants. *J Pediatr* 1983;**102**:918.

11. RUBELLA

Congenital rubella infection occurs as a result of rubella infection in the mother during pregnancy. The earlier in pregnancy the disease occurs, the more severely affected the fetus is likely to be—particularly during the first trimester.

The incidence of major anomalies—some of which may not be apparent immediately at birth—has been estimated to range from 20 to 60%. Therefore, it is essential that the rubella titer in a pregnant woman be determined. Vaccination is recommended prior to puberty.

Rubella should be considered in an infant with thrombocytopenia with petechiae or purpura, hepatitis, microcephaly, congenital heart disease (patent ductus arteriosus is the most common lesion), low birth weight for gestational age, cataracts, hepatosplenomegaly, myocarditis, and interstitial pneumonia. X-rays show characteristic longitudinal radiolucent areas in the distal metaphyses of long bones. Cultures of the infant's nasopharynx, throat secretions, and stool are usually positive, often for several weeks after delivery. Antibody titers, liver function tests, and long bone x-rays are needed.

No specific treatment is available. The prognosis is variable, depending on the degree of involvement of various organs. The highest incidence of severe involvement occurs with infection soon after conception. In these children, sequelae include mental retardation, behavioral disorders, and sensory handicaps. Nearly one-third have visual impairment because of cataracts, glaucoma, or retinitis. However, the most widespread problem in survivors, even with late-gestation infections, is hearing loss. In spite of these problems, up to 90% of survivors have been socially well adjusted and integrated into normal work or school settings.

American Academy of Pediatrics: Revised recommendations on rubella vaccine. *Pediatrics* 1980;**65:**1182.

Chess S, Fernandez P, Korn S: Behavioral consequences of congenital rubella. *J Pediatr* 1978;**93:**699.

Cooper LZ: Congenital rubella in the United States. Pages 1–22 in: *Infections of the Fetus and Newborn Infant*. Krugman S (editor). Year Book, 1975.

Kibrick S, Loria RM: Rubella and cytomegalovirus: Current concepts of congenital and acquired infection. *Pediatr Clin North Am* 1974;**21:**513.

Krugman S: Rubella immunization: Present status and future perspectives. *Pediatrics* 1980;**65:**1174.

Macfarlane DW et al: Intrauterine rubella, head size and intellect. *Pediatrics* 1975;**55:**797.

12. HERPESVIRUS INFECTION

Congenital or neonatal infection with herpesvirus hominis is now commonly recognized. Infant infection is usually secondary to genital infection in the mother, primarily with type 2 herpesvirus hominis. The spectrum of infection in the infant may extend from subclinical, with apparent recovery, to generalized multiple organ involvement and death. Skin vesicles are common and are sometimes present at birth. Central nervous system, eye, and generalized visceral involvement occurs frequently. Later handicaps are common in survivors, particularly when the central nervous system is affected.

The diagnosis is made by virus culture from maternal and infant lesions and by demonstrating inclusion bodies and positive fluorescent antibodies in cytologic preparations of cells from the margins of skin lesions. A rising antibody titer in the infant is confirmatory.

Treatment is supportive. Idoxuridine has been given, with variable results. Isolation techniques should be instituted to minimize spread to personnel and to other susceptible infants. If the mother is clinically well, it is best to have the infant room-in with her in a private room.

Prevention may be attempted by cesarean delivery when maternal genital lesions are present, thus avoiding fetal contact with the lesions during delivery. This is only effective if the cesarean section is done within 4 hours after rupture of membranes.

Hanshaw JB, Dudgeon JA: Herpes simplex infection of the fetus and newborn. Chap 5, pp 153–181, in: *Viral Diseases of the Fetus and Newborn*. Schaffer AJ, Markowitz M (editors). Saunders, 1978.

Whitley RJ et al: Vidarabine therapy of neonatal herpes simplex virus infection. *Pediatrics* 1980;**66:**495.

Yeager AS, Arvin AM: Reasons for the absence of a history of recurrent genital infections in mothers of neonates infected with herpes simplex virus. *Pediatrics* 1984;**73:**188.

13. TOXOPLASMOSIS

Toxoplasmosis is caused by the parasite *Toxoplasma gondii*. The clinical features of congenital toxoplasmosis closely resemble those of cytomegalic inclusion disease with a similar spectrum of degree of involvement. More severe clinical disease is associated with intrauterine growth retardation, microcephaly or hydrocephaly, microphthalmia, chorioretinitis, calcifications in skull x-rays, thrombocytopenia, and jaundice.

Diagnosis is confirmed by antibody titers that rise or persist in the infant. IgM in cord blood is usually elevated. The organism may be cultured, but this must be done in a laboratory with small animal or tissue culture capabilities, because *Toxoplasma* organisms are obligate intracellular parasites.

Many infants affected at birth die during the neonatal period. Those who survive are usually handicapped, with mental retardation, convulsions, neuromuscular disease, poor vision, and microcephaly or hydrocephaly.

Remington JS, Desmonts G: Toxoplasmosis. Chap 6, pp 191–332, in: *Infectious Diseases of the Fetus and Newborn Infant*. Remington JS, Klein JO (editors). Saunders, 1976.

Wilson CB et al: Development of adverse sequelae in children born with subclinical congenital *Toxoplasma* infection. *Pediatrics* 1980;**66**:767.

14. CONGENITAL SYPHILIS

The diagnosis must be suspected from the maternal history, since the infant is usually asymptomatic and full-term. The infant's serum is positive for IgM fluorescent antibody specific for syphilis. Darkfield examination of cerebrospinal fluid is positive for treponemes. X-rays of the long bones should be done. Cure is possible with adequate penicillin therapy. Good outcome depends on recognition and treatment of the infection in the neonatal period before symptoms appear. Otherwise, severe sequelae may occur, particularly involving the central nervous system.

Bryan EM, Nicholson E: Congenital syphilis: A study of physical and biochemical aspects. *Clin Pediatr* 1981;**20**:81.

15. GONOCOCCAL INFECTION

Gonococci may colonize an infant during passage through the infected mother's birth canal. Therefore, the obstetric diagnosis, if known or suspected by serum testing and positive histologic vaginal discharge, should be communicated to the infant's caretakers. Cord blood and a serum sample from the infant should be tested at 6–12 weeks for specific antibody titer. Conjunctivitis and keratitis are usually prevented with prophylactic eye care at birth. A common presentation of neonatal disease is copious purulent drainage from the eyes at 3–7 days. Affected infants require readmission for parenteral antibiotic therapy.

Segal S et al: Prophylaxis and treatment of neonatal gonococcal infections. *Pediatrics* 1980;**65**:1047.

16. TUBERCULOSIS

Tuberculosis in a pregnant woman can pose a serious threat to her offspring immediately after birth. If the mother is diagnosed with active cavitary tuberculosis at the time of delivery, she and her infant can either be kept together while both receive treatment or can be separated for 21 days while the mother receives treatment. It is much more common to have an asymptomatic but skin test-positive mother. These women should be placed on drug therapy and the infants carefully followed with skin tests for several months. The key to appropriate care is meticulous follow-up.

Hageman J et al: Congenital tuberculosis: Critical reappraisal of clinical findings and diagnostic procedures. *Pediatrics* 1980;**66**:980.

Myers JP et al: Tuberculosis in pregnancy with fatal congenital infection. *Pediatrics* 1981;**67**:89.

17. OTHER INFECTIONS

Echoviruses, coxsackieviruses, myxoviruses, and a variety of other viruses may cause congenital infection. They should be considered when meningoencephalitis, pneumonia, myocarditis, hepatitis, cataracts, or other unexplained disease is present.

Varicella may occur in a fetus or newborn if the mother develops the disease during her pregnancy. The infant will develop clinical disease—usually typical skin vesicles—after the usual incubation period of 2–3 weeks. The clinical course is usually modified in the infant, presumably by passive antibodies from the mother. The disease is contagious while active lesions are present.

Infants born to mothers who are hepatitis B antigen-positive are at high risk for becoming positive over the first several months of life. The illness is characterized by hepatomegaly, prolonged or recurrent jaundice, poor appetite, and failure to thrive. The best treatment is prevention; therefore, exposed infants should receive high-titer hepatitis B immune globulin within 72 hours of birth and every 6 weeks up to 6 months of age.

The most common cause of neonatal conjunctivitis is now *Chlamydia*. Clinical studies have shown that erythromycin will cure the infection if given for 10–14 days, but other commonly used ophthalmic antibiotics may exacerbate it.

Heggie AD et al: Topical sulfacetamide vs. oral erythromycin for neonatal chlamydial conjunctivitis. *Am J Dis Child* 1985;**139**:564.

Jhaveri R et al: High titer multiple dose therapy with HBIG in newborn infants of HBsAg positive mothers. *J Pediatr* 1980;**97**:305.

Monif GRG: Chap 3, pp 31–86, in: *Infectious Diseases in Obstetrics and Gynecology*. Harper & Row, 1974.

Shiraki K et al: Acute hepatitis B in infants born to carrier mothers with the antibody to hepatitis B e antigen. *J Pediatr* 1980;**97**:768.

GASTROINTESTINAL & ABDOMINAL SURGICAL CONDITIONS IN THE NEWBORN (See also Chapter 19.)

TRACHEOESOPHAGEAL FISTULA & ESOPHAGEAL ATRESIA

Tracheoesophageal fistula and esophageal atresia are usually diagnosed in the delivery room or nursery recovery area by the nurse or first attendant to the infant. The infant shows immediate onset of respiratory distress, cyanosis, excessive secretions in the oropharynx, and choking with feeding. Obstetric history usually includes polyhydramnios. Diagnosis can be made by x-ray following placement of a radiopaque catheter in the esophageal pouch. If the abdomen remains scaphoid and no bowel gas is seen on x-ray, there is no associated tracheoesophageal fistula. However, the most common type of tracheoesophageal fistula is the H type associated with esophageal atresia.

When fistula is present alone, the diagnosis may be difficult to confirm. Careful evaluation must be done in any infant who has respiratory symptoms, particularly coughing, choking, and cyanosis associated with feeding. The differential diagnosis includes pharyngeal muscle weakness, vascular rings, and esophageal diverticula.

Treatment varies depending upon the type of lesion and the degree of abnormality present. Frequent or continuous gentle suctioning of the upper pouch and pharynx will minimize tracheal aspiration of saliva. Generally, gastrostomy is performed early and the fistula ligated at that time. If the ends of the esophagus are too far apart for a direct anastomosis, the upper pouch is exteriorized. After a sufficient period of growth, during which time the infant is fed through the gastrostomy, a primary repair of the esophagus is made.

Careful attention to fluid, electrolyte, and caloric requirements, as well as infection, is important during preparation for surgery and in the postoperative period. Associated congenital anomalies, particularly vertebral, anal, cardiac, renal, and limb, may coexist. Evaluation for these should be made prior to surgery.

INTESTINAL OBSTRUCTION

A newborn infant with abdominal distention and vomiting must be suspected of having intestinal obstruction. The level of obstruction and the decision whether or not to undertake surgery can usually be made by careful review of the history and physical examination. A plain film of the abdomen is frequently all that is needed to confirm the clinical impression.

Immediate treatment consists of placing a soft, large-bore, red rubber catheter into the stomach and instituting intermittent mechanical suction. This will prevent further distention and decrease the risk of visceral perforation. The infant's temperature, vital signs, urine output, and electrolyte status should be monitored frequently. The infant should receive nothing by mouth, and intravenous fluids should be started. Additional colloid or crystalloid fluids may be needed prior to surgery if the infant is dehydrated or in shock.

Additional workup should be done only when needed to clarify the diagnosis or to aid in planning surgery. Unnecessary studies put the infant through needless procedures and delay definitive treatment. The infant may tolerate surgery better soon after birth than later. Needless delay must be avoided when vascular supply to the bowel may be compromised. Again, careful attention to the infant's needs in preparation for surgery and during the postoperative period is important.

Surgery may consist of definitive repair of the abnormality or may be palliative, ie, decompression of the bowel followed later by repair of the primary lesion. Total parenteral nutrition (TPN) may be a useful adjunct to care in the pre- and postoperative periods.

A high intestinal obstruction such as **duodenal atresia, midgut volvulus,** or **annular pancreas** will cause abdominal distention, vomiting, and feeding intolerance. Abdominal x-rays will show the level of obstruction because of the abrupt change from air-filled viscus to no visceral gas. In malrotation and volvulus, bile-stained emesis is the key symptom, and surgery is urgently needed to prevent vascular insufficiency and bowel necrosis. **Hypertrophic pyloric stenosis** usually causes symptoms of gastric distention, with projectile vomiting and excessive hunger presenting at 2–6 weeks of life.

Intestinal obstruction at lower levels along the gastrointestinal tract is often more difficult to diagnose. The infant will tolerate initial feedings, may not vomit, and will develop abdominal distention much later. X-rays may show nonlocalized distention of large and small bowel. **Meconium ileus** may be the presenting symptom of cystic fibrosis. In utero bowel perforation may have occurred, and x-rays may show abdominal calcifications. **Peritoneal bands, intussusception, Hirschsprung's disease (aganglionosis), meconium plug syndrome,** and **small left colon syndrome** can be diagnosed by barium enema. **Imperforate anus** can be recognized on physical examination. The abnormal anatomy varies from a thin rectal membrane to complete rectal atresia. Fistulas may exist between the terminal ileum and the perineum, bladder, or vagina.

The bowel may have multiple atresias, and therefore x-ray studies and surgical laparotomy should include consideration of the entire bowel. The differential diagnosis includes all causes of functional obstruction **(paralytic ileus).** Air-fluid levels are seen on x-ray, and abdominal distention, decreased bowel sounds, and vomiting may occur secondary to sepsis, urinary tract infection, respiratory distress syndrome, and central nervous system dysfunction. These problems resolve with proper medical treatment.

OTHER ABDOMINAL SURGICAL CONDITIONS

Appendicitis & Meckel's Diverticulum

These disorders may occur in the newborn period and always present difficult diagnostic problems. The infant will show general symptoms of illness and may have abdominal distention, decreased bowel sounds, and constipation. Fever and leukocytosis may not be present. Careful examination of the abdomen will usually show localizing findings of peritonitis. The appendix is often ruptured at the time of diagnosis. Meckel's diverticulum may present with sudden gastrointestinal bleeding.

Omphalocele

Omphalocele will be present at birth and requires immediate surgical consultation. Part or all of the intestine, as well as the liver and spleen, may be visible through the sac. In addition to the preoperative medical care detailed in the section on intestinal obstruction, sterile saline gauze packs and an occlusive plastic bandage should be used to cover the wound. Transport to a level 3 care center must be done without delay. Other anomalies, particularly of midline structures (brain and heart), should be ruled out.

Gastroschisis

Gastroschisis is a congenital defect of the abdominal wall that results in herniation of all or part of the abdominal organs into the amniotic sac. Because the bowel is exposed to amniotic fluid for a prolonged time during the gestation, it will be edematous, thickened, malrotated, and shortened. Preoperative care consists of all the procedures noted above with the addition of cultures and antibiotics. Postoperatively, bowel function returns slowly, and central alimentation is lifesaving.

Necrotizing Enterocolitis

This illness of the newborn infant most commonly occurs in the sick premature infant and the hyperviscous full-term infant. The pathogenesis includes infectious necrosis of an ischemic bowel wall. Pathophysiologic causes include excessive fluid administration, patent ductus arteriosus, and too rapid increases in volume and concentration of feedings. Infants present with abdominal distention, vomiting, positive Hematest or grossly bloody stools, and pneumatosis intestinalis on x-ray. Medical management consists of suction-decompression, septic workup and antibiotics, and aggressive blood pressure support. Metabolic acidosis and hyperkalemia are ominous signs of necrosing tissue. Early surgical consultation is indicated in all cases. (See also Epidemic Diarrhea, above.)

Ruptured Abdominal Viscera

A ruptured abdominal viscus will present with peritonitis and pneumoperitoneum if the stomach or bowel is perforated. Rupture of a solid viscus presents with hemoperitoneum, anemia, and shock.

Pneumoperitoneum

Pneumoperitoneum may occur spontaneously, particularly in very immature infants. The rupture is often in the large bowel along the hepatic flexure. In contrast to the findings of necrotizing enterocolitis, the bowel is entirely normal except for the perforation. Depending on when the perforation occurs, postoperative complications may be minimal, since the bowel contents are often sterile.

Pneumoperitoneum may also result from dissection by air along the mediastinum and through the diaphragm next to the esophagus, with rupture into the peritoneal cavity. This complication develops in infants receiving positive pressure ventilation with the respirator set at relatively high pressures. With positive pressure ventilation, air may accumulate rapidly in the peritoneal cavity, and continuous drainage of air from the peritoneum may be required to allow adequate movement of the diaphragm. Although the accompanying pneumomediastinum or pneumothorax is generally obvious, it occasionally may be inapparent.

Diaphragmatic Hernia

This congenital malformation consists of herniation of abdominal organs into the hemithorax (most commonly left) because of a defect in the diaphragm. Infants who present in the delivery room with severe respiratory distress, cyanosis, and failure to respond to oxygen and mask-bag ventilation may have associated hypoplasia of one or both lungs. The infant must be intubated to avoid further distention of the bowel with air, placed on ventilator support and suction-decompression, and transported directly to the level 3 care center for surgery. Survival depends on rapid surgical repair, excellent medical management, and the amount of lung tissue that developed in utero.

DeLuca FG, Wesselhoeft CW: Surgically treatable causes of neonatal respiratory distress. *Clin Perinatol* 1978;**5**:377.

Haller JA, Talbert JL: *Surgical Emergencies in the Newborn.* Lea & Febiger, 1972.

Lilly JR et al: *Pediatric Surgery: Case Studies.* Medical Examination Publishing Co., 1978.

HEMATOLOGIC DISORDERS (See also Chapter 16.)

BLEEDING DISORDERS

The most common causes of bleeding in the newborn infant are vascular accidents, clotting deficiencies (particularly vitamin K-dependent factors), thrombocytopenia, and disseminated intravascular coagulation.

Hemorrhagic Disease of the Newborn (Hypoprothrombinemia)

Vitamin K-dependent clotting factors (factors II, VII, IX, X) are normal at birth but decrease within 2–3 days. In vitamin K-deficient infants, these levels may be very low, resulting in prolonged bleeding times. Bleeding may occur into the skin or gastrointestinal tract, at the site of injection or circumcision, or at internal sites. Small amounts of vitamin K are sufficient to correct the clotting factor defects unless liver function is immature in a very sick or premature infant. All newborn infants should receive 1 mg of vitamin K intramuscularly on admission to the nursery.

Blood in Vomitus or Stool

Swallowing maternal blood during delivery is not uncommon. If enough has been ingested, the infant may vomit bright red or dark blood or may pass stool containing dark or bright red, fresh-appearing blood. Clinical evidence of acute blood loss is lacking, but a transient rise in blood urea nitrogen may occur. Blood of maternal origin may be differentiated from infant blood by testing for fetal hemoglobin, which is resistant to alkali denaturation. A small amount of red bloody stool or vomitus is mixed with 5–10 mL of water and centrifuged. To 5 parts of pink supernatant, add 1 part 0.25 N sodium hydroxide. If fetal hemoglobin is present, the solution remains pink; if adult hemoglobin is present, it becomes brown.

Gastrointestinal bleeding in the newborn may be due to trauma, peptic ulcer, duplication of bowel, Meckel's diverticulum, intussusception, volvulus, hemangioma or telangiectasia of the bowel, polyp, rectal prolapse, anal fissure (a common cause of a small amount of blood in the stool in infants), infection (especially salmonellae, shigellae), systemic bleeding disorders (particularly hemorrhagic disease of the newborn), and tumors.

If blood is of maternal origin, no treatment is needed. If bleeding is of fetal origin, treat as for acute blood loss with blood transfusions and supportive care and then proceed with diagnosis and treatment of the underlying disease. The most common intrinsic cause of bloody vomitus is a gastric ulcer, which seldom causes massive bleeding and perforation. The bleeding generally can be managed with frequent oral milk feedings alone. If blood loss has been significant but transfusion is not necessary, iron supplementation may be required during the first few months.

ANEMIA

Acute blood loss before or during delivery can occur into the maternal circulation, the amniotic sac, into a twin fetus in the twin-twin transfusion syndrome, or into the vagina. Acute blood loss after delivery may be external (gastrointestinal, circumcision site, umbilical stump) or internal (fracture site, cephalhematoma, central nervous system or pulmonary hemorrhage, soft tissue hematoma, injured internal organ). Anemia may be secondary to hemolysis (isoimmunization, acquired hemolytic disease, red cell metabolic abnormalities) or to congenital aplastic or hypoplastic anemia.

The degree of bleeding, which may occur at many sites during delivery (including muscle and skin), is frequently underestimated. In general, whenever there is serious doubt about the extent of bleeding in the fetus, the infant's blood volume should be expanded with plasma expanders or whole blood.

If severe anemia is chronic or due to acute hemolysis, transfusion may have to be done with sedimented red cells, using small volume exchange transfusions to avoid overloading the vascular space.

As more immature infants have survived, the issue of late "physiologic" anemia has become a bigger problem. The use of booster transfusions is appropriate for infants who begin to show symptoms such as tachycardia, tachypnea, failure to gain weight, or apnea. However, many infants tolerate hemoglobin levels as low as 7.5 mg/dL, and avoiding a transfusion certainly prevents exposure to hepatitis, cytomegalovirus, transfusion reactions, and thrombotic injuries.

POLYCYTHEMIA

Unusually high hematocrits are seen in newborn infants infrequently in some pediatric services and in as many as 5% of all births in others. Polycythemia results in increased blood viscosity, particularly when the hematocrit exceeds 70%. A peripheral hematocrit of 70% is an indication for performing a venous hematocrit. If the venous hematocrit is greater than 65%, hyperviscosity is present. The diagnosis should be suspected in infants who are postterm, small for gestational age, or large for gestational age or in twins (with fetofetal transfusion). Infants of diabetic mothers may be hyperviscous (owing to deformity of red blood cells) without polycythemia being present.

Hyperviscosity decreases effective perfusion of the capillary beds of the microcirculation and increases the work load of the heart. Clinical manifestations include an enlarged heart, pulmonary perihilar infiltrates, tachypnea, oxygen dependency, priapism, and central nervous system signs ranging from increased jitteriness to overt seizures.

Treatment is recommended for symptomatic infants. The acute symptoms of hypoglycemia, respiratory distress, and cardiac failure may be improved dramatically with treatment. Less serious symptoms of poor feeding, lethargy, and poor peripheral perfusion may also be improved but may not warrant the risks of catheter placement and partial plasma exchange. More serious symptoms of hyperviscosity, though rare, appear to be associated with ischemia of the kidneys and bowel. Treatment for asymptomatic infants is no longer recommended.

Treatment consists of administering a small isovolumetric exchange transfusion using plasma as the donor fluid. Phlebotomy should not be done for several reasons, partly because it reduces the hematocrit slowly and partly because reduction in circulating blood volume may cause additional undesirable problems.

Follow-up studies in which infants who had neonatal hyperviscosity were compared with controls have demonstrated that the former have delays in fine motor and language skills at 1 year of age and that there are gross motor delays and an increase in the number of neurologic diagnoses at 2 years of age. Partial exchange transfusions may decrease the incidence of these findings slightly, but they also appear to increase the acute risk of necrotizing enterocolitis. The effects of these early findings on school performance have not yet been determined.

Black VD, Lubchenco LO: Neonatal polycythemia and hyperviscosity. *Pediatr Clin North Am* 1982;**29:**1137.

Black VD et al: Gastrointestinal injury in polycythemic term infants. *Pediatrics* 1985;**76:**225.

Black VD et al: Neonatal hyperviscosity: Randomized study of effect of partial plasma exchange transfusion on long-term outcome. *Pediatrics* 1985;**75:**1048.

Blanchette VS, Zipursky A: Assessment of anemia in newborn infants. *Clin Perinatol* 1984;**11:**489.

Blank JP et al: The role of RBC transfusion in the premature infant. *Am J Dis Child* 1984;**138:**831.

Linderkamp O et al: Contributions of red cells and plasma to blood viscosity in preterm and full-term infants and adults. *Pediatrics* 1984;**74:**45.

Stockman JA, Clark DA: Weight gain: A response to transfusion in selected preterm infants. *Am J Dis Child* 1984;**138:**828.

Wirth FH, Goldberg KE, Lubchenco LO: Neonatal hyperviscosity: Incidence. *Pediatrics* 1979;**63:**833.

METABOLIC DISORDERS

HYPOGLYCEMIA

Glucose concentration is slightly lower in the umbilical cord blood than in the mother's blood. The glucose concentration in the infant's blood decreases during the hours after delivery (rarely decreasing below 30–40 mg/dL) and then stabilizes between 50 and 80 mg/dL when the infant is 6–12 hours of age. Concentrations below 40 mg/dL are considered abnormal.

Hypoglycemia is frequent in 2 extremes of altered intrauterine nutrition: the infant of the diabetic mother, who is well nourished, with abundant glycogen and fat stores; and the infant with intrauterine growth retardation, who is undernourished, with minimal glycogen and fat deposits. (These conditions are discussed separately below.) In addition, hypoglycemia is associated with Beckwith's syndrome, erythroblastosis fetalis, nesidioblastosis, leucine sensitivity, glycogen storage disease, and galactosemia. Hypoglycemia may occur in any sick infant and is frequent after birth asphyxia.

The manifestations of hypoglycemia in the newborn infant may be mild and nonspecific: lethargy, poor feeding, regurgitation, apnea, and twitching. As symptoms become more severe, the infant will develop pallor, sweating, cool extremities, and prolonged apnea and convulsions.

Blood glucose concentration should be measured frequently during the first few days of life in all infants at risk of hypoglycemia, particularly small-for-gestational-age infants, infants with erythroblastosis, those born of diabetic mothers, and those with asphyxia at birth. In all clinical conditions where hypoglycemia is likely to occur, it is important to follow the blood glucose concentration closely when the infant is weaned to milk feedings. Because milk feedings contain little glucose, a hypoglycemic infant will have to rely on gluconeogenesis in order to maintain adequate glucose. Thus, hypoglycemia may reappear in the susceptible infant at this time.

Infants of Diabetic Mothers

Infants of diabetic mothers have special problems because they are large for gestational age. Even in pregnant women whose diabetes has been under good control, the blood glucose concentration will vary more in a 24-hour period than in normal women. In addition, other compounds in the blood, such as free fatty acids and insulin, are present in abnormal amounts. Such findings contribute to the birth of large-for-gestational-age infants to mothers whose diabetes would appear to be relatively mild. Infants of diabetic mothers also have problems related to the diabetes in the mother. These infants may become hypoglycemic within the first hour after birth, and they should be tested with Dextrostix every 20 minutes and started on oral or intravenous glucose as soon as possible. Careful observation of glucose levels should be done during the next few days to ensure a smooth regulation of glucose homeostasis.

Infants With Intrauterine Growth Retardation

Infants with intrauterine growth retardation (small-for-gestational-age infants) can be born after normal uncomplicated pregnancies, but such infants usually are found in association with the maternal problems noted earlier in this chapter. Regardless of the cause of intrauterine growth retardation, these infants tend to be at increased risk of hypoglycemia.

Small-for-gestational-age infants should receive 10% glucose infusion, 100 mL/kg/d, to maintain blood glucose concentrations greater than 40 mg/dL. Dextrostix or some other means of measuring blood glucose concentrations should be used. Some infants will develop hypoglycemia in spite of this therapy, in which case the glucose concentrations or the flow rate of the infusion should be increased proportionately. In rare instances, small-for-gestational-age infants may develop marked hyperglycemia and a transient diabetes mellitus-like syndrome. Insulin therapy is rarely required and seldom need be given past the first week of life. The small-for-gestational-age infant with hypoglycemia and a very high hematocrit (capillary hematocrit > 75%) is likely to show the most severe clinical signs of hypoglycemia, presumably reflecting a reduction in cerebral plasma flow. A small exchange transfusion with plasma should be given to reduce the hematocrit and to correct the hypoglycemia.

Cowett RM, Stern L: Carbohydrate homeostasis in the fetus and newborn. Chap 26, pp 583–599, in: *Neonatology*, 2nd ed. Avery GB (editor). Lippincott, 1981.

Fluge G: Neurological findings at follow-up in neonatal hypoglycemia. *Acta Paediatr Scand* 1975;**64:**629.

Lubchenco LO, Bard H: Incidence of hypoglycemia in newborn infants classified by birth weight and gestational age. *Pediatrics* 1971;**47:**831.

Pagliara AS et al: Hypoglycemia in infancy and childhood. (2 parts.) *J Pediatr* 1973;**82:**365, 558.

HYPOCALCEMIA

The plasma of a fetus has a higher total calcium concentration and a higher calcium activity than that of a neonate or adult. In general, hypocalcemia in the newborn infant may be defined as a plasma concentration less than about 3.5 meq/L (7 mg/dL). Within the range of 3.2–4 meq/L, infants vary considerably in clinical hypocalcemic signs. Infants are generally symptomatic at levels below 3.2 meq/L. Hypocalcemia is most likely to occur at 2 times: shortly after birth and toward the end of the second or third week of life. Hypocalcemia occurring shortly after birth has been associated with infants of diabetic mothers, sepsis of the newborn infant, perinatal asphyxia, prematurity, and maternal hyperparathyroidism. Late-onset hypocalcemia usually appears in the healthy term infant at 3–4 days or later after milk feedings have been well established. This form often leads to seizures and may be life-threatening.

Clinical Findings

A. Symptoms and Signs: The infant may be twitchy, tremulous, or have frank convulsions, although many infants with low serum calcium levels are without apparent symptoms.

B. "Tetany of the Newborn": This is the late-onset disorder that occurs almost exclusively in infants fed proprietary milk formulas. Cow's milk formulas contain high concentrations of phosphates, which are not cleared adequately by the kidney. This leads to elevation of serum phosphorus, secondary lowering of serum calcium, and clinical tetany. It is not known why only a small number of infants are at risk.

Treatment

A. Oral Calcium: Oral administration of calcium lactate or gluconate is the preferred method of treatment. Calcium can either be given as a diluted solution or added to formula feedings several times a day in a dose of 0.5–1 g/kg/d.

In "tetany of the newborn," it is advisable to lower the solute and phosphorus loads as well as to provide extra calcium. This can be done by using one of the commercially available low-solute formulas.

B. Intravenous Calcium: Intravenous administration of calcium solutions may occasionally be necessary. The infusion must be given slowly, diluted with an equal amount of glucose in water. The heart rate is monitored carefully during the infusion and immediately afterward; cardiac slowing and arrest can occur as a result of rapid administration of calcium salts. The response to intravenous calcium is usually only transient. (***Note:*** Calcium salts cannot be added to intravenous solutions that contain $NaHCO_3$, since they will precipitate as calcium carbonate.)

Prognosis

A normal outcome is reported in nearly all infants who survive neonatal hypocalcemic seizures.

Brown DR, Tsang RC, Chen I: Oral calcium supplementation in premature and asphyxiated neonates. *J Pediatr* 1976;**89:**973.

Clark PCN: Hypocalcemic and hypomagnesemic convulsions. *J Pediatr* 1970;**70:**806.

Shaw JC: Evidence for defective skeletal mineralization in low-birthweight infants: The absorption of calcium and fat. *Pediatrics* 1976;**57:**16.

Tsang RC, Donovan EF, Steichen JJ: Calcium physiology and pathology in the neonate. *Pediatr Clin North Am* 1976;**23:**611.

LATE METABOLIC ACIDOSIS

Late metabolic acidosis may occur in preterm infants during the first weeks of life. Early findings consist of a diminished rate of weight gain (in spite of adequate intake) associated with a falling serum total CO_2 content and a relatively alkaline urine for the degree of metabolic acidosis present. This disease is usually transient and responds to the addition of $NaHCO_3$, 3 meq/kg/d, to formula feedings.

Schwartz GJ et al: Late metabolic acidosis: A reassessment of the definition. *J Pediatr* 1979;**95:**102.

INFANTS OF ADDICTED MOTHERS

1. NARCOTICS

Clinical Findings

Withdrawal symptoms occur in about two-thirds of infants born to mothers who are addicted to heroin, methadone, or related drugs. Symptoms consist primarily of increased tremors, irritability and hyperactivity, hypertonicity, sweating, yawning, sneezing, excessive hunger and salivation, nasal stuffiness, and regurgitation. Severely affected infants may have vomiting, diarrhea, respiratory distress, and convulsions. This clinical picture of increased activity—often frantic behavior—is typical enough to suggest the diagnosis even though a history of drug abuse had not been elicited prior to delivery. Infants may be small for gestational age. Confirmation can be obtained by doing a screening test for drug excretory products in the urine of mother or infant.

Treatment

Observe carefully for onset and progression of symptoms. Give no specific treatment until symptoms develop.

With onset of significant irritability, tremors, and hyperactivity, sedation is required. Phenobarbital, 5–10 mg/kg/d in divided doses every 4–6 hours, is recommended because of its safety and predictability of effect. The dose may need to be increased cautiously to provide adequate control of symptoms, but respiratory depression must be avoided. Phenobarbital blood levels should be obtained in infants treated near the limits of the therapeutic range, since phenobarbital plasma clearances in newborn infants vary considerably from one infant to another. Continue at the necessary dose until withdrawal symptoms subside—a few days or several weeks—and then gradually decrease the dose. In addition to sedation, swaddling the infant and using a pacifier may help control the excessive activity, allowing the infant to rest between feedings.

Prognosis

The prognosis is good for the immediate health of the infant. Careful evaluation of the family unit must be made in each case. The infant may be cared for by the mother, but continued interest and long-term support by the health team and the mother's active involvement with a drug treatment program are essential. Otherwise, arrangements for care of the infant by temporary placement must be considered.

Long-term outcome of these infants is somewhat more worrisome. Growth in all parameters may be skewed downward, as reported in follow-up studies of preschool children born to heroin-addicted mothers. Furthermore, these children have been rated as having more difficult behavior problems, and they have increased perceptual and organizational problems compared to control children born to nonaddicted mothers in equally high-risk social and drug environments.

Lifshitz MH et al: Factors affecting head growth and intellectual function in children of drug addicts. *Pediatrics* 1985;**75:**269.

Neumann LL, Cohen SN: The neonatal narcotic withdrawal syndrome: A therapeutic challenge. *Clin Perinatol* 1975; **2:**99.

Rothstein P, Gould JB: Born with a habit: Infants of drug-addicted mothers. *Pediatr Clin North Am* 1974;**21:**307.

Wilson GS et al: The development of preschool children of heroin-addicted mothers: A controlled study. *Pediatrics* 1979;**63:**135.

2. ALCOHOL

Clinical Findings

Recently, it has become clear that the use and abuse of alcohol in pregnancy is an important teratogen. In mothers with chronic alcoholism, there is an increased probability of fetal wastage and fetal alcohol syndrome. In fully manifest cases, these infants have severe intrauterine growth retardation, postnatal growth and developmental delays, short palpebral fissures, joint anomalies, and heart defects. In mothers who drink moderately, ie, 1–2 oz of absolute alcohol daily (1–2 mixed drinks containing one jigger of concentrated alcohol or 8–12 oz of wine), there is a 10–20% incidence of anomalies, mental deficiency, and growth retardation.

Treatment

Supportive care may be required in the immediate newborn period for infants of chronic alcohol users. More commonly, they will have the typical problems of small-for-gestational-age infants, ie, hypoglycemia, polycythemia, and hyperviscosity. These problems should be anticipated and prevented.

Prognosis

Infants who have features of the fetal alcohol syndrome at birth are very likely to show long-term sequelae. Growth deficiencies occur, and the degree of mental deficit correlates with the severity of dysmorphism at birth. Hyperactivity adds to the school problems. The severity of outcome is not influenced by socioeconomic background or educational opportunities.

Clarren SK, Smith DW: The fetal alcohol syndrome. *N Engl J Med* 1978;**298:**1063.

Davis PJM, Partridge JW, Storrs CN: Alcohol consumption in pregnancy: How much is safe? *Arch Dis Child* 1982; **57:**940.

Little RE: Moderate alcohol use during pregnancy and decreased infant birth weight. *Am J Public Health* 1977;**67:**1154.

Streissguth AP, Herman CS, Smith DW: Intelligence, behavior, and dysmorphogenesis in the fetal alcohol syndrome: A report on 20 patients. *J Pediatr* 1978;**92:**363.

Tennes K, Blackard C: Maternal alcohol consumption, birth weight, and minor physical anomalies. *Am J Obstet Gynecol* 1980;**138:**774.

3. TOBACCO SMOKING

Clinical Findings

Maternal smoking has been conclusively associated with decreased birth weight at every gestational age after 30 weeks, and it appears to follow a dose-response curve. With more detailed questioning, investigators have found that light smoking as well as heavy smoking, defined as less or more than 10 cigarettes per day, is associated with increased perinatal death. The increased rate of fetal death has been attributed to anoxia and prematurity. The physiologic responses to anoxia in smokers' infants are increased ratios of placental to fetal weight, increased carboxyhemoglobin levels, and a shift of the oxygen dissociation curve to the left. The differences in placental morphology and implantation may account for the increased incidences of bleeding, abruptio placentae, placenta previa, and premature rupture of membranes in smokers.

Treatment

Treatment consists of prevention. Infants of mothers who stop smoking completely during the last 3 months of pregnancy have no increased risk of perinatal death on that basis.

Prognosis

The Brazelton Assessment Scale in newborn infants of smoking mothers reveals decreased responses to auditory stimuli. Preliminary results of follow-up for 5 years have shown an increase in postneonatal deaths, hospital admissions, physical and mental impairments, and respiratory and skin diseases in children of smoking compared to nonsmoking mothers.

Meyer MB, Tonascia JA: Maternal smoking, pregnancy complications, and perinatal mortality. *Am J Obstet Gynecol* 1977;**128:**494.

Naeye RL: Abruptio placentae and placenta previa: Frequency, perinatal mortality, and cigarette smoking. *Obstet Gynecol* 1980;**55:**701.

Pedreira FA et al: Involuntary smoking and incidence of respiratory illness during the first year of life. *Pediatrics* 1985; **75:**594.

Rantakallio P: The effect of maternal smoking on birth weight and the subsequent health of the child. *Early Hum Dev* 1978;**2:**371.

Saxton DW: The behaviour of infants whose mothers smoke in pregnancy. *Early Hum Dev* 1978;**2:**363.

4. OTHER DRUGS

Many drugs are prescribed for therapy of maternal conditions or are abused at the time of conception and during pregnancy. Similarly, many drugs are used or abused during lactation. Before drugs are prescribed, benefits of therapy for the mother must be weighed against possible risks to the fetus or nursing infant. Nearly all drugs pass quickly through the placenta and, after birth, into the breast milk. The amount of drug transferred and the period in embryogenesis when the transfer occurs can influence the outcome in the fetus and newborn infant.

American Academy of Pediatrics Committee on Drugs: Psychotropic drugs in pregnancy and lactation. *Pediatrics* 1982; **69:**241.

Berkowitz RL, Coustan DR, Mochizuki TK: *Handbook for Prescribing Medications During Pregnancy.* Little, Brown, 1981.

Briggs GG et al: *Drugs in Pregnancy and Lactation: A Reference Guide to Fetal and Neonatal Risk.* Williams & Wilkins, 1983.

RENAL DISORDERS

The most common causes of renal failure in premature and full-term newborn infants are asphyxia and shock. The other renal problems that may be encountered in the nursery are infections and anomalies. For further discussion, see Chapter 21.

1. RENAL FAILURE

The normal urine output of a newborn infant is 1–2 mL/kg/h. After a severe intrapartum or neonatal asphyxial insult, there may be 2–3 days of anuria or oliguria, followed by polyuria and then gradual recovery. If glomerular damage has occurred, the urine will contain protein and red blood cells. If the damage is primarily tubular, the problems will be abnormal urine flow rates and electrolyte imbalances. If the insult is due to hypotension or prerenal failure, treatment should be early colloid administration followed by restriction of fluids to insensible losses plus urine output replacement. The infant should be weighed every 8–12 hours and given time to recover. Excessive fluid administration will lead to pulmonary edema, accumulation of extravascular water, and congestive heart failure. Hyperkalemia may lead to cardiac dysrhythmias and death and must be aggressively treated with intravenous calcium, bicarbonate, continuous insulin and glucose infusion, or cation-exchange resin enemas. Serial measurements of urine and serum electrolytes and osmolalities will be extremely useful in determining fluid and electrolyte management.

Another problem of the very low birth weight infant is glucosuria with obligate water and sodium losses and rapid dehydration. Therefore, we recommend that infants weighing less than 1200 g be started on 5% dextrose solutions.

2. URINARY TRACT INFECTIONS

Infants with prolonged jaundice, failure to thrive, and vomiting may have urinary tract infections. In the premature infant, this may be part of a generalized sepsis, whereas in the full-term infant, it is more commonly associated with an anomaly of the urinary tract.

3. URINARY TRACT ANOMALIES

The incidence rate of functionally significant anomalies of the kidneys or excretory tracts in newborn infants is around 0.8%. In infants who seem to be well, over 90% of these anomalies can be detected by careful abdominal palpation. Abnormal abdominal masses in the newborn must be diagnosed; in descending order of frequency, they are hydronephrosis, cystic kidney, renal artery or renal vein thrombosis, neuroblastoma, and Wilms' tumor. In infants with oligohydramnios and anuria, renal agenesis must be suspected. Syndromes with multiple anomalies or chromosomal abnormalities frequently include congenital renal abnormalities.

Anand SK: Acute renal failure in the neonate. *Pediatr Clin North Am* 1982;**29:**791.

Arant BS: Estimating glomerular filtration rate in infants. *J Pediatr* 1984;**104:**890.

Dauber IM et al: Renal failure following perinatal anoxia. *J Pediatr* 1976;**88:**851.

Guignard JP: Renal function in the newborn infant. *Pediatr Clin North Am* 1982;**29:**777.

Jain R: Acute renal failure in the neonate. *Pediatr Clin North Am* 1977;**24:**605.

Rahman N, Boineau FG, Lewy JE: Renal failure in the perinatal period. *Clin Perinatol* 1981;**8:**241.

Schwartz GJ, Feld LG, Langford DJ: A simple estimate of glomerular filtration rate in full-term infants during the first year of life. *J Pediatr* 1984;**104:**849.

BRAIN & NEUROLOGIC DISORDERS

Brain damage in newborn full-term infants is usually due to physical trauma at birth or to perinatal asphyxia; congenital anomalies and infections of the central nervous system are the next most common causes. (See also Chapter 23.) Most of the brain damage due to trauma or asphyxia is preventable, primarily through improved obstetric care and secondarily through improved neonatal care immediately following delivery.

1. PROLONGED & SEVERE HYPOXIA

Clinical Findings

Intrauterine hypoxia causes brief tachycardia in the fetus and increased fetal movement, followed by depression and bradycardia. Meconium may be passed into the amniotic fluid and subsequently aspirated. At delivery, the infant is hypotonic, cyanotic, and pale and makes little or no respiratory effort. The Apgar score is less than 3.

Hypoxia causes a redistribution of cardiac output, with the brain and the heart receiving increased blood flow, whereas the lung and certain other organs have markedly decreased blood flow even with relatively moderate degrees of hypoxia. If hypoxia is severe, other organs such as the skin, muscle, and gastrointestinal tract also have reduced blood flow and become underperfused with blood of low oxygen content. This state leads to an increasingly severe metabolic acidosis. Active resuscitation is indicated, and prolonged assisted ventilation may be necessary. After a variable period, the infant may make spontaneous respiratory efforts and gradually establish spontaneous respirations. A high-pitched and irritable cry, absent or poor Moro reflex, diminished or absent deep tendon reflexes, decreased muscle tone, and retinal hemorrhages are common.

By the second day of life, reflexes become hyperactive. There may be less spontaneous activity and a weak sucking reflex. The infant may remain hypotonic, become increasingly hypertonic with opisthotonos and spasticity, or regain normal tone and flexion posture. Recovery in the following days may be limited, gradual, or complete. It has been shown that in the infant, the brain stem is selectively more vulnerable than the cerebral cortex to anoxia. This may explain the types of disorders seen in severe asphyxia—ie, pinpoint pupils; absence of cough and gag reflexes; cranial nerve palsies; and disorders of muscle tone, temperature control, and regulation of breathing.

Trauma that may result in subarachnoid or cerebral hemorrhage is usually associated with a history of difficult delivery, often precipitous or breech. The infant may appear well after birth, but within a few hours develops clinical findings of irritability, increased muscle tone, high-pitched cry, respiratory distress, decreased or absent Moro and sucking reflexes, increased or asymmetric muscle tone, twitching, retinal hemorrhages, and dilated pupils. Convulsions may occur. Anemia and shock will occur if bleeding has been of sufficient volume. If bleeding is mild and does not recur, symptoms will begin to improve. The degree of permanent neurologic damage will depend on the extent and location of the injury.

Treatment

The infant who has sustained an injury to the central nervous system requires special care and observation. Good supportive care can reduce the risk of additional injury from hemorrhage, hypoglycemia, hypocalcemia, or aspiration pneumonia. This may include ventilatory and circulatory support until the extent of brain damage can be determined. Prediction of outcome is difficult in the first days of life and should be made with caution. Periodic reassessment and reevaluation are often needed. This should be explained to the parents. Parents need to know *and believe* that the physician and the rest of the health care team will continue to provide support, advice, and assistance during the difficult days of diagnosis and decision making.

Lumbar puncture, CT scanning, and ultrasonography are valuable adjuncts to the clinical examination in determining the extent of the insult and the onset of complications, specifically hydrocephalus.

Prognosis

The behavioral abnormalities that asphyxiated infants have in the immediate newborn period have been correlated with long-term sequelae. These include difficulty in feeding (which necessitates gavage), cyanotic or apneic spells, lethargy, seizures, temperature instability, high-pitched cry, and persistent vomiting. The recovery of muscle tone during the first few days of life in asphyxiated newborn infants has also been helpful in predicting outcome. Infants with behavioral abnormalities and hypotonia tend to have high mortality and morbidity rates, whereas those with increased or normal tone and normal behaviors may have only slight motor handicaps or be completely normal. In general, premature infants have a greater capacity to withstand severe hypoxic insults and recover than do full-term infants. Infants who suffer acute intrapartum or neonatal cardiorespiratory arrest have a high mortality risk, but if resuscitation leads to spontaneous breathing by 30 minutes, the morbidity risk is, surprisingly, as low as 25%.

Bergamasco B et al: Neonatal hypoxia and epileptic risk: A clinical prospective study. *Epilepsia* 1984;**25:**131.

Finer NN et al: Factors affecting outcome in hypoxic-ischemic encephalopathy in term infants. *Am J Dis Child* 1983;**137:**21.

Sarnat HB, Sarnat MS: Neonatal encephalopathy following fetal distress: A clinical and electroencephalographic study. *Arch Neurol* 1976;**33:**696.

Scott H: Outcome of very severe birth asphyxia. *Arch Dis Child* 1976;**51:**712.

Steiner H, Neligan G: Perinatal cardiac arrest: Quality of the survivors. *Arch Dis Child* 1975;**50:**696.

Volpe JJ: Perinatal hypoxic-ischemic brain injury. *Pediatr Clin North Am* 1976;**23:**383.

2. CONVULSIONS

Seizures occurring at the time of delivery or very shortly thereafter in the newborn infants of full-term, uncomplicated pregnancies are rare and should raise the possibility of intrauterine cerebral hemorrhage, pyridoxine dependency, or intoxication with local anesthetics. Common causes of neonatal seizures are discussed in Chapter 23.

Treatment

Phenobarbital is an excellent anticonvulsant in the newborn infant, giving a good anticonvulsive effect at doses that do not cause respiratory depression. For status epilepticus, give 5–10 mg/kg intravenously and repeat in 30 minutes until seizures are controlled or a total dose of 30 mg/kg has been given. Maintenance phenobarbital doses of 5–10 mg/kg/24 h should then be given. Serum levels of the drug may need to be checked at intervals to determine the optimal dosage. If breakthrough seizures occur, diazepam (Valium) may be given in a dose of 0.1–0.3 mg/kg intravenously. However, this drug may exacerbate respiratory depression and it has a half-life of around 15 minutes, so it has limited usefulness. Phenytoin (Dilantin) may be added in a dose of 5–15 mg/kg/24 h for more prolonged seizure control.

In all infants, diagnosis and treatment of the underlying cause of seizures are preferred. For seizures due to metabolic disorders, improvement may be dramatic and the need for anticonvulsants alleviated. For infants who have had central nervous system hemorrhage or infection, resolution of the insult must be achieved before the seizures can be controlled. When structural abnormalities of the brain or genetic diseases are the cause, lifelong drug therapy must be anticipated.

Prognosis

Long-term follow-up studies of children who have had neonatal seizures have shown that the outcome depends principally upon the cause. Thus, newborn infants with hypocalcemic seizures have a very good prognosis. On the other hand, infants with seizures due to anoxia or congenital anomalies have a poor prognosis. Infants with seizures associated with intracerebral hemorrhage or infection have a variable future. Long-term neurologic handicaps and seizure disorders are well predicted by abnormal electroencephalographic findings in the first 1–3 weeks of life.

Donn SM, Grasela TH, Goldstein GW: Safety of a higher loading dose of phenobarbital in the term newborn. *Pediatrics* 1985;**75:**1061.

Rose AL, Lombroso CT: Neonatal seizure states: A study of clinical, pathological, and electroencephalographic features in 137 full-term babies with a long-term follow-up. *Pedatrics* 1970;**45:**404.

Volpe J: Neonatal seizures. *N Engl J Med* 1973;**289:**413.

3. CENTRAL NERVOUS SYSTEM HEMORRHAGE OF THE PREMATURE INFANT

Prior to 35 weeks of gestation, the fetal brain has an immature vascular bed in the germinal matrix. Thus, the premature infant is susceptible to subependymal hemorrhage with rupture of blood into the ventricles and extension into the cerebral cortex.

Clinical Findings

In the past, autopsy studies have shown that premature infants dying between 3 and 7 days of age often had extensive central nervous system hemorrhage, and this was interpreted to mean a uniformly fatal disease. Recent investigators have reported that nearly 30% of infants with birth weights less than 1500 g will have hemorrhages, and two-thirds of these will be asymptomatic. The peak incidence of hemorrhage occurs in infants born at 26–32 weeks of gestation, and factors that appear to increase the likelihood of hemorrhage are male sex, twinning, hyaline membrane disease, ventilator support, and pneumothoraces.

Treatment

It is important to diagnose the extent of hemorrhage by obtaining an ultrasound or CT scan during the third to seventh day of life. If ventricular dilatation with blood is present, serial ultrasound examinations of the brain should be done at weekly intervals. In mild hemorrhages, the blood will resolve and no further ventricular dilatation will occur. In hemorrhages where intraventricular dilatation is marked, some may remain static but others will show progressive hydrocephalus. Research is currently under way to determine if serial lumbar punctures, aggressive osmotic diuresis, or early ventriculoperitoneal shunting is the therapy of choice.

Prognosis

One 2-year follow-up of survivors has shown a good outcome in infants who did not have hemorrhages extending into the cerebral parenchyma or causing ventricular dilatation. Poor outcome has been reported in infants with hydrocephalus in spite of early treatment and resolution on follow-up ultrasound scans. Close developmental follow-up and early intervention programs are indicated. The ability of children who have suffered central nervous system hemorrhages as premature infants to function adequately in school is still undetermined.

Chaplin ER et al: Posthemorrhagic hydrocephalus in the preterm infant. *Pediatrics* 1980;**65:**901.

Korobkin R, Guilleminault C: *Advances in Perinatal Neurology*. Vol 1. SP Medical and Scientific Books, 1979.

Kreusser et al: Serial lumbar punctures for at least temporary amelioration of neonatal posthemorrhagic hydrocephalus. *Pediatrics* 1985;**75:**719.

McDonald MM et al: Role of coagulopathy in newborn intracranial hemorrhage. *Pediatrics* 1984;**74:**26.

Ment LR et al: Intraventricular hemorrhage in the preterm neonate: Timing and cerebral blood flow changes. *J Pediatr* 1984;**104:**419.

Papile LA, Munsick-Bruno G, Schaefer A: Relationship of cerebral intraventricular hemorrhage and early childhood neurologic handicaps. *J Pediatr* 1983;**103:**273.

Papile LA et al: Incidence and evolution of subependymal and intraventricular hemorrhage: A study of infants with birth weights less than 1500 grams. *J Pediatr* 1978;**92:**529.

Tekolste KA, Bennett FC, Mack LA: Follow-up of infants receiving cranial ultrasound for intracranial hemorrhage. *Am J Dis Child* 1985;**139:**299.

Volpe JJ: Neonatal intraventricular hemorrhage. *N Engl J Med* 1981;**304:**886.

CONGENITAL ANOMALIES

Major congenital malformations are seen in 1.5% of live births and account for 22% of perinatal deaths, 18% of stillbirths, and 27% of neonatal deaths. This is one of the most difficult problems, medically and emotionally, in the newborn nursery. For the family, what was anticipated to be a happy event suddenly becomes a devastating experience. The parents must face the reality of the defect and the uncertainty of the infant's immediate needs and long-term prognosis. The parents need honest and sensitive direction from their health care providers, so that they feel involved in decisions made to provide the best possible care for their infant. (Specific congenital anomalies are discussed in Chapters 13, 22, 23, and 33.)

Diagnosis

Maternal, obstetric, and family histories should always be taken. Particularly relevant conditions are polyhydramnios, oligohydramnios, previous birth defects in the family, and previous pregnancy losses. Antepartum diagnosis using ultrasound or amniocentesis may be possible and may help in preparing for resuscitation, diagnostic procedures, and surgery for the infant during the immediate newborn period. Delivery of these infants at a tertiary care center may be critical to their survival.

Most structural defects, however, occur in full-term infants and are unexpected. For these infants, early recognition, stabilizing care, and transfer to an intensive care center are appropriate. Specific diagnostic tests are necessary for infants with significant congenital heart disease, metabolic disorders, and surgically correctable lesions.

Inborn errors of metabolism causing hyperammonemia are life-threatening and usually present unexpectedly in an infant who appears well during the first days of life. Early recognition and transfer to an intensive care center should be carried out so that diagnosis can be made and treatment begun. Peritoneal dialysis or hemodialysis is especially helpful in maintaining the infant, reducing seizures, and correcting electrolyte and serum ammonia levels while diagnostic tests are being done. The results of serum and urine tests for amino acids, organic acids, and urea cycle metabolites can be available within 24 hours. Proper therapy and ultimate prognosis are often dependent on the speed and accuracy with which the diagnosis is made and the severity of the enzymatic defect.

In addition, there are certain non-life-threatening defects that should be identified on the first day of life so that specific care can be initiated. Examples are cleft lip, cleft palate, hip dislocation, clubfoot, and the more life-threatening problems associated with myelomeningocele and chromosomal disorders. The diagnosis of these problems can usually be made by a complete and careful physical examination of the infant.

Treatment

Specific attention to an infant's congenital anomaly in the nursery will often prevent complications and enhance long-term outcome. For example, successful treatment of hip dislocation may be accomplished with merely 6–12 weeks of splinting that is initiated in the nursery. Special methods of feeding the infant with cleft lip or palate can help avoid regurgitation, aspiration, inflammation of nasal mucosa, and poor nutrition and growth. The workup and diagnosis of ambiguous genitalia and the determination of the child's sex are critical for care and for parent bonding.

Consultation with appropriate medical and surgical subspecialists should be done within the first few hours to days of life, depending on the urgency of the problem and the clinical course of the infant. In all cases, both specialty and routine care arrangements must be clearly planned with the parents prior to nursery discharge. The major role of the primary health caretakers of the infant involves communication with the parents. Many families will handle well the stress of an abnormal infant and their own emotional reactions simply with the counseling of a professional person whom they trust. If psychologic or social needs cannot be met, the primary caretaker may be the key person in assisting families to seek and accept professional psychiatric help.

Prognosis

Mortality rates vary depending on the individual anomalies. Infants with anomalies may die in utero, during the newborn period, or within the first year of life. If death seems likely, families should be prepared so that they can grieve appropriately and should be given their choice of having the infant in the hospital or at home. All families suffering stillbirths, neonatal deaths, or infant deaths need opportunities for follow-up discussions and counseling.

The long-term outcome of infants who survive with major congenital anomalies is dependent upon the medical nature of the problem and the family's emotional ability to cope with the infant. Intensive support and subspecialty care offer increasingly better chances for corrective treatment. Physical therapists, occupational therapists, developmental psychologists, and visual and auditory specialists are becoming increasingly available for children ages 0–3 years. The family's ability to find and use an appropriate program for their child is greatly enhanced by a close working relationship between the primary physician, subspecialists, and therapists. The ultimate goal is to provide an environment in which the child's full potential can be reached and to allow parents and siblings to develop their own lives fully and in a satisfying way.

Brown JV et al: Nursery-based interventions with prematurely born babies and their mothers: Are there effects? *J Pediatr* 1980;**97:**487.

Brunner RL, Jordan MK, Berry HK: Early-treated phenylketonuria: Neuropsychologic consequences. *J Pediatr* 1983; **102:**831.

Brusilow SW, Batshaw ML, Waber L: Neonatal hyperammonemic coma. Pages 69–103 in: *Advances in Pediatrics.* Vol 29. Barness LA (editor). Year Book, 1982.

Charney EB et al: Management of the newborn with myelomeningocele: Time for a decision-making process. *Pediatrics* 1985;**75:**58.

Duff RS: Counseling families and deciding care of severely defective children: A way of coping with Medical Vietnam. *Pediatrics* 1981;**67:**315.

Ferry PC: On growing new neurons: Are early intervention programs effective? *Pediatrics* 1981;**67:**38.

Fost N: Counseling families who have a child with a severe congenital anomaly. *Pediatrics* 1981;**67:**321.

Kulkarni P: Postneonatal infant mortality in infants admitted to a neonatal intensive care unit. *Pediatrics* 1978;**62:**178.

Leib S, Benfield DG, Guidubaldi J: Effects of early intervention and stimulation on the preterm infant. *Pediatrics* 1980;**66:**83.

Lewis E: Mourning by the family after a stillbirth or neonatal death. *Arch Dis Child* 1979;**54:**303.

Myers GJ: Myelomeningocoele: The medical aspects. *Pediatr Clin North Am* 1984;**31:**165.

Regemorter NV et al: Congenital malformations in 10,000 consecutive births in a university hospital: Need for genetic counseling and prenatal diagnosis. *J Pediatr* 1984;**104:**386.

Relman AS: Christian Science and the care of children. (Sounding Boards.) *N Engl J Med* 1983;**309:**1639.

Speck WT, Kennell JH: Management of perinatal death. *Pediatr in Rev* 1980;**2:**59.

Swan R: Faith healing, Christian Science, and the medical care of children. (Sounding Boards.) *N Engl J Med* 1983; **309:**1639.

Talbot NA: The position of the Christian Science church. (Sounding Boards.) *N Engl J Med* 1983;**309:**1641.

SELECTED REFERENCES

Avery GB (editor): *Neonatology: Pathophysiology and Management of the Newborn.* Lippincott, 1981.

Avery ME, Taeusch HW (editors): *Schaffer's Diseases of the Newborn,* 5th ed. Saunders, 1984.

Battaglia FC, Meschia G, Quilligan EJ: *Perinatal Medicine.* Vol 2. Mosby, 1978.

Boyd RDH, Battaglia FC: *Perinatal Medicine.* Butterworth, 1983.

Creasy RK, Resnik R (editors): *Maternal and Fetal Medicine: Princples and Practice.* Saunders, 1984.

Frankenburg WK, Camp BW: *Pediatric Screening Tests.* Thomas, 1975.

Hurt H (editor): Symposium on Continuing Care of the High-Risk Infant. *Clin Perinatol* 1984;**11:**3. [Entire issue.]

Kaminetzky HA, Iffy L: *Progress in Perinatology.* Stickley, 1977.

Moss AJ, Adams FH, Emmanoulides GC: *Heart Disease in Infants, Children, and Adolescents,* 2nd ed. Williams & Wilkins, 1977.

Osofsky JD: *Handbook of Infant Development.* Wiley, 1979.

Remington JS, Klein JO (editors): *Infectious Diseases of the Fetus and Newborn Infant,* 2nd ed. Saunders, 1983.

Solomon LB, Esterly NB: *Neonatal Dermatology.* Saunders, 1973.

Volpe JJ: *Neurology of the Newborn.* Saunders, 1981.

4 Normal Childhood Nutrition & Its Disorders

Donough O'Brien, MD, FRCP, & K. Michael Hambidge, MC, FRCP

GENERAL NUTRITIONAL REQUIREMENTS & COMPOSITION OF FOODS

Requirements for various nutrients change during childhood depending on the growth rates of different tissues; they also vary considerably with sex, stage of maturation, physical activity, and body build. The nutritional needs during any growth period will depend on the nutritional status of the child at that time and on whether or not a given nutrient can be stored by the body. The recommended daily allowances (Tables 4–1 and 4–2) may be used as guides; however, differences in needs should be recognized for each child. A child's general health and conformity to established growth percentiles are the best indices of nutritional status.

CALORIES

Total caloric requirements for children rise with age in a curve that roughly parallels the height and weight curves. Appetite is a reliable index of caloric needs of most healthy children. The recommended caloric intakes for males and females at different ages are given in Table 4–3, but they can be approximated by adding 100 kcal per year of age to a base of 1000 kcal.

Caloric excess can be as undesirable as caloric deficiency. Important factors in considering the quantity of food an infant will voluntarily consume are the bulk of the food and the energy needs of the child. Intake also depends to some extent on the caloric concentration of the feeding. Human milk and most commercial formulas average 20 kcal/oz, but higher caloric densities of 24 or 27 kcal/oz are available for the low-birth-weight infant.

CARBOHYDRATES

The normal diet consists of approximately 50% calories as carbohydrate, 35% calories as fat, and 15% calories as protein. Carbohydrate intake is often higher in the diets of people in the lower socioeconomic groups, where its consumption is associated with a higher incidence of obesity. Humans have no set requirement for carbohydrate, and it is not considered "essential." Carbohydrate provides about 4 kcal/g consumed. Starch and sucrose are the major carbohydrates ingested from plant foods. The former is a polysaccharide that must be hydrolyzed to glucose prior to absorption. Modified corn or tapioca starches that affect the texture of foods may make up 15% of calories in some formulas and a substantial part of the total solids in certain infant foods. The greater part of ingested starch is converted to maltose by salivary amylase working in the mouth and stomach and by pancreatic amylase, which has similar activity in the intestine. The disaccharides then enter the intestinal mucosa, where final hydrolysis and absorption or metabolism of the monosaccharides occurs.

The major disaccharides ingested are lactose (glucose + galactose), sucrose (glucose + fructose), and maltose (glucose + glucose). Milk contains primarily lactose, and intestinal lactase activity is highest in young infants. Lactase activity falls after infancy to lower levels than sucrase or maltase activity and is most easily compromised following diarrhea, malnutrition, or other gastrointestinal insults. Restriction of lactose-containing formulas in diarrhea is thus physiologically wise. Black children and American Indian children normally have a lessening of lactase activity before adolescence and are thereafter less able to tolerate large quantities of milk products. There is some evidence, however, that chronic lactase deficiency may be related to subclinical enteric infection rather than genetic factors. Premature infants may also have a reduced ability to hydrolyze lactose.

The term dietary fiber comprises certain inert carbohydrate polymers, eg, cellulose, pectin, guar gum. They appear to increase stool water, decrease intestinal transit time, and delay carbohydrate absorption. Children's diets in North America are low in fiber, but the significance of this is not known.

American Academy of Pediatrics: Plant fiber in the pediatric diet. *Pediatrics* 1981;**67**:572.

PROTEINS

In contrast to carbohydrate, protein is essential for growth and life. There are 8 essential amino acids

Table 4–1. Recommended dietary allowances of the Food and Nutrition Board, National Academy of Sciences–National Research Council.[1] (Revised 1980.)
Designed for the maintenance of good nutrition of practically all healthy people in the USA.

		Weight		Height			Fat-Soluble Vitamins			Water-Soluble Vitamins							Minerals					
	Age (Years)	(kg)	(lb)	(cm)	(in)	Protein (g)	Vitamin A (μg RE)[3]	Vitamin D (μg)[4]	Vitamin E (mg α-TE)[5]	Vitamin C (mg)	Thiamine (mg)	Riboflavin (mg)	Niacin (mg NE)[6]	Vitamin B_6 (mg)	Folacin[7] (μg)	Vitamin B_{12} (μg)	Calcium (mg)	Phosphorus (mg)	Magnesium (mg)	Iron (mg)	Zinc (mg)	Iodine (μg)
Infants	0–0.5	6	13	60	24	kg × 2.2	420	10	3	35	0.3	0.4	6	0.3	30	0.5[8]	360	240	50	10	3	40
	0.5–1	9	20	71	28	kg × 2	400	10	4	35	0.5	0.6	8	0.6	45	1.5	540	360	70	15	5	50
Children	1–3	13	29	90	35	23	400	10	5	45	0.7	0.8	9	0.9	100	2	800	800	150	15	10	70
	4–6	20	44	112	44	30	500	10	6	45	0.9	1	11	1.3	200	2.5	800	800	200	10	10	90
	7–10	28	62	132	52	34	700	10	7	45	1.2	1.4	16	1.6	300	3	800	800	250	10	10	120
Males	11–14	45	99	157	62	45	1000	10	8	50	1.4	1.6	18	1.8	400	3	1200	1200	350	18	15	150
	15–18	66	145	176	69	56	1000	10	10	60	1.4	1.7	18	2	400	3	1200	1200	400	18	15	150
	19–22	70	154	177	70	56	1000	7.5	10	60	1.5	1.7	19	2.2	400	3	800	800	350	10	15	150
	23–50	70	154	178	70	56	1000	5	10	60	1.4	1.6	18	2.2	400	3	800	800	350	10	15	150
	51+	70	154	178	70	56	1000	5	10	60	1.2	1.4	16	2.2	400	3	800	800	350	10	15	150
Females	11–14	46	101	157	62	46	800	10	8	50	1.1	1.3	15	1.8	400	3	1200	1200	300	18	15	150
	15–18	55	120	163	64	46	800	10	8	60	1.1	1.3	14	2	400	3	1200	1200	300	18	15	150
	19–22	55	120	163	64	44	800	7.5	8	60	1.1	1.3	14	2	400	3	800	800	300	18	15	150
	23–50	55	120	163	64	44	800	5	8	60	1	1.2	13	2	400	3	800	800	300	18	15	150
	51+	55	120	163	64	44	800	5	8	60	1	1.2	13	2	400	3	800	800	300	10	15	150
Pregnant[2]						+30	+200	+5	+2	+20	+0.4	+0.3	+2	+0.6	+400	+1	+400	+400	+150		+5	+25
Lactating[2]						+20	+400	+5	+3	+40	+0.5	+0.5	+5	+0.5	+100	+1	+400	+400	+150		+10	+50

[1] The allowances are intended to provide for individual variations among most normal persons as they live in the USA under usual environmental stresses. Diets should be based on a variety of common foods in order to provide other nutrients for which human requirements have been less well defined.

[2] The increased iron requirement during pregnancy cannot be met by the iron content of habitual North American diets or by the existing iron stores of many women; therefore, the use of 30–60 mg supplemental iron is recommended. Iron needs during lactation are not substantially different from those of nonpregnant women, but continued supplementation of the mother for 2–3 months after parturition is advisable in order to replenish stores depleted by pregnancy.

[3] Retinol equivalents: 1 μg retinol or 6 μg β-carotene = 1 RE.

[4] As cholecalciferol: 10 μg cholecalciferol = 400 IU vitamin D.

[5] α-Tocopherol equivalents: 1 mg D-α-tocopherol = 1 α-TE.

[6] Niacin equivalents: 1 mg niacin or 60 mg dietary tryptophan = 1 NE.

[7] The folacin allowances refer to dietary sources as determined by *Lactobacillus casei* assay after treatment with enzymes ("conjugases") to make polyglutamyl forms of the vitamin available to the test organism.

[8] The RDA for vitamin B_{12} in infants is based on average concentration of the vitamin in human milk. The allowances after weaning are based on energy intake (as recommended by the American Academy of Pediatrics) and consideration of other factors such as intestinal absorption.

Table 4–2. Estimated safe and adequate daily dietary intakes of additional selected vitamins and minerals.[1]

		Vitamins			Trace Elements[2]						Electrolytes		
	Age (Years)	Vitamin K (μg)	Biotin (μg)	Pantothenic Acid (mg)	Copper (mg)	Manganese (mg)	Fluoride (mg)	Chromium (mg)	Selenium (mg)	Molybdenum (mg)	Sodium (mg)	Potassium (mg)	Chloride (mg)
Infants	0–0.5	12	35	2	0.5–0.7	0.5–0.7	0.1–0.5	0.01–0.04	0.01–0.04	0.03–0.06	115–350	350–925	275–700
	0.5–1	10–20	50	3	0.7–1	0.7–1	0.2–1	0.02–0.06	0.02–0.06	0.04–0.08	250–750	425–1275	400–1200
Children and adolescents	1–3	15–30	65	3	1–1.5	1–1.5	0.5–1.5	0.02–0.08	0.02–0.08	0.05–0.1	325–975	550–1650	500–1500
	4–6	20–40	85	3–4	1.5–2	1.5–2	1–2.5	0.03–0.12	0.03–0.12	0.06–0.15	450–1350	775–2325	700–2100
	7–10	30–60	120	4–5	2–2.5	2–3	1.5–2.5	0.05–0.2	0.05–0.2	0.1–0.3	600–1800	1000–3000	925–2775
	11+	50–100	100–200	4–7	2–3	2.5–5	1.5–2.5	0.05–0.2	0.05–0.2	0.15–0.5	900–2700	1525–4575	1400–4200
Adults		70–140	100–200	4–7	2–3	2.5–5	1.5–4	0.05–0.2	0.05–0.2	0.15–0.5	1100–3300	1875–5625	1700–5100

[1] From Recommended Dietary Allowances, Revised 1980. Food and Nutrition Board, National Academy of Sciences–National Research Council. Because there is less information on which to base allowances, these figures are not given in the main table of the RDAs and are provided here in the form of ranges of recommended intakes.

[2] Since the toxic levels for many trace elements may be only several times usual intakes, the upper levels for the trace elements given in this table should not be habitually exceeded.

Table 4–3. Estimated safe and adequate daily dietary intake of calories.*

Individual	Age (yr)	Energy (kcal)
Infants	0.0–0.5	kg × 117
	0.5–1.0	kg × 108
Children	1–3	1300
	4–6	1800
	7–10	2400
Males	11–14	2800
	15–18	3000
	19–22	3000
	23–50	2700
	51+	2400
Females	11–14	2400
	15–18	2100
	19–22	2100
	23–50	2000
	51+	1800
Pregnant		+300
Lactating		+500

* From Recommended Dietary Allowances, Revised 1980. Food and Nutrition Board, National Academy of Sciences–National Research Council.

that cannot be synthesized by adults: isoleucine, leucine, lysine, methionine, phenylalanine, threonine, tryptophan, and valine. Histidine may be added to this list. Cysteine and tyrosine are considered partially essential because their rates of synthesis are limited and may be inadequate in certain circumstances. During early development, rates of synthesis of cysteine, tyrosine, and perhaps taurine do not provide sufficient amounts of these substances. Precise requirements for total and individual essential amino acids are not known; needs are relatively high in infancy and decrease with age. The essential amino acids in human milk provide about 45% of total amino acid requirements. If one essential amino acid is missing, body protein catabolism will temporarily supply the missing amino acid for necessary protein formation, and serum levels will rise coincidentally. Within 1–2 weeks, however, weight loss and protein malnutrition will follow. Protein malnutrition may also occur with seemingly adequate protein intake if caloric intake is low. Protein provides about 4 kcal/g consumed.

Pregnancy and lactation, rapid growth, infection, and tissue repair all increase protein needs. Athletic activity and heavy physical work increase caloric demands but probably not the need for protein.

Animal proteins contain essential amino acids in a ratio that meets human needs more closely than do plant proteins. Wheat, rice, and sorghum are deficient in lysine, and legume proteins are deficient in methionine and cystine. Appropriate mixtures of vegetable proteins may be necessary for maximal nutritional efficiency.

Proteins are hydrolyzed as a result of pepsin activity in the stomach, pancreatic trypsin digestion in the intestine, and peptidase digestion by the pancreatic and intestinal peptidases. The resultant amino acids may be further catabolized in the intestine or may be absorbed into the portal blood system. It is thought by some that the passage of large proteins through the intestinal mucosa results in allergies to those proteins. Protein malabsorption and leakage may occur in diseases such as intestinal lymphangiectasia.

FATS

Fats provide about 9 kcal/g of food consumed and represent both the most compact and most important energy stores because they are not solubilized in water. In addition, certain polyunsaturated fatty acids, primarily linoleic but also linolenic and arachidonic acids, are "essential" in that they cannot be synthesized by humans and must be provided in the diet of small infants as about 1% of calories to ensure normal growth and prevent desquamating dermatitis. Commercial formulas usually contain over 3% of calories as linoleic acid or greater than 300 mg/100 kcal. Formulas high in polyunsaturated fat and also in supplemental iron may cause an increased degree of red cell hemolysis in low-birth-weight infants if they do not also contain additional vitamin E. Vitamin E, 0.7 IU/100 kcal or 1 IU/g of linoleic acid, is recommended. Unsaturated fatty acids are present in only small amounts in animal fats but comprise over 50% of soy and corn oils. Coconut oil, however, contains less than 1.5% linoleic acid.

Linoleic acid is also important because it is the immediate substrate for the prostaglandins and for their derivatives, thromboxanes and prostacyclins. The latter are short-lived but important cell-regulatory substances. Finally, increased consumption of polyunsaturated fats—in combination with reducing cholesterol intake—has been shown to reduce blood cholesterol levels, which may diminish the chances of coronary heart disease.

Triglycerides are emulsified by bile salts in the presence of mono- and diglycerides. This provides a large surface area for the action of pancreatic lipase, which mainly acts to remove the 2 outer fatty acids in the 1 and 3 positions on the glycerol.

Long-chain fatty acids ($> C_{16}$) are absorbed in the free state or as monoglycerides into the mucosal cell, where they are resynthesized into triglyceride, coated with protein, and extruded into the lacteals as chylomicrons. Medium-chain (C_{10}–C_{16}) and short-chain ($< C_{10}$) fatty acids may be absorbed into mucosal cells in any form as mono-, di-, or triglycerides or in the free state. Resynthesized in the mucosal cell into triglyceride, they pass into the portal blood. Short-chain fatty acids also enter the portal blood and are attached to albumin.

Medium-chain triglyceride (MCT) preparations have an obvious role in patients who for a variety of reasons cannot absorb long-chain triglycerides.

Special restriction of dietary lipid in infancy is not indicated except in the obese.

Naismith DJ et al: Reappraisal of linoleic acid requirement of the young infant, with particular regard to use of modified cows' milk formulae. *Arch Dis Child* 1978;**53:**845.

VITAMINS

Vitamins are organic compounds which the body cannot make in adequate quantity for optimal health and which must be provided from external sources. The vitamins are divided into the fat-soluble vitamins—A, D, E, and K—and the water-soluble vitamins—vitamin C and the B complex. The fat-soluble vitamins are stored in the liver, and excess quantities can lead to toxicity. The water-soluble vitamins are not stored in the body in large amounts, and excess quantities—such as with vitamin C "megadosage" in cold prevention—just result in excessive excretion. Sources and recommended dietary allowances of the various vitamins are outlined in Tables 4–1 and 4–2.

MAJOR & TRACE ELEMENTS

Major elements required for adequate nutrition are sodium, potassium, chloride, calcium, phosphorus, and magnesium. Sulfur is also necessary for sulfur-containing amino acids. Important trace elements are iron (see Chapter 16), iodine, copper, zinc, and selenium. Other trace elements thought to be important are chromium, manganese, and molybdenum. Cobalt is an essential component of the vitamin B_{12} molecule. The extent to which humans may be at risk from nutritional deficiencies of these elements is not known, but it is apparent that specific trace element deficiencies are of clinical importance in a variety of circumstances.

Sodium, Potassium, & Chloride

High sodium intake or high ratios of sodium to potassium in infancy and childhood may cause poor health in later years, especially hypertension. Kidneys in normal full-term infants and children can process high sodium loads but may not be able to process the relatively high mineral content of cow's milk, so that the risk of dehydration and hypernatremia is increased whenever diarrhea or other conditions increase the demand for water. Therefore, the lower sodium content of human milk is preferable for both short- and long-term reasons. The ratio of sodium to potassium in formula should not exceed 1:1 and that of sodium and potassium to chloride should be at least 3:2. Metabolic alkalosis has occurred in infants receiving a soybean formula deficient in chloride.

Wolfsdorf JI, Senior B: Failure to thrive and metabolic alkalosis: Adverse effects of a chloride-deficient formula in two infants. *JAMA* 1980;**243:**1068.

Calcium, Phosphorus, & Magnesium

Calcium, phosphorus, and magnesium make up about 98% of total body mineral content. The greatest amount of these 3 substances is found in bone hydroxyapatite: calcium, 99%; phosphorus, 85%; and magnesium, 66%. Phosphorus is the major intracellular anion, and magnesium is the second most common intracellular cation (after potassium). Calcium, phosphorus, and magnesium all have important roles in cellular metabolism in addition to their structural function.

Calcium homeostasis is governed by the following: dietary content; passive intestinal absorption and absorption facilitated by 1,25-dihydroxycholecalciferol; renal excretion facilitated by parathyroid hormone; and bone absorption regulated and facilitated by parathyroid hormone and vitamin D. Phosphorus levels are governed by intake and by the contrary actions of parathyroid hormone and vitamin D within the renal tubules. Parathyroid hormone reduces renal tubular reabsorption of phosphorus. Vitamin D is thought to be required for renal tubular transport of phosphorus. Magnesium metabolism is less well understood, perhaps because clinical disorders are infrequent.

Milk and fortified cereals are the most important sources of calcium in infants and young children. In very small premature infants, calcium and phosphorus intake may be insufficient despite formula modification.

Forbes GB: Calcium, phosphorus and magnesium. Pages 111–121 in: *Pediatric Nutrition Handbook.* American Academy of Pediatrics, 1985.

INFANT FEEDING

BREAST FEEDING

Advantages & Disadvantages of Breast Feeding

A. Advantages: Breast feeding has been encouraged mainly for its psychologic advantages, economy, nutritional superiority, and immunologic benefits. For normal infants, the composition of human milk appears ideal and has the following advantages over cow's milk or formula: (1) The specific anti-infectious elements of colostrum and milk (including leukocytes, secretory IgA, lysozyme, lactoferrin, bifidus factor, and others) provide protection from gastrointestinal and upper respiratory tract disease and may play a role in the prevention of necrotizing enterocolitis. (2) A lower osmotic load, especially in regard to sodium, potassium, and phosphorus. (3) A more efficient absorption of nutrients such as iron and zinc.

(4) A lower protein content with a higher ratio of whey to casein. The importance of the higher taurine content is not yet fully understood. (5) A possible long-term advantage in the prevention of cardiovascular disease because the higher cholesterol content (compared to formula) may induce the production of enzymes required for cholesterol catabolism. (6) A higher vitamin C content. Nursing is of benefit to the mother in the postpartum period because it is associated with vigorous contraction of the uterine musculature and speeds the return of that organ to normal size and position.

B. Disadvantages and Contraindications: There are only a few absolute contraindications to breast feeding, eg. galactosemia in the infant and active tuberculosis in the mother. Breast feeding is not advisable if the mother has strong negative feelings about it.

There are temporary problems associated with nursing a weak, ill, or premature infant or one with cleft palate or lip. The mother may need to pump the milk from her breasts until the infant is able to nurse. Nursing mothers may experience discomfort from engorgement of the breasts and sore or cracked nipples in the first few days after delivery. Mastitis may occur in the nursing mother and is best managed by antibiotic therapy and continued nursing of the infant to keep the affected breast well emptied. If breast abscess occurs, surgical drainage is usually required, and temporary pump expression may be necessary on the affected side.

Breast feeding is not invariably successful and needs supervision. Even a contented infant may be undernourished. However, some decline in weight for age percentiles after 3 months should not necessarily be taken as an indication of inadequate nutrition, since the commonly used percentile charts have been constructed from data on infants who have been primarily formula-fed. Infants of vegan mothers are vulnerable to specific vitamin deficiencies, eg. vitamin B_{12}. Rarely, a woman does not secrete normal quantities of zinc into her milk. Only premature infants are affected. Human milk banks throughout the USA can provide milk for premature infants or for infants with immunodeficiency, allergy, or malabsorption syndrome. Strict microbiologic control is necessary.

Management of Breast Feeding

When a mother wishes to nurse her infant, success or failure is related to the amount of factual information given to her and the emotional support of physicians, nurses, and family. Organizations such as the La Leche League, the Nursing Mothers of Australia, and the Plunkett Society in New Zealand have been very effective in promoting breast feeding.

It is important for a mother to know that very few women are unable to nurse their babies. She should know that breast milk may look "weak or dilute," but if the infant is not satisfied the problem is one of supply and not quality. It is essential that she understand that milk production can be increased by frequent nursing and that the supply of milk lags behind the infant's demand for approximately 24–48 hours. She should know that if she substitutes supplementary feedings for nursing—especially in the first weeks after birth—the supply of milk will decrease. Many working mothers find it possible to nurse their infants once milk production is well established. They may need to express milk at work when separated from their infants.

The importance of breast feeding in third world countries has long been emphasized by WHO and UNICEF. Formula feeding without an adequate family income or a clean water supply can be hazardous.

Ovulation may be inhibited for a time in a woman who is breast feeding frequently, but if pregnancy must be avoided, other forms of contraception are recommended.

Technique of Nursing

A. Breast Preparation Before Delivery: It is thought by some that nipple soreness can be minimized by preparation of the breasts prior to delivery. The method recommended is as follows: Cup one breast from below with the palm of the hand and, with a soft washcloth, rub the nipple 4 or 5 times. Then gently pull the nipple several times. This can be done once or twice daily.

B. Preparation for Nursing: A daily bath is all that is necessary for cleanliness of the breasts. When nursing, the mother should assume a comfortable position lying down or sitting in a rocking or upright chair.

C. Nursing the Infant: The infant should be fed when signs of hunger appear and should be offered both breasts at each feeding for maximum milk production. The infant usually nurses for about 10 minutes on the first side, completely emptying this breast, and then finishes the feeding on the opposite breast. The infant should be expected to nurse 8–10 times in 24 hours during the first month, and the mother should be encouraged to rest in order to meet this schedule.

The rooting reflex is stimulated by touching the baby's cheek with the nipple (not pushing the mouth toward the breast). It is important to help the infant grasp sufficient areola and to have the nipple well back in the baby's mouth.

The breast may need to be held away from the infant's nostrils once sucking begins.

After 1 or 2 minutes of nursing, the letdown reflex occurs, and the infant may have difficulty swallowing the rapidly flowing milk. The letdown affects both breasts simultaneously.

After nursing, the infant usually releases the nipple. If not, suction should be broken by gently opening the baby's mouth before removing the breast. Burping the infant following feeding is usually done, but breast-fed infants do not swallow as much air as bottle-fed infants.

Colostrum

Colostrum is a yellow, alkaline breast secretion that may be present in the last few months of pregnancy and for the first 2–4 days after delivery. It has a higher specific gravity (1.040–1.060), a higher protein, vitamin A, and mineral content, and a lower carbohydrate and fat content than breast milk.

Transmission of Drugs & Toxins in Breast Milk

A. Factors Affecting Drug Excretion in Milk: Virtually all drugs consumed by the mother will appear in her milk to some degree, usually in homeopathic amounts. Drug excretion into milk is affected by the drug's ionization, lipid solubility, protein-binding qualities, molecular size, and other factors, so that generalizations are difficult to make. Effects on the infant also depend upon the method and time of drug intake by the mother, the dosage, the metabolites produced, and oral absorption of the drug by the infant. Nursing prior to drug ingestion is thought to help minimize milk levels of drugs at feeding times.

B. Drugs Presenting a Hazard to the Infant: Careful observation of a nursing infant whose mother is taking medication is warranted. Very few drugs are actually contraindicated, eg, radioactive compounds, antimetabolites, lithium, diazepam (Valium), chloramphenicol, and tetracycline. When a course of therapy of a potentially hazardous drug will be brief, the mother can temporarily interrupt breast feeding and express her milk to maintain her supply.

Weaning

There is no best time for weaning, which can take place according to the needs and desires of both infant and mother. Gradual weaning is preferred. Cup or bottle feedings are increased progressively over a period of several weeks as breast feedings are omitted.

American Academy of Pediatrics. Committee on Nutrition, and Canadian Paediatric Society Nutrition Committee: Breast feeding. *Pediatrics* 1978;**62:**591.

Bowes WA Jr: The effect of medications on the lactating mother and her infant. *Clin Obstet Gynecol* 1980;**23:**1073.

Jelliffe DB, Jelliffe EFP: *Human Milk in the Modern World.* Oxford Univ Press, 1979.

Neifert MR: Returning to breast feeding. *Clin Obstet Gynecol* 1980;**23:**1061.

Neville MC, Neifert MR (editors): *Lactation: Physiology, Nutrition, and Breast Feeding.* Plenum Press, 1983.

Roddey OF, Martin ES, Swetenburg RL: Critical weight loss and malnutrition in breast-fed infants. *Am J Dis Child* 1981;**135:**597.

Smith DS: Harmful chemicals and drugs in breast milk. *Pediatr in Rev* 1981;**2:**279.

Whitehead RG, Paul AA: Growth charts and the assessment of infant feeding practices in the Western world and in developing countries. *Early Hum Dev* 1984;**9:**187.

Zmora E, Gorodischer R, Bar-Ziv J: Multiple nutritional deficiencies in infants from a strict vegetarian community. *Am J Dis Child* 1979;**133:**141.

INFANT FORMULAS

A variety of satisfactory prepared formulas, modified from cow's milk, are available commercially (Table 4–4). Cow's milk itself is not now recommended for infant feeding because of its relatively high osmotic load, its low content of linoleic acid, and the poor availability of its iron content.

Proteins

Human milk contains 1.3–1.6 g of protein per 100 kcal, whereas cow's milk contains 5.1 g/100 kcal and most commercial formulas contain 2.3 g/kcal (Table 4–6). The protein requirement for a small premature infant is still a matter of debate, although recent studies indicate that weight gains are probably similar in infants receiving 2.25–5 g/kg/d. It has been suggested that growth in length and body maturation may be enhanced by a higher protein intake, whereas edema and low serum protein levels are more common with lower serum protein intake.

Fats

Both human milk and cow's milk contain approximately 3.5% fat, and fats account for about 50% of the calories in either human or cow's milk. Thus, fat malabsorption should be considered in infants who fail to thrive. Human milk has more fat (7% of calories) as the essential fatty acid linoleic acid than does cow's milk (1% of calories). Formulas should contain at least 3.3 g of fat per 100 kcal (30% of calories), including 300 mg of linoleic acid per 100 kcal.

Low-birth-weight infants are less able to absorb butterfat because of hepatic immaturity and decreased bile salt synthesis. Formulas containing vegetable oils or medium-chain triglycerides are therefore recommended initially.

Carbohydrates

Table 4–6 shows that a higher percentage of calories are derived from carbohydrate when breast milk is consumed compared to cow's milk. Human milk contains about 7% carbohydrate compared to 4.5% for cow's milk. Lactose (galactose-glucose) is the major sugar in both. Small premature infants may not have fully developed intestinal lactate activity and may develop osmotic diarrhea with a secondary low stool pH, dehydration, and acidosis. A mild form of incomplete lactose malabsorption can apparently also exist in premature infants without these symptoms.

Ash

The ash content of milk refers to the minerals and includes primarily sodium, potassium, chlorine, calcium, and phosphate. The osmolality of breast milk is about 116 mosm/L and that of cow's milk 307 mosm/L. The increased calcium and phosphorus content of formulas for premature infants protects against rickets.

Table 4–4. Normal and special infant formulas.*

	Protein Source	Carbohydrate Source	Fat Source	Indications for Use	Comments (Nutritional Considerations)
Milk and milk-based formulas					
Evaporated milk formulas Cow's milk	Milk protein: whey/casein ratio: 18:82	Lactose, sucrose	Butterfat	For full-term infants with no special nutritional requirements. Undiluted cow's milk after 6 months only.	Supplement with iron and vitamin C; also A and D if not fortified.
Commercial infant formulas					
SMA (Wyeth)	Nonfat cow's milk, demineralized whey: whey/casein ratio: 60:40	Lactose	Oleo, coconut, oleic, and soy oils	For full-term and premature infants with no special nutritional requirements.	Supplemented with iron, 12 mg/L.
Enfamil (Mead Johnson)	Nonfat cow's milk, demineralized whey: whey/casein ratio: 60:40	Lactose	Soy, coconut oils	For full-term and premature infants with no special nutritional requirements.	Available fortified with iron, 1 or 12 mg/L.
Similac (Ross)	Nonfat cow's milk: whey/casein ratio: 18:82	Lactose	Soy and coconut oils, mono- and diglycerides	For full-term and premature infants with no special nutritional requirements.	Available fortified with iron, 12 mg/L.
Similac With Whey (Ross)	Nonfat cow's milk and demineralized whey	Lactose	Soy and coconut oils	For full-term and premature infants with no special nutritional requirements.	Whey/casein ratio similar to human milk. Fortified with iron, 12 mg/L.
Milumil (Milupa)	Casein-predominant milk base	Lactose, corn syrup, cornstarch	Coconut oil (60%), soy oil (40%)	For full-term infants with no special nutritional requirements.	Fortified with iron, 10 mg/L. Low in lactose.
Products for premature infants					
Preemie SMA (Wyeth)	Milk protein, demineralized whey: whey/casein ratio: 60:40	Maltodextrins, lactose	Oleo, coconut, oleic, and soy oils, MCT (coconut source)	For low-birth-weight infants.	Protein, 2.5 g/100 kcal. Calcium/phosphorus ratio: 1.9:1.
Similac Special Care (Ross)	Nonfat cow's milk, demineralized whey solids: whey/casein ratio: 60:40	Corn syrup solids, lactose	MCT, corn and coconut oils	For low-birth-weight infants.	Calcium/phosphorus ratio: 2:1. Osmolality, 20 kcal/oz: 250 mosm/kg water; 24 kcal/oz: 290 mosm/kg water.
Enfamil Premature Formula (Mead Johnson)	Nonfat cow's milk, demineralized whey: whey/casein ratio: 60:40	Corn syrup solids	Corn oil, MCT (coconut source), coconut oil	For rapidly growing low-birth-weight infants and infants with special nutritional requirements.	Protein, 3 g/100 kcal. Calcium/phosphorus ratio: 2:1. Osmolality 300 mosm/kg water.
Similac 24 LBW (Ross)	Nonfat cow's milk	Corn syrup solids, lactose	MCT, coconut, and soy oils, mono- and diglycerides	For rapidly growing low-birth-weight infants and infants with special nutritional requirements.	Protein, 2.7 g/100 kcal. Osmolality 290 mosm/kg water
Products for milk protein-sensitive infants ("milk allergy")					
Prosobee (Mead Johnson)	Soy protein isolate	Corn syrup solids	Soy and coconut oils	With milk protein allergy, lactose intolerance, lactase deficiency, galactosemia.	Hypoallergenic. Zero band antigen. Lactose- and sucrose-free.
Isomil (Ross)	Soy protein isolate	Corn syrup, sucrose	Soy and coconut oils	With milk protein allergy, lactose intolerance, lactase deficiency, galactosemia.	Soy protein isolate. Lactose-free.

* Committee on Nutrition, American Academy of Pediatrics: Commentary on breast feeding and infant formulas including proposed standards for formulas. *Pediatrics* 1976;**57**:278. Committee on Nutrition, American Academy of Pediatrics: Nutritional needs of low-birth-weight infants. *Pediatrics* 1977;**60**:519.

Table 4–4 (cont'd). Normal and special infant formulas.*

	Protein Source	Carbohydrate Source	Fat Source	Indications for Use	Comments (Nutritional Considerations)
Products for milk protein-sensitive infants ("milk allergy") (cont'd)					
Nursoy (Wyeth)	Whey protein isolate	Sucrose	Safflower, soy, and coconut oils	With lactose intolerance, cow's milk protein allergy.	
Products for infants with malabsorption syndromes					
RCF (Ross)	Soy protein isolate		Soy and coconut oils	With carbohydrate intolerance.	Carbohydrate is added according to amount infant will tolerate.
Portagen (Mead Johnson)	Sodium caseinate	Corn syrup solids, sucrose	MCT (coconut source) and corn oil	For impaired fat absorption secondary to pancreatic insufficiency, bile acid deficiency, intestinal resection, lymphatic anomalies.	Fat: 87% MCT, 12% corn oil. Nutritionally complete.
Nutramigen (Mead Johnson)	Casein hydrolysate	Sucrose, modified tapioca starch	Corn oil	For infants and children intolerant to food proteins. Use in galactosemic patients.	Enzymatic hydrolysate of casein. Hypoallergenic formula. Nutritionally complete.
Pregestimil (Mead Johnson)	Casein hydrolysate and L-amino acids	Glucose polymerase, modified tapioca starch	Corn oil, MCT	Disaccharidase deficiencies, malabsorption syndromes, cystic fibrosis.	Nutritionally complete, easily digestible protein, carbohydrate, and fat.
Vital HN (Ross)	Partially hydrolyzed wheat, meat, and soy proteins; L-amino acids	Hydrolyzed cornstarch and sucrose	Safflower oil, MCT (coconut source)	With impaired digestion or absorption, cystic fibrosis.	Nutritionally complete hydrolyzed diet. Osmolality 460 mosm/kg water at 1 kcal/mL.
Specialty formulas					
Lonalac (Mead Johnson) Powder	Casein	Lactose	Coconut	For children with congestive cardiac failure.	For long-term management, additional sodium must be given. Supplement with vitamins C and D and iron. Na = 1 meq/L.
Similac PM 60/40 (Ross) Powder	Demineralized, delactosed whey	Lactose	Coconut, corn oils	For newborns predisposed to hypocalcemia and infants with impaired renal and cardiovascular functions.	Low phosphorus. Relatively low solute load. Na = 7 meq/L.
Amin-Aid (American McGaw)	Essential amino acids (including L-histidine)	Maltodextrin sucrose	Partially hydrogenated soybean oil, lecithin, mono- and diglycerides	Essential amino acid and energy supplement for nutritional support of patients with acute or chronic renal failure.	Low electrolyte content. Osmolarity 850 mosm/L at 2 kcal/mL.
Elemental diets for tube feeding					
Vivonex (Norwich Eaton)	L-Amino acids	Glucose oligosaccharides	Safflower oil	Used as general dietary supplement or as sole nutritional source in malabsorption.	Pure amino acid base. Osmolality 550 mosm/kg water at 1 kcal/mL. Also high in nitrogen.

* Committee on Nutrition, American Academy of Pediatrics: Commentary on breast feeding and infant formulas including proposed standards for formulas. *Pediatrics* 1976;**57**:278. Committee on Nutrition, American Academy of Pediatrics: Nutritional needs of low-birth-weight infants. *Pediatrics* 1977;**60**:519.

Table 4–4 (cont'd). Normal and special infant formulas.*

	Protein Source	Carbohydrate Source	Fat Source	Indications for Use	Comments (Nutritional Considerations)
Modular formulas					
Polycose (Ross)		Glucose polymers			Carbohydrate only. A powdered or liquid calorie supplement. Powder: 32 kcal/tbsp.
MCT Oil (Mead Johnson)			90% MCT (coconut source)	With fat malabsorption.	Fat only. 8.3 kcal/g. 115 kcal/tbsp (15 mL).
Propac (Biosearch)	Whey		(See comments)	Protein supplement. For enteral use.	Protein with lecithin. 1 package (19.5 g) provides 15 g protein, 1.6 g fat, and 78 kcal.
For infants with inborn errors					
Lofenalac (Mead Johnson)	Casein hydrolysate, L-amino acids	Corn syrup solids, modified tapioca starch	Corn oil	For infants and children with phenylketonuria.	80 mg phenylalanine per 100 g. Must be supplemented with other foods to provide mineral phenylalanine.
Phenyl-Free (Mead Johnson)	L-Amino acids	Sucrose, corn syrup solids, modified tapioca starch	Corn oil	For children over 1 year of age with phenylketonuria.	Phenylalanine-free. Permits increased supplementation with normal foods.
PKU 1 (Milupa)†	L-Amino acids	Sucrose		For infants with phenylketonuria. (Available as PKU 2 for children over 1 year of age.)	Phenylalanine- and fat-free. Contains vitamins, minerals, and trace elements. Must be supplemented with phenylalanine/protein, carbohydrate, and fat.
MSUD Diet (Mead Johnson) Powder	L-Amino acids	Corn syrup solids, modified tapioca starch	Corn oil	For children with branched-chain ketoaciduria.	Leucine-, isoleucine-, and valine-free; must be supplemented.
Product 80056 (Mead Johnson)		Corn syrup solids, modified tapioca starch	Corn oil	In formulation of special diets.	Protein-free; carbohydrate, fat, vitamin, and mineral mix.

* Committee on Nutrition, American Academy of Pediatrics: Commentary on breast feeding and infant formulas including proposed standards for formulas. *Pediatrics* 1976;**57:**278. Committee on Nutrition, American Academy of Pediatrics: Nutritional needs of low-birth-weight infants. *Pediatrics* 1977;**60:**519.

† Milupa makes other formulas for inherited metabolic diseases.

Supplements

Infants receiving prepared formula require no additional vitamin supplements. Those receiving evaporated milk formula should receive daily supplements of a multivitamin preparation, eg, Vi-Daylin/F ADC Drops (Ross). Supplemental vitamin D, most easily given as ADC Drops, is generally recommended for breast-fed infants. The American Academy of Pediatrics has also recommended the general adoption of iron-fortified formulas. Underweight or overweight infants generally have the same food requirements as do infants of the same age with a normal weight. Whole cow's milk should not be used before age 6 months.

Preparation of the Formula

Many companies that supply baby foods prepare instruction booklets setting forth the steps in preparation of the formula. The emphasis presently is on demand feeding, but the physician should make certain that the formulas are diluted correctly and that caloric needs are being met. An infant generally does

Table 4–5. Composition and schedule of milk feedings for infants up to 1 year of age.*

Age (months)	0	1	2	3	4	5	6	7	8	9	10	11	12
Calories (kcal) per day†	130–100/kg (60–45/lb)					110–100/kg (50–45/lb)				100–90/kg (45–40/lb)			
Fluid per day (mL)	130–200/kg (2–3 oz/lb)				130–165/kg (2–2½ oz/lb)						130/kg (2 oz/lb)		
Number of feedings per day‡	6 or 7		4 or 5				3 or 4					3	
Ounces per feeding	2½–4	3½–5	4–6	5–7	6–8	7–9							

* Modified and reproduced, with permission, from Silver HK et al: *Handbook of Pediatrics,* 15th ed. Lange, 1986.
† The larger amount should be used for the younger infant.
‡ Will vary somewhat with individual infants.

Table 4–6. The composition of milk (per 100 kcal).

Nutrient (Unit)	Minimum Level Recommended*	Mature Human Milk	Typical Commercial Formula	Cow's Milk (Mean)
Protein (g)	1.8†	1.3–1.6	2.3	5.1
Fat (g)	3.3‡	5	5.3	5.7
Carbohydrate (g)	. . .	10.3	10.8	7.3
Linoleic acid (mg)	300	560	2300	125
Vitamin A (IU)	250	250	300	216
Vitamin D (IU)	40	3	63	3
Vitamin E (IU)	0.3 FT 0.7 LBW 1 g linoleic	0.3	2	0.1
Vitamin K (μg)	4	2	9	5
Vitamin C (mg)	8	7.8	8.1	2.3
Thiamine (μg)	40	25	80	59
Riboflavin (μg)	60	60	100	252
Niacin (μg)	250	250	1200	131
Vitamin B_6 (μg)	15 μg/g protein	15	63	66
Folic acid (μg)	4	4	10	8
Pantothenic acid (μg)	300	300	450	489
Vitamin B_{12} (μg)	0.15	0.15	0.25	0.56
Biotin (μg)	1.5	1	2.5	3.1
Inositol (mg)	4	20	5.5	20
Choline (mg)	7	13	10	23
Calcium (mg)	5	50	75	186
Phosphorus (mg)	25	25	65	145
Magnesium (mg)	6	6	8	20
Iron (mg)	1	0.1	1.5 in fortified	0.08
Iodine (mg)	5	4–9	10	7
Copper (μg)	60	25–60	80	20
Zinc (mg)	0.5	0.1–0.5	0.65	0.6
Manganese (μg)	5	1.5	5–160	3
Sodium (meq)	0.9	1	1.7	3.3
Potassium (meq)	2.1	2.1	2.7	6
Chloride (meq)	1.6	1.6	2.3	4.6
Osmolarity (mosm)	. . .	11.3	16–18.4	40

* Committee on Nutrition, American Academy of Pediatrics.
† Protein of nutritional quality equal to casein.
‡ Includes 300 mg essential fatty acids.

not need more than 1 quart of milk per day. One pint of whole milk per day is adequate for the older child who is eating a reasonable diet.

Sterilization of bottles and formulas is not usually necessary. In most city homes, the opened can is stored in the refrigerator and each bottle is diluted as required, using warm tap water. Bottles and nipples are washed in soap and water, rinsed, and dried. Where the water supply may not be clean, boiled water should be used. In situations where cleanliness is more difficult to maintain, powdered milks should be used and dissolved in boiled water.

Feeding the Infant

The bottle should be held, not propped, for 3 reasons: (1) There is a higher incidence of acute and recurrent otitis media in infants who suck bottles in the horizontal position. The short, wide auditory tube of infants is at such an angle that mucus from rhinitis or nose allergy fills or obstructs the ducts to the middle ear very readily. Also, the auditory tube orifice is opened during swallowing. (2) Older infants may develop incisor caries due to bottle propping. (3) The emotional and physical satisfactions gained from being held are well known.

The nipple holes should be wide enough so that a drop of milk forms on the end of the nipple and drops off with little shaking of the cool bottle when turned upside down.

More water may be added to the formula if the infant consistently finishes each bottle, but be certain caloric intake is adequate.

The infant need not take all of every bottle.

The infant should be burped during and at the end of feeding.

The Introduction of Mixed Feeding

Mixed feeding should not be started until the infant is 4–6 months old. This will diminish the likelihood of specific food allergies and of overfeeding. One to 2 teaspoons of single-ingredient foods should be offered to begin with. Rice cereal is commonly introduced first, then fruits and vegetables and meats; wheat, soy, and egg foods are usually deferred because of a somewhat greater risk of inducing allergy. Commercial infant foods are convenient but expensive. Foods of similar consistency can be prepared at home and, if convenient, stored in suitable aliquots in the freezer. Parents should be instructed not to add salt or more than small amounts of sugar to solid foods.

Special Dietary Products

Dietary products designed to serve special therapeutic functions may be divided into 3 main categories:

A. Complete Formulas (Elemental Diets): These low-residue liquid products are complete foods that need no supplementation. They are variable mixtures of simple hexoses, hydrolysates or amino acid mixes, and oils with or without medium-chain triglycerides. They are low in residue and require a minimum of pancreatic enzymes for absorption. The high osmolality can be circumvented by substituting glucose polymers for the carbohydrate.

B. Special Dietary Products to Be Used Only Under Medical Supervision: The dietary management of inborn errors of metabolism is dependent on a variety of products in which one or more components, usually an amino acid, is restricted or deleted. Because they are deficient in one or more essential nutrients and may well need further supplementation—eg, with minerals and vitamins—they must be prescribed only under the strictest nutritional supervision and with appropriate laboratory monitoring.

C. Modular Diets: The provision of individual components of complete nutrition is increasingly possible. Examples include medium-chain triglyceride preparations for use in steatorrheas; amino acid mixtures such as Amin-Aid, a nitrogen supplement, for children on chronic dialysis with growth problems; and Polycose, a glucose polymer used for increasing calorie intake. Used under proper supervision, these items are useful in nutrition therapy, although their use in children is often restricted by their unattractive organoleptic properties.

Committee on Nutrition: *Pediatric Nutrition Handbook*. American Academy of Pediatrics, 1985.

Sherman JO, Hamly CA, Khachadurian AK: Use of an oral elemental diet in infants with severe intractable diarrhea. *J Pediatr* 1974;**86:**518.

ASSESSMENT OF NUTRITIONAL STATUS

Conformity to established height and weight percentiles and a simple history of an adequate and well-balanced intake are usually sufficient to determine that the child's nutritional status is normal. A clinical diagnosis of specific or generalized malnutrition should be supported by the dietary history and, when possible, by laboratory examinations. Normal and deficient biochemical levels are given in Chapter 39. Laboratory appraisals are of significant value in the detection of specific nutritional defects. In children whose nutritional needs are distorted by inborn errors, by illness, or by deprivation, appraisal by a nutritionist or dietitian may be needed. Caliper measurements of subcutaneous fat thickness may be useful in the assessment of obesity.

Dietary information may be collected by using a food record, 24-hour recall, or dietary history. Computer programs are now available for the detailed analysis of these data.

Food Record

The 3- to 7-day food record is a helpful aid for

teaching adequate nutrition, and conscientious parents are good reporters. However, if the parent has many responsibilities, valid information is hard to obtain from a food record. In addition, the parent may be ashamed of or may feel threatened by revealing the child's normal eating habits and may "exaggerate" the record or temporarily offer more or better foods if the facts are being recorded. In older children and adolescents with a tendency to overweight, conscientious recording may discourage overeating.

24-Hour Recall

The 24-hour recall is a verbal report of all foods eaten by the patient during the preceding 24 hours. The amounts of foods consumed in a typical day must be reported, including a detailed description (how cooked, what added, etc) and the times of the day. This is suitable only for group surveys or for individuals seen at frequent intervals.

Dietary History

The dietary history includes the questions "how often" and "how much" about all foods, including beverages, snacks, etc. The questions listed below are typically asked in taking a preliminary history. The answers may suggest the need for more detailed and complete data that can easily be acquired by a dietitian or nutritionist.

A. Formulas: What formula is the child now taking? Frequency of feeding? Amount per feeding? How is the formula mixed and put in the bottle?

B. Table Foods: What is the meal pattern (times and kinds of foods eaten throughout the day)? Particular likes and dislikes? Can the child eat without help? Interest shown in food? When did the child start cereal? fruit? vegetables? meat? Has the introduction of solid food been a problem?

OTHER FACTORS AFFECTING DIETARY INTAKE

Nutritional status and dietary intake are in part a function of the total family situation. The kind of food served in a family is affected by cultural influences, food economics, and food preferences. Available money and the amount budgeted for food influence the purchasing power of a family. The food allotment is frequently sacrificed when a financial crisis occurs. Fluctuations in price and demands for increased quantities are more acutely felt in poorer families. Food assistance programs are available from the United States Department of Agriculture to families with limited incomes. Finally, although choice of foods is determined by early experience in the family, new food habits may be acquired through association with peers and educational programs.

COMMON PROBLEMS IN NUTRITION

In Infancy

Power struggles are frequently set up around eating because it is one of the few areas in which a child can attempt to exercise control over the parents. The 2 major reasons for such problems are lack of consistency and lack of patience on the part of the parents.

Likes and dislikes of tastes as well as food consistency are already present in the 1-year-old. Thus, although encouragement should be given to try new foods, they should not be forced on a child. As a child gets old enough to reason, games can be made of trying new foods. Problems may arise if parents expect a young child to reason like an adult. A child who is convinced at the outset that a new food will be distasteful may like it immediately if allowed to try it without coercion. Even if not, most children have a few favorite vegetables, fruits, and meats, and these can be offered until new tastes develop.

It is important for the parent to be consistent. If a rule is made that dessert or snacks are not allowed unless a child tries the carrots or other food, it should be adhered to. If children learn that they can get more food later whether or not they eat dinner, the battle is lost.

Children who lead active lives fortunately have feelings of hunger. Thus, if nutritious foods are available, the child will choose some of these to eat. The parents' responsibility is to have nutritious foods available and to keep the child's consumption of "empty calorie" foods such as candy, soft drinks, and pastries at a minimum. If snacks are allowed, they should be foods with some nutritional value and not just calories. Fruits or vegetables are good snack foods. A plate of fresh carrot sticks, cantaloupe, or sliced apples offered to a group of children will often encourage children to try new foods.

In Adolescence

Adolescent nutritional problems have received increased attention in recent years. Perhaps the greatest cause of nutritional deficiencies in adolescents is their fast-moving and demanding society, which allows little time for regular meals. It is estimated that over half of North American teenagers eat little or no breakfast and have a generally inadequate diet. Studies show that children concentrate and learn better in school if they have had an adequate breakfast.

School breakfast and lunch programs are now providing an increasingly important portion of children's nutritional needs. This is particularly true among lower socioeconomic populations.

Diets for Athletes

The most effective diet for vigorous physical activity is a conventional balance of fat, protein, and carbohydrate, with breakfast providing one-fourth to one-third of the day's needs. Coaches have stressed high-protein diets in the past, but research indicates that protein is not the fuel for working muscles. During mild exercise, fat is the prime fuel. As physical activity increases, carbohydrate becomes more important. Under extreme muscular effort, all muscle energy comes from carbohydrate.

Maximum dietary preparation several days prior to an athletic event is a normal balance of protein and fat with a high carbohydrate intake. The high carbohydrate intake improves the capacity for prolonged exercise when given in addition to the balanced diet. Food eaten immediately prior to the event must be readily digested. Fat takes longer to digest and should be kept to a minimum. Liquid meals of approximately 1000 kcal providing 75% carbohydrate and 25% protein are preferable because they are more readily digested and will not induce vomiting, as a heavy protein and fat meal could.

Water should not be restricted during exercise, and players should be allowed to drink glucose in water or 0.2% sodium chloride solution throughout a game. Maintaining water balance is important for the athlete. One of the principal manifestations of dehydration is fatigue. This is true in cold as well as hot weather. The use of special commercial drinks for athletes has its basis in this fact.

Smith NH: *Food for Sport.* Bull Publishing Co., 1976.

Vegetarian & Fad Diets

Many peoples of the world subsist on a diet considered by the more affluent to be a vegetarian diet. However, young peole may try various types of vegetarian diets by choice. These diets may be categorized as **pure vegetarian,** or **vegan, diets,** which are not supplemented with any animal foods, dairy products, or eggs; **lactovegetarian diets,** which are supplemented with milk and cheese; or **lacto-ovo-vegetarian diets,** which are supplemented with milk, cheese, and eggs. The latter 2 diets can be quite adequate. The former, lacking complete proteins, may eventually prevent adequate nutrition, as may any extremely narrow choice of foods.

Young health food "addicts" are usually interested in nutrition but need enough basic knowledge to plan diets with their health foods and maintain a balance. Health food stores, though expensive, are a source of various vitamins and foods that are acceptable to these young people. They must be warned, however, that the fat-soluble vitamins can be taken in toxic amounts, since they are stored in the body. Table 4–1 can be used as a guideline for dosage limitations of these nutrients.

So-called health foods are often stocked in chain groceries at cheaper prices than at the health food store. Most vegetarians who take a variety of fruits, vegetables, unrefined cereals, legumes, seeds, nuts, and dairy products have adequate intakes. It is the narrow diet restricted to a few foods and high in carbohydrates that tends to be inadequate.

Committee on Nutrition, American Academy of Pediatrics: Nutritional aspects of vegetarianism, health foods, and fad diets. *Pediatrics* 1977;**59:**460.

Megavitamin Therapy

The use of nicotinamide adenine dinucleotide (NAD), riboflavin, ascorbic acid, pyridoxine, calcium pantothenate, vitamin B_{12}, folic acid, and trace minerals in doses considerably in excess of the RDA has been advocated for childhood autism and learning disabilities.

While there are a number of rare dependency syndromes for which large doses of specific vitamins are indicated (eg, vitamin D in certain types of rickets; vitamin B_6 in some cases of homocystinuria), megavitamin therapy for learning disabilities is not justified on the basis of existing documented clinical results.

Committee on Nutrition, American Academy of Pediatrics: Megavitamin therapy for childhood psychoses and learning disabilities. *Pediatrics* 1976;**58:**922.

Diseases & Nutrition

Most cases of severe malnutrition in the USA are secondary to the onset of other chronic diseases. Such diseases commonly include congenital bowel malformations or obstructions in infancy, malabsorption diseases such as cystic fibrosis, congenital heart disease, liver disease, ileitis or colitis, and many others. Intravenous hyperalimentation is being used with increased frequency in the treatment of neonatal bowel abnormalities. Elemental diets (Pregestimil, Vivonex), usually consisting basically of mixtures of amino acids, glucose, and medium-chain triglycerides for optimal absorption and utilization, can be helpful nutritional supplements for many patients. Nutritionists working in hospitals should advise on nutrition in patients with chronic diseases.

DISORDERS OF NUTRITION

OBESITY

Obesity is considered the most common nutritional disorder in the USA. However, the definition of obesity is arbitrary, and there are wide variations in estimates of the number of overweight individuals, depending on which criteria are used. Five to 10% of preadolescent school children and 10–15% of adolescents are more than 20% overweight. The prevalence is greater in females after infancy and increases with age in both sexes. Obesity is less common at the lower end of the economic scale, but this does not apply in urban communities. Obesity is also less common in black males but more common in adolescent and adult black females than in white males and females. Excessive weight gain at some stage during infancy is associated with increased risk of obesity in childhood. If there is also at least one obese parent, the risk is 50% or greater.

In a clinical setting, the exact assessment of body fat by densitometry is impractical. The diagnosis of obesity is essentially arbitrary, but diagnosis is not a problem in cases severe enough to require treatment. For those who want more exact definitions and for monitoring the effect of dietary restriction, triceps skinfold thickness measurements may be helpful. The American Academy of Pediatrics has published figures for use in childhood (Table 4–7), and there are other more complex calculations of body fat depending on height, weight, and skinfold thickness.

The newborn infant is about 14% fat, and this proportion increases during childhood. A 10-year-old boy is about 23% fat, whereas a girl of the same age is as much as 28% fat. By 18 years, the young man has lost body fat (12%) to a much greater extent than the young woman (25%).

Pathogenesis

The basic cause of obesity is an imbalance between energy intake and expenditure. Periods of rapid weight gain are triggered by excessive intake of food energy, which is stored as fat. Once obesity is established, no excess intake of energy is necessary to maintain the overweight state. Sedentary life-styles, which have become a common feature of Western industrialized society, are usually an important contributory factor. Normally, physical activity accounts for about one-third of energy expenditure. Food is now generally available in abundance in industrialized societies, and the intake of food is not usually governed by availability or by the physiologic mechanisms of hunger and satiety. Especially in the overweight individual, appetite phenomena override these more basic mechanisms, and eating meets emotional rather than nutritional needs of the child or the parent. Frequently, overeating is associated with a specific life situation such as school dissatisfaction and parental or peer disapproval. Overeating and obesity appear to be the best adaptations that some people can make in coping with life's problems. Life may become too threatening and unsatisfactory without the comfort of eating. Psychologic problems may frequently antedate obesity. Thus, early-onset obesity has been linked with failure of maternal recognition and satisfaction of infant needs. In children, a specific psychologic trauma is often associated with later-onset obesity. In a smaller group, obesity is one feature of a specific underlying psychiatric disorder.

Though emotional factors undoubtedly play a large role in the development of obesity, other factors probably make a significant contribution in some cases. For example, though familial patterns are largely explained by maternal infant and child feeding practices and other early conditioning by the family, genetic factors may play a role. Thus, monozygotic twins are more likely to have similar body weights and skinfold thicknesses than are dizygotic twins. Children of obese parents have been reported to have a lower energy requirement at rest than children of normal-weight parents. Though there is no conclusive evidence that obese children, or some obese children, have an impaired thermogenic response to food, there is growing interest in this topic. It appears that humans can normally adapt to food intake in excess of energy requirements with little gain in weight, because of increased thermogenesis. Factors thought to be important in thermogenesis include increased activity of the sodium pump; "futile metabolic cycles"; increased secretion of thyroid hormones; and, especially, the quantity of brown adipose tissue. However, the role of impaired functioning related to one or more of these factors in the pathogenesis of human obesity remains uncertain. In in vitro studies, decreased lipolytic response to epinephrine has been reported in adipocytes obtained from obese adipose tissue, and this effect persists after weight loss. The significance of this observation in vivo is not known. Certain metabolic abnormalities associated with obesity, notably hyperinsulinemia, are secondary to the obesity. Increased adipose tissue cellularity has received a great deal of attention but is probably only a marker for obesity.

Obese children as a group grow at a slightly faster rate and mature sexually earlier than nonobese children. Lean body weight is normal to moderately increased. Rarely, obesity can be attributed to a specific hormonal, central nervous system, or familial disease. Typically in these circumstances, bone age is delayed and growth is retarded. Obesity and mild hypertension together with delayed bone age and growth retardation may be the only diagnostic clinical features of hyperadrenocorticism in children. Thyroid deficiency should be excluded. Hypothalamic dysfunction secondary to central nervous system infection, tumor, or injury can cause obesity. Obesity and short stature are features associated with 4 heritable syndromes:

Table 4–7. Obesity standards in Caucasian Americans.

Age (Years)	Minimum Triceps Skinfold Thickness Indicating Obesity (mm)	
	Males	Females
5	12	14
6	12	15
7	13	16
8	14	17
9	14	18
10	16	20
11	17	21
12	18	22
13	18	23
14	17	23
15	16	24
16	15	25
17	14	26

Laurence-Moon-Biedl syndrome, Prader-Willi syndrome, Alström's syndrome, an pseudohypoparathyroidism.

Severe obesity can become a life-threatening condition in the pickwickian syndrome. The immediate clinical consequences of more moderate degrees of obesity are mainly social and psychologic, especially in adolescence. Disturbances of body image may occur, and lowered self-image impairs social functioning. Overweight infants appear to be at increased risk of infection. Various abnormalities of the immune system are associated with obesity. Obesity in childhood or adolescence frequently progresses to obesity in adulthood, with its attendant risks of diabetes, hypertension, and cardiovascular disease, although the latter diseases are more often associated with obesity starting in adulthood. If obesity continues throughout adolescence, there is only a 4% chance that it will disappear during adulthood. Sixty percent of moderately obese children and 84% of markedly obese children become obese adults. One-third of obese adults, including most severely obese adults, became obese during childhood.

Biochemical abnormalities associated with obesity in childhood include increased circulating levels of free fatty acids, glycerol, ketone bodies, and insulin. Carbohydrate intolerance and elevated levels of triglycerides and cholesterol are less common in childhood obesity than in adult obesity.

Prevention

Prevention of obesity is more desirable than treatment, especially in view of the disappointing results of the latter. The most effective prevention probably begins in infancy. Families in which one or both parents are obese and the infant is gaining excessive weight are of special concern. Simple preventive measures have general application. These include encouragement of breast feeding, discouragement of solids before 6 months of age, and counseling of mothers to give food when the infant is hungry and not as a pacifier. In some cases, it is desirable to reeducate families regarding nutrition and to encourage physical activity. Prevention should start at the first clinic visit of the well baby. In the management of infants who are already overweight, the aim is for weight control rather than weight reduction. Caloric density of the formula should be reduced. Skim milk and 2% fat milk should not be used, because of the high osmolar load.

Treatment

Treatment of obesity in the preadolescent child requires management of the whole family. Diet therapy has a major role in management. Though it is extremely difficult to achieve satisfactory compliance, diet therapy can be achieved more readily than regular exercise in many patients. The family must modify its eating behavior. Cooking only single helpings, using small plates, eating meals as a family, and using vegetable rather than high-calorie snacks are all useful habits. More extensive modification of family behavior is frequently necessary when one or both parents are obese, in which case their child may have been overfed from an early stage of development. The parents will need long-term encouragement and support from a nutritionist and pediatrician. Initially, the family should keep a 3-day or longer diet record. The family should be provided with and educated in the use of calorie counters and instructed in food labeling. The child, if old enough, and other family members should each calculate their caloric intake. Future dietary planning will depend on comparison of the initial and ongoing calculations with amount of weight gained. Caloric intake in excess of normal recommended energy intake should obviously be modified, and it may be desirable to restrict the intake to 800 kcal/24 h. However, linear growth should not be compromised, and in general, semistarvation diets should not be employed in young children or adolescents. A weight loss of one-half pound per week should be regarded as success, and the child and family should be continually encouraged. Obese patients are typically inactive, and exercise is an important component of management. Frequently, obesity in young children is precipitated by an emotional problem that should be the focus of therapy. More severe psychologic problems often underly severe, long-standing obesity. Efforts to achieve weight reduction in these cases are not only likely to be unsuccessful but may precipitate more severe emotional disturbances.

In the adolescent, particularly in the adolescent girl, treatment of obesity is both difficult and unrewarding. Appetite suppressant drugs and thyroid are of little if any use. Regular exercise is helpful, but sustained enthusiasm is hard to achieve. Weight reduction can realistically be achieved only by reducing food intake. Motivation is essential, and whether this be for cosmetic or health reasons or whether it results from the containment of emotional problems, patients need continuous help and encouragement to succeed. Group organizations such as Weight Watchers and special summer camps can help, but in the long run success depends on individual determination and the support of an experienced and sympathetic nutritionist. It is important that caloric restriction not lead to vitamin, mineral, or essential amino acid deficiencies and that the restricted diet remain attractive. In general, the degree of caloric restriction will vary with individuals, though adolescent girls should have less than 1200 kcal/24 h and boys less than 1500 kcal/24 h. Fasting and fad diets should not be advised. Surgery (eg, gastric stapling) may be needed in life-threatening obesity in the pickwickian syndrome.

Frerichs RR, Harsha DW, Berenson GS: Equations for estimating percentage of body fat in children 10–14 years old. *Pediatr Res* 1979;**13:**170.

DISEASES OF GENERALIZED UNDERNUTRITION

Undernutrition has long been recognized as the single most important problem in child health the world over. Occult undernutrition is not uncommon among the poor and usually takes the form of iron deficiency anemia. Vitamin A deficiency may be seen in special groups such as children of migrant farm workers, and vitamin C deficiency is encountered in children of American Indians. Severe malnutrition usually is a complex result of want and ignorance, with some element of child abuse. Morbidity from infections and diarrheal diseases as well as the overall mortality rate are increased in undernourished children.

National Center for Health Statistics: *Dietary Intake Findings: United States 1971–74*. Publication No. (HRA) 77–1647. US Department of Health, Education, and Welfare, 1977.

PROTEIN-ENERGY MALNUTRITION

Classification

There continues to be confusion about the nomenclature and causes of various forms of protein-energy malnutrition. All are caused by multinutritional deficiencies. There tends to be an absolute deficiency of most nutrients, with sodium being the exception, and only the relative magnitude of these deficiencies varies from case to case and area to area.

Kwashiorkor is characterized by edema, desquamating skin, discolored hair, hepatomegaly, and extreme apathy. The Wellcome classification includes patients who weigh less than 80% but more than 60% of ideal body weight and have edema. The marasmic child, who by definition is below 60% of ideal body weight, is classically wasted, with relatively normal skin, hair, liver, and affect. The term "marasmic kwashiorkor" denotes less than 60% of ideal body weight with edema. Subjects whose weight is less than 80% but greater than 60% of the ideal and who do not have edema are termed "underweight." In the USA, the term "failure to thrive" is used frequently for infants whose weight is within this range.

Etiology

Dietary deficiencies are the outstanding etiologic factor worldwide, but in Western countries, severe forms of undernutrition occur most frequently in association with other disease states (eg, anorexia, intestinal malabsorption, deranged intermediary metabolism, or excessive loss of nutrients). More moderate deficits are most commonly caused by the parents' ignorance, poverty, or emotional conflicts over the infant or child.

Marasmus may occur at any stage of life. Common causes in infants are inadequate preparation of formulas (due to ignorance or poverty) and inadequate breast feeding. Other causes include prematurity with difficulty in feeding, infections, obstructive diseases of the upper gastrointestinal tract, malabsorption syndromes, inborn errors of metabolism, serious organic diseases, and maternal anxiety and insecurity. Parental neglect and battering must be ruled out. In technologically underdeveloped countries, kwashiorkor classically occurs at the time of weaning from breast milk onto foods that are nutritionally inadequate.

Clinical Findings

A. Symptoms and Signs: The primary feature of mild or early generalized undernutrition is weight loss or reduced growth velocity. There may be decreased physical activity and apathy.

In marasmus, weight loss is extreme, with striking depletion of both fat and muscle tissue. Patients fall in the low percentiles of weight-for-height relationships. Loss of fat from the buccal fat pads gives the facies a wizened, old-man appearance. Psychomotor impairment is not nearly so marked as in kwashiorkor. There are no skin lesions or edema. Hepatomegaly is absent, and hair changes are absent or inconspicuous. The infant usually retains a good appetite. Frequently, associated infections and diarrhea are present. Growth of hair and nails is retarded, and many hair follicles are atrophic.

In kwashiorkor, there is typically some weight loss despite edema fluid, and most muscle and fat tissues are retained. The moon facies results from retention of the buccal fat pads and from edema. Anorexia and apathy are extreme. In severe cases, the child is introverted and almost catatonic. Emotional responses are abnormal—eg, the infant may submit to painful procedures without movement or sound but cry when the mother attempts to nurse or cuddle. In classic or acute-onset "sugar-baby" kwashiorkor, there is gross hepatomegaly owing to fatty infiltration. The patient has marked pallor and signs of anemia. In severe cases, hyperpigmented, hyperkeratotic, and spotty skin lesions develop on the trunk and limbs, especially where skin irritation occurs. These lesions may become confluent and appear as a mosaic with desquamation of large hyperpigmented scales and superficial ulcerations. Petechiae and ecchymoses may be present. There may be hair loss, or hair may be easily plucked out. Depigmentation of the hair may occur, so that light bands of hair are present (**flag sign**). Associated infections and diarrhea are frequently present.

Signs of severe vitamin and mineral deficiencies may be present or may become apparent only during rehabilitation. Severely malnourished infants or children are often seriously ill owing to water and electrolyte imbalance caused by cardiovascular and renal insufficiencies and to defects in the immune system. Death may result from bronchopneumonia; gram-negative septicemia; overwhelming infection; or acute cardiovascular, renal, or hepatic failure.

B. Laboratory Findings: Marasmus is diagnosed clinically. Laboratory measurements are of no value in establishing the diagnosis, though they may be helpful in determining the cause in certain circumstances. Dietary, family, and social data are more relevant, together with the response to appropriate dietary therapy.

Kwashiorkor is characterized by hypoproteinemia and hypoalbuminemia. Circulating levels of other hepatic proteins are also depressed (eg, retinol-binding protein, thyroxin-binding prealbumin), and these provide more sensitive indices in mild or early cases. The hypoalbuminemia does not appear to be attributable to protein deficiency. The edema results primarily from impaired renal handling of sodium and altered permeability of all cell membranes. The low transferrin levels contribute to the commonly seen anemia of kwashiorkor. The prothrombin time is prolonged in kwashiorkor, but not in marasmus. Other laboratory findings of interest in the pathogenesis and management of kwashiorkor include multiple deficits of the immune system and depletion of total body potassium. Serum sodium may be low or normal, but total body sodium is grossly increased owing to the high intracellular sodium concentrations. In the presence of hepatomegaly, circulating levels of very low density lipoproteins (VLDL) and of triglycerides are likely to be depressed. Hypoglycemia can be a severe complication of poorly managed protein-energy malnutrition.

Differential Diagnosis

The differential diagnosis of kwashiorkor includes other causes of edema and, possibly, of hepatomegaly. Although kwashiorkor is the most likely diagnosis in countries where severe malnutrition is common, the disease may not be considered in the USA. Patients may undergo liver biopsy and experience a prolonged period of mismanagement before the diagnosis of kwashiorkor is made. Kwashiorkor is sometimes the presenting clinicial finding of cystic fibrosis in infancy, even if the nutritional and social history do not support the possibility of severe malnutrition.

Treatment

Severely malnourished children, especially with kwashiorkor, succumb during early therapy because of too vigorous or misguided treatment. The capacity for homeostasis and the physiologic ability to respond to stress are lost, though the extent of these abnormalities cannot be measured accurately in clinical practice. Other major hazards include specific nutrient deficiencies and imbalances, especially loss of sodium-potassium homeostasis; infections; and poor gut motility. These problems must be carefully evaluated, and treatment must be determined according to each patient's status. The greatest caution and patience must be exercised so as not to provide additional stress or give more nutrients than can be handled until the reductive adaptations are reversed (1–2 weeks).

The following principles of management should be used in treatment of kwashiorkor, marasmic kwashiorkor, and severe marasmus: (1) Provide nutrients for specific deficiencies, especially potassium. (2) Treat infections. (3) Avoid hypoglycemia by giving frequent small feedings. (4) Allow time to reverse reductive adaptations and altered metabolism, eg, restoration of normal levels of protein synthesis, immune responses, cellular sodium pump activity, and basal metabolic rate. (5) *Only after the first 4 goals have been achieved,* replenish lost tissue rapidly. (Milder degrees of undernutrition [eg, failure to thrive] should be managed differently; adequate nutrients to accomplish rapid weight gain should be administered without delay.) (6) Finally, and ideally, restore normal body composition.

Early therapy is aimed at cautious restoration of blood volume. Except when the patient is in shock, administration of intravenous fluids is best avoided and is not necessary once correction of severe hypovolemia, severe electrolyte disturbance (especially of potassium), and severe anemia (hemoglobin $\leq$ 5 g/dL) has been achieved. Intravenous fluids can place stress on the compromised myocardium and should not be administered unless essential. It is especially important to avoid giving intravenous sodium, even when serum sodium levels are low, because intracellular sodium levels will only be further increased owing to compromised renal handling of sodium. (Even in normal circumstances, intravenous sodium is handled less efficiently than oral sodium by the kidneys.) As the reductive adaptations are reversed, large amounts of sodium enter the extracellular fluid from the cells. This is potentially dangerous and contributes to the edema of refeeding when renal function does not recover simultaneously.

Administration of intravenous nutrition should also be avoided. Large quantities of nutrients, especially when given intravenously, are contraindicated during the acute phase, because they will further compromise liver function. Small blood transfusions can be very beneficial in the presence of severe anemia. As soon as severe hypovolemia is corrected and urine output is established, large quantities of potassium (but not sodium) should be administered. Magnesium supplements may also be beneficial at this stage. Localized or generalized infections are usually present, though signs may be minimal or absent, and appropriate antibiotic therapy should be started without delay. Hypoglycemia is best avoided by continuous or frequent oral feeding.

Oral administration of clear fluids should be started immediately, and maintenance oral nutrition should be achieved by the second or third day. For the first 24 hours, a continuous slow nasogastric drip may be used, followed by frequent small feedings every 1–2 hours. Intensive nursing is necessary at this stage. Intervals between feedings can gradually be extended. Maintenance protein requirements for malnourished infants are only 0.6 g/kg/d; amounts greater than 1.5 g/kg/d should be avoided during management of the acute phase (usually 1–2 weeks). Maintenance energy requirements are 95 kcal/kg/d. In the USA, a non-lactose-containing formula such as Pregestimil is often used. However, in developing countries, formulas based on cow's milk are used with success, and it appears that the lactose deficiency is not usually sufficiently severe to cause unacceptable diarrhea. Additional fats and carbohydrates (eg, medium-chain triglycerides and glucose polymers) may need to be added to diluted formula to achieve the optimal ratio of energy to protein. Sucrose may aggravate hepatomegaly and should be avoided. Early administration of large quantities of protein may also provoke hepatomegaly. Early nutritional management includes the provision of generous quantities of vitamins, including vitamin K.

Careful clinical judgment is required to determine the optimal time for switching from a maintenance to a recovery diet. Helpful indications are the disappearance of edema and anorexia, which give way to the patient developing a voracious appetite. Edema will disappear satisfactorily with a diet that provides protein rates of only 0.6 g/kg/d. Causes of persistent anorexia are small bowel overgrowth, hepatomegaly, infection, and a specific nutrient deficiency (eg, of zinc). Recovery diets should provide at least 200 kcal/kg/24 h and protein rates of about 3.5 g/kg/24 h. Recovery diets must also contain abundant vitamins, minerals, and trace elements. Hospital treatment should be continued in many cases until the weight-for-height ratio reaches the 50th percentile.

The final aim of management—achievement of normal body composition—continues to elude clinicians. Following recovery, the body contains excessive fat relative to lean body tissue, and the height-for-age percentile tends to remain low. Better understanding of the optimal recovery diet, including optimal quantities of micronutrients, may lead to progress in this area.

Prognosis

Severe protein-energy malnutrition, especially severe acute kwashiorkor, has a mortality rate of 30% or higher during early therapy. Regrettably, this high mortality rate is attributable in part to overzealous and misguided management and to avoidable acute electrolyte imbalance or severe hypoglycemia. The long-term prognosis for full recovery depends on the severity and duration of malnutrition and age of the patient. Subsequent brain development is especially vulnerable to the effects of early severe marasmus.

Brooke OG, Wheeler EF: High energy feeding in protein-energy malnutrition. *Arch Dis Child* 1976;**51:**968.

Chase HP et al: Kwashiorkor in the United States. *Pediatrics* 1980;**66:**972.

Golden MH: Protein deficiency, energy deficiency, and the oedema of malnutrition. *Lancet* 1982;**1:**1261.

FAILURE TO THRIVE

The term "failure to thrive" is commonly applied to infants who, for a variety of reasons, show a striking lag in somatic growth. By far the most common cause is nutritional deprivation. Nutritional problems in turn may reflect ignorance, poverty, child abuse, or emotional conflicts over the child.

Organic causes for failure to thrive must also be considered. The list given in Table 25–1 for short stature can be used as a diagnostic guide.

VITAMIN DEFICIENCIES, DEPENDENCIES, & INTOXICATIONS

FAT-SOLUBLE VITAMINS

VITAMIN A

Vitamin A is a fat-soluble alcohol derived in the animal body from certain of the carotenoid plant pigments, of which β-carotene is the most important. β-Carotene has a unique and specialized role in the photochemical basis of vision. The photosensitive pigment rhodopsin is formed from vitamin A and a protein called opsin. The general effect of vitamin A on cellular function is to reduce the stability of lysosomes; it has some influence also on sulfur metabolism (by activating sulfate in mucopolysaccharide formation) and on steroid hormone production. It is considered important in the maintenance of epithelial membranes in the body.

Vitamin A is present in food primarily as the palmitate ester and is hydrolyzed to its free alcohol, retinol, in the intestine. Within intestinal cells, retinol is reesterified, primarily to palmitate, incorporated into the chylomicrons of the mucosa, and absorbed into the lymphatic system.

1. VITAMIN A DEFICIENCY

Clinical Findings

A. Symptoms and Signs: Night blindness and loss of visual acuity in poor light are early eye symptoms, followed by squamous metaplasia that produces dryness of the conjunctiva, xerophthalmia, and, very often, typical small gray-white patches called Bitot spots on the bulbar conjunctiva. As metaplasia progresses, the cornea becomes cloudy and soft (keratomalacia) and eventually secondarily infected and ulcerated, at which point corneal damage and loss of vision are irreversible except for the possibility of corneal transplant. Hypertrophy or atrophy of tongue papillae occurs early in vitamin A deficiency. Follicular hyperkeratosis on the buttocks and extensor surfaces of the extremities is common, as are skin and upper respiratory tract infections.

Mexican-American children—especially those of

parents who are migrant farm workers—are especially vulnerable to vitamin A deficiency (serum levels < 20 μg/dL). Vitamin A deficiency is common in children with kwashiorkor. Vitamin A levels are lower in sera of children born of mothers who have not received prenatal vitamin supplementation.

B. Laboratory Findings: The normal plasma vitamin A level in childhood has been suggested to be 20 μg/dL or more prior to age 6 months and 30 μg/dL or more thereafter. The mean value in preschool children in the USA has been determined to be 33 ± 7.6 μg/dL.

Serum carotene determination is a helpful test in cases of nutritional vitamin A deficiency or fat malabsorption. The normal levels are approximately 70 μg/dL at birth, rising to approximately 340 μg/dL at age 1. The levels fall to about 150 μg/dL at age 3½; thereafter, they are between 100 and 150 μg/dL. Since β-carotene is carried attached to β-lipoproteins, conditions in which β-lipoproteins are elevated, such as hypothyroidism, will be associated with high circulating levels of β-carotene.

Prevention & Treatment

The minimum daily requirement for vitamin A varies with age but is in the range of 2500 IU (750 μg) in the child under age 4 years and 5000 IU from age 4 on. Vitamin A has approximately equal concentrations in breast and cow's milk (53 and 34 μg/dL, respectively). Supplementation is of particular importance in premature infants with small intakes and poor hepatic stores. Table 4–8 lists the vitamin A content of some common foods. The recommended daily dose of vitamin A in cases of vitamin A deficiency is 25,000 IU for 1–2 weeks in conjunction with a high-protein diet. It is usually necessary to replenish liver stores of vitamin A before the serum levels increase, which may take several weeks. It is also possible to treat deficiency with single massive doses. In cases of malabsorption, a water-miscible vitamin A preparation is given in twice the daily recommended amount (5000–10,000 IU) as a minimum requirement. When xerophthalmia is present, vitamin A may be given as an injection intramuscularly in doses up to 25,000 IU daily for 3–4 days.

Prognosis

When xerophthalmia is part of a malabsorption syndrome and treatment is early, effective, and sustained, the prognosis is good. If vitamin A deficiency is associated with general malnutrition, scarring and secondary infection of the cornea have occurred and subsequent blindness is common.

Oomen HA: Vitamin A deficiency, xerophthalmia and blindness. *Nutr Rev* 1974;**32:**161.

Table 4–8. Vitamin A content of some common foods.

Liver (2 oz fried)	37,000 IU
Carrots (1 large or 2 small)	11,000 IU
Sweet potato (1 small)	8,100 IU
Spinach (½ cup cooked)	7,300 IU
Cantaloupe (½ cup)	4,100 IU
Milk (1 cup, whole fresh)	340 IU

2. VITAMIN A TOXICITY

The requirement of a doctor's prescription in order to obtain high-potency vitamin A preparations in recent years has diminished but not abolished the incidence of toxicity. Patients may show peeling of the skin, particularly over the fingers and hands. Long bone pain is marked over the distal extremities, and the child may refuse to walk. Loss of appetite, hypertrophy and hyperemia of gums, skin pigmentation, and alopecia are also found. Signs and symptoms of pseudotumor cerebri occur and can last for several months after vitamin A is discontinued. Radiologically, there is evidence of subperiosteal new bone formation.

The only treatment is discontinuation of excessive doses of vitamin A. Clinical improvement begins within a few days, but a return of the bones to normal may not occur for several months.

Committees on Drugs and on Nutrition, American Academy of Pediatrics: The use and abuse of vitamin A. *Pediatrics* 1971;**48:**655.

Mahoney CP et al: Chronic vitamin A intoxication in infants fed chicken liver. *Pediatrics* 1980;**65:**893.

VITAMIN D

Vitamin D is absorbed by the intestine in solution in triglyceride particles. It is then carried on an α_2-globulin to the liver, where it is converted to the more active forms 25-hydroxycholecalciferol and 25-hydroxyergocalciferol. These forms are essential to normal bone physiology and to the maintenance of adequate concentrations of calcium and phosphorus within the extracellular fluid. They also appear to enhance the enzymatic processes necessary for the calcification of the bone matrix. In the presence of parathyroid hormone, vitamin D promotes the reabsorption of phosphate by kidney tubules and may increase the tubular reabsorption of amino acids. Sunlight will also promote the endogenous synthesis of vitamin D.

The kidney in turn forms 1,25-dihydroxycholecalciferol, a derivative of 25-hydroxycholecalciferol that is specifically active in promoting the synthesis of the calcium transport protein in the intestinal villus.

Rickets is a disorder of the deposition of hydroxyapatite in bone matrix and in preosseous cartilage at the zone of provisional calcification. Essentially it is due to calcium or phosphorus deficiency during a period of active growth. A classification is given in Table 4–9. Simple dietary calcium deficiency is un-

Table 4–9. A classification of rickets.

Essential calcium deficiency
Responsive to normal doses of vitamin D_3 or calcitriol
Dietary vitamin D or calcium deficiency
Responsive to high doses of vitamin D_3 and to calcitriol
Fat malabsorption syndrome
Chronic renal disease
Vitamin D dependency:
Type 1: Defective 1α-hydroxylation
Type II: End-organ insensitivity
Resistant rickets of TPN
Essential phosphorus deficiency
Nutritional hypophosphatemic rickets
Renal tubular dystrophies, eg, cystinosis
Hypophosphatemic bone disease (rarely)
Phosphate depletion from overuse of aluminum hydroxide gels
X-linked vitamin D resistance
Oncogenous rickets
Essential calcium and phosphorus deficiency
Breast milk rickets
Essential matrix abnormalities
Metaphyseal dysostosis or chondrodysplasia
Hypophosphatasia and pseudohypophosphatasia

common in developed countries. More commonly, the deficiency is secondary to the formation of calcium soaps, with malabsorption in steatorrhea, or to deficiency, malabsorption, insensitivity to, or inadequate hydroxylation of vitamin D_3.

Rickets is very rare in full-term newborn infants, but there is some evidence that for optimum mineralization of bone, even the well-nourished mother should take the recommended daily allowance of vitamin D and that breast-fed infants should receive supplementation. Small premature infants, however, seem to be vulnerable to rickets and may develop late respiratory distress syndrome because of associated softening of the thoracic cage. There seem to be 2 reasons for this: (1) the low phosphorus content of both breast milk and conventional formulas and (2) immaturity of the mechanism responsible for the normal postnatal rise in serum 1,25-dihydroxycholecalciferol. Small infants receiving total parenteral nutrition (TPN) may also develop rickets.

Bosley AR, Verrier-Jones ER, Campbell MJ: Aetiological factors in rickets of prematurity. *Arch Dis Child* 1980;**55:**683.

Greer FR et al: Bone mineral content and serum 25-hydroxyvitamin D concentration in breast-fed infants with and without supplemental vitamin D. *J Pediatr* 1981;**98:**696.

Lovinger RD: Grand round series: Rickets. *Pediatrics* 1980;**66:**359.

1. RICKETS DUE TO VITAMIN D DEFICIENCY & VITAMIN D RESISTANCE

Essentials of Diagnosis

- History of insufficient dietary intake of vitamin D or of malabsorption.
- Listlessness, hypotonicity, and retarded motor development.
- Bony deformities clinically and on x-ray.
- Normal serum calcium, low serum phosphorus, elevated serum alkaline phosphatase.

General Considerations

Vitamin D-deficiency rickets continues to be a significant problem in those parts of North America where there is little direct sunlight and where the milk supply is not fortified with vitamin D. Minor degrees of clinical rickets are common in underprivileged groups such as migrant farm workers, especially those with darkly pigmented skins, in bedridden children in institutions, and in areas where cow's milk is unfortified. Calcium-deficiency rickets may be seen in families on vegan diets. Nowadays, however, the X-linked dominant form of vitamin D-resistant rickets is the commonest type seen clinically.

Clinical Findings

A. Symptoms and Signs: Findings include leg bowing in toddlers; beading of the ribs; widening of the wrists, knees, and ankles; frontal bossing; craniotabes; the development of Harrison's sulcus in the chest wall; and, very rarely, pathologic fractures. There also may be lethargy, hypotonicity, muscle pain, hyperextensibility of joints, and motor retardation followed, as the severity increases, by convulsions and tetany. A history of poor vitamin D intake or of exclusion from sunlight is usual. A family history of leg bowing is normally found in vitamin D-resistant rickets. Evidence of steatorrhea or of renal or liver disease is likely to be obvious.

B. Laboratory Findings: These include variable hypocalcemia and hypophosphatemia, depending on whether the cause is primarily one of calcium or phosphorus deficiency. Alkaline phosphatase levels are usually elevated except in generally malnourished children. Generalized aminoaciduria and some impairment of tubular hydrion excretion may also be present, as may minimal glycosuria. These findings apply to vitamin D deficiency. In vitamin D resistance, there is phosphaturia only. Levels of 24,25-dihydroxycholecalciferol and 25-hydroxycholecalciferol are low, and levels of 1,25-dihydroxycholecalciferol are low or normal.

C. X-Ray Findings: Cupping, fraying, and flaring are seen at the ends of the bones. Bony trabeculae lose their sharp definition, which accounts for the general decrease in skeletal radiodensity. In hypophosphatemic bone disease, there is coarse bone trabeculation and, rarely, evidence of rickets.

Differential Diagnosis

It should be possible on the basis of the history to differentiate rickets due to dietary deficiency of calcium or vitamin D or due to steatorrhea or chronic renal disease from that due to X-linked dominant phosphaturia. Other forms of phosphaturia (see Chapter 21) must of course be excluded, and the most common of these is cystinosis. A routine look for aminoaciduria and for cystine crystals in the lens or the bone marrow is wise. In hypophosphatasia and pseudohypophosphatasia, the bone changes are similar to those observed in rickets, serum calcium levels may be elevated, there is vitamin D resistance and phosphoethanolaminuria, and serum alkaline phosphatase levels are low or normal. In hereditary metaphyseal dysostosis, the bone changes are also similar, but there are no biochemical changes, no response to vitamin D even in large doses, and the children are essentially healthy, albeit stocky and bowlegged. This last condition is also sometimes associated with neutropenia, hair hypoplasia, and pancreatic insufficiency.

Prevention

The addition of vitamin D to fluid milk, to evaporated milk, and to special milk products and substitutes has helped eradicate vitamin D-deficiency rickets in the USA.

Treatment

Vitamin D-deficiency rickets is cured by vitamin D, 5000 IU orally every day for 4–5 weeks. Evidence of cure is rapid. Radiologic and biochemical signs of improvement appear after the first week of therapy. Vitamin D therapy may be ineffective in the presence of magnesium deficiency.

The disturbance of calcium absorption in malabsorption syndromes is secondary to enteric losses of vitamin D with stool fat. For this reason, doubling the recommended prophylactic dose of vitamin D is usually sufficient; however, in certain cases of hepatobiliary disease, a true resistance to vitamin D has been described. Vitamin D resistance must be treated with phosphate solutions and is relatively unresponsive to vitamin D_3 itself. Even without phosphate supplementation, good biochemical and growth responses to calcitriol (1,25-dihydroxycholecalciferol) may occur with doses of 20–80 ng/kg/d. Phosphate supplementation is still advisable, however.

Castile RG, Marks LJ, Stickler GB: Vitamin D deficiency rickets: Two cases with faulty infant feeding practices. *Am J* 16.2*Dis Child* 1975;**129:**964.

Chan JC, Lovinger RD, Mamunes P: Renal hypophosphatemic rickets: Growth acceleration after long term treatment with 1,25-dihydroxyvitamin D_3. *Pediatrics* 1980;**66:**445.

Goel KM et al: Florid and subclinical rickets among immigrant children in Glasgow. *Lancet* 1976;**1:**1141.

Kooh SW et al: Rickets due to calcium deficiency. *N Engl J Med* 1977;**297:**1264.

Reddy V, Sivakumar B: Magnesium-dependent vitamin D-resistant rickets. *Lancet* 1974;**1:**963.

2. BREAST MILK RICKETS

Modern laboratory methods show that the content of 1,25-dihydroxycholecalciferol in human breast milk is only 2.2 ± 0.1 pg/mL. Few breast-fed infants develop rickets, probably because of transplacental acquisition of 25-hydroxycholecalciferol and 24,25-dihydroxycholecalciferol. Infants who develop rickets—especially those who are premature—should receive supplements of 400 IU of vitamin D daily.

Human breast milk does not contain sufficient calcium and phosphorus for premature infants, and therefore calcium (about 100 mg/kg/d) and phosphorus (about 50 mg/kg/d) supplements should also be given.

Greer FR, Steichen JJ, Tsang RC: Calcium and phosphate supplements in breast milk-related rickets: Results in a very-low-birth-weight infant. *Am J Dis Child* 1982;**136:**581.

Weisman Y et al: Vitamin D metabolites in human milk. *J Pediatr* 1982;**100:**745.

3. VITAMIN D DEPENDENCY

Vitamin D-dependency rickets is a form of vitamin D-resistant disease that is probably due either to (1) a disorder in the formation or activity of 1,25-dihydroxycholecalciferol, which is the intestinally active polar dihydroxy form of 25-hydroxycholecalciferol; or (2) end-organ insensitivity to vitamin D. The forms are accordingly called type I and type II, respectively. The clinical features appear in the first year of life and mimic closely those of vitamin D-deficiency rickets. In type I, other siblings may be affected, and there is usually a history of normal vitamin D ingestion. There is a prompt response in type I to the administration of calcitriol (1,25-dihydroxycholecalciferol), starting with 0.25 μg/d and continuing until a biochemical response is achieved or a dose of 0.5–1.5 μg/d is reached. In type II, up to 600 ng/kg/d may be needed for a clinical response. The presence of hyperaminoacidemia and renal tubular acidosis distinguishes the condition from X-linked hypophosphatemic vitamin D-resistant rickets. Differentiation from the complex Fanconi syndrome may be difficult. However, the latter form of tubular disease is always secondary to some other condition (eg, cystinosis) and also requires phosphate supplementation as well as vitamin D for treatment.

There is some clincial heterogeneity in type II cases. Alopecia and bicarbonate-losing renal tubular acidosis may occur. High serum levels of 1,25-dihydroxycholecalciferol do not respond to pharmacologic doses of vitamin D_3.

Eil C et al: A cellular defect in hereditary vitamin D-dependent rickets type II: Defective nuclear uptake of 1,25-dihydroxyvitamin D in cultured skin fibroblasts. *N Engl J Med* 1981;**304:**1588.

Fraser D et al: Pathogenesis of hereditary vitamin-D-dependent rickets: An inborn error of vitamin D metabolism involving defective conversion of 25-hydroxyvitamin D to 1α,25-dihydroxyvitamin D. *N Engl J Med* 1973;**289:**817.

Sockalosky JJ et al: Vitamin D-resistant rickets: End organ unresponsiveness to 1,25 $(OH)_2D_3$. *J Pediatr* 1980;**96:**701.

4. HYPOPHOSPHATEMIC BONE DISEASE

Hypophosphatemic bone disease occurs sporadically or in familial distribution as an autosomal dominant. It is characterized by hypophosphatemia, osteomalacia without rickets, a normal fasting tubular reabsorption of phosphorus, and genu varum. Serum 1,25-dihydroxycholecalciferol levels are normal, but serum phosphorus levels and bone mineralization improve with the administration of up to 1 μg of calcitriol (1,25-dihydroxycholecalciferol) daily.

Scriver CR et al: Autosomal hypophosphataemic bone disease responds to 1,25-$(OH)_2D_3$. *Arch Dis Child* 1981;**56:**203.

5. VITAMIN D INTOXICATION

Two forms of vitamin D intoxication are recognized. In the first, relatively small daily ingestion of vitamin D, ie, 5000 IU/d or less from oversupplemented foods, appears to have led to idiopathic hypercalcemia (see Chapter 25) in sensitized children. The outbreaks occurred primarily in Britain, and the condition is now uncommon in infancy.

In persons not resistant to vitamin D, doses on the order of 1000–3000 IU/kg/d may lead to hypercalcemia with nausea, anorexia, constipation, polyuria, and transient nitrogen retention. Later, nephrocalcinosis and irreversible renal failure can occur.

Treatment consists of immediate discontinuation of vitamin D.

VITAMIN E DEFICIENCY

Vitamin E is important in stabilizing biologic membranes. Vitamin E is widely distributed in vegetable fats, plant seeds, nuts, egg yolk, and leafy vegetables.

Lack of vitamin E through dietary deficiency or secondary to steatorrhea has been shown to result in hemolytic anemia in premature infants. The syndrome appears around age 6 weeks with rhinorrhea, edema of the feet, legs, and scrotum, and anemia. The latter is associated with a reticulocytosis, anisocytosis and poikilocytosis, and red cell fragments and spherocytes in the peripheral smear.

Long-established vitamin E deficiency due to chronic liver disease or associated with abetalipoproteinemia may lead to a syndrome with impaired coordination and sensation and abnormal eye movements.

Premature infants fed on formulas with a vegetable oil fat source high in linoleic acid require vitamin E, 0.7 IU/100 kcal or 1 IU/g of linoleic acid. This is particularly important with iron-fortified preparations if hemolytic anemia is to be avoided.

Bieri JG et al: Medical uses of vitamin E. *N Engl J Med* 1983;**308:**1063.

Oski FA: Anemia in infancy: Iron deficiency and vitamin E deficiency. *Pediatr in Rev* 1980;**1:**247.

VITAMIN K

Vitamin K affects the rate of hepatic synthesis of prothrombin (factor II) and of factors VII, IX, and X. A large number of dietary components have biologic vitamin K activity, including green vegetables, soybeans, and fish. Intestinal bacteria also produce considerable quantities of vitamin K for absorption.

1. VITAMIN K DEFICIENCY

Vitamin K deficiency is most frequently found in newborn infants, particularly when breast-fed, since human milk contains only one-fourth (15 μg/L) the vitamin K found in cow's milk. The incidence of severe bleeding in newborn infants given vitamin K is 0.3% compared to 2–5% for infants not given vitamin K.

Diarrhea, oral antibiotics, fat malabsorption, some special formulas, and—since bile salts are important in vitamin K absorption—obstructive jaundice may lead to vitamin K deficiency. Bacterial colonization of the infant's intestine is frequently inadequate during the newborn period.

Newborn infants are usually given 1 mg of water-soluble vitamin K (eg, AquaMephyton) intramuscularly, which prevents the postnatal fall in factors II, VII, IX, and X and lessens the incidence of neonatal hemorrhage.

Committee on Nutrition, American Academy of Pediatrics: Vitamin K supplementation. *Pediatrics* 1971;**48:**483.

2. VITAMIN K TOXICITY

Either excessive administration of vitamin K or administration of the fat-soluble forms can result in hemolytic anemia. This may accentuate hyperbilirubinemia in the newborn infant.

WATER-SOLUBLE VITAMINS

Deficiencies of water-soluble vitamins are much less frequent in the USA because of the frequent fortification, particularly with B vitamins, of many foods. Most bread and wheat products are now routinely fortified with B vitamins.

There is less danger of toxicity from water-soluble vitamins because excesses can be excreted in the urine. However, deficiency states can also develop more quickly than with the fat-soluble vitamins because of the limited stores. Deficiencies of folate and vitamin B_{12} are discussed in Chapter 16.

Davis JR Jr, Goldenring J, Lubin BH: Nutritional vitamin B_{12} deficiency in infants. *Am J Dis Child* 1981;**135:**566.
Moran JR, Greene HL: The B vitamins and vitamin C in human nutrition. (2 parts.) *Am J Dis Child* 1979;**133:**192, 308.

THIAMINE DEFICIENCY

Thiamine (vitamin B_1) is an essential cofactor in the oxidative decarboxylation of pyruvic acid to acetyl-coenzyme A and of other α-keto acids. With magnesium, it activates transketolase in the regeneration of fructose 6-phosphate from ribulose 5-phosphate in the hexose monophosphate shunt. The vitamin is water-soluble and easily destroyed by heat; nevertheless, overt deficiency states are exceedingly rare in North America. Where deficiency does occur, the impact is predominantly on the heart and peripheral nerves. The myocardium shows fatty degeneration, and there is edema of the heart and interstitial tissues. Myelin and axonal degeneration is found in the peripheral nerves. Low red cell transketolase in 20% of underprivileged children in the USA offers some evidence of subclinical involvement in this group.

Clinical Findings

A. Symptoms and Signs: Symptoms are most likely to appear in early infancy, especially if the mother is providing thiamine-deficient breast milk. The infant becomes restless, has attacks of crying as though from abdominal pain, and may vomit breast milk. The vomiting may increase and be accompanied by abdominal distention, flatulence, constipation, and insomnia.

In the acute cardiac forms, there is tachycardia, gallop rhythm, dyspnea, cyanosis, cardiomegaly, hepatomegaly, and pulmonary edema. The condition is rapidly fatal unless treated. In endemic deficiency areas, cardiac failure of unknown cause should always be treated with thiamine. Less dramatic (but equally serious) is the meningitic form that starts with a bulging fontanelle, head retraction, and dilated pupils and may go on to convulsions and coma.

In older infants, a chronic form is common in which the symptoms are anorexia, weight loss, weakness, diarrhea, constipation, and edema. Peripheral palsies, which may include vocal cord paralysis, may be seen, and the stretch reflexes are usually absent. Ataxia is a common finding.

B. Laboratory Findings: A blood thiamine level under 4 μg/dL (normal, 10 ± 5 μg) is suggestive of thiamine deficiency, but perhaps the most helpful test is to show a level of thiamine in the milk below 7 μg/dL. A low red cell transketolase level is also diagnostically helpful.

Differential Diagnosis

The initial symptoms must be differentiated from pyloric stenosis and other high obstructions. The cardiac forms may be confused with fibroelastosis, congenital heart disease, Pompe's disease, and severe pneumonitis. A sterile cerebrospinal fluid culture excludes pyogenic meningitis. Chronic thiamine deficiency must be distinguished from lead poisoning.

Prevention & Treatment

The disease can be prevented by a normal diet containing at least 0.4 mg of thiamine daily. In acute deficiency states, 10 mg of thiamine should be given intravenously, followed by 10 mg intramuscularly twice daily for 3 days and 10 mg orally daily for 6 weeks.

Prognosis

Complete recovery is expected provided an adequate thiamine intake can be ensured.

Sandstead HH et al: Nutritional deficiencies in disadvantaged preschool children: Their relationship to mental development. *Am J Dis Child* 1971;**121:**455.

THIAMINE DEPENDENCY SYNDROMES

Anomalies of the branched-chain keto acid decarboxylase system (eg, maple syrup urine disease; see Chapter 33) are known to present as a number of traits. One of these is thiamine-dependent and responds to 10 mg of the hydrochloride daily.

Thiamine dependency has also been reported in a syndrome with optic atrophy and intermittent ataxia, lactic acidosis, and hyperalaninemia due to pyruvate decarboxylase deficiency.

Pueschel SM et al: Thiamine responsive intermittent branched-chain ketoaciduria. *J Pediatr* 1979;**94:**628.
Scriver CR: Vitamin-responsive inborn errors of metabolism. *Metabolism* 1973;**22:**1319.

RIBOFLAVIN DEFICIENCY

Riboflavin (vitamin B_2) is a constituent of a number of flavoprotein enzymes involved in intermediary metabolism. As riboflavin phosphate, it is incorporated into Warburg yellow enzyme, cytochrome c reductase, and D-amino acid dehydrogenase. As the flavin adenine nucleotide, it is the prosthetic group in glycine oxidase, xanthine oxidase, and diaphorase. Riboflavin is water-soluble and is a constituent of both animal and vegetable protein foods (eggs, meat, fish, beans, etc); therefore, riboflavin deficiency often accompanies protein malnutrition.

Breast milk and cow's milk provide adequate amounts of riboflavin; thus, the disorder appears only in children on restricted protein intakes or in those with protein malabsorption. However, because riboflavin is subject to photodegradation, infants undergoing phototherapy may need supplementation. The characteristic triad of signs is sore red lips, seborrheic skin lesions with fissuring of the nasolabial folds and extending from the angle of the mouth, and a purplish-red smooth tongue with enlarged papillae. Corneal injection may also occur at the limbus, with eye pain, tearing, photophobia, and, ultimately, interstitial keratitis. Excretion of less than 125 μg of riboflavin per gram of creatinine in a random urine sample is suggestive of riboflavin deficiency.

The deficiency state can be prevented by a diet containing 0.6 mg of riboflavin per 1000 kcal. Treatment consists of giving riboflavin, 2 mg intramuscularly daily for 2 days, followed by 10 mg intramuscularly daily for 3 weeks. Thereafter, a diet containing adequate amounts of riboflavin must be maintained.

NICOTINIC ACID DEFICIENCY (Pellagra)

Nicotinic acid (niacin) may be ingested from natural food sources or derived endogenously as one of the end products of the kynurenine pathway of tryptophan breakdown. The molecule is a component of nicotinamide adenine dinucleotide (NAD) and nicotinamide adenine dinucleotide phosphate (NADP), which act as hydrogen and electron transfer agents. Nicotinic acid is plentiful in most protein foods and grains. The only critical diet is one of highly milled maize, which also has a low tryptophan content. Niacin deficiency is seen in chronic diarrheas and in a variety of anorexic states.

Pellagra tends to be associated with a state of chronic, difficult to define ill health. The most typical lesions are found on the exposed parts of the skin and are aggravated by sunlight and sometimes confused with sunburn. The lesions start as an erythema which then becomes darkly pigmented and progresses to a rough, sharply demarcated, fissured, scaly dermatosis with little tendency to desquamate. The mouth and tongue become red and painful, and there is widespread gastrointestinal inflammation with dysphagia, nausea, vomiting, and attacks of diarrhea. Apathy is seen in childhood, but not the more severe psychoses that occur in adult pellagra.

The skin lesions may be confused with those of kwashiorkor. In kwashiorkor, however, the lesions tend not to be on the exposed extremities but around pressure sites in the groin and trunk. The diarrhea must be differentiated from that due to parasitic diseases (including amebiasis) and other infections.

The condition may be prevented by ensuring a nicotinamide intake of 6–10 mg/d orally, depending on age. Treatment consists of giving 10–25 mg of nicotinamide 3 times daily for 2 weeks, followed by a continuing adequate diet containing sufficient B complex vitamins.

PYRIDOXINE DEFICIENCY

Pyridoxine (vitamin B_6) deficiency was first produced artificially in 2 retarded infants. One developed a marked hypochromic anemia, and the other developed severe convulsions. Both infants responded promptly to intravenous pyridoxine and were stabilized on 150 μg/d orally. Shortly afterward, a group of infants given a proprietary liquid milk formula were observed to become hyperirritable between 6 weeks and 4 months of age. Generalized seizures followed and were treated successfully with oral pyridoxine or with a formula containing normal amounts of pyridoxine. A similar history was given by a mother whose breast milk was shown to contain unusually low amounts of pyridoxine. These infants all had normal interictal electroencephalographic findings, had no history of convulsions, and developed unexceptionally on a proper diet. Although pyridoxal phosphate is a coenzyme in a wide range of reactions, the key pyridoxal-dependent reaction in causing convulsions is thought to be that of the formation of gamma-aminobutyric acid from glutamic acid by glutamic acid decarboxylase.

In infancy, pyridoxal deficiency should be considered in any otherwise undiagnosed case of convulsions, anemia, or chronic diarrhea. Children receiving penicillamine for Wilson's disease or isoniazid or cycloserine for tuberculosis should be given pyridoxine, 2 mg/kg/d orally.

Complete recovery may be expected after the administration of 5 mg of pyridoxine intramuscularly followed by 0.5 mg daily by mouth for 2 weeks together with a normal dietary intake.

THE PYRIDOXINE (VITAMIN B_6) DEPENDENCY SYNDROMES

There are a number of rare inborn errors of metabolism in which the clinical picture or the abnormal biochemistry is ameliorated by large doses of pyridoxine given as the cofactor for the abnormal enzyme.

Some cases of infantile seizures respond promptly to 2–10 mg of pyridoxine orally, as do some cases of myoclonic epilepsy, although in the latter, treatment may have to be sustained with doses up to 100 mg/d orally.

Pyridoxine may also restore normal biochemical patterns in cases of homocystinuria, cystathioninuria, and kynureninase deficiency. It has recently been shown that pyridoxal phosphate may inhibit platelet aggregation and prolong clotting time, thus playing a role in entities such as hemolytic-uremic syndrome and in presenting vascular damage in hypercholesterolemia type II.

Is vitamin B_6 an antithrombotic agent? (Editorial.) *Lancet* 1981;**1:**1299.

BIOTIN DEFICIENCY

Biotin is a cofactor for carboxylases and other enzymes involved in CO_2 fixation. Biotin deficiency may occur with a diet of raw eggs, after prolonged parenteral alimentation, or with inborn errors of biotin metabolism or transport. Clinical features include an erythematous rash, keratoconjunctivitis, alopecia, and metabolic acidosis. Neurologic abnormalities range from mild hypotonia, irritability, and lethargy to frank ataxia. Response to biotin depends on the basic lesion.

Biotin deficiency. (Editorial.) *Lancet* 1981;**1:**1195.

Sweetman L et al: Clinical and metabolic abnormalities in a boy with dietary deficiency of biotin. *Pediatrics* 1981; **68:**553.

VITAMIN C DEFICIENCY

Essentials of Diagnosis

- Dietary history of an infant 6–12 months of age fed cow's milk and no citrus fruits or green vegetables.
- Fretfulness, anorexia, weight loss, and tenderness of the lower extremities. Legs held in the frogleg position.
- Hemorrhages in the gums, skin, or mucous membranes.

General Considerations

Structurally, ascorbic acid resembles monosaccharide sugars. Most animal species can synthesize ascorbic acid and thus have no dietary requirement for this vitamin. However, humans, other primates, and guinea pigs cannot metabolize glucose to ascorbic acid, because of the absence of the enzyme L-gulonolactone oxidase.

Ascorbic acid has many metabolic roles. Because of its reversible oxidation-reduction capacity, it is active in microsomal electron transport. It is important in preventing depolymerization of collagen and in maintaining the integrity of ground substance. Ascorbic acid presumably has an effect on hematopoiesis, since anemia usually accompanies scurvy.

By protecting the enzyme parahydroxyphenylpyruvic acid oxidase from inhibition by its substrate tyrosine, vitamin C plays an essential role in the metabolism of tyrosine in the newborn period.

Large doses of vitamin C have achieved some notoriety in the prophylaxis and amelioration of the common cold. A recent double-blind study showed some evidence of benefit in a group of school-age girls. However, excess vitamin C may cause renal stones as well as scurvy in infants of mothers receiving high doses in pregnancy.

Clinical Findings

Populations where breast feeding is in disfavor and where most newborns are fed cow's milk have a higher incidence of symptomatic scurvy. A history of a poor intake of fruits and vegetables is also suggestive. The time required for the development of scurvy after a grossly deficient diet is instituted is about 4–7 months. Certain groups such as the Navajo Indians are especially susceptible; otherwise, the condition is rare.

A. Symptoms and Signs: Nonspecific symptoms appear before any physical changes are evident. Irritability, weakness, anorexia, weight loss, and tenderness of the extremities, particularly of the legs, are common. In more advanced stages of the disease, the affected infant lies quietly in the frogleg position and may exhibit pseudoparalysis because the slightest motion causes severe pain. Small or large hemorrhages may occur anywhere in the body but are most frequent under the periosteum of the long bones, particularly the lower end of the femur and the proximal end of the tibia; this may not be detectable on x-ray until healing has begun with superficial calcification. Gastrointestinal, genitourinary, and meningeal bleeding have been reported occasionally in advanced stages. Hemorrhaging under the mucous membranes of the gums is common if teeth have erupted or are about to erupt. Conjunctival and tongue hemorrhagic lesions are also common. Costochondral beading, which differs from the rachitic rosary by its sharpness ("bayonet" deformity), often occurs.

B. Laboratory Findings: A fasting serum ascorbic acid level of below 0.1 mg/dL suggests scurvy. Samples must be assayed within 48 hours of collection.

C. X-Ray Findings: The earliest x-ray changes appear at the sites of most active growth, eg, the knees, and are characterized by thickening and irregularity at the epiphyseal lines with a subepiphyseal zone of rarefaction. There is thinning of bone cortices with atrophy of the trabecular structure, causing increased transparency ("ground glass" appearance). Shadows of the subperiosteal hemorrhages give the affected long bones a club shape; they become more clearly outlined after several days of treatment, when bone formation is initiated in the periphery.

Differential Diagnosis

If there are no gum hemorrhages, the signs may resemble those of acute pyogenic arthritis. However, the radiologic evidence is distinctive.

Prevention & Treatment

Breast-fed infants ingest ascorbic acid at a rate of 20–50 mg/d (4.3 mg/dL) unless the mother's diet is very inadequate. Cow's milk contains lesser amounts of vitamin C. Attempts at adding vitamin C to proprietary formulas have succeeded despite the fact that vitamin C is extremely susceptible to oxidation and heat.

The therapeutic dose of ascorbic acid is 100 mg 3 times a day for infants and children. Infants should receive—in formula, citrus fruit juice, or green vegetables—35 mg of ascorbic acid daily.

Prognosis

Dramatic clinical improvement occurs within 24 hours after therapy with vitamin C is started. X-ray signs show some degree of amelioration within 10 days of the onset of therapy.

Miller JZ et al: Therapeutic effect of vitamin C: A co-twin control study. *JAMA* 1977;**237:**248.

Moran JR, Greene HL: The B vitamins and vitamin C in human nutrition. 2. "Conditional" B vitamins and vitamin C. *Am J Dis Child* 1979;**133:**308.

TRACE ELEMENTS

Deficiencies of iron, iodine, zinc, copper, selenium, chromium, and molybdenum have been documented, and manganese deficiency has been reported.

COPPER DEFICIENCY

Copper deficiency may occur in the following circumstances: (1) in premature infants, especially those fed on low-copper milk preparations; (2) in association with more generalized malnutrition states; (3) in patients maintained on prolonged total parenteral alimentation without copper supplementation; and (4) secondary to intestinal malabsorption states or prolonged diarrhea. Milk is a poor source of dietary copper, and infants rehabilitated on a milk-based formula are at particular risk from copper deficiency.

Osteoporosis is an early finding. Later skeletal changes include enlargement of the costochondral cartilages, cupping and flaring of long bone metaphyses, and spontaneous fractures of the ribs. The radiologic findings, which are attributable in part to a lack of copper amine oxidases, may suggest a diagnosis of battering. Neutropenia and hypochromic anemia are other early manifestations. The anemia results in part from a lack of copper-containing ferroxidases, including ceruloplasmin, which are involved in the release of iron from body stores. The anemia is unresponsive to oral iron and in later stages to parenteral iron. Other clinical features that may be associated with copper deficiency include decreased pigmentation of skin and hair, dilated superficial veins, seborrheic dermatitis, anorexia, failure to thrive, diarrhea, hypotonia, and apneic episodes. Very severe central nervous system disease is present in Menkes' steely (kinky) hair syndrome, in which a profound copper deficiency state results from a specific X-linked inherited defect in the intestinal absorption of this element.

The diagnosis of nutritional copper deficiency is based on a combination of clinical findings (especially osteoporosis, neutropenia, and anemia), suggestive circumstances (eg, prematurity), and the presence of a low serum copper or ceruloplasmin level that is not attributable to other factors (eg, hypoproteinemia). Ceruloplasmin accounts for more than 90% of the circulating serum copper. Ceruloplasmin and, hence, serum copper are physiologically low in the neonate but increase to adult levels by 1–3 months of age. In the preterm infant, this increase does not commence until 40 weeks postconception.

Copper deficiency can be treated with a 1% solution of copper sulfate (2 mg of the salt or 500 μg of elemental copper per day for infants). Preventive measures include copper supplementation of parenteral alimentation solutions to provide copper at a rate of 20 μg/kg/d.

Ashkenazi A et al: The syndrome of neonatal copper deficiency. *Pediatrics* 1973;**52:**525.

Danks DM et al: Menkes' steely-hair (kinky-hair) disease: Further definition of the defect in copper transport. *Science* 1973;**179:**1140.

Karpel JT, Peden VH: Copper deficiency in long-term parenteral nutrition. *J Pediatr* 1972:**80:**32.

Naveh Y, Hazani A, Berant M: Copper deficiency with cow's milk diet. *Pediatrics* 1981;**68:**397.

ZINC DEFICIENCY

Zinc is an essential component of many metalloenzymes, including at least one in every major enzyme classification (eg, thymidine kinase, DNA and RNA polymerases, alkaline phosphatase, and carbonic anhydrase). Zinc is of importance in normal pre- and postnatal growth and development, at least in part because of its role in nucleic acid metabolism and protein synthesis. Zinc also appears to have an important though poorly defined role in essential fatty acid metabolism and prostaglandin synthesis. In zinc deficiency, the immune system is impaired because of defective chemotaxis and T cell function and thymic atrophy. Release of vitamin A hepatic stores into the circulation may be reduced as a result of diminished synthesis of retinol-binding protein. Because retinyl reductase is a zinc-dependent enzyme, night blindness in alcoholics may not improve with vitamin A supplements unless zinc is also given. Testosterone synthesis and insulin secretion can also be reduced.

Severe zinc deficiency has occurred in many infants and children receiving total parenteral nutrition. Prominent features include acro-orificial skin rash, diarrhea, cessation of weight gain, and depressed mood. Zn^{2+} in a dosage of 100 μg/kg/d intravenously is usually adequate, but if gastrointestinal fluid loss continues, a much larger dosage may be needed. Patients should be monitored with plasma zinc determinations or measurements of zinc balance. The premature infant fed intravenously should receive Zn^{2+} in a dosage of 300 μg/kg/d.

In the autosomal recessive disease acrodermatitis enteropathica, severe zinc deficiency causes similar clinical manifestations. The molecular defects in this disorder have not been identified, but they lead to a partial block in intestinal absorption of zinc. Clinical manifestations appear in early infancy, though usually not until after weaning in the breast-fed infant. Early features are similar to those described above for severe acquired zinc deficiency states, together with frequent bacterial and candidal infections. Without treatment, death usually occurs in later infancy or early childhood. Before the importance of zinc in the diet was recognized, partial remission occurred in some patients. Other complications in survivors for long periods included eye lesions, nail dystrophies, hypogonadism, and lethal congenital malformations in offspring. Rapid and sustained remission can usually be achieved with Zn^{2+}, 30–50 mg/d orally. Breast-fed premature infants may have severe zinc deficiency resulting from a rare defect in the maternal mammary gland that prevents the normal secretion of zinc into milk. Premature infants are particularly vulnerable because of their relatively high zinc requirements. Milder degrees of zinc deficiency appear to be common in premature infants. Severe zinc deficiency is confirmed by a plasma zinc concentration of less than 40 μg/dL and often less than 30 μg/dL.

Impaired zinc absorption leading to mild or moderate zinc deficiency may occur with many disease states, eg, generalized malabsorption syndromes or excessive losses of endogenous zinc via the gastrointestinal tract, kidneys, or sweat glands. Regional enteritis, celiac disease, and cystic fibrosis may result in poor zinc absorption. Excessive urine zinc losses occur in any catabolic state, some liver diseases, intravenous nutrition, diabetes mellitus, and sickle cell anemia. Protein-energy malnutrition is frequently associated with zinc deficiency and can delay recovery, cause thymic atrophy, and impair T cell function. The skin lesions of kwashiorkor are attributable in part to zinc deficiency. Features of moderate zinc deficiency include poor growth, lethargy, anorexia, impaired taste perception, and delayed sexual maturation. Plasma zinc concentrations are usually mildly to moderately depressed (40–60 μg/dL); however, levels in this range may occur without zinc deficiency in association with infection and other disorders.

There is evidence that mild nutritional zinc deficiency sufficient to depress growth and, in some cases, impair appetite is quite common in otherwise healthy infants and children in the USA. Plasma zinc levels may be normal or mildly depressed but are difficult to interpret, especially in infancy. Because of the nonspecific features and lack of reliable laboratory indices, confirmation of mild zinc deficiency states has depended primarily on carefully controlled trials of dietary zinc supplementation. Zinc deficiency must be considered in failure to thrive, especially if appetite is poor. If suspected, a trial regimen of Zn^{2+}, 0.5–1 mg/kg/d, should be given. Nutritional deficiency is rarely due to a total lack of dietary zinc but usually to poor zinc bioavailability in the diet. In general, bioavailability is greater in animal products than in vegetables and grains. Zinc is absorbed from breast milk much more easily than from cow's milk or infant formulas based on cow's milk or soy protein.

Hambidge KM: Zinc deficiency in the premature infant. *Pediatr in Rev* 1985;**6:**209.

Krebs NF, Hambidge KM, Walravens PA: Increased food intake of young children receiving a zinc supplement. *Am J Dis Child* 1984;**138:**270.

Neldner KN, Hambidge KM: Zinc therapy of acrodermatitis enteropathica. *N Engl J Med* 1975;**292:**879.

Walravens PA, Krebs NF, Hambidge KM: Linear growth of low-income preschool children receiving a zinc supplement. *Am J Clin Nutr* 1983;**38:**195.

Wolman SL et al: Zinc in total parenteral nutrition: Requirements and metabolic effects. *Gastroenterology* 1979;**76:**458.

IODINE DEFICIENCY

Endemic goiter due to iodine deficiency has been eradicated in North American and other industrialized countries by effective prophylactic measures. Though goiters still occur, it appears that these may be due primarily to unidentified goitrogens. Goiter continues to be a major health problem in many developing countries, particularly in mountainous areas such as the Andes and Himalayas and in parts of Africa, Southeast Asia, and Oceania. Goiter occurs when iodine intake or excretion in urine is less than 20 μg/d. Most goitrous persons are clinically euthyroid. Maternal iodine deficiency causes endemic cretinism in about 5–15% of neonates who develop endemic goiters.

"Neurologic" endemic cretinism is seen clinically in most regions. This is characterized by severe mental retardation, deaf-mutism, spastic diplegia, and strabismus. Clinical evidence of hypothyroidism is usually absent, and it is thought that the neurologic damage may be due to a direct effect of fetal iodine deficiency or to an imbalance between T_4 (low) and T_3 (normal or elevated). "Myxedematous" endemic cretinism predominates in some central African countries. Signs of congenital hypothyroidism are seen in this type. It is thought that milder neurologic damage may occur in many other cases of endemic neonatal goiter.

Use of iodized salt has been highly effective in preventing goiter in North American countries. In areas where endemic goiter occurs, intramuscular depot injections of iodized oil have also been used extensively for prevention.

Endemic goitre and cretinism. (Editorial.) *Lancet* 1979;**2:**1165.

From endemic goitre to iodine deficiency disorders. (Editorial.) *Lancet* 1983;**2:**1121.

OTHER TRACE METAL DEFICIENCIES

Trivalent **chromium** probably functions as a cofactor for insulin at the insulin-responsive cell membrane and is necessary for normal glucose tolerance. Chromium deficiency may be common, but information is limited, especially for children. Chromium supplementation in adults has resulted in improved glucose tolerance and significant increases in high-density lipoprotein (HDL) cholesterol. Children with insulin-dependent diabetes may have abnormal chromium levels, but the clinical significance is unclear. Chromium deficiency with resulting glucose intolerance has been reported in malnourished infants in some countries. Improvement occurred with a single dose of 180 μg of trivalent chromium administered as chromium chloride.

Selenium deficiency is the major etiologic factor in Keshan disease, which has occurred frequently in infants and young children in a large area of China. The major clinical feature was cardiomyopathy, now virtually eradicated with selenium supplementation. Selenium deficiency also appears to have caused fatal cardiomyopathy in an adult receiving prolonged intravenous nutrition. Low levels of selenium and low activity of erythrocyte glutathione peroxidase, a selenium enzyme, have occurred in children with inborn errors of amino acid metabolism given semisynthetic diets low in selenium. The clinical significance of these findings is not known.

One case of **molybdenum** deficiency has been documented in an adult receiving parenteral nutrition. Associated findings were central nervous system dysfunction and deficiencies of xanthine oxidase and sulfite oxidase, both of which contain molybdenum.

Low **manganese** levels have been reported in seizure disorders and malabsorption syndromes, but a causal relationship has not been demonstrated.

Abumrad NN et al: Amino acid intolerance during prolonged total parenteral nutrition reversed by molybdate therapy. *Am J Clin Nutr* 1981;**34:**2551.

Hambidge KM: Chromium nutrition in man. *Am J Clin Nutr* 1974;**27:**505.

Johnson RA et al: An occidental case of cardiomyopathy and selenium deficiency. *N Engl J Med* 1981;**304:**1210.

Keshan Disease Research Group of the Chinese Academy of Medical Sciences: Observations on effect of sodium selenite in prevention of Keshan disease. *Chin Med J [Engl]* 1979;**92:**471.

FLUORIDE SUPPLEMENTATION

When fluoride is incorporated into the hydroxyapatite matrix of dentine, it affords an inexpensive and effective means of helping to prevent dental caries. Fluoride is most effectively administered in the drinking water, but in infancy and childhood, fluoride in vitamin preparations or tablets serves the same purpose. The need for fluoride supplements depends on the amount in the water supply; infant formulas now contain no added fluoride. A dosage schedule as recommended by the American Academy of Pediatrics is given in Table 4–10.

Breast-fed infants should be given fluoride supplements after 6 months of age.

Table 4–10. Supplemental fluoride requirements (mg/d).

Age	Concentration of Fluoride in Drinking Water		
	< 0.3 ppm	0.3–0.7 ppm	> 0.7 ppm
2 weeks to 2 years	0.25	0	0
2–3 years	0.5	0.25	0
3–16 years	1.0	0.5	0

Committee on Nutrition: Fluoride supplementation: Revised dosage schedule. *Pediatrics* 1979;**63:**150.

UNSCIENTIFIC CLAIMS FOR TRACE ELEMENT SUPPLEMENTATION

The trace elements (like the vitamins) have been taken up by the "health food" industry and used for purposes of commercial exploitation without adequate scientific support for their value in the diet. The result is that many people are spending money needlessly for dietary supplements that cannot help and might hurt (eg, too much zinc can lead to copper deficiency). Claims of trace element deficiency are sometimes based on chemical analysis of the hair. The physician should encourage young people to insist on good evidence of need before they expend scarce financial resources on these useless products.

Hambidge KM: Hair analyses: Worthless for vitamins, limited for minerals. *Am J Clin Nutr* 1982;**36:**943.

ESSENTIAL FATTY ACID (EFA) DEFICIENCY

Deficiency of linoleic acid has come to be increasingly recognized in recent years, particularly with the increased survival of infants after major bowel surgery. Linoleic acid is referred to either as an 18:2ω6 fatty acid, meaning that it has 18 carbons and 2 double bonds with the first at the 6 position from the methyl (omega) end, or as an 18:2Δ9,16 fatty acid, meaning that the 2 double bonds are in the 9 and 16 positions from the carboxyl (delta) end. Linoleic acid cannot be synthesized in the body and is thus an "essential" nutrient. Linolenic acid (18:3ω3) is required by some mammals but not, so far as is known, by humans.

The classic studies of Hansen et al (1958) clearly demonstrated the need of human infants for linoleic acid. Infants were fed milks containing 0.04–7.3% linoleic acid, and all infants who received the lower quantity developed dry, scaly skin. Of 16 hospitalized infants, 4 of 5 with pneumonia, 3 of 4 with skin infections, and 6 of 7 with diarrhea were on fatty acid-deficient diets. Premature infants are most severely affected because of their rapid growth and low fat stores. Growth failure is a common feature of EFA deficiency, and thrombocytopenia and poor wound healing have been described. Older children with cystic fibrosis or other fat malabsorption problems may also be EFA-deficient.

Metabolism

Linoleic acid (18:2) is metabolized primarily first by desaturation and then by elongation to arachidonic acid (20:4). Prostaglandins are produced from arachidonic acid, and their importance in physiologic systems is the subject of great research interest at present.

Laboratory Diagnosis

The laboratory diagnosis of linoleic acid deficiency should be made by gas chromatography of plasma and red blood cell fatty acids. The latter represent membrane lipid and are more likely to be altered in chronic deficiency conditions such as cystic fibrosis. Normal values ± 2 SD are given below but should be determined for individual laboratories.

	Percentage of Total Fatty Acids (± 2 SD)	
	Linoleic Acid	**Arachidonic Acid**
Plasma	29.3 ± 10	9.4 ± 6
Red cells	14.1 ± 8	19.4 ± 7

Levels of 16:0 (palmitic), 18:0 (stearic), and 18:1 (oleic) acids are usually elevated with EFA deficiency. In addition, a peak for a 20:3ω9 (5,8,11-eicosatrienoic) fatty acid may be detected, which is considered diagnostic of linoleic acid deficiency. Prior to the availability of gas chromatography, EFA was often estimated using a triene:tetraene ratio, which is the ratio of the quantity of fatty acids with 3 double bonds to the quantity of fatty acids with 4 double bonds (primarily arachidonic acid). This ratio increases to a level above 0.6 with EFA deficiency as 20:3 compounds increase and arachidonic acid (made from linoleic acid) decreases.

Treatment

Three percent of calories should be provided as linoleic acid. Human milk has 5% of calories as linoleic acid, but cow's milk has only 1% and young infants may be borderline deficient if receiving only cow's milk. The deficiency is usually not great enough to impair growth or cause skin lesions. Safflower oil has 77% of fatty acids as linoleic acid, with corn oil at 57% and soy and cottonseed oils at 53%. Topical application of vegetable oils to the skin has been tried in some infants who could not ingest adequate quantities orally, but this is not always successful. When intravenous fat emulsion (Intralipid) is used to treat or prevent EFA deficiency, it should be remembered that it is usually used as a 10% solution and that 50% of the lipids are linoleic acid. Thus, 100 mL of a 10% solution would have 5 g of linoleic acid, or 45 kcal, which would be 3% of the calories for a child receiving 1500 kcal/d. It should also be remembered that vitamin E requirements are increased when more polyunsaturates are given, especially in iron-fortified formulas.

Elliott RB: A therapeutic trial of fatty acid supplementation in cystic fibrosis. *Pediatrics* 1976;**57**:474.

Friedman Z et al: Rapid onset of essential fatty acid deficiency in the newborn. *Pediatrics* 1976;**58**:640.

Hansen AE et al: Essential fatty acids in infant nutrition. 3. Clinical manifestations of linoleic acid deficiency. *J Nutr* 1958;**66**:565.

Holman RT: Essential fatty acid deficiency in humans. Page 127 in: *Dietary Lipids and Postnatal Development.* Raven, 1973.

PARENTERAL ALIMENTATION

Intravenous alimentation (total parenteral nutrition [TPN]) is indicated when it is not possible to deliver nutrients by the enteral route. The development of the cuffed Silastic small-bore (0.1 mm) Broviac subclavian catheter has made it possible to continue parenteral alimentation for months or even years after massive bowel resections.

COMPOSITION OF BASIC SOLUTION

The most commonly used solutions are based on free amino acids and glucose, with minerals and vitamins added. In the past, the composition of amino acid solutions was influenced by cost and by regulatory difficulties of making changes. Different solutions are now more easily obtainable, and ones with a composition resembling plasma are often used in small infants. Essential fatty acids must also be given (see discussion of Intralipid, below). The solution given here is one that can be easily dispensed in any well-equipped hospital pharmacy. Ideally, it should be prepared in 24-hour batches, since prescription changes may be required. When the procedure is carried out at home, however, as with the Broviac catheter, weekly dispensing is satisfactory if the solutions are refrigerated. A laminar airflow table should be used to ensure sterility. However, if such a unit is not available, solutions may be assembled using syringes with Millipore filter attachments. Table 4–11 shows the composition of a standard solution. When given in a volume of 130 mL/kg/24 h, this solution provides a protein equivalent of 2.2 g/kg/24 h (1.2 g of amino acid is equivalent to 1 g of protein) and about 62 kcal/kg/d when 10% glucose

Table 4–11. Composition of basic solution.

Component	Concentration per L	Volume (mL)
FreAmine III, 8.5%	20 g	235
Dextrose, 50%	100 g	200
Sodium chloride,* 4 meq/mL	10 meq	2.5
Potassium chloride,* 2 meq/mL	10 meq	5
Sodium acetate,* 2 meq/mL	17 meq	8.5
Potassium phosphate,* 4.4 meq/mL	15 meq	3.3
Magnesium sulfate, 50%	3 meq	0.75
Calcium gluconate, 10%	7.5 meq	16.3
Phytonadione, 2 mg/mL	100 μg	0.05
M.V.I.-12 (2-vial multivitamin infusion) (each vial)	5 mL	5
Zinc, 1 mg/mL	1 mg	1
Copper, 100 μg/mL	100 μg	1
Manganese, 5 μg/mL	5 μg	1
Chromium, 4 μg/mL	1.5 μg	0.375
Sterile water, qs ad		1000

* Total concentration of Na^+ = 30 meq/L, K^+ = 25 meq/L, and phosphorus = 12.5 mmol.

is used initially and 110 kcal/kg/d when 20% glucose is reached after about 2 weeks.

In small infants, the phosphate should be reduced from 12.5 mmol to 2.4 mmol, and initially lower concentrations of amino acids may be advisable.

TPN solutions do not contain iron. Where nutrition is sustained by this method for long periods, iron dextran injection (Imferon) may need to be given intravenously or intramuscularly. Elemental iron in a dose of 2.5 mg/kg will raise the hemoglobin level by 1 g/dL.

MANAGEMENT

Catheterization

Insertion of the catheter is a surgical procedure done under sterile conditions. A Silastic catheter with an inner diameter of 0.65 mm (0.025 inch) and an outer diameter of 1.2 mm (0.047 inch) is inserted into the external jugular vein and advanced until it reaches the junction of the superior vena cava and the right atrium. This position should be confirmed by fluoroscopy. The other end of the catheter is then drawn back through a subcutaneous tunnel to emerge through the skin in the right parietal area. The skin opening should be inspected daily.

Infusion & Monitoring

The following is an outline of management principles.

A. Infusion Apparatus:

1. Give nothing but the alimentation fluid through the catheter.

2. Do not add anything to the alimentation bottle.

3. Do not draw or infuse blood through the alimentation catheter.

4. Change the alimentation bottle and infusion set at least once every 24 hours.

5. Change the intravenous tubing, including the Buratrol and infusion pump tubing, once every 24 hours.

6. Change the dressing around the catheter, using sterile technique with gloves, at least every 2 days. Use povidone-iodine ointment around the catheter.

7. Procedure when the catheter is to be removed: (a) Draw a blood culture through the catheter prior to removal; (b) prepare the skin around the catheter with povidone-iodine, pull out the catheter, cut off the tip with sterile scissors, and send the tip in a culture tube for culture; and (c) draw a peripheral blood culture if infection is suspected on clincial grounds.

B. Clinical Course: See Table 4–12.

1. Strict intake and output records must be kept.

2. Each urine should be tested for specific gravity, sugar, acetone, and protein.

3. Dextrostix determinations should be done initially at every shift for 4 days. When changes in flow rate or of glucose concentration occur, Dextrostix testing should also be done at each shift. Thereafter, Dextrostix determinations should be performed daily.

4. Blood glucose concentrations should be measured daily for the first 4 days and 12 hours after any change in flow rate or carbohydrate concentration of the infusate. Blood glucose should also be assayed if the Dextrostix value exceeds 200 mg/dL or if 1% or more glycosuria occurs. In such situations, the flow rate of the infusate should be temporarily reduced by half and fluid requirements compensated by peripheral infusion. This avoids osmotic diuresis and dehydration. Suspicion of sepsis should also be entertained.

5. Electrolytes, blood urea nitrogen, and serum pH should be determined each day for the first 5 days and then every third day thereafter. These same parameters should be measured within 12 hours after any alteration in flow rate.

Table 4–12. Monitoring summary.*

Variables	Suggested Frequency	
	Week 1	**Week 2 On**
Growth variables		
Weight	Daily	Daily
Length	Weekly	Weekly
Occipitofrontal circumference	Weekly	Weekly
Metabolic variables		
Blood measurements		
Dextrostix and blood glucose	See text.	See text.
Plasma electrolytes	Daily for 5 days	Every 3 days
Blood acid-base status	Daily for 5 days	Every 3 days
Blood urea nitrogen	Daily for 5 days	Every 3 days
Ca^{2+}, P, Mg^{2+}	Days 1, 3, 6	Weekly
Total protein	Days 1, 3, 6	Weekly
Liver function tests†	Days 1, 3, 6	Weekly
Alkaline phosphatase	Days 1, 3, 6	Weekly
Ammonia	Clinical indications	Clinical indications
Urine measurements		
Volume	Daily	Daily
Glucose	Void	Twice a day
Specific gravity or osmolarity	Void	Twice a day
General measurements		
Infusate volume	Daily	Daily
Oral intake (if any)	Daily	Daily
Prevention and detection of infection		
Clinical observations (general status, temperature, etc)	Daily shift	Daily
Complete blood count with differential	Twice a week and on clinical indications	Clinical indications
Culture	Clinical indications	Clinical indications

* In very long term therapy, monthly laboratory checks are usually sufficient.
† AST (SGOT), ALT (SGPT), and LDH.

6. Serum or plasma calcium, phosphorus, magnesium, total protein, AST (SGOT), ALT (SGPT), LDH, and alkaline phosphatase determinations should be made at the time of initiating the infusion, on the third and sixth days of the infusion, and then once a week. The one exception is that 2 days after any change in flow rate, these values should again be measured.

7. Because of the difficulty of obtaining adequate samples, blood ammonia levels should be determined only on clinical indication. However, the physician should be alert to the possibility of ammonia intoxication in any infant with lethargy, pallor, temperature instability, poor growth, elevated liver enzymes, acidosis, azotemia, or a blood urea nitrogen below 6 mg/dL.

8. A complete blood count should be obtained twice weekly.

9. Administration of packed cells or whole blood should be done on clinical indication and to maintain a hematocrit greater than 30%. The routine or empiric administration of blood or plasma is not indicated.

10. Parenteral nutrition should be discontinued, if possible, with the patient on good oral intake and should be tapered gradually over 1–2 days. Careful observation for rebound hypoglycemia after abrupt termination of total parenteral nutrition is mandatory.

11. A thorough laboratory flow sheet must be maintained at the patient's bedside.

COMPLICATIONS

The complications of total parenteral nutrition can be divided into those related to the catheter itself and the metabolic problems associated with this method of management.

Catheter-Related Complications

Catheters may be initially malpositioned if fluoroscopic verification is not used, and they may become dislodged if not carefully protected. Clots may develop around the tip of the catheter, especially if there is any pump malfunction, and this in turn may lead to pulmonary embolization or superior vena caval thrombosis. Infection is a frequent complication usually due to some lapse in technique, eg, failure to change the tubing or to give proper attention to dressings.

If there is clinical evidence of infection of the catheter, it should be removed, the tip cultured, and a new one inserted. The organisms most often involved are from the normal body flora, ie, *Staphylococcus aureus, Streptococcus viridans, Proteus, Klebsiella,* and *Escherichia coli.* Saprophytes such as *Candida* and *Aspergillus* and weakly pathogenic organisms such as *Serratia* may also be involved.

Metabolic Complications

A. Glucose: Because many patients are already malnourished, with consequent glucose intolerance, it is wise to increase glucose concentrations gradually.

Hypoglycemia is also a complication that is most liable to occur if the rate of glucose administration is suddenly slowed. Therapy should always be discontinued slowly.

B. Nitrogen: Hyperammonemia is now rarer with the increased arginine intake. Azotemia may occur if the amino acid load is excessive. Changes may also be seen in the serum aminogram, with elevated levels of methionine and, less importantly, of threonine, valine, and glycine. Such changes do not seem to be harmful. The need for taurine in alimentation of small infants seems now to be established, even though this amino acid is still not generally included in the formulation.

C. Anemia: The constant infusion of a hypertonic solution may cause mild hemolytic anemia. This should be monitored by weekly blood counts. The presence of anisocytosis and serum haptoglobin saturation with hemoglobin are sensitive indications of hemolysis. Transfusions with packed cells may be required occasionally.

D. Psychologic Problems: Older children who have been encouraged to eat in order to maintain their nutritional status may be depressed at becoming dependent on intravenous nutrition. Psychiatric help to allow them to ventilate their feelings is often effective. Parents should be encouraged to hold infants receiving intravenous nutrition so that normal emotional attachments can develop.

E. Hepatic Complications: In premature infants, a progressive cholestasis, with portal tract fibrosis and infiltration, may accompany TPN and occasionally progress to liver failure. Abnormal liver function tests return to normal in 1–4 months after discontinuing the TPN.

F. Other Complications: Acidosis from the use of amino acid hydrochlorides, copper and zinc depletion, and biotin and essential fatty acid deficiencies all need to be watched for.

American Academy of Pediatrics Committee on Nutrition: Commentary on parenteral nutrition. *Pediatrics* 1983;**71:**547.

Kerner JA (editor): *Manual of Pediatric Parenteral Nutrition.* Wiley, 1983.

INTRAVENOUS FAT

Intralipid is a preparation of soybean oil emulsified with egg yolk phosphatide that is 10% fat, of which 50% is linoleic acid. Intravenous fat is a useful source of calories when only a peripheral vein is available that may be damaged by the high osmolality of isocaloric glucose solutions. Present evidence, however, shows that fat is somewhat less effective in protein sparing than glucose. Intravenous fat may also be used in the specific treatment of essential fatty acid deficiency.

Intralipid cannot be mixed with other infusates, because of the risk of breaking the emulsion. For this reason, it is usually given "piggyback" into a side arm of the infusion set just before the venous insertion. The rate of administration of fat should not exceed 3 g/kg/24 h (emulsion rate of 30 mL/kg/24 h). The actual requirement of Intralipid during long-term parenteral alimentation is not known; ideally, it should account for 5–10% of the daily caloric intake. Giving about 15% of calories once a week in Intralipid is more economical and appears to be satisfactory. The effectiveness of the cutaneous application of linoleic acid, 2–3 mg/kg/24 h, deserves to be further explored.

Intralipid should not be given to infants with respiratory problems, because it may diminish pulmonary perfusion, or to those with serum bilirubins greater than 8 mg/dL, because of the risk of bilirubin displacement from albumin by fatty acids.

Committee on Nutrition, American Academy of Pediatrics: Use of intravenous fat emulsions in pediatric patients. *Pediatrics* 1981;**68:**738.

SELECTED REFERENCES

Alfin-Slater RB, Kritchevsky D (editors): *Human Nutrition: A Comprehensive Treatise.* Vols 1–4. Plenum Press, 1979.

American Academy of Pediatrics: *Pediatric Nutrition Handbook.* American Academy of Pediatrics, 1985.

Center for Disease Control: *Ten-State Nutrition Survey, 1968–70.* Publication No. (HSM) 72-8134. US Department of Health, Education, and Welfare, 1972.

Composition of Foods. Agricultural Handbooks 8-1 to 8-6. US Department of Agriculture, 1976–1980.

Fomon SJ: *Infant Nutrition,* 2nd ed. Saunders, 1974.

McLaren DS, Burman D: *Textbook of Pediatric Nutrition.* Churchill Livingstone, 1976.

Neumann CG, Jelliffe DB (editors): Symposium on nutrition in pediatrics. *Pediatr Clin North Am* 1977;**24:**1. [Entire issue.]

Olsen RE: *Protein-Calorie Malnutrition.* Academic Press, 1975.

Owen GM et al: A study of nutritional status of preschool children in the United States 1968–1970. *Pediatrics* 1974;**53 (Suppl):**597.

Suskind RM: *Textbook of Pediatric Nutrition.* Raven Press, 1981.

Symposium on Nutrition. *Pediatr Clin North Am* 1985;**32:**273. [Entire issue.]

Tsang RC (editor): *Vitamin and Mineral Requirements in Preterm Infants.* Marcel Dekker, 1985.

Walker WA, Watkins JB (editors): *Nutrition in Pediatrics: Basic Science and Clinical Applications.* Little, Brown, 1985.

Immunization 5

Vincent A. Fulginiti, MD

All pediatric immunizations are planned to prevent specific infectious diseases or their toxic manifestations. Thus, to achieve maximum effectiveness, the vaccines must be administered to the appropriate populations at the appropriate times in life when the individual is immunologically capable and has not yet been exposed to the natural disease. "Routines" of immunization are designed to simplify ordinary practice and to permit reasonable immunization scheduling. However, exceptions to the routine are dictated by peculiar local epidemiologic circumstances (eg, epidemics or absence of a disease in the community) and by individual differences in immunologic response or susceptibility to the adverse effects of specific products. Each immunization should be viewed as a balance between the risk of that disease in the individual and population and the potential adverse effects of the immunizing procedure. This chapter will attempt to present the "routine" as well as the tempering influences for each product and schedule.

Administration of vaccines and other biologic agents is not without intrinsic risk. For all products utilized, there are expected side effects and occasional adverse reactions. Each physician may be considered responsible for informing patients and parents of the risk of a given biological as well as its benefits. The patient (as well as the parent) should also be informed about the risk of *no* immunization, ie, the risks of the natural disease. Although consent is implied in usual practice, some sentiment is developing for a requirement that written permission be obtained before any vaccine is administered. In some states, such written "consent" is required for some immunizations. The Centers for Disease Control (CDC) has developed standard information sheets for parental or patient use before written consent is obtained by the physician. To the author's knowledge, there is no single authoritative method for documenting so-called informed consent in these circumstances. The prudent physician should discuss each vaccine with the patient or parent, answer questions if there are any, and obtain some record of permission granted by patient or parent for administration of the vaccine. It is anticipated that specific routine procedures may be adopted locally or nationally in the future.

Of vital concern is the maximum utilization of routine immunizations. If more than 95% of preschool children can be reached, then it may be possible to eliminate most, if not all, of the usual communicable diseases. This responsibility is shared by the parent (patient) and physician. Physicians should make a diligent effort to identify unimmunized individuals under their care and administer vaccines on the schedule applicable to their age group. Parents should use a standard form for recording immunizations, adhere to the recommended schedules, and maintain the immunization record as they would a birth certificate, passport, or other important document.

Sources of Information

Recommendations for immunization change as experience accumulates and new products and new indications become available. Several sources of such information are available to the practitioner:

(1) The American Academy of Pediatrics' *Red Book.* A useful, comprehensive guide to immunization practices. Distributed free to all Fellows of the Academy and available to others from the Academy, PO Box 1034, Evanston, IL 60204. The *Red Book* is supplemented by special information published as needed in the *Academy Newsletter*.

(2) *Control of Communicable Diseases in Man,* 14th ed. Benenson AS (editor). American Public Health Assoc., Washington DC, 1985. Similar to the *Red Book,* this publication provides somewhat more detailed clinical and microbiologic information.

(3) *Morbidity and Mortality Weekly Report.* A weekly publication of the Centers for Disease Control, Atlanta, GA 30333, of the US Department of Health and Human Services. Useful reports of the major notifiable diseases supplemented periodically with specific immunization recommendations of the USPHS Advisory Committee on Immunization Practices.

(4) Local public health agencies—either through periodic publications or by special bulletins—make available immunization information, particularly of a local nature. Specific inquiry about requirements for foreign travel, special immunizations, etc, can be handled at these agencies.

(5) *Health Information for International Travel* is a useful booklet published yearly as a supplement to *Morbidity and Mortality Weekly Report* and can be obtained on request from the Centers for Disease Control, Building 1, Room SSB 253, Bureau of Epidemiology, Atlanta, GA 30333 (HEW Publication No. [CDC] 77–8280).

STERILITY & SAFETY OF INJECTABLE VACCINE ADMINISTRATION

Avoidance of Bacterial Infection & Hepatitis

Most of the "sterile" or aseptic precautions are recommended in order to prevent the introduction of unwanted infectious agents. Simple cleanliness and the use of sterilized equipment would suffice to prevent most bacterial infections. However, the more stringent precautions are designed to prevent hardier bacteria and the hepatitis agent from gaining access to the vaccinee.

The following steps are recommended:

A. Single-Unit Dosage: Where possible, single-unit disposable equipment should be used for immunizations. Plastic syringes or single-dose vaccine units are most desirable.

B. Sterilization of Equipment: If glass syringes are used, adequate sterilization procedures must be employed between individual patient usage. The following procedures are recommended by the American Academy of Pediatrics: (1) Autoclaving at a temperature of 121 °C (249.8 °F) for a period of 15 minutes at 15 lb pressure. (2) Dry heat for 2 hours at 170 °C (338 °F) or boiling for 30 minutes is also acceptable, but one must be certain that the time and temperature requirements are met.

C. Disinfection: For most procedures, it is sufficient to cleanse the intended injection site and the surface of the immunization container with a solution of 70% alcohol. Some prefer 2% tincture of iodine followed by 70% alcohol. Iodine burns have occurred when the tincture is not removed or is allowed to pool in contact with the skin.

Routes & Methods of Immunization

All adjuvant or "depot" antigens that contain alum, aluminum hydroxide or phosphate, mineral oil, etc, should be administered *intramuscularly only*. Subcutaneous injection results in considerable irritation and pain and may lead to the so-called sterile abscess.

Intramuscular injections should be given into the anterolateral thigh or into the deltoid or triceps muscle mass (older children and adults). This is to avoid sciatic nerve damage, which may follow intragluteal injections.

One should always aspirate prior to injection to avoid intravascular administration.

Aqueous vaccines can be given either intramuscularly or subcutaneously—or, on occasion, intracutaneously.

Live vaccines should be given on occasions separated by at least 1 month. This will minimize potential interference and additive effects such as fever, malaise, etc, and will clarify the cause of reactions should they occur. An exception to this practice is the use of *proved* live virus vaccine combinations. These preparations have been shown to be effective and safe, with no additive clinical effects. If immune globulin has been administered, live vaccines should be deferred for at least 12 weeks.

Host Factors in Safety of Immunizations

Only healthy children should be immunized. Febrile illnesses, incubation of a childhood exanthem, and any active infection are contraindications to immunization. The child who has a "cold" when it is time for routine immunizations poses a problem in completion of the primary series. There are 2 alternatives to achieve adequate protection: (1) Have the child return between regularly scheduled visits when well. (2) Administer the vaccine. This requires judgment, as the child may have a minimal upper respiratory tract illness and will tolerate the procedure quite well.

Chronic illnesses in themselves are not necessarily contraindications; they may make immunizations more desirable or even mandatory. Caution must be exercised if central nervous system disease is present and progressive. Ordinarily, static central nervous system lesions do not contraindicate immunization.

Immunologic deficiency states are an absolute contraindication to live virus immunization. Whether congenital or acquired, these deficiency diseases expose the host to the danger of dissemination of the vaccine virus. Malignant neoplasms of the lymphatic system are frequently overlooked as predisposing the host to such complications. More and more children are being treated with corticosteroids and immunosuppressive agents. These drugs may induce a state of lowered immunologic reactivity, and live virus immunization at such times may result in generalized and frequently fatal infections.

Siblings of individuals who are immunodeficient should not receive live poliovaccine, since it may spread vaccine virus from the vaccinee to the susceptible person. Inactivated poliovaccine should be substituted. Measles, mumps, and rubella live vaccines do not spread vaccine virus and should be administered to siblings in order to prevent the natural disease from occurring in the vaccinees and thereby prevent exposure of the immunodeficient family member to the natural virus.

Allergy to a component of the vaccine preparation is infrequent but often can be anticipated. Antibiotic allergies should be elicited by questioning, and the antibiotic composition of various viral vaccines should be ascertained. Live virus vaccines now contain trace amounts of neomycin, which rarely produces a delayed-type local reaction and even more rarely a systemic reaction. Egg-sensitive individuals should not receive egg-grown vaccines; currently, only influenza viruses are grown in eggs. In the past, fowl embryonic tissue culture vaccines were thought to be free of egg antigens; however, recent experience has shown that trace amounts of ovalbumin may be present and may provoke an anaphylactoid reaction in sensitized individuals. (For specific advice concerning the management of children with egg sensitivity, see Herman et al, 1983.)

Rarely, patients are sensitive to mercury included in some biologicals as a preservative. Mercury can accumulate during long-term gamma globulin treatment, resulting in acrodynia (pink disease).

THE IMMUNIZING ANTIGENS

Increasing numbers of vaccines, antisera, and gamma globulin preparations are becoming available. They differ significantly in their composition, form, stability, route of administration, and timing. It is essential that the practitioner carefully assess each preparation before administering it to a patient. The brochure provided with the preparation is almost always complete in its description of the product and its proper use.

"Typical" Composition

The typical vaccine does not exist, but the following categories of components are found. The list is presented to point out the complexities of some vaccines and the difficulty in attributing an unusual reaction to a specific component. Immunization involves administering a complex product to a complex individual, and the result of this administration is complex.

A. The Principal Antigen: This may be whole bacteria, bacterial products (toxins, hemolysins, etc), whole viruses, or substructures of viruses.

B. Host-Derived Antigens: Protein or other constituents of host tissue may be carried along with or intimately associated with the virus particles.

C. Altered Antigens: Distorted proteins and other substances may become incorporated into vaccines as a result of the complex changes associated with the effects of virus infection on the cells in which it is grown.

D. Preservatives and Stabilizers: A variety of chemical compounds are employed to prevent bacterial growth or to maintain the desired antigen in a stable form. Mercury compounds and glycine are typical examples.

E. Antibiotics: Trace amounts may be found in viral vaccines that must be prepared in antibiotic-containing media. Various antibiotics are employed, and the "same" vaccine prepared by different manufacturers may vary in the specific antibiotics used.

F. Menstruum: All vaccines are solutions or suspensions. The fluid phase may consist simply of saline solution or may be as complex as the tissue culture media employed in viral growth.

G. Unwanted or Unknown Constituents: Despite elaborate precautions in preparing vaccines, viruses or other antigens may be included that are not wanted or not even detectable.

H. Adjuvants: A varicty of substances may be used to enhance the antigenic effect of the principal antigen. Such materials as alum, aluminum phosphate, and aluminum hydroxide are currently in use, and others (mineral oil, peanut oil, etc) may be employed in the future. These materials retain the antigen at the depot site and release it slowly, thus enhancing the response by prolonging contact.

Properties of Antigens

Antigens vary in their ability to produce the desired immunologic response; some do so weakly, and some strongly. For a given antigen, the response may be variable, with some individuals responding poorly and a few not at all. One should be aware of this phenomenon in assessing the clinical effects of a preparation. Some children who receive optimal immunizations will simply not respond and may contract the disease if exposed naturally. This should not condemn the particular antigen for all children, as it may protect the vast majority of recipients.

Adjuvant Vaccines

In general, depot type vaccines are preferred, since they provide more prolonged immunity and greater antigenic stimulation and reduce the systemic effects observed with fluid antigens, which are rapidly absorbed. For example, DTP (diphtheria and tetanus toxoids and pertussis organisms) provides prolonged antitoxic immunity against both diphtheria and tetanus. In addition, it enhances the antibody response to pertussis, particularly in early infancy. Fluid or aqueous preparations may achieve earlier immunity and are less likely to produce local reactions at the site of injection.

Gamma Globulin Preparations

A variety of gamma globulins are available for clinical use. Whatever the label, they are all essentially the same. They consist of roughly a 16% solution of a limited spectrum of serum proteins in the gamma range of electrophoretic mobility. They differ in their antibody content to a significant degree. For example, tetanus immune globulin is a preparation obtained by pooling and concentrating donor plasma from individuals recently stimulated with tetanus toxoid, thus ensuring a higher level of antitoxin than is found in other gamma globulins obtained from donors irrespective of their tetanus immunization status. Each of the specifically labeled gamma globulins contains a standard level of the specific antibody desired, whereas randomly prepared lots do not.

Gamma globulins are now available in both intramuscular and intravenous forms. The intramuscular preparation must never be administered intravenously. The intravenous forms are provided by different manufacturers and have some differing characteristics. Each product must be administered strictly according to the guidelines provided by the manufacturer in the package insert.

The dosage of gamma globulin is not uniform but varies for each specific preparation and for the specific clinical circumstances of its use. One must learn these variables in order to use the antibody contained in the preparations effectively.

Intradermal testing with gamma globulin is unnecessary and may be misleading. The intradermal inoculation of gamma globulin may result in a wheal and flare reaction that does not indicate sensitivity to intramuscular administration. Thus, this method is not advised.

Whenever gamma globulin is administered simultaneously with an active immunizing antigen, one must be concerned about decreasing the effect of the antigen. This is due to the combination of the specific antibody in the gamma globulin with the antigen that occurs in the host after injection. It may be wise in some situations to administer additional doses of the antigen subsequently to ensure adequate stimulation. These special circumstances are pointed out in the specific immunization sections that follow.

Horse Serum Sensitivity

A major limiting factor in the use of antibody in the form of horse serum is the existence or development of horse serum sensitivity. This possibility must be considered each time the use of horse serum is contemplated. Appropriate medications to treat anaphylactic shock should be readily available. The possibility of serum sickness developing later should be borne in mind.

To test for preexistent horse serum sensitivity, the following steps should be taken:

A. Allergic History: Elicit a careful history of prior administration of horse serum products and of any allergic reactions. Allergy in general is an indication for caution in administering horse serum.

B. Sensitivity Tests: Skin or conjunctival tests should be performed, bearing in mind that severe reactions may occur from the testing procedure itself and that the physician must be prepared to intercede.

1. Skin test—Give intradermally 0.1 mL of a 1:100 saline dilution of the serum to be used. In allergic individuals, reduce the dose to 0.05 mL of a 1:1000 dilution. The appearance of a wheal in 10–30 minutes indicates hypersensitivity.

2. Conjunctival test—One drop of a 1:10 dilution in saline is placed in the lower conjunctival sac and 1 drop of saline solution in the other eye as a control. A positive reaction consists of conjunctivitis and tearing in 10–30 minutes.

C. Desensitization: Table 5–1 outlines the subsequent procedure to be followed.

Table 5–1. Desensitization procedure in horse serum sensitivity.

History	Sensitivity Test	Procedure
−	−	Intramuscular dose can be given. For intravenous use, give 0.5 mL serum in 10 mL fluid first; if there is no reaction in 30 minutes, give the remainder of the dose as a 1:20 dilution.
+ or −	− or +	If serum use is imperative, give 1 mL of 1:10 dilution subcutaneously; if there is no reaction, proceed with 1 mL undiluted and if still no reaction proceed as above.
+	+	Serum should only be used if there is no alternative and it may be lifesaving. Begin with 0.05 mL of a 1:20 dilution subcutaneously and increase every 15 minutes as follows if there is no reaction: 0.1 mL of 1:10, 0.3 mL of 1:10, 0.1 mL undiluted, 0.2 mL undiluted, 0.5 mL undiluted, and then the remainder of the dose. If an untoward reaction occurs at any stage, reduce the dose by half.

SPECIFIC IMMUNIZATIONS

DIPHTHERIA

Immunity against diphtheria is related to the levels of circulating antitoxin. Immunization may not prevent the carrier state. Occasionally, even well-immunized individuals develop the disease, although morbidity is less and mortality rates are lower in such cases than in the nonimmunized. Protection is in excess of 85%. The major significant reservoirs of diphtheria in the USA today are the unimmunized, particularly older individuals whose immunity has waned and underprivileged children who have received no immunizations.

Vaccines Available

A. Combined Diphtheria-Tetanus-Pertussis (DTP): See below.

B. Diphtheria Toxoid: This is recommended only when there is a specific contraindication to the combined preparations. It is usually given in 3 doses of 0.5 mL intramuscularly 4–6 weeks apart. A recall dose should be given 1 year later.

C. Diphtheria-Tetanus (DT) (Pediatric): This preparation contains full amounts of both diphtheria and tetanus toxoids and is indicated in those individuals who cannot be given pertussis vaccine. It is usually given in 3 doses of 0.5 mL intramuscularly 4–6 weeks apart with a booster 1–2 months later. Do not administer to adults, because severe reactions may occur.

D. Diphtheria-Tetanus (Td) (Adult): This preparation contains one-twentieth the amount of diphtheria toxoid contained in DTP or in pediatric DT. It is designed for use after the age of pertussis immunization. This amount of diphtheria toxoid elicits a booster response but results in far fewer local reactions. The dose is 0.5 mL intramuscularly.

E. Diphtheria Toxoid (Fluid): This is an infrequently used preparation that does not contain alum.

F. Diphtheria Toxin for Schick Test: Intradermal inoculation of 0.1 mL will result in 10 mm or more of erythema and induration approximately 4 days after injection. Pseudoreactions reach their peak earlier and fade by the third or fourth day. If a reaction occurs, it means that the individual has too little antibody to neutralize the toxin and is susceptible.

Schick test material may be difficult or impossible to obtain. If protection is questionable in a given individual, it is best to administer the vaccine.

Immunization Schedules

Diphtheria immunization should be initiated in early infancy. Three doses of toxoid, alone or in combination with tetanus and pertussis vaccines, are administered at 2, 4, and 6 months. A booster dose is required at 1½ years, at 4–6 years, at 14–16 years, and every 10 years thereafter (Table 5–2). If it is desired to avoid pertussis immunization, then 3 doses of pediatric DT should be administered to children younger than 7 years. Older individuals should receive 2 doses of adult Td 8 weeks apart. In all cases, a booster dose should be administered 1 year later and at 10-year intervals.

Precautions

Diphtheria toxoid is associated with few side effects in the pediatric age range. As it is a depot type vaccine, it should never be given by a route other than intramuscular. In older children and adolescents, a reduced dose of diphtheria toxoid will ensure a low reaction rate and still provide effective immunization.

Antibody Preparations

Diphtheria antitoxin (equine) is prepared by hyperimmunization of horses and is available in vials containing 1000, 10,000, 20,000, and 40,000 units.

Diphtheria antitoxin should be given as early as

Table 5–2. Recommended schedules of active immunization.

Normal infants and children	
2 months	DTP[1] and OPV[2]
4 months	DTP and OPV
6 months	DTP and (OPV)[3]
15 months	Measles, mumps, rubella[4]
~ 18 months	DTP and OPV
2 years	Hib[5]
4–6 years (school entry)	DTP and OPV
14–16 years	Td[6]
Every 10 years thereafter	Td
Those not immunized in infancy	
Less than 7 years of age	
Initial	DTP and OPV
1 month later	Measles, mumps, rubella
2 months later	DTP and OPV
4 months later	DTP
6–12 months later (or preschool)	DTP and OPV
Those not immunized in infancy	
Less than 7 years of age (cont'd)	
Anytime after 2 years	Hib
14–16 years of age	Td
Every 10 years thereafter	Td
7 years of age and older but less than 18 years	
Initial	Td and OPV
1 month later	Measles, mumps, rubella
2 months later	Td and OPV
6–12 months later	Td and OPV
14–16 years of age	Td
Every 10 years thereafter	Td
Older than 18 years	
Substitute IPV[7] for OPV and give boosters as directed by manufacturer.	

[1] **DTP:** Diphtheria and tetanus toxoid (alum-precipitated or aluminum hydroxide-adsorbed) combined with suspension of pertussis bacilli or extracted pertussis bacillary antigens—to be administered IM.

[2] **OPV:** Live polioviruses types 1, 2, and 3 in liquid form for oral administration. OPV is preferred vaccine (American Academy of Pediatrics, Committee on Infectious Diseases of USPHS, Special Institute of Medicine Poliovirus Immunization Review Panel).

[3] OPV optional. Should be administered in areas anticipating importation of poliovirus, eg, southwest border states in USA.

[4] **Measles, mumps, rubella:** All are live vaccines prepared in tissue culture and administered subcutaneously. Live measles vaccine may be administered alone (if preferred) or in commercially available combinations (see text). If these vaccines are given separately, a 1-month interval between them should be observed. The only live measles vaccine available is further attenuated, which should *not* be given with gamma globulin. Whenever possible, tuberculin testing should be performed prior to measles virus vaccine administration (see text).

[5] **Hib:** *Haemophilus influenzae* type b vaccine (see text).

[6] **Td:** Diphtheria-tetanus vaccine, adult preparation (see text).

[7] **IPV:** Inactivated polioviruses types 1, 2, and 3. Some experts feel IPV should be offered as a choice to all individuals. Most experts agree it is the preferred vaccine for the immunodeficient or immunosuppressed patient and as primary immunization for adults.

possible (half intramuscularly and half intravenously) in the following clinical situations: tonsillar infection, 20,000 units; anterior nares, 10,000–20,000 units; larynx, 20,000–40,000 units; nasopharynx, 40,000–75,000 units (dilute 1:20 in saline and administer slowly).

If the diagnosis has been delayed beyond 72 hours from the onset of symptoms and in very severe cases of diphtheria—especially those associated with considerable brawny edema of the neck—larger doses (80,000–120,000 units) should be employed.

The unimmunized individual exposed to diphtheria should receive 3000–10,000 units if follow-up cannot be ensured. Some experts prefer use of toxoid with culture and follow-up to use of horse serum antitoxin. Most experts recommend antimicrobial therapy in unimmunized contacts with any type of immunoprophylaxis.

Always test for horse serum sensitivity. Administer all antitoxin intravenously if symptoms are severe and the disease is life-threatening. The actual dose of antitoxin is less critical than early administration. If the patient has been ill more than 48 hours, increase the dose. ***Note:*** *Never substitute antibiotic therapy for antitoxin therapy.*

PERTUSSIS

Potent pertussis vaccines confer immunity upon infants given the full schedule. Attack rates can be reduced from 90% to less than 15%. One major problem is the need for early protection in infants, since little or no maternal immunity is transferred. Although schedules in which immunization is started at 6–8 weeks of life result in a lower level of antibody than those beginning after 6 months of age, it is vital to begin immunization early, accepting a somewhat lesser immunologic effect for the earlier protection afforded. Furthermore, booster doses eliminate the difference between the early-immunized and the later-immunized.

Considerable controversy about the alleged side effects of pertussis vaccine led to spontaneous reduction of its use in Great Britain and to cessation of its use in Japan. In Great Britain, at least 2 waves of pertussis occurred in the years following reduced utilization of vaccine; in Japan, more than 35,000 cases occurred, with 118 deaths from the disease. (The Japanese had originally halted their use of pertussis vaccine because of 2 deaths attributed to the vaccine—one from the "collapse" syndrome and one following encephalopathy.) After this resurgence of pertussis, vaccine utilization increased in both countries. In Great Britain, the standard vaccine was used; in Japan, a new acellular vaccine has been employed.

In the USA, there has also been controversy over the use of pertussis vaccine, and media attention has been focused on the issue of the risks involved. However, in view of the ratio of benefits to risks and in light of the experiences in Great Britain and Japan, most authorities urge that physicians continue to use the current vaccine (and observe the precautions discussed below) and that efforts be renewed to develop a safer but equally effective vaccine.

Pertussis vaccine has a predictable, very low rate of serious side effects and a much larger rate of annoying, temporary side effects with no residua. Pertussis vaccine is effective in reducing the risk of acquiring the disease and should continue to be used in routine immunization practice.

Vaccines Available

A. Plain Pertussis Vaccine (Without Alum): This is useful for rapid protection in epidemics. Administer 3 intramuscular doses of 0.5 mL each (4 NIH units) at monthly intervals. Vaccine is available only on request from the Michigan State Health Department.

B. Adjuvant Pertussis Vaccine (With Alum, Aluminum Phosphate, or Aluminum Hydroxide): Give 3 intramuscular doses of 0.5 mL each (4 NIH units) at monthly intervals for primary immunization. Within 8–12 months following primary immunization, whether with plain or adjuvant pertussis vaccine, a booster dose of adjuvant vaccine should be used.

C. Diphtheria-Tetanus-Pertussis (DTP): See below.

Immunization Schedules

Pertussis immunization is usually started at 8 weeks of age in combination with diphtheria and tetanus vaccine (DTP), but it may be begun at 6 weeks of age if convenient to scheduling of well-child visits in a particular practice. In areas of high endemicity, some physicians prefer to administer DTP at 2 weeks of age to initiate the series and then provide an extra booster dose at 9 months of age.

As shown in Table 5–2, 3 doses at bimonthly intervals complete primary immunization. Booster doses should be administered 8–12 months after completion of the primary series. Ordinarily, pertussis immunization is maintained by boosters at approximately 18 months and 4 years of life (prior to starting school).

Precautions

Since pertussis vaccine is usually a depot antigen, it should only be given intramuscularly. Local and systemic reactions (tenderness, induration, and fever) are common, and many physicians prescribe an antipyretic agent routinely for 2–12 hours following immunization. Severe reactions are less common and those involving the central nervous system least common. The occurrence of a severe febrile reaction or any central nervous system symptoms following pertussis immunization is an absolute contraindication to giving further doses. Pertussis vaccine should be administered to infants with central nervous system disease if their condition is static. If the central nervous system lesion is changing, do not give pertussis vaccine.

Recently, the *Red Book* Committee of the American Academy of Pediatrics recommended that DTP immunization in children with convulsions be delayed until they have had at least 6 months of freedom from convulsions or have reached 1 year of age and have seizures under control. At that time, a decision should be made as to whether pertussis vaccine is to be administered. If it is to be given, then DTP should be initiated and the usual schedule of intervals between doses followed. If pertussis vaccine is not to be given, then substitute DT and proceed with primary immunization.

Accurate statistics for reactions are scarce. A group of investigators in California found that local or transient systemic reactions (pain, erythema, induration, fever, irritability) occurred in 30–50% of recipients of DTP in contrast to a much smaller proportion of recipients of DT. Serious reactions included convulsions (1:1750 doses of DTP) and "collapse" (hypotonic-hyporesponsive reaction) in 1:1750 doses. None of the affected children suffered permanent sequelae.

Generalized urticaria has been reported in some children immunized with DTP and other vaccines containing these antigens in various combinations. It is not known whether this hypersensitivity reaction is caused by the primary antigens or some other agent in the vaccine. It is also possible that the urticarial reaction is unrelated to any component of the vaccine and just occurs coincidentally. In these instances, it is prudent to refer the patient to an allergist or immunologist for skin testing to determine if the vaccine evokes an immediate reaction. If the results of skin tests are positive, the physician may wish to consider desensitization, since vaccination is the only effective method to prevent diphtheria, tetanus, and pertussis.

A study of childhood encephalopathy in England placed the risk of postvaccine central nervous system involvement at 1:310,000 doses of vaccine.

Infantile myoclonic seizures (infantile spasms) and sudden infant death syndrome (SIDS) are *not* related to vaccine use, despite the fact that they occur in patients of the same age range as that in which DTP is administered. Several studies have shown that infantile spasms occur with the same frequency even if DTP is not initiated until 6 months of age and that they occur with equal frequency in vaccinated and unvaccinated infants. However, it does appear that DTP may elicit the illness in individuals destined to have it, since the onset of infantile spasms occurs more frequently in the first 7 days after DTP administration. Although there have been claims that SIDS is caused by pertussis vaccine, a large-scale study by the National Institutes of Health showed no such relationship. In the rare cases in which infants have been reported to die from the "collapse" syndrome (hypotonic-hyporesponsive reaction) after DTP administration, no causal relationship to pertussis vaccine has been established.

Prophylaxis

Pertussis immune globulin is no longer available commercially.

Although data are contradictory, some experts suggest the administration of erythromycin (40 mg/kg/d) to exposed infants. There is evidence that erythromycin can eradicate the organism in established disease without necessarily influencing the course of illness.

TETANUS

Tetanus vaccine is one of the best immunizing agents available, conferring almost 100% protection in a fully immunized individual. A prolonged period of adequate immunity follows primary immunization, and booster doses are required only 10 years apart. Military personnel who received primary immunization in the 1940s maintained adequate serum antitoxin levels or were easily "boosted" by a single dose as long as 20 years later.

Vaccines Available

A. Plain Tetanus Toxoid (Fluid): This preparation is rapidly absorbed, resulting in more rapid immunization, but it is rarely needed.

B. Tetanus Toxoid, Aluminum Phosphate Adsorbed: This is the usual "booster" toxoid. Administer 0.5 mL intramuscularly as a booster; 3 doses spaced at monthly intervals provide primary immunization.

C. Tetanus-Diphtheria Toxoid (Pediatric and Adult): See Diphtheria, above.

D. Diphtheria-Tetanus-Pertussis (DTP): See next section.

Immunization Schedules

Three doses of 0.5 mL of an adjuvant tetanus toxoid suffice for primary immunization. Booster doses should be given 1 year later and every 10 years thereafter.

Management of injuries requires (1) early treatment, (2) adequate surgical care of the wound, (3) antibiotic therapy, if indicated, and (4) tetanus immunoprophylaxis. With minor injuries, prophylaxis is not necessary, although this may be an opportunity to start tetanus immunization in an unimmunized individual. In the case of injuries involving heavy contamination or extensive tissue destruction or delay in treatment, it is desirable to employ both tetanus immune globulin and recall tetanus vaccine in the previously immunized. With lesser injuries, tetanus immune globulin should not be given, but a booster (0.5 mL) dose of toxoid should be administered if one has not been given in the past 5 years. In the unimmunized, both tetanus immune globulin and tetanus toxoid should be given. It is imperative that full immunization subsequently be completed in the unimmunized.

Precautions

Tetanus toxoid is one of the safest immunizing antigens in the pediatric age range. Reactions are very infrequent and usually mild when they do occur, consisting only of local erythema and tenderness. More severe local reactions, sometimes accompanied by fever, are encountered in older individuals with repetitive doses of toxoid. Reduction in dosage reduces the risk of such reactions.

Antibody Preparations

A. Tetanus Immune Globulin, Human (Hyper-Tet): This is the preparation of choice. It has virtually no side effects and is not immunologically removed from the circulation, ensuring prolonged antitoxin levels. It is supplied in 250-unit vials. The prophylactic dose is 250–500 units administered intramuscularly. The therapeutic dose is uncertain, but 3000–6000 units is the recommended initial dose. It is thought that this dose is sufficient, but in severe cases one may repeat it if the clinical response is unsatisfactory.

B. Tetanus Antitoxin, Equine: This preparation should not be used today, because of the dangers of horse serum sensitization. (Whenever possible, human tetanus immune globulin should be used.)

The equine preparation is supplied in 1500-, 3000-, 20,000-, and 40,000-unit vials. For prophylaxis against tetanus, give 5000–10,000 units. For therapy of tetanus, give 50,000–100,000 units—preferably half intravenously and half intramuscularly (given simultaneously)—after testing for horse serum sensitivity.

COMBINED DIPHTHERIA-TETANUS-PERTUSSIS (DTP)

The most common and most practical method for immunizing infants and young children is the combination of diphtheria and tetanus toxoids with pertussis vaccine (DTP). The combination has the advantages of triple immunization simultaneously and in one injection plus the enhancement of pertussis vaccine potency by the adjuvant effect of the toxoids. It has the disadvantage of confusing the cause of reactions, since all 3 antigens are given at once.

Vaccines Available

Diphtheria and tetanus toxoids and whole pertussis vaccine is a combination of the bacterial suspension of pertussis plus the 2 toxoids. It is usually distributed in multiple dose vials. The individual dose is 0.5 mL intramuscularly.

Immunization Schedules

Three 0.5-mL doses of vaccine are administered intramuscularly at bimonthly intervals, usually beginning at 2 months of age. A booster dose should be given at 18 months and again at 4–6 years. Thereafter, the pertussis component is eliminated and DT or Td preparations are utilized. (Exceptions are noted under Pertussis, above.)

Note: Recent data show that DTP can be administered simultaneously with some other vaccines injected at different sites. For example, simultaneous injections of DTP and M-M-R II (combined measles, mumps, and rubella vaccine) can be given to persons who find repeated visits to a physician inconvenient or who must receive multiple vaccinations over a short interval. In extreme cases, simultaneous DTP, M-M-R II, and OPV can be administered safely and effectively.

Precautions

See precautions for the individual components.

POLIOMYELITIS

Poliovaccines afford a high degree of protection to individuals adequately immunized against all 3 types of poliovirus. Both inactivated (killed, Salk) and attenuated (oral, live, Sabin) vaccines produce satisfactory immunity.

The advantages of inactivated vaccine (IPV) are that it cannot cause polio from the vaccine, the assurance that the vaccinee receives the vaccine, and simplicity of storage. The disadvantages include reduction in antibody titer and, presumably, immunity with the passage of time; the ability of wild poliovirus to grow in the intestinal tract of the vaccinee; and the need for repeated intramuscular injections.

The advantages of attenuated vaccine (OPV) include ease of administration (oral); prolonged immunity; intestinal immunity, which prevents wild poliovirus multiplication in the intestinal tract; a lesser risk of sensitization to vaccine constituents other than poliovirus; and its ability to limit epidemics by mass application. Its disadvantages include uncertainty of adequate immunization if the vaccinee vomits or if it is given early in life; the potential instability of types 3 and 1, which appear to have reverted to neurovirulence and have produced clinical polio in a few recipients or contacts of recipients; and the need for storage and maintenance at freezing temperatures.

The choice between IPV and OPV has been the subject of considerable controversy. This controversy erupted into the legislative and public domains, with the result that an expert committee of the Institute of Medicine was established to reconsider poliovaccine policy. The report issued in 1977 contains the following recommendations and findings:

(1) OPV should be continued as the principal vaccine.

(2) IPV should be provided for persons with heightened susceptibility to infection (immunodeficient children and their siblings, immunosuppressed persons, adults undergoing initial vaccination, adults traveling to areas of high incidence of disease).

(3) OPV is acceptable for adults who have previously been immunized or if circumstances do not permit adequate intervals for IPV administration.

(4) IPV should be provided to any individuals who elect to receive it after being informed of the

risks of OPV and the recommendation that it be administered. Such persons should be prepared to make a commitment to the full schedule of IPV immunization.

(5) One dose of OPV is recommended for all entrants into the seventh grade or equivalent. (Of course, a full series of trivalent OPV should be given to those who are unimmunized.)

(6) Any other immunization options were considered imprudent until at least 90% of persons are adequately immunized; federal support was urged to accomplish this.

(7) These recommendations should be reviewed.

(8) Current consent forms should be modified to reflect the above recommendations. Specifically mentioned were (a) more information on IPV and (b) a statement about a person's right to request IPV.

No further action has been taken on any of these proposals to date. The various recommending bodies still maintain that OPV is the vaccine of choice and are awaiting results of field trials with a more potent inactivated vaccine, alone and in combination with DTP, for primary immunization of infants. Preliminary results are encouraging, and thus recommendations may change in the future.

Within the pediatric age range, it would appear that attenuated vaccine in its trivalent form represents the safest, simplest, and most effective immunizing material. Until the issues are completely resolved, primary and so-called booster doses of poliovaccine should be the trivalent attenuated type.

In epidemics, monotypic vaccine corresponding to the epidemic type should be administered in a mass, short-term campaign. This method will result in limiting the epidemic but should be followed with efforts to provide protection against the nonepidemic types.

Early problems with inactivated vaccine manufacture that permitted live polio or simian viruses to remain in supposedly inactivated lots are no longer existent. Inactivated vaccines are now free of any demonstrable viral agent prior to release.

Vaccines Available

A. Inactivated Poliovaccine: This is a formaldehyde-inactivated virus containing all 3 types (1, 2, and 3). The viruses are grown on monkey kidney tissue culture containing minute amounts of penicillin. Neomycin is added during manufacture to ensure sterility. The vaccine does not contain alum or any other adjuvant. The vaccine is supplied in 9-mL vials. The usual dose is 1 mL intramuscularly.

IPV is available from Squibb/Connaught, Inc., Princeton, New Jersey.

B. Monovalent Attenuated Poliovirus Vaccine: This vaccine is no longer available. Its use is restricted to epidemics, and it is stockpiled at the Centers for Disease Control.

C. Trivalent Attenuated Poliovirus Vaccine: This preparation is similar to the monovalent preparation except that it contains all 3 types of poliovirus in a single dose. Each dose contains more types 1 and 3 polioviruses than type 2 in order to prevent inhibition of the other types by type 2. Current trivalent OPV is prepared in human fetal diploid cell culture.

Immunization Schedules

Scheduling of polio immunization has undergone many revisions, and a number of alternatives are available to the practitioner. A final and definitive schedule awaits long-term safety and immunity data. For the present, the following regimens are listed in the order of preference:

A. Trivalent Attenuated Vaccine Alone:

1. Infants—Three oral doses of trivalent vaccine are administered concurrently with DTP immunization at 2, 4, and 6 months of age. This regimen is followed by single doses of trivalent attenuated vaccine at 18 months and 4–6 years of age (just before entry into school).

2. Older children—Two orai doses of trivalent attenuated vaccine are administered 6–8 weeks apart. This regimen can be utilized in the unimmunized, in those whose previous immunization is uncertain, in those who have received monovalent attenuated vaccines, or in those previously immunized with inactivated vaccine. An additional dose of trivalent vaccine should be given at entry into school or nursery school if this is 12 months or more following the initial series.

B. Inactivated Vaccine:

1. Infants—Give three 1-mL doses intramuscularly at monthly intervals or as specified in the product insert. Booster doses have traditionally been given 12 months later and at approximately 2-year intervals thereafter for as long as protection is considered necessary, though the need for and timing of booster doses is currently a subject of dispute.

2. Older children, adolescents, and adults— If inactivated vaccine is the desired method of immunization, follow the recommendations in ¶ 1, but do not administer attenuated vaccine to individuals over age 18 as initial immunization. (See Institute of Medicine's recommendation, above.) Immunity may be maintained by 1 mL inactivated vaccine every 5 years, although exact schedules for booster doses are uncertain.

Precautions

Inactivated poliovaccine causes essentially no side effects. It is an aqueous product and does not contain alum.

OPV (attenuated vaccine) is associated with a remote risk of paralytic disease. In normal infants, the risk approximates one per 9 million doses. In siblings and other contacts of an immunized individual, the risk is somewhat higher, probably one per 3.5–4 million doses. Immunodeficient individuals may be at 10,000 times the risk of normal individuals.

Persons over 18 years of age should not receive the attenuated vaccine as an initial immunization. Known immunodeficient children or persons who are immunosuppressed should not receive OPV, nor should their siblings or children.

Antibody Preparations

Human gamma globulin is no longer used in the prevention of this disease. Although it is true that polio can be prevented by the prophylactic use of gamma globulin, there are no indications for its use for this purpose in modern medical practice.

MEASLES

Attenuated measles vaccine affords 95–100% protection against natural disease. Immunity appears to be long-lived—probably lifelong—but the exact duration will only be determined by continued observation.

Recent experience indicates that a sizable reservoir of susceptible persons exists despite the widespread use of measles vaccines in the last 24 years. Subpopulations in this reservoir include the following:

(1) Unimmunized persons at all ages. Over 90% of school-age children receive immunization. Younger children and those beyond high school age have a higher percentage of unimmunized persons.

In 1983, 1984, and 1985, measles outbreaks occurred on college campuses and among some high school groups. Almost one-third of all reported cases now occur in these aggregates. In some instances, the disease has been severe, and deaths have been reported. Sizable reservoirs existing in such localized communities favor transmission once a patient with measles exposes others to the disease.

(2) Individuals who received vaccine that was rendered inert by incorrect storage, handling, or administration. The size of this group is unknown.

(3) Individuals who received active live vaccine but failed to be immunized. There are several subgroups in this category:

(a) The 3–5% who fail to be immunized—so-called primary vaccine failures. This appears unavoidable with current vaccines, which are successful in 95–97% of the persons who receive them. There is no way of identifying such individuals.

(b) Infants immunized prior to 13 months of age, especially if gamma globulin was also administered. Failure of immunization in this group is probably the result of sustained maternal immunity. Estimates of the failure rate by age are as follows: 9 months of age, 35%; 12 months, 15–22%. There is controversy concerning the number of immunization failures at 12 months.

(c) Individuals given live vaccine after having received killed or inactivated vaccine. In many of these persons, the live vaccine was rendered inert in vivo by antibody developed after inoculation of killed virus.

(4) Recipients of inactivated vaccine, alone or in combination with live vaccine (so-called KKK or KL or KKL recipients). These children not only were unimmunized on a permanent basis but retain an unusual susceptibility to wild measles virus that causes severe disease on exposure ("atypical measles"). Several hundred thousand children received killed measles vaccine prior to 1968 in the USA and up to 1970 in Canada. Atypical measles has occurred as long as 16 years after receipt of killed measles vaccine.

These observations have led to revision of live measles vaccine recommendations, which are discussed below.

In recent years, the larger proportion of measles cases occurring in the USA has been in refugees or transmitted from refugees. Physicians should be alert to this when treating refugees or contacts who have a fever and a rash. Every effort should be made to administer measles vaccine to refugee children.

Vaccines Available*

A. Further Attenuated Measles Virus Vaccine (Moraten Strain): This product was prepared from Edmonston strain virus and passaged many times in chick embryo tissue culture. The result is further attenuation, with a lessened capacity for febrile and exanthematous reactions but apparent preservation of immunologic potency. The advantage of this vaccine is that it does not require simultaneous administration of measles immune globulin. The Moraten strain is the only currently available live virus vaccine in the USA.

B. Combined Vaccines: Measles (rubeola) vaccine has been combined with rubella (German measles) virus. It has also been combined with both rubella and mumps viruses.

Immunization Schedules

Attenuated measles vaccine should be administered at 15 months of age. If vaccine is given earlier, a significant number of individuals fail to be immunized, presumably as a result of sustained maternal immunity.

In communities with measles epidemics, infants pose special problems in immunization practice. Infants who are under 6 months of age and whose mothers had measles vaccine or the natural disease are probably protected from measles, since they have transplacental antibodies. From 6 months onward, the infant population has increasing susceptibility as maternal antibody wanes. If there is no risk of exposure, infants under 15 months of age should not receive measles vaccine. However, infants from 6–15 months of age who are likely to be exposed to measles should be offered protection. Administration of standard immune globulin (0.25 mL/kg intramuscularly)

* Inactivated measles virus vaccine: Two preparations were marketed for use; they are no longer available. One was prepared in monkey kidney tissue culture and the other in chick embryo tissue culture. The American Academy of Pediatrics has officially advised that children who were already immunized with these preparations be given a subsequent dose of attenuated vaccine (see Immunization Schedules).

will afford protection for 12 weeks or so, usually for the duration of most miniepidemics. When the younger infants in this group reach 15 months of age, they can be given live measles virus vaccine (M-M-R II). An alternative course of action favored by some physicians is to administer live measles virus vaccine instead of immune globulin. There are 2 potential problems with this procedure: (1) the infant may not be protected in time if exposure to measles has already occurred, and (2) the infant may develop immunologic tolerance to measles virus vaccine, which could result in less than optimal response upon reimmunization after 15 months of age. This latter phenomenon is controversial, with conflicting data in the literature. Because of these uncertainties, the use of immune globulin is recommended by the author.

Considerable confusion occurs as a result of varying recommendations by national advisory groups, local health departments, legislative statutes, and individual expert opinion. The major problems with the new recommendation of 15 months for initiating live measles virus vaccine are listed below with suggested courses of action:

(1) Should individuals immunized in the past at less than 15 months but on or after 12 months of age be reimmunized? Children who have received live virus vaccine at 12 months of age pose a dilemma for the clinician. Such children number in the millions, and it is deemed imprudent to reimmunize all of them because of the limited experience with 2 doses of live virus vaccine. However, in an epidemic situation, it is probably wise to reimmunize those who are at risk of exposure. It is hoped that this dilemma will be resolved by an intense immunization campaign that should reduce the incidence of minor epidemics of measles.

Routine reimmunization of all such individuals is not recommended for the following reasons:

(a) Millions of children are involved, and over 85% of them are already immune. To reach the approximately 15% who are not immune would require administration of a second dose of live vaccine to the 85% or more who are. Although second doses of live virus vaccine are thought to be safe, the data are insufficient to be certain.

(b) One modification of this negative recommendation is to reimmunize those at high risk of exposure to natural disease. Thus, if in a given year and a given community measles is epidemic, it may be prudent to administer live vaccine to individuals who received their primary immunization at 12 months of age.

(c) Another reason for not routinely immunizing such individuals is the controversy about the accuracy of the data implying failure of immunity in 15–22% of children immunized at 12 months of age. Some studies do not show this effect, and some experts dispute the new recommendation.

(2) Should individuals immunized prior to a specified year, usually 1965 or 1968, receive a second dose of live virus vaccine? This recommendation is being made by some health departments on the following bases: (a) Children immunized prior to these dates most likely received their primary immunization either at or before 12 months of age; or (b) gamma globulin was apt to have been administered with the live vaccine.

The routine use of a given year as the cutoff point for recommending reimmunization is not felt to be sound. Rather, the specific history (or records) of each child should be examined and a decision made based on the reasoning detailed above.

Gamma globulin administration is cited as a reason for reimmunization as a result of confused interpretation of the data. The following facts are known: (a) If gamma globulin was given with Edmonston virus (the original measles strain, not currently in use) at an appropriate dose and at a separate site, using a separate syringe, the child will be protected. This observation is supported by several long-term studies. (b) If gamma globulin was given in too large a dose, or mixed with live virus vaccine, or injected at the same site, it is possible that the vaccine was rendered ineffective. (c) If gamma globulin was given in the usual dose for the Edmonston strain but in conjunction with one of the further attenuated strains (Schwarz or Moraten), it is possible that the vaccine virus was inhibited. (d) If gamma globulin was given with live virus vaccine *prior to* 12 months of age, immunization may not have occurred.

Again, it is wise to review the specific record of each recipient in order to make a sound decision regarding the necessity for a second dose of live virus vaccine.

(3) Should rubella and mumps live virus vaccines also be given at 15 months of age? Although there is evidence that live mumps and rubella vaccines are fully effective when given at 12 months of age, for practical purposes it is recommended that they be given together with measles vaccine at 15 months of age. The advent of the combined vaccine for measles, mumps, and rubella (M-M-R II) has made this practical suggestion easy to implement. The physician can administer a single product at 15 months of age and accomplish protection against all 3 viruses in 95% or more of recipients.

(4) What should be done with children whose history is unknown or confused? The prudent course to follow in instances where exact information concerning the timing and nature of the vaccines given is not available is to administer the appropriate vaccines as if no immunization had been given. The single precaution is in the instance of possible prior receipt of killed (inactivated) measles vaccine. In this circumstance, a local or systemic reaction may result (see below).

For individuals older than 15 months of age, a single dose of attenuated vaccine is sufficient. If the child has had natural measles but this is not certainly known, attenuated vaccine administration causes no untoward effects. Susceptible adolescents and adults have been immunized with no greater clinical symptoms than those seen in infants and children.

Further attenuated vaccine administration results in fever (5–15%) and rash (5%).

A special use of attenuated measles vaccine is in the just-exposed child. If attenuated vaccine is administered just prior to or on the day of exposure to natural disease in a susceptible child, the disease may be prevented by successful immunization. This is because the incubation period of the vaccine is approximately 7 days, in contrast to a 10-day period for the natural disease. However, if exposure has occurred one or more days previously, it is best to administer a preventive dose of immune globulin and to administer live virus vaccine 12 weeks later.

Inactivated measles virus vaccine is no longer available. A state of altered immunologic reactivity to live virus, attenuated or wild, appears to be induced in some vaccinees. This will result in induration, erythema, and tenderness at the site of subsequent attenuated virus vaccine in 6–50% of previous recipients of inactivated vaccine. Additionally, upon exposure to natural disease months or years after receiving inactivated vaccine (the longest interval to date is 16 years), some children develop an atypical measles characterized by pneumonia with or without pleural effusion, a petechial rash, edema, and temperatures of 39.5–40.5 °C (103–104.9 °F). Because of the risk of atypical measles, children who have been immunized with inactivated vaccine should be given attenuated vaccine. Although this may result in a local reaction in some cases, the risk is acceptable in the face of potentially serious atypical measles.

A few instances of modified or atypical measles occur in children who have previously been immunized with live virus vaccine. Although this finding has led to questions about the permanence and quality of immunity following live measles virus vaccine, the incidence of such reactions is very low, and no firm recommendations can be derived at this time. Only continued observation of vaccinees and the passage of time will provide the definitive information needed to merit reappraisal of current policy. For the present, practice should be guided by the overwhelming accumulation of data that suggest that long-term, solid immunity follows the administration of live virus vaccine.

Central nervous system reactions after live measles virus vaccine appear to be unrelated to use of the vaccine, since the incidence of such reactions is the same in immunized and unimmunized individuals. Contrary to earlier concerns that use of live measles virus vaccine might lead to an increase in the incidence of slow measles virus infection (subacute sclerosing panencephalitis), all evidence to date indicates that use of the live vaccine has resulted in a significant reduction in the incidence of this illness.

Precautions

Because attenuated measles vaccine has been associated with febrile convulsions, a history of febrile convulsions is a contraindication to its use. As with any live vaccine, its administration to pregnant women and to infants and children with acquired or congenital immunologic deficiencies is contraindicated.

Individuals who are allergic to eggs and who have experienced an anaphylactic reaction to egg ingestion in the past may experience anaphylaxis upon receipt of a chick embryo-grown vaccine such as live measles virus vaccine. Such children should be skin tested and desensitized if the test is positive. (For details, see Herman et al, 1983.) With negative skin tests or positive tests without a history of reaction to egg, the risk of administration of live measles vaccine is minimal.

Antibody Preparations

Measles immune globulin is no longer available. The dose of ordinary immune globulin for use in attenuated measles virus immunization is 0.025 mL/kg. In the prophylaxis of measles following natural exposure of a nonimmune individual, the dose is 0.25 mL/kg. This is the so-called preventive dose. Prevention of measles depends upon administration of an adequate dose early in the incubation period, usually within 6 days of exposure. In unimmunized susceptible patients, it is best to attempt protection with immune globulin upon exposure and to administer attenuated vaccine 8–12 weeks later.

SMALLPOX

Smallpox immunization is no longer necessary or desirable. The last instance of natural smallpox occurred in 1977, and despite diligent search since then, no additional cases have occurred. The armed forces are still immunizing some individuals, but there is no indication for immunization of anyone today.

In the past, smallpox vaccine was used by some physicians in an attempt to treat and prevent recurrent herpes simplex infections. There is no rationale to this form of therapy, and, in fact, it can produce serious side effects from smallpox vaccine.

In the rare instance of a civilian in contact with military personnel who have been vaccinated and who develop a complication of smallpox vaccination, the involved physician should contact the Centers for Disease Control, Immunization Branch, for advice.

RUBELLA

Rubella is a benign disease of childhood. The major reason for immunization is to prevent rubella infection of pregnant women and subsequent fetal infection. In 1964, more than 20,000 infants died or were permanently handicapped as a result of intrauterine rubella infection.

Immunization is recommended by the various immunization advisory committees for all prepubertal children in the USA. In England and elsewhere, immunization is only recommended among women of childbearing age.

The efficacy of rubella immunization has been established. More than 96% of recipients develop demonstrable serum antibody, and exposure has demonstrated protection against disease. However, reinfection with mild rubella virus occurs in individuals previously immunized, and it is not known whether a previously immunized pregnant woman who is reinfected will transmit the virus to her fetus. Most virologists do not believe intrauterine infection will occur in the fetuses of previously immunized pregnant women, because viremia has not been demonstrated.

Rubella virus is recoverable from the throat in more than 75% of recipients of vaccine. The virus is present in low titers, and except in a few instances, transmission to a susceptible contact has not been observed. It thus appears unlikely that a susceptible pregnant woman will contract rubella from an immunized child.

Arthritis and arthralgia have been observed in recipients of rubella virus vaccine. In children, the frequency is low. In adolescents and adults, over 10–30% of recipients have had this manifestation of immunization, paralleling the incidence in natural disease.

Peripheral neuritis, resulting in prolonged and painful neuromuscular syndromes, has been observed rarely in children who have received rubella vaccine. Two forms are thus far recognized: one affecting the upper extremities with severe, recurrent pain; and another affecting the lower extremities, resulting in a peculiar crouching posture. The exact significance and the extent of these syndromes are not defined at present.

Vaccines Available

Only one type of vaccine is now commercially available. The reader is advised to consult the manufacturers' brochures concerning specific instructions for administration. All rubella vaccine preparations are of the human diploid strain (RA 27/3).

Two licensed products incorporate rubella virus with other viruses: with measles in one preparation (M-R-Vax II) and with measles and mumps in the other (M-M-R II). There is no loss of antigenicity in these combinations, and they appear to be safe.

Immunization Schedules

Current policy is to administer rubella vaccine routinely in infancy and to attempt immunization of all susceptible children prior to pubescence. In addition, some experts advise identification of rubella susceptibility in postpubescent girls by antibody testing and subsequent live virus administration. If this approach is to be used, the following should be observed:

(1) Inform patient (and parent, where applicable) of risks of vaccine, including the occurrence of arthralgia and arthritis and the potential risk of fetal infection if pregnancy is current or occurs within 2 months.

(2) Rule out pregnancy by administering a pregnancy test.

(3) Advise a medically sound program of contraception for at least 2 months following vaccine administration.

The Centers for Disease Control no longer recommend that these precautions be taken—only that the postpubescent girl be notified of the risks involved and cautioned against becoming pregnant for 3 months after vaccination.

Although rubella vaccine can be administered at 12 months of age, since the recommendation to change measles vaccine to 15 months has been made and since rubella vaccine is most practically (and frequently) given in combination with measles and mumps vaccine (M-M-R II), it is most practical to administer it at 15 months of age.

Precautions

The usual precautions concerning live virus vaccines apply to rubella virus vaccine also. (See Measles, above.)

Rubella virus immunization may result in arthritic symptoms or in peripheral neuritis syndromes. These conditions postdate immunization by as much as 70 days, and the association may not be apparent unless sought.

There is a potential risk of decidual or fetal infection if a woman is pregnant at the time of receipt of rubella virus vaccine or becomes pregnant shortly thereafter (see Immunization Schedules, above.) Recent data from the Centers for Disease Control suggest that this risk is not realized in practice.

Some experts recommend routine reimmunization of all preadolescents in order to diminish the pool of nonimmune adults. All advisory committees oppose this recommendation, because 90% of this group is already immune, and the vaccinations are costly and time-consuming and carry risk of complications.

Antibody Preparations

No specific rubella immune globulin preparation exists. Standard pooled adult immune globulin has been used in exposed pregnant women in an effort to prevent transplacental virus transmission. Results to date have been unpredictable with doses of 20–40 mL intramuscularly.

MUMPS

Mumps is generally a benign disease that in most children either is asymptomatic or causes only mild to moderate symptoms. Infection may be accompanied by aseptic meningitis, pancreatitis, or orchitis or oophoritis. The gonadal complications are the major reasons for protecting adolescents and adults against mumps. An attenuated vaccine has recently become available that induces antibody in 98% of susceptible vaccinees, and early studies indicate almost complete protection for 1 year and possibly for 2 years. Further data on the duration of immunity will become available with continuing observation of vaccinees.

Vaccines Available

A. Attenuated Mumps Vaccine, Jeryl-Lynn Strain: This vaccine is a chick embryo-adapted mumps virus to which neomycin has been added. It is supplied as a freeze-dried (lyophilized) powder to be reconstituted according to the manufacturer's directions. Its stability is such that reconstituted vaccine must be used within 8 hours, preferably immediately. Storage of the dry powder is at ordinary refrigerator temperatures. The vaccine is light-sensitive and should be protected from sunlight. The dosage is 0.5 mL intramuscularly.

B. Combined Vaccine: Mumps vaccine has been combined with measles and rubella virus vaccines. In the combined vaccine (M-M-R II), it appears to be antigenic and safe.

Immunization Schedules

Routine mumps vaccination in childhood is now recommended by the Committee on Infectious Diseases of the American Academy of Pediatrics. Mumps immunization has a lower priority than any of the others discussed above, but it is especially recommended that the following groups who have not had mumps should receive the vaccine: children approaching puberty; adolescents and adults, particularly males; institutionalized children; and children in large groups where epidemic mumps may disrupt normal routines. Routine use in children should be limited to those over age 1 and only after DTP and poliomyelitis immunizations are complete.

The introduction of combined measles-mumps-rubella vaccines has led to the practical abandonment of individual vaccine indications. For those physicians who choose not to use the triple vaccine routinely at 15 months of age, the separate products can be administered according to the specific recommendations listed for each component.

The susceptible exposed adolescent or adult poses a difficult problem. It has been estimated that oophoritis occurs in 5% of females with mumps and unilateral orchitis in 20–30% of males. Although sterility is an extremely uncommon result, the gonadal infection is an uncomfortable and incapacitating one. The best course appears to be to administer attenuated mumps vaccine prior to exposure. Vaccination at or following exposure will not prevent mumps, since antibody development requires 28 days, but it will protect from future exposures in case infection does not occur.

Precautions

As with other live vaccines, mumps vaccine should not be given to pregnant women, to children with congenital or acquired immunologic deficiencies, or to egg-sensitive individuals (see Measles, above). No untoward reactions have been observed in a small number of adults given the vaccine.

Antibody Preparations

Mumps immune globulin is no longer licensed or available.

HAEMOPHILUS INFLUENZAE TYPE b

Haemophilus influenzae type b (Hib) causes severe infections in more than 18,000 children in the USA each year: 10,000 cases of meningitis and 8000 cases of other invasive diseases (epiglottitis, cellulitis, pneumonia with or without empyema, septic arthritis, osteomyelitis, etc). For all but epiglottitis, the peak age is in infancy, with 70% of serious cases occurring in the first 2 years of life. Immunologically, young infants do not respond well, if at all, to the polysaccharide antigen of the capsule of Hib, and this immunologic inadequacy accounts in part for the virulence of the organism in such young infants.

The extracted, purified polyribophosphate capsular antigen has been concentrated into a vaccine and tested in several countries. The largest experience has been in Finland, where the vaccine was shown to be ineffective in infants under 18 months of age, paralleling the natural experience with the organism. However, children 2 years of age and older responded well to the vaccine and were shown to be protected against meningitis for at least 4 years after vaccination. Children in the age group of 18–23 months were few in number, and experts have interpreted their experience somewhat differently. Although the Finnish investigators believe that the vaccine is effective in this age group, some North American authorities do not feel confident, because of the small number of children involved and the lack of significant data to justify vaccination. Thus, recommendations differ for this age group, but all experts agree about the usefulness of the vaccine for children from 2 years old until the sixth birthday.

Under intensive investigation are methods to overcome the lack of responsiveness of infants under 18 months, the most vulnerable age group. The most promising method at present is the coupling of Hib vaccine with diphtheria toxoid, which in preliminary investigations appeared capable of stimulating antibody in young infants. Other initiatives include the coupling or combining of Hib vaccine with DTP and with other protein moieties and the use of outer membrane protein antigens as the major component of vaccine. Currently, the only vaccine available is the polysaccharide capsular antigen, but one of the other protein-linked antigens may become available in the near future.

Vaccines Available

One manufacturer has produced and marketed a concentrated, purified polyribophosphate (polysaccharide) capsular antigen vaccine that contains 25 μg of antigen per 0.5 mL dose. The vaccine is sterile and lyophilized and contains, in addition to the principal antigen, lactose in a concentration of 2.5 mg/0.5 mL, thimerosal (mercurial derivative) 1:10,000, and sodium chloride for isotonicity.

Immunization Schedules

A single 0.5-mL dose of Hib vaccine is recommended for all children at 2 years of age. Attempts should be made at this time to vaccinate between the ages of 2 years and the sixth birthday. The American Academy of Pediatrics also suggests that some children who are older than 6 years and at unusual risk of acquiring invasive Hib infections (eg, children who have sickle cell disease or have undergone or are about to undergo splenectomy) may also benefit from vaccination.

For children 18–23 months of age, there are conflicting recommendations. Some experts suggest that these children be immunized now and then reimmunized after 2 years of age. The Finnish investigators recommend immunization at age 18 months and again at age 3 years. The American Academy of Pediatrics does not recommend immunizing any children 18–23 months of age. The Centers for Disease Control advocate consideration of immunization of these children if they are at high risk of disease (eg, if attending a day-care center) or if they have anatomic or functional asplenia or cancer being treated with immunosuppressive drugs. In any case, before a child who is 18–23 months of age is immunized, the parents should be told that protection is not ensured. There is increasing immunogenicity of the vaccine from the 18th month of life through 24 months; approximate rates for successful immunization are 75% at 18 months and over 90% at 2 years of age and beyond.

Children under 18 months of age should not receive Hib vaccine.

Routine reimmunization or booster doses of Hib vaccine are not recommended in the USA at this time. Further recommendations may be made in the future, or a new vaccine may supplant the current one.

Although data are limited, it appears that administration of Hib vaccine at the same time as DTP (but in a different site) does not result in higher reaction rates than those expected with DTP alone. Many experts, including the author, suggest that Hib vaccine not be administered with DTP; separate immunizations will avoid confusion of any reactions between the 2 products.

Precautions

Serious adverse reactions are not anticipated with Hib vaccine. Among more than 48,000 recipients of this vaccine in Finland, only one child experienced an anaphylactic reaction, and the reaction was easily controlled and temporary. Local reactions (induration, tenderness) and mild fever occurred in 50% of the Finnish children, but high fever occurred in less than 1%. In trials in the USA, fewer local and febrile reactions were noted.

Sensitivity to any component of the vaccine would contraindicate its use in that individual.

Antibody Preparations

Standard immune globulin is not indicated in the prophylaxis or treatment of Hib infection except in those individuals with immunoglobulin-antibody deficiencies, in which case it is administered for reasons of deficiency and not specifically to prevent Hib infections. Trials are under way to determine if administration of immune globulin early in life can prevent Hib infection in highly susceptible populations, such as among Native American children, whose incidence of infection is much higher than that of other North American children.

SPECIFIC IMMUNIZATIONS FOR SPECIAL CIRCUMSTANCES

RABIES

In the USA, about 25,000 persons receive rabies immunization each year. The vast majority of these immunizations are unnecessary, but the disease is so feared and the circumstances surrounding many animal bites so uncertain that administration of the vaccine seems the safer course to follow. However, there is a predictable morbidity with rabies immunization, and if unnecessary immunizations are given too frequently, the risk of complications of the vaccine or antiserum will outweigh the potential benefits. The physician must know the epidemiology of rabies in the local region. A bite from a pet beagle is not equivalent to a bite from a stray street dog. In the first situation, rabies is exceedingly unlikely; in the second, it is a distinct possibility. Physicians are referred to their state health department and to the USPHS for local information about rabies epidemiology in their areas of practice.

Vaccines Available

Fixed rabies virus is grown in human diploid cell (HDC) cultures and inactivated to produce the vaccine (HDCV). Two products are in use throughout the world. One is prepared by Wyeth Laboratories (USA) and is inactivated with tri-N-butyl phosphate and β-propiolactone. The other is prepared by Merieux Institute (France) and is inactivated with β-propiolactone. Both are supplied as 1-mL single-dose lyophilized vaccine, with diluent provided to mix the vaccine.

Immunization Schedules

A. Preexposure Immunization:

1. Indications—All persons in high-risk groups should be considered for prophylaxis. These include veterinarians, animal handlers, laboratory workers, and children whose life-style or environment exposes them to species with known rabies (eg, foxes, skunks, bats, raccoons) and other wild animals or domestic animals with a high incidence of rabies. Preexposure prophylaxis should also be considered for persons who will reside for 1 month or longer in areas of the world where rabies is known to be endemic and where the risk of bites, scratches, or abrasions is highly likely.

Even if preexposure immunization was given, post-exposure prophylaxis may be necessary (see below).

2. Dosage of rabies vaccine—HDCV should be given in a 3-dose regimen on days 0, 7, and 28. Response has been so uniform to this regimen that postvaccination antibody titers need not be obtained, except in certain laboratory workers with continuous exposure (such as virology technicians working with the wild rabies virus). In the latter group, individuals should have antibody tested every 6 months, and booster doses should be given to maintain appropriate titers as specified by the Centers for Disease Control (1:5 or higher by the rapid fluorescent-focus inhibition test) or by the World Health Organization (0.5 IU). For other high-risk individuals with frequent exposure, such as veterinarians or animal handlers, antibody levels should be tested every 2 years, with booster doses administered as needed.

B. Postexposure Prophylaxis:

1. Treatment of wounds—All potentially infected wounds should be immediately and thoroughly washed with soap and water. Tetanus prophylaxis should be administered as indicated.

2. Indications for postexposure prophylaxis—Always consult local health authorities for the particular epidemiologic status of rabies in species endemic to the area. In general the following guidelines prevail:

a. For dog and cat bites in areas free of rabies in these species, no vaccine need be instituted. In areas where rabies is possible in dogs and cats, begin rabies vaccine (see dosage, below), and either quarantine the animal for 10 days or sacrifice the animal and examine the brain by fluorescent antibody technique. If results are negative, then discontinue therapy; if positive, complete the full course of vaccine.

b. For cattle, horses, rabbits, hares, and wild rodents, consult local authorities. Bites from squirrels or from pet hamsters, guinea pigs, and other domesticated rodents almost never require rabies prophylaxis.

c. Uncaptured animals always pose a problem. In areas free of rabies, the physician need not administer prophylaxis unless the circumstances of the bite are suspicious, eg, an unprovoked attack by an animal that appeared ill. In areas where rabies is possible in the particular species of animal, always institute and complete prophylaxis.

d. Wild animal bites, particularly by skunks and bats, are absolute indications for rabies prophylaxis. Frequently, therapy is delayed in the case of wild animal bites pending confirmation of rabies in the captured or killed animal. The author believes this is an unwise practice. Therapy should be started as soon after the bite as possible. The physician can always discontinue therapy if the animal is proved to be free of rabies, but lost time cannot be regained if the animal is rabid.

e. Pets seldom become infected unless exposed to a rabid animal. Pets with current rabies immunization are obviously not a risk.

f. Provoked bites in toddlers are seldom an indication for immunization, particularly if the animal is a pet.

g. Stray animals pose a special problem, since they frequently cannot be found. The physician must depend upon current epidemiologic information and balance the risks of immunizing against the possibility of rabies.

h. If in doubt and the animal is impounded, begin immunization and discontinue the series after 10 days if the animal remains healthy. If the animal sickens or dies, it is essential that adequate virologic examination be carried out by the local public health authorities.

3. Dosage of postexposure prophylactic agents—Individuals who require rabies vaccine should receive *both* rabies immune globulin (RIG) and HDCV as follows:

a. RIG—As soon after exposure as is possible—but even up to 8 days if medical care has been delayed—administer 20 IU/kg in an adequate muscle mass. If possible, give half of the dose by infiltration at and around the bite and the other half intramuscularly. (If RIG is unavailable, antirabies serum may be substituted; give 40 IU/kg.)

b. HDCV—As soon after the bite as is possible, administer 1 mL of HDCV intramuscularly. Inject it at a different site from that used for RIG, and use a different syringe. Additional doses of HDCV are given on days 3, 7, 14, and 28. It is not necessary to measure serum antibody titers after this regimen unless the patient is immunosuppressed. The World Health Organization recommends a sixth dose of vaccine, administered 90 days after the first dose.

Note: If the animal is captured and does not have rabies, as shown either by negative results in examination of the brain or by lack of symptoms after quarantine, then vaccine can be discontinued. Otherwise, the immunization schedule should be completed as outlined above.

Precautions

HDCV causes far fewer reactions than vaccines in vogue years ago. Local reactions (pain, redness, local irritation) are noted in 25%, and mild systemic reactions (headache, nausea, myalgia, abdominal pain, dizziness) occur in 20%. Rarely, Guillain-Barré syndrome has occurred within 12 weeks of HDCV immunization.

Immune complex reactions have been observed in as many as 6% of persons receiving booster doses of vaccine and very rarely have occurred during primary immunization. Within 2–21 days after HDCV use, generalized urticaria and other symptoms (myalgia, arthralgia, arthritis, nausea, vomiting, fever, malaise) may be seen. Rarely, angioedema has been reported.

Reactions to RIG are confined to local irritation for the most part, with an occasional report of low-grade fever. Antirabies serum causes serum sickness in almost half of the treated adults. Children appear to have a lower reaction rate (see section on horse serum).

If a full course of rabies prophylaxis is indicated, the presence of mild adverse reactions should not be a cause for discontinuation. Administration of appropriate anti-inflammatory agents will usually control such reactions. If there are severe reactions, especially those involving the central nervous system, the risks of adverse effects must be balanced against the risk of rabies, and individual decisions must be made about whether to continue rabies prophylaxis. Antibody titers should be measured and a specialist consulted as further aids in determining the correct course of action in this potentially difficult dilemma. For consultation from the Centers for Disease Control, telephone (404) 329–3095 or (404) 329–2888.

Antibody Preparations

Rabies immune globulin (RIG) is prepared from the plasma of human volunteers who have been actively immunized. In other aspects, it is identical to all human immune globulin preparations. This is the preferred preparation for use in rabies prophylaxis.

Antirabies serum is horse serum containing rabies neutralizing antibody, 1000 units/mL. Observe all precautions for horse serum administration.

INFLUENZA

Most experts estimate that protection in excess of 65–75% can be expected with influenza vaccine. Nonepidemic influenza is a relatively unimportant cause of serious childhood respiratory infections. Epidemic or pandemic influenza may result in significant morbidity in very young infants and in individuals with chronic cardiac, pulmonary, metabolic, renal, or neurologic disease. Furthermore, institutionalized children may constitute a unique epidemiologic setting in which rapid spread is facilitated. These groups should be immunized regularly, but especially in epidemic years. Pandemic spread may require more broad-scale immunization of healthy infants and children, particularly when a new antigenic strain appears.

As a result of experience in 1976–1977 with swine influenza immunization, much was learned of the safety and efficacy of influenza vaccines in children. Whole virus vaccine appears to be too toxic for use in children. However, preparations of inactivated vaccine that have been chemically treated to "split" the virus into its highly antigenic surface antigens are apparently both safe and effective.

Vaccines Available

Influenza vaccine is chemically inactivated virus. There are 2 principal forms. The first consists of the entire virus (whole virus vaccine) and is not further discussed, since it is not recommended for children.

Further treatment of whole virus vaccine produces a highly concentrated surface antigen product—the so-called split virus vaccine. This preparation currently contains antigens of the prevalent "A" strain of influenza and the expected "B" strains. The composition varies as the virus antigens change. Consult current recommendations for the year in which the vaccine is to be used.

The vaccine is an aqueous suspension and is administered intramuscularly.

Immunization Schedules

Routine immunization is not currently recommended. Only children at increased risk of influenza infection should receive the vaccine; these include children with chronic cardiovascular and respiratory diseases, malignant neoplasms, immunodeficiency syndrome, and immunosuppression. Other groups that may be eligible are those with chronic disabling neurologic or metabolic and renal diseases.

Precise dosage information is widely available.

Booster doses should be given yearly or at least within 3 years of primary immunization.

Side Effects

Three types of side effects and adverse reactions have been observed. They are more frequent with whole virus vaccine and negligible following split virus vaccine. Children with no prior influenza virus experience are more vulnerable to the toxic effects of influenza virus preparations.

(1) Toxic effects, presumably due to the viruses' innate toxicity, consist of fever, malaise, myalgia, etc, beginning 6–12 hours after immunization and lasting 1–2 days.

(2) Presumed allergic responses occurring within a short time after receiving the vaccine and consisting of immediate hypersensitivity or type I reactions (wheal and flare, urticarial lesions, and anaphylaxis) are very rare and may be related to egg sensitivity, although no such relationship has been proved.

(3) Neurologic reactions are much more common in adults. Guillain-Barré syndrome has been observed infrequently after influenza immunization, occurring at a rate of about 10 per million persons vaccinated. It also occurs in nonimmunized individuals. Permanent paralysis and even death have occurred.

Precautions

A history of severe reaction to influenza vaccine should preclude its readministration.

Egg-sensitive individuals should not receive the vaccine, as the virus is grown in hens' eggs.

Influenza vaccine is not absolutely contraindicated in pregnancy but should be avoided just like any procedure that is not essential.

PNEUMOCOCCAL DISEASE

Pneumococcal disease still accounts for many cases of otitis media, lower respiratory tract infection, and meningitis in infants and children. Although penicillin has resulted in marked reduction in morbidity and mortality rates from these diseases, some individuals are at very high risk. The immunodeficient child, the child with sicklemia, and the functionally and organically asplenic child all represent high-risk groups for abrupt, life-threatening pneumococcal disease. The disease encountered in these children is often fulminant and thus difficult to treat early and effectively. In addition, some pneumococci have been demonstrated to be resistant to penicillin and other commonly used antibiotics. These facts argue for the use of an effective vaccine, at least in selected groups of children.

In late 1977, a vaccine containing the purified capsular polysaccharide of 14 of the most common strains of pneumococci causing disease in humans was approved for use by the FDA. In 1983, a new preparation containing 23 strains was marketed.

Vaccine Available

Pneumovax 23 (Merck) and Pnu-Imune 23 (Lederle) are mixtures of capsular polysaccharides of 23 types of pneumococci, including those that account for almost 90% of blood isolates in humans. The vaccine contains 25 μg of each component antigen. *Consult product brochures for dosage and route of administration.* In experimental trials, children were given 0.5 mL subcutaneously.

Immunization Schedule

Pneumococcal vaccine cannot be recommended for routine use. The vaccine appears to be of low reactogenicity, although data in children are limited.

A single dose appears to be all that is required at present; the need for booster doses, if any, has not been established.

Currently, only children over 2 years of age with high risk of death following pneumococcal infections are candidates for vaccination. Amman et al (1977) suggest that patients with functional and anatomic asplenia as well as those with sicklemia can receive this vaccine safely and respond with demonstrable antibody titers. The immunized children with sicklemia, in addition, had significantly fewer serious bacteremic pneumococcal infections than unimmunized age-matched children with sicklemia (8 infections with 2 deaths compared to no infections).

Since infections have occurred in immunized children, both with strains of pneumococci contained in the vaccine as well as with some not present, prophylaxis with penicillin or ampicillin should still be undertaken. All infections in such children after immunization should be promptly and rigorously treated.

At present, the vaccine can only be recommended for children with sicklemia and functional or anatomic asplenia. Some experts add nephrosis and B cell immunodeficient states. More data are needed before recommendations can be made for other children.

Precautions

Adverse effects have been observed only rarely in the few children studied and reported thus far. Local pain and low-grade fever have been noted.

In 1981, development of anti-blood group A antibody was reported in some vaccinees, and pneumococcal vaccination of girls was therefore not recommended. A vaccine without group A substance has now replaced the earlier type of vaccine, and there is no longer any risk.

TUBERCULOSIS

BCG (bacille Calmette-Guérin) vaccine is an attenuated tuberculosis vaccine that is indicated for children in geographic areas or in social circumstances where the risk of infection is high. A positive tuberculin test indicates BCG will be ineffective and potentially dangerous. The vaccine should not be given to any child with acquired or congenital immunologic deficiency.

Immunization is accomplished by intracutaneous, superficial injection over the deltoid or triceps muscle. The dosage is 0.05 mL (newborns) or 0.1 mL (for all other children).

A large-scale, well-conducted trial of BCG in India did not demonstrate any protective effect.

CHOLERA

For infants and children traveling to or resident in cholera endemic areas, 3 intramuscular or subcutaneous injections at weekly (or longer) intervals are advised. The dosage is as shown below. Booster doses appropriate to age must be given as often as every 6 months to maintain immunity.

	6 Months–4 Years	5–9 Years	10 Years–Adult
First dose	0.1 mL	0.3 mL	0.5 mL
Second dose	0.3 mL	0.5 mL	1.0 mL
Third dose	0.1 mL	0.3 mL	0.5 mL

HEPATITIS B VIRUS

An inactivated vaccine containing killed hepatitis B virus surface antigen (HBsAg) is commercially available. It is prepared from human plasma and contains no known live agents of any type, including the putative agent of AIDS, HTLV-III. Hepatitis B virus vaccine is highly antigenic and affords 96% protection against infection with hepatitis B virus. It is recommended in a 3-dose regimen (at 0, 30, and 180 days) for individuals at high risk. Children in this category include (1) children in families with hepatitis B virus infection or chronic carriers (HBsAg-positive individuals); (2) children residing in institutions for the mentally retarded; and (3) children who receive frequent infusions of blood or blood products (eg, hemophiliacs, leukemic children). Other, more controversial indications include (1) close contacts of HBsAg-positive individuals who are not institutionalized and (2) infants born to mothers who are HBsAg-positive.

Efforts should be made to identify pregnant women at risk of transmitting hepatitis B virus to the infant. High-risk groups include women of Asian extraction (foreign or native born); sub-Saharan Africans; Haitians; dialysis patients or workers; contacts of dialysis patients; women with a history of hepatitis (during or before pregnancy); recipients of frequent transfusions of blood or blood products; women with numerous sexual partners; and intravenous drug abusers. Women in this group should be screened before delivery to determine if they are HBsAg-positive. The infants of those with positive results should be given hepatitis B immune globulin (HBIG), 0.5 mL intramuscularly, as soon after delivery as is possible, preferably in the delivery suite. The infant should then receive hepatitis B virus vaccine soon thereafter, again in 1 month, and finally at 6 months after the first dose. Serum antibody should be tested after the infant is 9 months old. If results of the antibody test are positive, nothing further need be done; if negative, test for hepatitis B surface antigen. If results of the antigen test are positive, the infant is probably chronically infected (up to 2.5% of infants are infected in utero, and infection cannot be prevented); if negative, administer another dose of vaccine, and retest for serum antibody 1 month later.

PLAGUE

Plague immunization is recommended for children residing in or traveling to endemic areas (particularly the Far East). Primary immunization is as follows:

	Age (in Years)			
	Less Than 1	1–4	5–10	Over 10
Day 0	0.1 mL	0.2 mL	0.3 mL	0.5 mL
Day 30	0.1 mL	0.2 mL	0.3 mL	0.5 mL
4–12 weeks later	0.04 mL	0.08 mL	0.12 mL	0.2 mL

YELLOW FEVER

Yellow fever vaccine is obtainable from certain public health facilities and is available commercially (YF-Vax). A single injection of 0.5 mL of a 1:10 dilution is given, with a similar booster dose every 6 years. For travel to certain areas, this immunization is mandatory. Consult authorities.

NEW, UNRELEASED VACCINES

Live Attenuated Varicella Vaccine

Varicella can be a serious, even lethal, infection in immunocompromised children, especially those with lymphatic cancer. Investigators in Japan developed an attenuated strain, OKA, that proved safe on administration to susceptible individuals with leukemia who were in remission. Investigators in the USA are exploring this vaccine as well as one developed in the USA. Normal children, some susceptible adults, and several hundred children with leukemia have received varicella vaccine thus far. Preliminary results in trials in the USA demonstrate efficacy and safety, and it is possible that one or more of these vaccines may be licensed for limited use in the near future.

Acellular Pertussis Vaccine

Researchers in Japan are investigating a vaccine containing 2 antigens derived from *Bordetella (Haemophilus) pertussis*. In small, preliminary trials, the vaccine appears effective in prevention of pertussis without significant side effects. If large-scale trials currently under way substantiate these preliminary results, the vaccine may be tested and licensed in the USA.

IMMUNE GLOBULIN PROPHYLAXIS & THERAPY

INTRAMUSCULAR IMMUNE GLOBULIN

All of the currently available human immune globulins for intramuscular use are similar in physical and chemical properties. All are prepared from pooled donor plasma (usually 1000 or more individual donors), are Cohn-fractionated, concentrated to a 16.5% solution, and have preservatives added. The generic term for such preparations is immune globulin (IG). Intramuscular IG contains principally IgG with only trace amounts of IgA, IgM, and other serum proteins. The IgG tends to aggregate on storage—a biologically significant phenomenon. Aggregated IgG behaves as antigen-antibody complexes and has produced anaphylaxis on entry into the bloodstream. For this reason, intramuscular IG preparations must only be administered intramuscularly, and great care must be exercised to avoid injection directly into a vessel.

Intramuscular IG can be very irritating because of its concentration. Doses larger than 5 mL must be split and injected deeply intramuscularly into separate large muscle masses.

The antibody content of a specific IG depends upon the pool from which it is derived. Ordinary IG contains those antibodies generally present in adults in large quantities—measles, hepatitis, pneumococcal, etc. IG that has been prepared from selected donor pools is termed special immune globulin (SIG) and is labeled with the name of the disease to be prevented or treated, eg, tetanus immune globulin, rabies immune globulin. SIG has carefully calibrated amounts of antibody directed against a specific infectious agent. The use of the various specific SIG preparations is discussed elsewhere in this chapter.

Adverse effects of IG or SIG are few. Pain on injection is usual, particularly with large doses. Rarely, so-called sterile abscesses may develop. Administration of intramuscular IG intravenously can result in anaphylactic shock due to aggregated IgG; rarely, anaphylaxis follows intramuscular administration of large doses if absorption is rapid. Individuals who receive IG may develop antibodies against some components. For example, individuals lacking serum IgA (one in 800 of the general population; a higher rate in some disease states) will develop anti-IgA antibody directed against the trace amounts of IgA present in IG. Subsequently, upon exposure to passive IgA such as occurs with blood transfusion, pyogenic reactions may occur. In similar fashion, antibody may develop against IgG in pooled IG that is genetically different from the recipient's IgG. Subsequent administration of "foreign" IgG may result in reactions.

A potential adverse effect of IG administration has not yet been demonstrated. Women who receive IG may develop antibody directed against those types of immunoglobulin genetically different from their own. If, during a subsequent pregnancy, a woman who has received IG has a fetus who possesses one of these different immunoglobulin types, it is conceivable that her preexistent antibody will suppress fetal immunoglobulin synthesis. Hypoimmunoglobulinemia may result in the fetus and be manifest after birth. This situation is analogous to Rh incompatibility. Thus far, this phenomenon has not been seen.

There are only 3 unequivocal indications for IG administration: (1) as replacement therapy in IgG-deficient states, (2) in the prevention of measles, and (3) in the prevention of hepatitis. All other uses are either unproved or unwarranted.

Replacement Therapy in IgG-Deficient States

Passive antibody can protect individuals incapable of IgG synthesis. Most conditions warranting such therapy are genetic immunodeficiencies; a few acquired states are associated with deficient IgG (see Chapter 17). The usual dose for initiating adequate IgG levels is 1.4 mL (220–240 mg)/kg as a single dose. Subsequent doses are for maintenance; 0.6–0.7 mL/kg every 3–4 weeks is usually sufficient. All of these doses are empiric, and some variation may be expected. The best guideline for adequacy of therapy is the absence of serious bacterial infections (eg, bacteremia, meningitis) in the individual patient. Serum immunoglobulin levels are unreliable in predicting the adequacy of IG therapy. Infections of the mucosal surfaces may not diminish with IG administration, since the individuals being treated usually have secretory IgA deficiencies that are not repaired by IG administration.

Administration of IG will not benefit patients with neutrophil dysfunction, lymphocyte-mediated immune deficiency, complement deficiency, or any other non-IgG deficient condition.

Measles Prevention

See discussion in the earlier section on measles.

Prevention of Hepatitis

Specific hepatitis B immune globulin (HBIG) is now available. Both HBIG and IG can be utilized in low-dose exposure such as needle sticks with contamination, mucosal exposure to contaminated blood, and intimate contact with an infected person (eg, sex partner relationship).

A. Infectious Hepatitis: Prophylaxis (using ordinary IG) against infectious hepatitis (type A hepatitis) should be offered family contacts and individuals experiencing heavy or continuous exposure.

1. Family contact exposure—This is defined as any relationship in which individuals share living, eating, and toilet facilities. This includes many babysitters or other caretakers, lodgers, and members of some sports teams as well as blood relatives living together. This category usually does not include schoolmates, members of social groups, or casual contacts. The dose is 0.02 mL/kg, and the expected duration of protection is 5 weeks.

2. Intense or continued exposure—This is defined as the kind of exposure experienced by persons who provide custodial care with maximal fecal exposure (eg, attendants in institutions for the mentally retarded or psychiatrically ill patients), health workers with repeated exposure to clinical cases, or travelers to endemic areas where hygienic facilities are primitive. The dose is 0.02 mL/kg. With continued exposure, the same dose is repeated in 5–6 months. Continuous exposure for this length of time is probably associated with infection during the passive protection period, and further doses of IG are unnecessary.

B. Serum Hepatitis: In the past, IG has proved unreliable in the prevention of serum hepatitis (type B HBsAg-positive hepatitis). IG prepared since 1972 appears to have higher effective antibody levels against serum hepatitis. This may be related to selection of donors only from antigen-negative donors.

Experts now suggest that post-1972 IG can protect against minimal exposure such as pricking one's finger with a needle known to be contaminated with antigen-positive blood. The suggested dose is 0.02 mL/kg.

Prophylactic use of HBIG in infants of HBsAg-positive mothers is discussed in the section on hepatitis B virus (see above).

INTRAVENOUS IMMUNE GLOBULIN

Recently, 2 intravenous IG preparations have been introduced in the USA. (Additional preparations of intravenous IG are in use throughout the world and may become available in the USA in the near future.) These 2 preparations have been treated chemically in order to reduce the risk of anaphylactic reactions and to maintain the antibody potency of the immune globulins. They are primarily IgG, with both IgA and IgM present in small amounts. All subclasses of IgG are represented, and concentrations of antibodies to a variety of pathogens are sufficient to enable intravenous IG use in replacement therapy.

Intravenous IG must be administered slowly through an ensured venous route, and specific instructions in the product brochures that accompany each preparation (dose, timing, rate of administration, and precautions) must be followed assiduously. Intravenous IG is useful as replacement therapy for those individuals in whom intramuscular IG has become uncomfortable or in whom it cannot be administered because of a concomitant bleeding diathesis. It has also been useful in the management of idiopathic thrombocytopenic purpura (see Chapter 16). Results of preliminary trials in Japan suggest that intravenous IG has some effect in preventing aneurysms in patients with Kawasaki disease.

UNPROVED, UNWARRANTED USE OF IMMUNE GLOBULIN

IG should not be given when it is not indicated, because it is painful and costly and in limited supply. The most common abuse is the administration of IG to children with frequent upper respiratory coryzal symptoms, most frequently due to allergic disease. Without demonstrable IgG or antibody deficiency, there is no indication for the use of IG in this common situation.

IG has no place in the treatment of asthma, allergic rhinitis, and other allergic diseases; recurrent herpes simplex (hominis) infections; recurrent group A hemolytic streptococcal infections; most established bacterial infections; in children who fail to thrive; or as a last resort in incurable diseases.

There are some uses for IG that are controversial or equivocal. Examples are patients with severe burns, susceptible varicella contacts, and pregnant women exposed to rubella. There are a few reports suggesting that IG administration might be beneficial in the prevention of *Pseudomonas* infection in severely burned young patients. Most available information does not support the use of IG in burned patients. Certain susceptible varicella contacts (newborn or young infants, patients with lymphatic malignant neoplasms) are given IG in large doses to prevent chickenpox. IG in large doses can modify varicella but does *not* prevent the disease. It is better to administer varicella-zoster immune globulin (VZIG) for this purpose (see Chapter 26). Pregnant women who are susceptible to rubella and exposed in the first trimester pose a frustrating problem. If therapeutic abortion is not contemplated, there is no way to make certain that the fetus will be protected. Large doses (20–40 mL) of IG have been administered, but there is no evidence that this protects the fetus and some data suggest that it does not.

SELECTED REFERENCES

American Academy of Pediatrics: *Report of the Committee on Infectious Diseases,* 20th ed. American Academy of Pediatrics, 1986.

American Academy of Pediatrics Committee on Infectious Diseases: *Hemophilus* type b polysaccharide vaccine. *Pediatrics* 1985;**76:**322.

American Academy of Pediatrics Committee on Infectious Diseases: Pertussis vaccine. *Pediatrics* 1984;**74:**303.

American Academy of Pediatrics Committee on Infectious Diseases: Prevention of hepatitis B infections. *Pediatrics* 1985;**75:**362.

American Academy of Pediatrics Committee on Infectious Diseases: Recommendations for using pneumococcal vaccine. *Pediatrics* 1985;**75:**1153.

Amman AJ et al: Polyvalent pneumococcal polysaccharide immunization of patients with sickle cell anemia and patients with splenectomy. *N Engl J Med* 1977;**297:**897.

Arbeter A et al: Varicella vaccine trials in healthy children. *Am J Dis Child* 1984;**138:**434.

Asano Y et al: Live varicella vaccine. *Pediatrics* 1985;**75:**667.

Barkin RM et al: Pediatric diphtheria and tetanus toxoid vaccine: Clinical and immunologic response when administered as the primary series. *J Pediatr* 1985;**106:**779.

Bart KJ et al: Elimination of rubella and congenital rubella from the United States. *Pediatr Infect Dis* 1985;**4:**14.

Brunell PA et al: Antibody responses following measles-mumps-rubella vaccine under conditions of customary use. *JAMA* 1983;**250:**1409.

Centers for Disease Control: Adverse events following immunization. *MMWR* 1985;**34:**43.

Centers for Disease Control: Prevention and control of influenza. *MMWR* 1985;**34:**262.

Centers for Disease Control: Rabies prevention: United States, 1984. *MMWR* 1984;**33:**393.

Centers for Disease Control: Recommendations for protection against viral hepatitis. *MMWR* 1985;**34:**313.

Cherry JD et al: Recurrent seizures after diphtheria, tetanus and pertussis immunization. *Am J Dis Child* 1984;**138:** 904.

Cody CL et al: Nature and rate of adverse reactions associated with DTP and DT immunization in infants and children. *Pediatrics* 1981;**68:**650.

Daum R, Granoff D: Vaccine against *Haemophilus influenzae,* type b, *Pediatr Infect Dis* 1985;**4:**355.

Frank JA et al: Major impediments to measles elimination. *Am J Dis Child* 1985;**139:**881.

Fulginiti VA: Immunization: Theory and practice. Chapter 3 in: *Practice of Pediatrics.* Kelley VC (editor). Harper & Row, 1984.

Fulginiti VA (editor): *Immunization in Clinical Practice.* Lippincott, 1982.

Fulginiti VA, Helfer RE: Atypical measles in adolescent siblings 16 years after killed measles virus vaccine. *JAMA* 1980;**244:**804.

Giebnick S: Preventing pneumococcal disease in children. *Pediatr Infect Dis* 1985;**4:**343.

Herman JJ et al: Allergic reactions to measles (rubeola) vaccine in patients hypersensitive to egg protein. *J Pediatr* 1983;**102:**196.

Hinman AR: Prevention of congenital rubella infection. *Pediatrics* 1985;**75:**1162.

Hinman AR et al: Pertussis and pertussis vaccine: Reanalysis of benefits, risks and costs. *JAMA* 1984;**251:**3109.

John TJ et al: Control of measles by annual pulse immunization. *Am J Dis Child* 1984;**138:**299.

Käyhty H et al: Serum antibodies after vaccination with *Haemophilus influenzae* type b capsular polysaccharide and responses to reimmunization. *Pediatrics* 1984;**74:**857.

Lampe R et al: Measles reimmunization in children immunized before 1 year of age. *Am J Dis Child* 1985;**139:**33.

Murphy JV et al: Recurrent seizures after diphtheria, tetanus and pertussis immunization. *Am J Dis Child* 1984;**138:**908.

Weller T: Poliomyelitis: Its global demise? *Pediatrics* 1984;**74:**442.

Ambulatory Pediatrics 6

Barton D. Schmitt, MD

This chapter offers guidelines for the conduct of 4 specific types of pediatric visit: (1) health maintenance care, (2) acute illness care, (3) chronic disease follow-up, and (4) consultation. Each type of visit requires a specific service that is different in many ways from the others. If the pediatrician and the office staff can mentally classify the patients in this way and vary their approach accordingly, the delivery of pediatric care will become more logical and consistent.

This organization of ambulatory care has 3 general advantages: (1) The quality of care improves, since the patient benefits from the comprehensiveness of care that only a systematic approach can ensure. (2) The practice of pediatrics becomes more enjoyable because the establishment of clear office guidelines and policies prevents many frustrations and much duplication of effort by the physician. (3) The cost of medical care is reduced by increasing the efficiency of health care delivery.

HEALTH MAINTENANCE VISITS

OBJECTIVES

Health maintenance or health supervision visits are the key to preventive pediatrics. These visits involve 3 people: the physician, the parent, and the child. Children should assume more active roles in their own health care with each passing year. The visit has multiple purposes: responding to the parent's or child's current concerns, presenting age-appropriate anticipatory guidance, assessing growth and development (see Chapter 2), performing a physical examination (Chapter 1), obtaining laboratory screening tests, and administering immunizations (Chapter 5). A natural outcome of these visits is a deepening of family-physician rapport.

PARENTAL CONCERNS

The first part of each well child visit should be directed toward dealing with the current concerns of the parent, usually the mother. Most expectant mothers have many questions that should be discussed with their pediatrician several weeks prior to delivery. The most frequent concerns include arguments for and against breast feeding and circumcision, preparation of the breasts if breast feeding is to be used, hospital policies about rooming-in and parent-infant contact in the delivery room, essential baby equipment, separation problems with other children during the mother's confinement, and ways of decreasing sibling jealousy. It has been traditional for the first newborn office visit to take place at 6 weeks, probably because 6 weeks is the traditional time for the mother's first postdelivery obstetric visit. However, most mothers—particularly primiparas—have many questions and concerns well before this traditional interval after birth. A 2-week postpartal office visit is much more logical.

A health maintenance visit without parental concerns is uncommon. Some mothers bring a list of questions, "How much should babies cry?" "How do I know he's getting enough to eat?" "Can I spoil her by picking her up too much?" "Is it all right to spank children?" "How old should Johnny be before I let him cross the street alone?" Many of the questions have no clear-cut answers. The seasoned pediatrician usually enjoys the challenge of these discussions and the satisfaction that comes with reassuring an anxious parent.

Anderson FP: Evaluation of the routine physical examination of infants in the first year of life. *Pediatrics* 1970;**45:**950.

Charney E: Counseling of parents around the birth of a baby. *Pediatr in Rev* 1982;**4:**167.

Heavenrich RM: Child health supervision: Is it worth it? (2 parts.) *Pediatrics* 1973;**54:**52, 272.

Hoekelman RA: What constitutes adequate well-baby care? *Pediatrics* 1975;**55:**313.

Korsch BM: How comprehensive are well child visits? *Am J Dis Child* 1971;**122:**483.

Liptak GS, Hulka BS, Cassel JC: Effectiveness of physician-mother interactions during infancy. *Pediatrics* 1977;**60:**186.

ANTICIPATORY GUIDANCE

Anticipatory guidance usually includes nutritional counseling, accident prevention, behavioral counseling, suggestions for developmental stimulation, sex education, dental recommendations, medical information, etc. Special counseling is in order for adolescents (see Chapter 9). A list of suggested topics to be discussed at particular ages is found on the health maintenance forms presented at the end of the chapter. A blank space or line on these forms indicates that a comment is required following that item. All anticipatory guidance advice is followed by the optimal age for discussion in parentheses. A check mark in the box that follows each of these advice items indicates that this counseling was done. These topics can be covered in a variety of ways. Some physicians prefer to discuss all the items with the parents personally; others prefer to delegate the discussion of these issues to an assistant, who might be either a nurse or a nonprofessional assistant; and still others use printed materials that can be supplemented by personal comments as the need arises.

Christopherson ER: Incorporating behavioral pediatrics into primary care. *Pediatr Clin North Am* 1982;**29:**261.

Feldman KW: Prevention of childhood accidents: Recent progress. *Pediatrics* 1980;**2:**75.

Lovejoy FH, Chafee-Bahamon C: The physician's role in accident prevention. *Pediatr in Rev* 1982;**4:**53.

Mack A: *Toilet Learning.* Little, Brown, 1978.

PHYSICAL EXAMINATION

A complete physical examination should be performed during most health maintenance visits (see Chapter 1). Height, weight, and head circumference should be measured and plotted on growth curves (see Chapter 2). During childhood, most chronic diseases will affect growth. Although these examinations are usually normal, they serve as a point of reference in evaluating future illnesses. Therefore, the extent of the examination should be carefully recorded. To save time, the checklist shown in Table 6–1 can be used. Elaboration is required only for the abnormal findings.

Some physical findings are silent—ie, they are not noticeable to parents and cause few if any symptoms. Of greatest concern are disorders that are treatable if detected early but potentially serious when not detected. A routine examination will diagnose most such conditions (eg, congenital heart disease). A few conditions are detected only by a detailed examination (eg, retinoblastoma [red fundus reflection test], strabismus [corneal light reflection test], congenital hip dislocation [Ortolani maneuver, or restricted abduction], scoliosis, coarctation of the aorta [femoral pulses], hypertension, lower urinary tract obstruction [inquire about urine stream], imperforate hymen, and labial adhesions). Visual deficits (eg, refractive errors or color blindness) and hearing deficits can also be missed if appropriate testing is not included. Dental caries may be overlooked by physicians who assume, not always rightly, that their patients are receiving periodic dental examinations (see Chapter 12). Early cancer detection can be improved by teaching self-examination of the breasts or testes.

Table 6–1. Checklist for physical examination.

	Normal	Abnormal
1. GENERAL APPEARANCE: well nourished, hydrated, alert		
2. SKIN: color, rash, swelling, hair, nails		
3. HEAD: shape, anterior fontanelle		
4. EYES: conjunctiva, cornea, pupils, extraocular movement		
5. EARS: pinnae, canals; tympanic membrane appearance, mobility		
6. NOSE: nares, turbinates		
7. MOUTH: tongue, teeth, oral mucosa, tonsils, pharynx		
8. NECK: thyroid, range of motion		
9. NODES: cervical, axillary, inguinal, other		
10. CHEST: symmetry, expansion, breasts		
11. LUNGS: rate, auscultation, percussion		
12. HEART: rate, rhythm, S_1, S_2, murmur, femoral pulses		
13. ABDOMEN: contour; palpation of liver, spleen, and kidney; mass; tenderness		
14. GENITALIA: ♀ external; ♂ penis, meatus, testes, hernia		
15. SPINE: curvature (scoliosis), sacral area		
16. EXTREMITIES: range of motion, tenderness, edema, clubbing		
17. NEUROLOGIC (SCREEN): cranial nerves 3, 4, 6, 7, and 12; gait; cerebellar function; motor system (strength, tone)		
18. NEUROLOGIC (COMPLETE): above plus other cranial nerves; sensory and motor systems (deep tendon reflexes, clonus)		

Strong WB, Linder CW: Preparticipation health evaluation for competitive sports. *Pediatr in Rev* 1982;**4:**113.

THE SCHOOL READINESS EXAMINATION

The preschool examination of the 4- or 5-year-old child should be designed to answer the basic question, "Is the child ready for school?" Auscultation of the heart and lungs at this time is probably far less important than noting any abnormalities of speech, hearing, or vision and determining if developmental age is commensurate with chronologic age, if attention span is adequate for learning, and if parents have adequately prepared the child for separation when entering school. These problems should also be investigated earlier, but they are of greatest significance at the preschool examination. A school readiness screening questionnaire is provided at the end of this chapter.

Vision

Five to 10% of preschool children have some kind of visual impairment. The illiterate E chart, Snellen chart, or Allen cards can be used for checking visual acuity, and each eye should be tested separately. The 5-year-old child should have a visual acuity of 20/30 (6/9) or better in both eyes, and there should be no more than a 2-line difference between the 2 eyes. Suppression amblyopia affects 2–5% of children and must be detected early before permanent loss of vision occurs. Amblyopia is often secondary to strabismus, which can be detected by noting the position where light is reflected off both corneas or by the cover test (see Fig 11–3).

Hearing

Hearing deficits occur in approximately 1% of young school children, and in 10% the loss is profound and bilateral. Most children with hearing loss have recurrent purulent otitis media or serous otitis media. Even children with a single episode of otitis media may have some degree of hearing impairment for 3–6 months after the acute episode. Although the losses are generally not too severe, if they occur at an inopportune time they may be sufficient to prevent an early school-age child from learning phonics; hence, the effect of the loss may be carried on and magnified throughout much of the school years (see Chapter 13). If such losses are detected before entry into school, some of the learning, behavior, and discipline problems that occur secondary to poor attention might be averted. Detection of such problems is as much a part of preventive pediatrics as is the immunization routine. Audiologic screening tests can be performed by nonprofessional technicians and should be a part of the preschool examination.

Speech

The child entering school should be able to speak distinctly and clearly without difficulty; should be able to answer questions; and, after a period of getting acquainted, should be able to carry on a conversation with the physician about recent events. Poor speech may impair performance in school. An easily administered screening articulation test has been developed to identify children who should be referred to a speech pathologist for definitive evaluation (see Drumwright reference, below, and Chapter 2).

Emotional Development & Behavior

The assessment of emotional development and behavior is an important part of the preschool examination. In one study, 42 physicians were observed conducting 673 well child clinic visits. On the average, they said fewer than 2 sentences per visit to the mother that were relevant to child behavior. Yet, when given the opportunity to respond to a questionnaire about behavior, 85% of mothers of preschool children (ages 1½–6 years) indicated one or more such concerns (mean of 3.5 concerns per child). A simple self-administered questionnaire (see Willoughby and Haggerty reference, below) is an effective and efficient device which not only indicates to the parent that the physician is interested in discussing behavioral problems and emotional growth but also helps the physician to concentrate on areas of guidance most relevant to the parent's concerns. The pediatric health maintenance forms (provided at the end of this chapter) stress anticipatory guidance and counseling for behavioral aspects of pediatrics.

Physical, emotional, and developmental maturation proceeds at different rates for different children. Some children are ready for school long before their fifth birthday; others are not nearly ready at that age. Some parents tend to push their children into experiences that are beyond their capacities at a given age. Children should begin their school experiences with successes; the child who starts with failure is often criticized and becomes discouraged and less interested in school, so that a pattern of failure may develop. The child may continue to lag behind and miss the early fundamentals of learning, which are the basis for further education. Many children develop behavioral disorders and truancy simply because they cannot read and so are unable to understand what is going on in the classroom. Part of the physician's role is to help parents recognize physical, emotional, and developmental lags early, so that corrective measures can be taken to prepare the child for school. A number of easily administered developmental tests are available. The Denver Developmental Screening Test (see Chapter 2) is extremely helpful in the younger age groups. If, despite intervention, the child is not ready for school, the physician must advise the parents appropriately.

American Academy of Pediatrics: Joint Committee on Infant Hearing: Position Statement of 1982. *Pediatrics* 1982;**70:**496.

Drumwright A et al: The Denver Articulation Screening Examination. *J Speech Hear Disord* 1973;**38:**3.

Gammon JA: Visual system screening in infants and young children. *Pediatr in Rev* 1982;**4:**71.

Grant WW: Health screening in school-age children. *Am J Dis Child* 1973;**125:**520.

Willoughby JA, Haggerty RJ: A simple behavior questionnaire for preschool children. *Pediatrics* 1964;**34:**798.

LABORATORY SCREENING TESTS

A health maintenance flow sheet (see example provided at the end of this chapter) is a helpful reminder to the nurse and physician that certain procedures, laboratory tests, developmental evaluations, and immunizations need to be done. All of these items can be initiated by the nurse or aide if the physician establishes the routine to be followed.

Blood

Iron deficiency anemia (see Chapter 16) is found more often in lower socioeconomic populations and has its highest incidence in infants between 9 and 24 months of age. A routine hemoglobin or hematocrit is recommended in this age group and is particularly important in the child whose diet is low in iron-containing foods.

Children with sickle cell disease (see Chapter 16) must be diagnosed before 6 months of age to prevent death due to sepsis or splenic sequestration (10–20% mortality rate). Do not wait for the routine hematocrit at age 9 months. It is strongly recommended that all black newborns have hemoglobin electrophoresis performed on cord blood or in conjunction with heelstick testing for phenylketonuria.

Screening for phenylketonuria (see Chapter 33) should be done by blood test in the hospital nursery prior to the infant's discharge, and in over 40% of states such a test is required by law. An infant with this disorder who failed to ingest sufficient milk protein may have a negative test in the first few days of life. Therefore, most centers recommend a repeat test at 10–14 days of age. Screening newborns for another treatable cause of mental retardation, congenital hypothyroidism, is also now recommended. A T_4 or TSH assay can be done using cord blood.

Screening for lead poisoning (see Chapter 30) is extremely important in areas where the child has access to lead-based paint or soil contaminated by lead. Children living in such neighborhoods should have a routine blood lead level performed at 18–24 months of age. This test should be repeated at 6-month intervals until age 3 years in children with pica or where there is an index case in their building.

Urine

Routine urinalysis has a low yield in the asymptomatic patient. In contrast to the adult population, it is unusual for a child to have asymptomatic diabetes, and proteinuria is a rare presenting sign for a renal abnormality in an asymptomatic child. Transient orthostatic proteinuria is common in adolescents but benign. We recommend that the urine dipstick test be performed only on symptomatic children.

In screening for asymptomatic urinary tract infection, microscopic examination of the urinary sediment is time-consuming and not reliable. Several inexpensive methods are available to screen a first morning specimen for bacteriuria (eg, nitrite or glucose detection strips), followed by a urine culture if the dipstick test is positive. Since untreated asymptomatic bacteriuria has an excellent prognosis and does not lead to renal damage, screening should be reserved for high-risk groups (eg, children with diabetes).

Many teenage girls are sexually active and will benefit from annual gonococcal cultures and Papanicolaou smears. Birth control counseling and sexuality counseling can also be offered at this time.

Bailey EN et al: Screening in pediatric practice. *Pediatr Clin North Am* 1974;**21:**123.

Buist NR, Jhaveri BM: A guide to screening newborn infants for inborn errors of metabolism. *J Pediatr* 1973;**82:**511.

Chisholm JJ: Screening for lead poisoning in children. *Pediatrics* 1973;**51:**280.

Gutgesell M: Practicality of screening urinalyses in asymptomatic children in a primary care setting. *Pediatrics* 1978;**62:**103.

Hein K et al: The need for routine screening in the sexually active adolescent. *J Pediatr* 1977;**91:**123.

Levy HL, Mitchell ML: Regional newborn screening for hypothyroidism. *Pediatrics* 1979;**63:**340.

North AF: Screening in child health care: Where are we now and where are we going? *Pediatrics* 1974;**54:**631.

Pless IB: Routine tests in pediatric practice: Things better left undone. *Pediatr Dig* (Aug/Sept) 1979;**21:**13.

Selkon JB et al: Covert bacteriuria in school girls in Newcastle upon Tyne. *Arch Dis Child* 1981;**56:**585.

IMMUNIZATIONS

A child's immunization status can be easily monitored on the health maintenance flow sheet (see example provided at the end of this chapter). In our clinic, the 15-month visit is for shots only. A record of the child's immunizations should also be given to the parents and updated by the nurse as additional immunizations are given.

The details of routine immunization of children are presented in Chapter 5.

PARTICIPATION OF PARAMEDICAL PERSONNEL

A number of other professionals (social workers, visiting nurses, nutritionists) as well as volunteers (community outreach workers) have been helping physicians take care of patients for many years. Only large clinics or group practices are able to employ and fully utilize such a variety of health workers. Some smaller pediatric offices employ a social worker one-half day a week to help patients with serious emotional and social problems, since such patients would otherwise take up an inordinate amount of physician time.

In the past 15 years, many programs have been initiated to train new types of allied health workers to help the pediatrician. Examples include pediatric nurse practitioners, chronic disease nurses, and community health workers. The pediatric nurse practitioner (PNP) is a graduate nurse who has been given additional training to improve nursing skills and history-taking skills, to perform a physical examination that includes use of an otoscope and stethoscope, and to give well child guidance and counseling. The role of the PNP is to help the physician deliver health maintenance care and to distinguish the sick child from the well child and the abnormal finding from the normal one. The PNP is well accepted by parents, is able to respond to parents' concerns about normal growth and development, and is trained to make accurate physical assessments. The time thus saved allows the pediatrician to spend more time with sick patients and to increase the total number of patients cared for.

In addition to these programs, Silver and others (see references, below) have trained an entirely new type of health worker: the child health associate. This allied health worker, who has completed a minimum of 2 years of college and 3 years of pediatric training, is licensed to deliver all well child care and to diagnose and treat (under a physician's supervision) most acute ambulatory illnesses. The child health associate's only responsibility for hospitalized patients involves healthy newborns. Help is thus available to the physician in caring for the expanding pediatric population.

DeAngelis C: Non-physician health care providers and community support services. *Pediatr Clin North Am* 1981;**28:**551.

Duncan B, Smith AN, Silver HK: Comparison of the physical assessment of children by pediatric nurse practitioners and pediatricians. *Am J Public Health* 1971;**61:**1170.

Silver HK, Igoe JB, McAtee PR: The school nurse practitioner: Providing improved health care to children. *Pediatrics* 1976;**58:**580.

Silver HK et al: Assessment and evaluation of child health associates. *Pediatrics* 1981;**67:**47.

ACUTE ILLNESS VISITS

The episodic office visit for the child with an acute illness places special demands on the physician.

OBJECTIVES

Diagnosis and treatment of the chief complaint is the first priority for the parents, patient, and physician. Extenuating circumstances (eg, a crowded waiting room) rarely justify an incomplete workup of an acute chief complaint. Detection of patients who have a chronic disease or an undiagnosed chronic complaint is of nearly equal importance to the physician.

COMMON TYPES OF ACUTE ILLNESSES

The following diagnoses or conditions are the acute illnesses most commonly seen in office practice, listed in approximate order of frequency. Any health care provider who sees children must master the evaluation and management of these disorders: common colds, acute otitis media, viral pharyngitis and tonsillitis, gastroenteritis, acute tracheitis and bronchitis, conjunctivitis, streptococcal pharyngitis, diaper rash, thrush, impetigo, chickenpox, viral maculopapular rashes, skin trauma, head trauma, sprains, urinary tract infection, pneumonia, croup, cellulitis and boils, and ingestions.

ASSESSING ACUTE ILLNESS

Optimal management of an acute illness mainly includes telephone triaging, office triaging, diagnosis, assessment of the need for hospitalization, home therapy, and a follow-up plan.

The detection of multiple health problems is best accomplished by using a brief screening questionnaire, which should be completed for any new patient. Some parents have only crisis care available to their families (eg, in rural areas). Other parents have access to comprehensive health care but use only crisis care. The screening questionnaire is unnecessary for patients already being followed for health maintenance care. The parent can complete the questionnaire while waiting to see the physician. If chronic physical, emotional, or school problems are detected, the doctor should strongly recommend a follow-up appointment for a complete evaluation.

Katcher AL: Efficient office practice. *Pediatrics* 1977;**59:**533.

1. TELEPHONE TRIAGING & ADVICE

Does the Patient Need to Be Seen?

The physician is the person best qualified to give medical advice, both in the office and over the phone. However, because talking with parents on the phone may take too much physician time, this function is usually delegated to another member of the office team. Most of the questions are routine ones that require only routine answers. An office nurse specifically trained for the role is probably the best person to take routine calls. Office policies about medical advice over the phone should be standardized. Routine instructions for handling minor infections, minor injuries, reactions to immunizations, infant feeding problems, newborn care, and prescription refills are easy to communicate to parents if they are written down in an office protocol book. The protocol book should also specify the point at which each problem requires an office visit. This decision depends on (1) the type of symptom, (2) the duration of the symptom, (3) the age of the patient, (4) whether or not the patient acts "very sick," (5) an assessment of the parents' anxiety, and (6) the presence of any underlying chronic disease. (For example, most patients under 1 year of age with diarrhea and vomiting need to be examined.) After telephone baseline data are gathered, the nurse must be able to decide whether the child needs an appointment or not; the nurse should err on the side of giving an appointment when in doubt. For patients not seen, any pertinent telephone data should be entered on a temporary log sheet. If an office visit later becomes necessary, the data should be transferred to the patient's chart.

It is helpful if parents understand 2 general telephone rules: (1) The nurse will screen all calls during office hours except emergency ones and (2) nighttime calls should be restricted to emergencies or urgent problems that cannot wait until morning. Most routine calls come from overanxious, insecure parents who need reassurance and acceptance, not brisk criticism and implied rejection. The conversation with the nurse should help to build up a young mother's confidence. The mother can be asked what she had considered doing, and that plan of action should be strongly endorsed if possible. If parents are helped to become more confident and independent in these matters, unnecessary visits will be less frequent, as will medical costs for society in general. However, the conversation should convey the message that telephone calls are an important aid in medical care and that the parent is free to call again.

The physician directly accepts some calls: (1) emergency calls from parents, (2) calls from physicians and other professionals, (3) calls regarding hospitalized patients, (4) long distance calls, (5) calls from a parent who "demands" to talk to the physician, and (6) calls where the nurse is unclear about what should be done. These exceptions to the rule are obvious. Parents reasonably expect that their child's personal physician or a designated substitute should be readily available for emergencies, even if the "emergency" exists only from their viewpoint. The physician must be conscientious about accepting calls after midnight, for they often relate to psychosocial crises or urgent medical problems that cannot be ignored even for a few hours.

There are 4 other possible methods of dealing with telephone calls, any of which may serve as an alternative to having an office nurse screen and give telephone advice: (1) The physician can accept calls continuously throughout the day. These interruptions are unacceptable to most physicians and parents. (2) The physician can have a telephone hour at the beginning, middle, and end of the day and accept only emergency calls at other times. The disadvantages of this approach are that some parents must then wait for answers to urgent questions, and the physician lengthens his or her day with many routine calls. (3) The physician may charge for telephone advice. This decreases the number of calls, but in the process it may discourage important calls and thus interfere with preventive pediatrics. High charges for nighttime calls may help control these calls; however, the cost of billing makes charges for calls during office hours impractical. (4) The physician can allow various nonmedical office personnel to accept telephone calls randomly themselves. This approach would result in inconsistent medical advice and could be dangerous. The physician is of course legally liable for any harm to a patient proximately caused by improper advice given over the phone by employees.

Brown SB, Eberle BJ: Use of the telephone by pediatric house staff: A technique for pediatric care not taught. *J Pediatr* 1974;**84:**117.

Katz, HP: *Telephone Manual of Pediatric Care*. Wiley, 1982.

Perrin EC, Goodman HC: Telephone management of acute pediatric illness. *N Engl J Med* 1978;**298:**130.

Schmitt BD: *Pediatric Telephone Advice*. Little, Brown, 1980.

Strain JE, Miller JD: The preparation, utilization, and evaluation of a registered nurse trained to give telephone advice in a private pediatric office. *Pediatrics* 1971;**47:**1051.

When Does the Patient Need to Be Seen?

Some patients must be seen immediately (eg, for a foreign body in the eye). Others can be seen later the same day (eg, for a cough that kept the patient awake much of the preceding night). Other patients can be scheduled 1–2 days later (eg, for recurrent epistaxis). The nurse can make these decisions.

Where Should the Patient Be Seen?

Most sick patients can be seen in the physician's office by appointment. The physician can keep the first and last hour of each day plus at least 15 minutes out of each hour reserved for acute problems. Most of the first-hour appointments will be given to parents who call the physician during the preceding evening.

Another facility where patients can be seen for medical care is the hospital emergency room. This routing applies to patients who are highly likely to be admitted (eg, for croup). Some physicians also send patients with poisonings, lacerations, or possible fractures to the nearest emergency room.

A third possibility is a house call. Most physicians consider this disadvantageous to themselves financially and to the patient medically, since laboratory services are not available. A rare indication for a house call might be a contagious disease that needs confirmation (eg, varicella). The physician could occasionally see such a patient in the office parking lot.

2. OFFICE TRIAGING & PROCEDURES

How Sick Is the Patient?

The nurse should screen all sick patients as soon as possible after they arrive at the office. They can be thought of in terms of 3 general groups: emergency, contagious, and minor illness. Most patients have a minor illness (eg, cold, accident, earache) and can be seen at their appointed time. Some patients are contagious until proved otherwise and should quickly be moved from the waiting room to an isolated examining room (eg, febrile illnesses with rashes, lice, jaundice, possible pertussis). An attempt should be made to keep children with bronchiolitis or croup away from infants. When an office emergency (eg, febrile seizures, respiratory distress) is recognized by the nurse, the physician should be notified immediately. The physician can take appropriate emergency action, stabilize the patient, and arrange for transfer to the hospital if necessary (eg, an acidotic, dehydrated infant). (See Chapter 8.)

Russo RM et al: Triage abilities of nurse practitioner vs pediatrician. *Am J Dis Child* 1975;**129**:673.

Preparation of the Patient for the Physician

The office aide can record the sick patient's temperature, height, and weight. The office nurse can record the chief complaint. Depending upon the symptom, the nurse can take vital signs and initiate the office's standing orders on laboratory procedures and symptomatic treatment listed below.

Initial Treatment & Laboratory Workup

Steps in initial management are listed below. Details of procedures are outlined elsewhere in the text.

A. Abdominal Pain: Take samples for urinalysis and urine culture; save stool specimen for occult blood testing.

B. Animal Bite: Wash out immediately with benzalkonium chloride for 10 minutes. Initiate the official reporting form, and call the county health department. Delay irrigation if culture is needed.

C. Cough: If present over 1 month, apply a tuberculin skin test.

D. Diarrhea: Take a sample for stool culture if the stool contains blood or mucus or if diarrhea has persisted for more than 1 week at any age. For children under age 2, give 180 mL (6 oz) of an oral electrolyte solution, and record the naked weight on each visit. If a child appears dehydrated, collect urine for specific gravity.

E. Earache: Give acetaminophen if in obvious pain. Obtain audiometrics if cooperative. If there is a possibility of mumps, isolate the patient.

F. Eye Injury: Test visual acuity if child is over age 3. Place eye tray in the examining room.

G. Fever Over 39 °C (102.2 °F): Give acetaminophen in age-appropriate dose. Put the child in an examining room and assist with undressing. Give a sponge bath if temperature exceeds 40 °C (104 °F) despite drugs and if the child is uncomfortable. Provide a bag for urine if the child is not toilet trained, and save urine in refrigerator for analysis and culture. If unexplained fever has been present over 24 hours, order a white count and differential. If the infant is under 2 months of age, notify the physician immediately.

H. Fractures: Notify physician immediately, obtain equipment to immobilize the site, and fill out the x-ray request.

I. Head Injury: Record vital signs and check pupils for equal size and reaction to light.

J. Infectious Hepatitis Exposure: Record weights of persons who have had intimate contact with the patient, and anticipate giving immune globulin, 0.03 mL/kg intramuscularly.

K. Lacerations: Wash thoroughly with hexachlorophene soap and water (at least 10 minutes). Check date of last tetanus shot and record. (The physician must decide if tetanus booster or antitoxin is needed.) Shave around the wound edges if necessary (but never shave eyebrows). Have parents sign consent for suturing.

L. Nosebleed: Instruct the parent or child on how to compress the bleeding site for 10 minutes. Check blood pressure and perform fingerstick for hematocrit.

M. Painful Urination (Burning or Frequency): Take sample for urinalysis, urine culture, nitrite dipstick, and a gram-stained smear of unspun drop.

N. Pinworms: Record the approximate weights of all family members if the infection is a recurrent one (for calculation of dosage of medication, see Chapter 28).

O. Sore Throat: Take material for throat culture (contraindicated if the patient has croup).

P. Streptococcal Sore Throat (Culture Positive): Inquire about penicillin allergy and record. Arrange for symptomatic family contacts to have throat cultures taken.

Q. Vomiting: Record exact weight. Give patient emesis basin and sips of iced cola drink while waiting. If patient appears dehydrated, collect urine for specific gravity.

3. THE WORKING DIAGNOSIS

The physician makes the final decision about the diagnosis and the severity of the disease. Emergency conditions not obvious to the nurse (eg, shock or meningitis) may be noted by the physician. History taking can be modified to emphasize the chief complaint. A history of recent contact with persons with contagious diseases is often important. Severity can be partially assessed by inquiries about playfulness, energy, ability to sleep, and the parent's feelings about how sick the child is this time compared to other times. If a family of sick children is brought in, the physician should ask the mother which children she considers the sickest. The physical examination should be mainly directed toward the chief complaint. A patient with a dog bite does not require a complete examination, but a patient with an earache must be checked for mastoid swelling and meningeal signs in addition to otoscopic examination.

Utilizing the conventional techniques of history, physical examination, and laboratory tests, the physician will correctly diagnose most acute chief complaints. However, a vigilant clinical mind is necessary in order not to miss a diagnosis of septicemia. Septic children usually present with unexplained fever, but (unlike children with acute viral fevers) they often will not smile or play, even with their parents. They frequently are physically exhausted and too weak to resist the physical examination, constantly irritable and unable to sleep, and respond paradoxically to cuddling by the mother. Irritability usually stems from pain or hypoxia. A less common finding in the toxic child is constant lethargy or sleepiness. This is difficult to assess because most sick children sleep more than normally. A child with suspected septicemia requires an intensive workup and therapy in a hospital setting. These more complicated acute illness evaluations can be expedited if the physician has studied appropriate decision-making algorithms (see Chapter 13).

Nelson KG: An index of severity for acute pediatric illness. *Am J Public Health* 1980;**70:**804.

Russo RM et al: Outpatient management of the severely ill child. *Am J Dis Child* 1972;**124:**235.

4. INDICATIONS FOR HOSPITALIZATION

For every acute problem, the physician must decide whether to treat the child at home or in the hospital.

Patients whose problems fit into one of the following 3 groups of indications should be hospitalized:

Major Emergencies

Some examples of obvious life-threatening conditions are shock, severe dehydration, coma, meningitis (bacterial or of unknown cause), respiratory distress, congestive heart failure, severe hypertension, acute renal failure, status epilepticus, and surgical emergencies.

Potentially Life-Threatening or Crippling Illnesses

Some patients are not in critical condition when first seen but require hospitalization because their problem may be rapidly progressive during treatment. If deterioration occurs in the hospital, emergency therapy can be rapidly instituted. Most of the entities in this group are caused by infection or trauma. Endogenous diseases rarely change this rapidly. Although absolute rules cannot be formulated for every situation, the following guidelines can be applied to most cases of acute illness. Obviously, these rules will have some exceptions such as when the emergency room has a 6-hour observation area. Also, the list is not complete (eg, chronic diseases are not listed).

These problems are listed according to body systems:

A. Skin:

1. Cellulitis if the patient is less than 2 months old; if there is buccal involvement or the cavernous sinus drainage area is involved; if underlying sinusitis or osteomyelitis is suspected; if cellulitis is secondary to a puncture wound in the foot; or if there is no response after 2 days of therapy.
2. Erysipelas, toxic epidermal necrolysis, or acute necrotizing fasciitis. Omphalitis if the patient is less than 2 months old.
3. Suspected thrombophlebitis.
4. Burns (second- or third-degree) involving more than 10% of surface area (> 15% if the patient is more than 1 year old); burns of perineal area, hand, or face if they might need grafting; all inhalation burns; and most electrical burns.
5. Pupura with fever, without fever but unexplained, or without fever but progressive.

B. Eyes:

1. Gonococcal conjunctivitis or bacterial keratitis.
2. Eye injury if visual acuity is decreased.
3. Papilledema.

C. Ears, Nose, and Throat:

1. Acute otitis media if the patient is less than 1 month old with fever, systemic symptoms, or no response after 2 days of therapy.
2. Mastoiditis.
3. Sinusitis if overlying redness or edema is present.
4. Nasal obstruction if the patient is less than 6 months old and an apneic episode has occurred.
5. Epistaxis if uncontrolled; if hypertension is present; if there is bleeding elsewhere; or if severe anemia is present.
6. Fluctuant tonsillar abscess.
7. Retropharyngeal abscess.
8. Diphtheria (any symptoms at any age).
9. Cervical adenitis if the patient is toxic, dehydrated, dysphagic, dyspneic, or less than 6 months old and needs treatment by incision and drainage.

D. Respiratory System:

1. Epiglottitis (all cases).
2. Viral laryngitis if there is stridor at rest, dyspnea, or drooling; if the child has repeatedly awakened from sleep with stridor; if the illness is currently progressive; if there is a history of a previous bout with rapid progression; if there are apneic or cyanotic episodes; or if the patient is less than 1 year old and the stridor is easily provoked (eg, occurs with any crying).
3. Pertussis if symptomatic and the patient is less than 1 year old; pertussis at any age if accompanied by apnea, respiratory distress, a whoop, or weight loss.
4. Bronchiolitis if the patient is dyspneic, has apneic or cyanotic episodes ($P_{O2} <$ 50), has poor fluid intake, or is unable to sleep.

5. Asthma if respiratory distress persists after 2 injections of epinephrine, one nebulized dose of a beta-agonist, or both.
6. Pneumonia if the patient is less than 1 month old; if bacterial pneumonia is suspected and the patient is less than 6 months old; if there is a history of apnea, cyanosis, or choking spells; if there is dyspnea (any age); if there is pleural effusion; if staphylococcal pneumonia is suspected (any age); if aspiration pneumonia is present; if fluid intake is poor; if there is underlying cystic fibrosis or congenital heart disease; or if there is no response after 2 days of therapy.
7. Suspected foreign body of the airway.
8. Hemoptysis if unexplained; if there is bleeding elsewhere; or if anemia is present.
9. Apnea in all cases except periodic breathing, breath-holding spells, or mild choking on food.

E. Cardiovascular System:

1. Suspected subacute bacterial endocarditis.
2. Any myocarditis or pericarditis.
3. Acute hypertension or shock.
4. Unexplained dysrhythmias.

F. Gastrointestinal System:

1. Vomiting with dehydration, delirium, or persistent abdominal pain.
2. Hematemesis if documented and not caused by swallowed blood.
3. Diarrhea if explosive in character; if accompanied by abdominal distention or associated Kussmaul respirations; if typhoid fever is suspected in a patient of any age; if acute *Shigella* infection is suspected in a patient less than 1 year old; or if staphylococcal enterocolitis is suspected in a patient less than 1 year old who has moderate dehydration or mild dehydration with vomiting.
4. Melena or unexplained bright-red blood mixed in the stools.
5. Suspected appendicitis, peritonitis, or intussusception.
6. Abdominal trauma if penetrating injury has occurred or if damage to the spleen, liver, kidneys, pancreas, or intestines is suspected.
7. Toxic ileus.

G. Urinary System:

1. Pyelonephritis if the patient is less than 2 months old, toxic, or unimproved after 2 days of therapy; if gram-negative sepsis is suspected; if underlying renal disease is present; or if recurrences have been frequent.
2. Acute edema, oliguria, or azotemia.
3. Hematuria with symptoms listed in (2), renal colic, and unexplained or posttraumatic gross hematuria.
4. Acute urinary retention.

H. Genitalia:

1. Vaginitis if associated with salpingitis.
2. Vaginal injury with sharp object.
3. Suspected testicular torsion.
4. Priapism.

I. Skeletal System:

1. Suspected osteomyelitis.
2. Arthritis if possibly septic or acute rheumatic fever.
3. Wringer injury if above the elbow; if a hematoma or avulsed skin is present; if a fracture or nerve injury is present; or if the peripheral pulse is diminished.

J. Nervous System:

1. Aseptic meningitis if the level of consciousness is depressed or there is a motor deficit.
2. Suspected tetanus.
3. Suspected epidural spinal abscess or brain abscess.
4. Febrile or afebrile seizures if they continue more than 30 minutes; if there are persistent neurologic signs; if the level of consciousness is decreased; or if serious underlying disease cannot be ruled out.
5. Head injury if the patient has been unconscious longer than 5 minutes; if there are persistent neurologic signs; if the level of consciousness is decreased; if a seizure has occurred; if cerebrospinal fluid rhinorrhea or otorrhea is present; if there is significant swelling over the middle meningeal artery; if there are retinal hemorrhages or progressive headaches; or if abnormal or irregular vital signs are present.
6. Skull fractures that are depressed or compound (ie, into air sinuses or overlying scalp laceration), fractures across the middle meningeal artery or venous sinus, occipital fracture into the rim of the foramen magnum, or any fracture with an underlying bleeding disorder.
7. Suspected spinal cord trauma.
8. Acute muscle weakness.
9. Acute cognitive deterioration, including delirium that is unexplained or persists longer than 2 hours.
10. Suspected increased intracranial pressure.

K. General:

1. Fever if the patient is less than 2 months old; if toxicity is evident and serious underlying disease cannot be ruled out; or if fever is due to heat stroke.
2. Poisoning if the patient is symptomatic (eg, respirations slow or irregular, drowsiness, etc); the agent or dosage is unknown; or the dosage is a potentially fatal one.

3. Suspected lead poisoning.
4. Unexplained mass.
5. Failure to thrive if severe or unexplained or if serious neglect is suspected.
6. Unexplained hypoglycemia.
7. Suspected anaphylactic reaction with laryngeal reaction, bronchospasm, hypotension, or dysrhythmias.

Duff RS et al: Use of utilization review to assess the quality of pediatric inpatient care. *Pediatrics* 1972;**49:**169.

Gururaj VJ: Short stay in an outpatient department. *Am J Dis Child* 1972;**123:**128.

Lovejoy FH et al: Unnecessary and preventable hospitalizations: Report on an internal audit. *J Pediatr* 1971;**79:**868.

Psychosocial Indications for Hospitalization

Patients with acute psychosocial problems now comprise a larger proportion of hospitalized children than was formerly the case. Until society can provide alternative facilities for these crises, hospitalization will continue to fulfill this need. These indications fall into 3 general groups: parent, child, and disease problems.

A. Parent Problems:

1. Child abuse (eg, battering, failure to thrive secondary to neglect, or incest).
2. Incipient battering (eg, the parent has made a homicidal threat against a child).
3. Absent parents (eg, abandonment, emancipated minors without caretakers, or the parents themselves are hospitalized).
4. Physically exhausted parents (eg, no sleep for 2 nights).
5. Severely overanxious parents (eg, if the parents remain immobilized and extremely anxious after a careful explanation of their child's illness).
6. Neglectful parents who seem uninterested in their child's illness or therapy (eg, neglected eczema). This is a rare situation compared to overly anxious parents.
7. Intellectually incompetent parents (eg, a mentally retarded mother who cannot reliably follow verbal or written instructions).
8. Emotionally disturbed parents who need psychiatric hospitalization and treatment for their own problems (eg, a floridly psychotic mother).
9. Parent who is alcoholic or drug abuser.

B. Child Problems:

1. Suicide attempt—A short hospital admission allows time for the mental health worker to make an evaluation and for the family to look seriously at their problems.
2. A destructive, dangerous child can be held on a pediatric ward pending placement. A dangerous adolescent will require a psychiatric care facility.
3. An incapacitating emotional symptom (eg, a severe conversion reaction such as paraplegia or blindness).

C. Disease Problems:

1. An incapacitating (but not life-threatening) physical disease (eg, severe Sydenham's chorea).
2. Initial diagnosis of a disease with a complex treatment regimen. The parents and patient deserve a careful, unhurried, and organized introduction to the complex home management of some chronic diseases (eg, diabetes mellitus).
3. Initial diagnosis of a fetal disease—This gives the family time to work through the impact phase (eg, leukemia).
4. Terminal care if the family does not want the child to die at home.
5. Chronic diseases that are exacerbated by family conflicts (eg, ulcerative colitis).
6. Hazardous home (eg, carbon monoxide or lead poisoning).

Unnecessary Hospitalization

In the USA, overhospitalization is currently a greater problem than underhospitalization. In recent studies, at least 20% of hospitalizations were judged to be unnecessary. Overhospitalization takes 3 general forms: (1) Hospitalization for an acute illness sometimes occurs because the primary physician is uncertain of the diagnosis and prognosis (eg, viral rashes). Reassurance in the face of such insecurity can often be gained by immediate consultation with a colleague. (2) Hospitalization is sometimes arranged for a diagnostic evaluation and tests because the patient has no outpatient insurance (eg, urinary tract infection). Unless the parents are in serious financial difficulty, this custom is unethical. It is to be hoped that more realistic insurance coverage will make ambulatory studies equally reimbursable. (3) Periodic hospitalizations sometimes are ordered for routine reevaluations of a chronic disease (eg, chronic glomerulonephritis). Even if the patient travels a great distance, this reevaluation can be done on an ambulatory basis if it is carefully planned in advance. The combined costs of the special studies plus hotel accommodations will be far less than hospitalization charges. In cases of elective hospitalization, preadmission evaluations can reduce hospital stays by 2 or 3 days.

The indications for hospitalization are becoming more selective. The time has passed when every child with infectious mononucleosis, hepatitis, pneumonia, gross hematuria, or a urinary tract infection is automatically admitted. Fewer than 10% of patients with these acute disorders require hospitalization. In fact, in emergency rooms with special observation units, children with moderate dehydration, diabetic ketoacidosis, status asthmaticus, etc, are treated and released in 3–6 hours.

Unnecessary hospitalization carries 5 main problems or risks, the last one probably being the most serious: (1) Children under 3 years of age can experience separation problems. (2) The parents' confidence in caring for a sick child themselves is undermined. (3) There is a danger of cross-infection to the patient and others. (4) There is a risk of medical error, such as the wrong medication or wrong dosage. (5) Society sustains an endlessly rising cost for medical care.

An acutely ill child can be observed in the office for several hours if it is not clear whether or not hospitalization is necessary. This will allow time for any reassurance given to the mother to take effect, and it permits the physician to compare the patient at 2 points in time and determine whether the condition is improving or getting worse. This interval also helps one decide what to do when the mother's history and the physical examination are inconsistent (eg, "recurrent vomiting" without dehydration, "no urination" without bladder distention). If necessary, another physician can be called in for consultation during this time.

Goldbloom RB, Macleod MU: Impact of preadmission evaluations on elective hospitalization. of children. *Pediatrics* 1984;**73**:656.

5. TREATMENT OF THE NONHOSPITALIZED PATIENT

Words are as necessary as drugs in the treatment of a sick child. The parents expect to be told their child's diagnosis and its causes, prognosis, and treatment. They also need to have their special concerns acknowledged and clarified. If this communication does not take place, the parents will often be dissatisfied with the quality of care being given, and their compliance with regard to medications, advice, and follow-up will probably be less than optimal.

If the child has a mild acute illness (eg, viral nasopharyngitis), the parent would be reassured by the following general types of comment:

Diagnosis

"David has a cold." The diagnosis should be conveyed in plain English, not in medical jargon. If the physician does not specifically state the diagnosis, the parents may assume none has been arrived at. (See also Ambiguous Diagnosis, below.)

Etiology

"It's due to a virus." This means to most parents that the infection is not serious. Some parents need an added statement that there was nothing they could have done to prevent it—eg, "Everyone is coming down with this."

Parents' Concerns

Mothers often do not listen to their physician's instructions until their own main concerns have been discussed. These concerns are easily elicited by Korsch's 3 questions: (1) "Why did you bring David to the clinic today?" (2) "What worried you most about him?" (3) "Why did that worry you?" After these concerns are out in the open, the physician is in a position to clarify misconceptions. Reassurance can be specific—eg, "He doesn't have meningitis," or, "It won't turn into leukemia."

Treatment

In self-limited disease, the goal of medication is to keep the patient comfortable. A useful list of commonsense approaches to management (sometimes overlooked) is as follows: (1) An antipyretic is useful if the patient's fever causes discomfort. (2) Sedatives (eg, chloral hydrate) should be prescribed more often for the acutely restless child, since the parent cannot function adequately as a nurse without some sleep. (3) Codeine can be freely used for acute cough that interferes with sleep. (4) Advice about diet, bed rest, isolation, and mood is also appreciated by the parent. The patient can usually be allowed to dictate the diet during periods of illness. (5) In most cases, the patient can also be allowed to decide whether to stay in bed, to be up in pajamas watching television, etc. (6) Isolation within the family structure is rarely indicated, since exposure has usually preceded the diagnosis. (7) Parents can be reassured about temporary emotional regression during an acute illness. A return to the previous level of maturity need not be encouraged until good health returns.

Prognosis

"David will probably feel better in 2 or 3 days. This is not a serious infection. If something new develops or his fever lasts over 3 days, give me a call." Nothing is gained by mentioning all the possible complications. Without promoting anxiety, the door to additional medical evaluation is quietly left open for any new problems that might arise.

Closing

"You're doing a fine job with David. Just hold the fort and he will be his old self in a few days." The visit should close on a positive note, even a compliment if possible. If David is older, an attempt can be made to boost his morale as well—eg, "This won't keep *you* out of action for long."

The Ambiguous Diagnosis

An unclear diagnosis presents special problems in communication with the parents. The physician must be honest about the inconclusive diagnosis and yet not unduly alarm the parents. "David's illness is not far enough along to be diagnosed exactly. Another day or so will be needed to pinpoint the problem. I can tell you a few things for certain. He is not in any serious trouble. He doesn't have meningitis. I definitely want to see him tomorrow. Call me sooner if there are any new developments."

Symptomatic therapy should also be prescribed.

Carey WB, Sibinga MS: Avoiding pediatric pathogenesis in the management of acute minor illness. *Pediatrics* 1972;**49**:553.

Korsch B et al: Practical implications of doctor-patient interaction analysis for pediatric practice. *Am J Dis Child* 1971;**121:**110.
Waller DA, Levitt EE: Concerns of mothers in a pediatric clinic. *Pediatrics* 1972;**50:**931.

6. FOLLOW-UP OF THE NONHOSPITALIZED PATIENT

Many children seen in an emergency room have conditions that require following (eg, asthma, bronchiolitis, croup, pneumonia, otitis media, burns, and seizures). If a child has an ambiguous diagnosis (eg, high fever of unknown origin) or an unpredictable course (eg, vomiting), daily follow-up is necessary. This protects both the patient and the physician. This follow-up can be accomplished by revisits, telephone calls, or a visiting nurse.

Revisits

Daily office visits are the best approach to the more serious problem. The weight of an infant with diarrhea and the degree of respiratory distress in a child with croup cannot be estimated over the phone. If a scheduled appointment is not kept, the office clerk should immediately notify the physician, and a phone call or home visit should be made on that same day. If transportation is a problem for the parent, a community service agency can usually help. If the late results of laboratory tests indicate that an illness is quite serious (eg, stool culture growing *Salmonella* in a 4-month-old infant) and reasonable attempts to locate the parents fail, the police may be asked to find and bring the patient to the clinic or office.

Telephone Calls

A daily telephone call will suffice for milder problems when only historical follow-up data are needed (eg, vomiting or lethargy). Since these calls are essential to proper management, the physician or nurse should make them. A daily telephone list can be kept and the charts pulled prior to calling. If the follow-up is felt to be important, parents should not be depended upon to initiate these calls. Telephone calls become the realistic choice of follow-up when long distances are a factor.

Home Visits

The evaluation of children with allergies, obesity, failure to thrive, recurrent accidents, recurrent ingestions, or behavior problems is enhanced by a home visit. The follow-up of early-discharge newborns is simplified by home visits. Dressing changes of burns or wounds can readily be done in the home. Most of these house calls are made by the public health nurse, but the office nurse or physician can also become involved. Mothers of large families who have both a baby-sitter problem and a transportation problem appreciate this type of follow-up. Mothers who have several sick children or who are themselves in poor health also benefit from home visits.

Berger LR, Samet KP: Home visits: Extending the boundaries of comprehensive pediatric care. *Am J Dis Child* 1981;**135:**812.
DeAngelis C, Fosarelli P: Assignment of follow-up appointments from an emergency room by pediatric residents. *Am J Dis Child* 1985;**139:**341.
Pearce T, O'Shea JS, Wessen AF: Correlations between appointment keeping and reorganization of hospital ambulatory pediatric services. *Pediatrics* 1979;**64:**81.
Weitzman M, Moomaw MS, Messenger KP: An after-hours pediatric walk-in clinic for an entire urban community. *Pediatrics* 1980;**65:**964.

MEDICOLEGAL PROBLEMS

The management of acute illness offers the greatest potential for malpractice litigation in pediatrics. Physicians are legally liable for damage proximately caused not only by their own mistakes but by the mistakes of their employees as well. Errors can be made in any of the areas previously discussed. An error in telephone triaging can result in a delay in diagnosis (eg, calling meningococcemia a viral exanthem, or arranging an appointment for the next day for scrotal pain that turns out to be testicular torsion). An error in underhospitalization can lead to death (eg, epiglottitis being treated on an outpatient basis). Errors in therapy may result in sciatic nerve palsy if an injection is given into an inappropriate quadrant of the buttocks or may result in acute rheumatic fever if penicillin is not given for a streptococcal sore throat because it was not cultured. Errors in follow-up can result in undiagnosed abdominal pain silently progressing to ruptured appendix.

The physician should obtain parent consent forms for all medical procedures (eg, lumbar puncture, suturing) unless an emergency exists. Consultation should be sought whenever a physician is uncertain about what is happening with an acutely and perhaps seriously ill patient.

The errors listed above are not difficult to prevent if the physician bases all medical decisions on what is best for the patient.

Brown RH: Consent. *Pediatrics* 1976;**57:**414.
Conkling WS (chairman): *An Introduction to Medical Liability for Pediatricians.* Task Force on Medical Liability of the Council on Pediatric Practice, 1975.
Markham BF: Legal issues for the practicing pediatrician. *Pediatr Clin North Am* 1981;**28:**617.

CHRONIC DISEASE FOLLOW-UP VISITS

At least 7.5% of children in the USA have one or more chronic illnesses; management of these patients is thus a major part of pediatric practice. Office visits for a child with known or potential chronic disease present special problems. There are 5 broad types of chronic disease, each being progressively more difficult to manage: (1) potential chronic disease (eg, the small premature infant, the newborn who has recovered from hypoglycemia, or the older child who has recovered from meningitis; (2) reversible chronic disease (eg, tuberculosis, eczema, or idiopathic thrombocytopenic purpura); (3) static chronic disease (eg, cerebral palsy, deafness, or dwarfism); (4) progressive chronic disease (eg, diabetes mellitus or sickle cell anemia); and (5) fatal disease (eg, leukemia or muscular dystrophy). Children with these problems usually receive excellent care when they are hospitalized. They should also receive the same thoughtful care when they do not occupy a hospital bed or have an interesting complication.

COMMON TYPES OF CHRONIC ILLNESSES

The following diagnoses or conditions are the chronic disorders most commonly seen in office practice: serous otitis media, hay fever, asthma, obesity, enuresis, recurrent abdominal pain, recurrent headaches, acne, developmental delays or mental retardation, seizures, learning disabilities, attention deficit disorder, menstrual problems, visual acuity defect, hearing defect, depression, child abuse, recurrent urinary tract infections, hypertension, congenital heart disease, failure to thrive, short stature, eczema, cerebral palsy, constipation or soiling, recurrent hematuria, scoliosis, chronic diarrhea, peptic ulcer, and diabetes mellitus.

OBJECTIVES

There are 2 primary objectives in the management of a chronic disease. The first is to counteract the effects of the disease to the extent possible. This requires the aggressive use of every available treatment measure that could be useful for the individual patient's problems. The second objective is to help the patient and parents make a suitable emotional adjustment to the treatment regimen and to the effects of the disease that cannot be controlled. Except for necessary restrictions imposed by the disease, the child should be reared just like other children. The goal of management is to enable the patient to live as normal a life as possible in all positive respects.

Chronic disease management is optimal when the following receive ongoing attention: continuity of care, frequent visits, problem-oriented records, chronic disease flow sheets, personal medical identification documents, a chronic disease patient registry kept in the office, and medical passport.

1. CONTINUITY OF CARE

The patient with a chronic disease may have multiple problems that are difficult to manage. If anyone deserves continuous medical care from one physician, this person does. Discontinuous care by several physicians (eg, in emergency rooms) often results in a confused and maladjusted patient. When the patient has a progressive or fatal disease, depression can occur. In such a situation, patients depend upon a single sustaining physician to help them maintain their tenuous hope for the child's survival. Fragmented medical care usually accentuates a poor psychologic adjustment. The physician who agrees to care for a patient with a chronic disease should be available by phone at all times, even when at home. If the physician cannot deal with a problem personally, arrangements can be made for the patient to be seen by another physician who has been fully briefed. If the physician must be away for any reason, a substitute physician who has been designated well in advance should be available.

Becker MH et al: Continuity of pediatrician: New support for an old shibboleth. *J Pediatr* 1974;**84:**599.

2. FREQUENT VISITS

The patient with a chronic disease should be contacted frequently. Monitoring the patient's disease and response to therapy is impossible without periodic visits or telephone communications. If the problem is stabilized, the patient should be seen personally at least every 6 months; 3-month intervals are better for progressive diseases. If the disease is in relapse, the patient may need to be seen daily.

3. PROBLEM-ORIENTED RECORDS

In addition to a personal physician, comprehensive care of the chronically ill patient depends upon good record keeping. No physician's memory is completely reliable, and in any case the patient must have accurate office records when the physician moves away from the city or dies. An excellent system of record keeping has been developed and refined in a practice setting (see references, below). It has 4 components: the initial data base, the active problem sheet, the plan for each problem, and the progress notes that contribute to the continually expanding data base and problem list.

Initial Data Base

The conventional present illness, review of systems, past medical history, family history, psychosocial history, physical examination, and laboratory screening tests comprise the data base. Information from all accessible sources is used. (See Chapter 1.)

Active Problem Sheet

The active problem list is the keystone of this system. It lists all of the patient's significant problems, including psychosocial ones. These problems are defined from the data base currently at hand. They can be expressed as an etiologic diagnosis (eg, rheumatic heart disease), a pathophysiologic state (eg, congestive heart failure), or a sign or symptom (eg, edema). When the therapy carries considerable risk, it should be defined as a problem (eg, corticosteroids or tracheostomy). An attempt is made to list the problems in order of priority. Each problem is then assigned a permanent number. Thereafter, this number should precede any entry in the chart concerning this problem. The active problem sheet should be kept in the front of the patient's chart as a table of contents. The dates should be date of onset or resolution. New problems are added as identified, and old problems are transferred to the "resolved or inactive" column when appropriate. Symptom problems should be re-identified as diagnosed problems when the data accumulated justify doing so. When a patient with multiple diseases is cared for by several physicians, the last column on the active problem list can be used to list the responsible physician for each problem. This technique is especially helpful for improving continuity of care in a large medical center.

The active problem list can become somewhat standardized if "#1" is always used for "health maintenance care" (or well child care) and "#2" is always used for "minor acute illnesses" (or temporary problems). The latter category is a convenient place to bury self-limited minor illnesses that do not warrant being given individual permanent numbers. Examples are colds, coughs, gastroenteritis, conjunctivitis, mumps, viral exanthems, impetigo, diaper rash, insect bites, minor trauma, etc. Acute illnesses that can be serious (eg, pneumonia) or recurrent (eg, otitis media) obviously should be given different numbers.

Plan for Each Problem

Each problem as listed in the active problem sheet needs an individual diagnostic, therapeutic, and educational plan. If the plans for all the problems are combined, omissions are likely to occur.

Progress Notes

Progress notes contain newly collected data, an analysis of the data, and a reassessment of the plan. These notes should always pertain to one of the problems on the active problem sheet and be so labeled both by number and by title, eg, as follows:

> **Seizures, grand mal:**
>
> **Subjective**—Two seizures last week, lasting 1 minute and 5 minutes. Occurred at 7:00 AM and 10:00 AM. No precipitating events apparent. Last seizure 3 months ago. No headaches or vomiting. Not drowsy from medication.
>
> **Objective**—Neurologic examination and fundi normal. No nystagmus.
>
> **Assessment**—Seizures still in poor control.
>
> **Plan**—Continue phenobarbital, 90 mg/d. Recheck blood level. Reviewed reasons for strict compliance.

Bjorn JC, Cross HD: *Problem-Oriented Practice*. Modern Hospital Press, 1970.

Gordon IB: Office medical records. *Pediatr Clin North Am* 1981;**28:**565.

4. THE CHRONIC DISEASE FLOW SHEET

There are many variables in the management of a chronic disease. The variables can become lost in the substance of the chart and relatively unavailable for comparison and interpretation. For a patient with a chronic disease or multiple problems, critical data from the progress note should be recorded on a chronic disease flow sheet which tabulates variables so that trends and correlations can be accurately determined. The long axis of the flow sheet has time intervals. Inpatient flow sheets maintained for a critically ill child usually monitor vital signs, intake and output, blood gases, and numerous chemical determinations. Outpatient flow sheets often contain none of the above. Although a specific flow sheet is designed for each chronic disease, the following variables are commonly present in the ambulatory management of most chronic diseases. An example of how to use a flow sheet for a patient with diabetes mellitus is provided at the end of this chapter.

Disease Status

One must monitor the activity level of the disease to know whether therapy is being effective or not. Such activity can be evaluated through the history, physical findings, laboratory data, consultations, and hospitalizations. Variables so determined can be tabulated on the flow sheet.

A. Symptom Data: Frequency of attacks and duration of attacks are the main determinants of the success of asthma therapy. Migraine headaches, seizure episodes, and psychogenic recurrent abdominal pain must also be monitored largely by attack rates.

B. Physical Findings: Childhood nephrosis must be followed by weighing the patient and observing the presence or absence of edema. Splenomegaly is an important variable in leukemia. Motor milestones are important in cerebral palsy.

C. Laboratory Data: Chest films are important for following tuberculosis, EEGs for seizures, liver enzyme levels for chronic active hepatitis, urine cultures for recurrent urinary tract infection, etc.

D. Data for Early Detection of Complications: Some chronic diseases have complications that are not preventable but respond much better to therapy if they are detected early. Warning signs of these complications should be listed on the flow sheet. Examples are (1) head circumference measurements to detect early subdural effusions or hydrocephalus after meningitis and (2) blood pressure measurements to detect early hypertension in chronic renal disease. Once hypertension is discovered, it is no longer an anticipated complication but an indicator of disease activity.

E. Consultations: One of the patient's problems may be managed by another specialist. The primary physician should record on the flow sheet, under the dates of these visits, the consultant's name and a brief note about that specialist's conclusions. The date will permit easy location of the consultation report in the chart when it is needed.

F. Hospitalizations: All hospitalizations should be recorded under the problem they were required for. They usually represent a marker of increased activity of the disease.

G. Emotional Status: Emotional maladjustments are a frequent and often unnecessary side effect of chronic diseases. The physician can prevent them in many instances by reviewing an emotional problem checklist on *every* visit. Some of the more common but unspoken maladjustments are necessary restrictions, overprotectiveness, favoritism, school phobia, underdiscipline, and teasing by peers. This subject is more fully discussed in Chapter 24.

Treatment Regimen

Therapy may or may not be responsible for improvements in clinical status. Examining the temporal relationship of one to the other allows the physician to decide if treatment has been effective. A chronic disease flow sheet should supply this information.

A. Medications: All medications and dosages should be listed with the dates when started, when discontinued, and when the dosage is changed. The dosage may be increased because the patient has outgrown it or because the problem is not under optimal control (eg, increasing the dosage of digoxin in persistent congestive heart failure). New drugs should be added when other drugs have been pushed to tolerance without adequate control (eg, adding metaproterenol to daily theophylline therapy in asthma). Any drug the patient is receiving should have at least one related variable listed under disease status that permits rapid assessment of the efficacy of the drug (eg, bowel movements per day recorded for the patient with ulcerative colitis who is taking sulfasalazine).

B. Toxicity: If drugs with side effects are being used, these problems should be anticipated. The bone marrow, kidney, or liver function tests that need monitoring should be recorded on the flow sheet, as well as the required frequency of testing. If the potential toxicity is high, the drug should also be recorded on the problem list. If suddenly discontinuing the drug could lead to a severe adverse reaction, this risk should be frequently discussed with the patient (eg, anticonvulsants).

C. Nondrug Therapy: Other methods of treatment besides drugs should be recorded on the flow sheet so that their effect on the course of the disease can be estimated. Examples are specific food avoidance in recurrent urticaria or bubble bath avoidance in recurrent urinary tract infection. In static diseases, compensatory devices (eg, braces in cerebral palsy or hearing aids in deafness) should be listed, as well as the recommended interval for routine checks of these devices. Reassurance and other forms of supportive psychotherapy will generally be given on every visit and need not be listed here.

D. Therapy for Prevention of Complications: Many chronic diseases have predictable complications that are preventable if therapy is instituted in advance. If these are listed in the flow sheet, the physician will be certain to remind the parent of them on each visit. Examples are performing daily range-of-motion exercises to prevent contractures in rheumatoid arthritis, requesting penicillin prophylaxis before dental procedures to prevent subacute bacterial endocarditis in congenital heart disease, avoidance of altitudes over 10,000 feet to prevent a crisis in sickle cell disease, and carrying an antihypoglycemic food in the pocket at all times in diabetes mellitus.

E. Compliance With Therapy: The best treatment regimen is useless unless the patient complies with it. A check on the patient's compliance can be performed by inquiring about the degree of satisfaction or dissatisfaction with the medical care received; by asking if the medications have been difficult to take; or in some cases by measuring blood or urine levels (eg, aspirin, penicillin).

F. Disease Education Reviews: Patients may not cooperate with a therapeutic plan until they are intellectually and emotionally committed to it. Unless the family fully understands what they are expected to do, they cannot do it. Unless they understand priorities, they may unknowingly discontinue some critical element in the treatment program when the program as a whole becomes frustrating. Optimal patient education is reached when patient and family know as much about the home treatment of the disease as the physician does and when they can make minor adjustments in treatment independently.

When facts regarding the disease and its treatment are reviewed, one should begin with basic information even though it has been covered many times before. After the first session, the subject is reviewed by asking the patient questions. In the early years, the facts are covered with the patient and both parents present. If the father does not share responsibility for medical care of the child, serious marital problems may develop. In the adolescent years, the review sessions should be done privately with the teenager. The patient's understanding of the problems should be explored approximately every 6 months. In the period immediately following diagnosis, it should be covered on every visit for a few months.

G. School Notification: Each fall the physician should notify the school nurse about any patient whose disease may become manifest or cause a problem of any sort at school. This notification will prevent emotional problems secondary to mishandling of the physical problem by the school. The patient with chronic heart or lung disease may need a gym excuse (no gym) or a modified gym status (eg, no gym on days of wheezing; no rope climbing). Both nurse and teacher need to know how to respond to a seizure or insulin reaction at school. The physician should have this listed on the flow sheet so it is never overlooked. The parents of the patient's closest friends should also have this information, as should the babysitters.

Paulson JA: Patient education. *Pediatr Clin North Am* 1981;**28:**627.

Schmitt BD: The chronic disease flow sheet in ambulatory pediatrics. *Pediatrics* 1973;**51:**722.

5. THE MEDICAL IDENTIFICATION CARD

The patient with a chronic disease should carry an identification card that sets forth the active problem list, medications being taken currently, the physician's telephone number, and the parents' telephone numbers at home and at work. If the disease can lead to sudden changes in consciousness (eg, insulin reaction in diabetes mellitus) or if an allergy is present that could be fatal if violated (eg, penicillin hypersensitivity), the patient should obtain a medical identification bracelet or necklace. These can be ordered from Medic Alert Foundation International, Turlock, CA 95380.

6. CHRONIC DISEASE PATIENT REGISTRY

Every effort should be made to keep certain patients from being "lost to follow-up." People with chronic diseases (eg, those with rheumatic heart disease receiving prophylactic penicillin) fall into this group. To prevent the disappearance of any of these patients, the physician should keep them listed in a chronic disease patient registry. Their charts should have a special mark placed on the corner of the cover to show that they are special high-risk patients. These patients should be sent a reminder card 1 week prior to appointments. If the parent cancels an appointment and promises to call back and make another one, the patient's name should be placed on a critical phone call list that automatically goes into effect if the appointment is not remade within 2 weeks. If the patient misses an appointment, the physician should be notified that same day and should call the patient. If the parent has no phone, a letter should be sent. If there is no response to the letter, a visiting nurse referral should be sent. This usually returns the patient to the physician or shows that the family has changed physicians. If the family does not wish further medical care from anyone and the patient's disease is life-threatening but treatable (eg, tuberculosis, chronic pyelonephritis), the physician should report the case to the local child protective services. Since this is an example of medical care neglect, a court order will be issued for treatment of the child. The physician should assume personal responsibility for following any high-risk patient until transfer of care occurs.

7. THE MEDICAL PASSPORT

Every year, 20% of North American families change residences. Some of them have children with chronic diseases. Nothing is more frustrating for a physician than to take a complicated new patient with no past records. Legally, the records belong to the physician; but morally, the records belong to the patient. The patient who moves should carry a copy of the active problem list, chronic disease flow sheet, health maintenance flow sheet, consultation reports, hospital discharge summaries, pertinent x-ray reports, and a covering letter. Original copies should never be sent, because they may be lost. The physician should also give the family the names of 2 or 3 pediatricians they might use in the city they are moving to. These may be personal acquaintances or selections made from the *Directory of Medical Specialists*.

CONSULTATIVE VISITS

The physician must know both how to serve as a consultant and how to seek consultation when it is called for. The practicing pediatrician is still the best consultant for most pediatric problems.

OBJECTIVES

The usual purpose of a consultation is the evaluation of an undiagnosed problem followed by therapeutic recommendations. Some referrals are for treatment advice only. A secondary goal of consultation is to provide the referring physician with a continuing medical educational experience.

THE PEDIATRICIAN IN THE ROLE OF CONSULTANT

Referring Source

A. Self-Referral: Although not technically a consultation, some problems require the same kind of intensive approach that is needed when consulting with a colleague. A problem requiring a careful diagnostic evaluation may be detected during a well child visit or a sick child visit. These "big" problems are often not mentioned by the parent until the end of the visit or may be detected by a screening questionnaire. The physician should arrange to see such patients again. These diagnostic evaluations can keep practice stimulating. If the physician is unsure about the workup of a particular problem, it will be necessary to review the literature ahead of time.

B. Physician Referral: Family practitioners or other specialists occasionally refer patients to a pediatrician for consultation. Within the pediatric community, some pediatricians refer patients to other physicians who have a subspecialty interest or expertise in a specific disease. This is more common within a group practice.

C. Nonphysician Referral: A physician who is well thought of receives referrals from dentists, school officials, psychologists, social workers, nurses, and other patients. Some of these referred patients will require a consultation type of visit.

Appointments

Consultations usually require 1-hour appointments. In some cases, 2 or more visits may be required to complete the evaluation. The average pediatrician will need to have 2–5 of these 1-hour appointments scheduled each week. The visit will be considerably more productive if a screening questionnaire is completed in advance (eg, using forms such as those presented at the end of this chapter). The questionnaire delineates the patient's physical, intellectual, and emotional problems and serves as an initial data base. The psychosocial portion is different for each of 4 age groups. The physician will then have a tentative problem list at hand when the patient is first seen.

These long appointments are easily arranged when the patient is referred by another professional, because a telephone call or letter usually precedes the patient. However, a patient with almost any problem requiring a careful evaluation can walk into a physician's office at any time. When the mother of a 10-year-old patient who is being seen for acute otitis media mentions that her child has experienced 4 years of encopresis or 6 months of "staring spells" at school, the busy physician may feel under some pressure to make a quick recommendation. The temptation may be strong to do a 5-minute workup and order some laboratory tests, or to hospitalize the patient for evaluation at greater leisure, or even to disregard the complaint or minimize its importance. Needless to say, these responses do not serve the patient's best interests. Long-standing diagnostic dilemmas require a comprehensive assessment that takes at least an hour. Most such evaluations can be done on an ambulatory basis. Shortcuts can lead to tentative conclusions, unconvinced parents, postponement of the indicated workup, "doctor shopping," secondary gain for the patient, and an unresolved problem.

The first visit can serve a useful purpose. One can tell the parents that the child's problem is complicated and demands a complete evaluation. A few screening laboratory tests such as a blood count and erythrocyte sedimentation rate may be ordered. The parent can fill out the screening data questionnaire. A release can be signed for hospital discharge summaries, prior consultation reports, laboratory test results (especially any tests that are dangerous, painful, or expensive), school reports, and growth information. These data will make the consultation visit more meaningful and avoid duplication of effort. In these consultations (unlike hospitalized consultations), an immediate appointment is rarely needed, and the patient can be rescheduled for the following week or later if more time is needed to accumulate data.

Extent of Services

When the patient is referred by the parents or a nonphysician, the request is usually for total care. When the patient is referred by a physician, there are 5 possible degrees of service the consulting physician can offer. If the referring physician does not specify precisely what is needed, the consulting physician may either ask for more specific details about what is wanted or may assume that this cannot be predicted in advance and must await the results of the evaluation.

A. Evaluation Only: The consultant can do a diagnostic evaluation on a patient and tell the parents nothing except that the findings will be discussed with their primary physician. Parents generally do not like this. They are paying for the consultation, and they want to hear something from the expert personally. Common courtesy suggests that they are right.

B. Evaluation and Interpretation: After the evaluation is completed, the consultant usually discusses the diagnosis and the causes of the problem with the family. Recommendations for therapy should be mentioned, if at all, only in very general terms and with the clear understanding that the referring physician will be coordinating the therapy. The patient should then be returned to the referring physician, who will make specific therapeutic recommendations to the family. A specific return appointment date with the referring physician should be given. This is the usual type of referral process for a patient with a chronic disease. The consultant may be called upon periodically to reassess the response to therapy and to offer revised recommendations.

C. Evaluation and Treatment of an Isolated Problem: Sometimes the referring physician wants the consultant to assume responsibility for management of the problem that is the subject of referral. This usually happens with treatable problems that will require only 3–6 visits (eg, recurrent headaches, breath-holding spells, ringworm, Sydenham's chorea). The consultant should clearly define and support the referring physician's role as the continuing provider of health supervision and acute illness care during this interval. When the problem is resolved, the patient should be returned to the referring physician for resumption of care.

D. Total Health Care: Occasionally, a physician refers a patient to a consultant for management of a specific problem plus all future medical care. This may occur when the family is moving to a new area or is unable for financial reasons to maintain the contact with a private physician. In the latter instance, referral should be to a community-based clinic rather than another private physician.

E. Evaluation and Referral for Additional Consultation: The patient's problem may require the expertise of a subspecialist (eg, pediatric hematologist). Before this step is taken, permission must be sought from the original physician for further consultation. The pediatrician's advice about where to seek further expert consultations will usually be heeded.

Barness LA et al: Computer-assisted diagnosis in pediatrics. *Am J Dis Child* 1974;**127:**852.

Swender PT et al: Computer-assisted diagnosis. *Am J Dis Child* 1974;**127:**859.

Communication With the Referring Source

Communication is the key to a satisfactory referral process. The consulting physician is mainly responsible for this aspect of consultation. The referring physician should not have to ask the consultant for the results. The following procedure serves as an appropriate format for completing the process diplomatically.

A. Acknowledge the Referral: As soon as a referral letter is received, the consulting physician should send the referral source a brief note acknowledging the referral. Additional information can also be requested at this time: "Thank you for your recent referral letter on David Jones. I have sent the parents a screening data questionnaire. As soon as it is returned, he will be scheduled for a full evaluation. I will be in contact with you regarding the results. Best regards."

B. Send a Consultation Report: This report should be sent promptly. The content of the final report depends on the referring source. School officials do not want to know medical details; they usually just want to know if the patient is physically healthy or, if not, what their responsibility is. A referring physician expects a full report that will be helpful in treating the patient. Recommendations should therefore be specific (drugs, dosages, other forms of therapy, duration of therapy, specific laboratory tests, the frequency of these tests, etc). A copy of or reference to a recent review article on the subject will also be appreciated.

This evaluation should be typed as a formal consultation report. It should not contain personal comments or resemble a letter. When written in this style, it can serve as an official evaluation report for anyone who might request a copy of it in the future. To make this communication to the referring physician more personal, it should be accompanied by a covering letter: "It was a pleasure to see David Jones today. A complete summary of his evaluation is included. The recommendations may need to be modified in the light of your previous experience with this family. As you know, the marital situation is very stormy. It would be a privilege to see David again if you feel the need arises."

C. Call the Referring Physician Selectively: Most referring physicians prefer a consultation report to a phone call because the former can become a permanent part of the patient's record. Some cases require a brief telephone report in addition to the written consultation report. These cases include situations where the patient needs to return to the referring physician before a consultation report can be sent, where the patient needs to be referred to an additional specialist, or where a question exists about proper disposition.

D. Arrange a Return Appointment With the Referring Physician: At the end of the consultation, the consultant should tell the parents when the patient should see the primary physician—usually in 1–2 weeks. Positive comments about the referring physician's competence and judgment should be made. The parents must feel confident that the primary physician can provide the necessary follow-up care. If the referring physician had tentatively made the correct diagnosis prior to referral, the consultant's corroboration should be made clear to the parents and recorded in the consultation report.

Fees for Services Rendered

Many pediatricians are reluctant to charge adequately for their time. This seems illogical, since an ambulatory consultation can prevent the high cost of an unnecessary hospital workup. Even if ambulatory insurance does not cover the full cost of such an evaluation, the pediatrician should bill for these evaluations as "office consultations" and charge for the time allotted. An hour is worth the same whether it is spent with one consultation or several well or sick children.

THE PEDIATRICIAN IN THE ROLE OF REFERRING PHYSICIAN

Indications for Referral

There are generally 8 indications for seeking consultation. The last 2 are primarily to help the parents deal with reality.

A. Uncertain Diagnosis: Referral for a diagnostic evaluation is a time-honored indication. The ambulatory consultation is preferable to hospitalization.

B. Treatment Requires Special Expertise: *Examples:* Surgery, cancer chemotherapy.

C. Treatment Is Nonmedical: *Examples:* Services of psychiatrists, psychologists, social workers, special teachers, speech therapists.

D. Treatment Is Complex: The treatment of some diseases is so complex that the physician unfamiliar with it should refer those patients. *Examples:* Cystic fibrosis, muscular dystrophy, leukemia.

E. Conventional Treatment Is Not Effective: When the patient is not doing as well as expected, 2 heads are better than one. Even with diseases the physician has successfully treated many times, an atypical problem may arise that requires a fresh opinion (eg, recalcitrant seizures). Phone consultation with the appropriate subspecialist will sometimes solve the problem.

F. Medicolegal Problems: Parents bring in children with injuries for which they are suing a physician or other person. The pediatrician's main task is to decide if the alleged disability or defect is real. If the injury proves to be significant, the physician can help the family find an expert consultant whose testimony will be received in court (eg, an orthopedist in the case of a hand injury). If it seems that the parents are exaggerating the disability for financial gain, the physician should declare the child healthy and recommend return to full activity without confronting the family with such suspicions.

G. Parents Insist on Overtreatment: The pediatrician can help the family avoid uselessly aggressive intervention by recommending consultation with experts known to have conservative views. Even though there are honest differences of opinion about the indications for tonsillectomy, "corrective shoes," hyposensitization, etc, it is often in the patient's best interests not to have to undergo further painful or protracted procedures with little chance of substantial benefit.

H. Parents Are Thinking About a Consultation: When the parents have to ask for a consultation or obtain one without telling the physician, the pediatrician has waited too long. Such an attitude should be suspected when the parents seem angry or critical or uncertain about following advice. The parents' tendency to deny an unfavorable prognosis can be anticipated with certain diseases (eg, fatal diseases and mental retardation). This denial should be respected if it does not interfere with therapy.

A rare or fatal disease is not as such an indication for referral. Some physicians automatically seek "confirmation" of a diagnosis they are already sure of or "approval" of a treatment regimen they are already familiar with. This practice is wasteful of medical resources and may undermine the family's confidence in the doctor.

Method of Referral

A. Obtain Permission From the Family: The family will usually agree to a referral if the reason for it is made clear. Patients sometimes feel that a referral means they are being abandoned by their physician. The referring physician's continuing availability for primary medical care must be made clear. The family should also be told in advance that the consultation will cost more than a regular visit but that it will be worth more.

B. Help the Family Choose a Consultant: The physician should maintain a file listing the best consultants locally and at the nearest medical center. The parents can be given the names of 2 or 3 competent physicians. If one is outstanding, the pediatrician should not be reluctant to state a preference. If the parents suggest someone they have heard of but who the physician feels is unqualified, the pediatrician should express doubts about that person's degree of expertise in this particular kind of case. It often happens that only one subspecialist is available in the community (eg, oncologist) and that no choice exists.

C. Make an Appointment for the Family: After the family has agreed to the referral, the physician's secretary should arrange an appointment. This increases compliance. If the case is particularly complicated, a long consultation visit should be requested.

D. Send a Referral Letter: A referral letter should be sent immediately so that it will arrive well in advance of the appointment with the consultant. All pertinent information, such as copies of previous evaluations, hospital discharge summaries, and laboratory results, should be included. If time is short, the consultant can be prepared for the visit by phone and pertinent data can be sent along with the patient.

E. Specify the Service Requested: The specific questions to be answered and the future role of the referring physician should be clarified if possible in the referral letter.

QUALITY CONTROL OF AMBULATORY PEDIATRIC CARE

The concept of peer review or medical audit can be implemented by any group of physicians for purposes of self-education as well as continuing improvement of quality. In a good hospital with an interested staff—especially where house staff are present—quality control is almost a built-in feature. Frequent reassessments of the inpatient's status by the physician, plus constant review by other medical and paramedical personnel, make "peer review" an ongoing process.

Care of ambulatory patients, on the other hand, usually is not reviewed systematically. The following is a suggestion for developing a program that will both improve the quality and cost-effectiveness of ambulatory practice and make it more challenging and satisfying. Physicians can attempt to schedule 1 hour a week for chart review. Several pediatricians should be present to make this a maximal learning experience. In group practice, the participants are already available. The pediatrician in solo practice can meet with the one or 2 pediatricians who share the responsibility for responding to night calls. The group can focus on random charts or on selected charts that cover a specific problem. The latter method requires an office data retrieval system.

CHART REVIEWS

Health Maintenance Chart Review

The delivery of comprehensive health maintenance care can be easily audited by reviewing the health maintenance flow sheet (see example provided at the end of this chapter). Since the nursing staff is primarily responsible for filling out these flow sheets, this type of review is largely a check on their ability to comply with office protocol and need not be done very often. The office protocols themselves require periodic review and revision.

Acute Illness Chart Review

Acute illness charts can be audited for completeness in diagnosis and therapy of the chief complaint. The following questions can be asked: (1) Was the diagnosis valid? Validity is substantiated if the chart contains adequate historical, physical, or laboratory data to document the diagnosis. (2) Was the therapy optimal? (3) Was the follow-up plan optimal? Charts of patients with a specific acute illness (eg, acute lymphadenitis, streptococcal pharyngitis, or infectious hepatitis) can be pulled and audited to test the group consensus about therapy and follow-up.

Chronic Disease Chart Review

Examination of the chronic disease flow sheet (see example provided at the end of this chapter) is an easy way to audit chronic disease management. If no such flow sheet exists for the patient, the variables recommended above for monitoring chronic disease can be assessed as one reviews the entire chart. This process could then result in the formation of a chronic disease flow sheet for that patient. Chart review sessions can be more educational if only one chronic disease is considered each time and if an "expert" on that disease is present. The expert can be an actual subspecialist or a member of the group who has reviewed the literature or attended a workshop on this disease.

Diagnostic Problem Chart Review

An easy way to review consultations is to criticize the consultation report. The following questions can be asked: (1) Was the data base adequate? (2) Were all of the active problems identified? (3) Was the diagnostic plan for each problem optimal? (4) Were the final diagnoses valid? (5) Was the recommended therapy for each diagnosis optimal? (6) Was the role of the referring physician clarified and honored? If these consultations are concerned with general pediatric problems, an outside consultant will usually not be required.

Brook RH, Appel FA: Quality-of-care assessment: Choosing a method for peer review. *N Engl J Med* 1973;**288:**1323.

Coulter LW: Peer review: Tutor or judge? *JAMA* 1974; **230:**1161.

Haggerty RJ: Quality assurance: The road to PSRO and beyond. *Pediatrics* 1974;**54:**90.

Meyers A: Audit of medical records from pediatric specialty clinics. *Pediatrics* 1973;**51:**22.

Osborne CE, Thompson HC: Criteria for evaluation of ambulatory child health care by chart audit: Development and testing of a methodology. *Pediatrics* 1975;**56(Suppl):**625.

Starfield B et al: Private pediatric practice: Performance and problems. *Pediatrics* 1973;**52:**344.

MEDICAL CARE COMPLIANCE

Correct diagnoses and optimal therapeutic recommendations can be ensured by the voluntary type of peer review discussed above. An aspect of the quality of care not easy to assess by chart review but which needs to be borne in mind is patient compliance. Superb recommendations do not guarantee anything. Medical care does not become effective until the parent accepts the diagnosis and carries out the therapeutic recommendations. The parent's compliance often reflects their degree of satisfaction with the care the child is getting. The physician must make an effort to find out why appointments are not kept, medications are not given, etc; otherwise, even the best-conceived therapeutic goals will often not be achieved.

Charney E: Patient-doctor communication: Implications for clinicians. *Pediatr Clin North Am* 1972;**19:**263.

Rogers KD: Effectiveness of aggressive follow-up on Navajo infant health and medical care use. *Pediatrics* 1974;**53:**721.

PRACTICAL TIPS FOR AMBULATORY CARE

FOREIGN BODIES

Metallic Foreign Body in the Soft Tissues

Tape a straight pin with the point over the site where the metallic object entered the skin. Then obtain an x-ray of the area. An exact measurement can then be obtained to locate the foreign body in relation to the straight pin. Located in this manner, the foreign body can be removed with minimal exploration.

Splinters Under the Nails

With a single-edged razor blade or a sharp thin scalpel, gently shave the nail over the distal end of the splinter until the splinter is exposed. The sliver can then be easily pulled out with a pair of fine-pointed tweezers.

Embedded Fishhook

Fishhooks can be removed (eg, from a finger) without wire cutters by bringing them back through their point of entry. For shallow wounds, the skin overlying the metal can be cut and the fishhook lifted out. For deeper wounds, a technique that does not include yanking is preferred. An 18-gauge needle is inserted into the wound through the point of entry.

After the needle bevel is locked firmly over the barb, the fishhook and needle can be slowly withdrawn through the original wound as a unit. Local anesthesia helps.

A technique that includes yanking is preferred by fishermen in remote areas. A piece of fishline is looped around the curve of the fishhook. The 2 ends of the fishline are wrapped tightly about the physician's forefinger about 1 foot from where it is looped around the hook. The patient's finger is held against a firm surface to stabilize it. The free shank of the fishhook is pressed against the patient's finger with the physician's free hand until the barb is disengaged and the barb's long axis is parallel to the line of intended expulsion. With the string in this same axis, a quick yank expels the hook immediately.

Friedenberg S: Removing an embedded fishhook. *Hosp Physician* (Aug) 1971;**7**:48.

Longmire WT: Another twist on a fishhook. *Emergency Med* (July) 1971;**3**:98.

Feasting Ticks

Grasp the tick as close to the skin surface as possible with tweezers. Pull straight upward with steady, even pressure. Do not twist or jerk the tick, as this may cause the mouth parts to break off. Wash the site of the bite and the hands thoroughly after removal. While traction is uniformly effective, covering the tick with petroleum jelly, fingernail polish, or rubbing alcohol is uniformly ineffective. Applying a hot match also fails to induce detachment.

Needham GR: Evaluation of five popular methods for tick removal. *Pediatrics* 1985;**75**:997.

The Zipper-Entrapped Foreskin

A young child in a hurry to urinate can inadvertently catch his foreskin in his zipper. A zipper is composed of 2 rows of zipper teeth plus a zipper fastener in the middle. The zipper fastener is composed of an upper and a lower plate. The plates are joined by a U-shaped median bar. This U-shaped bar should be cut with bone cutters or wire cutters. After this is done, the zipper fastener will come apart, and this will usually free the skin. If the skin remains attached to the zipper teeth, these can be separated by grasping them on both sides and using a circular motion, rotating the 2 sides away from each other. Use local anesthesia for initial pain.

Saraf P, Rabinowitz R: Zipper injury of the foreskin. *Am J Dis Child* 1982;**136**:557.

Ring on a Swollen Finger

In most cases, an attempt is made to save the ring. The key to removing the ring is reducing finger edema. At 5-minute intervals, the patient should alternate soaking the hand in ice water and holding it (fingers extended) high in the air. At 30 minutes (after the hand has been elevated for the third time), mineral oil or cooking oil can be applied to the finger. While the hand remains elevated, steady upward pressure can be applied until the ring slides off.

A string technique may work in some resistant cases. Pass a piece of string under the ring and then wind the distal end of the string in close loops tightly from the distal edge of the ring past the knuckle. Exert a slow, firm pull on the proximal end of the string. The edema passes underneath the ring, and the ring is slowly pulled distally as the cord unwinds.

As a last resort, the ring must be cut off. If there is a dentist's office nearby, have the dentist cut it off with a Carborundum disk attached to the drill. The flesh of the finger must be protected by an inserted strip (eg, a tongue blade segment). This method has the disadvantage of destroying the ring and possibly heating the ring enough to burn the finger.

Hair Wrapped Around a Digit

A piece of fine hair wrapped about an infant's digit and left unnoticed can cause severe edema or even amputation. Removal of the hair is usually difficult because it cannot be readily grasped. Application of a liquid hair remover (eg, Nair) will usually dissolve the hair within 15 minutes.

Douglas ED: (Correspondence.) *J Pediatr* 1977;**91**:162.

Gum in the Hair

An easy and nontraumatic way to remove gum from children's hair is by rubbing the gum with peanut butter until the hairs are freed from the gum. This technique is far superior to pulling or cutting the gum out of the hair.

Tar on the Skin

Tar can be removed by applying ice to it or soaking it in ice water for 1 or 2 minutes. The ice causes the tar to become hard and nonsticky, so that it can be easily peeled from the skin. Hydrocarbon solvents merely soften the tar and smear it around, and they are painful if a wound is present.

Fiberglass Spicules or Cactus Spines

The small glass spicules from fiberglass can be removed by applying a layer of facial gel or wax depilatory (hair remover). Either let it air dry for 5 minutes or accelerate the process with a hair dryer. Then peel it off. White glue can also be tried, but it is less effective. This treatment is also helpful for some plant stickers (eg, cactus, stinging nettle). A corticosteriod cream applied twice daily for 1–2 days may be helpful after the treatment.

LACERATIONS

Wound Cleaning in a Resistant Child

The wound can be covered with gauze saturated with 1% lidocaine for 15 minutes. This will cause only momentary discomfort. The area will then be relatively anesthetized, and vigorous wound cleaning will be tolerated. The subcutaneous injection of additional lidocaine after the wound is cleaned will also be better tolerated.

Avoiding Unwanted Tattoos

Dirty abrasions of the knee, face, and elbow can result in permanent tattooing if all foreign particulate matter, especially carbon particles, is not meticulously removed. The area should be anesthetized as described above and then scrubbed gently with an antibacterial cleanser and a soft surgical nail brush. Tar can usually be removed by rubbing with petrolatum. Some contaminated pieces of skin may need debridement.

Laceration Closure in a Frightened Child

Wounds can often be closed without local anesthesia or sutures by using microporous adhesive tape (Steri-Strip). The skin adjacent to the laceration is made tacky with tincture of benzoin. The ⅛-inch strips of tape are applied in either a parallel or crisscross pattern. This microporous tape is a decided improvement over "butterfly" tape.

Suture Removal

There is a way to avoid having to dig embedded sutures out of the skin of a struggling child. At the time the laceration is closed, a straight needle threaded with silk can be passed under each suture used for skin closure. The ends of this silk suture can be tied together, leaving a loose loop. At the time of removal, picking up this loose loop will lift the sutures that have been used to close the wound. The scissors can then be easily slid underneath the sutures for snipping. A new, inexpensive sterile stitch cutter makes suture removal easy.

Traumatic Amputations

When a patient loses a significant piece of skin (eg, a fingertip) in an accident, the skin should be placed in cold normal saline solution and sent with the patient to a plastic surgeon. A watchful waiting approach in children less than 10 years of age will usually result in spontaneous regeneration of the distal digit.

Rosenthal LJ, Reiner MA, Bleicher MA: Nonoperative management of distal fingertip amputations in children. *Pediatrics* 1979;**64:**1.

BLUNT TRAUMA

Subungual Hematomas

The painful pressure secondary to a subungual hematoma can easily be relieved by applying a red-hot paper clip or other thick wire to the nail surface. The paper clip is held by a clamp. A hole is quickly bored through the nail, and the blood is allowed to escape. This "hot iron" approach can be very frightening for a child. If there is a dentist's office nearby, it is preferable to have the dentist bore a hole quickly through the nail with a high-speed drill.

Traumatic Tooth Avulsion

Reimplantation of a tooth is possible only with the permanent teeth. The physician or parent should attempt to replace the avulsed tooth in its socket prior to going to the dentist. If this proves impossible, the tooth should be placed in cold normal saline solution and sent with the patient to the dentist. The deadline for successful replacement is 2 hours.

Bernick SM: What the pediatrician should know about children's teeth: Dental emergencies. *Clin Pediatr* 1970;**9:**487.

MISCELLANEOUS PROCEDURES

Genital Labial Adhesions

Labial adhesions can usually be separated by introducing a probe into any opening remaining in the introitus and then tearing the adhesions. This method is only acceptable for thin adhesions. An ointment should be applied to the newly separated surfaces for several days to prevent them from resealing. A nontraumatic method for separating thicker labial adhesions is application of estrogen cream (eg, Premarin) twice daily to the medial line for 3 or 4 days.

Hiccup

One teaspoonful of ordinary white granulated sugar swallowed "dry" will result in immediate cessation of hiccup in almost all patients. If the hiccups recur, this method will again be effective. Recalcitrant hiccups may respond to stimulation of the nasopharynx with a rubber catheter.

Engleman EG et al: (Correspondence.) *N Engl J Med* 1971;**285:**1489.

Inadvertent Subcutaneous Injections

When intramuscular agents are given subcutaneously by mistake, complications can result. The location of the needle point can be rapidly assessed by trying to wiggle it prior to injection. If it is in a muscle mass, the needle point will be relatively fixed. If it is in the subcutaneous fatty tissues, it can be felt to move freely.

Painful Bee Stings or Other Insect Bites

A dash of meat tenderizer (papain powder) and a drop of water massaged into the sting site for 5 minutes will quickly relieve the pain. If these ingredients are not available, an ice cube often helps.

Paraphimosis

In this condition, the foreskin has become retracted and trapped behind the corona. Manual reduction can usually be achieved by placing the tips of the index and middle fingers of one hand behind the swollen foreskin, the thumb of the other hand over the urethral meatus, and applying gradual pressure. The foreskin will usually return to its normal position after this technique has been applied continuously for 4–5 minutes. If this approach fails, a urologist should be consulted for an emergency dorsal slit.

Plastibell Circumcision Ring Paraphimosis

Sometimes the Plastibell circumcision ring slips behind the glans onto the shaft of the penis and cannot be slipped forward. Local swelling can be reduced by applying cold compresses for 10 minutes. The plastic ring can then be cut with a pair of scissors. Mineral oil can be applied to allow the scissors blade to slip easily under the ring. If the operator is worried about cutting the skin, a piece of a small feeding tube can be threaded under the ring and used as a guide for the scissors. This problem can be prevented if parents are told to call their physician if the ring has not fallen off by day 12.

Postcircumcision Skin Tags

Parents occasionally bring their infant in during the first month of life because the foreskin has an irregular skin tag. A clamp can be applied along the desired line of cleavage for 1 minute. After the clamp is removed, an iris scissors can be used to cut along the crushed skin line without causing any significant bleeding.

SELECTED REFERENCES

Ambulatory Pediatrics Association: *Educational Guidelines for Training in General/Ambulatory Pediatrics*. Ambulatory Pediatrics Association, 1984.

American Academy of Pediatrics: *Guidelines for Health Supervision*. American Academy of Pediatrics, 1985.

American Academy of Pediatrics: *Standards of Child Health Care*, 3rd ed. Council of Pediatric Practice, 1977.

Charney E: Primary care pediatrics. *Pediatr Clin North Am* 1974;**21**:3. [Entire issue.]

DeAngelis C (editor): *Pediatric Primary Care*, 3rd ed. Little, Brown, 1984.

Gordon IB, Paulson JA: Issues for the practicing pediatrician. *Pediatr Clin North Am* 1981;**28**:535. [Entire issue.]

Green M, Haggerty RJ (editors): *Ambulatory Pediatrics*. Vols 1, 2, and 3. Saunders, 1968, 1977, and 1984.

Helfer RE (editor): *Advances in Ambulatory Pediatrics*. Year Book, 1973.

Shelov SP et al: *Primary Care Pediatrics: A Symptomatic Approach*. Appleton-Century-Crofts, 1984.

PEDIATRIC HEALTH MAINTENANCE

Birth through 3 months

Parent's concerns

Newborn data base
Birth weight ____ Gestational age ____
Pregnancy or delivery problems Neonatal problems

Growth (comment on growth curve)

Feeding advice
Formula ____ oz/24 hours ____
Breast feeding: Frequency ____ min/feeding ____
Vitamins ____ Iron ____
Solids ____ Fluoride drops ____
Feeding problems ____
Advice: Introduce bottle in breast fed (2w) ☐ Introduce fluids other than milk (2m) ☐

Developmental status
Stimulation advice: Hold baby (2w) ☐ Talk to baby (2m) ☐

Child rearing advice
Sleep pattern ____
Crying or colic ____
Mother-child interaction ____
Sibling rivalry (2w) ____

Family status
Advice: Paternal involvement, family planning (2w) ☐ Utilize sitter (2m) ☐

Accident prevention advice
Car seats, crib safety (2w) ☐ Rolling over (2m) ☐ Smoke detector ☐

Medical advice
Demonstrate use of bulb syringe for nose (2w) ☐ Foreskin or circumcision care ♂ (2w) ☐
Temperature taking, Tylenol and fever handout (2m) ☐ Discuss when to call doctor (2m) ☐

Intercurrent illness

PEDIATRIC HEALTH MAINTENANCE

4 months through 14 months

Parent's concerns

Growth (comment on growth curve)

Feeding advice
Formula ____ oz/24 hours ____
Breast feeding: Frequency ____ min/feeding ____
Vitamins ____ Iron ____
Solids ____ Fluoride drops ____
Feeding problems ____
Advice: No bottles in bed; introduce solids, spoon, cup (4m) ☐
Confirm intake of iron-rich solids (6m) ☐ Introduce finger foods, confirm on 3 meals/day (9m) ☐
Entirely on table foods. Phase out bottle by 18m (12m) ☐

Developmental status
Stimulation advice: Toys for reaching (4m) ☐ Avoid confining baby equipment (6m) ☐
Repeat baby's sounds (9m) ☐ Name objects and pictures for baby (12m) ☐

Child rearing advice
Sleep pattern ____
Behavior problems ____
Advice: Sleeps through the night (4m) ☐ Normal separation anxiety (6m) ☐
Discipline: Use negative voice and eye contact rather than physical punishment (9m) ☐
Don't punish for normal exploratory behavior, discuss positive strokes for good behavior (12m) ☐

Family status

Accident prevention advice
Safe toys (4m) ☐ Stairs and gates, drowning in bathtub (9m) ☐
Electrical cords (6m) ☐ Ipecac and poison talk (12m) ☐

Medical advice
Teething myths (6m) ☐ Avoid expensive shoes (9m) ☐ Use of 911 (12m) ☐

Intercurrent illness

PEDIATRIC HEALTH MAINTENANCE

15 months through 3 years

Parent's concerns

Growth (comment on growth curve)

Diet

Milk ________ oz/24 hours

Eating problems ________

Advice: Entirely on table foods, off all bottles (18m) ☐

Normal decreased intake, iron intake (2y) ☐

Developmental status

Advice: Read to child (1½, 2) ☐ Listen to child (2) ☐ TV rules (3) ☐

Child rearing advice

Sleep problems ________

Behavior problems ________

Frequency of spanking ________

Advice: Don't punish for normal negativism, ignore temper tantrums (1½) ☐

Discuss toilet training and readiness (1½, 2, 3) ☐ Discuss positive "strokes" for good behavior (2) ☐

Emphasize consistency in discipline and use of time-out room (2, 3) ☐

Family status

Accident prevention advice

Scalds, aspiration foods (1½) ☐ Street/garage safety (2) ☐

Drowning in ditch and pools (3) ☐

Dental advice

Brushing frequency ________ Fluoride intake ________

Advice: Avoid snacks that cause cavities (1½) ☐ Benefits of fluoride toothpaste (2) ☐

Brushing techniques (3) ☐

Intercurrent illness

PEDIATRIC HEALTH MAINTENANCE

4 years through 5 years

To be completed by parent	Check correct answer	
School readiness:		
1. Does your child pay attention when being read to?	Yes	No
2. Can your child play quietly alone for over ½ hour?	Yes	No
3. Does your child mind adults and follow instructions?	Yes	No
4. Does your child speak clearly enough for others to understand?	Yes	No
5. Does your child object to being left with a sitter?	No	Yes
6. Can your child dress without help?	Yes	No
7. Does your child ever wet or soil him/herself during the day?	No	Yes

To be completed by physician or nurse

Parent's concerns

Growth (comment on growth curve)

Diet

School readiness

Problems detected by above questions ________

Development: PDQ (4, 5) Score ________ Weak category ________

DDST (if fails PDQ) Result ________

Articulation: DASE (4) Score ________ Percentile ________

Advice: Preschool if any problems (4) ☐

Accident prevention advice

Adult seat belts, petting dogs (4) ☐ Crossing street, trampoline (5) ☐

Dental advice

No daytime thumb-sucking (4) ☐ No nighttime thumb-sucking (5) ☐

Frequency of brushing ________ Type of toothpaste ________ Fluoride intake ________

Intercurrent illness

PEDIATRIC HEALTH MAINTENANCE

6 years through 11 years

Parent's concerns

Diet

School
Name of school ______ Grade ______
Academic performance ______
Attendance ______
Behavior ______
Advice: Child's responsibility for schoolwork (6) ☐ Adult at home before and after school (6, 10) ☐

Behavior
Behavior problems ______
Chores ______
Friends ______
Advice: TV less than 2 h/d (6) ☐ Understanding of death (6) ☐
One sport or club (8, 10) ☐ Smoking (10) ☐

Family status

Sex education
Discuss puberty and menarche before junior high school (10) ☐
Menstrual status (10 ♀) ______

Accident prevention advice
Bicycle safety (6) ☐ Swimming lessons (8) ☐
Fires, matches (10) ☐

Dental advice
Frequency of brushing ______ Type of toothpaste ______ Fluoride intake ______
Dental referral (6) ☐

Intercurrent illness

PEDIATRIC HEALTH MAINTENANCE

12 years through 18 years

Parent's concerns

Adolescent's concerns

Growth (comment on growth curve)

Diet

School
Name of school ______ Grade ______
Academic performance ______
Attendance ______
Behavior ______
Career plans ______

Behavior
Free time/friends ______
Chores/job ______
Person to confide in ______
Predominant mood ______
Advice: Discuss values of babysitting (12) ☐ Discuss drugs and alcohol (12, 16) ☐
Discuss smoking (14) ☐

Family status
Advice: Discuss independence and parent's trust (16) ☐

Sex education
Dating, masturbation (14) ☐ Marriage (18) ☐
Sexual activity, preventing pregnancy, venereal disease (14, 16, 18) ______

Accident prevention advice
Firearms (12) ☐ Cycling safety (14) ☐ Driving safety, water safety (16) ☐
Motorcycles, seat belts (18) ☐

Dental advice
Frequency of brushing ______ Type of toothpaste ______

Medical advice
Acne ☐ Personal hygiene (14) ☐ Teach self-examination of breasts (16♀) ☐

Intercurrent illness

University of Colorado Medical Center

PEDIATRIC OPD

Health Maintenance Flow Sheet

Name ______________________

Hosp. No. ______________________

Date of Birth ______________________

Directions: Record date only for all immunizations.
Record value for head circumference, height, weight, BP, and Hct.
Record N (normal) or ABN (abnormal) for all other items.

	NB	2 wk	2 mo	4 mo	6 mo	9 mo	12 mo	15 mo	18 mo	2 yr	3 yr	4 yr	5 yr	6 yr	8 yr	10 yr	12 yr	14 yr	16 yr	18 yr
Today's date																				
Head circ.																				
Height (cm)																				
Weight (kg)																				
BP																				
Dental caries screen																				
DTP (Td after 6 years)																				
OPV																				
Measles, mumps, rubella																				
Haemophilus influenzae type b vaccine																				
TB test																				
PDQ (DDST if fail PDQ)																				
Speech (DASE)																				
Hearing[1]																				
Vision[2]																				
Biochemical screen[3]																				
Hct																				
Sickle cell test (for black patients)[4]																				
VDRL/GC[5]																				
Pap smear[6]																				

[1] High-risk inquiry (NB)
Listens to soft sounds (2m)
Turns to sound (6m)
Audiometrics (4y and thereafter)

[2] Red reflex (NB or 2 w)
Regards smiling face (2m)
Follows past midline (4m)
Corneal light reflection test (6m)
Visual acuity (3y and thereafter)
Color vision (6y)

[3] PKU, T_4, galactosemia (newborn nursery)
PKU retest (2w) if first test done before 48 hours

[4] If not performed in newborn, perform at 9 months of age

[5] Sexually active patients

[6] If pelvic exam is done for other reason

University of Colorado Medical Center

DIABETES MELLITUS FLOW SHEET

Name ____________________
Hosp. No. ____________________
Date ____________________

Dates:	Baseline Data	22 Apr 85	6 May 85	10 June 85	5 Aug 85	7 Oct 85	13 Oct 85	4 Nov 85
DISEASE STATUS								
Hypoglycemia –frequency	3-4x/m.	"	2	0	3	1	1	1
–time of day	Usually 11 AM	"	11 AM 4 PM	—	Various	10 AM	11 AM	4 PM
–severity	Rarely a Seizure	"	Mild	—	Mild	Mild	Seizure	Mild
–pptg. event	?	"	Mother forbade snack	—	Exercise at camp	Gym	Took 10u. extra insulin	Sports
Ketosis –frequency	0-1x/m.	"	0	0	0	1	0	0
–duration	Days	"	—	—	—	8 hrs	—	—
–pptg. event	?	"	—	—	—	UTI	—	—
Weight (lbs)/BP	—	85 88/62	85 —	86 —	88 96/70	87 —	88 —	88 —
Fundi/liver (cm)	—	OK / 1	—	—	OK / 1	—	—	—
Urine gluc./acet.	—	0/0	1+/0	3+/0	1+/0	4+/large	1+/0	2+/0
Blood gluc./acet.	highly variable	—	—	—	—	410/small	—	—
Hospitalizations	5x in last 4yrs.	—	—	—	—	—	—	—
Emotional status	Depressed	"	"	Improved	Happy	OK	OK	OK
TREATMENT REGIMEN								
Insulin –type	Reg/NPH	"	"	"	"	"	"	"
–dosage	14/20	8/22	6/22	"	"	"	"	"
–SC dystrophy	buttocks hypertrophy	"	"	"	"	"	"	"
Rotates sites	all into buttocks	discontinue buttocks	Done	75% into Ⓑ thigh	OK	"	"	"
Diet type	ADA exchange	Unmeasured Diet	Mother resistant	OK	"	"	"	"
Snacks	Variable	3 snacks	Mother resistant	OK	"	Raisins before gym	OK	"
Carrying food/ Glucagon at home	No/Yes	Advice given/"	No/"	Yes/"	No/"	Yes/"	"/"	"/"
Rx compliance –gives shot	Mother gives 100%	Pt. to give shots	90% by pt.	10% by pt.	100% by pt. Camp helped	"	"	"
–checks urine	Yes	Same	"	"	"Forgot" records	Same	No	Only when symptomatic
Camp/ID card	No/No	Rec./given	—/Yes	Camp form/"	—/"	—/"	—/"	—/"
Education (time spent)	—	1 hour	1 hour	30 mins	15 mins	15 mins	20 mins	10 mins

Developmental Disorders 7

Bonnie W. Camp, MD, PhD

This chapter considers problems in development of cognitive and social competence. Competence is usually defined by comparing performance levels of an individual child with some norm derived from evaluating many children of the same age. Other standards of competence include comparison of the child's performance level with that of the adult norm and comparison of the child's present skills with skills needed to accomplish a given task or engage in a specific activity. Functional problems of mentally retarded children are discussed in this chapter; however, the main emphasis is on the larger group of children with learning and behavior problems that may or may not be associated with mental retardation.

Measurement of developmental competence is patterned on concepts of measuring intelligence. Although there is continued controversy over the extent to which heredity and environment determine intelligence, assessment of competence can be more usefully discussed independently of this issue. Assessment of competence hinges on the recognition that (1) children are able to perform increasingly more complex and difficult tasks as they get older; and (2) when tested at ages fairly close together, individual children tend to have a similar standing in relation to other children from one age to the next. By evaluating a child's performance on a variety of tasks requiring skills such as reasoning, abstract thinking, judgment, and planning and by determining how the child compares with other children of the same age, it is usually possible to predict school performance. Such assessments provide the basis for deriving an intelligence quotient and also may have implications for social behavior.

Measures of intelligence may be thought of as measures of general competence that attempt to determine what a child has learned in the process of exposure to an environment that provides unsystematic opportunities for learning that are grossly similar within a given culture. Anything that limits the breadth, variety, and depth of exposure or the ability of a child to profit from such exposure may place limits on the learning a given child will achieve in a given period. Anything that increases systematic exposure or increases breadth, variety, and depth of exposure potentially enhances learning.

Both biologic and psychosocial factors can increase or interfere with the growth-promoting effect of a child's general experience. Assessment of a child's general developmental or intellectual standing relative to other children sheds no light on the cause of the child's performance; consequently, it is important to determine whether an intelligence test gives a representative estimate of the child's usual functioning and whether other information might provide an explanation for low scores. Differences in experiential background often account for low scores of children from nondominant cultures given standard intelligence tests. Such explanations, however, do not necessarily alter the predictive value of scores from intelligence tests.

A variety of delays or deficiencies in the development of specific cognitive competence have also been identified and may or may not be associated with deficiencies in general competence. The most significant of these are associated with failure to acquire basic academic skills such as reading, writing, and arithmetic. Specific measures of competence are usually measures of achievement in areas where systematic instruction has been given (eg, music lessons, arithmetic lessons). Here again, both biologic and psychosocial factors (eg, "musical talent" or "math aptitude") may facilitate or interfere with development of competence in these specific areas. Measures of relative standing in specific areas of achievement correlate well with measures of intelligence. This correlation provides the basis for determining a child's expected level of achievement while the discrepancy between expected and actual levels of achievement is a key factor for differential diagnosis in children with developmental problems.

Traditionally, social and emotional aspects of development have not been conceptualized as a dimension of competence. However, it is increasingly recognized that social competence is an important concept for assessing some aspects of social and emotional development. This is particularly true for aspects of behavior and social interaction such as empathy, distractibility, activity level, and aggression, which show strong, regular progression with age and which are associated with what has traditionally been termed cognitive development.

GENERAL PRINCIPLES IN EVALUATING COGNITIVE & SOCIAL COMPETENCE

Developmental evaluation should include (1) data that demonstrate a child's level of cognitive and social competence in both general and specific areas; (2) data that will assist in making an etiologic diagnosis; and (3) data relevant to management planning. An interdisciplinary team is often employed to develop the data base and a plan for management; this is the most thorough and effective approach. In addition to the pediatrician, the team usually includes a psychologist, social worker, educational specialist, and speech and language specialist. Assistance is also often needed from health care specialists in nursing, physical therapy, occupational therapy, ophthalmology, audiology, nutrition, and dentistry. Where an organized, functioning team is not available, the primary care physician can achieve similar results by requesting consultations from various professionals and obtaining information from other sources such as school personnel. It is also possible for the primary care physician to develop the minimal data base needed for initial assessment with only limited reliance on outside sources. In the following discussion, suggestions are given for ways in which the primary care physician can do this through use of questionnaires and screening tests when assistance from other professionals is limited or unavailable.

History

A. Medical History: The medical history should focus on aspects of pregnancy, labor, and delivery that are likely to produce damage to the child's central nervous system (eg, use of drugs or x-rays during pregnancy; neonatal infections, asphyxia, and elevated bilirubin levels). Later evidence of central nervous system insults or injury, failure to thrive, chronic illnesses, hospitalizations, or abuse may also contribute significantly to a child's performance at school age. Neonatal records are often an important source of information, since they may reveal information forgotten by or unknown to parents. Recent studies have also focused on ways of combining psychosocial information about families from birth certificates to assess the risk for later problems in development.

B. Developmental History: This should include information about the age at which various milestones were passed, especially those pertaining to speech and language. Inability to use meaningful words other than "dada," "mama," "bye-bye," and "hello" by 18 months and inability to speak in short phrases by 24 months have been reported in association with specific learning disability as well as general slow learning and mental retardation. Development of motor skills is also important, particularly in assessing mental retardation, but deviance or delay in motor development may also be present in other conditions such as cerebral palsy and neuromuscular disorders. Information about sleep patterns, problems of temperament such as excessive crying or hyperactivity, and general problems may also be helpful.

C. Family History: Specific information regarding central nervous system disorders, mental retardation, epilepsy, or evidence of school problems or specific learning disabilities in other family members should be included. Details of the mother's pregnancy history, including stillbirths, deaths, and other problems, may also be helpful.

D. Educational and Learning History: In preschool children, considerable information can be obtained from a description of something the child has learned in an informal setting. If the child has been placed in a formal preschool setting, information should be obtained regarding the type of preschool and the child's relationships with other children and with teachers. Teachers can often give an excellent description of the child's performance and behavior in the classroom environment, and such assessments, even in the preschool period, are often as good as tests in predicting later problems.

Once a child has reached school age, the educational history should include details of grade placement, special educational evaluations and placement, repetition of grades, and other details of academic performance and participation in special programs. In the absence of a psychologist or educational specialist to provide this information, direct contact with school personnel is imperative for the primary care physician. Telephone conversations with the school nurse, teacher, social worker, or other professionals are very helpful in obtaining a clear picture of the child's performance and behavior in the school environment. Written reports from teachers using questionnaires that systematically address the most common types of learning problems can also be of great assistance.

E. Psychosocial History: Family problems and parental characteristics often interfere with development of both cognitive and social competence and foster deviant behavior in the child. Children of hostile, rejecting, highly authoritarian parents tend to be the most severely affected; these children often show advanced competence at 1 year of age but a progressive decline in competence beginning around 4 years of age. Children of nurturing parents with highly authoritarian parenting practices often do better; however, children of nurturing parents who are firm and verbal in providing guidance and setting standards without being rigidly authoritarian show advanced competence that increases with age. Parents who provide little nurturance or sense of belonging, who are too lax or too harsh in punishment, or who fail to supervise their children tend to have children who show early evidence of aggressive behavior problems that persist into adolescence and adulthood.

Because developmental and behavior problems in the child are often provoked by and associated with problems within the family or seem to be associated with a lack of family support for developing new skills, a good psychosocial history is an essential part of any developmental evaluation. Ideally, this should include assessment of the family's ability to promote cognitive and social development, which includes, as a minimum, information regarding the parents' linguistic and cultural background, quality of verbal interaction, disciplinary practices (use of positive reinforcement to shape behavior, reliance on physical punishment or limited use of reasoning or verbal explanations in discipline), ability to set standards, neglect or reliance on parenting practices that interfere with or inhibit development, family instability, marital discord, a hostile attitude toward the child, limitations in cognitive and social competence, depression, signs of maladjustment (eg, alcoholism, chronic unemployment, criminal or psychiatric problems), and general stress in the parents and chaos in the family that may contribute to and intensify developmental problems in the child.

In examining only the child, it is often difficult to distinguish behavior disorders associated with family problems from developmental disorders due to immaturity or alteration in development of the neurologic system. This difficulty has resulted in diagnosis by exclusion—ie, psychosocial assessment is used to determine whether there are social or emotional factors in the child's environment that can account for the observed learning or behavior problems. This is a practical approach in middle-class families, since it is often possible to ascertain that the family is reasonably stable and able to provide adequate support and stimulation to the child. Diagnosis by exclusion is, however, a very unsatisfactory approach for dealing with children from lower socioeconomic families, ie, the majority of children with behavior problems. The need for better assessment of these children is particularly acute, since they often have delays in both social and cognitive development and combinations of developmental delay and behavior problems. Ninety percent of the children who later show mental or emotional disorders are normal at birth and appear to be casualties of inadequate or pathologic environments.

At present, the most commonly used approach to family assessment is a global, clinical social history. Some of this information is usually included in the history obtained by the primary care physician. In most instances, however, a social worker will provide the most thorough and complete analysis. In preschool children, it is often helpful to supplement the usual clinical social history with the HOME (*h*ome *o*bservation for *m*easurcment of the *e*nvironment) interview assessment of Bradley and Caldwell (see references, below). This is the most thoroughly studied approach to the systematic evaluation of the growth-promoting aspects of the child's environment. This interview, which requires a home visit, is used to identify economically disadvantaged families unlikely to support development in their children. It may be performed by any trained person but is usually done by a social worker or nurse. A shorter, questionnaire version of the HOME interview, the Home Screening Questionnaire (HSQ), provides most of the information obtained from the longer interview version and can be administered and scored by the pediatrician during a clinic or office visit. Although it has not yet been studied widely enough to determine its clinical usefulness, the HSQ appears to be a promising tool for use by the primary care physician. Neither scale is expected to be useful in evaluating children from middle or upper socioeconomic families.

Badger E, Burne D, Vietze P: Maternal risk factors as predictors of development outcome in early childhood. *Infant Ment Health J* 1981;**2:**33.

Bradley RH, Caldwell BM: Pediatric usefulness of home assessment. In: *Advances in Behavioral Pediatrics.* Vol 2. Camp BW (editor). JAI Press, 1981.

Coons CE et al: *The Home Screening Questionnaire Reference Manual.* LADOCA Publishing Foundation, 1981.

Physical & Neurologic Examination

It is essential that a thorough physical and neurologic examination be performed. A number of children will demonstrate neurologic "soft signs," eg, clumsiness, right-left confusion, disordered temporal orientation, overflow phenomena, choreiform movements, and finger agnosia. Although "soft signs" are commonly associated with school learning and behavior problems, the significance of these signs is controversial because they are also found in children who have no other problems and because most appear to represent delay in maturation rather than dysfunction. PANESS (*p*hysical *a*nd *n*eurologic *e*xamination for *s*oft *s*igns), a standardized neurologic examination, has been studied and shows promising results.

In addition, recent studies linking minor physical anomalies with behavior disorders in childhood have prompted physicians to examine for the presence of dysmorphic features such as abnormal palmar creases, syndactyly, unruly hair, malformed ears, skin tags, and facial abnormalities. While these features are commonly seen in children with mental retardation, the implications of their presence in nonretarded children are not fully understood.

Holden EW, Tarnowski KJ, Prinz RJ: Reliability of neurobiological soft signs in children: Reevaluation of the PANESS. *J Abnorm Child Psychol* 1982;**10:**163.

Sensory Function

All children in whom developmental delay or mental retardation is suspected should be examined for visual and auditory problems. In infants and young children, sensory deficits may be mistaken for retardation. Retarded children often have sensory deficits in addition to their retardation, and this increases the complexity of their problem. In most nonretarded, school-aged children, vision and hearing can be satisfactorily evaluated by the usual screening methods and referral made to a specialist for further evaluation of children with abnormal screening results.

A variety of vision problems have been proposed as causes of reading problems, without substantial research support. Learning to read can be accomplished quite satisfactorily with limited peripheral visual acuity. Although it is important that visual defects be corrected to improve the child's overall functioning, it is generally agreed that learning problems are seldom linked to refractive errors.

Hearing loss, on the other hand, has a significant impact on language development and may be associated with severe learning and behavior problems. Intermittent hearing loss, such as that due to otitis media, has been implicated in learning disabilities. In the past, deaf children have often been mistakenly labeled retarded. In children, losses in the high-frequency range may be associated with problems in discriminating speech sounds necessary for school learning. Others may have problems differentiating speech sounds despite normal hearing.

Emotional & Social Behavior

Although some information can be obtained directly from the child through interviews, play, and projective testing, typically one must rely on interviews with parents and reports from school personnel to obtain a picture of the child's social competence. Much of this information is obtained by social workers, psychologists, or psychiatrists. In evaluating reports of problem behavior at home and at school, it is helpful to assess the degree of deviance by comparing an individual child's behavior with children in general. Large studies of normal children indicate that most children show a few signs of deviant behavior. The truly deviant child, however, usually demonstrates this in a variety of ways. It is especially important to seek information about positive attributes, because these appear to be more powerful indicators of later mental health than negative attributes are of later maladjustment. Three of the most important positive attributes are school attendance (irrespective of performance), positive peer relations, and nondelinquency.

General adaptation and development of self-help are often included in developmental assessments of preschool children. Beginning around age 4 years (when abstract reasoning becomes the dominant factor in measures of cognitive development), it becomes increasingly important to include some assessment of general adaptation in the differential diagnosis of mental retardation. Children from minority cultures who perform poorly on IQ tests often appear less retarded when general adaptation is evaluated.

Rating scales of behavior, such as Conners' Abbreviated Teacher's School Report (Table 7–1) for identifying children with attention deficit disorder, are important tools for assessing school behavior. The Conners scale has been used in many parts of the world, is readily acceptable to teachers, and can be used by primary care physicians to assess the need for and response to stimulant medication.

A scale for obtaining teacher ratings of general behavior is also useful for identifying children with deviant behavior other than distractibility and hyperactivity and for assessing the degree and amount of prosocial (positive) behavior. Several such scales are available for assessing children as early as the pre-

Table 7–1. Abbreviated teacher's school report (after Conners).*

Child's Name ______________ Birthdate ______________
Study Number ______________

Teacher's Observations

Information Obtained ______________ By ______________
Day Mo Yr

Beside each item below, indicate the degree of the problem by a check mark meaning . . .

Observation	0 = Not At All	1 = Just a Little	2 = Pretty Much	3 = Very Much
Restless or overactive				
Excitable, impulsive				
Disturbs other children				
Fails to finish things started, short attention span				
Constantly fidgeting				
Inattentive, easily distracted				
Demands must be met immediately—easily frustrated				
Cries often and easily				
Mood changes quickly and drastically				
Temper outbursts, explosive and unpredictable behavior				

Instructions for the abbreviated Conners scale: Score each item 0–3 as indicated at the top of each column. Add up all scores. Final score should be below 15 (normal = mean 4.3, SD 5.2). Use reverse side for other observations of teacher.

* Source: Conners CK: Rating scales for use in drug studies with children. In: *Psychopharmacology Bulletin.* Special issue—Pharmacotherapy of children. DHEW Publication No. (HSM) 73-9002. US Government Printing Office, 1973.

school period, and some include rating scales to be completed by parents as well as the teacher.

Family & Social Resources

The type, extent, and cost of educational and counseling services available to the child and family, the family's ability to support and carry through with treatment plans, and other community resources should be assessed early in the evaluation. These factors often limit or modify the treatment plan developed for a child. Sixty percent of families presenting children for evaluation of learning problems have clear-cut social and emotional problems that need to be assessed and addressed as an integral part of treatment planning for the child. Social services are usually the principal sources of information in this area, and much of this information will be derived from the psychosocial history. In addition, however, the primary care physician should become familiar with resources in the community.

Intelligence

Measures of intelligence attempt to describe a child's general cognitive competence in relation to other children of the same age. The tests provide an increasingly difficult set of problems, and questions tend to tap general knowledge, reasoning, judgment, and organization of analytic skills that are expected to develop in the course of experiences encountered by most children in the process of growing up. Where children have grossly different experiences from those in the standard population, their scores may be expected to vary upward or downward. Originally, the IQ score obtained from such tests represented the percentage of expectancy a child had reached at a given age. This was derived by the formula (mental age ÷ chronologic age) × 100. Scores on most modern tests can still be reported in terms of MA/CA, but the most important tests yield IQ scores that represent a child's relative distance from the average child in standard score units.

In the preschool period, the principal diagnostic tests in general use are the Bayley Scales of Infant Development (for children under 30 months of age), the Stanford-Binet Intelligence Scale, and the McCarthy Scales of Children's Abilities (for children 3 years of age and older). These are all individually administered tests, given by trained personnel. The screening tests used most commonly in the preschool period are the Revised Denver Developmental Screening Test (Frankenberg); the Revised Developmental Screening Inventory (Knobloch et al); and, among older preschool children, the Cooperative Preschool Inventory (Caldwell).

The Wechsler scales (Wechsler Adult Intelligence Scale [WAIS], Wechsler Intelligence Scale for Children, Revised [WISC-R], and Wechsler Preschool and Primary Scale of Intelligence [WPPSI] and the Stanford-Binet Intelligence Scale are the most widely used individual intelligence tests for school-age and older children. The Stanford-Binet test is a highly verbal test with nonverbal items intermingled; results are reported as a single IQ score. The Wechsler scales are subdivided into 6 verbal and 6 nonverbal tests so that a verbal IQ and performance IQ can both be obtained as well as an IQ based on the full test (full-scale IQ). It is commonly thought that intelligence tests can reveal the potential for higher functioning, especially when scatter (the pattern of high and low scores) is examined carefully, and the Wechsler scales lend themselves particularly well to this task.

Both the Stanford-Binet test and the Wechsler scales require extensive training for proper administration and are usually administered by trained psychologists. The Slosson Intelligence Test, however, is an abbreviated version of the Stanford-Binet test and is designed for use by nonprofessionals, including office assistants and primary care physicians. It is probably the most suitable screening test for estimating intelligence in children over 4½ years of age.

A number of briefer screening tests, such as the Peabody Picture Vocabulary Test and the Quick Test, are also suitable for use in office settings. These measure vocabulary skills alone, based on the fact that vocabulary has the best correlation with overall estimates of intelligence. A variety of other short screening tools are available, some of which rely on parent reporting or a combination of parent reporting and observation, but these often suffer from limited information regarding standardization data.

Achievement

Achievement usually refers to performance in specific school-related areas where a child has received instruction. In the preschool period, achievement is seldom distinguished from general development. By the time the child enters kindergarten, however, a variety of procedures are available for assessing readiness. In a child with a mental age of 6 years, 2 of the best predictors for readiness to enter the first grade are the ability to engage in sustained task-oriented behavior and the knowledge of letter names and sounds. A number of procedures are available to assess school readiness, and in recent years, testing programs have been specifically designed for early identification of children with learning disabilities. Although results of these programs appear to be about as accurate as teacher assessments of kindergarten performance, many feel that the programs represent an important advance. Most of the early identification testing programs are designed for use in schools or by psychologists. Several procedures are also available for use by primary care physicians in screening for school readiness at the time of well child visits in the 4½- to 5½-year age range. These include the developmental screening tests described previously and the preschool portions of the Wide Range Achievement Test (WRAT; see below).

For school-age children, scores on a variety of achievement tests are often available through routine classroom testing done at school, and results of such testing should be included in the educational history.

Where low scores are obtained on group testing of achievement, individual testing should be performed before accepting the results as representative of the child's ability. Many school systems with special education services can administer individual tests of achievement and give the test scores to the primary care physician; unfortunately, however, many children who are referred to a pediatrician for evaluation have no current achievement test scores in their school records. This is particularly true for children referred because of behavior problems. When an educational specialist or psychologist is unavailable to provide this information, the primary care physician may wish to make his or her own assessment through use of a screening test such as WRAT.

WRAT is a rapid screening test for assessing achievement in reading, spelling, and arithmetic. It is suitable for testing children from kindergarten through college, and norms (available from the National Health Survey, as well as the publisher) are based on results in children from a representative sample of ethnic and economic groups throughout the country. The reading test covers only the accuracy of word reading and tends to yield higher scores than more thorough and comprehensive procedures do. However, WRAT is a simple and easy test to administer, and scores are reported in grade equivalents, percentiles, and standard scores that are comparable to many IQ test scores. In addition, the copying portions of the spelling test can be used to attain a rapid assessment of visual-motor coordination (discussed below).

Perceptual-Motor Function

In the early school years, a number of children with delays in copying and drawing skills will also demonstrate problems in learning to read. These problems have been variously termed visual-perceptual and visual-motor problems, and their presence in children beyond 7–9 years of age has often been thought to indicate the existence of central nervous system dysfunction, although this is controversial. While there is a relationship between visual-perceptual problems and reading problems in the early school years, reading achievement becomes more and more related to intelligence as children get older, whether or not the perceptual problems persist. Furthermore, perceptual problems are common among children from families in lower socioeconomic groups and even among children whose only history is confinement to bed for more than 2 months during the preschool years.

Since performance on tests of copying skills are highly correlated with intelligence, they are most useful when there is a discrepancy between developmental level on visual-perceptual tests and general intelligence. Methods for assessing the degree of this discrepancy are not as well developed as for assessing the discrepancy between IQ and achievement. At a practical level, however, these problems may be severe enough to interfere with learning the skills of printing and writing. In this latter case, it is usually more helpful to analyze the child's writing, but several visual-perceptual tests are commonly used to examine copying skills per se.

Speech & Language

Speech and language delays are common in mentally retarded children but may also occur in children with average or above-average intelligence. A number of children who appear to have specific learning problems will, on closer evaluation, show evidence of delay in language development or an articulation problem (or both). These problems can limit academic achievement in areas that depend on verbal skills (eg, reading). Speech and language delays in preschool children and methods for evaluating them have been discussed previously (see Chapter 2).

Most children should reach the adult proficiency level in language by 7–8 years of age, at which time evaluation of language skills typically becomes merged with evaluation of verbal intelligence. Scores on tests such as the Wechsler scale, the Stanford-Binet test, or the Slosson test will reflect language skills as well as intelligence. Specialized tests for assessing components of receptive and expressive language and language-processing skills are also available.

Motivation

Clinical assessment of motivation has received little attention despite mounting evidence that motivation is a key factor in determining how a child will use whatever time and help are provided for learning new skills. Studies of achievement motivation have suggested that 2 main motivational types can be identified, ie, those who are challenged by moderately difficult tasks and respond to success and those who are primarily motivated to avoid failure and will only attempt very easy tasks, where failure is unlikely, or very difficult ones, where failure carries no stigma. One of the major shifts that occurs in the age range of 5–7 years is from motivational dependence on social and external rewards to internal motivation for mastery of skills. Some children make this shift poorly or not at all and will fail to learn in the usual academic climate, which emphasizes mastery and competition. Often these are the children who seem primarily motivated to avoid failure and who need liberal support from external sources (praise, concrete incentives) just for trying. While motivational immaturity is seldom the principal problem, it is often a major determinant of how well a child will respond or progress in an educational program.

Beery KE: *Revised Administration, Scoring, and Teaching Manual for the Developmental Test of Visual-Motor Integration.* Modern Curriculum Press, 1982.

Caldwell M: *Preschool Inventory (Revised).* Educational Testing Service, 1970.

Frankenburg WK: *Denver Developmental Screening Test Reference Manual (Revised).* LADOCA Foundation, 1975.

Jastak JF, Jastak S: *Wide Range Achievement Test.* Jastak Associates, 1978.

Knobloch H, Steven F, Malone AF: *Manual of Developmental Diagnosis*. Harper, 1980.
Slosson RL: *Slosson Intelligence Test for Children and Adults*. Slosson Educational Publications, 1981.

EVALUATING THE DISCREPANCY BETWEEN INTELLIGENCE & ACHIEVEMENT

The differential diagnosis of competency problems necessitates an evaluation of the significance of the discrepancy between expected achievement based on measures of general competence (intelligence) and actual achievement in specific areas of academic performance. The following material presents 2 methods of calculating the degree of discrepancy between IQ and achievement, based on grade equivalents and standard scores.

The United States Office of Education defines the discrepancy between achievement and IQ as significant when achievement is below 50% of expected grade level. The lowest level of achievement commensurate with age and intelligence is calculated by the following formula:

Age [(IQ/300) + 0.17] − 2.5 = Lowest grade equivalent score which is commensurate with age and intelligence

For an 8-year-old child with an IQ of 100, this formula indicates that a grade level of 1.5 is the lowest score that would be commensurate with age and intelligence. If this child's achievement test scores are below grade level 1.5, then there is a significant discrepancy. If they are at grade level 1.5 or higher, the discrepancy is not significant.

The following formula utilizes the direct correlation between intelligence test and achievement test scores to calculate the smallest difference between IQ and achievement test score needed to represent a significant discrepancy (D):

$D = 1.96\ SD\sqrt{1-r^2}$ where SD = Standard deviation of scores on achievement test
r = correlation between IQ and achievement test scores

This formula can be used to compare an IQ obtained from a test such as the Slosson test with a standard score obtained from the WRAT. The Slosson test manual provides the information that the correlation coefficient with the WRAT is 0.72, and the WRAT manual provides the information that the standard deviation of scores on the WRAT is 15. According to this calculation, a difference of 20 points between IQ and achievement test score is needed before a difference between these 2 tests is significant at the $p = .05$ level of confidence or better.

Both of these approaches call attention to the fact that some difference between expected and actual achievement represents normal variation, while a significant discrepancy is defined in terms of an unusual degree of difference. Individual school districts are free to adopt their own criteria for this discrepancy which must be met to be eligible for special services.

TEMPERAMENTAL TRAITS & REACTIONS TO DEVELOPMENTAL CRISES

During the ages of 5–7 years and 10–13 years, major developmental changes occur in most children. In the 5- to 7-year period, children enter school, begin to develop operational thought, and shift from associative thinking to use of verbal mediation activity in learning and thinking. The 10- to 13-year period heralds the onset of puberty, entrance into junior high school, and development of formal operational thought. Inflections in the growth curve for intelligence occur during both periods, and there is a dramatic increase in a cluster of behavior problems that appear to be phase-specific reactions to the developmental changes occurring during these periods. These problems include restless sleep, disturbing dreams, physical timidity, irritability, overdependence, and jealousy. Emotional turbulence during one of these periods may or may not be associated with turbulence during the other period, and its occurrence in either does not seem to be indicative of serious long-term problems.

Often there is overlap between these phase-specific reactions and temperamental traits, which include characteristics such as shyness, oversensitiveness, somberness, and reserve. Both phase-specific reactions and temperamental traits may be a source of conflict between parents and children, but they do not in themselves indicate the presence of serious emotional disturbance. They usually resolve with support, and the child does not need treatment.

Kohlberg L, LaCrosse J, Ricks D: The predictability of adult mental health from childhood behavior. In: *Manual of Child Psychopathology*. Wolman BB (editor). McGraw-Hill, 1972.

DISORDERS IN DEVELOPMENT OF COGNITIVE COMPETENCE

SPECIFIC LEARNING DISORDERS

Essentials of Diagnosis

- Significant discrepancy between estimated intelligence (usually verbal) and achievement in one or more areas.

- Achievement commensurate with intelligence in one or more academic areas.
- No evidence of sensory deficits.
- Behavior problems may or may not be present (and often are not present).

General Considerations

Specific problems may be experienced in any area of academic achievement, but the most common problems involve reading or spelling (dyslexia). Frequent but less common problems are specific to arithmetic (dyscalculia) or writing (dysgraphia). Intelligence is usually average or above average, but the key element in making the diagnosis is demonstrating a discrepancy between actual achievement and expected achievement in a specific area.

Descriptive Classification

A. Reading and Spelling Disorders (Developmental Dyslexia): Dyslexia is the most common type of specific learning disorder. It occurs more frequently in boys than in girls (3:1), and in 34% of cases there is a strong history, especially among the men in the family. Speech and language problems and problems in sequencing are the most common developmental problems associated with specific reading disorder. A variety of developmental problems such as clumsiness and incoordination, directional confusion, right-left confusion, disordered temporal orientation, and difficulties in naming colors and in recognizing the meaning of pictures have been reported in children with specific reading problems. These are of lesser importance than the speech and language problems and may be more related to intelligence than to reading disorder per se. A history of delays in speech and language development is present in at least one-third of cases. This involves delays such as failure to use meaningful words other than "mama," "dada," "hello," and "bye-bye" until after 18 months of age and failure to use 3-word phrases before 24 months of age. Although evidence of associated neurologic deficit or differential use of the right versus the left hemisphere can be demonstrated in some children, such results of neurologic investigations have generally contributed little to treatment or prognosis.

Traditionally, the definition of specific reading disorder (dyslexia) included failure to learn to read despite adequate sensory apparatus, conventional instruction, average intelligence, and sociocultural opportunity. Such diagnosis by exclusion was an attempt to distinguish between "unexpected" reading failure and reading failure that could be explained by a more general or pervasive factor, such as mental subnormality, cultural or educational deprivation, sensory defects, or emotional disturbance. With this approach, most children with reading problems tend to be excluded from the diagnosis of specific reading disorder—ie, their reading problems are attributed to the fact that they are slightly below average in intelligence, come from economically disadvantaged homes, or have emotional and behavior problems. Yet many in this large group show reading achievement below expectancy for their mental age; and in neurologic status, cognitive functioning, and other areas of achievement they are indistinguishable from the group defined in the traditional sense as having specific reading disorder. In addition, the presence of a significant discrepancy between actual and expected achievement is the only characteristic that is common to members of highly specific etiologic groups such as those with genetic dyslexia diagnosed on the basis of linkage studies.

Consequently, current thinking endorses the concept that subtypes of reading disability should first be described in terms of clear-cut characteristics irrespective of etiologic considerations. There have been 2 major approaches to this subtyping. One approach attempts to distinguish among different problems on the basis of analysis of reading and spelling errors; this has led to subtyping into 2 groups based on whether performance indicates heavier reliance on auditory-sequential-phonologic skills (auditory reader) or on visual-spatial-imagery (visual reader). The other approach uses associated disabilities such as those in language, perceptual-motor skills, and memory to distinguish the following probable subtypes: (1) a language disorder group with defects in understanding and expression of oral language; (2) a dyscoordination group with defects in speech articulation, copying skills, and understanding of oral language; (3) a visual-spatial-perceptual disorder group with visual, perceptual, and visual-constructive problems but intact oral language; and (4) a group with dysphonemic sequencing disorder.

B. Mathematics Disorders (Developmental Dyscalculia): Mathematics disorders have been studied primarily in relation to the developmental Gerstmann syndrome (dyscalculia, right-left disorientation, and finger agnosia) and often have been considered to be part of a reading disorder. However, limited studies of school children who demonstrate a significant discrepancy between actual and expected achievement in arithmetic suggest that a specific syndrome of mathematical disability does exist and affects approximately 6% of the population. Developmental disorder is distinguished from acquired disorder by the absence of clearly defined brain damage and neurologic findings in the former.

Several forms have been described and are characterized by difficulty in verbalizing, writing, reading, manipulating, or understanding mathematical operations. In individuals whose difficulties are confined to performance on numerical tests, signs of neurologic abnormalities tend to be few. In those who are unable to read or write numbers, the disorder may be associated with general disorders in reading and writing as well as mathematics so that a learning disorder specific to mathematics may be difficult to demonstrate.

C. Writing Disorders (Developmental Dysgraphia): Children with reading problems often have illegible handwriting as well as spelling problems. In younger children, problems due to immature perceptual-motor development (eg, mirror writing, reversal of letters, and poor construction of letters) are common. Some children will have problems confined to illegible handwriting, inaccurate copying, or inability to transmit sequences of verbal information to paper. In some of these instances, illegibility is associated with mild cerebral palsy or general problems in fine motor coordination. Whether encountered alone or in combination with reading or math disability, specific training is often required to correct the penmanship problems.

A common syndrome seen in students during late elementary and junior high school involves not only elements of poor handwriting (slow, illegible, poor spatial organization) but also deficits in memory, expressive language, organization of ideas, and fluency. This has been termed "developmental output failure"; it is usually manifested by overall reduced productivity, with refusals to complete work, failure to submit assignments, and "forgetting" to do homework.

Left-handed children deserve special attention because they have frequently had poor instruction. In most instances, their problems in penmanship will improve with appropriate instruction. Despite common belief to the contrary, there is little evidence associating left-handedness with any kind of deficiency.

Etiologic Classification

Both psychobiologic and sociopsychologic factors appear to play a major causative role in specific learning disabilities. The group of children who fail to learn despite conventional instruction, adequate familial-cultural opportunity, and adequate intelligence have generally been thought to represent an idiopathic or genetically based syndrome. This group has been distinguished from children with emotionally, educationally, or culturally based limitations on the one hand and those with disorders secondary to sensory defects, brain damage, or mental retardation on the other.

In the idiopathic group, the term minimal brain dysfunction (MBD) has often been applied when neurologic "soft signs," poor motor coordination, and distractibility are present along with learning problems in children of average or above-average intelligence. The term has also been applied indiscriminately to children who show any one of these features alone, but the clinical picture of children with the full picture described above provides the most convincing evidence for attributing the problem to some type of neurologic handicap. However, since extensive research has failed to provide substantial evidence of dysfunction and since many of the characteristics are common in preschool children and tend to be present only in younger learning-disabled children, many have abandoned the concept of minimal brain damage altogether in favor of the view that the neurologic problem is one of immaturity.

Clinical Findings

A family history often reveals affected family members, especially among the males. Findings on physical examination are usually normal, and those on neurologic examination are normal except for the presence of "soft signs." Behavior problems may or may not be present. Intelligence test results often indicate average or above-average intelligence on nonverbal tests and may or may not show some decrease in verbal IQ. In contrast, achievement in the affected area of learning is significantly below nonverbal intelligence and sometimes below verbal intelligence. Achievement in nonaffected areas tends to progress normally. Vision and hearing are usually normal, although deficits in processing auditory sequential information are often noted on extensive testing.

No special tests are useful in evaluation of this problem. Electroencephalography, CT scanning, and a variety of other procedures have been used in the past with little or no success.

Differential Diagnosis

The term "specific learning disability" is primarily a descriptive one that distinguishes between specific learning disorder, general learning disorder (slow learner), or mental retardation. Etiologic diagnosis is more difficult. The most important distinction is whether there is a strong family history, inadequate educational background, or sociocultural disadvantage.

Treatment

The principal treatment for specific learning disorders is individualized instruction. Most of the children are best viewed as "hard to teach," and ultimate outcome will usually depend upon the child's access to individual instruction with an experienced and knowledgeable teacher and motivation to use the time and help provided. There have been many claims that instruction should be tailored to the subtype of reading disorder, but research has generally failed to support this claim. In part, this may result from the fact that discussions of reading instruction often deal only with questions of content. In this regard, there are basically 4 ways of altering the content of reading materials: (1) presentation of the whole word approach (look-say); (2) use of phonics (intrinsic or extrinsic); (3) use of a syllabary (or rebus); and (4) orthographic changes, eg, use of a modified alphabet such as the Initial Teaching Alphabet or use of words in color.

It is evident from considering the various structures of the reading programs and strategies used in teaching that the number of possible approaches to reading instruction is quite large. With the variety of approaches available, selection of the best approach for a particular child may require a series of learning trials. Most children will begin to demonstrate learning after 4–6 lessons. General principles for promoting progress, however, include introduction of some phonics or word attack skills at some level of teaching;

mastery of early, less difficult material before proceeding to more difficult material; and continuation of instruction over a long enough period for results to be long-lasting. Approximately 40 lessons are required before most children will register a substantial and enduring gain in reading skills. More rapid increases are sometimes reported, but these can often be attributed to spuriously depressed initial scores.

A minority of children will fail to learn despite appropriate individual instruction. Special programs are needed to help these children profit from school attendance.

Several approaches to drug therapy for children with reading disability have been proposed, but none have yet received adequate study to warrant their recommendation. Furthermore, drug therapy prescribed for attention deficit disorder, if successful, may be expected to alter impulsive and distractible behavior but typically does not "cure" the learning problems if these are present. At best, the climate for learning is improved, but educational progress will still depend primarily on the quality and amount of instruction provided to the child.

Prognosis

With or without individual instruction, only a minority of children remain nonreaders into adulthood. There are, however, many adolescents and adults who read poorly. Ultimate level of skill usually depends on the child's intelligence, the type and amount of individual instruction provided, the severity of retardation, the age at which remediation is begun, motivation, and several other factors including the child's general emotional state. In some adults, poor spelling may be the only stigma of a childhood reading problem, while other adults may continue to show evidence of problems in reading and general language skills as well. Even with individual instruction, progress is often slow, sometimes slower than progress being made by children described as slow learners. In children with specific learning disorder, however, progress in nonaffected areas of achievement tends to proceed at a normal pace.

Benton AL, Pearl D (editors): *Dyslexia: An Appraisal of Current Knowledge*. Oxford Univ Press, 1978.

Kosc L: Developmental dyscalculia. *J Learning Disabilities* 1974;**7**:164.

Schain RJ: *Neurology of Childhood Learning Disorders*. Williams & Wilkins, 1972.

SLOW LEARNER

Essentials of Diagnosis

- Achievement below average.
- Not mentally retarded but IQ often below average.
- No significant discrepancy between IQ and achievement.
- Usually poor in all subjects.
- School progress may be at a slower rate than average, but progress is continuous.

General Considerations

The average IQ of children in this group tends to be in the 80s. Approximately 11% have definite evidence of neurologic dysfunction, 25% show questionable neurologic findings, and 60% have difficulty in copying forms. Clumsiness, motor impersistence, and right-left confusion are twice as common in this group as in children with specific learning disorders. Forty percent tend to have at least one sign of language delay (eg, first phrases after 24 months). The frequency of neurodevelopmental problems increases in children with lower IQs.

Clinical Findings

The most important characteristic is the lack of a significant discrepancy between intelligence and achievement. These children are often low average to borderline in intelligence, and achievement is slow but commensurate with mental age. Usually the child is slow in all areas of achievement, but achievement in one area may be slower than in others. The lower the child's intelligence, the more one is likely to find evidence of neurodevelopmental problems and associated behavior problems. The history often reveals evidence of developmental delays, especially in the language area. A family history of school problems may or may not be present. In the absence of a positive family history, problems during the pregnancy, advanced maternal age, or difficulties in the newborn period are often cited as possible causes of early brain damage that might explain the appearance of such a child in a well-educated family. In many instances, however, the mother's educational and cognitive level will be consistent with that of the child whether signs of neurodevelopmental delay are present or not.

Treatment

Educational programming is the principal approach to this problem. Often, however, a major task is to help the family recognize and accept the fact that a child is a slow learner. This may require counseling or short-term psychotherapy to deal with the family's denial and their wish to find some explanation for the slowness that would relieve their feelings of guilt. Often the school has developed an appropriate educational plan for the child, and treatment needs to be directed toward helping the family accept the school's plan.

Prognosis

Given an appropriate educational opportunity to progress at their own rate, slow learners tend to make steady progress commensurate with their mental age. In many instances, long-term follow-up may show that these children actually make better progress in their areas of deficiency than do children with specific learning disorders.

NONSPECIFIC & EMOTIONALLY BASED LEARNING DISORDERS

Essentials of Diagnosis

- Usually, average or above-average intelligence.
- Significant discrepancy between intelligence and achievement, often in more than one academic area.
- Often associated with emotional or behavior problems.
- Frequent among children from culturally disadvantaged homes and large families.

General Considerations

Included in this group are the large numbers of children with learning disorders in association with psychiatric disorders and familial-cultural problems of motivation. A significant discrepancy between intelligence and achievement may exist in one or more areas, or the child may be generally slow. Family problems are usually apparent, and children frequently come from culturally disadvantaged homes and large families. These children have many of the same educational needs as children with more specific problems—and often more—but they have, unfortunately, been excluded from federal funding for education of the learning disabled.

Differential Diagnosis

Differentiation from specific learning disabilities is made primarily on the basis of motivational and emotional problems and a lack of specificity of learning problems in children with average or above-average intelligence. Slow learners or mentally retarded children with emotional problems may be indistinguishable. The most difficult differential diagnosis is between specific reading disabilities in an emotionally disturbed child and an emotionally based learning disability concentrated in the language area.

Treatment

Despite the problem in differential diagnosis, treatment for emotional and learning problems is indicated in all groups demonstrating both types of disturbance. Some schools provide special classrooms for children with emotional disturbances and behavior disorders. Often the severity of the emotional or behavior problem will be the final criterion for planning the child's educational program.

MENTAL RETARDATION

Essentials of Diagnosis

- Significantly limited intelligence (≥ 2 SD below average [IQ below 70]).
- Significantly below age level in adaptation.
- Sensory defects may be present but not responsible for delay.
- Begins in the developmental period.

General Considerations

Mental retardation is a descriptive term defined as significantly subaverage intellectual functioning existing concurrently with deficits of adaptive behavior and manifested during the developmental period. Significantly subaverage intelligence is defined as 2 SD or more below average (IQ below 70 on the Wechsler scales or below 69 on the Stanford-Binet test) and by definition affects approximately 2–3% of the general population. An additional 6% are considered borderline in intelligence (IQ of 70–79). Adaptive deficiency is less easily evaluated.

About 10% of the retarded population are identified during infancy and early childhood. The majority fall in the moderate to profound retardation group (IQ below 50), and most of them have clear-cut evidence of brain damage, genetic disorder, or other pathologic conditions. Moderate to profound retardation is distributed equally among different socioeconomic groups but is more common in males than in females.

The remaining 90% of the retarded population tend to be mildly retarded (IQ of 50–69), and most are not identified before entering school, partly because limited efforts are made at earlier identification. The great majority of those with mild handicaps are diagnosed as cultural-familial retardates. They have no symptoms of central nervous system injury, and they come from families characterized by low intelligence and low socioeconomic status. Many who are mildly handicapped and identified primarily during the school years eventually blend into society and become at least marginally adequate citizens. There is a preponderance of males at all levels of retardation, except for those with organic disorders that are diagnosed after age 5 years.

Etiologic Considerations

Mental retardation is a descriptive diagnosis with a wide variety of causes. Many of the causative factors that can be identified are essentially untreatable. The basic data base will be helpful in deciding how far to pursue an etiologic diagnosis.

A. Genetic:

1. Inborn errors of metabolism—Aminoacidopathies, cerebral lipidoses, mucopolysaccharidoses, disorders of carbohydrate metabolism.

2. Chromosome disorders—Autosomal disorders, sex chromosome disorders.

B. Intrauterine: Congenital infections, placental-fetal malfunction, complications of pregnancy (maternal malnutrition, preeclampsia-eclampsia, use of drugs or radiation, intrauterine growth retardation).

C. Perinatal: Prematurity, postmaturity, metabolic disorders (hypoglycemia, hyperbilirubinemia).

D. Postnatal: Endocrinopathies, metabolic disorders, trauma, infections, poisoning, abuse.

E. Cultural-Familial: Low family intelligence, low socioeconomic status, environmental deprivation.

Clinical Findings

A. History: In infants and preschool children with developmental delays, there may be evidence of a genetic syndrome or factors in the prenatal or perinatal period that can account for delay. Often, however, there will also be evidence of maternal deprivation or neglect, particularly among children who are only mildly or moderately delayed. The older the child at the time of diagnosis, the more likely that retardation will be explained by deficiencies in early experience or by familial-cultural factors. Even when there are other family members with similar problems, a genetic basis for the retardation cannot be established unequivocally. Children who are not diagnosed until after entering school will often have a history of normal development in the first 2 years, and siblings may show a similar decline in relative competency as they get older. Children who come from nondominant cultural backgrounds will often show adequate functioning on measures of adaptation despite poor performance on standard intelligence tests. If behavior problems, especially disruptive and antisocial behavior, are absent, children who show relatively better adaptability than intelligence tend to blend into society after leaving school.

B. Symptoms and Signs: In mental retardation, the developmental or intellectual performance is at least 2 SD below the mean, and there is accompanying evidence of significant limitations in adaptability. In preschool children, developmental delay on screening tests may be the principal presenting finding. Sensory defects are also common, as are speech and language problems, motor handicaps, neurodevelopmental delays, seizure disorders, and behavior problems. Serious family problems are also common, and frequently the mentally retarded child merely appears to be enough slower than other members of the family to be identified as retarded rather than borderline or dull normal. If the child is examined adequately, signs of significant developmental delay including deficiencies in adaptation will often be evident by age 2 years.

Once the child reaches school age, general adaptation and achievement in all areas tend to be low but commensurate with mental age. Children with low IQs who are not retarded on measures of adaptation should not be diagnosed as mentally retarded. Occasionally, a mildly retarded or borderline child will show a significant discrepancy between actual and expected achievement in one academic area more than in others. This may technically represent a specific learning disability; however, if the child's overall intelligence is low enough (IQ below 70), special education will be indicated anyway. Idiot savants have been described as showing extraordinary ability in a circumscribed area while functioning on a mentally retarded level in all other ways. Neglect, abuse, and other family experiences damaging to growth may result in bizarre forms of behavior and emotional disturbance that are difficult to distinguish from autistic or psychotic behavior. Mentally retarded children are often transparent mirrors of disturbances going on within the family. The appearance of unusual behavior, sexual acting out, or bizarre activity in an otherwise stable retarded child is often an indication of a disturbance in the family.

C. Special Studies: General rules for ordering tests include (1) laboratory testing for treatable conditions when an etiologic diagnosis is unknown, eg, use of an amino acid or organic acid screen; and (2) ordering other tests such as electroencephalography, skull films, and chromosome studies only if clinical findings suggest specific syndromes or problems.

Differential Diagnosis

Once a descriptive diagnosis is made, the basic data base should provide enough information so that a decision can be made on how far to pursue an etiologic diagnosis. It is particularly important to distinguish the deaf, blind, and orthopedically handicapped from the mentally retarded. This is often difficult, since many retarded children also have sensory and orthopedic handicaps. It is also often difficult to differentiate between autism and retardation in very young children, particularly when family and social background indicates deprivation or neglect. Usually, however, the young retarded child shows delay in all areas of development, while the autistic child may be quite normal in motor development but show bizarre behavior and serious delays in language development.

Management

Mental retardation usually is diagnosed only after a significant period of developmental delay has been observed. The older the child at the time of diagnosis, the less the likelihood of reversing the signs of retardation even when a treatable cause can be identified. Prevention is therefore the only significant approach to treatment at present. A screening program for early detection of inborn errors of metabolism and institution of treatment before significant damage to the nervous system can occur represents the model approach to the problem of mental retardation. This same model has been used in developing preventive programs for children at risk for familial-cultural retardation. Controlled studies of stimulation programs for infants in sociocultural groups with high rates of mental retardation have shown significant long-range results after termination of the program when (1) parents have been involved in the program, (2) the infant participated in the program frequently (once every 2 weeks or more), and (3) the program continued for at least 2 years. Headstart has also been shown to decrease the number of children in special education classes and to increase the number of children from high-risk populations who remain in school.

In most instances, however, management of the retarded child does not involve treatment of the retardation per se but must be directed toward (1) assessing the impact on the family and providing support and psychotherapy, (2) providing protection for the child, (3) providing education and rehabilitation to maximize the child's potential, and (4) providing treatment of associated medical, emotional, and behavior problems.

A. Impact on the Family: The diagnosis of mental retardation is a disaster for which few families are prepared. Often parents can assess the mental age of their child within a few months but still refuse to accept the implications of this information. The tact and sensitivity with which the initial discussion of developmental delay is broached can determine how early the family will allow appropriate treatment, education, and rehabilitation to be started; thus, the primary care physician should be alert to parents' initial questions about developmental delay. A second opinion or repeated evaluation is almost mandatory when the impression of significant developmental delay arises unexpectedly from screening tests or school observations. Once the diagnosis is confirmed, the family will need continued assistance and support in adjusting to the diagnosis and in making contact with community resources.

Retarded children and adults can successfully remain within the family in most instances, but they usually require a host of family and community support services. These often include social services, infant education programs, and occupational and physical therapy programs and services for handicapped infants that begin as early as the newborn period. In school-age children, most services are organized through the public school systems, but the primary care physician may be called on to assist in difficult situations.

Once a severely handicapped child is "accepted" by the family, family resources may be totally consumed by care of the child, often to the detriment of normal siblings. Professionals involved with these families should provide help in developing priorities and alleviating parental guilt at being unable to do everything everyone suggests for the child. Less severely handicapped children are often less acceptable to the family, with resulting conflict and emotional disturbance as parents attempt to deny or seek more ego-syntonic diagnoses and explanations for the child's delays. Parental difficulty in accepting evidence of mild retardation often leads them to seek more than one evaluation as they pass through a mourning process and eventually develop more realistic expectations for the child. Parent support groups have been particularly helpful to families with retarded children.

B. Protection, Education, and Rehabilitation: Although they seldom alter the diagnosis, early intervention programs for developmentally delayed infants and young children are often associated with improved development of language, ambulation, and self-care. An emphasis on family life, whether within the biologic family, a foster family, or a group home, has been associated with a generally improved level of social competence and a decrease in the incidence of emotional and behavior problems.

Mildly retarded children (IQ of 50–69) usually are considered educable and in many instances are able to blend into society with minimal or no protective custody. Moderately retarded children (IQ of 30–49) are considered trainable but require protective care (sheltered workshop, guardian, institutionalization). More recently, the public schools have been required to provide services to members of this group who are ambulatory. Severely to profoundly retarded children (IQ below 30) usually require institutional care, and this group often includes the most severely deformed, nonambulatory, and minimally communicative individuals.

C. Treatment of Associated Medical, Emotional, and Behavior Problems: Sensory, motor, and orthopedic handicaps and other medical problems should be treated appropriately. The most controversial area of management concerns the use of psychotropic medication for treatment of emotional and behavior problems, especially in institutionalized retarded children. Although most of these medications are approved primarily for use in treatment of psychotic conditions, the phenothiazines in particular have been employed extensively in behavioral management of retarded persons.

Psychotropic medication practices have often resulted in too much being given for too long a time to too many institutionalized children. Frequently, several psychotropic drugs are given at the same time. Some children may be so heavily drugged that they are unable to respond maximally to educational and rehabilitative programs. These practices are often based on claims that the response to neuroleptic and psychotropic medications is altered in retarded children, but other evidence supports the interpretation that psychotropic medication often represents a "chemical straitjacket" that is used as a substitute for adequate personnel to provide more appropriate care. It is uncertain whether attention deficit disorder in mentally retarded children should be treated with stimulant medication. Some children appear to become worse with treatment (as do many psychotic children), whereas stimulant medication appears to be the treatment of choice for others. As children are withdrawn from heavy medication with phenothiazines and other major psychotropic drugs, symptoms such as dyskinesia may emerge, ie, withdrawal emergent symptoms, which require diagnosis and treatment in themselves. The most serious of these is tardive dyskinesia, which may also appear during treatment with tranquilizers.

To avoid misuse of psychotropic medication in the mentally retarded, (1) a diagnosis of the emotional behavior problem should be made and an appropriate drug and dosage selected on the basis of the diagnosis; and (2) the patient's response to the medication should be carefully monitored by the physician through direct evaluation and observation as well as review of reports provided by custodial personnel.

MOTOR HANDICAPS

A variety of nonspecific problems in development of motor coordination have been observed in children with learning disorders and also as isolated problems. Mental retardation, cerebral palsy, or a neuromuscular disorder is also present in many cases. A larger group, estimated at about 6–7% of the population, shows clumsiness, awkwardness, choreiform movements, or generally poor coordination but no signs of systemic disease except for an increased incidence of other "soft signs" on neurologic examination. Many of the children in this group also show evidence of learning problems, and the motor problems have been cited as evidence of a neurologic basis for the learning problems. However, as with "soft signs" in general, this interpretation is controversial.

Clumsiness and awkwardness have also been reported in association with attention deficit disorder. In this instance, treatment with stimulant medications has frequently been accompanied by improvement in motor coordination. Occupational and physical therapy are often recommended for these children, though there are no adequately controlled studies with data to support the efficacy of these approaches for improving educational achievement. There is clear evidence that instruction in reading is better than perceptual-motor training in improving reading ability irrespective of the child's motor status. The whole area of mild motor disability has received so little formal scrutiny, however, that much is yet to be learned about ways of identifying and ameliorating developmental impairments in motor skills.

Connolly K: Motor development and motor disability. In: *Developmental Psychiatry*. Rutter M (editor). Heinemann, 1980.

Henderson A: Research in occupational therapy and physical therapy with children. In: *Advances in Behavioral Pediatrics*. Vol. 2. Camp BW (editor). JAI Press, 1981.

DEVELOPMENTAL-ADAPTATIONAL PROBLEMS

Developmental-adaptational problems are behavior problems that in normal children decline steadily with age either from infancy or from their appearance in the preschool years. Manifestations include fears, distractibility, hyperactivity, destructiveness, lying, negativism, temper tantrums, enuresis, and thumbsucking. Children with these manifestations often show no maladjustment later in life; absence of these manifestations does not rule out later maladjustment. The gradual decline in these behavior problems is associated with maturation of cognitive competency, including not only intelligence but moral maturity and ego development as well. When deficiencies in social character and cognitive adaptability persist in children beyond the early school years, they are more likely to have a poor prognosis.

ATTENTION DEFICIT DISORDER

Essentials of Diagnosis

- Distractibility or short attention span.
- Present longer than 6 months.
- Not associated with psychosis.
- May or may not be associated with hyperactivity, retardation, or aggressive behavior.

General Considerations

Attention deficit disorder is characterized by heightened distractibility, short attention span, and impulsiveness. The rate of incidence is about 5%, and the disorder is more common in boys than in girls. Most of the children previously labeled hyperactive or said to have minimal brain dysfunction are children with attention deficit disorder. In normal children, attention span and ability to concentrate on cognitive tasks increase throughout childhood. Ability of preschool children to engage in sustained task-oriented behavior is one of the most reliable predictors of later school performance. Some evidence suggests that even in infants, attention span may be an early indication of later cognitive performance. In older children, attentiveness is one of the major characteristics of competent children with good peer relations.

The child who persists in immature forms of attentional behavior after age mates have matured is noticeably out of phase in cognitively stressful situations such as school. In these circumstances, children may appear driven to aimless, purposeless activity. Some children also show hyperactive behavior at home, on the playground, and in the physician's office, as well as in the classroom; others may only show problems under cognitive stress. Some children with attention deficit disorder have also been described as hypoactive rather than hyperactive.

In evaluating behavior problems, it is important to determine whether aggressive behavior problems or conduct disorders are also present. This mixture of behavior problems is common. It is not clear whether the presence of aggressive behavior alters the short-term response to treatment. However, long-term prognosis is poorer in those who have a mixed disorder than in those whose behavior problems are confined to distractibility, impulsiveness, and short attention span.

The causes of attention deficit disorder are not well understood, although there is evidence of a genetic or constitutional basis for the problem in many children. The diagnosis is largely descriptive, but it carries the implication that specific causes of distractibility and short attention span (eg, neurologic insult or injury, emotional trauma, psychosis, depression) have been eliminated. Immaturity in development of the central nervous system is one of the most likely underlying causes of the problem. However, children who show the functional disorder may or may not have evidence of "soft signs" on neurologic examination or abnormal findings on electroencephalography. The presence of neurodevelopmental signs has not been consistently related to treatment outcome.

Clinical Findings

A. History: The most important diagnostic information comes from a description of behavior in the classroom and teacher ratings on the abbreviated Conners report (Table 7–1). Ratings more than 2 SD above the mean (ie, ratings of 15 or higher for children 6–10 years of age in the USA) are significant. In the absence of high scores on this scale, it is very unlikely that the child has attention deficit disorder. Physicians worried about teacher bias in completing the rating will often find that ratings obtained from several teachers will show similar results. However, ratings completed by parents may or may not show deviance. It is useful to obtain one of the general teacher rating scales as well as the abbreviated Conners report, since many children will also show other behavior or learning problems. The most common other behavior problem encountered among children with attention deficit disorder is aggressive behavior or conduct disorder. The family history is often positive for similar problems in childhood, particularly among male relatives. Children with attention deficit disorder are frequently described as active, colicky infants, and typically parents can recall many incidents indicating distractibility and hyperactivity in the preschool period. Attention deficit disorder is usually first recognized as a problem after a child enters school. The diagnosis can sometimes be made with great confidence in preschool children, but many of these children are primarily in need of improved parental management.

B. Symptoms and Signs: The neurologic examination may or may not show signs of neurologic immaturity. There are usually no sensory impairments. A significant number of children also have learning problems that may be general or specific, usually depending on the child's level of intelligence. Attention deficit disorder occurs at all intellectual levels, but among children of average intelligence with behavior problems confined to the attention deficit disorder syndrome, achievement is often adequate despite teacher complaints that the child is "not learning." When a learning problem accompanies a behavior problem, the problems should be addressed separately.

Family problems may continue to attention deficit disorder and increase the difficulty of treatment, especially in children who show aggressive behavior. Attention deficit disorder is excluded when a diagnosis of childhood psychotic disorder has been made, but the diagnosis may be made in mentally retarded children.

C. Special Studies: There are no special tests that aid in diagnosis. If there is a question of seizure disorder or clear-cut evidence of neurologic disorder, investigation of these conditions is indicated.

Treatment

Two major effective forms of treatment are behavior modification programs in the classroom and stimulant drugs (methylphenidate [Ritalin], dextroamphetamine [Dexedrine; many others], and pemoline [Cylert]). Drug treatment, if effective, tends to have more dramatic results than behavior modification.

Approximately 50–80% of children with attention deficit disorder are responsive to stimulant drug therapy. Dose-response studies on methylphenidate suggest that a dose of 0.3 mg/kg produces optimal cognitive improvement (concentration) as well as significant improvement in social behavior (reflected by Conners' scale). Greater improvement in social behavior can be achieved with higher doses, but this occurs at the expense of some loss in concentration. Peak action usually occurs 2 hours after ingestion, and most effects have dissipated after 6 hours. The usual regimen is to start with an early morning dose, followed by a dose at noon if needed. Morning activities often require the most concentration, and the noon dose may be unnecessary. If problems at home are also severe, a third dose may be given in the late afternoon. Medication on weekends and during school holidays should be tailored to the needs of the child and family. Dextroamphetamine and methylphenidate are quite similar in onset and duration of action, and most children who respond to one will respond to the other. Pemoline appears to be somewhat different in onset of action, and doses often require adjustment over a longer period of time.

Drug "holidays" are an important part of chronic drug therapy with psychotropic drugs. Medication should be withdrawn for at least 2 weeks of each year to determine whether therapy needs to be continued. Two convenient times for this are summer vacations and spring holidays. In the latter case, a week at home without medication can precede a week at school without medication.

Monitoring for side effects should be continuous. Weekly teacher reports (Conners' scale) during the first month are helpful for monitoring and evaluating treatment. The child should be reevaluated at 1 month to determine if the response is sufficient to justify continuing with medication.

Behavior modification programs are often tailored to an individual child's situation. Planning an individualized program usually involves the services of a psychologist or educational specialist. Think Aloud, a general cognitive behavior modification program for improving self-control in children 6–8 years of age, can be used in an office setting. Typically, it has been carried out by special teachers, psychologists, social workers, or other mental health workers but can be used by an intelligent parent or interested physician.

Prognosis

With or without treatment, the long-term outcome is better in the more intelligent children with stable families and uncomplicated attention deficit disorder. These children often require only short-term treatment (usually 2 years or less).

Camp BW, Bash MAS: *Think Aloud: Increasing Social and Cognitive Skills—A Problem Solving Program for Children.* Research Press, 1981.

Whalen CK, Henker B (editors): *Hyperactive Children: The Social Ecology of Identification and Treatment.* Academic Press, 1980.

AGGRESSIVE ANTISOCIAL BEHAVIOR PROBLEMS

Essentials of Diagnosis

- Fighting and physically attacking other children or adults.
- Often boisterous, disruptive, and argumentative, with a ''chip on the shoulder'' attitude.
- Usually associated with evidence of family disturbance or disharmony.
- Often accompanied by poor achievement in children over 10 years of age.
- More common among less intelligent children.

General Considerations

Destructive, aggressive behavior is common in preschool children but declines significantly with the developmental shift at 5–7 years of age. Nevertheless, it is one of the most malignant behavior problems of childhood. It is more common in boys than in girls. By age 6–8, most normal children have shown a marked decrease in aggressive behavior. A significant number of those who continue to show aggressive behavior after 8 years of age will be aggressive in adolescence. Aggressive behavior is less likely to persist in children who identify with the values of one or both parents. Family disharmony and disturbance are the most important contemporaneous instigators of aggressive behavior problems at school.

Clinical Findings

A. History: Active destructive behavior is often seen at an early age and is frequently accompanied by risk-taking and other forms of behavior that make the child difficult to manage. The parents are often characterized as too strict or too lax, providing the child with little supervision or sense of belonging, and often openly rejecting the child. Aggressive behavior by the parents often complicates the diagnosis, since the child may be merely imitating the parents' behavior. Aggressive children of aggressive parents, however, often reject the parents' values even as they imitate the parents' behavior.

B. Symptoms and Signs: The most important information is from teacher, parent, and other reports of aggressive, antisocial, or disruptive behavior. Since some aggressive behavior is present in most children, only teacher and parent rating scales for general behavior that show increases of at least 1.5 SD above normal in amount of aggressive behavior should be considered significant. Neurologic examination usually shows normal results. Intelligence may be average or above average, but aggressive problems occur more frequently in children with lower IQs. Achievement may be average in the first few years of school but shows a steady decline after third grade, frequently accompanied by truancy. Learning delays in all areas are common in the aggressive delinquent adolescent, but 26% show evidence of specific learning disorders. (Most children with specific learning disability are not aggressive, however.) In early school years, the cognitive pattern of aggressive boys tends to show more impulsiveness and less verbal mediation activity than that of normal boys. By adolescence, the typical antisocial, aggressive boy shows a characteristic pattern of decreased verbal intelligence relative to nonverbal, impulsive stereotyped thinking and immaturity in ego development.

Treatment

Large-scale delinquency prevention programs for young aggressive boys have been unsuccessful even when they provided remedial reading instruction as well as counseling and family support. Small-scale behavior modification programs have had some success in normalizing cognitive and social behavior or slowing the increase in delinquent behavior. Psychotherapy and other methods of treatment have met with more modest success.

Behavior modification or other treatment programs are typically designed and monitored by psychologists or child psychiatrists. For younger children (6–8 years of age), the Think Aloud program has been used successfully by teachers, psychologists, social workers, and other mental health workers to help normalize both cognitive and social behavior at school.

When attention deficit disorder accompanies aggressive behavior problems, stimulant medication is sometimes helpful in decreasing general disruptive behavior as well as impulsiveness and distractibility, but the response may be quite variable.

Camp BW, Ray RS: Aggression. In: *Cognitive Behavior Therapy for Children.* Meyers A, Craighead LW (editors). Plenum Press, 1984.

Lefkowitz MM et al: *Growing Up to Be Violent.* Pergamon Press, 1977.

SELECTED REFERENCES

Levine MD et al: *Developmental and Behavioral Pediatrics.* Saunders, 1983.

Mussen PH (editor): *Carmichael's Manual of Child Psychology.* Vols 1–4. Wiley, 1983.

Thompson RJ Jr, O'Quinn AN: *Developmental Disabilities: Etiologies, Manifestations, Diagnoses, and Treatments.* Oxford Univ Press, 1979.

8 Emergencies & Accidents

Roger M. Barkin, MD, MPH, & John D. Burrington, MD

CARDIOPULMONARY ARREST

Cardiopulmonary arrests in children are primarily respiratory in origin, resulting from obstruction or hypoxia. The precipitating causes are often preventable or identifiable prior to the arrest.

Resuscitation should be initiated when peripheral pulses are not palpable or severe bradycardia exists. Irreversible central nervous system damage occurs within 4 minutes if circulation is not restored.

Principles of Management

A. Verification of Unconsciousness: Establish unresponsiveness or respiratory difficulty. Gently shake the patient to determine consciousness. If resuscitation is required, position the patient for basic life support without subjecting the patient to further injury. Call for help.

B. Airway: Airway management must reflect the nature of precipitating causes of respiratory difficulty and the potential for cervical spine injury.

1. Clear the upper airway by one of the following methods:

a. Lift the occiput slightly off the bed or flat surface by placing a towel roll or hand under the occiput.

b. With one hand under the neck and the other on the forehead, lift the neck slightly and tip the head backward with gentle pressure on the forehead (head tilt and neck lift method; Fig 8–1A).

c. Extension of the neck can also be maintained by pressure on the forehead while the tips of the fingers of the hand that had been under the neck are used to lift the bony part of the jaw (chin) forward (head tilt and chin lift method).

2. Maintain patency of the airway. Adjuncts to management include the following:

a. Suction and clear debris as necessary. Remove loose teeth.

b. An oropharyngeal or nasopharyngeal airway may be useful in maintaining patency. The oropharyngeal airway (Fig 8–2) is poorly tolerated in the conscious patient.

c. Endotracheal intubation provides a stable airway and is indicated if there is continued obstruction or if assisted ventilation will be required on a prolonged basis. The choice of oral or nasal route depends upon the expertise of the clinician. The size of the tube to be used may be estimated by selecting a tube that approximates the size of the patient's little finger. The following guidelines for tube size may also be useful: newborns, 1.5–3.5 mm; 1 month, 3.5 mm; 1 year, 4 mm; 2–3 years, 4.5 mm; 4–5 years, 5–6 mm; 6–8 years, 6–6.5 mm; 10–12 years, 7 mm; and 14 years, 7.5–8.5 mm. Uncuffed tubes are used for children under 7–8 years of age.

d. Cricothyroidotomy is indicated in children over 3 years in very rare circumstances where acute airway obstruction cannot be otherwise relieved.

C. Breathing: Check for spontaneous breathing by observing movement of the chest and abdomen or by feeling air movement at the mouth.

1. If the patient is not breathing, begin ventilation by mouth-to-mouth resuscitation, covering both the nose and mouth in infants or pinching the nostrils closed in children (Fig 8–1).

2. Initially, give 4 quick breaths to check for airway patency.

3. Continue ventilating at a cardiac compression to ventilation ratio of 5:1 in infants and children.

4. Subsequently—or initially, if equipment is available—use a self-inflating resuscitation bag (Fig 8–3). Effective positive pressure ventilation can be achieved by applying the mask firmly over the nose and mouth and squeezing the bag, which expands spontaneously when released. Oxygen should be administered by attaching the tubing to the air intake valve at the end of the bag.

D. Circulation: Assess circulation by checking brachial, femoral, or carotid pulses. If there is no

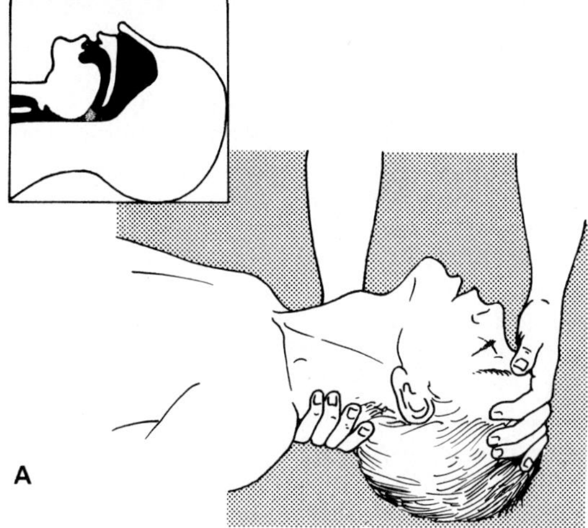

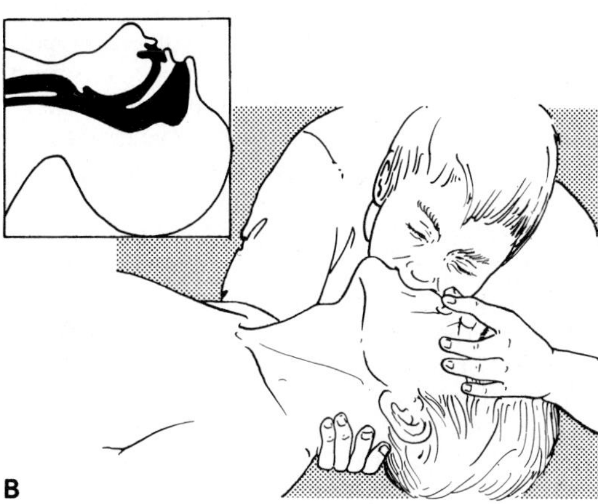

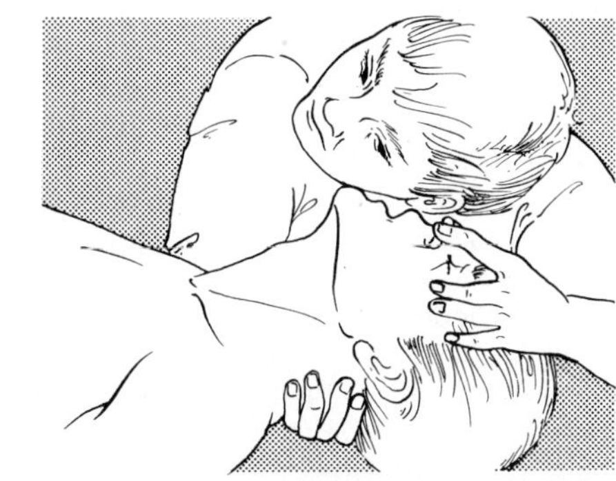

Figure 8–1. Proper performance of mouth-to-mouth resuscitation. *A:* Open airway by positioning neck anteriorly in extension. Inserts show airway obstructed when the neck is in resting flexed position and opening when neck is extended. *B:* Rescuer should close victim's nose with fingers, seal mouth around victim's mouth, and deliver breath by vigorous expiration. *C:* Victim is allowed to exhale passively by unsealing mouth and nose. Rescuer should listen and feel for expiratory air flow.

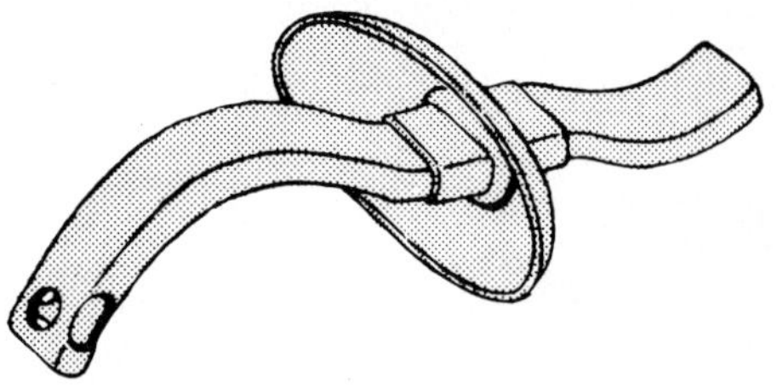

Figure 8–2. Airway for use in mouth-to-mouth insufflation. The larger airway is for adults. The guard is flexible and may be inverted from the position shown for use with infants and children.

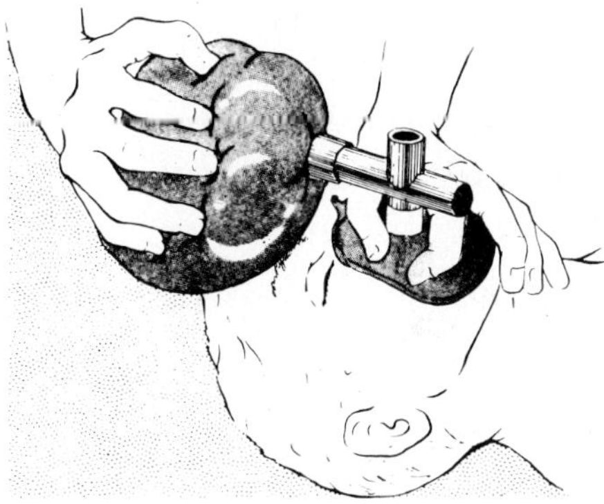

(1) Lift the victim's neck with one hand.
(2) Tilt head backward into maximum neck extension. Remove secretions and debris from mouth and throat, and pull the tongue and mandible forward as required to clear the airway.
(3) Hold the mask snugly over the nose and mouth, holding the chin forward and the neck in extension as shown in diagram.
(4) Squeeze the bag, noting inflation of the lungs by the rise of the chest wall.
(5) Release the bag, which will expand spontaneously. The patient will exhale, and the chest will fall.
(6) Repeat steps 4 and 5 approximately 12–20 times per minute depending on the patient's age.

Figure 8–3. Self-inflating resuscitation bag.

pulse, begin external chest compression. Pulses and blood pressure should be monitored during compression.

1. For children under 1 year of age, use both hands to encircle the chest, and deliver 100 compressions per minute with a 5:1 ratio of compressions to ventilations.

2. For children over 1 year of age, use the heel of the hand to compress the lower third of the sternum (Fig 8–4), displacing the sternum 1–1½ inches in children 1–8 years of age and 1½–2 inches in older children. Deliver 60–80 compressions per minute with a 5:1 ratio of compressions to ventilations.

E. Intravenous Access and Fluids: Intravenous cannulation must be achieved rapidly. The size and type of catheter depend upon the expertise of

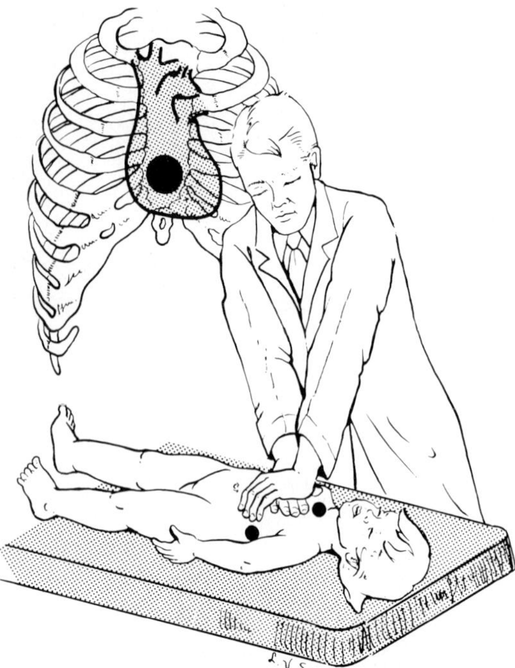

Figure 8–4. Technique of closed chest cardiac massage. (Heavy circle in heart drawing shows area of application of force. Circles on supine figure show points of application of paddles for defibrillation.)

the clinician and availability of sites. If venous access is difficult, a venous cutdown should be done early in the resuscitation. Initial fluid management should reflect the cause of cardiopulmonary arrest. If there is any question of hypovolemia, give a rapid infusion of normal saline solution or lactated Ringer's injection, 20 mL/kg over 20–30 minutes. If there is no response and the patient remains in shock following restoration of volume, rhythm, and ventilation, consider vasopressor agents (see below).

F. Medications: Virtually all patients should receive oxygen, and those who do not respond to relief of airway obstruction should receive first-line cardiac drugs.

1. Sodium bicarbonate—Give 1–2 meq/kg intravenously every 5–15 minutes, and monitor arterial blood gases if possible. Acidosis should be corrected, since it has a negative effect on cardiac function and efficacy of adrenergic drugs. Following cardiac arrest, the reduction of Pa_{CO_2} levels by adequate ventilation may partially reduce acidosis. Hyperventilation of the patient will further improve the pH.

2. Sympathomimetic drugs—These drugs stimulate the α- and β-adrenergic receptors; their effects vary depending upon the relative balance of stimulation achieved. The primary effect of α-adrenergic drugs is vasoconstriction; β_1-adrenergic drugs, tachycardia and increased myocardial contraction; and β_2-adrenergic drugs, vasodilation and bronchodilation. The following drugs are commonly used:

a. Epinephrine—Give epinephrine (1:10,000 solution), 0.1 mL/kg intravenously or intratracheally every 5–10 minutes as needed. Epinephrine stimulates both α- and β-adrenergic receptors and increases heart rate, force of myocardial contraction, and vascular resistance. It is utilized in cases of ventricular standstill or fine ventricular fibrillation to convert the latter to coarse fibrillation.

b. Dopamine—Give 5–20 μg/kg/min intravenously by continuous drip. Dopamine stimulates α- and β-adrenergic receptors as well as specific dopaminergic receptors that maintain renal and mesenteric blood vessel dilatation at low doses (< 20 μg/kg/min). At higher doses, α-adrenergic effects become prominent. The drug is particularly useful for treatment of cardiogenic shock as well as for maintenance of renal perfusion. It is not indicated for treatment of hypovolemic shock.

c. Isoproterenol—Initially, give 0.1 μg/kg/min intravenously by continuous drip, and increase slowly in increments up to 1.5 μg/kg/min as required. Isoproterenol is a pure β-receptor agonist. It increases heart rate and myocardial contraction and produces vasodilation. The blood pressure is usually maintained by greater cardiac output. It is particularly useful in cases of bradycardia unresponsive to atropine.

3. Atropine—Give 0.01–0.03 mg/kg (minimum, 0.1 mg per dose; maximum, 0.5 mg per dose) intravenously or intratracheally every 5 minutes as needed. Atropine has vagolytic action, with increased sinoatrial node discharges and increased atrioventricular node conduction, and is useful in cases of symptomatic severe bradycardia as well as in cases of organophosphate overdose.

4. Calcium chloride—Give a 10% solution of calcium chloride, 20–30 mg/kg (0.02–0.03 mL/kg; maximum, 500 mg per dose) intravenously every 10 minutes as needed. Administer the drug slowly, and monitor the patient. Calcium chloride is useful in cases of ventricular standstill, electromechanical dissociation, and hyperkalemia. Give with caution in patients receiving digitalis. Do not mix with sodium bicarbonate.

5. Antiarrhythmic drugs—These are rarely needed in children, since the incidence of dysrhythmia is relatively low.

a. Lidocaine—Give a loading dose of 1 mg/kg intravenously, followed by 20–50 μg/kg/min by intravenous infusion. Lidocaine is indicated for ventricular dysrhythmia and for cardiac arrest secondary to ventricular fibrillation.

b. Bretylium—Give a loading dose of 5 mg/kg intravenously, followed by 10 mg/kg intravenously every 10 minutes as needed (maximum, 30 mg/kg total dose). Bretylium is used if the patient with dysrhythmia fails to respond to lidocaine.

G. Defibrillation: Defibrillation, employing a shock of 1–2 J/kg as needed, is indicated primarily for ventricular fibrillation. One electrode is placed in the second intercostal space of the right sternal border, and a second electrode is placed in the fourth intercostal space of the left midaxillary line (Fig 8–4). Adequate electrode paste should be applied, and personnel should be warned not to touch the patient or the bed at the time of defibrillation. If a single shock is ineffective, a second shock in rapid succession may be successful. Defibrillation is used for ventricular fibrillation, while synchronized cardioversion is appropriate for ventricular tachyarrhythmias.

SHOCK

Shock occurs when there is acute circulatory dysfunction associated with inadequate tissue perfusion to meet metabolic requirements. Compensatory mechanisms initially sustain cellular function, but with progression of shock, cellular metabolic changes result in further tissue injury and cell death.

Clinical Findings

Compensated shock, the early stage of shock, is marked by maintenance of normal vital signs through intrinsic mechanisms. The effectiveness of these mechanisms is dependent upon the preexisting cardiac and pulmonary status and on the volume and rate of blood loss. Orthostatic changes are the most sensitive indicators of volume status, and acidosis may be the earliest sign of impaired tissue perfusion.

Uncompensated shock follows compensated shock and is characterized by cardiovascular dysfunction and impairment of microvascular perfusion. Hypotension, tachycardia, and decreased cardiac output commonly progress to cardiovascular collapse.

Newborns in shock appear lethargic, with pale, mottled, and slightly gray skin. Late shock is manifested by a decrease in skin temperature, particularly of the extremities.

Classification

Three major types of shock may occur, each requiring a different management approach:

Hypovolemic shock is due to a reduction in circulating blood volume.

Cardiogenic shock is secondary to depressed cardiac output from myocardial insufficiency or obstruction of venous return or cardiac outflow.

Vasogenic (distributive) shock is due to abnormal distribution of blood secondary to vasomotor paralysis and increased venous capacitance. Typically, vasogenic shock is anaphylactic, septic, or neurogenic in origin.

General Principles of Management

(1) Establish a stable airway, and administer oxygen by mask, hood, or cannula.

(2) Give a fluid push of normal saline solution or lactated Ringer's injection, 20 mL/kg, unless the patient is hypervolemic, as determined by clinical examination or central venous pressure measurement. (See also p 1069.)

(3) Establish a central venous pressure monitor if the patient does not respond to the initial fluid push.

(4) Insert a urinary catheter to monitor output.

(5) Measure electrolytes, pH, and complete blood count. Correct fluid and electrolyte imbalance as outlined in Chapter 36.

(6) Insert a nasogastric tube.

Treatment of Specific Types of Shock

A. Hypovolemic Shock:

1. Administer normal saline solution or lactated Ringer's injection intravenously at a rate of 20 mL/kg over 20–30 minutes. If there is no response, repeat the infusion while continuing to monitor urine output, blood pressure, pulse, and perfusion rates.

2. If there is no response after 2 infusions, measure central venous pressure and consider other causes of shock, such as pericardial tamponade or tension pneumothorax.

3. If hemorrhage is the cause of hypovolemia, give type-specific or cross-matched blood following the initial crystalloid infusion. Whole blood is useful for massive acute bleeding; packed red blood cells may be used if there has been extensive crystalloid infusion in the relatively stable patient or if bleeding is chronic.

4. Following massive blood transfusions, give fresh frozen plasma and platelets if indicated. Monitor coagulation.

5. Colloid is not indicated in severe capillary leak syndromes such as burns, sepsis, or terminal shock. It may be useful in hypovolemia accompanied by renal, cardiac, or respiratory failure.

6. If the hypovolemic patient does not respond to fluid therapy, use the appropriate pediatric size of pneumatic antishock trousers (MAST suit). ***Caution:*** MAST suits should only be used by experienced clinicians.

7. After the patient's condition is stable, replace fluid losses and deficits as discussed in Chapter 36. Replacements must reflect the type and degree of dehydration.

8. Crystalloid solution is the initial fluid of choice in burn therapy, as discussed below.

9. Vasopressor agents are not indicated in the treatment of hypovolemic shock. Fluids are the treatment of choice.

B. Cardiogenic Shock:

1. A fluid push may improve cardiac output by increasing filling pressure, particularly if the central venous pressure is 15 cm of water or below. Give normal saline solution or lactated Ringer's injection carefully (because of salt load) at a rate of 5 mL/kg over 30 minutes, and monitor the response.

2. Sodium bicarbonate, 1–2 meq/kg intravenously, is often indicated either empirically or by acid-base measurements.

3. An ECG and chest x-ray are mandatory. Echocardiography is also a useful tool in assessing function as well as excluding cardiac tamponade.

4. Dysrhythmia requires emergency treatment. Predisposing factors, including electrolyte abnormalities, acidosis, alkalosis, drugs, fever, pericardial disease, ischemia, and hypoxia, should be excluded.

5. Inotropic agents are usually indicated, optimally following evaluation of preload and ejection time by echocardiography or central venous pressure measurement. If peripheral perfusion is poor and quantitative measurements are not possible, consider giving a crystalloid fluid push to test the response prior to initiating pharmacologic therapy with dopamine, 5–20 μg/kg/min intravenously by continuous drip.

6. Vasodilators are indicated if there is peripheral hypoperfusion and the patient is hypervolemic or there is outflow obstruction secondary to arteriolar vasoconstriction. Give nitroprusside, 0.5–10 μg/kg/min intravenously by continuous drip, and monitor the blood pressure closely because of the drug's potent vasodilator effect. Nitroprusside is sensitive to light.

7. Pericardiocentesis may be used to exclude pericardial tamponade. Thoracentesis may be used to treat tension pneumothorax.

8. Measurement of central venous pressure or pulmonary artery wedge pressure (by Swan-Ganz catheter) is usually necessary to monitor fluids and efficacy of pharmacologic therapy.

C. Vasogenic (Distributive) Shock:

1. Septic shock—The patient with septic shock presents with fever, toxicity, and concurrent shock. There is often a history of infection preceding shock. Complete blood count, platelet count, and blood cultures should be obtained.

a. Crystalloid solution should be infused to maintain an adequate central venous pressure but will rarely be adequate as the only therapy.

b. Inotropic agents are usually required. Dopamine, 5–20 μg/kg/min intravenously by continuous drip, should be given.

c. Corticosteroids are usually initiated, although their efficacy has not been substantiated. Either hydrocortisone or methylprednisolone may be used. The dosage of hydrocortisone (Solu-Cortef) is 50 mg/kg intravenously; that of methylprednisolone (Solu-Medrol) is 30–50 mg/kg intravenously.

d. Antibiotics should be initiated after obtaining appropriate cultures. The choice may be determined by a specific clinical presentation (eg, meningococcemia), or broad-spectrum antibiotics may be given initially as follows; ampicillin, 200–300 mg/kg/24 h every 4 hours intravenously plus chloramphenicol, 100 mg/kg/24 h every 6 hours intravenously. An alternative is ampicillin, given as above, plus a third-generation cephalosporin, eg, cefotaxime (150 mg/kg/24 h every 4–6 hours intravenously) or ceftriaxone (75–100 mg/kg/24 h every 12 hours intravenously).

e. Naloxone (Narcan) serves as an endorphin antagonist and may have some efficacy in the treatment of gram-negative sepsis.

f. Coagulopathies should be treated appropriately.

g. Human antiserum to mutant *Escherichia coli* has been used successfully in the treatment of gram-negative bacteremia in adults.

2. Anaphylactic shock—Anaphylactic shock is an extreme reaction to allergy or hypersensitivity. Anaphylaxis represents a wide spectrum of reactions, ranging from only mild distress to true respiratory insufficiency and cardiovascular collapse. Upper airway laryngospasm and lower airway bronchospasm may be present in association with urticaria.

a. Initial attention must be focused on the airway. Oxygen is always required, and intubation is rarely necessary.

b. In the presence of shock, epinephrine (1:10,000 solution), 0.1 mL/kg, should be administered intravenously.

c. Diphenhydramine (Benadryl), 2 mg/kg parenterally, is given initially, followed by a parenteral dose of 5 mg/kg/24 h every 6 hours.

d. Corticosteroids should be given, although the benefits are delayed. Either hydrocortisone (Solu-Cortef), 4–5 mg/kg, or methylprednisolone (Solu-Medrol), 1–2 mg/kg, may be given intravenously every 6 hours.

e. Hypotension is treated with fluids and dopamine.

f. If possible, a tourniquet should be applied proximal to the site of injection.

3. Neurogenic shock—Neurogenic shock is usually due to interruption of normal neuronal control, resulting in impaired vascular tone. There is usually a history of exposure to anesthetic agents; spinal cord injuries; or ingestion of barbiturates, narcotics, or tranquilizers.

a. Fluids should be administered to maintain a central venous pressure of 5–8 cm of water.

b. Vasopressors are usually required. Many prefer norepinephrine (Levophed), 0.1–1 μg/kg/min intravenously by continuous drip, because of its prominent vasoconstrictive action.

D. Refractory Shock: Shock unresponsive to normal therapy is unusual in children but requires a rapid evaluation of potential complicating conditions, including multiple organ failure, outflow or filling obstruction (eg, tension pneumothorax or pericardial tamponade), coagulopathy, sepsis, respiratory failure, and exsanguinating blood loss.

EVALUATION & STABILIZATION OF THE TRAUMATIZED CHILD

The traumatized patient requires expert medical care combined with reassurance and a special sensitivity to the emotional support needed by the child and family. Establishment of appropriate treatment priorities is crucial to the management of such patients.

An aggressive and deliberate approach must be the basis for caring for the patient and should be individualized to reflect the extent of injury. Victims of major accidents should be considered to be seriously injured until their condition is proved stable. Treatment must often be initiated on the basis of clinical findings and cannot await diagnostic confirmation. The assessment and management must be individualized, but the multiply traumatized patient will benefit from the following approach.

Primary Assessment

Primary assessment must focus on the airway, ventilation, adequacy of circulation and perfusion, and management of cervical spine injury or exsanguinating hemorrhage.

A. Airway: Assure patency of the airway by clearing debris (especially chewing gum) and positioning the head to minimize any obstruction. In all patients with head trauma or multiple injuries, specific attention must be directed toward stabilizing the cervical spine to avoid further injury.

B. Ventilation: Ventilation must be assessed to determine its adequacy and ensure that breath sounds are symmetric, with consideration given to the presence of pneumothorax, hemothorax, flail chest, or pulmonary contusion. Evaluate for evidence of respiratory distress, cyanosis, tracheal deviation, and bony crepitus.

C. Cervical Spine Injuries: Cervical spine injuries should be considered in all multiply traumatized patients as well as those with head injuries or impaired sensorium. If there is any question of injury, the head should be immobilized with sandbags and secured in position until a series of x-rays of the cervical spine can be completed. A cross-table lateral neck film will detect 80–90% of injuries.

D. Circulation: Circulation may be rapidly assessed by determining adequacy of perfusion and by measuring blood pressure. Up to 25% of blood volume may be lost before hypotension is detected in patients in the supine position. Orthostatic changes occur early. In the absence of external trauma, the major body cavities that require evaluation are the chest, abdomen, and retroperitoneum.

Major blood loss may occur secondary to orthopedic injuries.

Head trauma does not cause shock unless there is massive bleeding with spreading of sutures in the infant or avulsion of the scalp. Other causes of posttraumatic shock to consider are cardiac contusion or rupture, lacerations, vascular injury, and underlying disease; these causes should be detectable on physical examination.

Initial Resuscitation

Initial management must focus on eliminating life-threatening conditions and ensuring that a number of technical activities are completed as appropriate.

(1) Oxygen should be administered to all patients. If there is any question of airway patency, the patient should be intubated. Nasotracheal intubation is preferred if cervical spine injury is suspected and there are no facial injuries present. If there is no evidence of spinal injury or if the cross-table lateral x-ray shows negative results, oral intubation may be attempted. Cricothyroidotomy is rarely indicated.

(2) Active intervention may be necessary to control ventilation following stabilization of the airway. If there is evidence of pneumothorax or hemothorax, a chest tube should be inserted, often on the basis of clinical examination in the unstable patient.

(3) External hemorrhage must be controlled, usually by direct pressure. Be careful of pressure over the neck or eyes, since pressure may cause an increase in vagal tone.

(4) An intravenous line must be placed; the number and size of lines should reflect the severity of the injury. If shock is present, a bolus of normal saline solution or lactated Ringer's injection (20 mL/kg) should be given intravenously as rapidly as possible. Subsequent administration of crystalloid and blood must reflect the response to this initial infusion. In general, once a total of 40–50 mL of crystalloid per kilogram has been given, blood is required if hypovolemic shock is still present. Type- and cross-matched blood should be given if possible.

(5) If significant shock is present, pediatric pneumatic antishock trousers should be inflated after the lower extremities, back, and abdomen have been examined for injury. Once inflated, pneumatic trousers should not be removed until some stability has been achieved. At that time, the compartments of the trousers should be deflated one at a time, starting with the abdomen, and vital signs and acid-base status should be carefully monitored.

(6) If blood is present at the urethral meatus, immediate urologic consultation is necessary and radiologic examination required. Urinary catheters should usually be inserted after ensuring that there is no blood at the urethral meatus. Dipstick tests should be done; if positive, a microscopic examination should follow.

(7) A nasogastric tube should be inserted after the cervical spine is proved stable. Aspirate should be obtained and tested for blood.

(8) Cardiac monitoring should be initiated and an ECG done.

(9) Immediately after intravenous catheters are placed, blood should be drawn for hematocrit, complete blood count, typing and cross-matching, and arterial blood gas measurements. Electrolyte, glucose, and blood urea nitrogen determinations and urine and serum toxicology screens should be ordered if appropriate.

(10) X-rays should include a complete series of cervical spine films as well as chest and pelvic films. X-rays of the abdomen and extremities may be done,

if indicated, after the patient's condition is stable. Portable films are useful in the unstable patient.

(11) All of the patient's clothing should be removed so that the patient can be examined thoroughly. This prevents overlooking an injury. A complete examination is necessary; do not stop the examination when one major injury has been detected.

(12) The initial history must be sufficient to determine the nature of the injury, with particular attention to measures of severity (eg, in the case of an accident, the extent of damage to the automobile and its speed) as well as the time elapsed since the accident. Past medical problems, allergies, use of medications, and other relevant medical data should be ascertained rapidly.

(13) Once the priority areas have been evaluated and treatment initiated, the patient should be reassessed. If no further immediate therapy is required, a more complete secondary examination can be initiated and a detailed history obtained.

Secondary Assessment & Treatment

The secondary assessment must include a systematic examination and initiation of appropriate therapeutic procedures.

A. Head and Nerve Injuries: A rapid but complete neurologic examination should be performed (see Chapter 23), with assessment of the following:

1. Level of consciousness.

2. Movement of the body—Determine symmetry, position, and posturing.

3. Pupils—Dilated fixed pupils are a reliable sign of the site of the lesion unless drug ingestion has occurred. For example, in cerebral mass lesions, there is ipsilateral dilatation of the pupil with contralateral hemiparesis.

4. Extraocular movement—A hemispheric lesion will cause the eyes to deviate toward the lesion, but a brain stem lesion will cause the eyes to deviate away from the lesion.

5. Reflexes.

6. Tympanic membrane and nose—Determine if hematotympanum or otorrhea is present.

7. Rectal examination—Determine muscle tone. Absence of rectal tone in a comatose patient may be the only evidence of spinal cord injury.

8. Head and scalp.

Frequent serial examinations of neurologic function are indicated to determine progression of deficits.

Diagnostic procedures include cervical spine x-rays, as discussed above. The cross-table lateral spine x-ray is an excellent screening mechanism that detects 80–90% of injuries. It is indicated in any patient with decreased sensorium, neck trauma, or tenderness of the neck following trauma, as well as in patients with major trauma and an unknown or unreliable medical history.

Skull x-rays are indicated in patients with an abnormal sensorium following trauma if there was a significant loss of consciousness, a neurologic defect, or increasing or persistent headache; in patients with head trauma, especially trauma due to a depressing force, such as a shoe or hammer; and in cases in which CT scans are necessary and a delay in obtaining their results is anticipated.

CT scan is the definitive test and should be done following trauma if there is a localized neurologic defect, deteriorating neurologic status, evidence of skull depression on x-ray or clinical examination, or any evidence of increased intracranial pressure.

B. Face and Mouth Injuries: The patient should be assessed for lacerations, fractures, malocclusion, and loose teeth.

Most linear lacerations or punctures of the buccal mucosa, tonsillar pillars, or posterior pharynx in children result from falling with a lollipop stick, pencil, ruler, or other object in the mouth. These injuries usually require no therapy beyond antibiotics. They heal as well without sutures as they do with them. The specific indications for examination and possible suturing under anesthesia are (1) deep puncture of the soft palate, (2) the presence of a flap of mucoperiosteum lifted off the hard palate, and (3) crepitus of the neck, indicating deep puncture.

Tongue lacerations usually result from penetration by the incisors. These, too, will heal without sutures in most cases. Lacerations through the edge of the tongue, producing a triangular flap, are best sutured with an absorbable suture.

Treatment of traumatic injuries to the teeth must reflect the degree of displacement or mobility and whether primary or secondary teeth are involved. In general, displacement or evulsion of a permanent tooth requires emergency care after the patient's condition is stable. The tooth should be reinserted and held in place until a dentist can see the patient. Injuries to primary teeth should be seen but on a less urgent basis.

C. Neck Injuries: The patient should be assessed for tracheal deviation, vein distention, ecchymosis, and evidence of penetrating injuries. Injuries may be indicative of chest disorders or cervical spine damage. Lesions that penetrate the platysma usually require surgical exploration.

D. Chest Injuries: The chest should be reexamined more thoroughly, and response to initial measures for stabilization should be evaluated. Chest x-ray and determination of arterial blood gases may be indicated if the patient is stable and findings on examination remain equivocal.

1. Rib fracture—Pleuritic pain (sharp pain exacerbated with breathing), localized severe pain with pressure at the fracture site, crepitus with respiration, pain with compression of the sternum or lateral chest, or pleural friction rub may be present. Patients should be examined for hemothorax or pneumothorax. Rib fractures are unusual in younger children and indicate a severe traumatic injury. Fractures of ribs 1 and 2 may be associated with a vascular injury. Fractures of ribs 10–12 often accompany abdominal injuries.

2. Flail chest—If 3 or more adjacent ribs are

fractured at 2 points, the chest may move paradoxically with respiration—ie, the chest moves inward with inspiration and outward with expiration. Flail chest is characterized by pain, dyspnea, and respiratory distress. The respiratory distress is primarily due to the underlying pulmonary injury. Stabilization of the flail chest is necessary, often by mechanical means. Intubation may be required if respiratory distress is present or there are massive injuries with accompanying pathologic disorders. Positive pressure ventilation will stabilize the chest.

3. Pulmonary contusion—This results when there is lung parenchymal damage. Chest trauma causes hemorrhage over the contused area of lung, often with a rapid deceleration injury. Respiratory distress develops with significant hypoxia, usually within 4–6 hours of the injury. Increased pulmonary shunting leads to a progressive rise in Pa_{CO2} and fall in Pa_{O2} levels. Chest x-ray demonstrates alveolar infiltrates progressing on occasion to consolidation. The findings may be delayed.

Patients with pulmonary contusion require oxygen by mask and pulmonary support. Intubation and ventilation may be necessary, with accompanying use of positive end-expiratory pressure.

4. Pneumothorax—Pneumothorax is classically characterized by dyspnea, cyanosis, and absence of breath and voice sounds on the involved side. In cases of tension pneumothorax, pulsus paradoxus is seen.

a. Spontaneous pneumothorax—In older children, there is usually rupture of a bleb, with leakage of air into the pleural cavity; the source of the leak usually heals spontaneously. Spontaneous pneumothorax is characterized by the sudden onset of dyspnea, pleuritic pain, hyperresonance, and absent breath and voice sounds over the involved lobe. Symptoms and signs do not progress. The condition may complicate an asthmatic attack or cystic fibrosis.

b. Tension pneumothorax—Failure of the lung leak to seal may produce a one-way valve effect leading to an increase of air in the pleural space with each breath. This results in mediastinal shift, rapidly progressive dyspnea and cyanosis, and typical physical findings. Tension pneumothorax may result from trauma such as a penetrating or blunt injury or may accompany spontaneous pneumothorax. This is a life-threatening condition and requires immediate decompression by needle or chest tube (usually preceding chest x-ray).

c. Open pneumothorax—Open pneumothorax is characterized by the presence of an open wound and severe respiratory distress with cyanosis and audible sucking sounds. The opening should be closed at once and covered with an occlusive dressing (eg, petrolatum gauze). A chest tube is required.

5. Hemothorax—Signs of pleural fluid include absent fremitus, loss of resonance, absent breath and voice sounds, and tracheal shift, together with evidence of hemorrhage into the chest. Hemothorax is often associated with pneumothorax. Use of a chest tube is definitive therapy and should follow chest x-ray if the patient is stable.

6. Penetrating wounds of the chest—

a. Closed wounds—A minute point of entry may be associated with extensive intrathoracic damage. The patient should be assessed for pneumothorax, hemothorax, subcutaneous or mediastinal emphysema, cardiac contusion, or cardiac tamponade and treated appropriately on the basis of findings.

b. Open wounds—Open wounds inevitably produce critical pneumothorax (see above).

E. Cardiac Injuries: Patients should be examined for evidence of anterior chest wall trauma, which may be the only evidence of cardiac contusion. Tachycardia may also be present, consistent with cardiac contusion or evidence of ischemia. Fullness of the jugular vein should be ascertained and the point of maximal impulse determined.

1. Cardiac contusion—Cardiac contusion results from blunt trauma to the anterior mid chest. Chest pain may be present initially or may be delayed. Findings on ECG demonstrate tachycardia or nonspecific ST–T wave changes. Dysrhythmia may be present.

2. Pericardial tamponade—This results from penetrating wounds of the chest and accumulation of blood in the pericardial sac, progressing to limitation of diastolic filling of the heart and subsequent narrowing of pulse pressure, increased pulse rate, paradoxic pulse, engorged neck veins with high central venous pressure, and hypotension. Pericardiocentesis is the treatment of choice (see Chapter 35).

F. Abdominal Injuries: In children, abdominal injuries are primarily blunt in origin. The ability to obtain an accurate history is often compromised by the clinical condition of the patient, the age of the child, the presence of intracranial injuries, or drug or alcohol use. Tenderness is usually present in patients with abdominal disorders and alert mental status. It may be localized or diffuse. Bowel sounds may be absent, and distention may develop. After consultation and with the advice and assistance of a surgical consultant, peritoneal lavage should be performed if indicated. A modified open technique is usually preferred. Helpful x-ray studies that may be done, depending upon the stability of the patient, include plain films, contrast studies, a liver-spleen scan, and a CT scan.

1. Nonpenetrating abdominal injuries—Injuries with significant hypotension and cardiovascular collapse usually require immediate laparotomy. Stable patients with equivocal results of examination may be observed or undergo peritoneal lavage, depending upon the condition of the child and the facilities and expertise available to care for the patient.

a. Splenic rupture—Manifestations are due to hemorrhage and shock. Splenic rupture is characterized by a history of injury followed immediately or with some delay (subcapsular hemorrhage) by left upper quadrant and shoulder pain, rebound tenderness, muscle rigidity, signs of bleeding, a mass in the left upper quadrant, and shock. Spontaneous rupture may occur with leukemia, infectious mononucleosis, or malaria.

b. Liver rupture—Manifestations are due to hemorrhage, shock, and possibly bile peritonitis. Liver rupture is characterized by a history of injury followed immediately or after a few hours by right upper quadrant pain, tenderness, and signs of hemorrhage. Shock and rapid exsanguination may occur.

c. Pancreatic and duodenal injuries—Because they are retroperitoneal, signs and symptoms are often obscure and delayed. Pancreatic injuries may be associated with diffuse midepigastric, abdominal, or back pain. Amylase levels may be elevated. Pancreatic pseudocysts may develop. Intramural duodenal hematomas cause proximal intestinal obstruction.

d. Intestinal rupture—Manifestations are due to localized peritonitis, anemia, or gangrene of the bowel following injury or mesenteric tear and impairment of blood supply. Upright x-rays show free air under the diaphragm and ileus and free fluid in the abdomen. Amylase levels may be elevated.

e. Kidney rupture—Manifestations are due to perirenal bleeding and urinary extravasation or intrarenal bleeding. Kidney rupture is characterized by a history of bleeding or injury followed by flank pain, hematuria, local costovertebral angle tenderness, swelling, muscle spasms, a palpable mass, nonshifting flank dullness, shock, and ecchymoses. An intravenous urogram is important for confirmation and determination of the extent of injury. Hematuria may not be present with renal vascular thrombosis, renal pedicle injury, or complete transection of the ureter.

f. Bladder rupture—Bladder rupture occurs from blunt trauma and may be intraperitoneal or extraperitoneal, thereby determining the nature of the signs and symptoms. The trauma usually occurs when the patient has a full bladder. Patients develop persistent pain, suprapubic tenderness, ileus, and inability to void. Signs of free fluid in the peritoneal cavity may be present, and a boggy suprapubic mass may be felt if the diagnosis is delayed. Radiologic examination is the most dependable test for bladder injury and should include a pelvic x-ray to rule out concurrent fractures.

g. Urethral rupture—Manifestations depend upon the segment of the urethra involved. Urine or blood extravasates around the bladder, prostate, or perineum or in the anterior perineal wall. An abdominal or perineal injury followed by pain, blood at the urethral meatus, difficulty in voiding, and signs of extravasation requires immediate evaluation. Urologic consultation should be obtained immediately (before inserting a urinary catheter).

2. Penetrating abdominal injuries—Penetrating injuries must be explored locally and the patient examined thoroughly. Minute wounds may mask extensive internal damage. If there is any evidence of intraperitoneal penetration on local wound exploration, peritoneal lavage should be performed if the patient is stable and laparotomy if the patient is deteriorating.

G. Perineal Injuries: Perineal injuries most often result from falls on a bicycle (impact of the bicycle seat), falls in a bath tub, or sexual assault.

Injuries to the labia often cause bruising, edema, and urinary retention. Have the child attempt to urinate while sitting in a tub of warm water. Catheterization is rarely necessary.

Vaginal injuries in the young child require examination under sedation or anesthesia.

Penile, scrotal, and testicular injuries will reflect the nature of the insult. A urologist should usually be consulted. Superficial lacerations may be closed with absorbable suture. Deeper wounds require operative exploration.

H. Orthopedic Injuries: See Chapter 22.

Committee on Trauma, American College of Surgeons: *Advanced Trauma Life Support Course*. American College of Surgeons, 1981.

Gratz JR: Accidental injury in childhood: A literature review on pediatric trauma. *J Trauma* 1979;**19**:551.

Jorden RJ: Evaluation and stabilization of multiply traumatized patients. In: *Emergency Pediatrics*. Barkin RM, Rosen P (editors). Mosby, 1984.

ENVIRONMENTAL INJURIES*

BURNS

Initial assessment and management of the patient with a burn are the most important determinants of morbidity and ultimate survival.

Initial Assessment

Initial evaluation must include information about the nature of the injury and the patient's age, weight, and underlying medical problems. Special attention must focus on the presence and extent of associated injuries, eg, evidence of significant smoke inhalation associated with hoarseness, cough, singed nasal hairs, oral burns, carbonaceous sputum, wheezing, rhonchi, and cyanosis. Burns should be classified according to their depth and extent.

A. Classification by Depth of Burn:

1. First-degree burns—Superficial partial-thickness (first-degree) burns involve the epidermis only. The skin area is pink or red, blanches with pressure, and is painful to touch. Causes include sunburn, scalds, and distant flash fires.

2. Second-degree burns—Partial-thickness (second-degree) burns involve the epidermis and corium. The skin is red, blistered, or moist with exudate

* Drowning is discussed in Chapter 14.

and is painful to pinprick or touch. Causes include scalds and flash fires.

3. Third-degree burns—Full-thickness (third-degree) burns involve the entire dermis and sometimes fat, muscle, or bone. The skin is white, dry or charred, and painless. Causes include scalds from steam, open flame burns, and contact with chemicals or electric current.

B. Classification by Extent of Burn: The body surface area affected in infants and children can be estimated using the percentages depicted in Fig 8–5.

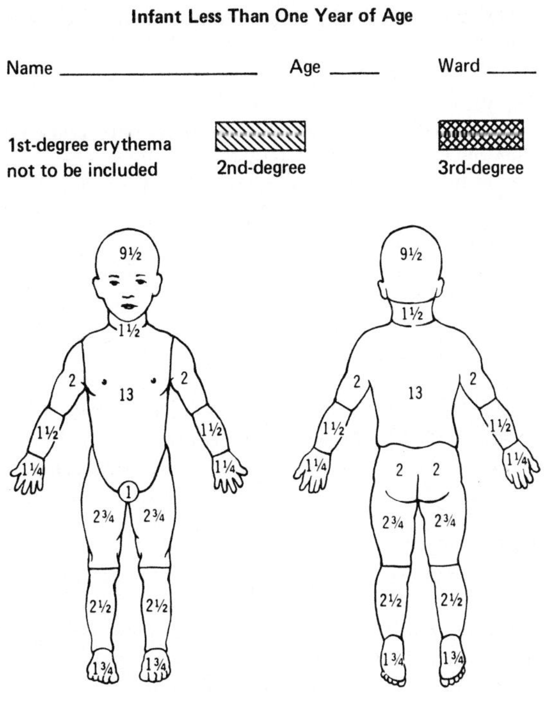

Variations From Adult Distribution in Infants and Children (in Percent).

	Newborn	1 Year	5 Years	10 Years
Head	19	17	13	11
Both thighs	11	13	16	17
Both lower legs	10	10	11	12
Neck	2	These percentages remain constant at all ages.		
Anterior trunk	13			
Posterior trunk	13			
Both upper arms	8			
Both lower arms	6			
Both hands	5			
Both buttocks	5			
Both feet	7			
Genitalia	1			
	100			

Figure 8–5. Lund and Browder modification of Berkow's scale for estimating extent of burns. (The table under the illustration is after Berkow.)

In adults, the "rule of nines" is easy to remember: head and neck (9%), anterior trunk (18%), posterior trunk (18%), each leg (18%), each arm (9%), and anorectal area (1%).

1. Major burns—Burns are classified as major if any of the following are present: (a) partial-thickness burns involving more than 25% of the body surface area in adults or more than 20% in children; (b) full-thickness burns involving more than 10% of the body surface area; (c) burns involving the hands, face, eyes, ears, feet, or perineum; (d) inhalation injuries, electrical burns, or burns complicated by fractures or other major trauma; and (e) burns in poor-risk patients.

2. Moderate uncomplicated burns—These include (a) partial-thickness burns involving 15–25% of the body surface area in adults or 10–25% in children; and (b) full-thickness burns involving less than 10% of the body surface area.

3. Minor burns—These include (a) partial-thickness burns involving less than 15% of the body surface area in adults or less than 10% in children; and (b) full-thickness burns involving less than 2% of the body surface area.

Initial Management

A. Minor Burns and Rare Moderate Burns:

1. Initially, place a cool cloth on the burned area. Burns should be debrided where appropriate. Intact blisters should be left unbroken unless they are present in flexion creases. Partial-thickness burns should be treated with 1% silver sulfadiazine cream (Silvadene) if they involve more than 5% of the body surface area. Smaller burns may be similarly treated, or a fine-mesh gauze impregnated with water-soluble cream or antibiotic cream may be applied. Very small burns may be left exposed.

2. Have the patient return in 24 hours for a dressing change and then every 2–3 days unless the affected areas become malodorous, painful, hot, or red.

B. Major Burns and Most Moderate Burns:

1. Assess the airway and ventilation, and administer oxygen to all patients. Pulmonary complications may be delayed up to 24 hours.

2. Immediately begin fluid replacement with lactated Ringer's injection containing 5% dextrose, given intravenously by 1 or 2 large-bore catheters. The amount is calculated as follows: 4 mL of fluid × the patient's weight (in kilograms) × the percentage of body surface area involved. This is given over a 24-hour period, with half infused over the first 8 hours. Maintenance requirements are given in addition to the amount calculated. No potassium should be added to the fluid.

3. Monitor urine output and specific gravity; the latter is one of the most sensitive indicators of adequacy of fluid therapy.

4. Insert a nasogastric tube.

5. Monitor electrolyte, hematocrit, and arterial blood gas levels.

6. Treat the wounds as follows:

a. Using sterile technique (gown, gloves, cap, and mask), remove burned clothes and examine the patient. Gently scrub the wound with povidone-iodine (Betadine) soap diluted in saline or water. All dead material should be debrided. Intact blisters should not be touched unless they are present in flexion creases.

b. Obtain surgical consultation immediately.

c. Apply 1% silver sulfadiazine cream liberally to wounds, and cover them with a bulky dressing consisting of several layers of absorbent material held in place with a gauze wrapping. Burns on the face and perineum are usually left open after application of the cream.

d. Consider skin grafting after early (1–4 days) wound excision.

7. Give penicillin if there is evidence of group A streptococcal infection.

8. Give a tetanus toxoid booster if the child is immunized, or give tetanus immune globulin if the child is unimmunized.

9. Give antacid therapy.

10. Pain medication may be used once vital signs have stabilized.

11. Parenteral nutrition is often required.

12. Emotional support of the family should be initiated early. Child abuse must be considered.

Barkin RM: Burns. In: *Emergency Pediatrics.* Barkin RM, Rosen P (editors). Mosby, 1984.

Dimick HR: Triage of burn patients. *Top Emerg Med* 1981;**3:**17.

Moncrief JA: Burns. 1. Assessment. 2. Initial management. *JAMA* 1979;**242:**72, 179.

ANIMAL BITES

Animal bites are common in children, dog bites being the most frequently encountered. *Pasteurella multocida* is the most common pathogen, while *Staphylococcus aureus* is often a secondary invader. Rabies is an unusual pathogen but must be considered in any case of animal bite (see Chapter 26). Rodents (rats, mice, gerbils, hamsters, squirrels, etc) rarely carry rabies.

Treatment

Irrigation and debridement of the wound are of paramount importance. Local or regional anesthesia may be required. Irrigation should be done extensively with 1% povidone-iodine (Betadine) solution. All devitalized tissue should be excised to give clear, square edges.

Suturing is indicated for cosmetic or functional reasons and should only be done after thorough irrigation and debridement. Hand injuries and puncture wounds should never be sutured. The wound should be left open if there is any question about the extent of the wound and the adequacy of irrigation or if follow-up difficulties are anticipated.

The risk of infection in patients with animal bites is very high, particularly if wounds are on the hands or feet or if wounds have been sutured. Antibiotics (penicillin or a cephalosporin) should be given in these specific cases.

If indicated, tetanus toxoid should be administered (see Chapter 27) and rabies prophylaxis initiated (see Chapter 26).

HUMAN BITES

Human bites usually cause more tissue damage and carry a higher risk of infection than do bites inflicted by other animals. The most common injury results from a clenched fist striking an opponent's teeth.

Treatment

Irrigation and debridement are of primary importance, as in other bites. The wound should never be sutured but should be soaked and debrided regularly during the healing phase. Antibiotics (cephalosporin) should be initiated, and tetanus immunization should be given if needed. Close follow-up is essential.

HYPERTHERMIA

Exposure to environmental heat without appropriate preparation and protective equipment may lead to one of several preventable illnesses, including heat cramps, exhaustion, and stroke.

Heat Cramps

Heat cramps are caused by prolonged or excessive exercise in an environment with high temperatures and low humidity. The patient sweats profusely and may try to relieve thirst by drinking fluids that do not contain salt. The condition is characterized by severe cramps in skeletal muscles that were subjected to intense work, most commonly those of the legs. Patients are alert and oriented, with normal or slightly elevated temperatures.

If cramps are mild, an oral salt solution (1 tsp of salt in 500 mL of water) can be given. If they are severe, normal saline solution (20 mL/kg) may be given intravenously over 1–2 hours.

Heat Exhaustion

Heat exhaustion results from exposure to high temperatures and continued sweating in the absence of appropriate replenishment of water and salt. The condition is liable to occur in children with unusual salt losses, eg, those with cystic fibrosis or salt-losing renal disease. It may occur in healthy active children who replace sweat losses with inappropriate fluids.

With water depletion, patients develop hypernatremic dehydration and are thirsty, irritable, fatigued, and disoriented. Salt depletion is more common and presents with fatigue, headache, nausea, vomiting, diarrhea, and muscle cramps. Temperatures are normal with either water or salt depletion.

Treatment must reflect the underlying cause. The patient should be removed from heat and sun, and the extracellular fluid volume should be restored, usually after normal saline solution, 20 mL/kg, is given intravenously over 45 minutes. Chapter 36 outlines this approach to rehydration in depth.

Heat Stroke

Although rare, heat stroke results from the inability of the body to dissipate heat. Factors associated with heat stroke include underlying diseases (eg, cystic fibrosis), large body surface areas (eg, in the newborn), and ingestion of drugs (eg, phenothiazines, anticholinergic agents, β-blocking drugs, and ethanol). Although strenuous activity may produce heat stroke, the condition may occur without excess exertion.

Patients present with headache, dizziness, fatigue, confusion, or disorientation, which may progress to coma. The skin is red, hot, and dry, and temperatures over 40 °C (104 °F) are common.

Multiple complications may occur, including coma, acute tubular necrosis, acidosis, dysrhythmia, hepatic damage, and disseminated intravascular coagulation.

Treatment must be initiated immediately, since heat stroke is life-threatening. After the patient is removed from the heat source, the airway should be stabilized, clothing removed, and the patient immersed in cool water. Use of cold compresses may be necessary. The patient should be placed in an ice bath until the temperature reaches 38.5 °C (about 101 °F), and extremities should be massaged. Intravenous fluids should be given to maintain the fluid and electrolyte balance after normal saline solution, 20 mL/kg intravenously, is administered initially over 45–60 minutes. Patients with heat stroke require meticulous medical support and intensive monitoring of vital signs, input and output, and urine specific gravity.

HYPOTHERMIA

Hypothermia is characterized by an internal (core) temperature of 35 °C (95 °F) or less. In children, it usually results from prolonged exposure to the cold. Special rectal thermometers are needed for reading of low temperatures.

Clinical Findings

Patients must be carefully examined for underlying medical problems and trauma associated with or preceding the exposure. The severity of clinical findings reflects the degree and duration of hypothermia and the nature of the exposure. There may be progressive deterioration in mental status, with eventual loss of consciousness, dysrhythmia, coma, and cardiopulmonary arrest. Infants with hypothermia have decreased appetite; lethargy; and cold, erythematous, and scleremic (hardened) skin. Bradycardia and abdominal distention may be observed. Metabolic acidosis, hypoglycemia, and hyperkalemia are usually present.

Frostbite may develop in patients with hypothermia. The severity depends upon the following factors: (1) the intensity of exposure to cold (a function of temperature and wind velocity) as well as increased rates of heat loss from the tissues owing to contact with water or metal and restrictive or tight clothing proximal to the involved areas; (2) the duration of exposure to cold; and (3) the rate of rewarming. Frostbite injury is characterized by loss of sensation of affected parts and white, cold skin over affected areas.

Classification of Cold Injury

A. First-Degree Injury (Frost Nip): Erythema of the skin and edema of the affected part but without blister formation. No significant tissue damage.

B. Second-Degree Injury: Formation of blisters and bullae.

C. Third-Degree Injury: Necrosis of the thick layers and subcutaneous tissues without loss of the affected part.

D. Fourth-Degree Injury: Complete necrosis with gangrene and loss of the affected part.

Complications

Complications include necrosis of the affected area and bacterial infection through broken skin. Late sequelae involving frostbitten areas and lasting months to years have included persistent pain, hyperhidrosis, skin tenderness, cold sensitivity, and retarded epiphyseal growth.

Treatment

A. Frost Nip: Treat by local warming.

B. Superficial and Deep Frostbite:

1. Loosen any garments that restrict blood flow.
2. Remove any wet garments in contact with the skin.
3. Cover the involved area with dry bulky garments.
4. Elevate the affected area.
5. Protect the part from trauma. Do not rub frostbitten tissue or pack with snow, because this macerates the area and causes further damage.
6. Transport the patient to a warm environment, and rewarm the frostbitten area by immersion in a large volume of water preheated to 38–41 °C (about 100–105 °F) for about 20 minutes. Do not rewarm if there is any chance of refreezing during transport. Rewarming with an oven, fire, or other source of dry heat should *not* be attempted, since unequal exposure will result in tissue burns. Analgesics may be required during the rewarming period.
7. Place the patient at bed rest with the part elevated.
8. Maintain local hygiene by whirlpool baths twice a day for 20 minutes at body temperature.

9. Avoid all surgical procedures on cold-injured skin. Do not remove or puncture bullae or blisters.

10. Sympathectomy and paravertebral block are of little value.

11. Amputation of a necrotic limb should be postponed 2–3 months until optimal healing has occurred. If uncontrolled infection supervenes, early amputation may be required.

C. Hypothermia:

1. Initial stabilization must focus on the priorities of airway, breathing, and circulation. The patient should be moved to a warm environment. Treat the underlying disease.

2. Patients with temperatures above 32 °C (89.6 °F) should be rewarmed with external passive measures such as blankets. If there is no increase in temperature, the patient should be evaluated for underlying disease.

3. Temperatures below 32 °C require active rewarming at about 0.5 °C/h.

a. If the cardiovascular system is stable, active external rewarming using warmed blankets and water bottles is appropriate.

b. If the cardiovascular system is unstable, spinal injury exists, or diabetic ketoacidosis is present, initiate active external rewarming combined with the use of humidified heated (40.5 °C [104.9 °F]) oxygen, warmed intravenous fluids, and, lastly, hemodialysis. (Hemodialysis is controversial.) Dysrhythmias should be aggressively treated.

Reuler JB: Hypothermia: Pathophysiology, clinical setting and management. *Ann Intern Med* 1978;**89**:519.

Stine, RJ: Heat illness. *JACEP* 1979;**8**:154.

ELECTRIC SHOCK & ELECTRIC BURNS

The danger of injury from electric shock depends upon the voltage and the frequency. Alternating current is more dangerous than direct current. At a frequency of 25–300 cycles, voltages below 230 volts can produce ventricular fibrillation. High voltages (which may be encountered in television circuits) produce respiratory failure. Faulty wiring of home appliances may lead to electric shock. In homes with young children, it is advisable to install occlusive safety outlets in the play area.

Electric Shock

Consciousness is rapidly lost. If the current continues, death from asphyxia due to ventricular fibrillation or respiratory arrest occurs within a few minutes.

Interrupt the power source or knock the wire away from the skin with a dry piece of wood or other nonconducting material, and institute external cardiac massage or mouth-to-mouth respiration, depending on whether asphyxia is cardiac or respiratory. Supply oxygen if available, and institute appropriate treatment for shock.

Electric Burns

Momentary contact, particularly with a high-voltage outlet, will lead to localized, sharply demarcated, painless gray areas without associated inflammation of the skin. The examiner should search for a second area of grayness where the current has left the body. Sloughing occurs after a few weeks. With simple burns, the skin should be cleansed and a dry dressing applied. Deeper burns should be treated with 1% silver sulfadiazine cream (Silvadene) under an occlusive dressing. Management is the same as for other types of burns. Infection occurs less often with electric burns, but reconstructive surgery for scarring after healing may be required.

Toddlers and young children often sustain electric burns of the mouth by biting an electric cord. They are rarely electrocuted, because the circuit is completed locally in the mouth. There is a local slough of tissue that may lead to brisk bleeding. The defect should be allowed to heal by scarring and the corner of the mouth revised later. Hospitalization is usually indicated.

Orgel MG, Brown HC, Woolhouse FM: Electrical burns of the mouth in children: A method for assessing results. *J Trauma* 1975;**18**:285.

IRRADIATION REACTIONS

The effects of radiation may develop during or after the course of therapeutic x-ray or radium administration or after any exposure to ionizing radiation (eg, x-rays, neutrons, gamma rays, alpha or beta particles). The harmful effects of radiation are determined by the degree of exposure, which in turn depends upon not only the quantity of radiation delivered to the body but also the type of radiation, the duration of exposure, and which tissues of the body are exposed. Three hundred to 500 R (400–600 rads) of x-ray or gamma radiation applied to the entire body at one time would probably be fatal. (For purposes of comparison, a routine chest x-ray delivers about 0.3 R.) Tolerance to radiation is difficult to define, and there is no firm basis for evaluating radiation effects for all types and levels of irradiation.

ACUTE (IMMEDIATE) RADIATION EFFECTS ON NORMAL TISSUES

Diagnosis

A. Injury to Skin and Mucous Membranes: Irradiation causes erythema, depilation, destruction of fingernails, or epidermolysis, depending upon the dose.

B. Injury to Deep Structures:

1. Hematopoietic tissues—Injury to the bone marrow may cause diminished production of blood elements. Lymphocytes are most sensitive and erythrocytes least sensitive. Damage to the blood-forming organs may vary from transient depression of one or more blood elements to complete destruction.

2. Blood vessels—Smaller vessels (capillaries and arterioles) are more readily damaged than larger blood vessels. If injury is mild, recovery occurs.

3. Gonads—In males, small single doses of radiation (200–300 R) cause temporary aspermatogenesis, and larger doses (600–800 R) may cause sterility. In females, single doses of 200 R may cause temporary cessation of menses, and 500–800 R may cause permanent infertility. Moderate to heavy radiation of the embryo in utero results in injury to the fetus or in embryonic death and abortion.

4. Lungs—High or repeated moderate doses of radiation may cause pneumonitis.

5. Salivary glands—The salivary glands may be depressed by radiation, but relatively large doses may be required.

6. Stomach—Gastric secretion may be temporarily (occasionally permanently) inhibited by moderately high doses of radiation.

7. Intestines—Inflammation and ulceration may follow moderately large doses of radiation.

8. Central nervous system—The brain and spinal cord may be damaged by high doses of radiation, owing to impaired blood supply.

9. Resistant structures—The normal thyroid, pituitary, liver, pancreas, adrenals, and bladder are relatively resistant to radiation. Peripheral and autonomic nerves are highly resistant to radiation.

C. Systemic Reaction (Radiation Sickness): The basic mechanisms of radiation sickness are not known. Anorexia, nausea, vomiting, weakness, exhaustion, lassitude, and (in some cases) prostration may occur, singly or in combination. Radiation sickness associated with x-ray therapy is most likely to occur when the therapy is given in large dosage to large areas over the abdomen, less often when given over the thorax, and rarely when given over the extremities. With protracted therapy, this complication is rarely significant. The patient's emotional reaction to the illness or to the treatment plays an important role in aggravating or minimizing such effects.

Prevention

Persons handling radiation sources can minimize exposure to radiation by recognizing the importance of exposure time, distance, and shielding. Areas housing x-ray and nuclear materials must be properly shielded. Untrained or poorly trained personnel should not be permitted to work with x-ray and nuclear radiation. Any unnecessary exposures, diagnostic or therapeutic, should be avoided. X-ray equipment should be periodically checked for reliability of output, and proper filters should be employed. When feasible, it is advisable to shield the gonads, especially of young persons. Fluoroscopic examination should be performed as rapidly as possible, using an optimal combination of beam characteristics and filtration; the tube-to-table distance should be at least 45 cm, and the beam size should be kept to a minimum required by the examination. Special protective clothing may be necessary to protect against contamination with radioisotopes. In the event of accidental contamination, removal of all clothing and vigorous bathing with soap and water should be followed by careful instrument (Geiger counter) check for localization of ionizing radiation.

Treatment

There is no specific treatment for the biologic effects of ionizing radiation. The success of treatment of local radiation effects will depend upon the extent, degree, and location of tissue injury. Treatment is supportive and symptomatic.

A systemic radiation reaction following radiation therapy (radiation sickness) is preferably prevented, but when it does occur, it is treated symptomatically and supportively. Antinauseant drugs, eg, dimenhydrinate (Dramamine), 100 mg 1 hour before and 1 hour and 4 hours after radiation therapy, may be of value. Whole blood transfusions may be necessary if anemia is present. Transfusion of marrow cells has been employed recently. Disturbances of fluid and electrolyte balance require appropriate treatment. Antibiotics may be of use for secondary infection.

DELAYED (CHRONIC) EFFECTS OF EXCESSIVE DOSES OF IONIZING RADIATION

Diagnosis

A. Somatic Effects:

1. Skin scarring and atrophy may occur. Late effects include telangiectases, obliterative endarteritis, pulmonary fibrosis, and intestinal stenosis.

2. Cataracts may occur following irradiation of the lens.

3. Leukemia may occur, perhaps only in susceptible individuals, many years following radiation.

4. The incidence of neoplastic disease is increased in persons exposed to large amounts of radiation, particularly in areas of heavy damage.

5. Microcephaly and other congenital abnormalities may occur in children exposed in utero, especially if the fetus was exposed during the first 4 months of pregnancy.

B. Genetic Effects: Alteration of the sex ratio at birth (fewer males than females) suggests genetic damage. The incidence of congenital abnormalities, stillbirths, and neonatal deaths when conception occurs after termination of radiation exposure is apparently not increased.

Treatment

See treatment of acute radiation reactions.

SELECTED REFERENCES

Barkin RM, Rosen P (editors): *Emergency Pediatrics*. Mosby, 1984.

Mills J et al (editors): *Current Emergency Diagnosis & Treatment*, 2nd ed. Lange, 1985.

Rosen P et al: *Emergency Medicine: Concepts and Clinical Practice*. Mosby, 1983.

Adolescence 9

Elizabeth R. McAnarney, MD, & Donald E. Greydanus, MD

Anyone who wishes to understand a process as complex as health care of teenagers should start with a review of the normal developmental processes of adolescence and puberty. Teenagers are a special group of individuals with some unique medical problems who yet share common health care concerns with children and with adults. They are undergoing a dramatic series of changes that will take them from childhood to adulthood. Puberty thrusts the child—willing or not, prepared or not—into a new phase of growth and development. The individual must within a finite span of years evolve into an autonomous adult capable of functioning intellectually, vocationally, and sexually in ways acceptable to society. The young person must confront complex issues, including physical changes, anticipated separation from parents, peer group influences, emerging sexuality, increasing educational requirements, and socioeconomic problems of success or simply survival in an uncertain and perhaps inhospitable economic environment. Past experiences combine with ongoing adolescent processes to determine what kind of adult the individual will become.

Workers in the health care system have a responsibility to help young people survive this uncertain journey. Those who provide health care to teenagers must recognize that these patients are no longer children and not yet adults, but unique individuals at various psychophysiologic stages depending on many factors in addition to chronologic age. Thus, not all adolescents of a given age are at the same stage of development, and an understanding of the psychologic, physiologic, and cognitive stages of adolescent development is essential in approaching any patient in this age group. This chapter will address various issues that confront the clinician whose patients include teenagers. It begins with a demographic perspective of adolescence and goes on to discuss the problems of adolescence in sections on puberty, behavioral and psychologic aspects of adolescence, and gynecologic disorders of adolescents.

DEMOGRAPHIC PERSPECTIVE OF ADOLESCENT DISORDERS

There are over 40 million teenagers in the USA, constituting 20% of the population, and the number is expected to exceed 54 million by the year 2000. Up to 75% of teenagers live in urban areas. While the sex ratio is nearly equal, the number of male teenagers is slightly greater. Worldwide, there will be over 1 billion young people (ages 15–24) by the year 2000, with most residing in non-Western parts of the world. In this chapter, the terms teenager and adolescent will refer to those ages 10–19 years.

Despite the impression that teenagers are a "healthy" group, significant rates of disease and death are reported in adolescents, and the health care needs of this large and diverse group are considerable.

Chronic Illnesses & Physical Handicaps

About 5 million adolescents (12%) suffer from chronic illnesses or handicaps. Of over 1 million North Americans with **epilepsy,** 90% of cases are diagnosed by age 20 years. The incidence of seizure disorders during adolescence is high: 24.7 per 100,000 population in those 10–14 years of age and 18.6 per 100,000 in those 15–19 years of age. The risk of **diabetes mellitus** during adolescence is also high. With a general incidence of 5.8–10 per 100,000 population, there are currently over 100,000 diabetics under age 20 years in the USA. **Asthma** is reported in 3% of school children 6–16 years of age and represents the most common medical reason for school absenteeism.

Other common disorders in adolescents include dental problems, especially **dental caries,** with the average 15-year-old having 10 "diseased" teeth (ie, teeth missing, decayed, or filled); mild to severe **acne vulgaris,** which is noted in over 80% of teenagers; **hypertension,** recurrent **migraine headaches,** or severe **dysmenorrhea,** noted in about 10% of teenagers; and **eating disorders,** including obesity (10% of adolescents) and anorexia nervosa (1% of teenage girls 16–17 years of age).

Sensory handicaps reported in adolescents include **visual and hearing deficits.** Refractive errors are noted in 20% of older teenagers, but most of these are correctable with glasses or contact lenses. Unfortunately, about 100,000 school children have partial or limited vision. Adolescents with severe hearing deficits comprise about 10% of the 15 million cases reported in the USA. At birth, 1 of every 1000 infants is profoundly deaf and 24 of every 1000 have moderate to severe hearing loss. Various ear disorders during childhood and adolescence increase the number of hearing deficits in the general population.

The incidence of **mental retardation** (IQ below

70) in the general population is about 3%; since 100,000 individuals are born annually with mental deficits, this number is increasing. Currently, over 1 million teenagers in the USA have mental deficits. Many of these teenagers are ambulatory and able to function in society, since 80% are mildly retarded (IQ range of 50–69) and 12% are moderately retarded (IQ range of 35–49).

Of the 125,000 individuals with **paraplegia** in the USA, most are male adolescents 15–24 years of age. As a result of car accidents, sports injuries, and other causes, the number of paraplegics increases by about 10,000 per year. Less severe accidents are frequent in the millions of teenagers participating in various sports programs.

Death

In teenagers 15–19 years of age, the leading causes of death (in order of incidence) in males are **accidents, homicide, suicide,** and **cancer;** in females, they are accidents, cancer, suicide, and homicide.

Accidents, the primary cause of death in teenagers of all ages, account for over 25,000 deaths per year. Most of these are due to car accidents, many of which are precipitated by drug use.

Each year, over 5000 teenagers commit suicide and over 5000 are murdered. The number who attempt suicide is not known, but annual estimates range from 250,000 to over 1 million. Suicide rates have doubled since 1960.

The incidence of cancer in teenagers is over 16 per 100,000 population. The primary sites of cancer are the blood, lymph nodes, bone, and brain.

Behavioral Problems

Psychologic and emotional difficulties during adolescence are diverse and frequently reflect failure to conform to societal standards. **School phobia** and **school (academic) failure** are major problems for many teenagers. On any given day, up to 30% of urban school children are reported absent, and 8% of these are consistently absent from school. School phobia has been estimated to occur in 17 of every 1000 school-age children, and 20% of urban teenagers simply drop out of school after age 14–15 years. The reasons for these school-related problems are numerous and complex, but school failure clearly places the individual at a tremendous disadvantage, especially in a job market requiring increasingly advanced and technical skills.

Studies of **juvenile delinquency** in the USA indicate that 1 of every 9 teenagers (1 of every 6 male adolescents) is referred to juvenile court before age 18, and 3% are declared guilty of a crime. Teenagers up to age 18 are responsible for 40% of all serious crimes; this figure swells to over 60% when individuals 18–21 years of age are included. Each year, as many as one-half million from this group are serving jail sentences.

Other evidence of the tremendous unhappiness noted in today's teenagers is the estimated 1 million or more **runaway adolescents** reported in larger cities. Long-standing psychosocial problems and conflicts usually prompt their leaving home. Unfortunately, many of these teenagers subsequently develop additional psychosocial problems and sometimes medical illnesses, and thus initial problems are worsened. Estimated prevalences of significant psychiatric illnesses in young people range from 12 to 20%, with 50% or more originating in the first decade of life.

Drug and alcohol use and abuse are classic sociocultural phenomena in teenagers. Though many experiment with cigarettes, 11% and 13% of male and female teenagers, respectively, are regular smokers (10 or more cigarettes per day). The effect on rates of illness and death in this cohort during later life is tremendous. Many adolescents experiment with marihuana, and 10% are regular users, with significant detrimental effect on overall adjustment to adolescence. The majority of teenagers (70% or more) try alcohol, and many are regular users. Studies reveal that 25% of high school seniors (17–18 years of age) are intoxicated at least once a month. The negative effects of such alcohol abuse on achievement in adulthood are considerable.

Consequences of Adolescent Sexuality

Studies show that over half of teenagers have experienced coitus by age 19. Though exact numbers are not known, it is clear that millions of teenagers are sexually active, often without sufficient knowledge of the consequences. There are over 1 million teenage **pregnancies** each year, including 30,000 in girls under age 14. These pregnancies result in over 600,000 births, 400,000 abortions, and a maternal death rate of 8.5 per 100,000 live births.

In addition, the adolescent population accounts for millions of cases of **sexually transmitted disease** each year, covering over 20 different disorders. One-fourth of cases of gonorrhea are reported in adolescents, and it is estimated that 5000 female teenagers are absent from school each day because of gonorrhea. In 1980, **gonorrhea** rates were reported as 460 cases per 100,000 general population and 930 cases per 100,000 male teenagers 15–19 years of age. Female teenagers account for 30% or more of the 1 million cases of **pelvic inflammatory disease** each year. About 70% of cases of pelvic inflammatory disease are seen in individuals 25 years of age or less. Each decade, over 1 million cases of infertility due to sexually transmitted disease are reported, and many of these are in adolescents. Some investigators estimate that 10% or more teenagers will become infertile as a consequence of sexually transmitted disease.

Psychosocial problems related to sexual abuse are considerable. Sexual abuse accounts for 12% of child abuse, and each year there are over 5000 cases of reported incest and 60,000 cases of rape. These figures considerably underestimate the actual numbers, since such problems usually go unreported.

Bennett DL: Young people and their health needs: A global perspective. *Semin Adolesc Med* 1985;**1:**1.
Centers for Disease Control: Annual summary 1980: Reported morbidity and mortality in the United States. *MMWR* 1981;**29:**38.
Cohen MI: Adolescent health: Concerns for the eighties. *Pediatr in Rev* 1982;**4:**4.
Hofmann AD, Greydanus DE (editors). *Adolescent Medicine.* Addison-Wesley, 1983.
Strasburger VC: Who speaks for the adolescent? *JAMA* 1983;**249:**1021.

GROWTH & DEVELOPMENT

PUBERTY

A biologic hallmark of adolescence is the specific central nervous system maturation climaxing at the end of latency, producing the physiologic process termed puberty. The hypothalamus produces gonadotropin-releasing hormone (GnRH), which stimulates the maturing anterior pituitary to secrete 2 important hormones: follicle-stimulating hormone (FSH) and luteinizing hormone (LH). Low levels of these hormones can be measured during latency. During very early adolescence, periodic increases in secretion of LH (and FSH to some extent) occur during sleep. By early to middle adolescence, there is a major, more regular secretion of both hormones, resulting in a complex series of pubertal events: In general, LH stimulates secretion of the main male hormone, testosterone, from the testicular Leydig cells. LH also causes ovulation of a mature ovum in the menstruating female. FSH aids spermatogenesis in males, aids maturation of ova in females, and causes secretion of the main female hormone, estradiol. Involved in this process are a series of feedback loops in which testosterone appears to inhibit GnRH and LH activity, while FSH activity is inhibited by a poorly understood protein, inhibin, which is a product of the Sertoli cells.

The mechanism activating the hypothalamic-pituitary-adrenal-gonadal axis, or "pubertal" axis, is unclear. Phenomena thought to trigger pubertal changes include maturation of the amygdala, pineal gland deterioration, adrenal androgen secretions (androstenedione and dehydroepiandrosterone), reduced sensitivity of the hypothalamus to testosterone or estrogen, attainment of a critical weight, and the midcycle LH surge.

Although the pubertal axis is intact in utero and during childhood, it is normally activated between the ages of 8 and 15 years. The appearance of secondary sex characteristics before 8–8½ years of age in girls or before 9–10 years in boys constitutes precocious puberty; development after 14–14½ years in girls or after 15–15½ years in boys constitutes delayed puberty (see Chapter 25).

PHYSICAL CHANGES DURING ADOLESCENCE

The age at onset of physical changes varies among individuals; however, puberty usually proceeds in a sequential pattern once it begins. In girls, the first sign of puberty is the budding of breasts (thelarche). This is sequentially followed by pubic hair growth (pubarche), height velocity peak (9 ± 1 cm per year), onset of menses (menarche), axillary hair growth, and final pubertal changes. In boys, the sequence is early testicular growth, pubarche, further testicular growth, penile growth, nocturnal emissions, height velocity peak (10.2 ± 1.5 cm per year), marked voice change, axillary and facial hair growth, and other final pubertal changes. Once puberty has started, it usually takes 2–4 years for male and female adolescents to reach adult height (25% increase from adolescence) and weight (50% increase). During this time, lymph node tissue regresses, major organs show a 2-fold increase, and there are continuing changes in the genital system.

Sexual Maturity Rating (Tanner Staging)

Tanner's sexual maturity rating system categorizes male and female genital changes (Tables 9–1 and 9–2) by stage, with stage I representing the prepubertal level; stage II, the early pubertal level; stage V, the adult level; and stages III and IV, the intermediate levels of genital changes during puberty. The advantages of this rating scale for clinical use are that it includes age ranges of normal for each level as well as specific descriptions of changes. Thus, the patient is not evaluated merely on the basis of chronologic age. A number of important clinical correlations with this rating scale have been described.

As seen in Table 9–1, girls who are in stage I beyond 14½–15 years of age have delayed puberty and should be evaluated. Height velocity peak in girls often occurs between stages II and III, but its timing is dependent on when stage II occurs. Menarche often occurs in late stage III or early stage IV, 1–3 years after thelarche. There is limited height gain postmenarche, during which time axillary hair develops (stages III–V). Correlating pubertal events with breast stages has proved to be more useful than correlating them with pubic hair stages.

The onset of male puberty is signaled by testicular growth. If the testes have not grown beyond 2.5 cm by age 15, delayed puberty is diagnosed (Table 9–2) and a thorough evaluation begun. Gynecomastia usually occurs during stages II and III. Height velocity peak in boys occurs between stages III and IV or IV and V, in contrast to this phenomenon occurring between stages II and III in girls. This accounts for the discrepancies in height seen in a classroom group

Table 9–1. Sexual maturity rating (Tanner staging) in female adolescents.*

Stage	Breast Growth	Pubic Hair Growth	Other Changes	Age Range (Yr)
I	Preadolescent.	None.	Preadolescent.	0–15
II	Breast budding (thelarche); areolar hyperplasia with small amount of breast tissue.	Long, downy pubic hair near the labia, often appearing with breast budding or several weeks or months later.	Peak growth velocity often occurs soon after stage II.	8 or 8½–15
III	Further enlargement of breast tissue and areola, with no separation of their contours.	Increase in amount and pigmentation of hair.	Menarche occurs in 25% of girls in late stage III.	10–15
IV	Separation of contour; areola and nipple form secondary mound above breast tissue.	Adult in type but not in distribution.	Menarche occurs in most girls in stage IV, 1–3 years after thelarche.	10–17
V	Larger breast with single contour.	Adult in distribution.	Menarche occurs in 10% of girls in stage V.	12½–18

* Slightly modified and reproduced, with permission, from Greydanus DE, McAnarney ER: Adolescence. In: *Survey of Clinical Pediatrics,* 7th ed. Wasserman E, Gromisch DS (editors). McGraw-Hill, 1981.

of children 12–13 years old—ie, there appear to be many tall girls and short boys. The 14-year-old boy in stage II–III often has good potential for growth (if familial genetics allow), while the 14-year-old boy in stage IV–V usually has limited potential, since his growth spurt is probably over.

The Tanner scales can also be used to more accurately predict the course of certain orthopedic disorders (eg, scoliosis, Osgood-Schlatter disease, slipped capital femoral epiphysis), which will worsen during phases of rapid growth. Screening and evaluation of these and other disorders should take into account the sexual maturity rating as well as the chronologic age, since not all adolescents of the same chronologic age share the same characteristics. The application of the rating scale in placing adolescents of the same age into different sports groups is another practical example of the scale's use.

Barnes HV: Physical growth and development during puberty. *Med Clin North Am* 1975;**59:**1305.

Daniel WA Jr: Growth at adolescence: Clinical correlates. *Semin Adolesc Med* 1985;**1:**15.

Table 9–2. Sexual maturity rating (Tanner staging) in male adolescents.*

Stage	Testes Growth	Penis Growth	Pubic Hair Growth	Other Changes	Age Range (Yr)
I	Preadolescent; testes ≤ 2.5 cm.	Preadolescent.	None.	Preadolescent.	0–15
II	Enlargement of testes; increased stippling and pigmentation of scrotal sac.	Minimal or no enlargement.	Long, downy hair, often appearing several months after testicular growth; variable pattern noted with pubarche.	. . .	10–15
III	Further enlargement.	Significant enlargement, especially in length.	Increase in amount; curling.	. . .	10½–16½
IV	Further enlargement.	Further enlargement, especially in diameter.	Adult in type but not in distribution.	Axillary hair and some facial hair develop.	Variable (12–17)
V	Adult in size.	Adult in size.	Adult in distribution (medial aspects of thighs; linea alba).	Body hair continues to grow, and muscles continue to increase in size for several months to years. Peak growth velocity is reached by 20% of boys.	13–18

* Slightly modified and reproduced, with permission, from Greydanus DE, McAnarney ER: Adolescence. In: *Survey of Clinical Pediatrics,* 7th ed. Wasserman E, Gromisch DS (editors). McGraw-Hill, 1981.

Finkelstein JW: The endocrinology of adolescence. *Pediatr Clin North Am* 1980;**27:**53.

Long TJ et al: Basic issues in adolescent medicine. *Curr Probl Pediatr* 1984;**14:**1.

Root AW: Hormonal changes in puberty. *Pediatr Ann* (Oct) 1980;**9:**365.

Tanner JM: *Growth at Adolescence,* 2nd ed. Blackwell, 1962.

BEHAVIORAL & PSYCHOLOGIC CHANGES DURING ADOLESCENCE

Adolescence is a period of transition from dependent childhood to independent adulthood. The transition is characterized by gradual separation from the family, development of rational thought, formation of intimate relationships, and choice of vocation.

Adolescence does not represent a homogeneous stage of development. The rate of psychologic maturation does not always parallel the rate of physical changes, and the psychologic development of adolescents of a specific chronologic age may not adhere specifically to the substages outlined below. For example, some 13-year-olds may be closer to preadolescent development, while others may be closer to middle adolescent development.

Early Adolescence

Early adolescence (10–14 years of age) is marked by an ambivalent attitude toward independence. The adolescent beginning to gain independence from the family may regress and become clinging and dependent when independent actions are challenged. The adolescent's identity at this stage is primarily focused on physical identity—ie, "Who am I as a physically changing person?" Time is spent standing in front of the mirror, examining body parts and becoming acquainted with the changing body. The thoughts of most young adolescents are still oriented toward the present and are on the concrete operational level. A 14-year-old may show some evidence of formal operational thinking, but because use of logic is often tenuous and uncertain, the adolescent may revert to concrete operational thinking. Since most adolescents in this stage are not psychologically mature enough to engage in long-term, intimate, heterosexual relationships, they may form fleeting and undifferentiated (often labeled "homosexual") relationships (see below). This undifferentiated sexuality provides the experience upon which future heterosexual, intimate relationships are formed and usually does not imply that these young people will choose a homosexual life-style as adults.

Middle Adolescence

Middle adolescence (15–16 years of age) is the stage most adults consider to be the most difficult one of adolescent development, since psychologic changes are often rapid. It is the stage of maximal striving for independence from the family. Adolescents in this stage have increased verbal and cognitive skills and often use them to challenge, argue, and debate with adults. In addition, they often have access to automobiles, motorcycles, and public transportation, which facilitates breaking away from the family. Their identity is focused on the question "Who am I as a person and what makes me different from or the same as others in my life?" Quests for independence and identity are reflected in experimental behavior patterns such as testing limits and imposed restrictions, experimenting in sexual behavior, and using cigarettes, alcohol, and drugs. ("I wouldn't know what it felt like unless I tried it.")

During middle adolescence, most young people develop the capacity for formal operational thinking—the ability to "think about thoughts," utilize abstract thinking, and think ahead. As adolescents begin to understand others' thought processes, they become concerned with how others view them. The belief that everyone else is highly interested in the adolescent's thoughts and appearance is part of the general egocentrism, or self-centeredness, of adolescence. This major change from the concrete operational thinking of early adolescence to the formal operational thinking of middle adolescence is dramatic and causes the adolescent to begin to consider the needs of others and to engage in more intimate behavior with others. Even though the heterosexual experimentation and relationships in which these adolescents engage may be of short duration, they provide the background against which mature and intimate adult relationships are built.

Late Adolescence

Late adolescence (17–20 years of age) is the period characterized by establishing independence from the family, becoming more comfortable with personal and sexual identity, and using acquired skills of formal operational thinking to plan for the future and choose a vocation. During this stage, young people often develop lasting sexual relationships.

It is important for pediatricians to remember that although these adolescents look like adults, they are still developing individuals and thus need continuing support and guidance.

Elkind D: *Children and Adolescents: Interpretive Essays on Jean Piaget,* 2nd ed. Oxford Univ Press, 1974.

Hamburg BA: Early adolescence: A time of transition and stress. *Postgrad Med* 1985;**78:**158.

Rutter M et al: Adolescent turmoil: Fact or fantasy? *J Child Psychol Psychiatry* 1976;**17:**35.

Sahler OJZ, McAnarney ER: *The Child From Three to Eighteen.* Mosby, 1981.

SEXUALITY IN ADOLESCENCE

Human sexuality involves physical and psychologic changes that begin prior to birth and continue throughout life, with major changes occurring during adolescence. Not only do the reproductive organs mature, but adolescents become capable of developing intimate relationships, since they are able to move beyond egocentric needs and express and feel genuine concern about others. The pediatrician's and parents' concerns for the child's sexuality should begin during the neonatal period and continue through adolescence.

Early Adolescence

During early adolescence (10–14 years of age), the major focus is on the rapidly changing physical and sexual self. Girls become conscious of their broadening hips and their breast and pubic hair development. Menarche signifies their sexual maturity and reproductive capability. Boys become conscious of testicular and penile growth, darkening and stippling of the scrotal sac, and pubic hair development.

In this stage, adolescents may participate in some fleeting, undifferentiated, playful sexual behavior as an antecedent to future heterosexual behavior. Although this behavior is referred to as "homosexual" behavior, it differs from the homosexual behavior of older adolescents, which may represent a commitment to a homosexual partner and homosexual lifestyle. Masturbation, either alone or in groups of young people, also serves as a preparation for future heterosexual exploration.

Health education in the pediatrician's office may include asking patients to use the Tanner ratings to stage themselves, which adolescents do remarkably accurately. Every adolescent should be taught about both male and female sexual development. Variations of normal, such as leukorrhea and asymmetric breast development in girls and gynecomastia in boys, should also be discussed during early adolescence.

Middle Adolescence

By middle adolescence (15–16 years of age), the major physical changes in the male and female reproductive systems have occurred. Most girls have experienced menarche, and most boys are experiencing seminal emissions and are capable of penile erections.

Sexual behavior is directed toward dating heterosexual partners, first as part of a group; next, with several other couples; and, finally, with the couple alone. Exploratory, experimental heterosexual behavior is common. Such behavior includes holding hands initially, followed by kissing, petting, genital manipulation, and, ultimately, for some adolescents, coital activity. Not all adolescents proceed sequentially through dating and sexual behavior patterns; some may engage in coitus early in the relationship, while others may consciously decide to postpone coitus and engage in less intimate behavior such as petting.

The exploratory sexual behavior of adolescents in this stage differs from the mature sexual relationships of older adolescents and adults. Intimate adult sexual behavior is predicated on a secure sense of self-identity and the ability to move beyond egocentric needs and to care about another. Erikson refers to this young adult stage as one of intimacy versus isolation.

Health education in the pediatrician's office should focus on the adolescent's growing comfort with and responsibility for the body. Those coitally active should understand the consequences of their sexual decisions and should be aware of methods of contraception. Breast self-examination and testicular self-examination should also be taught. (The incidence of carcinoma of the breast is less than that of the testicles.)

Late Adolescence

During late adolescence (17–20 years of age), sexual concerns often focus on a current heterosexual relationship and thoughts about the future. Since adolescents in this stage have acquired formal operational thinking skills, they begin to consider the future in terms of vocational and educational choices as well as sexual life-style choices (heterosexual versus homosexual) and plans about marriage and family. Some adolescents may plan to start their families early and to follow their parents' vocation. Others may choose to pursue their education prior to having a family.

Emphasis of health education should be placed on consideration of sexual and personal responsibilities. Sexually active adolescents who wish to delay an untimely pregnancy should be advised in the use of contraception.

One national survey reported that in 1979, 46% of "never-married" female adolescents 15–19 years of age had engaged in coitus: 22% of 15-year-olds surveyed, 38% of 16-year-olds, 48% of 17-year-olds, 57% of 18-year-olds, and 69% of 19-year-olds. The numbers for male adolescents in each age group are thought to be higher. These figures indicate that a large number of adolescents in this age group are at risk for pregnancy and sexually transmitted diseases.

Doyle KLL, Cassell C: Teenage sexuality: The early adolescent years. *Obstet Gynecol Annu* 1981;**10**:423.

Greydanus DE, Dewdney D (editors): Adolescent sexuality and pregnancy. (2 parts.) *Semin Adolesc Med* 1985;**1**:97, 152.

Jones R, Shearin R: Communicating with adolescents and young adults about sexuality. *Pediatr Ann* 1982;**11**:733.

Satterfield S: Common sexual problems of children and adolescents. *Pediatr Clin North Am* 1975;**22**:643.

BEHAVIORAL & PSYCHOLOGIC ASPECTS OF PROBLEMS DURING ADOLESCENCE

Interview

Knowledge of adolescent psychologic development, an appreciation of the importance of the interview as a major source of data gathering, and interviewing experience with many adolescents all facilitate a thorough understanding of the individual adolescent seeking care.

A good interview should sound like a relaxed conversation. Ensuring privacy and comfort and explaining guidelines for confidentiality will optimize the quality of the interview.

A. Privacy and Comfort: Privacy is important from both the adolescent's and the pediatrician's perspectives, since it decreases distractions from the environment and also provides an atmosphere in which personal information can be shared without concern for random disclosure to others. Comfort of the interviewer and the adolescent is critical. Because adolescents may be frightened in the initial interview, a statement such as "It is not unusual for young people to be scared initially when they come here" may be helpful in decreasing anxiety.

B. Confidentiality: Before the interview begins, it is important to discuss guidelines for confidentiality, since the adolescent will only share what are often painful and frightening experiences if trust is established. Both adolescents and their parents may question whether what they tell the pediatrician will be repeated to other family members.

An initial statement such as the following may be offered: "Mary, you may wonder whether I plan to discuss the content of our interviews with your parents. I will not be discussing what we talk about, unless in my judgment your parents must know. If that were to happen, I would let you know, and then you would have the choice of telling them yourself in my presence or having me tell them." The same guidelines are discussed with the parents, assuring them that their discussions will remain confidential unless that would not be in their or their child's best interests.

At times, it becomes necessary to disclose interview data, such as when a suicidal adolescent girl will not tell her parents about her suicidal thoughts but feels frightened by them and isolated from others; in this case, it is important for her parents to know about her thoughts, and the adolescent will often want someone else to tell them and feel relieved when the parents know.

C. Approach to Interviewing: A thorough understanding of the differences between early, middle, and late adolescence is critical for acquiring optimal information. Open-ended, exploratory statements such as "Tell me about your problems" may elicit a blank stare from the patient in early adolescence who has not yet developed formal operational thinking skills or the ability to utilize abstract thinking. Adolescents who have concrete operational thinking skills should be asked specific questions for which specific answers can be given. The interview may begin with questions about pets, hobbies, sports, and other topics familiar to the patient before problems are discussed.

The challenge in interviewing patients in middle adolescence is determining whether they are closer to early adolescence or middle adolescence in their thinking skills. Teenagers in middle adolescence may, in fact, vacillate from concrete to formal operational thinking, depending upon when and under what circumstances they are being interviewed.

Most patients in late adolescence have formal operational thinking skills and can handle open-ended interviews well. The open-ended interview is often effective in eliciting a wide range of responses that supplement factual information. (See also Chapter 24.)

Cohen MI: The Society for Behavioral Pediatrics: A new portal in a rapidly moving boundary. *Pediatrics* 1984;**73**:791.

Felice M, Friedman SB: The adolescent as a patient. *J Cont Educ Pediatr* 1978;**20**:15.

Rapp CE: The adolescent patient. *Ann Intern Med* 1983;**99**:52.

Smith J, Felice M: Interviewing adolescent patients: Some guidelines for the clinician. *Pediatr Ann* (June) 1980;**9**:238.

DEPRESSION DURING ADOLESCENCE

Symptoms and signs of depression in adolescents may differ from those in adults, and thus depression often goes unrecognized. While depression in adults is usually characterized by stated feelings of sadness and changes in mood, appetite, sleep patterns, and sexual drive, that of adolescents may take the form of behavioral disturbances such as suicidal behavior, functional pain, conversion symptoms, eating disorders, school problems, acting-out behavior, and other problems discussed in sections below. Since depression may precede the onset of these behavioral disorders, their effective management includes the treatment of depression.

Depression during adolescence may be the first symptom of serious psychiatric conditions such as schizophrenia or affective disorders.

Presentation

The presentation of depression during adolescence will reflect the adolescent's stage of development. Patients in early adolescence may not recognize their sadness and may present with one or more of the following "depressive equivalents": (1) boredom and restlessness; (2) fatigue and preoccupation with bodily functions, most often reflected in multiple somatic complaints (eg, headache, abdominal pain, and dizziness) that are vague and poorly defined; (3) difficulty in concentrating, most often reflected in poor school performance; (4) acting-out behavior (eg, temper tantrums, conflicts with authority figures, running away from home); and (5) flight to or from people, manifested either as clinging to an adult or close friend or as complete isolation from others. Young adolescents may even cling to a family pet, since the pet makes fewer demands than humans. When asked whether he or she is sad, the young adolescent may deny this feeling, primarily because concrete operational thinking skills are not adequate for full understanding of feelings. Since early adolescence is probably the major stage during which depression is undiagnosed, the pediatrician should closely follow patients in whom depression is suspected.

Depression during middle adolescence may reflect a mixed presentation of the "depressive equivalents" of early adolescence and the adultlike presentation of late adolescence. The presentation of depression is closely related to the level of cognitive development.

Depression during late adolescence, when the young person is fully capable of formal operational thinking, is likely to be similar in presentation to depression in adults: stated feelings of sadness, tearfulness, abdominal pain or headaches, appetite disturbances (eg, overeating, undereating), sleep difficulties (eg, early morning wakefulness, disrupted or prolonged sleep), and changes in sexual behavior (eg, withdrawal, promiscuity). Most older adolescents comprehend the meaning of "feeling sad" and acknowledge this feeling when asked directly.

Diagnosis

Acute depression is usually reactive, resulting from a real or fantasized loss. The history is commonly one of normal growth and development, with onset of depression after the loss of a family member or friend through illness, death, or divorce or in anticipation or fear of such a loss. Even the death of a pet may trigger depression. Adolescents with acute depression are basically healthy and are responding normally to a real or imagined loss, much the way others would respond to such circumstances. The depression is often of short duration (eg, 6 months).

Chronic depression often has an indolent course. It may result from environmental stress or deprivation, or it may have a genetic basis (eg, manic-depressive illness). The dexamethasone suppression test may be helpful in diagnosis of endogenous chronic depression. The history is usually one of long-term sadness and never having experienced joy, and the patient often relates that symptoms are similar to those of other family members. (See also Chapter 24.)

Treatment

In acute depression, recognizing and discussing the adolescent's sense of loss, giving reassurances that such feelings are normal, and mobilizing family support may help resolve feelings of sadness and depression. Adolescents who are chronically depressed may benefit from psychiatric referral and possibly from antidepressant medication.

Aylward GP: Understanding and treatment of childhood depression. *J Pediatr* 1985;**107:**1.

Herzog GB, Rathburn JM: Childhood depression. *Am J Dis Child* 1982;**136:**115.

Puig-Antich J: Clinical and treatment aspects of depression in childhood and adolescence. *Pediatr Ann* 1984;**13:**37.

Schowalter JE: Depression in children and adolescents. *Pediatr Rev* 1981;**3:**51.

SUICIDAL BEHAVIOR DURING ADOLESCENCE

Suicidal behavior during adolescence, either threatened or actual, should always be taken seriously as a "cry for help." Suicide is the third leading cause of death among young people 15–24 years of age and follows accidents and homicide in that order. The rates of suicide for males and females have at least doubled since 1960. The majority of suicidal adolescents are depressed, and some may have more serious psychologic disorders, such as psychosis.

Contrary to earlier beliefs that suicidal behavior was a "surprise" behavior, most professionals now agree that suicidal behavior during adolescence usually has several antecedents, often detailed in a careful interview. These antecedents include (1) a long-term history of problems such as environmental deprivation or generally poor coping ability during periods of stress; (2) escalation of personal problems (eg, home problems, school problems); (3) progressive isolation from other people who might be able to help the adolescent; (4) short-term or long-term inability to recover from real or fantasized losses, especially the loss of an individual upon whom the adolescent has relied in the past (eg, a family member, an adult who is particularly important to the adolescent, or a close friend who has broken off friendship or has moved away); and (5) serious consideration of suicide as a solution to problems and as a means of expressing anguish to others.

Presentation

The adolescent may be referred to the physician after talking of suicide or after an attempt at suicide, or suicidal behavior may be noted incidentally during examination for another problem (eg, depression). In the latter case, the patient may find thoughts of self-destructive behavior so frightening that he or she has never admitted or discussed them. The professional who suspects the adolescent is suicidal may say: "I am concerned about you, because you seem sad. When people are sad, they sometimes consider hurting themselves or killing themselves. Have you had thoughts of killing yourself?"

Diagnosis

In the diagnosis of suicidal behavior, the clinician should determine the nature and duration of suicidal thoughts and actions, the patient's history of depression, and the family history of depression and suicidal behavior. It should also be determined whether the behavior represents a **suicidal gesture,** a serious **suicidal attempt,** or a **suicidal gamble.**

Suicidal gestures are more frequent in females than in males and most often involve ingestion of a toxic substance after minimal planning. There is usually some prior communication of plans either through a telephone call to a friend or the placement of a note where others will find it. The gesture often represents the first time the adolescent has shown suicidal behavior and is frequently a response to the real or fantasized loss of a special person. The patient may be mildly or moderately depressed but commonly has a history of good interpersonal relationships. The family usually responds in a concerned and consistent, caring manner.

Suicidal attempts are more frequent in males than in females and commonly involve violent methods such as use of firearms or hanging—methods meant to kill. Although ingestants may be used, they are less likely to be used by young people with serious intentions of suicide. The suicidal attempt is usually carefully planned to occur without intervention (eg, when other members of the family are away from home), and there is usually no prior communication (notes, telephone calls) about the suicidal act. The patient commonly has a history of chronic depression and poor interpersonal relationships and may be psychotic. The family may respond to the suicide attempt with minimal distress, ignoring the gravity of the adolescent's behavior.

Suicidal gambles share some of the characteristics of suicidal gestures and suicidal attempts and may be considered the middle ground between gestures and attempts. Those taking a gamble leave it to chance circumstances to determine whether they live or die. Adolescents who make suicidal gambles usually are females who exhibit suicidal behavior more than once to draw attention to their distress.

Treatment

Psychologic evaluation follows medical treatment for ingestion of a toxic substance or for wounds. The evaluation focuses on the dynamics of the suicidal act; determination of whether the act represents a suicidal gesture, attempt, or gamble; and the diagnosis of premorbid depression or psychosis.

Most adolescents who have made suicidal gestures can be followed on an outpatient basis, as long as one health care professional assumes full responsibility for following the patient and contacting the patient if he or she fails to return for an appointment. Failure to keep an appointment may be the adolescent's way of asking "Do you care about me?"

Adolescents who make serious suicide attempts need psychiatric inpatient treatment. They often show continued determination to kill themselves and may well act on their impulses if they do not receive adequate psychiatric care and appropriate protection (usually not available in general medical wards).

Adolescents who make suicidal gambles often require hospitalization (in an adolescent unit or a general medical ward) to clarify the patient's history and details of the action and to determine whether the behavior represents a gamble or an attempt. Hospitalization also serves to emphasize the gravity of the problem to the adolescent and the family.

Adolescents who are talking of or thinking of suicide also may warrant hospitalization as a means of prevention and as a statement of the health care professional's concern for the young person's distress.

The ideal approach to suicidal behavior during adolescence is a preventive one: early recognition and treatment of depression before the adolescent needs to "cry for help." These young people often wonder whether anyone cares about them and their fate. An empathic, caring professional can often provide reassurance and stability in their lives. (See also Chapter 24.)

Committee on Adolescence, American Academy of Pediatrics: Teenage suicide. *Pediatrics* 1980;**66:**144.

Hodgman CH: Recent findings in adolescent depression and suicide. *Dev Behavior Pediatr* 1985;**6:**162.

Marks A: Management of the suicidal adolescent on a nonpsychiatric adolescent unit. *J Pediatr* 1979;**95:**305.

Seiden RH: Death in the West: A regional analysis of the youthful suicide rate. *West J Med* 1984;**140:**969.

FUNCTIONAL PAIN DURING ADOLESCENCE

Pain of nonorganic cause is common during adolescence. The major sites of functional pain are the abdomen and head. Pain in the back or joints is also reported.

Presentation

Functional abdominal pain or headaches usually occur as vague, diffuse, chronic, recurrent symptoms. When asked where the pain is located, the adolescent usually indicates that pain is all over the abdomen or the head. Functional pain usually does not wake the adolescent from sleep. These symptoms of functional pain are in marked contrast to those of organically caused pain, which may be localized (eg, classic appendicitis, with pain in the right lower quadrant) and may wake the adolescent from sleep.

Diagnosis

The interview should elicit information about the onset, duration, severity, and location of the pain, with particular emphasis on information needed for differentiating nonorganic from organic pain. Questions should be directed toward conditions that exacerbate or relieve the pain (eg, foods, certain positions). The psychosocial history should include school history (appropriateness of grade level for chronologic age, marks in school, recent change in performance level, absenteeism secondary to the pain, and behavioral changes noted by school personnel); family history (recent change in family structure, in health of the parents and siblings, or in parents' jobs or financial status); and peer history (activities with peers and recent changes in peer relationships). Adolescents with functional pain often show signs of psychosocial dysfunction.

Physical examination of the adolescent with abdominal pain should focus on abdominal, chest, and gynecologic examinations, which may reveal abdominal distention, hyperactive bowel sounds, or abdominal mass; rales, suggestive of pneumonia; or pelvic mass. Appropriate tests should be performed if the history or examination suggests ulcers, chronic inflammatory bowel disease, cholecystitis, cholelithiasis, urinary tract infection, menstrual cramps, ovarian dysfunction, pelvic inflammatory disease, or other diseases possibly causing the pain.

Physical examination of the adolescent with headaches should focus on neurologic and ophthalmoscopic examinations, which may reveal impaired cranial nerve function, decreased visual field (detected by confrontation), asymmetric or impaired reflexes, or cerebellar signs. Organic causes of headache, such as seizures, brain tumor, migraine, or vascular malformation, should be ruled out.

In cases of back and joint pains, arthritis should be ruled out.

For adolescents with pain of probable functional origin, the minimal laboratory evaluation should include a complete blood count to screen for leukocytosis and anemia and an erythrocyte sedimentation rate, particularly for adolescents with abdominal pain, to screen for chronic inflammatory bowel disease. A normal erythrocyte sedimentation rate does not rule out chronic inflammatory bowel disease, since some adolescents with this disease have normal rates.

Treatment

Functional pain is real pain, and this must be acknowledged to the adolescent and the adolescent's family. The pediatrician should not underestimate the therapeutic value of a complete history and physical examination, including screening tests, for adolescents who may fear they have a life-threatening condition such as cancer. Treatment should be directed toward determining why the adolescent has the pain and what the symptom means to the adolescent and toward a return to normal function (in school, peer, and other activities) as soon as possible. Many adolescents benefit from a series of counseling sessions in which the major focus is on problem solving and not on pain. In fact, in order to decrease the adolescent's secondary gain of having the pain (eg, increased attention), some practitioners choose not to discuss the pain unless the adolescent initiates the discussion.

It is important not to terminate follow-up care as soon as symptoms resolve. If treatment is terminated too soon, the adolescent may again become symptomatic in order to continue the secondary gain of seeing the professional. As the adolescent becomes asymptomatic, the frequency of the contacts may be decreased gradually. Adolescents who feel ready to terminate their contacts with the health professional often cancel appointments on their own.

Hall RCW et al: Physical illness presenting as psychiatric disease. *Arch Gen Psychiatry* 1978;**35:**1315.

Hughes MJ: Recurrent abdominal pain and childhood depression. *Am J Orthopsychiatry* 1984;**54:**146.

Masek BJ, Russo DC, Varni JW: Behavioral approaches to the management of chronic pain in childhood. *Pediatr Clin North Am* 1984;**31:**1113.

Routh DK, Ernst AR: Somatization disorder and relatives of children and adolescents with functional abdominal pain. *J Pediatr Psychol* 1984;**9:**427.

CONVERSION SYMPTOMS DURING ADOLESCENCE

Conversion symptoms during adolescence may be difficult to distinguish from functional pain. Engel (1970) has described conversion as a "psychic mechanism whereby an idea, fantasy, or wish is expressed in bodily rather than verbal terms and is experienced by the patient as a physical rather than a mental symptom."

Presentation

There are a number of presentations of conversion, the most common of which are abdominal pain, headache, chest pain, paresthesias, inability to walk, paralysis of an extremity, syncope, and dizziness. As with functional pain, the symptoms are often vague and do not fit the criteria for diagnosis of an organic condition. (See also Chapter 24.)

Diagnosis

Diagnosis is based on the inclusion of criteria for conversion and should *not* be based solely on exclusion of organic causes—ie, "We've completed every test we can think of and the results are all normal, so the patient must have conversion symptoms."

The history, physical examination, and laboratory evaluation are similar to those for functional pain (see above).

Criteria for the diagnosis of conversion (Friedman, 1973) include the following:

(1) Symptoms have symbolic meaning—eg, an adolescent who masturbates and feels guilty may develop paralysis of the arm.

(2) Symptoms offer a primary gain such as reduction of anxiety—eg, paralysis of the arm prevents masturbation and reduces anxiety or conflicting feelings about masturbation.

(3) Symptoms offer secondary gains that aid the adolescent in coping—eg, symptoms justify absence from school and gain increased attention from parents, friends, and health care professionals.

(4) Symptoms are not limited to but are more common in adolescents with hysterical personalities. Adolescents with hysterical personalities often are theatrical in the way they describe their symptoms (eg, the stomach pain is like a lightning bolt), and their behavior with individuals of the opposite sex is often seductive.

(5) There may be an apparent indifference or lack of concern about the symptoms (*la belle indifférence*), even though the person complains bitterly of the symptoms. At times, it is difficult to differentiate *la belle indifférence* from boredom resulting from the repetition of describing the symptoms to numerous interviewers.

(6) Symptoms often become manifest at times of

personal or family stress. Some adolescents are very sensitive to family stress, particularly financial problems and marital problems, and the adolescent's symptoms may be a "cry for help" for the entire family.

(7) The parents are often overprotective of their children and continue to be overprotective, even after the children are mature and fully capable of independent functioning.

(8) The family members often are very health-oriented and discuss their health concerns in family settings, such as at the dinner table.

(9) There is a model for the symptom. The question "Whom else do you know with this problem?" gives approval to the fact that someone else has the symptom and is more likely to elicit an accurate history than the question "Do you know anyone else with the same symptoms?" for which the answer is usually "No."

(10) There is often a history of unexplained symptoms in the past and may be a history of surgical procedures for abdominal symptoms.

Fulfillment of the majority of these criteria is critical to the diagnosis of conversion symptoms.

The diagnosis is usually made from results of outpatient interviews and examinations. However, hospitalization may be indicated to confirm the diagnosis, in which case the length of hospitalization should be as short as possible. Prolonged hospitalization during diagnosis may provide additional secondary gain and thus reinforce the symptoms.

Treatment

Treatment includes discussion of the diagnosis with the adolescent and parents and careful follow-up by the primary care professional or referral to a specialist. In most cases, we recommend that the adolescent be followed by the primary care professional, so if the nature of the symptoms changes, appropriate reevaluation for organic causes of the symptoms can occur in the context of a supportive relationship.

Treatment is similar to that outlined for functional pain (see above) and should focus on problem solving and coping with stress. Discussions about and reinforcement of the conversion symptom should be avoided. Short, frequent sessions are often more successful than long, infrequent contacts.

Engel G: Conversion symptoms. Page 650 in: *Signs and Symptoms.* Macbryde C, Blacklow R (editors). Lippincott, 1970.

Friedman S: Conversion symptoms in adolescents. *Pediatr Clin North Am* 1973;**20:**873.

Lazare A: Conversion symptoms. *N Engl J Med* 1981;**305:**745.

Maloney MJ: Diagnosing hysterical conversions in children. *J Pediatr* 1980;**97:**1016.

Oberfield RA, Rueben RN, Burkes LJ: Interdisciplinary approach to conversion disorders in adolescent girls. *Psychosomatics* 1983;**24:**983.

OTHER HYSTERICAL SYMPTOMS DURING ADOLESCENCE

Some adolescents express their anxiety as a response to stress through one of several dramatic conditions such as hyperventilation, syncope, or seizures.

Hyperventilation

Symptoms may include tingling and numbness of the extremities, syncope, chest tightness and a sensation of smothering, palpitations or a "racing" heart, and weakness. Some adolescents will acknowledge that they breathe very quickly prior to the onset of symptoms, and the symptoms can often be reproduced by asking the adolescent to hyperventilate.

A thorough understanding of the reasons for the adolescent's anxiety is imperative. Counseling should be directed toward constructive problem solving with the adolescent and often the family. It may be helpful for some patients to use a rebreathing bag when they begin to experience feelings of anxiety. Although this may prevent or alleviate the symptoms of hyperventilation, the primary goal of treatment is relief of the adolescent's stress and anxiety.

Syncope

Syncope may be considered a conversion symptom, since it often represents expression of an idea or fantasy in bodily rather than mental terms. Hysterical syncope is seen more commonly in female adolescents, and its presentation is similar to that of a "swoon," usually occurring in the presence of others and in a manner that avoids injury. The patient most often collapses from either a standing or sitting position and may or may not lose consciousness. If the patient's eyes are closed during syncope, the examiner may encounter resistance to opening them.

Diagnosis is based on a negative history of seizure diathesis (no aura, incontinence, jerking movements of the extremities, or postictal state) and normal findings on neurologic examination. Observation of an episode of syncope, with documentation of its nature, is critical. The adolescent's reactions to and perceptions of the episodes are also important. If it is difficult to determine the nature of the episode, a short hospitalization may be warranted to allow the examiner to observe the syncope.

Treatment is directed toward determining the reasons for syncope and what meaning syncope has for the patient. Counseling should be directed toward solving conflicts experienced by the adolescent.

Psychogenic Seizures

Psychogenic seizures, with complete blackout and amnesia to the time of the seizure, are more commonly seen in female adolescents. Bodily injury is usually avoided.

Diagnosis is based on a negative history of seizure diathesis (see above), normal electroencephalographic findings, and normal blood glucose and serum electrolyte levels. In most cases, seizures are a response to circumstances from which the patient is trying to escape, eg, separation from or death of a loved one, or divorce of the parents.

Treatment is similar to that of syncope. (See also Chapter 23.)

Goodyer IM: Epileptic and pseudoepileptic seizures in childhood and adolescence. *J Am Acad Child Psychiatry* 1985;**24:**3.

Gross M: Pseudoepilepsy: A study in adolescent hysteria. *Am J Psychiatry* 1979;**136:**210.

Herman SP, Stickler GB, Lucas AR: Hyperventilation syndrome in children and adolescents: Long-term follow-up. *Pediatrics* 1981;**67:**183.

Missri J, Alexander S: Hyperventilation syndrome. *JAMA* 1978;**240:**2093.

PREGNANCY DURING ADOLESCENCE

About 46% of never-married women who are 15–19 years of age report having had coitus, and each year about 1 million women under 20 years of age become pregnant. In the majority of these pregnancies, the male partner is also an adolescent. Thus, close to 2 million adolescents are affected each year by teenage pregnancy.

Presentation

Although some adolescents may immediately state concern about being pregnant, younger ones may believe the pediatrician will "guess" that they are pregnant and, thus, may present with vague complaints, such as headache or abdominal pain; only when the menstrual history is taken does it become clear that the patient is amenorrheic.

Diagnosis

The history should include age at menarche, last and past menstrual periods, and symptoms of vaginal spotting, nausea or vomiting, or breast tenderness or polyuria. Physical examination should include pelvic evaluation for uterine enlargement. Pregnancy may be confirmed by a urine test, but false-negative results have been reported up to 6 weeks after the missed period. Serum pregnancy tests based on radioimmunoassay of human chorionic gonadotropin may be positive as early as 7 or 8 days following conception.

Treatment

The pediatrician has a clear role in the diagnosis of the pregnancy and in outlining options for disposition of the pregnancy. Some pediatricians will also choose to provide supportive counseling for the pregnant adolescent.

Once pregnancy is confirmed, determination of the gestational age of the fetus is a priority, since it will influence the options available to the pregnant woman. Thus, referral of the adolescent to an obstetrician or specialist in an adolescent maternity program must be expedited.

If the fetus is less than 20 weeks of age, the options are continuation of the pregnancy, with subsequent self-parenting or adoption of the child, or termination of the pregnancy. Abortion is legally possible in some situations up to 23 weeks, but there is increasing argument regarding the use of abortion in the 20th–23rd weeks. The actual age of fetal viability remains extremely controversial. The decision to continue or terminate the pregnancy is ideally made by the adolescent and those with close emotional ties, ie, the parents and boyfriend. Although disposition of the pregnancy ultimately is the adolescent's decision, the degree of influence of others will vary, depending upon the adolescent's developmental age and the degree of parental and partner participation in the decision-making process. If the patient is in early adolescence, her parents may be more actively involved in decision making; if she is in late adolescence, her partner may be more influential than her parents.

In any case, a review of the decision-making process is warranted to determine that all options have been carefully considered and the patient is not making a premature decision about a matter that has lifelong implications.

McAnarney ER: Adolescent pregnancy and child-bearing: New data, new challenges. *Pediatrics* 1985;**75:**973.

McAnarney ER (editor): *Premature Adolescent Pregnancy and Parenthood.* Grune & Stratton, 1983.

Stuart IR, Wells CF (editors): *Pregnancy in Adolescence: Needs, Problems, and Management.* Van Nostrand-Reinhold, 1982.

Teenage pregnancy and fertility trends: United States 1974 and 1980. *JAMA* 1985;**253:**3064.

EATING DISORDERS DURING ADOLESCENCE

Eating disorders during adolescence are becoming an area of increasing concern to pediatricians, who are frequently faced with the problem of determining "how thin is too thin." Classic anorexia nervosa is seen in 4.6 of 1000 school-age girls, but the incidence of the variants of anorexia nervosa, such as thinness associated with active exercising (jogging, preparation for sports such as football, ballet dancing) and forced vomiting, is less clear.

1. ANOREXIA NERVOSA

The exact cause of anorexia nervosa has not been determined, but the condition is believed to be influenced by physiologic and psychologic factors. Anorexia is seen in 9 times as many females as males and occurs primarily among those of middle to upper socioeconomic status. The classic picture is that of a hyperactive, emaciated female who, despite her inanition, denies being thin.

Diagnosis

The diagnosis of anorexia nervosa is based upon several criteria.

A. Voluntary Dieting: The typical history is one of voluntary dieting, weight loss, and subsequent inability to stop dieting and losing weight. There is often a family history of chronic dieting.

B. Weight Loss: A weight loss of greater than 20% of the average body weight is usually considered diagnostic, but this standard is controversial. The weight loss is often denied by the anorectic patient.

C. Forced Vomiting or Catharsis: Some adolescents will admit to use of forced vomiting or laxatives to rid themselves of nutrients after eating.

D. Preoccupation With Food: Some anorectic adolescents cook for the family, despite their lack of interest in eating. Others choose food-related careers. Most have an extensive understanding of calories and dietary requirements and are often more knowledgeable about foods than the health professionals who are providing their care.

E. Hypometabolic Symptoms:

1. Amenorrhea follows weight loss in the majority of cases; however, it may precede weight loss in some instances.

2. Hypothermia, bradycardia, and hypotension are present in adolescents who have lost significant amounts of weight. The patient often complains of feeling cold. Shaking hands with the patient usually reveals that skin is cool to touch, and the hands may appear cyanotic. Patients with significant weight loss and severe hypometabolic symptoms are at risk for cardiac dysrhythmia and cardiac arrest.

F. Laboratory and X-ray Evaluation:

1. Pancytopenia, anemia, leukopenia, and thrombocytopenia are common.

2. Serum levels of cholesterol and glutamic-oxaloacetic transaminase may be increased, while total protein and albumin levels may be decreased or normal.

3. Decreased alkaline phosphatase levels may be found.

4. Changes in hormonal profile may include decreased levels of luteinizing hormone and follicle-stimulating hormone, loss of diurnal variation in cortisol levels, decreased triiodothyronine levels, normal or increased growth hormone levels, and flattened glucose tolerance curves.

5. Dehydration may be reflected in elevated levels of blood urea nitrogen and elevated specific gravity of urine.

6. CT scans reveal dilated ventricles in some anorectic adolescents.

G. Psychosocial Aspects:

1. Most anorectic adolescents have a distorted body image.

2. Most have been described as "good children" with high academic achievement.

3. Most pursue their thinness in a compulsive manner that is similar to the way in which they exercise and study.

4. Many show signs of depression. Contrary to earlier studies indicating that anorectic adolescents were not depressed, we have more recently found that many of these patients show signs of depression on admission to our inpatient facilities. It is difficult to determine whether depression is secondary to the biologic effects of starvation or whether it is primary and present before the adolescent begins dieting.

5. Family relationships are often distorted, and there may be major conflicts within the family involving separation, control, independence, and individuation.

6. Most anorectic adolescents avoid close heterosexual relationships. This is thought to be an attempt by the adolescent to regress sexually or not to mature at all. Even though some patients do achieve heterosexual intimacy, many engage in superficial, hysterical interactions.

Differential Diagnosis

Hypopituitarism, hypothyroidism, chronic inflammatory bowel disease, and depression with secondary anorexia should be considered.

Treatment

There is no universal treatment for anorexia in adolescents. Treatment can only begin when the symptomatic patient and the family recognize the need for treatment. Some families delay seeking treatment until the adolescent shows marked physical signs of debilitation, which is often a poor prognostic sign.

The pediatrician's primary role is the improvement and maintenance of the adolescent's physical well-being. The role is shared with the psychiatrist or psychologist.

The authors utilize inpatient care freely, as it often communicates to the adolescent and family our concern for the patient's well-being. Inpatient care also allows for complete and structured medical and psychologic evaluations.

If the adolescent does not begin to eat during hospitalization, behavior modification techniques are employed. A "contract" outlining the goals (amount of weight gain, schedule for gaining weight, etc) is negotiated, and rewards are based on fulfilling the contract and gaining weight. All staff members are informed of the contract terms to ensure that inappropriate behavior is not reinforced. In the authors' inpatient setting, nurses play a major role in developing and managing the contract with the adolescent.

Adolescents with severe (30% or more) weight loss are at risk for electrolyte imbalance, fluid overload, and cardiac failure if caloric intake is increased too quickly. Thus, initial daily intake is restricted to 1500 kcal and then gradually increased by 200–300 kcal every 3–4 days.

Close communication between the pediatrician and psychiatrist is vital, so that decisions are clear and manipulation of the health professionals by the adolescent is minimized.

After hospital discharge, the patient is followed

on an outpatient basis. Treatment is directed toward maintaining the weight mutually agreed upon by the adolescent and the health professional and within the range of standardized weight and height charts. If the weight drops below this level, the patient is rehospitalized. (See also Chapter 24.)

Balaa MA, Drossman DA: Anorexia nervosa and bulimia: The eating disorders. *DM* 1985;**31:**9.

Crisp AH: *Anorexia Nervosa: Let Me Go.* Grune & Stratton, 1980.

McSherry AJ: The diagnostic challenge of anorexia nervosa. *Am Fam Physician* 1984;**29:**141.

Swift WS: The long-term outcome of early onset anorexia nervosa. *J Am Acad Child Psychiatry* 1982;**21:**38.

2. BULIMIA & FORCED VOMITING

There is an increasing number of adolescent females who gorge themselves with food, often foods high in carbohydrates, and then force vomiting. The exact cause of this disorder is unknown.

Presentation

Young people, often those in the stage of late adolescence, may present with this complaint, either because they are tired of the ritualistic cycle of "gorging and purging" or because their parents or friends have discovered their behavior. It is important to inquire whether the adolescent engages in this behavior alone or with a group (eg, at a social function in a college dormitory). The isolated adolescent who participates in this behavior needs help.

Diagnosis

Diagnosis is based primarily on history. Some adolescents will have sustained a weight loss; others will not. Frequently, there are signs of changes in the dental enamel due to the effects of contact with acidic stomach contents. Serum electrolyte determinations may reveal hypochloremia and metabolic alkalosis.

Treatment

Treatment is based on resolution of emotional conflicts associated with bulimia and forced vomiting. These conflicts may be sexual in nature, particularly directed toward heterosexual partners or sexual conflicts with the family.

Bailey S: Diagnosing bulimia. *Am Fam Physician* 1984;**29:**161.

Brown NW: Medical consequences of eating disorders. *South Med J* 1985;**78:**403.

Harris RT: Bulimarexia and related serious eating disorders with medical complications. *Ann Intern Med* 1983;**99:**800.

3. THINNESS & EXERCISE

More research is needed to determine "how thin is too thin" for adolescents who become thin from ritualistic exercising. However, pediatricians should be concerned about an adolescent who has been losing weight over time and is below the third percentile for age.

Gayle C: The female athlete. Chap 5, pp 59–74, in: *Sports Medicine: Health Care for Young Athletes.* Smith NJ (editor). American Academy of Pediatrics, 1983.

Meyer H: The underweight adolescent. *Clin Pediatr* 1980; **19:**820.

Pugliese MJ et al: Fear of obesity. *N Engl J Med* 1983;**309:**513.

4. EXOGENOUS OBESITY

Obesity is seen more frequently in female than male adolescents and occurs primarily in those of lower socioeconomic status. Overeating is the cause of obesity in about 90% of overweight adolescents.

Presentation

Obese adolescents may seek medical care for the condition, or their parents may take them for treatment—a point of critical importance to whether treatment is successful. Treatment is more likely to succeed if the adolescent seeks help than if the parents force the adolescent to be treated.

Diagnosis

Diagnosis is based primarily on the history and the adolescent's physical appearance of being overweight. The degree of obesity can be determined by plotting the adolescent's weight and height on the standard growth curves or by caliper measurement of skinfold thickness.

The history often reveals that one or both parents are obese and that the adolescent has irregular eating habits, often munching on high-calorie snacks while watching television. Obese adolescents often exercise little, if at all, and are frequently isolated from peers and have poor self-esteem. A minority of obese adolescents actually view their obesity as a positive attribute and are popular and recognized by peers as being special.

If there is reason to suspect an endogenous cause of obesity (eg, pituitary tumor, hypothyroidism, Cushing's syndrome, genetic disorder) on the basis of the history and physical examination, appropriate laboratory examinations should be done. The treatment of these conditions differs from treatment of exogenous obesity.

Treatment

Successful treatment is largely predicated on the adolescent's desire and motivation to lose weight.

New approaches to weight loss include the use of group therapy and behavior modification programs. Consistent restriction of daily intake to 1400–1600 kcal, a structured and consistent exercise program, and positive reinforcement of weight loss are central to the weight loss program. In some cases, the eating habits of the family must be modified before the patient will lose weight.

Treatment failures are frequent. However, recent studies suggest that some adolescents who fail in initial treatment may succeed in losing weight a few years later. (See also Chapters 4 and 24.)

Barnes HV: An approach to the obese adolescent. *Med Clin North Am* 1975;**59:**1507.

Forbes GB: Obesity. In: *Ambulatory Pediatrics II*. Saunders, 1977.

Freedman DS: Relationship of changes in obesity to serum lipids and lipoprotein changes in childhood and adolescence. *JAMA* 1985;**254:**515.

Garn SM: Continuities and changes in fatness from infancy through adulthood. *Curr Probl Pediatr* 1985;**15:**5.

Hervey GR: The physiological background of obesity. *Pediatr Ann* 1984;**13:**543.

Weil W: Obesity in children. *Pediatr in Rev* 1981;**3:**180.

SCHOOL PROBLEMS DURING ADOLESCENCE

1. SCHOOL PHOBIA (School Withdrawal)

The diagnosis of school phobia is based on the history of persistent absence from school despite parents' and professionals' efforts to encourage the adolescent to return to school.

Presentation

Adolescents who present with school phobia usually have a previous history of unexplained school absences and may also have functional pain (abdominal pain or headaches) and a chronic history of difficulties separating from the family.

Diagnosis

The medical history should focus on physical complaints such as symptoms of illness or sensory impairments that may affect school attendance. Physical examination should screen for visual and hearing deficits as well as for evidence of delayed growth, a sensitive concern to some adolescents.

The psychosocial history should focus on the adolescent's school history: days of absence during current and previous years; pattern of absence (eg, absence on certain days, which may indicate dislike for a particular subject or teacher); observations by school personnel of the adolescent's classroom and social behavior, particularly in comparison with that of peers at the same grade level; number and nature of visits to the school nurse; and academic achievement and results of formal testing. The adolescent and the parents should be asked to sign a consent form for the release of school records to the pediatrician. If the pediatrician plans to visit the school, both the adolescent and the parents should know the time and purpose of the visit and which school personnel will be involved.

The family history should include details of recent or anticipated changes in the family structure or environment, such as divorce, moving to a new home, and illness in the family. Some adolescents are afraid to leave home and think they can prevent events such as these from occurring; others wish to avoid a condition at school over which they have little or no control. A history of how the parents respond to the adolescent's school absence is also critical, since lonely, frightened parents may either directly or indirectly encourage the adolescent to remain home. Data should also be elicited on the adolescent's ability to cope with separation from the family in early years (responses to attending kindergarten, camp, etc), secondary gains for remaining at home (eg, maintenance of a dependent state, increased attention, reinforcement from parents or peers), school attendance and performance records of the adolescent's siblings, and the adolescent's relationships with siblings.

The peer history should include information about friends whom the adolescent names, the activities in which the adolescent participates with friends, and the amount of time spent with friends in relation to the time spent with the family, particularly the parents.

Treatment

School phobia during childhood and early adolescence has a better prognosis than school phobia during middle adolescence. We usually refer an adolescent over 14 years of age for mental health evaluation if school absence has persisted for more than 4–6 weeks and there is a chronic history of difficulties in separating from the family. The pediatrician's role is to emphasize that the adolescent is physically healthy but requires assistance from a mental health professional, the family, and school personnel to return to school. These adolescents are the most difficult to treat.

Immediate return to school is indicated for the physically healthy patient in the early stage of adolescence. The help of parents and school personnel in enforcing the return to school is vital. The longer adolescents remain out of school, the more anxious they become and the more difficult their return to school becomes. The pediatrician must decide whether he or she or another professional will undertake efforts to determine why the adolescent does not want to go to school and begin efforts to solve or minimize the underlying problems. (See also Chapter 24.)

Nader PR, Bullock D, Caldwell B: School phobia. *Pediatr Clin North Am* 1975;**22:**605.

Sahler OJZ, McAnarney ER: Pages 145–151 in: *The Child From Three to Eighteen*. Mosby, 1981.

2. SCHOOL FAILURE (Academic Failure)

Presentation

School (academic) failure is common during adolescence. In some instances, adolescents with limited intellectual abilities or learning disabilities are no longer able to meet the increasing academic demands that high school places on them, even though they kept up with demands in late elementary or junior high school. In other cases, underachievement may be due to emotional problems or to physical causes such as visual or hearing disability, chronic disease (eg, anemia), or neurologic dysfunction.

Diagnosis

Determining the cause of school failure requires a thorough history, physical examination, and laboratory evaluation by the pediatrician.

The medical history includes details of any chronic illness or condition (eg, visual or hearing impairment, anemia) that might affect school attendance or impede learning. The details of the school history, including school attendance, grades over several years, and formal intellectual testing results, can be obtained from school personnel with the adolescent's and parents' permission. The family history is directed toward eliciting information on school problems in other family members, such as the parents or siblings, and determining how and if they were resolved.

Physical examination includes visual and hearing tests as well as a neurologic evaluation. Laboratory examination includes at least a complete blood count and urinalysis.

Differentiation between school failure due to limited intellectual ability and that due to learning disability is based on the psychosocial history and results of intelligence tests performed by a psychologist trained in psychometric testing. Adolescents with learning disability may be found to have normal general intelligence (normal IQ) but (1) difficulty in acquiring skills in a specific academic area (eg, reading, spelling) or (2) attention deficit disorder, characterized by difficulty paying attention for any length of time, impulsiveness, disorganization, and inability to delay gratification. Special educational testing is indicated.

In adolescents with normal intelligence and no specific learning disabilities, the reasons for educational underachievement should be identified. Underachievement may be related to depression, hostility, or (more seriously) an affective disorder, any of which can impede learning.

Treatment

Treatment depends upon the cause of school failure. Adolescents with limited intelligence need appropriate educational placement. Those with learning disabilities in specific academic areas require remedial tutoring. Adolescents whose academic failure is associated with underachievement and behavioral or emotional problems may need psychologic treatment directed toward resolution of the problems, depending upon the severity of the problems. In this latter group, the pediatrician may counsel the adolescent and the family or may refer the adolescent to a mental health professional for treatment.

Hartzell HE, Compton C: Learning disability: Ten-year follow-up. *Pediatrics* 1984;**74:**1058.

Lewis DO: The neuropsychiatric assessment of the adolescent. *Pediatr Ann* 1984;**14:**378.

Oberklaid F, Levine MD: Precursors of school failure. *Pediatr in Rev* 1980;**2:**5.

Sahler OJZ: The teenage with failing grades. *Pediatr in Rev* 1983;**4:**293.

Weitzman M et al: School absence: A problem for the pediatrician. *Pediatrics* 1982;**69:**739.

Wender EH: Learning disabilities in children. *Pediatr in Rev* 1981;**3:**91.

ACCIDENTS DURING ADOLESCENCE

Accidents are the leading cause of death among adolescents. Each year, there are an estimated 15,000–18,000 deaths from automobile accidents. The number of hospitalizations from these accidents, as well as sports injuries and work-related injuries, is also high, and prolonged hospitalization often affects educational progress and other aspects of growth and development. Prevention of accidents during adolescence is a particular challenge to the pediatrician.

One of the hallmarks of middle adolescence is experimental behavior, which often involves taking risks that most adults would avoid. An adolescent who has one or 2 accidents may be among this group of "experimenters" who believe that they will escape unharmed from their activities. After surgical or medical care is initiated, the pediatrician should investigate the circumstances of the accident; how many accidents the adolescent has had; how the adolescent is doing at home, in school, and in relationships with peers; and other factors that will determine what measures need to be taken to prevent injury.

If the adolescent has a history of recurrent accidents and appears to use poor judgment frequently, there is often an underlying problem. Adolescents who are depressed, have low self-esteem, or have little respect for themselves or others may take risks to gain attention, exert their power and strength, or challenge authority, eg, by driving under the influence of drugs or alcohol and driving at excessive speeds. Such underlying problems must be explored and resolved so that accidents can be prevented. Referral of the adolescent for mental health evaluation may be indicated. (See also Chapter 8.)

CHRONIC ILLNESS DURING ADOLESCENCE

About 5 million adolescents suffer from chronic illness. The number continues to grow as a result of increased survival rates for childhood diseases such as cystic fibrosis, renal disease, and diabetes mellitus. In general, young people who are born with or acquire their illness during early childhood are able to cope better with their illness than those who acquire the illness during adolescence. Children with consistent and caring family support show better adjustment than those with inconsistent or no support. Young people with obvious (visible) handicaps that do not severely limit their activities may cope better than those who have minimal external evidence of illness but whose illness makes them unable to keep up with their peers.

Each adolescent adjusts in a unique manner to his or her chronic illness. Some adolescents grow and develop optimally despite their chronic illness, while others experience considerable problems. This section will consider adjustment to chronic illness during adolescence as a stage related phenomenon.

Chronic Illness During Early Adolescence

Early adolescence is normally characterized by ambivalence toward independence. In chronically ill adolescents, a combination of physical and emotional factors may delay or prevent independence. The adolescent may be overly dependent on the parents, or the parents may be overprotective. The illness itself may delay onset of puberty. The general identity question "Who am I as a physically changing person?" may be viewed as "Who am I as a physically changing person who has trouble walking, breathing, etc?" The development of formal operational thinking skills may also be delayed, since the illness with its daily regimen of medications, exercises, or other forms of treatment tends to focus the adolescent's thoughts on the present and reinforce concrete operational thinking patterns.

Chronic Illness During Middle Adolescence

Middle adolescence normally is the time when the young person is striving maximally for independence from the family. As is true during early adolescence, the chronically ill adolescent in this stage may be unable to gain independence because of physical limitations or lack of freedom to experiment with various experiences upon which independence is built. Some adolescents who are physically ill become reckless in their strivings for independence, either in an effort to deny their limitations or as a statement that they are capable of normal adolescent experiences. The general identity question "Who am I as a person?" may take the form of "Who am I as a sick person?" Cognitive development may be somewhat delayed as the chronically ill adolescent copes with daily problems related to the illness and follows strict daily treatment regimens that reinforce concrete operational thought processes.

Chronically ill adolescents who do well during this stage often have a history of adjusting well to their illness over time, usually have families who are supportive of their growing need for independence, and often are experiencing stability of their illness.

Chronic Illness During Late Adolescence

Late adolescence normally is the time when the young person individuates from the family and leaves home. The severity of illness may determine whether the adolescent is capable of living independently. Families often express concern that the condition will worsen under the stressful circumstances of a new setting. The close bond that has developed between the adolescent and the physician also may be terminated if the adolescent leaves home, and this may be a source of anxiety for the adolescent, the family, and the physician. Some adolescents may decide to break away gradually, eg, by attending a college close to home for the first 2 years and then moving away from home for the second 2 years after adjusting to partial independence. (See also Chapter 24.)

Blum R: *Chronic Illness and Disabilities in Childhood and Adolescence*. Grune & Stratton, 1984.

Coupey S, Cohen MI: The adolescent with chronic disease. *Paediatrician* 1981;**10:**183.

Easson WM: The seriously ill or dying adolescent: Special needs and challenges. *Postgrad Med* 1985;**78:**183.

Kellerman J et al: Psychological effects of illness in adolescence. *J Pediatr* 1980;**97:**126.

ACTING-OUT BEHAVIOR DURING ADOLESCENCE

Drug abuse, alcohol abuse, truancy, juvenile delinquency, and other forms of acting-out behavior are frequently seen in adolescents with behavioral problems evident since childhood, in those with acute or chronic depression, and in those with affective disorders. The role of the pediatrician is usually one of defining the problem, determining its cause, and making appropriate referral for definitive treatment.

1. DRUG ABUSE

In 1977, it was estimated that 54% of high school seniors had used an illicit drug. In 1979, studies of teenagers 12–17 years of age estimated that about 7 million in this group had tried marihuana and 4 million were currently using marihuana. The number of adolescents who abuse drugs varies according to age.

Increased or continued use of marihuana may be associated with placement of greater value on independence than on academic achievement, lower expectations for academic achievement, decreased religious beliefs, greater tolerance of deviance from the norm, decreased compatibility between friends and parents, greater influence of friends and lesser influence of parents, and greater tendency toward other problem behavior such as excessive drinking. Increased marihuana use may be part of a syndrome of adolescent problem behavior of which alcohol abuse may also be a part. (See also Chapter 24.)

Diagnosis

The following categories may be helpful in differentiating drug users from drug abusers: (1) adolescents who experiment with the drug to satisfy curiosity and conform to peer group behavior; (2) adolescents who use drugs as a form of recreation and who become regular users and sometimes overindulge; and (3) adolescents who are compulsive users and who have a physical or psychologic dependence on the drug (drug abusers).

Evaluation of the adolescent includes a history of drug use and physical and psychologic evaluations.

A. History of Drug Use: Data should include onset of drug use; what drug or drugs were initially or are currently being used; initial and current frequency of use; circumstances under which drugs are used (in a group, alone, etc); reasons for use; desire to continue or discontinue drug use; and effects of drug use on the adolescent's life. Untoward effects may include physical problems (eg, infected injection sites, anorexia), psychologic problems (eg, hallucinations), legal problems (arrests), family problems (discord with parents, placement outside the home), and school or work problems (attendance, achievement, and ability to get along well with peers, coworkers, teachers, and employers).

B. Psychologic Evaluation: The adolescent should be evaluated for evidence of depression, psychotic behavior, hallucinations, lack of clarity of thinking, and confusion or disorientation. A family history of manic-depressive illness or other psychologic problems should be elicited, and efforts should be made to determine whether drug abuse is part of a larger picture of behavioral dysfunction, eg, psychopathic or sociopathic tendencies.

C. Physical Examination: Examination should include evaluation of height, weight, and general physical appearance. Evidence of bronchitis, hepatitis, malnutrition, and intravenous needle ("track") marks should be noted.

Treatment

Treatment will depend upon the pattern of drug use. Adolescents using drugs for recreational purposes with a group of friends are basically healthy. With guidance from their parents and other adults, they will escape major physical or psychologic consequences of their drug use. Young people abusing drugs often have major psychologic problems and may have physical problems such as malnutrition. They clearly need medical and psychologic care. Some may be frightened of health care or afraid that the physician will disclose their drug abuse to the legal authorities. Others will respond positively to the pediatrician's offer to provide medical care but may be reluctant to receive psychologic counseling. Over time, the physician may help them recognize their need for psychologic care. The success of treatment depends on the adolescent's motivation, psychologic status, and emotional support from family and friends. (See also Chapter 24.)

Bachman JG, Johnston JD, O'Malley P: Smoking, drinking, and drug use among American high school students: Correlates and trends, 1975–1979. *Am J Public Health* 1981;**71**:59.

Committee on Drugs, American Academy of Pediatrics: Marijuana. *Pediatrics* 1980;**65**:652.

Dyment PG: Drugs and the adolescent athlete. *Pediatr Ann* 1984;**13**:602.

Jalai B, Jalai M, Crocetti G: Adolescents and drug use: Toward a more comprehensive approach. *Am J Orthopsychiatry* 1981;**51**:121.

Jones R: Substance use and abuse. *Semin Adolesc Med* 1985;**1**:235.

Schwartz RH: Frequent marihuana use in adolescence. *Am Fam Physician* 1985;**31**:201.

2. ALCOHOL ABUSE

Alcohol is the substance most frequently abused by adolescents, and alcohol abuse is reported in about 3 million adolescents each year. Studies in 1979 showed that 16.4 million teenagers 12–17 years of age had tried alcohol and that 8.7 million were currently using alcohol. Other studies have estimated that 70–90% of high school students have had some experience with alcohol by 18 years of age and have indicated that more boys than girls drink, the amount and frequency of drinking increase with adolescent age, and drinking habits of parents and peers influence adolescent drinking patterns. Many of the 15,000–18,000 deaths of adolescents in automobile accidents are attributed to drinking and driving.

Diagnosis

The following may be helpful in classifying the drinking habits of adolescents:

(1) Abstainers: No drinking, or drinking less than once a year (27%).

(2) Infrequent or light drinkers: Drinking at most once a month (33%).

(3) Moderate drinkers: Drinking any amount at least once a week, or drinking 3–4 times per month with 2–4 drinks per time (15%).

(4) Moderate drinkers to heavy drinkers: Drinking at least once a week (2–4 drinks), or drinking 3–4 times per month (5–12 drinks) (14%).

(5) Heavy drinkers: Drinking at least once a week (5–12 drinks) (11%).

The history of drinking behavior during adolescence should include data similar to that for drug abuse (see above).

Chronic alcoholism in other family members may suggest a genetic predisposition to depression or manic-depressive illness, in which case a psychiatric referral should be seriously considered.

Findings on physical examination may include malnutrition, cirrhosis of the liver, vitamin deficiencies, and, in some severe cases, peripheral neuropathy.

Treatment

Treatment will depend upon whether the adolescent is experimenting with alcohol or abusing alcohol. Adolescents abusing alcohol often have major psychologic problems and may have severe medical problems. Their response to appropriate medical and psychologic care is dependent upon their motivation, psychologic status, and emotional support from family and friends. Some alcohol-abusing adolescents may require institutionalization for withdrawal from alcohol and subsequent treatment.

Aten M, McAnarney E: Pages 88–89 in: *A Behavioral Approach to the Care of Adolescents*. Mosby, 1981.

Stephenson JN et al: Treating the intoxicated adolescent. *JAMA* 1984;**252:**1884.

Stern M et al: Father absence and adolescent problem behaviors: Alcohol consumption, drug use, and sexual activity. *Adolescence* 1984;**19:**302.

Wesson DR: Substance abuse. *JAMA* 1985;**252:**2286.

3. TRUANCY

Truancy is absenteeism from school on a regular basis without permission from the school authorities or the parents. It is more common in adolescents whose families are of lower socioeconomic status and whose parents have minimal educational aspirations for their children.

Diagnosis

The diagnosis of truancy is usually made by school or legal authorities and is based upon the pattern of school inattendance (number of full days missed, number of classes missed, etc).

It is important for the pediatrician to differentiate truancy from school phobia and absenteeism based on underachievement and failure. Unlike the adolescent who has school phobia and remains at home, the truant adolescent leaves home each morning but either does not arrive at school or is absent from one or more classes during the day. The parents are usually unaware of where the adolescent is when school is missed. The adolescent's behavior may be otherwise normal, or there may be evidence of other antisocial behavior and failure to conform to societal norms. Thus, in addition to attendance and scholastic records, school data solicited should include documentation of the adolescent's overall behavior and any evidence of lying to school authorities, cheating on examinations, or stealing.

The attitudes of the parents toward the truancy should also be explored, since the adolescent's behavior may be reflecting the parents' attitude that school attendance is not important—eg, "When John is 16, he'll quit school anyhow." The parents may have a history of showing minimal interest in working with professionals to encourage the adolescent to return to school.

Treatment

Since truant adolescents and their families often view the school curriculum as irrelevant to the adolescent's future, the educational goals of the adolescent should be evaluated and the adolescent referred for formal educational testing to determine areas of interest and talent. If a particular adolescent is talented in industrial arts and wants to work in this field after high school, the individual educational program may be adjusted to make school training relevant to these strengths and aspirations. Many truant adolescents eventually drop out of school at 16 years of age. Those entering the work world unprepared may repeat their truant behavior at work.

Sahler OJZ: The teenager with failing grades. *Pediatr in Rev* 1983;**4:**293.

Sahler OJZ, McAnarney E: Pages 163–168 in: *The Child From Three to Eighteen*. Mosby, 1981.

Wallerstein J: Children of divorce: Long-term outcome. *Med Asp Hum Sex* 1985;**19:**132.

4. JUVENILE DELINQUENCY

Delinquency is defined as "the violation of legally established codes of conduct." One author estimates that each year 2.9% of North American adolescents 10–17 years of age appear in juvenile court for other than traffic offenses. Weiner (1975) divided juvenile delinquents into three categories:

(1) Sociologic delinquents usually use adaptive forms of behavior rather than maladaptive forms. These young people commit acts of delinquency in the context of a supportive group (eg, a gang). They usually have close interpersonal relationships with other members of the family but may lack close supervision of their activities during adolescence. Recreational programs may provide these young people opportunities to direct their energies toward productive ends.

(2) Characterologic delinquents have asocial personalities and no close interpersonal ties. They are often loners and have chronic histories of behavioral dysfunction. These delinquents need intensive, long-term psychotherapy.

(3) Neurotic delinquents are trying to communicate their feelings and needs as "cries for help," and thus they may leave evidence to ensure their identification as perpetrators of the crime. Their delinquency is an acute rather than a chronic behavioral problem. These adolescents are frequently depressed and need active intervention. The pediatrician's role is either to provide supportive help or to refer the adolescent for mental health care.

Diagnosis

The history should be directed toward determining

whether the juvenile delinquency is sociologic, characterologic, or neurotic in nature. Information should include reasons for committing the act of delinquency; whether the adolescent has participated in such activities previously; attitudes toward the act (happiness, remorse, fear, anxiety); and responses of authorities (legal, school, etc). This information will help the pediatrician determine whether the delinquent act is an acute response to the adolescent's internal needs (neurotic) or part of an asocial pattern of behavior (characterologic).

Treatment

Treatment is based on the nature of the juvenile delinquency. As indicated above, sociologic delinquents can be encouraged to divert their energies through participation in recreational programs; characterologic delinquents should be referred for intensive psychotherapy; and neurotic delinquents require acute intervention aimed at problem solving and resolving feelings of depression.

Copoulos E, Hein K: Delinquency and the pediatrician. *Pediatr in Rev* 1982;**4**:156.

Owens JWM: Incarcerated youths: Urgent needs. *Pediatrics* 1985;**75**:539.

Schowalter JE: Running away. *Pediatr in Rev* 1983;**4**:213.

Webster-Stratton C: Comparison of abusive and nonabusive families with conduct disordered children. *Am J Orthopsychiatry* 1985;**55**:59.

Weiner I: Juvenile delinquency. *Pediatr Clin North Am* 1975;**22**:673.

BREAST DISORDERS DURING ADOLESCENCE

Breast Examination

Examination of the breasts is a vital but infrequently performed aspect of the physical examination. Questions can be raised and answers given regarding breast development and sexuality in general, about which the adolescent usually has very limited knowledge.

Over 25% of women in the reproductive years will develop some type of breast disorder requiring medical attention. Breast cancer, though rare in adolescence, is the leading cause of cancer-induced death in older women. Thus, it is important to teach teenage girls principles of self-examination of the breasts. This will encourage them to learn about their own bodies, improve their self-image and health care knowledge, allow them the opportunity to ask further questions, and prepare them to detect disorders in the future.

If specific concerns about a possible breast disorder are raised by the patient or parent, a careful history and evaluation are warranted. The history should include onset of local and systemic symptoms (lesion, pain, discharge, etc) and rate of breast growth or change. The patient should also be asked whether trauma preceded the symptoms and whether any drugs are being taken. Physical examination should include determining the Tanner stage of sexual maturity (Table 9–1), checking for lymphadenopathy, and breast and abdominal examination.

The American Cancer Society recommends a very detailed breast examination to detect cancer, involving evaluation of the patient in both sitting and supine positions. Although some modification of this detailed approach can be used to lessen the natural embarrassment of the patient, the evaluation should be thorough enough to observe the Tanner stage of each breast, asymmetry of breasts, palpable lesions (in each quadrant), nipple discharge, skin changes, and lymphadenopathy (axillary or supraclavicular).

Onset & Progression of Breast Changes

A major milestone in the growing girl's life is the onset of breast development (thelarche). This signals to her, her family, and others that adolescence has begun. Although thelarche usually occurs between 11 and 11½ years of age in girls in the USA, a normal range of 8–15 years is noted. The term premature thelarche refers to breast development in the absence of other signs of puberty, often in children 1–4 years of age. A careful evaluation is warranted if breast development or puberty is precocious or delayed (see Chapter 25). Occasionally, a congenital anomaly such as amastia (absence of a breast), athelia (absence of a nipple), polymastia, or polythelia is noted in teenagers. Inverted nipples may also occur. Surgical correction is recommended when breast growth is complete. A complication of surgery is inability to breast-feed.

Thelarche begins with breast budding, characterized by subareolar hyperplasia or smooth, firm swelling under the areola. Unilateral development is not rare, and asymmetric breast development, though often of concern to the patient, is a very common phenomenon. Absence of the pectoralis major muscle and other chest wall anomalies may accompany breast hypoplasia or amastia (as noted in Poland's syndrome). Bilateral breast hypoplasia may occur in various disorders causing delayed puberty (eg, Turner's syndrome). Biopsy of a unilateral breast bud should be avoided, since this will preclude further breast development. The breasts usually appear more symmetric in later adolescence, and unilateral breast augmentation is available if asymmetry persists. Breast development is usually complete 2–4 years after thelarche, but variations do occur. Correlation of various pubertal events with breast stages is a helpful clinical tool (Table 9–1).

Breast size is always of concern to young girls and adolescents, and counseling about breast growth may be necessary. The normal variation in breast size should be stressed, and counseling should take into account the Tanner stage of development of the individual patient. Many teenagers remain in stage III of breast development until pregnancy, and they should be assured that small breasts do not affect ability to reproduce or to breast-feed.

After thelarche, breast atrophy may occur in association with weight loss secondary to dieting, anorexia nervosa, or other illnesses.

Idiopathic breast hypertrophy may occur at any time during life. However, if it occurs during adolescence, it is usually termed virginal or juvenile hypertrophy. The exact cause of this process of massive unilateral or bilateral breast enlargement is not known. It may be due to increased breast tissue sensitivity to hormones secreted at puberty, endogenous production of hormones within the breast tissue cells, or an abnormality of the interaction with exogenous estrogen. This condition often causes considerable anxiety and embarrassment for both the patient and family. Although breast reduction procedures are available and may be urged by the parents, it is usually best to delay such surgery until later adolescence to allow the patient to decide if she really wishes smaller breasts. However, extreme embarrassment, severe neck or back pain, or breast tissue necrosis may indicate the need for surgery. Subcutaneous mastectomy with prosthesis is currently preferable to reduction mammoplasty, since there is a high failure rate with the latter procedure. In patients who have undergone surgery, breast feeding is often not possible. Danazol has been tried as an alternative to surgery.

Benedek EP, Poznanski E, Mason S: A note on the female adolescent's psychological reactions to breast development. *J Am Acad Child Psychiatry* 1979;**18**:537.

Goldbloom RB: Self-examination by adolescents. *Pediatrics* 1985;**76**:126.

Jimerson GK: The adolescent breast: Disorders and evaluation. *Med Asp Hum Sex* 1985;**19**:66.

Marchant DJ: History, physical examination, and breast self-examination. *Clin Obstet Gynecol* 1982;**25**:359.

Small EC: Psychosocial issues in breast disease. *Clin Obstet Gynecol* 1982;**25**:447.

FIBROADENOMA

Fibroadenoma, the most common breast mass in teenagers, is noted in 70–90% of biopsied breast lesions. The cause of this benign tumor is unknown, but sensitivity to hormones secreted at puberty has been postulated.

Clinical Findings

Fibroadenoma presents as an encapsulated, rubbery, nontender mass that slowly enlarges. It may be 3–4 cm at discovery but can reach or exceed 12 cm in rare cases. Fibroadenoma may occur in any breast quadrant but is often found in the upper, outer breast tissue. Although a single lesion is usually found, lesions may be multiple and recurrent (25% of cases).

In pregnant or lactating women, fibroadenoma characteristically does not change in size during cessation of the menstrual cycle.

The presence of any breast lesion requires careful evaluation to rule out cancer.

Differential Diagnosis

Classic fibroadenoma should be differentiated from its atypical variants as well as from virginal hypertrophy (see above), cysts, abscesses, adenocarcinoma, and other lesions listed in Table 9–3.

Fibroadenomatosis is characterized by multiple and recurrent lesions.

Giant or juvenile fibroadenoma is a rare variant in which there is very rapid enlargement of an encapsulated mass, sometimes resulting in compression of adjacent normal breast tissue. The condition is painless and benign and may be bilateral. Surgical excision is usually indicated.

Cystosarcoma phylloides, a painless and rapidly growing tumor of epithelial and stromal elements, also occurs in teenagers. It may present with bloody nipple discharge and is malignant in about 10% of cases. Early surgical excision is important.

Cancer of the breast (adenocarcinoma) is very rare in teenagers but has been reported in both male and female adolescents. It presents as a hard, nonmovable lesion with overlying skin changes and axillary lymphadenopathy.

Treatment

Most clinicians will observe the lesion during 1–2 menstrual cycles and then biopsy it if it remains suspicious. Others advocate immediate biopsy with surgical removal. Repeated biopsy of recurrent fibroadenomas is usually not warranted.

Dewhurst J: Breast disorders in children and adolescents. *Pediatr Clin North Am* 1981;**28**:287.

Goldstein DP, Miller V: Breast masses in adolescent females. *Clin Pediatr* 1982;**21**:17.

Ligon RE et al: Breast masses in young women. *Am J Surg* 1980;**140**:779.

Schydlower M: Breast masses in adolescents. *Am Fam Physician* (Feb) 1982;**25**:141.

Table 9–3. Causes of breast masses.

Fibroadenoma (classic or juvenile)
Breast abscess
Breast cyst (including fibrocystic breast disease)
Cystosarcoma phylloides
Breast carcinoma
Intraductal papilloma
Fat necrosis
Lipoma
Hemangioma
Lymphangioma
Idiopathic (virginal or juvenile) hypertrophy
Miscellaneous (intraductal granuloma, interstitial fibrosis, sclerosing adenosis, granular cell myoblastoma, keratoma of the nipple)

Seashore JH: Breast enlargements in infants and children. *Pediatr Ann* (Oct) 1975;**4:**8.

Teasdale C, Baum M: Breast cancer in a schoolgirl. *Lancet* 1976;**2:**627.

Turbey WJ, Buntain WL, Dudgeon DL: The surgical management of pediatric breast masses. *Pediatrics* 1975;**56:**736.

Greenblatt RB et al: Fibrocystic disease of the breast. *Clin Obstet Gynecol* 1982;**25:**365.

Hutter RVP: Good-bye to "fibrocystic disease." *N Engl J Med* 1985;**312:**179.

Pietsch J: Breast disorders. Chap 8, pp 96–104, in: *Pediatric and Adolescent Obstetrics and Gynecology.* Lavery JP, Sanfilippo JS (editors). Springer-Verlag, 1985.

BREAST ABSCESS

Breast abscess may be seen in teenagers. Precipitating factors include skin infection, trauma, breast feeding, general body weakness (eg, with chronic illness), and epidermal cysts.

Clinical Findings

Breast abscess may present with single or multiple lesions that are painful and fluctuant or cystic. The overlying skin is erythematous and warm to touch.

Culture usually reveals *Staphylococcus aureus,* but *Escherichia coli* and *Pseudomonas* have been reported in as many as 25% of cases. Severe cellulitis of overlying skin is associated with gram-negative infectious agents.

Differential Diagnosis

Other single or multiple cysts may occur in teenagers, including galactoceles, blue dome (blood-filled cysts), and, occasionally, cysts resembling fibrocystic breast disease. Fibrocystic disease occurs more commonly in women 35–60 years of age, is frequently bilateral, and is characterized by sterile cysts containing brownish or bloody fluid. Lesions may be very tender premenstrually and may change in size during various phases of the menstrual cycle. Breast examination usually reveals generalized cordlike nodularities in both breasts.

There is considerable controversy about the definition of fibrocystic disease; however, most authorities believe that the disease is uncommon during adolescence. The term mastodynia denotes breast tenderness and engorgement that are often cyclic and respond to treatment with ibuprofen or vitamin E (α-tocopherol). Aspiration or excisional biopsy may be necessary to diagnose fibrocystic breast disease or other cystic diseases.

Treatment

Incision, with drainage and culture of exudate, is usually recommended if the breast abscess becomes fluctuant. Following drainage, oral antibiotics (eg, dicloxacillin, nafcillin, erythromycin, or ampicillin) may be given for 1–2 weeks. Culture results guide the choice of antibiotics.

If trauma precipitated the abscess, application of ice packs to the area for the first 24 hours may relieve pain; thereafter, heat applied to the area may be helpful.

Recurrences are reported in as many as 50% of cases. Scarring may occur, especially if trauma precipitated the abscess or if abscesses recur.

GALACTORRHEA

Galactorrhea refers to inappropriate secretion of fluid from the breasts, ie, secretion that is not related to postpartum conditions (birth or abortion) or breast feeding. Hyperprolactinemia may be present. Although galactorrhea in teenagers is usually of a benign nature, a careful evaluation to determine the underlying cause is necessary.

Galactorrhea may be due to increased intercostal nerve stimulation (eg, from herpes zoster or following thoracic surgery); increased central nervous system stimulation resulting from hypothalamic injury (as noted in infection, tumor, or surgery) or related to the effects of emotional stress such as depression or anxiety; endocrine disorders, especially hypothyroidism; use of drugs such as reserpine, phenothiazine, methyltestosterone, estrogen, spironolactone, and oral contraceptives; or nipple stimulation due to jogging. Although occasionally reported, the association between galactorrhea and chronic marihuana abuse has not been proved. Galactorrhea in association with amenorrhea and hyperprolactinemia may indicate the presence of a hypothalamic or pituitary prolactin-producing tumor.

Treatment of galactorrhea depends on the underlying cause and should be directed by the gynecologist.

Rohn RD: Galactorrhea in the adolescent. *J Adolesc Health Care* 1984;**5:**37.

Taylor SJ et al: Case-control study of galactorrhea and its relationship to oral contraceptives. *Obstet Gynecol* 1985;**65:**665.

GYNECOMASTIA

Idiopathic gynecomastia (breast enlargement in the male teenager) is a transient phenomenon noted in half to two-thirds of adolescents. Elevated prolactin levels, abnormal serum binding protein levels, an abnormal ratio of testosterone to estrogen, and other causes have been suggested but not proved.

Clinical Findings

Idiopathic gynecomastia usually presents as a unilateral, firm, subareolar enlargement (type 1) in a boy in Tanner stage II–III of sexual development. The mass may be tender and is not usually over 3–4 cm in diameter. Bilateral involvement is seen in 20% of cases. Type 2 gynecomastia describes a generalized breast enlargement, and the term macromastia is applied to breasts at Tanner stage III or greater.

Table 9–4. Disorders associated with gynecomastia.

Klinefelter's syndrome
Traumatic paraplegia
Male pseudohermaphroditism
Testicular feminization syndrome
Reifenstein's syndrome
17-Ketosteroid reductase deficiency
Endocrine tumors (seminoma, Leydig cell tumor, teratoma, feminizing adrenal tumor, hepatoma, leukemia, hemophilia, bronchogenic carcinoma, leprosy, etc)
Hypothyroidism
Hyperthyroidism
Cirrhosis
Herpes zoster
Friedreich's ataxia

Differential Diagnosis

A careful evaluation is necessary to rule out various disorders associated with gynecomastia (Table 9–4). A drug history should also be obtained, since gynecomastia can be induced by a variety of drugs (Table 9–5). The association of marihuana and gynecomastia has been suggested but not proved. Exposure to estrogen by mouth, injection, or inhalation (eg, hairspray particles) can induce breast enlargement.

Differential diagnosis also includes pseudogynecomastia, which may be due to an excess of fatty tissue or to increased development of the pectoral muscles.

Gynecomastia is usually considered idiopathic if the patient is in early puberty, there is no history of drug ingestion or evidence of Klinefelter's syndrome, and findings on general medical screening are normal.

Treatment

If idiopathic gynecomastia is suspected, reassurance is given and the patient followed periodically until satisfactory regression occurs. Resolution may take several months to 2 years. Surgery should be offered early to those with macromastia or to any adolescent with severe psychologic maladjustment. Danazol or clomiphene has been used to treat gynecomastia, but the efficacy of these drugs in teenagers is not yet proved.

Carlson HE: Gynecomastia. *N Engl J Med* 1980;**303:**795.

Knorr D, Bidlingmaier F: Gynecomastia in male adolescents. *Clin Endocrinol Metab* 1975;**4:**157.

Table 9–5. Drugs implicated in gynecomastia.

Amphetamines	Human chorionic gonadotropin
Birth control pills (rare)	Insulin
Busulfan	Isoniazid
Cimetidine	Marihuana (controversial)
Clomiphene	Methadone
Corticosteroids	Reserpine
Digitalis	Spironolactone
Estrogens	Testosterone
Ethionamide	Tricyclic antidepressants

Marynick SP et al: Persistent pubertal macromastia. *J Clin Endocrinol Metab* 1980;**50:**128.

CONTRACEPTION & GYNECOLOGIC DISORDERS DURING ADOLESCENCE

The major gynecologic concerns of adolescents include contraception, vulvovaginitis, pelvic inflammatory disease, and menstrual disorders (reviewed in this section) and pregnancy (discussed in an earlier section). The majority of gynecologic problems and concerns can and should be managed by the pediatrician or family physician. Serious problems, as identified in this section, should then be referred to appropriate specialists.

CONTRACEPTION

Currently, there are millions of teenagers in the USA who are sexually active. The high incidence of sexually transmitted diseases among teenagers and the large number (1.3 million) of adolescent pregnancies reported each year indicate an increasing need for education and counseling about adolescent sexuality. The pediatrician or family physician is usually in the best position to offer this education to teenagers—both male and female—who express interest in contraception or indicate that sexual activity is contemplated or has begun.

The choice of a specific contraceptive method (Table 9–6) depends on several factors, including the adolescent's stage of cognitive development, moral (religious) attitudes, knowledge of available methods, and results of medical screening tests.

Table 9–6. Methods of contraception.

A. Abstinence
B. Barrier methods:
   1. Vaginal diaphragm
   2. Condom
   3. Vaginal spermicides
   4. Vaginal collagen sponge
C. Oral contraceptives:
   1. Estrogen and progestin combinations
   2. Progestin alone ("minipill")
D. Intrauterine contraceptive devices (IUD or IUCD)
E. Injectable hormonal contraceptives
F. Miscellaneous:
   1. Postcoital contraceptives
   2. Periodic abstinence ("rhythm" methods)
   3. Coitus interruptus
   4. Lactation
   5. Masturbation
   6. Sterilization
   7. Abortion

Table 9–7 outlines a suggested approach for interviewing and screening in teenage girls who wish to use contraception, especially oral contraception. Prescription of contraceptives is dependent on thorough screening and pelvic examination.

Pelvic Examination

The pelvic examination is the core of the physical evaluation for use of contraceptives. Other indications for pelvic examination in teenagers include periodic screening for sexually transmitted disease in sexually active individuals; evaluation of patients with symptoms suggestive of sexually transmitted disease, pelvic disorders, or pregnancy; determination of the cause of vaginal discharge or bleeding; and differential diagnosis of abdominal pain of possible pelvic origin.

There is debate regarding when the first pelvic examination should be performed in asymptomatic teenage girls who are not sexually active. In such cases, we generally recommend a pelvic examination between the ages of 14 and 16 years. The time to prepare the patient for this first examination is long before she presents with symptoms of pelvic problems; and under most circumstances, the examiner should be her pediatrician or family physician—not a gynecologist.

In patients who have had pelvic examinations previously, any anxiety or difficulty with this procedure should be openly discussed before it is performed again.

Begin the examination by careful inspection of the external genitalia, utilizing good lighting. Have all the necessary equipment and materials available—speculum, lubricant jelly, cotton swabs, culture me-

Table 9–7. Suggested plan to evaluate adolescents for birth control pills.*

I. History
- A. Does the patient need and want contraception?
- B. Does she understand what methods of contraception are available?
- C. What is her menstrual history?
  1. Age at menarche?
  2. Are menstrual periods regular? For at least 1 year?
  3. Date of last menstrual period?
  4. Previous pregnancies or abortions?
- B. Does she need or wish additional counseling about sexuality?
- E. Is she willing to use a barrier method (diaphragm with contraceptive foam or condom with contraceptive foam)?
- F. After discussion of the various options, has she chosen the birth control pill? What concerns does she have about birth control pills?
- G. Will she take these pills on a daily basis?
- H. Are there absolute contraindications to birth control use?
  1. Thrombophlebitis, thromboembolism, or thrombotic disease
  2. Breast cancer
  3. Estrogen-producing neoplasia
  4. Undiagnosed uterine bleeding
  5. Pregnancy
  6. Active acute or chronic liver disease
- I. Are there relative contraindications to birth control pill use?
  1. Hypertension
  2. Migraine headaches
  3. Hyperlipidemia
  4. Sickle cell disease (trait or anemia)
  5. Uncontrolled epilepsy
  6. Poorly controlled diabetes mellitus
  7. Significant chest pain of unknown cause
  8. Optic nerve or retinal disease
  9. Clotting abnormalities or coagulation defects
  10. Melasma or "mask of pregnancy"
  11. Collagen vascular disorders
  12. Uterine fibroids
  13. Lactation
  14. Oligomenorrhea
  15. Depression
  16. Cholelithiasis
  17. Inflammatory bowel disease
  18. Major organ disease (eg, heart, lung, or kidney disease)
  19. Chorea
  20. Porphyria
  21. Erythema nodosum
  22. Other (acne vulgaris or candidal vaginitis, which may worsen with birth control pill use; use of contact lenses, which may be affected by pill use; use of drugs such as anticonvulsants and antibiotics, which may render the pill less effective; etc)

I. Complete physical examination with emphasis on the following:
- A. Tanner staging of sexual maturity (should be stage IV or V)
- B. Blood pressure
- C. Eye examination (jaundice, visual defects)
- D. Thyroid examination
- E. Breast examination
- F. Cardiovascular system evaluation
- G. Liver evaluation (size, tenderness, stigmas of hepatitis or chronic liver disease)
- H. Skin evaluation (acne vulgaris, melasma, xanthoma)
- I. Complete pelvic examination

III. Laboratory tests
- A. Urinalysis, including a microscopic examination
- B. Liver function tests if liver status is in doubt
- C. Screening for *Neisseria gonorrhoeae* and *Chlamydia trachomatis* (cervical culture) and other sexually transmitted diseases
- D. Papanicolaou smear
- E. Triglyceride and cholesterol screen if there is a family history of hyperlipidemia
- F. Other tests as indicated by history and physical examination

* Adapted, with permission, from Greydanus DE, McAnarney ER: Contraception in the adolescent: Current concepts for the pediatrician. *Pediatrics* 1980;**65:**1.

dia, glass slides, etc. A long, thin, Huffman speculum is suitable for most patients, including virginal adolescents. Sexually active teenagers may tolerate the thicker Pedersen speculum, while multiparous women can tolerate the wider Graves speculum. Whether to have a chaperone or the mother present should be decided by the patient and the examiner.

Gently explain each step of the procedure. Keep the speculum in a posterior position, avoiding the sensitive urethra and clitoris. If pain or discomfort develops, stop and reevaluate the technique. It is important to avoid creating a negative experience for the patient. Evaluate for bleeding, ulcers, discharge, tenderness, and other evidence of genital disorders. A cervical culture for *Neisseria gonorrhoeae* and *Chlamydia trachomatis* and a Papanicolaou smear (from the endocervix and posterior vaginal fornix) are routine procedures in screening for contraceptive use. Other tests may be indicated if vaginitis or cervicitis is suspected—eg, a saline preparation may be used to detect "clue cells" (epithelial cells studded with organisms) or *Trichomonas vaginalis,* and a potassium hydroxide preparation may be used to detect spores and hyphae if *Candida albicans* infection is suspected (see Vulvovaginitis, below).

After the speculum examination, a manual examination of the uterus and adnexal structures is done to evaluate for tenderness, enlargement, or other signs of disease. A rectal examination is not usually necessary in teenagers, unless better delineation of the pelvic structures is necessary or symptoms of rectal disorders are noted.

When the procedure is completed, information should be clearly presented to the patient (and parents, if appropriate). Emphasize how well the patient has done and, if appropriate, stress that findings are normal. After the medical history and physical examination have been completed and the patient is fully dressed, questions about sexuality and contraception can be answered. The use of audiovisual aids is helpful, especially for young patients.

The clinician should explain the various methods of contraception and help the patient decide which method is best suited for her. It is helpful to include the male partner in the final decision.

Contraceptive Methods (Table 9–6)

A. Abstinence: Discussions of contraception should always include the topic of abstinence. Many adolescents are not sexually active, and their abstinence can be encouraged. Those who are sexually active can be reminded of the risks of pregnancy and sexually transmitted diseases.

B. Barrier Methods: The first recommendation of a contraceptive for sexually active teenagers is a barrier method, ie, condom or vaginal diaphragm with vaginal spermicides.

1. Vaginal diaphragm—The diaphragm, a rubber cap with metallic rim, is used in combination with contraceptive jelly. It is placed in the vagina prior to coitus and left in place for 6 hours after coitus. Its contraceptive effectiveness is variable; however, when used correctly, pregnancy rates have been reported to be as low as 2.4–6 per 100 woman years. A coil-spring or flat-spring diaphragm works well for most adolescents, and the proper size (ranging from 50 to 105 mm) can be determined, using diaphragm fitting rings, during a routine pelvic examination. Contraindications to diaphragm use include pelvic abnormalities preventing its proper fit (between the external cervical os and pubic symphysis) and allergy to rubber or spermicide. Most teenagers do not choose to use the diaphragm as a contraceptive method; some dislike the forethought and preparation for sexual activity, the procedure for inserting the diaphragm, and the need to introduce additional contraceptive jelly each time prior to coitus. There have been reports of toxic shock syndrome and cystitis in diaphragm users.

2. Condom—The condom is an effective barrier method with no side effects except for rare allergy to latex. It can be purchased without prescription, provides some protection against sexually transmitted disease, may prevent premature ejaculation, and allows the male partner to share in responsibility for contraceptive use. Many types of condoms are available, including lubricated types with reservoir tips. Condoms can be used in combination with contraceptive foam, cream, or jelly to increase contraceptive effectiveness.

3. Vaginal spermicides—Spermicidal preparations are available in gel, cream, paste, foam, and suppository forms. These preparations can be purchased without a prescription, are relatively inexpensive, can be used to reduce dyspareunia, have few side effects, and provide some protection against sexually transmitted diseases. Their effectiveness is enhanced when used in combination with a condom or diaphragm; very high pregnancy rates result if they are used alone. There is no evidence that use of these agents is linked to spontaneous abortions or congenital malformations in offspring.

4. Vaginal collagen sponge—Recently, a vaginal collagen sponge has been introduced, but its usefulness for teenagers has not yet been determined. Its contraceptive potential does not exceed that of the diaphragm, while its complications include vaginal malodor and a possible increased risk of toxic shock syndrome.

C. Oral Contraceptives: Oral contraceptives are safe and effective for sexually active teenagers who are carefully screened and followed.

1. Estrogen and progestin combinations—Oral contraceptives currently used in the USA consist of an estrogen (either ethinyl estradiol or mestranol) and a progestin (norgestrel, levonorgestrel, ethynodiol diacetate, norethindrone, norethindrone acetate, or norethynodrel). This combination of hormones inhibits ovulation and produces thinning of the endometrium and thickening of the cervical mucus. The concentration of estrogen and progestin is the same in each pill to be taken daily for 21 days, with a placebo given for 7 days to complete the 28-day course. Use of pills containing 30–50 μg of estrogen and 0.15–1.5 mg of progestin is currently recommended.

Another type of combination pill—the "triphasic pill" in which estrogen and progestin concentrations are changed 3 times over a 21-day cycle—has been introduced in Europe and the USA. The triphasic pill, which seems to more closely simulate a natural menstrual cycle, is an effective contraceptive. Because its use may result in fewer cases of breakthrough bleeding and acne than the traditional combination pills, the triphasic pill may become popular in the near future.

2. Progestin alone (the "minipill")—Adolescents with diabetes, cyanotic heart disease, hypertension, and other conditions in which combination oral contraceptives are contraindicated may benefit from use of the minipill (Micronor, Nor-QD, Ovrette), which contains progestin alone. Its contraceptive action is based on its ability to cause thinning of the endometrium (which prevents blastocyst implantation), thickening of the cervical mucus (which makes it impervious to sperm penetration), and an increase in ovum transport. If taken daily, the minipill is effective for most women. However, since progestin does not reliably inhibit ovulation, pregnancy rates are higher: 2–5 per 100 woman years with the minipill versus fewer than 1 per 100 with combination oral contraceptives. Breakthrough bleeding and amenorrhea are common for individuals using the minipill.

3. Indications and contraindications—Table 9–7 outlines a plan to evaluate adolescents for use of birth control pills. The pill should never be prescribed if any of the 6 absolute contraindications are noted and should be avoided or at least carefully considered if the relative contraindications are present. Clinical judgment and knowledge of the pill's side effects, as well as an understanding of the risks of pregnancy, are important in determining whether the pill can be used if these medical conditions are noted in sexually active teenagers.

Risks and benefits should be discussed with the patient. She should be advised of possible side effects such as acne, candidal vaginitis, weight gain (2–5 kg), edema, and changes in blood pressure (rises of 5–6 mm Hg and 1–2 mm Hg in systolic and diastolic pressures, respectively, are common), as well as the risks associated with smoking and pill use. In adult women, studies indicate that pill use provides a protective effect against cancer of the breasts, endometrium, and ovaries. Pill use has not been linked to pituitary cancer. The only pill-associated neoplasm is benign hepatic cell adenoma, which occurs annually in 3.4 cases per 100,000 pill users. Pill use may be one of several factors related to cervical cancer; these other factors include early onset of coitus, multiple sex partners, and infection with sexually transmitted diseases (eg, herpes simplex and condyloma acuminatum). Further study is needed to establish the precise link (if any) between cervical cancer and pill use. An annual Papanicolaou smear is thus recommended. The effect of the pill on pelvic inflammatory disease is discussed in a subsequent section.

If the patient is certain that she does not want to use a barrier method and chooses to use birth control pills, oral contraceptives containing 30 μg of estrogen (28-day packet) are recommended. The patient should be advised to take the first pill on day 5 of the menstrual period and use other contraceptive methods for the first 7 days of taking the pill. (Starting on the first menstrual day is the official recommendation in England.) If one pill is missed, she should take it as soon as it is remembered and take the next one in the proper sequence. Controversy exists over the procedure to follow if 2 or more pills are missed. Some believe that another method of contraception should be used until 5 days after the next menstrual cycle; others indicate that missing 2 pills in a row does not reduce the contraceptive effectiveness but that a new pill cycle should be begun after 7 pill-free days if 3 or more pills are missed. The patient should be encouraged to contact the physician if questions or problems arise or if breakthrough bleeding is noted.

In cases of breakthrough bleeding, tablets containing 50 μg of estrogen should be used.

If symptoms suggestive of excess estrogen develop (eg, nausea, vomiting, edema, dysmenorrhea, elevated blood pressure, headaches), pills with a lower estrogen level should be prescribed (eg, 30 μg instead of 50 μg).

4. Follow-up—Careful and frequent follow-up is important for teenagers taking birth control pills. Monthly follow-ups for 3 months and then appointments every 3–6 months, with cervical cultures for *N gonorrhoeae* and Papanicolaou smears every 6–12 months, are recommended. There are no data on how long the pill can be safely used by teenagers, but its use should be reconsidered after 4–5 years.

Most teenagers do very well taking the pill, and pregnancy is avoided when the pills are taken as directed. If it appears that directions for use are not being followed or the patient fails to return for periodic monitoring, other methods of contraception should be discussed.

D. Intrauterine Contraceptive Devices (IUD or IUCD): An IUD such as the copper T or copper 7 device can provide a very effective means of contraception for carefully screened teenagers. The device must be placed in the uterus by a trained professional, usually during the patient's menstrual period.

IUD use is contraindicated in patients with severe forms of anemia, menorrhagia, and dysmenorrhea (conditions that are worsened with IUD use); patients at risk for bacterial endocarditis; and patients with cervical or uterine hypoplasia.

The primary concern of most clinicians regarding use of IUDs by teenagers is the major risk (3–9 times greater risk) of severe pelvic inflammatory disease. For this reason, its use should be considered only for adolescents at very low risk of pelvic inflammatory disease.

E. Injectable Hormonal Contraceptives: Medroxyprogesterone acetate is a very effective contraceptive agent that may be given intramuscularly in cases when oral contraceptives are contraindicated (in sexually active teenagers with thrombotic disease, cyanotic heart disease, sickle cell anemia, etc) or not feasible to use (eg, in psychotic or mentally retarded teenagers who are at high risk for pregnancy).

When 150 mg of medroxyprogesterone acetate is given intramuscularly every 3 months on a regular basis, the pregnancy rate is equivalent to that of oral contraceptives, ie, 1 per 100 woman years. Side effects include the eventual development of irregular menses or amenorrhea in two-thirds of patients. The FDA has expressed some concern over its use, noting its theoretical link to breast cancer and chromosomal damage. However, there is no direct evidence for this, and medroxyprogesterone acetate is considered safe by many clinicians. The Committee on Drugs for the American Academy of Pediatrics has recommended its use as a method of contraception in carefully selected adolescents.

F. Miscellaneous Contraceptive Methods: For rape victims at risk of pregnancy (see Chapter 8), **postcoital contraceptives** can be given. The use of diethylstilbestrol (DES) is controversial, since it may increase the risk of carcinoma of the vagina, breasts, and endometrium. A currently accepted method is to give birth control pills containing 50 μg of ethinyl estradiol and 0.5 mg of norgestrel (Ovral), 2 tablets orally within 72 hours of the rape and 2 more tablets 12 hours later. To reduce nausea and vomiting, also give an antiemetic. Alternative postcoital contraceptives can be used: (1) 0.1 mg of ethinyl estradiol and 1 mg of dl-norgestrel, 2 doses 12 hours apart; (2) ethinyl estradiol, conjugated estrogens, or conjugated estrone sulfate, given for 5 days; or (3) postcoital insertion of an IUD.

Periodic abstinence, or "rhythm" methods, are dependent on avoiding sexual activity during the periovulatory period. The popular Billings ovulation method teaches avoidance of coitus when cervical mucus becomes the nature of raw egg whites (spinnbarkeit formation). Most adolescents are not motivated or aware enough of their own bodies to utilize this method effectively; however, it remains an option for a few.

Coitus interruptus, or withdrawal of the penis before ejaculation, is associated with a high rate of pregnancy and is not recommended for teenagers.

Lactation does provide some measure of contraceptive protection, but concurrent use of other contraceptives, such as barrier types, is recommended. The rate of pregnancy increases after 6 months of lactation, and nearly all women ovulate 9–12 months postpartum.

Masturbation and other forms of noncoital sexual activity used as substitutes for sexual activity may be acceptable to some adolescents.

Sterilization is not usually an option for teenagers and should not be considered as a contraceptive method for this group.

Abortion, though legally available to many adolescents, should not be regarded as a contraceptive method. Dilation and curettage or suction curettage is usually done within the first trimester in teenagers seeking abortion. Intra-amniotic injection of an oxytocic agent (hypertonic saline, urea, or prostaglandins) is usually recommended for those in the second trimester but is often used after the 16th week of gestation. Each of the many abortion methods has its own risks and must be done by a well-trained clinician.

Bracken MD: Spermicidal contraceptives and poor reproductive outcomes: The epidemiologic evidence against an association. *Am J Obstet Gynecol* 1985;**151**:552.

Chvapil M et al: Collagen sponge as vaginal contraceptive barrier: Critical summary of 7 years of research. *Am J Obstet Gynecol* 1985;**151**:325.

Gilchrist MJR, Rauh JL: Office microscopic examination for sexually transmitted diseases. *J Adolesc Health Care* 1985;**6**:311.

Committee on Drugs, American Academy of Pediatrics: Medroxyprogesterone acetate (Depo-Provera). *Pediatrics* 1980;**65**:74A.

Greydanus DE: Contraception. Chap 18, pp 234–261, in: *Pediatric and Adolescent Obstetrics and Gynecology*. Lavery JP, Sanfillipo JS (editors). Springer-Verlag, 1985.

Haspels AA, Van Santen MR: Postcoital contraception. *Pediatr Adolesc Gynecol* 1984;**2**:63.

Kols A et al: Oral contraceptives in the 1980s. *Popul Rep* [*A*] 1982;**10**:189.

Leppert PC: Adolescent anxiety at first pelvic examination. *Med Asp Hum Sex* 1985;**19**:24.

Mishell DR Jr: Current status of intrauterine devices. *N Engl J Med* 1985;**312**:984.

Turetsky RA, Strassburger VC: Adolescent contraception: Review and recommendations. *Clin Pediatr* 1983;**22**:337.

VULVOVAGINITIS

Vulvovaginitis (Table 9–8), one of the most frequent gynecologic disorders of adolescence, is often associated with physiologic changes and changes in the normal flora of the vagina at puberty. The vulvovaginal tissues of children are characteristically thin and have an alkaline pH, no superficial or cornified cells (polygonal cells with small pyknotic nuclei), less than 20% intermediate cells, and 80–100% parabasal cells (round or oval cells with large vesicular nuclei). Estrogen secretion at puberty causes major changes in the vulvovaginal and lower genital tract tissues, including development of a longer, thicker vagina and cervix; production of an acid pH; and a marked change in vaginal cytology, characterized by 60% superficial cells, 40% intermediate cells, and no parabasal cells. At puberty, lactobacilli (Döderlein's bacilli) are present in the vagina and contribute to the maintenance of acid pH through the production of lactic acid from carbohydrates, particularly glycogen. This acidic pH offers some protection from vagi-

Table 9–8. Causes of vulvovaginitis.

Physiologic leukorrhea
Vaginitis
Trichomonas vaginalis infection
Gardnerella (Haemophilus) vaginalis infection
Candida albicans infection
Cervicitis
Neisseria gonorrhoeae infection
Herpes simplex virus infection
Chlamydia trachomatis infection
Miscellaneous
Foreign body vaginitis
Allergic vulvovaginitis
Vulvar ulcerations and erosions (syphilis, herpes simplex virus infection, chancroid, granuloma inguinale, lymphogranuloma venereum, amebiasis, Behçet's syndrome, regional enteritis, lichen simplex chronicus, bullous diseases [eg, pemphigus], tuberculosis, filariasis, schistosomiasis, Reiter's syndrome [very rare in females], etc)
Vulvitis (psoriasis, tinea infection, molluscum contagiosum, condyloma acuminatum, scabies, pediculosis, furunculosis, pruritus vulvae, etc)

nal infection. At puberty, columnar epithelium extends to the ectocervix, giving it a reddened appearance. This phenomenon, previously called cervical erosion, is a normal part of pubertal change but may account for the susceptibility of adolescents to infection with *Neisseria gonorrhoeae* and *Chlamydia trachomatis*. Further extension of the epithelium may be seen in women who are pregnant or taking birth control pills.

Although vaginitis in children tends to be nonspecific, vaginitis in adolescents is usually due to infection with a specific organism. It is often difficult to identify the organism, since the normal flora in the vagina includes lactobacilli, diphtheroids, streptococci, staphylococci, *Bacteroides fragilis, Neisseria sicca, Branhamella catarrhalis, Escherichia coli,* other *Enterobacteriaceae,* yeasts, and other organisms. Some organisms are carried in the vagina without causing symptoms until changes occur in the vaginal flora. Many (though not all) cases of vulvovaginitis in adolescents are diagnosed as sexually transmitted diseases. Unfortunately, the number of sexually transmitted diseases in children and adolescents is increasing as coital activity among teenagers and sexual abuse of children and adolescents have increased. Because sexually active teenagers are also at increased risk for cervical intraepithelial neoplasia, a Papanicolaou smear should be taken each year.

Altchek A: Vulvovaginitis, vulvar skin disease and pelvic inflammatory disease. *Pediatr Clin North Am* 1981;**28:**397.

Cates W Jr, Rauh JO: Adolescents and sexually transmitted diseases: An expanding problem. *J Adolesc Health Care* 1985;**6:**257.

Gibbs RS: Sexually transmitted diseases in the female. *Med Clin North Am* 1983;**67:**221.

Hurd JK Jr: Vaginitis. *Med Clin North Am* 1979;**63:**423.

Jones DED et al: Cervical intraepithelial neoplasia in adolescents. *J Adolesc Health Care* 1984;**5:**243.

Russo JF, Jones DED: Abnormal cervical cytology in sexually active adolescents. *J Adolesc Health Care* 1984;**5:**269.

Schneider GT: Vaginal infections. *Postgrad Med* (Feb) 1983;**73:**255.

Sexually transmitted diseases: Treatment guidelines, 1982. *MMWR* 1982;**31:**33S.

1. PHYSIOLOGIC LEUKORRHEA

A normal increase in vaginal discharge is noted in early to middle adolescence, often beginning several weeks or months prior to menarche. It is due to estrogen secretion, which stimulates vulvovaginal and cervical glands (sebaceous, sweat, Bartholin's, and other glands). There may also be some fluid transudation through vaginal walls.

Physiologic leukorrhea occurs transiently in some newborn females, reflecting estrogen stimulation; the estrogen source is the mother.

Clinical Findings

A. Symptoms and Signs: Vaginal discharge is usually clear, sticky, and nonirritating. It is characteristic of the perimenarcheal period and may cease (or decrease in amount) once menarche occurs. A similar increase in discharge may be noted later in life during sexual excitement and during pregnancy. Poor hygiene and various infections may complicate this basic condition.

B. Laboratory Findings: The history of vaginal discharge in a young non-sexually active teenage girl is usually sufficient for the diagnosis of physiologic leukorrhea. Microscopic examination of the saline preparation (wet preparation) in which a drop of vaginal secretion is added to a drop of saline usually reveals many superficial cells and few leukocytes or bacteria. Cultures are not necessary if the patient is not sexually active.

Treatment

The patient should be reassured that leukorrhea is associated with normal changes of puberty and does not represent any disease state or injury. Frequent changes of absorbent cotton undergarments and proper perineal hygiene are recommended. Medications (eg, vaginal creams) are not recommended, since they may cause an allergic reaction (dermatitis medicamentosa) and offer no therapeutic advantage.

2. *TRICHOMONAS VAGINALIS* VAGINITIS

Trichomonas vaginalis, a unicellular, flagellate protozoon, is one of the most common causes of sexually transmitted disease in adolescents and adults. Classically, it causes a primary infection of the cervix and vagina, along with a secondary infection of the vulva. The bladder, urethra, paraurethral (Skene's) glands, and Bartholin's glands may also be affected.

Although sexual activity is the usual mode of transmission, fomite transmission also occurs. The incubation period is variable, ranging from a few days to 3 or 4 weeks. The carrier state may last for months or possibly years. *T vaginalis* infection may be concurrent with *Neisseria gonorrhoeae* infection and condylomata acuminata.

Clinical Findings

A. Symptoms and Signs: Pain, erythema, and intense pruritus of the vulvovaginal area are typical. The discharge is often copious, malodorous ("fishy"), frothy, and gray-green in color and may be purulent, mucopurulent, or seropurulent. There may also be cervicovaginal ecchymoses ("strawberry marks"), swollen vaginal papillae, and excoriation of the vulva and inner thigh. The cervix and vagina may be friable, bleeding easily when touched. The vaginal pH is 5 or higher.

As with most sexually transmitted diseases, tremendous variability in clinical manifestations is characteristic. Symptoms of cystitis or urethritis may be intense. Chronic carrier states (without symptoms) are common, while postpartum infection may cause considerable fever and endometritis. Chronic infection may cause menorrhagia and dysmenorrhea. About 10–15% of severe cases also present with low abdominal pain, which subsides after adequate treatment. The cause of this abdominal pain is unclear, but it may be a low colon inflammation such as that noted with *Campylobacter* or *Yersinia* infection.

B. Laboratory Findings: Vaginal discharge in a sexually active adolescent should be evaluated for *Trichomonas* (and other organisms), even if it does not appear to be characteristic of sexually transmitted disease. Purulent discharge or friable cervix may be caused by a variety of organisms, including *N gonorrhoeae, Chlamydia trachomatis,* and herpes simplex. However, redness of the cervix may simply represent normal cervical erosion (growth of the endocervical columnar epithelium into the external cervical os) with physiologic leukorrhea.

Microscopic examination of the discharge in saline preparation often reveals the presence of *T vaginalis* organisms, which appear as moving, pear-shaped, flagellate organisms whose size is usually twice that of a white blood cell. Saline preparations may yield negative results if the patient is a chronic carrier or recently used a chemical douche. Organisms may also be noted in urine samples and Papanicolaou smears. *T vaginalis* can be cultured from specimens of discharge, but cultures are not routinely performed in most laboratories.

Treatment

The treatment of choice is metronidazole, 2 g in a single oral dose. An alternative dosage schedule, 250 mg 3 times daily for 7 days, can be used, but more side effects (Table 9–9) are reported with this dosage. Patients should be instructed to avoid alcohol consumption while taking metronidazole, since alcohol may induce a disulfiramlike reaction causing nausea and vomiting. Fears of metronidazole causing cancer have not been supported by recent studies.

Table 9–9. Side effects of metronidazole.

Nausea	Dermatitis
Vomiting	Dry mucous membranes
Dizziness	Bitter aftertaste
?Depression	Transient neutropenia
Headaches	Disulfiramlike effect with alcohol
Drowsiness	Teratogenic effects
Candidal vaginitis	

Because of its teratogenic effects, metronidazole should not be given during pregnancy (especially the first trimester). Lactating women should be given 2 g of metronidazole in a single dose and then stop breast feeding for at least 24–30 hours. Pregnant women may be given clotrimazole (100-mg vaginal tablet at night for 7 nights); this improves the symptoms but has a low cure rate.

Candidal vaginitis may occur after treatment with metronidazole, especially if the 7-day regimen is used. In such cases, vaginitis is usually easily cured with common antifungal agents.

Resistance to metronidazole is rare. "Recurrences" are nearly always due to failure to take the medication or to reinfection from the sexual partner. There are 2 general rules to follow when treating an adolescent with a sexually transmitted disease: Treat the sexual partner in addition to the patient, and look for concomitant infections in both.

Fouts AC, Kraus SJ: *Trichomonas vaginalis:* Reevaluation of its clinical presentation and laboratory diagnosis. *J Infect Dis* 1980;**141:**137.

Goldman P: Metronidazole. *N Engl J Med* 1980;**303:**1212.

Hager WD et al: Metronidazole for vaginal *Trichomonas:* Seven-day versus single-dose regimens. *JAMA* 1980;**244:** 1219.

Lefrock JL, Molavi A: Metronidazole. *Am Fam Physician* (July) 1981;**24:**185.

3. *CANDIDA ALBICANS* VAGINITIS

Candida albicans is a common part of the normal vaginal flora. Vaginitis may result from endogenous overgrowth of this yeastlike fungus or from its spread by sexual contact. Although *Candida* may be found alone, it is found in combination with other organisms in over half of the cases of vaginitis.

Factors precipitating infection are shown in Table 9–10. Some precipitants promote overgrowth of *C albicans* by removal of other normal flora (eg, broad-spectrum antibiotics, metronidazole); some encourage *C albicans* growth by increasing epithelial cell glycogen content (eg, pregnancy, oral contraceptives, dia-

Table 9–10. Factors precipitating candidal vaginitis.

Diabetes mellitus
Pregnancy
Broad-spectrum antibiotics
Oral contraceptives
Obesity
Tight nylon undergarments
Sexual activity (oral and genital)
Contaminated soaps, douche bags, and other objects
Large reservoir of organisms in the gastrointestinal tract, vagina, mouth, semen, or skin
Corticosteroids
Factors lowering host defenses (cancer, immunosuppressive drugs, anemia, etc)
Endocrinopathies
Drug addiction (eg, heroin)

betes); and some work by lowering general defense mechanisms (eg, severe iron deficiency anemia, drug addiction, chronic illness, cancer, corticosteroid use). Constant exposure to infected sources (eg, an infected sexual partner, contaminated soaps) or a large intestinal reservoir of *C albicans* may cause infection or reinfection. Obesity, exposure to heat, and wearing occlusive clothing (eg, tight nylon undergarments, tight jeans) also encourage *C albicans* growth.

About 10% of cases of candidal vaginitis are chronic or resistant to usual therapy; therefore, careful evaluation for underlying precipitating factors is important.

Clinical Findings

A. Symptoms and Signs: Clinical manifestations may include a thick, white, cheeselike vaginal discharge; pH of 3.8–5.0; vulvovaginal erythema; intense pruritus; dysuria and frequency; and dyspareunia. Severe or chronic infection may lead to perineal erythema, fissuring, lichenification, and secondary bacterial infection that can be extensive, often involving the perianal, inguinocrural, and intercrural regions. Pruritic, sterile lesions (''id reactions'') are occasionally noted on the sides of fingers and hands.

B. Laboratory Findings: A potassium hydroxide preparation or culture (on Sabouraud's, Nickerson's, or similar medium) may be used to support the clinical impression of candidal vaginitis. A drop of the vaginal secretion is mixed with a drop of 10–20% potassium hydroxide solution, covered with a coverslip, and examined microscopically for the presence of both hyphae and spores. Because the results of the preparation are not always positive in cases of candidal infection, treatment may be instituted on clinical grounds alone. Cultures are supportive but take several days or more to yield results.

Treatment

Acute vulvitis responds to warm sitz baths (with baking soda, Burow's solution, etc) and local application of corticosteroid cream or antifungal medication. Vaginitis may be treated with miconazole nitrate vaginal cream (at bedtime for 7 nights) or clotrimazole (100-mg vaginal tablet at bedtime for 7 nights). Nystatin vaginal tablets can be used, but the dose of one tablet (100,000 units) twice daily must be continued for 2 full weeks. New therapies for candidiasis include 2% butoconazole nitrate cream (6 mL given once intravaginally for 3 days) and ketoconazole vaginal tablets (variable doses). The latter has been successful for the treatment of chronic or recurrent disease. Chronic or recurrent infection warrants a careful evaluation for underlying factors (Table 9–10).

Droegmueller W et al: Three-day treatment with butoconazole nitrate for vulvovaginal candidiasis. *Obstet Gynecol* 1984;**64:**530.

Felman YM, Nikitas JA: Trichomoniasis, candidiasis, and *Corynebacterium vaginale* vaginitis. *NY State J Med* 1979; **79:** 1563.

Miles MR, Olsen L, Rogers A: Recurrent vaginal candidiasis: Importance of an intestinal reservoir. *JAMA* 1977;**238:**1836.

Sobel JD: Management of recurrent vulvovaginal candidiasis with intermittent ketoconazole prophylaxis. *Obstet Gynecol* 1985;**65:**435.

4. *GARDNERELLA VAGINALIS* VAGINITIS

Infection with *Gardnerella vaginalis* is thought to be the cause of most cases of what was previously called ''nonspecific'' vaginitis. This gram-negative organism (formerly called *Corynebacterium vaginale* or *Haemophilus vaginalis*) has caused considerable controversy but is now generally accepted as a common pathogen of sexually transmitted disease. As is true in cases of *Trichomonas* or *Candida* infection, the male sexual partner is usually asymptomatic.

Clinical Findings

A. Symptoms and Signs: Infection causes a gray-white, homogeneous, nonpruritic, and malodorous leukorrhea with a pH of 5.0–5.5. It is a ''surface'' infection, and in contrast to *Trichomonas* vaginitis, gross vulvovaginal changes are rare. The presence of other organisms (mixed infection) may alter the classic findings. Transient *G vaginalis* bacteremia has been reported, mostly related to delivery or abortion.

B. Laboratory Findings: A saline preparation or gram-stained smear of vaginal secretion often reveals ''clue cells''—epithelial cells studded with many small gram-negative bacilli—with areas between the epithelial cells relatively devoid of observable bacteria. In the less reliable amine test, a ''fishy'' odor of released amines is noted when 10% potassium hydroxide is mixed with the vaginal secretion. A specific fluorescent antibody test for *G vaginalis* may also be performed. Culture of a vaginal specimen for anaerobic and aerobic microbes usually reveals *G vaginalis* and anaerobic bacteria (eg, *Bacteroides* and *Peptococcus* species).

Treatment

Treatment is aimed at reducing the number of

Table 9–11. Treatment regimens for *Gardnerella* vaginitis.

Metronidazole, 500 mg orally 2 times daily for 7 days
Ampicillin, 500 mg orally 4 times daily for 7 days
Cephradine, 250 mg orally 4 times daily for 7 days
Cephalexin, 500 mg orally 4 times daily for 7 days
Tetracycline, 500 mg orally 4 times daily for 7 days

anaerobic bacteria so that a more normal flora can be established. Table 9–11 outlines several treatment modalities that have been advocated. *G vaginalis* is considered to be a normal part of the vaginal flora, and thus treatment is not recommended unless there are overt symptoms. The most effective regimen is metronidazole given in a 7-day course (see dosage in Table 9–11); this regimen was found to result in an 86% cure rate versus a 67% cure rate with a single 2-g dose of metronidazole. Ampicillin is recommended by the Centers for Disease Control for treatment of pregnant women, although it is not as effective as metronidazole. Treatment of asymptomatic carriers of *G vaginalis* is not recommended by the Centers for Disease Control, and therapy for male sexual partners is controversial.

Amsel R et al: Non-specific vaginitis. *Am J Med* 1983;**74:**14.

Bump RC et al: The prevalence, 6-month persistence and predicted values of laboratory indicators of bacterial vaginosis (nonspecific vaginitis) in asymptomatic women. *Am J Obstet Gynecol* 1984;**150:**917.

Gardner HL: *Haemophilus vaginalis* vaginitis after 25 years. *Am J Obstet Gynecol* 1980;**137:**385.

Malouf M et al: Treatment of *Haemophilus vaginalis* vaginitis. *Obstet Gynecol* 1981;**57:**711.

Purdon A Jr et al: An evaluation of single-dose metronidazole treatment for *Gardnerella vaginalis* vaginitis. *Obstet Gynecol* 1984;**64:**271.

Reimer LG, Reller LB: *Gardnerella vaginalis* bacteremia: A review of 30 cases. *Obstet Gynecol* 1984;**64:**170.

Spiegel CA et al: Anaerobic bacteria in non-specific vaginitis. *N Engl J Med* 1980;**303:**601.

5. *NEISSERIA GONORRHOEAE* CERVICITIS

Gonorrhea, a sexually transmitted disease, is a major problem in sexually active teenagers. In the USA, an estimated one-half million cases per year occur in teenagers. Although the 20- to 24-year-old age group traditionally has a higher incidence of gonorrhea than teenagers, the 15- to 19-year-old age group often has a higher incidence of gonococcal complications, owing to a delay in seeking treatment. While a male sexual partner has a 25% chance of acquiring gonorrhea from an infected female partner, the female sexual partner has nearly a 100% chance of acquiring the male partner's infection. The majority of women with gonococcal infection of the cervix are asymptomatic. *Neisseria gonorrhoeae* has a predilection for the cervical columnar epithelium and the urethra, where it can remain for months (or even years). Thus, periodic gonococcal screening in sexually active adolescents is important. Endocervicitis (infection of the cervical columnar epithelium) is primarily caused by *N gonorrhoeae, Chlamydia trachomatis,* or herpes simplex virus. Because of its characteristic mucopurulent discharge, it is often referred to as mucopurulent cervicitis.

Clinical Findings

A. Symptoms and Signs: A yellow-green, purulent or mucopurulent vaginal discharge is the classic presentation of symptomatic gonorrhea. Gonorrhea in prepubertal children usually presents as vaginitis, while that in pubescent adolescents presents as cervicitis. Dysuria, frequency, or irregular vaginal or menstrual bleeding is noted in some cases. Variable cervical tenderness, urethritis, bartholinitis, or skenitis (inflammation of paraurethral, or Skene's, glands) may be observed. Bartholinitis is characterized by a tender unilateral mass, 2–7 cm in diameter, in the labia majora. Mild proctitis may occur owing to the close anatomic relationship of the rectum to the vagina; this is due to a "backwash" phenomenon and usually only causes serious infection when rectal coitus occurs with an infected male partner. Septicemia occurs in 2–3% of untreated adolescents, with resultant dermatitis, arthritis, and other complications; gonococcal perihepatitis may also occur (see Chapter 27). Pelvic inflammatory disease is noted in 10–20% of patients with untreated gonococcal cervicitis.

B. Laboratory Findings: Asymptomatic gonorrhea can only be diagnosed by culture of a cervical specimen. The presence of purulent or mucopurulent discharge in a sexually active individual warrants suspicion for gonorrhea as well as other sexually transmitted diseases. A gram-stained smear of cervical secretions may reveal numerous gram-negative, kidney-shaped diplococci in polymorphonuclear leukocytes. A positive culture on Thayer-Martin medium is considered definitive. The culture specimen is usually obtained directly from the cervix; however, since rectal cultures are positive in 5% of cases in which cervical cultures are negative, rectal specimens should also be obtained. Pharyngeal specimens are cultured when there is a history of orogenital sexual activity or suspicion of gonococcal throat infection. In such cases, the patient is normally screened for syphilis as well.

Since *C trachomatis* and other organisms are commonly found in patients with gonorrhea, specimens should be carefully examined for mixed infections.

Treatment

Tables 9–12 and 9–13 outine the standard treatment regimens for uncomplicated gonorrhea and penicillinase-producing *N gonorrhoeae.* A 10- to 14-day course of a broad-spectrum antibiotic (eg, tetracycline) is often added to the treatment regimen to reduce the risk of postgonococcal pelvic inflammatory disease. Because of the high prevalence of mixed infections with *N gonorrhoeae* and *C trachomatis,* some

Table 9–12. Treatment regimens for gonococcal urethritis (cervicitis).

Aqueous procaine penicillin G (4.8 million units IM) plus probenecid (1 g orally)
Ampicillin (3.5 g orally) or amoxicillin (3 g orally) plus probenecid (1 g orally)
Tetracycline (500 mg 4 times daily for 5 days) in patients allergic to penicillin
Doxycycline (100 mg twice daily for 5 days)
Erythromycin (500 mg 4 times daily for 5 days)
Cefoxitin (2 g IM) plus probenecid (1 g orally)
Cefotaxime (1 g IM)
Spectinomycin (2 g IM)

clinicians treat gonococcal cervicitis with a 7-day course of tetracycline (500 mg 4 times daily) or doxycycline (100 mg twice daily). A 5-day course is effective treatment for gonorrhea and a 7-day course for chlamydial infections. The regimens shown in Tables 9–12 and 9–13 (except for spectinomycin) will effectively treat incubating syphilis as well.

Recent evidence suggests that a new extended-spectrum cephalosporin, ceftriaxone (in a single 125-mg intramuscular dose), may become the drug of choice for uncomplicated gonorrhea and for pharyngeal, anorectal, and pencillinase-producing forms of gonorrhea.

Pregnant adolescents with gonorrhea may be given amoxicillin or ampicillin with probenecid (Tables 9–12 and 9–13). Erythromycin (500 mg 4 times daily for 7 days) may be used for pregnant adolescents with mixed gonorrhea and chlamydial infections.

The male sexual partner should also be evaluated and treated.

Brown ER, Nair V: Laboratory identification of sexually transmitted diseases. *J Reprod Med* 1985;**30:**237.

Britigan BE, Cohen MS, Sparling PF: Gonococcal infection: A model of molecular pathogenesis. *N Engl J Med* 1985;**212:**1683.

Fiumara NJ: Treating gonorrhea. *Am Fam Physician* (May) 1981;**23:**123.

Judson FN, Ehret JM, Handsfield HH: Comparative study of ceftriaxone and spectinomycin for treatment of pharyngeal and anorectal gonorrhea. *JAMA* 1985;**253:**1417.

McGregor JA: Adolescent misadventures with urethritis and cervicitis. *J Adolesc Health Care* 1985;**6:**286.

Wiesner P, Thompson SE: Gonococcal diseases. *DM* (Feb) 1980;**26:**3.

Table 9–13. Treatment regimens for penicillinase-producing gonorrhea.

Spectinomycin* (2 g IM)
Cefoxitin (2 g IM) plus probenecid (1 g orally)
Cefotaxime (1 g IM)
Trimethoprim (80 mg) plus sulfamethoxazole (400 mg), 9 tablets orally in one dose for 5 days for treatment of pharyngeal gonorrheal infection

* Drug of choice. Tetracycline can be added to treat coexisting chlamydial infection.

6. HERPES SIMPLEX CERVICITIS

Herpes simplex infections are common in adolescents. Type 1 virus, which causes herpes labialis, keratitis, eczema herpeticum, and gingivostomatitis, is not considered a sexually transmitted disease and is commonly seen in children. In teenagers, only 10% of genital herpesvirus infections are due to herpes simplex virus type 1; the remainder are due to type 2 virus, which is commonly spread by sexual contact. Initial infection occurs after a variable incubation period (days to weeks) and is more severe than subsequent episodes. Recurrence is common, and the reservoir for infection is probably the cervix.

The highest incidence of genital infection may be in the 15- to 19-year-old age group; studies have noted that 3–12% of sexually active female teenagers have positive cultures for herpes simplex. The active lesions are very infectious, with a 30–60% infectivity rate. It is not currently possible to predict the risk of transmission of infection by asymptomatic patients.

A link between herpes infection and cervical cancer in adult life has been suggested. The association of herpes infection with fetal infection and death is well known.

Clinical Findings

A. Symptoms and Signs: Cervicitis and vulvar ulcerations are classic findings in sexually active teenagers with genital herpesvirus infection. Hyperesthesia or pruritus is followed shortly by the appearance of vulvar vesicles, which tend to occur in small groups on erythematous bases. The vesicles break down within 24–30 hours to form multiple ulcers that are small, shallow, and painful. After 3–14 days, lesions clear, usually without scarring. Ulcers may also be seen on the cervix and periurethral areas; occasionally, the vagina, urethra, thighs, and buttocks are involved. Mucopurulent cervical discharge and inguinal lymphadenopathy are often noted.

B. Laboratory Findings: Cultures of the vesicles or ulcers may reveal herpes simplex virus type 1 or 2. Although the following tests are also used in diagnosis, cultures are preferred. Giemsa-stained or Wright-stained smears (Tzanck test) of scrapings from vesicles or ulcers may reveal "balloon" cells with intranuclear inclusion bodies or multinucleated giant cells. A Papanicolaou smear may also show multinucleated giant cells, but these cells can be noted with herpes zoster and varicella infections as well. Viral herpetic particles can be seen with electron microscopy. Viral serologic studies and specific immunofluorescence techniques are also available.

Differential Diagnosis

The diagnosis of genital herpes is difficult unless the typical pattern of ulceration is seen, since vulvar ulceration occurs with other infections (Table 9–8). Diagnosis may also be difficult if complications (eg, radiculomyelitis) develop before classic features.

Syphilis should always be considered in the differential diagnosis of any genital ulcer. Rarely, syphilis and herpes simplex are found concurrently. Secondary bacterial infection of herpetic lesions occurs more commonly.

Complications

Complications reported to occur with herpesvirus infection include radiculomyelitis (with acute urinary retention), hepatic failure, aseptic meningitis, ascending myelitis, and erythema multiforme. Herpes encephalitis secondary to genital herpes is rare.

Treatment

In general, treatment is preventive and symptomatic. Some relief of symptoms may occur with the use of warm sitz baths, povidone-iodine solution, topical lidocaine (eg, Xylocaine jelly), or petroleum jelly. Recent studies indicate that topical use of 5% acyclovir ointment may be helpful for treatment of initial herpes infection. It is applied to the lesions every 3 hours, 6 times daily, for 7 days. Acyclovir ointment appears to limit the shedding of virus and may shorten the duration of symptoms with primary infection if it is started within 6 days of onset of symptoms. It does not prevent recurrences and has not been tested in pregnant or lactating women. Oral and parenteral use of acyclovir is under current investigation. Recent studies indicate that oral acyclovir can shorten the duration of primary infection but has minimal effect for preventing recurrent infection. Some clinicians have limited its use to cases of severe recurrent disease. Intravenous acyclovir may be more promising, but further studies are needed.

Treatment of secondary bacterial infection with broad-spectrum antibiotics may be necessary. Sexual activity should be avoided when the patient is symptomatic, and use of condoms during asymptomatic periods is recommended by some clinicians. Classic herpesvirus infection recurs at variable, unpredictable times after the initial infection. Patients with a history of infection should have a Papanicolaou smear done each year, and if the patient becomes pregnant, she should inform the obstetrician of the history of herpesvirus infection.

Becker TM et al: Genital herpes infections in private practice in the United States, 1966–1981. *JAMA* 1985;**253:**1601.

Corey L: Diagnosis of genital herpes simplex virus infection. *J Reprod Med* 1985;**30:**262.

Rauh JL, Brookman RR, Schiff GM: Genital viral surveillance among sexually active adolescent girls. *J Pediatr* 1977;**90:**844.

Rubin MH, Ward DM, Painter CJ: Fulminant hepatic failure caused by genital herpes in a healthy person. *JAMA* 1985;**253:**1299.

Rosenberg M, Lefrock JL: Drug therapy for sexually transmitted diseases. *Am Fam Physician* 1985;**31:**257.

Oral acyclovir for genital herpes simplex infection. *Med Lett Drugs Ther* 1985;**27:**41.

Sexually transmitted diseases: Treatment guidelines, 1982. *MMWR* 1982;**31:**33S.

Table 9–14. Disorders caused by *Chlamydia trachomatis* infections.

Females
Cervicitis
Urethral syndrome
Pelvic inflammatory disease
Peritonitis
Perihepatitis (Fitz-Hugh–Curtis syndrome)
Bartholinitis
Arthritis
Endocarditis
Ectopic pregnancy
Postpartum endometritis
Males
Nongonococcal urethritis
Epididymitis
? Reiter's syndrome
Pharyngitis
Penile edema
Proctitis
Prostatitis

7. *CHLAMYDIA TRACHOMATIS* CERVICITIS

The role of *Chlamydia trachomatis* as a major pathogen in sexually transmitted disease is discussed in Chapter 27. Table 9–14 outlines disorders caused by *C trachomatis* in males and females. Recent studies indicate it is a major cause of cervicitis, urethral syndrome, postpartum endometritis, perihepatitis, and pelvic inflammatory disease. This organism is often found concurrently with *Neisseria gonorrhoeae* but frequently is the sole agent of disease.

Clinical Findings

Symptoms of chlamydial cervicitis are variable, but common findings include purulent or mucopurulent cervical discharge; hypertrophic, friable cervix; and abnormal findings on the Papanicolaou smear, indicating inflammation or infection. Special serologic tests and cultures for *C trachomatis* can be performed but are not available in most laboratories. Negative cultures for *N gonorrhoeae* may implicate *C trachomatis* as the infecting organism.

Treatment

Treatment regimens for chlamydial infection are listed in Table 9–15. Tetracycline or doxycycline may be used for nonpregnant women and erythromycin for pregnant women. Posttreatment follow-up and

Table 9–15. Treatment regimens for chlamydial urethritis or cervicitis.*

Tetracycline, 500 mg 4 times daily orally for 7–14 days
Doxycycline, 100 mg 2 times daily orally for 1–2 weeks
Erythromycin, 500 mg 4 times daily orally for 1–2 weeks

* Penicillin, ampicillin, amoxicillin, metronidazole, and cephalosporins are ineffective.

treatment of the sexual partner are important, as for all sexually transmitted diseases.

Bump RC: *Chlamydia trachomatis* as a cause of prepubertal vaginitis. *Obstet Gynecol* 1985;**65:**384.

Chacko MR, Lovchik J: *Chlamydia trachomatis* infection in sexually active adolescents: Prevalence and risk factors. *Pediatrics* 1984;**73:**836.

Faro S: *Chlamydia trachomatis* infection in women. *J Reprod Med* 1985;**30:**273.

Golden N et al: Prevalence of *Chlamydia trachomatis* cervical infection in female adolescents. *Am J Dis Child* 1984;**138:** 562.

Judson FN: Assessing the number of genital chlamydial infections in the United States. *J Reprod Med* 1985;**30:**269.

Schachter J: Chlamydial infections. *N Engl J Med* 1978; **298:**490.

Shafer MA et al: Chlamydial endocervical infections and cytologic findings in sexually active adolescents. *Am J Obstet Gynecol* 1985;**151:**765.

8. MISCELLANEOUS CAUSES OF VULVOVAGINITIS

Foreign Body Vaginitis

After several days, a forgotten menstrual tampon or other object in the vagina can produce leukorrhea that persists until the foreign body is removed. Vaginal discharge may be bloody or purulent and is usually intensely malodorous. Urethritis and cystitis occasionally occur. Vulvar pruritus, backache, and dyspareunia are noted less frequently. Removal of the object and proper perineal hygiene are effective treatment.

Allergic or Contact Vaginitis

Erythema of vulvar and vaginal tissues, accompanied by pain, edema, pruritus, and leukorrhea, may occur upon contact with allergens such as feminine hygiene deodorants, chemical douches, vaginal contraceptives (eg, foam, cream), sanitary napkins, perfumes, and fabric softeners. Treatment consists of applying hydrocortisone ointment or cream, avoiding the allergen, and avoiding use of tight nylon undergarments (which worsen the symptoms).

Variants of allergic or contact vaginitis do occur. For example, vaginitis has been reported in association with hay fever or seasonal rhinitis. Allergic vaginitis has also been noted (rarely) upon contact with sperm; this is termed familial allergic seminal vulvovaginitis. Antihistamine cream and the use of a condom are helpful in such cases.

Salivary Vulvitis

Orogenital sexual activity may produce unusual vulvar symptoms. Infection with β-hemolytic streptococci, *Haemophilus influenzae, Candida albicans,* and other microbes may cause a "nonspecific" vulvitis with minimal vaginocervical symptoms. This has been termed salivary vulvitis. Treatment involves cessation of orogenital activity and use of drugs effective against the specific organisms cultured.

Syphilis

Infection due to *Treponema pallidum* is discussed in Chapter 27. Any sexually active individual with genital ulcers should be screened for syphilis. Table 9–8 lists other causes of ulcerous lesions that should be considered. Screening for syphilis involves serial darkfield examinations (on 3 successive days) and serial serologic tests (at initial presentation, in 6 weeks, and in 3 months).

Altchek A: Recognizing and controlling vulvovaginitis in children. *Contemp Pediatr* (May) 1985;**4:**59.

Olansky S, Rogers WG, Anthony WC: Diagnosis of anogenital ulcers. *Cutis* 1976;**17:**705.

Schneider GT: Vaginal infections. *Postgrad Med* (Feb) 1983; **73:**255.

Tanowitz HB: Parasitic gynecologic diseases. *Med Asp Hum Sex* 1974;**8:**45.

Treatment of sexually transmitted diseases. *Med Lett Drugs Ther* 1984;**26:**5.

Young AW, Tovell HMM, Sadri K: Erosions and ulcers of the vulva: Diagnosis, incidence and management. *Obstet Gynecol* 1977;**50:**35.

PELVIC INFLAMMATORY DISEASE

Pelvic inflammatory disease refers to an infection of the uterus, uterine (fallopian) tubes, and contiguous tissues in menstruating women. It has been linked to several factors, including surgery, instrumentation, pregnancy, cancer, and sexually transmitted diseases. This section focuses on pelvic inflammatory disease as a sexually transmitted disease.

There are over 1 million cases of pelvic inflammatory disease each year in the USA, with 25–50% requiring hospitalization. The incidence of pelvic inflammatory disease is about 10–13 per 1000 women 15–39 years of age and 20 per 1000 women 20–24 years of age. Most patients are under age 25, most are nulliparous, and nearly one-third are under age 19. Risk factors include young age, multiple sexual partners, history of previous pelvic inflammatory disease, and presence of an intrauterine contraceptive device. The infection is less common during pregnancy. It may occur after an abortion if agents causing sexually transmitted disease are present.

Initial causes of pelvic inflammatory disease are usually *Neisseria gonorrhoeae, Chlamydia trachomatis,* and (less frequently) *Mycoplasma hominis.* Continued infection, often with uterine tube injury, leads to infection with multiple bacteria, as listed in Table 9–16. Polymicrobial infection leads to severe sequelae and complicates treatment. How often *N gonorrhoeae* initiates the infection is unclear, but it is cultured in 30–60% of cases studied. Classic studies also report that 10–17% of cases of untreated cervical gonorrhea eventually develop into pelvic inflammatory disease, and about two-thirds of cases of gonococcal pelvic inflammatory disease occur within 7 days of the menstrual period. Adolescents may be more susceptible

Table 9–16. Microbial causes of pelvic inflammatory disease.

Neisseria gonorrhoeae
Chlamydia trachomatis
Mycoplasma hominis (possibly *Ureaplasma urealyticum* as well)
Neisseria meningitidis
Group A β-hemolytic streptococci
Haemophilus influenzae
Actinomyces israelii
Secondary invaders:
Coliform bacteria
Streptococcus faecalis
Bacteroides fragilis
Gardnerella vaginalis
Other aerobic and anaerobic bacteria

to pelvic inflammatory disease than adults because of limited exposure (and thus decreased immunity) to infecting organisms and a higher tendency for cervical growth of *N gonorrhoeae* and *C trachomatis* (due to more visible columnar epithelium in the adolescent cervix). Recent evidence suggests that the use of oral contraceptives offers some protection against gonococcal disease but may enhance chlamydial disease by encouraging cervical growth of this organism. The presence of sperm and *Trichomonas vaginalis* may also be a risk factor for the development of clinical disease.

Clinical Findings

A. Symptoms and Signs: Pelvic inflammatory disease must be suspected in any sexually active adolescent with low abdominal pain. Most have cervical and adnexal tenderness, but only 50% present with overt leukorrhea. The symptoms are variable, depending on which organism or organisms are present and how long the condition has continued. A combination of leukorrhea, adnexal tenderness, fever, leukocytosis, and elevated erythrocyte sedimentation rate is found in only 20% of gonococcal-induced cases. Palpable adnexal swelling is noted in only 25% and tubo-ovarian abscess in 10%. Pelvic inflammatory disease precipitated by *Chlamydia* has fewer classic features and may even be silent.

B. Laboratory Findings: An elevated leukocyte count is often not present, while an elevated erythrocyte sedimentation rate usually is noted. Specific culture results depend on the site (cervix, rectum, uterine tube, or peritoneum) and the duration of symptoms. Gonococci may not be cultured from the cervix several days after the symptoms are noted, yet the exotoxin-induced uterine tube injury may have occurred already, with resultant polymicrobial infection. Negative results in the serum pregnancy test reduce the likelihood of an ectopic pregnancy.

C. Special Examinations: Culdocentesis and ultrasonography may be useful in some cases of pelvic inflammatory disease. Most clinicians currently agree that laparoscopy is the diagnostic procedure of choice, especially in atypical or silent cases. Diagnosis is based on classic findings of abdominal pain, cervical and adnexal tenderness, and one or more of the following: temperature over 38 °C, white blood count over 10,500, increased erythrocyte sedimentation rate, purulent material in specimens from culdocentesis, or an inflammatory mass noted on ultrasonography. The laparoscope can be used to verify the diagnosis, determine the severity of disease, and identify a tubo-ovarian cyst or other abscess.

Differential Diagnosis

The differential diagnosis of pelvic inflammatory disease is listed in Table 9–17. The diagnosis of pelvic inflammatory disease is difficult even for the most experienced clinician. Misdiagnosis occurs in 35% or more of cases if the diagnosis is made only on the basis of the history, abdominal examination, and pelvic examination.

Complications

Early diagnosis and treatment are essential for preventing the many sequelae of pelvic inflammatory disease. Many adolescents develop tubal occlusion, with resultant infertility. Classic studies note a 13% infertility rate after one severe episode of pelvic inflammatory disease; this rises to 35% with the second episode and to 50–70% with 3 or more episodes. Disease is recurrent in 20% of cases; thus, the risk of infertility is high. In the USA, pelvic inflammatory disease has caused sterilization in an estimated 300,000 teenage girls over the past 15 years. The number of cases of ectopic pregnancy has recently tripled, and this increase has been associated with an increase in pelvic inflammatory diseases. Other sequelae include Fitz-Hugh–Curtis syndrome, chronic abdominal pain, dyspareunia, dysmenorrhea, dysfunctional uterine bleeding, pelvic adhesions, psychologic problems, and surgical complications. *Chlamydia* may cause chronic asymptomatic oophoritis, which can lead to severe premenstrual tension syndrome and ovulation dysfunction.

Table 9–17. Differential diagnosis of pelvic inflammatory disease.

Appendicitis
Mesenteric lymphadenitis
Acute pyelonephritis
Torsion of ovarian cyst
Rupture of ovarian cyst
Ectopic pregnancy
Endometriosis
Acute pancreatitis
Various nonsurgical causes of severe abdominal pain
Inflammatory bowel disease
Diabetic ketoacidosis
Food poisoning
Gastroenteritis (eg, due to *Yersinia enterocolitica* or *Campylobacter fetus*)
Henoch-Schönlein syndrome
Hemolytic-uremic syndrome
Acute intermittent porphyria

Treatment

Various treatment regimens have been proposed. Determining the best regimen to use is difficult, since the exact microbial etiologic agents are not usually known. Therapy is designed to deal with 3 classifications of pelvic inflammatory disease: gonococcal, chlamydial, and polymicrobial.

A. Outpatient Therapy: Outpatient therapy for mild cases is aimed at treating gonorrhea or chlamydial infections (discussed in previous sections). Additional treatment for continued infection includes the combination of metronidazole (500–750 mg 3 times daily) with either tetracycline (500 mg 4 times daily) or doxycycline (100 mg twice daily) for 7–14 days.

B. Inpatient Therapy: Patients who fail to respond to oral regimens and those with severe pelvic inflammatory disease should be hospitalized. Other reasons for hospitalization include adnexal mass, pregnancy, peritoneal signs or toxicity, and uncertain diagnosis.

Hospitalized adolescents may be treated with one of the following regimens for at least 4 days, or until 2 days after improvement:

1. Ampicillin, 500 mg intravenously every 6 hours.
2. Tetracycline, 250–500 mg intravenously every 6 hours.
3. Aqueous crystalline penicillin G, 20 million units/d intravenously, plus gentamicin or tobramycin, 2 mg/kg intravenously initially, followed by 1.5 mg/kg intravenously 3 times daily. Clindamycin, 600 mg intravenously every 6 hours, may be added immediately or in 1–2 days if clinical improvement does not occur.
4. Doxycycline, 100 mg intravenously every 12 hours, plus cefoxitin, 2 mg intravenously every 6 hours. Clindamycin or metronidazole may also be used with this regimen, in which case 15 mg/kg is given intravenously as a loading dose, followed by 7.5 mg/kg given intravenously every 6 hours.
5. Doxycycline, 100 mg intravenously every 12 hours, plus metronidazole, 1 g intravenously every 12 hours. Another suggested dosage schedule for metronidazole is given in (4), above.

Coverage for the various etiologic agents or pelvic inflammatory disease must be ensured. Metronidazole has become popular recently, owing to its superior bactericidal activity against anaerobes, including *Bacteroides fragilis.*

Patients released from the hospital may be given oral antibiotics (eg, doxycycline or tetracycline) to complete a 10- to 14-day course of total therapy. Careful follow-up evaluation and early consultation with a gynecologist are recommended. Treatment of the patient's sex partner should also be instituted.

Friberg J: Diagnosis of genital *Mycoplasma* and *Ureaplasma* infections. *J Reprod Med* 1985;**30:**258.

Handsfield HH: Sexually transmitted diseases. *Hosp Pract* (Jan) 1982;**17:**99.

Mead PB: Pelvic inflammatory disease: Use of appropriate antibiotics. *Clin Obstet Gynecol* 1985;**28:**405.

Sexually transmitted diseases: Treatment guidelines, 1982. *MMWR* 1982;**31:**33S.

St. John RK, Brown ST (editors): International Symposium on Pelvic Inflammatory Disease. *Am J Obstet Gynecol* 1980;**138:**845.

Washington AE, Sweet RL, Shafer MB: Pelvic inflammatory disease and its sequelae in adolescents. *J Adolesc Health Care* 1985;**6:**293.

Washington AE et al: Oral contraceptives, *Chlamydia trachomatis* infection, and pelvic inflammatory disease: A word of caution about protection. *JAMA* 1985;**253:**2246.

MENSTRUAL DISORDERS

The average age for onset of menstruation (menarche) in the USA is 12.6–12.9 years, while the normal range is 10–17 years, depending on when thelarche occurs. It may take 1–3½ years for menarche to follow thelarche, and it takes an average of 20 months for normal menstrual cycles to become established following menarche.

Variation in "normal" menstruation is noted, since "normal" cycles may be 21–35 days in length, with a 2- to 8-day flow and a 2- to 3-day individual variation. Blood flow may vary from 20 to 50 mL each cycle, and tremendous variation may occur during the immediate postmenarcheal time. These variations must be kept in mind when teenagers with menstrual concerns are evaluated.

The menstrual process is characterized by a complex series of events. The hypothalamus secretes gonadotropin-releasing hormone (GnRH), which stimulates the anterior pituitary to secrete follicle-stimulating hormone (FSH) and luteinizing hormone (LH). FSH stimulates preovulatory growth as well as estrogen production by the developing ovarian follicle. LH stimulates ovulation and enhances progesterone production by the corpus luteum. Estrogen and progesterone are then produced in increased amounts over the next 7–10 days. In the absence of fertilization and implantation, the corpus luteum begins to regress, which leads to rapid decline in secretion of these hormones and then menstruation due to endometrial sloughing. This entire process, which occurs several hundred times during the lifetime, is regulated by complex negative and positive feedback systems that require fine coordination of activities of the hypothalamus, pituitary, thyroid, adrenals, ovaries, and uterus. Thus, it is not surprising to note many variations of normal and to note specific disease processes affecting this intricate system. This section will outline 2 basic menstrual disorders: dysmenorrhea and dysfunctional uterine bleeding. Amenorrhea is discussed in Chapter 25.

Comerci GD: Symptoms associated with menstruation. *Pediatr Clin North Am* 1982;**29:**177.

Eisenberg E: Menarche: The transition from childhood to womanhood. *Adv Pediatr* 1984;**31:**359.

Greydanus DE, McAnarney ER: Menstruation and its disorders in adolescence. *Curr Probl Pediatr* (Aug) 1982;**12:**1.

Gysler M, Cowell CA: Gynaecological endocrinology of the paediatric and adolescent age group. *Clin Endocrinol Metab* 1982;**11:**233.

Koff E, Rierdan J, Jacobson S: The personal and interpersonal significance of menarche. *J Am Acad Child Psychiatry* 1981;**20:**148.

McDonough PG, Gambrell RD Jr: The adolescent gynecological patient and her problems. *Clin Obstet Gynecol* 1979;**22:**491.

Sanfilippo JS, Yussman MA: Gynecologic problems of adolescence. Chap 6, pp 61–83, in: *Pediatric and Adolescent Obstetrics and Gynecology*. Lavery JP, Sanfilippo JS (editors). Springer-Verlag, 1985.

1. AMENORRHEA (See Chapter 25.)

2. DYSMENORRHEA

Painful menstrual cramps are noted in over half of adolescents with regular menstruation, and perhaps as many as 10% must alter their daily routines because of incapacitating pain. Previous studies associated menstrual cramps with psychologic causes, but current studies clearly implicate physiologic mechanisms: Increased sensitivity and increased synthesis of endometrial prostaglandins (especially prostaglandin $F_{2\alpha}$) cause increased uterine spasms, increased endometrial ischemia, and more pain. Cold temperature may worsen dysmenorrhea by causing vasoconstriction of myometrial arterioles and release of more prostaglandin $F_{2\alpha}$. Most cases of menstrual cramps in adolescents are primary dysmenorrhea, but other factors should be considered in the evaluation, since secondary dysmenorrhea also occurs in this age group.

The cause of premenstrual tension syndrome is unknown; proposed causes include a deficiency of β-endorphins, progestin, or pyridoxine; an excess of estrogen or prolactin; hypoglycemia; electrolyte disturbances; prostaglandin abnormalities; and abnormal levels of methoxyhydroxyphenylglycol (a central nervous system metabolite of norepinephrine).

Clinical Findings

Primary dysmenorrhea usually occurs 6–20 months after menarche, ie, once a more regular menstrual pattern develops. It usually implies that ovulation is occurring, with increased progesterone secretion and then increased prostaglandin synthesis. Menstrual cramps commonly begin around or shortly after the time of bleeding and are usually centered in the low to mid abdomen, with pain sometimes radiating to the back or thighs. This process may last 1–3 days. Some adolescents also have premenstrual tension syndrome in which additional symptoms develop a few days before the cramps and continue for a variable time, often lasting through menstruation. These symptoms may include nausea, vomiting, breast swelling or tenderness, headache, abdominal bloating, gastrointestinal dysfunction, hyperphagia, weight gain secondary to sodium and water retention, insomnia, acne, edema, mood changes, and a tendency toward violence.

A careful history and physical examination, with pelvic examination to rule out secondary dysmenorrhea, should be performed in adolescents with severe dysmenorrhea.

Differential Diagnosis

Table 9–18 lists causes of secondary dysmenorrhea, some of which are also associated with increased prostaglandin synthesis.

Endometriosis should always be considered as a cause of severe dysmenorrhea, especially in cases unresponsive to medical therapy. Endometrial tissue developing outside the uterus produces various symptoms, including irregular vaginal bleeding, progessive dysmenorrhea, other types of chronic pelvic pain, and gastrointestinal dysfunction. The pelvic examination may be normal in early stages of endometriosis. The diagnosis is based on symptoms and results of laparoscopy and is confirmed by tissue biopsy. Therapy consists of various medications to suppress ovulation (eg, oral contraceptives or danazol); surgery may be indicated.

Severe refractory dysmenorrhea may also have primary or secondary psychologic features, as is true for any case of chronic pain, which can lead to chronic pain syndrome. Thus, attention to psychologic factors is necessary in some cases.

Treatment

In patients with primary dysmenorrhea, mild cramps may respond to common analgesics, local heat application, and rest. Exercise plans to improve muscular tone are of unproved benefit. If the patient is sexually active, oral contraceptives (tablets containing 30–50 μg of estrogen) are often effective. Birth control pills can also be used for non-sexually active adolescents, but sometimes objections are raised by the parent and patient about the "sexual aura" associated with their use. An excellent alternative is to use one of several available prostaglandin synthesis inhibitors (Table 9–19). These agents are absorbed quickly, and most individuals do well if the medication is started when cramps begin (usually before or on the first day of menstrual bleeding) and continued for 3–5 days. Recent evidence indicates that mefenamic acid may be somewhat more effective than the other agents listed in Table 9–19. A 3-month

Table 9–18. Causes of secondary dysmenorrhea.

Pelvic inflammatory disease
Intrauterine contraceptive device
Endometriosis
Congenital anomalies of the genital tract
Uterine neoplasms (including fibroids)
Dermoid cysts
Pelvic adhesions

Table 9–19. Prostaglandin synthesis inhibitors for treatment of primary dysmenorrhea.

Ibuprofen (Motrin), 400 mg 4 times daily orally (not to exceed 2400 mg/d) for 3–5 days
Naproxen sodium (Anaprox), 550 mg orally as a loading dose and then 275 mg 4 times daily orally (not to exceed 1375 mg/d) for 3–5 days
Naproxen (Naprosyn), 500 mg orally as a loading dose and then 250 mg 4 times daily orally (not to exceed 1250 mg/d) for 3–5 days
Mefenamic acid (Ponstel), 500 mg orally as a loading dose and then 250 mg 4 times daily for 3–5 days
Aspirin, 650 mg 4 times daily orally (weak inhibitor) for 3–5 days

cycle of any of these agents can be tried, and if it is not effective, another drug from this group is used. About 70–90% of patients are reported to have significant reduction of pain. Side effects are minimal and are usually limited to gastrointestinal dysfunction.

If significant relief does not occur with use of a prostaglandin inhibitor or birth control pills for 4–6 months, a reevaluation is needed. Secondary dysmenorrhea should be reconsidered and gynecologic consultation obtained. These agents listed in Table 19–9 may be effective in relieving pain associated with secondary dysmenorrhea as well.

Treatment of premenstrual tension syndrome is controversial, and no agent has proved to be generally effective. Methods traditionally used include rest, a low-salt diet, diuretics, mild tranquilizers, and progestins (vaginal or rectal). Other medications have included vitamin B_6, oral contraceptives, bromocriptine mesylate, clonidine, antidepressants, and verapamil. Much research is needed to establish the actual causes and effective treatment of premenstrual tension syndrome.

Anersch B, Milsom I: An epidemiologic study of young women with dysmenorrhea. *Am J Obstet Gynecol* 1982;**144:**655.

Dawood MY: Dysmenorrhea. *J Reprod Med* 1985;**30:**154.

Drugs for dysmenorrhea. *Med Lett Drugs Ther* 1979;**21:**81.

Huffman JW: Endometriosis in young teenage girls. *Pediatr Ann* (Dec) 1981;**10:**44.

O'Brien PMS: The premenstrual syndrome: A review. *J Reprod Med* 1985;**30:**113.

Owen PR: Protaglandin synthetase inhibitors in the treatment of primary dysmenorrhea. *Am J Obstet Gynecol* 1984; **146:**96.

Ylikorkala O, Dawood MY: New concepts in dysmenorrhea. *Am J Obstet Gynecol* 1978;**130:**833.

3. DYSFUNCTIONAL UTERINE BLEEDING

Irregular menstrual bleeding patterns during the first 2–4 years after menarche are usually associated with physiologic immaturity. There may be metrorrhagia (bleeding of normal amount at irregular intervals), menometrorrhagia (excessive bleeding at irregular intervals), oligomenorrhea (menstrual cycles 40 days or more apart), polymenorrhea (menstrual cycles less than 21 days apart), or other irregularities.

Dysfunctional uterine bleeding is defined as abnormal uterine bleeding due to hormonal variations. The numerous causes of abnormal bleeding patterns in adolescents are outlined in Table 9–20.

Dysfunctional uterine bleeding often implies anovulatory bleeding. Typically, the amount and timing of estrogen secretion are abnormal, with no midcycle LH surge and thus no ovulation. In the absence of

Table 9–20. Causes of abnormal uterine bleeding.*

Pregnancy complications
Spontaneous or induced incomplete abortion
Ectopic pregnancy (tubal pregnancy)
Hydatidiform mole
Blood dyscrasias
Iron deficiency anemia
Factor VIII deficiency
Von Willebrand's disease
Idiopathic thrombocytopenic purpura
Leukemia
Scurvy
Pathologic disorders of the cervix
Polyps
Erosion
Sarcoma botryoides
Mixed mesodermal sarcoma
Vaginal disorders
Adenosis (exposure to diethylstilbestrol)
Adenocarcinoma (exposure to diethylstilbestrol)
Uterine disorders
Polyps
Fibroids
Congenital anomalies
Carcinoma
Endometriosis
Ovarian disorders
Stein-Leventhal syndrome
Tumor
Persistent corpus luteum cyst (Halban's disease)
Adrenal disorders (hyperadrenocorticism)
Pituitary tumor (eg, craniopharyngioma)
Malnutrition
Obesity
Sudden weight changes (eg, due to excessive exercise)
Pelvic inflammatory disease
Vulvovaginitis (eg, due to *Trichomonas vaginalis* or *Neisseria gonorrhoeae*)
Tuberculosis
Trauma (eg, from coitus, foreign body, intrauterine contraceptive device)
Organ failure (cardiac, liver, renal)
Diabetes mellitus
Hypothyroidism (rarely, hyperthyroidism)
Chronic illness
Premature menopause
Medications (eg, warfarin, oral contraceptives, diet pills, phenothiaznes, anticholinergics)
Emotional factors

* Modified and reproduced, with permission, from Greydanus DE: Menstrual disorders. In: *Bedside Pediatrics.* Ziai M (editor). Little, Brown, 1983.

ovulation, the corpus luteum fails to function, and there is no late-cycle progesterone secretion. Progesterone is necessary to inhibit growth of the estrogen-stimulated endometrial lining. Thus, there is continued estrogen stimulation of the endometrium, which causes bleeding at irregular, unpredictable intervals.

Dysfunctional uterine bleeding may occur despite the presence of ovulation, but this hormonal variation is less common in young teenagers.

Clinical Findings

Irregular, painless bleeding is commonly noted in teenagers during the 2–4 years after menarche. Bleeding may be mild or life-threatening, and acute or chronic anemia may be noted. Typical findings in cases of anovulatory bleeding include no history of mittelschmerz, no rise in basal body temperature, and no dysmenorrhea. Indirect measures of ovulation include blood levels of progesterone, urinary levels of pregnanediol (a metabolite of progesterone), and identification of secretory endometrium by biopsy.

Differential Diagnosis

A careful evaluation is necessary to determine other causes of bleeding (Table 9–20). Severe bleeding, especially at or shortly after menarche, may be due to a bleeding disorder; therefore, coagulation screening tests are indicated.

Pregnancy complications must be ruled out in any sexually active adolescent. Ectopic pregnancy classically presents with a history of a delayed menstrual cycle, uterine bleeding, abdominal or pelvic pain, adnexal mass, or a combination of these findings. The serum pregnancy test is positive in cases of ectopic pregnancy.

Spontaneous abortion and sexually transmitted diseases (eg, gonorrhea, trichomoniasis) must also be considered in sexually active teenagers.

Certain genital abnormalities (eg, vaginal adenosis) related to in utero exposure to diethylstilbestrol (DES) may cause abnormal bleeding. Screening of all female teenagers who were exposed to DES is necessary, beginning at menarche or by age 14 if menarche has not started, or any time vaginal bleeding is noted.

Abnormal bleeding may be due to coital trauma, endometritis, complications of contraceptive use (IUD or oral contraceptives), thyroid disease, drug reactions, or other causes shown in Table 9–20.

Treatment

Although mild anovulatory bleeding may not require treatment, the patient should be observed until ovulation with regular menstruation occurs, which may take several months or longer. Mildly anemic patients may benefit from oral iron supplements.

Bleeding that is prolonged or severe requires hormone regulation. In some cases, immediate hospitalization, intense evaluation, and use of parenteral hormones (intravenous estrogen with oral or intramuscular progesterone) may be indicated.

Treatment regimens are outlined in Tables 9–21 and 9–22. Oral progestins can be used, but they are not as fast-acting or effective as estrogens in some women who bleed heavily. In general, the clinician uses one of these regimens to stop the bleeding (it usually stops within 12–30 hours) and then begins another regimen 7 days later to regulate the menstrual pattern over the following several weeks or months.

Hormone regulation is usually continued for 3–6 months, during which time the menstrual patterns are evaluated. Adolescents who continue to bleed severely require gynecologic consultation, as do those whose abnormal bleeding continues beyond 3–4 years after menarche. Many adolescents with chronic bleeding abnormalities develop endometrial cystic glandular hyperplasia, Stein-Leventhal syndrome, endometrial cancer, or infertility in adulthood.

Table 9–21. Hormonal therapy for anovulatory dysfunctional uterine bleeding.*

Regimens to stop severe bleeding
Estrogen and progestin combination† oral contraceptives (eg, Norinyl 2 mg, Demulen, Ortho-Novum-2, Enovid 5, Ovulen, Ovral, Ortho-Novum 1/50), 1–2 tablets orally immediately; then 1 tablet orally 4 times daily for 4–6 days
Norethindrone (Norlutin), 30–40 mg orally daily until bleeding stops; then 10 mg orally daily for 14 days
Norethindrone acetate (Norlutate), 15–20 mg orally daily until bleeding stops; then 10 mg orally daily for 14 days
Medroxyprogesterone acetate (Provera), 30–40 mg orally daily for 3–4 days; then 10 mg orally daily for 14 days
Progesterone in oil, 50–100 mg IM; may be repeated in 4–8 hours
Emergency treatment: Conjugated estrogens (Premarin), 20–60 mg IV every 2–6 hours for 12–36 hours
Megestrol acetate (Megace), 20 mg orally 2–4 times daily for 7–10 days
Hydroxyprogesterone caproate in oil (Delalutin), 250 mg IM; repeat in 3 days
Regimens to regulate the menstrual cycle
Estrogen and progestin combination† oral contraceptives daily for 3–6 menstrual cycles‡
Norethindrone (Norlutin), 5–20 mg orally either on menstrual days 21–26, 5–25, or 1–7 each month for 3–6 months, and sometimes longer
Norethindrone acetate (Norlutate), 2.5–10 mg orally as per the schedule for Norlutin
Medroxyprogesterone acetate (Provera), 10–20 mg orally as per the schedule for Norlutin

* Modified and reproduced, with permission, from Greydanus DE, McAnarney ER: Menstruation and its disorders in adolescence. *Curr Probl Pediatr* (Aug) 1982;**12:**1.

† See Table 9–22 for estrogen and progestin contents of oral contraceptives.

‡ The cycles are regulated hormonally until further physiologic maturity occurs and causes self-regulation and more normal menstrual cycles with less bleeding. This can take 3–6 months, or even 2 or more years.

Table 9–22. Estrogen and progestin contents of oral contraceptives used for acute treatment of dysfunctional uterine bleeding.

Oral Contraceptive	Estrogen	Progestin
Norinyl 2 mg	100 μg mestranol	2 mg norethindrone
Demulen	50 μg ethinyl estradiol	1 mg ethynodiol diacetate
Ortho-Novum-2	100 μg mestranol	2 mg norethindrone
Enovid 5	75 μg mestranol	5 mg norethynodrel
Ovulen	100 μg mestranol	1 mg ethynodiol diacetate
Ovral	50 μg ethinyl estradiol	0.5 mg norgestrel
Ortho-Novum 1/50	50 μg mestranol	1 mg norethindrone

Altcheck A: Dysfunctional uterine bleeding in adolescence. *Clin Obstet Gynecol* 1977;**20:**633.

Claessens EA, Cowell CA: Acute adolescent menorrhagia. *Am J Obstet Gynecol* 1981;**139:**277.

Frank AR et al: Regression of cervicovaginal abnormalities in DES-exposed women. *J Reprod Med* 1985;**30:**400.

Goldfarb JM, Little AB: Abnormal vaginal bleeding. *N Engl J Med* 1980;**302:**666.

Herbst AL: Diethylstilbestrol exposure: 1984. *N Engl J Med* 1984;**311:**1433.

Reindollar RH, McDonough PG: Adolescent menstrual disorders. *Clin Obstet Gynecol* 1983;**26:**690.

Southam AL, Richart RM: The prognosis for adolescents with menstrual abnormalities. *Am J Obstet Gynecol* 1966;**94:**637.

Spellacy WN: Abnormal bleeding. *Clin Obstet Gynecol* 1983;**26:**702.

SELECTED REFERENCES

American Psychiatric Association: *Diagnostic and Statistical Manual of Mental Disorders (DSM-III),* 3rd ed. American Psychiatric Association, 1980.

Barnes HV (editor): Symposium on adolescent medicine. *Med Clin North Am* 1975;**59:**1279.

Betts JM, Eichelberger M (editors): Symposium on pediatric and adolescent sports medicine. *Clin Sports Med* 1982;**1:**341.

Blum RW (editor): *Adolescent Health Care: Clinical Issues.* Academic Press, 1982.

Blum RW (editor): *Chronic Illness and Disabilities in Childhood and Adolescence.* Grune & Stratton, 1984.

Christopherson ER (editor): Symposium on behavioral pediatrics. *Pediatr Clin North Am* 1982;**29:**235.

Hofmann AD, Greydanus DE (editors): *Adolescent Medicine.* Addison-Wesley, 1983.

Holmes KK et al (editors): *Sexually Transmitted Diseases.* McGraw-Hill, 1984.

Huffman JW, Dewhurst CJ, Capraro VJ: *The Gynecology of Childhood and Adolescence,* 2nd ed. Saunders, 1981.

Lavery JP, Sanfilippo JS (editors): *Pediatric and Adolescent Obstetrics and Gynecology.* Springer-Verlag, 1985.

Levine M et al (editors): *Developmental Behavioral Pediatrics.* Saunders, 1983.

Litt IF (editor): Symposium on adolescent medicine. *Pediatr Clin North Am* 1980;**27:**1.

McAnarney ER (editor): *Premature Adolescent Pregnancy and Parenthood.* Grune & Stratton, 1983.

Prugh DJ: *The Psychosocial Aspects of Pediatrics.* Lea & Febiger, 1983.

Sahler OJZ, McAnarney ER: *The Child From Three to Eighteen.* Mosby, 1981.

Smith NJ (editor): *Sports Medicine: Health Care for Young Athletes.* American Academy of Pediatrics, 1983.

Stuart IR, Wells CF (editors): *Pregnancy in Adolescence: Needs, Problems, and Management.* Van Nostrand-Reinhold, 1982.

Skin 10

William L. Weston, MD

GENERAL PRINCIPLES OF DIAGNOSIS

Examination of the skin requires that the entire surface of the body be inspected in good light and palpated. The skin offers many clues to internal disorders and must be scrutinized with the same care required for auscultation of diastolic murmurs. The onset and duration of each symptom should be recorded.

Examination of the Skin

Examination of the skin should consist of identification of a primary lesion followed by description of secondary changes, color, configuration, and distribution of the lesions. The sometimes difficult language of dermatology prevents many students of medicine from accurately describing cutaneous eruptions. The word "rash" is too vague to be useful and should be qualified appropriately. The following terminology should be mastered by all practitioners.

A. Primary Lesions (the First to Appear):

1. Macule—Any circumscribed color change in the skin that is flat. *Examples:* White (vitiligo), brown (café au lait spot), purple (petechia).

2. Papule—A solid, elevated area > 1 cm in diameter whose top may be pointed, rounded, or flat. *Examples:* Acne, warts, small lesions of psoriasis.

3. Plaque—A solid, circumscribed area < 1 cm in diameter, usually flat-topped. *Example:* Psoriasis.

4. Vesicle—A circumscribed, elevated lesion > 1 cm in diameter and containing clear serous fluid. *Example:* Blisters of herpes simplex.

5. Bulla—A circumscribed, elevated lesion < 1 cm in diameter and containing clear serous fluid. *Example:* Bullous erythema multiforme.

6. Nodule—A deep-seated mass with indistinct borders that elevates the overlying epidermis. *Examples:* Tumors, grauloma annulare. If it moves with the skin on palpation, it is intradermal; if the skin moves over the nodule, it is subcutaneous.

7. Wheal —A circumscribed, flat-topped, firm elevation of skin resulting from tense edema of the papillary dermis. *Example:* Urticaria.

B. Secondary Changes:

1. Pustule—A vesicle containing a purulent exudate. *Examples:* Acne, folliculitis.

2. Scales—Dry, thin plates of keratinized epidermal cells (stratum corneum). *Examples:* Psoriasis, ichthyosis.

3. Lichenification—Dry, leathery thickening of skin with deep and exaggerated skin lines and a shiny surface resulting from chronic rubbing of the skin. *Example:* Atopic dermatitis.

4. Erosion and oozing—A moist, circumscribed, slightly depressed area representing a blister base with the roof of the blister removed. *Examples:* Burns, bullous erythema multiforme. Most oral blisters present as erosions.

5. Crust—Dried exudate of plasma on the surface of the skin following acute dermatitis. *Examples:* Impetigo, contact dermatitis.

6. Fissure—A linear split in the skin extending through the epidermis into the dermis. *Example:* Angular cheilitis.

7. Scar—A flat, raised, or depressed area of fibrotic replacement of dermis or subcutaneous tissue. *Examples:* Acne scar, burn scar.

8. Atrophy—Depression of the skin surface due to thinning of one or more layers of skin.

C. Color: The lesion should be described as red, yellow, brown, tan, or blue. Particular attention should be given to the blanching of red or brown lesions, eg, petechiae.

D. Configuration of Lesions: Clues to diagnosis may be obtained from the characteristic morphologic arrangement of primary or secondary lesions.

1. Annular (circular)—Annular nodules represent granuloma annulare; annular papules are more apt to be due to dermatophyte infections.

2. Linear (straight line)—Linear papules represent lichen striatus; linear vesicles, incontinentia pigmenti; linear papules with burrows, scabies.

3. Grouped—Grouped vesicles occur in herpes simplex or zoster.

E. Distribution: It is useful to note whether the eruption is generalized, acral (hands, feet, buttocks, or face), or localized to a specific skin region.

F. Description of Skin Lesions: Skin lesions are described in reverse order from that of their identification. One begins with distribution, configuration, color, secondary changes, and then primary lesion; eg, guttate psoriasis could be described as generalized discrete, red, scaly papules.

GENERAL PRINCIPLES OF TREATMENT OF SKIN DISORDERS

PERCUTANEOUS ABSORPTION & THE ROLE OF WATER

Some skin disorders can be treated in different ways by different practitioners and with varying degrees of success. In this section we will deliberately exclude many therapies, including a few time-honored ones, in order to present a rational approach to the treatment of skin disease.

Treatment should be simple and aimed at preserving or restoring the physiologic state of the skin. It is essential to keep in mind that one is treating the child and not the anxious parent or grandparent. Topical therapy is often preferred because medication can be delivered in optimal concentrations at the exact site where it is needed.

Water is an important therapeutic agent that is often forgotten (it is the active ingredient in Burow's solution, calamine lotion, potassium permanganate, and tannic acid soaks). When the skin is optimally hydrated, it is soft and smooth (Table 10–1). This occurs at approximately 60% environmental humidity. Since water evaporates readily from the cutaneous surface, the skin (stratum corneum of the epidermis) is dependent on the water concentration in the air, and sweating contributes little. However, if sweat is prevented from evaporating (eg, in the axilla, groin), the environmental humidity is increased and so is the hydration of the skin. As environmental humidity falls below 15–20%, the stratum corneum shrinks and cracks; the epidermal barrier is lost and allows irritants to enter the skin and induce an inflammatory response. Replacement of water will correct this if the water is not allowed to evaporate. Therefore, in treating dry and scaly skin, one would soak the skin in water for 5 minutes and then add a barrier to prevent evaporation. Oils and ointments prevent evaporation for 8–12 hours. Thus, oils and ointments must be applied once or twice a day. In areas already occluded (axilla, diaper area), ointments or oils will merely increase retention of water and should not be used.

Overhydration (maceration) can also occur. As environmental humidity increases to 90–100%, the number of water molecules absorbed by the stratum corneum increases and the tight lipid junctions between the cells of the stratum corneum are gradually replaced by weak hydrogen bonds (water); the cells eventually become widely separated, and the epidermal barrier falls apart. This occurs in immersion foot, diaper areas, axillas, etc. It is desirable to enhance evaporation of water in these areas. Exposure to less humidity and the use of powders (talcum) that take up extra water are indicated in maceration.

Table 10–1. Bases used for topical preparations.

Base	Combined With	Uses
Liquids		Wet dressings: relieve pruritus, vasoconstrict.
	Powder	Shake lotions, drying pastes: relieve pruritus, vasoconstrict.
	Grease and emulsifier; oil in water	Vanishing cream: penetrates quickly (10–15 minutes) and thus allows evaporation.
	Excess grease and emulsifier; water in oil	Emollient cream: penetrates more slowly and thus retains moisture on skin.
Grease		Ointments: occlusive (hold material on skin for prolonged time) and prevent evaporation of water.
Powder		Enhances evaporation.

(1) Most greases are triglycerides (eg, Aquaphor, petrolatum, Eucerin).
(2) Oils are fluid fats (eg, Alpha Keri, olive oil, mineral oil).
(3) True fats (eg, lard, animal fats) contain free fatty acids that increase in amount upon standing and cause irritation.
(4) Ointments (eg, Aquaphor, petrolatum) should not be used in intertriginous areas such as the axillas, between the toes, and in the perineum, because they increase maceration. Lotions or creams are preferred in these areas.
(5) Oils and ointments hold medication on the skin for long periods of time and are therefore ideal for barriers or prophylaxis and for dried areas of skin. Medication gets into the skin more slowly from ointments.
(6) Creams carry medication into skin and are preferable for intertriginous dermatitis.
(7) Solutions, gels, or lotions should be used for scalp treatment.

Evaporation of water is also cooling, vasoconstrictive ("gets the red out"), and antipruritic—all desirable objectives in the management of itchy, red skin. Water applied frequently to the skin and allowed to dry will result in drying of the skin surface.

WET DRESSINGS

By placing the skin in an environment where the humidity is 100% and allowing the moisture to evaporate to 60%, pruritus is relieved. Evaporation of water stimulates cold-dependent nerve fibers in the skin—thereby, theoretically, tying up the circuits so that the itching sensation coming through the pain fibers will not reach the central nervous system. It also is vasoconstrictive, which helps reduce the erythema and also decreases the inflammatory cellular response.

Gauze of 20/12 mesh is commonly used for wet dressings. Parke-Davis 4-inch gauze comes in 100-yard rolls, and 5 yards is usually sufficient for application to the extremities. Curity 18-inch gauze can be used for application to the trunk. An alternative is to use the "2 long johns" technique, in which a pair of wet cotton long-sleeved and long-legged underwear is covered by a dry pair.

Warm but not hot water is used, and the gauze or long johns are soaked in the water and then wrung out until no more drops come out. The dressings are then wrapped around the extremities and fastened with a safety pin. The wet dressings are then covered with dry flannel or dry long johns, which will slow down the evaporation process but not completely retard it, so that the wet dressings need only be changed every 3 or 4 hours.

TOPICAL GLUCOCORTICOSTEROIDS

Topical glucocorticosteroids (Table 10–2) can be used under wet dressings. Fluocinolone acetonide cream (Fluonid, Synalar 0.01%) is made specifically for this purpose. If these steroids are to be used, the wet dressings are removed completely and the medication is replaced every 4–6 hours. Treatment for 24, 48, or 72 hours is usually sufficient to completely clear a severe generalized dermatitis. Prolonged use of this treatment will result in a significant systemic absorption of steroids. Establishing a higher concentration of corticosteroid drug in the skin by topical rather than systemic therapy will result in marked clearing. Because of the high concentration of steroids remaining in the skin, the mainstay of treatment of chronic forms of atopic dermatitis is application of topical glucocorticosteroid preparations (Table 10–2) twice daily.

Table 10–2. Topical glucocorticosteroids.

	Concentrations (Percent)
Low potency = 1	
Hydrocortisone	1.0
Desonide	0.05
Moderate potency = 5–10	
Triamcinolone acetonide	0.025 and 0.1
Fluocinolone acetonide	0.01 and 0.025
Hydrocortisone valerate	0.2
Flurandrenolide	0.025
Flumethasone pivalate	0.03
Betamethasone valerate	0.1
Betamethasone acetate	0.2
Betamethasone dipropionate	0.05
Methylprednisolone acetate	0.25
Betamethasone benzoate	0.025
Desoximetasone	0.25
Diflorasone diacetate	0.05
High potency = 10–100	
Fluocinonide	0.05
Halcinonide	0.025 and 0.1

Fritz KA, Weston WL: Topical glucocorticosteroids. *Ann Allergy* 1983;**50:**68.

DISORDERS OF THE SKIN IN NEWBORNS

TRANSIENT DISEASES IN THE NEWBORN

No treatment is required for any of these disorders, though treatment may be given as noted below.

Milia

Multiple white papules 1 mm in diameter scattered over the forehead, nose, and cheeks are present in up to 40% of newborn infants. Histologically, they represent superficial epidermal cysts filled with keratinous material associated with the developing pilosebaceous follicle. Their intraoral counterparts are called Epstein's pearls and are even more common than facial milia. All of these cystic structures spontaneously rupture and exfoliate their contents.

Esterly NB, Solomon LM: *The Skin in Neonatal-Perinatal Medicine.* Fanaroff AA, Martin RJ (editors). Mosby, 1983.

Jorgenson RJ et al: Intraoral findings and anomalies in neonates. *Pediatrics* 1982;**69:**577.

Sebaceous Gland Hyperplasia

Prominent yellow macules at the opening of each pilosebaceous follicle, predominantly over the nose, represent overgrowth of sebaceous glands in response to the same androgenic stimulation that occurs in adolescence.

Acne Neonatorum

Open and closed comedones, erythematous papules, and pustules identical in appearance to adolescent acne may occur in infants over the forehead, cheeks, and chin. The lesions may be present at birth but usually do not appear until 3–4 weeks of age. Spontaneous resolution occurs over a period of 6 months to a year. Rarely, neonatal acne may be a manifestation of a virilizing syndrome.

Duke EMC: Infantile acne associated with transient increases in plasma concentrations of luteinising hormone, follicle-stimulating hormone and testosterone. *Br Med J* 1981;**282:**1275.

Lucky AW: Endocrine aspects of acne. *Pediatr Clin North Am* 1983;**30:**511.

Harlequin Color Change

A cutaneous vascular phenomenon unique to neonates occurs when the infant (particularly one of low birth weight) is placed on one side. The dependent half develops an erythematous flush with a sharp demarcation at the midline, and the upper half of the body becomes pale. The color changes usually subside within a few seconds after the infant is placed supine but may persist for as long as 20 minutes.

Mortenson O, Stougard-Andresen P: Harlequin color change in the newborn. *Acta Obstet Gynecol Scand* 1959;**38**:352.

Mottling

A lacelike pattern of dilated cutaneous vessels appears over the extremities and often the trunk of neonates exposed to lowered room temperature. This feature is transient and usually disappears completely upon rewarming.

Erythema Toxicum

Up to 50% of term infants develop erythema toxicum. Usually at 24–48 hours of age, blotchy erythematous macules 2–3 cm in diameter appear, most prominently on the chest but also on the back, face, and extremities. These are occasionally present at birth but rarely have their onset after 4–5 days of life. The lesions vary in number from 2–3 up to as many as 100. Incidence is much higher in term infants than in premature ones. The macular erythema may fade within 24–48 hours or may progress to develop urticarial wheals in the center of the macules or, in 10% of cases, pustules. Examination of a Wright-stained smear of the lesion will reveal numerous eosinophils. This may be accompanied by peripheral blood eosinophilia of up to 20%. All of the lesions fade and disappear by 5–7 days. A similar eruption in black newborns has a neutrophilic predominance and leaves hyperpigmentation.

Carr JA et al: Relationship between toxic erythema and infant maturity. *Am J Dis Child* 1966;**112**:129.

Ramamurthy RS, Esterly NB: Transient neonatal pustular melanosis. *J Pediatr* 1976;**88**:831.

Sucking Blisters

Bullae, either intact or in the form of an erosion representing a blister base without inflammatory borders, may occur over the forearms, wrists, thumbs, or upper lip. These presumably result from vigorous sucking in utero. They resolve without complications.

Miliaria

Obstruction of the eccrine sweat ducts occurs often in neonates and produces one of 2 clinical pictures depending upon the level of obstruction. **Miliaria crystallina** is characterized by tiny (1–2 mm) superficial grouped vesicles without erythema over intertriginous areas and adjacent skin (eg, neck and upper chest). Obstruction occurs in the stratum corneum portion of the eccrine duct. More commonly, obstruction of the eccrine duct deeper in the epidermis results in erythematous grouped papules in the same areas and is called **miliaria rubra.** Rarely, these may progress to pustules. Heat and high humidity predispose to eccrine duct pore closure. Removal to a cooler environment is the treatment of choice.

Harpin VA, Rutter N: Sweating in preterm babies. *J Pediatr* 1982;**100**:614.

Subcutaneous Fat Necrosis

Reddish or purple, sharply circumscribed, firm nodules occurring over the cheeks, buttocks, arms, and thighs and occurring between day 1 and day 7 in infants represent subcutaneous fat necrosis. Cold injury is thought to play an important role. These lesions resolve spontaneously over a period of weeks, although, like all instances of fat necrosis, they may calcify.

Sclerema

Premature newborns, especially those who suffer metabolic alterations (eg, metabolic acidosis, hypoglycemia, hypothermia), are susceptible to a diffuse hardening of the skin that makes the skin look shiny and feel tight. Severe cold injury in undernourished infants is assumed to be the cause.

Treatment consists of protecting the infant from undue exposure to cold and repairing metabolic and nutritional deficiencies.

Anagnostakis A et al: Sclerema neonatorum. *Pediatrics* 1974;**53**:24.

BIRTHMARKS

Birthmarks may involve an overgrowth of one or more of any of the normal components of skin: pigment cells, blood vessels, lymph vessels, etc. A nevus is a hamartoma of highly differentiated cells that retain their normal function.

Note: All tissue excised should be submitted for pathologic examination.

1. PIGMENT CELL BIRTHMARKS

Mongolian Spot

A blue-black macule found over the lumbosacral area in 90% of American Indian, black, and Oriental infants is called a mongolian spot. These spots are occasionally noted over the shoulders and back and may extend over the buttocks. Histologically, they consist of spindle-shaped pigment cells located deep in the dermis. The lesions fade somewhat with time, but some traces may persist into adult life.

Jacobs A, Walton R: The incidence of birthmarks in the neonate. *Pediatrics* 1976;**58**:218.

Café au Lait Spot

A café au lait spot is a light brown, oval macule (dark brown on black skin) that may be found anywhere on the body. Ten percent of white and 22% of black children have café au lait spots greater than 1.5 cm in their longest diameter. These lesions persist throughout life and may increase in number with age. The presence of 6 or more café au lait macules greater than 1.5 cm in their longest diameter may represent a clue to neurofibromatosis. Patients with Albright's syndrome also have increased numbers of café au lait macules. Although it has been suggested that the melanocytes of café au lait macules in neurofibromatosis contain giant pigment granules, this is not often the case in children, and their absence does not rule out neurofibromatosis.

Riccardi VM: Pathophysiology of neurofibromatosis. *J Am Acad Dermatol* 1980;**3:**157.

Junctional Nevus & Compound Nevus

Dark brown or black macules, usually few in number at birth but becoming more numerous with age, represent junctional nevi. Histologically, these lesions are large clones of melanocytes at the junction of the epidermis and dermis. With aging, they may become raised (papules) and contain intradermal melanocytes, creating a compound nevus. Often the surface becomes irregular and roughened.

There is controversy about whether junctional and compound nevi are precancerous. Seventy to 80% of melanomas arise on skin that previously contained no pigmented lesion, so the question is not whether junctional nevi are more likely to produce melanoma than normal skin but whether the pigmented lesion really is a junctional nevus or has been a melanoma all along.

Lesions with variegated colors (red, white, blue), notched borders, and nonuniform, irregular surfaces should arouse a suspicion of melanoma. Ulceration and bleeding are advanced signs of melanoma.

If melanoma is a possibility, excisional biopsy for pathologic examination should be done as the treatment of choice.

Rhodes AR: Pigmented birthmarks and precursor melanocytic lesions of cutaneous melanoma identifiable in childhood. *Pediatr Clin North Am* 1983;**30:**435.

Intradermal Nevus & Blue Nevus

Brown to blue solitary papules with smooth surfaces represent intradermal nevi. When pigmentation is present deeper in the dermis, the lesions appear blue or blue-black and are called blue nevi.

Spindle & Epithelioid Cell Nevus (Juvenile Melanoma)

A reddish-brown solitary nodule appearing on the face or upper arm of a child represents a spindle and epithelioid cell nevus. The name melanoma is misleading because this tumor is biologically benign. Histologically, it consists of pigment-producing cells of bizarre shape with numerous mitoses.

Treatment consists of excision.

Coskey RJ, Mehregan A: Spindle cell nevi in adults and children. *Arch Dermatol* 1973;**108:**535.

Giant Pigmented Nevus (Bathing Trunk Nevus)

An irregular dark brown to black plaque over 10 cm in diameter represents a giant pigmented nevus. Often the lesions are of such size as to cover the entire trunk (bathing trunk nevi). Histologically, they are compound nevi. Transformation to malignant melanoma has been reported in as many as 10% of cases in some series, although the true incidence is probably somewhat less. Malignant change may occur at birth or at any time thereafter.

Because of the possibility of melanoma, it is currently recommended that the entire lesion be excised if feasible. The risk of melanoma and the potential for cosmetic improvement should be carefully evaluated for each patient.

Alper J et al: Birthmarks with serious medical significance: Nevocellular nevi, sebaceous nevi and multiple café-au-lait spots. *J Pediatr* 1979;**95:**696.

Castilla EE, Graca Dutra M, Orioli-Parreiras IM: Epidemiology of congenital pigmented naevi. 1. Incidence rates and relative frequencies. *Br J Dermatol* 1981;**104:**307.

The management of congenital melanocytic nevi: Special symposium. *Pediatr Dermatol* 1984;**2:**143.

2. VASCULAR BIRTHMARKS

Flat Hemangioma

Flat vascular birthmarks can be divided into 2 types: those that are orange or light red (salmon patch) and those that are dark red or bluish red (port wine stain).

A. Salmon Patch: The salmon patch (nevus flammeus) is a light red macule found over the nape of the neck, upper eyelids, and glabella. Fifty percent of infants have such lesions over their necks. Eyelid lesions fade completely within 3–6 months and glabellar lesions by age 5 or 6; those on the nape of the neck fade somewhat but may persist into adult life.

B. Port Wine Stain: Port wine stains are dark red or purple macules appearing unilaterally on the side of the face or an extremity. A port wine stain over the face may be a clue to **Sturge-Weber syndrome,** which is characterized by seizures, mental retardation, glaucoma, and hemiplegia. Most infants with unilateral port wine stains do not have Sturge-Weber syndrome. If the angioma is in the distribution of the ophthalmic branch of the trigeminal nerve or hemihypertrophy of that side of the face exists, Sturge-Weber syndrome is more likely.

Similarly, a port wine hemangioma over an extremity may be associated with hypertrophy of the soft tissue and bone of that extremity **(Klippel-Trenaunay syndrome).**

The only treatment for port wine stain is the use

of cosmetic coverings such as Covermark. Laser therapy should be delayed until after age 20.

Barsky SH et al: The nature and evolution of port wine stains: A computer-assisted study. *J Invest Dermatol* 1980;**74:**154.
Jacobs AH, Walton RG: The incidence of birthmarks in the neonate. *Pediatrics* 1976;**58:**218.

Strawberry Hemangioma

A red, rubbery nodule with a roughened surface is a strawberry nevus. The lesion is often not present at birth but is represented by a permanent blanched area on the skin that is supplanted at 2–4 weeks of age by red nodules. Histologically, these are often mixtures of capillary and venous elements, and although a deep nodule (cavernous hemangioma) may be part of the strawberry lesion, the biologic behavior is the same. Fifty percent resolve spontaneously by age 5; 70% by age 7; 90% by age 9; and the rest by adolescence.

Strawberry hemangiomas resolve, leaving only redundant skin, and uncomplicated ones are best treated by watchful waiting. Complications include superficial ulceration and secondary pyoderma, which are treated by topical antiseptics and observation.

Complications that require treatment are (1) thrombocytopenia due to platelet trapping within the lesion **(Kasabach-Merritt syndrome);** (2) airway obstruction (hemangiomas of the head and neck are often associated with subglottic hemangiomas); (3) visual obstruction (with resulting amblyopia); and (4) cardiac decompensation (high-output failure). In these instances, the treatment of choice is prednisone, 1–2 mg/kg orally daily or every other day for 4–6 weeks.

Esterly NB: Kasabach-Merritt syndrome in infants. *J Am Acad Dermatol* 1983;**8:**504.
Sasaki GH, Pang CY, Witliff JL: Pathogenesis and treatment of infant skin strawberry hemangiomas: Clinical and in vitro studies of hormonal effects. *Plast Reconstr Surg* 1984;**73:**359.

Lymphangioma

Lymphangiomas are rubbery, skin-colored nodules occurring in the parotid area **(cystic hygromas)** or on the tongue. They often result in grotesque enlargement of soft tissues.

Surgical excision is the only treatment available, although the results are not satisfactory.

Flanagan BP, Helwig EB: Cutaneous lymphangioma. *Arch Dermatol* 1977;**113:**14.
Peachey RDG, Lim CC, Whimster IW: Lymphangioma of skin: A review of 65 cases. *Br J Dermatol* 1970;**83:**519.

3. EPIDERMAL BIRTHMARKS

Nevus Unius Lateris & Ichthyosis Hystrix

Linear or groups of linear, warty, papular, unilateral lesions represent overgrowth of epidermis since birth. These areas may range from dirty yellow to brown or may be darkly pigmented. The histologic features of the lesions include thickening of the epidermis and elongation of the rete ridges and hyperkeratosis. Clinically, the lesions may be associated with focal motor seizures, mental subnormality, and skeletal anomalies.

Treatment once or twice daily with topical tretinoin 0.05% (retinoic acid [Retin-A]) will keep the lesions flat.

Hurwitz S: Epidermal nevi and tumors of epidermal origin. *Pediatr Clin North Am* 1983;**30:**483.

Nevus Comedonicus

The lesion known as nevus comedonicus consists of linear groups of widely dilated follicular openings plugged with keratin, giving the appearance of localized noninflammatory acne. The treatment of choice is surgical removal. If this is not feasible, topical retinoic acid is helpful.

Cantu JM, Gomez-Bustamente MO, Gonzalez-Mendoza A: Familial comedones. *Arch Dermatol* 1978;**114:**1807.

Nevus Sebaceus

The nevus sebaceus of Jadassohn is a hamartoma of sebaceous glands and underlying apocrine glands that is diagnosed by the appearance at birth of a yellowish, hairless, smooth plaque in the scalp or on the face. The lesion may be contiguous with an epidermal nevus on the face and constitute part of the linear epidermal nevus syndrome.

Histologically, nevus sebaceus represents an overabundance of sebaceous glands without hair follicles. At puberty, with androgenic stimulation, the sebaceous cells in the nevus divide, expand their cellular volume, and synthesize sebum, resulting in a warty mass.

Because 15% of these lesions become basal cell carcinomas after puberty, excision is recommended before puberty.

Domingo J, Helwig EB: Malignant neoplasms associated with nevus sebaceous of Jadassohn. *J Am Acad Dermatol* 1979;**1:**545.
Lovejoy FH Jr, Boyle WE Jr: Linear nevus sebaceous syndrome: Report of 2 cases and a review of the literature. *Pediatrics* 1973;**52:**382.

4. CONNECTIVE TISSUE BIRTHMARKS (Juvenile Elastoma, Collagenoma)

Connective tissue nevi are smooth, skin-colored papules 1–10 mm in diameter that are grouped on the trunk. A solitary, larger (5–10 cm) nodule is called a **shagreen patch** and is histologically indistinguishable from other connective tissue nevi that show thickened, abundant collagen bundles with or without associated increases of elastic tissue. Although the shagreen patch is a cutaneous clue to tuberous sclerosis, the other connective tissue nevi occur as isolated events.

These nevi remain throughout life, and no treatment is necessary.

Uitto J, Santa Cruz DJ, Eisen AZ: Connective tissue nevi of the skin. *J Am Acad Dermatol* 1980;**3:**441.

HEREDITARY SKIN DISORDERS

The Ichthyoses

Ichthyosis is a term applied to several heritable diseases characterized by the presence of excessive scales on the skin. The nomenclature of this group of diseases is confusing. Major categories are listed in Table 10–3. X-linked ichthyosis is related to cholesterol sulfatase deficiency.

Control scaling with α-hydroxy acids, eg, 5% pyruvic, citric, lactic, or salicylic acid in petrolatum applied once or twice daily. Restoring water to the skin is also very helpful.

Elias PM: Epidermal lipids, membrances and keratinization. *Int J Dermatol* 1981;**20:**1.

Elliott SJ: X-linked ichthyosis: A metabolic disease. *J Am Acad Dermatol* 1979;**1:**139.

Williams ML: The ichthyoses—pathogenesis and prenatal diagnosis: A review of recent advances. *Pediatr Dermatol* 1983;**1:**1.

Epidermolysis Bullosa

The diagnostic feature of this group of diseases is the formation of hemorrhagic blisters in response to slight trauma. They can be divided into scarring and nonscarring types (Table 10–4).

Treatment usually consists of systemic antibiotics for infection, protective dressings of petrolatum or zinc oxide, and cooling the skin. If hands and feet are involved, reducing skin friction with 5% glutaraldehyde every 3 days is helpful. In recessive dystrophic epidermolysis bullosa, phenytoin (Dilantin), 3 mg/kg/d, has reduced new blister formation in most cases.

Cooper TW, Bauer EA: Epidermolysis bullosa: A review. *Pediatr Dermatol* 1984;**1:**189.

Eady RAJ, Tidman MJ: Diagnosing epidermolysis bullosa. *Br J Dermatol* 1983;**108:**621.

Incontinentia Pigmenti

Linear blisters in the newborn represent incontinentia pigmenti. These are replaced by hypertrophic, linear, warty bands within several months, followed by swirling brown hyperpigmentation. Most cases are thought to be X-linked dominant, lethal to the male. Mental retardation and seizures were reported in as many as 30% of cases in one series, but the true incidence is probably much less.

Carney RG Jr: Incontinentia pigmenti. *Arch Dermatol* 1976;**112:**535.

COMMON SKIN DISEASES IN INFANTS, CHILDREN, & ADOLESCENTS

ACNE

Clinical Findings

The common forms of acne in pediatric patients occur at 2 ages: in the newborn period and in adolescence. Neonatal acne is a response to maternal androgen, first appearing at 4–6 weeks of age and lasting until 4–6 months of age. It is characterized by inflam-

Table 10–3. Four major types of ichthyosis.*

Name	Age at Onset	Clinical Features	Histology	Inheritance
Ichthyosis with normal epidermal turnover				
Ichthyosis vulgaris	Childhood	Fine scales, deep palmar and plantar markings	Decreased to absent granular layer, hyperkeratosis	Autosomal dominant
X-linked ichthyosis	Birth	Palms and soles spared; thick scales that darken with age; corneal opacities in patients and carrier mothers	Hyperkeratosis	X-linked
Ichthyosis with increased epidermal turnover				
Epidermolytic hyperkeratosis	Birth	Verrucous, yellow scales in flexural areas and palms and soles	Hyperkeratosis, vacuolated reticular spaces in epidermis	Autosomal dominant
Lamellar ichthyosis	Birth; collodion baby	Erythroderma, ectropion, large coarse scales; thickened palms and soles	Hyperkeratosis, many mitotic figures	Autosomal recessive

* Reproduced, with permission, from Frost P, Weinstein GD: Ichthyosiform dermatoses. In: *Dermatology in General Medicine.* Fitzpatrick TB (editor). McGraw-Hill, 1971.

Table 10–4. Types of epidermolysis bullosa.

Name	Age at Onset	Clinical Features	Histology	Inheritance
Nonscarring types				
Epidermolysis bullosa simplex	Birth	Hemorrhagic blisters over the lower legs; cooling prevents blisters	Disintegration of basal cells	Autosomal dominant
Recurrent bullous eruption of the hands and feet (Weber-Cockayne syndrome)	First few years of life	Blisters brought out by walking	Cytolysis of suprabasal cells; keratotic cells	Autosomal dominant
Junctional bullous epimatosis (Herlitz disease)	Birth	Erosions on legs, oral mucosa; severe perioral involvement	Separation between plasma membrane of basal cells and PAS-positive basal lamina	Autosomal recessive
Scarring types				
Epidermolysis bullosa dystrophica, dominant	Infancy	Numerous blisters on hands and feet; milia formation	Separation of PAS-positive basal lamina; anchoring fibrils lost	Autosomal dominant
Epidermolysis bullosa dystrophica, recessive	Birth	Repeated episodes of blistering, secondary infection and scarring—"mitten hands and feet"	Separation below PAS-positive basal lamina; anchoring fibrils lost	Autosomal recessive

matory papules with all lesions in the same stage at the same time. The lesions are primarily on the face, upper chest, and back, in a distribution similar to that seen in adolescent acne. It has been hypothesized but not proved that infants who have severe neonatal acne will develop severe adolescent acne.

The onset of adolescent acne is between ages 8 and 10 in 40% of children. The early lesions are usually limited to the face and are primarily closed comedones (whiteheads; see below). Eventually, 85% of adolescents will develop some form of acne.

Acne occurs in sebaceous follicles, which, unlike hair follicles, have large, abundant sebaceous glands and usually lack hair. They are located primarily on the face, upper chest, back, and penis. Obstruction of the sebaceous follicle opening produces the clinical lesion of acne. If the obstruction occurs at the follicular mouth, the clinical lesion is characterized by a wide, patulous opening filled with a plug of stratum corneum cells. This is the open comedo, or blackhead. Open comedones are the predominant clinical lesion in early adolescent acne. The black color is due not to dirt but to oxidized melanin within the stratum corneum cellular plug. Open comedones do not often progress to inflammatory lesions. Closed comedones, or whiteheads, are caused by obstruction just beneath the follicular opening in the neck of the sebaceous follicle, which produces a cystic swelling of the follicular duct directly beneath the epidermis. The stratum corneum produced accumulates continuously within the cystic cavity. The resultant lesion is an enlarging sphere just beneath the skin surface. Most authorities believe that closed comedones are precursors of inflammatory acne. If open or closed comedones are the predominant lesions on the skin in adolescent acne, it is called **comedonal acne.**

In typical adolescent acne, several different types of lesions are present simultaneously, eg, open and closed comedones and inflammatory lesions such as papules, pustules, and cysts. Inflammatory lesions may also rarely occur as interconnecting, draining sinus tracts. Adolescents with cystic acne require prompt medical attention, since ruptured cysts and sinus tracts result in severe scar formation. New acne scars are highly vascular and have a reddish or purplish hue. Such scars return to normal skin color after several years. Acne scars may be depressed beneath the skin level, raised, or flat to the skin. In adolescents with a tendency toward keloid formation, keloidal scars can occur following acne lesions, particularly over the sternal area.

Differential Diagnosis

Consider rosacea, nevus comedonicus, flat warts, the angiofibromas of tuberous sclerosis, miliaria, and molluscum contagiosum.

Pathogenesis

The primary event in acne formation is obstruction of the sebaceous follicle. Ordinarily the lining of such follicles contains one or 2 layers of stratum corneum cells, but in acne the stratum corneum is overproduced. This phenomenon is androgen-dependent in adolescent acne. The sebaceous follicles contain an enzyme, testosterone 5α-reductase, which converts plasma testosterone to dihydrotestosterone. This androgen is a potent stimulus for nuclear division of the follicular germinative cells and subsequently of excessive cell production. Thus, obstruction requires the presence of both circulating androgens and the converting enzyme. After the production or the administration of androgens, there is a delay until cellular proliferation occurs and follicular obstruction subsequently appears.

The pathogenesis of inflammatory acne is not well understood. Undoubtedly, physical manipulation of a closed comedo could lead to rupture of the cavity contents into the dermis with a subsequent inflammatory response. Spontaneous inflammation also occurs in obstructed follicles, but the reason for this is unclear. An attractive hypothesis is that overgrowth of gram-positive bacteria in the obstructed follicle (either *Propionibacterium acnes* or *Staphylococcus epidermidis*) might produce enzymes or other factors that initiate inflammation. Overproduction of sebum and free fatty acid formation seem unlikely as causes of inflammation in acne as presently understood.

Adolescent acne may result from several external causes. Frictional acne due to headbands, football helmets, or tight-fitting brassieres or other garments occurs predominantly underneath the area where the garment is worn. Oil-base cosmetics may be responsible for predominantly comedonal acne, and hair sprays may produce acne along the hair margin.

Drug-induced acne should be suspected in teenagers if all lesions are in the same stage at the same time and if involvement extends to the lower abdomen, lower back, arms, and legs. Drugs responsible for acne include corticotropin (ACTH), glucocorticoids, androgens, hydantoin, and isoniazid.

Treatment

A. Topical Keratolytic Agents: The mainstay of acne therapy is the use of potent topical keratolytic agents applied to the skin to relieve follicular obstruction. Two classes of potent keratolytic agents are available: retinoic acid and benzoyl peroxide gel. These have been found to be the most efficacious agents in the treatment of acne. Either agent may be used once daily, or the combination of retinoic acid cream applied to acne-bearing areas of the skin once daily in the evening and a benzoyl peroxide gel applied once daily in the morning may be used. This regimen will control 80–85% of adolescent acne.

B. Topical Antibiotics: Topical antibiotics are used to avoid the side effects caused by systemic antibiotics. Topical antibiotics are less effective than systemic antibiotics and at best are equivalent in potency to 250 mg of tetracycline orally once a day. One percent clindamycin phosphate solution is the most efficacious of all topical antibiotics. Some percutaneous absorption may occur rarely with this drug, resulting in diarrhea and colitis; 1.5% and 2% topical erythromycin solutions are effective; 1% topical tetracycline solution is minimally effective.

C. Systemic Antibiotics: Antibiotics that are concentrated in sebum, such as tetracycline and erythromycin, are very effective in inflammatory acne. The usual dose is 0.5–1 g taken once or twice daily on an empty stomach (nothing to eat 1 hour before or after the medication). Tetracycline or erythromycin should be continued for 2–3 months until the acne lesions are suppressed.

D. Oral Retinoids: An oral retinoid, 13-*cis*-retinoic acid (isotretinoin; Accutane), offers the most efficacious treatment of severe cystic acne. The precise mechanism of its action is unknown, but decreased sebum production, decreased follicular obstruction, decreased skin bacteria, and general anti-inflammatory activites have been described. The initial dosage is 40 mg once or twice daily. This drug is not effective in comedonal acne or other mild forms of acne. Side effects include dryness and scaliness of the skin, dry lips, and, occasionally, dry eyes and dry nose. Up to 10% of patients experience mild, reversible hair loss. Elevated liver enzymes and blood lipids have rarely been described. Isotretinoin is teratogenic. Use in young women of childbearing age is not recommended.

E. Other Acne Treatments: There is no convincing evidence that dietary management, mild drying agents, abrasive scrubs, oral vitamin A, ultraviolet light, cryotherapy, or incision and drainage have any beneficial effects in the management of acne.

F. Avoidance of Cosmetics and Hair Spray: Acne can be aggravated by a variety of external factors that result in further obstruction of partially occluded sebaceous follicles. Discontinuing the use of oil-base cosmetics, face creams, and hair sprays may alleviate the comedonal component of acne within 4–6 weeks.

Patient Education & Follow-Up Visits

It is important to explain the mechanism of acne and the treatment plan to adolescent patients. Time should be set aside at the first visit to answer the patient's questions. Explain that there will not be much improvement for 4–8 weeks. Establish guidelines for ideal control, and explain that the best the patient might achieve is one or 2 new pimples a month. No drug is available that will prevent an adolescent from ever having another acne lesion. A written education sheet is most useful.

Follow-up visits should be made every 4–6 weeks. The criterion for ideal control is a few lesions every 2 weeks. Explain again what medications are being used and what the treatment is intended to achieve, and question the patient to determine whether the medications are being used properly.

Lucky AW: Endocrine aspects of acne. *Pediatr Clin North Am* 1983;**30:**395.

Schachner L: The treatment of acne: A contemporary review. *Pediatr Clin North Am* 1983;**30:**501.

BACTERIAL INFECTIONS OF THE SKIN

Impetigo

Erosions covered by honey-colored crusts are diagnostic of impetigo. Staphylococci and group A streptococci are important pathogens in this disease, which histologically consists of superficial invasion of bacteria into the upper epidermis, forming a subcorneal pustule.

Although topical antibiotics may effect a clinical cure, parenteral penicillin or oral penicillin for 10 days is necessary to eradicate streptococci. The risk of nephritogenic strains varies considerably from area to area, but active treatment of patients and contacts with systemic penicillin will significantly reduce the incidence of acute glomerulonephritis in endemic areas. Dicloxacillin or other antistaphylococcal antibiotics are used when staphylococcal infection is suspected.

Tunnesen WW Jr: Cutaneous infections. *Pediatr Clin North Am* 1983;**30:**515.

Ecthyma

Ecthyma is a firm, dry crust, surrounded by erythema, that exudes purulent material. It represents deep invasion by the streptococcus through the epidermis to the superficial dermis.

Treatment is with systemic penicillin.

Kelly C, Taplin D, Allen A: Streptococcal ecthyma. *Arch Dermatol* 1971;**103:**306.

Cellulitis

Cellulitis is characterized by erythematous, hot, tender, ill-defined plaques accompanied by regional lymphadenopathy. Histologically, this disorder represents invasion of microorganisms into the lower dermis and sometimes beyond, with obstruction of local lymphatics. Streptococci and staphylococci are common offending organisms, although a bluish cellulitis is diagnostic of *Haemophilus influenzae.*

Septicemia is common, and treatment with the appropriate systemic antibiotic is indicated.

Fleisher G et al: Cellulitis: Bacterial etiology, clinical features and laboratory findings. *J Pediatr* 1980;**97:**591.

Folliculitis

A pustule at a follicular opening represents folliculitis. If the pustule occurs at eccrine sweat orifices, it is correctly called **poritis.** Staphylococci and streptococci are the most frequent pathogens.

Treatment consists of measures to remove follicular obstruction—either cool wet compresses for 24 hours or keratolytics such as are used for acne.

Abscess

An abscess occurs deep in the skin, at the bottom of a follicle or an apocrine gland, and is diagnosed as an erythematous, firm, acutely tender nodule with ill-defined borders. Staphylococci are the most common organisms.

Treatment consists of incision and drainage and systemic antibiotics.

Scalded Skin Syndrome

This entity consists of the sudden onset of bright red, acutely painful skin, most obvious periorally, periorbitally, and in the flexural areas of the neck, the axillas, the popliteal and antecubital areas, and the groin. The slightest pressure on the skin results in severe pain and separation of the epidermis, leaving a glistening layer (the stratum granulosum of the epidermis) beneath. The disease is due to a circulating toxin (exfoliatin) elaborated by group II staphylococci (types 71, 55, 3A, 3B, and 3C). The site of action of exfoliatin is the intercellular area of the granular layer, resulting in a separation of cells.

Scalded skin syndrome includes **Ritter's disease** of the newborn, toxic epidermal necrolysis, and the mildest form, staphylococcal scarlet fever. (See also Bullous Impetigo, below.) In all of the forms of this entity, the causative staphylococci may not be isolated from the skin but rather from the nasopharynx, an abscess, blood culture, etc.

Treatment consists of systemic administration of antistaphylococcal drugs, eg, dicloxacillin, 25–50 mg/kg/d orally, or methicillin, 200–300 mg/kg/d intravenously. No topical therapy is necessary or warranted except in the newborn, where silver sulfadiazine or other burn therapy is used.

Bullous Impetigo

A fourth form of scalded skin syndrome is bullous impetigo. All impetigo is bullous, with the blister forming just beneath the stratum corneum, but in "bullous impetigo" there is, in addition to the usual erosion covered by a honey-colored crust, a border filled with clear fluid. Staphylococci may be isolated from these lesions, and systemic signs of circulating exfoliatin are absent. "Bullous varicella" is a disorder that represents bullous impetigo in varicella lesions.

Treatment with dicloxacillin, 25–50 mg/kg/d orally for 5–6 days, is effective. Application of cool compresses to debride crusts is a helpful symptomatic measure.

Hansen RC: Staphylococcal scalded skin syndrome, toxic shock syndrome and Kawasaki disease. *Pediatr Clin North Am* 1983;**30:**533.

FUNGAL INFECTIONS OF THE SKIN

1. DERMATOPHYTE INFECTIONS

Essentials of Diagnosis

- Red, scaly, round lesions.
- Hair loss with or without scaling in tinea capitis.

General Considerations

Dermatophytes become attached to the superficial layer of the epidermis, nails, and hair, where they proliferate. They grow mainly within the stratum corneum and do not invade the lower epidermis or dermis. Release of toxins from dermatophytes, especially those whose natural host is animals or soil, eg, *Microsporum canis* and *Trichophyton verrucosum,* results in dermatitis. Fungal infection should be suspected with any red and scaly lesion.

Classification & Diagnosis

A. Tinea Capitis: Thickened, broken-off hairs with erythema and scaling of underlying scalp are the distinguishing features (Table 10–5). Pustule formation and a boggy fluctuant mass on the scalp occur in *M canis* and *Trichophyton tonsurans* infections. This mass, called a **kerion,** represents an exaggerated host response to the organism. Fungal culture should be performed in all cases of suspected tinea capitis.

B. Tinea Corporis: Tinea corporis presents either as annular marginated papules with a thin scale and clear center or as an annular confluent dermatitis. The most common organisms are *Trichophyton mentagrophytes* and *M canis*. The diagnosis is made by scraping thin scales from the border of the lesion, dissolving them in 20% KOH, and examining for hyphae.

C. Tinea Cruris: Symmetric, sharply marginated lesions in inguinal areas are seen with tinea cruris. The most common organisms are *Trichophyton rubrum, T mentagrophytes,* and *Epidermophyton floccosum*. Scrapings taken from the border should be examined under the microscope with 20% KOH for dermatophytes.

D. Tinea Pedis: The diagnosis of tinea pedis in a prepubertal child must always be regarded with skepticism; atopic feet or contact dermatitis is a more likely diagnosis in this age group. Tinea pedis is seen most commonly in postpubertal males with blisters on the instep of the foot. Fissuring between the toes is occasionally seen. Microscopic examination of thin scales or the undersurface of the blister roof confirms the diagnosis.

E. Tinea Unguium (Onychomycosis): Loosening of the nail plate from the nail bed (onycholysis), giving a yellow discoloration, is the first sign of fungal invasion of the nails. Thickening of the distal nail plate then occurs, followed by scaling and a crumbly appearance of the entire nail plate surface. *T rubrum* and *T mentagrophytes* are the most common causes. The diagnosis is confirmed by KOH examination. Usually one or 2 nails are involved. If every nail is involved, psoriasis or lichen planus is a more likely diagnosis than fungal infection.

Table 10–5. Clinical features of tinea capitis.

Most Common Organisms	Clinical Appearance	Microscopic Appearance in KOH
Trichophyton tonsurans (60%)	Hairs broken off 2–3 mm from follicle; "black dot"; no fluorescence	Hyphae and spores within hair
Microsporum canis (39%)	Thickened broken-off hairs that fluoresce yellow-green with Wood's lamp*	Small spores outside of hair; hyphae within hair
Microsporum audouini (1%)	Thickened broken-off hairs that fluoresce yellow-green with Wood's lamp*	Small spores outside of hair; hyphae within hair

* Select fluorescent hairs for examination in KOH and culture.

Treatment

The treatment of dermatophytosis is quite simple: *If hair or nails are involved, griseofulvin is the treatment of choice*. Topical antifungal agents do not enter hair or nails in sufficient concentration to clear the infection. The absorption of griseofulvin from the gastrointestinal tract is enhanced by a fatty meal; thus, whole milk or ice cream taken with the medication increases absorption. The dosage of griseofulvin is 10–20 mg/kg/d. With hair infections, it should be continued for a minimum of 6 weeks; in nail infections, for a minimum of 3 months. It is supplied in capsules containing 250 mg or as a suspension containing 125 mg/5 mL. The side effects are few, and the drug has even been used successfully in the newborn period.

The treatment of kerion includes suppression of the exaggerated inflammatory response with corticosteroids. Prednisone, 1.5 mg/kg/d orally for 7–10 days, is recommended for prevention of scarring and alopecia.

Tinea corporis, tinea pedis, and tinea cruris can be treated effectively with topical medication after careful inspection to make certain that the hair and nails are not involved. The most consistently effective topical agent is tolnaftate (Tinactin) cream or 1% powder, applied 2–3 times a day until the eruption has cleared. Treatment should be continued for 1 week after the eruption has disappeared. Haloprogin (Halotex), miconazole (Micatin), and clotrimazole (Lotrimin) are useful alternatives.

Provost T: The rise and fall of fluorescent tinea capitis. *Pediatr Dermatol* 1983;**1**:127.

Rockoff AS: Fungus cultures in a pediatric clinic. *Pediatrics* 1979;**63**:276.

Stein DH: Superficial fungal infections. *Pediatr Clin North Am* 1983;**30**:545.

2. TINEA VERSICOLOR

Tinea versicolor is a superficial infection caused by *Pityrosporon orbiculare* (also called *Malassezia furfur*), a yeastlike fungus. It characteristically causes polycyclic connected hypopigmented macules and very fine scales in areas of sun-induced pigmentation. In winter, the polycyclic macules appear reddish-brown.

Treatment consists of application of selenium sulfide (Selsun), full-strength suspension, or 25% sodium thiosulfate (Tinver). Selenium sulfide should be applied to the whole body and left on overnight. Treatment can be repeated again in a week and then monthly thereafter. It tends to be somewhat irritating, and the patient should be warned about this difficulty.

Faergemann J, Fredriksson T: Tinea veriscolor: Some new aspects of etiology, pathogenesis and treatment. *Int J Dermatol* 1982;**21:**8.

3. *CANDIDA ALBICANS* INFECTIONS

In addition to being a frequent invader in diaper dermatitis, *Candida albicans* also infects the oral mucosa, where it appears as thick white patches with an erythematous base **(thrush);** the angles of the mouth, where it causes fissures and white exudate **(perlèche);** and the cuticular region of the fingers, where thickening of the cuticle, dull red erythema, and distortion of growth of the nail plate suggest the diagnosis of candidal paronychia. *C albicans* is able to penetrate the stratum corneum layer and locally activate the complement system.

Nystatin (Mycostatin) is the drug of first choice for *C albicans* infections. It is supplied as an ointment or a cream, as an oral suspension, and as vaginal tablets. In diaper dermatitis, the cream form can be applied every 3–4 hours. In oral thrush, the suspension should be applied directly to the mucosa with the parent's finger or a cotton-tipped applicator, since it is not absorbed and acts topically. In candidal paronychia, nystatin is applied over the area, covered with occlusive plastic wrapping, and left on overnight after the application is made airtight.

Haloprogin, miconazole, econazole nitrate, or clotrimazole is an effective alternative.

Carter VH, Olansky S: Haloprogin and nystatin therapy for cutaneous candidiasis. *Arch Dermatol* 1974;**110:**81.

Ray TL, Wuepper KD: Recent advances in cutaneous candidiasis. *Int J Dermatol* 1978;**17:**683.

VIRAL INFECTIONS OF THE SKIN

Herpes Simplex

Grouped vesicles or grouped erosions suggest herpes simplex. The microscopic finding of epidermal giant cells after scraping the vesicle base with a No. 15 blade, smearing on a slide, and staining with Wright's stain (Tzank smear) suggests herpes simplex or varicella-zoster. In infants, lesions due to herpes simplex type 1 are seen on the gingiva and lips, periorbitally, or on the thumb in thumb suckers. Recurrent erosions in the mouth are usually aphthous stomatitis in children rather than recurrent herpes simplex. Herpes simplex type 2 is seen on the genitalia and in the mouth in adolescents. Herpes simplex infection of the genitalia is now the second most common veneral disease. Cutaneous dissemination of herpes simplex occurs in patients with atopic dermatitis **(eczema herpeticum, Kaposi's varicelliform eruption).**

In severe disseminated infection, oral acyclovir may be helpful.

Chadwick EG et al: Advances in antiviral therapy: Acyclovir. *Pediatr Dermatol* 1984;**2:**64.

Kibrick S: Herpes simplex infection at term: What to do with mother, newborn, and nursery personnel. *JAMA* 1980; **243:**157.

Spruance SL et al: The natural history of recurrent herpes labialis. *N Engl J Med* 1977;**297:**69.

Varicella-Zoster

Grouped vesicles in a dermatome on the trunk or face suggest herpes zoster. Zoster in children is not painful and usually has a mild course. In patients with compromised host resistance, the appearance of an erythematous border around the vesicles is a good prognostic sign. Conversely, large bullae without a tendency to crusting imply a poor host response to the virus. Varicella-zoster and herpes simplex lesions undergo the same series of changes: papule, vesicle, pustule, crust, slightly depressed scar. Varicella appears in crops, and many different stages of lesions are present at the same time.

Itching is usually the only symptom, and cool baths as frequently as necessary or drying lotions such as calamine lotion are sufficient to relieve symptoms. In immunosuppressed children, intravenous or oral acyclovir should be considered.

Balfour HH et al: Acyclovir halts progression of herpes zoster in immunosuppressed patients. *N Engl J Med* 1983;**308:** 1448.

Luby JP: Varicella-zoster virus. *J Invest Dermatol* 1973;**61:**212.

Rogers RS, Tindall JP: Herpes zoster in children. *Arch Dermatol* 1972;**106:**204.

Virus-Induced Tumors

A. Molluscum Contagiosum: Molluscum contagiosum consists of umbilicated, white or whitish-yellow papules in groups on the genitalia or trunk. They are common in sexually active adolescents as well as in infants and preschool children. Crushing a lesion between glass slides followed by microscopic examination after staining with Wright's stain will demonstrate epidermal cells with inclusions. Molluscum contagiosum is a poxvirus that induces the epidermis to proliferate, forming a pale papule.

Removal of the lesion with a sharp curet or knife is curative. This therapy may leave a small scar, and one must weigh the advantage of removal of lesions that will disappear in 2 or 3 years.

B. Warts: Warts are skin-colored papules with irregular (verrucous) surfaces. They are intraepidermal tumors caused by infection with human papilloma virus. This DNA virus induces the epidermal cells to proliferate, thus resulting in the warty growth. If the wart virus stimulus is small, the result is a flat wart. If the stimulation is great, the cells proliferate and thicken, causing the skin to fold upon itself and giving rise to an irregular (verrucous) surface—as seen on the isolated wart on the body (verruca vulgaris), the plantar wart (verruca plantaris), and, often, the veneral wart (condyloma acuminatum).

No therapy for warts is ideal, and some types of therapy should be avoided because the recurrence rate of warts is high. Flat warts generally require no treatment. They may be considered a mild wart virus infection, and since they usually disappear within 6–9 months they are best left alone. This holds true especially for all flat warts on the face. A good response to 0.05% tretinoin (Retin-A) cream, applied once daily for 3–4 weeks, has been reported.

The best treatment for the solitary **common ("vulgaris") wart** is to freeze it with liquid nitrogen. The liquid nitrogen should be allowed to drip from the cotton-tipped applicator onto the wart without pressure. Pressure exaggerates cold injury by causing vasoconstriction and may produce a deep ulcer and scar. Liquid nitrogen is applied by drip until the wart turns completely white and stays white for 20–25 seconds. Small plantar warts usually need not be treated. Large and painful ones are treated most effectively by applying 40% salicylic acid plaster cut with a scissors to fit the lesion. The sticky brown side of the plaster is placed against the lesion, taped on securely with adhesive tape, and left on for 5 days. The plaster is then removed, and the white necrotic warty tissue can be gently rubbed off with the finger and a new salicylic acid plaster applied. This procedure is repeated every 5 days, and the patient is seen every 2 weeks. Most plantar warts resolve in 2–4 weeks when treated in this way.

Sharp scalpel excision, electrosurgery, and radiotherapy should be avoided, since the resulting scar often becomes a more difficult problem than the wart itself and there may be recurrence of the wart in the area of the scar.

Condyloma acuminatum is best treated with 25% podophyllum resin (podophyllin) in alcohol. This should be painted on the lesions and then washed off after 4 hours. Re-treatment in 7–10 days may be necessary. A condyloma not on the vulvar mucous membrane but on the adjacent skin should be treated as a common wart and frozen.

For isolated warts and periungual warts, cantharidin (Cantharone) is effective and painless in children. It causes a blister and sometimes is difficult to control. An undesirable complication is the appearance of warts along the margins of the cantharidin blister. Cantharidin is applied to the skin, allowed to dry, and covered with occlusive tape such as Blenderm for 24 hours.

No wart therapy is immediate and definitive, and recurrences are reported in 20–30% of cases even with the best care.

Binney ML et al: Warts. *Br J Dermatol* 1976;**94:**667.

Briggaman RA, Wheeler CE Jr: Immunology of human warts. *J Am Acad Dermatol* 1979;**4:**297.

Postlewaite R: Molluscum contagiosum: A review. *Arch Environ Health* 1970;**21:**432.

Pyrhonen S, Johansson E: Regression of warts. *Lancet* 1975;**1:**92.

INSECT INFESTATIONS (Zoonoses)

Essentials of Diagnosis

- Discrete red papules, nodules, and S-shaped burrows on skin.
- Hand and foot involvement common.

Scabies

Scabies is suggested by the appearance of linear burrows about the wrists, ankles, finger webs, areolas, anterior axillary folds, genitalia, or face (in infants). Often, there are excoriations, honey-colored crusts, and pustules from secondary infection. Identification of the female mite or her eggs and feces is necessary to confirm the diagnosis. Slice off an unscratched papule or burrow with a No. 15 blade and examine microscopically in either immersion oil or 10% KOH to confirm the diagnosis. In a child who is often scratching, scrape under the fingernails. Examine the parents for unscratched burrows.

Lindane (gamma benzene hexachloride; Kwell) is an excellent scabicide. However, since lindane is concentrated in the central nervous system and central nervous system toxicity from systemic absorption in infants has been reported, the following restricted use of this agent is recommended: (1) For adults and older children, one treatment of lindane lotion or cream applied to the entire body and left on for 4 hours, followed by shower, is sufficient. (2) Infants tend to have more organisms and many more lesions and may have to be re-treated in 7–10 days. All family members should be treated simultaneously. Crotamiton (Eurax) may be substituted for lindane in infants.

Fernandez N, Torres A, Ackerman AB: Pathologic findings in human scabies. *Arch Dermatol* 1977;**113:**320.

Hurwitz S: Scabies in babies. *Am J Dis Child* 1973;**126:**226.

Solomon LM et al: Gamma benzene hexachloride toxicity. *Arch Dermatol* 1977;**113:**353.

Pediculoses (Louse Infestations)

Excoriated papules and pustules with a history of severe itching at night suggest infestation with the human body louse. This louse may be discovered in the seams of underwear but not on the body. In the scalp hair, the gelatinous nits of the body louse adhere tightly to the hair shaft. The pubic louse may be found crawling among pubic hairs, or blue-black macules may be found dispersed through the pubic region (maculae ceruleae). The pubic louse is often seen in the eyelashes of newborns.

Lindane (gamma benzene hexachloride; Kwell) has been the treatment of choice. Since this agent is concentrated in the central nervous system and central nervous system toxicity from systemic absorption in infants has been reported, the following modification in its use is recommended: For head lice, a shampoo preparation is left on the scalp for 5 minutes and rinsed out thoroughly. The hair is then combed with a fine-tooth comb to remove nits. This may be repeated in 7 days. Lindane cream or lotion applied to the body for 4 hours may be necessary for body lice, but washing the clothing in boiling water followed by ironing the seams with a hot iron usually eliminates the organisms. Malathion (Prioderm) is recently approved for head lice.

Lindane cream or lotion applied to the pubic area for 24 hours is sufficient to treat pediculosis pubis. It may be repeated in 4–5 days.

Honig PJ: Bites and parasites. *Pediatr Clin North Am* 1983; **30:**563.

Taplin D et al: A comparative trial of three treatment schedules for the eradication of scabies. *J Am Acad Dermatol* 1983;**9:**550.

Papular Urticaria

Papular urticaria is characterized by grouped erythematous papules surrounded by an urticarial flare and distributed over the shoulders, upper arms, and buttocks in infants. These lesions represent delayed hypersensitivity reactions to stinging or biting insects and can be reproduced by patch testing with the offending insect. Dog and cat fleas are the usual offenders. Less commonly, mosquitoes, lice, scabies, and bird and grass mites are involved. The sensitivity is transient, lasting 4–6 months.

The logical therapy is to remove the offending insect. Topical corticosteroids and oral antihistamines will control symptoms.

Massie FS: Papular urticaria: Etiology, diagnosis and management. *Cutis* 1974;**13:**980.

DERMATITIS*
(Eczema)

Essentials of Diagnosis

- Red skin with disruption of skin surface.
- Vesicles, crusting, or lichenification may be present.

General Considerations

The terms dermatitis and eczema are currently used interchangeably in dermatology, although the etymologic implication of eczema is "a boiling over" and the term originally denoted an acute weeping dermatosis. All forms of dermatitis, regardless of cause, may present with acute edema, erythema, and oozing with crusting, mild erythema alone, or lichenification. Lichenification is diagnosed by thickening of the skin with a shiny surface and exaggerated, deepened skin markings. It is the response of the skin to chronic rubbing or scratching.

Although the lesions of the various dermatoses are histologically indistinguishable, clinicians have nonetheless divided the disease group called dermatitis into several categories based on known causes in some cases and differing natural histories in others.

Atopic Dermatitis

Atopic dermatitis is not a clearly defined clinical entity but a general term for chronic superficial inflammation of the skin that can be applied to a heterogeneous group of patients. Many (not all) patients go through 3 clinical phases. In the first, infantile eczema, the dermatitis begins on the cheeks and scalp and frequently expresses itself as oval patches on the trunk, later involving the extensor surfaces of the extremities. The usual age at onset is 2–3 months, and this phase ends at age 18 months to 2 years. Only one-third of all infants with atopic eczema progress to phase 2—childhood or flexural eczema—in which the predominant involvement is in the antecubital and popliteal fossae, the neck, the wrists, and sometimes the hands or feet. This phase lasts from age 2 years to adolescence. Some children will have involvement of the soles of their feet *only,* with cracking, redness, and pain—the so-called **atopic feet.** Only a third of children with typical flexural eczema will progress to adolescent eczema, which is usually manifested by hand dermatitis only. Atopic dermatitis is quite unusual after age 30.

Atopic dermatitis has no known cause, and despite the high incidence of asthma and hay fever in these patients (30%) and their families (70%), evidence for allergy beyond this hereditary association is limited to testimonials. The case for food and inhalant allergens as causes of atopic dermatitis is not strong enough to warrant further discussion in this text.

A few patients with atopic dermatitis have immunodeficiency with recurrent pyodermas, unusual susceptibility to herpes simplex and vaccinia virus, hyperimmunoglobulinemia E, defective neutrophil and monocyte chemotaxis, and impaired T lymphocyte function.

A faulty epidermal barrier may predispose the patient with atopic dermatitis to itchy skin. Inability to hold water within the stratum corneum results in rapid evaporation of water, shrinking of the stratum corneum, and "cracks" in the epidermal barrier. Such skin forms an ineffective barrier to the entry of various irritants—and, indeed, it may be clinically useful to regard atopic dermatitis as a primary irritant contact dermatitis and simply tell the patient, "You have sensitive skin." Chronic atopic dermatitis is frequently secondarily infected with *Staphylococcus aureus* or *Streptococcus pyogenes.*

A. Treatment of Acute Stages: Application of wet dressings and topical corticosteroids is the treatment of choice for acute, weeping atopic eczema. Fluocinolone (Synalar), 0.01% cream, designed for

* From the perspective of a dermatologist. See also the discussion of atopic dermatitis in Chapter 32.

use under wet dressings, is applied 4 times daily and covered with wet dressings as outlined at the beginning of this chapter. Systemic antibiotics chosen on the basis of appropriate skin cultures may be necessary, since lesions in the acute stages are often secondarily infected with *S aureus* or streptococci.

B. Treatment of Chronic Stages: Treatment is aimed at avoiding irritants and restoring water to the skin. No soaps or harsh shampoos should be used, and the patient should avoid woolen clothing or any rough clothing. Restoring water to the skin is important in atopic dermatitis. This can be accomplished by 2 "drip-dry" baths daily, less than 5 minutes each, after which lubricating oils or ointments are applied. Alpha Keri bath oil or Keri lotion (both lanolin-base preparations) will suffice, as will Nutraderm or Lubriderm lotion (oil-in-water emulsion bases). Plain petrolatum and lards are often too greasy and may cause considerable sweat retention. Liberal use of Cetaphil lotion as a soap substitute 4 or 5 times a day according to the modified Scholtz regimen is also satisfactory as a means of lubrication. A bedroom humidifier is often helpful. Topical corticosteroids should be limited to the less potent ones. Hydrocortisone ointment, 1% twice daily, is often sufficient. There is *never* any reason to use high-potency corticosteroids in atopic dermatitis. In superinfected atopic dermatitis, systemic antibiotics for 10–14 days (erythromycin, 40 mg/kg/d; dicloxacillin, 50 mg/kg/d) are necessary.

Treatment failures in chronic atopic dermatitis are most often due to patient noncompliance. This is a frustrating disease for parent and child.

Marsh DG, Meyers DA, Bias WB: The epidemiology and genetics of atopic allergy. *N Engl J Med* 1981;**305:**1551.

Vickers CFH: The natural history of atopic eczema. *Acta Derm Venereol (Stockh)* 1980;**92(Suppl):**113.

Yates VM, Kerr REI, MacKie RM: Early diagnosis of infantile seborrheic dermatitis and atopic dermatitis: Clinical features. *Br J Dermatol* 1983;**108:**633.

Nummular Eczema

Nummular eczema is characterized by numerous symmetrically distributed coin-shaped ("nummular") patches of dermatitis, principally on the extremities. These may be acute, oozing, and crusted or dry and scaling. The disease lasts 9 months to 2 years. The differential diagnosis should include tinea corporis and atopic dermatitis.

The same topical measures should be used as for atopic dermatitis, though treatment is often more difficult.

Primary Irritant Contact Dermatitis (Diaper Dermatitis)

Contact dermatitis is of 2 types: primary irritant and allergic eczematous. Primary irritant dermatitis develops within a few hours, reaches peak severity at 24 hours, and then disappears. Allergic eczematous contact dermatitis (see below) has a delayed onset of 18 hours, peaks at 48–72 hours, and often lasts as long as 2 or 3 weeks, even if exposure to the offending antigen is discontinued.

Diaper dermatitis, the most common form of primary irritant contact dermatitis seen in pediatric practice, is due to prolonged contact of the skin with urine and feces, which contain irritating chemicals such as urea and intestinal enzymes. The diagnosis of diaper dermatitis is based on the picture of erythema and thickening of the skin in the perineal area and the history of skin contact with urine or feces. In 80% of cases of diaper dermatitis lasting more than 4 days, the affected area is colonized with *Candida albicans* even before the classic signs of a beefy red, sharply marginated dermatitis with satellite lesions appear.

Treatment consists of changing diapers frequently. Because rubber or plastic pants serve as occlusive dressings and prevent the evaporation of the contactant and enhance its penetration into the skin, they should be avoided as much as possible. Talcum powder as a hygroscopic agent is useful in taking up irritant from the skin.

Treatment of long-standing diaper dermatitis should include application of nystatin (Mycostatin) cream with each diaper change. In extremely inflammatory diaper dermatitis, 1% hydrocortisone cream may be alternated with nystatin cream at every other diaper change.

Leyden JJ, Kligman AM: The role of microorganisms in diaper dermatitis. *Arch Dermatol* 1978;**114:**371.

Weston WL et al: Diaper dermatitis: Current concepts. *Pediatrics* 1980;**66:**532.

Lichen Simplex Chronicus (Localized Neurodermatitis)

Lichen simplex chronicus is a sharply circumscribed single patch of lichenification, usually found on the back of the neck in adolescent girls. The patients produce the morphologic skin changes by chronic rubbing and scratching.

Treatment of the thickened lesions is with topical corticosteroids. Because the epidermal barrier has thickened, penetration of topical corticosteroids is poor. Penetration can be enhanced in several ways. Airtight occlusion with plastic dressings (eg, Saran Wrap) overnight over topical corticosteroids is useful, or flurandrenolide (Cordran) tape impregnated with corticosteroids will penetrate the lesion. Covering the lesion will also prevent scratching of the area.

Allergic Eczematous Contact Dermatitis (Poison Ivy Dermatitis)

Children often present with acute dermatitis with blister formation, oozing, and crusting. Blisters are often linear and of acute onset. Plants such as poison ivy, poison sumac, and poison oak cause most cases of allergic contact dermatitis in children.

Allergic contact dermatitis has all the features of

delayed type (T lymphocyte-mediated) hypersensitivity. Although many substances may cause such a reaction, nickel sulfate (metals), potassium dichromate, thimerosal (an antiseptic [Merthiolate] and a preservative in cosmetics and cream), neomycin, and formaldehyde (in clothing) are the most common causes. The true incidence of allergic contact dermatitis in children is not known.

Treatment of contact dermatitis in localized areas is with topical corticosteroids. In severe generalized involvement, prednisone, 1–2 mg/kg/d orally for 14–21 days, can be used.

Weston WL, Weston JA: Allergic contact dermatitis in children. *Am J Dis Child* 1984;**138:**932.

Seborrheic Dermatitis

Seborrheic dermatitis consists of an erythematous scaly dermatitis accompanied by overproduction of sebum occurring in areas rich in sebaceous glands, ie, the face, scalp, and perineum. This common condition occurs predominantly in the newborn and at puberty, the ages at which hormonal stimulation of sebum production is maximal. Although it is tempting to speculate that the overproduction of sebum causes the dermatitis, the exact relationship is unclear.

Seborrheic dermatitis on the scalp in infancy is often confused with atopic dermatitis, and only after other areas are involved or flexural involvement occurs is it clear that the diagnosis is atopic dermatitis. Psoriasis also occurs in seborrheic areas in older children and should always be considered in the differential diagnosis.

Seborrheic dermatitis responds well to topical corticosteroids; 1% hydrocortisone cream 3 times daily is often sufficient to control this disorder.

Dandruff

Physiologic scaling or mild seborrhea, in the form of greasy scalp scales, can easily be treated by daily or alternate-day shampoos with cream rinse shampoos or selenium sulfide.

Leyden JJ et al: Role of microorganisms in dandruff. *Arch Dermatol* 1976;**112:**333.

Dry Skin (Asteatotic Eczema, Xerosis)

Newborns and older children who live in arid climates are susceptible to dry skin, characterized by large cracked scales with erythematous borders. The stratum corneum is dependent upon environmental humidity for its water, and below 30% environmental humidity the stratum corneum loses water, shrinks, and cracks. These cracks in the epidermal barrier allow irritating substances to enter the skin, predisposing to dermatitis.

Treatment consists of increasing the water content of the skin's immediate external environment. House humidifiers are very useful. Two 5-minute baths a day with immediate application of oils (Alpha Keri, Domol) or ointments (petrolatum, Aquaphor) after the bath will allow the skin to retain water. Frequent soaping of the skin impairs its water-holding capacity and serves as an irritating alkali, and all soaps should therefore be avoided. Frequent use of emollients (eg, Cetaphil, Eucerin, Lubriderm, Nutraderm) should be a major part of therapy.

Keratosis Pilaris

Follicular papules containing a white inspissated scale characterize keratosis pilaris. Individual lesions are discrete and may be red. They are prominent on the extensor surfaces of the upper arms and thighs and on the buttocks and cheeks. In severe cases, the lesions may be generalized. Such lesions are seen frequently in children with dry skin and have also been associated with atopic dermatitis and ichthyosis vulgaris.

Treatment is with keratolytics such as topical retinoic acid cream followed by skin hydration.

Pityriasis Alba

White, scaly macular areas with indistinct borders are seen over extensor surfaces of extremities and on the cheeks in children. Suntanning exaggerates these lesions. Histologic examination reveals a mild dermatitis. These lesions may be confused with tinea versicolor.

There is no satisfactory treatment.

Polymorphous Light Eruption

The appearance of vesicular, eczematous, or urticarial lesions in sun-exposed areas (cheeks, nose, chin, dorsum of the hands and arms) in the springtime should suggest a diagnosis of polymorphous light eruption. Confirmation can be made by skin biopsy demonstrating dense lymphocytic infiltrates in the dermis or by reproducing the lesion by daily exposure to artificial ultraviolet light. In American Indians, it is inherited as an autosomal dominant. Onset is usually at age 5 or 6, and spontaneous improvement occurs at puberty. The first rays of sunlight of sufficient energy reaching the earth's surface in early spring induce the disease. As summer progresses, the skin thickens in response to sunlight, less ultraviolet energy enters the skin, and the disease subsides. The differential diagnosis includes erythropoietic protoporphyria, in which patients experience severe pain and itching after 5 or 10 minutes of exposure to the sun but do not develop significant skin lesions except for small papules over the dorsum of the hand; and photodermatitis from plants (psoralens) or drugs, eg, thiazide diuretics, antihistamines, phenothiazine tranquilizers, tetracyclines, and sulfonamides.

Treatment of the dermatitis with topical corticosteroids, eg, 1% hydrocortisone cream to the face 3 times daily, and daily use of sunshield (5% PABA; PreSun) applied at bedtime and each morning are sufficient.

Ramsay CA: Photosensitivity in children. *Pediatr Clin North Am* 1983;**30:**687.

COMMON SKIN TUMORS

If the skin moves with the nodule on lateral palpation, the tumor is located within the dermis; if the skin moves over the nodule, it is subcutaneous. Table 10–6 lists the tumors according to these categories.

Knight BJ et al: Superficial lumps in children: What, when and why? *Pediatrics* 1983;**72:**147.

Granuloma Annulare

Circles or semicircles of nontender intradermal nodules found over the lower legs and ankles, the dorsum of the hands and wrists, and the trunk, in that order, suggest granuloma annulare. Histologically, the disease appears as a central area of tissue death (necrobiosis) surrounded by macrophages and lymphocytes.

No treatment is necessary. Lesions resolve spontaneously within 1 or 2 years.

Muhlbauer JE: Granuloma annulare. *J Am Acad Dermatol* 1980;**3:**217.

Pyogenic Granuloma

Rapid growth of a dark red papule with an ulcerated and crusted surface over 1–2 weeks following skin trauma suggests pyogenic granuloma. Histologically, this represents excessive new vessel formation with or without inflammation (granulation tissue). It is neither pyogenic nor granulomatous but should be regarded as an abnormal healing response.

Excision is the treatment of choice.

Leyden JJ, Master GH: Oral cavity pyogenic granuloma. *Arch Dermatol* 1973;**108:**226.

Epidermal Inclusion Cysts

Epidermal inclusion cysts are smooth, dome-shaped nodules in the skin that may grow to 2 cm in diameter. In infants they may be found about the eyes and in older children and adolescents on the chest, back, or scalp. They are the most common superficial lumps in children.

Treatment, if desired, is surgical excision.

Keloids

Keloids are scars raised above the skin surface with many radial projections of scar tissue. They continue to enlarge over several years. They are often found on the face, earlobes, neck, chest, and back. Keloids show no racial predilection. Treatment includes intralesional injection with triamcinolone acetonide, 20 mg/mL, or excision and injection with glucocorticosteroids.

Murray JC et al: Keloids: A review. *J Am Acad Dermatol* 1981;**4:**461.

PAPULOSQUAMOUS ERUPTIONS (See Table 10–7.)

Pityriasis Rosea

Erythematous papules that coalesce to form oval plaques preceded by a large oval plaque with central clearing and a scaly border (the herald patch) establish the diagnosis of pityriasis rosea. The herald patch has the appearance of ringworm and is often treated as such. It appears 1–30 days before the onset of the generalized papular eruption. The oval plaques are parallel in their long axis and follow Langer's lines of skin cleavage. In whites, the lesions are primarily on the trunk, accentuated in the axillary and inguinal areas. In blacks, lesions are primarily on the extremities. This disease is common in school-age children and adolescents and is presumed to be viral in origin. It lasts 6 weeks and may be pruritic the first 7–10 days. The major differential diagnosis is secondary syphilis, and a VDRL test should be done if syphilis is suspected. A chronic variant of this disease may last 2 or 3 years and is called **chronic parapsoriasis** or **pityriasis lichenoides chronicus.**

Exposing the skin to sunlight until a mild sunburn occurs (slight redness) will hasten the disappearance of lesions. Ordinarily, no treatment is necessary.

Arndt KA et al: Treatment of pityriasis rosea with ultraviolet radiation. *Arch Dermatol* 1983;**119:**381.
Vollum DI: Pityriasis rosea in the African. *Trans St Johns Hosp Dermatol Soc* 1973;**59:**269.

Psoriasis

Psoriasis is characterized by erythematous papules

Table 10–6. Common skin tumors.

Intradermal	Intradermal (cont'd)
Granuloma annulare	Lymphangioma
Dermatofibroma	Hemangioma
Epidermal inclusion cyst	Hair and sweat gland hamartomas
Neurofibroma	**Subcutaneous**
Neuroma	Lipoma
Leiomyoma	Rheumatoid nodule
Calcifying epithelioma	Osteoma
Melanocytic nevus	
Pyogenic granuloma	

Table 10–7. Papulosquamous eruptions in children.

Psoriasis
Pityriasis rosea
Secondary syphilis
Lichen planus
Chronic parapsoriasis
Pityriasis rubra pilaris
Tinea corporis
Dermatomyositis
Lupus erythematosus

covered by thick white scales. Guttate (droplike) psoriasis is a common form in children that often follows an episode of streptococcal pharyngitis by 2–3 weeks. The sudden onset of small (3–8 mm) papules, which are seen predominantly over the trunk and quickly become covered with thick white scales, is characteristic of guttate psoriasis. Chronic psoriasis is marked by thick, large (5–10 cm) scaly plaques over the elbows, knees, scalp, and other sites of trauma. Pinpoint pits in the nail plate are seen as well as yellow discoloration of the nail plate resulting from onycholysis. Thickening of all 20 fingernails and toenails is an uncommon feature. The sacral and seborrheic areas are commonly involved. Psoriasis has no known cause and demonstrates active proliferation of epidermal cells with a turnover time of 3–4 days versus 28 days for normal skin. These rapidly proliferating epidermal cells are producing excessive stratum corneum, giving rise to thick opaque scales. Papulosquamous eruptions that present problems of differential diagnosis are listed in Table 10–7.

All therapy is aimed at diminishing epidermal turnover time. Sunlight or artificial ultraviolet light (UVL) alone will produce some improvement. Coal tar enhances the effect of UVL and hastens the disappearance of psoriatic lesions. Bathing with a bath product containing tar (eg, Balnetar) at night, followed by UVL the next day, may be sufficient in mild cases. In more severe psoriasis, 2% crude coal tar in petrolatum should be applied after the bath. The newer tar gels (Estar gel, psoriGel) do not cause staining and are most efficacious. They are applied twice daily for 6–8 weeks.

Crude coal tar therapy is messy and stains bedclothes, and patients may prefer to use topical corticosteroids. Penetration of topical corticosteroids through the enlarged epidermal barrier in psoriasis requires that more potent preparations be used, eg, fluocinonide (Lidex, Topsyn), 0.05%, or triamcinolone (Aristocort, Kenalog), 0.5%, 4 times daily. A successful alternative is to add a keratolytic agent to the topical corticosteroid to help remove scales and enhance penetration of the steroid. A cream consisting of salicylic acid, 2%, in fluocinonide, 0.05%, 4 times daily, is effective.

Anthralin therapy is also useful. Anthralin is applied to the skin for a short contact time (eg, 20 minutes once daily) and is then washed off with a neutral soap (eg, Dove). A 6-week course of treatment is recommended.

Scalp care using a tar shampoo (Polytar, Zetar, many others) requires leaving the shampoo on for 5 minutes, washing it off, and then shampooing with commercial shampoo to remove scales. It may be necessary to shampoo daily until scaling is reduced.

More severe cases of psoriasis are best treated by a dermatologist using the Goeckerman regimen.

Menter MA et al: Resistant childhood psoriasis: An analysis of patients seen in a day care center. *Pediatr Dermatol* 1984;**2**:8.

Nyfors A: Psoriasis in children. *Acta Derm Venereol (Stockh)* 1981;**95**:47.

Perlman SG: Psoriatic arthritis in children. *Pediatr Dermatol* 1984;**1**:283.

Lichen Planus

Lichen planus consists of pruritic, light purple, flat-topped, many-sided papules, predominantly on the lower legs, penis, wrists, and arms. A white lacy pattern in the buccal mucosa is often seen. Pruritus may be severe.

If pruritus is mild, no treatment is necessary, and the disease will disappear in 6–12 months. With severe pruritus, a trial of antihistamines, eg, diphenhydramine, 5 mg/kg/d, or hydroxyzine, 2 mg/kg/d orally, is warranted. Rapid relief of pruritus and disappearance of the lesions can be achieved by administering prednisone, 1 mg/kg/d orally for 3–4 weeks.

Black MM, Wilson-Jones E: The role of the epidermis in the histopathogenesis of lichen planus. *Arch Dermatol* 1972; **105**:81.

HAIR LOSS (Alopecia)

Hair loss in children (Table 10–8) imposes great emotional stress on the parent and doctor—often more so than on the child. A 60% hair loss in a single area is necessary before hair loss can be detected clinically. Examination should begin with the scalp to determine if there are color changes or infiltrative changes. Hairs should be examined microscopically for breaking and structural defects and to see if growing or resting hairs are being shed. Placing removed hairs in mounting fluid (Permount) makes them easy to examine. Three diseases account for most cases

Table 10–8. Other causes of hair loss in children.*

Hair loss with scalp changes
- Nodules and tumors:
  - Nevus sebaceus
  - Epidermal nevus
- Thickening:
  - Linear scleroderma (morphea) (en coup de sabre)
  - Burn
- Atrophy:
  - Lupus erythematosus
  - Lichen planus

Hair loss with hair shaft defects (hair fails to grow out enough to require haircuts):
- Monilethrix—alternating bands of thin and thick areas
- Trichorrhexis nodosa—nodules with fragmented hair
- Trichorrhexis invaginata (bamboo hair)—intussusception of one hair into another
- Pili torti—hair twisted 180 degrees, brittle
- Pili annulati—alternating bands of light and dark pigmentation

* Price VH: Office diagnosis of hair shaft defects. *Cutis* 1975;**15**:231.

of hair loss in children: alopecia areata, tinea capitis, and trichotillomania.

Alopecia Areata

Loss of every hair in a localized area is called alopecia areata. This is the most common cause of hair loss in children. An immunologic pathogenetic mechanism is suspected because dense infiltration of lymphocytes precedes hair loss. Ninety-five percent of children with alopecia areata completely regrow their hair within 12 months, though as many as 40% may have a relapse in 5 or 6 years. A rare and unusual form of alopecia areata begins at the occiput and proceeds along the hair margins to the frontal scalp. This variety, called **ophiasis,** often results in total scalp hair loss **(alopecia totalis).** The prognosis for regrowth in ophiasis is poor.

No treatment is indicated for alopecia areata. Systemic corticosteroids given to suppress the inflammatory rsponse will result in hair growth, but the hair will fall out again when the drug is discontinued. In children with alopecia totalis, a wig is most helpful.

Rook A, Dawber R: *Diseases of the Hair and Scalp.* Blackwell, 1982.

Trichotillomania

Traumatic hair pulling causes the hair shafts to be broken off at different lengths, an ill-defined area of hair loss, petechiae around follicular openings, and a wrinkled hair shaft on microscopic examination. This may be merely habit or the result of severe anxiety in the child. Eyelashes and eyebrows rather than scalp hair may be pulled out. Such episodes are best considered a nervous habit. Oiling the hair to make it slippery is an aid to behavior modification.

Price VH: Management of hair problems. *Int J Dermatol* 1979;**18:**95.

REACTIVE ERYTHEMAS

Erythema Multiforme

Erythema multiforme begins with papules that later develop a dark center and then evolve into lesions with central blisters and the characteristic target lesions (iris lesions) with 3 concentric circles of color change. Primary injury is to endothelial cells, with later destruction of epidermal basal cells and blister formation. Erythema multiforme has sometimes been diagnosed in severe mucous membrane involvement, but **Stevens-Johnson syndrome** is the usual term for severe involvement of conjunctiva, oral cavity, and genital mucosa.

Many causes are suspected, particularly herpes simplex virus, sulfonamide drugs, and *Mycoplasma* infections. Recurrent erythema multiforme is usually associated with reactivation of herpes simplex virus. In the mild form, spontaneous healing occurs in 10–14 days, but Stevens-Johnson syndrome may last 6–8 weeks if untreated.

Treatment is symptomatic in uncomplicated erythema multiforme. Removal of offending drugs is an obvious necessary measure. Oral antihistamines such as hydroxyzine, 2 mg/kg/d orally, are useful. Cool compresses and wet dressings will relieve pruritus.

Edmond BJ, Huff JC, Weston WL: Erythema multiforme. *Pediatr Clin North Am* 1983;**30:**631.

Huff JC et al: Immunofluorescent identification of a herpes simplex viral antigen in skin lesions of erythema multiforme. *Ann Intern Med* 1984;**101:**48.

Erythema Nodosum

Erythema nodosum consists of painful, erythematous nodules on the anterior lower legs. In streptococcal infections, coccidioidomycosis, histoplasmosis, and tuberculosis, the onset of erythema nodosum parallels the appearance of cell-mediated immunity. Streptococcal infections and birth control pills are the most common causes of this panniculitis in the USA.

Treatment consists of removal of the offending drug or eradication of infection. Topical corticosteroids afford some relief, but prednisone, 1–2 mg/kg/d orally, may be necessary for 2–3 weeks.

Blomgren SE: Conditions associated with erythema nodosum. *NY State J Med* 1972;**72:**2302.

Drug Eruptions

Drugs may produce urticarial, morbilliform, scarlatiniform, or bullous skin eruptions. Urticaria may appear within minutes after drug administration, but most reactions begin 7–14 days after the drug is first administered. Drugs commonly implicated in skin reactions are listed in Table 10–9.

MISCELLANEOUS SKIN DISORDERS ENCOUNTERED IN PEDIATRIC PRACTICE

Aphthous Stomatitis

Recurrent erosions on the gums, lips, tongue, palate, and buccal mucosa are often confused with herpes simplex. A smear of the base of such a lesion stained with Wright's stain will aid in ruling out herpes simplex by the absence of epithelial giant cells. A culture for herpes simplex is also useful in this difficult differential diagnostic problem. It has been shown that recurrence of aphthous stomatitis correlates positively with lymphocyte-mediated cytotoxicity.

There is no specific therapy for this condition. Rinsing the mouth with liquid antacids will provide relief in most patients. Topical corticosteroids in a base that adheres to mucous membrane (Kenalog in Orabase) may provide some relief. In severe cases that interfere with eating, prednisone, 1 mg/kg/d orally for 3–5 days, will suffice to abort an episode.

Table 10–9. Common skin reactions associated with frequently used drugs.

Drug	Common Reactions
Aspirin	Urticaria rarely; purpuric eruptions.
Anti-infective agents	
Erythromycin	Urticaria.
Griseofulvin	Exanthematous eruptions; rarely, cold urticaria or photodermatitis.
Lincomycin (Lincocin)	Urticaria or exanthematous eruptions.
Penicillin and synthetic penicillins	Serum sickness, urticaria, exanthematous eruptions, anaphylactic shock. Ampicillin causes a high incidence of exanthematous eruption in patients with infectious mononucleosis.
Streptomycin	Exanthematous eruptions, urticaria, stomatitis.
Sulfonamides	Urticaria, erythema multiforme, exanthematous eruptions, Stevens-Johnson syndrome, photodermatitis.
Tetracycline	Exanthematous eruptions, urticaria; rarely, bullous eruptions. Demeclocycline (Declomycin) can cause phototoxic reactions.
Antihistamines	Exanthematous eruptions, urticaria, photodermatitis.
Barbiturates	Maculopapular eruptions, urticaria, erythema multiforme, Stevens-Johnson syndrome, bullous eruptions.
Chlorothiazides	Exanthematous eruptions, urticaria, photodermatitis, hemosiderosis of the lower extremities, leading to development of petechiae with resultant pigmentation (Schamberg's phenomenon).
Cortisone and derivatives	Acneiform drug reactions on trunk—pustular, purpuric eruptions.
Insulin	Urticaria, erythema at injection site.
Iodides (cough syrups, antiasthma preparations)	Acneiform pustules over trunk, granulomatous reaction.
Phenytoin	Exanthematous eruptions usually in first 3 weeks of treatment; gingival hyperplasia, hypertrichosis; pseudolymphoma syndrome.
Prochlorperazine	Urticaria, pruritus, photosensitive dermatitis.

Schachner L, Press S: Vesicular, bullous, and pustular disorders in infancy and childhood. *Pediatr Clin North Am* 1983; **30:**609.

Corns & Calluses

Thickened areas of epidermis in response to repeated or prolonged friction or pressure are called either corns or calluses. Corns are clearly demarcated and painful, whereas calluses have ill-defined margins and are not tender. A painful corn may overlie an exostosis, and one should get an x-ray of that digit.

Treatment begins with removing the cause of friction or pressure, if possible, such as ill-fitting shoes. Local therapy consists of paring down the lesion with a razor blade or No. 15 knife blade and covering it with a cut-to-size piece of 40% salicylic acid plaster. Cover firmly with adhesive tape to prevent loosening due to sweating. The plaster should not be allowed to get wet. It can be removed every 5 days and the dead skin gently removed. The plaster may then be put in place.

Bennett RG, Gammer S: Painful callus of the thumb due to phalangeal exostosis. *Arch Dermatol* 1973;**108:**826.

Morphea (Linear Scleroderma)

Morphea is characterized by the appearance, anywhere on the body, of well-circumscribed, shiny, white, firmly adherent skin. It is particularly cosmetically deforming on the face. A light purple border is indicative of an early lesion or continuing activity. Skin biopsy reveals replacement of subcutaneous fat with thickened collagen fibers. The lesions tend to burn themselves out in 3–5 years. It may be difficult to differentiate morphea from lichen sclerosis et atrophicus, which has similar white patches that occur primarily on the upper back and genitalia. Histopathologic differentiation is often necessary and may be difficult. Recently, it has been noted that linear scleroderma in children may progress to severe systemic lupus erythematosus after several years.

Lesions that are not cosmetically disturbing should not be treated. Lesions on the face may be cleared by injections of repository corticosteroids, eg, triamcinolone acetonide diluted 1:4 with saline to make 2.5 mg/mL and injected through a 30-gauge needle. Less than 1 mL should be injected. Complications of local corticosteroid injection include atrophy, depigmentation, ulceration, and infection; therefore, this therapy should be reserved for unusual circumstances.

Mackel S et al: Concurrent linear scleroderma and systemic lupus erythematosus. *J Invest Dermatol* 1979;**73:**368.

Necrobiosis Lipoidica Diabeticorum

A depressed yellow area with telangiectasia surrounded by an erythematous nodular border found on the anterior lower leg is diagnostic of necrobiosis lipoidica diabeticorum. Histopathologic findings in-

Table 10–10. Cutaneous signs of systemic disease in infants and children.

Sign	Disease
Acnelike erythematous papules in mid face and white ash-leaf macules on trunk, shiny thickened patch on back, subungual fibromas	Tuberous sclerosis
Pruritic blisters on buttocks, elbows, knees, and scapula	Dermatitis herpetiformis (celiac disease)
Café au lait macules	Neurofibromatosis, Albright's disease
"Chicken skin"—yellow rows of soft papules with wrinkled valleys in between in neck, axillas, groin	Pseudoxanthoma elasticum
"Dirty" neck and axillas (hyperpigmented, velvety flexural papules)	Acanthosis nigricans and obesity (endocrinopathies)
Eczematous erosions around the mouth, eyes, perineum, fingers, and toes; alopecia and diarrhea	Acrodermatitis enteropathica (zinc deficiency)
Erythematous isolated papules on elbows, knees, buttocks, face	Papular acrodermatitis (antigen-positive hepatitis)
Erythematous truncal macules with central pallor	Juvenile rheumatoid arthritis
Erythematous flat-topped papules over knuckles	Dermatomyositis
Hemorrhagic (1–2 mm) macules on lips, tongue, palms (epistaxis, gastrointestinal bleeding)	Hereditary hemorrhagic telangiectasia (Osler-Weber-Rendu syndrome)
Hyperpigmentation in palmar creases, knuckles, scars, buccal mucosa, linea alba, scrotum	Addison's disease
Linear or oval vesicles on hands or feet, erosions on soft palate, tonsillar pillars	Hand, foot, and mouth syndrome (Coxsackie A16 and others)
Palpable purpura	Vasculitis
Pigmented macules on oral mucosa	Peutz-Jeghers disease (benign small intestinal polyps)
Purpuric lakes	Purpura fulminans—disseminated intravascular coagulation
Purpuric pustules on hands and feet	Gonococcemia
Purpuric (petechiae) seborrheic dermatitis	Histiocytosis X
Sebaceous (multiple) cysts on face and trunk	Gardner's syndrome (premalignant polyps of colon and rectum)
Stretchy skin; healing with large purple scars	Ehlers-Danlos syndrome
Tight, hard skin, telangiectases, hypo- and hyperpigmentation	Scleroderma
Ulcers with undermined, liquifying borders	Pyoderma gangrenosum (ulcerative colitis, regional enteritis, rheumatoid arthritis)
Vitiligo (completely depigmented macules with hyperpigmented borders)	Pernicious anemia, Hashimoto's thyroiditis, Addison's disease, diabetes mellitus
Yellow papules (lower eyelids, joints, palms)	Xanthomas, hyperlipidemias

clude atrophy of the epidermis and a palisading granuloma of lymphocytes and macrophages surrounding an area of homogenized devitalized dermis. Lesions are most often found in diabetics but can be seen in nondiabetic children. There is no satisfactory treatment.

SELECTED REFERENCES

Hurwitz S: *Clinical Pediatric Dermatology*. Saunders, 1981.

Weston WL: *Practical Pediatric Dermatology*, 2nd ed. Little, Brown, 1985.

11 Eye

Philip P. Ellis, MD

GROWTH & DEVELOPMENT OF THE EYE

Although the eye is not completely developed at birth, it is a relatively large functioning sensory organ in the newborn. The postnatal growth of the eye and the brain are comparable. By the end of the fourth year, the eye has attained about 70% of its adult volume. Subsequent growth is much slower, until about age 10–12 years, when adult proportions are reached.

The average anteroposterior diameter of the newborn infant's eye is approximately 16.5 mm (the average adult diameter of the eye is slightly over 24 mm). The cornea is comparatively large, with an average transverse diameter of 10 mm; by the second year of life, the average adult corneal diameter of 12 mm is reached. The cornea in the newborn is relatively flat, and the iris contains little pigment and appears to have a bluish color. As pigment forms, the color of the iris becomes more distinct. By the age of 6 months, it is usually possible to determine whether the irides will become brown or remain blue.

The lens in the newborn infant's eye is quite spherical compared to that in the adult eye. This helps to overcome some of the hyperopia (farsightedness) resulting from the comparative shortness of the eyeball and the relative flatness of the cornea. At birth, approximately 75–80% of children are hyperopic. Hyperopia may increase for the first 7 or 8 years of life and then frequently diminishes. This contrasts to myopia (nearsightedness), which does not usually develop until age 8–10 and then increases until 20–30 years of age.

The macula in the retina is poorly developed at birth, and this is a major factor in the poor vision of newborns. Full development of the macula does not occur until about 6 months of age. The periphery of the retina is not as well developed as the remainder. Peripheral vascularization is not complete until about the time of term delivery.

Myelinization of the optic nerve is incomplete at birth; further myelinization continues until about the fourth month of life. The sclera is relatively thin, and the underlying uvea is what causes the blue color of the newborn sclera. Scleral fibers soon thicken to give a whiter appearance to the eye.

The orbit is almost round at birth. By the first year of life, orbital volume is doubled, and by the sixth year it is redoubled. The lacrimal gland is poorly developed at birth, which accounts for the paucity of tears when the newborn cries. The nasolacrimal duct is usually patent at birth, but in many infants the distal end remains plugged for several months (see discussion under lacrimal apparatus).

Coordinated movement of the eyes is not well developed for the first few months of life, although many full-term infants establish ocular alignment within 4 weeks of birth. Binocular visual responses begin to develop between the ages of 3 and 6 months and become firmly established during the second 6 months of life. Persistent deviation of an eye should always be investigated by an ophthalmologist.

Visual acuity in infants is much better than previously estimated. At the age of 5 months, it is about 20/100; at 2 years, about 20/60; and at 4–5 years, almost 20/20.

Crawford JS, Morin JD (editors): *The Eye in Childhood.* Grune & Stratton, 1983.

Harley RD (editor): *Pediatric Ophthalmology,* 2nd ed. 2 vols. Saunders, 1983.

Hoyt CS, Nickel B, Billson FA: Ophthalmological examination of the infant: Developmental aspects. *Surv Ophthalmol* 1982; **26:**177.

GENERAL PRINCIPLES OF DIAGNOSIS

A careful history is essential in establishing an accurate diagnosis of an ocular disorder. The history should include time and rate of onset of the presenting symptoms, associated symptoms, past history of eye disorders and treatment, and pertinent family and social history. However, many eye problems, such as poor vision in one eye, are asymptomatic and are discovered only on testing of visual acuity or other objective diagnostic methods.

COMMON NONSPECIFIC SYMPTOMS & SIGNS

Redness

Redness is a common finding in many ocular disorders. It is produced by dilatation of conjunctival and superficial scleral vessels in response to inflammation, infection, or irritation. The differential diagnosis of redness of the eye is presented in Table 11–1.

Tearing

In infants, tearing is usually due to nasolacrimal duct obstruction. Tearing may also be associated with local inflammatory, allergic, and viral diseases and with congenital glaucoma.

Discharge

Purulent discharge is usually associated with bacterial infections. Mucoid discharge is usually associated with chemical irritations, some viral infections, or allergic conditions; it may be secondary to obstructions of the nasolacrimal duct.

Pain

Pain in or about the eye may be due to foreign bodies in the cornea or conjunctiva, corneal abrasions, acute infections of the lid, orbital cellulitis, acute dacryocystitis, acute iritis, or glaucoma. Refractive errors seldom produce headaches in young children. Large refractive errors or poor convergence may produce headaches in older children, particularly those who read a good deal.

Poor Vision

In infants, poor vision is usually due to a serious ophthalmologic or neurologic disorder such as congenital nystagmus, corneal or lenticular opacities, disorders of the retina, optic nerve and central nervous system abnormalities, or very high myopia. In older children, the development of poor vision is often associated with refractive errors. Unilateral poor vision is usually associated with strabismus or large unequal refractive errors between the 2 eyes (anisometropia).

Leukocoria

A white spot in the pupil is a serious finding that may be due to congenital cataract, retrolental fibroplasia, retinal dysplasia, intraocular infection, retinoblastoma, or persistence and hyperplasia of primary vitreous.

EXAMINATION

Visual Acuity

Routine testing of visual acuity should be part of every general physical examination. It is the single most important test of visual function. In children 4 years of age or older, satisfactory visual acuity tests can usually be obtained with the use of Snellen test charts. In children 2½–3 years old, vision can often be tested with the use of Allen or E cards. Objects familiar to the child (eg, animals, trees, houses) are

Table 11–1. Differential diagnosis of redness of the eye in pediatric patients.

	Acute Conjunctivitis	Acute Iritis	Acute Glaucoma*	Corneal Abrasion
Incidence	Very common.	Uncommon.	Rare.	Fairly common.
Etiology	Usually bacterial; may be viral, fungal, or allergic.	Usually unknown; may be associated with juvenile rheumatoid arthritis.	Developmental defects or obstruction of aqueous drainage channels.	Foreign body; abrasion.
Redness	Diffuse injection of conjunctiva; greater toward fornices.	Purple-red; circumcorneal injection.	Often diffuse injection of bulbar conjunctiva.	Diffuse injection of conjunctiva.
Discharge	Moderate to heavy; mucoid or mucopurulent.	None.	None; tearing.	Watery.
Visual acuity	Normal.	Decreased.	Decreased.	Decreased.
Corneal transparency	Clear.	Clear or some haze.	Hazy; cornea enlarged in congenital form.	Variable haze.
Anterior chamber depth	Normal.	Normal; cloudy.	Shallow; deep in congenital form.	Normal.
Pupil size	Normal.	Constricted.	Dilated.	Normal.
Intraocular pressure	Normal.	Usually normal; may be low or elevated.	Elevated.	Normal.
Conjunctival smear results	Causative organisms identified; numerous polymorphonuclear neutrophils found in bacterial infection; numerous mononuclear cells found in viral infection.	Normal.	Normal.	Normal.

* Primary narrow-angle glaucoma is very rare in children. Congenital glaucoma may not produce redness of the eye.

depicted on the Allen cards in graduated sizes. When E cards are used, the child is asked to point in the direction of the "feet" of the figure E. Because of distractions in the office, children are sometimes unable to perform this test adequately; special illiterate E cards may be sent home so that the parents can test the vision at home under better circumstances. The parent can repeat the test at leisure, and the final result is usually more accurate than testing done in the office by the pediatrician or the nurse.

Visual acuity is difficult to evaluate in infants. One can observe whether an infant will follow a light or a bright attractive toy in different directions of gaze. Each eye is tested separately. If the infant fails to respond to such testing, one can observe the pupillary responses for reaction to direct light stimulus. These responses depend upon a functioning retina and optic nerve. However, cortical blindness can exist with preservation of pupillary light reflexes. Optokinetic nystagmus (slow pursuit movements in the direction of a moving stimulus and quick saccadic movements in the reverse direction or "railway nystagmus") indicates that there are functioning neural receptors in the retina and intact neural pathways. Visual acuity can be estimated on the basis of optokinetic responses to different sizes of stimuli and their presentation at slower and faster paces. The measurement of visual evoked potential (recording electrical activity of the visual cortex after ocular stimulation by a flash of light) is a sophisticated method of evaluating vision in an infant in whom blindness is suspected. Another technique is forced-choice preferential looking. This involves showing the infant 2 visual stimuli of equal luminance: a solid gray screen and a screen with gratings of black and white stripes that can be varied in width. Acuity is estimated by determining the narrowest width of stripes that can be differentiated from the solid gray screen.

Infants can also be tested by alternately covering each eye. If visual acuity is poor in one eye, the infant will resist actively when the good eye is covered and vision is disturbed but will be much less affected when the eye with decreased vision is covered.

Poor visual acuity due to refractive errors in older children can be differentiated from poor vision due to other diseases by a pinhole test. If the reduced visual acuity is due to a refractive error, placement of a pinhole before this eye in line with the pupil will result in improved vision.

External Examination

External examination should include general inspection of the lids and eyeballs, noting their prominence, size, and position as well as any growths, inflammations, discharge, or vascular injection. Forward protrusion (exophthalmos) or retraction (enophthalmos) of the globe should be noted. Unusual size of the globes as indicated by megalocornea or microphthalmos should be noted. The positions of the lids in relation to the globe and the coverage of the lids over the closed eyes should be observed. Normally, with the eyes open, the lower lid margin is at the lower border of the cornea in the forward position of gaze, and the upper lid should cover approximately 2 mm of the cornea. Any drooping of the upper lid (ptosis) or retraction of the eyelids should be noted. The lid margins should be inspected to see if they are against the globes in proper alignment or if there is ectropion (turning outward of the lid margins) or entropion (turning inward). The distribution of the lashes and their position should be studied. The lid margins should be inspected for inflammation, crusting, and patency of the lacrimal puncta.

If a conjunctival foreign body is suspected, the lids should be everted and the palpebral and bulbar conjunctivae inspected. The upper lid may be everted by pulling the lid forward (grasping the lashes), placing a small applicator behind the tarsal area, and gently pressing down on the lid (Fig. 11–1). The maneuver is facilitated if the patient looks downward. If a corneal abrasion or foreign body is suspected or if there is sudden unexplained pain in the eye, sterile fluorescein solution should be instilled into the conjunctival cul-de-sac and the cornea observed to see if there is any staining. Observation of staining is enhanced with the use of a blue light. Pupillary light reflexes should be tested for each eye, and both direct and consensual reflexes should be noted.

Corneal sensitivity may be tested by touching the cornea gently with a fine wisp of cotton. If corneal sensation is intact, a brisk blink reflex will result.

Extraocular Muscles

The position of the eyes should be observed by inspection. As a rule, there is little difficulty in telling whether gross strabismus is present. A quick estimation of the alignment of the eyes can be made by the corneal light reflection technique (Hirschberg test). The light reflection should come from corresponding parts of each cornea when a light is shone

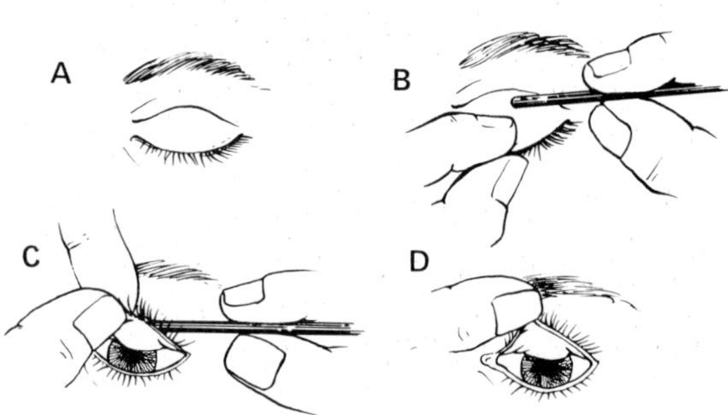

Figure 11–1. Eversion of the upper lid. **A:** The patient looks downward. **B:** The fingers pull the lid down, and a rod is placed on the upper tarsal border. **C:** The lid is pulled up over the rod. **D:** The lid is everted. (Redrawn ano reproduced with permission, from Liebman SD, Gellis SS [editors]: *The Pediatrician's Ophthalmology*. Mosby, 1966.)

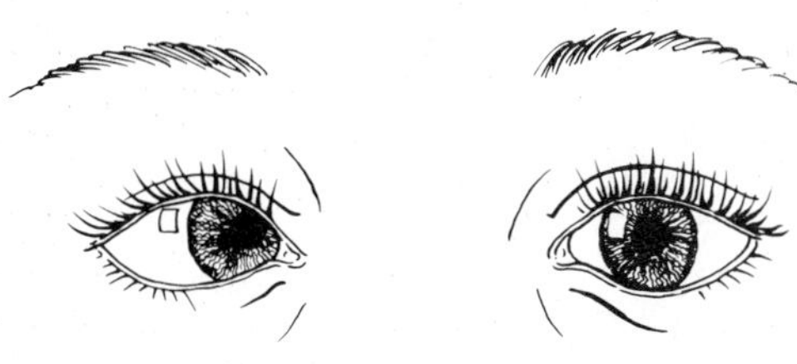

Figure 11–2. Lateral displacement of light reflection showing esotropia (internal deviation) of the right eye. Nasal displacement of the reflection would show exotropia (outward deviation).

into the eyes. If there is lateral displacement of the light reflection, esotropia (internal deviation) of the eye is present (Fig 11–2). If the light reflection is displaced nasally, exotropia (outward deviation) is present. A more refined method of judging alignment of the eyes is by means of the cover test. In this test, the patient is instructed to look at an object and one eye is then covered. If the uncovered eye has been looking straight forward at the object, there will be no shift in movement of this eye. If, however, the eye has been turned either inward or outward, then a corresponding corrective movement will be made with this eye to align the object in the visual gaze (Fig 11–3). The other eye is then similarly tested. The eye under cover should also be observed to see whether there is inward or outward movement, indicating the presence of a phoria, or a tendency for ocular deviation. If the eye remains in the deviated position after removing the occluder, a tropia (deviation of the eyes not corrected by the fusion mechanism) rather than a phoria (deviation that is corrected by the fusion mechanism) is present.

The cardinal positions of gaze should be checked. An object or light is shown to the infant, and the ability to follow the movement of the object in different directions is tested. If marked strabismus or muscle paralysis is present, there may be limitation of movement in one direction of gaze. To determine if true paresis of an extraocular muscle is present, the nondeviating eye should be covered and the ocular movement of the uncovered eye tested in all directions of gaze.

Nystagmus

If nystagmus is present, its characteristics should be observed and the movements classified, first by rate or variation in rate of movement and then by direction. **Pendular (undulatory) nystagmus** consists of excursions that are equal in each direction of gaze; this type of nystagmus is usually observed in children with poor vision and is usually ocular in origin. **Jerking (rhythmic) nystagmus** is characterized by a slow component followed by a quick corrective component; it may be congenital, physiologic (at the extreme positions of gaze), due to inner ear disease, or secondary to central nervous system disease. **Congenital nystagmus** is a type of jerking nystagmus that is usually not associated with other neurologic disorders. The nystagmus is present in all directions of gaze, but it is usually minimized when the patient's eyes are turned slightly to one side or the other. This type of nystagmus usually decreases when the eyes converge. **Latent nystagmus** is manifest only when one eye is covered.

Nystagmus is further classified according to the direction of movement (horizontal, rotatory, vertical, or mixed). Rotatory and vertical nystagmus result from brain stem disorders. Spasmus nutans is a rare disorder in which vertical head nodding is associated with nystagmus; the nystagmus is usually horizontal but may be vertical. An anomalous head tilt is often present. The condition occurs in small infants and usually disappears within the first 2 years of life. Rarely, spasmus nutans is associated with a central nervous system disorder.

Measurement of Intraocular Pressure

The only satisfactory method of measuring ocular pressure is with a tonometer. Tactile tension, particularly in infants, is totally unreliable.

If glaucoma is suspected because of unexplained tearing or enlarged and hazy corneas, the intraocular pressure should be measured with a tonometer. In infants, general anesthesia is usually required, although in selected cases chloral hydrate sedation and topical corneal anesthesia may be used. At age 6–7 years, intraocular pressure can usually be measured with a tonometer after topical anesthesia. Intraocular pressures should be measured with any enlarged or hazy corneas or traumatic hyphema (blood in the anterior chamber).

Ophthalmoscopic Examination

Satisfactory ophthalmoscopic examination of the infant eye can be accomplished only after pupillary dilation. The combination of 1% tropicamide (Mydriacyl) or 2–5% homatropine with 2.5% phenylephrine or that of 0.2% cyclopentolate with 1% phenylephrine (Cyclomydril) instilled 2–3 times at intervals of 10–15 minutes usually gives satisfactory pupillary dilation. In children 2 years of age and older, 1% cyclopentolate (Cyclogyl) gives good pupillary dilation; a second dose may be necessary in children with dark irides.

When an ophthalmoscope is held 30–45 cm (12–18 inches) in front of the eye and the eye is observed through a plus 10 or 15 lens, an orange-red reflection of light (the "red reflex") is observed through the pupil. If the red reflex is not present or dark spots are noted in the reflected light, an opacity of the cornea, lens, or vitreous is probably present. If red reflexes from both eyes are different (eg, irregular or distorted), refractive errors in one or both eyes should be suspected.

Ophthalmoscopic study should include all structures of the eye, such as the cornea, lens, vitreous,

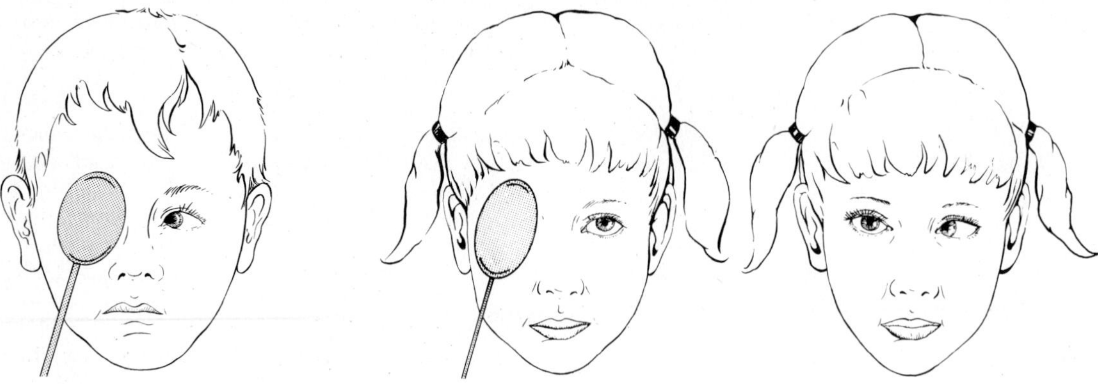

The eyes of a child with severe amblyopia may not be able to fixate an object even when the good eye is covered. Vision of such an eye is 20/200 or less.

If the child with an amblyopic eye will fixate an object only when the good eye is covered but does not hold fixation when the cover is removed, vision of the poor eye is usually from 20/100 to 20/50.

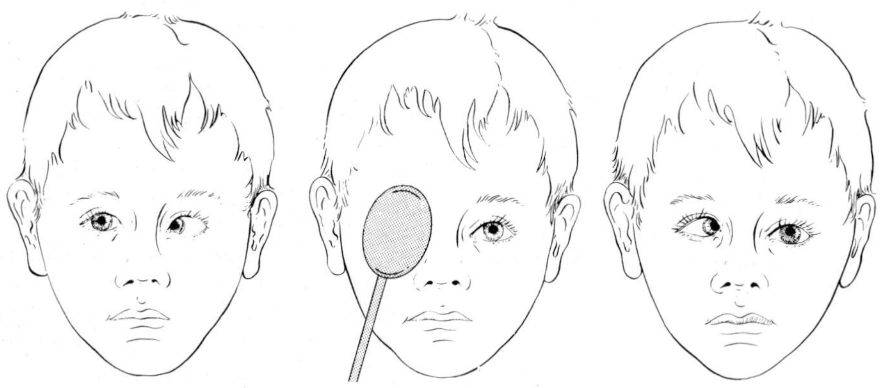

If covering the fixing eye causes fixation with the other eye, and if this second eye maintains fixation for some time even when the cover is removed, the second eye will usually have vision between 20/50 and 20/30.

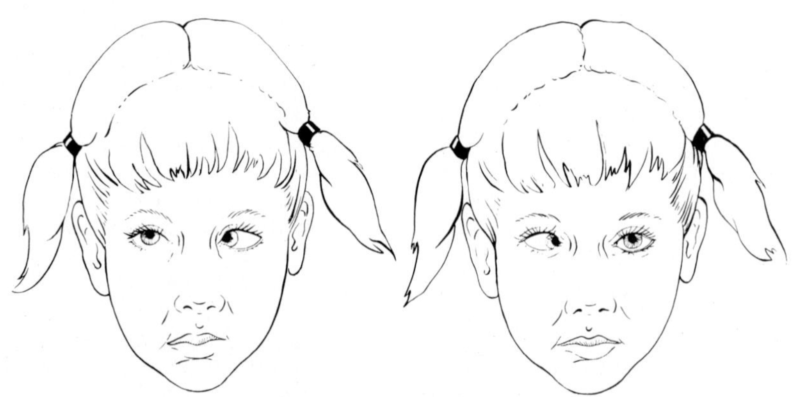

Spontaneous alternation of fixation between the 2 eyes occurs if vision is equal (no suppression amblyopia).

Figure 11–3. Estimation of visual acuity in amblyopia. (Modified slightly. Redrawn and reproduced, with permission, from Havener WH: *Synopsis of Ophthalmology*, 5th ed. Mosby, 1979.)

optic disk, and retina. In the infant, the optic disk appears paler than in the adult. The foveal light reflection is absent. The periphery of the fundus is gray. The peripheral retinal vessels are not well developed.

Refraction Test for Glasses

Cycloplegia is necessary to perform satisfactory refractions in infants and small children. The topical instillation of 1% cyclopentolate (Cyclogyl) or 5% homatropine is usually adequate. More complete cycloplegia can be obtained with 0.5–1% atropine instilled 2–3 times a day for 3 days, but this is seldom necessary. Retinoscopy is used to determine the refractive error in children up to 7–8 years of age. Subsequently, subjective methods of refraction are also used.

Visual Fields

It is virtually impossible to judge visual fields in infants. One can sometimes estimate gross restriction of peripheral visual fields by covering one eye and directing the infant's gaze to an object. A second object is brought in from the side, and the infant is observed to see when the direction of the gaze is first shifted to the new object. Different types of toys and colored lights can be used for the visual test objects.

Perimetry examination of visual fields in children is easier to perform than tangent screen examination. At age 6 or 7 years, satisfactory perimetry examinations can usually be performed. Attractive toys and large objects are brought in along the perimetry arm.

Fulton AB, Hansen RM, Manning KA: Measuring visual acuity in infants. *Surv Ophthalmol* 1981;**25:**325.

Harley RD (editor): *Pediatric Ophthalmology,* 2nd ed. 2 vols. Saunders, 1983.

Harrington DO: *The Visual Fields: A Textbook and Atlas of Clinical Perimetry,* 5th ed. Mosby, 1981.

Helveston EM, Ellis FD: *Pediatric Ophthalmology Practice.* Mosby, 1980.

Hoyt CS: The clinical usefulness of the visual evoked response. *J Pediatr Ophthalmol Strabismus* 1984;**21:**231.

Hoyt CS, Nickel B, Billson FA: Ophthalmological examination of the infant: Developmental aspects. *Surv Ophthalmol* 1982;**26:**177.

Lavery MA et al: Acquired nystagmus in early childhood: A presenting sign of intracranial tumor. *Ophthalmology* 1984;**91:**425.

Mayer DL, Fulton AB, Rodier D: Grating and recognition acuities of pediatric patients. *Ophthalmology* 1984;**91:**947.

GENERAL PRINCIPLES OF TREATMENT OF OCULAR DISORDERS

For diseases of the anterior segment of the eye, topical medication is effective. For diseases of the posterior segment of the eye and of the orbit, systemic medication is necessary. In many instances (eg, severe intraocular infections or uveitis), a combination of topical and systemic medications is required.

The intraocular penetration of topically applied drugs depends upon their solubility in fat and water. The epithelium of the cornea presents a barrier to medications that are not fat-soluble. The alkaloids, the corticosteroids, and some of the anesthetics penetrate the eye quite easily after topical application to the cornea. Most antibiotics do not penetrate the eye in therapeutic concentrations when topically applied.

The degree of intraocular penetration of systemically administered drugs depends upon their ability to pass the blood-aqueous and blood-vitreous barriers. In the normal eye, most systemically administered antibiotics do not penetrate the barriers. In the inflamed eye, the barriers are broken down, and drugs penetrate in much better concentrations. Systemically administered corticosteroids penetrate the eye quite easily. Certain drugs such as mannitol and glycerol do not cross the blood-aqueous barrier and therefore are valuable in the temporary treatment of acute glaucoma because an osmotic gradient is produced in which the blood is hypertonic to the aqueous and vitreous.

Solutions Versus Ointments

Topical ophthalmic preparations may be administered either as solutions or as ointments. In children, ointments have several advantages over solutions: They are not washed away with the tears; they are quite comfortable upon initial instillation; there is less absorption into the lacrimal passage; and since the contact time in the eye is much longer, they can be used less frequently. The chief disadvantage of ointments is that they produce a film over the eye and thus interfere with vision. The advantages of solutions are that they do not interfere with vision and they cause fewer contact dermatitis reactions than ointments; the chief disadvantage is that they must be instilled frequently.

Topical Corticosteroids

The corticosteroids are effective in many eye diseases, including allergic blepharitis and conjunctivitis, vernal conjunctivitis, phlyctenular keratoconjunctivitis, mucocutaneous conjunctival lesions, contact dermatitis of the eyelid and conjunctiva, interstitial keratitis, and many forms of iritis and iridocyclitis. Weaker corticosteroid preparations such as 1% medrysone, 0.5–1.5% hydrocortisone, and 0.125% prednisolone are usually adequate for the management of allergic reactions of the conjunctiva and eyelid.

Many complications follow long- and short-term administration of topical corticosteroids. Among these are increased incidence or aggravation of herpes simplex keratitis and fungal ulcers of the cornea, decreased healing of corneal abrasions and wounds, glaucoma, and cataract formation. The incidence of complications increases with the use of the more potent corticosteroid preparations such as 0.1% dexamethasone, 1% prednisolone, 0.1% triamcinolone, and 0.1% betamethasone. The use of these agents generally should be reserved for the treatment of severe intraocular inflammation. Any eye disorder severe enough to require prolonged topical corticosteroid therapy should be treated by an ophthalmologist.

Topical Antibiotics & Chemotherapeutic Agents

Ideally, the infecting organism should be identified and its antibiotic sensitivity established before specific antibiotic therapy is started. This is often impractical, however, and topical antibiotics are in most cases instituted empirically. Topical use of antibiotics that are seldom employed systemically will decrease the risk of hypersensitivity reactions. For this reason, neomycin, bacitracin, and polymyxin (or mixtures) are frequently used in the treatment of conjunctivitis. Broad-spectrum antibiotics and sulfacetamide or sulfisoxazole seldom produce sensitivity. Topical penicillin therapy should be avoided if possible.

In Tables 11–2 and 11–3 are listed the commonly used topical chemotherapeutic and antibiotic ophthalmic agents.

Mydriatics & Cycloplegics

Mydriatics are agents that dilate the pupil without paralyzing the ciliary muscle of accommodation. They are useful for ophthalmoscopic examination and in preventing and breaking posterior synechiae (adhesions of the iris to the lens). The commonly used mydriatics are phenylephrine, 2.5–10%, and hydroxyamphetamine, 1%. The duration of effect of the mydriatics is only a few hours.

Cycloplegic drugs are agents that produce paralysis of accommodation as well as pupillary dilation. They are used in refraction and in the treatment of acute inflammatory conditions of the iris and ciliary body. The more commonly used cycloplegics are atropine, 0.25–2%; homatropine, 2–5%; scopolamine, 0.2%; cyclopentolate, 1–2%; and tropicamide, 1%.

Atropine is the most powerful cycloplegic; its effect may last for as long as 14 days. Scopolamine has an effect that lasts 2–5 days, whereas the effects of homatropine are usually gone within 48 hours. Cyclopentolate and tropicamide produce more rapid cycloplegia than the other agents, but their effect is usually gone within 24 hours.

Topical Anesthetics

The most commonly used local anesthetics are proparacaine, 0.5%; benoxinate, 0.4%; and tetracaine, 0.5%. Topical anesthetics may be used before the removal of a conjunctival or corneal foreign body. They may be necessary to relieve the blepharospasm induced by a chemical injury before satisfactory irrigation and examination of the eye can be accomplished. They should never be prescribed for home use, since they might mask a serious ocular disorder or result in corneal ulceration.

Sterility of Topical Medication

Any ophthalmic medication may become contaminated. This is particularly true of solutions of fluorescein, which frequently become infected with *Pseudomonas aeruginosa*. It is well to discard all old ophthalmic solutions and any container whose tip has been touched by the examiner's hand or by the patient's eyelids. In the case of fluorescein, single-

Table 11–2. Topical chemotherapeutic and antibiotic agents.

Drug	Trade Name	Solution	Ointment
Amphotericin B	Fungizone	0.5–1.5 mg/mL*	
Bacitracin	Baciguent	2000–10,000 units/mL†	500 units/g
Chloramphenicol	Antibiopto, Chloromycetin, Chloroptic, Econochlor, Ophthochlor	1.6–5 mg/mL	10 mg/g
Colistin	Coly-Mycin S	1.2–5 mg/mL*	
Erythromycin	Ilotycin	5 mg/mL*	5 mg/g
Gentamicin	Garamycin, Genoptic	3 mg/mL	3 mg/g
Neomycin	Myciguent	1.75–3.5 mg/mL†	3.5 mg/g
Natamycin	Natacyn	50 mg/mL	
Polymyxin B		5000–16,250 mg/mL†	5000–10,000 units/g†
Streptomycin		50 mg/mL*	
Sulfacetamide sodium	Many	100–300 mg/mL	100 mg/g
Sulfisoxazole	Gantrisin	40 mg/mL	40 mg/g
Tetracycline group	Many	5–10 mg/mL	10–30 mg/g
Tobramycin	Tobrex	3 mg/mL	3 mg/g

* Not commercially available.
† Available commercially only in combined drug preparations.

Table 11–3. Combinations of anti-infective drugs.

Drugs	Trade Name
Bacitracin and polymyxin B	Polysporin
Bacitracin (gramicidin), neomycin, and polymyxin B*	Mycitracin, Neosporin
Chloramphenicol and polymyxin B	Chloromyxin
Oxytetracycline and polymyxin B	Terramycin-Polymyxin B
Neomycin and polymyxin B	Statrol

* Some commercial preparations utilize gramicidin in place of bacitracin.

use disposable solution or impregnated filter paper strips should be employed.

Systemic Absorption of Topical Medication

Since absorption of topical eye medication into the circulation may occur in sufficient quantity to produce systemic side effects, the total dosage should be carefully considered. For example, each drop of 1% atropine contains 0.5 mg of atropine. If 1% atropine drops were instilled into each eye and total absorption occurred, a toxic reaction would result in children. Other drugs most likely to produce toxicity include scopolamine, cyclopentolate, echothiophate iodide, and 10% phenylephrine (the latter should never be used in infants and small children).

When medication is instilled into the eye of an infant, pressure should be exerted over the lacrimal sac for a minute to prevent the drug from reaching the nasal mucosa, where it could be absorbed. Alternatively, the head may be tipped temporally to the side of the treated eye so that the excess medication will run out of the outer corner of the eye.

Ellis PP: *Ocular Therapeutics and Pharmacology,* 7th ed. Mosby, 1985.

Fraunfelder FT, Roy FH (editors): *Current Ocular Therapy,* 2. Saunders, 1985.

Palmer EA: Risks of dilating a child's pupils. *Trans Pac Coast Otoophthalmol Soc Annu Meet* 1982;**63:**141.

Timewell RM et al: Safety and efficacy of tobramycin and gentamicin sulfate in the treatment of external ocular infections of children. *J Pediatr Ophthalmol Strabismus* 1983; **20:**22.

OCULAR INJURIES

FOREIGN BODIES

Conjunctival Foreign Body

A conjunctival foreign body can usually be removed with a moist cotton applicator. A common site for foreign bodies is the furrow immediately behind the margin of the upper lid. Eversion of the upper lid, as described above, is necessary to visualize these foreign bodies.

Corneal Foreign Body

Superficial corneal foreign bodies usually can be removed without difficulty. A sterile topical anesthetic should be instilled into the eye and an attempt made to wipe away the foreign body with a moist cotton applicator. If this is not successful, a blunt spud or small, sterile, dull hypodermic needle (No. 20) can be used. Care must be taken not to injure the deeper layers of the cornea; if the foreign body is deeply embedded in the stroma, the patient should be referred to an ophthalmologist. Rust rings of foreign bodies should be removed primarily. An antibiotic ointment should be instilled, and the eye should be patched until epithelialization of the cornea has occurred. The patient should be reexamined within 24 hours to make certain that infection has not occurred.

Intraocular Foreign Body

Intraocular foreign bodies are serious injuries that may not be suspected on initial examination. The usual history is that the patient was pounding on a metallic object with a hammer when something flew up into the eye. Examination may show a perforating wound of the cornea, a hole in the iris, an irregular or "peaked" pupil, and an opaque lens. However, the foreign body may be so small that little evidence of penetration is seen. X-rays of the eye may be necessary to rule out the possibility of foreign body. If there is any question of a foreign body, the patient should be referred to an ophthalmologist, since removal of these foreign bodies is extremely difficult. The visual prognosis is guarded.

Benson WE: Intraocular foreign bodies. Chapter 15 in: *Clinical Ophthalmology.* Vol 5. Duane TD (editor). Harper & Row, 1984.

De Juan E Jr, Sternberg P Jr, Michels RG: Penetrating ocular injuries: Types of injuries and visual results. *Ophthalmology* 1983;**90:**1318.

Deutsch TA, Feller DB: *Paton & Goldberg's Management of Ocular Injuries,* 2nd ed. Saunders, 1985.

Freeman HM (editor): *Ocular Trauma.* Appleton-Century-Crofts, 1979.

Gombos GM: *Handbook of Ophthalmologic Emergencies,* 2nd ed. Medical Examination Publishing Co., 1977.

INJURIES OF THE EYELIDS

Ecchymosis

Severe ecchymosis of the eyelids should be treated first with cold compresses to reduce hemorrhage and swelling. After 24–48 hours, hot packs will speed absorption of extravasated blood.

Lacerations

Lacerations of the eyelids should be sutured primarily. When the laceration involves the lid margin, particularly the lower lid, it is imperative that the margins be sutured as evenly as possible to prevent development of a notch. In such cases, the patient should be referred to an ophthalmologist. Lacerations involving the medial portion of the eyelids should be examined to rule out injury to the lacrimal canaliculi. If the canaliculi are cut, they should be repaired at the time of primary closure of the lid laceration, since delayed attempts to repair cut canaliculi are less successful.

Baylis HI, Axelrod R: Repair of lacerated canaliculus. *Ophthalmology* 1978;**85:**1271.

Billson FA, Taylor HR, Hoyt CS: Trauma to the lacrimal system in children. *Am J Ophthalmol* 1978;**86:**828.

Deutsch TA, Feller DB: *Paton & Goldberg's Management of Ocular Injuries,* 2nd ed. Saunders, 1985.

Gombos GM: *Handbook of Ophthalmologic Emergencies,* 2nd ed. Medical Examination Publishing Co., 1977.

Harley RD: Ocular manifestations of child abuse. *J Pediatr Ophthalmol Strabismus* 1980;**17:**5.

Tenzel RR: Trauma and burns. *Int Ophthalmol Clin* (Spring) 1970;**10:**55.

CORNEAL INJURIES

Corneal Abrasions

Corneal abrasions usually produce severe discomfort. The diagnosis is made by instilling fluorescein into the eye and observing the cornea for staining.

Treatment consists of the instillation of a mild cycloplegic such as 5% homatropine or 1% cyclopentolate (Cyclogyl), the application of antibiotic ointments, and firm patching of the eye for 24–48 hours or until the epithelium has healed.

Corneal Lacerations

Patients with corneal lacerations should be referred to an ophthalmologist for primary suturing. The patient should be observed for the development of intraocular infection. Systemic antibiotics and tetanus toxoid are indicated if the perforation occurred with a contaminated object.

Gombos GM: *Handbook of Ophthalmologic Emergencies,* 2nd ed. Medical Examination Publishing Co., 1977.

Deutsch TA, Feller DB: *Paton & Goldberg's Management of Ocular Injuries,* 2nd ed. Saunders, 1985.

HYPHEMA

Hyphema (blood in the anterior chamber) is a common contusion injury in children. It is a serious injury, often requiring hospitalization. Secondary bleeding is frequent and occurs usually within 6 days after the primary bleeding. Patients with hyphema should be examined for the development of glaucoma. Ophthalmoscopy should also be attempted to ascertain whether there has been more extensive injury to the posterior part of the eye. Black children with hyphema should be tested for sickle cell disease, because if the disease is present, they are more likely to develop complications.

Treatment consists of bed rest, eye bandages, and sedatives. Binocular bandages are advisable, but if they produce excitement they may be omitted. Recent studies have suggested that bed rest and monocular patches are as effective as binocular patches in mild or moderate hyphemas. However, in severe hyphemas, binocular patches are preferred. No pupillary dilating (mydriatic) or pupillary constricting (miotic) drops should be used. If glaucoma develops, the use of carbonic anhydrase inhibitors, intravenous urea or mannitol, or oral glycerol is indicated initially. If this does not control the glaucoma, surgical removal of the blood clot by irrigation or with a cryoprobe or vitrectomy instrument is indicated. To reduce the incidence of rebleeding, some authors have recommended the use of systemic aminocaproic acid (Amicar) for 5 days after the initial hemorrhage.

Another complication of hyphema is blood staining of the cornea. This occurs only if the hemorrhage remains for a long period; it may occur whether or not glaucoma develops.

Deutsch TA, Feller DB: *Paton & Goldberg's Management of Ocular Injuries,* 2nd ed. Saunders, 1985.

Fritch CD: Traumatic hyphema. *Ann Ophthalmol* 1976;**8:**1223.

Gombos GM: *Handbook of Ophthalmologic Emergencies,* 2nd ed. Medical Examination Publishing Co., 1977.

Lattin DE, Ellis PP: Aminocaproic acid in the management of hyphema. *Trans Pac Coast Otoophthalmol Soc Annu Meet* 1982;**63:**185.

McGetrick JJ et al: Aminocaproic acid decreases secondary hemorrhage after traumatic hyphema. *Arch Ophthalmol* 1983;**101:**1031.

Pilger IS: Medical treatment of traumatic hyphema. *Surv Ophthalmol* 1975;**20:**28.

Read J, Goldberg MF: Comparison of medical treatment for traumatic hyphema. *Trans Am Acad Ophthalmol Otolaryngol* 1974;**78:**799.

Wilson FM II: Traumatic hyphema: Pathogenesis and management. *Ophthalmology* 1980;**87:**910.

BURNS

Burns of the eyelids should be treated in essentially the same way as burns of the skin elsewhere. It is important to protect the eyeballs from infection and exposure. Since burns frequently become contaminated with *Pseudomonas* organisms that can produce severe corneal ulceration, an antibiotic preparation containing either colistin, gentamicin, tobramycin, or polymyxin B should be instilled into the eyes 3–4 times a day. As the burns begin to heal, cicatricial ectropion with corneal exposure may develop. To prevent corneal exposure, ointments should be applied inside the eyelids. Plastic surgery often is necessary to correct cicatricial ectropion.

Chemical burns of the cornea and conjunctiva

should be treated initially with thorough irrigation with any clean nonirritating fluid. This may be tap water, saline or boric acid solution, or whatever is available. In no case should a delay occur because of attempts to obtain a particular irrigating solution. It may be necessary to instill topical anesthetics into the eye to relieve blepharospasm before irrigation can be accomplished. Adequacy of the irrigation can be judged by testing the conjunctival fluid for neutrality with pH test paper. After irrigation, the eye should be inspected for retained chemical particles, which can be removed with a moist cotton applicator. The extent of the damage is then determined. If the burn involves the cornea, the pupil should be dilated with 1% atropine or 5% homatropine after irrigation to provide comfort. An antibiotic ointment should be instilled and the eye patched. Any patient who has suffered a severe chemical burn of the eye should be hospitalized and should be seen by an ophthalmologist.

Ultraviolet burns of the cornea usually cause severe pain and tearing. There is a history of exposure to ultraviolet light (eg, a welder's arc, snow on the ski slopes, sunlamp or treatment lamp). Symptoms develop 10–12 hours after exposure. Examination shows superficial corneal edema and pinpoint areas that stain with fluorescein. Treatment consists of the application of a topical anesthetic every 5–10 minutes until the pain is relieved. After pain has subsided, an antibiotic or an antibiotic-corticosteroid ointment is instilled into the eye and the eye is patched. Systemic analgesics and sedatives are then prescribed. Recovery is usually prompt and complete within 48 hours. (***Note:*** Topical anesthetics should never be sent home with the patient.)

Retinal burns with permanent loss of vision may occur as a result of exposure to strong infrared light such as from observing an eclipse. If this is suspected, the patient should be referred to an ophthalmologist.

Deutsch TA, Feller DB: *Paton & Goldberg's Management of Ocular Injuries*, 2nd ed. Saunders, 1985.

Guy RJ et al: Three-years' experience in a regional burn center with burns of the eyes and eyelids. *Ophthalmic Surg* 1982;**13:**383.

Havener WH: *Ocular Pharmacology*, 5th ed. Mosby, 1983.

Pfister RR: Chemical injuries of the eye. *Ophthalmology* 1983;**90:**1246.

Pfister RR, Paterson CA: Ascorbic acid in the treatment of alkali burns of the eye. *Ophthalmology* 1980;**87:**1050.

FRACTURES OF THE ORBIT

Fractures of the orbit with any degree of displacement of the bones should be surgically reduced. The techniques of surgery depend upon the location and extent of the fracture. If the fractures are not satisfactorily reduced, complications occur that include displacement of the globe, enophthalmos, and diplopia. Any injury severe enough to cause an orbital fracture may cause further skull fractures and intracranial and intraocular damage. The patient should be studied for these possibilities.

Blowout fractures generally result from blunt injury such as a blow from a ball or fist. The bones of the orbital rim usually remain intact, but there is a blowout of the floor of the orbit (rarely, the medial wall of the orbit) with herniation of the orbital contents into the blowout site. Blowout fractures should be suspected if there is evidence of diplopia in any direction of gaze or if there is limitation of ocular movement, particularly upward. Hypesthesia of the skin in the distribution of the infraorbital nerve is present in about 30% of patients. Subcutaneous emphysema may be present. Weakness of ocular movement, particularly downward gaze, and enophthalmos may be present initially or develop later. Blowout fractures are not always seen on routine x-rays of the orbit. Tomograms and other special diagnostic radiologic techniques, including CT scans, are sometimes necessary to demonstrate this fracture. Surgical treatment is often required.

Beyer CK, Fabian RL, Smith B: Naso-orbital fractures: Complications and treatment. *Ophthalmology* 1982;**89:**456.

Hawes MJ, Dortzbach RK: Surgery on orbital floor fractures: Influence of time of repair and fracture size. *Ophthalmology* 1983;**90:**1066.

Smith B, Nightingale JD: Fractures of the orbit: Blowout and nasoorbital fractures. *Int Ophthalmol Clin* (Fall) 1978; **18:**137.

Wilkins RB, Havins WE: Current treatment of blow-out fractures. *Ophthalmology* 1982;**89:**464.

CONTUSIONS OF THE GLOBE

In addition to the hyphema mentioned above, contusions of the globe may result in dislocation of the lens, hemorrhage into the vitreous, retinal edema and hemorrhage, retinal detachment, choroidal hemorrhage, choroidal rupture, and rupture of the eyeball. The diagnosis of these conditions is based upon (1) changes in visual acuity and (2) direct observation with the ophthalmoscope and slit lamp. If the fundus can be visualized well and if visual acuity is good, there is little likelihood that any significant damage to the posterior part of the eye has occurred. However, complications such as retinal detachment or dislocation of the lens may not appear until weeks after the initial injury.

Cherry PMH: Rupture of the globe. *Arch Ophthalmol* 1972;**88:**498.

Eagling EM: Ocular damage after blunt trauma to the eye: Its relationship to the nature of the injury. *Br J Ophthalmol* 1974;**58:**126.

Gombos GM: *Handbook of Ophthalmologic Emergencies*, 2nd ed. Medical Examination Publishing Co., 1977.

Harley RD: Ocular manifestations of child abuse. *J Pediatr Ophthalmol Strabismus* 1980;**17:**5.

Holt JE, Holt GR, Blodgett JM: Ocular injuries sustained during blunt facial trauma. *Ophthalmology* 1983;**90:**14.

REFRACTIVE ERRORS

Myopia (nearsightedness) is easily diagnosed; distant objects are blurred. Near vision is not usually impaired except in very high myopia. Frequently, the patient squints in order to form a physiologic pinhole to improve visual acuity.

The diagnosis of **hyperopia (farsightedness)** in children is more difficult. Children are able to accommodate much more effectively than adults and thus overcome their hyperopia. Sometimes there are associated symptoms of eyestrain or headaches after prolonged periods of close work. Children with severe farsightedness may have internal deviations of the eyes (accommodative esotropia).

Astigmatism produces distorted vision. Children will attempt to overcome the blurry vision by squinting their eyes and forming a pinhole. Children with severe astigmatism may complain of eyestrain and headaches.

Anisometropia is a difference in refractive errors of the 2 eyes. Severe anisometropia may cause amblyopia.

Treatment of significant refractive errors consists of the proper fitting of lenses. Small degrees of hyperopia need not be corrected in children. Full correction of myopia is indicated. The use of bifocals in myopic children does not appear to prevent the progressive type of myopia. Other forms of treatment such as the use of "eye exercises" or certain diets do not appear to influence the progression of myopia. Long-term use of atropine drops may reduce progression of myopia, but this therapy is impractical and not usually recommended.

Contact lenses are seldom indicated in children. The exception is the child with unilateral aphakia (absence of the lens), severe anisometropia, corneal scarring producing an irregular astigmatism, or keratoconus. Contact lenses have been purported to reduce the progression of myopia, but there is little evidence for this view.

Abrams D: *Duke-Elder's Practice of Refraction,* 9th ed. Churchill Livingstone, 1978.

Kivlin JD, Flynn JT: Therapy of anisometropic amblyopia. *J Pediatr Ophthalmol Strabismus* 1981;**18:**47.

Michaels DD: *Visual Optics and Refraction: A Clinical Approach,* 2nd ed. Mosby, 1980.

Prakash P, Agarwal LP, Gupta SB: Refractive error in children. *J Pediatr Ophthalmol* 1971;**8:**42.

Saunders RA, Ellis FD: Empirical fitting of hard contact lenses in infants and young children. *Ophthalmology* 1981;**88:**127.

STRABISMUS (Squint)

Approximately 5% of children have strabismus. The eyes may deviate inward (esotropia), outward (exotropia), upward (hypertropia), or downward (hypotropia). Strabismus is comitant if the same degree of deviation exists in all fields of gaze and noncomitant if the angle of deviation changes in the various directions of gaze. The terms tropia and phoria are both used to describe abnormal positions of the eye; tropias are manifest deviations, whereas phorias are latent deviations that become manifest only if fusion or binocular vision is blocked.

Nonparalytic strabismus is usually first observed either shortly after birth or at the age of 2–3 years; rarely, the onset is at a later age. Infants do not develop coordinated eye muscle movements until about 3–5 months of age. An occasional infant is observed to have temporary deviation of the eyes, and realignment subsequently occurs. Any child who has a deviation that persists for several weeks or who develops a deviation after the age of 6 months should be investigated for the cause of the strabismus.

The diagnosis of strabismus is frequently made by simple inspection. If the eyes are deviated considerably, the diagnosis is evident. If there is only a slight deviation or if there is a questionable deviation because of wide epicanthal folds (pseudostrabismus) with more of the white of the eye being exposed temporally than nasally, the diagnosis is established by the corneal light reflection technique (Fig 11–2) or the cover test (Fig 11–3), as described above. Strabismus may also be suspected on the basis of marked reduced visual acuity in one eye. Children with a persistent head tilt or face turn may have strabismus with very little apparent displacement of the eyes.

During visual development, diplopia occurs if alignment of the eyes is such that the object viewed does not fall on corresponding parts of the retina. To avoid diplopia, the child learns to suppress the vision in the deviating eye. If one eye continually deviates, then suppression is always in this eye, with the result that macular vision never develops. This condition is called **amblyopia ex anopsia** or **suppression amblyopia.** Visual screening examination of preschool children is important in diagnosing early suppression amblyopia.

Paralytic or noncomitant strabismus may result from central nervous system diseases or anatomic maldevelopments of the ocular muscles. The sudden onset of paralytic strabismus in any child should prompt examination for central nervous system disease.

Treatment

Children do not outgrow strabismus. Early treatment is important and should be given by an ophthalmologist. Treatment is directed toward the development of good visual acuity in each eye, realignment of the eyes in good cosmetic position, and functional cures with the establishment of binocular vision. The following steps are considered in the treatment of strabismus: (1) careful ophthalmoscopic examination to rule out an organic intraocular cause for the deviation, eg, congenital cataracts, tumors, optic nerve atrophy; (2) cycloplegic refraction and prescription of lenses; (3) occlusion of the good eye to develop macular vision in the bad eye; and (4) surgery to align the eyes if glasses are unsuccessful in correcting the deviation.

Early surgery (ages 6–24 months) with alignment of the eyes is more likely to result in a functional cure than surgery performed at age 4–5 years or later.

Orthoptic exercises are of value in establishing binocular vision if the visual axes are nearly aligned. They are also of value in certain forms of intermittent strabismus.

Dale RT: *Fundamentals of Ocular Motility and Strabismus.* Grune & Stratton, 1982.

Ing MR: Early surgical alignment for congenital esotropia. *J Pediatr Ophthalmol Strabismus* 1983;**20:**11.

Mohindra I et al: Development of acuity and stereopsis in infants with esotropia. *Ophthalmology* 1985;**92:**691.

Parks MM: *Atlas of Strabismus Surgery.* Lippincott, 1983.

Reinecke RD, Miller D: *Strabismus: A Programmed Text,* 2nd ed. Appleton-Century-Crofts, 1977.

Von Noorden GK: *Burian-von Noorden's Binocular Vision and Ocular Motility,* 2nd ed. Mosby, 1979.

PTOSIS

Ptosis is a drooping of the upper eyelid. It may be congenital or acquired and unilateral or bilateral. Ptosis may be associated with anisometropia.

Congenital ptosis usually results from incomplete development of the levator muscle. Occasionally, it is associated with third cranial nerve trauma at the time of birth or congenitally misdirected third cranial nerve fibers, in which case other abnormalities of ocular movement are often present.

Acquired ptosis may be traumatic in origin, may follow inflammation or scarring of the eyelids, or may present as a sign of some neurologic disorder. When ptosis is a sign of myasthenia gravis, an injection of edrophonium chloride (Tensilon) will produce prompt improvement. (See discussion of myasthenia gravis in Chapter 23.)

The treatment of congenital ptosis is surgical. The operation is usually performed at the age of 3–4 years. Rarely, the surgery should be done earlier if the eyelid covers the pupil completely and prevents development of normal vision. Unequal refractive errors between eyes may be associated with ptosis. The treatment of acquired ptosis depends upon the origin, but primary consideration should be directed toward treating any basic underlying disease.

Beard C: *Ptosis,* 3rd ed. Mosby, 1980.

Crawford JS, Iliff CE, Stasior OG: Symposium on congenital ptosis. *J Pediatr Ophthalmol Strabismus* 1982;**19:**245.

Fox SA: *Surgery of Ptosis.* Williams & Wilkins, 1980.

Wobig JL: Congenital ptosis and levator resection. *Trans New Orleans Acad Ophthalmol* 1982;**86.**

GLAUCOMA

Primary Glaucoma

Primary congenital glaucoma (hydrophthalmos) is due to an abnormal development of the aqueous drainage structures; it may be present at birth or may develop within the first 2 years of life. Diagnosis is based upon (1) enlarged corneas that are frequently edematous and show linear white opacities (breaks in Descemet's membrane), (2) symptoms of photophobia and tearing, (3) increased intraocular pressure, and (4) enlarged cupping of the optic disk. Since the coats of the eye of an infant are not as rigid as those of an adult, increased intraocular pressure results in stretching of the corneal and scleral tissues.

Early surgery is essential. Medical therapy is of little value. Surgery is successful in controlling intraocular pressure in about 75% of cases. Without treatment, permanent blindness occurs at an early age.

Glaucoma may be associated with other developmental anomalies. These include aniridia, posterior embryotoxon (failure of reabsorption of the mesodermal tissue in the periphery of the iris and drainage angle), Sturge-Weber disease, Lowe's syndrome, Marfan's syndrome, Hurler's syndrome, Pierre Robin syndrome, Rubinstein-Taybi syndrome, neurofibromatosis, homocystinuria, congenital rubella syndrome, and trisomy 13 (D) or 18 (E_1).

Secondary Glaucoma

Secondary glaucoma may be due to many causes. The mechanism of this type of glaucoma is usually an obstruction of the aqueous outflow channels. The various causes include lens dislocation, hemorrhage into the eye, iritis, tumors (including retinoblastoma), retrolental fibroplasia, and xanthogranulomas in the iris. Treatment of these conditions is complicated, and the patient should be referred to an ophthalmologist.

Beauchamp GR, Parks MM: Filtering surgery in children: Barriers to success. *Ophthalmology* 1979;**86:**170.

Chandler PA, Grant WM: *Glaucoma,* 2nd ed. Lea & Febiger, 1979.

Goethals M, Missotten L: Intraocular pressure in children up to five years of age. *J Pediatr Ophthalmol Strabismus* 1983;**20:**49.

Kolker AE, Hetherington J Jr: *Becker-Shaffer's Diagnosis and Therapy of the Glaucomas,* 5th ed. Mosby, 1983.

Kwitko ML: *Glaucoma in Infants and Children.* Appleton-Century-Crofts, 1973.
McPherson SD, Berry DP: Goniotomy versus external trabeculotomy for developmental glaucoma. *Am J Ophthalmol* 1983;**95:**427.
Quigley HA: Childhood glaucoma: Results with trabeculotomy and study of reversible cupping. *Ophthalmology* 1982; **89:**219.

CATARACTS

A cataract is an opacity of the lens; it consists of precipitated lens protein. Cataracts may be unilateral or bilateral and partial or complete; considerable variation exists in the extent, position, shape, and density of cataract formation. They may be congenital and associated with other congenital anomalies. They can occur as a result of maternal rubella during the first trimester of pregnancy. Cataracts may be secondary to ocular trauma or associated with systemic diseases such as diabetes mellitus, galactosemia, atopic dermatitis, Marfan's syndrome, or Down's syndrome. They may also be due to long-term systemic corticosteroid therapy.

The symptoms vary considerably according to location and extent. Vision may be affected very slightly, or considerable reduction in vision can occur. White spots may be observed in the pupil. In a few cases, strabismus or pendular nystagmus is present.

The diagnosis is made by inspection with a flashlight or by examination with an ophthalmoscope or slit lamp. In some cases, cataracts can be observed only when the pupils are dilated.

Surgical lens extraction (within the first few weeks of life) is indicated if the cataracts are bilateral and sufficiently dense that vision cannot develop. If cataracts are not dense enough to interfere with visual development, surgery should be deferred, since some congenital cataracts do not progress. Surgery is indicated when visual loss is a serious handicap to the child.

In the past, the results of surgical treatment of unilateral congenital cataracts were poor. More recently, there has been an attempt to improve results with early surgery (as soon as the diagnosis is made) and fitting of contact lenses within a few days after surgery. Most ophthalmologists do not favor intraocular lens implantation in children.

Ciba Foundation: *Symposium on Human Cataract Formation.* Pitman, 1984.
Gelbart SS et al: Long-term visual results in bilateral congenital cataracts. *Am J Ophthalmol* 1982;**93:**615.
Hiles DA (editor): Infantile cataract surgery. *Int Ophthalmol Clin* (Winter) 1977;**17:**1. [Entire issue.]
Jaffe NS: *Cataract Surgery and Its Complications,* 4th ed. Mosby, 1984.
Kwitko ML: *Surgery of the Infant Eye.* Appleton-Century-Crofts, 1979.
New Orleans Academy of Ophthalmology: *Symposium on Cataracts.* Mosby, 1979.
Parks MM: Visual results in aphakic children. *Am J Ophthalmol* 1982;**94:**441.

DISLOCATED LENS

Dislocation (luxation) or partial dislocation (subluxation) of the lens may result from blunt trauma to the eye and orbit. It may also be observed in patients with genetic dwarfism, scleroderma, Rieger's syndrome, and other hereditary disorders, including Marfan's syndrome and Marchesani's syndrome (with the lens usually dislocated superiorly) and homocystinuria (lens usually dislocated inferiorly).

Glaucoma is a common complication of dislocated lenses. All children with dislocated lenses should be evaluated by an ophthalmologist.

Crawford JS, Morin JD (editors): *The Eye in Childhood.* Grune & Stratton, 1983.
Nelson LB, Maumenee IH: Ectopia lentis. *Surv Ophthalmol* 1982;**27:**143.
Seetner AA, Crawford JS: Surgical correction of lens dislocation in children. *Am J Ophthalmol* 1981;**91:**106.

DISEASES OF THE EYELIDS

HORDEOLUM

External hordeolum (sty) is a staphylococcal abscess of the sebaceous glands of the lid margin. Symptoms consist of localized tenderness, redness, and swelling. Internal hordeolum is an acute infection of the meibomian glands that usually points conjunctivally.

Treatment of both types consists of warm moist compresses 3–4 times a day. Instillation of an antibiotic or sulfonamide ophthalmic ointment 4–5 times a day is useful during the acute stage. To reduce the likelihood of a recurrence, treatment should be continued for several days after the lesion has subsided.

Spontaneous rupture frequently occurs, but if it does not, the lesion should be incised when it becomes large and pointed. The removal of an eyelash may promote drainage of an external hordeolum.

Fedukowicz HB, Stenson S: *External Infections of the Eye,* 3rd ed. Appleton-Century-Crofts, 1985.
Vaughan D, Asbury T: *General Ophthalmology,* 10th ed. Lange, 1983.

CHALAZION

Chalazion is a granulomatous inflammation of the meibomian glands. The cause is not known. Symptoms consist of slight discomfort in the eyelid and a slight redness and a lump on the conjunctival surface of the lid overlying the involved meibomian gland. Local excision is often necessary, but chalazions may disappear after treatment with warm moist compresses. Corticosteroid injection into the chalazion is often effective.

Perry HD, Serniuk RA: Conservative treatment of chalazia. *Ophthalmology* 1980;**87:**218.

Vaughan D, Asbury T: *General Ophthalmology,* 10th ed. Lange, 1983.

Watson AP, Austin DJ: Treatment of chalazions with injection of a steroid suspension. *Br J Ophthalmol* 1984;**68:**833.

BLEPHARITIS (Granulated Eyelids)

Chronic inflammation of the lid margins may be seborrheic (nonulcerative), staphylococcal (ulcerative), or a combination of the 2 types. Symptoms are redness, burning, itching, and crusting of the lid margins. In the staphylococcal type, the scales are dry; small ulcerative lesions of the skin are observed; and the eyelashes may fall out. In the seborrheic type, the scales are oily; seborrhea of the scalp is usually present as well.

Treatment of staphylococcal blepharitis consists of the instillation of antibiotic or sulfonamide ophthalmic ointment into the eye twice a day. Treatment should be continued for a week or so after all symptoms have disappeared. The crusts on the lids should be gently removed with a moist cotton applicator before the ointment is instilled. Occasionally, systemic antibiotics are required in severe cases of staphylococcal blepharitis.

The treatment of seborrheic blepharitis consists of controlling scalp seborrhea if it exists, removing the scales along the lid margins with a moist cotton applicator, and instilling sulfacetamide or an antistaphylococcal antibiotic ophthalmic ointment.

Seborrheic blepharitis can often be controlled by scrubbing the edge of the eyelids twice a day with a cotton applicator moistened in a bland, half-strength baby shampoo that does not irritate the eye.

Fedukowicz HB, Stenson S: *External Infections of the Eye,* 3rd ed. Appleton-Century-Crofts, 1985.

Feman SS, Reinecke RD (editors): *Handbook of Pediatric Ophthalmology.* Grune & Stratton, 1978.

Scheie HG, Albert DM: *Textbook of Ophthalmology,* 9th ed. Saunders, 1977.

DISEASES OF THE CONJUNCTIVA

CONJUNCTIVITIS

Conjunctivitis is the most common of all pediatric ocular disorders. It is usually due to bacterial, viral, or fungal infections. Less commonly, it may result from an allergic reaction or physical or chemical irritation. Symptoms consist of redness of the conjunctiva, foreign body sensation, a mucoid or purulent discharge, and sticking together of the eyelids in the morning. Vision is not affected. The cornea, anterior chamber, and intraocular pressure are normal.

Bacterial Conjunctivitis

The most common causes of bacterial conjunctivitis are the pneumococcus, *Staphylococcus aureus,* Koch-Weeks bacillus, and hemolytic streptococci. There may be associated bacterial infections elsewhere in the body. Conjunctival membranes (diphtheritic conjunctivitis) or pseudomembranes (streptococcal conjunctivitis) may be present. Discharge, usually a prominent feature of bacterial conjunctivitis, is purulent or mucopurulent in character.

The causative organism should be identified, if possible, by obtaining smears and cultures. Empiric treatment with broad-spectrum antibiotics or sulfonamide ophthalmic ointments instilled into the eye 4–5 times a day usually results in improvement within 48–72 hours. If improvement does not occur, it is important to make an etiologic diagnosis if this has not been done earlier. Bacterial conjunctivitis is usually a self-limited disease, but secondary corneal infection and ulceration occur rarely.

Inclusion Conjunctivitis (Swimming Pool Conjunctivitis)

This disease is caused by the same chlamydial organism that produces inclusion conjunctivitis in the newborn. It is characterized by conjunctival redness, clear or mucoid discharge, and follicles in the lower palpebral conjunctiva. Treatment consists of the systemic administration of either sulfonamides, a tetracycline (but not to infants or young children), or erythromycin. Topical application of these drugs is not as effective as systemic treatment.

Trachoma

Trachoma is infection of the conjunctiva with a bacterium formerly thought to be a large atypical virus but now reclassified as a bacterium of the genus *Chlamydia.* The disease is usually associated with poor hygiene and poor economic conditions. It is a major cause of blindness in the world but is rare in the USA except among American Indians.

In the early stages, trachoma is characterized by a catarrhal type of reaction with diffuse redness, mild irritation, and a thin watery discharge. Subsequently, the conjunctiva becomes thickened, with papillary hypertrophy and formation of follicles, particularly in the tarsal region of the upper lids. Scarring of the conjunctiva develops later, and there is corneal vascularization and opacification.

Local therapy can probably control trachoma adequately, but systemic therapy is usually recommended also. Systemic sulfonamides, tetracyclines, and erythromycin are the agents most commonly used. For children over 9 years of age in whom dentition is complete, a 3- to 4-week course of oral tetracycline is given. Doxycycline is preferred, since administration is required only once a day. For children under age 9, the drug of choice is sulfisoxazole (Gantrisin), 100 mg/kg/d orally in 4 divided doses for 1 week, followed by 60 mg/kg/d for an additional 2 weeks. It is sometimes necessary to repeat this treatment after 1 week without medication. Alternatively, a 3- to 4-week course of oral erythromycin may be given. The local treatment of choice is 1% tetracycline ointment applied twice a day, 6 days a week for 10 weeks. Since recurrences are common, follow-up evaluation is important.

Viral Conjunctivitis

Viral conjunctivitis is frequently due to infection with adenovirus type 3, 4, or 7 and may be associated with pharyngitis and preauricular adenopathy. The conjunctiva is quite hyperemic and shows follicular reaction. There is a thin watery discharge. The condition usually lasts 12–14 days. No treatment is of value. Sulfonamide preparations or broad-spectrum antibiotics are instilled locally to prevent secondary infection.

Epidemic keratoconjunctivitis is highly contagious, is usually due to infection with adenovirus type 8 or 19, and is often spread by the fingers of physicians during their examination of the eye or through contaminated instruments or eye drops. Conjunctivitis is followed in 5–14 days by photophobia and epithelial keratitis. Corneal subepithelial opacities may persist for months but will eventually fade without sequelae. While corticosteroids may relieve acute symptoms, their use should be avoided because of their many potential complications.

Leptothrix Conjunctivitis

Leptothrix conjunctivitis is characterized by small gray necrotic lesions on the palpebral conjunctiva. There is usually a history of contact with a cat. The course is protracted. Improvement may follow local excision of the necrotic areas.

Actinomyces Infections

Actinomyces species may produce conjunctivitis. The conjunctivitis is usually on the nasal side of the conjunctiva and is frequently associated with inflammation of the lacrimal canaliculi. The organisms are susceptible to penicillin and broad-spectrum antibiotics. If an infection exists in the canaliculi, this must be cleared before cure can result.

Allergic Conjunctivitis

Allergic conjunctivitis produces symptoms of itching, lacrimation, mild redness, and a stringy mucoid discharge. Eosinophils may be seen on scrapings from the conjunctiva. For acute cases of conjunctivitis, use of topical weak ophthalmic corticosteroid drops (eg, 0.125% prednisolone) instilled 5–6 times a day or use of 1.5% hydrocortisone ophthalmic ointment or its equivalent instilled 3–4 times a day is quite effective. For chronic forms of allergic conjunctivitis, an attempt should be made to isolate the offending allergen and to eliminate contact with it. Desensitization to the allergen can be carried out if elimination of contact is not possible. Temporary symptomatic relief may be obtained with the use of topical ophthalmic solutions containing vasoconstricting agents and antihistamines.

Phlyctenular Keratoconjunctivitis

Phlyctenular keratoconjunctivitis appears as elevated clear nodules, situated near the limbus, with surrounding hyperemia. The disease has been associated with a hypersensitivity reaction to tuberculin; phlyctenules may also develop as a hypersensitivity reaction to other bacterial products or other antigens.

Treatment consists of the local application of corticosteroids. Systemic tuberculosis should be ruled out.

Vernal Conjunctivitis

This form of conjunctivitis is seen in patients ages 5–20. It tends to be seasonal and becomes less severe with age. Symptoms consist of lacrimation, itching, stringy discharge, and giant "cobblestone" papillary hypertrophy in the tarsal conjunctiva or grayish elevated areas at the limbus. Many eosinophils are seen in the scraping of the lesions.

Treatment consists of the local application of corticosteroid ointment several times a day. Topical solutions of 4% cromolyn sodium (Opticrom) applied several times a day often provide relief from symptoms. Severe cases may require more extensive therapy, but this should be conducted by an ophthalmologist.

Ophthalmia Neonatorum

Ophthalmia neonatorum is inflammation of the conjunctiva of the newborn. It may be due to bacterial infection (gonococcal, staphylococcal, pneumococcal, or chlamydial [inclusion blennorrhea]) or to chemical irritation (silver nitrate). Bacterial conjunctivitis appears 2–5 days after birth; chlamydial conjunctivitis appears 5–10 days after birth. Conjunctivitis associated with silver nitrate usually is evident within the first 24–48 hours after birth. A definite diagnosis is established by smears and cultures of the material taken from the conjunctiva. Conjunctivitis due to silver nitrate is sterile, although secondary bacterial infections may occur.

In most states in the USA, chemical (1% silver nitrate) or antibiotic prophylaxis of the newborn eye is required. These laws are highly variable in the different states. Various antibiotics such as penicillin, tetracyclines, or bacitracin are currently used for prophylaxis of gonococcal ophthalmia.

It is most important to treat gonococcal conjunctivitis vigorously, since in untreated or inadequately treated cases corneal ulceration and perforation can occur. The treatment of gonococcal conjunctivitis consists of instilling penicillin, erythromycin, or tetracycline drops into the eye every 1–2 hours and giving penicillin G, 50,000 units/kg intravenously daily. If one eye is uninvolved, it should be covered with a shield to prevent contamination from the involved eye. The purulent discharge should be irrigated from the conjunctiva with normal saline and allowed to drain toward the outer edge of the eyelids away from the other eye. Cold compresses may be of value in relieving the marked swelling of the eyelids.

Other types of bacterial conjunctivitis of the newborn should be treated by the instillation of appropriate antibiotic ointments 4 times a day. Chlamydial conjunctivitis is treated by the local instillation of 0.5% erythromycin or 1% tetracycline ointment 4 times a day for 3 weeks or by use of oral erythromycin for 14 days.

In all cases of conjunctivitis, treatment should be continued for a few days after the symptoms have subsided; this will prevent early recurrences.

Brook I, Martin WJ, Finegold SM: Effect of silver nitrate application on the conjunctival flora of the newborn and the occurrence of clostridial conjunctivitis. *J Pediatr Ophthalmol Strabismus* 1978;**15:**179.

Chandler JW: Ophthalmia neonatorum: An update. *Trans Pac Coast Otoophthalmol Soc Annu Meet* 1982;**63:**161.

Darrell RW: *Viral Diseases of the Eye*. Lea & Febiger, 1985.

Foster CS, Duncan J: Randomized clinical trial of topically administered cromolyn sodium for vernal keratoconjunctivitis. *Am J Ophthalmol* 1980;**90:**175.

Stenson S, Newman R, Fedukowicz H: Conjunctivitis in the newborn: Observations on incidence, cause and prophylaxis. *Ann Ophthalmol* 1981;**13:**329.

Wilson LA (editor): *External Diseases of the Eye*. Harper & Row, 1979.

MUCOCUTANEOUS DISEASES

Conjunctival lesions may be associated with mucocutaneous diseases, including erythema multiforme, Stevens-Johnson syndrome, Reiter's syndrome, and Behçet's syndrome. The conjunctival involvement consists of erythema, vesicular lesions that frequently rupture, membrane formation, and the development of symblepharon (adhesion) between the raw edges of the bulbar and palpebral conjunctivae. Goblet cells in the conjunctiva are destroyed in the cicatricial process. This decreases the mucus secretion that is essential for the spread of tears over the cornea. Keratitis sicca (corneal drying) may result.

Treatment of the conjunctival lesions associated with these conditions is symptomatic, ie, soothing eye drops and compresses. Topical corticosteroids are helpful in the acute stages in diminishing the intensity and complications of the acute inflammatory phase. Antibiotics are of no benefit except for prevention of secondary infection. Erythema multiforme and Stevens-Johnson disease may be precipitated by sulfonamide and antibiotic therapy. Topical antibiotic therapy may be used when secondary bacterial infection occurs; care must be taken to choose an antibiotic to which the patient is not sensitive. The use of topical lubricants and the application of soft contact lenses may prevent corneal drying and ulceration.

Arstikaitis MJ: Ocular aftermath of Stevens-Johnson syndrome. *Arch Ophthalmol* 1973;**90:**376.

Grayson M: *Diseases of the Cornea,* 2nd ed. Mosby, 1983.

Sampson WG et al: Symposium on soft contact lenses. *Trans Am Acad Ophthalmol Otolaryngol* 1974;**78:**383.

Wilson LA (editor): *External Diseases of the Eye*. Harper & Row, 1979.

DISEASES OF THE CORNEA

CORNEAL ULCERS

Corneal ulcers are serious ocular disorders. They may follow corneal injury or conjunctivitis or may be associated with systemic infections. Corneal ulcers are usually diagnosed by simple inspection. There is loss of anterior substance of the cornea, with surrounding opaque gray or white necrosis. Corneal ulcers may be peripheral or central. Several ulcers may be present in the same eye. The area of ulceration stains with fluorescein. A serious effort should be made to determine the etiology of any corneal ulcer. Cultures and scrapings should be taken, and sensitivity tests should be performed if bacterial organisms are found.

Bacterial Corneal Ulcers

Central bacterial corneal ulcers are due to infections with pneumococci, hemolytic streptococci, *P aeruginosa,* and, less commonly, gram-positive and gram-negative rods. Marginal corneal ulcers may develop as a result of bacterial sensitivity, most commonly to staphylococcal infections.

Treatment should be started immediately, before sensitivity tests are completed. Subsequently, the antibiotic can be changed if necessary. For mild superficial bacterial ulcers, the topical use of antibiotic drops or ointment at frequent intervals is usually satisfactory. Until the susceptibility of the organism is known, treatment can be started with an ophthalmic antibiotic preparation that includes neomycin, bacitracin, and polymyxin B or with a broad-spectrum antibiotic. Cycloplegic drops should be used to relieve the iridocyclitis that accompanies bacterial ulcers. In more severe corneal ulcers that involve the deeper portions of the stroma, more intensive antibiotic therapy should be given. Antibiotics should also be given subconjunctivally and systemically. Corticosteroids should not be given topically in these cases, since they interfere with the healing process and might exaggerate an infection that was not susceptible to the treatment being used.

Marginal corneal ulcers respond to topical corticosteroids. If a staphylococcal infection of the conjunctiva or eyelid is present, it should be treated with appropriate antibiotics.

Viral Corneal Ulcers

A. Herpes Simplex Ulcer (Dendritic): Herpes simplex keratitis is becoming a more common corneal disease in children. Lesions in the cornea may or may not be associated with herpes labialis. Corneal involvement is frequently precipitated by the topical application of corticosteroids and less commonly with the systemic use of corticosteroids. In the initial infection, the lesion has the appearance of a dendrite (Fig 11–4) that may be easily identified after the instillation of fluorescein. There are one or more branching vesicular lesions involving the anterior part of the cornea. These vesicles rupture. Subsequently, deeper involvement of the cornea may occur. Iritis may also develop as a complication.

Treatment of acute herpes infections of the cornea consists of topical application of antiviral medication: idoxuridine (IDU), vidarabine, or trifluridine. Idoxuridine is applied in 0.5% ointment (Stoxil) 4 times a day or in 0.1% solution (Herplex, Stoxil) hourly during the day and every 2 hours at night. Vidarabine in 3% ointment (Vira-A) is applied 5 times a day. Trifluridine is applied in 1% solution (Viroptic) every 2 hours up to 9 times a day. Acyclovir in 3% ointment is currently under investigation for the treatment of herpes keratitis. No commercial preparation for ophthalmic use is available in the USA. Because of the difficulty in effectively administering drops to young children, an ointment is often a better means to ensure compliance with therapy. The eye is usually more comfortable if the pupil is kept dilated with 1% atropine or 5% homatropine.

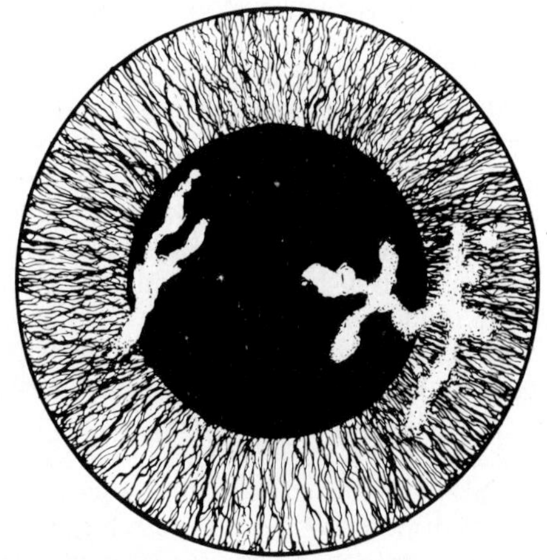

Figure 11–4. Dendritic type of lesion seen in herpes simplex keratitis. (Reproduced, with permission, from Vaughan D, Asbury T: *General Ophthalmology,* 8th ed. Lange, 1977.)

Mechanical denuding of the infected corneal epithelium is also an effective method of treating fresh cases of superficial herpes simplex keratitis. This may be done alone or in conjunction with topical antiviral therapy. A cotton-tipped applicator is used to gently remove infected epithelium without disrupting the basement membrane, which must remain intact for reepithelialization. This should be performed by an ophthalmologist.

Deeper involvement of the cornea may represent a hypersensitivity reaction, and the use of topical corticosteroids in conjunction with an antiviral medication sometimes improves the condition. However, this type of therapy should be undertaken only by an ophthalmologist, since the use of corticosteroids in an active herpes infection can lead to rapid deterioration of the cornea.

B. Herpes Zoster Infection: Herpes zoster keratitis is associated with zoster infection of the first branch of the trigeminal nerve. Corneal involvement may be superficial or deep and accompanied by uveitis. Topical and systemic acyclovir are often effective. Topical corticosteroids are used for the management of deep corneal involvement with uveitis. Relief is obtained with the use of topical corticosteroids. Cycloplegic drops should be used for relieving the iridocyclitis that accompanies herpes zoster infection. The physician must be certain of the diagnosis of herpes zoster before employing topical corticosteroids, since other viral diseases of the cornea are aggravated by these agents.

Fungal Corneal Ulcers

Mycotic corneal infections are difficult to diagnose. There is usually a history of recent trauma or foreign body. Frequently, the ulcerated cornea shows surrounding satellite lesions; hypopyon (pus in the anterior chamber) may be present. Fungal corneal ulcers are rare, but their incidence seems to be increasing, possibly from the widespread use of topical corticosteroid and broad-spectrum antibiotic medications. Whenever a diagnosis of mycotic corneal ulceration is suspected, cultures and sensitivity tests should be obtained.

The only commercially available topical medication for fungal keratitis is natamycin (Natacyn). It is applied in 5% suspension every 1–4 hours, depending on the severity of the disease. It is effective against a broad spectrum of fungi, including filamentous forms of fungi and *Candida albicans*. Amphotericin B, although not commercially available as an ophthalmic preparation, may be prepared in concentrations that are effective topically (0.5–1.5 mg/mL). For deeper infections, amphotericin B may be used subconjunctivally but is extremely irritating; rarely, intravenous administration is utilized in severe cases. Topical application of 1% miconazole (Monistat), prepared from the intravenous product, is frequently effective. Flucytosine (Ancobon) may be given orally in doses of 50–150 mg/kg/d for deep ocular infections; it is most effective against *Candida*.

Baum J, Barza M: Topical vs subconjunctival treatment of bacterial corneal ulcers. *Ophthalmology* 1983;**90:**162.

Jones BR: Principles in the management of oculomycosis. *Am J Ophthalmol* 1975;**79:**719.

Jones DB: Initial therapy of suspected microbial corneal ulcers. 2. Specific antibiotic therapy based on corneal smears. *Surv Ophthalmol* 1979;**24:**97.

Kaufman HE: Update on antiviral agents. *Ophthalmology* 1985;**92:**533.

Leibowitz HM: *Corneal Disorders: Clinical Diagnosis and Management*. Saunders, 1984.

Liesegang TJ: Corneal complications from herpes zoster ophthalmicus. *Ophthalmology* 1985;**92:**316.

Pavan-Langston D et al: Acyclovir and vidarabine in the treatment of ulcerative herpes simplex keratitis. *Am J Ophthalmol* 1981;**92:**829.

Poirier RH: Herpetic ocular infections of childhood. *Arch Ophthalmol* 1980;**98:**704.

ALLERGIC REACTIONS

Allergic reactions in the cornea may involve either the superficial epithelial or deeper stromal layers. Most forms of deep keratitis probably represent hypersensitivity reactions. The allergen may be airborne, or it may enter the cornea by way of the circulation in the limbus. Treatment consists of determining the offending agent, if possible, and then eliminating its contact with the patient. Cold compresses and the use of mild, commercially available vasoconstrictor drops that contain either naphazoline 0.05%, phenylephrine 0.125%, or tetrahydrozoline 0.05% provide relief in mild cases. Topical corticosteroids are required in more severe cases. They should be used only under the supervision of an ophthalmologist. Topical corticosteroids usually give considerable relief.

Interstitial Keratitis

Interstitial keratitis is an acute immune reaction in the cornea, usually associated with congenital syphilis. Symptoms consist of intense photophobia, tearing, pain, and decreased vision. On examination, the cornea has a diffuse opaque appearance. Fine vessels may be noted in the stroma. There may be aggregates of these vessels, which appear as orange-red areas (salmon patches). Other evidence of congenital syphilis may also be present. Serologic tests are often negative.

Interstitial keratitis may be associated with other diseases such as tuberculosis and the autoimmune disorders, and any such contributing condition should be ruled out.

Treatment consists of the use of topical corticosteroids and cycloplegics for relief of symptoms. If active syphilis is present, it should be appropriately treated.

Grayson M: *Diseases of the Cornea,* 2nd ed. Mosby, 1983.

Smolin G, O'Connor GR: *Ocular Immunology.* Lea & Febiger, 1981.

Theodore FH, Bloomfield SE, Mondino BJ: *Clinical Allergy and Immunology of the Eye.* Williams & Wilkins, 1983.

Thygeson P: The immunology and immunopathology of corneal infection. *Trans Pac Coast Otoophthalmol Soc Annu Meet* 1976;**57:**357.

Waring GO et al: Alterations in Descemet's membrane in interstitial keratitis. *Am J Ophthalmol* 1976;**81:**773.

Wilson LA (editor): *External Diseases of the Eye.* Harper & Row, 1979.

CORNEAL DRYING & EXPOSURE

Keratoconjunctivitis Sicca

This condition is rare in children and results from a lacrimal gland insufficiency. The treatment of choice is tear replacement with artificial tear solutions as necessary to keep the cornea moist. Bland ophthalmic ointments (Duolube, Duratears, Lacri-Lube) may also be used, particularly at bedtime.

Xerophthalmia

Severe vitamin A deficiency reduces conjunctival secretion of mucus, and this leads to conjunctival and corneal drying and keratinization. The cornea may become soft and necrotic (keratomalacia), and corneal perforation may occur. The conjunctival changes are characterized by a foamy, triangular lesion that is usually on the temporal side and has its base at the limbus (Bitot's spot). The conjunctival and corneal changes together are known as xerophthalmia.

Patients are treated with systemic vitamin A. Topical antibiotic drops may be indicated to prevent secondary infection.

Exposure Keratitis

Exposure keratitis may develop after facial nerve palsies or after a period of unconsciousness during which the eyes are exposed. Treatment is similar to that described above.

Neuroparalytic Keratitis

Neuroparalytic keratitis is seen after damage to the ophthalmic division of the trigeminal nerve. It is treated by tear replacement (see Keratoconjunctivitis Sicca, above).

Familial Dysautonomia (Riley-Day Syndrome)

In this condition, there is a deficiency of tears,

and corneal drying can occur. Tear replacement (see Keratoconjunctivitis Sicca, above) is indicated.

Gasset AR, Kaufman HE: Hydrophilic lens therapy of severe keratoconjunctivitis sicca and conjunctival scarring. *Am J Ophthalmol* 1971;**71:**1185.

Katz JI et al: Slow-release artificial tears and the treatment of keratitis sicca. *Ophthalmology* 1978;**85:**787.

Lemp MA: Artificial tear solutions. *Int Ophthalmol Clin* (Spring) 1973;**13:**221.

Levine MR: Medical and surgical treatment of the dry eye. *Int Ophthalmol Clin* (Fall) 1978;**18:**101.

Sommer A, Sugana T: Corneal xerophthalmia and keratomalacia. *Arch Ophthalmol* 1982;**100:**404.

Wilson LA (editor): *External Diseases of the Eye.* Harper & Row, 1979.

CORNEAL INVOLVEMENT IN OTHER SYSTEMIC DISEASES

The cornea is involved in many systemic diseases. Small calcium deposits may be observed in the corneas of patients with hyperparathyroidism. Cystine crystals are observed in patients with renal rickets (cystinosis). Excessive intake of vitamin D may lead to calcification of the anterior part of the cornea in a band opacity of the exposed portion of the cornea. Deficiency of vitamin A may lead to drying (xerosis) and softening (keratomalacia) of the cornea. Corneal ulceration may occur in patients with severe debilitating diseases such as dysentery. Corneal opacities may occur in children with Hurler's disease (gargoylism) and other mucopolysaccharide disorders.

In all of these conditions, it is important to recognize the underlying disease and treat appropriately.

Grayson M: *Diseases of the Cornea,* 2nd ed. Mosby, 1983.

Poirier RH, Hyndiuk RA: Diagnosis and therapy of corneal disease. In: *Gordon's Management of Ocular Disease,* 2nd ed. Dunlap EA (editor). Harper & Row, 1976.

Sugar J: Corneal manifestations of systemic mucopolysaccharidoses. *Ann Ophthalmol* 1979;**11:**531.

Wilson LA (editor): *External Diseases of the Eye.* Harper & Row, 1979.

Zimmerman TJ, Hood I, Gasset AR: Adolescent cystinosis. *Arch Ophthalmol* 1974;**92:**265.

UVEITIS

Inflammation of the uveal tract may present anteriorly as iritis or cyclitis (inflammation of the ciliary body) or as posterior inflammations (choroiditis). Uveitis may be associated with other ocular diseases, such as corneal ulceration, keratitis, hypermature cataracts, necrotic intraocular tumors, or optic neuritis.

Uveitis may be classified as exogenous or endogenous. Exogenous uveitis follows the accidental introduction of pathogenic organisms or a foreign substance into the eye. Endogenous uveitis is a result of various systemic processes.

Uveitis may also be classified as suppurative or nonsuppurative according to the type of tissue reaction. Nonsuppurative uveitis, which is the more common form, may further be divided into granulomatous and nongranulomatous types. Nongranulomatous uveitis usually involves the iris and ciliary body and produces symptoms of photophobia, pain, redness, and blurred vision. The pupil is small and often irregular. There is circumcorneal injection. On examination with a slit lamp, cells in the anterior chamber and fine precipitates on the posterior surface of the cornea may be observed. Granulomatous uveitis may involve the iris, ciliary body, or choroid. Pain, redness, and photophobia are not so prominent as in the nongranulomatous form. Vision may be markedly disturbed, particularly if the involvement is in the macular area. On ophthalmoscopy, the vitreous may be quite hazy. Active lesions of choroiditis may be seen as swollen, white, indistinct irregular patches. As the choroiditis subsides, pigmentary changes may take place.

Uveitis presents a complex problem. The endogenous nonsuppurative form may be associated with systemic disease. In children, the most common associated disease is juvenile rheumatoid arthritis. Other common associated diseases are toxoplasmosis; histoplasmosis; tuberculosis; sarcoidosis, polyarteritis, rheumatoid arthritis, and other collagen diseases; bacterial infections of the sinuses or teeth; food and pollen allergies; and viral diseases such as mumps, measles, chickenpox, influenza, herpes simplex, and herpes zoster. The relationship between systemic disease and uveitis may be incidental. There is pathologic evidence that the choroid and retina may be invaded with *Toxoplasma* and *Mycobacterium tuberculosis.* However, aside from these specific instances, causative organisms have not been found to enter the uveal tissue. There is accumulating evidence that most cases of uveitis are due to an immune reaction.

Treatment

If systemic disease is present, it should be appropriately treated. However, successful treatment of systemic disease does not always result in a cure of the uveitis. Nonspecific treatment of uveitis consists of the use of cycloplegics to dilate the pupil and to relieve the ciliary and iris spasm. Atropine, 1–2% solution, or scopolamine, 0.25% solution, should be used 2–3 times daily. In addition, the topical use of 10% phenylephrine hydrochloride is indicated to widely dilate the pupil. Corticosteroids should be used unless they are contraindicated by the presence of a specific bacterial or viral infection. For inflammations of the anterior uveal tract, topical and subconjunctival corticosteroids are useful in reducing the inflammation. For posterior uveitis, systemic corticosteroids should be used.

The management of uveitis is difficult. Many complications can occur, including glaucoma, cataract, and retinal detachment. Therefore, these cases should be managed by an ophthalmologist.

Char DH: *Immunology of Uveitis and Ocular Tumors.* Grune & Stratton, 1978.

Friedman AH, Luntz M, Henley WL: *Diagnosis and Management of Uveitis: An Atlas Approach.* Williams & Wilkins, 1982.

Giles CL, Schlaegel TF Jr: Childhood uveitis. *Int Ophthalmol Clin* (Fall) 1977;**17:**75.

Schlaegel TF: Etiologic diagnosis of uveitis. In: *Clinical Ophthalmology.* Vol 4. Duane TD (editor). Harper & Row, 1981.

Schlaegel TF Jr: *Ocular Toxoplasmosis and Pars Planitis.* Grune & Stratton, 1978.

Smith RE, Nozik RM: *Uveitis: A Clinical Approach to Diagnosis and Management.* Williams & Wilkins, 1983.

SYMPATHETIC OPHTHALMIA

Sympathetic ophthalmia is a special form of bilateral granulomatous uveitis. It follows a penetrating ocular injury of the uveal tract. It may occur at any time from 10 days after injury to many years later, but it usually presents within the first 2–4 months after initial injury. The etiology of sympathetic ophthalmia is not understood, but it probably represents a hypersensitivity response to uveal pigment. The diagnosis is based on a history of an injury to one (exciting) eye with the subsequent development of uveitis in the other (sympathizing) eye.

Treatment consists of the use of systemic and topical corticosteroids and topical cycloplegics. Immunosuppressive agents also are employed in resistant cases. Long-term therapy is usually necessary, and maintenance doses of corticosteroids are usually indicated to prevent a flare-up of this condition. The disease can be averted by early enucleation of the eye that has received a severe injury to the ciliary body and has become visually useless.

Jakobiec FA et al: Human sympathetic ophthalmia: An analysis of inflammatory infiltrate by hybridoma-monoclonal antibodies, immunochemistry, and correlative electron microscopy. *Ophthalmology* 1983;**90:**76.

Lubin JR, Albert DM, Weinstein M: Sixty-five years of sympathetic ophthalmia: A clinicopathologic review of 105 cases (1913–1978). *Ophthalmology* 1980;**87:**109.

Makley TA, Azar A: Sympathetic ophthalmia: A long-term follow-up. *Arch Ophthalmol* 1978;**96:**257.

DISEASES OF THE RETINA

HEREDITARY RETINAL DISORDERS

Hereditary retinal disorders may be evident shortly after birth or not until the second decade of life. Many of these disorders involve primarily one layer of the retina (eg, the pigment epithelium, the rod and cone layer, or the ganglion cell layer), but other layers of the retina are usually secondarily involved.

Retinitis pigmentosa is a bilateral hereditary disease involving chiefly the retinal rods or the retinal pigment epithelium. Symptoms of night blindness usually begin early in the second decade. Restriction of visual fields subsequently occurs; this generally progresses, so that by middle age the visual fields are markedly contracted and the visual acuity severely depressed. However, certain forms of the disease are less severe, especially in the early stages. Ophthalmoscopic examination may reveal only some incipient pigmentary abnormalities in the midperiphery of the ocular fundus. The diagnosis may be confirmed by electroretinography, which shows markedly reduced or unrecordable activity. As the disease progresses, additional changes occur: narrowing of the retinal arteries and veins, waxy appearance of the optic disk, and "bone corpuscle" pigment deposits. Retinitis pigmentosa may be associated with many systemic diseases: renal abnormalities, deafness, convulsions and obesity, hypogenitalism, polydactyly, mental retardation (Laurence-Moon-Biedl syndrome), and abetalipoproteinemia. There is no satisfactory treatment for retinitis pigmentosa. The mode of inheritance varies. Genetic counseling is advisable for prospective parents with this disorder.

Fundus flavimaculatus consists of multiple round and fishtail-like yellow-white lesions of the posterior and midperipheral fundus. The onset is in the first or second decade of life. Some patients with this disorder develop atrophic changes in the macula with severe visual loss (Stargardt's disease); others may retain good macular function and visual acuity.

Coats's disease is an exudative retinopathy characterized by hemorrhagic and exudative lesions and by telangiectatic vessels. The onset is usually within the first few years of life; males are affected more often than females. Usually only one eye is involved; vision is often severely impaired. The disorder may cause a white pupillary reflex (leukocoria) and must be differentiated from other causes of leukocoria, such as cataracts, persistent hyperplastic primary vitreous, and retinoblastoma.

Vitelliruptive degeneration (Best's disease) is a disorder of the retinal pigment epithelium that occurs in the macular region at or shortly after birth. Ophthalmoscopically, the macula has a yellow deposit resembling a "sunny side up" fried egg. During the first or second decade of life, the lesion changes; the sunny side up egg yolk becomes scrambled, and scarring and pigmentary changes may lead to loss of central vision.

Leber's congenital amaurosis is characterized by congenital blindness or reduced vision. Initially, the ocular fundus appears normal or there may be some mild pigmentary changes. With time, the disk becomes atrophic, and pigmentary changes become more obvious. Electroretinographic testing shows changes similar to those seen in retinitis pigmentosa.

Color vision abnormalities are common, with approximately 7% of males and 0.5% of females affected. Many of the tests used clinically are not sensitive enough to detect small changes. Color vision is a retinal cone function; each cone has 3 distinct photosensitive pigments, with spectral sensitive patterns maximal at red, green, or blue. Hereditary color vision defects result from a deficiency or absence of one or more of the 3 cone photosensitive pigments. Patients with defects of color vision are classified as follows:

(1) Anomalous trichromats: In these individuals, all cone pigments are present, but there is a deficiency of one of them. Protanomalous trichromats have decreased sensitivity to the red-sensitive pigment. Deuteranomalous trichromats have decreased sensitivity to the green-sensitive pigment and tritanomalous trichromats to the blue-sensitive pigment. Anomalous trichromats constitute the largest group of patients with color vision defects.

(2) Dichromats: These persons have 2 of the 3 cone pigments. They may be subdivided into 3 groups: Protanopes lack the red-sensitive pigment and are red blind; deuteranopes lack the green-sensitive pigment and are green blind; tritanopes lack the blue-sensitive pigment and are blue blind.

(3) Monochromats: These individuals have only one cone-sensitive pigment and are truly color blind. They have decreased vision, photophobia, irregular pigmentation in the retina, and nystagmus. This is an extremely rare condition, occurring in only about 1:1,000,000 of the male population.

Breton ME, Nelson LB: What do color blind children really see? Guidelines for clinical prescreening based on recent findings. *Surv Ophthalmol* 1983;**27:**306.

Fishman GA: Retinitis pigmentosa: Visual loss. *Arch Ophthalmol* 1978;**96:**1185.

Mollon JD: Color vision. *Annu Rev Psychol* 1982;**33:**41.

Tasman W, Shields JA: *Disorders of the Peripheral Fundus.* Harper & Row, 1980.

RETINOPATHY OF PREMATURITY (Retrolental Fibroplasia)

Retinopathy of prematurity is a primary bilateral retinal vascular disorder of premature infants. The disease occurs almost exclusively in those with a birth weight under 1500 g who have received excessive amounts of oxygen therapy during the first 10–14 days of life. Infants at highest risk are those born under 32 weeks' gestation and with a birth weight under 1000 g. For several years, after the role of oxygen in the development of retinopathy of prematurity was established, the disease became almost extinct. Recently, therapy employing high concentrations of oxygen to treat respiratory distress syndrome in premature infants has again been used and, possibly as a result, retrolental fibroplasia is being seen with increasing frequency.

In general, peripheral vascularization of the retina is not complete until about 2 weeks after full-term birth. However, this is variable; some eyes have complete vascularization at 8 months' gestational age. Until retinal vascularization is complete, the peripheral immature vessels, which are immediately posterior to the demarcation site of vascular to avascular retina, are extremely sensitive to hyperoxia and respond by vasoconstriction and obliteration. When oxygen concentrations are subsequently reduced, the retinal vessels in the posterior pole often dilate as a result of peripheral vascular shunts formed near the site of vaso-obliteration. These shunts may take the form of neofibrovascular membranes on the surface of the retina or may extend into the vitreous cavity. Tractional retinal detachments may occur. In advanced stages, the retrolental space is filled with fibrovascular and retinal tissues, the anterior chambers are shallow, and the eyes are small and blind. In incomplete forms, myopia and strabismus are often observed; retinal detachment may occur as a late complication in the teenage years. Up to 85% of acute cases of retrolental fibroplasia regress as vascularization to the peripheral aspect of the retina is completed in a nearly normal manner.

It is essential that pediatricians be aware of the relationship of oxygen therapy to the development of retinopathy of prematurity—not only the concentration of oxygen but also the duration of oxygen treatment and the degree of prematurity. The generally accepted safe concentration of oxygen is less than 40%, but this is subject to the other variables noted above. Many experts believe an arterial blood oxygen level over 70 mm Hg is inadvisable.

All premature infants receiving high concentrations of oxygen therapy should be followed as closely as possible to make certain that arterial blood oxygen levels do not remain excessively high for any period of time. Changes in the immature retinal vessels appear to be related not only to high arterial blood oxygen levels but also to the duration of hyperoxia. The value of the early administration of vitamin E (an antioxidant) in diminishing the severity of retinopathy of prematurity or in preventing its occurrence is under investigation.

All premature infants should have a careful ophthalmoscopic examination by the sixth week of life, at which time severe forms of retinopathy are more common. If signs of the disease are present, a follow-up ophthalmoscopic examination is needed after discharge, and the parents should be counseled. Refraction should be an essential part of this follow-up examination, since amblyopia (associated with strabismus and refractive errors) is common and treatable. Surgical treatment of retinal detachment is sometimes indicated. Cryotherapy of the retina in rapidly advancing cases has been advocated.

Biglan AW et al: Blood oxygen, carbon dioxide and pH levels prior to diagnosis of retinopathy of prematurity. *J Pediatr Ophthalmol Strabismus* 1985;**22:**44.

Flynn JT et al: Retrolental fibroplasia: Clinical observations. *Arch Ophthalmol* 1977;**95:**217.

Kalina RE, Karr DJ: Retrolental fibroplasia: Experience over two decades in one institution. *Ophthalmology* 1982;**89:**91.

Kingham JD: Acute retrolental fibroplasia. *Arch Ophthalmol* 1977;**95:**39.

Kushner BJ et al: Retrolental fibroplasia: Pathologic correlation. *Arch Ophthalmol* 1977;**95:**29.

Mousel DK: Retinopathy of prematurity in the intensive care nursery. *J Pediatr Ophthalmol Strabismus* 1978;**15:**147.

Patz A: Current therapy of retrolental fibroplasia: Retinopathy of prematurity. *Ophthalmology* 1983;**90:**425.

Pulkin JE, Simon RM, Ehrenkranz RA: Influence on retrolental fibroplasia of intramuscular vitamin E administration during respiratory distress syndrome. *Ophthalmology* 1982;**89:**96.

Shahinian L, Malachowski N: Retrolental fibroplasia: A new analysis of risk factors based on recent cases. *Arch Ophthalmol* 1978;**96:**70.

Silverman WA: *Retrolental Fibroplasia.* Grune & Stratton, 1980.

RETINAL DETACHMENT

Detachment of the retina in children is usually associated with severe ocular trauma or with high myopia. In the latter condition, there are degenerative changes in the periphery of the retina that lead to subsequent separation of the retina. The diagnosis is established by a history of progressively more severe blurred vision. The visual disturbance may start with the sensation of flashing lights, or the patient may observe a dark cloud coming in from one section of the visual field. On ophthalmoscopy, the area of detachment appears elevated and gray. The retinal vessels appear darker, and the retina is seen with increased convex dioptric power in the ophthalmoscope.

The only treatment is surgical repair.

Arentsen JJ, Welch RB: Retinal detachment in the young individual: A survey of 100 cases seen at the Wilmer Institute. *J Pediatr Ophthalmol* 1974;**11:**198.

Benson WE: *Retinal Detachment.* Harper & Row, 1980.

Tasman W (editor): *Retinal Diseases in Children.* Harper & Row, 1971.

RETINOBLASTOMA

Retinoblastoma is a comparatively rare malignant tumor of children. It usually appears before the third year of life, although rare cases have been reported with onset in adolescence. Retinoblastoma is a hereditary disease that is due to mutation of an autosomal dominant gene. A family history of retinoblastoma is found in less than 10% of cases. The vast majority are new, sporadic mutations. Approximately 25% of cases are bilateral. Patients who have survived bilateral retinoblastoma or who have a family history of retinoblastoma have about a 50% chance of transmitting the disease to their offspring. Genetic counseling is advisable for survivors of retinoblastoma as well as for parents of children with retinoblastoma.

The presenting symptom is usually a white spot in the pupil. Strabismus may be present. If the tumor becomes very large, glaucoma may occur, with a steamy cornea and red eye. Occasionally, retinoblastoma ruptures through the globe and results in a painful red eye. The diagnosis is usually made by ophthalmoscopic examination. To accomplish ophthalmoscopy, wide pupillary dilation is essential; general anesthesia is often necessary. The tumor appears as a solid yellow or white elevated mass. A small section of the eye may be involved, or the entire eye may be filled with tumor.

Treatment consists of enucleation of the involved eye in unilateral cases, although in selected cases small tumors are sometimes treated with x-ray or cryotherapy. If there is involvement of both eyes, the more severely involved eye should be enucleated and the other eye treated with x-ray therapy together with chemotherapy. Cryotherapy is sometimes employed for treatment of small peripheral lesions.

For parents who have an affected child but no previous family history of retinoblastoma, the risk of retinoblastoma in a second child is 1%. Patients who have had retinoblastoma have an increased risk of developing a second primary neoplasm later in life.

Abramson DH et al: The management of unilateral retinoblastoma without primary enucleation. *Arch Ophthalmol* 1982;**100:**1249.

Abramson DH et al: Treatment of bilateral groups I through III retinoblastoma with bilateral radiation. *Arch Ophthalmol* 1981;**99:**1761.

Ellsworth RM: Retinoblastoma. Chapter 35 in: *Clinical Ophthalmology*. Vol 3. Duane TD (editor). Harper & Row, 1982.

Francois J, DiBie S, Matton-Van Leuren MT: The Costenbader Memorial Lecture: Genesis and genetics of retinoblastoma. *J Pediatr Ophthalmol Strabismus* 1979;**16:**85.

Kobrin JL, Blodi FC: Prognosis in retinoblastoma: Influence of histopathologic characteristics. *J Pediatr Ophthalmol Strabismus* 1978;**15:**278.

Peyman GA, Apple DJ, Sanders DR: *Intraocular Tumors.* Appleton-Century-Crofts, 1977.

Reese AB: *Tumors of the Eye,* 3rd ed. Harper & Row, 1976.

OPTIC NEURITIS

Optic neuritis may involve only the head of the nerve (papillitis) or the orbital portion of the nerve (retrobulbar neuritis). Optic neuritis may occur in association with generalized infectious diseases, demyelinating diseases, blood dyscrasias, or metabolic diseases or may be due to exposure to toxins or drugs or extension of inflammatory disease such as sinusitis or meningitis. Clinically, there is an acute loss of vision. Involvement may be of one or both eyes; in children, the disease is frequently bilateral. Central visual defects are present. There may be some discomfort in the eyes on movement of the globes. On ophthalmoscopic examination, papilledema may be present or the disks may appear normal.

Optic neuritis in children often follows viremia and is usually a self-limited disease. The visual prognosis is generally favorable. If the cause can be determined, it should be treated. Systemic corticosteroid therapy has been advocated, but its effectiveness has not been established.

The presence of papilledema may be a sign of increased intracranial pressure. The differentiation between optic neuritis and papilledema secondary to increased intracranial pressure is not always easy. In general, papilledema due to increased intracranial pressure does not produce a severe loss of vision, and there often are associated neurologic signs.

Burde RM et al: Optic neuritis: Etiology? *Surv Ophthalmol* 1980;**24:**307.
Glaser JS (editor): *Neuro-Ophthalmology*. Harper & Row, 1978.
Miller NR: *Walsh and Hoyt's Clinical Neuro-Ophthalmology*, 4th ed. 2 vols. Williams & Wilkins, 1982.
Walsh TJ: *Neuro-Ophthalmology: Clinical Signs and Symptoms*. Lea & Febiger, 1978.

DISEASES OF THE ORBIT

ORBITAL CELLULITIS

Orbital cellulitis is a serious illness characterized by proptosis; swelling, redness, and congestion of the eyelids, orbital tissues, and bulbar conjunctiva; discomfort; and, frequently, fever. A distinct magenta discoloration of the skin of the eyelids is present in cases of *Haemophilus influenzae* infection. In children, orbital cellulitis is usually due to bacterial infection. There may be associated infections elsewhere in the body, particularly in the sinuses. Treatment consists of hot packs and the vigorous use of systemic (primarily intravenous) antibiotics; a favorable response is usually obtained within 48–72 hours.

Jones IS, Jakobiec FA (editors): *Diseases of the Orbit*. Harper & Row, 1979.
Macy JI, Mandelbaum SH, Minckler DS: Orbital cellulitis. *Ophthalmology* 1980;**87:**1309.
Watters EC et al: Acute orbital cellulitis. *Arch Ophthalmol* 1976;**94:**785.
Weiss A et al: Bacterial periorbital and orbital cellulitis in childhood. *Ophthalmology* 1983;**90:**195.

ENDOCRINE EXOPHTHALMOS

Endocrine exophthalmos is relatively uncommon in children. It may be unilateral or bilateral. In addition to exophthalmos, there may be retraction of the upper lids or swelling of the lids. Injection and swelling of the conjunctiva may be present, and there may also be some extraocular muscle weakness.

Treatment consists of management of the underlying thyroid disturbance. Severe ocular involvement in the form of exposure keratitis, glaucoma, or decreased visual acuity should be treated by an ophthalmologist.

Chumbley LC: *Ophthalmology in Internal Medicine*. Saunders, 1981.
Kramar P: Management of eye changes of Graves' disease. *Surv Ophthalmol* 1974;**18:**369.
Uretsky SH, Kennerdell JS, Gutai JP: Graves' ophthalmopathy in childhood and adolescence. *Arch Ophthalmol* 1980;**98:**1963.
Young LA: Dysthyroid ophthalmopathy in children. *J Pediatr Ophthalmol Strabismus* 1979;**16:**105.

ORBITAL TUMORS

Orbital tumors are rare in children. The most common primary tumors are hemangiomas, neurofibromas, gliomas of the optic nerve, dermoids, rhabdomyosarcomas, and tumors of the lacrimal gland. Neuroblastoma and lymphoma may spread into the orbit. The presenting symptoms are exophthalmos, congestion and ecchymosis of the globe and lids, extraocular muscle weakness, and displacement of the globe. Optic nerve gliomas may show enlargement of the optic foramen on x-ray examination.

Each case should be carefully evaluated. Treatment includes surgical removal, x-ray therapy, or the use of chemotherapy in certain cases. For certain benign tumors, it is often better not to attempt total removal of the lesion.

Howard GM: Tumors of the orbit in children. *Trans Pac Coast Otoophthalmol Soc Annu Meet* 1978;**59:**115.
Jones IS, Jakobiec FA (editors): *Diseases of the Orbit*. Harper & Row, 1979.
Rosenthal AR: Ocular manifestations of leukemia: A review. *Ophthalmology* 1983;**90:**899.
Rush JA et al: Optic glioma: Long-term follow-up of 85 histopathologically verified cases. *Ophthalmology* 1982;**89:**1213.
Sagerman RH, Tretter P, Ellsworth RM: Orbital rhabdomyosarcoma in children. *Trans Am Acad Ophthalmol Otolaryngol* 1974;**78:**602.
Shields JA: *Diagnosis and Management of Intraocular Tumors*. Mosby, 1983.

ORBITAL PSEUDOTUMOR

Pseudotumor of the orbit is uncommon in children. It is an inflammation of the orbital tissues, sometimes granulomatous in character but usually unrelated to any specific granulomatous disease. The histopathologic picture is highly variable but often shows lymphocytic aggregates, perivascular inflammation, and plasma cells. As a rule only one orbit is affected, but in about 25% of cases the other orbit is involved also. The symptoms may develop suddenly or slowly over a period of months. Swelling of the eyelid and conjunctiva often precedes the development of proptosis and diplopia. The diagnosis is usually made by exclusion of other causes of swelling and proptosis: neoplasms, endocrine exophthalmos, orbital cellulitis, etc. Spontaneous remission often occurs. However, dramatic improvement usually follows systemic corticosteroid therapy.

Heersink B, Rodrigues MR, Flanagan JC: Inflammatory pseudotumor of orbit. *Ann Ophthalmol* 1977;**9:**17.

Mottow LS, Jakobiec FA: Idiopathic inflammatory orbital pseudotumor in childhood. *Arch Ophthalmol* 1978;**96:**1410.

DISEASES OF THE LACRIMAL APPARATUS

DACRYOSTENOSIS

In a significant number of infants, the nasolacrimal duct fails to completely canalize at the time of birth; the obstruction is usually at the nasal end of the duct. Symptoms consist of persistent tearing and, often, mucoid discharge in the inner corner of the eye.

Most cases subside without treatment. The obstruction usually opens spontaneously, and relief of symptoms occurs. Massage over the lacrimal sac with expression toward the nose may be helpful in establishing the patency. If a cure does not result within the first few months of life, probing of the nasolacrimal duct should be performed by an ophthalmologist.

Kushner BJ: Congenital nasolacrimal system obstruction. *Arch Ophthalmol* 1982;**100:**597.

Paul TO: Medical management of congenital nasolacrimal duct obstruction. *J Pediatr Ophthalmol Strabismus* 1985;**22:**68.

Sevel D: Development and congenital abnormalities of the nasolacrimal apparatus. *J Pediatr Ophthalmol Strabismus* 1981;**18:**13.

Veirs ER: *Lacrimal Disorders: Diagnosis and Treatment.* Mosby, 1976.

Wilson LA (editor): *External Diseases of the Eye.* Harper & Row, 1979.

DACRYOCYSTITIS

Inflammation of the tear sac (dacryocystitis) is usually secondary to obstruction of the nasolacrimal duct. There is resultant stasis of the tears in the sac, with secondary bacterial infection. Symptoms consist of tearing and mucopurulent discharge. There may be acute inflammation in the region of the lacrimal sac. Occasionally, the sac may rupture to the skin surface.

If possible, cultures should be obtained and the organism identified. For mild cases, expression of the contents of the lacrimal sac followed by instillation of topical antibiotics in the region of the lacrimal puncta may be effective. More severe cases should also be treated with systemic antibiotics. Irrigation of the canaliculi and lacrimal sac with antibiotic solution is a more successful method of delivering adequate concentrations of antibiotics to the area of infection. Once the infection has subsided, an attempt should be made to establish the passage of tears. The nasolacrimal duct should be probed under general anesthesia if the system does not permit passage of fluid irrigated through the canaliculi.

Harris GJ, Di Clementi D: Congenital dacryocystocele. *Arch Ophthalmol* 1982;**100:**1763.

Veirs ER: *Lacrimal Disorders: Diagnosis and Treatment.* Mosby, 1976.

DACRYOADENITIS

Inflammation of the lacrimal gland may be associated with systemic disorders such as mumps or sarcoidosis. More rarely, infections of the lacrimal gland may be secondary to tuberculosis or syphilis.

Treatment should be directed toward the specific disease, if present; otherwise, symptomatic treatment should be used. Local applications of heat or cold over the lacrimal gland may give relief. Bed rest and salicylate analgesics are also useful. Systemic corticosteroids may reduce inflammation, but the use of corticosteroids in any viral infection is risky.

Darrell RW: *Viral Diseases of the Eye.* Lea & Febiger, 1985.

Jones IS, Jakobiec FA (editors): *Diseases of the Orbit.* Harper & Row, 1979.

Obenauf CD et al: Sarcoidosis and its ophthalmic manifestations. *Am J Ophthalmol* 1978;**86:**648.

SELECTED REFERENCES

Crawford JS, Morin JD (editors): *The Eye in Childhood.* Grune & Stratton, 1983.

Duane TD (editor): *Clinical Ophthalmology.* 5 vols. Harper & Row, 1984.

Ellis PP: *Ocular Therapeutics and Pharmacology,* 7th ed. Mosby, 1985.

Ernest JT (editor): *Year Book of Ophthalmology.* Year Book, 1983.

Feman SS, Reinecke RD (editors): *Handbook of Pediatric Ophthalmology*. Grune & Stratton, 1978.

Fraunfelder FT, Roy FH (editors): *Current Ocular Therapy 2*. Saunders, 1985.

Gittinger JW Jr: *Ophthalmology: A Clinical Introduction*. Little, Brown, 1984.

Harley RD (editor): *Pediatric Ophthalmology*, 2nd ed. 2 vols. Saunders, 1983.

Havener WH: *Ocular Pharmacology*, 5th ed. Mosby, 1983.

Havener WH: *Synopsis of Ophthalmology*, 5th ed. Mosby, 1979.

Helveston RM, Ellis FD: *Pediatric Ophthalmology Practice*. Mosby, 1980.

Miller D: *Ophthalmology: The Essentials*. Houghton Mifflin, 1979.

Miller NR: *Walsh and Hoyt's Clinical Neuro-Ophthalmology*, 4th ed. 2 vols. Williams & Wilkins, 1982.

Moses RA (editor): *Adler's Physiology of the Eye: Clinical Applications*, 7th ed. Mosby, 1981.

Nelson LB: *Pediatric Ophthalmology*. Saunders, 1984.

Newell FW: *Ophthalmology: Principles and Concepts*, 6th ed. Mosby, 1986.

Peyman GA, Sanders DR, Goldberg MF: *Principles and Practice of Ophthalmology*. 3 vols. Saunders, 1980.

Robb RM: *Ophthalmology for the Pediatric Practitioner*. Little, Brown, 1981.

Scheie HG, Albert DM: *Textbook of Ophthalmology*, 9th ed. Saunders, 1977.

Vaughan D, Asbury T: *General Ophthalmology*, 11th ed. Lange, 1986.

Wybar K, Taylor D (editors): *Pediatric Ophthalmology: Current Aspects*. Marcel Dekker, 1983.

Teeth

12

Gary K. Belanger, DDS, & Paul S. Casamassimo, DDS, MS

THE ORAL CAVITY

Included in the oral cavity are the teeth (20 primary, 32 permanent), the maxillary and mandibular jaws, hard and soft palates, tongue, and salivary glands (major and minor). Each tooth is composed of an enamel crown; a dentin body and roots, with cementum covering the root surfaces; and a pulp cavity containing connective tissue, nerves, lymphatics, and blood vessels that branch off larger structures in the jaw and enter the root tip in a bundle. (See Fig 12–1.)

The teeth are supported in bone via ligaments that connect the cementum-covered root surfaces to the bone. Like the teeth, the periodontal ligament is innervated. The gingivae are attached to alveolar bone and to the teeth on the alveolar process. The area where gingiva meets tooth is called the gingival epithelial attachment, which is usually at the neck of the tooth. Attached gingiva is normally pink and stippled in children.

Primary teeth are usually smaller, whiter, and more bulbous than permanent ones. Below each primary tooth normally rests a permanent successor in a crypt of bone. The developing permanent tooth is susceptible to systemic disorders and local problems affecting the overlying primary tooth, such as dental caries and trauma.

ERUPTION OF TEETH

Cellular development of primary teeth begins during the sixth week of embryogenesis, with calcification beginning during the second trimester. A few permanent teeth also begin to develop by birth, but very little calcification occurs. Table 2–12 summarizes the timing of calcification, eruption, and exfoliation of primary and permanent teeth.

Although the pattern of tooth eruption is easily observed, it may not be a good predictor of general growth and development or other physical parameters. Many local factors influence eruption of teeth, and the pattern can be affected by normal variation, systemic conditions, and genetic tendencies.

Normal Patterns of Eruption

Primary teeth should erupt within 6 months of their average expected time. According to the "rule of 4s," 4 teeth will erupt beginning at about 7 months of age, and 4 more will erupt approximately every 4 months thereafter. Another general guide is that there will be no teeth at 6 months, 6 teeth at 12 months, and 12 teeth at 18 months of age. Primary teeth erupt in the following sequence: central incisors, lateral incisors, first molars, cuspids, and second molars. The exfoliation sequence is more variable (see Table 2–12).

As the primary teeth near gingival penetration, infants begin **teething.** They may become more restless and irritable, and they drool and place their fingers in their mouths more frequently. Most studies have discounted teething as a cause of systemic disturbances, diarrhea, fever, seizures, or an altered hematocrit. Although the incidence of fever, rhinitis, gastrointestinal upset, upper respiratory tract infections, and dermatitis may increase coincidentally with tooth eruption, a causal relationship is equivocal. Many normal changes in the infant's environment are thought to contribute to these illnesses, including diet changes, increased exposure to infections, and loss of maternal antibodies.

Use of a soft cloth, a teething ring, or dry abrasive toast may hasten eruption and provide relief of pain. Gingival incision is rarely indicated to allow eruption of primary teeth, although some extremely delayed permanent teeth may benefit from this procedure. Tooth eruption is a process associated with gingival inflammation that may be made worse as oral bacteria inoculate soft tissues surrounding the erupting tooth. Molars occasionally erupt with a tissue flap of gingiva

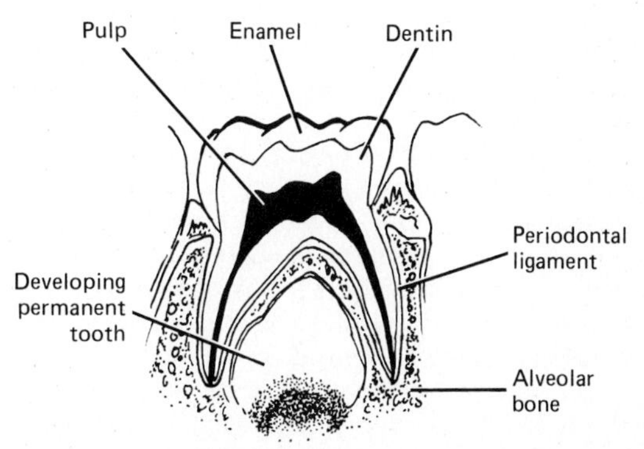

Figure 12–1. Cross-sectional view of a primary tooth and underlying tooth bud.

over them, and this operculum can trap food debris and cause localized discomfort.

Since plaque forms on all teeth—including newly erupted ones—parents should be encouraged to initiate an oral hygiene program as soon as the first tooth erupts. Oral hygiene is reviewed in the section on dental caries (see below).

Abnormal Patterns of Eruption

A. Precocious Eruption: Teeth present at birth are called **natal teeth,** and teeth erupting within the first month of life are called **neonatal teeth.** Their precocious eruption has been attributed to hormonal imbalances and to their development immediately below the gingival surface rather than deep in bone. They occur in about one out of 2000–3000 infants and most frequently are found in the lower incisor region. Most are the normal mandibular primary incisors, but occasionally they may be extra (supernumerary) teeth. A dental radiograph is necessary to make this distinction and usually also shows very little or no root development of the erupted teeth. Natal and neonatal teeth are typically hypermobile and have the potential of being detached. Supernumerary teeth should definitely be removed because they may be aspirated, may contribute to nursing difficulties, or may cause traumatic ulceration of the ventral surface of the tongue (Riga-Fede disease). These same concerns are present for normal primary incisors that have erupted early, but their removal may lead to later dental arch collapse. Blood coagulation tests should be performed before natal or neonatal teeth are removed.

B. Delayed Eruption: Premature loss of a primary tooth can cause either accelerated or delayed eruption of the underlying secondary tooth. Early eruption occurs if the permanent tooth is beginning its active eruption and the overlying primary tooth is removed. This generally occurs when the primary tooth is within 1 year of its normal time of exfoliation. If, however, loss of the primary tooth occurs more than a year from expected exfoliation, the permanent tooth will likely be delayed in its eruption, owing to healing that results in filling in of bone and gingiva over the permanent tooth. The loss of a primary tooth may cause adjacent teeth to tip into the space and impact the underlying permanent tooth. A space maintainer should be placed by a dentist to prevent this possibility.

Other local factors delaying or preventing eruption include supernumerary teeth, cysts, tumors, overretained primary teeth, ankylosed primary teeth, and impaction. A generalized delay in eruption may be due to endocrinopathies (hypothyroidism, hypopituitarism) or other systemic conditions (cleidocranial dysplasia, rickets, trisomy 21).

C. Ectopic Eruption: Ectopic eruption occurs if the position of an erupting tooth is abnormal. In severe instances, the order in which teeth erupt is affected. If the dental arch provides insufficient room for permanent teeth, they may erupt abnormally. In the mandible, lower incisors may be lingually placed to such an extent that the primary incisors do not exfoliate. The parents' concern about a "double row of teeth" may be the reason for the child's first dental visit. If the primary teeth are not loose, they should be removed by the dentist. If they are loose, they should be allowed to exfoliate naturally. In the maxilla, inadequate room for eruption of the permanent first molar may cause resorption of the distal root structures of the second primary molar. If the problem is severe, the permanent molar may even become caught under the unresorbed enamel crown of the deciduous molar and thus require extraction of the primary tooth and orthodontic repositioning of the permanent first molar after it has erupted. If it is not repositioned, the second premolar is likely to become impacted. If problems are detected early, the dentist may be able to favorably redirect the permanent molar's eruption pathway so that the permanent first molar correctly erupts and the second primary molar is not lost.

D. Impaction: Impaction occurs when a tooth is prevented from erupting for any reason. The teeth most often affected are the third molars and the maxillary canines. Because patients with impacted third molars are at risk for developing ameloblastomas or dentigerous cysts if these teeth are not surgically removed, the impacted third molar (along with its opposing third molar) should be removed after it has been determined that eruption will not be possible. Maxillary canines, however, should not be extracted, because of their aesthetic importance and key role in dental occlusion. They can often be brought into correct alignment through surgical exposure and orthodontic treatment.

E. Other Variations: Failure of teeth to develop—a condition sometimes called **congenitally missing teeth**—is quite rare in the primary dentition. However, it occurs in about 5% of permanent dentitions (exclusive of third molars), and one or more of the third molars is missing in about 25% of all individuals. The incidence of congenitally missing teeth varies among different genetic groups, but the most frequently missing are maxillary lateral incisors and mandibular second premolars.

Occasionally, there are **extra teeth,** most typically an extra (fourth) molar or extra (third) bicuspid. **Mesiodentes,** which are peg-shaped supernumerary teeth situated at the maxillary midline, are seen in about 5% of individuals and may interfere with eruption of permanent incisors. Mesiodentes should be considered for removal even if they do not erupt.

EPITHELIAL INCLUSION CYSTS

Many infants are born with single or lobulated white elevations that are approximately 1–5 mm in diameter and present in different areas of the mouth. These elevations are sometimes erroneously thought to be dental structures. Three different terms have been used to describe them: Epstein's pearls, Bohn's nodules, and dental lamina cysts. **Epstein's pearls** are found along the palatine raphe and often occur in multiples; they represent trapped excesses of epithelium and keratin related to midline fusion. **Bohn's nodules** are often lobulated and occur along the buccal or lingual sides of the gum pads; they are thought to arise from mucous glands. **Dental lamina cysts** occur on the crest of the upper or lower ridges and are excess epithelium derived from the underlying dental lamina. Although the 3 terms are sometimes used interchangeably and the clinical appearance of the elevated areas may be similar, they differ in histology and location.

ANKYLOGLOSSIA

In young children, the lingual frenum may appear to be short (as if attached to the tip of the tongue) and heart-shaped when elevated. Some investigators consider this a normal developmental finding that will resolve within a few years. Others express concern about a potential for speech problems, interference with sucking, and inability to cleanse the buccal sides of upper teeth. Surgical lingual frenectomy is sometimes performed to correct the situation.

HYPERTROPHY OF THE MAXILLARY FRENUM

Hypertrophy of the maxillary midline frenum may appear to be the cause of spacing between central incisors. However, this spacing (diastema) is normal in primary dentition (before 6 years of age) and in mixed dentition (6–11 years of age). The flaring of all 4 maxillary permanent incisors is not abnormal and may contribute to spacing between these teeth. The frenum often appears to diminish with age as a consequence of its insertion remaining fixed while the maxilla grows vertically. Surgical intervention is indicated only if the hypertrophied frenum and diastema persist after eruption of the maxillary canines (around 12 years of age). Even after a maxillary frenectomy, orthodontic closure of the diastema may be necessary. The condition is more prevalent among blacks.

DISCOLORATION OF TEETH

Staining of teeth can occur on the outside surface of enamel (extrinsic) or within the tooth structure (intrinsic).

Certain foods and other agents taken orally can cause **extrinsic staining,** and poor oral hygiene (inadequate plaque removal) exacerbates the problem. In young children, plaque adhering to the gingival third of the teeth may take on a greenish-gray, black, or orange discoloration. Regular doses of iron can produce a tenacious black external staining. In almost all cases, professional polishing can remove the stain. If the stain reflects chronic neglect of oral hygiene, there may be areas of decalcification under the stained plaque.

Agents that can be incorporated directly into the tooth structure and cause **internal discoloration** include tetracycline, fluoride in excess amounts, bilirubin, and hemolytic breakdown products. Genetic disorders and environmental conditions affecting developing teeth can cause extra dentin to be deposited in the pulp or can cause hypoplasia or hypomineralization of enamel. Very little can be done to prevent internal discoloration due to the above causes—with the notable exception of tetracycline administration. Extreme care should be taken to avoid prescribing any form of the drug from birth until age 12 years. Pregnant women should not be treated with tetracycline, since the drug can traverse the placenta and be deposited in the calcifying teeth of the fetus. In some patients with tetracycline-stained teeth, dental bleaching procedures result in cosmetic improvement. In others, veneering or complete crowning of affected teeth may be the only satisfactory treatment.

MALOCCLUSION

Classification

Edward Angle's system for classifying molar occlusion (Fig 12–2) was developed at the beginning of this century and still serves as the foundation for describing malocclusions. In class I ("normal") occlusion, the first (mesiobuccal) cusp of the upper first permanent molar is aligned in the major (buccal) groove of the lower first permanent molar. In class II occlusion (distal occlusion, distoclusion), the lower molar aligns in a posterior position, causing lower jaw retrognathia. In class III occlusion (mesio-occlusion, mesioclusion), the lower molar aligns in an anterior position, causing lower jaw prognathism.

Very few individuals develop an "ideal" dental occlusion or bite. Other features occurring independently or in combination can contribute to malocclusion and should be noted in the clinical description: skeletal interrelationships of the cranium and upper and lower jaws; position of teeth relative to the supporting jaws; vertical relationship of teeth (open or deep bite); spacing or crowding of teeth; position of individual teeth (rotated in any direction, overlapping, etc); muscular imbalances; and habits that may affect alignment of teeth (eg, sucking the thumb or fingers).

Management

Malocclusion does not carry with it the pctential for grave consequences if left untreated. Nonetheless, most individuals want to present the best possible appearance, and measures can be taken to prevent,

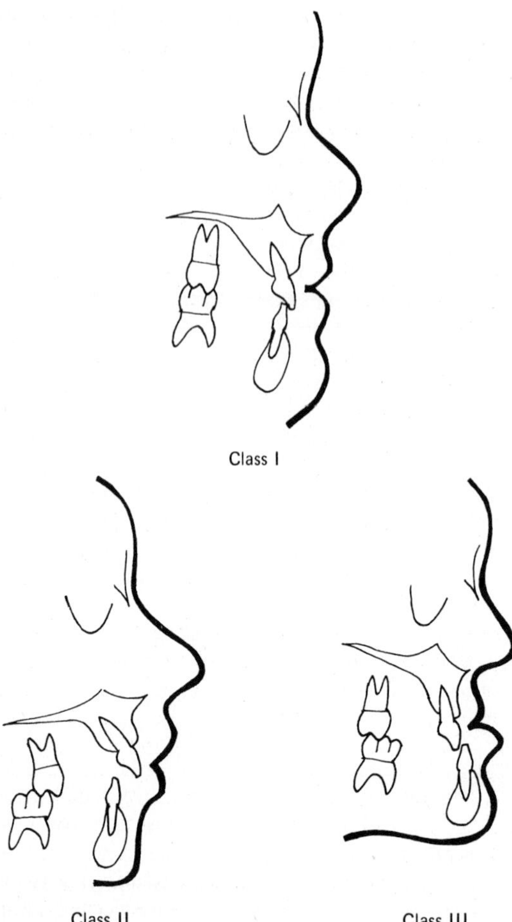

Figure 12–2. Angle's classification of malocclusion based on first permanent molar position. Facial profile is straight in class I, retrognathic in class II (receding chin), and prognathic in class III (jutting chin).

intercept, or correct common problems related to inadequate room for proper alignment of permanent teeth.

A. Preventive Orthodontics: The fundamental goal of preventive orthodontics is to maintain normal occlusion by detecting and treating abnormalities in the eruption and exfoliation of teeth (eg, overretained primary teeth, ectopic eruption, extra teeth, impaction) before they contribute to malocclusion. A critical component of preventive orthodontics is the placement of space maintainers to prevent tipping of adjacent teeth into spaces left by large interproximal cavities, such as occurs when primary teeth are lost early.

The elimination of deleterious oral habits (eg, sucking the thumb, fingers, or lips; thrusting the tongue) can prevent or minimize some malocclusion problems. Thumb-sucking is not considered a serious dental problem until the maxillary permanent central incisors begin to erupt. At this point, irreversible bone movement and poor alignment of the teeth can occur. Dental appliances, myofunctional exercises, or both may help some children stop these habits, but each child should be professionally evaluated before such measures are taken.

B. Interceptive Orthodontics: Interceptive orthodontic treatment is indicated if there are factors whose elimination would result in a return to normal occlusion. The interceptive procedures produce maximum benefit for the growing child before complete establishment of the permanent dentition at about age 12 years. Some of the more common treatments include (1) restoring teeth to their proper position if they have drifted and will prevent other teeth from assuming their intended positions; (2) using headgear to move teeth or to inhibit growth of the maxilla (to allow mandibular growth to "catch up"); (3) correcting crossbites in anterior or posterior teeth; (4) eliminating pernicious oral habits; (5) sequentially extracting certain primary teeth or reducing their width to allow space for erupting permanent teeth; and (6) directing forces to counter undesirable jaw relationships that may be developing.

Various mechanical appliances can be used to change the position of the teeth, jaws, or oral musculature. Traditional orthodontic braces, extraoral appliances (eg, headgear), or removable acrylic appliances with orthodontic wires can be used successfully to make minor tooth movements. In the USA, there is a developing popularity for the use of a functional appliance that evolved in Europe after World War II. Bands around teeth have generally been supplanted by plastic brackets bonded to the teeth with resin.

C. Corrective Orthodontics: It is preferable to prevent or intercept developing malocclusion, but this is not always possible. Some children do not have the benefit of preventive services at the most effective time, and others have sufficiently severe problems that can only be treated by corrective orthodontics.

Corrective orthodontics employs many of the treatment methods used in interceptive orthodontics, but treatment is more aggressive and comprehensive. In many instances, all teeth will require treatment. In some patients with small dental arches, there may not be sufficient area to accommodate the permanent teeth. Extraction of permanent teeth is becoming increasingly controversial, and strategies to expand dental arches without extraction are gaining popularity.

DENTAL CARIES

Dental caries is one of the most common infectious diseases. It affects both primary and permanent dentitions and can occur at any age. The disease is characterized by decalcification of the tooth, beginning with the enamel and progressing to the dentin and cementum. If untreated, the carious process can reach the pulp and cause severe tooth pain and abscess formation.

The initiation of dental caries requires 3 factors: (1) acidogenic bacteria, eg, *Streptococcus mutans;* (2) a source of nutrient carbohydrate, usually sugar;

and (3) a tooth that is susceptible to decalcification. Research has identified a genetic component to dental caries, but the infectious nature of the disease makes environment far more significant than heredity.

The human body's natural protection against dental caries rests mainly in the saliva. Immunoglobulins, minerals, and the cleansing effect of saliva contribute some degree of natural resistance. The process involved is described as remineralization, a dynamic equilibrium in which new carious lesions are constantly developing and being arrested by the action of saliva. Low levels of fluoride seem to push the equilibrium to the side of recalcification.

Prevention

Public health measures such as water fluoridation, improved access to care, better public education, and better diets have caused a general decrease in the rate of caries in children and adolescents. A vaccine against caries is currently being developed, but large-scale human application is far in the future.

A. Oral Hygiene: Oral hygiene is directed at removing plaque from teeth before it becomes cariogenic. The bacteria in plaque require 18–24 hours to produce acid to decalcify teeth.

Parents should be encouraged to start cleaning the child's teeth as soon as they erupt. A toothbrush and toothpaste are not necessary, since a washcloth, piece of cotton gauze, or cotton-tipped applicator is adequate for wiping away plaque on newly erupted teeth. Subsequent tooth cleaning is best done with a soft toothbrush, and parents should take responsibility for tooth cleaning until the child demonstrates proficiency. A basic scrub technique suffices for primary dentition and mixed dentition, and its aim is mechanical removal of plaque and gentle stimulation of gingivae. Whether or not a child's teeth should be flossed will depend on the presence of interdental caries, tight contact between teeth, and the efficacy of toothbrushing alone for that child. Flossing removes plaque between teeth where toothbrush bristles cannot reach. Parents should assist in flossing, since a child may not have the desire to floss or the dexterity to prevent injury to gingivae.

Irrigating devices ("water picks") tend to remove loose food debris but not plaque. Therefore, they are of limited value for tooth cleaning in children. Gingival damage has been noted when irrigation devices are used improperly with the spray directed into the gingival sulci. They may be a useful adjunct to regular brushing procedures in individuals wearing orthodontic appliances.

Devices to clean teeth can be adapted with extensions or special grips to meet the individual needs of the physically handicapped child. Adult participation is crucial to success.

Tooth brushing is mainly responsible for the removal of plaque. Dentifrice itself plays a minor role in tooth cleaning in the young child, but the fluoride in it is beneficial. Some children find the taste of toothpaste offensive. The preparation used should be one approved by the American Dental Association, should contain fluoride to provide maximal topical benefit, and should be pleasant-tasting to encourage the child to brush. Since toothpaste is often ingested by young children, only a small amount is recommended for brushing.

Professional cleaning is recommended when calculus (tartar) or stain develops on the teeth. Tooth polishing at checkups and prior to a fluoride treatment is no longer considered routine and should be done only as frequently as determined by the dentist.

B. Diet and Nutrition: Removal or lessening of carbohydrate substrate prevents bacteria from producing the mucopolysaccharides that form plaque and the acid that decalcifies teeth. Studies in animals have shown that dental caries cannot occur without fermentable carbohydrate. Although no consistent relationship exists between the amount of carbohydrate consumed and the rate of caries, research has demonstrated that the frequency of carbohydrate ingestion, the consistency of the carbohydrate ingested (eg, stickiness, liquid form), and the timing of carbohydrate ingestion in relation to ingestion of other foods are important factors in the process of caries formation.

A nutritious diet of essential nutrients contributes to the development of healthy teeth and helps prevent caries. Control of refined carbohydrate in the diet is the major aspect of dietary control of dental caries. Restriction of the amount of sugar consumed is a general dietary goal. Several aspects of controlled sugar intake benefit dental health: (1) Decreasing the frequency of carbohydrate ingestion reduces the number of exposures of oral plaque to fermentable substrate and consequently reduces the time teeth are exposed to acid. (2) Ingestion of liquid rather than solid or sticky carbohydrate allows more rapid clearance of sugar from the oral cavity. (3) If carbohydrate ingestion is followed by brushing the teeth, by drinking noncariogenic liquids, or by eating fibrous foods, the time teeth are exposed to acid is decreased. (4) Control of carbohydrate intake by changes in the way they are consumed rather than by food substitution is preferred in children, since alternative snacks or foods may be high in sodium, fat, and artificial additives. Current nutritional counseling should approach sugar restriction with attention to overall diet, energy requirements, family resources, and cooperation of the parents and child.

C. Fluoride: Fluoride is the single most effective anticariogenic measure known. It has 3 important mechanisms of action: (1) its incorporation into the developing tooth's enamel, which makes apatite more resistant to acid produced by bacteria; (2) its interference in bacterial metabolism; and (3) its enhancement of remineralization, which arrests developing carious lesions. Systemic fluoride can benefit children while teeth are developing, and topical fluoride is helpful after teeth have erupted.

1. Systemic fluoride—Fluoride contained in water, food, and prescribed supplements is absorbed in the blood and distributed to the bones and developing teeth. Fluoride is deposited in the enamel as fluorapetite, which has a greater resistance to acid.

Both primary and permanent dentitions benefit from systemic fluoride. Water fluoridation at a fluoride level of 0.7–1.2 parts per million (ppm) is considered optimal. There is no proved efficacy of prenatal fluoride therapy, in which a pregnant woman ingests fluoride to benefit her child's primary dentition; therefore, this is not an accepted procedure. Fluoride supplementation in children can begin at birth or as late as 6 months of age to provide protection to the primary and permanent teeth. The average child requires a fluoride intake of 0.05 mg/kg/d for fluoride to provide maximum benefit. If the child's water supply provides less than 0.7 ppm of fluoride, supplementation should be considered.

Table 12–1 shows supplemental fluoride dosage recommendations for children under 15 years of age. At 15 years, systemic fluoride is no longer considered beneficial. As indicated in the table, dosages are based on the level of fluoride in the local water. Well water or water from municipal supplies of unknown fluoride content should be tested by a public health department or private laboratory. Breast-fed infants and infants receiving premixed formula (formula not made to be mixed with tap water) should be assumed to be receiving no fluoride. The appropriate form of supplemental fluoride (vitamin-fluoride compound, tablet, or drop) is based on the child's age and life-style. Supplementation should be reassessed annually.

2. Topical fluoride—Topical fluoride benefits teeth as long as they are subject to decay. Dentifrice and water containing fluoride, foods processed or prepared with fluoridated water, and topical fluoride treatment all help reduce susceptibility to dental caries. Factors to be considered in determining the need for professionally applied fluoride treatments include the child's overall fluoride exposure, extent of dental caries, and presence of risk factors such as a handicapping condition or orthodontic appliances. The combination of topical and systemic fluoride treatment offers increased protection against dental caries.

Over-the-counter topical fluoride rinses can also supplement a systemic treatment program. Inadvertent ingestion of these products and fluoridated dentifrices can result in fluorosis, a white or brown intrinsic staining of teeth. A dentist should be consulted to determine the fluoride program for a child, based on all sources of fluoride.

D. Sealants: Sealants are plastic coatings designed to be applied by dental professionals on newly erupted or caries-susceptible teeth, usually recently erupted permanent or primary molars and permanent premolars. They are applied to the pits and fissures of the biting surfaces of teeth, which are areas in which fluoride has little effect. Sealants form a barrier to bacterial penetration. Ten-year follow-up studies have shown a high rate of protection. The decision to apply sealant to a tooth should be based on the child's susceptibility to caries, the length of time the tooth has been in the mouth, and the presence of decay on other surfaces of the tooth.

Diagnosis & Treatment

A. Specific Types of Dental Caries: Dental caries can occur any time after eruption of the first primary tooth. **"Nursing bottle caries"** is caused by prolonged access to the bottle, usually at night or nap time. The carbohydrate-containing liquid (milk, formula, carbonated beverage, or fruit juice) pools on the teeth and is metabolized by bacteria to form acid. The decreased saliva flow and the oral muscular activity during sleep contribute to the process. Oral hygiene practices are often lacking. Characteristically, maxillary primary incisors are decayed (with or without abscesses) and mandibular anterior teeth unaffected. Tooth cleaning, topical fluoride application, restoration or extraction of teeth, and sedation or general anesthesia may be needed to treat the infant. Prevention of nursing bottle caries involves either eliminating use of the bottle at night and nap time or substituting water for other liquids in the bottle.

Incipient (beginning) caries involves the early decalcification of enamel. Opaque white areas are the result of changes in the light-transmitting qualities of enamel. Incipient caries often occurs at the gum line under long-standing plaque. Good hygiene and fluoride application can often stop the process before cavitation occurs.

Rampant caries is characterized by rapidly progressing tooth decay in a child or adolescent who may have been free of or minimally affected in the past. The teeth are often cavitated or decayed to the alveolar ridge. Painful abscesses may be present. The dentin

Table 12–1. Supplemental fluoride dosage recommendations.*

Fluoride Content of Drinking Water	Dosage of Oral Fluoride		
	Age 0–2 Years	Age 2–3 Years	Age 3–14 Years
< 0.3 ppm	0.25 mg/d	0.5 mg/d	1 mg/d
0.3–0.7 ppm	0 mg/d	0.25 mg/d	0.5 mg/d

* Approved by the American Academy of Pediatrics and the American Dental Association. Fluoride supplementation is unnecessary if the fluoride content of drinking water is over 0.7 ppm or if the patient is 15 years of age or older.

is often yellow or orange and is soft, indicating active decay. Therapy involves extensive restoration, pulpal treatment, dietary measures, and fluoride supplementation.

Radiation caries can occur in children who have head and neck neoplasia and have undergone irradiation of salivary glands. The decay pattern is much like rampant decay. These children should receive careful follow-up by a dentist.

Caries associated with bulimia is a generalized process that often results in enamel erosion due to regurgitation of acidic stomach contents. Teeth may have a frosted rather than glossy look and may appear to be ground down. There may be gingival recession and areas of dark tooth decay, frequently at the gum line. Treatment is often difficult; therefore, prevention is critical.

B. General Guidelines for Dental Referral: Dark staining of grooves, large accumulations of plaque with or without white decalcification, dark pits, and a history of discomfort to hot, cold, or sweets suggest caries. Frank cavitation, destruction of crowns of teeth, gingival swelling, significant and prolonged pain with or without facial swelling, and broken fillings indicate the need for professional attention.

The prognosis for untreated dental caries is poor. Some carious lesions may turn black as exposed dentin picks up food stains. Most often, the caries process progresses to the pulp of the tooth, causing pain, pulpitis, abscess, and loss of the tooth through coronal destruction or extraction.

Secondary prevention involves early intervention by a dental professional. The time of the first dental visit by a child remains controversial. Pediatric dentists recommend an initial preventive and educational visit within 6 months of eruption of the first primary tooth, especially if the child has known or suspected developmental delays, lives in a community without fluoridated water, or has a family history of poor dental health. Data indicate that up to 50% of 2-year-olds have some tooth decay, so an initial exam by 18–24 months of age should be beneficial.

The dentist's treatment of dental caries has remained essentially the same, with use of silver amalgam, steel crowns, and plastic fillings as the main elements. Current data support the safety of mercury-silver amalgam as a filling material. Tooth-colored composite resins can also be used for both anterior and posterior teeth. In some cases, these resins can be affixed to teeth without drilling; prior to affixing them, the tooth surface is treated with mild acid, which creates microscopic projections that aid in the binding process.

TOOTHACHE

The most common cause of toothache is pulpal stimulation due to dentin exposure or direct pulpal exposure secondary to dental caries. In some cases, pain is related to infection in the space between the tooth and supporting bone. Toothache secondary to caries or periodontal infection is usually accompanied by one or more of the following: swelling of adjacent gingival tissues, purulence from the gingival sulcus, mobility, elevation from the socket, and a large cavity. If these are lacking, the physician or dentist should suspect a traumatic injury, either chronic (eg, bruxism, or grinding of teeth) or acute (eg, a blow to the teeth); systemic illness; sinusitis; neoplasia; or referred pain. In children, most tooth pain is related to dental caries and subsequent infection.

TRAUMATIC INJURIES

Traumatic injuries to the primary and permanent teeth of children often cause the immediate problems of pain and hemorrhage and can cause long-term sequelae, including loss of damaged teeth, malposition of injured primary teeth or their permanent successors, discoloration of the crowns of injured teeth (due to hemolytic pigments), destruction of the enamel of permanent successors to injured primary teeth, delayed exfoliation of the primary teeth, and possible displacement of an underlying permanent tooth bud.

Factors of concern in cases of traumatic injury are whether the affected teeth are primary or permanent, the type of injury, the time elapsed since the injury occurred, and whether or not any treatment was rendered in that interim. Injuries may involve the teeth or the alveolar bone and tooth-supporting structures. In traumatic injuries, the physician should render immediate care to ensure retention of the teeth (Table 12–2) and make an appropriate dental referral.

Tooth injuries most often involve some type of fracture of the crown, with or without exposure of pulp. When pulpal tissues are exposed, time becomes an important element in management. The longer the pulpal tissues are exposed to the environment, the more likely it is that necrosis and death of the pulp will occur and result in ultimate loss of the tooth. Referral is urgent in these cases.

Injuries that involve dislocation or avulsion of the tooth from the socket are even more urgent. As time elapses, repositioning of dislocated teeth becomes more difficult owing to swelling and clot formation. Although an intruded tooth should be repositioned only by the dentist, other dislocated teeth should be repositioned immediately and stabilized.

An avulsed permanent tooth should be treated as an emergency, since immediate reinsertion is critical to saving the tooth. The tooth should be located, placed in the socket, and stabilized until the patient can reach a dentist. Stabilization can be achieved by having the patient bite on a piece of gauze or by having the patient or someone else hold the tooth in. If the tooth cannot be reinserted owing to poor visibility or the presence of foreign material, it should be placed in milk, saliva, or normal saline solution and then transported with the patient to the dentist. Under no circumstances should the tooth be washed

Table 12–2. Management of traumatic injuries of the teeth and supporting bone.

	Tooth Fracture	Tooth Dislocation or Avulsion
Primary teeth	**No pulp exposed:** Refer to dentist within 24 hours. **Pulp exposed:** Refer to dentist immediately.	**Intrusion:** Do not reposition the tooth. Refer to dentist immediately. **Dislocation:** Reposition the tooth and refer to dentist immediately. **Avulsion:** Do not reinsert the tooth. Refer to dentist immediately.
Permanent teeth	**No pulp exposed:** Refer to dentist within 24 hours. **Pulp exposed:** Refer to dentist immediately.	**Intrusion:** Do not reposition the tooth. Refer to dentist immediately. **Dislocation:** Reposition the tooth and refer to dentist immediately. **Avulsion:** Either (1) reinsert the tooth and refer to dentist immediately; or (2) place the tooth in milk, saliva, or normal saline solution and transport it with the patient to the dentist (urgent).

or scrubbed prior to reimplantation. Cleaning should be confined to gentle rinsing in an isotonic solution. Critical to successful reimplantation is maintenance of the viability of the cells on the root surface, and cleaning the root with other than osmotically neutral fluid causes death of these cells.

Reimplantation of primary teeth is usually not recommended, since it is difficult to keep the reinserted tooth stable in a young child and thus reimplantation is unsuccessful.

Antibiotics are not usually required for reimplantation and do not appear to affect the outcome of reimplantation when they are used for other related injuries.

GINGIVAL & PERIODONTAL CONDITIONS

Gingivitis & Periodontitis

Gingivitis is caused by accumulations of plaque and is a common condition in children, especially when oral hygiene is poor. The disease is by definition confined to soft tissues and does not involve the alveolar bone supporting the teeth. Clinical findings include redness around the gingival margins and swelling of the interdental papillae. The disease can occur at any age and does not necessarily progress to periodontitis.

Periodontitis is an infection of the supporting periodontal ligament and bone. Unlike gingivitis, which is reversible with improved hygiene, periodontitis causes irreversible destruction of tissues. Young children are rarely affected by periodontitis. Prepubescent children with **juvenile periodontitis** have rapid and severe loss of supporting bone, usually around permanent molars and incisors. *Actinobacillus actinomycetemcomitans* is thought to be the cause. Diagnosis without radiographs is difficult, since the bone destruction occurs below the gingival margin and inflammation is often lacking. Teeth may or may not be loose.

Both gingivitis and periodontitis are considered infections, and both are caused by bacterial plaque, which produces toxins that destroy tissue. Thus, prevention and treatment are based on removal of the bacterial plaque and calculus (tartar) and institution of good oral hygiene practices (tooth cleaning, gingival stimulation, and flossing). In cases of juvenile periodontitis, tetracycline is given. Some patients with periodontitis also require surgery to remove the diseased tissue and restore tissue to its normal contour so that plaque is less likely to accumulate. The teeth may need to be splinted together for support.

Herpetic Gingivostomatitis

Herpetic gingivostomatitis in children is due to primary infection with herpes simplex virus. Although most children with primary herpetic infection are asymptomatic, a few present with acute and painful symptoms that last for 10–14 days and include fever, malaise, lymphadenopathy, and lesions occurring on the lips, attached gingivae, hard palate, and dorsum of the tongue. The lesions begin as vesicles and soon rupture to form ulcers. By the time the child is seen, the infection is often well established. Therapy consists of palliative measures. Hydration during the more painful period of infection is a major concern in the very young. Cold fluids and ice cubes or Popsicles can be used to maintain hydration and numb the mouth to permit eating. Topically applied local anesthetic can also be used but should not be ingested. A mixture of one part diphenhydramine (Benadryl), one part kaolin and pectin (Kaopectate), and one part water can provide topical relief as well. In rare instances, intravenous fluids and hospitalization may be needed to prevent severe dehydration. Recurrent herpes is usually manifested as herpes labialis with minor discomfort.

Acute Necrotizing Ulcerative Gingivitis

Acute necrotizing ulcerative gingivitis, also called trench mouth, is thought to be caused by spirochete-fusiform symbiosis. The classic signs and symptoms are fetid breath, pain, and necrotic desquamation of interdental gingival papillae with pseudomembrane formation over the areas of destruction. The infection is often related to stress and tends to occur in the adolescent age group. Treatment consists of gentle debridement of affected tissues and administration of an antibiotic such as penicillin. Oxygenating agents applied topically can also help. Acute necrotizing ulcerative gingivitis can be differentiated from herpetic stomatitis by its odor and classic lesions and by its predilection for older children.

Aphthous Stomatitis

Aphthous stomatitis can also be mistaken for herpetic stomatitis but is thought to be caused by bacterial agents. The lesions are ulcers that tend to occur on an unattached mucous membrane such as the buccal mucosa, soft palate, or undersurface of the tongue. Treatment is palliative, and the infection lasts from 10–14 days. Aphthous ulcers can recur as isolated lesions, often in response to eating acidic foods.

Premature Bone Loss

Bone loss in primary dentition is a rare occurrence. If primary teeth become loose well ahead of their scheduled exfoliation, the following causes should be considered: mercury poisoning, radiation toxicity, juvenile periodontitis, Papillon-Lefèvre syndrome, scurvy, acatalasia, hypophosphatasia, diabetes mellitus, Gaucher's disease, leukemia, neutropenia, histiocytosis X, Wiskott-Aldrich syndrome, and neutrophil dysfunction.

OTHER INTRAORAL LESIONS

A **mucocele** is a benign whitish or light blue swelling that most often occurs on the lower lip but is sometimes seen on the palate, cheek, or floor of the mouth. The lesion, which indicates a blocked minor salivary gland, can rupture and re-form. Treatment is excision.

A **parulis,** or **gumboil,** is the intraoral manifestation of a periapical (pulpal) infection of a tooth. The parulis is the site of fistulation of an abscess at the root tip, which is usually either the result of dental caries that has progressed to the pulp and caused its necrosis or the consequence of a traumatic injury. The lesion can appear as a finely pointed white pimple or a larger yellowish-red elevation, usually on the buccal gingiva at a level approximating the location of the tooth's root. The adjacent tooth often has a large cavity. The parulis may or may not be associated with gingival swelling, pain, or tooth mobility, depending on its duration. Treatment is directed at the offending infection.

An **eruption cyst** is a purple swelling (hematoma) that occurs over the crown of an erupting tooth. Tooth eruption is accompanied by the rupture of small vessels that hemorrhage into the eruption capsule. No treatment is needed, since the cyst will resolve spontaneously.

Gingival overgrowth is common in children whose seizure disorders are being treated with phenytoin. The growth represents both hypertrophy and hyperplasia of gingival cells. Although the response to phenytoin therapy is variable, children tend to have more overgrowth than adults do. Meticulous oral hygiene may lessen the extent of overgrowth, but discontinuance of the medication is the only sure way to prevent it. Surgery is required to remove excess tissue.

Cellulitis of the face can result from disseminated tooth abscess and should be treated with antibiotics. Extraction of the offending tooth may also be indicated. Hot packs to the face are contraindicated, since they may cause external pointing of the abscess and result in scarring. Untreated cellulitis can progress to a more severe problem such as brain abscess, cavernous sinus thrombosis, or Ludwig's angina.

SELECTED REFERENCES

Andreasen JO: *Traumatic Injuries to the Teeth.* Saunders, 1981.

Baer PN, Benjamin SD: *Periodontal Disease in Children and Adolescents.* Lippincott, 1974.

Braham R, Morris M: *Textbook of Pediatric Dentistry,* 2nd ed. Williams & Wilkins, 1985.

Budnick SD: *Handbook of Pediatric Oral Pathology.* Year Book, 1981.

McDonald RE: *Dentistry for the Child and Adolescent,* 4th ed. Mosby, 1983.

Moyers RE: *Handbook of Orthodontics,* 4th ed. Year Book, 1983.

Stewart RE, Barber TK (editors): *Pediatric Dentistry.* Mosby, 1981.

Wei HY (editor): *Pediatric Dental Care: An Update for the Dentist and Pediatrician.* Medcom, 1978.

13 Ear, Nose, & Throat

Barton D. Schmitt, MD, & Stephen Berman, MD

THE EAR: DISEASES & DISORDERS

OTITIS MEDIA

Otitis media, defined as an inflammation of the middle ear, is usually associated with an effusion or collection of fluid in the middle ear space. Otitis media with effusion is classified by its duration (acute if present < 3 weeks; subacute if present from 3 weeks to 3 months; and chronic if present > 3 months) and by the characteristics of the effusion. The effusion is purulent in acute otitis media, is a transudate in serous otitis media, and is thick and tenacious in mucoid (secretory) otitis media. Chronic effusions may be purulent, serous, or mucoid, and it is often difficult to identify the type of effusion by otoscopy. Chronic effusions may develop by multiple pathways. The purulent effusion of acute otitis media may persist through the subacute phase or may evolve into a serous or mucoid effusion. Serous effusions may persist, evolve into mucoid effusions, or become reinfected and present as another episode of acute purulent otitis media. Mucoid effusions generally persist but can also become reinfected.

In clinical practice, about one-fourth of the pediatrician's time is spent in the diagnosis and management of otitis media. By the time children reach 3 years of age, more than two-thirds of them have experienced one episode of otitis media, and one-third have had 3 or more episodes. More children present with otitis media in the winter months, when respiratory syncytial virus and other viruses are present in the community. These upper respiratory tract infections adversely affect auditory (eustachian) tube function and predispose the child to middle ear effusion. Since young children have shorter, more compliant and more horizontally placed auditory tubes than older children and adults, colds in young patients will produce more severe auditory tube dysfunction. This dysfunction prevents middle ear secretions from draining and results in negative pressure in the middle ear space. Negative pressure predisposes the patient to periodic aspiration of contaminated nasopharyngeal secretions, which causes bacterial infection.

The diagnosis of otitis media with effusion is based on specific otoscopic findings, which include the appearance of the tympanic membrane and an assessment of its mobility. In recent years, tympanometry has also become a useful technique in documenting middle ear effusions in children and infants older than 7 months. Unfortunately, it does not identify early acute otitis media prior to the development of an effusion. In pediatric practice, tympanometry is useful for screening patients uncooperative to examination, clarifying questionable otoscopic findings, and providing an objective measurement to follow the course of persistent effusions. Otoscopy and tympanometry are discussed on p 322.

Bluestone CD: State of the art: Definitions and classifications. In: *Proceedings of the Third International Symposium: Recent Advances in Otitis Media With Effusion*. Lim DJ (editor). Decker & Co., 1984.

Henderson FW et al: A longitudinal study of respiratory viruses and bacteria in the etiology of acute otitis media with effusion. *N Engl J Med* 1982;**306:**1377.

Howie VM, Schwartz RH: Acute otitis media: One year in general pediatric practice. *Am J Dis Child* 1982;**137:**155.

1. ACUTE OTITIS MEDIA

Essentials of Diagnosis

- Earache or irritability.
- Ear discharge.
- Red, bulging, immobile tympanic membrane.

General Considerations

In a review of numerous case reports of acute purulent otitis media, Schwartz (1981) summarized bacteriologic findings in middle ear aspirates as follows: *Streptococcus pneumoniae,* 31% of cases; *Haemophilus influenzae,* 27%; group A streptococci, 2%; *Staphylococcus aureus,* 2%; and others (including enteric gram-negative organisms, *Branhamella catarrhalis,* and anaerobic organisms), 4%. In 33% of cases, aspirates were either sterile or grew presumed nonpathogens such as *Staphylococcus epidermidis* and diphtheroids.

Recently, *B catarrhalis* has been more commonly recognized as a causative agent of acute purulent otitis media. *H influenzae* remains an important pathogen in cases throughout childhood and into early adulthood.

Attempts to isolate respiratory viruses or *Mycoplasma pneumoniae* from ear aspirates have generally been unsuccessful. However, using enzyme-linked immunosorbent assay (ELISA) techniques, investigators have recently reported that viral antigens (usually of respiratory syncytial virus) were identified in one-fourth of 53 cases of acute purulent otitis media.

In about 5% of cases, multiple pathogens are isolated from a single specimen of middle ear effusion. In children with bilateral acute otitis media, different pathogens can be recovered from each ear in 5–10% of cases. The most frequently found pathogenic organisms that are resistant to ampicillin or amoxicillin include β-lactamase-producing *H influenzae* (5% of cases), *S aureus* (2%), and *B catarrhalis* (5–20%).

The microbiologic causes of acute otitis media in early infancy differ from those in later life. The risk of gram-negative enteric infection is especially high in infants who are under 6 weeks of age and have been hospitalized in a neonatal intensive care nursery. In normal infants seen during the first 3 months of life, acute otitis media is often caused by *S aureus, Chlamydia trachomatis, S pneumoniae,* or *H influenzae.*

Clinical Findings

A. Symptoms and Signs: Acute otitis media often presents with pain in association with symptoms of upper respiratory tract infection (eg, rhinorrhea, stuffy nose, and cough) or purulent conjunctivitis. While older children may complain of earache, young children demonstrate pain by crying, increased irritability, or difficulty in sleeping. Irritability may be related to hearing loss as well as pain. Tugging at the ears sometimes is a useful sign, though it can be falsely positive. Fever is present in less than half of cases, and high fever is rarely seen. Facial palsy or ataxia may occur in the rare case.

The tympanic membrane appears either red or yellow, depending on the degree of inflammation and the amount of purulent material in the middle ear space. In early cases, bulging may be limited to the pars flaccida. Later, the entire eardrum bulges outward, giving a doughnutlike appearance. Tympanic membrane mobility is absent or markedly diminished. If the eardrum has spontaneously ruptured, cloudy to purulent discharge will be present in the ear canal, making examination of the tympanic membrane difficult. Cerumen that has melted with high fever or tears and is present in the ear canal can cause confusion with middle ear discharge.

Occasionally, bullae form between the outer and middle layers of the tympanic membrane and produce acute bullous myringitis. This entity should be considered a form of acute purulent otitis media and is described in detail in the next section.

B. Laboratory Findings: Nasopharyngeal and throat cultures are not useful, because *S pneumoniae* and nontypeable *H influenzae* are often present in well children and thus of no significance. If perforation has occurred, it is useful to culture the discharge, using a nasopharyngeal culture swab. If the discharge has been present for over 8 hours, the likelihood of demonstrating the organism is small, since it frequently is overgrown with saprophytes.

Beyond the neonatal period, acute otitis media infrequently presents with signs of systemic toxicity; therefore, blood cultures, urine culture, and lumbar puncture are indicated in the child with acute purulent otitis media who also appears toxic or has signs of meningeal irritation.

Differential Diagnosis

Not all earaches are caused by acute otitis media. Mumps, toothaches, otitis externa, a foreign body in the ear canal, an ear canal furuncle, ear canal trauma, hard cerumen, etc, can all present with a chief complaint of earache. Injected vessels at the drum periphery and along the malleus are frequently overdiagnosed as "early otitis media." These can occur with fever or crying, both of which can cause a flushed tympanic membrane as well as a flushed face. Cleaning wax from the ear canal can cause reactive hyperemia of the same vessels. This degree of injection is also seen in the common cold. Such an eardrum may be red, but it will be mobile and not require treatment. Since acute otitis media is the most common complication of a cold, an infant with a cold and fever must never be sent home without examination of the eardrums. Cerumen removal (see below) will often be necessary.

Complications

The most common complication associated with acute otitis media is a hearing loss of 20–35 dB, which may persist for several months. The tympanic membrane may rupture spontaneously because of pressure necrosis and produce a sizable perforation. Acute otitis media may also cause labyrinthitis and ataxia, facial paralysis, cholesteatoma, mastoiditis, ossicular necrosis, pseudotumor cerebri (otitic hydrocephalus), or cerebral thrombophlebitis.

Treatment

An algorithm for the management of acute purulent otitis media is shown in Fig 13–1.

A. Specific Measures:

1. Systemic antibiotics—The drug of choice for acute otitis media in children of all ages is amoxicillin, 40 mg/kg/d in 3 divided doses, continued for 10 days.

Patients allergic to penicillin can be treated adequately with an oral 10-day course of erythromycin, 40 mg/kg/d, plus sulfisoxazole, 150 mg/kg/d in 4 divided doses. Another alternative is trimethoprim, 10 mg/kg/d, with sulfamethoxazole, 50 mg/kg/d. Tetracyclines are contraindicated for ear infections, because about 50% of pneumococci and streptococci are resistant to these drugs and because they cause staining of the tooth enamel.

If symptoms such as fever, earache, irritability, vomiting, or lethargy persist beyond 48 hours of therapy, the patient should be reevaluated. After 2 weeks of therapy, about 50% of children are cured, 40%

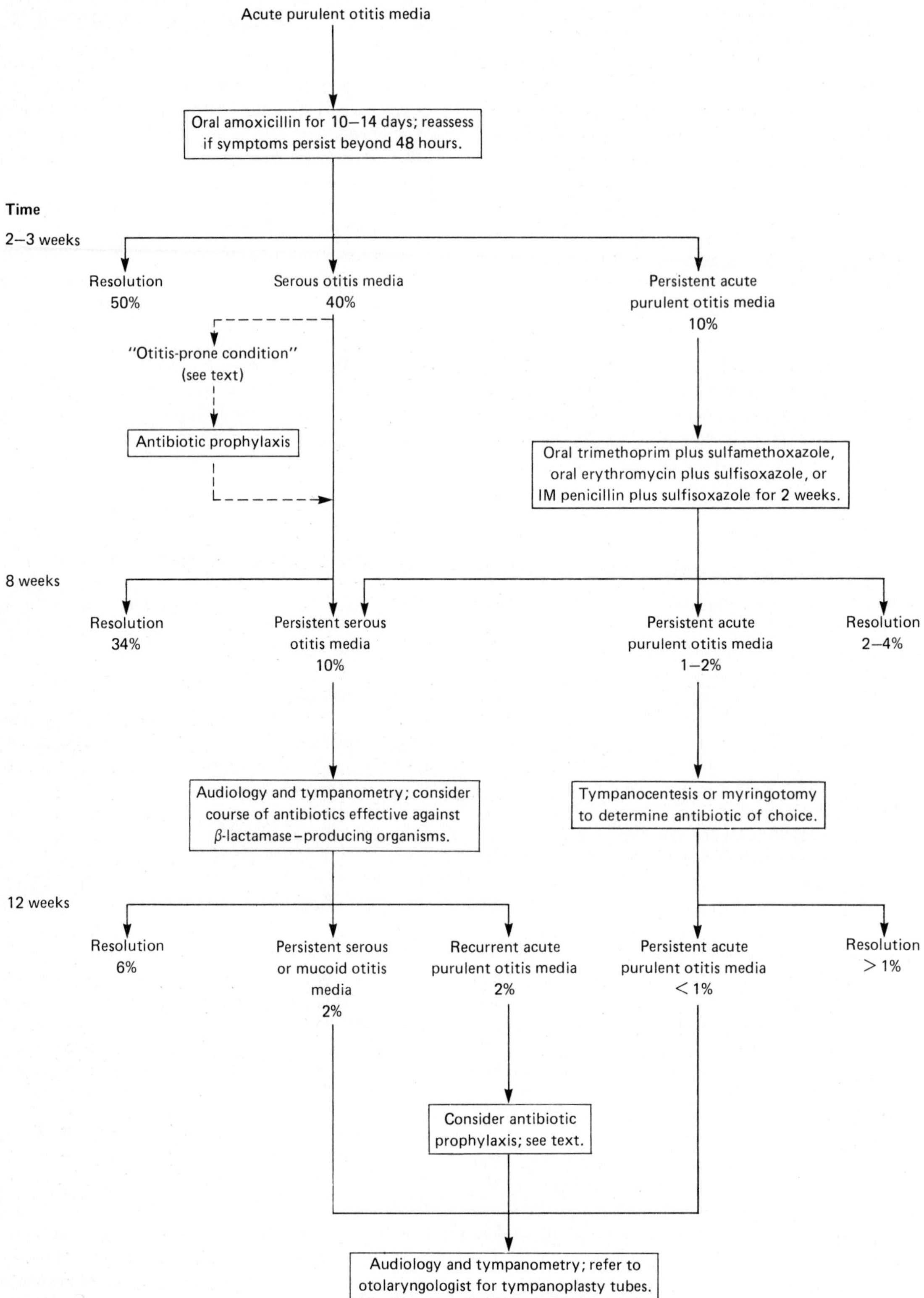

Figure 13–1. Algorithm for the management of otitis media with effusion. For prophylaxis in children with recurrent acute purulent otitis media, see text.

still have residual middle ear effusion, and 10% still have persistent acute infection. Teele (1981) reported that the majority (57%) of children who failed to respond after 36–48 hours of initial therapy with either amoxicillin, trimethoprim plus sulfamethoxazole, or erythromycin plus sulfisoxazole had sterile effusions. Organisms resistant to initial therapy were identified in 19% of repeated cultures of middle ear aspirates. Resistant isolates from children initially treated with amoxicillin were sensitive to trimethoprim plus sulfamethoxazole or erythromycin plus sulfisoxazole and vice versa. Children with persistent infection after a 10- to 14-day course of amoxicillin should receive a full 14-day course of trimethoprim plus sulfamethoxazole or erythromycin plus sulfisoxazole. If the physician is concerned about compliance, the patient can be treated with an intramuscular injection of penicillin G benzathine and procaine combined (Bicillin C-R) and oral sulfisoxazole. If the acute infection still persists after this second course of antibiotics, myringotomy or tympanocentesis should be performed and middle ear secretions cultured to determine the most appropriate antibiotic therapy. Failure of acute otitis media to resolve after a third course or antibiotic therapy requires referral to an otolaryngologist for possible placement of tympanostomy tubes.

Infants less than 2 months of age can be treated with amoxicillin if they are outpatients and mildly ill. These children should be reexamined at 24 and 48 hours. If their condition worsens during this time period, they should be hospitalized. Infants who present with systemic symptoms or who fail to respond to outpatient management require tympanocentesis, blood culture, and usually a lumbar puncture. Ampicillin plus either gentamicin or cefotaxime should be initiated pending results of culture.

Because the risk of infection with a gram-negative enteric organism is high in neonatal intensive care units, hospitalized infants with acute otitis media require tympanocentesis and blood culture.

2. Antibiotic ear drops—If the eardrum has been perforated, there is usually a cloudy to watery material in the ear canal, and antibiotic ear drops are not required. However, the child with considerable purulent drainage from the ear may profit from this adjunctive therapy. The purulent material should be removed by gentle suction, using a syringe and a short plastic tubing such as can be made by cutting a scalp vein needle set. Normal saline solution can be instilled without force and then removed. After this type of cleansing has eliminated the pus, antibiotic-corticosteroid ear drops (eg, Cortisporin Otic) can be instilled 3 times a day. The child should be held with head sideways and stationary for a few minutes after drops are instilled. Cotton plugs are contraindicated.

B. General Measures:

1. Analgesics and antipyretics—An irritable child with an earache requires acetaminophen or even codeine in order to sleep through the first night while on treatment. Young children can be given codeine, 0.5 mg/kg/dose, up to 4 times a day. Codeine is available in several cough medicines in a concentration of 10 mg/tsp. Antipyretics for fever control may be required during the first 1 or 2 days.

2. Oral decongestants—Antihistamine-decongestant combinations have proved to be ineffective in the treatment of otitis media.

3. Reassurance—Some parents are overly concerned about ear infections and their complications. Reassurance should be given as required. There is little danger of permanent hearing loss as long as the prescribed medicines are taken as directed. The child can be allowed to go outside, and the ears need not be covered. Mountain travel is permitted. Swimming is permitted if perforation is not present.

4. Unwarranted measures—Vasoconstrictor nose drops are of no value, since it is nearly impossible to deliver them to the entrance of the auditory tube. Analgesic ear drops have not proved effective for the relief of pain and have the disadvantage of obscuring the field of vision if the tympanic membrane needs to be reexamined.

C. Myringotomy and Tympanocentesis: A common pitfall in therapy is not performing myringotomy or tympanocentesis when it is indicated (see p 322). In a child with an acutely bulging eardrum, myringotomy is indicated if the patient has severe pain (as evidenced by inconsolable screaming) or if recurrent vomiting or ataxia is associated with the ear infection. In these circumstances, myringotomy is more effective than analgesics or antiemetics. Unfortunately, myringotomy does not appear to prevent the development of persistent residual effusions.

Prognosis

With treatment, suppurative complications such as mastoiditis are rare. Temporary hearing loss is common, permanent conductive hearing loss is less common, and permanent sensorineural hearing loss is rare.

Berman SA, Balkany TJ, Simmons MA: Otitis media in infants less than 12 weeks of age: Differing bacteriology among in-patients and out-patients. *J Pediatr* 1978;**93**:453.

Berman SA, Lauer BA: A controlled trial of cefaclor versus amoxicillin for treatment of acute otitis media in early infancy. *Pediatr Infect Dis* 1983;**2**:30.

Blumer JL, Bertino JS, Husak MP: Comparison of cefaclor and trimethoprim-sulfamethoxazole in the treatment of acute otitis media. *Pediatr Infect Dis* 1984;**3**:25.

Boder FF: Conjunctivitis-otitis syndrome. *Pediatrics* 1982; **69**:695.

Chang MJ et al: *Chlamydia trachomatis* in otitis media in children. *Pediatr Infect Dis* 1982;**1**:95.

Klein BS, Dollete FR, Yolken RH: The role of respiratory syncytial virus and other viral pathogens in acute otitis media. *J Pediatr* 1982;**101**:16.

Klein JO, Teele DW: Isolation of viruses and *Mycoplasma* from middle ear effusions: A review. *Ann Otol Rhinol Laryngol* 1976;**85**:140.

Paradise JL: Otitis media in infants and children. *Pediatrics* 1980;**65**:917.

Randall JE, Hendley JO: A decongestant-antihistamine mixture in the prevention of otitis media in children with colds. *Pediatrics* 1979;**63:**483.

Rodriguez WJ et al: Erythromycin-sulfisoxazole for persistent acute otitis media due to ampicillin-resistant *Haemophilus influenzae. Pediatr Infect Dis* 1983;**2:**27.

Schaefer C et al: Illnesses in infants born to women with *Chlamydia trachomatis* infection. *Am J Dis Child* 1985;**139:**127.

Schwartz RH: Bacteriology of otitis media: A review. *Otolaryngol Head Neck Surg* 1981;**89:**444.

Schwartz RH, Rodriguez WJ, Schwartz DM: Office myringotomy for acute otitis media: Its value in preventing middle ear effusion. *Laryngoscope* 1981;**91:**616.

Shurin PA et al: *Branhamella catarrhalis* in otitis media. *Pediatr Infect Dis* 1983;**2:**34.

Shurin PA et al: Trimethoprim-sulfamethoxazole compared with ampicillin in treatment of acute otitis media. *J Pediatr* 1976;**88:**646.

Teele DE et al: Bacteriology of acute otitis media unresponsive to initial antimicrobial therapy. *J Pediatr* 1981;**98:**537.

2. ACUTE BULLOUS MYRINGITIS

In acute bullous myringitis, bullae form between the outer and middle layers of the tympanic membrane. In the past, this was considered to be always due to viral infections. More recent studies demonstrate that 50–75% of affected patients have an underlying acute purulent otitis media. The organisms isolated in cases of acute bullous myringitis are similar to those found in acute otitis media. A causative role for *Mycoplasma pneumoniae* or viruses in cases of bullous myringitis is not confirmed.

The patient usually complains of ear pain on the involved side. Examination of the ear reveals 1–3 bullae that may cover 20–90% of the drum surface. They are thin-walled and often sagging in appearance, and they often contain a straw-colored fluid. There is minimal erythema.

Antibiotics are prescribed as for acute otitis media. Analgesics are sometimes indicated. The bullae do not have to be opened unless they are causing significant pain. They can be easily opened by nicking with a myringotomy knife or spinal needle.

Follow-up care is the same as that described for acute purulent otitis media.

Klein JO, Teele DW: Isolation of viruses and *Mycoplasma* from middle ear effusions: A review. *Ann Otol Rhinol Laryngol* 1976;**85:**140.

Roberts DB: The etiology of bullous myringitis and the role of *Mycoplasma* in ear disease: A review. *Pediatrics* 1980;**65:**761.

3. SEROUS OTITIS MEDIA

Essentials of Diagnosis

- Painless hearing loss of 15–20 dB.
- Dull, immobile tympanic membrane.

General Considerations

Serous otitis media results when the auditory tube fails to clear secretions present in the middle ear space. The effusion resembles serum transudate, and histopathologic examination of the middle ear shows subepithelial edema. The effusion is usually associated with a low-grade (15–20 dB) conductive hearing loss. Serous effusions may either precede or follow purulent otitis media. Acute serous otitis media can occur in association with transient auditory tube dysfunction in the absence of a middle ear infection. This phenomenon usually occurs during colds or bouts of allergic rhinitis. It can also follow overly vigorous nose blowing. In older children and adolescents, the serous effusion usually resolves in 4–7 days. Residual serous otitis media following appropriate antibiotic therapy for acute otitis media occurs in 40–50% of children. These residual effusions clear spontaneously within 2 months in 85% of cases.

Persistent serous effusions may be associated with a low-grade bacterial infection, especially infection with β-lactamase-producing organisms such as *Haemophilus influenzae, Branhamella catarrhalis, Staphylococcus aureus,* and penicillin-resistant *Streptococcus pneumoniae*. Clinical resolution of acute otitis media may not correlate well with bacteriologic cure. In aspirates of serous effusions obtained during the surgical placement of tympanoplasty tubes, organisms are isolated in about 50% of cases. The most common pathogenic organisms isolated are *H influenzae* (25% of cases), *S pneumoniae* (10%), and *S aureus* (7%). Many of the *H influenzae* strains (45%) are β-lactamase-positive.

Clinical Findings

Children with serous otitis media are usually asymptomatic and have hearing loss. The patient may complain of a feeling of fullness in the ear. An older patient may compare the feeling with "talking inside a barrel." In the preverbal child, hearing loss should be suspected if irritability, inattentiveness, or increased behavior problems are noted. Unlike acute purulent otitis media, there is minimal pain.

The tympanic membrane may appear mildly infected and dull or have a normal appearance. Mobility is diminished or absent. When fluid levels or air bubbles are visualized, the effusion is in a stage of resolution, with auditory tube function improving. When auditory tube dysfunction results in persistent negative pressure in the middle ear space, the tympanic membrane appears retracted, and the position of the short process of the right malleus changes from 7 o'clock to 9 o'clock. Tympanic membrane mobility is altered; ie, the membrane may move only when negative pressure is applied.

The most common complication of serous otitis media is conductive hearing loss, which may adversely affect language development, intellectual functioning, and academic performance. The presence of a serous effusion predisposes the child to another episode of acute otitis media. In some children with recurrent acute otitis media, effusion persists in the middle ear between episodes and causes a cycle of acute otitis media alternating with serous otitis media.

Treatment

Management of serous otitis media is outlined in Fig 13–1. When serous otitis media has persisted longer than 6 weeks, institute a 14-day course of one of the following regimens to treat β-lactamase-producing organisms: trimethoprim plus sulfamethoxazole; erythromycin plus sulfisoxazole; cefaclor alone; or ampicillin plus clavulanic acid.

The efficacy of oral decongestants and antihistamines in preventing or treating serous effusions is controversial. Most studies report that these drugs are not effective.

Healy GB: Antimicrobial therapy for chronic otitis media with effusion. In: *Proceedings of the Third International Symposium: Recent Advances in Otitis Media With Effusion.* Lim DJ (editor). Decker & Co., 1984.

Lim DJ: Pathogenesis of otitis media with effusion. *Pediatr Infect Dis* 1982;**1(Suppl 5):**S14.

Marchant CD et al: A randomized controlled trial of cefaclor compared with trimethoprim-sulfamethoxazole for treatment of acute otitis media. *J Pediatr* 1984;**105:**633.

Marks NJ, Mills RP, Shaheen OH: A controlled trial of cotrimoxazole therapy in serous otitis media. *J Laryngol Otol* 1981;**95:**1003.

Moran DM et al: The use of an antihistamine-decongestant in conjunction with an anti-infective drug in the treatment of acute otitis media. *J Pediatr* 1982;**101:**132.

Olson AL et al: Prevention and therapy of serous otitis media by oral decongestant: A double-blind study in pediatric practice. *Pediatrics* 1978;**61:**679.

4. MUCOID OTITIS MEDIA

Essentials of Diagnosis

- Dull, immobile tympanic membrane.
- Hearing loss of 25–50 dB.
- Type B pattern on tympanogram (Fig 13–3).

General Considerations

Bacteria have been isolated from approximately 50% of mucoid effusions at the time of insertion of tympanoplasty tubes. The most common pathogenic organisms isolated from these effusions are *Haemophilus influenzae* (25% of cases), *Streptococcus pneumoniae* (10%), and *Staphylococcus aureus* (7%). Many of the *H influenzae* strains (45%) are β-lactamase-positive. *Staphylococcus epidermidis* and diphtheroids are isolated in 35% of effusions. Evidence supporting the pathogenic role of these organisms includes the findings of type-specific antibody; studies in animals also suggest that the middle ear space should be sterile. Pathogenic factors that may contribute to the persistence of middle ear effusions include the adverse effects of gram-negative endotoxins on the middle ear space as well as the chronic inflammatory response secondary to persistent bacterial infection.

Mucoid (secretory) otitis media is characterized by a thick and tenacious middle ear effusion that contains high levels of immunoglobulin. The otitis appears to be related to type 1 and type 3 allergic reactions associated with recurrent low-level exposure to bacterial antigens. Evidence supporting a type 1 reaction includes the documentation of a higher level of IgE in mucoid effusions than in blood and the presence of IgE plasma cells in effusions. A type 3 reaction is supported by findings of B cells, specific antibacterial antibody, and depressed total hemolytic complement levels in mucoid effusions.

Most cases of mucoid otitis media are due to primary congenital auditory tube dysfunction. On occasion, a contributing factor such as the following may be uncovered.

(1) Allergic rhinitis can precipitate mucoid otitis media and is diagnosed by the presence of frequent episodes of clear nasal discharge, sneezing, nasal itching, and over 20% eosinophils on a stained smear of nasal discharge.

(2) Persistent acute purulent otitis media, if inadequately treated, may convert to mucoid otitis media.

(3) Bottle feeding in a supine position predisposes the child to persistent serous and mucoid otitis media. Bottle-propping should be discontinued and the child fed in a more erect posture.

(4) Certain congenital malformations can lead to recurrent ear problems. Chronic mucoid otitis media is seen in 90% of children with cleft palate and 40% of children with submucous clefts. Cystic fibrosis, trisomy 21, hypothyroidism, and Turner's syndrome also predispose to recurrent ear problems.

(5) Marked adenoidal hyperplasia can occasionally block the exit of the auditory tubes.

(6) Nasopharyngeal neoplasms can also produce auditory tube obstruction.

(7) The child's risk of developing mucoid effusion may be increased if the parents smoke.

When mucoid otitis media has been present for 3 months, the contributing factors mentioned above should be investigated.

Clinical Findings

Like patients with serous otitis media, those with mucoid otitis media are usually asymptomatic or complain of a feeling of fullness in the ear. The tympanic membrane commonly appears dull and opaque; in severe cases, it may have a bluish tint. Tympanic membrane mobility is usually markedly diminished.

Complications

Children with mucoid otitis media are at increased risk of developing retraction pockets, which predispose to cholesteatoma and other complications such as necrosis of the ossicles and cholesterol granuloma.

Mucoid otitis media is associated with a hearing loss of 25–50 dB, which may persist for a prolonged period of time. A persistent, moderate hearing loss early in life is likely to result in delays in language development and adversely affect intellectual functioning.

Treatment

A. Medical Measures: If mucoid otitis media has persisted longer than 8 weeks, institute a 2- to 4-week course of one of the following regimens to treat β-lactamase-producing organisms: trimethoprim plus sulfamethoxazole; erythromycin plus sulfisoxazole; cefaclor alone; or ampicillin plus clavulanic acid.

The role of systemic corticosteroids in the treatment of mucoid otitis media is unclear at this time and requires further investigation. Oral decongestants and antihistamines have not proved to be effective for treatment.

B. Surgical Treatment: If manifestations of mucoid otitis media (ie, documented effusion, hearing loss >20 dB, and abnormal findings on tympanogram) have failed to resolve after a 3-month period despite a course of antibiotics, the patient should be referred to an otolaryngologist for insertion of tympanoplasty tubes. A child with signs of partial resolution noted on otoscopy, audiogram, or tympanogram should be followed for another month prior to referral. A child whose tympanic membrane is severely retracted and whose tympanogram shows a peak at negative pressure should be followed for the development of persistent retraction pockets. Persistent retraction pockets should also be treated with tympanoplasty tubes.

Myringotomy followed by insertion of tympanoplasty tubes (polyethylene flanged ventilation tubes) has given excellent results in this disorder as long as the tubes are in place. The tubes permit pressure equalization and drying of the middle ear cavity without a functional auditory tube. The hearing returns to normal with the tube in place. This procedure can be done in an outpatient setting by an otolaryngologist. The long-term efficacy of tympanoplasty tubes has not been well evaluated. One study from Great Britain with bilateral chronic serous otitis media failed to show a significant postsurgical difference in hearing after 6 months to 5 years between the ear in which a tube was inserted and the control ear. Possible side effects of tympanoplasty tubes are persistent perforations, cholesteatoma, secondary infection, mastoiditis, tympanic membrane scarring or atrophy, retraction pockets, dislocation of the tube into the middle ear cavity, and the risks of anesthesia. Removal of the adenoids is rarely helpful.

Fraser JG, Menta M, Fraser PM: The medical treatment of secretory otitis media: A clinical trial of three commonly used regimens. *J Laryngol Otol* 1977;**91:**757.

Grundfast KM: A review of the efficacy of systemically administered decongestants in the prevention and treatment of otitis media. *Otolaryngol Head Neck Surg* 1981;**89:**432.

Healey GB, Smith HG: Current concepts in the management of otitis media with effusion. *Am J Otolaryngol* 1981;**2:**138.

Kilby D, Richards SH, Hart G: Grommets and glue ears: Two-year results. *J Laryngol Otol* 1972;**86:**881.

Paradise JL: Tympanostomy tubes: Rationale, results, reservations, and recommendations. *Pediatrics* 1977;**60:**86.

Schwartz RH: Otitis media with effusion: Results of treatment with a short course of oral prednisone or intranasal beclomethasone aerosol. *Otolaryngol Head Neck Surg* 1981;**89:**386.

Sorri et al: Can secretory otitis media be prevented by oral decongestants? *Acta Otolaryngol [Suppl]* 1982;**386:**115.

5. RECURRENT OR PERSISTENT OTITIS MEDIA WITH EFFUSION (The "Otitis-Prone Condition")

Essentials of Diagnosis

- Two episodes of acute otitis media in a patient under 12 months of age.
- Three episodes of acute otitis media within a 6-month period in a patient over 12 months of age.
- Middle ear effusion persisting 3 months or longer.

General Considerations

Specific conditions that cause auditory tube dysfunction and predispose children to early and recurrent otitis media include viral upper respiratory tract infections, allergic and vasomotor rhinitis, trisomy 21, cystic fibrosis, hypothyroidism, and anatomic abnormalities such as cleft palate, obstructing adenoids, and nasopharyngeal tumors. It is likely that auditory tube dysfunction and abnormalities in immune response are interrelated and that a primary disturbance in one area results in a secondary disorder in the other.

Infants who experience their initial episode of otitis media in the first 2 or 3 months of life are more likely to have bilateral chronic otitis media or recurrent episodes of acute otitis media during the first year. Recurrence or persistence of disease places infants and children at risk for permanent ear damage and fluctuating or persistent hearing loss. Studies have shown that the amount of time effusion is present during the first 6–12 months of life has the strongest correlation with delays in language development at 3 years of age. Therefore, early identification of otitis-prone infants and children is essential for prevention of adverse sequelae.

Management

A. Identification and Monitoring of Otitis-Prone Infants and Children: The criteria for identifying otitis-prone children are listed above (see Essentials of Diagnosis). Because episodes of acute otitis media in infancy are frequently asymptomatic, high-risk infants require close monitoring and follow-up. Tympanometry can be used as an adjunctive method to monitor those over 7 months of age. Audiologic testing should be performed, and patients with conductive hearing loss that persists for longer than 3 months should be referred to an otolaryngologist. Language development should be evaluated at 18, 24, and 36 months by use of the Early Language Milestone (ELM) scale. An appropriate home language stimulation program and guidelines for the management of behavior problems related to conductive hearing loss should be instituted for all infants and children with impaired hearing. (See Detection and Management of Hearing Deficits, below.)

B. Antibiotic Prophylaxis: Prophylaxis with sulfisoxazole, 30–40 mg/kg orally twice daily, should be started following the resolution of the second episode of acute otitis media in infants under 1 year of age and the third episode within a 6-month period after 1 year of age. Sulfisoxazole should be continued for 3 months. During the next 3–6 months, it is often helpful to advise parents to restart the antibiotic at the first sign of a cold and give it for a minimum of 1 week or until cold symptoms resolve. This program of prophylaxis has reduced the frequency of acute otitis media from 20 to 5.6%.

C. Management of Chronic Effusions: Infants in whom middle ear effusion has persisted for 2 months and who have not received a second course of antibiotics should be given appropriate antibiotic treatment to cover β-lactamase-producing organisms. Treatment consists of a 14-day course of one of the following regimens: erythromycin plus sulfisoxazole; trimethoprim plus sulfamethoxazole; ampicillin plus clavulanic acid; or cefaclor alone.

The value of a course of systemic corticosteroids (prednisone, 1–2 mg/kg/d) in combination with an antibiotic is controversial. If hearing loss or middle ear effusion persists for 3 months or if antibiotic prophylaxis fails to prevent recurrent acute episodes, refer the patient to an otolaryngologist for insertion of tympanoplasty tubes.

Berman S: Otitis media with effusions: Its relationship to language development, intellectual functioning and academic performance. *Adv Behav Pediatr* 1981;**2:**129.

Berman S, Murphy JR: Persistent and recurrent otitis media: A review of the "otitis-prone" condition. *Primary Care* 1984;**11:**407.

Biedel CW: Modification of recurrent otitis media by short-term sulfonamide therapy. *Am J Dis Child* 1978;**132:**681.

Gebhart DE: Tympanostomy tubes in the otitis media prone child. *Laryngoscope* 1978;**91:**849.

Howie WM et al: Use of pneumococcal polysaccharide vaccine in preventing otitis media in infants: Different results between racial groups. *Pediatrics* 1984;**73:**79.

Liston TE et al: The bacteriology of recurrent otitis media and the effect of sulfisoxazole chemoprophylaxis. *Pediatr Infect Dis* 1984;**3:**20.

Marchant CD et al: Course and outcome of otitis media in early infancy: A prospective study. *J Pediatr* 1984;**104:**826.

Perrin JM et al: Sulfisoxazole as chemoprophylaxis for recurrent otitis media. *N Engl J Med* 1974;**291:**644.

Teele DW et al: Otitis media with effusion during the first three years of life and development of speech and language. *Pediatrics* 1984;**74:**282.

Varsano I et al: Sulfisoxazole prophylaxis of middle ear effusion and recurrent acute otitis media. *Am J Dis Child* 1985;**139:**632.

ACUTE BAROTITIS

Sudden changes in barometric pressure, as can occur with diving or flying, can lead to an acute serous effusion into the middle ear cavity. The history itself is diagnostic. The patient presents with complaints of severe pain and loss of hearing in the affected ear. Otoscopic examination usually reveals a hemorrhagic tympanic membrane.

The process is self-limited, lasting for 2–3 days. The principal therapeutic agent is an analgesic, usually codeine. Decongestants are also prescribed, but antibiotics are not necessary. The prognosis is excellent. The patient should be taught techniques for prevention, such as use of a nasal decongestant spray before descent and autoinflation maneuvers during descent.

ACUTE TRAUMA TO THE MIDDLE EAR

Head injuries, a blow to the ear canal, sudden impact with water, blast injuries, or the insertion of pointed instruments into the ear canal can lead to perforation of the tympanic membrane or hematoma of the middle ear. One study reported that 50% of serious penetrating wounds of the tympanic membrane were due to parental use of a cotton-tipped swab.

Treatment of middle ear hematomas consists mainly of watchful waiting. Prophylactic antibiotics are not necessary unless signs of superimposed infection appear. The prognosis for unimpaired hearing depends upon whether or not the ossicles are dislocated or fractured in the process. The patient needs to be followed by audiometrics until hearing has returned to normal.

Traumatic perforations of the tympanic membrane often do not heal spontaneously and should be referred to an otolaryngologist. Perforations caused by a foreign body must be seen immediately, whereas those due to impact can be seen within 24 hours. Early debridement and placement of a graft virtually ensure closure.

Silverstein H et al: Penetration wounds of the tympanic membrane and ossicular chain. *Trans Am Acad Ophthalmol Otolaryngol* 1973;**77:**125.

CHRONIC PERFORATION OF THE TYMPANIC MEMBRANE

Essentials of Diagnosis

- Painless otorrhea, intermittent or persistent.
- Perforated tympanic membrane.
- Conductive hearing loss of 20–40 dB.

General Considerations

A perforation of the tympanic membrane can be considered chronic if it lasts for longer than 1 month. Most perforations seen with acute otitis media heal within 2 weeks. Chronic perforations usually can be prevented by aggressive early treatment of acute otitis media. Reinfections of the exposed middle ear cavity are the most common finding in this disorder.

Clinical Findings

A. Symptoms and Signs: A perforation is always present. If no infection is present, the middle ear cavity is seen to contain thickened, inflamed mucosa. If superimposed infection is present, serous or purulent drainage will be seen, and the middle ear cavity may contain granulation tissue or even polyps. A conductive hearing loss will usually be present depending on the size of the perforation.

The site of perforation is important. Central perforations are usually relatively safe from cholesteatoma formation. Peripheral perforations, especially in the pars flaccida, impose a risk for development of cholesteatoma because the ear canal epithelium adjacent to the perforation may invade it. The condition is almost always painless.

B. Laboratory Findings: Any discharge present should be cultured before treatment is initiated. Sensitivity tests are often necessary because the most common organisms are *Pseudomonas, Escherichia coli,* and staphylococci. A PPD test should be done to rule out tuberculosis.

C. X-Ray Findings: Mastoid films are helpful if a superimposed mastoiditis is suspected.

Complications

This disorder can have serious complications, but they are rare with proper therapy. They occur mainly in unattended cases of superinfected, chronically perforated eardrums. Cholesteatoma is the most common complication and can be suspected if the discharge is foul-smelling and if a white, oily mass is seen within the perforation. The associated perforation may be pinpoint in size. If the discharge does not respond to 2 weeks of aggressive therapy, mastoiditis or granulations are probably present. Serious central nervous system complications such as extradural abscess, subdural abscess, brain abscess, meningitis, labyrinthitis, or lateral sinus thrombophlebitis can occur with extension of this process. Therefore, patients with facial palsy, vertigo, or other central nervous system signs should be referred immediately to an otolaryngologist. Otogenous tetanus is another possible sequela.

Treatment

A. Specific Measures: If a serous or purulent discharge is present, antibiotic-corticosteroid ear drops (eg, Coly-Mycin S Otic, Cortisporin Otic) should be instilled 3 times daily. This should be continued for 1 week after the discharge has resolved. Both products contain polymyxin and neomycin. *Pseudomonas* is sensitive to the former. Gentamicin ear drops are also useful. The ear drops will not be effective unless the ear canals are aspirated before the drops are instilled. If the discharge is purulent or foul-smelling or if systemic signs are present, systemic antibiotics should also be prescribed. A cephalosporin can be given at the outset and another drug substituted depending on the culture results. This can be continued for 2 weeks. If there is any recurrence of discharge, antibiotic ear drops should be instilled immediately.

B. Surgical Treatment: Repair of the defect in the tympanic membrane is rarely successful during the time period when children have frequent colds and recurrent auditory tube dysfunction. Therefore, tympanoplasty is usually deferred until age 9–12. The perforated eardrum can be repaired earlier if the nonperforated one remains free of infection and effusion for a year. If drainage persists despite treatment, the patient must be referred to an otologist to rule out cholesteatoma, mastoiditis, or other complication.

C. Follow-Up Care: The patient should be seen once a week until the discharge has cleared and about once every 3 months until surgery has been done. This follow-up is imperative to prevent any serious complications.

D. Prevention of Recurrences:

1. Prophylactic ear drops—For the 1-month period following any flare-ups of otorrhea, ear drops consisting of povidone-iodine solution (not tincture) should be instilled in each ear once daily.

2. Bathing—Before bathing and hair washing, cotton plugs should be put in the ear and the surface completely covered with petrolatum ointment.

3. Swimming—Swimming should be discouraged unless it is a matter of great importance to the patient, in which case it can be continued using custom-fitted ear molds plus a bathing cap for girls or a scuba cap for boys. Diving, jumping into the water, and underwater swimming are absolutely forbidden.

4. Unwarranted measures—The constant use of a cotton plug in the ear canal will increase the risk of superinfection. Exposure to air is helpful in the treatment.

Prognosis

With treatment, 80–90% of perforations heal spontaneously by 1 year. The remainder require careful follow-up. With proper care, these patients will be in good condition for tympanoplasty at age 9–12.

Fairbanks DN: Antibiotic ear drop use in the nonintact tympanic membrane. *Pediatr Ann* 1984;**13:**411.

Felder H: Chronic otitis media in children. *Pediatr Ann* 1976;**5:**474.

Fischer GW et al: Otogenous tetanus: Sequelae of chronic ear infections. *Am J Dis Child* 1977;**131:**445.

MacAdam AM et al: Tuberculous otomastoiditis in children. *Am J Dis Child* 1977;**131:**152.

MASTOIDITIS

Infection of the mastoid antrum and air cells may follow an episode of untreated or improperly treated acute otitis media. The most common etiologic agents are *Streptococcus pyogenes, Streptococcus pneumo-*

niae, and *Staphylococcus aureus*. *Haemophilus influenzae* causes mastoiditis much less frequently than expected. Other agents that can cause this disease include *Pseudomonas, Mycobacterium,* and enteropathic gram-negative rods. Anaerobic organisms appear to play a role in chronic mastoiditis; however, there are no data on how frequently they cause acute mastoiditis.

Mastoiditis is unusual before age 2, when air cells begin to develop.

Clinical Findings

The principal complaints are usually postauricular pain and fever. On examination, the mastoid area is often swollen and reddened. In the late stage, it may be fluctuant. The earliest finding is severe tenderness upon mastoid percussion. Acute otitis media is almost always present. Late findings are a pinna that is pushed forward by postauricular swelling and an ear canal that is narrowed in the posterior superior wall because of pressure from the mastoid abscess. In infants less than 1 year of age, the swelling occurs superior to the ear and pushes the pinna downward rather than outward.

Mastoiditis is a clinical diagnosis. It cannot be diagnosed on the basis of x-rays alone. In the acute phase, there is diffuse inflammatory clouding of the mastoid cells as in every case of acute purulent otitis media. Only later is there evidence of bony destruction and resorption of the mastoid air cells.

Complications

Meningitis is a complication in about 9% of cases of acute mastoiditis. This infection should be suspected when a child has high fever, stiff neck, severe headache, or other meningeal signs. A lumbar puncture should be performed to accurately diagnose this condition. Brain abscess occurs in 2% of cases and may be associated with persistent headache, recurring fever, or changes in sensorium. A CT scan should be performed.

Treatment & Prognosis

The patient must be hospitalized because this disorder represents osteitis at this site. Before therapy is initiated, myringotomy (see below) should be performed in order to obtain material for culture and also to relieve the pressure in the middle ear-mastoid space.

The initial management of uncomplicated acute mastoiditis includes intravenous antibiotic therapy and possibly surgery. Results of gram-stained smears taken during tympanocentesis may help in the choice of antibiotics. Ampicillin and nafcillin appear to be a reasonable initial choice. Indications for immediate surgery include the clear evidence of a major complication such as meningitis, brain abscess, cavernous sinus thrombosis, acute suppurative labyrinthitis, or facial palsy. Some otolaryngologists consider the destruction of septal bone (osteitis) and resorption of the mastoid air cells an indication for surgery.

Oral antibiotics should be continued for 4–6 weeks after the patient is discharged.

The prognosis is good if treatment is started early and continued until the process is inactive.

Brook I: Aerobic and anaerobic bacteriology of chronic mastoiditis in children. *Am J Dis Child* 1981;**135**:478.

Ginsburg CM, Rudoy R, Nelson JD: Acute mastoiditis in infants and children. *Clin Pediatr (Phila)* 1980;**19**:549.

Macadam AM, Rubio T: Tuberculous otomastoiditis in children. *Am J Dis Child* 1977;**131**:152.

Meyerhoff WL, Gates GA, Montalbo PJ: *Pseudomonas* mastoiditis. *Laryngoscope* 1977;**87**:483.

Ostfeld E, Rubinstein E: Acute gram-negative bacillary infections of middle ear and mastoid. *Ann Otol Rhinol Laryngol* 1980;**89**:33.

Shaffer HL, Gates GA, Meyerhoff WL: Acute mastoiditis and cholesteatoma. *Otolaryngology* 1978;**86**:394.

Venezio FR et al: Complications of mastoiditis with special emphasis on venous sinus thrombosis. *J Pediatr* 1982; **101**:509.

CONGENITAL EAR MALFORMATIONS

Agenesis of the external ear canal results in deafness that requires evaluation in the first month of life by hearing specialists and an otolaryngologist.

"Lop ears" (Dumbo ears) lead to much teasing and ridicule. To prevent the secondary emotional problems, these can be corrected at age 5 or 6 by plastic surgery. The ear is of approximately adult size by then, and there is little risk of affecting growth.

An ear is low-set if the upper pole is below eye level. This condition is often associated with renal malformations (eg, Potter's syndrome), and an intravenous urogram is helpful.

Preauricular tags, ectopic cartilages, fistulas, sinuses, or cysts require surgical correction, mainly for cosmetic reasons. Most preauricular pits are asymptomatic. If one should become infected, it should be treated with antibiotics and referred to an otolaryngologist for eventual resection. Children with any of the above findings should have their hearing tested.

Jaffe BF: Pinna anomalies associated with congenital conductive hearing loss. *Pediatrics* 1976;**57**:332.

OTITIS EXTERNA

Otitis externa is an inflammation of the skin lining the ear canals. The most common cause is accumulation of water in the ear, leading to maceration and desquamation of the lining and conversion of the pH from acid to alkaline (eg, from swimming or frequent showers). Swimming pools are worse than lakes because the chlorine kills the normal ear flora. Other causes are trauma to the ear canal from using cotton-tipped applicators to clean it or poorly fitted ear plugs for swimming; contact dermatitis due to hair sprays, perfumes, or self-administered ear drops; and chronic drainage from a perforated tympanic membrane. The superimposed infections are often due to *Staphylococcus aureus* or *Pseudomonas aeruginosa.*

Clinical Findings

There is pain and itching in the ear, especially with chewing or pressure on the tragus. Movement of the pinna or tragus causes considerable pain. Drainage is minimal. The ear canal is grossly swollen, and the patient resists any attempt to insert an ear speculum. Debris is noticeable in the canal. It is often impossible to visualize the tympanic membrane. Hearing is normal unless complete occlusion has occurred.

Treatment

Topical treatment usually suffices. The crucial initial step is removal of the desquamated epithelium and moist cerumen. This debris can be irrigated out or suctioned out using warm half-strength white vinegar or Burow's solution (1 packet of Domeboro Powder to 250 mL tap water). Once the ear canal is open, a combination of antibiotic-corticosteroid ear drops (eg, Cortisporin Otic) is given 3–4 times daily. The corticosteroid is needed to reduce the severe inflammatory response. The insertion of a wick is painful and usually unnecessary. A follow-up visit in 1 week to document an intact tympanic membrane is imperative.

Oral antibiotics are indicated if any signs of invasiveness are present, such as fever, cellulitis of the auricles, or tender postauricular lymph nodes. Penicillin is an appropriate initial drug while awaiting the results of culture of the ear canal discharge. Systemic antibiotics alone without topical treatment will not clear up otitis externa. Analgesics—sometimes codeine—may be required temporarily. Children predisposed to this problem should instill 2–3 drops of 1:1 white vinegar/70% ethyl alcohol into their ears before and after swimming. During the acute phase, swimming should be avoided if possible. A cotton earplug is not helpful and may be harmful.

Marcy SM: Infections of the external ear. *Pediatr Infect Dis* 1985;**4:**192.

EAR CANAL FOREIGN BODY

Numerous objects can be inserted into the ear canal by a child. An insect in the ear should be killed with alcohol solution (gin will do for telephone advice). The patient should be immobilized on a papoose board with the head firmly grasped by an assistant.

An attempt should be made first to remove a foreign body by straightening the ear canal by pulling on the pinna and gently shaking the child's head. If a smooth object such as a bead is present, a cotton-tipped applicator with warmed dental wax or collodion should be inserted and placed against the object for 1–2 minutes, after which time it can be removed. An object with an irregular surface can perhaps be removed with a bayonet forceps. A steel object (eg, ball bearing) can sometimes be removed with a magnetic probe. A right-angled hook or custom-designed paper clip can sometimes be inserted past the object and withdrawn, pushing the object ahead of it.

If these methods fail, irrigation can be attempted. The tube should be inserted past the object so the stream rebounds against the tympanic membrane and flushes the object out. Another approach for smooth objects is to use a suction machine. The end of the rubber tubing forms a better seal with the foreign body if it is first coated with petrolatum.

Irrigation with water is contraindicated with vegetable materials because they swell on contact with water. They can be irrigated with a 70% alcohol solution. Wet tissue paper is also difficult to remove.

If the object is large or wedged in place, the patient should be referred to an otolaryngologist early rather than risk damage to the eardrum or ossicles.

Cunningham DG, Zanga JR: Myiasis of the external auditory meatus. *J Pediatr* 1974;**84:**857.

Stool SE, McConnell CS: Foreign bodies in pediatric otolaryngology: Some diagnostic and therapeutic pointers. *Clin Pediatr (Phila)* 1973;**12:**113.

EAR CANAL FURUNCLE

A furuncle in the outer cartilaginous portions of the ear canal is most often caused by *Staphylococcus aureus*. The patient usually complains of pain in the outer part of the ear opening and resists insertion of a speculum. A small red lump will be noticed by simply looking through the otoscope with a large speculum that is not inserted. Treatment consists of topical bacitracin ointment. When the furuncle has pointed, incision and drainage should be carried out, usually with a needle. Spread of this infection is rare; if it occurs, dicloxacillin, 25 mg/kg/d orally, should be added to the regimen. Recurrences point to manipulation of the ear canal (eg, with dirty fingernails, paper clips, hairpins, or cotton swabs).

EAR CANAL TRAUMA

Children may insert sticks or other objects into the ear canal. This normally results in abrasion of the ear canal, with more bleeding than might be suspected. Parents cause similar injuries by overzealous attempts to remove earwax. It is mandatory that the tympanic membrane be examined. If it is free of injury, no treatment is necessary, since the abrasions heal readily.

HEMATOMA OF THE PINNA

Trauma to the earlobe can result in the formation of a hematoma between the perichondrium and cartilage. The hematoma appears as a boggy purple swelling of the upper half of the earlobe. If this is unattended, it can cause pressure necrosis of the underlying cartilage and result in a boxer's "cauliflower ear." To prevent this cosmetic handicap, patients should all be referred to a surgeon for aspiration and the application of a carefully molded pressure dressing.

PIERCED EAR PROBLEMS

The most common complication of ear piercing is superimposed infection, usually with *Staphylococcus aureus*. A small abscess develops at the site, and purulent material drains from both sides of the perforation. The infection usually stems from the use of contaminated needles or posts (eg, keeping the channel open with a piece of straw). This localized infection can occasionally progress to life-threatening staphylococcal septicemia. Other potential complications are viral hepatitis, erysipelas, and keloid formation.

Treatment of a primary infection requires removal of the foreign body (the earring); administration of dicloxacillin, 25 mg/kg/d orally for 5 days while culture is being performed; and use of local bacitracin ointment. Infections acquired later can often be aborted with bacitracin ointment applied to the posts and reinserted 3 times a day.

Especially if they are made of nickel, earrings can occasionally cause dermatitis of the earlobe. If this is suspected, the earrings should be removed and replaced with 14 K gold or stainless steel earrings and topical corticosteroids applied to the posts several times a day.

A serious complication of pierced ears is to have the earring post grasped by a child in play and completely pulled through the earlobe, leaving a jagged laceration. The scar that develops can lead to deformity of the earlobe and may require plastic surgery. Another potential complication in infants is removal of the earring and putting it in the mouth, which may cause choking or aspiration. For this reason, the ears should not be pierced until the child is at least 8 years of age. Ideally, the child should give consent for this procedure and be a teenager before it is performed. The physician can train the office nurse to pierce ears under aseptic conditions with equipment purchased from a surgical supply house. This would prevent the majority of primary infections that occur.

Cortese TA, Dickey RA: Complications of ear piercing. *Am Fam Physician* (Aug) 1971;**4:**66.

Johnson CJ et al: Earpiercing and hepatitis. *JAMA* 1974; **227:**1165.

Lovejoy FH: Life-threatening staphylococcal disease following ear piercing. *Pediatrics* 1970;**46:**301.

THE EAR: DIAGNOSTIC & THERAPEUTIC PROCEDURES

DETECTION & MANAGEMENT OF HEARING DEFICITS*

Hearing deficits are classified as conductive, sensorineural, or mixed. Conductive hearing loss results from a blockage of the transmission of sound waves from the external auditory canal to the inner ear and is characterized by normal bone conduction and reduced air conduction hearing. In children, conductive losses are most often caused by middle ear effusion. Sensorineural hearing loss occurs when the auditory nerve or cochlear hair cells are damaged. Mixed hearing loss is characterized by components of both conductive and sensorineural loss. The criteria for normal hearing levels in children are lower than those in adults, since children are in the process of learning language. In children, a hearing loss of 15–30 dB is considered mild, 31–50 dB moderate, 51–80 dB severe, and 81–100 dB profound.

Conductive Hearing Loss

About 70% of children under 3 years of age will have one or more episodes of otitis media, and by far the greatest number of conductive hearing losses during childhood are caused by otitis media and its sequelae. Other causes include atresia, stenosis, or collapse of the ear canal; furuncle, cerumen, or foreign body in the ear; aural discharge; bony growths; otitis externa; perichondritis; middle ear anomalies (eg, stapes fixation, ossicular malformation); and cleft palate.

The average hearing loss due to middle ear effusion (whether serous, purulent, or mucoid) is 27–31 dB, the equivalent of a mild hearing loss. This loss may be intermittent in nature and may occur in one or both ears, and this accounts for the wide variability of the effects of ear disease on language development in children. A large-scale prospective study documented a correlation between the presence of middle ear effusion in the first 6–12 months of life and lower language scores at 3 years of age. The effect of effusion on language was more severe when the first attack of otitis media occurred before 6 months of age.

The American Academy of Pediatrics recommends that hearing be assessed and language development

* Contributed by Dewey Walker, MD, Marion Downs, MA, and Jerry Northern, PhD.

skills be monitored in children who have frequently recurring acute otitis media or middle ear effusion persisting longer than 3 months. The effects of hearing loss may be insidious and may not be discernible until the explosive phase of expressive language development occurs between 16 and 24 months of age; therefore, the optimal times for screening very young children are 18 and 24 months. An acceptable tool for language screening at these ages is the Early Language Milestone (ELM) scale. Children 3, 4, and 5 years of age should also be screened for language delays.

To mitigate the likelihood of a communication disorder developing, the physician should inform the parents of a child with middle ear disease that the child's hearing may not be normal and should instruct the parents to (1) turn off sources of background noise (eg, televisions, radios, dishwashers) when speaking to the child; (2) focus on the child's face and gain his or her direct attention before speaking; and (3) speak slightly louder than usual.

Sensorineural Hearing Loss

Sensorineural hearing loss arises from a lesion in the cochlear structures of the inner ear or in the neural fibers of the auditory nerve (cranial nerve VIII). Most sensorineural losses in children are congenital, with an incidence of one in 750 live births. Causes of congenital deafness include perinatal infections, problems related to premature birth, and autosomal recessive and dominant inheritance of various deafness syndromes. In some hereditary diseases (eg, Alport's syndrome), hearing loss is progressive and becomes apparent later in childhood. The incidence of acquired sensorineural loss in children has decreased since the advent of effective immunization programs (eg, against rubella and mumps) and the control of erythroblastosis fetalis with RH_O (D) immune globulin. Meningitis remains the most common cause of acquired hearing loss, with deafness occurring in 10.3% of children with bacterial meningitis.

In the past, the effect of unilateral deafness on school performance was thought to be insignificant. However, studies now show that more than one-third of affected children fail one or more grades in school. Therefore, merely recommending preferential classroom seating for these children is no longer sufficient; they should be referred for full evaluation of their hearing needs.

Learning language skills is more severely affected by bilateral than unilateral sensorineural hearing loss. The earlier the deafness occurs, the graver the consequences for language development; the earlier a sensorineural loss is detected and treated (by sound amplification and language habilitation), the better the chances of a good outcome. For example, detection of deafness in a 3-month-old infant and treatment by 4 months of age will result in an optimal outcome. Unfortunately, an average of 2.7 years lapses between the time a hearing loss is recognized and treatment is instituted. The alert physician can eliminate this time lag by utilizing the screening techniques described below.

Screening for Hearing Deficits

Screening procedures are essential for early detection and diagnosis of hearing deficits. The procedures used will vary according to the child's age.

A. Screening of Newborns: During either the hospital stay or the infant's first office visit, records of the infant's neonatal course and family history should be reviewed to determine if the infant is at risk for hearing deficits. According to the Joint Committee on Infant Screening, the following factors place infants at high risk: (1) a family history of childhood hearing impairment; (2) perinatal infections (eg, cytomegalovirus, rubella, herpes simplex, toxoplasmosis, syphilis); (3) anatomic malformations involving the head or neck (eg, dysmorphic appearance, including syndromic and nonsyndromic abnormalities of the pinna); (4) birth weight less than 1500 g; (5) hyperbilirubinemia at levels exceeding indications for exchange transfusion; (6) bacterial meningitis; and (7) signs of severe asphyxia at birth (eg, Apgar scores of 0–3, failure to show spontaneous respiration by 10 minutes after birth, hypotonia persisting to 2 hours of age). If any of these risk factors are present, the infant should be screened by an audiologist, preferably prior to 3 months of age but not later than 6 months after birth. The ideal screening test utilizes brain stem-evoked response audiometry. If results of the screening test are positive for hearing deficit, the audiologist should do further diagnostic testing.

B. Screening of Infants: In the past, the parents' report of their infant's behavior was considered an adequate assessment of the infant's hearing. However, a deaf infant's behavior can appear normal and mislead the parents as well as the professional, especially if the infant has autosomal recessive deafness and is the firstborn child of carrier parents. The following office screening techniques should identify gross hearing losses, but they may or may not detect less severe hearing losses due to otitis media.

1. From birth to 4 months—In response to a sudden loud sound (70 dB or more) produced by a horn, clacker, or special electronic device, the infant should show a startle reflex or blink the eyes.

2. From 4 months to 2 years—While the infant is distracted with a toy or bright object, a noisemaker is sounded softly outside of the field of vision at the child's waist level. Normal responses are as follows: at 4 months, there is a widening of the eyes, a cessation of previous activity, and possibly a slight turning of the head in the direction of the sound; at 6 months, the head turns toward the sound; at 9 months or older, the child should usually be able to locate a sound originating from below as well as turn to the appropriate side; after 1 year, the child should be able to locate sound whether it comes from below or above. After responses to these soft sounds are noted, a loud horn or clacker should be used to produce an eye blink or startle reflex. This last maneuver is necessary because deaf children are often very visually alert and scan the environment so actively that their scanning can be mistaken for an appropriate response to the softer noise test. A deaf child will not blink in response to the loud sound. Children who fail to respond appropriately should be referred for audiologic assessment.

C. Screening of Older Children: When children reach 3 years of age, their hearing can be tested by earphones and pure tone audiometry. The test frequencies for screening are 1000 Hz, 2000 Hz, and 4000 Hz, with the same tone presented at each frequency. Normally, the screening level is 20 dB. If a soundproof room is not available, the screening may be done at 25 dB. If the child does not respond at any one of the test frequencies in either ear, the test should be repeated within 1 week. Failures on rescreening should be referred for audiologic evaluation.

High-risk categories in older children include osteogenesis imperfecta and syndromes associated with deafness, such as Waardenburg's syndrome, Hurler's syndrome, Alport's syndrome, Treacher Collins syndrome, Klippel-Feil syndrome, and fetal alcohol syndrome. Children with these disorders should receive an audiologic evaluation as part of the complete workup. In addition, before any child is labeled as having mental retardation, autism, or severe behavioral problems, the adequacy of his or her hearing must be determined. If a developmental speech delay is diagnosed, hearing should be tested as the first step in evaluating the language problem.

Referral

In addition to the referrals for audiologic testing described above, a child with confirmed hearing loss should be referred to an otolaryngologist for evaluation and further management. Any child failing the language screen should be referred to a speech pathologist for language evaluation. Home language enrichment programs for children with mild language delays can be directed by the physician or by a speech pathologist. Programs for the deaf child vary from aural to total communication; the latter includes elements of aural programs plus signing. Each program should be thoroughly scrutinized for its relevance to the deaf child's age and hearing level.

Prevention

Appropriate pediatric care may help prevent many causes of hearing deficits. Erythroblastosis fetalis can be prevented by the use of RH_O (D) immune globulin, and hyperbilirubinemia can be controlled by phototherapy and exchange transfusions. Congenital rubella infections can be prevented by the use of rubella vaccine, and immunizations for other childhood diseases (eg, mumps) effectively prevent hearing losses from those conditions.

Aminoglycosides are potentially ototoxic and should be used judiciously and monitored carefully, especially in premature infants and in patients with renal insufficiency.

Reduction of exposure to loud noise in the child's environment will prevent high-frequency hearing losses. Repeated exposure to loud music, firecrackers, or shots from guns or cap pistols can impair hearing.

American Academy of Pediatrics: Policy statement by the Joint Committee on Infant Hearing. *Pediatrics* 1982;**70:**496.

American Speech and Hearing Association, Committee on Audiometric Evaluation: Guidelines for identification audiometry. *ASHA* (Feb) 1985;**17:**94.

Bess FH, Tharpe AM: Unilateral hearing impairment in children. *Pediatrics* 1984;**74:**206.

Gerkin KP: The high-risk register for deafness. *ASHA* (March) 1984;**26:**17.

Northern JL, Downs MP: *Hearing in Children*, 3rd ed. Williams & Wilkins, 1984.

Roeser RJ, Downs MP: *Auditory Disorders in School Children.* Thieme-Stratton, 1981.

Teele DW et al: Otitis media with effusion during the first three years of life and development of speech and language. *Pediatrics* 1984;**74:**282.

CERUMEN REMOVAL

Cerumen removal is an essential skill for anyone who treats ear problems. Cerumen often prevents adequate visualization of the tympanic membrane. Impacted cerumen can also cause itching, pain, hearing loss, or otitis externa. If cerumen impinges on the eardrum, a chronic cough may be triggered and will persist until the cerumen is removed. The most common cause of impacted cerumen is the use of cotton-tipped swabs by parents in misguided attempts to clean the ear canal. Parents should be advised that earwax protects the ear (cerumen contains lysozymes and immunoglobulins that curtail infection) and will come out by itself; therefore, they should never put anything into the ear canal to hurry the process.

The technique of removal depends on the consistency of the earwax. All the procedures described below require careful immobilization to prevent injury of the ear canal.

(1) Very soft cerumen: Semiliquid earwax can be removed with cotton twisted on toothpicks or paper clips. Several passages with clean cotton are usually necessary. Nasopharyngeal culture swabs are an expensive substitute.

(2) Average cerumen: Sticky cerumen will adhere to an ear curet. A piece of this consistency can sometimes be removed by embedding the ear curet in it. If this technique fails, irrigation as described below should be instituted.

(3) Hard cerumen: Very hard cerumen may adhere to the ear canal wall and cause considerable pain or bleeding if one attempts to remove it with a curet. This type of wax should be softened before irrigation with Cerumenex or a few drops of detergent. After 20 minutes, irrigation can be started with water warmed to 35–38 °C (95–100.4 °F) to prevent vertigo.

An easy-to-assemble ear syringe consists of a 12-mL plastic syringe plus a piece of small plastic tubing. The tubing can be made from any scalp vein needle set by cutting off the needle about 3 inches from the female connector. The front end of the tubing is placed in the canal, behind the cerumen if possible, and the water is ejected with maximal pressure on the syringe plunger. The advantage of this technique is that the very small tubing may be inserted into the ear canal itself and the water stream is thus directed in the proper direction without interfering with reflux.

A commercial Water Pik is also an excellent device for removing cerumen, but it is important to set it at a low power (2 or less) to prevent any damage to the intact tympanic membrane.

A perforated tympanic membrane is a contraindication to any form of irrigation.

Kravitz H et al: The cotton-tipped swab: A major cause of ear injury and hearing loss. *Clin Pediatr (Phila)* 1974; **13:**965.

OTOSCOPY

Removal of cerumen (see above) may be necessary for adequate visualization of the ear and for assessment of the mobility of the tympanic membrane by pneumatic otoscopy.

The tympanic membrane is divided into 4 sections, based on the position of the long process of the malleus and the umbo, as shown in Fig 13–2. The anterosuperior quadrant contains the short process of the malleus; the posterosuperior quadrant, the incus and pars flaccida; the posteroinferior quadrant, the round window; and the anteroinferior quadrant, the pars tensa and light reflex. To assess mobility of the tympanic membrane, a pneumatic otoscope with a rubber suction bulb and tube is used. The speculum inserted into the patient's ear canal must be large enough to provide an airtight seal. When the rubber bulb is squeezed, the tympanic membrane will flap briskly if no fluid is present (normal finding); however, if fluid is present in the middle ear space, the mobility of the tympanic membrane will be diminished.

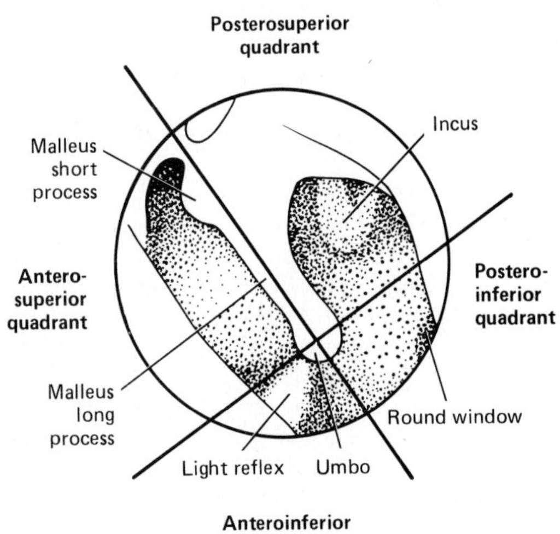

Figure 13–2. Schematic diagram of the left tympanic membrane. (Courtesy of the Department of Otolaryngology, University of Pittsburgh School of Medicine, and Eli Lilly and Co.)

TYMPANOMETRY

Tympanometry utilizes an electroacoustic impedance bridge to measure tympanic membrane compliance and display it in graphic form. Compliance is determined at specific air pressures (from +200 to −400 mm H_2O air pressure) that are created in the hermetically sealed external ear canal. The existing middle ear pressure can be measured by determining the ear canal pressure at which the tympanic membrane is most compliant. Since total visualization of the tympanic membrane is not necessary, tympanometry does not require removal of cerumen unless the canal is completely blocked.

Tympanograms can be classified into 3 major patterns, as shown in Fig 13–3. The type A pattern, characterized by maximum compliance at normal atmospheric pressure (0 mm H_2O air pressure), indicates a normal tympanic membrane, good auditory tube function, and absence of effusion. The type B pattern identifies a nonmobile tympanic membrane, which may be associated with middle ear effusion, perforation, patent ventilation tubes, or excessive and hard-packed cerumen. The type C pattern indicates an intact mobile tympanic membrane with poor auditory tube function and excessive negative pressure (> -150 mm H_2O air pressure) in the middle ear. Middle ear effusion is present in about 20% of patients with a type C pattern.

Northern JL: Advanced techniques for measuring middle ear function. *Pediatrics* 1978;**61:**761.

MYRINGOTOMY & TYMPANOCENTESIS

Tympanocentesis (placement of a needle through the tympanic membrane) is mainly a diagnostic procedure, since the hole closes over quickly and provides little sustained drainage. Tympanocentesis is helpful in (1) acute otitis media in a hospitalized newborn, because the pathogens may be gram-negative; (2) acute otitis media in a patient with compromised host resistance, because the organism may be unusual; (3) painful bullae of the tympanic membrane; (4) a complete workup for presumed sepsis or meningitis; and (5) acute purulent otitis media that is unresponsive to therapy after courses with 2 different antibiotics.

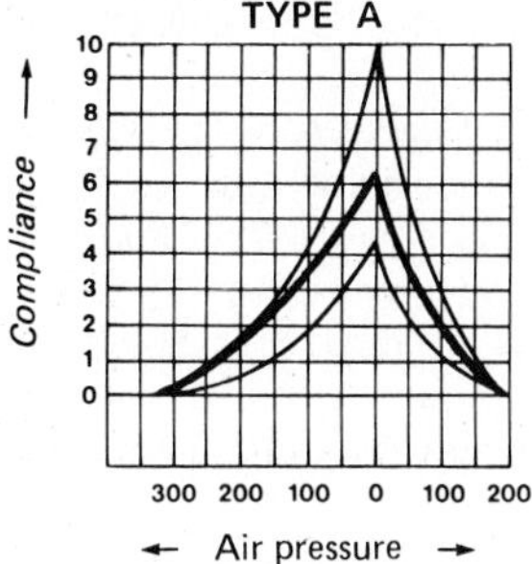

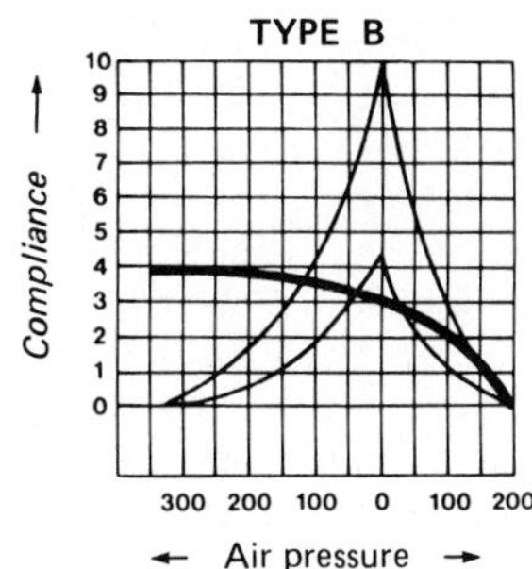

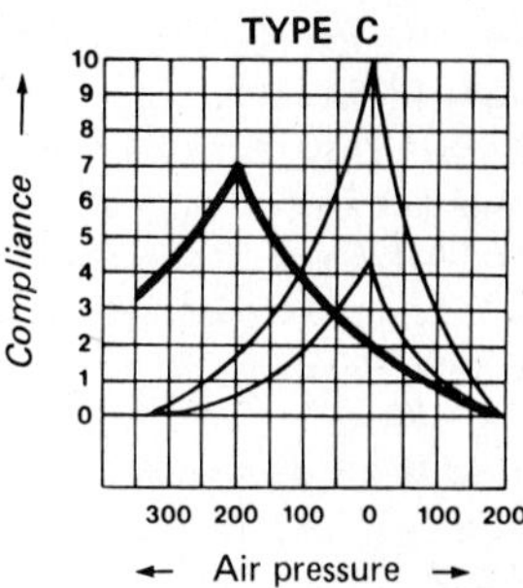

Figure 13–3. Type A tympanograms are characterized by maximum compliance at normal atmospheric pressure (0 mm H_2O air pressure). Type B tympanograms show little or no change in compliance of tympanic membrane as air pressure in external ear canal is varied. Type C tympanograms show near-normal compliance with significant negative middle ear pressures (typically more severe than −150 mm H_2O). (Reproduced, with permission, from Northern JL. Advanced techniques for measuring middle ear function. *Pediatrics* 1978;**61**:761.)

Myringotomy involves incision of the drum with a myringotomy knife, leaving a flap through which drainage fluid may escape. This procedure is helpful for both diagnostic and therapeutic purposes. Myringotomy is indicated (1) when a patient on an initial visit with bulging acute purulent otitis media has severe pain or vomiting, since both symptoms are relieved by myringotomy; (2) when pain and fever fail to resolve after 48 hours of appropriate antibiotic treatment, since a middle ear abscess or resistant organism may exist; and (3) for acute mastoiditis, because it is important to permit drainage as well as to identify the particular organism.

Technique of Myringotomy

A. Premedication: In the conditions mentioned, the pain from a myringotomy is only slightly greater than the pain that already exists from acute inflammation of the tympanic membrane. Therefore, no premedication is generally indicated. The patient who is extremely difficult to hold may be premedicated with meperidine, 1 mg/kg intramuscularly. Some recommend applying Bonain's solution (equal parts cocaine, phenol, and menthol) to the tympanic membrane with a calcium alginate swab.

B. Restraint: The patient must be completely immobile while the incision is being made. A papoose board or a sheet can be used to immobilize the body. An extra attendant is required to hold the patient's head steady.

C. Site: With an open-headed operating otoscope, the operator carefully selects a target. This is generally in the posteroinferior quadrant. This site prevents disruption of the ossicles during the procedure.

D. Incision: The knife is lowered slowly until it touches the surface of the tympanic membrane at the chosen site. A quick 2- to 3-mm incision in the anterior direction is then made, leaving a curved flap in the area indicated (eg, from 8 o'clock to 4 o'clock on the right eardrum).

E. Culture: The myringotomy knife tip should be wiped on a cotton swab moistened with a few drops of normal saline. The material is then placed on a sheep blood agar plate, chocolate agar plate, and a slide for Gram staining.

Technique of Tympanocentesis

Steps A, B, and C are as described above.

In this procedure, the operator needs an assistant to hold the patient's head immobile. An 8.8-cm spinal needle (No. 18 or No. 20) with a short bevel is attached to a 1-mL syringe. The plunger is removed from the syringe, and a 3-way stopcock is inserted into the syringe opening. A piece of extension tubing is attached to the exposed end of the 3-way stopcock, and the other end is kept in the operator's mouth for suction. The spinal needle is bent at a slight angle so that its end is out of the operator's line of vision. The operator moves the needle toward the posteroinferior quadrant, inserting it through the tympanic membrane, and aspirates the middle ear effusion into the syringe.

Kaplan SL, Feigen RD: Simplified technique for tympanocentesis. *Pediatrics* 1978;**62**:418.

THE NOSE & PARANASAL SINUSES

RHINITIS

1. ACUTE VIRAL RHINITIS (Common Cold)

The common cold is the most frequent infectious disease of humans, and the incidence is higher in early childhood than in any other period of life. Closely similar upper respiratory infections may be caused by perhaps 100 different viruses such as rhinovirus, coronavirus, adenovirus, influenza virus, parainfluenza virus, respiratory syncytial virus, coxsackievirus, etc. Minor epidemics occur during the winter months and spread rapidly among susceptible people. The peak month (September) coincides with the opening of schools.

Clinical Findings

The patient usually experiences a sudden onset of clear or mucoid rhinorrhea plus a fever. The main symptoms are usually profound congestion of the nose and sinuses. Mild sore throat and cough also frequently develop. Although the fever is usually low-grade in older children, in the first 5 or 6 years of life it can be as high as 40.6 °C (105 °F). The nose and throat are usually inflamed. Several members of a family are often sick simultaneously.

Complications

Acute otitis media is the most common complication and is often heralded by return of fever or crying. Other complications due to superinfection are purulent sinusitis, purulent conjunctivitis, pneumonia, and pyogenic adenitis. Common nonpyogenic complications are viral sinusitis, bronchitis, croup, and bronchiolitis.

The onset or presence of a cold or upper respiratory tract infection in a child scheduled for surgery may require postponement of the operation. The primary physician can use the following guidelines when screening children for elective surgery: Surgery is usually postponed if fever or cough is present. Surgery can proceed if the child has only a runny nose, sore throat, or ear infection. If anesthesia will not require intubation (eg, as for placement of tympanoplasty tubes), surgery can be permitted even if the child has a cough (as long as findings on chest film are normal).

Treatment

Treatment is largely symptomatic. Aspirin or acetaminophen is helpful for fever, sore throat, or muscle aches. A stuffy, congested nose can be treated with normal saline nose drops, 3 drops in each nostril; the patient should be in the supine position with the neck hyperextended. After several minutes, a suction bulb can be used to remove the secretions of the infant unable to blow its nose. If this fails and the stuffy nose still interferes with feeding or sleep, phenylephrine (Neo-Synephrine), 0.125%, or xylometazoline (Otrivin), 0.05%, 2 drops every 4 hours as necessary, can be used in children under 2 years of age. Children over 2 years of age can use 0.25% phenylephrine drops. Drops should be discontinued after 1 week to prevent a rebound chemical rhinitis. If there is significant rhinorrhea, an antihistamine decongestant can be used but is of unproved value.

Antibiotics do not prevent superinfection and should not be used. Vaporizers and humidifiers have no proved value and should not be routinely prescribed, especially if the parents cannot easily afford them.

Colds account for many unnecessary visits to the physician. Parents are often unduly worried about how many colds their children have or are overconcerned about noisy breathing, which they fear indicates pneumonia. Most colds can be assessed and treated by telephone.

The prognosis is excellent. In the usual cold, the fever lasts for less than 3 days and the other symptoms persist for 1–2 weeks.

Douglas R: Pathogenesis of rhinovirus common colds in human volunteers. *Ann Otol Rhinol Laryngol* 1970;**79:**563.

Lampert RP et al: A critical look at oral decongestants. *Pediatrics* 1977;**55:**550.

West S et al: A review of antihistamines and the common cold. *Pediatrics* 1975;**56:**100.

2. ACUTE PURULENT RHINITIS

Purulent yellow discharge that persists for several days usually represents purulent sinusitis or other bacterial superinfection of a common cold. Any purulent discharge that is profuse and continuous for over 1 day probably should be treated. The common cold may also be associated with some mucopurulent discharge, but discharge is usually intermittent and worse upon awakening in the morning. The most likely organisms are pneumococci, *Haemophilus influenzae*, β-hemolytic streptococci, and *Staphylococcus aureus*. Rare causes are diphtheria and syphilis. The β-hemolytic streptococci are the most likely organisms if there is crusting around the nares that resembles impetigo, redness of the skin below the nares, or a blistering distal dactylitis.

Without treatment, this process can progress to acute otitis media, purulent sinusitis, pneumonitis, or even septicemia.

Oral amoxicillin for 10 days will cure most of these patients. Occasionally, dicloxacillin will be needed because of culture results. The purulent material should be removed as completely as possible with a suction bulb or cotton-tipped applicators and a washcloth and soap. Bacitracin ointment should be applied if nasal impetigo exists.

If the problem recurs after adequate treatment, the patient should be referred to an otolaryngologist to rule out the possibility of a foreign body. If the discharge is foul-smelling and unilateral, this becomes especially likely. The response to treatment is excellent in the majority of cases.

Hays GC, Mullard JE: Can nasal bacterial flora be predicted from clinical findings? *Pediatrics* 1972;**49:**596.

3. PERSISTENT RHINITIS IN NEWBORNS

Rhinorrhea or nasal congestion in a young infant may be due to various causes.

About half of newborns are obligate nasal breathers, and if the nose becomes congested, they have difficulty with air exchange and may become irritable and dyspneic. The problem is worse during feeding because the infant's oral airway is then completely useless. These infants gradually learn to become mouth breathers as well as nasal breathers by age 5 or 6 months.

Differential Diagnosis & Treatment

A. Transient Idiopathic Stuffy Nose of the Newborn: Many infants have unexplained, transient (about 3 weeks) stuffy noses with mucoid or clear discharge that bubbles during feeding. The cause is not known. The diagnosis is made by exclusion. Normal saline nose drops can be instilled and, after several minutes, removed with cotton-tipped applicators or gentle suction on a rubber bulb syringe. If the problem interferes with feeding, this can be preceded by 2 drops of 0.125% phenylephrine (Neo-Synephrine) no more than 4 times a day for several days.

B. Reserpine Side Effects: If the mother is taking reserpine and the drug is in her blood at an effective level during labor, the newborn may have a profoundly stuffy nose. Treatment is as above.

C. Chemical Rhinitis: This may be due to overtreatment of idiopathic stuffy nose with topical vasoconstrictors. The irritative nose drops should be discontinued. The patient can be helped with oral decongestants for a few days.

D. Pyogenic Rhinitis: Infants with pyogenic rhinitis can have a clear or mucoid discharge rather than the purulent discharge seen in older children. The diagnosis is based on cultures of nasal discharge. Treatment is as outlined above.

E. Congenital Syphilis: The onset is usually before 6 weeks of age. The diagnosis is established by checking the serology done on the mother during the prenatal period. If other signs besides the nasal discharge exist, such as an unresponsive skin rash or hepatosplenomegaly, additional serologic testing should be performed on the infant. Treatment is discussed in Chapter 27.

F. Hypothyroidism: See Chapter 25.

G. Choanal Atresia: This occurs bilaterally in 25% of affected children and unilaterally in 75%. Bilateral cases can cause severe respiratory distress—even apnea at birth if the child is an absolute nasal breather. Both types eventually present with a chronic nasal discharge because the normal sinus and nasal secretions can escape only anteriorly. A No. 8 soft rubber catheter should be passed through the nose and visualized in the oropharynx. If this cannot be accomplished, a diagnosis of choanal atresia should be confirmed by radiographic study.

An oral airway should be placed immediately if the infant has bilateral choanal atresia. A dentist can fashion a comfortable airway to tide the patient over until mouth breathing is established. Feeding by syringe or medicine dropper is preferred. An otolaryngologist should decide on the optimal timing for definitive surgery, but it is usually 1 year of age.

H. Nasal Fracture Secondary to Birth Trauma: Physical examination should reveal subluxation of the nasal septum occluding the nasal passages. The infant should be referred to an otolaryngologist for reduction.

I. Allergic Rhinitis Associated With Cow's Milk: An allergic reaction to cow's milk can cause noisy breathing and increased production of nasal and oral mucus in infants 1–2 months of age. The symptoms resolve 24–48 hours after eliminating cow's milk from the diet, and they return promptly if the infant is rechallenged with milk.

4. RECURRENT RHINITIS IN THE OLDER CHILD

This problem is all too frequent in the office practice of pediatrics. A child is brought in with the chief complaint that he or she has "one cold after another," has "constant colds," or "is always sick." Such a patient may be in the office on almost a weekly basis. Although the problem is frustrating, the differential diagnosis is rather simple.* Approximately two-thirds of these children have recurrent colds, and another one-third have allergic rhinitis.

Differential Diagnosis & Treatment

A. Common Cold: The most common cause of recurrent runny nose is repeated viral upper respiratory infections. The onset is usually after 6 months of age. The bouts of rhinorrhea are usually accompanied by fever. Cultures are negative for bacteria. There is some evidence for contagion within the family or peer group in most of these cases. The nasal mucosa during attacks is often inflamed.

The most common reason for presentation is that the parents are overly concerned because they do not understand that the average child has approximately 8 colds a year in the preschool period. Or the patient may be overly exposed to viruses as a result of close contact with a sibling at school who brings home many pathogens or by frequently being left with large numbers of children at a day-care center or with a baby-sitter.

Treatment consists of specific reassurance and con-

**Note:* An excessively ordered test is serum immunoelectrophoresis. Children with immune defects do not have an increased number of colds. Therefore, immunoglobulin tests are worthless unless the patient suffers from recurrent pneumonia, recurrent sinusitis, recurrent adenitis, or other recurrent severe infections.

cerned follow-up. The parents can be told that their child's general health is good, as evidenced by adequate weight gain and a robust activity level; that the prognosis is good in that this number of colds will not persist for more than a few years; that the body's exposure and response to colds is building up an antibody supply; and that this problem is not their fault and that they are doing a good job as parents.

B. Allergic Rhinitis: The onset of "hay fever" is usually after 2 years of age—after the child has had adequate exposure to allergens. There is no fever or contagion among close contacts. The attacks include frequent sneezing, rubbing of the nose, and a profuse clear discharge. The nasal turbinates are swollen. The nasal smear demonstrates over 20% of the cells to be eosinophils. (Nasal eosinophilia may be normal during the first 3 months of life.) Nasal secretions should be collected only when the patient is symptomatic. Between attacks or after receiving antihistamines, the eosinophil smear may be falsely negative.

Oral decongestants and antihistamines should be tried until the right drug and dosage are found to give the optimal effect. Avoidance of allergens (especially pets) should be encouraged and environmental controls initiated. If the symptoms persist, the patient should be referred to an allergist for evaluation and possibly for treatment with beclomethasone nasal spray or hyposensitization.

A full discussion of allergic rhinitis is found in Chapter 32.

C. Chemical Rhinitis: Prolonged use of vasoconstrictor nose drops beyond 7 days results in a rebound reaction and secondary nasal congestion (rhinitis medicamentosa). The offending nose drops should be discontinued.

D. Vasomotor Rhinitis: Some children react to sudden changes in environmental temperature with prolonged congestion and rhinorrhea. Air pollution (especially tobacco smoke) may be a factor. Oral decongestants can be used periodically to give symptomatic relief.

Complications

Because this problem is such a nuisance, iatrogenic overtreatment is the most common complication.

Giving immune globulin injections is the most common error made in this disorder. The injections may be initiated without determining the serum IgG level or as a consequence of misinterpreting the results by comparing them with adult levels rather than with norms for age. Many studies show that immune globulin injections do not benefit patients with frequent upper respiratory infections. In addition to being painful and expensive, they may cause anaphylaxis or isoimmunization. Other worthless approaches to this problem include bacterial vaccines, prophylactic antibiotics, and tonsillectomy and adenoidectomy. The effectiveness of high doses of vitamin C in reducing the symptoms and duration of colds is promising but still controversial. Patients are not infrequently kept home from school, trips, athletic practices, parties, etc, with little indication. As long as they do not have a fever or severe symptoms, they can attend these functions. They should be given suitable medications for symptomatic relief of mild symptoms so that they can participate normally in these important events of childhood. The risk to other children is almost irrelevant because these infections are contagious even during the incubation period and the best time to have them and develop immunity is during childhood.

Coulehan JL et al: Vitamin C prophylaxis in a boarding school. *N Engl J Med* 1974;**290:**6.

McCammon RW: Natural history of respiratory tract infection patterns in basically healthy individuals. *Am J Dis Child* 1971;**122:**232.

Miller DL et al: Allergic diseases of the nose and middle ear in children. *Pediatr Ann* 1976;**5:**482.

Miller RE et al: The nasal smear for eosinophils: Its value in children with seasonal allergic rhinitis. *Am J Dis Child* 1982;**136:**1009.

MOUTH BREATHING SECONDARY TO NASAL OBSTRUCTION

A child is sometimes brought in with the complaint that "He always breathes through his mouth," "He snores," etc. With the mouth covered, each nostril should be tested individually for patency. One or both nostrils may be so severely occluded that adequate air exchange cannot occur. Even when the nasal passages are not completely occluded, the patient may prefer to breathe through the mouth because it is more comfortable. With complete obstruction, a constant nasal discharge ensues because the normal sinus and nasal secretions can escape only anteriorly. The sense of smell is also reduced.

Differential Diagnosis

A. Large Adenoids: Large adenoids can be suspected if the soft palate is depressed or has limited elevation, the patient has hyponasal speech, or possibly if the tonsils are huge. They can be diagnosed more precisely by digital palpation or by lateral soft tissue films of the nasopharynx.

B. Nasal Polyps: Polyps appear as glistening, gray to pink, jellylike masses that are prominent just inside the anterior nares and occur singly or in clusters. They are most common in severe allergic rhinitis. They also occur in cystic fibrosis. One must be careful not to mistake the turbinates for polyps.

C. Recurrent Sinusitis: See below.

D. Allergic Rhinitis: See above.

E. Chemical Rhinitis: See above.

F. Other Causes: Persistent mouth breathing may be due to obstruction by nasopharyngeal tumor or by meningocele or encephalocele herniated into the nasal cavity. If unilateral nasal obstruction and epistaxis are frequent, juvenile angiofibroma should be suspected.

Complications

Most children with prolonged mouth breathing eventually develop dental malocclusion and what has been termed an adenoidal facies. The face is pinched and the maxilla narrowed because the molding pressures of the orbicularis oris and buccinator muscles are unopposed by the tongue. If nasopharyngeal tumors, meningoceles, or encephaloceles are not diagnosed early, they can cause considerable destruction or may even become incurable. Children with severe snoring may also develop sleep apnea or pulmonary hypertension.

Treatment

Allergic rhinitis usually responds to antihistamines or to intranasal cromolyn or corticosteroids. Sinusitis usually resolves with antibiotics. All other patients with documented chronic mouth breathing should be referred to an otolaryngologist for definitive evaluation and treatment. Polyps should never be removed until a meningocele has been ruled out.

Bresolin D et al: Facial characteristics of children who breathe through the mouth. *Pediatrics* 1984;**73:**622.

Myer CM et al: Nasal obstruction in the pediatric patient. *Pediatrics* 1983;**72:**766.

Sessions RB et al: Juvenile nasopharyngeal angiofibroma. *Am J Dis Child* 1981;**135:**535.

SINUSITIS

1. ACUTE SINUSITIS

Essentials of Diagnosis

- Purulent rhinorrhea.
- Malodorous breath.
- Cough and congestion.
- Facial pain.
- Percussion tenderness over the sinuses.
- Postnasal drip.

General Considerations

Sinusitis occurs when the sinus ostia are occluded and the sinus secretions accumulate. If the obstruction is intermittent, the sinus secretions drain periodically. The most common cause is the common cold, which results in edema and obstruction of the sinus ostia. In some cases, there is no superinfection of the sinus secretions. In cases in which superinfection occurs, the organisms are *Streptococcus pneumoniae, Haemophilus influenzae* (nontypeable), *Branhamella catarrhalis,* and β-hemolytic streptococci. Anaerobic bacterial infections can cause fulminant frontal sinusitis. Sinusitis is also commonly seen during pollen season in children with allergic rhinitis.

The ethmoid sinus is the only one that is significantly developed at birth. The maxillary sinus is rudimentary at birth and visible on x-ray by 6 months. The frontal sinus is not visible until 3–9 years of age. Clinical ethmoiditis does not usually occur until 6 months of age. About half of cases occur between 1 and 5 years of age, during which time the most common presenting sign is periorbital cellulitis. The maxillary sinus is the principal site of disease, probably because its ostia do not drain by gravity. Maxillary sinusitis is seen clinically after 1 year of age. Frontal sinusitis is unusual before 10 years of age.

Clinical Findings

A. Symptoms and Signs: The most common finding is a sense of fullness or facial pain overlying the involved sinus. Ethmoiditis causes retro-orbital pain; maxillary sinusitis causes upper molar or zygomatic pain; and frontal sinusitis causes pain above the eyebrow. The patient usually also complains of nasal congestion, an intermittent, profuse discharge persisting after resolution of the upper respiratory infection, a postnasal drip on swallowing, and halitosis. A history of periorbital swelling on awakening (especially swelling of the upper eyelid) is common in patients with ethmoiditis.

Physical examination reveals percussion tenderness overlying the sinusitis. In ethmoiditis, the tenderness is elicited by pressing medially on the inner canthus of the eye. Tenderness of the eyeball may also be present. Maxillary sinusitis reveals percussion tenderness over the maxillary bone. Frontal sinusitis reveals tenderness when pressing upward on the floor of the supraorbital ridge. If the sinus is partially open, a convincing piece of evidence for the presence of retained sinus secretions is the reaccumulation of nasal secretions every time the patient sniffs or the drainage is aspirated. This finding can be accentuated by the introduction of a vasoconstrictor. The oropharynx reveals a purulent discharge after each swallow. Fever is occasionally present. Transillumination of the sinuses is difficult to perform and not very helpful unless it is grossly asymmetric. In those cases in which the sinuses are superinfected, fever and purulent rhinitis are usually present. Sinusitis precipitates intractable wheezing in some children with reactive airway disease. Vigorous treatment of the sinusitis eliminates the wheezing and the need for bronchodilators in 80% of these children.

B. Laboratory Findings: A culture of fresh discharge is obtained by blowing the nose. Microscopic examination of secretions will show sheets of neutrophils and bacteria in bacterial sinusitis, few neutrophils in viral sinusitis, and sheets of eosinophils in allergic sinusitis. Sinus aspiration should be performed for diagnostic purposes in patients with complications and in those with an immunosuppressive disease. If the patient is hospitalized because of complications, a blood culture should be obtained.

C. X-Ray Findings: In most cases, the clinical findings are so classic that x-rays are not needed. Positive x-ray films will show opacification of the involved sinuses, air-fluid levels if the obstruction is intermittent, or mucosal thickening of greater than 5 mm. It is notable that x-ray findings positive for sinusitis may be found in asymptomatic patients with colds or nasal allergies. Sinus x-rays are mainly indicated in children with facial swelling of unknown cause; acute sinusitis that is unresponsive to 48 hours of therapy; undocumented chronic or recurrent sinusitis; and chronic asthma. A CT scan should be performed if bony erosions are present. Ultrasonography can also be used to document sinusitis.

Differential Diagnosis

In the infant, acute ethmoiditis may go undiagnosed for several days with a fever of unknown origin. Recognition occurs when overlying redness appears. In older children, the main diagnostic problem is confusion with headaches due to other causes. An uncommon cause of maxillary sinusitis is extension of a periapical abscess of an upper molar.

Complications

Untreated ethmoiditis not uncommonly presents as an abscess of the inner canthus or a periorbital abscess. Occasionally, this can progress to a retroorbital abscess or even cavernous sinus thrombosis, which has a dire prognosis. The most common complication of frontal sinusitis is osteitis of the frontal bone, but serious intracranial complications such as subdural empyema, brain abscess, and meningitis can occur. The most common maxillary complication is cellulitis of the cheek.

Treatment

A. Specific Measures:

1. Topical decongestants—The key to good therapeutic results in most cases of sinusitis without superinfection is adequate drainage of the sinus.

The application of long-acting vasoconstrictor nose drops every 12 hours can often induce adequate drainage. In the older child, the nose should first be cleared by sniffing; a nasal aspirator may be used for infants. The nose drops must be delivered to the sinus ostia. The correct position for the child to be in when the nose drops are placed is with the head low and turned slightly toward one side. A nasal spray does not provide adequate delivery of the medication. Vasoconstrictor nose drops should be used sparingly (ie, only when the nose is very congested). Also, this medication cannot be used for more than 7 days, because of the risk of rebound edema.

Some patients with allergy require beclomethasone nasal spray for relief.

2. Oral decongestants—Systemic decongestants combined with antihistamines may provide an added measure of relief for closed ostia. These are especially helpful for patients with underlying allergies. They should be continued for 2 days after symptoms have subsided.

3. Oral antibiotics—In those cases where superinfection is suspected, amoxicillin should be added to the treatment regimen in a dosage of 50 mg/kg/d orally for 2–3 weeks.

4. Treatment of complications—Patients with evidence of invasive infection or any of the complications listed above should be immediately hospitalized. Intravenous therapy with nafcillin plus cefotaxime or with chloramphenicol alone should be initiated until culture results become available.

B. General Measures: A patient will often need aspirin or even codeine temporarily to permit sleep until drainage of the obstructed sinus is achieved. The application of ice over the sinus may help to relieve pain.

Dryness of the mucous membranes—as occurs in many overheated homes in the winter if adequate humidification is not provided—can contribute to the obstruction. A humidifier in the patient's room and periodic warm showers may be of value. A child with sinusitis can be permitted to swim. Diving should be temporarily restricted unless nose plugs are used.

C. Surgical Treatment:

1. Lavage of the sinuses—If there is incapacitating initial pain or persistence of significant pain beyond several days, refer the patient to an otolaryngologist for lavage of the involved sinus.

2. External drainage—In complicated cases admitted to the hospital, an otolaryngologist should always be consulted. Sinus aspiration is helpful in many cases. For sinus intraorbital or intracranial complications, some feel that external drainage of the abscess is as important as antibiotic therapy.

D. Follow-Up Care: The patient should be seen at least once a week after treatment has been started. If the drainage has become purulent, a sample should be taken for culture and the patient started on antibiotics. If the sinusitis is unresponsive but considered sterile, the patient should be referred to an otolaryngologist for lavage and other measures.

Prognosis

Acute sinus congestion is usually a mild, self-limited condition that lasts for less than 1 week. Therapy as outlined above usually provides partial to complete relief of symptoms during that week. When bacterial superinfection occurs, the initiation of antibiotics usually relieves fever and pain in 48 hours.

Brook I et al: Complications of sinusitis in children. *Pediatrics* 1980;**66:**568.

Kovatch AL et al: Maxillary sinus radiographs in children with nonrespiratory complaints. *Pediatrics* 1984;**73:**306.

Sable NS et al: Acute frontal sinusitis with intracranial complications. *Pediatr Infect Dis* 1984;**3:**58.

Wald ER: Acute sinusitis in children. *Pediatr Infect Dis* 1983;**2:**61.

Wald ER et al: Acute maxillary sinusitis in children. *N Engl J Med* 1981;**304:**749.

Wald ER et al: Treatment of maxillary sinusitis in childhood: A comparative study of amoxicillin and cefaclor. *J Pediatr* 1984;**104:**297.

2. RECURRENT SINUSITIS

Frequent episodes of sinusitis occur in a small group of patients. The most common cause is allergic rhinitis. The second most common cause—especially of frontal sinusitis—is diving or jumping into water feet first. The remaining cases are caused by pressure against the ostia by a septal deviation, nasal malformation, a polyp, or a foreign body. In cases of recurrent pyogenic pansinusitis, poor host resistance (eg, an immune defect, Kartagener's syndrome, or cystic fibrosis) must be ruled out by immunoglobulin studies, cilia studies, and a sweat chloride test. If allergies and diving do not offer a sufficient explanation for the problem, the patient should be referred to an otolaryngologist for complete evaluation.

Jaffe BF: Chronic sinusitis in children. *Clin Pediatr (Phila)* 1974;**13**:944.

Rachelefsky GS et al: Chronic sinus disease associated with reactive airway disease in children. *Pediatrics* 1984;**73**:526.

RECURRENT EPISTAXIS

Most children have a few isolated nosebleeds, but recurrent nosebleed usually warrants a visit to the pediatrician. The nose is a very vascular structure. In most cases, epistaxis is due to mild trauma to the anterior portion of the nasal septum (Kiesselbach's area), sometimes as a result of falls or fistfights but usually due to vigorous nose rubbing, nose blowing, or nose picking.

Clinical Findings

A. Symptoms and Signs: The frequency of nosebleeds may be once a month to several times a day. If they are profuse, subsequent hematemesis or tarry stools may be reported. Examination of Kiesselbach's area reveals a red, raw surface with fresh clots or old crusts. There will often be blood under the fingernails.

B. Laboratory Findings: A baseline hematocrit is indicated in most patients. The true degree of anemia following a severe nosebleed may not be evident until 6–12 hours after bleeding has ceased.

Most patients do not need a bleeding workup, but bleeding tests are indicated if any of the following are present: a family history of a bleeding disorder, a past medical history of easy bleeding, spontaneous bleeding at other sites, bleeding that lasts for over 20 minutes or will not clot with direct pressure by the physician, onset before age 2, or a drop in the hematocrit due to epistaxis.

Differential Diagnosis

Although most cases of epistaxis occur following trauma to the normal nose, several contributing factors must be ruled out. If they are present, specific treatment will be needed.

A. Allergic Rhinitis: Boggy, inflamed mucosa is predisposed to epistaxis. This diagnosis is confirmed by a nasal smear for eosinophils. In such a case, antihistamines may help to decrease the amount of nasal pruritus and subsequent rubbing.

B. Chronic Bleeding Disorder: Numerous bleeding disorders (eg, von Willebrand's disease, thrombocytopenia) may present as recurrent epistaxis. A history of easy bleeding with circumcision, tonsillectomy, lacerations, venipuncture, or tooth eruption points to this type of disorder. A family history of hemophilia or other bleeding tendencies is suggestive. A history of spontaneous bleeding at other sites—gastrointestinal tract, hemarthrosis, menorrhagia, petechiae with crying, etc—or current physical findings of bleeding at other sites is suggestive. The presence of hepatomegaly or splenomegaly is also suggestive. These patients require bleeding screens.

C. Aspirin: Recent studies reveal that ingestion of normal doses of aspirin can interfere with platelet aggregation or adhesiveness and cause prolonged bleeding. The abnormal bleeding time is confirmatory.

D. Vascular Malformation: Kiesselbach's area must be carefully examined for telangiectasia, hemangiomas, or varicosities.

E. Hypertension: High blood pressure may predispose to prolonged nosebleeds.

F. Nasopharyngeal Angiofibroma: This tumor of adolescent males often presents with epistaxis. Bleeding confined to the back of the throat makes the elimination of this diagnosis mandatory. Lateral soft tissue films of the nasopharynx are diagnostic.

Complications

Unless an underlying bleeding disorder exists, the only complication of nosebleed is mild anemia. The latter is unusual and responds to iron therapy.

Treatment

A. Immediate Treatment: The following approach can be carried out in the office or given as phone advice: The patient should sit up and lean forward so as not to swallow the blood. The nose is pinched, with pressure over the bleeding site being maintained for 10 minutes by the clock. If bleeding continues, pressure is not being applied to the right spot, and it should be changed.

If this is not effective, clots should be removed by suction or blowing the nose. A pledget wet with 0.25% phenylephrine (Neo-Synephrine) nose drops, 1% lidocaine (Xylocaine) with 1:1000 epinephrine—or the most potent topical vasoconstrictor of all, 1% cocaine—is inserted into the nose. Pressure is again applied for 10 minutes. Rarely does this technique fail.

Two different approaches involve the insertion of a small piece of gelatin sponge (Gelfoam) or topical thrombin over the bleeding site or the insertion of a wedge of salt pork into the bleeding nostril.

B. Preventive Treatment: The friability of the nasal vessels can be decreased with daily application of petrolatum by cotton-tipped applicator. The lubricant is applied daily until 5 days have passed without a nosebleed, then weekly for 1 month, and resumed only if the nosebleeds recur. In a very dry environment, humidification of the patient's room may be helpful. Aspirin should be avoided.

C. Reassurance: Parents need reassurance regarding the amount of blood lost. It always looks like more than it actually is. A normal hematocrit is usually comforting to the parents. The child should not be blamed regarding this problem. The parents should be told that simply rubbing a blocked nose or picking out dried mucus can cause nosebleeds.

D. Unwarranted Treatment: Electrocautery is contraindicated because it is painful and frightening to the child. Both electrocautery and chemical cautery can cause destruction of the septal tissue, resulting in scarring and an increased tendency for later bleeding.

Prognosis

Once home treatment and prophylaxis are mastered, nosebleeds become an insignificant problem for most families. In unusual cases where posterior bleeding occurs, the child must be referred to an otolaryngologist for a posterior pack, evaluation for nasopharyngeal lesions, and possibly a transfusion.

Chanin A: Prevention of recurrent nosebleeds in children. *Clin Pediatr (Phila)* 1972;**11:**684.

Hathaway WE: Bleeding disorders due to platelet dysfunction. *Am J Dis Child* 1971;**121:**127.

NASAL FURUNCLE

A nasal furuncle is an infection of a hair follicle in the anterior nares. Hair plucking or nose picking can provide a route of entry. The most common organism is *Staphylococcus aureus*. The diagnosis is made by finding an exquisitely tender, firm, red lump in the anterior naris. Treatment includes dicloxacillin, 50 mg/kg/d orally for 5 days, to prevent spread. The lesion should be gently incised and drained as soon as it points, usually with a needle. Topical bacitracin ointment may be of additional value. Since this lesion is in the drainage area of the cavernous sinus, the patient should be followed closely until healing is complete. Parents should be advised never to pick or squeeze a furuncle in this location, nor should the physician. Associated cellulitis or spread requires hospitalization for intravenous antibiotics.

Some patients with recurrent skin abscesses as well as nasal furuncles are nasal carriers of *S aureus*. The skin problem will often not resolve until the nasal carrier state is eradicated by systemic antibiotics, topical antibiotics, and recolonization of the nasal mucosa with nonpathogenic staphylococci.

NASAL SEPTUM SUBLUXATION

About 5% of newborn infants have a subluxation of the quadrangular cartilage of the septum. The tip of the nose deviates to one side, and the inferior septal border deviates to the other. There is also leaning of the columella and instability of the nasal tip. In the delivery room, reduction should be accomplished by lifting up the inferior border of the septum and replacing it in the septal groove of the floor of the nose. If any question regarding the procedure exists, an otolaryngologist should be consulted. This disorder must be distinguished from the more common transient flattening of the nose caused by the birth process.

Jazbi B: Nasal septum deformity in the newborn. *Clin Pediatr (Phila)* 1974;**13:**953.

Silverman SH et al: Dislocation of the triangular cartilage of the nasal septum. *J Pediatr* 1975;**87:**456.

NASAL FRACTURE

Most blows to the nose result in swelling and hematoma without a fracture. A persistent nosebleed after trauma suggests nasal fracture. Crepitus or instability of the bones in the nasal bridge is diagnostic of fracture, as is marked deviation of the nose to one side. However, septal injury can only be ruled out by a careful intranasal examination. If the parents feel that the appearance of the nose remains abnormal after the edema has resolved (usually 3–4 days), this should be taken as strong evidence for fracture. X-rays are not usually helpful, since they are negative in half of fractures. In general, they are warranted only in patients who have clinical suggestion of a fracture.

Patients with suspected nasal fractures should be referred to an ear, nose, and throat surgeon for definitive therapy. Resetting of the nasal fracture can be postponed up to 1 week without causing difficulty.

Goode RL, Spooner TR: Management of nasal fractures in children. *Clin Pediatr (Phila)* 1972;**11:**526.

Olsen KD, Carpenter RJ, Kern EB: Nasal septal trauma in children. *Pediatrics* 1979;**64:**32.

NASAL SEPTUM HEMATOMA

After nasal trauma, it is essential to examine the inside of the nose with a nasal speculum. Hematoma of the nasal septum imposes a considerable risk of pressure necrosis and resorption of the cartilage, leading to septal perforation or a saddle-back nose in adulthood. This diagnosis is confirmed by the abrupt onset of nasal obstruction following trauma and the presence of a widened nasal septum.

Treatment consists of prompt referral to an otolaryngologist for evacuation of the hematoma and packing of the nose.

NASAL SEPTUM ABSCESS

A nasal septal abscess usually follows nasal trauma or a nasal furuncle. The symptoms include fever, nasal tenderness, and nasal occlusion. Physical findings reveal a fluctuant gray septal swelling, usually bilateral. The possible complications are the same as for nasal septal hematoma plus septicemia, meningitis, or cavernous sinus thrombosis.

Treatment consists of immediate hospitalization, incision and drainage by an otolaryngologist, and intravenous antibiotics.

Segal S et al: Bacterial meningitis secondary to abscess of the nasal septum. *Pediatrics* 1977;**60:**102.

FOREIGN BODIES IN THE NOSE

Most objects inserted into the nose are detected by the parent soon after insertion, and the child is brought in immediately. Occasionally, a nasal foreign body is detected only after unilateral purulent rhinitis occurs. Commonly inserted objects are pussy willow buds, beads, buttons, bullets, nuts, and marbles. To prepare for removal, the nose should be suctioned and opened fully with a topical vasoconstrictor. The child's head should be held firmly to prevent movement and secondary injury during the removal. The position of the head should be forward to prevent aspiration of the foreign body into a bronchus. A nasal speculum is sometimes helpful. Suction can be used to remove the layer of mucus that hides the object.

There are many ways to remove nasal foreign bodies. The obvious first maneuver is vigorous nose blowing if the child is old enough. If the object is round, such as a bead, collodion on a cotton-tipped applicator can be placed against it and left there for 1 or 2 minutes, after which it will usually be dry enough to remove the object. Irregular objects can sometimes be grasped with a bayonet forceps. If there is room to go past the object, a right-angled hook can be inserted and withdrawn, pushing the object ahead of it. If these techniques are not successful and there is some space between the object and the side of the nose, a lubricated No. 8 Bardex Foley catheter can be inserted. When the balloon is past the object, it can be inflated and then used to extract the object.

With the head tilted over a large basin, the noninvolved nostril can be flushed rapidly with normal saline from a nasal bulb syringe. The wave of fluid will wash around to the involved side and in most cases will force the object out. Closing the uninvolved nostril and placing one's mouth over the patient's mouth to administer a sudden blast of air will force the foreign body out if enough pressure is exerted. If the object seems inaccessible, is wedged in, or is quite large, the patient should be referred to an otolaryngologist without worsening its position through futile attempts.

Goff WE: "Tip of the Month." *Consultant* (Jan) 1973;**13:**144.
Rees AC: "Tip of the Month." *Consultant* (Feb) 1970;**10:**12.
Stool SE, McConnell CS: Foreign bodies in pediatric otolaryngology. *Clin Pediatr (Phila)* 1973;**12:**113.

THE THROAT

ACUTE STOMATITIS

Recurrent Aphthous Stomatitis ("Canker Sore")

The main finding is multiple (1–4) small (3–10 mm) ulcers on the inside of the lips and throughout the remainder of the mouth. There is usually no associated fever or cervical adenopathy. The ulcers are very painful and last 1–2 weeks. They may recur numerous times throughout a patient's life span. The cause is not known, although an allergic or autoimmune basis is suspected. It is important to rule out any offending agents that could be avoided (chocolate, nuts, tomatoes, etc). These lesions are commonly misdiagnosed as herpes simplex.

Treatment consists of topical corticosteroids, either in a dental paste—eg, triamcinolone acetonide, 0.1% (Kenalog in Orabase)—or in a mouthwash administered 4 times a day. Pain can be symptomatically improved by a bland diet, avoiding salty or acid foods, switching from a bottle to a cup in infants, 2% viscous lidocaine (Xylocaine) prior to meals, and aspirin or even codeine at bedtime. In children not old enough to expectorate the lidocaine, it must be used sparingly to prevent side effects. Some patients gain pain relief from chemical cautery of the ulcers (eg, with silver nitrate). Measures that are unwarranted and sometimes harmful are smallpox vaccine, systemic antibiotics, and *Lactobacillus*-containing agents.

Herpes Simplex Gingivostomatitis

Approximately 1% of children who have their first encounter with the herpes simplex organism develop multiple (10 or more) small (1–3 mm) ulcers of the buccal mucosa, anterior pillars, inner lips, tongue, and especially the gingiva, with associated fever, tender cervical nodes, and generalized inflammation of the mouth. The children are commonly under 3 years of age. This disorder lasts 7–10 days. Severe dysphagia interferes with eating and drinking. The primary disorder does not recur; herpes simplex recurs only in the form of cold sores that are found mainly at the labial mucocutaneous juncture. A throat culture is recommended to rule out streptococcal infection and a white blood cell count to rule out agranulocytic mucosa lesions.

Treatment is symptomatic as described for recurrent aphthous stomatitis (see above), with the exception that corticosteroids are contraindicated because they may result in spread of the infection. The patient must be followed closely. Dehydration occasionally ensues despite liberal offerings of cold fluids, in which case the patient must be hospitalized so that intravenous fluids can be administered. Herpetic laryngotracheitis is a rare complication.

Stevens-Johnson Syndrome

The bullous form of erythema multiforme should be considered whenever there are vesicles and ulcers of the lips and oral mucosa with similar lesions on the conjunctivae and genitalia. In addition, most affected patients have a generalized erythema multiforme rash plus high fever and severe prostration. (For full discussion, see Chapter 10.)

Thrush of Mouth

Oral candidiasis mainly affects bottle-fed infants and occasionally older children in a debilitated state. *Candida albicans* is a saprophyte that normally is not invasive unless the mouth is abraded. The use of broad-spectrum antibiotics may be a contributing factor. The symptoms include soreness of the mouth and refusal of feedings. Lesions consist of white curd-like plaques predominantly on the buccal mucosa. These plaques cannot be washed away after a water feeding.

Specific treatment consists of use of nystatin (Mycostatin) oral suspension, 1 mL 4 times a day for 1 week. This should be preceded by attempts to remove any large plaques with a moistened cotton-tipped applicator. The child should be fed temporarily with a spoon and cup to eliminate pain, continued abrasion, and possible contamination from nipple feedings.

Oral Syphilis

The primary chancre can occur on the lips or in the oral cavity. Secondary syphilis can present as mucous patches on any part of the oral cavity. These have a gray, slimy, concentric appearance and can occur in various sizes. Both of these lesions can be diagnosed by darkfield examination. By the time mucous patches are present, the serologic test for syphilis will be positive. Syphilis is discussed more fully in Chapter 27.

Traumatic Oral Ulcers

Ulcers are a nonspecific response of the oral mucosa to trauma. Mechanical trauma most commonly occurs on the buccal mucosa secondary to accidentally biting it with the molars. Thermal trauma, eg, from very hot foods, can also cause ulcerative lesions. Chemical ulcers can be produced by mucosal contact with aspirin, caustics, etc. Oral ulcers can also occur with leukemia or on a recurrent basis with cyclic neutropenia.

These lesions usually need no treatment. The pain subsides in 2 or 3 days.

Dilley DH, Blozis GG: Common oral lesions and oral manifestations of systemic illnesses and therapies. *Pediatr Clin North Am* 1982;**29:**585.

Fermaglich DR, Fermaglich LF: Tracheostomy in primary herpetic gingivostomatitis. *J Pediatr* 1973;**82:**884.

Goldberg MP: The oral mucosa in childhood. *Pediatr Clin North Am* 1978;**25:**239.

Wright JM: A review of the oral manifestations of infections in pediatric patients. *Pediatr Infect Dis* 1984;**3:**80.

ACUTE VIRAL PHARYNGITIS & TONSILLITIS

Over 90% of cases of sore throat and fever in children are due to viral infections. Most children develop associated rhinorrhea and mild cough and in fact are having a cold and nothing more. The findings seldom give any clue to the particular viral agent, but 6 types of viral pharyngitis are sufficiently different to permit the clinician to make an educated guess about the specific cause.

Clinical Findings

A. Infectious Mononucleosis: The findings are an exudative tonsillitis, generalized cervical adenitis, and fever, usually in a teenage patient. A palpable spleen or axillary adenopathy adds weight to the diagnosis. The presence of more than 20% atypical lymphocytes on a peripheral blood smear or a positive mononucleosis spot test (Monospot) confirms the diagnosis. This diagnosis is often not considered until a patient with a presumptive diagnosis of streptococcal pharyngitis has failed to respond to 48 hours of treatment with penicillin.

B. Herpangina: Herpangina ulcers, 2–3 mm in size, are found on the anterior pillars and sometimes on the soft palate and uvula. There are no ulcers in the anterior mouth as seen in herpes simplex. Fever is present. The disease lasts up to a week. Herpangina is caused by several members of the coxsackie A group of viruses, and a patient can have up to 5 bouts of herpangina in a lifetime.

C. Lymphonodular Pharyngitis: The classic finding is small, yellow-white nodules in the same distribution as the small ulcers in herpangina. In this condition, which is caused by coxsackievirus A10, the nodules do not ulcerate.

D. Hand, Foot, and Mouth Disease: This entity is caused by coxsackieviruses A5, A10, and A16. Ulcers occur on the tongue and oral mucosa. Vesicles, which usually do not ulcerate, are found on the palms, soles, and interdigital areas.

E. Pharyngoconjunctival Fever: This disorder is caused by an adenovirus. Exudative tonsillitis, conjunctivitis, and fever are the main findings.

F. Rubeola: The prodrome of measles looks like any nonspecific viral respiratory infection until one closely examines the buccal mucosa and the inner aspects of the lower lip. Small white specks the size of salt granules on an erythematous base (Koplik's spots) found at these sites are pathognomonic of measles.

Treatment

The treatment of acute viral pharyngitis is strictly symptomatic. Older children can gargle with warm hypertonic salt solution. Younger children can suck on hard candy (especially butterscotch). Analgesics and antipyretics are sometimes helpful. Antibiotics are contraindicated.

ACUTE STREPTOCOCCAL PHARYNGITIS & TONSILLITIS

Approximately 10% of children with sore throat and fever have a streptococcal infection. Untreated streptococcal pharyngitis can result in acute rheumatic fever, glomerulonephritis, and suppurative complications (eg, cervical adenitis, peritonsillar abscess, otitis media, cellulitis, and septicemia). Vesicles and ulcers are suggestive of viral infection, whereas cervical adenitis, petechiae, a beefy-red uvula, and a tonsillar exudate are suggestive of streptococcal infection; the only way to make a definitive diagnosis is by obtaining a throat culture. A throat culture can be read 18 hours after being placed in an incubator. The bacteriology involved is simple, and an inexpensive office incubator is available. Office throat cultures are essential to the rational treatment of pharyngitis. A fuller discussion of the diagnosis and treatment of streptococcal infections is found in Chapter 27.

Other bacterial causes of acute pharyngitis are *Corynebacterium diphtheriae, Neisseria gonorrhoeae,* group C streptococci, meningococci, *Chlamydia,* and *Mycoplasma pneumoniae*. *Staphylococcus aureus* and *Streptococcus pneumoniae* may play a role in debilitated patients (eg, patients with cystic fibrosis).

Battle CU, Glasgow LA: Reliability of bacteriologic identification of β-hemolytic streptococci in private offices. *Am J Dis Child* 1971;**122:**134.

Hable KA et al: Bacterial and viral throat flora. *Clin Pediatr (Phila)* 1971;**10:**199.

Sprunt K et al: Identification of *Streptococcus pyogenes* in a pediatric outpatient department. *Pediatrics* 1974;**54:**718.

RECURRENT PHARYNGITIS

School-age children are occasionally brought to a physician with a complaint of recurrent or persistent sore throat. Fever and other systemic manifestations are usually absent. There are 3 common causes of this problem: mouth breathing, postnasal drip, and school phobia.

Mouth breathing leads to dryness and irritation of the throat, especially in areas of low humidity. Occasionally, children will even complain upon awakening that their lips are stuck to their teeth. The causes of mouth breathing (see p 326) should be investigated. Symptomatic treatment consists of good hydration and environmental humidification.

Postnasal drip due to chronic sinusitis can lead to continuous irritation of the throat. Examination reveals mucopurulent secretions descending from the nasopharynx after the patient sniffs. The irritation is largely due to repeated clearing of the throat. Treatment is described on p 328.

Children with **school phobia** are brought in repeatedly for sore throats, but physical examination reveals a normal oropharynx and tonsillar area. The diagnosis is made by asking the parent if the problem has been interfering with the child's school attendance. The answer will be affirmative and completely out of keeping with the degree of symptoms. Management is described in Chapter 24.

PERITONSILLAR ABSCESS (Quinsy)

Tonsillar infection occasionally penetrates the tonsillar capsule, spreads to the surrounding tissues, and causes peritonsillar cellulitis. If untreated, necrosis occurs and a tonsillar abscess forms. This can occur at any age. The most common cause is β-hemolytic streptococci.

The patient complains of a severe sore throat even before the physical findings become marked. A high fever is usually present. The process is almost always unilateral. The tonsil bulges medially, and the anterior pillar is prominent. The soft palate and uvula on the involved side are edematous and displaced medially toward the uninvolved side. In severe cases, there is trismus, dysphagia, and, finally, drooling. The quality of the voice is severely impaired by the fixation of the soft palate. On palpation, the tonsil is firm and exquisitely tender. A serious complication of inadequately treated peritonsillar abscess is a lateral pharyngeal abscess. This leads to fullness and tenderness of the lateral neck, as well as torticollis. Without intervention, the abscess eventually threatens life by airway obstruction or carotid artery erosion.

Aggressive treatment in early cases of peritonsillar cellulitis will usually abort the process and prevent suppuration. The treatment of choice is procaine penicillin by daily injection plus oral penicillin 4 times a day in high doses. Daily follow-up is critical to detect possible abscess. If the initial swelling is marked, fluctuation develops, a neck mass develops, or symptoms fail to respond to 48 hours of antibiotics, the patient should be hospitalized for intravenous antibiotics. An otolaryngologist should be consulted to perform incision and drainage. To locate the space, a needle is introduced into the abscess at the point of maximal swelling of the soft palate, and the incision is then made along the needle shaft. This procedure should be done with the patient's head in a lowered position to prevent aspiration of the purulent drainage. Material should be taken for culture. Recurrent peritonsillar abscesses are so uncommon (7%) that routine tonsillectomy for a single bout is not indicated. Hospitalized patients can be discharged on oral antibiotics when the fever is resolved for 24 hours and they can swallow easily.

Rubinstein E, Onderdonk AB, Rahal JJ Jr: Peritonsillar infection and bacteremia caused by *Fusobacterium gonidiaformans*. *J Pediatr* 1974;**85:**673.

Schuit KE, Johnson JT: Infection of the head and neck. *Pediatr Clin North Am* 1981;**28:**965.

RETROPHARYNGEAL ABSCESS

Retropharyngeal nodes drain the adenoids and nasopharynx and can become infected. The most common cause is β-hemolytic streptococci. If this pyogenic adenitis goes untreated, a retropharyngeal abscess forms. The process occurs almost exclusively during the first 2 years of life. Beyond this age, retropharyngeal abscess usually results from superinfection of a penetrating injury of the posterior wall of the oropharynx.

The diagnosis should be strongly suspected in an infant with fever, respiratory symptoms, and neck hyperextension. Dysphagia, dyspnea, and gurgling respirations are also found and are due to the impingement by the abscess. Prominent swelling on one side of the posterior pharyngeal wall confirms the diagnosis. Swelling usually stops at the midline because a medial raphe divides the prevertebral space. Lateral neck soft tissue films provide additional confirmation if needed.

Retropharyngeal abscess is a surgical emergency. Immediate hospitalization is required. A surgeon should incise and drain the abscess to prevent its extension. The head should be kept down during incision to prevent aspiration of purulent material. Intravenous hydration and antibiotics should be instituted before surgery. Penicillin is the drug of choice pending the results of stained smear examination.

Janecka IP, Rankow RM: Fatal mediastinitis following retropharyngeal abscess. *Arch Otolaryngol* 1971;**93:**630.

McCook TA, Felman AH: Retropharyngeal masses in infants and young children. *Am J Dis Child* 1979;**133:**41.

LUDWIG'S ANGINA

Ludwig's angina is a rapidly progressive cellulitis of the submandibular space. The submandibular space extends from the mucous membrane of the tongue to the muscular and fascial attachments of the hyoid bone. The initiating factor in over half of cases is dental disease, including abscesses and extraction. Some patients have a history of lacerations and injuries to the floor of the mouth. Group A streptococci are the most common organisms identified, but other pathogens have been recovered.

The presenting symptoms are fever and tender swelling of the floor of the mouth. The tongue can become enlarged as well as tender and erythematous. Upward displacement of the tongue may cause dysphagia and drooling. Laboratory evaluation includes blood cultures and hypopharyngeal aspiration to attempt to identify the specific pathogen.

Treatment consists of giving high dosages of intravenous ampicillin and methicillin until the results of cultures and sensitivity tests are available. Since the most common cause of death in Ludwig's angina is sudden airway obstruction, the patient must be followed closely in the intensive care unit and intubation provided for any progressive respiratory distress.

Barkin RM et al: Ludwig angina in children. *J Pediatr* 1975;**87:**563.

Gross SJ et al: Ludwig angina in childhood. *Am J Dis Child* 1977;**131:**291.

ACUTE CERVICAL ADENITIS

Essentials of Diagnosis

- Large, tender, unilateral cervical mass.
- Fever.
- Moderate to marked leukocytosis.

General Considerations

Local infections of the ear, nose, and throat can spread to the regional node and cause a secondary inflammation there. The most commonly involved node is the jugulodigastric node, which drains the tonsillar area. The problem is most prevalent among preschool children.

A classic case involves a large, unilateral, solitary, tender node. About 70% of these cases are due to β-hemolytic streptococci, 20% are due to staphylococci, and the remainder may be due to viruses. *Haemophilus influenzae* has rarely been reported as the cause. Surgeons report a higher incidence of staphylococcal infection, but they see a greater proportion of atypical cases that have failed to respond to penicillin therapy and thus require incision and drainage.

The most common site of invasion is from pharyngitis or tonsillitis. Other entry sites for pyogenic adenitis are periapical dental abscess (usually producing a submandibular adenitis), facial impetigo (infected cuts or bug bites), infected acne, and otitis externa (usually producing a preauricular adenitis).

Clinical Findings

A. Symptoms and Signs: The patient is brought

in with the chief complaint of a swollen neck or face. There is usually sustained high fever, especially in staphylococcal infections. The mass is often the size of a walnut or even an egg. It is taut, firm, and exquisitely tender. If left untreated, it may develop an overlying erythema. The exact size of the node should be measured for future follow-up. Each tooth should be examined for a periapical abscess and percussed for tenderness. A protective torticollis is sometimes present.

B. Laboratory Findings: The white blood cell count is usually about 20,000/μL with a shift to the left. The combination of leukocytosis and a positive throat culture or an elevated ASO titer identifies streptococci in about two-thirds of streptococcal cases. A tuberculin skin test should be given. Aspirated material from fluctuant nodes should be gram-stained and cultured.

Differential Diagnosis

The causes of cervical adenopathy are numerous. Five general categories can be distinguished on the basis of the clinical findings.

A. Acute Unilateral Cervical Adenitis: See above.

B. Acute Bilateral Cervical Adenitis: Painful and tender nodes are present on both sides, and the patient usually has fever.

1. Infectious mononucleosis—This diagnosis can be aided by the findings of splenomegaly, over 20% atypical cells on the white blood cell smear, and a positive mononucleosis spot test (Monospot). Toxoplasmosis and cytomegalovirus infections can imitate this disorder.

2. Tularemia—There will be a history of wild rabbit or deerfly exposure.

3. Diphtheria—This only occurs in nonimmunized children.

C. Subacute or Chronic Adenitis: In this condition, an isolated node usually exists, but it is smaller and less tender than the acute pyogenic adenitis described previously.

1. Nonspecific viral pharyngitis—This accounts for about 80% of cases in this category.

2. β-Hemolytic streptococcal infection—Streptococci can occasionally cause a low-grade cervical adenitis; staphylococci never do.

3. Cat-scratch fever—The diagnosis is aided by the finding of a primary papule in approximately 60% of cases. Cat contact or scratches are present in over 90% of cases. The node is usually mildly tender. The cat-scratch skin test is helpful and relatively safe.

4. Atypical mycobacterial infection—The node is generally nontender and submandibular (occasionally preauricular). The nodes become fluctuant after several months. Affected patients are usually 1–5 years of age. A history of drinking unpasteurized milk is helpful. A mildly positive PPD is suggestive. A PPD-standard gives 5–10 mm of induration, whereas the PPD-Battey gives greater than 10 mm of induration. If skin tests for atypical mycobacteria are not available, the OT (old tuberculin) test can be substituted for screening.

D. Cervical Node Tumors: Malignant tumors usually are not suspected until the adenopathy persists despite treatment. Classically, the nodes are painless, nontender, and firm to hard in consistency. They may occur as a single node, unilateral multiple nodes in a chain, bilateral cervical nodes, or generalized adenopathy. Cancers that may present in the neck are Hodgkin's disease, lymphosarcoma, fibrosarcoma, thyroid cancer, leukemia, and cancers with an occult primary in the nasopharynx (eg, rhabdomyosarcoma). A benign tumor that presents as enlarged cervical nodes is sinus histiocytosis.

E. Imitators of Adenitis: Several structures in the neck can become infected and resemble a node. The first 3 masses are of congenital origin and are listed in order of frequency.

1. Thyroglossal duct cyst—When superinfected, this congenital malformation can become acutely swollen. Helpful findings are the fact that it is in the midline, located between the hyoid bone and suprasternal notch, and moves upward on sticking out the tongue or swallowing. Occasionally, the cyst develops a sinus tract and opening just lateral to the midline.

2. Branchial cleft cyst—When superinfected, this can become a tender mass, 3–5 cm in diameter. Aids to diagnosis are the fact that the mass is located along the anterior border of the sternocleidomastoid muscle and is smooth and fluctuant as a cyst should be. Occasionally, it is attached to the overlying skin by a small dimple or a draining sinus tract.

3. Cystic hygroma—Most of these lymphatic cysts are located in the posterior triangle just above the clavicle. The mass is soft and compressible and can be transilluminated. Over 60% are noted at birth, and the remainder usually present by 2 years of age. If cysts become large enough, they can compromise swallowing and breathing.

4. Mumps—The most common pitfall in diagnosis is mistaking mumps for adenitis. However, mumps crosses the angle of the jaw, is associated with preauricular percussion tenderness, and is bilateral in 70% of cases, and there is frequently a history of exposure to mumps. Submandibular mumps can present a diagnostic dilemma.

5. Ranula—This sublingual retention cyst can be mistaken for a submental node (see p 339).

6. Sternocleidomastoid muscle hematoma—This cervical mass is noted at 2–4 weeks of age. On close examination it is found to be part of the muscle body and not movable. An associated torticollis is usually confirmatory.

Complications

The most common complication in the untreated case is suppuration of the node, with eventual pointing and exterior drainage. In the preantibiotic era, extension sometimes occurred internally, resulting in jugular vein thrombosis, carotid artery rupture, septicemia, and compression of the esophagus or larynx. Poststreptococcal acute glomerulonephritis and bacteremia have also been reported.

Treatment

A. Specific Measures: Unless the patient has recently been exposed to β-hemolytic streptococci, dicloxacillin or erythromycin is usually started initially. The antibiotic can be changed to penicillin if it is not well tolerated and the throat culture is positive for streptococci. Dicloxacillin must be started initially if the patient is under 6 months of age or the node is already fluctuant or erythematous. The patient should be referred to a dentist if a periapical abscess is suspected. Patients should also be given prophylactic penicillin therapy to prevent associated facial cellulitis or submandibular adenitis.

B. General Measures: Analgesics (even codeine) are necessary during the first few days. Patients may receive significant relief from application of cold compresses or an ice cube to the inflamed node.

C. Surgical Treatment: Early treatment with antibiotics prevents many cases of pyogenic adenitis from progressing to suppuration. However, once fluctuation occurs, antibiotic therapy alone is not sufficient treatment. When fluctuation or pointing is present, the primary physician should incise and drain the abscess. This can easily be done as an office procedure or in an ambulatory surgery unit. Hospitalization is required only if the patient is toxic, dehydrated, dysphagic, dyspneic, or less than 6 months of age.

D. Follow-Up Care: The patient must be seen daily. A good response includes resolution of the fever and improvement in the tenderness after 48 hours of treatment. Reduction in size of the nodes may take several more days. The antibiotic should be continued for 10 days. If there is no improvement in 48 hours and the PPD test is negative, the node should be aspirated with an 18-gauge needle and 0.5 mL of normal saline in the syringe to obtain material for gram-stained smear, culture, and sensitivity tests. Aspirated material should be cultured aerobically and anaerobically.

E. Treatment of Nonpyogenic Adenitis:

1. Cat-scratch fever and atypical mycobacterial infection—Treatment is described in Chapter 27.

2. Persistent unexplained node—As previously mentioned, cancer of the cervical node is usually asymptomatic. The patient with a cervical node that has been enlarging for more than 2 weeks despite treatment or is still large and unchanged in size for more than 2 months should be referred to a surgeon for biopsy.

3. Branchial cleft cyst and thyroglossal duct cyst—If superinfected, these lesions should be treated with penicillin for 10 days. After the infection clears, the patient should be referred to a surgeon for definitive excision of the cyst.

Prognosis

With appropriate treatment, the prognosis is excellent. After the infection clears, the node may remain palpable for several months but will gradually decrease in size unless it is scarred. Recurrent pyogenic adenitis is rare. When it occurs, it is usually due to diseases such as chronic granulomatous disease of childhood or an immunologic disorder.

Barton LL, Feigin RD: Childhood cervical lymphadenitis: A reappraisal. *J Pediatr* 1974;**84:**846.

Boyce JM et al: Nosocomial staphylococcal cervical lymphadenitis in infants: Report of an outbreak. *Pediatrics* 1976;**57:**854.

Buckingham JM, Lynn HB: Branchial cleft cysts and sinuses in children. *Mayo Clin Proc* 1974;**49:**172.

Jaffe BF, Jaffe N: Head and neck tumors in children. *Pediatrics* 1973;**51:**731.

May M: Neck masses in children: Diagnosis and treatment. *Pediatr Ann* 1976;**5:**517.

Novack AH: Lumps and bumps in the neck. *Pediatr Dig* 1979;**21:**15.

Pounds LA: Neck masses of congenital origin. *Pediatr Clin North Am* 1981;**28:**841.

Zitelli BJ: Neck masses in children: Adenopathy and malignant disease. *Pediatr Clin North Am* 1981;**28:**813.

TONSILLECTOMY & ADENOIDECTOMY (T&A)

Removal of the tonsils and adenoids has been described as a North American ritual. Although about 30% of children in the USA have their tonsils and adenoids removed, only 1–2% of children have adequate medical indications for this procedure.

Besides being usually unnecessary, the procedure is costly and carries considerable risk. The mortality rate under good conditions is still one death per 15,000 operations. Postoperative bleeding on the fifth to eighth day occurs in approximately 5% of cases and requires transfusion or suturing of the tonsillar bed. Some children with previously normal speech develop hypernasal speech. The emotional hazards of hospitalization and surgery in a child under 5 years of age have been well documented. There are still questions regarding the role of tonsils in immunologic response and disease prevention.

Invalid Reasons for T&A

The following conditions account for the removal of over 95% of tonsils and adenoids.

A. "Large Tonsils": Many parents feel that large tonsils mean bad tonsils. It is unfortunate that the peak incidence of infections correlates so well with tonsillar size. Normal lymphoid atrophy occurs spontaneously after age 8. The parent should be reassured that the patient's tonsils are within normal range. It is very important at well child checkups not to call a child's tonsils "big" or "bad."

B. Recurrent Colds and Sore Throats: T&A

does not decrease the incidence of viral respiratory infections. Parents must be reassured that these infections are a natural event at this age and that contacts eventually give the patient increased immunity.

C. Recurrent Streptococcal Pharyngitis: At one time, repeated episodes of "strep throat" were considered an indication for tonsillectomy. However, it has been shown in several studies that the incidence of streptococcal infections does not decrease after the tonsils have been removed unless 7 or more attacks occur per year. Moreover, the future diagnosis of streptococcal infections is made difficult by the lack of tonsillar exudates.

D. Recurrent Otitis Media: Most cases of recurrent purulent otitis media can be treated with prophylactic antibiotics. Most cases of chronic serous otitis media eventually resolve or require tympanoplasty tubes.

E. Parental Pressure: Some parents place great demands on their doctor for a T&A and must be skillfully reeducated.

F. School Absence: For the child who misses school for vague symptoms, removing the tonsils will not relieve the school phobia.

G. "Chronic Tonsillitis": It is unclear whether this condition even exists. If it does, it is certainly very rare. The tonsil is allegedly so diseased that even antibiotics cannot eliminate the infections.

H. Miscellaneous Conditions: Poor appetite, allergic rhinitis, asthma, unexplained fevers, and halitosis are not indications for tonsillectomy.

Indications for Adenoidectomy

A. Persistent Nasal Obstruction and Mouth Breathing: Mouth breathing can have many causes (see p 000). However, if this problem is due to large adenoids, they should be removed to prevent an adenoidal facies. Removal should be preceded by a 2-week trial of penicillin to rule out enlargement from subacute adenoiditis.

B. Snoring: The adenoids should be removed if they appear to be the cause of continual nighttime snoring and daytime snorting.

C. Hyponasal Speech: Large adenoids can cause hyponasal speech that leads to poor communication as well as teasing. On examination, large adenoids are found to be preventing the uvula from moving upward normally.

Indications for Tonsillectomy

A. Persistent Oral Obstruction and Dysphagia: Intermittent oral obstruction and dysphagia can occur as a result of inflammation and swelling of the tonsils. If the problem is persistent and the tonsils are seen to almost touch in the midline, tonsillectomy should be performed. This is especially likely to happen in people who have small oral cavities.

B. Recurrent Peritonsillar Abscess: This problem implies that the tonsil is no longer inhibiting the spread of infection and needs to be removed. About 20% of peritonsillar abscesses recur.

C. Recurrent Pyogenic Cervical Adenitis: Again, the tonsil is no longer acting as an effective barrier to the spread of infection.

D. Suspected Tonsillar Tumor: The prominent unilateral tonsil, especially if it is rapidly enlarging, may be removed with the presumptive diagnosis of tonsillar neoplasm. On palpation, these tumors are usually firm and fixed. This is a grave diagnosis to miss.

Indications for Combined T&A

A. Cor Pulmonale: A patient with adenoidal hypertrophy can develop chronic hypoxia that leads to pulmonary hypertension and finally to cor pulmonale and right-sided heart failure. This is a rare but serious complication that is definitely helped by T&A, sometimes on an emergency basis.

B. Sleep Apnea Syndrome: Affected chidren all have loud snoring interrupted by 30- to 60-second apneic and cyanotic episodes. Many are referred because of excessive daytime sleepiness and worsening school performance. Acquired pectus excavatum has also been reported in some of these children. Their symptoms are reversed by T&A.

C. Recurrent Aspiration Pneumonia: The patient with huge tonsils, muffled speech, and gurgling respirations may occasionally present with repeated aspiration pneumonia.

Contraindications to T&A

A. Short Palate: Adenoids should not be removed in a child with a cleft palate, submucous cleft palate, or bifid uvula, because of the risk of aggravating the velopharyngeal incompetence and causing hypernasal speech and nasal regurgitation.

B. Bleeding Disorder: If a chronic bleeding disorder is present, it must be diagnosed and compensated for before a T&A.

C. Acute Tonsillitis: T&A should be postponed until an acute tonsillitis is resolved. This guideline may prevent a superinfection of the wound.

D. Polio Season: T&A during polio season in a susceptible population leads to an increased risk of bulbar poliomyelitis. Wide-scale use of poliovaccine can eliminate this hazard.

Management of Parental Pressure

If parents are dissatisfied with the kind of treatment they are receiving, they can "doctor-shop" until they find someone who will remove their child's tonsils. This can be prevented by the following approach:

The parents' complaint must be taken seriously. All of the reasonable indications for T&A must be competently investigated. The ear, nose, and throat examination must be performed carefully, and the parents must be assured that there are some valid reasons to take out the tonsils but only when the benefit outweighs the risk, discomfort, inconvenience, and expense.

The parents can then be reassured that their child is basically healthy. The prognosis for spontaneous involution of the tonsils and adenoids and a lower incidence of respiratory infections in years to come can be offered. In addition, it can be mentioned that the risk of taking the tonsils out is considerably greater than the risk of leaving them in.

If the parents are still unconvinced, a consultation is in order. Since it is in the child's best interest, an otolaryngologist should be chosen who shares the pediatrician's viewpoint on this subject.

Guilleminault C et al: Sleep apnea in eight children. *Pediatrics* 1976;**58**:23.

Paradise JL: Tonsillectomy and adenoidectomy. *Pediatr Clin North Am* 1981;**28**:881.

Paradise JL et al: Efficacy of tonsillectomy for recurrent throat infection in severely affected children. *N Engl J Med* 1984;**310**:674.

Shaikh W et al: A systematic review of the literature on evaluative studies of tonsillectomy and adenoidectomy. *Pediatrics* 1976;**57**:401.

DISORDERS OF THE LIPS*

Labial Sucking Tubercle

A small baby may present with a small callus in the mid upper lip. It usually is asymptomatic and disappears after cup feeding is initiated.

Swollen Lip

Allergy can cause the sudden onset of angioedema of the lip. Possible causes include foods, contact dermatitis to lipstick, and insect bites. Treatment includes avoidance of the cause, cold compresses, and oral antihistamines.

Cheilitis

Dry, cracked, scaling lips are usually due to sun or wind exposure. Contact dermatitis from mouthpieces of various woodwind or brass instruments has also been reported. Licking the lips accentuates the process, and the patient should be warned of this. Liberal use of lip balms gives excellent results.

Perlèche

The angle of the mouth may become fissured and raw. This most commonly happens in children who drool or lick the sides of the mouth, establishing a macerated area. The most common pathogen is *Candida albicans*. Sores at the corners of the mouth can also be due to use of wide teething rings with rough edges. Riboflavin deficiency is a rare cause. The lesions respond well to nystatin (Mycostatin) cream. Occasionally, a corticosteroid must be added.

* Herpetic lesions are discussed in Chapter 26.

Inclusion Cyst

Inclusion cysts, or retention cysts, are due to the obstruction of mucous glands or other mucous membrane structures. In the newborn, they occur on the hard palate or gums and are called Epstein's pearls. These small cysts resolve spontaneously in 1–2 months. In older children, inclusion cysts usually occur on the palate, uvula, or tonsillar pillars. They appear as taut, yellow sacs varying in size from 2 to 10 mm. They spontaneously resolve in several months to a year without requiring incision and drainage. They can be rechecked in 1 month to confirm that they are not enlarging rapidly and thereafter reevaluated only during regular visits. Occasionally, a mucous cyst on the lower lip (mucocele) will require drainage for cosmetic reasons. Minor salivary glands are present at this site, and biting the lip may sever their ducts and initiate the problem.

DISORDERS OF THE TONGUE

Geographic Tongue (Benign Migratory Glossitis)

This condition of unknown cause is marked by circular or elliptical smooth areas on the tongue devoid of papillae and surrounded by a narrow ring of hyperkeratosis. The pattern can change from day to day. The lesions are painless and may last months to years. This puzzling disorder is benign, uncommon after age 6, and requires no treatment.

Fissured Tongue (Scrotal Tongue)

This condition is marked by numerous irregular fissures on the dorsum of the tongue. It occurs in approximately 1% of people and is usually a dominant trait. It is also frequently seen in children with trisomy 21 and other retarded patients who have the habit of chewing on a protruded tongue.

Coated Tongue (Furry Tongue)

The tongue normally becomes coated if mastication is impaired and the patient is on a liquid or soft diet. Mouth breathing, fever, or dehydration can accentuate the process.

Macroglossia

Tongue hypertrophy and protrusion may be a clue to Beckwith's syndrome, glycogen storage disease, cretinism, Hurler's syndrome, lymphangioma, or hemangioma. In trisomy 21, the normal-sized tongue protrudes because the oral cavity is small.

Acute Bacterial Glossitis

Reported causes of acute suppurative glossitis include *Haemophilus influenzae* type b, *Streptococcus haemolyticus*, and *Pseudomonas*. This rare disease is characterized by fever and rapid swelling and tenderness of the tongue. Intravenous antibiotics are required.

Edwards MS, Reynolds GES: Acute glossitis due to *Hemophilus influenzae* type b. *J Pediatr* 1978;**93**:532.

ORAL TRAUMA

Puncture wounds of the floor of the mouth and soft palate are not uncommon in children. Most could be prevented if children were forbidden to play with sticks or pencils in their mouths. Treatment includes a tetanus booster if one has not been given in the previous 5 years. Prophylactic antibiotics are not helpful, but the patient should be seen after 48 hours to rule out the possibility of superinfection. Puncture wounds of the anterior pillar or posterior pharynx should be followed closely for carotid thrombosis or retropharyngeal abscess, respectively.

Lacerations of the lip require precise closure and alignment of the mucocutaneous juncture. Lacerations of the buccal mucosa usually heal without suturing. Most tongue lacerations heal without suturing; if they involve the edges of the tongue and are large enough to cause gaping of the wound, black silk sutures must be placed, sometimes under general anesthesia.

HALITOSIS

"Bad breath" is a puzzling and distressing complaint. In most cases, it is due to acute stomatitis, pharyngitis, or sinusitis. In children, there are 2 common causes of chronic halitosis: continual mouth breathing and thumb-sucking or blanket-sucking. Unusual causes of foul breath are a nasal foreign body, esophageal diverticulum, gastric bezoar, bronchiectasis, and lung abscess. In older children, the presence of orthodontic devices or dentures can cause halitosis if good dental hygiene is not maintained. Also, offensive skin odors (eg, dirty feet) of long duration can become absorbed and excreted through the lungs. Mouthwashes and chewable breath fresheners give limited improvement. The cause must be uncovered to help the patient with chronic halitosis.

SALIVARY GLAND DISORDERS*

Suppurative Parotitis

Pyogenic parotitis is an unusual clinical disorder found predominantly in newborns and debilitated older patients. The parotid gland is swollen, tender, and often reddened. The diagnosis is made by expression of purulent material from Stensen's duct. The material should be smeared and cultured. Fever and leukocytosis may be present.

Treatment includes hospitalization and intravenous methicillin because the most common causative organism is *Staphylococcus aureus*. If fluctuation occurs and drainage through Stensen's duct is impaired, aspiration of the pus with an 18-gauge needle can avoid the necessity for incision and drainage. This may have to be repeated 3 or 4 times.

Recurrent Idiopathic Parotitis

Some children experience repeated episodes of parotid swelling that lasts 1–2 weeks and then resolves spontaneously. There is usually mild pain and often no fever. The process is most often unilateral, which weighs heavily against an autoimmune process as the underlying cause and points instead to some sort of obstructive process. Serum amylase is normal, which speaks against a diagnosis of viral parotitis as can occur with mumps, parainfluenza, and other viral infections. As many as 10 episodes may occur from age 2 on. The problem usually resolves spontaneously at puberty.

Treatment includes analgesics if pain is present. A 4-day course of corticosteroids can be recommended if it can be initiated early in an attack (see Gellis reference, below). A second attack of parotid swelling without fever should result in referral to an otolaryngologist for a sialogram to rule out calculus of Stensen's duct. The usual finding is sialectasis. The sialogram seems to improve as the recurrence rate diminishes.

Pneumoparotitis

Children with pneumoparotitis complain of a sudden onset of pain and swelling in the parotid area. A history of playing a musical wind instrument or blowing up balloons confirms the diagnosis. The cause of this transient condition is inflation of the parotid gland secondary to sudden increased intraoral pressure.

Tumors of the Parotid

Mixed tumors and hemangiomas can present in the parotid gland as a hard or persistent mass. The patient should be referred to a surgeon.

Ranula

A ranula is a retention cyst of a sublingual salivary gland. It is found on the floor of the mouth to one side of the lingual frenulum. Ranula has been described as resembling a frog's belly, since it is thin-walled and contains a clear bluish fluid. Referral to an otolaryngologist for marsupialization is indicated.

David RB et al: Suppurative parotitis in children. *Am J Dis Child* 1970;**119**:332.

Gellis SS: Editorial on recurrent parotitis. Page 169 in: *Yearbook of Pediatrics*. Year Book, 1970.

Habel DW: Recurrent swelling of the parotid gland. *Postgrad Med* (Aug) 1970;**48**:116.

* Mumps is discussed in Chapter 26.

Leake D et al: Neonatal suppurative parotitis. *Pediatrics* 1970;**46:**202.
Saunders HF: Wind parotitis. *N Engl J Med* 1973;**289:**689.

ORAL CONGENITAL MALFORMATIONS

Tongue-Tie

The tightness of the lingual frenulum varies greatly among normal people. A short frenulum prevents both protrusion and elevation of the tongue. A puckering of the midline of the tongue occurs with tongue movement. The condition in no way interferes with the ability to nurse. It is unlikely that it interferes with the ability to speak, since even children with ankyloglossia have normal speech.

Treatment consists of reassurance. Although there is no evidence to support it, clipping of the frenulum is sometimes recommended if the tongue does not protrude beyond the teeth or gums. If this degree of tongue-tie is associated with impairment of rapid articulation, the patient should be referred to an otolaryngologist for correction. Casual frenulum clipping can result in significant bleeding from a cut lingual artery or injury to the orifices of Wharton's duct.

Catlin FI, DeHaan V: Tongue-tie. *Arch Otolaryngol* 1971; **94:**548.

Cleft Lip & Cleft Palate

Cleft lip, cleft palate, or both conditions are found in one in 800 live births. They are readily diagnosed in the newborn nursery. Treatment requires a multidisciplined team approach—plastic surgeons, otolaryngologists, audiologists, speech therapists, orthodontists, and prosthodontists. Cleft lip repair is usually withheld until the child weighs over 5 kg. Cleft palate repair is usually performed at 18 months of age; this is essential to permit normal speech development, which should begin at this time. Occasionally, the palate is short and results in nasal speech. A permanently constructed flap of tissue from the posterior pharyngeal wall may be of benefit.

Cleft palate causes eating problems and poor weight gain due to nasal regurgitation or lung aspiration of milk. Best results are obtained by feeding the baby with a cup or special compressible feeder (see Paradise reference, below). The sitting position is optimal for feeding. Cleft palate nipples are usually no more effective than standard nipples. Approximately 90% of children with cleft palate have chronic otitis media and must be carefully followed for this problem. Some otolaryngologists recommend prophylactic tympanoplasty tubes.

Bergstrom L, Hemenway WG: Otologic problems in submucous cleft palate. *South Med J* 1971;**64:**1172.
Paradise JL, McWilliams BJ: Simplified feeder for infants with cleft palate. *Pediatrics* 1974;**53:**566.
Schilli W et al: A general description of 315 cleft lip and palate patients. *Cleft Palate J* 1970;**7:**573.

Bifid Uvula

A bifid uvula can be a normal finding. However, there is a close association between this and submucous cleft palate. A submucous cleft can be diagnosed by palpation of the hard palate. In this condition, the posterior bony portion of the hard palate is absent. Affected children have a 40% risk of developing chronic serous otitis media. They also are at risk of incomplete closure of the palate, resulting in hypernasal speech.

High-Arched Palate

A high-arched palate is usually a genetic trait of no consequence. It is also seen in children who are chronic mouth breathers. Some rare causes of high-arched palate are congenital disorders such as Marfan's syndrome, Treacher Collins syndrome, and Ehlers-Danlos syndrome.

Pierre Robin Syndrome

This congenital malformation is characterized by the triad of micrognathia, cleft palate, and glossoptosis. Affected children present as emergencies in the newborn period because of infringement on the airway by the tongue. The main objective of treatment is to prevent asphyxia until the mandible becomes large enough to accommodate the tongue. In some cases, this can be achieved by leaving the child in a prone position while unattended. In severe cases, a custom-fitted oropharyngeal airway or large suture through the base of the tongue that is anchored to the soft tissue in front of the mandible is required. The child requires close observation until the problem is outgrown.

Gunter G et al: Early management of the Pierre Robin syndrome. *Cleft Palate J* 1970;**7:**495.
Hawkins DB, Simpson JV: Micrognathia and glossoptosis in the newborn. *Clin Pediatr (Phila)* 1974;**13:**1066.
Shprintzen JJ: Morphologic significance of bifid uvula. *Pediatrics* 1985;**75:**553.

SELECTED REFERENCES

Bluestone CD: *Pediatric Otolaryngology.* 2 vols. Saunders, 1983.
Stool SE, Belafsky ML: *Pediatric Otolaryngology: Current Problems in Pediatrics.* Year Book, 1971.
Strome M: *Differential Diagnosis in Pediatric Otolaryngology.* Little, Brown, 1976.

Respiratory Tract & Mediastinum

14

John G. Brooks, MD

The diagnosis and treatment of pulmonary diseases in children are enhanced by an understanding of the relevant pathophysiology. The basics of normal and abnormal anatomy and physiologic mechanisms are outlined in this chapter, and the diseases are classified according to the structures they involve.

ANATOMY & DEVELOPMENT

The air-containing compartment of the respiratory system includes the upper airway (above the glottis), larynx, trachea, bronchi, bronchioles (characterized by the absence of cartilage and bronchial mucous glands in the wall), terminal bronchioles (the smallest airways supplied primarily by the bronchial circulation), respiratory bronchioles (largest airways into which alveoli open directly, and the largest airways perfused primarily by the pulmonary circulation), alveolar ducts, and alveoli. The embryonic lung bud arises from the primitive endodermal tube in the fourth week of gestation and progresses by asynchronous dichotomous branching to form all conducting airways (terminal bronchioles and all larger airways) by the end of the fourth month of gestation. By about the 25th–28th weeks of gestation, after further airway growth and pulmonary capillary proliferation, the juxtaposition of terminal air spaces and pulmonary capillaries creates the potential for enough gas exchange to support life. Subsequently, terminal airway stability, which is dependent on the presence of surfactant, becomes the principal respiratory factor limiting viability. Although birth initiates major changes in respiratory function, its impact on lung morphology is minor. Between the end of the third trimester and early adolescence, all alveoli are formed. Subsequently, there are further increases in alveolar complexity and size until about age 18 years. During infancy and childhood, cartilaginous support of the larynx, trachea, and bronchi continues to develop along with airway smooth muscle and pathways for collateral ventilation. During this period also, the upper airway becomes better stabilized (less vulnerable to spontaneous obstruction by the tongue and other pharyngeal tissues); the larynx becomes 1–2 cervical vertebrae lower, the respiratory muscles stronger and more fatigue-resistant, and the chest wall less compliant. Functional changes in the respiratory system include the end of obligate nasal breathing at about age 2–4 months and a change of the part of the airway with the smallest cross-sectional area from the level of the cricoid cartilage to the level of the vocal cords at about age 5 years. Some of these alterations, with the relatively small diameter of all airways in infants and young children, partially explain the tendency of these patients to develop significant respiratory distress with diseases such as croup, which would usually cause far fewer signs and symptoms in adults. Because of the sparseness of airway smooth muscle in normal young infants, bronchospasm is rare in the first 6 months of life, although it can occur.

Hodson WA (editor): *Development of the Lung*. Dekker, 1977.

Inselman LS, Mellins RB: Growth and development of the lung. *J Pediatr* 1981;**98:**1.

Murray JF: *The Normal Lung: The Basis for Diagnosis and Treatment of Pulmonary Disease*. Saunders, 1976.

Polgar G, Weng TR: The functional development of the respiratory system: From the period of gestation to adulthood. *Am Rev Respir Dis* 1979;**120:**625.

Scarpelli EM: *Pulmonary Physiology of the Fetus, Newborn, and Child*. Lea & Febiger, 1975.

PHYSIOLOGY

The caliber of airways and pulmonary vessels is controlled by mechanical, humoral, and neural reflex mechanisms. Changes in caliber may or may not be uniform throughout the lung. When only some of the airways and blood vessels are involved, the distribution may be either regional or anatomic (ie, affecting only certain sizes or types of airways or vessels). All intrapulmonary structures are connected by a connective tissue network that is important for transmitting mechanical forces throughout the lung (eg, negative pleural pressure opens alveoli and other airways during inspiration). This network (especially the elastic tissue) exerts radial traction on airway walls (and to a lesser extent the vessel walls), and this tethering action is important in maintaining normal lumen patency. The greatest alterations of airway caliber usually result from humoral or neural influences on airway smooth muscle. There is normally some resting tone of airway smooth muscle. Some endogenous bronchoconstrictors are acetylcholine; histamine; bradykinin; prostaglandin $F_{2\alpha}$; leukotrienes C, D, and E; serotonin; and significant hyper- or hypocapnia. Bronchodilatation is caused by β-adrenergic agonists and prostaglandins of the E series. Stimulation of pulmonary irritant receptors, which are located very superficially in the respiratory mucosa throughout most of the conducting airways, causes bronchoconstriction by a vagally mediated reflex. The irritant receptors may be stimulated by ether, cigarette smoke, sulfur dioxide, ammonia, dust particles, or mechanical deformation by a catheter, bronchoscope, or endotracheal tube or by rapid inflations or deflations of the lung. Most changes in pulmonary vascular tone are humorally mediated. There are various endogenous pulmonary vasoconstrictors, including histamine, angiotensin, fibrinopeptides, prostaglandin $F_{2\alpha}$, and alveolar hypoxia. Pulmonary vasodilatation may be caused by bradykinin, glucagon, E series prostaglandins, β-adrenergic agonists, and acetylcholine.

Airway secretions are generally increased by irritant stimulation through a vagally mediated reflex or directly by parasympathomimetic agonists.

Dawson CA: Role of pulmonary vasomotion in physiology of the lung. *Physiol Rev* 1984;**64:**544.

Nadel JA (editor): *Physiology and Pharmacology of the Airways.* Dekker, 1980.

Nadel JA, Barnes PJ: Autonomic regulation of the airways. *Annu Rev Med* 1984;**35:**451.

Paintal AS: Thoracic receptors connected with sensation. *Br Med Bull* 1977;**33:**169.

Sullivan CE et al: Regulation of airway smooth muscle tone in sleeping dogs. *Am Rev Respir Dis* 1979;**119:**87.

DIAGNOSTIC AIDS

1. PHYSICAL EXAMINATION OF THE RESPIRATORY SYSTEM

The appropriate physical examination of the respiratory system of a child depends to some extent upon the age and cooperation of the patient. For example, chest percussion is of limited value in infants but is an important part of the chest examination in older children. In general, however, every examination should include inspection, percussion, and auscultation. One should inspect the nares for patency (passing a small soft catheter through the nares into the posterior pharynx rules out choanal atresia), the posterior pharynx for obstructing lesions (eg, large or displaced tonsils), and the neck for masses, use of accessory muscles of respiration, and central position of the trachea. The chest should be observed for abnormal shape (eg, pectus excavatum or carinatum, scoliosis, or increased anteroposterior diameter), asymmetry, and chest wall retractions. The nail beds, the lips, and the mucous membranes of the mouth should be inspected for pallor or cyanosis, and the digits should be examined for clubbing. The patient's height and weight should be carefully measured and plotted on a growth chart.

By means of auscultation, the examiner should assess the amount and symmetry of air entry and the character of breath sounds. An early sign of airway obstruction may be relative prolongation of expiratory sounds. Rhonchi (coarse, discontinuous, and low-pitched) indicate large airway obstruction, usually by mucus. Rales (high-pitched, fine crackles) are usually inspiratory and indicate narrowing of small airways. Expiratory wheezes can be due to narrowing of large or small airways.

Cardiac auscultation should be performed to detect murmurs or increased intensity of the pulmonary valve closure sound (P_2), indicating pulmonary hypertension. Increased lung volume due to trapped gas often lowers the diaphragm and causes the edge of the liver to be palpable below the right costal margin.

Godfrey S et al: Clinical and physiological associations of some physical signs observed in patients with chronic airways obstruction. *Thorax* 1970;**25:**285.

Scarpelli EM: Examination of the lung (physiologic and anatomic basis). Chap 1, pp 1–69, in: *Pulmonary Disease of the Fetus, Newborn, and Child.* Scarpelli EM, Auld PAM, Goldman HS (editors). Lea & Febiger, 1978.

Waring WW: The history and physical examination. Chap 3, pp 57–78, in: *Disorders of the Respiratory Tract in Children,* 4th ed. Kendig EL, Chernick V (editors). Saunders, 1983.

2. PULMONARY FUNCTION TESTING

Pulmonary function testing can provide important diagnostic and prognostic information in the management of children with pulmonary disease. Such studies are helpful in differentiating obstructive from restrictive lung disease (Table 14–1). Obstructive lung disease is far more common than restrictive lung disease in children. Pulmonary function testing is useful in determining the site of obstruction as well as its reversibility. The effects of a specific respiratory challenge (eg, antigen or exercise) or of a particular therapeutic regimen can be quantitatively evaluated with pulmonary function testing. Such tests are also helpful in objectively following the course and severity of

Table 14–1. Pulmonary function tests in obstructive airway disease and restrictive lung disease. (N = normal.)

	Obstructive	Restrictive
Forced vital capacity (FVC)	↓	↓
Total lung capacity (TLC)	N or ↑	↓
Residual volume (RV)	↑	N or ↓
Forced expiratory volume in 1 second (FEV_1) as % of FVC	↓	N
Forced expiratory flow from 25 to 75% of FVC (FEF_{25-75})	↓	N or ↓

many pulmonary diseases. Finally, preoperative pulmonary function evaluation of patients with lung disease can help evaluate the risk of anesthesia as well as assist in the planning of postoperative respiratory care.

The most useful pulmonary function tests are measurements of arterial blood gases, lung volumes, and maximal expiratory flow rates. The first is appropriate in any age group; the latter 2, like other more sophisticated pulmonary function tests, require a cooperative subject and therefore are clinically feasible only in children over age 5–7 years.

Spirometry provides a measure of the vital capacity, ie, the maximum volume of air that can be taken into or forced out of the lungs; the forced expired volume exhaled in the first second of a maximum expiration (FEV_1), usually expressed as a percent of the total forced vital capacity (normal, $\geq$ 80%); and maximal flow rates at a variety of lung volumes. The maximum flow rate at high lung volumes (peak expiratory flow rate, PEFR) is an indication of respiratory muscle strength, degree of effort and cooperation, and large airway caliber. FEV_1 is primarily an index of larger airway caliber. Small airway function is reflected in the contour of the flow volume loop and the maximum flows at low lung volumes, eg, the average forced expiratory flow over the middle half of expiration (FEF_{25-75}). Absolute lung volumes (functional residual capacity, FRC; residual volume, RV), measured either by gas dilution techniques or body plethysmography, are often elevated with small airway disease and are usually decreased in restrictive lung disease. The carbon monoxide diffusing capacity of the lung is a general reflection of pulmonary blood volume and is most useful when destruction of pulmonary capillaries is suspected in the absence of significant airway disease.

One approach to interpreting pulmonary function tests is to determine first whether the vital capacity is normal or diminished. If diminished, is the abnormality due to a decrease in total lung capacity (TLC), as would be seen in restrictive disease; or is it due to elevation of RV owing to obstructive disease? A summary of pulmonary function test results in obstructive and restrictive lung disease is presented in Table 14–1. After the initial distinction between restrictive and obstructive disease is made, it is important to inspect the remainder of the pulmonary function results for internal consistency. If obstructive disease is suggested, there must be other evidence of small airway disease such as a decrease in the FEF_{25-75}. In contrast, in restrictive lung disease the maximum expiratory flow rates should be relatively normal. Inconsistency in the results of the different tests may indicate a poor or inconsistent effort on the part of the patient or a combination of respiratory problems. Failure to expire to a true residual volume is one of the most common sources of error due to lack of cooperation among pediatric patients. If obstructive disease is identified, the patient should inhale a bronchodilator, and pulmonary function tests should be repeated after about 20 minutes to look for evidence of reversibility of the airway obstruction. The most reliable pulmonary function tests in young children are probably arterial blood gas measurements and FEV_1.

Arterial Blood Gases

Measurement of arterial oxygen tension (P_{aO_2}), CO_2 tension (P_{aCO_2}), and pH is an excellent means of assessing the gas exchange function of the lungs. Arterial sites for obtaining blood percutaneously, in decreasing order of desirability, are the radial, brachial, dorsalis pedis, posterior tibial, and femoral arteries. In order to minimize the deviation from steady-state conditions caused by the arterial puncture, the site should be infiltrated with local anesthesia about 5–10 minutes before the arterial sample is drawn. When direct arterial sampling is not possible, "arterialized" capillary blood can be obtained. If the patient has adequate peripheral perfusion and if proper technique is used, the values are quite reliable for pH, P_{CO_2}, and base excess. The reliability of this oxygen measurement depends on the P_{aO_2}. The proper technique for a capillary sample from the heel involves heating the extremity with warm towels for 10 minutes prior to the puncture and then making a sufficiently deep stab wound to ensure good blood flow. The free-flowing blood should be collected in a capillary tube as close as possible to the bleeding site without air bubbles collecting in the tube.

Normal blood gas values for sea level and for Denver, Colorado (altitude 5280 feet) are listed in Table 14–2. The amount of fixed shunting (including both intrapulmonary and intracardiac shunts) can be estimated by measuring P_{aO_2} with the patient breathing 100% oxygen.

Measurements of transcutaneous P_{O_2} and oxygen saturation (by ear oximetry) allow for continuous monitoring of steady-state blood gases. The new pulse oximeters have a high degree of accuracy and provide assessments of steady-state oxygenation that are generally as reliable as those derived from indwelling arterial catheters. Transcutaneous CO_2 monitors are available but are less accurate.

American Thoracic Society Medical Devices Committee: Snowbird workshop on standardization of spirometry. *Am Rev Respir Dis* 1979;**119:**831.

Bates DV, Macklin PT, Christie RV: *Respiratory Function and Disease*. Saunders, 1971.

Cherniack RM: Pitfalls in pulmonary function testing. *Respir Care* 1983;**28:**434.

Table 14–2. Normal arterial blood values with F_{IO_2} = 0.21 (room air).

	P_{aO_2} (mm Hg)	P_{aCO_2} (mm Hg)	pH
Sea level	85–95	36–42	7.38–7.42
Denver	65–75	35–40	7.36–7.40

Dull WL et al: The efficacy of isoproterenol inhalation for predicting the response to orally administered theophylline in chronic obstructive pulmonary disease. *Am Rev Respir Dis* 1982;**126:**656.

Froese AB: Preoperative evaluation of pulmonary function. *Pediatr Clin North Am* 1979;**26:**645.

Huch A, Huch R, Lubbers D: *Transcutaneous* P_{O2}. Thieme-Stratton, 1981.

Hunt CE: Capillary blood sampling in the infant: Usefulness and limitations of 2 methods of sampling compared with arterial blood. *Pediatrics* 1973;**51:**501.

Lemen RJ: Pulmonary function testing in the office and clinic. Chap 6, pp 125–134, in: *Disorders of the Respiratory Tract in Children,* 4th ed. Kendig EL, Chernick V (editors). Saunders, 1983.

McBride JT, Wohl MEB: Pulmonary function tests. *Pediatr Clin North Am* 1979;**26:**537.

Polgar G, Promadhat V: *Pulmonary Function Testing in Children.* Saunders, 1971.

Ries, AL, Farrow JT, Clausen JL: Accuracy of two ear oximeters at rest and during exercise in pulmonary patients. *Am Rev Respir Dis* 1985;**132:**685.

Sly RM: Assessing lung function in children. *J Respir Dis* 1984;**5:**51.

3. COLLECTION OF MATERIAL FOR CULTURE

Many pediatric pulmonary diseases are due to infections. A variety of techniques are available for collection of material suitable for culture. There is a poor correlation between organisms grown from cultures of the nose or throat and those infecting the lower airway. Therefore, material from below the larynx should be obtained for culture to identify organisms in the lower airways. Expectorated sputum is the easiest material to obtain in cooperative patients, although it will be contaminated with upper airway organisms. A smear of sputum or other material collected should be prepared, appropriately stained, and examined with a microscope for the presence of organisms and inflammatory cells. Sputum expectoration may be encouraged or increased by chest percussion and postural drainage or by inhalation of ultrasonic mist for 10–15 minutes. In patients who are unable to expectorate sputum for collection, direct tracheal suction is useful—performed either blindly or under direct vision using a laryngoscope or a bronchoscope. The protected specimen-brush catheter provides a sample from the lower respiratory tract that is less contaminated than samples from the older open-end brush-in-catheter system. A transtracheal route (percutaneous introduction of the catheter through the cricothyroid membrane) is usually not recommended in children. Brush biopsy and transbronchial biopsy are additional methods by which to obtain material for culture from the lower airway, using a bronchoscope. These latter techniques are most applicable in older children.

Direct needle aspiration of the lung is a useful procedure in children of all ages. Following local anesthesia of the appropriate area of the chest wall, aspiration is performed with a short-bevel No. 20- to 22-gauge needle attached to a glass syringe rinsed with nonbacteriostatic normal saline to create an airtight seal. Rapid introduction, over the top of the rib, into the affected lung parenchyma and aspiration during withdrawal of the needle will recover enough material for culture. The patient should refrain from breathing during the brief period while the needle is in the chest. An area of relatively acute disease should be identified on the chest x-ray, and an effort should be made to aspirate from that area if it is accessible and not adjacent to another major organ such as the heart or liver. Fluoroscopy can be helpful in directing the needle. The major complications of this procedure are hemoptysis and pneumothorax, but these are uncommon when the procedure is performed properly. Patients with pulmonary hypertension or obstructive airway disease with hyperaeration are at increased risk of morbidity.

Bartlett JG: Diagnostic accuracy of transtracheal aspiration bacteriologic studies. *Am Rev Respir Dis* 1977;**115:**777.

Chastre J et al: Prospective evaluation of the protected specimen brush for the diagnosis of pulmonary infections in ventilated patients. *Am Rev Respir Dis* 1984;**130:**924.

Congeni B, Mankervis G: Diagnosis of pneumonia by counterimmunoelectrophoresis of respiratory secretions. *Am J Dis Child* 1978;**132:**684.

Garcia D et al: Lung puncture aspiration as a bateriologic diagnostic procedure in acute pneumonias of infants and children. *Clin Pediatr* 1971;**6:**346.

Mimica I et al: Lung puncture in the etiologic diagnosis of pneumonia: The study of 543 infants and children. *Am J Dis Child* 1971;**122:**278.

Murray P, Washington J: Microscopic and bacteriologic analysis of expectorated sputum. *Mayo Clin Proc* 1975;**50:**339.

4. RADIOGRAPHIC PROCEDURES

The chest x-ray is important in diagnosis and management of pediatric lung disease, and high-speed exposure techniques significantly reduce the radiation exposure from such films. Both frontal and lateral chest x-rays should be obtained in most cases for optimal interpretation and localization. Hyperaeration, for example, is best assessed on a lateral film by loss of diaphragmatic convexity. Lateral decubitus chest x-rays are useful in assessing the presence, extent, and mobility of pleural air or fluid. Forced expiratory chest x-rays can demonstrate localized obstruction to expiration (trapped air), as can be caused by an aspirated foreign body. Such trapped air may show no abnormality on inspiratory chest x-ray, whereas on a forced expiratory film there may be mediastinal shift toward the contralateral side and relatively greater radiolucency over the affected area. The forced expiratory film can be obtained even in young uncooperative subjects if a technician wearing a lead glove presses on the immobilized child's epigastrium as the child exhales. The barium swallow is useful for evaluation of possible vascular rings, the H type of tracheoesophageal fistula, chalasia, achalasia, and pharyngeal incoordination. The larger airways and the upper airway can be effectively evaluated by higher-penetration x-rays, ie, air contrast studies of the airway, often done in association with fluoroscopy. Evaluation of intrathoracic masses may be enhanced by conventional tomograms of the chest, CT scans, or magnetic resonance imaging. Ventilation and perfusion scans using radioactive xenon- and technetium-labeled albumin, respectively, provide crude assessments of regional ventilation and perfusion. Regional differences in wash-in and wash-out rates of ventilation can be assessed in this manner. A much more precise evaluation of the pulmonary vascular bed is obtained with a pulmonary angiogram.

Bronchography is associated with a high morbidity rate in the pediatric range and is rarely indicated.

Bergeson PS et al: Committee on hospital care: Preoperative chest radiographs. *Pediatrics* 1983;**71:**858.

Caffey J: *Pediatrics X-Ray Diagnosis,* 8th ed. Year Book, 1985.

Culham JAG: Special procedures in pediatric chest radiology. *Pediatr Clin North Am* 1979;**26:**661.

Felson B: The chest roentgenologic workup: What and why? Conventional methods. *Respir Care* 1980;**25:**955.

Fletcher BD: Diagnostic radiology of the respiratory tract. Chap 5, pp 96–124, in: *Disorders of the Respiratory Tract in Children,* 4th ed. Kendig EL, Chernick V (editors). Saunders, 1983.

VanMoore A, Putman CE: Radiologic diagnosis of chest disease. *Surg Clin North Am* 1980;**60:**715.

Wood RA, Hoekelman RA: Value of the chest x-ray as a screening test for elective surgery in children. *Pediatrics* 1981;**67:**447.

GENERAL METHODS OF THERAPY FOR LUNG DISEASE

Effective treatment of lung disorders is enhanced by good understanding of the physiologic alterations that occur during the disease process. Several general therapeutic and prophylactic modes of therapy, each directed toward a particular physiologic function or malfunction, are discussed below.

Lough MD et al (editors): *Pediatric Respiratory Therapy,* 2nd ed. Year Book, 1979.

Mellins R: Respiratory care in infants and children: Report of Ad Hoc Committee, American Thoracic Society. *Am Rev Respir Dis* 1972;**105:**461.

Proceedings of the Conference on the Scientific Basis of Inhospital Respiratory Therapy Held in Atlanta, Georgia, on November 14–16, 1979. *Am Rev Respir Dis* 1980;**122(5–Part 2):**1. [Entire issue.]

Scarpelli EM, Auld PAM, Goldman HS (editors): *Pulmonary Disease of the Fetus, Newborn, and Child.* Lea & Febiger, 1978.

OXYGEN THERAPY

Oxygen therapy is defined as delivering an inspired oxygen concentration of greater than 21%. It is indicated when arterial blood gas determinations show that the arterial oxygen tension is low. The inspired gas, delivered by nasal cannula, mask, hood, endotracheal tube, or tent, should be sufficiently enriched with oxygen to maintain an arterial oxygen tension of 65–85 mm Hg. Such inspired gas should always be humidified and should usually be warmed; supersaturation is usually not desirable. Oxygen tents are usually not able to deliver concentrations of oxygen greater than 25–30% unless the tent is tightly sealed, which interferes with nursing care.

Nasal prongs are useful for children. For infants, a nasal cannula can be constructed from a soft rubber or polyvinyl tubing that should be taped with the tip just outside or, for higher inspired oxygen concentration, just inside the nares (Fig 14–1). With nasal prongs or a nasal catheter, an effective inspired oxygen concentration of up to 30–40% can usually be maintained. When nasal obstruction is present or a higher concentration of oxygen is required, a face mask or some other mode of delivery is necessary. The flow through a nasal catheter or prongs usually should not exceed 3 L/min in children and less in infants to avoid excessive drying and irritation of the nasal mucosa. The lowest effective amount of increased inspired oxygen should be delivered in order to minimize the risk of pulmonary oxygen toxicity.

Systemic oxygenation must be assessed directly by arterial blood gas measurements or indirectly, eg, by ear oximeter, in all patients receiving oxygen therapy. Some infants and children with chronic lung disease (eg, bronchopulmonary dysplasia or end-stage

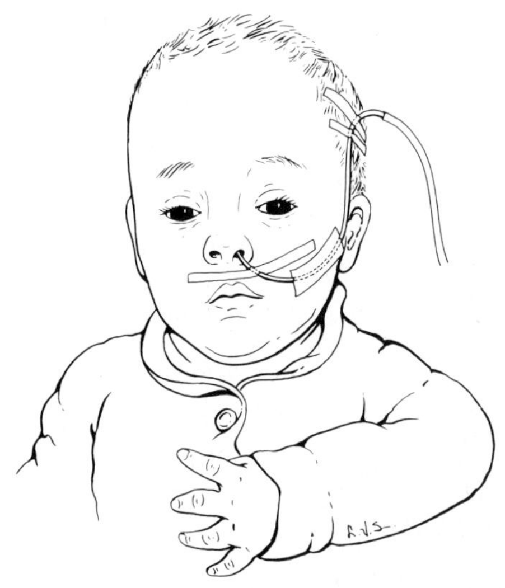

Figure 14–1. Nasal cannula for oxygen administration to infants.

cystic fibrosis) can be treated at home with low-flow oxygen if the family can understand and accept certain responsibilities and possible complications. Continuing need for and adequacy of the oxygen therapy must be documented at regular intervals in both inpatients and outpatients.

Anthonisen NR: Hypoxemia and O_2 therapy. *Am Rev Respir Dis* 1982;**126:**729.

Bland RD: Special considerations in oxygen therapy for infants and children. *Am Rev Respir Dis* 1980;**122(5–Part 2):**45.

Deneke SM, Fanburg BL: Normobaric oxygen toxicity of the lung. *N Engl J Med* 1980;**303:**76.

Friedman SA et al: Oxygen therapy, evaluation of various air-entraining masks. *JAMA* 1974;**228:**474.

Petty TL: Who needs home oxygen? *Am Rev Respir Dis* 1985;**131:**930.

MIST THERAPY

The most effective and safe expectorant and mucolytic agent for airway secretions is water given systemically. Small amounts of water may be deposited in the lower airway by inhalation of air of high humidity or by ultrasonic aerosol. However, the small possible benefits of delivering extra water by the airway are overshadowed by the potential complications such as bronchoconstriction or increased cough (although under some circumstances stimulation of a cough may be desirable) secondary to stimulation of irritant receptors in the upper and large airways, infection of the airway by organisms growing in the mist-producing equipment, or fluid overload in small patients. Although mist therapy is not suggested for lower airway disease, it is important that no completely dry gases be delivered to the airway, since they also are irritating and, particularly if delivered through an endotracheal tube, can interfere with normal function of airway cilia. Mist aerosol therapy is a treatment of choice for acute inflammatory laryngeal or subglottic obstruction due to viral or postextubation croup.

Brain JD: Aerosol and humidity therapy. *Am Rev Respir Dis* 1980;**122 (5–Part 2):**17.

Harris TM et al: An evaluation of bacterial contamination of ventilator humidifying systems. *Chest* 1973;**63:**922.

Rosenblut M, Chernick V: Influence of mist tent therapy on sputum viscosity and water content in cystic fibrosis. *Arch Dis Child* 1974;**49:**606.

Sasaki CT, Suzuki M: The respiratory mechanism of aerosol inhalation in the treatment of partial airway obstruction. *Pediatrics* 1977;**59:**689.

Taussig LM: Mists and aerosols: New studies, new thoughts. *J Pediatr* 1974;**84:**619.

BRONCHODILATOR INHALATION THERAPY

Bronchoconstriction and the resultant impaired respiratory function can result from a wide variety of intrinsic and extrinsic stimuli. Many bronchodilator agents are available, and those which are most used clinically can be divided into 4 classes: (1) β-adrenergic agonists, (2) methylxanthines, (3) parasympatholytic agents, and (4) corticosteroids. These drugs are used most commonly in the treatment of asthma (see Chapter 32), but some patients with other types of acute (eg, bronchiolitis) or chronic (eg, cystic fibrosis) lung disease may benefit from bronchodilator therapy.

The remainder of this discussion will deal only with inhaled adrenergic agonist drugs. Aerosolized adrenergic agonist agents may be delivered from a prepackaged pressurized canister (most include a fluorocarbon propellant, which may increase myocardial sensitivity to the potential arrhythmogenic complications of these agents). Such canisters have the disadvantage of being very easy for the patient to abuse by too frequent use, thus risking overdosage and death. A safer but less convenient means of delivery is by a reusable nebulizer (eg, DeVilbiss No. 40), where the drug solution is aerosolized by continuous gas flow from a tank of compressed gas or from a portable gas compressor. The nebulized drug should be inhaled slowly and deeply through the mouth. For many patients, the nebulizer should be driven by 40% or 100% oxygen to counteract the potential or real arterial hypoxemia caused by the pulmonary vasodilating effect of the adrenergic agonists and the resultant increase in venous admixture from increased perfusion of poorly ventilated areas of the lung. When possible, an improvement in pulmonary function after bronchodilator inhalation should be quantitatively documented before initiating a regular program of bronchodilator therapy. Such pulmonary function studies should include measurement of both maximal expiratory flow rates and absolute lung volumes, since improvement may be evident in only one of these categories. Bronchodilator inhalation is frequently used prior to chest percussion.

Infants or uncooperative children may be given the necessary few breaths of aerosol by placing a feeding nipple with the tip cut off over the end of a canister nebulizer, holding the nose, and administering the drug at the beginning of an inspiration, usually when the child cries. The use of "spacer" tubes between the canister and the mouthpiece may facilitate delivery of the bronchodilator. Continuous breathing of an aerosolized 1:4 or 1:8 mixture of bronchodilator in distilled water is also effective and can be administered by face mask or mouthpiece depending on the age and degree of cooperation of the patient. There is no evidence that better distribution of the aerosol can be obtained with delivery by intermittent positive pressure breathing (IPPB) than with active deep breathing. A patient who will not cooperate for active breathing is unlikely to cooperate for IPPB. Delivery of a drug by inhalation by any means has the disadvantages that most of the aerosol is deposited in the upper airway, and the aerosol that does reach the smaller airways is preferentially directed toward the well-ventilated areas and away from those which are poorly ventilated, ie, those in most need of bronchodilation. Whichever delivery system is used, the patient must be carefully instructed in correct technique, and the patient's technique must be reviewed at regular intervals.

All currently available β-adrenergic agonists have both β_1 activity (eg, inotropic and chronotropic cardiac effects; decreased intestinal motility) and β_2 activity (eg, relaxation of airway and arteriolar smooth muscle; skeletal muscle tremor), although some newer agents such as metaproterenol, terbutaline, and albuterol (salbutamol) have more β_2 selectivity than isoproterenol and isoetharine. In addition, these newer agents have longer durations of action (3–5 hours). Further discussion of other bronchodilator agents is included in the section on asthma (see Chapter 32).

Brain JD, Valberg PA: Deposition of aerosol in the respiratory tract. *Am Rev Respir Dis* 1979;**120:**1325.

Gross NJ, Skorodin MS: Anticholinergic, antimuscarinic bronchodilators. *Am Rev Respir Dis* 1984;**129:**856.

Harper TB, Strunk RC: Techniques of administration of metered-dose aerosolized drugs in asthmatic children. *Am J Dis Child* 1981;**135:**218.

Murray JF: Indications for mechanical aids to assist lung inflation in medical patients. *Am Rev Respir Dis* 1980;**122(5–Part 2):**121.

Nelson HS: Beta adrenergic agonists. *Chest* 1982;**82:**33S.

Paterson JW et al: Bronchodilator drugs. *Am Rev Respir Dis* 1979;**120:**1149.

Tabachnik E, Levison H: Clinical application of aerosols in pediatrics. *Am Rev Respir Dis* 1980;**122(5–Part 2):**97.

PULMONARY PHYSIOTHERAPY

Postural drainage and chest percussion are used to aid in the removal of material such as mucus and aspirated matter from the lungs. They are accomplished by positioning a patient so that the involved segment is uppermost. The therapist then percusses over the involved area with a cupped hand and relaxed wrist and elbow. There is a slightly different optimal body position for drainage of each lung segment into a major airway. It is important that the therapist be aware of normal lung anatomy and position the patient accordingly. For generalized disease, percussion should be done with the patient in the different positions shown in Fig 14–2. While infants and small children can often be effectively positioned in the therapist's lap or across the therapist's legs, pillows, padded boards, sturdy ironing boards, or beanbag chairs are effective for positioning older children. Some material such as a shirt or towel over the skin being percussed will minimize chest wall tenderness. Care should be taken to avoid trauma to the liver, kidneys, or spleen. The time spent percussing each lung area depends on the extent of lung involvement and the cooperation and tolerance of the child. When there is widespread lung disease, each of the areas of the lungs (9 different body positions) should be percussed for 1–2 minutes, not to exceed a total of about 20–25 minutes for the whole treatment. If only one lung area is involved, 2–3 minutes in that position is sufficient. The frequency of treatments may vary from every 2 hours to once or twice daily. If possible, treatments given only once daily should be given in the morning shortly after the patient awakens.

When the cough reflex is weak or absent, mechanical suction should be readily available in order to assist with removal of secretions from the upper airways. All patients should be encouraged to expectorate the sputum rather than swallow it. In patients with significant lung disease, body positioning and chest percussion may cause significant decreases in arterial oxygenation; these patients should receive supplemental inspired oxygen during and for short periods before and after such treatments.

Regular exercise is encouraged in patients with chronic lung disease, as the associated deep breathing may precipitate cough and enhance removal of lung secretions. Mechanical chest percussors are available and are useful for self-administered pulmonary physiotherapy in older children and adults.

There are several ways to stimulate a child to cough and breathe deeply. The best ways are simply for a parent or nurse to verbally encourage the child, to assist the child by frequent changes of position, and to position the child's hands so that the expansion of the chest can be perceived. This takes time, patience, and imagination. Devices that may be helpful in encouraging large inspirations to counteract atelectasis are blow bottles, balloons, and incentive spirometers. Large forced inspirations or forced expirations will often stimulate cough and thus enhance clearance of mucus. "Huff coughing," the rapid and forced expulsion of air through an open glottis, is effective in clearing the airways of secretions.

Blow bottles consist of a closed system of 2 bottles connected by a tube that nearly reaches the bottom of each bottle. Colored fluid in one bottle is transferred to the other bottle when the patient blows on a second tube emerging from the top of the bottle. The child must be encouraged to inhale and exhale as fully as possible, since little is gained by exhaling in short puffs. Some supervision and instruction are essential. Balloons are used in the same way as blow bottles.

In some patients who cough poorly, deep pharyngeal suctioning may stimulate cough and assist in removal of secretions from the large airways. This method, as well as direct tracheal suctioning, can cause laryngospasm and thus should be used only in intensive care units by experienced personnel.

De Boeck C, Zinman R: Cough versus chest physiotherapy: A comparison of the acute effects on pulmonary function in patients with cystic fibrosis. *Am Rev Respir Dis* 1984;**129:**182.

Desmond KJ et al: Immediate and long-term effects of chest physiotherapy in patients with cystic fibrosis. *J Pediatr* 1983;**103:**538.

Kigin CM: Chest physical therapy for the post-operative or traumatic injury patient. *Phys Ther* 1981;**61:**1724.

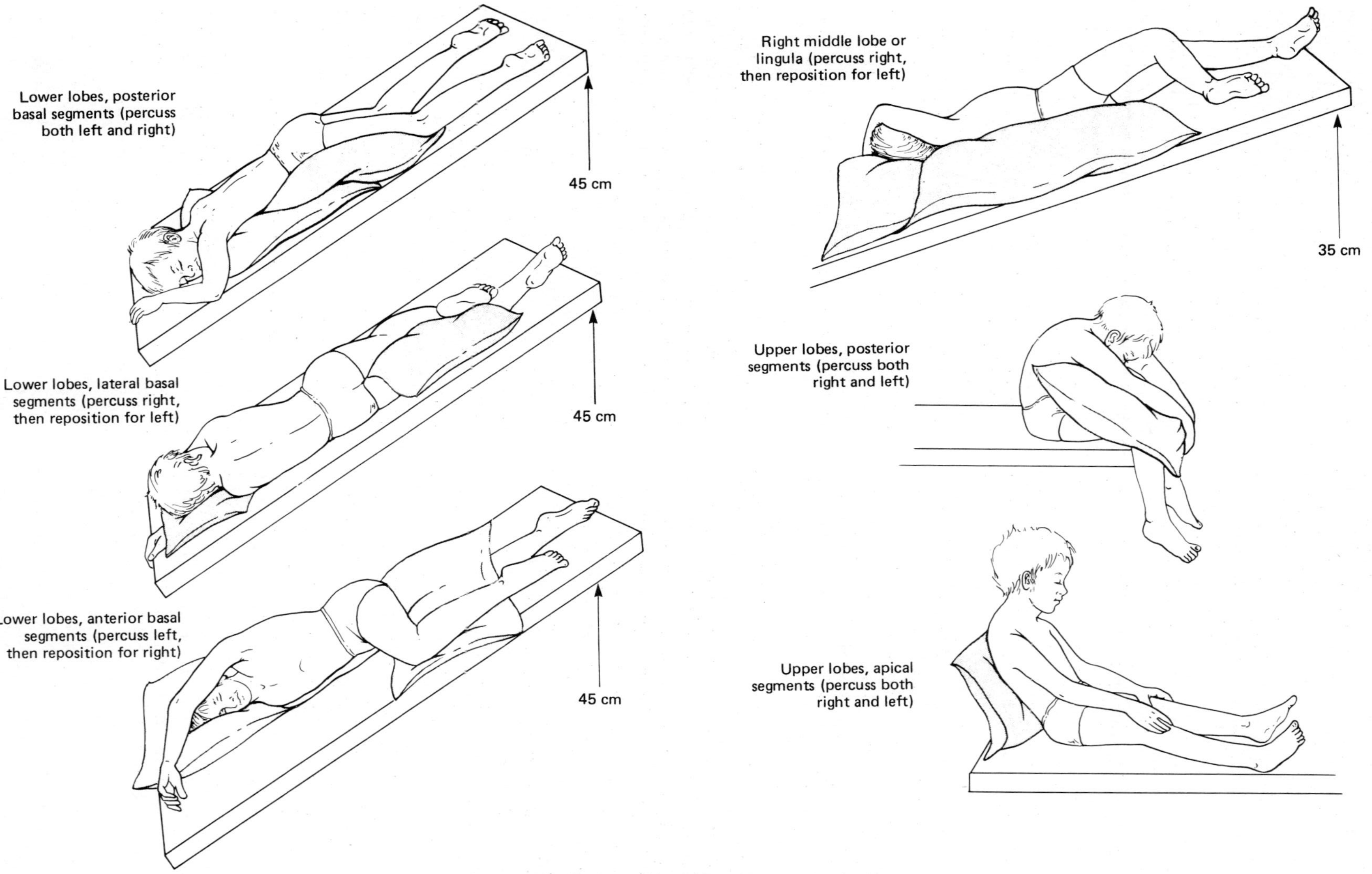

Figure 14–2. Body positions for pulmonary drainage.

Menkes H, Britt J: Rationale for physical therapy. *Am Rev Respir Dis* 1980;**122(5–Part 2):**127.
Pinney M: Postural drainage for infants: A better approach. *Nursing* 1972;**2:**45.
Pryor JA et al: Evaluation of the forced expiration technique as an adjunct to postural drainage in treatment of cystic fibrosis. *Br Med J* 1979;**2:**417.
Wanner A: Does chest physical therapy move airway secretions? (Editoral.) *Am Rev Respir Dis* 1984;**130:**701.

MECHANICAL VENTILATION

Most mechanical ventilators can be classified as either volume-limited or pressure-limited. The volume-limited ventilator produces a preset volume, and that entire volume minus the compression volume (the volume "lost" as a result of gas compression in the ventilator tubing circuit) is transferred to the patient provided there are no leaks in the ventilator circuit. When very high inspiratory pressures are required because of markedly decreased lung compliance or increased airway resistance, a volume-limited ventilator may be necessary for adequate ventilation of the patient. Volume-limited ventilators do not compensate for variable leaks in the circuit (eg, around the endotracheal tube) but do deliver a constant tidal volume in patients with changing lung mechanics.

The pressure-limited ventilator inflates the patient's lung to a certain preset pressure; once this pressure is reached, expiration may begin or the inspiratory pressures may be held constant, but there is no further lung inflation. This type of ventilator will compensate for changing leaks in the circuit but will not deliver a constant tidal volume with changing lung mechanics; ie, for a given ventilator setting, if the lung compliance falls (stiffer lungs), a smaller tidal volume will be delivered. Most patients can be adequately ventilated with either a pressure-limited or a volume-limited ventilator. The pressure-limited ventilators with a continuous flow through the circuit are generally less expensive and often more versatile, particularly with small patients.

All mechanical ventilation systems should have an apparatus for humidification and adjustments of oxygen concentration in the inspired gas as well as appropriate high- and low-pressure alarms for the patient circuit. It is essential that an accurate pressure gauge be properly functioning and easily visible to display a continuous recording of the patient circuit pressure. Finally, it is essential that safety pressure popoffs be available and properly set.

Techniques of setting up the ventilator and attaching the patient are as follows:

(1) Set up the ventilator as described below, while assisting the patient's ventilation with a manual resuscitation device as necessary.

(2) Adjust the tidal volume or inspiratory and expiratory pressure levels to the estimated requirement. An average starting tidal volume setting is 10–15 mL/kg. For patients with normal lungs, inspiratory and expiratory pressures of 16–18 cm water and 2 cm water, respectively, are appropriate starting pressures. These settings must be increased or decreased depending on the arterial blood gases.

(3) Adjust inspiratory and expiratory time to produce the desired respiratory rate. An appropriate beginning respiratory rate for a patient with normal lungs would be 14–24 breaths/min, depending on the patient's age. A normal inspiratory time is about 0.3–0.6 second, also depending on age. Prolonged inspiratory times are likely to improve arterial oxygenation but may interfere with pulmonary circulation and cardiac output. It is important that adequate time (at least 0.4–0.5 second) be available for expiration. A longer expiratory time is required when there is significant airway obstruction.

(4) Adjust inspired oxygenation concentration.

(5) Fill and set humidifier.

(6) Adjust inspiratory flow rate. Slower rates should be used for smaller patients and for patients with significant obstructive airway disease.

(7) Make sure that all warning devices and safety popoffs are set and working.

(8) Attach patient to the ventilator.

(9) Observe movement of patient's chest and auscultate to check for good ventilation of both lungs.

(10) Measure arterial blood gases and pH regularly.

The different modes of mechanical ventilation are discussed below. Some recently described techniques of high-frequency ventilation (eg, high-frequency jet ventilation, high-frequency oscillations) are still experimental, and their clinical safety and indications for use have not been adequately evaluated.

Controlled Ventilation

The ventilator controls both the rate and depth of ventilation, and the patient is unable to take spontaneous breaths between the mandatory delivered breaths. For this reason, there may be incoordination of the patient's spontaneous breathing attempts and the ventilator-delivered breaths. This can only be remedied by decreasing the patient's respiratory drive or ability to breathe. The former is achieved by mildly hyperventilating the patient or by the administration of narcotics to depress the respiratory center. The latter method involves administration of muscular blocking agents (eg, pancuronium). Paralysis of patients being mechanically ventilated should be performed only when very close observation of the patient is available, because of the risk of ventilator failure or the patient becoming disconnected from the respirator.

Assist Controlled Ventilation

The small negative pressure generated by the beginning of a patient's respiratory effort triggers the delivery of a full preset tidal volume or inspiratory pressure to the patient. Thus, the patient controls the rate but not the depth of ventilation. Incoordination of ventilator effort and patient effort is less likely with this mode of ventilation, but hyperventilation is a relatively common problem.

Intermittent Mandatory Ventilation (IMV)

The ventilator is set to deliver a certain rate and depth of mandatory breaths. In addition, however, there is a mechanism to provide fresh gas in the patient's circuit to allow the patient to take spontaneous breaths of any rate or depth in between the mandatory breaths. Some ventilators have synchronized IMV (SIMV), meaning that the mandatory breaths are delivered at the time of an inspiratory effort by the patient if such an effort is made within the appropriate time period for a mandatory breath. This is helpful in gradually decreasing the rate of mandatory breaths (''weaning'' the patient from the ventilator) as less ventilatory support is required and the patient is able to perform more effective spontaneous ventilation. This is the most effective mode of ventilation for most patients.

Positive End-Expiratory Pressure (PEEP)

A positive end-expiratory pressure can be maintained throughout the expiratory period when a patient is receiving mechanical ventilation by any of the 3 above modes. PEEP helps minimize alveolar volume loss during expiratory pauses and thus decreases the tendency toward atelectasis and the resultant venous admixture. PEEP is indicated in most conditions where mechanical ventilation is required for alveolar or small airway instability or collapse.

Continuous Positive Airway Pressure (CPAP)

CPAP refers to a relatively constant positive airway pressure in the absence of any mandatory, mechanically delivered tidal volumes. The indications are similar to those for PEEP. Nasal prongs, a nasopharyngeal tube, or a face mask can be used instead of an endotracheal tube for application of the positive airway pressure.

Negative Pressure Ventilation

Negative pressure modes of mechanical ventilation analogous to those positive pressure methods listed above can be used for respiratory support in infants and children. Negative pressure ventilation using some modern version of the iron lung avoids the complications of endotracheal intubation but has the disadvantage of making nursing care and other access to the patient more difficult, and it is difficult to generate large transpulmonary pressures. Temperature control and actual trauma to the patient are problems in very small infants.

Boros SJ et al: Neonatal high-frequency jet ventilation: Four years' experience. *Pediatrics* 1985;**75:**657.

Chang HK, Harf A: High-frequency ventilation: A review. *Respir Physiol* 1984;**57:**135.

Chatburn RL: High-frequency ventilation: A report on a state of the art symposium. *Respir Care* 1984;**29:**839.

Frates RC et al: Outcome of home mechanical ventilation in children. *J Pediatr* 1985;**106:**850.

Lough MD, Schuchardt B: Mechanical ventilation. Chapter 7 in: *Pediatric Respiratory Therapy*. Lough MD et al (editors). Year Book, 1979.

Mushin WW et al: *Automatic Ventilation of the Lungs*, 3rd ed. Blackwell, 1980.

Nugent S et al: Pharmacology and use of muscle relaxants in infants and children. *J Pediatr* 1979;**94:**481.

Pollack MM et al: Cardiopulmonary parameters during high PEEP in children. *Crit Care Med* 1980;**8:**372.

ENDOTRACHEAL INTUBATION

Endotracheal tubes are available in a variety of shapes and sizes. The sizes refer to the internal diameter of the tube and range from about 2.5 to 9.5 mm. Only tubes made of inert polyvinyl chloride should be used. The correct tube size is that which comfortably passes the vocal cords and the cricoid cartilage. Generally, a tube that will pass through the external nares will also pass through the cords and subglottic area. For an approximate guide to the endotracheal tube sizes appropriate for infants and children, see Table 14–3. The appropriate length of the tube should be estimated by holding the tube alongside the patient's airway; before the intubation, the tube should be shortened, leaving only a little extra length. Tubes of 5 mm internal diameter or larger are available with or without cuffs. A cuffed tube is indicated in a patient with excessive upper airway secretions or hemorrhage to prevent the spread of these materials into the lung, or, when very high pressures may be required for ventilation, to minimize the air and pressure leak around the tube. The cuff does not prevent spread of infection to the lower airway. Only tubes with soft, low-pressure cuffs should be used. When cuff inflation is necessary, the smallest possible volume of air should be used. All intubationsshould be performed by experienced personnel. The following equipment should be available for successful intubation:

(1) Suction machine producing an adequate nega-

Table 14–3. Recommended endotracheal tube sizes.

Age	Internal Diameter (mm)
Premature (<1 kg)	2.5
Premature (1–2.5 kg)	3.0
Newborn (2.5–4 kg)	3.5
1–12 months	4.0
1–3 years	4.5
3–10 years	5–5.5

tive pressure, equipped with a tonsil suction and a wide-bore suction catheter.

(2) Self-inflating bag capable of delivering 100% oxygen.

(3) Laryngoscope in good working order. Prior to intubation, the bulb and battery should be checked and the bulb tightened.

(4) Either a straight or curved laryngoscope blade may be used depending on the preference of the intubator. At least 2 sizes of blades should be available.

(5) McGill forceps if nasal intubation is to be performed.

(6) A cardiac monitor or stethoscope to monitor heart rate and rhythm during intubation.

(7) Endotracheal tube of the correct diameter and length (Table 14–3) and a tube smaller than the estimated size should also be available. If it is possible that the airway might be severely obstructed (as in croup), a very small tube should be available.

(8) Tape for securing the tube in place.

(9) Very flexible stylet.

Intubation Technique

When all equipment has been assembled and checked, the patient should be positioned so the intubator can be at the patient's head, with the patient's head and shoulders aligned straight in the neutral position. The person performing the procedure should be sitting or kneeling in a comfortable position so that his or her head is just above the head of the patient. The patient's head (not the shoulders) must be placed on a small pillow or roll in the "sniff position" (Fig 14–3). The position of the head on the pillow depends on the patient's age. In the adult, the head is rotated back; in the child, the head is in a more horizontal position; and in the infant, the glottis can often be observed better with the neck slightly flexed. Either the oral or the nasotracheal route may be used depending on the preference and skills of the intubator. Intubation should usually be performed with the patient awake and breathing spontaneously. The patient should breathe 100% oxygen for several minutes prior to the intubation attempt. The posterior pharynx should be maximally suctioned and the patient then reoxygenated. It is sometimes helpful to put some tape on the convex surface of the laryngoscope blade in order to minimize the chance of the tongue slipping across the blade. In addition, a small catheter or feeding tube can be taped along the outside of the closed side of the laryngoscope blade and attached to an oxygen source delivering 1–3 L/min to improve oxygen delivery to the patient during the intubation procedure. The laryngoscope blade is introduced on the right side of the patient's mouth and then brought into the mid position. It is very important to identify the anatomy of the larynx and observe the endotracheal tube pass through the vocal cords. If there is difficulty observing the larynx, gentle external pressure on the thyroid cartilage will often improve visualization. The tube should be passed through the larynx to a distance approximately midway between the vocal cords and the carina. After intubation, several breaths of positive pressure ventilation should be delivered while the chest is auscultated to ensure equal breath sounds in each hemithorax. It is best to listen in each axilla and then over the stomach to rule out accidental esophageal intubation. If breath sounds are decreased on the left side, the tube should be slowly withdrawn, with continuous auscultation until the breath sounds improve on the left, unless there is some intrinsic problem of the left lung that would cause decreased breath sounds. When it is properly positioned, the endotracheal tube should be securely fastened in place. A variety of methods are available for fastening both oral and nasotracheal tubes, perhaps the quickest being a piece of tape that totally encircles the head. If this method is used, it is useful to apply backing to part of the tape so that it does not stick to the hair. Finally, tube placement should be verified by chest x-ray.

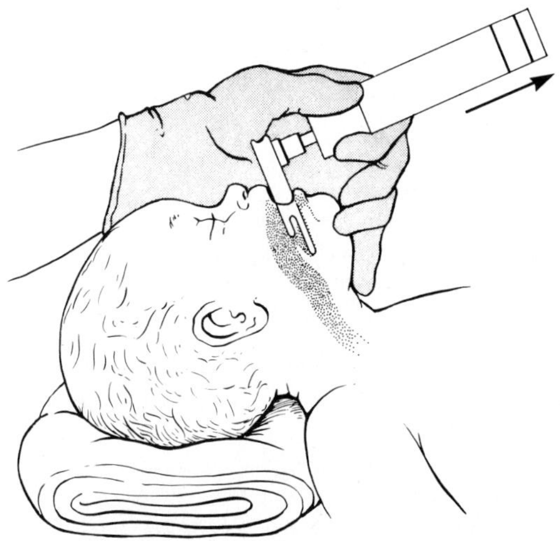

Figure 14–3. Position of head and neck for intubation.

Since an endotracheal tube bypasses the normal humidification and filtering functions of the upper airway, any air administered through an endotracheal tube must be cleaned, warmed, and humidified.

The major complications of endotracheal intubation are (1) tube obstruction or displacement (either too far into the airway, so that the left lung is no longer ventilated, or out of the trachea, so that no effective ventilation is performed); and (2) local tissue damage due to infection or pressure necrosis in the nose, oral cavity, larynx, or subglottic trachea. Key aspects of endotracheal tube care that minimize the risk of complications are frequent tube suctioning, optimal mouth care, secure fixation of the tube, and keeping the tube in neutral position as it emerges from the mouth or nose to avoid unnecessary tissue pressure. Endotracheal tube cuffs should be inflated only when necessary, and then with no more than the minimum effective pressure.

Aberdeen E, Downes JJ: Artificial airways in children. *Surg Clin North Am* 1974;**54:**1155.
Jennings PB, Alden ER, Brenz RW: Teaching pediatric intubation. *Pediatrics* 1974;**52:**284.
Redding GJ et al: Partial obstruction of endotracheal tubes in children: Incidence, etiology, significance. *Crit Care Med* 1979;**7:**227.
Spitzer AR, Fox WW: Postextubation atelectasis: The role of oral versus nasal endotracheal tubes. *J Pediatr* 1982; **100:**806.
Stauffer JL: Tracheal intubation. Chapter 2 in: *Pulmonary Emergencies.* Sahn SA (editor). Churchill Livingstone, 1982.
Stauffer JL et al: Complications and consequences of endotracheal intubation and tracheotomy: A prospective study of 150 critically ill adult patients. *Am J Med* 1981;**70:**65.

TRACHEOSTOMY

Whenever possible, tracheostomy should be performed as an elective procedure over a previously placed endotracheal tube under controlled conditions, preferably in an operating room. Occasionally, tracheostomy is required as an urgent lifesaving procedure.

Emergency Cricothyroidotomy

An incision is made between the cricoid and thyroid cartilages into the trachea in the subglottic area. A tracheostomy tube or other improvised airway is then introduced. Such a tube placed through the cricothyroid membrane is within a few millimeters of the true vocal cords, so it must be removed within 24 hours and replaced by a regular tracheostomy performed under optimal conditions. A well-designed instrument for cricothyroidotomy is the cricothyroidotomy scissors.

Elective Tracheostomy

This procedure requires that an airway first be established by endotracheal tube or bronchoscope. The procedure should be done in the operating room with adequate light, suction, instrumentation, and anesthesia. If an attempt is made to perform this procedure over an obstructed airway, pneumomediastinum and pneumothorax may result because of the marked negative intrathoracic pressure.

Local anesthesia may be adequate, since the agitated, hypoxic child usually goes to sleep following placement of the endotracheal tube or bronchoscope. The diameter of a tracheostomy tube should be approximately two-thirds that of the trachea. Teflon tubes are best for general use. The advantages of the Teflon tube over the older silver tube are its movable flange, which decreases the chance of accidental extubation, and its softness, which decreases the risk of tissue erosion or necrosis. The smaller sizes of Teflon tube have no inner cannula.

Tracheostomy Care

Constant vigilance by experienced nurses is necessary in the acute care of children with tracheostomies. Tracheostomy tubes may become displaced from the trachea into the soft tissues of the neck. This problem must be recognized immediately and the tube replaced, although effective ventilation through the upper airway by means of a bag and mask can be lifesaving before the tube is replaced. "Stay" sutures placed in the tracheal cartilage at the time of tracheostomy aid greatly in locating the stoma in cases of accidental decannulation of a fresh tracheostomy.

The necessary equipment (adequate suction, sterile suction catheter and glove, self-inflating resuscitation bag, appropriate-sized face mask, and extra, appropriate-sized tracheostomy tube) and personnel must be at hand if tracheostomy in small children is to successfully reduce the number of childhood deaths due to upper respiratory problems. Infants under 1 year of age are at increased risk of tracheostomy tube obstruction and death. Regular tube suctioning, good humidification of inspired gas, and careful stabilization of the tube to prevent accidental extubation are of key importance to minimize this risk.

Decannulation

In decannulation, the tube should be replaced with progressively smaller sizes and finally blocked for 24 hours before completely removing the tube. The external fistula closes within several days. Painstaking and persistent effort is necessary in decannulation of children under 1 year of age.

Aberdeen E, Downes JJ: Artificial airways in children. *Surg Clin North Am* 1974;**54:**1155.
Aradine C: Home care for young children with long-term tracheostomies. *Am J Maternal Child Nursing* 1980;**5:**121.
Foster S, Hoskins D: Home care of the child with a tracheotomy tube. *Pediatr Clin North Am* 1981;**28:**855.
Rodgers BM et al: Pediatric tracheostomy: Long-term evaluation. *J Pediatr Surg* 1979;**14:**258.
Sasaki CT, Gaudet PT, Peerless A: Tracheostomy decannulation. *Am J Dis Child* 1978;**132:**266.

DISORDERS OF THE CONDUCTING AIRWAYS

Abnormalities of the conducting airways (pharynx, larynx, trachea, bronchi, and bronchioles) produce signs and symptoms secondary to airway obstruction. The major signs of airway obstruction are stridor, rhonchi, wheezing, and prolongation of inspiratory or expiratory time. Obstruction of the extrathoracic airway results in greater obstruction to inspiration than to expiration (eg, croup), while obstructive lesions of the intrathoracic airway cause greater expiratory than inspiratory obstruction (eg, asthma). The increase in obstruction is due to dynamic compression of the airways during that phase of respiration. Therefore, an assessment at the time of physical examination and history taking of the relative severity of airway obstruction during inspiration as compared to expiration can be very helpful in localizing the primary obstructive disorder.

CONGENITAL ABNORMALITIES OF THE LARYNX

With the exception of atresia, laryngeal malformations are characterized by the development of a weak, sometimes hoarse cry and varying degrees of stridor. Congenital obstructive laryngeal lesions may cause symptoms of primarily inspiratory obstruction from the time of birth, or the infant may be relatively free of symptoms until the first upper respiratory infection occurs. The additional airway narrowing due to the infectious inflammation of the respiratory epithelium may precipitate significant respiratory difficulty. The clinical findings in patients with congenital laryngeal malformations are likely to include inspiratory stridor, intercostal and supraclavicular retractions that are worse with crying, and a hoarse cry. The diagnostic evaluation should include a careful history and physical examination, anteroposterior and lateral x-rays of the chest, lateral soft tissue x-rays of the neck, and fluoroscopic examination of the upper airway and of the contrast-filled esophagus to rule out an anomalous vessel that might be compressing the upper trachea. Pulmonary function tests performed on patients with fixed upper airway narrowing who are old enough to cooperate (ie, over age 6 years) demonstrate decreased peak flow rates (more marked on inspiration than on expiration). The definitive diagnosis is usually made by direct laryngoscopy or bronchoscopy. Treatment of congenital laryngeal malformations is usually directed at correction of the primary abnormality when possible and maintenance of an adequate airway at all times. Inspiratory obstruction due to a wide variety of causes is likely to be ameliorated by placing the infant in a prone position. Other congenital causes of inspiratory stridor that should be considered in the differential diagnosis include macroglossia, micrognathia, upper airway cysts, nasal obstruction, and congenital subglottic stenosis or subglottic hemangioma.

Cotton RT, Richardson MA: Congenital laryngeal anomalies. *Otolaryngol Clin North Am* 1981;**14:**203.

Ferguson CF: Congenital abnormalities of the infant larynx. *Otolaryngol Clin North Am* 1970;**3:**185.

Healy GB et al: Surgical advances in the treatment of lesions of the pediatric airway: The role of the carbon dioxide laser. *Pediatrics* 1978;**61:**380.

Landing BH: Congenital malformations and genetic disorders of the respiratory tract (larynx, trachea, bronchi, and lungs). *Am Rev Respir Dis* 1979;**120:**151.

1. CONGENITAL LARYNGEAL STRIDOR (Laryngomalacia)

Congenital laryngeal stridor is a usually benign entity due to minor developmental variations of the larynx. There may be an unusually shaped (''omega-shaped'' [Ω]) and long epiglottis that falls posteriorly during inspiration, causing partial obstruction; particularly short aryepiglottic folds; or unusually large, mobile arytenoid cartilages that move forward during inspiration and cause obstruction. The diagnosis is made by exclusion and by direct laryngoscopy. Congenital laryngeal stridor accounts for more than 75% of all laryngeal problems of infants. The onset of the inspiratory stridor is usually within the first week of life, although it may be delayed for several months. The stridor has usually disappeared by 12–18 months, although occasionally it may persist for several years. Such infants are usually not hoarse and only very rarely become cyanotic. There may be feeding difficulties (vomiting after feeding) and an increased incidence of early speech problems.

Since this is usually a benign, self-limited disorder, specific treatment is rarely required. Some infants may require hospitalization at the time of an upper respiratory infection owing to increased severity of the respiratory obstruction. In the very unusual case, tracheostomy is required because of chronic upper airway obstruction, usually during the second year of life.

Cox MA et al: Reversible pulmonary hypertension in a child with respiratory obstruction and cor pulmonale. *J Pediatr* 1975;**87:**190.

Lane RW et al: Laryngomalacia: A review and case report of surgical treatment with resolution of pectus excavatum. *Arch Otolaryngol* 1984;**110:**546.

Macfarlane PI, Olinsky A, Phelan PD: Proximal airway function 8 to 16 years after laryngomalacia: Follow-up using flow-volume loop studies. *J Pediatr* 1985;**107:**216.

McSwiney PF, Cavanagh NPC, Languth P: Outcome in congenital stridor (laryngomalacia). *Arch Dis Child* 1977;**52:**215.

2. LARYNGEAL WEB

A laryngeal web is a triangular membrane, often concave posteriorly, in the anterior portion of the larynx. The membrane is usually attached to the superior surface of the true vocal cords. In other instances, apparent fusion of the anterior part of the true or false cords produces a weblike structure.

The onset of inspiratory stridor, if the web is large enough, is usually at birth. Affected infants have weak, occasionally hoarse cries.

Conservative treatment is usually adequate. Repeated gentle dilation with laryngeal dilators may be appropriate. The physician should always be prepared to perform a tracheostomy following each dilation, since the procedure may precipitate increased laryngeal edema and further obstruction. Simple incision of the web may be followed by re-formation. In older children, a thin sheet of Teflon can be placed within the larynx and between the ''leaves'' of the divided web. This is attached to the thyroid cartilage and allowed to remain in place until complete epithelialization has taken place.

3. LARYNGOCELE

This congenital lesion is seldom clinically apparent at birth. A defect in the muscular wall of the larynx allows the inflation of an air-filled cyst. This cyst may present in the neck when the intralaryngeal pressure is elevated and may cause upper airway obstruction.

4. LARYNGEAL CYSTS

A true laryngeal cyst is differentiated from laryngocele because it secretes fluid. It is rare in infancy but may present in the neck as a localized swelling that increases with crying or may impinge on the airway from the laryngeal ventricle. The cyst is usually sessile, with a thin glistening wall. In addition to the signs and symptoms of inspiratory obstruction, there may be dysphagia. Laryngeal cysts must be differentiated from internal thyroglossal duct cysts at the base of the tongue. Occasionally, laryngeal cysts may be eliminated by repeated aspiration, but much more frequently surgical removal of the cyst wall, as completely as possible, is necessary to eliminate recurrence.

Shackelford GD, McAlister WH: Congenital laryngeal cyst. *Am J Roentgenol* 1972;**114:**289.

5. LARYNGOTRACHEO-ESOPHAGEAL CLEFT

This unusual congenital anomaly results from failure of posterior cricoid fusion during embryologic formation of the tracheoesophageal septum, leaving the larynx and part of the trachea open posteriorly. Affected patients are likely to have inspiratory stridor owing to poor laryngeal support and frequent aspiration of secretions and food. The cry is often very weak; there may be frequent cyanotic episodes due to aspiration; and recurrent or persistent pneumonitis is common. Weight gain is poor as a result of severe feeding problems and chronic lung disease.

The diagnosis of this entity can be very difficult. The diagnostic workup should include a barium swallow with fluoroscopy, direct laryngoscopy, esophagoscopy, and bronchoscopy. These patients should be fed by gastric tube. Corrective surgery has been successful in a few patients. Before surgery is attempted, the patient's nutritional status should be carefully attended to and intensive pulmonary therapy instituted. Tracheostomy or gastrostomy may be helpful in rehabilitation.

Beazer R et al: Laryngotracheo-esophageal cleft. *Arch Dis Child* 1973;**48:**912.

Novak RW: Laryngotracheoesophageal cleft and unilateral pulmonary hypoplasia in twins. *Pediatrics* 1981;**67:**732.

6. VOCAL CORD PARALYSIS

Vocal cord paralysis may be unilateral or bilateral and congenital or acquired. Vocal cord paralysis at birth is usually a laryngeal manifestation of a significant anomaly of another organ system. Bilateral cord paralysis may rarely be an isolated finding in an otherwise normal infant but more frequently is associated with birth trauma, cerebral agenesis, severe retardation, or meningomyelocele. Unilateral cord paralysis, whether congenital or acquired, is more common on the left than on the right because of the longer course of the left recurrent laryngeal nerve in the thorax and its anatomic proximity to major thoracic structures. The clinical presentation is similar to that of other congenital obstructive lesions of the upper airway. The amount of obstruction depends primarily on the severity of the paresis or paralysis. An artificial airway is rarely required with unilateral paralysis but frequently is required with bilateral paralysis. The diagnosis is established by direct laryngoscopy. The prognosis depends primarily on the associated anomalies.

Cormier Y et al: Upper airways obstruction with bilateral vocal cord paralysis. *Chest* 1979;**75:**423.

Holinger PC et al: Respiratory obstruction and apnea in infants with bilateral abductor vocal cord paralyses, meningomyelocele, hydrocephalus, and Arnold-Chiari malformation. *J Pediatr* 1978;**92:**368.

CROUP SYNDROME

Croup syndrome consists of inspiratory stridor and cough, usually of relatively acute onset. There may be associated hoarseness. This syndrome may be caused by a variety of inflammatory conditions of the upper airway in the region of the larynx. There may be underlying noninflammatory abnormalities of the upper airway such as vocal cord paralysis or congenital laryngeal stridor. Occasionally, the syndrome is caused entirely by noninflammatory problems such as an aspirated foreign body lodged in the extrathoracic airway, most likely at the level of the larynx or the cricoid cartilage. Croup syndrome can be due to hypocalcemic laryngeal tetany, or it may be one manifestation of the more generalized allergic response, as in angioneurotic edema. There may be a truly allergic form of croup (spasmodic) in the absence of other atopic symptoms. However, infection is the cause of croup syndrome in most cases (Table 14–4). Viral croup is most common, and bacterial croup is most serious. Rubeola and diphtheria can cause significant croup, but this is rarely seen.

Brooks JG: Upper airway obstruction. Chapter 3 in: *Pulmonary Emergencies*. Sahn SA (editor). Churchill Livingstone, 1982.

Davis HW et al: Acute upper airway obstruction: Croup and epiglottitis. *Pediatr Clin North Am* 1981;**28:**859.

Grunebaum M: Respiratory stridor: A challenge for the pediatric radiologist. *Clin Radiol* 1973;**24:**485.

Hamilton AG et al: Laryngeal edema due to hereditary angioedema. *Anaesthesia* 1977;**32:**265.

McBride JT: Stridor in childhood. *J Fam Pract* 1984;**19:**782.

1. VIRAL CROUP (Laryngotracheobronchitis)

Viral croup most commonly affects children between ages 3 months and 3 years, characteristically occurs during the late fall or early winter, and is usually caused by parainfluenza virus type 1. It can also be caused by parainfluenza virus 2 or 3, respiratory syncytial virus, influenza virus, rubeola virus, adenoviruses, or *Mycoplasma pneumoniae*. Although there is likely to be inflammation of the respiratory mucosa of all the conducting airways, the major cause of symptoms is inflammation and edema in the subglottic area, particularly at the level of the cricoid cartilage, which can cause significant narrowing of the airway at that point.

Table 14–4. Croup syndrome.

	Bacterial Croup (Epiglottitis)	Viral Croup (Laryngotracheobronchitis)
Common cause	*Haemophilus influenzae*	Parainfluenza virus
Most common age range	3–7 years	Less than 3 years
Seasonal occurrence	None	Late fall, winter
Clinical onset	Rapidly, acutely ill	Preceded by rhinitis and cough for several days
Dysphagia	Marked; may be drooling	None
Fever	> 39.4 °C (103 °F)	Variable, usually < 39.4 °C (103 °F)
White blood count	High (>18,000/μL)	Usually normal
Criteria for diagnosis	"Cherry-red" epiglottis on direct visualization	Clinical presentation and exclusion of other diagnoses
Treatment	Chloramphenicol intravenously, artificial airway	Cool mist; racemic epinephrine
Complications	Pneumonia, cervical lymphadenitis, exudative tonsillitis, otitis media, pulmonary edema, respiratory failure	Pneumonia, pulmonary edema, respiratory failure, cardiac failure

Clinical Findings

A. Symptoms and Signs: The onset is usually gradual, with a history of several days of symptoms of upper respiratory tract infection prior to the onset of barking cough and then inspiratory stridor. There are generally only mild elevations of temperature and white blood count, and the child does not appear toxic. If the lower respiratory tract is significantly involved, wheezing may be present. As the laryngeal obstruction progresses, stridor becomes associated with suprasternal, subcostal, and intercostal retractions. Auscultation may reveal decreased breath sounds. The child may become anxious and restless as hypoxemia and hypercapnia develop. There is a significant inverse correlation between respiratory rate and arterial oxygen tension. Cyanosis is a late sign and may herald complete airway obstruction. A decrease in the intensity of the inspiratory stridor may indicate improvement or may indicate significant deterioration of the patient with decreased inspiratory effort or increased inspiratory obstruction.

B. Laboratory Findings: The white blood cell count seldom increases to greater than 15,000/μL, and there is usually no significant leftward shift. Virus isolation studies have epidemiologic but not diagnostic usefulness. Blood cultures are rarely positive.

C. X-Ray Findings: X-rays of the cervical trachea demonstrate fixed circumferential subglottic narrowing but are of greatest use to rule out epiglottitis. Chest x-ray is usually normal.

Complications

The principal complication in patients with viral croup is asphyxia secondary to subglottic obstruction. Other complications are related to misadventures in attempting to introduce an artificial airway in an emergency situation and complications associated with management of a tracheostomy or endotracheal tube after an airway has been provided. A particularly traumatic tracheal intubation may convert a reversible subglottic narrowing into a fixed, nonreversible subglottic stenosis. There may be associated pneumonia or pulmonary edema.

Treatment

A. Outpatient Management: Most patients have the characteristic barking cough but no inspiratory stridor and may be treated at home. The parents should be instructed about the signs and symptoms of increasing airway obstruction (eg, tachypnea, cyanosis, increased retractions, or increased anxiety). Cool mist is a useful home treatment for mild croup. A heavy mist generated by running the shower in the bathroom with the doors closed will often afford significant relief. A walk in cool night air may also provide relief.

B. Hospital Management: Any patient with an acute onset of persistent inspiratory stridor at rest should be admitted to the hospital for therapy and close observation. Hospitalization is required in 1–2% of patients with croup. Cool mist therapy is the most generally accepted treatment for viral croup and can be administered in either a high-humidity room or a clear plastic mist tent. Large particle mist is probably most effective. Some croup patients have such severe dyspnea that they do not take adequate fluids orally, and in such cases intravenous hydration is necessary. It is helpful to monitor the urine specific gravity and daily weights to ensure normal hydration without overhydration, as this may contribute to pulmonary edema. All patients should be closely observed for signs of increasing hypoxia and impending respiratory failure. It is important to minimize any unnecessary anxiety, since increased anxiety results in increased inspiratory effort, which in turn increases the airway obstruction (dynamic compression) and increases oxygen consumption, all of which may worsen the patient's condition. Significant persistent inspiratory stridor can often be transiently ameliorated or eliminated by inhalation of nebulized racemic epinephrine. The solution for nebulization is prepared by adding 0.5 mL of racemic epinephrine to 3.5 mL of preservative-free sterile water. Since significant inspiratory stridor may return 1–2 hours after racemic epinephrine treatment, such therapy is appropriate only for hospitalized patients.

All croup patients who have significant obstruction have some degree of hypoxemia. For this reason, 25–30% oxygen is often administered. Occasionally, the administration of oxygen may be associated with marked calming of the patient because of a marked decrease in respiratory effort, resulting in hypoventilation. Thus, any patient with significant croup should be observed very closely for the first few minutes of oxygen administration.

Pharmacologic sedation should not be given to patients with viral croup unless an artificial airway is in place. Having the mother or some other familiar person close to the young patient is often the most effective form of sedation.

The use of corticosteroids is controversial. However, a brief course of dexamethasone (Decadron) or comparable agent—eg, 0.5 mg/kg/d in 4 divided doses for 1–3 days—may be beneficial in cases of *severe* croup, particularly in patients who have become unresponsive to racemic epinephrine.

If the usual medical measures are unsuccessful in relieving respiratory distress and if the patient remains restless and agitated and has progressively increasing cyanosis and decreasing air entry, an artificial airway must be provided. Some centers use arterial or "arterialized" capillary blood gas analysis as an indication of the need for an artificial airway. However, the author has generally avoided blood gas measurements because the procedure increases the agitation of the patient and usually does not provide steady-state results unless drawn through an indwelling arterial catheter.

Endotracheal intubation is the recommended means of establishing an artificial airway. Intubation should be performed under controlled and optimal circumstances, as discussed in an earlier section. A small endotracheal tube should be used to reduce trauma to the glottis and the subglottic area. Optimal endotracheal tube care is mandatory and consists of careful tube stabilization and suctioning, postural drainage and chest percussion, and humidification of inspired air. The patient can usually be extubated in 3–5 days, when able to breathe easily around the endotracheal tube.

Prognosis

Most children do not progress beyond the stage of cough, stridor, and mild retractions, and the disease usually resolves completely in 3–7 days. When tested in later childhood, children with a history of croup in infancy have an increased occurrence of airway hyperreactivity (eg, bronchospasm with exercise).

Denny FW et al: Croup: An eleven-year study in a pediatric practice. *Pediatrics* 1983;**71:**871.

Fogel JM et al: Racemic epinephrine in the treatment of croup: Nebulization alone versus nebulization with intermittent positive pressure breathing. *J Pediatr* 1982;**101:**1028.

Gurwitz D, Corey M, Levison H: Pulmonary function and bronchial reactivity in children after croup. *Am Rev Respir Dis* 1980;**122:**95.

Mills JL et al: The usefulness of lateral neck roentgenogram in laryngotracheobronchitis. *Am J Dis Child* 1979;**133:**1140.

Tunnessen WW, Feinstein AR: The steroid-croup controversy: An analytic review of methodologic problems. *J Pediatr* 1980;**96:**751.

Welliver RC, Sun M, Rinaldo D: Defective regulation of immune responses in croup due to parainfluenza virus. *Pediatr Res* 1985,**19:**716.

Westley CR, Cotton EK, Brooks JG: Nebulized racemic epinephrine by IPPB for the treatment of croup. *Am J Dis Child* 1978;**132:**484.

Zach M et al: Croup, recurrent croup, allergy, and airways hyperreactivity. *Arch Dis Child* 1981;**56:**336.

2. EPIGLOTTITIS (Bacterial Croup)

Epiglottitis is the most serious form of croup syndrome and generally affects children between ages 3 and 7 years, with no particular seasonal distribution. The course is rapidly progressive and fulminant. The most common pathogen is *Haemophilus influenzae* type b, although β-hemolytic streptococci and pneumococci have been implicated in rare cases. See Table 14–4 for a comparison of the clinical presentation of epiglottitis with that of viral croup.

Clinical Findings

A. Symptoms and Signs: The onset is abrupt

over a period of only a few hours. Young children often present with high fever and respiratory distress; older children may appear toxic and in addition complain of difficulty in swallowing and severe sore throat. Because of extreme dysphagia and pharyngeal hypersecretion, pooling of secretions in the posterior pharynx and drooling are prominent signs. Since the marked inflammation involves primarily the epiglottis and arytenoid cartilages, the patient may have a muffled voice but is usually not hoarse. There is usually a high fever (> 39.4 °C [103 °F]), and the patient appears toxic or even in shock. Within a few hours after the onset of symptoms, the child may be in marked respiratory distress with severe inspiratory stridor and retractions. The pharynx is likely to be inflamed, and there may be excessive pharyngeal secretions. The diagnosis is made by direct visualization of the markedly enlarged, friable, "cherry-red" epiglottis with a tongue blade or laryngoscope. Any attempt to visualize the laryngeal area should be preceded by preparation for introduction of an artificial airway and administration of 100% oxygen to the patient. Direct visualization must be undertaken with great caution because stimulation of the epiglottis has produced abrupt laryngeal obstruction and death. The tongue blade is less invasive and can be used with the patient in the characteristic sitting position with the neck extended, which is the position of choice for these patients in order to maximize the patency of the upper airway. The disadvantage of the tongue blade method is that it is impossible to visualize the arytenoid cartilages, and occasionally the inflammation may be localized to this site. Direct visualization with a laryngoscope or bronchoscope has the advantage that the anatomy can be much more clearly seen (especially the arytenoid cartilages), but this method may precipitate laryngospasm and is usually performed with the patient supine, which may cause the epiglottis to totally obstruct the airway. No throat culture should be obtained until epiglottitis has been ruled out or until an artificial airway is in place, since this maneuver may also precipitate laryngeal obstruction.

B. Laboratory Findings: Leukocytosis (> 15,000 white blood cells/μL) and a leftward shift of the differential count are usually present. Blood cultures are usually positive for *H influenzae* type b.

C. X-Ray Findings: Lateral x-rays of the soft tissues of the neck may be of value in confirming the enlargement of the epiglottis without resorting to direct visualization. This technique is particularly applicable when experts in intubation are not immediately available. The patient with suspected epiglottitis should always be accompanied to the x-ray department for such an examination, since total airway obstruction can develop at any time. All x-rays must be taken with the patient in the upright position, since the airway may obstruct if the patient lies down.

Treatment

When the diagnosis of epiglottitis is suspected, one of the above methods of confirming the diagnosis should be employed. Once the diagnosis is established, steps should be taken to introduce an artificial airway. Based on personnel and facilities available, each medical center must devise a protocol for optimal management of patients with suspected epiglottitis. Preparations should be made for controlled intubation, preferably in an operating room, with a tracheostomy set available. Because of the marked swelling and friability of the tissue, intubating such a patient is extremely difficult. The person most skilled in performing intubation should perform this procedure. A smaller than usual endotracheal tube should be used for this difficult intubation. While preparation is being made for controlled intubation, an intravenous line should be established and antibiotic therapy started by that route. Chloramphenicol, 100 mg/kg/d in 4 divided doses, is the treatment of choice.

Neither racemic epinephrine nor corticosteroids are appropriate treatment for epiglottitis.

Prognosis

The inflammation usually subsides rapidly after the initiation of antibiotic therapy. The patient should be extubated when able to breathe around the endotracheal tube and when direct visualization demonstrates marked decrease in the epiglottic swelling. This usually occurs after 24–72 hours of intubation. If an artificial airway and antibiotics are not provided promptly, the mortality rate may be as high as 50%.

Faden HS: Treatment of the *Haemophilus influenzae* type B epiglottitis. *Pediatrics* 1979;**63:**402.

Lazoritz S et al: Management of acute epiglottitis. *Crit Care Med* 1979;**7:**285.

Molteni RA: Epiglottitis: Incidence of extraepiglottic infection. Report of 72 cases and review of the literature. *Pediatrics* 1976;**58:**526.

Rapkin RH: Simplicity and reliability of radiograph of the neck in the differential diagnosis of the croup syndrome. *J Pediatr* 1972;**80:**96.

3. BACTERIAL TRACHEITIS

Bacterial tracheitis, usually due to *Staphylococcus aureus* (or, less frequently, *Haemophilus influenzae*), presents with inspiratory stridor and brassy cough but with a higher temperature and more pronounced leftward shift of the differential white blood count than occurs with viral croup. The incidence is unknown but may be slightly higher than that of bacterial epiglottitis. The age of most reported patients varies from infancy to 10 years. These patients tend to lie flat, in contrast to the preference for the sitting position in the patient with epiglottitis. The diagnosis is usually made after patients fail to respond to conventional croup therapy. They require antistaphylococcal or other appropriate antibiotic therapy and often tracheal intubation for removal of profuse, thick, purulent tracheal secretions.

Henry RL, Mellis CM, Benjamin B: Pseudomembranous croup. *Arch Dis Child* 1983;**58:**180.
Jones R et al: Bacterial tracheitis. *JAMA* 1979;**242:**721.
Liston SL et al: Bacterial tracheitis. *Arch Otolaryngol* 1981;**107:**561.
Sofer S, Chernick V: Increased need for tracheal intubation for croup in relation to bacterial tracheitis. *Can Med Assoc J* 1983;**128:**160.

OTHER ACQUIRED ABNORMALITIES OF THE EXTRATHORACIC AIRWAY

1. UPPER AIRWAY OBSTRUCTION DUE TO ENLARGED TONSILS & ADENOIDS

The syndrome of chronic hypoventilation, particularly during sleep, and cor pulmonale, sometimes associated with daytime somnolence in children, is most commonly caused by marked enlargement of tonsillar and adenoidal lymphoid tissue in the posterior pharynx. A similar clinical picture can rarely develop with other causes of chronic upper airway obstruction such as laryngomalacia, micrognathia, or macroglossia. The marked upper airway obstruction results in a great increase in the work of breathing and the gradual development of hypoventilation with CO_2 retention and associated hypoxemia. The low oxygen saturation causes pulmonary vasoconstriction, increased right ventricular work, and, eventually, cor pulmonale. Most children with this problem are between the ages of 3 months and 9 years; there is predominance of males over females of 3:1, and patients often have a history of recurrent pulmonary infections, somnolence, snoring, and mouth breathing.

Clinical Findings

Patients usually have a rattly, low-pitched inspiratory stridor that worsens in supine position. Tonsillar and adenoidal tissues are enlarged. There are likely to be accentuations of the pulmonary valve component of the second heart sound, a cardiac gallop, and often a cardiac murmur (especially of tricuspid insufficiency). Ten percent of these patients have digital clubbing. Systemic hypertension may be present.

Chest x-ray demonstrates an enlarged cardiac silhouette, and there is often pulmonary edema. Such patients are often misdiagnosed as having myocarditis. X-rays of the soft tissues of the neck and direct visualization of the oropharynx and nasopharynx demonstrate in many cases large tonsils and adenoids that significantly narrow the airway.

Electrocardiography may demonstrate right axis deviation, right atrial hypertrophy, and right ventricular hypertrophy.

Arterial blood gases may demonstrate CO_2 retention and hypoxemia, and there may be an elevated serum bicarbonate concentration as compensation for the chronic respiratory acidosis.

When this diagnosis is suspected in outpatients, it is appropriate to examine a chest x-ray and ECG and determine the serum bicarbonate to look for any indirect evidence of chronic hypoventiliation or hypoxemia.

Treatment

If the significance of the upper airway obstruction is in doubt, a nasopharyngeal airway can be placed, and this should afford significant relief. The definitive treatment is tonsillectomy and adenoidectomy. Oxygen therapy and sedation should be used very cautiously, since there may be depressed ventilatory drive. Assisted ventilation may be necessary for several days after surgery, because of excessive secretions, upper airway edema, and persistent congestive heart failure.

Prognosis

There is great clinical improvement after tonsillectomy and adenoidectomy; gradual increase in respiratory drive is probable. The pulmonary hypertension is probably completely reversible in most cases.

Brouillette R et al: A diagnostic approach to suspected obstructive sleep apnea in children. *J Pediatr* 1984;**105:**10.
Brouillette RT et al: Obstructive sleep apnea in infants and children. *J Pediatr* 1982;**100:**31.
Fan L, Murphy S: Pectus excavatum from chronic upper airway obstruction. *Am J Dis Child* 1981;**135:**550.
Remmers JE: Obstructive sleep apnea: A common disorder exacerbated by alcohol. *Am Rev Respir Dis* 1984;**130:**153.
Rowland TW et al: Chronic upper airway obstruction and pulmonary hypertension in Down's syndrome. *Am J Dis Child* 1981;**135:**1050.
Slovis TL: Non-invasive evaluation of the pediatric airway: A recent advance. *Pediatrics* 1977;**59:**872.

2. SUBGLOTTIC STENOSIS

Narrowing of the subglottic airway (from the level of the cricoid cartilage up to just below the vocal cords) can be either congenital, due to an abnormality of development, or acquired. Infants with congenital subglottic stenosis usually have inspiratory stridor from the time of birth, although milder cases of congenital or acquired stenosis may only have recurrent attacks of "croup." In any case, the voice and cry are usually normal except for inspiratory stridor. Acquired stenosis is usually secondary to trauma associated with the insertion or presence of an endotracheal tube. There is an increased risk of developing subglottic stenosis when the traumatized subglottic area is or becomes infected. The risk is minimized by using a small endotracheal tube, performing controlled gentle intubation, using an endotracheal tube made of polyvinyl chloride, and providing optimal tube stabilization and mouth care.

The treatment of subglottic stenosis may involve

tracheostomy, repeated dilation or cauterization of the narrowed airway (or both), or, occasionally, surgical resection. The differential diagnosis, particularly when there is asymmetric or unilateral narrowing, should include subglottic tumors such as hemangioma.

Couriel JM, Phelan PD: Subglottic cysts: A complication of neonatal endotracheal intubation? *Pediatrics* 1981;**68:**103.

Downing TB, Johnson DG: Excision of subglottic stenosis with the urethral resectoscope. *J Pediatr Surg* 1979;**14:**252.

Healy GB et al: The use of the carbon dioxide laser in the pediatric airway. *J Pediatr Surg* 1979;**14:**735.

Marshak G, Grundfast KM: Subglottic stenosis. *Pediatr Clin North Am* 1981:**28:**941.

Ratner I, Whitfield J: Acquired subglottic stenosis in the very low birth weight infant. *Am J Dis Child* 1983;**137:**40.

3. LARYNGEAL FRACTURE

Laryngeal fractures and soft tissue injuries in children are commonly the result of the child's being hurled against the dashboard of a car as the result of sudden deceleration. If the larynx is crushed, the airway may be completely obstructed so that immediate tracheostomy is required to prevent death. If the child survives the immediate postinjury period, careful observation is necessary during the ensuing 48 hours, since edema and expansion of hematomas may compromise the airway.

After attention has been paid to the airway, the important considerations in these injuries are debridement and closure of lacerations and treatment of intracranial complications. The physician is commonly misled at this point by the inclination to be conservative. Expectant treatment is just as inappropriate for the fractured larynx as it is for fracture-dislocation of the tibia. If normal function is to be restored, reduction of laryngeal fractures is usually necessary.

Myers EN: Assessing and repairing laryngeal injuries. *J Respir Dis* 1982;**3:**43.

4. GLOTTIC & SUBGLOTTIC TUMORS

Papilloma and subglottic hemangioma are the most common tumors of the laryngeal area in infants and young children. Both may be present at birth and may present with inspiratory stridor. Subglottic lymphangioma can also occur but is very rare.

Papilloma

The most common laryngeal tumor in pediatrics is papilloma. It most often presents between ages 2 and 4 years. It is histologically benign, consisting of proliferation of stratified squamous epithelium with a central core of connective tissue and very little vascular supply. There are usually multiple papillomas, and they typically disappear about the time of puberty. If they do persist into adulthood, spontaneous remission becomes less likely and the possibility of malignant degeneration exists. The papillomas most commonly involve the cords and the anterior commissure but may extend to other glottic and subglottic structures and occasionally farther down the airway.

A typical presentation is with croupy cough and persistent hoarseness. There is progressive evidence of upper airway obstruction and occasionally lower airway obstruction when there is more extensive distribution of the papillomas.

Treatment consists of repeated superficial excision until the problem spontaneously subsides. These tissue growths do not metastasize but do tend to recur frequently even after repeated excision. It is of key importance to maintain an adequate airway at all times.

McDonald GA, Strong MS: Respiratory papillomatosis: Keeping it under control. *J Respir Dis* 1984;**5:**36.

Mehta P, Harold N: Regression of juvenile laryngobronchial papillomatosis with systemic bleomycin therapy. *J Pediatr* 1980;**97:**479.

Smith L, Gooding CA: Pulmonary involvement in laryngeal papillomatosis. *Pediatr Radiol* 1974;**2:**161.

Steinberg BM et al: Laryngeal papillomarvirus infection during clinical remission. *N Engl J Med* 1983;**308:**1261.

Subglottic Hemangioma

Hemangiomas of the larynx in the infant are usually subglottic and tend to present early in life with signs of airway obstruction, usually without hoarseness. The hemangioma is sessile, soft and compressible, and usually not notably blue or red. In half of patients with subglottic hemangioma, there are associated skin hemangiomas. Over 90% of isolated subglottic hemangiomas present before age 6 months.

Most subglottic hemangiomas tend to regress and totally disappear within the first several years of life. Tracheostomy may be required while waiting for the hemangioma to regress spontaneously or with therapy. Some advocate corticosteroid therapy to reduce the size of the subglottic hemangioma. Successful treatment of severe subglottic hemangiomas with carbon dioxide laser has been reported.

Dillard RG: Subglottic hemangioma: A new approach to management. *Am J Dis Child* 1979;**133:**753.

Healy GB et al: The use of the carbon dioxide laser in the pediatric airway. *J Pediatr Surg* 1979;**14:**735.

INTRATHORACIC AIRWAY OBSTRUCTION*

1. FOREIGN BODY ASPIRATION

Essentials of Diagnosis

- Sudden onset of coughing and wheezing.
- Localized wheezing, hyperresonance, and decreased air entry.

* Status asthmaticus is discussed in Chapter 32.

- Localized air trapping on forced expiratory chest x-ray.

General Considerations

Children between ages 6 months and 4 years are at particularly high risk for aspiration of any small object to which they have access, such as seeds, grasses, nuts, beads, pins, or pebbles. The key to making this diagnosis, once it is suspected, is to take a very careful history in order to document the episode of choking associated with the onset of wheezing and chronic cough. There is often a history of playing with or near (or eating) some small object.

Clinical Findings

Aspiration of the foreign body classically precipitates an acute episode of choking, gagging, coughing, and wheezing, which in some instances may be associated with severe respiratory distress depending on the location of the foreign body in the airway. If the foreign body is not coughed out or removed, a period of several hours or days with diminished symptoms may occur followed by recurrence of wheezing and persistent cough. The foreign body initially functions as a ball valve obstruction, which may cause localized hyperinflation; later, however, the foreign body and the associated mucosal inflammation may completely obstruct the airway, causing distal atelectasis. Trapping of secretions behind the foreign body may occur at any time, and they may become infected. Recurrent or persistent pneumonia, always occurring in the same area of the lung, may be due to a retained foreign body. Bronchiectasis or lung abscess may develop in the distal airways if the foreign body remains in the airway for a long period with persistent pneumonia.

A. Symptoms and Signs: Physical examination of the chest will usually reveal asymmetric auscultatory findings, ie, decreased breath sounds over the affected lung, often associated with inspiratory rhonchi and expiratory wheezing, particularly in the first few hours after aspiration. There may be increased or decreased resonance to percussion over the affected area. Occasionally, the foreign body lodges in the larynx or trachea and causes signs of severe respiratory distress. When the foreign body comes to rest in a lower airway, there may be tracheal shift and asymmetric chest movement and aeration.

B. X-Ray Findings: The foreign body itself is usually radiolucent and therefore not seen on chest x-ray. If, as in the early stages after aspiration, the foreign body is functioning primarily as a ball valve obstruction, there may be localized hyperinflation. In such cases, however, the chest x-ray is often normal if taken during full inspiration, but a film during forced expiration will show localized hyperinflation (greater radiolucency) with mediastinal shift away from the affected side. A forced expiratory film can be obtained in a patient of any age by manual pressure on the abdomen during a spontaneous expiration. If the foreign body has completely obstructed an airway, there will be distal resorption of air with resultant atelectasis and volume loss seen on the chest x-ray. This is particularly likely if the foreign body has been in place for several weeks. In such cases, there will be no localized hyperinflation on the forced expiratory chest x-ray. Fluoroscopic examination of the chest is an alternative method for detecting air trapping and mediastinal shift. There may be no roentgenologic signs of asymmetry of aeration within the chest if the foreign body becomes lodged above the carina. If the signs, symptoms, and history are strongly suggestive of an aspirated foreign body, this diagnosis should be pursued by bronchoscopy even if repeated inspiratory and expiratory chest films are normal.

Prevention

Small objects such as beads, buttons, and certain foods (nuts, seeds, popcorn) must be kept out of the reach of small children. It is important to prevent children from running with foods or other small objects in their mouths and to discourage siblings from force-feeding infants in play.

Treatment

All patients with suspected acute foreign body aspiration should be admitted to the hospital. Improvements in bronchoscope optics have made rigid bronchoscopy a much safer procedure and therefore, with general anesthesia, the treatment of choice for aspirated foreign bodies. Bronchoscopy for foreign body in children is, however, a difficult and potentially hazardous procedure and therefore must be performed by an experienced and skilled bronchoscopist. The urgency with which treatment must be initiated and the recommended treatment depend to some degree on the location of the foreign body in the airway and the degree of the patient's respiratory distress. A foreign body located at or above the carina requires immediate emergency bronchoscopy. When the foreign body is lodged in a main stem bronchus, bronchoscopy should be performed as soon as convenient and certainly within 12–24 hours. Chest physiotherapy should not be used as the initial mode of therapy for removal of foreign bodies lodged in the trachea or large bronchi, because of the real danger of the foreign body being dislodged from its original site and moving to completely obstruct the trachea or larynx or the other main stem bronchus, leaving the patient with extreme respiratory insufficiency.

Once the foreign body has been removed, pulmonary physiotherapy should be administered until physical examination and chest x-ray show that a normal physiologic and anatomic status has been restored.

Prognosis

The chance of complete recovery is excellent if the patient survives the acute episode and if the foreign body is removed promptly. Foreign bodies that remain in place for many weeks can cause distal bronchiectasis or lung abscess.

Blazer S et al: Foreign body in the airway. *Am J Dis Child* 1980;**134:**68.
Greensher J, Mofenson HC: Emergency treatment of a choking child. *Pediatrics* 1982;**70:**110.
Kosloske AM: Tracheobronchial foreign bodies in children: Back to the bronchoscope and a balloon. *Pediatrics* 1980; **66:**321.
Law D, Kosloske AM: Management of trachael bronchial foreign bodies in children: A reevaluation of postural drainage and bronchoscopy. *Pediatrics* 1976;**58:**326.

2. ANATOMIC NARROWING OF THE INTRATHORACIC TRACHEA & BRONCHI

The intrathoracic airway can be narrowed by intrinsic tumors, granulation or inflammatory tissue, acquired or congenital fixed stenosis, extrinsic compression by aberrant blood vessels, or dynamic compression from altered transmural pressure gradients across the airway wall due to primary obstruction of more peripheral airways. Extrinsic compression of the airway can also be caused by mediastinal masses (Table 14–5).

Clinical Findings

Patients with fixed narrowing of the larger intrathoracic airways may present with a crouplike cough and, generally, more expiratory than inspiratory difficulty. An expiratory wheeze is frequently heard. There is often a history of recurrent pneumonia (often localized to the area distal to the obstruction) and increased respiratory distress with apparently mild respiratory infections. Chest x-ray may show localized or diffuse parenchymal infiltrates and possibly a mediastinal mass. (Many mediastinal masses do not cause airway narrowing.) Tomograms of the airway, thoracic CT scan, and high-kilovoltage x-rays that better delineate the tracheobronchial air column may demonstrate a localized airway narrowing. When the airway obstruction is due to functional dynamic compression and not to a fixed anatomic narrowing, the small lumen may be demonstrable only during a forced expiratory maneuver. Pulmonary function tests may demonstrate decreased maximal inspiratory and expiratory flow rates if the narrowing is fixed. When the intrathoracic narrowing is due to dynamic compression, the peak expiratory flow will be decreased much more than the peak inspiratory flow. If localized intrinsic narrowing is strongly suspected but cannot be demonstrated by noninvasive techniques, diagnostic bronchoscopy may be indicated. The presence of a bronchoscope in the airway may significantly alter intrapulmonary pressure gradients, so that a significant functional dynamic compression of the airway may not be evident. Bronchography is a potentially dangerous procedure in young children and is only rarely necessary. An esophagogram or systemic or pulmonary angiogram may be helpful in defining the cause of some types of large airway obstruction.

Table 14–5. Differential diagnosis of mediastinal mass according to anatomic location.

Superior mediastinum	Anterior mediastinum
Cystic hygroma	Thymoma
Vascular tumors	Thymic hyperplasia
Neurogenic tumors	Thymic cyst
Thymic tumors	Teratoma
Teratoma	Vascular tumors
Hemangioma	Lymphoma
Mediastinal abscess	Intrathoracic thyroid
Aortic aneurysm	Pleuropericardial cyst
Intrathoracic thyroid	Lymphadenopathy
Esophageal lesions	
Middle mediastinum	**Posterior mediastinum**
Lymphoma	Neurogenic tumors
Granuloma	Gastrointestinal tract duplications
Hypertrophic lymph nodes	Thoracic meningocele
Bronchogenic cyst	Aortic aneurysm
Gastrointestinal tract duplication	
Metastases	
Pericardial cyst	
Aortic aneurysm	
Anomalies of great vessels	

Treatment

The appropriate treatment depends on the specific type of airway obstruction. Some intrinsic obstructions to the larger intrathoracic airways, such as acquired tracheal or bronchial stenosis, can be successfully treated by endoscopic electrocoagulation or by total resection and end-to-end reanastomosis of the proximal and distal airway segments.

Gamsu G et al: Structure and function in tracheal stenosis. *Am Rev Respir Dis* 1980;**121:**519.
Healy GB, McGill T, Strong MS: Surgical advances in the treatment of lesions of the pediatric airway: The role of the carbon dioxide laser. *Pediatrics* 1978;**61:**380.
Kim SH, Hendren WH: Endoscopic resection of obstructing airway lesions in children. *J Pediatr Surg* 1976;**11:**431.
Landing BH: Congenital malformations and genetic disorders of the respiratory tract (larynx, trachea, bronchi, and lungs). *Am Rev Respir Dis* 1979;**120:**151.
Silverman NA, Sabiston DC: Mediastinal masses. *Surg Clin North Am* 1980;**60:**757.

3. TRACHEOMALACIA

The trachea of the newborn and young infant is significantly more compliant and therefore more compressible than that of the adult because of incomplete development of airway cartilage and other supportive tissue. Nonetheless, pathologic tracheomalacia in the absence of other lung disease is probably very rare. Tracheal collapse may occur in any patient with obstruction in smaller airways that necessitates forced expiration to empty the lungs. The positive intrathoracic pressure thus developed causes "dynamic compression" of the larger intrathoracic airways. Other causes of tracheal compression (eg, vascular ring) must be ruled out. There are rare cases of acquired or congenital defects of one or more tracheal rings that can cause a true isolated tracheomalacia.

Treatment in most cases of tracheomalacia, ie, those secondary to other airway disease, should be directed toward correction of the small airway disease. An artificial airway is rarely required.

Davies MRQ, Cywes S: The flaccid trachea and tracheoesophageal congenital anomalies. *J Pediatr Surg* 1978;**13:**363.

Feist JH et al: Acquired tracheomalacia: Etiology and differential diagnosis. *Chest* 1975;**68:**340.

4. VASCULAR RING

Tracheobronchial compression by anomalous or enlarged blood vessels will usually cause symptoms within the first year of life if at all. There may be associated congenital cardiac disease. The symptoms of the obstruction are most commonly a persistent expiratory wheeze and noisy breathing, often with recurrent pneumonias and persistent cough. Patients with vascular rings may assume an opisthotonos position to optimize the airway. Rarely, such compression of the airway may present with apneic episodes. There may be associated difficulty with swallowing. The chest x-ray is likely to show persistent or recurrent increased bronchovascular markings, and occasionally there may be evidence of airway indentation. An esophagogram is diagnostic in the great majority of cases of vascular ring. Bronchoscopy and pulmonary or systemic angiography are usually indicated to confirm or clarify the diagnosis. The more common vascular anomalies that may compress the trachea are (1) right aortic arch with left ligamentum arteriosum or patent ductus arteriosus, (2) double aortic arch, (3) anomalous innominate or left carotid artery, and (4) aberrant right subclavian artery.

All patients in whom vascular ring causes significant symptoms should have surgical correction if possible. Many infants have prolonged persistence of symptoms of expiratory obstruction even after surgical correction, suggesting a permanent abnormality of airway development, possibly secondary to the initial presence of the vascular anomaly.

Ashraf H, Subramanian S: Identifying the hallmarks of vascular rings in children. *J Respir Dis* 1985;**6:**31.

Keith HH: Vascular rings and tracheobronchial compression in infants. *Pediatr Ann* 1977;**6:**91.

Rheuban KS et al: Pulmonary artery sling: A new diagnostic tool and clinical review. *Pediatrics* 1982;**69:**472.

Zdesbska E et al: Early diagnosis and surgical treatment of children with congenital vascular ring and accompanying heart lesions. *J Pediatr Surg* 1977;**12:**121.

5. BRONCHITIS

Bronchitis may be acute or chronic, infectious (viral, bacterial [including mycoplasmal], or fungal), or due to chemical or mechanical irritation of the bronchial epithelium. Bronchitis as an isolated clinical entity is uncommon in childhood.

Clinical Findings

A. Symptoms and Signs: There is generally a dry, hacking, nonproductive cough for the first 4–6 days, after which the cough is likely to become productive. Fever, if present, is usually low-grade. Chest pain aggravated by coughing may develop. There are likely to be diffuse rhonchi, particularly during expiration. After 7–10 days, mucus production usually decreases and the cough gradually disappears.

B. Laboratory Findings: The white blood cell count is apt to be normal or only slightly elevated. Pulmonary function tests reveal a variable amount of airway obstruction that is usually not reversible with bronchodilator inhalation.

C. X-Ray Findings: The chest x-ray shows increased bronchovascular markings in chronic bronchitis and in some cases of acute bronchitis, but it may be normal.

Treatment

The general treatment for all types of bronchitis includes postural drainage and chest percussion preceded by bronchodilator inhalation, avoiding inhalation of irritants such as cigarette smoke and significant environmental pollution. Expectorants have no proved benefit. Cough suppressants are contraindicated, since coughing is necessary to clear secretions. Mist or high humidity offers symptomatic relief but does not shorten the course of the disease. Antibiotics should be used in bronchitis due to bacterial infection.

Adams L et al: Respiratory impairment induced by smoking in children in secondary schools. *Br Med J* 1984;**288:**891.

Colley JRT, Reed DD: Urban and social origins of childhood bronchitis in England and Wales. *Br Med J* 1970;**2:**213.

Fergusson DM et al: Parental smoking and respiratory illness in infancy. *Arch Dis Child* 1980;**55:**358.

Leeder SR: Role of infection in the cause and course of chronic bronchitis. *J Infect Dis* 1975;**131:**731.

Taussig LM et al: Chronic bronchitis in childhood: What is it? *Pediatrics* 1981;**67:**1.

6. BRONCHIECTASIS

Essentials of Diagnosis

- Chronic cough and sputum production (worse in morning).
- Persistent localized pulmonary abnormality.

General Considerations

Bronchiectasis is chronic dilatation and infection of one or more bronchi. It usually begins in early childhood and may be generalized or localized to one or 2 lobes. The incidence in the general population is less than 0.5%. The lower lobes are more commonly affected than the upper lobes. The disease may be classified as cylindric, varicose, or saccular depending on the nature and severity of the bronchiectatic changes on bronchography or histologic examination. The prognosis in terms of reversibility of the lesions relates to this classification. In cylindric bronchiectasis, the bronchi are dilated but retain regular, smooth outlines. In varicose bronchiectasis, both irregular dilatation and constriction of bronchi are seen. In saccular bronchiectasis, which carries the worse prognosis, the bronchi are widely dilated with increasing diameter in more distal airways. The airways tend to end in large blind sacs.

Bronchiectasis may occur in association with a variety of primary abnormalities or may be secondary to different lung insults. Some episodes of acute pneumonia due to adenovirus type 7 or 21, rubeola, pertussis, and, less frequently, *Haemophilus influenzae* type b, pneumococci, or *Staphylococcus aureus* may be followed by chronic recurrent symptoms of bronchiectasis rather than the usual resolution. Tuberculous pneumonia may also cause bronchiectasis.

Bronchiectasis may develop secondary to chronic or recurrent lower respiratory tract infections in patients with cystic fibrosis, immunodeficiency syndromes, abnormal respiratory cilia, recurrent aspiration, bronchial stenosis, congenital deficiencies of bronchial cartilage, pulmonary lobar sequestration, or bronchogenic cyst. Occasionally, localized bronchiectasis develops in a lobe that is chronically collapsed owing (for example) to an unrecognized aspirated foreign body, a mucus plug, or right middle lobe syndrome.

Some cases are probably congenital in origin and may result from an arrest of bronchial development, leading to the formation of cysts that become infected.

The association of bronchiectasis and sinusitis with dextrocardia is known as **Kartagener's syndrome.** Some patients with this syndrome have been shown to have anatomically and functionally abnormal cilia. The complete syndrome has a familial incidence but appears in only one generation.

Clinical Findings

A. Symptoms and Signs: The severity of the clinical manifestations of bronchiectasis varies widely. Most children with this disease appear healthy. There is likely to be a chronic productive cough, worse in the morning, which is often triggered by vigorous exercise. The sputum varies from white to gray in color, and in older children it may be foul-smelling and purulent. There may be a history of recurrent lower respiratory tract infections and dyspnea on exertion. Some children develop hemoptysis and bronchospasm. Digital clubbing appears in 25–50% of patients and does not necessarily relate to severity. There may be associated sinusitis, producing copious nasal and postnasal drainage and headache. There are likely to be recurrent or low-grade persistent fevers and moist rales over the involved area of lung. There may also be rhonchi, decreased air entry, and dullness to percussion over the bronchiectatic area.

B. Laboratory Findings: Sputum culture usually reveals a mixed flora of bacteria, with *H influenzae* being the most common. Pulmonary function testing reveals decreased maximal expiratory flow rates (particularly at lower lung volumes), elevated pulmonary resistance, and increased residual volume indicating gas trapping. These findings not only reflect the localized disease but also indicate that many patients have generalized small airway disease. A ciliary defect is best diagnosed by electron microscopic examination of material from a nasal or bronchial mucosal biopsy.

C. X-Ray Findings: The plain chest film is almost always abnormal in patients with bronchiectasis. Radiologic abnormalities may range from mildly increased bronchovascular markings to cystic changes or complete lobar collapse. Bronchograms may help determine whether disease is localized or diffuse; however, a normal bronchogram does not necessarily rule out bronchiectasis. Since bronchograms can be very dangerous in children, they should be performed with great care and only if surgery is seriously considered, ie, to support an impression of localized disease. They should not be performed until the patient has received maximal medical therapy for at least 3–6 months. A bronchogram will allow for classification of the bronchiectasis as cylindric, varicose, or saccular. In some cases, high-penetration chest x-rays will allow for the diagnosis of bronchiectasis without a bronchogram. An esophagogram may be helpful in patients suspected of having chalasia with gastroesophageal reflux and recurrent aspiration.

Complications

Complications include brain or lung abscess, emphysema, bronchopleural fistula, hemoptysis, cor pulmonale, and amyloidosis.

Prevention

Pneumonia should be treated with appropriate antibiotics in adequate dosages and vigorous pulmonary physiotherapy. All children should receive adequate immunizations for pertussis and rubeola.

Treatment

A thorough search for underlying causes of bronchiectasis should include repeated sputum cultures, evaluation of the immune system, sweat test, Mantoux test, sinus x-rays, and, in some cases, forced expiratory chest films, respiratory mucosal biopsy, and bronchoscopy. Systemic antibiotics should be selected on the basis of bacterial culture results and administered for at least 2–4 weeks. Optimal pulmonary physiotherapy is essential and consists of bronchodilator inhalation followed by postural drainage and chest percussion to the affected lobe or lobes. This should be performed at least 2–4 times daily. Patients with evidence of acute reversibility of airway obstruction following bronchodilator inhalation may benefit from chronic aminophylline therapy. Sinusitis, if present, should be vigorously treated.

Surgical removal of one or 2 lobes that have severe saccular bronchiectasis may be indicated if optimal medical therapy for at least 9–12 months has been without benefit and if the rest of the lung appears to be entirely normal. Only very few children with bronchiectasis are appropriate candidates for lobectomy.

Prognosis

The prognosis for patients with bronchiectasis depends on the cause, the severity, and the distribution of the bronchiectasis. Cylindric bronchiectasis is potentially reversible and is frequently present transiently after acute episodes of pneumonia, even in normal patients. The saccular type of bronchiectasis involves irreversible tissue destruction. Some patients will improve significantly after lobectomy or treatment of sinusitis, and most patients will show some improvement with optimal medical management. Most children with this disease are quite well controlled and lead relatively normal lives. In some cases, the disease clears entirely by adolescence. Patients in whom the bronchiectasis is associated with immunologic deficiency or cystic fibrosis have the poorest prognosis.

Carson JL, Collier AM, Hu SS: Acquired ciliary defects in nasal epithelium of children with acute viral upper respiratory infections. *N Engl J Med* 1985;**312:**463.

Chipps BE, Talamo RC, Winkelstein JA: IgA deficiency, recurrent pneumonias and bronchiectasis. *Chest* 1978;**73:**519.

Davis PB et al: Familial bronchiectasis. *J Pediatr* 1983;**102:**177.

McBride JT, Brooks JG: Sinobronchial syndrome. *Ear Nose Throat J* 1984;**63:**177.

Sanderson JM et al: Bronchiectasis: Results of surgical and conservative management: A review of 393 cases. *Thorax* 1974;**29:**407.

Turner JAP et al: Clinical expression of immotile cilia syndrome. *Pediatrics* 1981;**67:**805.

Whitelaw A et al: Immotile-cilia syndrome: A new cause of neonatal distress. *Arch Dis Child* 1981;**56:**432.

7. ACUTE BRONCHIOLITIS

Essentials of Diagnosis

- Rhinitis, cough, and expiratory wheeze.
- Tachypnea.
- Pulmonary hyperaeration on chest x-ray.

General Considerations

Acute bronchiolitis is a potentially serious disease that characteristically occurs during the winter months in children under age 2 years. The widespread bronchiolar inflammatory exudate, mucosal edema, and resultant narrowing of the airway can be due to infection or a combination of allergy and infection. An allergic component is particularly likely to be present in infants with recurrent acute bronchiolitis or a strong personal or family history of allergy. Respiratory syncytial virus (RSV) is by far the most frequent causative organism, but parainfluenza viruses, adenoviruses, and influenza viruses can cause the same clinical picture. All patients have some degree of hypoxemia, which may become severe. Occasionally, there is CO_2 retention. Hypoxemia may persist for 4–6 weeks after the child has begun to improve clinically.

Clinical Findings

A. Symptoms and Signs: After 1–2 days of mild rhinitis, the infant gradually develops increasing cough, expiratory wheeze, and respiratory distress. The respiratory rate becomes rapid, with shallow respiratory excursions. There may be nasal flaring, intermittent cyanosis, and intercostal, subcostal, and suprasternal retractions on inspiration. Chest auscultation reveals diffuse rales, expiratory wheezes, decreased breath sounds, and prolonged expiratory time. Pulmonary hyperinflation due to air trapping may produce an increase in chest diameter and depression of the diaphragm, resulting in displacement of the edge of the liver below the right costal margin. The easily palpable liver should not cause diagnostic confusion with cardiac failure, which is only rarely present.

Some infants with respiratory syncytial virus infection may present with significant apneic episodes early in the course of the disease, requiring mechanical ventilation. Coexisting or subsequent findings of bronchiolitis are usual in these patients.

B. Laboratory Findings: The white blood cell count is usually normal—an important point in the differentiation of acute bronchiolitis from pneumonia and pertussis. In allergic infants, nasal and peripheral eosinophilia may be present. Immunofluorescent staining of nasal secretions is likely to be positive for respiratory syncytial virus.

C. X-Ray Findings: The chest x-ray reveals hyperinflation (loss of posterior diaphragmatic upward convexity on lateral x-ray and increased lucency of lung fields). There may be increased bronchovascular markings and very mild infiltrates.

Differential Diagnosis

In small infants, it may be difficult to differentiate bronchiolitis from bronchopneumonia. Respiratory syncytial virus causes both bronchiolitis and pneumonia in infants. Both the temperature and the neutrophil count may be high in bacterial bronchopneumonia. Pertussis may be clinically similar to bronchiolitis except that white blood cell counts over 15,000/μL and marked lymphocytosis are unusual in bronchiolitis but common with pertussis.

Asthma can occur in infants, though it is rare before 6 months of age, and the differentiation from bronchiolitis may be impossible at the time of the first illness. A positive family history of allergy, repeated attacks, nasal or peripheral eosinophilia, and immediate response to a bronchodilator suggest that an allergy may be partly responsible for the wheezing.

In severe cases, an erroneous diagnosis of heart failure may be made. Growth retardation, enlarged heart (rare in bronchiolitis), and cardiac murmurs indicate heart disease.

Complications

The principal complication is secondary bacterial infection. Pneumothorax, mediastinal emphysema, and apnea and respiratory failure may occur.

Treatment

Hospitalization is recommended for infants with bronchiolitis who meet *any* of the following criteria: (1) younger than age 2 months, (2) a history or presence of cyanosis or apnea, (3) a history of a previous severe attack of wheezing, (4) a resting respiratory rate of 60/min or more, (5) arterial P_{CO2} exceeding 45 mm Hg, or (6) arterial P_{O2} under 60 mm Hg with the infant breathing room air. The intellectual and social situation of the family also influences the decision about hospitalization. Patients with bronchiolitis who are hospitalized for one of the above indications will be hypoxemic, so it is important to measure arterial blood gases or transcutaneous oxygen tension regularly. The inspired gas should be humidified and enriched with sufficient oxygen to maintain an arterial P_{O2} greater than 60 mm Hg. Infants with bronchiolitis may be dehydrated owing to inadequate fluid intake. The treatment should be directed toward achieving and maintaining a state of normal hydration, carefully following fluid intake and urine output as well as urine specific gravity. It is important to avoid overhydration, since this might contribute to pulmonary edema and thus further impair respiratory function. Chest percussion and postural drainage preceded by bronchodilator inhalation may be helpful in some patients with bronchiolitis.

Since allergic mechanisms may be responsible for part of the airway obstruction in some infants with acute bronchiolitis, a trial of an inhaled β-adrenergic agonist (eg, metaproterenol), with or without theophylline, 2–4 mg/kg orally every 6–8 hours, may be helpful in patients with significant airway obstruction.

Ribavirin, an antiviral agent (see Chapter 38), is reported to be clinically effective in many cases of bronchiolitis due to respiratory syncytial virus. Antibiotic therapy is indicated in more severe cases of bronchiolitis and those where secondary bacterial infection is strongly suspected. High fever, significant infiltrates on chest x-ray, significant elevation of the white cell count with a leftward shift of the differential count, respiratory failure, or positive bacterial cultures are indications for parenteral antibiotics.

Endotracheal intubation and mechanical ventilation are required for occasional infants who develop respiratory failure. Apnea, respiratory acidosis with a pH of less than 7.25, or inability to maintain the arterial P_{O2} above 60 mm Hg with $F_{I_{O2}}$ of 0.8–1.0 or more is a generally accepted indication for intubation and ventilation. The time course and progression of the disease may necessitate modification of these guidelines.

Corticosteroid therapy is not generally indicated in infants with bronchiolitis; however, there is a report of clinical efficacy of the combination of intramuscular dexamethasone with oral or inhaled albuterol. Pharmacologic sedation should not be used unless the patient is intubated and receiving assisted ventilation.

Prognosis

Acute symptoms of bronchiolitis usually last 2–7 days, with total resolution of the clinical disease by 7–10 days. With prompt optimal therapy, the prognosis is usually excellent. Far fewer than 1% of all infants with bronchiolitis will die of respiratory failure; however, the mortality rate exceeds 50% in patients who have congenital heart disease (especially with pulmonary hypertension) and an untreated respiratory syncytial virus infection of the lower respiratory tract. About half of infants with bronchiolitis will have subsequent episodes of wheezing and are very likely atopic.

Church NR et al: Respiratory syncytial virus-related apnea in infants: Demographics and outcome. *Am J Dis Child* 1984;**138:**247.

Hall CB et al: Ribavirin aerosol treatment of infants with respiratory syncytial virus pneumonia. *N Engl J Med* 1983;**308:**1443.

MacDonald NE et al: Respiratory syncytial viral infection in infants with congenital heart disease. *N Engl J Med* 1982;**307:**397.

McConnochie K et al: Normal pulmonary function measurements and airway reactivity in childhood after mild bronchiolitis. *J Pediatr* 1985;**107:**54.

Stokes GM et al: Lung function abnormalities after acute bronchiolitis. *J Pediatr* 1981;**98:**871.

Tabachnik E, Levison H: Infantile bronchial asthma. *J Allergy Clin Immunol* 1981;**67:**339.

Tal A et al: Dexamethasone and salbutamol in the treatment of acute wheezing in infants. *Pediatrics* 1983;**71:**13.

Wohl MEB, Chernick V: Bronchiolitis. *Am Rev Respir Dis* 1978;**118:**759.

8. BRONCHIOLITIS OBLITERANS (Bronchiolitis Fibrosa Obliterans)

Bronchiolitis obliterans, quite rare in children, can be diagnosed with certainty only by microscopic examination of lung tissue. A major insult to the lower respiratory tract is the most common cause, and the chief pathologic features are extensive damage to the bronchiolar wall with obstruction of the lumen by organized exudate and polypoid masses of granulation tissue. Distal to the bronchiolar obstruction, there may be air trapping or marked accumulation of fat-filled phagocytes. Ultimately, the involved bronchioles may be replaced by fibrous scars. There may be an associated interstitial pneumonia.

Bronchiolitis obliterans may occur following inhalation of toxic gases, lower respiratory tract infections (influenza, rubeola, pertussis, and adenovirus type 21), or inhalation of foreign bodies. In some cases, the cause is not known.

The most common symptoms are cough, dyspnea, chest pain, malaise, sputum production, and, sometimes, hemoptysis. Rales are commonly heard on chest auscultation. Chest x-ray abnormalities are variable and may include nodular densities, alveolar opacities, or, occasionally, hyperinflation. Pulmonary function studies may demonstrate either restrictive or obstructive disease.

Some children with bronchiolitis obliterans may benefit from corticosteroid therapy. In some cases, antibiotic therapy is indicated.

Becroft DMO: Bronchiolitis obliterans, bronchiectasis, and other sequelae of adenovirus type 21 infection in young children. *J Clin Pathol* 1971;**24:**72.

Epler GR et al: Bronchiolitis obliterans organizing pneumonia. *N Engl J Med* 1985;**312:**152.

Gosnick BB, Friedman PJ, Liebow AA: Bronchiolitis obliterans: Roentgenologic-pathologic correlation. *Am J Roentgenol* 1973;**117:**816.

9. ATELECTASIS

Nonaeration of part of the lung is usually due either to complete obstruction of a conducting airway, with resorption of all distal air, or to instability and collapse of terminal air spaces, often associated with inadequate surfactant, as in hyaline membrane disease or "shock lung." The extent of nonaeration or lung collapse may vary from one entire lung or more to involvement of only very distal air spaces in localized or diffuse distribution. With segmental or lobar atelectasis, the primary larger airway obstruction may be either intrinsic or extrinsic. Intraluminal obstruction of a major airway may be caused by a mucus plug, tumor, inflammatory tissue, or aspirated food, foreign body, or vomitus. Airway obstruction due to extrinsic compression is usually due to an enlarged lymph node, usually associated with infection or cancer. Enlarged or aberrant major blood vessels occasionally cause marked extrinsic compression of an airway sufficient to result in distal atelectasis. In addition, atelectasis can occur as a result of direct local parenchymal compression (eg, secondary to lobar emphysema or pleural effusion), chronic shallow respiration (eg, secondary to diaphragmatic paralysis or muscular dystrophy), or endobronchial tuberculosis. Atelectasis is a common finding in patients with cystic fibrosis and asthma. Allergic children have a tendency toward right middle lobe atelectasis, which may be chronic or recurrent. Atopy is the most common cause of persistent right middle lobe atelectasis. Postoperative atelectasis is not uncommon, particularly when the anesthesia time is prolonged or if the surgery involves the thorax or a major abdominal operation.

Clinical Findings

A. Symptoms and Signs: The clinical findings associated with atelectasis depend on its distribution and extent. Patients may present with persistent cough or fever. Physical examination may reveal tachypnea, rales or wheezing, or a localized decrease in breath sounds. In patients with chronic atelectasis, the volume loss in the affected area may be so complete that no localized dullness to percussion or decreased breath sounds can be detected on physical examination. If there is infection in the atelectatic lung or elsewhere, there may be a temperature elevation.

B. Laboratory Findings: There may be no abnormal laboratory findings. A Mantoux test should be performed. If infection is present, there may be an elevation of the white blood count. In older patients with significant atelectasis, it may be possible to measure a decrease in lung volumes by pulmonary function testing. Most patients with significant atelectasis, particularly those with reactive airway disease (asthma), will also have decreased maximal expiratory flow rates on pulmonary function testing.

C. X-Ray Findings: Chest x-ray may show diffuse patchy, lobar, or linear infiltrates; signs of unilateral or more localized volume loss (eg, unilateral diaphragmatic elevation, mediastinal shift, hilar elevation, or elevated or lowered fissure lines); or areas of compensatory hyperinflation. When the areas of atelectasis are small, there may be difficulty in distinguishing atelectasis from pneumonia.

Treatment

Therapy should include vigorous treatment of any underlying lung disease plus vigorous chest percussion and postural drainage combined with bronchodilator administration (inhaled, oral, or both). The pulmonary physiotherapy should be directed toward the affected area. If a localized lobar or segmental atelectasis persists for 1–2 months despite optimal medical therapy, bronchoscopy may be indicated for diagnosis and treatment. Lobectomy is indicated only after failure to expand the lung with at least 1–2 years of optimal therapy. There is no evidence that intermittent positive pressure breathing is effective long-term therapy for atelectasis due to large airway obstruction. If foreign body aspiration is a possibility, bronchoscopy should be performed after 1–2 weeks of medical therapy or sooner depending on the likelihood of this diagnosis. Children with right middle lobe atelectasis should be evaluated for asthma and, if appropriate, treated with chronic bronchodilator therapy.

Mak H et al: Recurrent wheezing and massive atelectasis in an adolescent. *J Pediatr* 1983;**102:**955.

Marini JJ: Management of lobar atelectasis. *Respir Care* 1983;**28:**204.

Marini JJ: Postoperative atelectasis: Pathophysiology, clinical importance, and principles of management. *Respir Care* 1984;**29:**516.

Marini JJ et al: Acute lobar atelectasis: A prospective comparison of fiberoptic bronchoscopy and respiratory therapy. *Am Rev Respir Dis* 1979;**119:**971.

10. BRONCHOPULMONARY DYSPLASIA

Bronchopulmonary dysplasia consists of chronic requirement for increased inspired oxygen in infants, usually following severe acute clinical hyaline membrane disease. The clinical and pathologic findings are characteristic. Bronchopulmonary dysplasia occurs in approximately 20–30% of infants with clinical hyaline membrane disease who require mechanical ventilation; most bronchopulmonary dysplasia patients were born prematurely.

Clinical Course & Manifestations

The disease has been divided into 4 stages as follows:

Stage 1 (days 1–3) is a period of acute hyaline membrane disease with a characteristic chest x-ray revealing air bronchograms and reticular granularity of the lung fields. During this period, there are findings of tachypnea, hypoxemia due to shunting through the areas of widespread alveolar atelectasis, and, often, hypercapnia. As a result of deficiency of surfactant that causes diffuse microatelectasis, the lungs are stiff and the functional residual capacity low. Histologically, there is diffuse collapse of terminal air spaces, but the larger airways are entirely normal. Most patients with clinical hyaline membrane disease begin to improve after 2–3 days and are normal by 5–10 days. In contrast, those who will develop bronchopulmonary dysplasia are likely to continue to worsen over the first several days of life, requiring mechanical ventilation.

Stage 2 (days 4–10) is the period of initial regeneration. There is a marked increase in oxygen requirement, with failure to improve clinically. Histologic examination shows early regeneration and metaplasia of the alveolar epithelium and some necrosis of the bronchiolar epithelium.

During **stage 3** (days 11–28), the period of transition to chronic disease, oxygen dependence persists, though the patient may no longer need mechanical ventilation. The chest x-ray demonstrates a "honeycomb lung," with multiple small, round, radiolucent areas. Histologic examination reveals regeneration and metaplasia of the bronchiolar epithelium, with increased airway mucus secretion and an inflammatory cell response. There are alternating areas of emphysema and atelectasis.

Stage 4 (after 4 weeks) is the period of true chronic lung disease. There may be a requirement for increased inspired oxygen for several months, although there is usually slow but progressive decrease of this requirement. There may be diffuse rales and wheezing on physical examination of the chest, with chest wall retractions, and increased chest circumference due to expiratory obstruction. The chest x-ray typically shows enlargement of the previously small radiolucent areas, beginning in the lung bases, with progression to generally radiolucent, hyperinflated lung fields with fibrous and atelectatic streaks. The histologic picture during this phase is characterized by alternating areas of atelectasis and emphysema, metaplasia of the bronchiolar epithelium, hypertrophy of smooth muscle in the walls of pulmonary arterioles and airways, and dilatation of pulmonary lymphatics. There may also be interstitial edema and, eventually, fibrosis.

These 4 stages are useful in understanding progression of the disease; however, stages are not usually distinctive but rather occur as a continuum, with different parts of the lung in different phases at any given time. In many patients, stages 2, 3, and 4 appear only as nonspecific streaky markings on x-ray, with areas of atelectasis alternating with areas of emphysema.

Differential Diagnosis

The chronic lung disease following some viral pulmonary infections (especially adenovirus) or occasionally following chronic congestive heart failure due to patent ductus arteriosus may be very similar, both clinically and pathologically, to bronchopulmonary dysplasia.

Prevention

It is likely that high positive airway pressures (barotrauma), high inspired oxygen concentrations (oxygen toxicity), and pulmonary immaturity contribute to the development of this iatrogenic disease, although the relative importance of these factors has not yet been determined. Great care should be taken during the treatment of acute clinical hyaline membrane disease to minimize the patient's exposure to high airway pressure (> 30 cm water) and high oxygen concentrations (> 60% oxygen). There is no evidence that prophylactic vitamin E administration influences the incidence or severity of bronchopulmonary dysplasia.

Treatment

Treatment of infants with bronchopulmonary dysplasia, both in the hospital and at home, is largely supportive. Even in the absence of overt signs of heart failure, some infants may benefit from diuretic therapy, particularly during acute exacerbations, because of an increased permeability of pulmonary capillaries that leads to pulmonary edema. Since excessive airway secretions and necrotic cellular debris may contribute to airway obstruction and since normal lung clearance mechanisms are not likely to be functioning properly, chest percussion and postural drainage may help these patients. In patients requiring chronic oxygen therapy, it is important to maintain an adequate hemoglobin concentration (≥ 14 g/dL) to maximize the oxygen-carrying capacity. It is helpful to follow the ECG for signs of increasing right ventricular hypertrophy, which may indicate increasing or chronic persistent hypoxemia. Increased serum bicarbonate may indicate chronic hypercapnia. Adequate nutrition is also of key importance, and the caloric needs of these patients may be significantly greater than normal. Occasional patients benefit from chronic bronchodilator therapy. There is no proved role for corticosteroid therapy in patients with bronchopulmonary dysplasia, although corticosteroids are occasionally administered in the most severely affected infants. Under some circumstances, it is appropriate to discharge the patient from the hospital before the oxygen requirement has returned to normal. This can be done by arranging for home oxygen administration through a nasal cannula (see Oxygen Therapy, above). Infants with bronchopulmonary dysplasia are likely to require several rehospitalizations for increasing respiratory distress and increased oxygen requirement, often precipitated by a mild viral infection.

Prognosis

Most patients with bronchopulmonary dysplasia will demonstrate slow but progressive improvement of lung function over the first few years of life.

Avery GB et al: Controlled trial of dexamethasone in respirator-dependent infants with bronchopulmonary dysplasia. *Pediatrics* 1985;**75:**106.

Berman W et al: Evaluation of infants with bronchopulmonary dysplasia using cardiac catheterization. *Pediatrics* 1982; **70:**708.

Logvinoff MM et al: Bronchodilators and diuretics in children with bronchopulmonary dysplasia. *Pediatr Pulmonol* 1985;**1:**198.

McCarthy K et al: Pathogenic factors in bronchopulmonary dysplasia. *Pediatr Res* 1984;**18:**483.

Merritt TA et al: Newborn tracheal aspirate cytology: Classification during respiratory distress syndrome and bronchopulmonary dysplasia. *J Pediatr* 1981;**98:**949.

Sauve RS, Singhal N: Long-term morbidity of infants with bronchopulmonary dysplasia. *Pediatrics* 1985;**76:**725.

Smyth JA et al: Pulmonary function and bronchial hyperactivity in long-term survivors of bronchopulmonary dysplasia. *Pediatrics* 1981;**68:**336.

Taghizadh A, Reynolds EOR: Pathogenesis of bronchopulmonary dysplasia following hyaline membrane disease. *Am J Pathol* 1976;**82:**241.

11. CYSTIC FIBROSIS

Essentials of Diagnosis

- Elevated sweat chloride (> 60 meq/L).
- Recurrent pulmonary infections or steatorrhea or family history of cystic fibrosis.

General Considerations

Cystic fibrosis is a genetically transmitted autosomal recessive disease characterized by widespread involvement of the exocrine glands. Approximately 5% of the Caucasian population are carriers of the recessive gene, and one in 2000 infants is affected. Multiple organ systems are involved: lungs, gastrointestinal tract, sweat glands, and testes.

In the lungs, there is production of abnormally viscous mucus. The respiratory cilia are unable to effectively clear this tenacious mucus. As a consequence, there is progressive obstruction of the airways, beginning with the small bronchioles, leading to air trapping and atelectasis. Secondarily acquired lung infection occurs and predisposes to destruction of the respiratory epithelium and airways, resulting in bronchiectasis. The bacteria most commonly cultured from expectorated sputum are *Pseudomonas aeruginosa, Staphylococcus aureus,* and *Haemophilus influenzae.* In addition, patients may be particularly vulnerable to viral lower respiratory tract infections.

There is a wide variability in the clinical presentation and course; some patients are severely affected as infants, and others remain asymptomatic until adolescence. Any patient with malabsorption problems or repeated pulmonary infections should be suspected of having cystic fibrosis.

Clinical Findings

A. Symptoms and Signs: In severe disease, patients have foul-smelling, bulky, frequent fatty stools, failure to thrive, and frequent pulmonary infections with marked exercise limitation and chronic cough productive of purulent sputum. Ten percent of newborns with cystic fibrosis present with intestinal obstruction secondary to inspissated meconium (meconium ileus). Infants with mild disease may present at an older age with symptoms resembling those of asthma. Occasional patients have no significant symptoms until early adulthood.

Physical examination may be normal or may reveal signs of pulmonary involvement and malnutrition. Manifestations of the associated lung disease include hyperexpansion of the thoracic cage with use of the auxiliary muscles of respiration, rales, rhonchi, wheezes, unevenly decreased breath sounds in different parts of the chest, cyanosis, and digital clubbing. The liver edge may be palpable well below the right costal margin, but this is probably due to a flattened diaphragm, lowering the liver, although it occasionally can be caused by cor pulmonale, and in that case would usually be associated with cardiac gallop rhythm. Patients with moderate to severe lung disease may have significant accentuation of the pulmonary component of the second heart sound. Physical signs of malabsorption include poor growth (weight gain is usually significantly more impaired than linear growth) and decreased subcutaneous tissue and muscle mass.

B. Laboratory Findings: The earliest laboratory signs of the associated pulmonary disease are a decrease in arterial oxygen tension and abnormalities of pulmonary function tests of small airway patency such as the forced expiratory flow rate from 75% to 25% of vital capacity (FEF_{25-75}), the flow volume loop, and the single breath oxygen test. With progression of pulmonary disease, pulmonary function testing demonstrates increasing obstructive lung disease with further decreased maximal flow rates and vital capacity and increased absolute lung volumes (first residual volume, then functional residual capacity, then total lung capacity are increased) and airway resistance. With very severe lung disease, in the preterminal period, there may be a decrease in total lung capacity.

A sweat test should be performed using the pilocarpine iontophoresis technique. Other types of sweat testing are not satisfactory. A sweat chloride concentration exceeding 60 meq/L is diagnostic if at least 50 mg of sweat have been collected. A concentration under 50 meq/L is normal. Patients with sweat chloride concentrations between 50 and 60 meq/L present diagnostic problems, although most of them will not have cystic fibrosis.

There is likely to be increased fat excretion in stool. No reliable methods are available for screening stool in newborns, for intrauterine diagnosis of cystic fibrosis, or for detection of the heterozygote; however, recent advances in localization of the cystic fibrosis gene by genetic linkage studies greatly enhance the likelihood of successful techniques for prenatal diagnosis.

With more severe lung disease, electrocardiography and echocardiography may demonstrate right ventricle abnormalities due to pulmonary hypertension.

Although liver involvement is histologically demonstrable at an early stage in the disease, laboratory evidence of liver involvement (increased liver enzymes and decreased liver-dependent clotting factors) does not appear until relatively late.

C. X-Ray Findings: The earliest abnormalities on chest x-ray are mild hyperinflation, best seen as loss of diaphragmatic doming on the lateral chest x-ray, and increased bronchovascular markings, particularly in the upper lobes. Later, there are diffuse infiltrates, marked hyperinflation, and areas of atelectasis interspersed with areas of "emphysema," giving an appearance of cystic lung changes. Sinus x-rays demonstrate a high incidence of sinusitis, and x-rays of the long bones may demonstrate pulmonary osteoarthropathy in patients with severe pulmonary disease.

Differential Diagnosis

Cystic fibrosis must be differentiated from allergic lung diseases, immunologic deficiency diseases, α_1-antitrypsin deficiency, anatomic airway abnormalities (eg, airway stenosis), recurrent aspiration, other causes of malabsorption, and failure to thrive.

Complications

Cardiopulmonary complications include pneumothorax, pulmonary abscess, allergic bronchopulmonary aspergillosis, hemoptysis, empyema, nasal polyps, sinusitis, pulmonary hypertension, cor pulmonale, respiratory failure, and pulmonary osteoarthropathy. Complications involving the intestinal tract include intussusception, impaction, rectal prolapse, recurrent abdominal pain, portal hyertension, esophageal varices, hematemesis, and failure to thrive. Nearly all males are sterile.

Treatment

A vigorous long-term multidisciplinary treatment program with good follow-up and continuity is extremely important in the treatment of patients with cystic fibrosis. In the USA, there is a network of more than 100 cystic fibrosis centers providing care, information, and consultation for affected patients. Contact the National Cystic Fibrosis Foundation, 6000 Executive Boulevard, Suite 510, Rockville, MD; telephone (301) 881–9130.

A. Pulmonary Therapy: Since all patients with cystic fibrosis probably have impaired lung clearance mechanisms and therefore accumulate viscous mucus in the airways, postural drainage and chest percussion in 9 different positions should be done at least once daily, especially in the morning (Fig 14–2). In many patients, it is helpful to precede the chest percussion by bronchodilator inhalation. All episodes of acute increases in cough, sputum production, dyspnea, or fever should be treated with oral or parenteral antibiotics depending on the severity of the acute and chronic illness as well as an increase in the frequency of pulmonary physical therapy. Antibiotics may be selected on the basis of sputum cultures and organism sensitivities, although any child with advanced cystic fibrosis will harbor *H influenzae, S aureus,* and *P aeruginosa*. The most effective oral antibiotics are trimethoprim-sulfamethoxazole (Bactrim, Septra), 8–20 mg/kg/d (trimethoprim) plus 40–100 mg/kg/d (sulfamethoxazole) in 2–3 divided doses; dicloxicillin, 25–50 mg/kg/d in 3–4 divided doses; chloramphenicol, 50 /kg/d in 3–4 divided doses; clindamycin, 10–25 mg/kg/d in 4 divided doses; and, for older children, tetracycline, 20–40 mg/kg/d in 3–4 divided doses. The most appropriate antibiotic regimen for intravenous administration is tobramycin, 3–5 mg/kg/d in 3 divided doses, plus either ticarcillin, 200–300 mg/kg/d in 4–6 divided doses, or nafcillin, 150 mg/kg/d in 4 divided doses. Larger doses of aminoglycoside antibiotics may be necessary to achieve adequate serum drug concentrations, since patients with cystic fibrosis have increased clearance rates of these drugs. It is usual to give one aminoglycoside and one synthetic penicillin for intravenous antibiotic therapy. Severely affected patients may have some degree of biventricular cardiac failure and may occasionally benefit from either diuretic or digitalis therapy. Oral bronchodilator therapy (theophylline, 4–6 mg/kg/dose in 3–4 daily doses) is of benefit to some patients with cystic fibrosis.

The efficiency of and indications (if any) for inhaled antibiotics and oral corticosteroids are currently under investigation. Home use of antibiotics, usually after hospitalization, is appropriate for some patients.

There is an increased incidence of atopy in children with cystic fibrosis, and some of these patients will benefit from intermittent antihistamine therapy. However, antihistamines must be used cautiously and with careful evaluation of effect in each patient, because they may increase viscosity of respiratory secretions.

Oxygen therapy is often indicated to maintain adequate arterial oxygen tension during acute exacerbations. In addition, severely affected patients may benefit from chronic oxygen administration at home, particularly at night. Recurrent morning headaches will often disappear when nighttime oxygen therapy is initiated.

Chemical pleurodesis (eg, with tetracycline) should be considered for patients with pneumothorax, particularly when the air leak is recurrent. Minor blood streaking of expectorated sputum is common in advanced disease. More significant hemoptysis should be treated with vitamin K and more aggressive antibiotic therapy, since hemoptysis is often associated with exacerbations of respiratory tract infections. Hospitalization is usually appropriate for hemoptysis other than blood-streaked sputum. Massive hemoptysis (eg, > 250 mL in 24 hours) may necessitate blood transfusion; in some cases, bronchial artery embolization may be appropriate.

B. Intestinal Tract Therapy:

1. Meconium ileus in the newborn—Intestinal obstruction due to uncomplicated meconium ileus in the newborn can usually be relieved by diatrizoate sodium (Gastrografin) or acetylcysteine (Mucomyst) enemas. When surgery is necessary, intestinal atresia or volvulus requiring resection may be found proximal to the meconium ileus.

2. Meconium ileus equivalent (fecal impaction) and intussusception in older children—These causes of intestinal obstruction and abdominal pain in older children can often be relieved without surgery. The inspissated feces can sometimes be softened by oral acetylcysteine, liquids, or mineral oil. Intussusception can usually be reduced by enemas, although surgery is occasionally required.

3. Pancreatic insufficiency—A number of pancreatic extract preparations are commercially available (eg, Cotazym-S, Pancrease, Viokase) in capsule, tablet, or powder form to be taken at mealtime. The dosage of pancreatic enzyme replacement should be individualized to produce 1–2 formed stools daily. One or 2 capsules are often indicated with snacks. The enzymes may be mixed with some form of fruit (eg, applesauce). The requirement for replacement enzymes may either decrease or increase with age.

Persistence of marked diarrhea in the face of seemingly adequate replacement therapy should make one suspect other causes. Disaccharidase deficiencies and celiac disease have been reported in rare patients with cystic fibrosis.

The diet should be high in protein and carbohydrate, and some attempt should be made to avoid excessively fatty foods. Small infants and occasionally older children may benefit from diets containing supplemental medium-chain triglycerides (eg, Portagen). Glucose polymers and high-protein snacks are also useful in caloric supplementation. Some infants with cystic fibrosis, particularly those receiving soybase formulas, may present with hypoproteinemic edema due to difficulty in absorbing the protein. Regular multivitamins and water-soluble vitamin E preparations (approximately 100–200 units/d) should probably be given to all cystic fibrosis patients. Supplemental vitamin A, D, or K should be given only to patients showing indications of a possible deficiency of the specific vitamin. Patients exposed to conditions that may cause heavy sweat loss (eg, hot weather, fever) and patients with hyponatremia should have 1 g of salt added to the daily diet up to age 2 years and 2 g/d over age 2 years.

C. Psychosocial Support: Cystic fibrosis imposes many extra psychologic, social, and financial burdens on the patient and family. Skilled counsel is an important aspect of care, particularly around the time the diagnosis is made and in the weeks before and after death.

Prognosis

Life expectancy for patients with cystic fibrosis has improved significantly in recent years, probably as a result of more aggressive therapy and more frequent diagnosis of patients with milder disease. Fifty percent of patients will survive to 20 years of age.

diSant'agnese PA, Davis PB: Cystic fibrosis in adults: 75 cases and a review of 232 cases in the literature. *Am J Med* 1979;**66**:121.

Kelly HW, Lovato C: Antibiotic use in cystic fibrosis. *Drug Intell Clin Pharm* 1984;**18**:772.

Levy LD et al: Effects of long-term nutritional rehabilitation on body composition and clinical status in malnourished children and adolescents with cystic fibrosis. *J Pediatr* 1985;**107**:225.

Lloyd-Still JD: *Textbook of Cystic Fibrosis*. PSG Inc., 1983.

Moss AJ: The cardiovascular system in cystic fibrosis. *Pediatrics* 1982;**70**:728.

Quinton PM, Bijman J: Higher bioelectric potentials due to decreased chloride absorption in the sweat glands of patients with cystic fibrosis. *N Engl J Med* 1983;**308**:1185.

Shay GF, Newth CJL: Cystic fibrosis update: Your patient's outlook is better than ever. *J Respir Dis* 1985;**6**:33.

Stern RC et al: Treatment and prognosis of lobar and segmental atelectasis in cystic fibrosis. *Am Rev Respir Dis* 1978; **118**:821.

Taussig LM: *Cystic Fibrosis*. Thieme-Stratton, 1984.

Taussig LM et al: Neonatal screening for cystic fibrosis: Position paper. (Committee Report.) *Pediatrics* 1983;**72**:741.

Wang EEL et al: Association of respiratory viral infections with pulmonary deterioration in patients with cystic fibrosis. *N Engl J Med* 1984;**311**:1653.

Wisnieski JJ et al: Immune complexes and complement abnormalities in patients with cystic fibrosis: *Am Rev Respir Dis* 1985;**132**:770.

DISEASES OF THE ALVEOLI & PULMONARY INTERSTITIUM

BACTERIAL PNEUMONIA

Essentials of Diagnosis

- History of mild upper airway infection.
- Abrupt rise in temperature to 39.5–40.5 °C (103.1–104.9 °F).

- Tachypnea and cough.
- Chest auscultation may be normal, or there may be generalized or localized signs of rales, dullness to percussion, and increased voice transmission.
- Specific etiologic diagnosis depends upon cultures of blood and respiratory secretions.

General Considerations

The characteristic lobar involvement found in adult bacterial pneumonia is less common in children. In infants and children, involvement is generally more diffuse and the airway more involved (bronchial pneumonia). It is not usually possible to reliably predict the causative organism from the clinical findings. Therefore, for successful treatment, an educated guess about the causative organism is of greatest therapeutic importance.

Patients with recurrent or persistent pneumonia should be evaluated for immunologic deficiency disease, cystic fibrosis, aspirated foreign body, allergy, bronchiectasis, recurrent aspiration, and other anatomic abnormalities of the airways.

Clinical Findings

A. Symptoms and Signs: The onset is usually quite rapid and is often preceded by an upper respiratory infection. Fever and tachypnea are the most important findings, especially in infants, in whom the physical examination may be otherwise normal. Any infant under age 6 weeks with cough should be assumed to have pneumonia until this is ruled out by chest x-ray. Chest wall retractions may be seen in infants and children. Older children may also experience chills.

Physical signs may include areas of depressed breath sounds, inspiratory rales and rhonchi, wheezing, dullness to percussion, tubular breath sounds, chest wall splinting, and cyanosis. Older children may complain of chest or abdominal pain. Rales may not be heard until the disease is resolving. Abnormal physical findings in the chest may precede chest x-ray abnormalities. Friction rubs are rare.

B. Laboratory Findings: The white blood cell count is likely to be elevated to 18,000–40,000/μL, mostly polymorphonuclear leukocytes. White blood cell counts under 10,000/μL with a shift to the left carry a poor prognosis in patients with bacterial pneumonia.

Streptococcus pneumoniae is the most common cause of bacterial pneumonia, but other infectious agents must be considered. *Haemophilus influenzae* can cause an identical clinical picture but may not respond to penicillin alone. Pneumonia due to group A β-hemolytic streptococci is uncommon but can be very severe. Empyema, if present, is more liquid than in *S pneumoniae* or staphylococcal disease. Group A streptococcal infection also has a greater tendency to ulcerate the trachea than *S pneumoniae* disease, and there may be a higher incidence of empyema. Staphylococcal infection is more apt to cause abscess formation and pneumatoceles than are other organisms. Tuberculosis should be considered in any case of pneumonia that fails to respond to usual antibiotic therapy.

C. X-Ray Findings: Chest x-ray abnormalities are likely to consist of patchy infiltrates and increased bronchovascular markings (bronchopneumonia) and, occasionally, lobar consolidation.

Differential Diagnosis

Bacterial pneumonia may resemble meningitis and acute abdominal disorders. Staphylococcal pneumonia may present with ileus due to a specific toxin.

Complications

Complications of bacterial pneumonia include septicemia, pneumatocele, lung abscess, pleural effusion, empyema, bronchiectasis, respiratory failure, pneumothorax, lung hemorrhage, septic shock, pyopneumothorax, and heart failure.

Treatment

A. Specific Measures: Any infant under age 2–3 months with pneumonia should be admitted to the hospital for at least a brief observation. Hospitalization of older infants and children depends on the severity of their illness and the most appropriate route for antibiotics. Appropriate antibiotics should be selected on the basis of the clinical presentation, with the assistance of a gram-stained smear of expectorated sputum; culture of aspirated tracheal secretions; counterimmunoelectrophoresis of urine or blood; or culture of material taken from the lung by needle aspiration when available. Specimens should be taken prior to initiating antibiotic therapy. Antibiotics may be given orally or parenterally depending on the severity of the illness but in severe cases should always be given intravenously. Penicillin is the drug of choice for pneumonia due to *S pneumoniae,* group A streptococci, and penicillin-sensitive staphylococci. Ampicillin should be used in *H influenzae* pneumonia. In resistant staphylococcal infections, intravenous sodium methicillin or nafcillin should be given. A percutaneous lung aspiration is indicated when an unusual organism is suspected or when the patient's condition is continuing to deteriorate despite usual therapy.

B. General Measures: Supportive measures such as humidified oxygen, pulmonary physiotherapy, and intravenous fluids are indicated in more severe cases. Tracheal intubation and mechanical ventilation are indicated for respiratory failure.

Prognosis

With adequate therapy, sequelae are rare; however, if staphylococcal, streptococcal, or *H influenzae* pneumonia is not adequately treated, the incidence of lung abscess and empyema may be high.

Asmar BI et al: *Haemophilus influenzae* type B pneumonia in 43 children. *J Pediatr* 1978;**93:**389.

Bartlett JG: Anaerobic bacterial pneumonitis. *Am Rev Respir Dis* 1979;**119:**19.

Chartrand SA, McCracken GH: Staphylococcal pneumonia in infants and children. *Pediatr Infect Dis* 1982;**1:**19.

Commers JR, Robichaud KJ, Pizzo PA: New pulmonary infiltrates in granulocytopenic cancer patients being treated with antibiotics. *Pediatr Infect Dis* 1984;**3:**423.

Mills EL: Viral infections predisposing to bacterial infections. *Annu Rev Med* 1984;**35:**469.

Paisley JW et al: Pathogens associated with acute lower respiratory tract infection in young children. *Pediatr Infect Dis* 1984;**3:**14.

Rubin BK: The evaluation of the child with recurrent chest infections. *Pediatr Infect Dis* 1985;**4:**88.

Wald ER: Management of pneumonia in outpatients. *Pediatr Infect Dis* 1984;**3(3 Suppl):**S21.

CHLAMYDIAL PNEUMONIA

In 1977, Beem and Saxon described a clinical pulmonary disease associated with *Chlamydia trachomatis* infection in infants under age 12 weeks. The symptoms and signs are those of interstitial pneumonia. The infants are afebrile and generally have symptoms confined to the respiratory tract. Tachypnea and a staccato type cough may be associated with mucoid rhinorrhea. X-ray usually reveals only hyperinflation; in some infants, diffuse interstitial and patchy alveolar infiltrates are noted. A history of conjunctivitis in the newborn period is often obtained.

Hypoxia and rales are often noted, although air entry remains good. Expiratory wheezing is unusual. Apneic episodes have been observed in a few infants.

Peripheral blood eosinophilia (> 300/mL) and hyperimmunoglobulinemia (IgM, IgG) are often present. Isolation of the agent and specific serologic tests are useful diagnostic tools when available.

The course of the disease is protracted; symptoms persist for weeks, and x-ray changes and physical findings may take a month or more to resolve.

Both the duration of shedding of the organism and the duration of clinical symptoms may be shortened by treatment with either sulfisoxazole (150 mg/kg/d) or erythromycin ethylsuccinate (40 mg/kg/d) for about 2 weeks.

Beem MO, Saxon E, Tipple MA: Treatment of chlamydial pneumonia of infancy. *Pediatrics* 1979;**63:**198.

Black SB et al: Serologic evidence of chlamydial infection in children. *J Pediatr* 1981;**98:**65.

Stutman HR, Rettig PJ, Reyes S: *Chlamydia trachomatis* as a cause of pneumonitis and pleural effusion. *J Pediatr* 1984;**104:**588.

Tipple MA, Beem MO, Saxon EM: Clinical characteristics of the afebrile pneumonia associated with *Chlamydia trachomatis* infection in infants less than six months of age. *Pediatrics* 1979;**63:**192.

VIRAL PNEUMONIA

Viral pneumonia is a relatively common and potentially serious disease, particularly in infants. The viruses that most commonly cause pneumonia in the pediatric age range are respiratory syncytial virus, adenoviruses, influenza and parainfluenza viruses, and rubeola virus. Viral lung disease usually involves both the conducting airways and the alveoli.

The onset of clinical findings is often preceded by an upper respiratory infection and is generally more insidious, with slower progression than in pneumonia due to bacteria. Tachypnea, cough, chest wall retractions, rales, wheezing, decreased breath sounds, and cyanosis may be present. The white blood cell count and temperature may be normal or slightly elevated. Additional clinical and serologic characteristics of the infecting viruses are discussed in Chapter 26.

Complications of viral pneumonia are atelectasis, bronchiectasis, interstitial fibrosis, hyperlucent lung (Swyer-James syndrome), and bronchiolitis obliterans. The pneumonia due to respiratory syncytial virus or adenovirus may resolve only very slowly over 3–12 months or may leave permanent obliterative and fibrotic changes. Respiratory syncytial virus infection may first present with apnea.

Therapy is similar to that for bacterial pneumonias (humidified oxygen, vigorous pulmonary physiotherapy, and tracheal intubation and mechanical ventilation if necessary to prevent respiratory acidosis more severe than pH 7.25, or for adequate oxygenation), although antibiotics are not indicated unless secondary bacterial infection is suspected. Ribavirin has been used in more severe cases of viral pneumonia.

Church NR et al: Respiratory syncytial virus-related apnea in infants: Demographics and outcome. *Am J Dis Child* 1984;**138:**247.

Glezen WP, Denny FW: Epidemiology of acute lower respiratory disease in children. *N Engl J Med* 1973;**288:**498.

Hall CB et al: Ribavirin aerosol treatment of infants with respiratory syncytial virus pneumonia. *N Engl J Med* 1983;**308:**1443.

Henderson SW et al: The etiologic and epidemiologic spectrum of bronchiolitis in pediatric practice. *J Pediatr* 1979;**95:**183.

James AG et al: Adenovirus type 21 bronchopneumonia in infants and young children. *J Pediatr* 1979;**95:**530.

MacDonald NE et al: Respiratory syncytial viral infection in infants with congenital heart disease. *N Engl J Med* 1982;**307:**397.

Sly PD et al: Factors predisposing to abnormal pulmonary function after adenovirus type 7 pneumonia. *Arch Dis Child* 1984;**59:**935.

Smith SD et al: Pulmonary involvement with cytomegalovirus infections in children. *Arch Dis Child* 1977;**52:**441.

MYCOPLASMAL PNEUMONIA (Primary Atypical Pneumonia)

Mycoplasma pneumoniae is the most common cause of lower respiratory tract infection in children over age 5 years. The clinical disease is usually mild and self-limiting, beginning with upper respiratory symptoms and fever and typically progressing to a dry cough, often associated with chills, headache, sore throat, and malaise. The cough may be severe and last for several weeks. Physical findings in the chest may be minimal, or there may be harsh breath sounds and rhonchi. Chest x-ray findings include an increase in bronchovascular markings with some areas of atelectasis, often more marked in the lower lobes. Diagnosis is established by culturing the organism from upper airway secretions or sputum or by demonstrating a rise in specific complement fixation antibodies. Serum cold agglutinins are not sufficiently specific to be useful for diagnosis of this infection. Occasional patients develop illness of greater severity, with high fever, pleural effusion, respiratory distress, and pleuritic pain. This has been noted particularly in patients with sickle cell disease.

Erythromycin (also tetracycline in older children) is effective treatment. The illness may be protracted, but nearly all patients recover completely.

Fernald GW et al: Respiratory infection due to *Mycoplasma pneumoniae* in infants and children. *Pediatrics* 1975;**55:**327.

Keitel WA, Couch RB: Mycoplasmal pneumonia: In the differential all year. *J Respir Dis* 1985;**6:**119.

Solanki DL, Berdoff RL: Severe mycoplasma pneumonia with pleural effusions in a patient with sickle cell-hemoglobin C(SC) disease: Case report and review of the literature. *Am J Med* 1979;**66:**707.

Stevens D et al: *Mycoplasma pneumoniae* infections in children. *Arch Dis Child* 1978;**53:**38.

PULMONARY TUBERCULOSIS

Essentials of Diagnosis

- Family history of tuberculosis or history of recent contact.
- Usually asymptomatic, especially in primary form.
- Miliary and progressive pulmonary disease: fever, anorexia, apathy, weight loss.
- Hilar lymph node involvement (may cause respiratory symptoms if the airway is obstructed).
- Positive tuberculin tests and chest x-ray findings.

General Considerations

In the USA, tuberculosis is primarily a disease of adults and is seen less frequently in children now than at any time previously. Spread of tuberculosis is by respiratory droplets. Since infected children usually have low counts of tubercle bacilli and noncavitary disease, they are less likely than adults to transmit tuberculosis. Disease in adults is contagious, and all children exposed to adults with known disease and also those detected by routine tuberculin testing should undergo further investigation. Severe disease, which can be fatal in early infancy and adolescence, is seen in the impoverished and undernourished, in patients with immunodeficiency diseases, and in individuals receiving immunosuppressive drugs.

The American Thoracic Society uses the following classification system for tuberculosis: **category 0**—no exposure to tuberculosis, noninfected, negative skin test reaction; **category I**—exposure to tuberculosis, no evidence of infection, negative skin test reaction; **category II**—infection without disease, positive skin test reaction, negative cultures, no lesions on x-ray; and **category III**—infection with disease, clinically evident lesion, positive skin test reaction, culturable organisms. The term "tuberculosis suspect" is used during diagnostic workup.

Clinical Findings

A. Symptoms and Signs: Classic adult symptoms are rare in children. Children with active tuberculosis (categories II and III) may be asymptomatic or may present with fever of unknown origin or with typical acute pneumonic symptoms and signs (cough, fever, rales, chest pain). Pulmonic lesions may be the source for extrapulmonic spread, such as to the meninges or in a generalized form (miliary tuberculosis).

B. Laboratory Findings: Tuberculin testing (tine, Mantoux) is the most useful diagnostic tool. The tine is a good screening test, but if the diagnosis is suspected, the Mantoux test (intradermal injection of Tween-stabilized PPD) should be used; it has the basic advantage that the severity of the reaction relates to the severity of the disease. The standard dose of PPD-tuberculin is 5 tuberculin units (TU) in 0.1 mL of solution, injected intracutaneously. In suspect cases, the test should be read in 48–72 hours by an experienced observer and recorded as millimeters of induration. A positive test result is an induration of greater than 10 mm. Skin sensitivity develops within 2–10 weeks after infection.

Isolation of *Mycobacterium tuberculosis* is best done from gastric contents, and morning washes should be repeated 3 times. When possible, antibiotic sensitivity studies should be done on the organisms recovered.

C. X-Ray Findings: Chest x-ray in primary disease may be normal. X-ray will vary with the extent of infection from slight infiltration and hilar node invasion to atelectasis and diffuse involvement, as in miliary spread. The primary pulmonary focus is more commonly found in the right than the left lung and only rarely occurs in the apices.

Differential Diagnosis

Pulmonary tuberculosis must be differentiated from mycoplasmal pneumonia, bacterial pneumonia, leukemia or other cancers, malnutrition, tumors, asthma, cystic fibrosis, and Löffler's syndrome.

Complications & Sequelae

Infants and adolescents are more likely to develop complications from pulmonary tuberculosis than people in other age groups. Complications include miliary spread, meningitis, cavitation (adolescents), atelectasis (airway obstruction due to endobronchial tuberculosis), lymph node involvement outside of the chest (cervical lymph nodes), epididymitis, renal involvement, osteomyelitis of the spine, retroperitoneal and abdominal involvement, and pleurisy. Severe pleural reactions can cause the lung to become restricted or trapped.

Prevention & Treatment

See discussion in Chapter 27.

Prognosis

The prognosis with proper therapy is excellent. If the organisms are resistant to the antituberculosis drugs, the prognosis is poor.

Chaparas SD et al: Tuberculin test: Variability with the Mantoux procedure. *Am Rev Respir Dis* 1985;**132:**175.

Glassroth J et al: Tuberculosis in the 1980's. *N Engl J Med* 1980;**302:**1441.

Harrison LH: Current aspects of the surgical management of tuberculosis. *Surg Clin North Am* 1980;**60:**883.

Jacobs RF, Abernathy RS: The treatment of tuberculosis in children. *Pediatr Infect Dis* 1985;**4:**513.

Miller FJW: *Tuberculosis in Children: Evolution, Epidemiology, Treatment, Prevention.* Churchill Livingstone, 1982.

Smith MHD: What about short course and intermittent chemotherapy for tuberculosis in children? *Pediatr Infect Dis* 1982;**1:**298.

Steiner P et al: Primary drug-resistant tuberculosis in children: Correlation of drug-susceptibility patterns of matched patient and source case strains of *Mycobacterium tuberculosis. Am J Dis Child* 1985;**139:**780.

ASPIRATION PNEUMONIA

A variety of aspiration syndromes may occur in pediatric patients. These can be classified in several different categories depending on the clinical presentation and course: (1) aspiration of toxic fluids (eg, gastric acid, hydrocarbons, meconium); (2) aspiration of bacteria; and (3) aspiration of particulate matter (eg, food, meconium). Most frequent in the pediatric age range are aspiration of particulate matter (see p 359 for discussion of aspirated foreign body; p 66 for meconium aspiration syndrome of the newborn) and aspiration of toxic fluids. Aspiration of gastric acid is most common in patients with reduced levels of consciousness and in patients with disorders of the esophagus or the cardioesophageal sphincter. Hydrocarbon aspiration is a relatively common problem in pediatrics and should be suspected in any patient who has ingested hydrocarbons. Hydrocarbon aspiration typically produces a generalized chemical pneumonitis, whereas other forms of aspiration generally involve primarily the dependent portions of the lung. In the supine position, this would include the posterior segments of upper lobes and superior segments of lower lobes; in the upright position, the basal segments of the lower lobes are dependent.

Aspiration of Gastric Acid

The aspiration of gastric acid may be subclinical and recurrent, especially during sleep, producing a chronic obstructive bronchitis that may progress to pulmonary fibrosis (this entity is associated with chalasia and gastroesophageal reflux), or there may be a single, larger episode of aspiration that produces the rapid onset of fever, tachypnea, diffuse rales, and severe hypoxemia. In this latter form, there may also be cough, cyanosis, wheezing, apnea, and shock. The severity of this clinical syndrome is related to the acidity and volume of the aspirate as well as the general condition of the patient and probably the specific lung defense capabilities. The rapid onset of symptoms in this entity helps distinguish it from other forms of pneumonia. Radiographic abnormalities develop over the first 24–36 hours, showing diffuse or localized mottled infiltrates with or without atelectasis. A small percentage of affected patients die soon after the aspiration. The remainder show relatively rapid clinical and radiologic improvement, usually between days 2 and 5 postaspiration, but some of these will develop signs of secondary bacterial infection in the form of clinical deterioration associated with new or increasing chest x-ray infiltrates, reappearance of fever, leukocytosis, and recovery of pathogens from tracheal aspirates. This latter course is associated with a significantly worse prognosis.

Appropriate treatment for aspiration of gastric acid and other toxic fluids depends on the volume of aspirate and the clinical condition of the patient. Humidified oxygen is usually indicated to maintain adequate arterial oxygenation; tracheal intubation and suctioning should be performed immediately if significant aspiration is suspected; vigorous pulmonary physiotherapy should be administered; and mechanical ventilation may be indicated in severely affected patients. Bronchodilator therapy may be of benefit. There is no evidence to support the routine use of corticosteroids or antibiotics in such patients, although some prefer to routinely treat any patient who has had a significant aspiration episode. Any sign of secondary bacterial infection should be treated with appropriate antibiotics. The prognosis for the majority of patients who do not develop secondary bacterial infection is excellent if there is no repeated aspiration. Some patients with recurrent subclinical aspiration due to chalasia, causing chronic lung disease, may benefit from medical treatment or surgical correction of the incompetent cardioesophageal sphincter, although complications and failures of such operations are not uncommon. The presence of gastroesophageal reflux on barium swallow in a patient with chronic lung disease does not indicate whether the lung disease or the reflux is the primary disease. The finding of fat-filled macrophages in tracheal aspirate material suggests chronic recurrent aspiration.

Aspiration of Hydrocarbons

Hydrocarbon aspiration may cause immediate choking, coughing, dyspnea, and cyanosis, with intercostal retractions and fever developing shortly thereafter. Respiratory symptoms develop usually within the first few hours, if at all, although chest x-ray abnormalities may first appear at any time within the first 12 hours. Chest auscultation may reveal coarse or decreased breath sounds. Initial chest x-ray abnormalities may consist of mottled perihilar densities with extension into the mid lung fields, basal pneumonitis, or atelectasis. With time, the mottled densities may coalesce into larger, patchy infiltrates. There may be peripheral obstructive emphysema and, ultimately, development of pneumatoceles and lung cysts. Clinical symptoms and x-ray abnormalities tend to begin to improve 2–5 days after aspiration. There may be high fever and an elevated white blood count.

Children who are symptomatic at the time of initial medical evaluation and those who develop symptoms within 6–8 hours of presentation must be hospitalized. General therapeutic measures of humidified oxygen, vigorous pulmonary physiotherapy, and mechanical ventilation, if necessary, are appropriate. There is no definite evidence to support the routine use of corticosteroids or antibiotics in all cases of hydrocarbon aspiration; however, in debilitated patients or in patients with more significant pneumonia, antibiotics are widely used. Some patients may benefit from bronchodilator therapy. Available data suggest a good prognosis for complete recovery if the patient survives the initial aspiration.

Aspiration of Pathogenic Bacteria

Aspiration of pathogenic bacteria is differentiated from that of toxic fluids by the initial presentation with high fever, purulent sputum, and a less fulminant initial process. The aspirated organisms are generally those from the oropharyngeal secretions, and the main pathogenic organisms are anaerobic streptococci, fusobacteria, and *Bacteroides melaninogenicus*. Patients hospitalized at the time of aspiration are at additional risk of colonization with enteric gram-negative bacilli (*Escherichia coli, Klebsiella,* etc), *Pseudomonas,* or *Staphylococcus aureus*. Antimicrobial therapy should be based on, or supported by, cultures of reliable material. While waiting for the results of such cultures, it is appropriate to start giving penicillin for aspiration pneumonia acquired outside the hospital and gentamicin and nafcillin or another penicillinase-resistant antibiotic for bacterial aspirations that occur in the hospital. Other measures, such as oxygen, pulmonary physiotherapy, circulatory support, and mechanical ventilation, are appropriate when indicated.

Anas N et al: Criteria for hospitalizing children who have in gested products containing hydrocarbons. *JAMA* 1981; **246:**840.

Brook I, Feingold SM: Bacteriology of aspiration pneumonia in children. *Pediatrics* 1980;**65:**1115.

Corwin RW, Irwin RS: The lipid-laden alveolar macrophage as a marker of aspiration in parenchymal lung disease. *Am Rev Respir Dis* 1985;**132:**576.

Goitein KJ, Rein AJ, Gornstein A: Incidence of aspiration in endotracheally intubated infants and children. *Crit Care Med* 1984;**12:**19.

Platzker ACG et al: Aspiration hazards to the developing lung. *Am Rev Respir Dis* 1985;**131:**S1.

Wynne JW, Modell JH: Respiratory aspiration of stomach contents. *Ann Intern Med* 1977;**87:**466.

HYPERSENSITIVITY PNEUMONITIS

Hypersensitivity pneumonitis is the result of a type 1 (immediate, IgE-mediated) or type 3 (Arthus) allergic response to an inhaled organic antigen. Examples of hypersensitivity pneumonitis are farmer's lung, bird-breeder's lung, humidifier lung, and allergic bronchopulmonary aspergillosis. The antigen exposure is usually intermittent, and the disease may be acute, subacute, or chronic. The acute form is characterized by sudden onset of a nonproductive cough, chest tightness, fever, chills, malaise, and dyspnea beginning 4–6 hours after antigen exposure. After recurrent exposures, there may be weight loss. Cyanosis, tachypnea, and basilar rales, usually without wheezing, are characteristic. Leukocytosis is common. The chest x-ray may be normal, or there may be diffuse small nodules or patchy interstitial infiltrates. Most of these findings with the acute form begin to resolve within 12–24 hours after termination of antigen exposure.

A more insidious onset of progressive dyspnea with eventual cyanosis and digital clubbing characterizes chronic hypersensitivity pneumonitis, which usually occurs after a prolonged, often intense antigen exposure. The chest x-ray shows a progressive increase in interstitial markings, and ultimately there may be a cystic appearance with decreased lung volume.

In the acute form, pulmonary function tests are initially indicative of restrictive disease, although with recurrent exposure an obstructive component may also become apparent. The signs of obstructive lung disease may predominate in the chronic form of hypersensitivity pneumonitis. Precipitins (precipitating antibodies) to specific molds or other offending organic antigens may be found in the patient's serum.

The optimal treatment for both acute and chronic forms is avoidance of the antigen. Both forms may be helped by cromolyn sodium and corticosteroids.

Chiron C et al: Lung function in children with hypersensitivity pneumonitis. *Eur J Respir Dis* 1984;**65:**79.

Kohler PF et al: Humidifier lung: Hypersensitivity pneumonitis related to thermotolerant bacterial aerosols. *Chest* 1976; **69:**294.

Roberts RC, Moore VL: Immunopathogenesis of hypersensitivity pneumonitis. *Am Rev Respir Dis* 1977;**116:**1075.

Rosenberg M et al: Clinical and immunologic criteria for the diagnosis of allergic bronchopulmonary aspergillosis. *Ann Intern Med* 1977;**86:**405.

Schatz M, Patterson R, Fink J: Immunologic lung disease. *N Engl J Med* 1979;**300:**1310.

Wang JLF et al: Allergic bronchopulmonary aspergillosis in pediatric practice. *J Pediatr* 1979;**94:**376.

IDIOPATHIC PULMONARY FIBROSIS (Fibrosing Alveolitis)

Idiopathic pulmonary fibrosis refers to a spectrum or continuum of disease characterized by varying combinations of (1) cuboidalization of alveolar lining cells and the presence of large mononuclear cells within the alveolar spaces and (2) thickening of alveolar walls by fibrosis and inflammatory cells. The alveolar process probably represents an earlier stage of this disease, which later progresses to become primarily interstitial. Different stages of this process have previously been called desquamative interstitial pneumonitis and usual interstitial pneumonitis. The interstitial fibrosis described by Hamman and Rich in 1935 was probably a rapidly progressive and severe form of idiopathic pulmonary fibrosis. In most pediatric cases, the cause is unknown, although antecedent infections may initiate this process in some patients. In adults, drug exposure or connective tissue disorders may be causative factors. The onset of symptoms is usually after the first few weeks of life but within the first year in the reported pediatric cases.

The most common clinical findings are dyspnea, tachypnea, cough, poor weight gain, and, later, rales, digital clubbing, and cyanosis. Pulmonary hypertension and respiratory and cardiac failure develop in more severely affected patients. Electrocardiography may demonstrate signs of right ventricular hypertrophy. Pulmonary function studies show decreased vital capacity and total lung capacity (indicating restrictive lung disease) and a diminished pulmonary diffusing capacity. In adults, the amount of hypoxemia on exercise is a good indication of the amount of interstitial fibrosis. Lung compliance is decreased. Gallium scintigraphy and analysis of cells obtained by bronchoalveolar lavage may help in predicting the outcome and in selecting and assessing treatment.

During the course of the disease, the chest x-ray progresses from an initial diffuse ground-glass appearance with fine mottling to more coarse mottling, then to the appearance of linear markings, which are usually perihilar, and finally to the end-stage chest x-ray of increased linear markings associated with hyperlucent areas, particularly at the lung bases, which may progress to a honeycomb lung pattern. The progression of this pattern generally extends over a period of 2–6 years. Cardiomegaly may be apparent on chest x-rays in severely affected patients.

There are no reported cases of spontaneous remission in children. All survivors have been treated with corticosteroids. Prednisone in a daily dose of at least 2 mg/kg should be given for 2 months. If there is improvement, corticosteroid withdrawal should be very slow so that at least 1 year of treatment will be completed. Cytotoxic agents have occasionally been beneficial. The mean survival of reported cases is 4–6 years.

Carrington CB et al: Natural history and treated course of usual and desquamative interstitial pneumonia. *N Engl J Med* 1978;**298:**801.

Crystal RG et al: Interstitial lung disease of unknown cause: Disorders characterized by chronic inflammation of the lower respiratory tract. (2 parts.) *N Engl J Med* 1984;**310:**154, 235.

Hewitt CJ et al: Fibrosing alveolitis in infancy and childhood. *Arch Dis Child* 1977;**52:**22.

Keogh BA et al: Effect of intermittent high dose parenteral corticosteroids on the alveolitis of idiopathic pulmonary fibrosis. *Am Rev Respir Dis* 1983;**127:**18.

Tal A et al: Fatal desquamative interstitial pneumonia in three infant siblings. *J Pediatr* 1984;**104:**873.

Turner-Warwick M et al: Cryptogenic fibrosing alveolitis: Response to corticosteroid treatment and its effect on survival. *Thorax* 1980;**35:**593.

EOSINOPHILIC PNEUMONIA

Eosinophilic pneumonia refers to pulmonary infiltrates on chest x-ray associated with eosinophilic infiltration in the lung seen on histologic examination, which may or may not be associated with eosinophilia of the peripheral blood. Crofton describes 5 types of pulmonary eosinophilia, most of which probably represent some form of hypersensitivity reaction.

Usually of shortest duration, and most benign, is simple pulmonary eosinophilia, or Löffler's syndrome, which consists of migratory pulmonary infiltrates associated with minimal (if any) respiratory symptoms and fever. This entity is distinguished from prolonged pulmonary eosinophilia primarily by the duration of symptoms, which is less than 1 month with simple pulmonary eosinophilia and over 1–2 months with prolonged pulmonary eosinophilia. The prolonged variety is usually associated with high fever, malaise, productive cough, and chest pain. A third category is transient or prolonged eosinophilic infiltrations of the lung in the course of chronic asthma. This may last for 3–4 months or for years.

Tropical eosinophilia is the association of fever, expiratory obstruction, and weight loss with diffuse, finely nodular radiographic infiltrates. This is usually associated with a marked peripheral eosinophilia and may be due to filarial infestation. Finally, there may be pulmonary eosinophilia associated with polyarteritis nodosa and Wegener's granulomatosis, where the primary involvement is in the pulmonary blood vessels, but other organs are apt to be involved also. Patients with this type of eosinophilia have quite severe symptoms and usually a fatal outcome.

Corticosteroids should be given if symptoms warrant treatment except in the case of tropical eosinophilia, which is best treated with the antifilarial drug diethylcarbamazine.

Burrows B et al: Epidemiologic observations on eosinophilia and its relation to respiratory disorders. *Am Rev Respir Dis* 1980;**122:**709.

Lynch JP, Flint A: Sorting out the pulmonary eosinophilic syndromes. *J Respir Dis* 1984;**5:**61.

Middleton WJ et al: Asthmatic pulmonary eosinophilia: A review of 65 cases. *Br J Dis Chest* 1977;**71:**115.

PULMONARY ALVEOLAR PROTEINOSIS

Pulmonary alveolar proteinosis is a rare, usually fatal childhood disease of unknown cause characterized histologically by marked accumulation within the alveoli and bronchioles of an eosinophilic, granular PAS-positive material. It often presents with fever followed by dyspnea, productive cough, chest pain, and poor weight gain. There may be yellow sputum production and cyanosis in older children, and death usually occurs after several months. Physical findings are generally sparse but may include scattered fine rales, occasional digital clubbing, and eventual cyanosis. The onset in children is usually before age 1 year. The chest x-ray demonstrates bilateral, symmetric, fine, soft, diffuse perihilar densities similar to those associated with pulmonary edema. PAS-staining material and birefringent crystals may be present in the sputum; however, most cases are diagnosed by lung biopsy or at autopsy.

No treatment has been uniformly successful. Lung lavage with heparinized saline has been beneficial in some cases.

Colon AR et al: Childhood pulmonary alveolar proteinosis (PAP). *Am J Dis Child* 1971;**121:**481.

Mazyck EM et al: Pulmonary lavage for childhood pulmonary alveolar proteinosis. *J Pediatr* 1972;**80:**839.

Teja K et al: Pulmonary alveolar proteinosis in four siblings. *N Engl J Med* 1981;**305:**1390.

Weiss ST, Mark EJ: Pulmonary reticulonodular disease with consolidation and abscess formation. *N Engl J Med* 1983;**308:**1147.

PULMONARY ALVEOLAR MICROLITHIASIS

Pulmonary alveolar microlithiasis, an often familial disease of unknown cause, is characterized by extensive intra-alveolar deposits of calcium carbonate seen on x-ray. At the time of diagnosis, there may be no symptoms; however, dyspnea, cough, cyanosis, and, eventually, digital clubbing and cor pulmonale develop subsequently. The diagnosis is most often made by chance on a routine chest x-ray that demonstrates fine, sandlike mottling distributed uniformly throughout both lung fields. In rare cases, a description of "sand" in the sputum may lead to the diagnosis.

There is no effective treatment, and the prognosis is variable.

WILSON-MIKITY SYNDROME

Wilson-Mikity syndrome is a poorly defined clinical syndrome characterized by gradually progressive respiratory distress and increased inspired oxygen requirement in small premature infants who have had minimal or no previous lung disease. The clinical pattern of increasing tachypnea, chest wall retractions, and cyanosis typically begins several weeks after birth. Physical examination of the chest may be normal, or there may be rales and wheezing. The cause is not known, although it may be related to viral infection or immaturity of the lung. Microscopically, the lungs are characterized by thickened alveolar septa and mononuclear cell infiltration. Chest x-rays show a widespread reticular pattern resembling that of stage 3 bronchopulmonary dysplasia, with small radiolucent areas (cysts) scattered throughout the lung fields. These changes become more prominent as the disease progresses.

Treatment consists of supportive care and oxygen. Mechanical ventilatory assistance is rarely needed. Antibiotics have not appeared to influence the course.

Although the course is prolonged and there is extensive lung involvement, only 10–15% of infants with this disorder die of respiratory failure or right heart failure. The others recover after several months.

The differential diagnosis includes bronchopulmonary dysplasia, viral pneumonia, patent ductus arteriosus with pulmonary congestion due to increasing left-to-right shunts, and chronic pulmonary insufficiency of prematurity (CPIP), which may be the direct consequence of the lung volume loss due to periodic breathing of prematurity.

Coates AL et al: Long-term pulmonary sequelae of the Wilson-Mikity syndrome. *J Pediatr* 1978;**92:**247.

Krauss AN et al: Chronic pulmonary insufficiency of prematurity (CPIP). *Pediatrics* 1975;**55:**27.

Krauss AN et al: Physiologic studies on infants with Wilson-Mikity syndrome. *J Pediatr* 1970;**77:**27.

Wilson MG, Mikity VG: A new form of respiratory distress in premature infants. *J Dis Child* 1960;**99:**489.

EMPHYSEMA

Essentials of Diagnosis

- Localized or generalized hyperexpansion of lungs.
- Distention and destruction of alveoli as shown on histologic examination.

General Considerations

Emphysema consists of loss of the elastic properties of the lung and is characterized by distention of alveoli with or without destruction of alveolar walls, resulting in air trapping. On x-ray, emphysema is seen as hyperinflation of all or part of the lung. Emphysema may be obstructive or compensatory. Compensatory emphysema occurs when normal lung expands to fill the space of collapsed lung (atelectasis) or absent lung.

Localized obstructive emphysema occurs when a bronchus is partially obstructed so that air entry past the obstruction is accomplished more easily than air exit. A whole lung, one lobe of one lung, or only one lobule may be involved. The obstruction may be intrinsic or extrinsic. In congenital or infantile lobar emphysema (see p 390), severe respiratory distress may develop in the neonatal period or in early infancy as a result of compression of normal lung by the emphysematous lobe. In older children with localized emphysema, conditions involving the airway must be considered, such as asthma, foreign body, tumor, vascular ring, and local inflammation due to viral or bacterial infection.

General obstructive emphysema may occur if there is widespread disease of bronchioles. It may be present in a wide range of clinical conditions, including cystic fibrosis, asthma, and bronchiolitis.

Familial emphysema due to α_1-antitrypsin deficiency is characterized by an onset of emphysema at a relatively early age (usually early adulthood) and progressive dyspnea in the absence of clinical bronchitis in the early stages of the disease. The sex incidence is equal. Diffuse panacinar emphysema is seen microscopically on lung sections. It is likely that the absence of α_1-antitrypsin allows naturally occurring proteolytic enzymes as well as proteolytic enzymes released from leukocytes destroyed during infection to slowly digest the structural protein of normal lung, leading to emphysema.

Alpha$_1$-antitrypsin deficiency is inherited as an autosomal recessive trait. Although some homozygous individuals report no pulmonary symptoms, they are usually symptomatic by the third or fourth decade; isolated cases of onset in adolescence and one case involving a young girl whose symptoms began at age 18 months have been reported. Heterozygous individuals may have an increased incidence of pulmonary disease. It is estimated that about 5% of the population are carriers of the gene, and one in 2000 births is a homozygous recessive. Alpha$_1$-antitrypsin deficiency has also been associated with a severe form of juvenile hepatic cirrhosis.

The diagnosis may be suspected by the absence of the α_1-globulin peak in routine protein electrophoresis. Specific assay of antitrypsin activity suggests the diagnosis, although Pi (protease inhibitor) typing is most definitive.

Clinical Findings.

A. Symptoms and Signs: The symptoms and signs depend upon the extent of involvement. The cardinal finding is dyspnea. In addition, cough, tachypnea, cyanosis, hyperresonant percussion sounds over the involved area, shift of cardiac impulse, and high-pitched wheezing are apt to be present. In localized or lobar involvement, the child may be asymptomatic, but careful examination of the chest will indicate poor air entry in the involved area. With increasing severity, progressive respiratory distress will be evident. Increased resonance on percussion, shift of the heart and trachea, wheezing, or absence of breath sounds indicates that the pulmonary involvement is sufficient to cause air trapping.

B. X-Ray Findings: Chest x-ray of fluoroscopic examination in the generalized disease shows increased radiolucency, depressed diaphragms, and horizontal ribs. Chest x-ray is an important diagnostic procedure but does not establish the diagnosis.

Treatment

The treatment of obstructive emphysema is directed toward the underlying cause. In infantile lobar emphysema, which is associated with significant respiratory distress, lobectomy may be a lifesaving measure in the neonatal period. In general, only supportive measures are helpful.

Patients with any type of emphysema should take extra care to avoid exposure to environmental pollutants, especially active and passive exposure to cigarette smoke.

Bruce RM et al: Collaborative study to assess risk of lung disease in Pi MZ phenotype subjects. *Am Rev Respir Dis* 1984;**130:**386.

Morse JO: Alpha$_1$-antitrypsin deficiency. *N Engl J Med* 1978;**299:**1045.

Ostergaard PA: Alpha$_1$-antitrypsin levels and clinical symptoms in forty-eight children with selective IgA deficiency. *Eur J Pediatr* 1984;**142:**276.

Sveger T: Alpha$_1$-antitrypsin deficiency in early childhood. *Pediatrics* 1978;**62:**22.

Sveger T: Prospective study of children with alpha$_1$-antitrypsin deficiency: Eight-year-old follow-up. *J Pediatr* 1984;**104:**91.

Vance JC et al: Heterozygous alpha$_1$-antitrypsin deficiency and respiratory function in children. *Pediatrics* 1977;**60:**263.

DISEASES OF THE PUMONARY CIRCULATION

PULMONARY HEMORRHAGE

Acute pulmonary hemorrhage and hemoptysis may be associated with bronchiectasis (especially in patients with cystic fibrosis), lung abscess, traumatic lung injury, foreign body aspiration, tuberculosis, heart disease, esophageal duplication, or coagulation disorders or may occur as idiopathic pulmonary hemosiderosis. Therapy is most cases involves treatment of the underlying disorder, and bed rest and blood transfusions may be indicated.

PULMONARY HEMOSIDEROSIS

Idiopathic pulmonary hemosiderosis refers to the accumulation of hemosiderin in the lung, particularly within alveolar macrophages, as a result of chronic or recurrent hemorrhage, usually from pulmonary capillaries. Nonidiopathic causes of a similar entity are myocarditis, polyarteritis nodosa, systemic lupus erythematosus, rheumatoid arthritis, rheumatic fever, Wegener's granulomatosis, and heart disease causing elevated pulmonary capillary or pulmonary venous pressure (especially mitral stenosis). Pulmonary hemosiderosis in association with glomerulonephritis is called **Goodpasture's syndrome.** Some infant patients with pulmonary hemosiderosis have had positive intradermal tests to cow's milk and improvement of symptoms on a milk elimination diet. This possible association between milk allergy and recurrent pulmonary hemorrhage is called **Heiner's syndrome.**

Idiopathic pulmonary hemosiderosis usually begins in the first decade of life (as early as age 4 months) and affects males and females equally. Goodpasture's syndrome affects mostly men in the late teens or older and has a more rapid downhill course.

Clinical Findings

A. Symptoms and Signs: Idiopathic pulmonary hemosiderosis typically begins as continuous mild pulmonary bleeding with a chronic nonproductive cough, fatigue, poor weight gain, and iron deficiency anemia. There may be intermittent blood staining of the sputum and occasional heme-positive stools. The first severe pulmonary hemorrhage is likely to occur after several weeks or months and may cause substernal pain, fever, rales, and dullness to percussion over the affected area. Twenty-five percent of patients with idiopathic pulmonary hemosiderosis eventually develop digital clubbing.

The pulmonary hemorrhage of Goodpasture's syndrome is often preceded by an initial upper respiratory tract infection and is usually less severe than with idiopathic pulmonary hemosiderosis. The hemorrhage usually precedes by weeks or months the onset of acute glomerulonephritis.

During acute episodes of pulmonary hemorrhage, there may be significant dyspnea, wheezing, cyanosis, hemoptysis, tachycardia, and shock if the blood loss is extremely large. After chronic pulmonary hemorrhage, some patients may develop jaundice and hepatosplenomegaly.

B. Laboratory Findings: There is a microcytic hypochromic anemia that responds to oral administration of iron salts with an elevation of the reticulocyte count. Peripheral eosinophilia is present in 10–25% of cases. The stool guaiac test may be positive. Hemosiderin-laden macrophages are present in the gastric contents and may be found in tracheal washings. These iron-containing cells are nonspecific indications of pulmonary hemorrhage. Lung biopsy shows alveolar epithelial hypoplasia, degeneration, and shedding with large numbers of hemosiderin macrophages and variable amounts of interstitial fibrosis. Biopsy may be necessary in order to establish the diagnosis, and open biopsy is preferred.

Pulmonary function studies demonstrate a reduction of lung volumes (restrictive lung disease), decreased lung compliance, reduced oxygen saturation, and, in some patients, a decreased pulmonary diffusing capacity for carbon monoxide.

C. X-Ray Findings: The abnormalities on chest x-ray may vary from none to mild perihilar transient infiltrates to marked parenchymal involvement with infiltrates, atelectasis, emphysema, and mediastinal adenopathy.

Treatment

Any underlying disease process should be appropriately treated. Oxygen and blood transfusion may be required during acute severe bleeding episodes. Most patients benefit from oral iron therapy. Corticosteroids and immunosuppressive agents such as azathioprine have been used, but there is no convincing evidence that they are always effective in either idiopathic pulmonary hemosiderosis or Goodpasture's syndrome. In rare infants with characteristic findings of milk allergy (Heiner's syndrome), milk elimination should be tried.

Course & Prognosis

Idiopathic pulmonary hemosiderosis is characterized by intermittent episodes of acute intrapulmonary hemorrhage separated by asymptomatic intervals. After some years, there may be chronic symptoms such as exertional dyspnea and anemia in the intervals between the acute episodes of hemorrhage. The long-term course is variable, and about 50% of patients die within 5 years of the onset of the clinical disease. Most patients with Goodpasture's syndrome die of renal failure within weeks to months after the diagnosis is established. Occasional patients with Goodpasture's syndrome and idiopathic pulmonary hemosiderosis have spontaneous complete recoveries.

Gong H, Salvatierra C: Clinical efficacy of early and delayed fiberoptic bronchoscopy in patients with hemoptysis. *Am Rev Respir Dis* 1981;**124:**221.

Kjellman B et al: Idiopathic pulmonary haemosiderosis in Swedish children. *Acta Paediatr Scand* 1984;**73:**584.

Leatherman JW, Davies SF, Hoidal JR: Alveolar hemorrhage syndromes: Diffuse microvascular lung hemorrhage in immune and idiopathic disorders. *Medicine* 1984;**63:**343.

Loughlin GM et al: Immune complex-mediated glomerulonephritis and pulmonary hemorrhage simulating Goodpasture's syndrome. *J Pediatr* 1978;**93:**181.

Metz SJ, Rosenstein BJ: Uncovering the cause of hemoptysis in children. *J Respir Dis* 1984;**5:**43.

PULMONARY EMBOLISM

Pulmonary embolism is rare in children and is usually due to venous stasis or trauma. Pulmonary emboli can occasionally occur as a complication of sickle cell anemia, rheumatic fever, infective endocarditis, schistosomiasis, long bone fractures, dehydration, polycythemia, atrial fibrillation, nephrotic syndrome, or ventriculovenous shunts for hydrocephalus. Pulmonary emboli can be single or multiple, large or small. The clinical presentation depends on the amount of the pulmonary vascular bed that is obstructed. Large pulmonary emboli may cause the acute onset of dyspnea, chest pain, chest splinting, cyanosis, tachycardia, rales with or without pleural friction rub, and, occasionally, hemoptysis. The chest x-ray may be normal or may show a peripheral infiltrate, small pleural effusion, or elevated diaphragm. The ECG is usually normal but may demonstrate right heart strain with very large pulmonary emboli. Pulmonary function tests usually show normal lung volumes and flow rates, with decreased pulmonary diffusing capacity for carbon monoxide and lowered arterial CO_2 and O_2 tension. Lactic dehydrogenase is usually elevated. A lung perfusion scan will show single or multiple localized perfusion defects. If either the lung scan or the arterial P_{O2} is normal, it is extremely unlikely that the patient has had an acute pulmonary embolism.

Therapy includes the administration of oxygen and often sedation and attempts to prevent venous stasis or any extension of thrombosis by the use of anticoagulant therapy. Survival of the acute embolic period depends on the size of the embolus. Thrombolytic therapy should be considered early in patients with massive pulmonary embolism or unstable hemodynamics (eg, systemic hypotension) due to the pulmonary embolism. The long-term prognosis in patients who survive the acute episode is related to the underlying disease.

Bell WR et al: The clinical features of submassive and massive pulmonary emboli. *Am J Med* 1977;**62:**355.

Cheely R et al: The role of non-invasive tests versus pulmonary angiography in the diagnosis of pulmonary embolism. *Am J Med* 1981;**70:**17.

Hull R et al: Adjusted subcutaneous heparin versus warfarin sodium in the long-term treatment of venous thrombosis. *N Engl J Med* 1982;**306:**189.

McMahon DP, Aterman K: Pulmonary hypertension due to multiple emboli: Clinical-pathological conference. *J Pediatr* 1978;**92:**841.

Rosenow EC et al: Pulmonary embolism. *Mayo Clin Proc* 1981;**56:**161.

Szucs MM et al: Diagnostic sensitivity of laboratory findings in acute pulmonary embolism. *Ann Intern Med* 1971;**74:**161.

PULMONARY EDEMA

Pulmonary edema results when the rate of accumulation of extravascular lung water exceeds the capability of the pulmonary lymphatic system to remove this fluid. Edema fluid initially accumulates in the interstitial space, first in the area surrounding small vessels and airways. The development of pulmonary edema is due to a change in hydrostatic or oncotic pressure gradients across the pulmonary vessel walls or increased permeability of the pulmonary capillary endothelium. Thus, it may be associated with heart disease, a wide variety of infectious and toxic lung insults (including a high level of inspired oxygen), and hypoproteinemia. "Neurogenic" pulmonary edema may develop following severe central nervous system injury or insult. Mild pulmonary edema may cause only tachypnea, mild rales and expiratory wheezes, and slight hypoxemia. More severe pulmonary edema causes dyspnea, chest wall retraction, cyanosis, and CO_2 retention. Chest x-ray may demonstrate prominent pulmonary vascularity, often with a diffuse haziness of the lung fields. Mild pulmonary edema, especially when associated with another underlying lung disease, may be difficult to identify but may contribute to the patient's respiratory difficulty.

Appropriate therapy depends on the severity of the pulmonary edema, the underlying disease, and the age of the patient but is likely to include supplemental oxygen, diuretics, restriction of fluid and salt intake, and, in some cases, morphine, phlebotomy, rotating tourniquets on the extremities, placing the patient in a semierect position, and digitalis therapy for cardiogenic pulmonary edema. Any underlying disease should be vigorously treated.

Colice GL et al: Neurogenic pulmonary edema. *Am Rev Respir Dis* 1984;**130:**941.

Fein A et al: The value of edema fluid protein measurement in patients with pulmonary edema. *Am J Med* 1979;**67:**32.

Milley JR et al: Neurogenic pulmonary edema in childhood. *J Pediatr* 1979;**94:**706.

Staub N: The pathogenesis of pulmonary edema. *Prog Cardiovasc Dis* 1980;**23:**53.

Staub NC: Pulmonary edema: Physiologic approaches to management. *Chest* 1978;**74:**559.

ADULT RESPIRATORY DISTRESS SYNDROME (Shock Lung)

Essentials of Diagnosis

- Acute respiratory failure.
- Progressive severe hypoxemia.
- Markedly decreased lung compliance (stiff lung).

General Considerations

Adult respiratory distress syndrome (ARDS) is the nonspecific reaction of the lung to a variety of severe insults. It is characterized by a severe progressive hypoxemia (despite inhalation of oxygen in high concentrations) as a result of diffuse increased permeability of the pulmonary capillary endothelium causing pulmonary edema. The alveoli and small airways are filled with edema fluid, tenacious exudates, hyaline membranes, and blood, resulting in marked right-to-left intrapulmonary shunting and very stiff lungs. Subsequently, there may be proliferation of type II cells and, eventually, thickening of the alveolar septa with inflammation and fibrosis. Causes of adult respiratory distress syndrome include extensive viral pneumonia, widespread fat emboli, inhalation or aspiration of corrosive chemical substances, near drowning, severe shock, severe trauma, sepsis, fluid overload, and oxygen toxicity.

Clinical Findings

A. Symptoms and Signs: Adult respiratory distress syndrome usually develops in patients with no history of pulmonary disease, and its onset is usually 24–48 hours after serious trauma or illness. The onset is marked by tachypnea, chest retraction, and cyanosis. There is often relentless progression of acute respiratory failure despite all therapeutic efforts.

B. Laboratory Findings: Blood gas determinations will reveal hypoxemia and metabolic acidosis early in the course of the disease. As the process progresses, CO_2 retention develops. Calculated alveolar to arterial oxygen gradients will become progressively greater, reflecting an increasing right-to-left shunt. Because of the marked pulmonary edema and surfactant deficiency, the lungs become very stiff and the tidal volumes quite small.

C. X-Ray Findings: Initial x-rays may be normal. With the onset of symptoms of respiratory failure, bilateral patchy infiltrates will appear and eventually coalesce as lung aeration deteriorates.

Treatment

Optimal resuscitation and treatment of the underlying condition are important in minimizing the risk and severity of adult respiratory distress syndrome. General therapeutic measures should include careful monitoring of fluid intake and output in an attempt to minimize the amount of extravascular lung water (ie, minimize intravascular volume when possible), careful monitoring of intravascular pressures (a Swan-Ganz catheter is often helpful), filtering of any blood administered through a 25- to 40-μm filter to remove any microaggregates, vigorous chest physiotherapy and postural drainage, and attempts to maintain caloric support. Diuretics such as furosemide may be helpful. Antibiotics should be used if specific infections are suspected, but not indiscriminately or prophylactically. Early and aggressive ventilator support should be initiated when a patient requires oxygen in a concentration greater than 60% to maintain a satisfactory arterial P_{O2}. A volume ventilator is usually desirable, since very high pressures may be required for adequate ventilation. Initially, continuous positive airway pressure may be sufficient to improve oxygenation. When assist breaths are initiated, positive end-expiratory pressure, sometimes to very high levels, should be employed. Short-term treatment with corticosteroids in high doses is widely used and may be beneficial in some cases.

Extracorporeal membrane oxygenators have been used in some patients with severe respiratory failure due to adult respiratory distress syndrome, but the results are discouraging and the financial burden extreme, so this treatment is not recommended.

Prognosis

The prognosis is generally poor because of the severity of the pulmonary insufficiency and the often severe associated precipitating insult. Skillful use of ventilators, pulmonary physiotherapy, continuous positive airway pressure, and fluid management may improve the outlook. Patients recovering from adult respiratory distress syndrome probably have persistence of some degree of interstitial lung disease, although there is progressive normalization of lung volumes and compliance.

Fanconi S et al: Long-term sequelae in children surviving adult respiratory distress syndrome. *J Pediatr* 1985;**106:**218.

Flick MR, Murray JF: High-dose corticosteroid therapy in the adult respiratory distress syndrome. *JAMA* 1984;**251:**1054.

Fowler AA et al: Adult respiratory distress syndrome: Prognosis after onset. *Am Rev Respir Dis* 1985;**132:**472.

Iannuzzi M, Petty TL: Adult respiratory distress syndrome: Update for 1984. *J Respir Dis* 1984;**5:**118.

Lyrene RK, Truog WE: Adult respiratory distress syndrome in a pediatric intensive care unit: Predisposing conditions, clinical course and outcome. *Pediatrics* 1981;**67:**790.

Montgomery AB et al: Causes of mortality in patients with the adult respiratory distress syndrome. *Am Rev Respir Dis* 1985;**132:**485.

Pepe PE, Hudson LD, Carrico CJ: Early application of positive end-expiratory pressure in patients at risk for the adult respiratory distress syndrome. *N Engl J Med* 1984;**311:**281.

Pfenninger J et al: Adult respiratory distress syndrome in children. *J Pediatr* 1982;**101:**352.

Rinaldo JE, Rogers RM: Adult respiratory distress syndrome: Changing concepts of lung injury and repair. *N Engl J Med* 1982;**306:**900.

CONGENITAL PULMONARY LYMPHANGIECTASIS

Congenital dilatation of the pulmonary lymphatics is a rare disease that usually causes respiratory failure and death within the first few days of life. The frequency in males is twice that in females. Lymphatic dilatation is usually secondary to a primary developmental defect of the pulmonary lymphatics or to pulmonary venous obstruction; occasionally, it is part of a syndrome of generalized (especially intestinal) lymphangiectasia. The onset of symptoms is usually at the time of birth, with cyanosis and severe respiratory distress. Occasionally, the onset of respiratory distress is delayed for a few days or weeks after birth. The diagnosis is definitively established by an open lung biopsy that demonstrates marked, irregular cystic dilatation of pulmonary lymphatic vessels and often some interstitial fibrosis. A chest x-ray demonstrates hyperaeration and diffuse nodular or reticular parenchymal lesions. If survival is prolonged, bullous changes may appear on chest x-ray. The differential diagnosis includes respiratory distress syndrome, aspiration pneumonitis, pulmonary hemorrhage, fulminant pneumonia, and, in patients who survive the newborn period, chronic lung disease, pulmonary edema, and cystic fibrosis.

There is no effective therapy for this disorder,

but oxygen, digitalis, and diuretics may provide some symptomatic relief.

Feldman AH, Rhatigan RM, Pierson KK: Pulmonary lymphangiectasia: Observation in 17 patients and proposed classification. *Am J Roentgenol* 1972;**116:**548.

France NE, Brown RJK: Congenital pulmonary lymphangiectasis. *Arch Dis Child* 1971;**46:**528.

Scott-Emuakpor AB et al: Familial occurrence of congenital pulmonary lymphangiectasis. *Am J Dis Child* 1981; **135:**1532.

DISORDERS OF THE CHEST WALL

Normal function of the chest wall (rib cage and diaphragm) is essential for effective ventilation. The 2 components of the chest wall serve both a passive supportive and an active bellows function. A relatively normal chest wall configuration and size are required for normal lung growth. The diaphragm contains the major respiratory muscles in newborns and infants.

A variety of abnormalities of the rib cage and spine can interfere with normal lung function and growth. Some congenital abnormalities such as severe asphyxiating thoracic dystrophy, which may or may not be associated with other major congenital abnormalities such as achondroplasia and cerebrocostomandibular syndrome, may be incompatible with life.

Bergofsky EH: Respiratory failure and disorders of the thoracic cage. *Am Rev Respir Dis* 1979;**119:**643.

Hull D, Barnes ND: Children with small chests. *Arch Dis Child* 1972;**47:**12.

Juan G et al: Effect of carbon dioxide on diaphragmatic function in human beings. *N Engl J Med* 1984;**310:**874.

Muller NL, Bryan AC: Chest wall mechanics and respiratory muscles in infants. *Pediatr Clin North Am* 1979;**26:**503.

Oberklaid F et al: Asphyxiating thoracic dysplasia: Clinical, radiological and pathological information on ten patients. *Arch Dis Child* 1977;**52:**758.

Rochester DF: Respiratory disease: Attention turns to the air pump. *Am J Med* 1980;**68:**803.

Roussos C, Macklem PT: The respiratory muscles. *N Engl J Med* 1982;**307:**786.

Stokes DC et al: Respiratory complications of achondroplasia. *J Pediatr* 1983;**102:**534.

Viires N et al: Effects of aminophylline on diaphragmatic fatigue during acute respiratory failure. *Am Rev Respir Dis* 1984;**129:**396.

EVENTRATION OF THE DIAPHRAGM

Eventration of the diaphragm is abnormal elevation of one or both leaves of the diaphragm. It may be due to congenital maldevelopment of diaphragmatic muscular or tendinous structures or acquired abnormality of the phrenic nerve. In congenital eventration, the diaphragmatic abnormality may be complete or only localized and is characterized by inadequate or absent muscularization, leaving only a translucent membrane separating the thoracic and abdominal cavities.

A variety of different processes may interfere with phrenic nerve conduction, thereby causing diaphragmatic paralysis or eventration. Some causes of phrenic nerve dysfunction are neuritis, which can be on an infectious, toxic, or allergic basis; compression of the nerve roots at the level of the cervical spine; central nervous system diseases; and peripheral phrenic nerve damage due to surgical or other trauma, pressure, or inflammation. Phrenic nerve palsy in the newborn is usually the result of birth trauma, particularly after breech or forceps deliveries. In such cases, the diaphragmatic paralysis is often associated with ipsilateral Erb's palsy. Phrenic nerve palsy is not infrequently caused by surgical trauma, particularly during correction of congenital heart lesions. Both congenital and acquired eventrations are more common on the left than on the right.

Clinical Findings

A. Symptoms and Signs: Clinical manifestations of diaphragmatic eventration are a result of decreased intrathoracic volume (decreased functional residual capacity) and of inefficient ventilation due to paradoxic movement of the abnormal diaphragm with associated mediastinal mobility. Typical clinical findings are tachypnea, cyanosis, sternal retraction, asymmetric chest movement, and subcostal retractions. There may be decreased breath sounds and dullness to percussion at the base of the affected lung. Recurrent fevers may result from bronchopneumonia due to ineffective cough and persistent atelectasis. Most patients with diaphragmatic eventration have minimal or no symptoms after the first year or 2 of life. In the neonatal period and during the first year of life, the above symptoms are more common and may be associated with recurrent respiratory infections, poor feeding, and failure to thrive.

B. X-Ray Findings: The diagnosis can usually be firmly established with regular anteroposterior and lateral chest x-rays and fluoroscopy. Complete or partial elevation of the abnormal diaphragm will be evident on regular chest x-rays. The amount of paradoxic diaphragm movement and mediastinal shift is best evaluated by fluoroscopy. In some cases of congenital eventration, there may be no paradoxic movement of the diaphragm, because of the presence of some muscles in all parts of the diaphragm. Occasionally, it is difficult to distinguish between a partial eventration and a low thoracic mass. Injection of a small amount of nonirritating radiopaque fluid or air into the peritoneal cavity will help outline the diaphragm and make the differential diagnosis.

Treatment

Asymptomatic eventration requires no treatment. Diaphragmatic plication significantly improves lung function and therefore is indicated for patients with significant disability (eg, prolonged increased oxygen or ventilator requirement, recurrent lower respiratory tract infections, feeding problems, or failure to thrive). Patients with acquired diaphragmatic eventration (eg, due to birth trauma or surgical injury of the phrenic nerve) may show significant improvement of diaphragmatic function over the first month or more postoperatively. If there has been no improvement at all in the first 2–4 weeks after the injury was acquired, plication is indicated if the patient has significant requirements for enriched oxygen or assisted ventilation. If the patient has milder manifestations of the eventration, a longer time for potential spontaneous recovery of diaphragmatic function should be allowed before surgical intervention. Vigorous chest physiotherapy should be administered to all patients with less than normal diaphragmatic function.

Booker PD et al: Congential diaphragmatic hernia in the older child. *Arch Dis Child* 1981;**56:**253.

Brouillette RT et al: Phrenic nerve pacing in infants and children: A review of experience and report on the usefulness of phrenic nerve stimulation studies. *J Pediatr* 1983;**102:**32.

Glenn WWL et al: Ventilatory support by pacing of the conditioned diaphragm in quadriplegia. *N Engl J Med* 1984;**310:**1150.

Greene W et al: Paralysis of the diaphragm. *Am J Dis Child* 1975;**129:**1042.

Lynn AM et al: Diaphragmatic paralysis after pediatric cardiac surgery: A retrospective analysis of 34 cases. *Crit Care Med* 1982;**11:**280.

Schwartz MZ, Filler RM: Plication of the diaphragm for symptomatic phrenic nerve paralysis. *J Pediatr Surg* 1978;**13:**259.

SCOLIOSIS

Congenital scoliosis is likely to be severe and is often associated with other anomalies as well as persistent respiratory failure or recurrent respiratory infections. Alveolar development is impaired. Idiopathic scoliosis is usually acquired during later childhood or adolescence and is quite common. Acquired scoliosis may also be secondary to neuromuscular disorders or congenital or acquired unilateral absence of lung volume (eg, due to pneumonectomy). Mild scoliosis has no effect on pulmonary function, but as the spinal curvature increases, patients may develop restrictive lung disease and—though usually not until adulthood—cor pulmonale and respiratory failure. Thus, surgical correction of moderately severe scoliosis is indicated to avoid these serious sequelae.

Cooper DM et al: Respiratory mechanics in adolescents with idiopathic scoliosis. *Am Rev Respir Dis* 1984;**130:**16.

Leech JA et al: Cardiorespiratory status in relation to mild deformity in adolescent idiopathic scoliosis. *J Pediatr* 1985;**106:**143.

Mezon BL: Sleep breathing abnormalities in kyphoscoliosis. *Am Rev Respir Dis* 1980;**122:**617.

Shneerson JM: Cardiac and respiratory responses to exercise in adolescent idiopathic scoliosis. *Thorax* 1980;**35:**347.

Wiers PWJ et al: Cuirass respirator treatment of chronic respiratory failure in scoliotic patients. *Thorax* 1977;**32:**221.

PECTUS EXCAVATUM (Funnel Chest)

Minor degrees of pectus excavatum are a common and insignificant occurrence; severe deformity is rare. There is often a positive family history, and occasionally this deformity is associated with Marfan's syndrome or homocystinuria. While no abnormalities of cardiac or pulmonary function are consistently associated with pectus excavatum, there may be a physiologic basis for respiratory symptoms in some patients with very severe deformity. The major difficulty is the psychologic impact of the cosmetic deformity, and this is most significant during the adolescent years.

Because the usual indication for surgical correction is cosmetic, surgery should usually be delayed until the patient is old enough to make the decision. Physiologic indications for corrective surgery have not been established, but in rare cases the potential or real interference with cardiopulmonary function may justify surgical correction. Careful respiratory support and vigorous chest physiotherapy are extremely important in the postoperative period in order to prevent progressive respiratory failure due to the effect of flail chest.

Beiser GD et al: Impairment of cardiac function in patients with pectus excavatum, with improvement after operative correction. *N Engl J Med* 1972;**287:**267.

Castile RG et al: Symptomatic pectus deformities of the chest. *Am Rev Respir Dis* 1982;**126:**564.

Fan L. Murphy S: Pectus excavatum from chronic upper airway obstruction. *Am J Dis Child* 1981;**135:**550.

Singh SV: Surgical correction of pectus excavatum and carinatum. *Thorax* 1980;**35:**700.

NEUROMUSCULAR DISORDERS

A wide variety of diseases that cause weakness of the respiratory muscles can result in chronic hypoventilation and inability to effectively clear secretions and maintain normal lung volumes and may ultimately progress to respiratory failure. Affected patients are particularly at risk for developing recurrent pneumonia. Examples of such causes of neuromuscular weakness are myasthenia gravis, Guillain-Barré syndrome, muscular dystrophy, cervical spinal cord injury, Werdnig-Hoffman disease, poliomyelitis, and iatrogenic disorders such as respiratory paralysis associated with polymyxin therapy. As involvement becomes more severe, patients will be noted to have decreased breath sounds, rhonchi, rales, wheezes, and dullness to percussion at the lung bases. Chest x-ray will demonstrate elevated diaphragms and often increased bronchovascular markings with infiltrates. Arterial blood gases will demonstrate hypoxemia and, at a later stage, CO_2 retention with respiratory acidosis that may or may not be compensated. Pulmonary function studies demonstrate decreased functional residual capacity, maximum expiratory flow rates, and lung compliance. It is important to periodically measure the tidal volume and vital capacity of these patients, since a vital capacity less than twice the tidal volume indicates that the patient will be unable to produce an effective cough and may require intubation for pulmonary toilet and prevention of respirator failure. All such patients will benefit by vigorous chest physiotherapy at regular intervals with postural drainage and chest percussion. The appropriateness of introduction of an artificial airway and initiation of mechanical ventilation should be considered in light of the prognosis of the underlying disease when respiratory failure appears imminent. Correct timing of this added support is particularly important when the neuromuscular disease may be reversible, as in Guillain-Barré disease and poliomyelitis. In these cases, elective intubation should be considered when the vital capacity decreases to a value approaching twice the tidal volume or if pharyngeal secretions become a significant problem. The prognosis depends on the cause of the muscular weakness.

Alderson SH, Warren RH: Ventilatory management of muscular dystrophy patients following spinal fusion. *Respir Care* 1984;**29:**829.

Brooks JG, Swisher CN: Respiratory dysfunction in pediatric neurologic disorders. In: *Respiratory Dysfunction in Primary Neurologic Disease.* Weiner WJ (editor). Futura, 1980.

Inkley SR, Aldenburg FC, Vignos PJ: Pulmonary function in Duchenne muscular dystrophy related to stage of disease. *Am J Med* 1974;**56:**297.

Lavigne JM: Respiratory care of patients with neuromuscular disease. *Nurs Clin North Am* 1979;**14:**133.

Newsaine JK: Intubation for acute respiratory failure in Guillain-Barré syndrome. *JAMA* 1979;**242:**1650.

DISORDERS OF THE PLEURA & PLEURAL CAVITY

There is normally no gas and only a very small amount of fluid between the parietal and visceral pleural surfaces, so the pleural cavity is only a potential space. The rapid uptake of fluid and gas by the pulmonary circulation out of the pleural cavity maintains the 2 pleural surfaces in apposition under normal circumstances. Most pediatric diseases of the pleura and pleural cavity involve the abnormal accumulation of air (pneumothorax), fluid (effusion), pus (empyema), contents of the lymphatic drainage system (chylothorax), blood (hemothorax), inflammatory tissue, or some combination of these within the pleural space.

Black LF: The pleural space and pleural fluid. *Mayo Clin Proc* 1972;**47:**493.

Kulkarni PB, Dorand RD: Hydrothorax: A complication of intracardiac placement of umbilical venous catheter. *J Pediatr* 1979;**94:**813.

Rudnick MR et al: Acute massive hydrothorax complicating peritoneal dialysis: Report of 2 cases and a review of the literature. *Clin Nephrol* 1979;**12:**38.

PLEURISY, PLEURAL EFFUSION, & EMPYEMA

Pleurisy may be either dry (plastic), serofibrinous (pleural effusion), or purulent (empyema). Dry pleurisy occurs most often with viral pneumonia (especially coxsackievirus pneumonia) and occasionally with upper respiratory tract infection, bacterial (especially pneumococcal) respiratory tract infection, tuberculosis, rheumatic fever, subacute infective endocarditis, systemic lupus erythematosus, pulmonary embolism, inflammatory lesions of the abdominal or chest walls, subphrenic abscess, and trauma to the chest wall. Serofibrinous pleurisy or pleural effusion most frequently accompanies infections of the lung (especially *Streptococcus pneumoniae* or tuberculous) or abdomen. In addition, pleural effusions may occur in association with metastatic lesions, rheumatic fever, polyarteritis nodosa, systemic lupus erythematosus, hypoproteinemia, congestive heart failure, ascites, pancreatitis, or pulmonary infarction. Empyema is usually secondary to bacterial pneumonia, most commonly due to staphylococci. *S pneumoniae* and *Haemophilus influenzae* are slightly less commonly the causative agents. Empyema due to group A β-hemolytic streptococci is unusual but can be very severe and prolonged. Empyema may occasionally develop as a result of trauma or rupture of a lung abscess or as a complication of primary pulmonary tuberculosis. Empyema is distinguished from pleural effusion by the presence of pus in the pleural space.

Clinical Findings

A. Symptoms and Signs: Depending on the severity of the involvement, all 3 types of pleurisy may present with chest pain (especially with deep breathing or coughing), guarded and grunting respirations, diminished respiratory excursions on the affected side, dyspnea, and, occasionally, abdominal pain. The child may lie on the affected side. In addition, when there is an abnormal collection of material in the pleural cavity, as with effusion or empyema, there may be dullness to chest percussion and decreased breath sounds over the effusion, cyanosis, and mediastinal shift away from the involved hemithorax. A pleural friction rub is heard most often in patients with dry pleurisy. Small effusions may produce no symptoms. Patients with empyema are most likely to be severely ill, and often there has been a secondary rise in temperature or persistence of high fever during the course of pneumonia.

B. Laboratory Findings: With any of the 3 types of pleurisy, pulmonary function testing may demonstrate loss of lung volume (restrictive lung disease). Other pulmonary function abnormalities may be caused by coexistent lung disease. There are not likely to be any other laboratory abnormalities due primarily to the pleural involvement in dry pleurisy. Patients with empyema usually have an elevated white blood cell count and often a positive blood culture.

Thoracentesis (see Chapter 35) is necessary to distinguish between empyema and serofibrinous effusions. The amount and mobility of pleural fluid should be evaluated before thoracentesis by a lateral decubitus chest x-ray (performed with the affected side in the dependent position) or by ultrasonography. Material obtained at thoracentesis should be cultured for aerobic and anaerobic organisms and tubercle bacilli and submitted for cell count and differential, Gram's and acid-fast stains, counterimmunoelectrophoresis, and determinations of specific gravity, glucose, protein, pH, and lactate dehydrogenase (LDH). If appropriate, the hematocrit and the amylase content of recovered fluid should be determined and cytologic examination performed. Serum samples obtained at the same time as thoracentesis should be analyzed for protein, glucose, LDH, and, if appropriate, amylase and pH.

Recovered fluid is considered an exudate if the pleural fluid protein to serum protein ratio is greater than 0.5, the pleural fluid LDH exceeds 200 IU, or the pleural fluid LDH to serum LDH ratio is greater than 0.6. An exudate results from disease (usually inflammation) of the pleural surface, as may occur with tuberculosis, pneumonia, cancer, pancreatitis, pulmonary infarction, or systemic lupus erythematosus. It may be infected or sterile. A transudate is usually a clear, sterile, yellow fluid that does not meet the above criteria for exudate and may result from a decrease in plasma oncotic pressure, increase in capillary permeability, or increase in pulmonary or systemic intravascular hydrostatic pressure, as in congestive heart failure, renal disease, or malnutrition.

C. X-Ray Findings: In patients with dry pleurisy, the chest x-ray may be normal, or there may be thickening of the pleural shadow along the thoracic wall. Pleural effusion and empyema cannot be distinguished from one another on chest x-ray. Nonetheless, any patient in whom these diagnoses are suspected should have chest x-rays taken both in the upright position and lying on the affected side. The pleural fluid will appear as a uniform density that completely or partially obscures the underlying lung. Small collections of fluid may only blunt the costophrenic or cardiophrenic angles or may widen the interlobar septa. The fluid is apt to accumulate in the most dependent part of the pleural space, but loculated fluid may not move with changes in body position. Purulent pleural exudates are usually loculated except in the early stages of infection. Large collections of pleural fluid may cause compressive atelectasis of adjacent lung tissue and shift of the mediastinal structures toward the contralateral hemithorax. The underlying lung may show radiologic abnormalities due to the primary disease process. Ultrasonography can be of great value in defining the volume and mobility of any effusion, as well as precisely defining its location.

Treatment & Prognosis

A tuberculosis skin test should be performed in all cases, and any underlying disease should be appropriately treated. Analgesics should be given for chest pain in patients with dry pleurisy. Thoracentesis is indicated in most patients who have significant amounts of pleural fluid, both for diagnosis and as treatment when the presence of the pleural fluid is causing respiratory distress. When an effusion reaccumulates, drainage is performed either by repeated needle aspirations or by insertion of a chest tube for closed system drainage.

All empyemas should be treated by continuous closed-system drainage using a large chest tube, particularly if the pH of the fluid is less than 7.0 or if the glucose concentration is less than 40 mg/dL. Treatment should be initiated promptly after the diagnosis is established. Several chest tubes may be required simultaneously or sequentially to drain loculated areas. Chest tubes are rarely required or effective for more than 1–2 weeks. In patients with empyema, appropriate systemic antibiotics should be selected on the basis of the Gram stain and culture of the material obtained by thoracentesis. Instillation of antibiotics into the pleural cavity is indicated only in the most severe cases (if ever). Thoracotomy with open drainage is very rarely necessary to treat chronic empyema, and pleural decortication is almost never necessary in children.

The prognosis for pleurisy depends upon the extent of involvement and the underlying disease. In general, the prognosis for pleural effusion is very good, as is that for empyema if appropriate therapy is initiated promptly. Empyema can be a very serious disease, especially in young children, and the chest x-ray may not return to normal for 6–12 months.

Untreated tuberculous empyema can progress to fibrothorax with contraction scarring of the pleura and marked restriction or "trapping" of the lung.

Adelman M et al: Diagnostic utility of pleural fluid eosinophilia. *Am J Med* 1984;**77**:915.

Freij BJ et al: Parapneumonic effusions and empyema in hospitalized children: A retrospective review of 227 cases. *Pediatr Infect Dis* 1984;**3**:578.

Light RW: Postoperative pleural effusion: Pathophysiology, clinical importance, and principles of management. *Respir Care* 1984;**29**:540.

Light RW et al: Parapneumonic effusions. *Am J Med* 1980;**69**:507.

McLaughlin FJ et al: Empyema in children: Clinical course and long-term follow-up. *Pediatrics* 1984;**73**:587.

Murphy D et al: Pneumococcal empyema: Outcome of medical management. *Am J Dis Child* 1980;**134:**659.

HEMOTHORAX

Hemothorax is defined as the accumulation of whole blood in the pleural space. It is most commonly caused by surgical or accidental trauma but can also be due to a coagulation defect or tumors of the pleura or lung. It may also be iatrogenic, associated with subclavian vein cannulation. Bleeding may be rapid or slow. Symptoms are related to blood loss or compression of pulmonary parenchyma by the pleural accumulation of blood. Hemothorax is often associated with pneumothorax in cases due to trauma. There is a significant risk of developing a hemoempyema. In many cases of uncomplicated hemothorax, thoracotomy tube drainage may not be necessary, since blood is absorbed from the pleural space spontaneously.

Chetty KG, Davidson PT: A guide to the management of hemothorax. *Hosp Med* (June) 1975;**11:**25.

CHYLOTHORAX

Chylothorax is accumulation of chyle in the pleural cavity, usually as a result of accidental or surgical trauma to the thoracic duct. In the newborn, chylothorax may be congenital or secondary to birth trauma. Occasionally, this rare disorder is caused by a spreading cancer or by obstruction of the thoracic duct due to enlarged lymph nodes. There may be a 2- to 10-day latent period between the injury to the thoracic duct and the appearance of chyle in the pleural cavity. The symptoms depend upon the amount of accumulated fluid. There is no associated pain, but tachypnea and dyspnea are likely with large accumulations of chyle. Other physical and radiologic findings are similar to those with pleural effusion. A white oily or milky fluid obtained at thoracentesis justifies the specific diagnosis. The fluid will appear grossly similar to a pleural effusion in patients who have no oral fat intake. Chylothorax must be differentiated from the accumulation of fatty material in a chronic pleural effusion. This distinction can be made by demonstrating the appearance in the pleural fluid of a fat-soluble dye ingested by the patient. Repeated therapeutic aspirations are usually required to treat the associated respiratory distress. Continuous removal of repeated reaccumulations of chyle can frequently cause significant depletion of the patient's protein and lymphocytes.

Spontaneous closure of the defect in the thoracic duct occurs in about half of cases. Therefore, every case should be treated conservatively for about 4–6 weeks. Conservative therapy consists of continuous chest tube drainage, first discontinuing all oral feedings and then reinitiating feedings with medium-chain triglyceride fats; hyperalimentation is often necessary to avoid significant protein malnutrition. If 4–6 weeks of conservative therapy are not successful in decreasing or stopping the accumulation of chyle, an attempt should be made to ligate the thoracic duct or to locate and close the site of leakage in the thoracic duct. This surgery is often unsuccessful.

Holm AL, Soderlund S: Experiences of postoperative chylothorax in children. *Pediatr Radiol* 1974;**4:**10.

Kosloske AM et al: Management of chylothorax in children by thoracentesis and medium chain triglyceride feedings. *J Pediatr Surg* 1974;**9:**365.

McWilliams BC et al: Transient T-cell depression in postoperative chylothorax. *J Pediatr* 1981;**99:**595.

Seriff NS et al: Chylothorax: Diagnosis by lipoprotein electrophoresis of serum and pleural fluid. *Thorax* 1977;**32:**98.

Teba L et al: Chylothorax review. *Crit Care Med* 1985;**13:**49.

PNEUMOTHORAX, PNEUMOMEDIASTINUM, PNEUMOPERICARDIUM, & PULMONARY INTERSTITIAL EMPHYSEMA

Pneumothorax is not common in pediatric patients except in newborns; term infants have an incidence of 1–2%, and the incidence is higher in premature infants. Pneumothorax may be spontaneous but more commonly is associated with birth trauma, positive pressure ventilation, or continuous positive airway pressure in newborn infants or with trauma, restrictive or obstructive lung disease (eg, asthma, cystic fibrosis, pneumonia), bronchopleural fistula, or rupture of pseudocysts in older children. It may also occur as a complication of a tracheostomy in older children. Especially in the newborn infant, pulmonary interstitial emphysema usually precedes other manifestations of air leak such as pneumomediastinum, pneumopericardium, pneumoperitoneum, subcutaneous emphysema, and pulmonary pseudocyst. Large accumulations of extrapulmonary air can cause significant interference with normal venous return, thus decreasing cardiac output and blood pressure, and can cause secondary atelectasis, shunting, and hypoventilation. Some patients with or without underlying lung disease may have recurrent pneumothoraces. About 20% of cases of spontaneous pneumothorax will recur, most of them within 1 year. Patients with 2 or 3 recurrences of pneumothorax in the same hemithorax, particularly those with no apparent underlying cause, should be considered for chemical pleurodesis or a pleural stripping operation in order to eliminate the pleural space.

Clinical Findings

A. Symptoms and Signs: Any type of air leak can be asymptomatic, or there may be cyanosis, tachypnea, and evidence on physical examination of gas trapping in the thorax. Tension pneumothorax presents with rapid onset of marked respiratory distress, particularly in newborns, in whom it may be associated with significant hypotension. There may be physical evidence of impaired venous return and shift of the cardiac impulse and trachea toward the unaffected side. A decrease in breath sounds is usually noted over the affected side in both newborns and older children. The older child is likely to experience sudden sharp chest pain, and there may be hyperresonance on percussion of the involved hemithorax. With pneumopericardium, there may be muffled heart sounds and severe circulatory insufficiency, not infrequently causing death by cardiac tamponade. In most cases, an isolated pneumomediastinum causes no symptoms other than mild tachypnea. Rarely, severe tension pneumomediastinum may develop, causing symptoms similar to those of tension pneumothorax.

B. X-Ray Findings: The definitive diagnosis of any type of air leak is by chest x-ray. Cross-table lateral and lateral decubitus x-rays (with affected side up) are best for demonstrating pneumothorax. Occasionally, the extrapulmonary intrathoracic air may not shift with changes in body position, because of loculation within the pleural space or localization of the air beneath the visceral pleura. Pneumomediastinum usually appears as a radiolucent line following the contour of the mediastinum. Pneumopericardium is best distinguished from pneumomediastinum by the fact that the radiolucent line is continuous along the diaphragmatic cardiac border. Pulmonary interstitial emphysema appears on x-ray as a collection of small linear, reticular, or cystic radiolucencies that tend to be wider in the more peripheral lung tissue. Particularly in the newborn infant, increased transillumination of the involved hemithorax using a high-intensity light source may strongly suggest the presence of tension pneumothorax.

Differential Diagnosis

The differential diagnosis of pneumothorax on chest x-ray is usually not difficult. Occasionally, there is some difficulty distinguishing between pneumothorax and diaphragmatic hernia, lung cysts, localized lung hyperinflation (eg, pulmonary interstitial emphysema, lobar emphysema), or artifact due to overlying skin folds or clothing.

Treatment

Tension pneumothorax in a newborn or young infant requires immediate emergency needle aspiration of pleural air followed by chest tube insertion and underwater closed-system drainage for several days (see also Chapter 35). Needle aspiration should be performed using a needle or catheter of appropriate size for the patient (20- to 22-gauge in newborn infants), inserting it into the second intercostal space in the midclavicular line. Pneumopericardium usually requires emergency treatment, which consists of aspirating the pericardial air through a needle introduced in the subxiphoid or left parasternal position. A drainage tube should be placed in the pericardial sac if there is repeated reaccumulation of pericardial air. Pneumomediastinum rarely requires aspiration. The air in the mediastinum is usually loculated into multiple cysts and therefore cannot be effectively removed by needle or mediastinal tube. There is no proved way to remove the abnormal air accumulation in pulmonary interstitial emphysema, although selective intubation of the contralateral bronchus has been associated with absorption of interstitial air in carefully selected neonates. Any patient with an air leak who requires resuscitation or assisted ventilation should be treated with the lowest possible inflation pressures. Small pneumothoraces (less than about 20% of the hemithorax) in stable patients of any age can be treated conservatively with bed rest. Conservative therapy would almost never be appropriate for a patient with an air leak who is receiving mechanical ventilation. In some cases, "spontaneous" resorption of pleural air can be hastened by having the patient breathe 100% oxygen. This is usually not appropriate in newborn infants, because of the risk of retrolental fibroplasia. Conservative therapy while awaiting spontaneous resorption is more often indicated in older patients. A chest tube may be indicated for patients with chronic small pneumothorax in order to cause some pleural reaction to seal the air leak. Surgical procedures are occasionally indicated for a persistent air leak such as a bronchopleural fistula. Significant respiratory distress is always an indication for chest tube drainage of the pleural air.

Albelda SM et al: Ventilator-induced subpleural air cysts: Clinical, radiographic and pathologic significance. *Am Rev Respir Dis* 1983;**127:**360.

Brooks JG et al: Selective bronchial intubation for the treatment of severe localized pulmonary interstitial emphysema in newborn infants. *J Pediatr* 1977;**91:**648.

Dattwyler RJ et al: Pneumomediastinum as a complication of asthma in teenage and young adult patients. *J Allergy Clin Immunol* 1979;**63:**412.

DeVries WC, Wolfe WG: The management of spontaneous pneumothorax and bullous emphysema. *Surg Clin North Am* 1980;**60:**851.

Plenat F et al: Pulmonary interstitial emphysema. *Clin Perinatol* 1978;**5:**351.

Rothberg AD et al: Understanding the Pleurevac. *Pediatrics* 1981;**67:**482.

Sahn SA, Good GAT: The effect of common sclerosing agents on the rabbit pleural space. *Am Rev Respir Dis* 1981;**124:**65.

Wilson WG, Aylsworth AS: Familial spontaneous pneumothorax. *Pediatrics* 1979;**64:**172.

DISORDERS OF THE MEDIASTINUM

MEDIASTINITIS

Acute suppurative mediastinitis is usually secondary to esophageal perforation occurring either iatrogenically during surgery, endoscopy, or attempted tracheal intubation or as a result of a swallowed foreign body. Spontaneous esophageal perforation, when it occurs, is usually due to vomiting. Nontraumatic mediastinal infection is rare.

The initial signs and symptoms of acute suppurative mediastinitis may be vague, with gradual onset of substernal pain, fever, chills, toxemia, and dysphagia. Under some circumstances, there may be a brassy cough, dyspnea, and sternal tenderness. The white blood cell count is usually high. Occasionally, the mediastinal process causes obstruction of venous return and venous distention. There may be a characteristic respiratory pattern of spasmodic or "halting" inspiration, sometimes accompanied by grimacing, thought to result from pain due to stretching of inflamed mediastinal structures during inspiration. The chest x-ray is characterized by widening of the upper mediastinum by a dense shadow bulging outward. The lateral x-ray may show anterior displacement of the trachea and the esophagus. There may be associated pleural effusion or pyopneumothorax and mediastinal emphysema. The key to therapy is the immediate initiation of parenteral broad-spectrum antibiotic therapy after obtaining appropriate cultures. In the absence of appropriate treatment, this disease can be rapidly progressive and death can occur. If a mediastinal abscess develops, surgical drainage may be indicated, although this is usually not necessary in the newborn if prompt antibiotic therapy is instituted. Tracheal obstruction may occur, requiring prompt creation of an artificial airway.

Engelman RM et al: Mediastinitis following open heart surgery: Review of two years' experience. *Arch Surg* 1973;**107:**772.

Enquist RW et al: Non-traumatic mediastinitis. *JAMA* 1976;**236:**1048.

Feldman R, Gromisch DS: Acute suppurative mediastinitis. *Am J Dis Child* 1971;**121:**79.

North J, Emanuel B: Mediastinitis in a child caused by perforation of pharynx. *Am J Dis Child* 1975;**129:**962.

MEDIASTINAL MASSES

Most mediastinal masses are asymptomatic and are discovered during routine chest x-ray. Symptoms may develop as a result of pressure on sensitive structures. Respiratory symptoms are more common in children than in adults. Most types of mediastinal masses tend to be localized to a specific mediastinal compartment, thus enhancing the accuracy of preoperative diagnosis. Some masses, however, can appear in different or several mediastinal compartments or may actually be intrapulmonary, although they appear to be in the mediastinum. The superior mediastinum includes the area above the pericardium and is bordered inferiorly by a line connecting the manubrium to the fourth thoracic vertebra posteriorly. The anterior mediastinum is the space between the sternum anteriorly and the pericardium posteriorly. The posterior mediastinum is bordered by the pericardium and diaphragm anteriorly and the lower 8 thoracic vertebrae posteriorly. The mid mediastinum is bounded by the other 3 compartments. The masses that are found in each compartment are listed in Table 14–5.

Mediastinal lymph nodes may be enlarged in benign or malignant disease. Benign cysts are usually abnormalities of embryologic development. An enlarged thymus is the most common mediastinal mass in children.

Clinical Findings

A. Symptoms and Signs: Respiratory symptoms, if present, result from pressure on airways, causing cough; incomplete airway obstruction, with wheezing or air trapping (or both); complete obstruction, with atelectasis; or compression of lung parenchyma, causing atelectasis. Pressure on the left recurrent laryngeal nerve may cause hoarseness due to paralysis of the left vocal cord. Pressure on the esophagus may cause dysphagia. Dilatation of neck vessels may occur as a result of superior vena caval obstruction. Physical findings are usually absent except when a very large mass is present.

B. Laboratory Findings: Although most information is usually gained by x-ray, a variety of other tests may be helpful when certain diagnoses are being considered. Such a workup might include an ECG, echocardiogram, thoracic ultrasound, fungal and mycobacterial skin tests, urinary catecholamine assay, peripheral lymph node biopsy, and mediastinoscopy.

C. X-Ray Findings: A variety of radiologic techniques may be used to define the contour, contents, and location of the mediastinal mass. Regular frontal and lateral chest x-rays, tomograms, thoracic CT scans, magnetic resonance imaging, high-kilovoltage x-rays to better delineate the tracheobronchial air column, esophagograms, and, occasionally, pulmonary or systemic angiograms (or both) and thyroid scans may be informative.

Treatment

Appropriate treatment depends on the type of mediastinal mass, although surgery is usually required either for diagnosis or treatment.

Filler RM et al: Mediastinal masses in infants and children. *Pediatr Clin North Am* 1979;**26:**677.

Halpren S et al: Anterior mediastinal masses: Anesthesia hazards and other problems. *J Pediatr* 1983;**102:**407.

Kelley MJ, Mannes EJ, Ravin CE: Mediastinal masses of vascular origin: A review. *J Thorac Cardiovasc Surg* 1978;**76:**559.

Schuster SR, Gang DL: A one-week-old girl with a thoracic mass. *N Engl J Med* 1984;**310:**36.

Silverman NA, Sabiston DC: Mediastinal masses. *Surg Clin North Am* 1980;**60:**757.

CONGENITAL ABNORMALITIES OF THE LUNG

Congenital abnormalities of the respiratory tract, some of which have been discussed above, may present with clinical signs or symptoms at any time between birth and adulthood depending on the type and severity of the lesion, while others may never cause symptoms.

PULMONARY AGENESIS, APLASIA, & HYPOPLASIA

Absence or incomplete development of one or both lungs can be classified by the degree of developmental arrest. **Agenesis** refers to the complete absence of one or both lungs; **aplasia** is the absence of any pulmonary tissue beyond a rudimentary bronchus; and greater development than this but failure of the pulmonary tissue to fully develop is referred to as **hypoplasia.** Agenesis and aplasia are rare occurrences of unknown cause that are often associated with other congenital anomalies. On clinical examination, there will be a shift of the cardiac impulse toward the affected side, where there is a decrease in air entry. There is likely to be decreased anteroposterior diameter of the chest on the affected side associated with decreased movement of that hemithorax with inspiration. Chest x-ray demonstrates total or partial opacification of one hemithorax, with mediastinal shift toward the affected side. Some of the contralateral lung may enter the affected hemithorax across the midline. The absence of pulmonary arteries and airways may be documented by pulmonary angiography and bronchography. Pulmonary function testing reveals decreased forced expiratory volume, decreased forced vital capacity, and small absolute lung volume as well as limited exercise tolerance. The only appropriate treatment is vigorous therapy (physiotherapy and antibiotics) for any infections in the "normal" lung. An ongoing physical therapy program should be directed toward preventing or delaying the onset of secondary scoliosis. The prognosis is worse when the aplasia or agenesis occurs on the right. This may be due to the normally larger volume of the right lung or to the fact that agenesis of the right lung is more frequently associated with congenital cardiac abnormalities. Most patients with right-sided agenesis die within months. With agenesis of the left lung, the chance for survival is better unless it is associated with other serious congenital abnormalities.

Pulmonary hypoplasia, or a small lung with relatively normal bronchial anatomy, may be an isolated finding or may be associated with congenital diaphragmatic hernia or eventration, renal agenesis **(Potter's syndrome),** abnormal chest wall development (eg, congenital scoliosis or asphyxiating thoracic dystrophy), or abnormal pulmonary arterial and venous anatomy of the right lung **(scimitar syndrome).** Unilateral pulmonary hypoplasia is apt to be associated with normal somatic growth and an increased frequency of lower respiratory tract infection in some young patients, whereas other patients may be totally free of symptoms. Physical examination may reveal decreased air entry on the affected side combined with a small hemithorax. Chest x-ray may show a small hemithorax with mediastinal shift.

A full workup is warranted before making a firm diagnosis of pulmonary underdevelopment in order to avoid misdiagnosing an acquired loss of lung volume—eg, due to airway obstruction by an aspirated foreign body or tumor.

Goldstein JD, Rein LM: Pulmonary hypoplasia resulting from phrenic nerve agenesis and diaphragmatic amyoplasia. *J Pediatr* 1980;**97**:282.

Helms P, Stocks J: Lung function in infants with congenital pulmonary hypoplasia. *J Pediatr* 1982;**101**:918.

Landing BH: Congenital malformations and genetic disorders of the respiratory tract (larynx, trachea, bronchi, and lungs). *Am Rev Respir Dis* 1979;**120**:151.

Levin DL: Primary pulmonary hypoplasia. *J Pediatr* 1979;**95**:550.

Page DV, Stocker JT: Anomalies associated with pulmonary hypoplasia. *Am Rev Respir Dis* 1982;**125**:216.

PULMONARY SEQUESTRATION

Pulmonary sequestration is a congenital malformation in which a small to large area of lung tissue is detached from the remaining lung. This multicystic tissue, composed of poorly developed alveoli and airways, is supplied by one or several systemic arteries arising from the thoracic or abdominal aorta. There is usually no communication—or only a deficient communication—with the rest of the bronchial tree. The venous drainage is to the pulmonary veins. Most commonly, the sequestered tissue is within the normal lung (intralobar) in one of the posterobasal segments of one of the lower lobes, especially the left. Occasionally, the sequestration is not surrounded by normal lung but is extralobar, with its own pleural covering. In this type, usually located between the diaphragm and the lower lobe, there are frequently venous connections to the caval or azygos veins. The sequestration may become the site of infection or cyst formation and thus may present at any age with recurrent or chronic localized pulmonary infection or infiltrate. Often, however, the sequestration may be discovered as an incidental asymptomatic finding of a cystic or consolidated density on a routine chest x-ray. Extralobar sequestration may appear as a wedge-shaped radiodense area in the retrocardiac area on the left or paravertebrally on the right. The anatomy can be defined by angiography, bronchoscopy, and bronchography. When infection occurs, there is usually some connection between the sequestration and surrounding airways. About one-third of affected patients become symptomatic in the first decade of life.

The differential diagnosis includes foregut cysts, atelectasis (eg, due to retained foreign body), congenital bronchogenic cysts, tumors, lung abscesses, eventration of the diaphragm, and adenomatoid malformation of the lung.

Sequestered lung tissue should be surgically removed in order to eliminate an actual or potential site of recurrent infection. Careful definition of the vascular supply to the sequestration should be obtained before surgery in order to avoid severing one of the related systemic arteries. The prognosis following surgery is good.

Enge I, Friestad O: Pulmonary sequestration. *Scand J Thorac Cardiovasc Surg* 1973;**7:**181.

Iwai K et al: Intralobar pulmonary sequestration with special reference to developmental pathology. *Am Rev Respir Dis* 1973;**107:**911.

Savic B et al: Lung sequestration: Report of 7 cases and review of 540 published cases. *Thorax* 1979;**34:**96.

Telander RL et al: Sequestration of the lung in children. *Mayo Clin Proc* 1976;**51:**579.

INFANTILE LOBAR EMPHYSEMA (Congenital Lobar Emphysema)

Infantile lobar emphysema is progressive overdistention of lung tissue, usually a single lobe, producing respiratory distress within the first 6 months of life, especially during the first 2 weeks. The left upper lobe and right middle lobe are most commonly affected. There is usually no identifiable cause, although localized bronchial cartilage deficiency causing a ball valve obstruction has been reported in some cases. Other causes of a similar clinical picture include bronchogenic cysts or mucoceles, aberrant or large pulmonary arteries (especially those associated with large left-to-right shunts), mucus plugs, foreign bodies, and redundant bronchial mucosa. Sometimes the airway obstruction is present at birth, and early chest x-rays may demonstrate localized delayed clearance of fetal lung fluid (ie, increased opacity) from the affected area. During the first week of life, this is usually replaced by air, and there is gradual development of increasing hyperinflation of the affected lung. Respiratory distress classically increases within the first days or weeks of life, with tachypnea, retractions, chest asymmetry, intermittent cyanosis, expiratory wheezing, and localized decreased air entry.

The chest x-ray will demonstrate localized hyperinflation with compression of adjacent lung and mediastinal shift toward the contralateral hemithorax. With progressive hyperinflation, there may be anterior herniation of the abnormal lung into the contralateral hemithorax. Barium swallow and pulmonary angiography may be helpful in the workup to look for the presence of enlarged or aberrant vessels. In addition to the causes mentioned above, the differential diagnoses include lung cyst, pneumatocele, localized pulmonary interstitial emphysema, diaphragmatic hernia, and localized pneumothorax. Lobectomy is the treatment of choice for patients with significant respiratory symptoms if symptoms cannot be relieved by any other method. Postoperatively, many patients will have persistence of recurrent cough and wheezing episodes. Approximately 10% will develop hyperinflation of another lobe at some time in the future.

Man DWK et al: Congenital lobar emphysema: Problems in diagnosis and management. *Arch Dis Child* 1983;**58:**709.

McBride JT et al: Lung growth and airway function after lobectomy in infancy for congenital lobar emphysema. *J Clin Invest* 1980;**66:**962.

Reid LM, Mark EJ: Hyperinflation of the left upper lobe in a five-year-old boy. *N Engl J Med* 1979;**301:**829.

Wall MA et al: Congenital lobar emphysema in a mother and daughter. *Pediatrics* 1982;**70:**131.

CYSTIC ADENOMATOID MALFORMATION

In cystic adenomatoid malformation, a rare congenital anomaly of the lung, there is a multicystic mass of pulmonary tissue containing disordered, polypoid proliferation of respiratory epithelium and bronchiolar structures that may or may not communicate with normal airways. The cysts are lined by cuboidal or columnar epithelium. Affected infants are often born prematurely and usually begin to experience respiratory distress at birth or within the first weeks of life. The cystic mass, which may occur in any lobe of the lung and occasionally in more than one lobe, produces symptoms of tachypnea, cyanosis, and retractions of enlargement, with secondary compression of normal lung tissue. Chest x-rays demonstrate an intrapulmonary mass that may be variably radiodense and radiolucent, with sharp, irregular borders There is often a shift of the mediastinum as the abnormal area becomes hyperinflated.

If the infant is symptomatic and if the abnormality appears to be localized to one lobe or lung, prompt surgical resection is indicated to avoid further compression of normal lung.

Buntain WL et al: Lobar emphysema, cystic adenomatoid malformation, pulmonary sequestration, and bronchogenic cyst in infancy and childhood: A clinical group. *J Pediatr Surg* 1974;**9:**85.

Stocker JT, Madewell JE, Drake RM: Congenital cystic adenomatoid malformation of the lungs: Classification and morphologic spectrum. *Hum Pathol* 1977;**8:**155.

PULMONARY CYSTS

Pulmonary cysts may be congenital or acquired, associated with the trachea or main bronchi (ie, extrapulmonary) or with the smaller airways or alveoli (ie, intrapulmonary), and symptomatic or asymptomatic. Distinguishing between congenital and acquired (usually postinfectious) causes may often be difficult but is of great importance, since surgery is usually indicated in the former category and generally contraindicated in the latter. The differential diagnosis of pulmonary cyst includes congenital cysts, cystic adenomatoid malformation, pneumatoceles, lung abscess, pulmonary sequestration, loculated pyopneumothorax, infantile lobar emphysema, diaphragmatic hernia, foreign body aspiration, a variety of mediastinal masses (Table 14–5), and localized pulmonary interstitial emphysema.

CONGENITAL LUNG CYSTS

True congenital parenchymal lung cysts are probably very rare. Most cysts seen in newborns and young infants are ultimately reversible and therefore likely to be acquired cysts resulting from infection. The most common forms of true congenital pulmonary cysts are bronchogenic cysts and congenital cystic adenomatoid malformation.

BRONCHOGENIC CYSTS

Congenital bronchogenic cysts characteristically occur adjacent to the airway near the tracheal bifurcation. Those at the carina are usually most serious, causing obstructive respiratory symptoms, often from birth, due to tracheobronchial compression. Hilar cysts attached to one of the main or lobar bronchi are more common in older children or adults and are very likely to be asymptomatic, diagnosed only as incidental findings on chest x-ray. There is little relationship between the size of the cyst and the degree of resultant respiratory distress. The cysts are thin-walled, occasionally multilocular, white or pearly gray, and contain clear mucoid fluid. The contents of the cyst may become infected, or the airway compression by the cyst may cause the distal lung parenchyma to become hyperinflated, atelectatic, or infected. The cysts are frequently adjacent to the esophagus and may cause dysphagia. Occasionally, an infected cyst develops a communication with a bronchus, resulting in hemoptysis, purulent sputum, and associated fever. Chest x-ray may be normal or may demonstrate the cyst, obstructive emphysema, atelectasis, mediastinal shift, or, in young newborns, an opacified hemithorax due to delayed clearance of fetal lung fluid. An esophagogram may demonstrate the presence of the cyst even when it is not apparent on the plain chest x-ray. The cyst is often positioned between the esophagus and the trachea. Bronchography is rarely indicated. Occasionally, a fluid level is evident in a cyst, indicating communication with the tracheobronchial tree.

Appropriate treatment is surgical resection and vigorous pulmonary physiotherapy.

Bronchial cysts. (Editorial.) *Br Med J* 1973;**2:**501.

ACQUIRED PULMONARY CYSTS

Pneumatocele

Pneumatoceles are round or oval radiolucent areas with thin, well-demarcated borders that appear on the chest x-ray during the course of pneumonia, usually due to staphylococcal infection or measles. Pneumonias due to infection with other viruses, tubercle bacilli, klebsiellae, group A streptococci, *Pseudomonas aeruginosa, Escherichia coli, Streptococcus pneumoniae,* or hydrocarbon aspiration may also be associated with pneumatoceles.

Pneumatoceles are characterized clinically by sudden appearance, rapid changes in size and position, and potential for rapid disappearance. They typically cause no symptoms unless very large, and they usually regress over a period of several weeks or months. The prognosis is excellent for eventual complete resolution with conservative therapy, which consists of chest percussion and postural drainage with appropriate antibiotic therapy for pneumonia. Bronchoscopic or surgical treatment is indicated only in the very rare case where the pneumatocele becomes infected and filled with purulent material or when it is life-threatening because of its size or location. Very rarely, rupture of a pneumatocele may cause pneumothorax and bronchopleural fistula with empyema.

Bergeson PS et al: Pneumatoceles following hydrocarbon ingestion: Report of three cases and review of the literature. *Am J Dis Child* 1975;**129:**49.

Boisset GF: Subpleural emphysema complicating staphylococcal and other pneumonias. *J Pediatr* 1972;**81:**259.

Stocker JT, McGill LC, Orsini EN: Post-infarction peripheral cysts of the lung in pediatric patients: A possible cause of idiopathic spontaneous pneumothorax. *Pediatr Pulmonol* 1985;**1:**7.

Lung Abscess

Lung abscesses are localized areas of suppuration associated with destruction of lung parenchyma. They may be multiple (especially in chronic lung disease, such as cystic fibrosis) or solitary. They may occur as a complication of bacterial pneumonia (eg, due to *Staphylococcus, Klebsiella, S pneumoniae,* or group A β-hemolytic streptococci) or a septic infarction in patients with congenital heart disease; secondary to aspiration of a foreign body or infected material or penetrating chest trauma; or because of infection of a pulmonary sequestration, atelectatic lung, pneumatocele, or congenital cyst. There is likely to be a rapid development of fever, dyspnea, cough, chest pain, and leukocytosis. The abscess appears on chest x-ray as a radiodense spherical structure that may have an air-fluid level if the abscess communicates with the airway. If the abscess is in peripheral lung tissue, there may be a pleural reaction; occasionally, the abscess ruptures into the pleural space, producing empyema and a bronchopleural fistula. If the abscess develops communication with the airways, there may be production of foul-smelling purulent sputum and, occasionally, hemoptysis.

Optimal treatment consists of appropriate parenteral antibiotics, vigorous pulmonary physical therapy with particular attention to postural drainage, and bronchoscopy to obtain material for culture, to rule out foreign body aspiration, and to drain the abscess. If there is no significant improvement after about 1 month of optimal medical therapy (repeated bronchoscopy and antibiotic coverage for anaerobic organisms may be required), lobectomy should be considered. With vigorous optimal therapy, in the absence of chronic underlying disease, the prognosis is good for complete recovery.

Alexander JC, Wolfe WG: Lung abscess and empyema of the thorax. *Surg Clin North Am* 1980;**60:**835.

Asher MI et al: Primary lung abscess in childhood: The long-term outcome on conservative management. *Am J Dis Child* 1982;**136:**491.

Brook I, Finegold SM: Bacteriology and therapy of lung abscess in children. *J Pediatr* 1979;**94:**10.

Irwin RS et al: Sampling lower respiratory tract secretions in primary lung abscess: A comparison of the accuracy of four methods. *Chest* 1981;**79:**559.

Levison ME et al: Clindamycin compared with penicillin for the treatment of anaerobic lung abscess. *Ann Intern Med* 1983;**98:**466.

Siegel JD, McCracken GH: Neonatal lung abscess: A report of six cases. *Am J Dis Child* 1979;**133:**947.

PULMONARY TUMORS

Primary tumors of the airway and parenchyma are very rare in pediatrics. Most intrathoracic tumors occur in the mediastinum (Table 14–5). Benign pulmonary tumors that have been reported in the respiratory tract of children are hamartomas, bronchial adenomas, papillomas, angiomas, leiomyomas, lipomas, and neurogenic tumors. Although very rare, the most frequent category of malignant pulmonary tumors in children is bronchogenic carcinoma, which carries a very poor prognosis. In addition, fibrocarcinomas and leiomyosarcomas have been reported. Leukemic pulmonary infiltrates can occur. Tumors that may metastasize to the lung are Wilms' tumor, chondrosarcoma, osteogenic sarcoma, Ewing's tumor, reticulum cell sarcoma, and soft tissue sarcoma. Tumors may be asymptomatic and detected on routine chest x-ray or may present with cough, hemoptysis, weight loss, malaise, anemia, or anorexia. Tests that may be appropriate in the workup of such problems include frontal and lateral chest x-rays, fluoroscopy, tomograms, CT scan, angiography, sputum culture and cytology, tuberculin and fungal skin tests, bone marrow analysis, lymph node biopsy, mediastinoscopy, bronchoscopy, lung biopsy, and thoracotomy. Appropriate therapy depends on the type of tumor.

Brooks JW: Tumors of the chest. Chapter 43 in: *Disorders of the Respiratory Tract in Children,* 4th ed. Kendig EL, Chernick V (editors). Saunders, 1983.

Gibbs AR, Seal RME: Primary lymphoproliferative conditions of lung. *Thorax* 1978;**33:**140.

Nitu Y et al: Lung cancer (squamous cell carcinoma) in adolescents. *Am J Dis Child* 1974;**127:**108.

DROWNING

Drowning is the third most common cause of accidental death in children in the USA. Groups at particularly high risk include teenage boys, all toddlers, and patients with seizure disorders. The acute differences between saltwater and freshwater near drownings have little clinical significance except that hypovolemia may be a problem in the former, whereas fresh water interferes more with pulmonary surfactant and atelectasis is a more significant problem. Although electrolyte abnormalities may occur in both types of near drowning, they are generally mild and do not require specific therapy.

Hypoxemia begins within seconds of submersion, and ineffective circulation begins about 2–4 minutes later (Fig 14–4). After 3–6 minutes of ineffective circulation, irreversible microscopic central nervous system changes begin. Laryngospasm begins early in this sequence, probably when the first water enters the posterior pharynx; aspiration of larger amounts

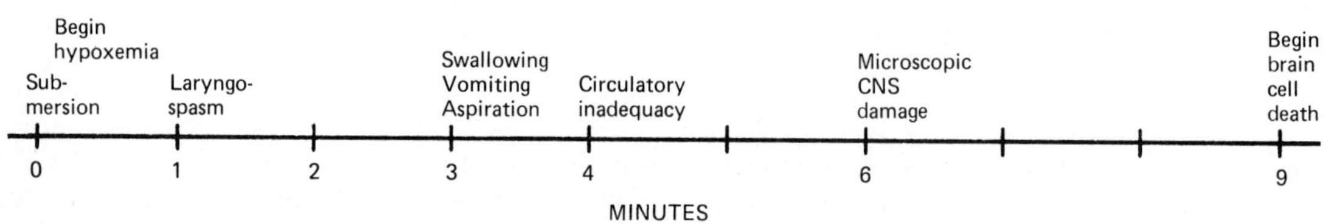

Figure 14–4. Time course of events during submersion (drowning).

of water generally occurs several minutes later, although 10% of victims die without ever aspirating. Thus, after 4–6 minutes of submersion, irreversible central nervous system changes begin. This time sequence may be delayed somewhat if the victim is submerged in very cold water or if the victim has ingested significant amounts of barbiturates.

The clinical presentation of near drowning victims varies widely. Patients with pulmonary edema will have tachypnea and rales, often accompanied by frothy sputum and cyanosis and sometimes by apnea. Initial chest x-rays may be normal or may demonstrate patchy, fluffy infiltrates. More severe cases will show some degree of central nervous system depression with or without seizures. Shock and severe metabolic acidosis may cause peripheral vasoconstriction with cool, mottled extremities.

The key to on-scene resuscitation of near drowning victims is to initiate ventilation (usually mouth-to-mouth) as early as possible. This may be in a rescue boat or when the swimming rescuer reaches shallow water. Prior to beginning mouth-to-mouth resuscitation, any foreign material should be quickly removed from the mouth and posterior pharynx with the rescuer's finger, but no time should be wasted in trying to "drain water" from the lungs. If there is no palpable heartbeat, external cardiac massage should be initiated and, with mouth-to-mouth ventilation, continued in transit to the hospital. If oxygen is available, it should be given at the earliest possible moment. Upon arrival at the emergency room, cardiopulmonary resuscitation should be continued if required while an intravenous line is inserted for administration of fluid, cardiotonic drugs, and bicarbonate. In addition to the profound hypoxemia, any severely depressed near drowning victim will have a marked metabolic acidosis. Initially, lactated Ringer's solution with 10% dextrose, 20 mL/kg, should be given. Subsequently, packed red blood cells may be more appropriate for freshwater victims, whereas plasma may be the best choice for saltwater victims.

All near drowning victims should be hospitalized for a minimum of overnight observation even if they appear normal at first. In mild cases, an initial chest x-ray and arterial blood gas determination or noninvasive oximetry should be performed while the patient breathes room air. Vital signs should be monitored frequently during the night, and arterial blood gas determination or oximetry should be repeated prior to discharge.

The major therapeutic efforts in the hospitalized near drowning victim are directed toward the cardiopulmonary and central nervous systems. Dysrhythmias, especially ventricular fibrillation, tend to occur early, and ventricular fibrillation is probably the major cause of immediate drowning deaths. Acute tubular necrosis occasionally develops, probably secondary to the period of shock and not as a result of the hemoglobinuria.

General management of the hospitalized near drowning victim includes monitoring serum electrolytes, hemoglobin, fluid intake and output, and chest x-ray. Diuretic therapy should be considered early if there is significant fluid overload without hypotension. Careful attention is required to maintain normal body temperature. Hypothermic patients must be rewarmed while under close observation, at a rate not to exceed 0.5 °C/h. Oxygenation is a major problem in these patients owing to the stiff, edematous lungs with widespread alveolar collapse or consolidation. If the inspired oxygen requirement exceeds 50% oxygen, positive end-expiratory pressure (PEEP) delivered by mask or endotracheal tube should be initiated to maintain alveolar patency and decrease the amount of intrapulmonary shunting. If PEEP is not adequate to maintain oxygenation, intermittent mandatory ventilation (IMV) should be initiated. Because of their stiff lungs, these patients may require high ventilatory pressures. In addition, obtunded or comatose near drowning victims may require intubation for pulmonary toilet (specifically for prevention of aspiration of secretions) or for CO_2 retention or apnea. Because of the alveolar instability resulting from surfactant deficiency, it is important not to withdraw the mechanical ventilation too early. A minimum of 1–2 days is likely to be required before discontinuing the ventilator. The aspirated material may precipitate bronchospasm in some patients, necessitating bronchodilator therapy (aminophylline or corticosteroids). Prophylactic antibiotics are not indicated. If pulmonary infiltrates on chest x-ray persist past 24–48 hours or if the patient's pulmonary status deteriorates, there may be a secondary bacterial infection that would warrant the institution of antibiotic therapy. Some signs of secondary infection such as fever, atelectasis, leukocytosis, and tachycardia can be a direct result of the near drowning and may not indicate infection unless appearance is delayed. Corticosteroids are not indicated for the lung disease in near drowning victims.

Advances in cerebral resuscitation have lagged behind those of cardiopulmonary resuscitation, so that today one is more likely to have a successful cardiopulmonary resuscitation and be left with a patient with significant irreversible neurologic deficit. The central nervous system changes are probably due chiefly to the asphyxia during submersion and secondary central nervous system insult during and after resuscitation and not to electrolyte abnormalities. Neurologic treatment consists of intravenous diazepam (Valium) for seizures, corticosteroids (eg, dexamethasone, 1 mg/kg/d), osmotic diuresis, and mechanical hyperventilation for cerebral edema in the semicomatose or comatose patient. Continuous measurement of intracranial pressure has been advocated by some for severely affected patients, in order to aid in appropriate manipulation of cerebral perfusion. Fluid administration should be decreased to two-thirds of maintenance, after initially establishing adequate circulation, in order to decrease cerebral and pulmonary edema due to the shock-damaged capillaries in these organs. Any subsequent neurologic deterioration in the hospitalized patient is usually preceded by pulmonary deterioration.

Although ultimate restoration of normal pulmonary function can be expected in survivors, the prognosis for subsequent neurologic function is not as good. Patients requiring cardiopulmonary resuscitation in the emergency room have an extremely high likelihood of permanent neurologic sequelae if they survive. Other findings on arrival in the emergency room that are associated with poor prognosis include coma and initial serum pH less than 7.0. Vigorous, rapid cardiopulmonary resuscitation should be performed in the emergency room if a child is brought in unconscious after a drowning accident, but the outlook for useful survival becomes less hopeful after 5–10 minutes of unsuccessful resuscitation.

Brooks JG: Marginal comment: Near drowning. *Am J Dis Child* 1981;**135:**998.

Conn AW et al: Cerebral resuscitation in near-drowning. *Pediatr Clin North Am* 1979;**26:**691.

Gilbert J, Puckett J, Smith RB: Near drowning: Current concepts of management. *Respir Care* 1985;**30:**108.

Gisvold SE, Safar P: Systematic studies of cerebral resuscitation potentials after global brain ischemia. *Crit Care Med* 1982;**10:**466.

Hoff B: Multisystem failure: A review with special reference to drowning. *Crit Care Med* 1979;**7:**310.

Orlowski JP et al: Submersion accidents in children with epilepsy. *Am J Dis Child* 1982;**136:**777.

Pearn JH et al: Neurologic sequelae after childhood near-drowning: A total population study from Hawaii. *Pediatrics* 1979;**66:**187.

Sarnaik AP et al: Intracranial pressure and cerebral perfusion pressure in near-drowning. *Crit Care Med* 1985;**13:**224.

RESPIRATORY FAILURE

Acute, severe respiratory failure is a life-threatening situation and requires immediate therapy. There is no universally accepted definition of respiratory failure, but it can be presumed to be present when the arterial CO_2 is elevated (eg, $P_{aCO2} > 50$ mm Hg) or when a moderate to severe degree of hypoxemia (eg, $P_{aO2} < 50$ mm Hg) exists.

Causes of Respiratory Failure

Respiratory failure may be caused by or secondary to (1) central nervous system disorders, eg, head injury; (2) neuromuscular diseases, eg, myasthenia gravis, poliomyelitis, or Guillain-Barré syndrome; (3) lung or airway diseases, eg, asthma, croup, foreign body aspiration, or peripheral lung disease such as respiratory distress syndrome: (4) heart disease, eg, cyanotic congenital heart disease; (5) pulmonary vascular bed disorders, eg, pulmonary edema or vasoconstriction; or (6) chest wall disorders, eg, flail chest or asphyxiating thoracic dystrophy.

Principles of Treatment

Treatment is aimed at restoring arterial oxygen and CO_2 tensions to normal. Low arterial oxygen tension can be treated by increasing the concentration of inspired oxygen and, in some cases, by the application of continuous distending pressure to the lung. In the presence of severe chronic hypercapnia and hypoxia, the predominant respiratory drive may be the hypoxic stimulus; administration of oxygen under these circumstances may result in hypoventilation or apnea, but this is a rare occurrence in the pediatric age group. It should always be borne in mind that lack of oxygen rapidly "wrecks the machinery," and severe hypoxia is not a situation that can be tolerated for long. Increased CO_2 tension is an indication that alveolar ventilation is decreased, and the only way the excess CO_2 can be eliminated is by increasing alveolar ventilation. This may require assisted ventilation.

Assisted ventilation may be administered by manual resuscitating devices or by mechanical ventilators. In general, the indications for assisted ventilation are as follows: (1) arterial oxygen tension that cannot be maintained at or near normal levels by increasing the inspired oxygen concentration; (2) elevated CO_2 tension (> 65 mm Hg); and (3) apnea. Excessive work of breathing leads to physical exhaustion, and severe respiratory failure may occur suddenly. The oxygen consumption related to excessive work of breathing may reach 40% of the total oxygen requirement.

Assisted ventilation may occasionally be indicated in the presence of normal blood gases. For example, in a patient with Guillain-Barré syndrome, when the vital capacity is reduced to twice the tidal volume, assisted ventilation may be indicated because of inability to cough and sigh effectively.

Gregory GA: *Respiratory Failure in the Child.* Churchill Livingstone, 1981.

The management of acute respiratory failure: Proceedings of a conference held November 4–6, 1982, at Cancun, Mexico. *Crit Care Med* 1983;**28:**517.

Newth CJL: Recognition and management of respiratory failure. *Pediatr Clin North Am* 1979;**26:**617.

Pingleton SK: Tailoring nutritional support in acute respiratory failure. *J Respir Dis* 1985;**6:**27.

Pontoppidan H: Acute respiratory failure in the adult. *N Engl J Med* 1972;**287:**690.

SUDDEN INFANT DEATH SYNDROME ("Crib Death")

Sudden infant death syndrome (SIDS) is defined as the sudden death of any infant or young child in whom the death is unexpected by history and a thorough postmortem examination fails to demonstrate an adequate cause for death. This entity has been known for centuries but has become of more interest recently as other causes of infant mortality are decreasing. The incidence of SIDS is 2:1000 live births (about 7500 SIDS deaths per year) in the USA. This is the largest single cause of infant death after the neonatal period. The peak incidence is at 2–4 months after birth, and 91% of SIDS deaths occur within the first 6 months of life. Less than 1% occur in the first 2 weeks.

The death characteristically occurs during sleep, particularly between midnight and 6:00 AM. Affected infants are previously entirely healthy or may have had findings of a mild upper respiratory infection. The incidence is increased in the winter months, in lower income groups, and in low-birth-weight infants. Males are affected more frequently than females in a 3:2 ratio. The death is silent. Groups at increased risk for SIDS include infants of drug-addicted mothers, very low birth weight infants, and infants who have experienced life-threatening episodes requiring resuscitative intervention.

In addition to the history, characteristic autopsy findings are necessary to establish a diagnosis of SIDS. Intrathoracic petechiae (especially on the thymus, pleura, and pericardium) are present in 87% of cases. There is usually some pulmonary edema; there may be pulmonary vascular congestion and mild pulmonary inflammation. Nonpolioviruses are isolated from 23–42% of SIDS victims at autopsy, but there are no consistent histologic changes to document a pathogenic role for viruses. Studies have demonstrated histologic findings compatible with previous chronic or recurrent hypoxia, suggesting that these victims may have had chronic or intermittent cardiopulmonary abnormalities for some time prior to death and, therefore, that SIDS victims are not always "previously normal" infants. The autopsy is of great importance to rule out other specific causes of sudden death in infants, such as meningitis, myocarditis, and intracranial hemorrhage.

Numerous causes have been suggested for the death of these patients, but none have been proved. It is probable that a number of causes may be responsible for the deaths in different cases. The upper airway probably plays an important role in the cause of death by one of several possible mechanisms. Subclinical gastric reflux stimulating apnea-inducing receptors in the region of the larynx is a possible cause. In animals, stimulation of such receptors can cause fatal apnea. This mechanism may combine with actual upper airway obstruction—to which the infant upper airway is particularly vulnerable—to cause a combined obstructive and central apnea in some infants. Some victims probably have persistent or intermittent weak respiratory drive and possibly weak arousal responses, which increase their susceptibility to fatal apnea. One group of investigators has documented the rare familial occurrence of prolonged sleep apneas during rapid eye movement sleep, and some of these affected infants have subsequently succumbed to apparent SIDS deaths.

Extensive psychosocial support is mandatory for families who have experienced the sudden infant death syndrome. This should be provided by trained personnel, who should also work to educate both lay and professional groups about the syndrome. The National Sudden Infant Death Syndrome Foundation, a private organization providing assistance to parents and information for public education about SIDS, can be of help. Telephone (301) 459–3388, or write to the Foundation at the following address: 8240 Professional Place, Suite 205, Landover, MD 20785.

Brooks JG: Relationship of apnea of infancy to SIDS. *Perinat Neonat* 1984;**8:**15.

Carpenter RG et al: Multistage scoring system for identifying infants at risk of unexpected death. *Arch Dis Child* 1977;**52:**606.

Guntheroth WG: *Crib Death: Sudden Infant Death Syndrome.* Futura Publishing Co., 1982.

Irgens LM, Skjaerven R, Peterson DR: Prospective assessment of recurrence risk in sudden infant death syndrome siblings. *J Pediatr* 1984;**104:**349.

Kelly DH, Shannon DC: Sudden infant death syndrome and near sudden infant death syndrome: A review of the literature, 1964–1982. *Pediatr Clin North Am* 1982;**29:**1241.

Shannon DC, Kelly DH: SIDS and near SIDS. (2 parts.) *N Engl J Med* 1982;**306:**959, 1022.

Tildon T et al: *Sudden Infant Death Syndrome.* Academic Press, 1983.

APNEA OF INFANCY ("Near Miss SIDS")

Infants who experience an episode of apnea of infancy may be at increased risk of sudden infant death syndrome (SIDS). Apnea of infancy may be defined as (1) an unexplained and frightening episode of cessation of breathing for 20 seconds or longer or (2) a shorter respiratory pause associated with bradycardia, cyanosis, or pallor. A variety of causes of such episodes have been proved or suggested, including laryngeal chemoreceptor apnea associated with chalasia, seizure disorders, respiratory tract infections due to *Bordetella pertussis* or respiratory syncytial virus, cardiac disease, upper airway obstruction, breath-holding spells, and sleep apnea.

While the risk of SIDS in infants with severe apneic episodes is increased in comparison with the general population, only a small proportion of SIDS victims, probably less than 5%, have been noted to experience apneic episodes before death.

Any infant presenting with a history of a recent significant episode of apnea should be hospitalized for evaluation and observation. A complete history should be taken and physical examination performed, focusing particularly on the above-mentioned possibilities for underlying causes of apnea of infancy. The minimum in-hospital laboratory evaluation should include a complete blood count, measurement of serum bicarbonate, and continuous cardiorespiratory monitoring throughout the hospital stay. In some cases, no specific cause is suggested, and it is appropriate to institute home monitoring for diagnostic and preventive reasons (see below). If episodes of significant apnea or bradycardia occur during hospitalization, the following studies may be helpful: chest x-ray, electroencephalography, electrocardiography, measurement of serum electrolytes and calcium, and appropriate cultures. Depending on the particular case, it may be appropriate to institute other studies, such as esophagography, arterial blood gas analysis, fluorescent antibody tests for *B pertussis* and respiratory syncytial virus, esophageal pH monitoring, and further evaluation of the heart and upper airway. Although recordings of cardiorespiratory patterns have been advocated, their value is limited because of lack of normal, age-adjusted data and the day-to-day variability in respiratory patterns. In addition, such recordings cannot predict a given infant's risk of succumbing to SIDS.

Although there are no clearly proved modes of therapy for preventing subsequent death in infants who experience episodes of apnea, a reasonable approach to treatment includes (1) instruction of those caring for the infant in cardiopulmonary resuscitation; (2) specific treatment of proved underlying causes when appropriate (eg, anticonvulsants, surgery such as tracheostomy or correction of congenital heart defects); and (3) a trial of low-dose aminophylline therapy (2 mg/kg 2–3 times daily) for patients with apparent immature respiratory centers.

Continuous electronic cardiorespiratory monitoring in the home can alert the parents to an episode of bradycardia or apnea, but the efficacy of this expensive mode of preventive therapy has not been clearly established. It clearly interferes with the normal parent-infant relationship but, in general, is received by the parents as a welcome alternative to the constant uncertainty of caring for an infant they fear may die suddenly. Monitoring should probably be initiated only for the most severely involved infants or for infants with a history of apnea who have a family history of SIDS. Monitoring should be initiated only where complete technical, medical, and psychosocial support for such a program is available. In most cases, monitoring of infants who have experienced severe apparent life-threatening episodes should not be discontinued until all of the following criteria are met: (1) the infant is at least 6 months of age; (2) at least 2 months have passed without an apneic or bradycardiac episode requiring intervention; and (3) the infant has experienced an upper respiratory infection without recurrence of significant episodes.

Ariagno RL, Brooks JG, Kelly D: Using home monitors for infant apnea. *Patient Care* (June) 1984;**18:**56.

Ariagno RL et al: "Near miss" for sudden infant death syndrome infants: A clinical problem. *Pediatrics* 1983;**71:**726.

Brooks JG: Apnea of infancy and sudden infant death syndrome. *Am J Dis Child* 1982;**136:**1012.

Brooks JG: The relationship of apnea of infancy to the sudden infant death syndrome. *Perinat Neonat* 1984;**8:**15.

Little GA et al: Prolonged infantile apnea: 1985. *Pediatrics* 1985;**76:**129.

McBride JT: Infantile apnea. *Pediatr in Rev* 1984;**5:**275.

Rein AJ et al: Symptomatic sinus bradycardia in infants with structurally normal hearts. *J Pediatr* 1985;**107:**724.

Southall DP et al: Prolonged apnea and cardiac arrhythmias in infants discharged from neonatal intensive care units: Failure to predict an increased risk for sudden infant death syndrome. *Pediatrics* 1982;**70:**844.

Spitzer AR et al: Awake apnea associated with gastroesophageal reflux: A specific clinical syndrome. *J Pediatr* 1984;**104:**200.

SELECTED REFERENCES

Avery ME et al: *The Lung and Its Disorders in the Newborn Infant,* 4th ed. Saunders, 1981.

Burgess WR, Chernick V: *Respiratory Therapy in Newborn Infants and Children.* Thieme-Stratton, 1981.

Comroe JH: *The Physiology of Respiration.* Year Book, 1970.

Cotes JE: *Lung Function: Assessment and Application in Medicine,* 4th ed. Blackwell, 1980.

Crofton J, Douglas A: *Respiratory Disease,* 3rd ed. Blackwell, 1981.

Fishman AP (editor): *Pulmonary Diseases and Disorders.* McGraw-Hill, 1980.

Fraser RG, Pare JAT: *Diagnosis of Diseases of the Chest,* 2nd ed. Saunders, 1979.

Kendig EL, Chernick V: *Disorders of the Respiratory Tract in Children,* 4th ed. Saunders, 1983.

Kerrebjin KF et al: Chronic nonspecific respiratory disease in children: A five year follow-up study. *Acta Paediatr Scand* [*Suppl*] 1977; **No. 261:**3.

Kryger M: *Pathophysiology of Respiration.* Wiley, 1981.

Levin DL et al: *A Practical Guide to Pediatric Intensive Care,* 2nd ed. Mosby, 1983.

Sahn SA: *Pulmonary Emergencies.* Churchill Livingstone, 1982.

Scarpelli EM, Auld PAM, Goldman HS (editors): *Pulmonary Disease of the Fetus, Newborn, and Child.* Lea & Febiger, 1978.

Smalhout B, Hill-Vaughan AB: *The Suffocating Child. Bronchoscopy: A Guide to Diagnosis and Treatment.* C. H. Boehringer Sohn, 1980.

Strang LB: *Neonatal Respiration: Physiological and Clinical Studies.* Blackwell, 1977.

Williams HE, Phelan PD: *Respiratory Illness in Children.* Blackwell, 1975.

Cardiovascular Diseases 15

Robert R. Wolfe, MD, & James W. Wiggins, Jr., MD

Cardiovascular disease is a significant cause of death and chronic illness in the pediatric population. In North America, more than 1% of newborn infants have congenital heart disease, usually due to multifactorial causes. It is becoming obvious that the prevention of adult heart disease must begin in childhood (eg, prevention of atherosclerosis by diet modification). Preventive medicine is the most important aspect of pediatric practice, and the goal of prevention pervades all aspects of cardiovascular disease. But prevention requires an understanding of the causes of disease, and in this there are wide discrepancies ranging from significant accomplishments in the case of rheumatic fever to the very tentative steps being taken to understand the causes of congenital heart disease, atherosclerosis, and essential hypertension.

CLUES TO THE PRESENCE OF HEART DISEASE

Although there are traditional signs and symptoms suggesting the presence of heart disease in an infant or child, it is necessary to know how to weigh clinical findings to determine which findings are significant and require immediate attention and which findings are insignificant. The presence of a heart murmur, for example, may suggest the possibility of heart disease in an infant, or the murmur may be a functional or innocent murmur (see below). All serious cardiovascular disorders are not accompanied by an easily detectable murmur.

The most important clues to the presence of heart disease requiring prompt attention are congestive heart failure and cyanosis. These clinical conditions will be discussed in more detail in subsequent sections.

DIAGNOSTIC EVALUATION

As in the diagnosis of diseases of any other organ system, an orderly sequence of evaluation is followed: (1) history, (2) physical examination, (3) electrocardiography, (4) chest x-ray, (5) echocardiography, and (6) cardiac catheterization (with angiography).

HISTORY

In obtaining the history from the family or the patient, one must keep in perspective the age and relative activity of that patient. A history of increasing feeding difficulties and diaphoresis is the most common feature of early congestive heart failure.

Family History

Since most cardiac diseases are familial, one of the first clues to the cause of cardiovascular disease in the child is a history of heart disease in a first-degree relative. A careful history should include details of early adult cardiovascular problems. These details might suggest the need to evaluate the child for hyperlipidemia.

Pregnancy

The history of pregnancy should elicit information regarding first-trimester exposure to illness or medications, which places infants at high risk for congenital heart disease. A history of significant problems related to labor and delivery, such as perinatal stress or asphyxia at birth, suggests causes of myocardial dysfunction in the neonate.

Growth & Development

Major cardiac problems frequently affect a child's ability to grow. There may be a history of poor feeding (early fatigue, vomiting, lethargy) or of failure to thrive despite adequate caloric intake. Gross motor development may also be delayed in children with significant congestive heart failure or cyanosis, although other aspects of development are less frequently affected.

Tachypnea

Parents frequently notice rapid or abnormal breathing in the child. Although infants at rest rarely breathe faster than 40 respirations per minute, infants in congestive heart failure usually have respiratory rates in excess of 60 (and often as rapid as 80–100). Tachypnea may be considered the cardinal sign of left-sided heart failure in the pediatric patient. Thus, the child should be evaluated before the physician gives the often unwarranted reassurance that "all infants breathe fast."

Cyanosis

The physiologic basis of cyanosis and the medical

and surgical approaches to the cyanotic patient will be discussed later. What should be noted here is that, curiously, many parents do not readily recognize cyanosis—nor do many physicians. The infant with a cyanotic heart lesion may be more gray than blue (and may have no heart murmur). Cyanotic heart disease may go unrecognized because of lack of appreciation of the subtleties of diagnosing cyanosis.

Hypoxemic Spells

It is important to determine if the patient with a cyanotic heart lesion such as tetralogy of Fallot is having hypoxemic spells, because prompt surgical intervention may be required. These spells usually occur on morning awakening or after a feeding or bowel movement; the infant begins breathing fast, becomes progressively more gray or blue, and cries as if having severe pain. Such a spell rarely may progress to unconsciousness, paresis, or even death.

Other Clinical Clues

Orthopnea, dyspnea, easy fatigability, growth failure, sweating, squatting, and pneumonia are frequent clues to the presence of various forms of heart disease.

PHYSICAL EXAMINATION

Careful and thorough examination of the patient frequently offers the best clues to significant cardiac problems. A systematic approach to the entire child will frequently lead to the probable diagnosis. The presence of other congenital abnormalities, particularly chromosomal disorders, increases the probability of congenital heart disease.

The examination should begin with a careful general inspection to note activity (agitation, lethargy) and skin perfusion and color. Vital signs, including temperature, pulse rate, respiratory rate, and particularly blood pressure (in all 4 extremities in symptomatic infants), can reflect the overall status of the patient. Auscultation of the heart and lungs should be performed early in the overall examination, since the infant's crying limits the physician's ability to hear even pronounced cardiac sounds. Abdominal examination for position and size of organs is also important.

1. CARDIOVASCULAR EXAMINATION

Inspection & Palpation

Conformation of the chest can give clues to past or present cardiomegaly. Prominence of the precordial chest wall is frequently seen in infants and children with cardiomegaly. Increased cardiac activity is often noted on inspection.

Palpation may reveal the presence of precordial activity, right ventricular lift, or left-sided heave; a diffuse point of maximal impulse; or the presence of a thrill due to a loud murmur. Thrills are typically located where the murmur is most intense and can sometimes be felt at the point of radiation, as in a suprasternal notch or carotid thrill with aortic stenosis. In patients with severe pulmonary hypertension, palpable pulmonary closure is frequently noted, usually at the mid to upper left sternal border.

Auscultation

To detect and differentiate abnormal heart sounds, one must be familiar with the pattern and timing of normal heart sounds.

A. Normal Heart Sounds: S_1 (the first heart sound) is the sound of atrioventricular valve closure. It is best heard at the lower left sternal border and is usually medium-pitched. Although 4 components of S_1 can be detected by phonocardiography, only one or 2 of these are usually heard when a stethoscope is used.

S_2 (the second heart sound) is the sound of semilunar valve closure. It has a higher pitch than S_1 and is best heard along the lower and upper left sternal border. S_2 has 2 component sounds, A_2 and P_2 (aortic and pulmonary valve closure). A_2 is best appreciated at the mid and lower left sternal border, while P_2 is best heard at the upper left sternal border and is normally softer than A_2. Splitting of S_2 varies with respirations, widening with inspiration and narrowing with expiration, and is best heard at the second left intercostal space at the sternal border.

S_3 (the third heart sound) is the sound of rapid filling of the left ventricle. It occurs in early diastole, after S_2, and is a medium- to low-pitched thud. In normal children, the sound will diminish or disappear when there is a change from the supine to the sitting or standing position; it is usually also intermittent.

S_4 (the fourth heart sound) is associated with atrial contraction and increased atrial pressure and has a low pitch similar to that of S_3. It occurs just prior to S_1 and is not normally audible.

B. Abnormal Heart Sounds: Findings of abnormalities in splitting or intensity of the component sounds of S_2 can be helpful in the diagnosis of major heart problems. With inspiration, there is a decrease in the intrathoracic pressure; this decrease causes increased filling of the right side of the heart, thereby prolonging the ejection time and delaying closure of the pulmonary valve. Normal intrathoracic pressure changes have little effect on the filling of the left side of the heart. Widening of splitting can be a clue to right-sided volume overload, while narrowing may indicate increased pulmonary artery pressure. A single S_2 is often heard in cases of malposition of the great vessels or severe pulmonary hypertension.

Ejection clicks are high-pitched and are usually related to dilated great vessels or valve abnormalities (or both). They can be heard throughout the ventricular systole and are classified as early, mid, or late. Early ejection clicks at the upper left sternal border are usually of pulmonary origin. Aortic clicks are heard in a wider distribution but best at the apex.

Widespread clicks originating or loudest at the apex can be mitral or aortic in origin. The mid to late ejection click at the apex is most typically mitral valve prolapse. Early clicks may also be heard in spontaneous closure of ventricular septal defects.

S_3 can be a functional sound in childhood, although it often is associated with cardiac abnormalities.

S_4 is not normally audible; its finding on auscultation is almost always associated with cardiac abnormalities.

C. Murmurs: Murmurs are the most common cardiovascular finding. The presence of a murmur in a child almost always causes alarm in the parents, who associate murmurs with major heart disease. However, most children have murmurs, and, fortunately, these are usually normal functional or innocent murmurs.

1. Characteristics—Murmurs can be evaluated on the basis of the following characteristics:

a. Location and radiation—Where the murmur is best heard and where the sound extends.

b. Relationship to cardiac cycle and duration—Systolic (with the pulse), diastolic, continuous, or to-and-fro.

c. Intensity—Classified as grade I, soft and heard with difficulty; grade II, soft but easily heard; grade III, loud but without a thrill; grade IV, loud and associated with a precordial thrill; grade V, loud, with thrill, and audible with the edge of the stethoscope off the chest; or grade VI, very loud and audible with the stethoscope off the chest or with the naked ear.

d. Quality—Harsh, musical, or rough; high, medium, or low in pitch.

e. Variation with position—Audible when patient is supine, sitting, standing, or squatting.

2. Functional murmurs—Most functional murmurs change or disappear with a change in position. The 7 most common functional murmurs heard in childhood can be classified as follows:

a. Newborn murmur—As the name implies, this murmur is frequently heard within the first few days of life. Typically, it is located at the lower left sternal border, without significant radiation. It is a soft, short, vibratory grade I–II/VI early systolic murmur that often subsides when mild pressure is applied to the abdomen. Newborn murmur usually disappears by 2–3 weeks of age.

b. Functional murmur of peripheral arterial pulmonary stenosis—This murmur is frequently heard in the premature infant, often after ligation of a patent ductus arteriosus. It is secondary to branching of the pulmonary artery. Typically, it is heard with equal intensity at the upper left sternal border, back, and in both axillas. It is a soft, short, high-pitched, grade I–II/VI systolic ejection murmur and usually disappears by 6 months of life. This murmur must be differentiated from true peripheral arterial pulmonary stenosis (rubella syndrome), coarctation of the thoracic aorta, valvular pulmonary stenosis, and atrial septal defect. These entities should, however, have other findings to suggest their organic nature.

c. Still's murmur—Probably the most common murmur of early childhood, this murmur can be heard in infancy, although it is most typically heard from the age of 2 years until adolescence. Classically, it is loudest midway between the apex and the lower left sternal border, and often it may be transmitted (depending on loudness) to the remainder of the precordial area. Still's murmur is a musical or vibratory, short, high-pitched, grade I–III early systolic ejection murmur. It is loudest when the patient is in the supine position; it diminishes or disappears when the patient sits or stands or during Valsalva's maneuver. It may be louder in patients with fever or tachycardia.

d. Pulmonary outflow ejection murmur—This murmur may be heard throughout childhood. It is usually a soft, short, systolic ejection murmur, grade I–III in intensity and well localized to the upper left sternal border. It becomes louder when the patient is in the supine position or when cardiac output is increased and softens with standing or during Valsalva's maneuver. Pulmonary outflow ejection murmur must be differentiated from other murmurs, such as that of pulmonary stenosis, which radiates to the back and has an associated click; atrial septal defect, which is characterized by a persistently split S_2 and tricuspid flow rumble; and peripheral arterial pulmonary stenosis, which is transmitted throughout the entire chest.

e. Venous hum—This very common murmur of childhood is usually heard after 3 years of age. The murmur is located at the upper right and left sternal borders and in the lower neck. It is described as a continuous musical hum of grade I–II intensity, and it may be accentuated in diastole and with inspiration. This murmur always disappears when the patient is placed in a supine position or when the jugular vein is compressed. Venous hum is thought to be produced by turbulence in the subclavian and jugular veins.

f. Innominate or carotid bruit—This murmur is more common in the older child and adolescent. It is heard in the right supraclavicular and neck areas. This is a long systolic ejection murmur, somewhat harsh and of grade II–III intensity. It can be accentuated by light pressure on the carotid artery and must be differentiated from all types of aortic stenosis.

g. Hemic murmur—Hemic murmurs are heard whenever anemia, fever, stress, or any increase in cardiac output is present. Typically, they are heard best in the aortic and pulmonary areas. These systolic ejection murmurs are of grade I–II intensity and are high-pitched. They disappear with normalization of cardiac output.

Frequently, an experienced listener is able to ascertain that a murmur is functional without performing extensive and expensive laboratory evaluations. When functional murmurs are found in a child, the physician should assure the parents that these are normal heart sounds of the developing child and that they represent no abnormality of the heart.

3. Organic murmurs—Organic murmurs are evaluated on the basis of the characteristics outlined above (location, intensity, etc). These murmurs will be discussed in relationship to specific lesions later in this chapter.

2. NONCARDIAC EXAMINATION

Femoral Pulse

Assessment of the femoral pulse is an essential part of the physical examination of every infant and child. The femoral pulse should be readily palpable and equal in amplitude and time of appearance with the brachial pulse. A femoral pulse that is absent or weak or one that is delayed in comparison with the brachial pulse suggests coarctation of the aorta. An absent or diminished femoral pulse may be the only clue to the cause of a life-threatening problem.

Arterial Pulse

A. Rate and Rhythm: Cardiac rate and rhythm are usually determined by palpation of the radial or brachial pulse. Throughout infancy and childhood, the rate is subject to great variation. Multiple determinations must be made under properly evaluated conditions before conclusions can be drawn about their significance. This is particularly important in infants.

Marked variations in heart rate occur with activity; therefore, the resting heart rate may be most accurately determined during sleep. In older children, exercise and emotional factors have a marked effect upon the heart rate. This should be taken into account when examining the child, since many children are apprehensive and may react emotionally to the initial phases of the examination. It is possible for normal infants to have heart rates of 180 or 190 during the activity associated with a physical or electrocardiographic examination. Average resting heart rates range from 120 in infants to 80 in older children.

In the pediatric age group, the rhythm may be regular or there may be a phasic variation in the heart rate (sinus dysrhythmia). Variations occasionally occur without relation to the respiratory cycle. Sinus dysrhythmia is a normal finding.

B. Quality and Amplitude of Pulse: Examination of the cardiovascular system should always include a careful examination and comparison of the pulses of the upper and lower extremities. A bounding pulse is characteristic of patent ductus arteriosus or aortic regurgitation. Narrow or thready pulses are found in patients with congestive heart failure or severe aortic stenosis.

Examination of the suprasternal notch should always be included. A visible pulsation in the suprasternal notch is usually abnormal, although it may be seen in patients who are emotionally excited. A prominent pulsation is found in aortic insufficiency, patent ductus arteriosus, and coarctation of the aorta. A palpable thrill in the suprasternal notch is characteristic of aortic stenosis and is occasionally found with valvular pulmonary stenosis, coarctation of the aorta, and patent ductus arteriosus.

Arterial Blood Pressure

Blood pressures should be obtained in the upper and lower extremities. Systolic pressure in the lower extremities determined by the auscultatory technique is usually higher than that found in the upper extremities in patients *over age 1 year*. In normal infants, the pressure in the arms may be higher. The cuff must cover the same relative area of the arm and leg, and this usually means that a larger cuff must be used for the leg than for the arm.

A. Procedures: Because of variation of blood pressure with respiration and slower rhythmic variations (Mayer or Traube-Hering waves), pressure obtained by any method should be repeated several times.

1. Auscultatory method—The auditory recognition of Korotkoff's sounds utilizing a stethoscope and sphygmomanometer is the most commonly used method of obtaining blood pressure in children and correlates well with direct intra-arterial measurements. However, despite its widespread application as the standard method of indirect blood pressure measurement, many factors grossly affect its accuracy. Among these are the dimensions of the inflatable bag within the cuff. The length of the bag should be 100% and the width 50% of the circumference of the limb. A cuff that is too narrow or too short will produce a blood pressure reading that is higher than the true pressure.

2. Palpatory method—This method can be used when the application of a stethoscope head to a small limb is awkward or impossible. Palpation of the pulse characteristics distal to the occluding cuff provides an approximation of the systolic blood pressure in the infant.

3. Flush method—The flush method is also useful in small infants. The distal foot or hand is blanched by manual squeezing or application of an elastic bandage, and the cuff is inflated above the systolic pressure. The extremity is then observed as the cuff pressure is slowly reduced, and the observed flush corresponds to a value approximating that of the systolic pressure. Simultaneous application of the cuffs to the upper and lower extremities and observation of flushing is a useful technique for assessing coarctation of the aorta.

4. Doppler ultrasonic method—Most recently, the combination of a small ultrasound transducer with earphones and a sphygmomanometer has proved to be especially applicable to the small infant. Considerations of cuff dimensions are still critical, however.

B. Pulse Pressure: Pulse pressure is determined by subtracting the diastolic pressure from the systolic pressure. Normally, the pulse pressure is less than 50 mm Hg or less than half the systolic pressure. A widened pulse pressure (which is associated with a bounding pulse) is present in aorticopulmonary shunt (eg, patent ductus arteriosus), aortic insufficiency, fever, anemia, and complete heart block. A narrow pulse pressure is seen in congestive heart failure, severe aortic stenosis, and pericardial tamponade.

Venous Pressure & Pulse

The level of the distended jugular vein above the suprasternal notch when the patient is at a 45-degree angle is a determinant of venous pressure in older children and adults. Normally, one may observe the level of the transition between collapse and distention of the jugular vein approximately 1–2 cm above the notch. Because of the short, fat neck in infants and young children, this is frequently not too helpful in this age group. In addition to the level of the pulse, the wave pattern should be observed. Two waves can frequently be seen: (1) The *a* wave, due to right atrial contraction, is a rather sharply rising wave and therefore occurs immediately before or with the first heart sound or point of maximum impulse. (2) The *v* wave, caused by filling of the right atrium during ventricular systole, is a more slowly rising wave and occurs toward the end of ventricular systole.

Extremities

Cyanosis of the extremities usually indicates congenital heart disease, but severe pulmonary disease must be excluded. Cyanosis is characterized by a bluish discoloration of the nails, but the entire distal portion of the extremity may be involved.

A. Clubbing of Fingers and Toes: Clubbing implies fairly severe cyanotic congenital heart disease. It usually does not appear until approximately age 1, although occasionally, in patients with severe cyanosis, it may occur earlier. The first sign of clubbing is softening of the nail beds. This is followed by rounding of the fingernails and then by thickening and shininess of the terminal phalanx, with loss of creases.

Cyanosis is by far the most common cause, but clubbing occurs also in patients with infective endocarditis, severe liver disease, and lung abscess.

B. Edema: Edema of the lower extremities is characteristic of right ventricular heart failure in older children and adults. However, in infants and younger children, peripheral edema is more likely to affect first the face, then the presacral region, and eventually the extremities.

Abdomen

Hepatomegaly is the cardinal sign of right heart failure in the infant and child. Presystolic pulsation of the liver may occur with right atrial hypertension and systolic pulsation with tricuspid insufficiency. Congestive splenomegaly may be present in patients who have had long-standing congestive heart failure. Enlargement of the spleen is one of the characteristic features of subacute infective endocarditis. Ascites is occasionally present in right heart failure.

Keith JD: Chaps 2 and 3, pp 14–31, in: *Heart Disease in Infancy and Childhood,* 3rd ed. Keith JD, Rowe RD, Vlad P (editors). Macmillan, 1978.

Nelson WP, Egbert AM: How to measure blood pressure accurately. *Primary Cardiol* (Sept) 1984;**10:**14.

Nora JJ: Etiologic aspects of heart diseases. Chap 1, pp 2–10, in: *Heart Disease in Infants, Children, and Adolescents,* 3rd ed. Adams FH, Emmanouilides GC (editors). Williams & Wilkins, 1983.

ELECTROCARDIOGRAM & VECTORCARDIOGRAM (ECG & VCG)

Certainly the ECG is to be considered an essential part of the evaluation of the cardiovascular system, and frequently the information gained from this study is very useful. The ECG is the sine qua non for the diagnosis of dysrhythmias and may offer the best clue to the specific diagnosis of congenital lesions (eg, left axis deviation in a blue baby, suggesting tricuspid atresia). Inversely, the ECG may provide little or no help (as in assessing right ventricular hypertrophy in the newborn or left ventricular hypertrophy in the child with congenital aortic stenosis).

It is not possible, within the limitations of this presentation, to teach the interpretation of the ECG, but a few basic facts and definitions should help to orient the student.

A. Propagation of Electrical Force: As shown in Fig 15–1, a wave of electrical force traveling toward an electrode inscribes a positive (upward) deflection; away from an electrode, a negative deflection; and perpendicular to an electrode, a low-voltage, isodiphasic complex. These forces are inscribed as loops on the VCG, and abnormalities are manifested as alterations in direction and duration of force or as increased or decreased electrical force (amplitude of QRS complex on ECG or loop on VCG).

B. Age-Related Variations: The ECG and VCG

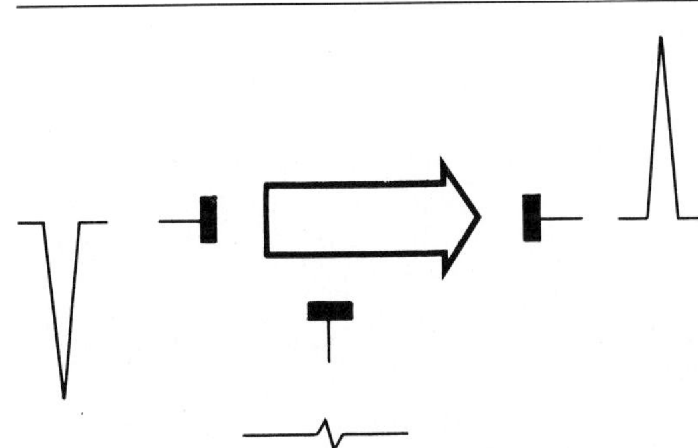

Figure 15–1. Depolarization of the myocardium. The arrow represents the wave of electrical force. As it travels toward the electrode, it inscribes a positive (upward) deflection; away from the electrode, a negative (downward) deflection; perpendicular to the electrode, a low-voltage, isodiphasic deflection.

evolve with the age of the patient. The rate gradually decreases and intervals generally increase with age. There is also progressive change in dominance of ventricles from right ventricular dominance in the young infant to left ventricular dominance in the older infant, child, and adult. The normal ECG of the 1-week-old would be highly abnormal for a 1-year-old, and the ECG of a 5-year-old would not be normal for an adult.

C. ECG Interpretation: Fig 15–2 defines the events recorded on the ECG. The sequence of recording the findings of the ECG is usually as follows: rate, rhythm, P wave, PR interval, QRS complex (including axis, amplitude, and duration), QT interval, ST segment, T wave, and impression.

1. Rate—The paper speed at which ECGs are usually taken is 25 mm/s. Each small square is 1 mm and each large square 5 mm. Therefore, 5 large squares represent 1 second, one large square 0.2 second, and one small square 0.04 second. A common method of estimating the ventricular rate is to count the number of large squares between 2 QRS complexes: If QRS complexes appear at a rate of one per large square (5/s), the ventricular rate is 300; if QRS complexes appear every 2 squares, the ventricular rate is 150, etc. The formula is to divide the number of large squares between QRS complexes into 300 and roughly interpolate for fractions of large squares.

2. Rhythm—Cardiac rhythm is a difficult subject that does not yield easily to oversimplification. However, a working definition of normal sinus rhythm must be offered even if it is not entirely satisfactory: a normal P wave followed by a normal PR interval and a normal QRS complex.

3. P wave—The P wave represents atrial depolarization. In the pediatric patient, it is normally not taller than 2.5 mm or more than 0.08 second in duration.

4. PR interval—This interval is measured from the beginning of the P wave to the beginning of the QRS complex. It increases with age and with slower rates. The PR interval ranges from a minimum of 0.11 second in infants to a maximum of 0.18 second in older children with slow rates. The PR interval is commonly prolonged in rheumatic heart disease and by digitalis.

5. QRS complex—This represents ventricular depolarization, and its amplitude and direction of force (axis) reveal the relative size of (viable) ventricular mass in hypertrophy, hypoplasia, and infarction. Abnormal ventricular conduction (eg, right bundle branch block, anterior fascicular block) is also revealed. Interpretation of the QRS complex is one of the most important aspects of cardiologic diagnosis.

6. QT interval—This interval is measured from the beginning of the QRS complex to the end of the T wave. The QT duration is affected by drugs such as digitalis and electrolyte imbalances such as hypocalcemia and hypokalemia (really QU interval prolongation). The normal duration is rate-related.

7. ST segment—This short segment lying be-

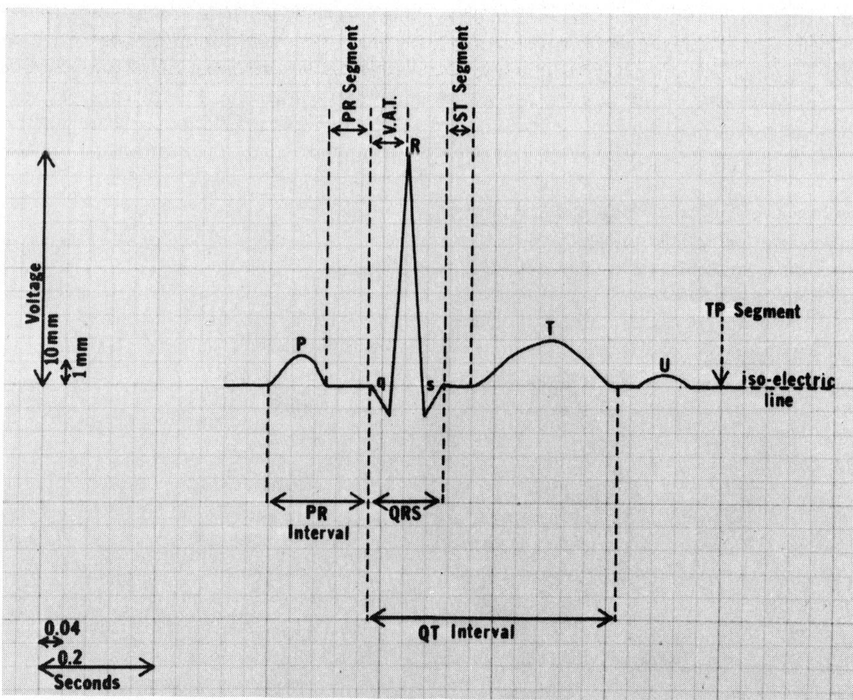

Figure 15–2. Complexes and intervals of the electrocardiogram.

tween the end of the QRS complex and the beginning of the T wave is affected by drugs and electrolyte imbalances and reflects myocardial injury.

8. T wave—The T wave represents myocardial repolarization and is altered by electrolytes, myocardial hypertrophy, and ischemia.

9. Impression—The ultimate impression of the ECG is derived from a systematic analysis of features such as those described above as compared with expected normal values for the age of the child.

D. VCG Interpretation: The VCG reveals much of the same information as the ECG. In fact, it is possible to draw the QRS loop of the VCG with considerable accuracy from QRS complexes of the ECG. Fig 15–3 displays the ECG and VCG of the same patient. The vector interpretation of the ECG (eg, direction and shape of loop) derived by looking at the ECG is perhaps the major contribution of vectorcardiography. It is usually not necessary to obtain an actual VCG to know what the loops look like.

Garson A Jr, Gillette PC, McNamara DC: *A Guide to Cardiac Dysrhythmias in Children.* Grune & Stratton, 1980.

Goldman MJ: *Principles of Clinical Electrocardiography,* 12th ed. Lange, 1986.

Liebman J, Plonsey R, Gillette PC: *Pediatric Electrocardiography.* Williams & Wilkins, 1982.

CHEST X-RAY

The chest x-ray, along with all other tests performed in pediatric patients, requires systematic evaluation. Accurate conclusions about the presence or absence of congenital heart defects and bone abnormalities can only be drawn if the proper procedures were followed—eg, the penetration of x-ray was adequate, and the films were obtained on adequate inspiration (distortions due to inadequate inspiration may look like cardiomegaly and increased vascular markings). The size of the heart, as seen on the chest x-ray, must be evaluated in relationship to the age and size of the patient. Chest films of the normal newborn will show a greater heart size and more pronounced vascular markings than those of the normal older child. These factors must all be taken into consideration in evaluating heart size and configuration and lung fields. The standard posteroanterior and left lateral chest films are usually adequate for this evaluation (Fig 15–4). If there is suspicion of vascular ring or mediastinal mass, multiple-view films with barium swallow are indicated.

Daves ML: *Cardiac Roentgenology.* Year Book, 1981.

Moes ACF et al: Chap 5, pp 45–51, in: *Heart Disease in Infancy and Childhood,* 3rd ed. Keith JD, Rowe RD, Vlad P (editors). Macmillan, 1978.

ECHOCARDIOGRAPHY & DOPPLER ULTRASONOGRAPHY

Echocardiography is now the major noninvasive method for diagnosis of congenital heart defects and is used to define anatomy, function, chamber and vessel size, and valve abnormalities. The use of M mode and 2-dimensional echocardiography will in most instances allow accurate diagnosis. These methods, along with Doppler ultrasonography (either pulsed or continuous wave ultrasound measurements) can now be used to predict cardiac output, valve gradients, and pulmonary artery pressure. Interpretation of the results of these studies requires the skill of the pediatric cardiologist, and in cases of major heart disease, cardiac catheterization should also be performed.

Feigenbaum H: *Echocardiography,* 3rd ed. Lea & Febiger, 1980.

Goldberg SJ, Allen HD, Sahn DJ: *Pediatric and Adolescent Echocardiography: A Handbook,* 2nd ed. Year Book, 1980.

Meyer RA: Echocardiography. Chap 4, pp 58–82, in: *Heart Disease in Infants, Children, and Adolescents,* 3rd ed. Adams FH, Emmanouilides GC (editors). Williams & Wilkins, 1983.

NUCLEAR CARDIOLOGY

Current use of radionuclide tracers in infants and children includes detection and quantification of left-to-right and right-to-left intracardiac shunting, quantification of cardiac output at rest and during exercise using gated blood pool scintigraphy, and myocardial imaging with thallium-201 for ischemia or infarction. In the older child, the latter method can be enhanced by exercise stress testing. These tests yield more objective data for evaluation of children with heart disease.

Hurwitz PA, Treves ST: Nuclear cardiology. Chap 6, pp 101–107, in: *Heart Disease in Infants, Children, and Adolescents,* 3rd ed. Adams FH, Emmanouilides GC (editors). Williams & Wilkins, 1983.

NUCLEAR MAGNETIC RESONANCE

Nuclear magnetic resonance (NMR) techniques, which are just being introduced in pediatric medicine, provide yet another method for noninvasive imaging of normal and abnormal cardiovascular structures. ^{31}P magnetic resonance spectroscopy appears to hold great promise as a clinical research tool for investigation of myocardial metabolism.

Friedman BJ et al: Comparison of magnetic resonance imaging and echocardiography in determination of cardiac dimensions in normal subjects. *J Am Coll Cardiol* 1985;**5:**1369.

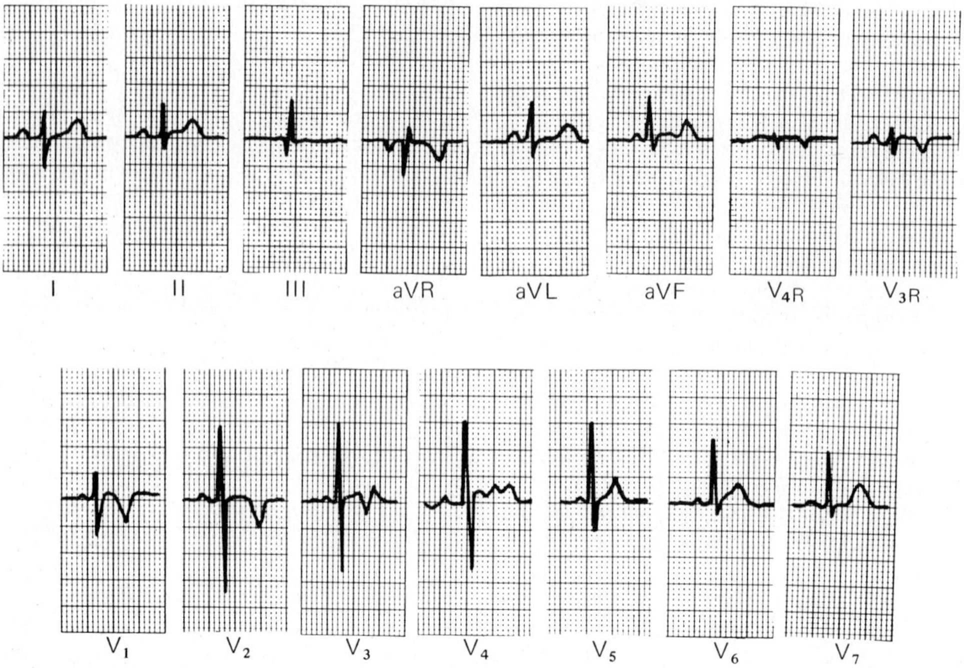

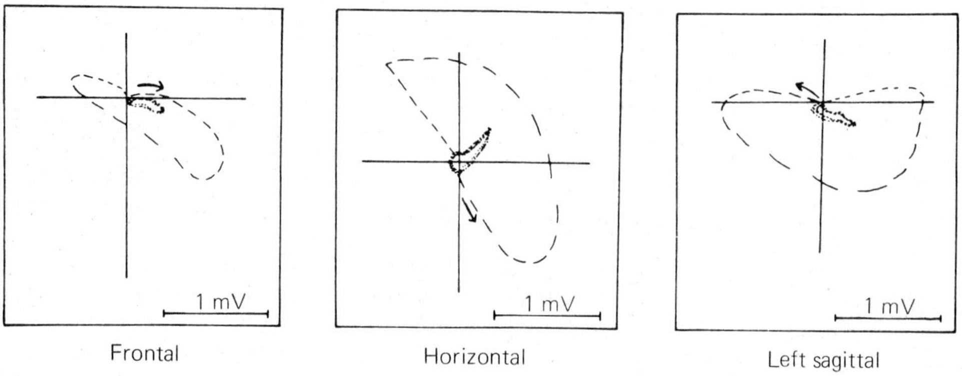

Figure 15–3. Electrocardiographic and vectorcardiographic findings in the same 10-month-old infant. The direction, duration, and magnitude of electrical force are comparable in each tracing.

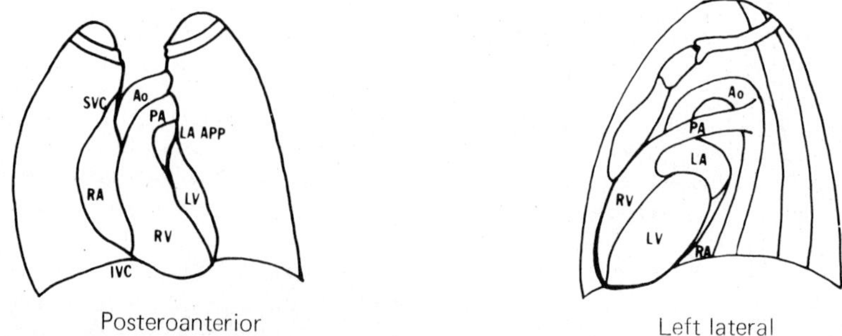

Figure 15–4. Position of cardiovascular structures in principal x-ray views. RA = right atrium; RV = right ventricle; LA = left atrium; LA APP = left atrial appendage; LV = left ventricle; Ao = aorta; PA = pulmonary artery; SVC = superior vena cava; IVC = inferior vena cava.

Leonard JC et al: Nuclear magnetic resonance. *J Pediatr* 1985;**106:**756.

Taegtmeyer H: Cardiovascular imaging: The biochemical basis. *Hosp Pract* (June) 1984;**19:**137.

ERGOMETRY

Pediatric ergometry is a newly evolving technique. It has long been hampered by lack of appreciation of its applications and availability of normal data. Most children with heart disease are capable of normal activity, and exercise data are essential to prevent overprotection. The response to exercise is valuable in determining the need for cardiovascular surgery and its timing. Bicycle ergometers or treadmills can often be employed to test children as young as 6 years. Important exercise parameters include stress ECGs, conditioning, and performance data. Significant stress ischemia or dysrhythmias warrant physical restrictions or appropriate therapy. Children demonstrating poor performance with suboptimal conditioning benefit from an exercise prescription. The pre- and postoperative child can then be objectively guided into appropriate recreational and competitive activities and given prevocational guidance.

James FW: Ergometry. Chap 7, pp 107–115, in: *Heart Disease in Infants, Children, and Adolescents,* 3rd ed. Adams FH, Emmanouilides GC (editors). Williams & Wilkins, 1983.

ARTERIAL BLOOD GASES (Arterial P_{O2}, Systemic O_2 Saturation)

Because cyanosis is difficult to measure (and sometimes to recognize) by inspection of the patient, objective laboratory determinations are required. The quantitative response of arterial P_{O2} or O_2 saturation (eg, by earpiece oximetry) to administration of 100% oxygen is one of the most useful methods of distinguishing cyanosis produced by heart disease from cyanosis related to lung disease in sick infants. In cyanotic heart disease, P_{aO2} increases very little from values obtained while breathing ambient room air as compared with values during 100% oxygen administration. However, there is usually a very significant increase in P_{aO2} when oxygen is administered to a patient with lung disease. Continuous noninvasive methods for monitoring arterial P_{O2} include the new transcutaneous O_2 monitor. Inherent limitations have prevented their general substitution for direct arterial sampling in this evaluation, but they are valuable in overall cardiopulmonary care of the sick infant. Table 15–1 illustrates the sort of response one might expect following at least 10 minutes of 100% oxygen administration to cyanotic infants with heart disease versus lung disease.

Table 15–1. Examples of responses to 10 minutes of 100% oxygen in lung disease and heart disease.

	Lung Disease		Heart Disease	
	Room Air	100% O_2	Room Air	100% O_2
Color	Blue →	Pink	Blue →	Blue
Oximetry	60% →	99%	60% →	62%
P_{aO2} (mm Hg)	35 →	120	35 →	38

OTHER NONINVASIVE LABORATORY STUDIES

In children of all ages, but particularly in the infant and newborn, many metabolic abnormalities can have a major influence on the performance of the cardiovascular system. In evaluating the symptomatic infant, it is important to rule out infection, hypoglycemia, hypocalcemia, hypovolemia, hyperkalemia, inborn errors of metabolism, anemia, etc. Likewise, severe cardiovascular problems may be accompanied by some of these abnormalities.

CARDIAC CATHETERIZATION & ANGIOCARDIOGRAPHY

The definitive anatomic and physiologic study of infants and children with heart disease is cardiac catheterization. It is essential for the primary physician to distinguish those infants and children who require the specialized diagnostic and therapeutic facilities of the pediatric cardiac center from those who may be safely managed without such facilities and consultation. On the basis of the preceding steps of diagnostic evaluation—history, physical examination, ECG, chest x-ray, and other noninvasive laboratory studies—the consulting pediatric cardiologist has a rather precise assessment of the anatomic and physiologic abnormalities in simple malformations and considerable useful information about complex malformations.

Indications & Objectives

A. Infants:

1. Indications—

a. All infants with cyanosis presumed to be cardiovascular in origin should be catheterized as soon as a reasonably stable clinical condition can be achieved—not only for diagnosis of the anatomic and physiologic abnormality but also for possibly lifesaving procedures such as the Rashkind balloon septostomy (which takes place in the cardiac catheterization laboratory).

b. Infants in severe congestive heart failure that does not respond promptly and satisfactorily to anticongestive measures.

c. Infants in whom early operation for congenital heart disease is contemplated.

d. Infants in whom the anatomic and physiologic

abnormality is sufficiently vague that appropriate medical management is not possible.

e. Infants who have evidence of complicating or potentially progressive problems, such as pulmonary hypertension and moderate to severe aortic stenosis, which will require precise longitudinal physiologic data.

2. Objectives—(In descending order of importance.)

a. To perform the study with the lowest possible rate of death or serious complications. This requires pediatric cardiologists and pediatric cardiac catheterization laboratories with experience in studying infants—to gain meaningful information promptly; to care for the critically ill infant with temperature and pH control, fluid management, and all essential pediatric treatment; and to anticipate and handle life-threatening crises.

b. To gain information which is not available by other methods and which will provide the basis for therapeutic decisions (medical or surgical).

c. To provide therapeutic intervention (eg, Rashkind septostomy).

d. To obtain sufficient physiologic and anatomic data so that repeat catheterization to complete the study will not be necessary.

B. Children:

1. Indications—

a. All children for whom heart surgery is contemplated (with the occasional exception of children with unequivocal patent ductus arteriosus and no evidence of an associated cardiovascular problem).

b. All children in whom there is question about the anatomic or physiologic abnormality which would significantly influence management and which cannot be completely answered by noninvasive methods.

c. Children with progressive lesions that require careful physiologic monitoring (such as aortic stenosis and pulmonary hypertension).

d. Children who have had cardiovascular surgery and require assessment of the adequacy of the repair.

e. Children with mild to moderate cardiovascular lesions when important information about the natural history is required. This should only be done in the setting of a well-designed protocol and fully informed consent.

2. Objectives—It goes without saying that conducting the study with the lowest possible risk is the most important objective of cardiac catheterization of the child as well as the infant; and the risk to the child (< 0.2%) is certainly much less than to the sick infant (2%). Therapy is not an objective of catheterization of the child, as it frequently is in the infant. Complete anatomic and physiologic data are more important objectives of catheterization in children than in infants. No physician or laboratory should undertake the catheterization of a child unless prepared to obtain a completely informative study and unless physicians and surgeons are available who are capable of proceeding with whatever medical or surgical therapy may be indicated.

Contraindications

Cardiac catheterization is contraindicated in infants and children who present with no clinical urgency and none of the indications listed above. It should not be done if personnel and facilities fail to meet high standards of patient safety and clinical diagnostic and therapeutic expertise.

Cardiac Catheterization Data

Fig 15–5 shows oxygen saturation (in percent) and pressure (in mm Hg) values obtained at cardiac catheterization from the chambers and great arteries of the heart. These values would be within the normal range for a child.

A. Oxygen Content and Saturation; Pulmonary and Systemic Blood Flow (Cardiac Output): In most laboratories, evidence of left-to-right shunt is determined by changes of blood oxygen content or saturation during passage of the catheter through the right side of the heart. A significant increase in oxygen content or oxygen saturation from one chamber to another indicates the presence of a left-to-right shunt at the site of the increase. The oxygen saturation of the peripheral arterial blood should always be determined during cardiac catheterization. Normal arterial oxygen saturation is 91–97%. A decrease (at sea level) below 91% suggests the presence of a right-to-left shunt, underventilation, or pulmonary disease.

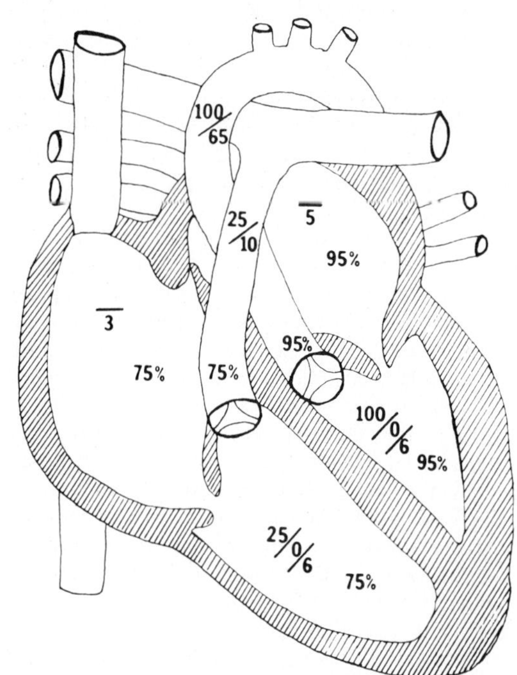

Figure 15–5. Pressures (in mm Hg) and oxygen saturation (in percent) obtained by cardiac catheterization in a normal child. 3 = mean pressure of 3 mm Hg in right atrium; 5 = mean pressure of 5 mm Hg in left atrium.

The size of a left-to-right shunt is usually expressed as a ratio of the pulmonary to systemic blood flow or as liters per minute as determined by the Fick principle:

$$\text{Cardiac output (L/min)} = \frac{\text{Oxygen consumption (mL/min)}}{\text{Arteriovenous difference (mL/L)}}$$

B. Pressures: Pressures should be determined in all chambers and vessels entered. Pressures should always be recorded when a catheter is pulled back from a distal chamber or vessel into a more proximal chamber. It is not normal for systolic pressure in the ventricles to exceed systolic pressure in the great arteries or mean diastolic pressure in the atria to exceed end-diastolic pressure in the ventricles. If a "gradient" in pressure does exist, it means that there is obstruction, and the severity of the gradient is one criterion for the necessity of operative repair. A right ventricular systolic pressure of 100 mm Hg and a pulmonary artery systolic pressure of 20 mm Hg yield a gradient of 80 mm Hg. In this case, the patient would be classified as having severe pulmonary stenosis requiring repair.

C. Pulmonary and Systemic Vascular Resistance: The vascular resistance is calculated from the following formula and reported in units or in dynes-sec-cm^{-5}/m^2:

$$\text{Resistance} = \frac{\text{Pressure}}{\text{Flow}}$$

Pulmonary vascular resistance equals mean pulmonary artery pressure divided by pulmonary blood flow per square meter of body surface area. (Pulmonary blood flow is determined from the Fick principle, as noted previously.) **Systemic vascular resistance** equals mean systemic arterial pressure divided by systemic blood flow.

Normally, the pulmonary vascular resistance ranges from 1 to 3 units or 80 to 240 dynes. If pulmonary resistance is above 10 units or the pulmonary/systemic resistance ratio is above 0.7, all other diagnostic findings should be reviewed carefully to confirm the presence of pulmonary hypertension that is so severe as to render the patient inoperable.

D. Special Techniques: Special techniques are frequently employed during the course of cardiac catheterization. These include the following:

1. Hydrogen electrode catheter—Used to determine the presence of very small left-to-right shunts, this technique enables the operator to detect such shunts even in the absence of any increase in oxygen saturation.

2. Indicator dilution curves—This involves injection of an indicator, such as indocyanine green (Cardio-Green), at specific places in the heart and detection of the dye downstream, usually in a peripheral artery. This technique permits the detection of both right-to-left and left-to-right shunts at the specific points within the cardiovascular system. Cardiac output is frequently determined by this method.

3. Selective angiocardiography and cineangiocardiography—In this technique, contrast material is injected in a specific chamber or vessel and the course of the contrast material followed by serial large film x-rays (angiocardiography) or by motion pictures (cineangiocardiography).

4. Contrast echocardiography—Saline or indocyanine green is rapidly injected via the cardiac catheter, and downstream "clouding" is imaged with either M mode or 2-dimensional echocardiography. Dynamic spatial or structural relationships of chambers, valves, and vessels are visualized; this may be done repetitively without the risk of radiation.

5. Balloon angioplasty—Specially designed balloon catheters are currently being evaluated for their efficacy and safety in children. Their use has been reported in cases of stenosis of the pulmonary valve and arteries, coarctation of the thoracic aorta, aorticopulmonary shunts, and arteriovenous fistula.

Jarmakani JM: Catheterization in angiocardiography. Chap 5, pp 83–100, in: *Heart Disease in Infants, Children, and Adolescents,* 3rd ed. Adams FH, Emmanouilides GC (editors). Williams & Wilkins, 1983.

Stanger P et al: Complications of cardiac catheterization of neonates, infants, and children: A three year study. *Circulation* 1974;**50:**595.

PRENATAL & NEONATAL CIRCULATION

Fetal Circulation

In the fetus, the placenta serves as the organ of respiration and for exchange of waste products for nutritive material. Oxygenated blood (80% saturated) passes from the placenta through the umbilical vein to the heart. As it flows toward the heart, it mixes with blood from the inferior vena cava and from the portal vein, so that blood entering the right atrium is approximately 65% saturated. A considerable amount of this blood is shunted immediately across the foramen ovale into the left atrium. The venous blood derived from the upper part of the body is much less saturated (approximately 30%), and most of it enters the right ventricle through the tricuspid valve. Thus, the blood in the right ventricle is a mixture of both relatively highly saturated blood from the umbilical vein and desaturated blood from the venae cavae. This mixture results in a blood oxygen saturation of approximately 50% in the right ventricle.

The blood in the left atrium is derived from the blood shunting across the foramen ovale and the blood returning from the pulmonary veins. A great deal of the left ventricular output goes to the head, whereas the lower portion of the body is supplied by blood both from the right ventricle, through the patent ductus arteriosus, and from the left ventricle.

Physiologic Changes at Birth & in the Neonatal Period

At birth, 2 dramatic events that affect the cardiovascular and pulmonary system occur: (1) the umbilical cord is clamped, removing the placenta from the circulation; and (2) breathing commences. As a result, marked changes in the circulation occur. During fetal life, the placenta offers little resistance to the flow of blood, so that the systemic circuit is a low-resistance one. On the other hand, the pulmonary arterioles are markedly constricted and offer strong resistance to the flow of blood into the lung. Clamping the cord causes a sudden increase in resistance to flow in the systemic circuit. As the lung becomes the organ of respiration, the oxygen tension (P_{O2}) increases in the vicinity of the small pulmonary arterioles, resulting in a release of the constriction and thus a significant decrease in the pulmonary arteriolar resistance. Indeed, the pulmonary vascular resistance shortly after birth is less than that of the systemic circuit.

Because of the changes in resistance, the great majority of the right ventricular outflow now passes into the lung rather than through the ductus arteriosus into the descending aorta. In fact, functional closure of the ductus arteriosus begins to develop shortly after birth. Recent studies have demonstrated that the ductus arteriosus remains patent for a variable period, usually 24–48 hours. During the first hour after birth, there is a small right-to-left shunt (as in the fetus). However, after 1 hour, bidirectional shunting occurs, with the left-to-right direction predominating. In most cases, right-to-left shunting completely disappears by 8 hours. However, in patients with severe hypoxia (in respiratory distress syndrome), the pulmonary vascular resistance remains quite elevated, resulting in a continued right-to-left shunt. The cause of the functional closure of the ductus arteriosus is not completely known. However, recent evidence indicates that the increased P_{O2} of the arterial blood causes spasm of the ductus. Anatomically, however, the ductus arteriosus does not close until approximately age 3 months.

In fetal life, the foramen ovale serves as a one-way valve, permitting shunting of blood from the inferior vena cava through the right atrium into the left atrium. At birth, because of the changes in the pulmonary and systemic vascular resistance and the increase in the quantity of blood returning from the pulmonary veins to the left atrium, the left atrial pressure rises above that of the right atrium. This functionally closes the flap of the one-way valve, essentially preventing flow of blood across the septum. It has been shown, however, that a small right-to-left shunt does continue for the first week of life. Although the foramen ovale remains functionally closed throughout life, it remains patent in about 25% of patients.

A clinical syndrome has been recognized that is characterized in term infants by onset of tachypnea, cyanosis, and clinical evidence of pulmonary hypertension during the first 8 hours after delivery. These infants have massive right-to-left ductal or foramen shunting or both for 3–7 days because of the high pulmonary vascular resistance. The clinical course is generally one of progressive cor pulmonale, hypoxia, and acidosis, terminating in early death unless the pulmonary resistance can be lowered. The resistance can usually be reversed by instituting appropriate means to increase alveolar P_{O2} hyperventilation and by intravenous administration of tolazoline. At postmortem, the only findings are increased thickness of the pulmonary arteriolar media, which is felt to represent persistence of the fetal circulation.

Changes in the First Year of Life

The most significant changes occur at birth and within the neonatal period. However, pulmonary vascular resistance and the pulmonary arterial pressure continue to fall during the first year of life. This results from the involution of the pulmonary arteriole from a relatively thick-walled, small-lumen vessel to a thin-walled, large-lumen vessel. Adult levels of resistance and pressure are usually achieved by age 6 months to 1 year.

Adams FH: Fetal circulation and alterations at birth. Chap 2, pp 511–517, in: *Heart Disease in Infants, Children, and Adolescents,* 2nd ed. Moss AJ, Adams FH, Emmanouilides GC (editors). Williams & Wilkins, 1977.

Drummond WH et al: The independent effects of hyperventilation, tolazoline, and dopamine on infants with persistent pulmonary hypertension. *J Pediatr* 1981;**98:**603.

MAJOR CLUES TO HEART DISEASE IN INFANTS & CHILDREN

CONGESTIVE HEART FAILURE

There are many levels of definition of congestive heart failure. At the clinical level, a simple definition is failure of the heart to meet the circulatory and metabolic needs of the body. Congestive heart failure is one of the 2 major clues to the presence of important heart disease. (The other is cyanosis; see below.) It has been estimated that congestive heart failure begins before age 1 year in over 90% of infants and children who ever develop the disorder in the pediatric age period—and most of these patients are less than 6 months of age.

Congestive heart failure beginning in infancy may persist throughout childhood until operation relieves the underlying malformation (unless surgery is not possible). Other infants with moderately severe heart failure in the first few months of life may gradually compensate (for a variety of reasons) and not require medical intervention after age 12 or 18 months even though their congenital heart lesions are still unrepaired.

Clinical Findings

The symptoms and signs of congestive heart failure have been discussed in the preceding sections on history and physical examination. Certain findings will be reviewed again here for purposes of emphasis and organization.

It may be said that the 3 cardinal signs of congestive heart failure in the pediatric patient are cardiomegaly (the sine qua non), tachypnea (left side), and hepatomegaly (right side).

Cardiomegaly represents a homeostatic (compensatory) mechanism that maintains adequate cardiac output by enlarging the capacity of the pump. This mechanism is frequently referred to as Starling's law of the heart. Up to a point, the enlarging heart can deliver a greater stroke volume output, but limits are soon reached (the descending limb of Starling's curve). Fig 15–6 shows a family of ventricular performance curves. The curve at the right depicts a damaged myocardium; the curve in the center, a normal myocardium; and the curve at the left, a myocardium under inotropic stimulation. One should be very cautious about the diagnosis of congestive heart failure in the absence of an enlarged heart (an exception being a condition such as total anomalous venous return below the diaphragm, which will for a short period of time be characterized by other signs of congestive heart failure without an enlarged heart). Cardiomegaly without other signs of congestive failure may well be taken as early or homeostatically compensated congestive heart failure.

Tachypnea may be considered the cardinal sign of left-sided heart failure. It may be present for a short time before hepatomegaly occurs, although pure left-sided or pure right-sided heart failure does not commonly exist independently for long.

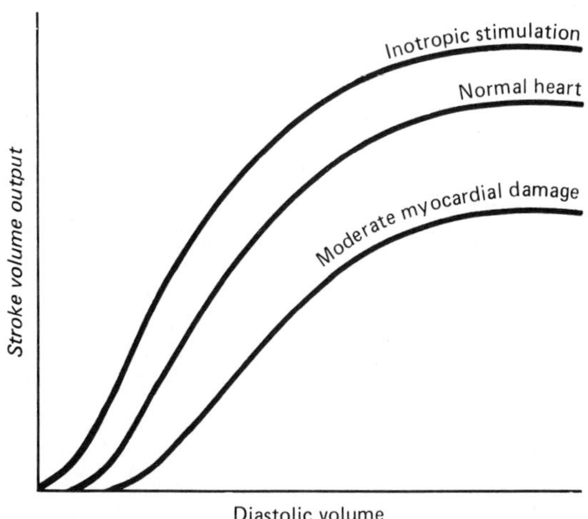

Figure 15–6. Ventricular performance curves.

Hepatomegaly is the cardinal sign of right-sided heart failure. The liver is capable of trapping relatively large amounts of edema fluid in the infant that would be more evident as peripheral edema in the older child and adult. It is therefore common rather than unusual for the infant in moderately severe heart failure to have an enlarged liver with no pretibial or even presacral or facial edema. Peripheral edema is found in infants only in the most severe cases of congestive heart failure.

Additional signs and symptoms of congestive heart failure are feeding difficulties, dyspnea, restlessness, easy fatigability, weak pulses, pallor, rales, peripheral edema, weight gain from fluid accumulation, tachycardia, sweating, pneumonia, orthopnea, and growth failure.

Underlying Causes of Heart Failure in the Pediatric Age Group

By far the most common cause of congestive heart failure in the pediatric patient is congenital heart disease. Causes in infancy and childhood appear in the outline below:

A. Heart Failure in Infancy:

1. Cardiovascular causes—Congenital heart disease (producing volume overload, obstruction, myocardial impairment), congenital vascular disease (eg, coarctation of the aorta, peripheral arteriovenous shunts), acquired myocardial disease (eg, myocarditis), dysrhythmias, rheumatic fever (very rare in infants in the USA).

2. Noncardiovascular causes—Acidosis, respiratory disease, central nervous system disease, anemia, sepsis, hypoglycemia.

B. Heart Failure in Childhood: Cardiovascular causes are potentially the same as in infancy except that rheumatic fever plays a more important role in childhood. Noncardiovascular causes become less important with increasing age—especially such mechanisms as acidosis and hypoglycemia.

Treatment

The physician undertaking the responsibility of caring for children must have facility with routine measures and familiarity with some emergency measures for treating congestive heart failure.

A. Routine Measures:

1. Digitalis—Digitalis is the keystone of the treatment of congestive heart failure. The major effect that is sought is improvement in myocardial performance (inotropic effect). This may be visualized as shifting the patient to a more efficient ventricular performance curve in the family of curves shown in Fig 15–6. The preparation most widely used in pediatrics is digoxin, which may be administered (in order of rapidity of onset of effect) intravenously, intramuscularly, or orally. The clinical urgency of the individual case dictates how quickly digitalization should be accomplished. Although there are general guidelines, the ultimate dosage (on a milligram per kilogram basis) must be individualized for each patient.

a. Protocols for digitalization—

(1) In hospital—

Age	Parenteral	Oral
Premature	0.035 mg/kg	0.04 mg/kg
2 weeks to 2 years	0.05 mg/kg	0.07 mg/kg
Under 2 weeks or over 2 years	0.04 mg/kg	0.06 mg/kg

Use of the elixir (0.05 mg/mL) is advisable even in older children because the bioavailability of the tablet preparations is unreliable.

The routine schedule consists of giving one-fourth the digitalizing dose intramuscularly or orally every 6 hours for 4 doses. For rapid digitalization, give half the digitalizing dose intravenously or intramuscularly and repeat in 4–6 hours. For very rapid digitalization, give the full digitalizing dose intravenously with very close monitoring. For maintenance, give one-fourth to one-third the oral digitalizing dose daily (divided in morning and evening doses).

(2) Digitalization of outpatients—Give the maintenance dose of digoxin (see above) divided in morning and evening doses. In less than a week, adequate digitalization is obtained without running the risk of a parent inadvertently failing to revert to a maintenance dosage schedule and continuing a high digitalizing dose to the point of toxicity (even death).

b. Digitalis toxicity—Slowing of the heart rate below 100 in infants, below 80 in young children, and below 60 in older children is often taken as a guide to reducing the dosage of digoxin. Any dysrhythmia that occurs during digitalis therapy should be attributed to the drug until proved otherwise, although ventricular bigeminy and various degrees of atrioventricular block are characteristic of digitalis toxicity. Age-specific serum levels suggestive of toxicity during maintenance therapy are as follows: newborn, over 4 ng/mL; 1 month to 1 year, over 3 ng/mL; after 1 year, over 2 ng/mL.

c. Digitalis poisoning—This is an acute emergency that must be treated *without delay*. The sooner the stomach is emptied, the better the prognosis, but even if many hours have passed, the stomach should still be emptied. Attention must then be paid to maintaining an adequate cardiac rate and output and to controlling the dysrhythmia. A useful basic intravenous solution is 10% glucose in water to which KCl (3 meq/kg/d) and regular insulin (20 units/1000 mL) have been added. KCl must be used with caution in patients with electrocardiographic high-grade block. It should be given in amounts not to exceed the maintenance requirement per 24 hours for the weight or surface area of the patient. To this solution may be added isoproterenol (in the calibrated administration set) titrated in quantities appropriate to maintain adequate heart rate and output in the face of complete heart block. Phenytoin (Dilantin) may be administered through the intravenous tubing to treat dysrhythmias by beginning with a 1-mg/kg slow intravenous push followed every 5–10 minutes with doubling doses to a maximum total combined dose of 15 mg/kg. If medical management is unsuccessful, temporary transvenous pacemakers are indicated.

2. Diuretics—If digitalis alone is inadequate to achieve satisfactory compensation, diuretics may be required. For rapid inpatient diuresis, give furosemide intravenously or intramuscularly; for maintenance therapy, give thiazides or furosemide orally daily along with spironolactone.

The dosages are as follows:

a. Furosemide—

(1) Intravenously or intramuscularly, 1 mg/kg as a single dose. Do not repeat more than once in a day, and be cautious about using on consecutive days.

(2) Orally, 2–5 mg/kg/d.

b. Thiazides—These drugs should be given daily with spironolactone. Do not give daily for prolonged periods unless spironolactone is being given also and serum electrolytes are being monitored periodically.

(1) Chlorothiazide suspension (250 mg/tsp), 20 mg/kg/d.

(2) Hydrochlorothiazide tablets, 2 mg/kg/d.

c. Spironolactone—Give 2–4 mg/kg/d in 2 divided doses.

3. Rest and sedation—The decompensated and mildly distressed patient requires rest; the severely distressed and anxious infant or child requires sedation. Parenteral morphine, 0.1 mg/kg, is useful for sedation as well as for control of acute pulmonary edema, but it should only be given with good airway control.

4. Oxygen—Oxygen will not make a patient with cyanotic heart disease pink, but it will raise the systemic P_{aO_2} in patients with severe congestive heart failure, overcoming the capillary-alveolar block of pulmonary edema and alleviating the hypoxemic contribution to congestive failure.

5. Salt restriction—Salt restriction must be approached with caution in infants and children. Treatment of the disease entity known as low-salt congestive heart failure is one of the more hazardous undertakings in medical management. Our feeling is that there is no place for salt-free formulas in the treatment of congestive failure in infants. Standard SMA or Similac 60/40 has about the same sodium content as human milk and about half the sodium content of cow's milk and other prepared formulas. Most cases of "low-salt failure" are largely due to overly vigorous salt restriction (sometimes combined with the other major factor, overly vigorous diuretic therapy). Clearly salty foods such as potato chips and bacon should be avoided, and no salt should be used beyond what is normally used in cooking. It is important that food be palatable enough to eat for a child, who may already be undernourished as a consequence of chronic, poorly compensated heart failure.

B. Emergency and Heroic Measures: The acute emergencies of congestive heart failure are usually related to fluid retention with pulmonary edema and low cardiac output. Some emergency therapeutic measures that may be lifesaving include the following:

1. Morphine—For acute pulmonary edema, give 0.1 mg/kg intravenously or subcutaneously.

2. Diuretics—Furosemide or ethacrynic acid may be given intravenously in an initial dosage of 1 mg/kg to produce a rapid diuresis.

3. Positive pressure breathing—Pulmonary edema may sometimes be managed by intubation or mask with bag-breathing or a respirator to raise the alveolar pressure above pulmonary capillary pressure.

4. Peritoneal dialysis—Although furosemide has largely met the need for the extremely rapid relief of fluid retention, there are 3 specific instances where peritoneal dialysis with a hypertonic solution may be indicated: (1) when fluid retention (especially pulmonary edema) is life-threatening and diuretics are unsuccessful; (2) in low-salt congestive heart failure when both the fluid retention and the electrolyte imbalance require correction; and (3) in the early postoperative care of an infant who may have an element of transient renal failure with both fluid retention and hyperkalemia.

The advantages of hypertonic peritoneal dialysis are that the procedure promptly (within minutes) draws fluid into the peritoneal cavity, where it is subject to immediate removal, while simultaneously correcting the electrolyte imbalance, whether it is low-sodium, high-potassium, or both. A suitable method is to introduce dialyzing solution (7% glucose with balanced salt) into the peritoneal cavity, using a pediatric dialysis trocar and catheter; 50 mL/kg should be administered slowly over a 10-minute period, allowed to remain for another 10 minutes, and withdrawn by gravity drainage. More than one "run" with hypertonic solution in 12 hours should be approached with caution, but in the presence of pulmonary edema, the hypertonic solution is required to withdraw fluid. If the major problem is electrolyte imbalance, such as potassium retention, a hypertonic solution is not required and the usual "isotonic" dialyzing fluid is indicated.

5. Afterload reduction—A relatively new form of therapy for "pump" failure is to effect afterload reduction by decreasing systemic vascular resistance with an intravenous infusion of vasodilators. Experience in children is limited. The procedure has been used largely in postoperative patients with reduced cardiac output and peripheral vasoconstriction. Agents such as nitroprusside have been lifesaving but must be used in a setting where central venous pressure, arterial pressure, cardiac output, etc, can be carefully monitored.

Arnold SB et al: Long-term digitalis therapy improves left ventricular function in heart failure. *N Engl J Med* 1980;**303:**1443.

Beckman RH, Rocchini AP, Rosenthal A: Hemodynamic effects of nitroprusside in infants with a large ventricular septal defect. *Circulation* 1981;**64:**553.

Beckman RH et al: Vasodilator therapy in children. *Pediatrics* 1984;**73:**43.

Driscoll D et al: Dopamine in children. *J Pediatr* 1978;**92:**309.

Epstein SE (editor): Calcium channel blockers: Present and future directions. *Am J Cardiol* 1985;**55:**1. [Entire issue.]

Smith TW: Digitalis in the management of heart failure. *Hosp Pract* (March) 1984;**19:**67.

Zaritsky A, Chernow B: Use of catecholamines in pediatrics. *J Pediatr* 1984;**105:**341.

CYANOSIS

One of the 2 major clues to the presence of heart disease in the infant and child is cyanosis. (The other is congestive heart failure; see above.)

Cyanosis represents an increased concentration (4–5 g/dL) of reduced hemoglobin in the blood. Bluish discoloration is usually, but not always, a sign. Patients with anemia and cyanosis may not appear blue; patients with polycythemia may appear cyanotic, even though true cyanosis is not present. Visible cyanosis accompanies low cardiac output, hypothermia, and systemic venous congestion, even in the presence of adequate oxygenation.

In patients with true central cyanosis, the cause of cyanosis (cardiac, pulmonary, hematologic, or central nervous system disorder) must be determined. Most often, the physician is faced with differentiating between cardiac and pulmonary problems. Evaluation of arterial blood gases (see above) is one of the easiest ways to differentiate between lung and heart disease. Cyanosis in heart disease is also related to pulmonary blood flow. In some "cyanotic" congenital heart defects, the decrease in pulmonary blood flow is minimal and results in minimal cyanosis. Presence of pulmonary hypertension also influences pulmonary blood flow, and thus oxygen therapy may cause a partial increase in oxygen saturation; the increase is usually much less in patients with heart disease than in those with pulmonary disease.

Evaluation for methemoglobinemia may be necessary to rule out hematologic causes. If the cause of cyanosis is a disease of the central nervous system, the patient will usually respond to oxygen therapy.

Cyanotic heart disease is usually a medical emergency, most often requiring palliative or corrective surgery.

CONGENITAL HEART DISEASE

Congenital heart disease is present in about 1% of recently studied North American and British populations, making this the most common category of congenital structural malformation. Curative or palliative surgical correction is now available for over 90% of patients with congenital heart disease.

The customary division of congenital heart diseases into noncyanotic and cyanotic types is useful if one understands the basis for it. By convention, patients with right-to-left shunts fall into the cyanotic category whether they have readily recognizable cyanosis or not; patients who do not have right-to-left shunts—even if they are cyanotic for other reasons, such as low cardiac output—are placed in the noncyanotic category. The physiologic basis of cyanosis has been discussed above. It should be remembered that whatever brings 4–5 g of unsaturated hemoglobin to the capillary bed produces cyanosis; if 4–5 g of unsaturated hemoglobin is not present (as in a patient with a cyanotic heart lesion, but with anemia), cyanosis is not present.

Etiologic Considerations

The incidence of congenital heart disease is high (1% of live births). Only 8% of all congenital heart defects are known to be associated with single mutant gene or chromosome abnormalities, and the remainder are due to various other causes. Multiple environmental factors, including diabetes, alcohol consumption, progesterone use, certain viruses, and other teratogens, are now associated with an increased incidence of malformations. These factors probably represent environmental triggers in persons susceptible or predisposed to congenital heart defects. The effect of rubella virus is probably independent of hereditary factors and consequently predisposes to patent ductus arteriosus and pulmonary artery branch stenosis. Acquired heart diseases, such as rheumatic fever, appear to have much stronger environmental influence. Atherosclerosis clearly can have distinct familial patterns but in some circumstances can be influenced by diet, drugs, or life-style.

In dealing with families of children with congenital heart disease, the physician must often answer the question of risk to future pregnancies. Table 15–2 outlines the risk for certain lesions in patients with one affected first-degree relative. Recent studies indicate that the incidence in children of affected mothers may be as high as 10–15%. With more than one affected first-degree relative, recurrence is also much higher, and some families may have a hereditary predisposition to congenital heart disease.

Nora JJ, Nora AH: *Genetics and Counseling in Cardiovascular Diseases*. Thomas, 1978.

Whittemore R, Hobbins JC, Engle MA: Pregnancy and its outcome in women with and without surgical treatment of congenital heart disease. *Am J Cardiol* 1982;**50:**641.

Table 15–2. Observed and expected recurrence risks in siblings of 1478 probands with congenital heart lesion.*

Anomaly	Probands	Affected Siblings No.	Percent	Exp. (√ p)
Ventricular septal defect	212	24/543	4.4	5.0
Patent ductus arteriosus	204	17/505	3.4	3.5
Tetralogy of Fallot	157	9/338	2.7	3.2
Atrial septal defect	152	11/342	3.2	3.2
Pulmonary stenosis	146	10/345	2.9	2.9
Aortic stenosis	135	7/317	2.2	2.1
Coarctation of aorta	128	5/272	1.8	2.4
Transpositions of great vessels	103	4/209	1.9	2.2
Atrioventricular canal	73	4/151	2.6	2.0
Tricuspid atresia	51	1/96	1.0	1.4
Ebstein's anomaly	42	1/96	1.1	0.7
Truncus arteriosus	41	1/86	1.2	0.7
Pulmonary atresia	34	1/77	1.3	1.0
Total	1478	95/3376		

* Reproduced, with permission, from Nora JJ: Etiologic factors in congenital heart disease. *Pediatr Clin North Am* 1971;**18:**1059.

NONCYANOTIC HEART DISEASE

ATRIAL SEPTAL DEFECT OF THE OSTIUM SECUNDUM VARIETY

Essentials of Diagnosis

- S_2 widely split and usually fixed.
- Grade I–III/VI ejection systolic murmur at pulmonary area.
- Widely radiating systolic murmur mimicking peripheral pulmonary artery stenosis (common in infancy).
- Diastolic flow murmur at lower left sternal border (if shunt is significant in size).
- ECG with rsR′ in lead V_1.

General Considerations

An atrial septal defect is an opening in the atrial septum permitting the shunting of blood between the 2 atria. There are 3 major types: (1) The ostium secundum type (discussed here) is the most common and is in an intermediate position. (2) The sinus venosus type is positioned high in the atrial septum, is the least common, and is frequently associated with partial anomalous venous return. (3) The ostium primum type is low in position and is a form of endocardial cushion defect; it is discussed in that section.

Atrial septal defect of the ostium secundum variety

occurs in approximately 10% of patients with congenital heart disease and is twice as common in females as in males. Diagnosis in infancy is becoming more common.

Pulmonary hypertension and growth failure are increasingly recognized in infancy and childhood. After the third decade, an increased pulmonary vascular resistance develops, the left-to-right shunting decreases, and right-to-left shunting begins.

Clinical Findings

A. Symptoms and Signs: Infants may present with congestive heart failure often unresponsive to medical management, necessitating early total corrective surgery. However, children with atrial septal defects often have no cardiovascular symptoms. Some patients remain asymptomatic throughout life; others develop easy fatigability as older children or adults. Cyanosis does not occur until pulmonary hypertension develops. This may never occur; if it does, it is not seen until after the third decade of life. Congestive heart failure is uncommon in infants and young children.

The arterial pulses are normal and equal throughout. In the usual case, the heart is hyperactive, with a heaving impulse felt best at the lower left sternal border and over the xiphoid process. There are usually no thrills. S_2 at the pulmonary area is widely split and sometimes fixed. The pulmonary component is normal in intensity. A grade I–III/VI, blowing, ejection type systolic murmur is heard best at the left sternal border in the second intercostal space. An additional murmur of relative peripheral pulmonary artery stenosis may be heard, more commonly in infants. A middiastolic murmur can often be heard in the fourth intercostal space at the left sternal border. This murmur is due to increased blood flow across the tricuspid valve during diastole (tricuspid flow murmur). The presence of this murmur suggests a high flow (pulmonary to systemic blood flow ratio greater than 2:1).

B. X-Ray Findings: Chest x-rays usually demonstrate cardiac enlargement. The main pulmonary artery may be dilated. The pulmonary vascular markings are increased as a result of increased pulmonary blood flow.

C. Electrocardiography and Vectorcardiography: The usual ECG shows right axis deviation with a clockwise loop in the frontal plane. In the right precordial leads, there is usually an rsR′ pattern.

D. Echocardiography: M mode echocardiography shows (1) paradoxic motion of the ventricular septal wall (moving in the same direction rather than the direction opposite to that of the free left ventricular wall) and (2) dilated right ventricular cavity with increased tricuspid valve excursion. Two-dimensional echocardiography for direct visualization of the defect in the mid portion of the atrial septum ensures the diagnosis.

E. Cardiac Catheterization: Oximetry reveals evidence of a significant increase in oxygen saturation at the atrial level. The pulmonary artery pressure is usually normal. The right ventricular pressure is occasionally greater than the pulmonary artery pressure, owing to "flow." Pulmonary vascular resistance is usually normal. The ratio of pulmonary to systemic blood flow may vary from 1.5:1 to 4:1. A catheter can easily be passed across the atrial septum into the left atrium. Contrast echocardiography and nuclear angiocardiography have enhanced the accuracy of diagnosis and quantifications of left-to-right shunts.

Treatment

Surgical closure is generally recommended for ostium secundum type atrial septal defects in which the ratio of pulmonary to systemic blood flow is greater than 2:1. Operation is usually performed electively in patients between ages 2 and 4 years. The death rate for surgical closure is less than 1%. When surgical intervention is early, late complications of right ventricular dysfunction and significant dysrhythmias may be avoided or diminished. Early surgery is also indicated in infants presenting with congestive heart failure or significant pulmonary hypertension.

Course & Prognosis

Patients with atrial septal defects usually tolerate them very well in the first 2 decades of life, and an occasional patient may live a completely normal life without symptoms. Frequently, however, pulmonary hypertension and reversal of the shunt develop by the third or fourth decade. Heart failure may also occur at this time. Subacute infective endocarditis is a very rare complication. Spontaneous closure occurs rarely and is sometimes associated with an aneurysm of the atrial septum. Exercise tolerance and oxygen consumption in surgically corrected children are generally normal, and physical limitations are unnecessary.

Cockerham JT et al: Spontaneous closure of secundum atrial septal defect in infants and young children. *Am J Cardiol* 1983;**52:**1267.

Marx GA et al: Transatrial septal velocity: Measurement by Doppler echocardiography in atrial septal defect. *Am J Cardiol* 1985;**55:**1162.

Meyer RA et al: Long-term follow-up study after closure of secundum atrial septal defects in children. *Am J Cardiol* 1982;**50:**143.

VENTRICULAR SEPTAL DEFECTS

Essentials of Diagnosis

Small- to moderate-sized left-to-right shunt without pulmonary hypertension:

- Acyanotic, relatively asymptomatic.
- Grade II–IV/VI pansystolic murmur, maximal along the lower left sternal border.
- P_2 not accentuated.

Large left-to-right shunt:

- Acyanotic.

- Easy fatigability.
- Congestive heart failure in infancy (often).
- Hyperactive heart; biventricular enlargement.
- Grade II–V/VI pansystolic murmur, maximal at lower left sternal border.
- P_2 usually accentuated.
- Diastolic flow murmur at apex.

Insignificant left-to-right shunt or bidirectional shunt with pulmonary hypertension:

- Quiet precordium with right ventricular lift.
- Palpable P_2.
- Short ejection systolic murmur along left sternal border; single accentuated S_2.
- Systemic arterial oxygen desaturation may be present; pulmonary arterial pressure and systemic arterial pressures are equal; little or no oxygen saturation increase at right ventricular level by catheterization.

General Considerations

Simple ventricular septal defect (without other lesions) is the single most common congenital heart malformation, accounting for about 25% of all cases of congenital heart disease. Defects in the ventricular septum can occur both in the membranous portion of the septum (most common) and in the muscular portion.

There are 5 different courses that patients with ventricular septal defect may follow:

A. Spontaneous Closure: Thirty to 50% of all ventricular septal defects close spontaneously. The small defects close in 60–70% of cases. Larger defects may occasionally also close spontaneously, and there are many documented examples of spontaneous closure of ventricular septal defects in the second and third decades of life. Half of the defects that do not close become functionally or anatomically smaller.

B. Shunts Too Small to Justify Repair: Asymptomatic patients with hearts normal in size (as seen on x-ray) and without pulmonary hypertension are generally not subjected to surgical repair. In those who have had cardiac catheterization, the ratio of pulmonary to systemic blood flow is usually found to be less than 2:1, and serial cardiac catheterizations demonstrate that the shunts get progressively smaller.

C. Disease Severe Enough to Require Surgery: The time of surgery depends upon the nature of the disease. Patients may require surgery in infancy because of intractable congestive heart failure; surgery before 2 years of age because of progression of pulmonary hypertension; or surgery between 2 and 5 years of age as an elective procedure.

D. Defect Inoperable Because of Pulmonary Hypertension: The vast majority of patients with inoperable pulmonary hypertension will develop this condition progressively. The combined data of the multicenter National History Study indicate that most cases of irreversible pulmonary hypertension can be prevented by surgical repair of the defect before 2 years of age.

E. Development of Infundibular Pulmonary Stenosis: Approximately 5% of infants with large left-to-right shunts will develop progressive infundibular obstruction effecting an outflow gradient and diminution of the shunt. A small proportion of these infants have precyanotic tetralogy of Fallot, as evidenced by coexistent right aortic arch or abnormal spatial orientation of the infundibulum.

Clinical Findings

A. Symptoms and Signs: Patients with small or moderate left-to-right shunts usually have no cardiovascular symptoms. There may be a history of frequent respiratory infections in infancy and early childhood. Patients with large left-to-right shunts frequently are sick early in infancy. Such patients have frequent respiratory infections, including bouts of pneumonitis. They grow slowly, with very poor weight gain. Dyspnea, exercise intolerance, and fatigue are quite common. Congestive heart failure may develop between 1 and 6 months of age. Patients who survive the first year usually improve, although easy fatigability may persist. With severe pulmonary hypertension (Eisenmenger's syndrome), cyanosis is present.

1. Small left-to-right shunt—There are usually no lifts, heaves, thrills, or shocks. The first sound at the apex is normal, and the second sound at the pulmonary area is split physiologically. The pulmonary component is normal. A grade II–IV/VI, medium- to high-pitched, blowing pansystolic murmur is heard best at the left sternal border in the third and fourth intercostal spaces. There is slight radiation over the entire precordium. No diastolic murmurs are heard.

2. Moderate left-to-right shunt—Slight prominence of the precordium is common. There is a moderate left ventricular thrust. A systolic thrill is palpable at the lower left sternal border between the third and fourth intercostal spaces. The second sound at the pulmonary area is most often split but may be single. A grade IV/VI, harsh pansystolic murmur is heard best at the lower left sternal border in the fourth intercostal space. A diastolic flow murmur is heard and indicates that the pulmonary venous return across the mitral valve is large and that the pulmonary to systemic blood flow ratio is at least 2:1.

3. Very large ventricular septal defects with pulmonary hypertension—The precordium is prominent, and the sternum bulges. A left ventricular thrust and a right ventricular heave are palpable. A shock of the second sound can be felt at the pulmonary area. A thrill may or may not be present at the lower left sternal border. A second heart sound is usually single or narrowly split, with accentuation of the pulmonary component. The murmur ranges from grade II to grade V/VI and is usually harsh and pansystolic. Occasionally, when the defect is large, very little murmur can be heard. A diastolic flow murmur may or may not be heard depending on the size of the shunt.

B. X-Ray Findings: X-rays of the chest vary depending upon the size of the shunt. In patients with small shunts, x-rays may be normal. The heart is normal in size, and the pulmonary vascular markings may be just beyond the upper limits of normal. Patients with large shunts usually show significant cardiac enlargement involving both the left and right ventricles and the left atrium. The aorta is usually small to normal in size, and the main pulmonary artery segment is dilated. The pulmonary vascular markings are significantly increased in patients with large shunts.

C. Electrocardiography: There is some correlation between the electrocardiographic and the hemodynamic findings. The ECG is normal in patients with small left-to-right shunts and normal pulmonary arterial pressures. Left ventricular hypertrophy is usually found in patients with large left-to-right shunts and normal pulmonary vascular resistance. Combined ventricular hypertrophy (both right and left) is found in patients with pulmonary hypertension due to increased flow, increased resistance, or both. Pure right ventricular hypertrophy is found in patients with pulmonary hypertension due to pulmonary vascular obstruction.

D. Echocardiography: The diagnosis of ventricular septal defect cannot reliably be made by M mode techniques. Two-dimensional echocardiography provides visualization of defects that are 4 mm or larger in about 65–75% of cases and often can pinpoint the anatomic location.

E. Cardiac Catheterization and Angiocardiography: Oxygen saturation is increased at the right ventricular level. The pulmonary artery pressure may vary from normal to that in the systemic arteries. Left atrial pressure (pulmonary capillary pressure) may be normal to increased. Pulmonary vascular resistance varies from normal to markedly increased. The ratio of pulmonary to systemic blood flow may vary from 1.1:1 to 4:1. Hydrogen electrode curves and dye dilution curves may indicate a shunt at the ventricular level. Angiocardiographic examination defines the number, size, and location of the defects.

Treatment

A. Medical Management: Patients who develop congestive heart failure should be treated vigorously with anticongestive measures (see Congestive Heart Failure, above). If the patient does not respond to vigorous anticongestive measures or shows signs of progressive pulmonary hypertension, surgery is indicated without delay.

B. Surgical Treatment: The age for elective surgery is becoming progressively earlier in most centers (range, < 2 years to 5 years). Patients with cardiomegaly, poor growth, poor exercise tolerance, or other clinical abnormalities who have cardiac catheterization findings of significant shunt ($\geq 2:1$) without significant pulmonary hypertension (> 10 units of resistance) are candidates for surgery. In general, patients with mean pulmonary artery pressures equal to systemic pressure who are unresponsive to oxygen administration, with little or no left-to-right shunt or bidirectional shunting, and pulmonary resistance calculated to be greater than 10 resistance units (or pulmonary/systemic resistance ratios > 0.7) are considered inoperable. There are patients who have pulmonary hypertension of lesser degree who remain operable, but there is a progressively greater risk with increasing pulmonary hypertension (from 1% risk for patients without pulmonary hypertension to 25% for those at the upper limits of operability).

In order to prevent pulmonary hypertension from reaching inoperable levels, early surgical intervention is recommended for patients who have increased pulmonary resistance. In centers with the capability of doing total correction on infants with or without deep hypothermia, complete repair before 2 years of age is recommended. The presence of multiple muscular defects in a tiny symptomatic infant is still considered to be an indication for pulmonary artery banding as an initial palliative procedure.

Course & Prognosis

Significant late dysrhythmias are uncommon. Functional exercise capacity and oxygen consumption are usually normal, and physical restrictions are unnecessary.

Cheatham JP, Latson LA, Gutgesell HP: Ventricular septal defect in infancy: Detection with two-dimensional echocardiography. *Am J Cardiol* 1981;**47:**85.

Yeager SB et al: Primary surgical closure of ventricular septal defect in the first year of life: Results in 128 infants. *J Am Coll Cardiol* 1984;**3:**1269.

ENDOCARDIAL CUSHION DEFECTS

Essentials of Diagnosis

- Murmur often inaudible in neonates.
- Loud pulmonary component of S_2.
- Common in infants with Down's syndrome.
- ECG with left axis deviation.

General Considerations

An endocardial cushion defect is a congenital cardiac abnormality that results from incomplete fusion of the embryonic endocardial cushions. The endocardial cushions help to form the lower portion of the atrial septum, the membranous portion of the ventricular septum, and the septal leaflets of the tricuspid and mitral valves. These defects are not very common. They account for about 4% of all cases of congenital heart disease. The incidence of this abnormality is 20% in patients with Down's syndrome.

Endocardial cushion defects may be divided into incomplete and complete forms. The complete form, also known as persistent common atrioventricular canal, consists of a high ventricular septal defect, a low atrial septal defect of the ostium primum variety that is continuous with the ventricular septal defect, and a cleft in both the septal leaflet of the tricuspid valve and the anterior leaflet of the mitral valve. In the incomplete form, any one of these components may be present. The most common partial form of endocardial cushion defect is the ostium primum type of atrial septal defect with a cleft in the mitral valve.

The complete form (persistent common atrioventricular canal) results in large left-to-right shunts at both the ventricular and atrial levels, tricuspid and mitral regurgitation, and marked pulmonary hypertension, usually with some increase in pulmonary vascular resistance. When the latter is present, the shunts may be bidirectional. The hemodynamics in the incomplete form are dependent upon the lesions present.

Clinical Findings

A. Symptoms and Signs: The clinical picture varies depending upon the severity of the defect. In the incomplete form, these patients may be indistinguishable from patients with the ostium secundum type of atrial septal defect. They are often asymptomatic. On the other hand, patients with atrioventricular canal usually are severely affected. Congestive heart failure often develops in infancy, and recurrent bouts of pneumonitis are common.

In the complete form, the murmur may be inaudible in the neonate. After 4–6 weeks, a nonspecific systolic murmur develops; the murmur is usually not as harsh as that of an isolated ventricular septal defect. The heart is significantly enlarged (both right and left sides), and a systolic thrill may be palpated at the lower left sternal border. The second heart sound is split, with an accentuated pulmonary component. A pronounced diastolic flow murmur may be heard at the apex and lower left sternal borders.

When severe pulmonary vascular obstruction is present, there is evidence of dominant right ventricular enlargement. A shock of the second sound can be palpated at the pulmonary area. No thrill is felt. The second sound is markedly accentuated and single. A nonspecific short systolic murmur is heard at the lower left sternal border. No diastolic flow murmurs are heard. Cyanosis is detectable in severe cases with predominant right-to-left shunts.

The physical findings in the incomplete form depend upon the lesions. In the most common variety (ostium primum atrial septal defect with mitral regurgitation), the findings are similar to those of the ostium secundum type of atrial septal defect with or without findings of mitral regurgitation.

B. X-Ray Findings: Cardiac enlargement is present depending on the degree of specific anatomic defect and the severity. In the complete (canal) form, there is enlargement of all 4 chambers. The pulmonary vascular markings are increased. In patients with pulmonary vascular obstruction, only the main pulmonary artery segment and its branches are prominent. The peripheral markings are usually decreased.

C. Electrocardiography: In all forms of endocardial cushion defect, left axis deviation with a counterclockwise loop in the frontal plane is present. The mean axis varies from approximately −30 to −90 degrees. Since left axis deviation is present in all patients with this defect, the ECG is a very important diagnostic tool. First-degree heart block is present in over 50% of cases. Right, left, or combined ventricular hypertrophy is present depending upon the particular type of defect and the presence or absence of pulmonary vascular obstruction.

D. Echocardiography: Many suggestive patterns have been found on M mode echocardiography, but excursion of the atrioventricular valve through the plane of the interventricular septal defect is characteristic. The anatomy can be directly visualized by 2-dimensional echocardiography; the sensitivity of this method is equal to that of selective cineangiography.

E. Cardiac Catheterization and Angiocardiography: The results of cardiac catheterization vary depending upon the type of defect present. When catheterization is performed from the leg, the catheter is easily passed across the atrial septum in its lowest portion and frequently enters the left ventricle directly. This is a result of the very low atrial septal defect and the cleft in the mitral valve. Increased oxygen saturation in the right ventricle or right atrium identifies the level of the shunt. Angiocardiography reveals a characteristic "gooseneck" deformity in the complete canal form. Contrast echocardiography is extremely useful in identifying the subgroups of endocardial cushion defects.

Treatment

Treatment consists of anticongestive measures and eventual surgical correction. In the incomplete form, surgery is associated with a relatively low death rate (2–5%). The complete form is associated with a significantly higher death rate (about 15–25%), but complete correction in the first year of life, prior to the onset of irreversible pulmonary hypertension, is advisable.

Pulmonary artery banding procedures are contraindicated in infants with shunts predominantly at the atrial level. They are less effective in patients with predominantly ventricular level shunts than in patients with simple ventricular septal defect.

Kawashima Y et al: Surgical treatment of complete atrioventricular canal defect with an endocardial cushion prosthesis. *Circulation* 1983;**68:**1421.

Sato B et al: Angiography of atrioventricular canal defects. *Am J Cardiol* 1981;**48:**492.

PATENT DUCTUS ARTERIOSUS

Essentials of Diagnosis

- Variable murmur, with active percordium and full pulses, in premature infants.
- Continuous murmur and full pulses in past prematures.

General Considerations

Patent ductus arteriosus is the persistence in extrauterine life of the normal fetal vessel that joins the pulmonary artery to the aorta. It is a common abnormality, accounting for about 12% of all cases of congenital heart disease. It is very common in children born to mothers who had rubella during the first trimester of pregnancy. There is a higher incidence of patent ductus arteriosus in infants born at high altitudes (over 10,000 feet). It is twice as common in females as in males. In intensive care premature nurseries where infants who would die with less aggressive management are salvaged, the frequency of patent ductus arteriosus may be as high as 20–60%.

The defect occurs as an isolated abnormality, but associated lesions are not infrequent. Coarctation of the aorta, patent ductus arteriosus, and ventricular septal defect are commonly associated. Even more important to recognize is the fact that patients with murmurs of patent ductus and without readily apparent findings of other associated lesions are being kept alive by the patent ductus. One would not wish to ligate a patent ductus in a patient with pulmonary atresia or merely follow such a patient with outpatient visits; the child should receive immediate precise diagnosis and appropriate treatment.

Clinical Findings

A. Symptoms and Signs: The clinical findings and the clinical course depend on the size of the shunt and the degree of pulmonary hypertension.

1. Typical patent ductus arteriosus—The pulses are bounding, and pulse pressure is widened (pulse pressure is greater than half of the systolic pressure). The first heart sound is normal. The second heart sound is usually narrowly split and very rarely (when the shunt is maximal) paradoxically split (ie, the second sound closes on inspiration and splits on expiration). The paradoxic splitting is due to the maximal overload of the left ventricle and the prolonged ejection of blood from this chamber.

The murmur is quite characteristic. It is a very rough "machinery" murmur that is maximal at the second intercostal space at the left sternal border and under the left clavicle. It begins shortly after the first heart sound, rises to a peak at the second heart sound, and passes through the second heart sound into diastole, where it becomes a decrescendo murmur and fades and disappears before the first heart sound. The murmur tends to radiate fairly well over the lung fields anteriorly but relatively poorly over the lung fields posteriorly. A diastolic flow murmur is often heard at the apex. Depending on the pulmonary artery pressure, the murmur may be only systolic in time. This should be fully appreciated when trying to reach a diagnosis of patent ductus arteriosus in infants. If the shunt is small, congestive failure is absent; if the shunt is large, congestive failure becomes important.

2. Patent ductus arteriosus with pulmonary hypertension—The physical findings depend upon the cause of the pulmonary hypertension. If pulmonary hypertension is due primarily to a marked increase in blood flow and only a slight increase in pulmonary vascular resistance, the physical findings are similar to those listed above. The significant difference is the presence of an accentuated pulmonary component of S_2. Bounding pulses and a loud continuous heart murmur are present. In patients with pulmonary vascular resistance and predominant right-to-left shunt, the findings are quite different. There may be evidence of cyanosis. The second heart sound is single and quite accentuated, and there is no significant heart murmur. The pulses are normal rather than bounding.

3. Patent ductus arteriosus in the premature neonate with associated IRDS—A premature neonate during or after the clinical course of infant respiratory distress syndrome (IRDS) may have a significant associated patent ductus arteriosus that is paradoxically difficult to detect clinically but is often threatening in magnitude. A soft nonspecific systolic murmur or no murmur is more common than the classic continuous murmur. The peripheral pulse and precordium are often bounding but typically are not characteristic for several days after the onset of a large left-to-right shunt. An early sign indicating the presence of a significant left-to-right shunt with concomitant congestive heart failure is increasing dependence on oxygen and respiratory support. In addition, increasing radiographic cardiomegaly and pulmonary edema plus increasing echocardiographic evidence of a left-to-right shunt differentiate this clinical and laboratory picture from bronchopulmonary dysplasia.

B. X-Ray Findings: In simple patent ductus arteriosus, the x-ray appearance depends upon the size of the shunt. If the shunt is relatively small or moderate in size, the heart is not enlarged. If the shunt is large, there is evidence of both left atrial and left ventricular enlargement. In both cases, the aorta is prominent, as is the main pulmonary artery segment.

C. Electrocardiography: The ECG may be normal or may show left ventricular hypertrophy, depending on the size of the shunt. In patients with pulmonary hypertension due to increased blood flow, there is usually biventricular hypertrophy. In those with pulmonary vascular obstruction, there is pure right ventricular hypertrophy. An anterior ST depression (V_1) of 2 mm suggests subendocardial ischemia due to a diastolic "steal" from the coronary arteries via the ductus; this finding indicates the need for closure.

D. Echocardiography: Enlargement of the left atrium as measured by M mode echocardiography is an important clue to the presence of congestive heart failure and is especially useful in diagnosing patent ductus arteriosus in the premature infant. A left atrial to ascending aorta ratio of less than 1.2 or 1.3 is considered evidence of a sizable left-to-right ductal shunt. Premature infants with patent ductus arteriosus who are undergoing medical or surgical therapy for closure should have a complete 2-dimensional echocardiographic evaluation to rule out associated heart disease, especially ductus-dependent lesions. The use of pulsed Doppler ultrasonography and 2-dimensional echocardiography can provide visualization of the ductus and confirmation of the direction and degree of shunting.

E. Cardiac Catheterization and Angiocardiography: Cardiac catheterization will reveal increased oxygen content or saturation at the level of the pulmonary artery. Hydrogen electrode curves are positive in the pulmonary artery and negative in the right ventricle. The catheter can often be passed through the ductus from the pulmonary artery into the descending thoracic aorta. Arteriograms taken following injection of contrast material into the aortic arch show a shunt at the level of the ductus. If catheterization is not performed, the cardiologist must be completely satisfied that there is neither an associated lesion nor pulmonary hypertension. One should not have to tie off more than one ductus in a patient with pulmonary atresia or interrupted aortic arch to be extremely cautious about sending patients with presumptive diagnoses of patent ductus arteriosus to surgery without cardiac catheterization.

Patients with patent ductus arteriosus and pulmonary hypertension due to large left-to-right shunts show a marked increase in oxygen saturation at the pulmonary artery level and normal systemic arterial saturation. Those with marked pulmonary vascular obstruction show little or no increase in oxygen content at the pulmonary artery and a decrease in systemic arterial saturation. In both cases, a catheter may be passed through the ductus into the descending thoracic aorta.

Cardiac catheterization is rarely indicated in the premature infant with symptomatic ductus.

Treatment

Treatment consists of surgical correction except in patients with pulmonary vascular obstruction. Patients with large left-to-right shunts and pulmonary hypertension should be operated on very early (even under the age of 1 year) to prevent the development of progressive pulmonary vascular obstruction. Simple patent ductus arteriosus should be corrected after the child reaches age 1, though the operation may be delayed until later without increasing the risk of death.

Patients with nonreactive pulmonary vascular obstruction who have resistance greater than 10 units and a pulmonary/systemic resistance ratio greater than 0.7 should not be operated upon. These patients are made worse by closure of the ductus, since the ductus serves as an escape route and limits the degree of pulmonary hypertension.

The premature infant with symptomatic ductus presents a special and controversial problem. At some institutions, it is customary to operate on virtually all premature infants weighing under 1200 g. At other institutions, surgery is rarely done, and most infants receive a maximum of 3 doses of either oral indomethacin (0.1–0.3 mg/kg every 8–24 hours) or parenteral indomethacin (0.1–0.3 mg/kg every 12 hours) if adequate renal, hematologic, and hepatic function are demonstrated. Contraindications to indomethacin treatment include hyperbilirubinemia of 12 mg/100 mL or greater, renal failure, shock, necrotizing enterocolitis, intracranial hemorrhage, hemorrhagic disease, and evidence of a spontaneously closing ductus. Efficacy and safety of indomethacin use are enhanced by the careful monitoring of serum levels of indomethacin. A serum level of less than 250 ng/mL is associated with treatment failure. Conventional conservative management includes fluid restriction with or without diuretics and ligation only if these fail. Factors to be considered in making a rational decision on modality of therapy include a high rate of spontaneous ductus closure without therapy and an extremely low surgical risk in experienced centers; the inability of most laboratories to monitor serum levels of indomethacin may influence the decision.

Course & Prognosis

Patients with simple patent ducus arteriosus and small to moderate shunts usually do quite well even without surgery. However, in the third or fourth decade of life, symptoms of easy fatigability, dyspnea on exertion, and exercise intolerance appear, usually as a consequence of the development of pulmonary hypertension or congestive heart failure.

Spontaneous closure of a patent ductus arteriosus may occur within the first year of life. This is especially true in infants who were born prematurely. After age 1, spontaneous closure is rare. Since subacute infective endocarditis is a potential complication, surgical ligation is recommended if the defect persists beyond age 1 year.

Patients with large shunts or pulmonary hypertension do much less well. Poor growth and development, frequent episodes of pneumonitis, and the development of congestive heart failure are not uncommon in patients with large left-to-right shunts. If these patients do not succumb to congestive heart failure in early infancy, they frequently go on to develop pulmonary vascular obstruction in later childhood or adolescence. Life expectancy is markedly reduced, and these patients often die in their second or third decade. Those rare patients with pulmonary vascular obstruction from very early infancy are actually less symptomatic than those with pulmonary hypertension without obstruction.

Dudell GG, Gersony WM: Patent ductus arteriosus in neonates with severe respiratory disease. *J Pediatr* 1984;**104:**915.

Gersony WM et al: Effects of indomethacin in premature infants with patent ductus arteriosus: Results of a national collaborative study. *J Pediatr* 1983;**102:**895.

Serwer GA, Armstrong BE, Anderson PA: Continuous wave Doppler ultrasonographic quantitation of patent ductus arteriosus flow. *J Pediatr* 1982;**100:**297.

Way GL et al: ST depression suggesting subendocardial ischemia in neonates with respiratory distress syndrome and patent ductus arteriosus. *J Pediatr* 1979;**95:**609.

MALFORMATIONS ASSOCIATED WITH OBSTRUCTION TO BLOOD FLOW ON THE RIGHT SIDE OF THE HEART

1. VALVULAR PULMONARY STENOSIS WITH INTACT VENTRICULAR SEPTUM

Essentials of Diagnosis

- No symptoms with mild and moderately severe cases.
- Cyanosis and a high incidence of right-sided congestive heart failure in very severe cases.
- Right ventricular lift; systolic ejection click at the pulmonary area in mild to moderately severe cases.
- S_2 widely split with soft to inaudible P_2; grade I–VI/VI obstructive systolic murmur, maximal at the pulmonary area.
- Dilated pulmonary artery on posteroanterior chest x-ray.

General Considerations

Obstruction of right ventricular outflow at the pulmonary valve level accounts for about 10% of all cases of congenital heart disease. In the usual case, the cusps of the pulmonary valve are fused to form a membrane or diaphragm with a hole in the middle that varies from 2 mm to 1 cm in diameter. Occasionally, there may be a fusion of only 2 cusps, producing a bicuspid pulmonary valve. Very frequently, especially in the more severe cases, there is secondary infundibular stenosis. The pulmonary valve ring is usually small. There is usually moderate to marked poststenotic dilatation of both the main and left pulmonary arteries. Patent foramen ovale is fairly common.

Obstruction to blood flow across the pulmonary valve results in an increase in pressure developed by the right ventricle to maintain an adequate output across that valve. Pressures greater than systemic are potentially life-threatening and are associated with "critical" obstruction. As a consequence of the increased work required of the right ventricle, severe right ventricular hypertrophy and eventual right ventricular failure can occur. In contrast to patients with right ventricular outflow obstruction, patients with this obstruction who also have a large ventricular septal defect (ie, tetralogy of Fallot) are not at great risk for heart failure; because of the septal defect, there is communication between the ventricles, which limits the amount of pressure developed in the right ventricle (pressure is equal to systemic pressure) and thereby makes heart failure extremely uncommon.

When the obstruction is severe and the ventricular septum is intact, a right-to-left shunt will often occur at the atrial level through a patent foramen ovale. Accordingly, patients with this condition may have a varying degree of cynosis. The presence of cyanosis indicates a relatively severe degree of valvular obstruction.

Clinical Findings

A. Symptoms and Signs: The history depends upon the severity of the obstruction. Patients with a mild or even a moderate degree of valvular pulmonary stenosis are completely asymptomatic throughout infancy, childhood, and adolescence. Patients with a more severe type of valvular obstruction may develop cyanosis and congestive heart failure very early—even in the neonatal period. Hypoxemic spells characterized by a sudden onset of marked cyanosis and dyspnea are much less common than in tetralogy of Fallot.

Patients with mild to moderate obstruction are acyanotic. Patients with severe or critical stenosis usually show evidence of central cyanosis. These patients are usually well developed and well nourished. They often have a round face and widely spaced eyes. The pulses are normal and equal throughout. Clubbing may occur in severe cases in which cyanosis has persisted for a long time. On examination of the heart, there may be prominence of the precordium. A heaving impulse of the right ventricle can frequently be palpated. A systolic thrill is often palpated in the pulmonary area and occasionally in the suprasternal notch. The first heart sound is normal. In patients with mild to moderate stenosis, a prominent ejection click of pulmonary origin is heard best at the second left intercostal space. This click varies with respiration. It is much more prominent during expiration than inspiration. In patients with severe stenosis, the click tends to merge with the first heart sound. The second heart sound also varies with the degree of stenosis. In mild valvular stenosis, the second heart sound is normally split and the pulmonary component is normal in intensity. In moderate degrees of obstruction, the second heart sound is more widely split and the pulmonary component is softer. In severe pulmonary stenosis, the second heart sound is single, since the pulmonary component cannot be heard. An ejection type, rough, obstructive systolic murmur is best heard at the second interspace at the left sternal border. It radiates very well to the back. No diastolic murmurs are audible. In older children, a prominent "A" wave is seen in the jugular venous pulse. If there is congestive heart failure, the liver is enlarged.

B. X-Ray Findings: In the mild form of pulmonary stenosis, the heart may be normal in size. Poststenotic dilatation of the main pulmonary artery segment and the left pulmonary artery is often present. In moderate to severe cases, there may be a slight right ventricular enlargement and there may or may not be poststenotic dilatation of the main pulmonary artery. In patients who are cyanotic, the pulmonary vascular markings are decreased; otherwise, they are normal.

C. Electrocardiography: Electrocardiographic findings are usually normal in patients with mild obstruction. Right ventricular hypertrophy is present in patients with moderate to severe valvular obstruction. In severe obstruction, right ventricular hypertrophy and the right ventricular strain pattern (deep inversion of the T wave) are seen in the right precordial leads. In the most severe form, right atrial hypertrophy is also present. Right axis deviation is also seen in the moderate to severe forms. Occasionally, the axis is greater than +180 degrees.

D. Echocardiography: M mode echocardiography reveals atrial contraction and elevated right ventricular diastolic pressure causing early opening of the pulmonary valve (ie, opening prior to the onset of ventricular systole). The pulmonary valve appears to be unusually echo-dense. The pulmonary valve image on 2-dimensional echocardiography shows a thickened structure with less than normal excursion.

E. Cardiac Catheterization and Angiocardiography: There is no increase in oxygen saturation or oxygen content in the right side of the heart. In the more severe cases, there is a right-to-left shunt at the atrial level. Pulmonary artery pressure is normal in milder cases and quite low in moderately severe to severe cases. Right ventricular pressure is always higher than pulmonary artery pressure. The gradient across the pulmonary valve varies from 10 to 200 mm Hg. In severe cases, the right atrial pressure is often elevated, with a predominant "A" wave. Cineangiocardiography with injection of contrast material into the right ventricle shows thickening of the pulmonary valve and the very narrow opening of the pulmonary valve. This produces a "jet" of contrast from the right ventricle into the pulmonary artery. Infundibular hypertrophy may be present. This is seen as a marked narrowing of the right ventricular outflow track during ventricular systole followed by a widening during diastole.

Treatment

Elective valvotomy is recommended for children with right ventricular pressures of greater than 50 mm Hg or higher than two-thirds of systemic pressure. Immediate correction is indicated for patients with systemic or greater right ventricular pressure. Percutaneous balloon valvuloplasty can also be performed to relieve the valvular obstruction.

The need for additional surgical resection of associated infundibular hypertrophy is controversial. Because additional surgery increases the risk and because the outflow obstruction usually regresses, many centers perform only the valvotomy.

Course & Prognosis

Patients with mild pulmonary stenosis live a normal life and have a normal life span. Those with stenosis of moderate severity usually show symptoms of easy fatigability and dyspnea on exertion, which may be progressive. Those with severe valvular obstruction may develop severe cyanosis and congestive heart failure in early life.

Postoperative follow-up suggests that most patients with right ventricular pressure equal to or less than systemic pressure who were treated surgically early in life have good voluntary maximum exercise capacity. Physical restriction is unwarranted in these patients.

Edwards BS et al: Morphologic changes in the pulmonary arteries after percutaneous balloon angioplasty for pulmonary artery stenosis. *Circulation* 1985;**71:**195.

Griffith BP et al: Pulmonary valvulotomy alone for pulmonary stenosis: Results in children with and without muscular infundibular hypertrophy. *J Thorac Cardiovasc Surg* 1982;**83:** 577.

Kan JS et al: Percutaneous balloon valvuloplasty: A new method for treating congenital pulmonary valve stenosis. *N Engl J Med* 1982;**307:**540.

2. INFUNDIBULAR PULMONARY STENOSIS WITHOUT VENTRICULAR SEPTAL DEFECT

Pure infundibular pulmonary stenosis is rare. One should suspect infundibular pulmonary stenosis where there is evidence of mild to moderate pulmonary stenosis and intact ventricular septum and (1) no pulmonary ejection click is audible and (2) the murmur is maximal in the third and fourth intercostal spaces rather than in the second intercostal space. Otherwise, the clinical picture may be identical.

3. DISTAL PULMONARY STENOSIS

Supravalvular Pulmonary Stenosis

Supravalvular pulmonary stenosis, a relatively rare condition, is due to coarctation of the body of the main pulmonary artery. The clinical picture may be identical with that of valvular pulmonary stenosis, although the murmur is maximal in the first intercostal space at the left sternal border and in the suprasternal notch. No ejection click is audible. A second heart sound is usually narrowly split, and the pulmonary component is quite loud as a result of closure of the pulmonary valve under high pressure. The murmur radiates extremely well into the neck and over the lung fields.

Peripheral Pulmonary Branch Stenosis

In peripheral pulmonary branch stenosis, there are multiple small coarctations of the branches of the pulmonary artery in the periphery of the lung. Systolic murmurs may be heard over both lung fields, both anteriorly and posteriorly. The transient pulmonary branch stenosis murmurs of infancy (previously described under heart murmurs) are innocent. Pulmonary artery branch stenosis murmurs may be the most audible murmurs in atrial septal defects in infancy and early childhood. The most common cause of significant pulmonary artery branch stenosis is maternal rubella. Several types of supravalvular aortic stenosis syndromes may be found in association with this condition.

Surgery is often unsuccessful. Transvenous angioplasty is currently being assessed but does not appear to be as efficacious in patients with peripheral pulmonary branch stenosis as in patients with pulmonary valvular stenosis.

Absence of a Pulmonary Artery

Absence of a pulmonary artery may be an isolated malformation or may occur in association with other congenital heart diseases. It is occasionally seen in patients with tetralogy of Fallot.

Dunkle LM, Rowe RD: Transient murmur simulating pulmonary artery stenosis in premature infants. *Am J Dis Child* 1972;**124:**666.

Lock JE et al: Balloon dilatation angioplasty of hypoplastic and stenotic pulmonary arteries. *Circulation* 1983;**67:**962.

MALFORMATIONS ASSOCIATED WITH OBSTRUCTION TO BLOOD FLOW ON THE LEFT SIDE OF THE HEART

1. COARCTATION OF THE AORTA

Essentials of Diagnosis

- Pulse lag in lower extremities.
- Blood pressure of 20 mm Hg or pressure greater in upper than in lower extremities.
- Blowing systolic murmur in left axilla.

General Considerations

Coarctation is a common cardiac abnormality accounting for about 6% of all cases of congenital heart disease. Three times as many males as females are affected. In the vast majority of cases, coarctation occurs in the thoracic portion of the descending aorta. The abdominal aorta is very rarely involved. Coarctations are usually in the juxtaductal position rather than the pre- or postductal position. The term **coarctation of aorta syndrome** is a useful concept, since most symptomatic infants will have associated patent ductus arteriosus, tubular hypoplasia of the aortic isthmus (frequently erroneously termed a coarctation), ventricular septal defect, and bicuspid aortic valve. The tubular hypoplasia of the aortic isthmus is probably related to paucity of blood flow in the fetus and often spontaneously enlarges with postnatal growth.

Clinical Findings

A. Symptoms and Signs: Patients with coarctation may or may not have cardiovascular symptoms in infancy, childhood, and adolescence. Congestive heart failure may develop in early infancy, and symptoms of decreased exercise tolerance and fatigability may appear in childhood.

The important physical finding is diminution or absence of femoral pulses. However, a significant number of infants will initially have equal upper and lower extremity pulses until the coexistent patent ductus arteriosus closes. Normally, the blood pressure in the upper extremities is slightly higher than in the lower extremities during the first few months of life. After 1 year of age, blood pressure higher in the arms than in the legs is suggestive of coarctation of the aorta. The actual level of blood pressure in the arms may be only moderately elevated, even in severe coarctation, or it may be significantly elevated. In the presence of severe congestive heart failure, the differences in pulses in the upper and lower extremities may not be readily apparent, but with compensation, the pulses in the arms are palpably stronger than those of normal infants; the pulses in the legs remain diminished or absent in affected infants. The left subclavian artery is occasionally involved in the coarctation, in which case the left brachial pulse is weak. If the coarctation is uncomplicated, the heart sounds are normal. The aortic component of the second heart sound is occasionally increased in intensity. An ejection systolic murmur of grade II/VI intensity is often heard at the aortic area and the lower left sternal border. The pathognomonic murmur of coarctation is heard in the interscapular area of the back, over the area of the coarctation. This murmur is usually systolic in timing. If the coarctation is complicated by other malformations, murmurs associated with these other abnormalities will be audible.

B. X-Ray Findings: In the older child, the heart may be normal in size, although there is usually some evidence of left ventricular enlargement. The ascending aorta is usually normal in size. On barium swallow, the esophagus has a characteristic E shape. The first arc of the E is due to dilatation of the aorta just proximal to the coarctation. The second arc is due to poststenotic dilatation of the aorta. The middle bar of the E is due to the coarctation itself. In older children, notching or scalloping of the ribs caused by marked enlargement of the intercostal collaterals can be seen.

In infants in congestive heart failure, there is evidence of marked cardiac enlargement and pulmonary venous congestion.

C. Electrocardiography: ECGs in children may be normal or may show evidence of slight left ventricular hypertrophy. In infants with or without congestive heart failure, the ECG usually demonstrates right ventricular hypertrophy.

D. Echocardiography: M mode echocardiography reveals only secondary evidence of the coarctation. In infants with congestive heart failure, dilated right and left ventricles are noted. A striking posterior displacement of the mitral valve in the left ventricular cavity with poor excursion is common. Real-time 2-dimensional echocardiography may visualize the coarctation directly.

E. Cardiac Catheterization and Angiocardiography: These studies demonstrate the position, anatomy, and severity of the coarctation and will assess the adequacy of the collateral circulation.

Treatment

Infants with coarctation of the aorta and congestive heart failure require vigorous anticongestive measures. Dilation of the associated patent ductus arteriosus with a constant infusion of prostaglandin E_1 may stabilize the critically ill infant until operation can be performed. Many with isolated coarctation and no associated lesions respond well and do not require surgery in infancy. In infants with striking congestive heart failure and without associated cardiovascular abnormalities, severe systemic hypertension is often a contributing factor. Reduction of afterload with intravenous nitroprusside or propranolol followed by chronic oral propranolol is often lifesaving and allows deferral of definitive correction until a more optimal age.

Infants with associated intracardiac defects sometimes need immediate surgery but frequently require revision of the recoarctation later in life. Modification of the surgical technique utilizing a subclavian flap anastomosis reduces the likelihood of this late complication. This technique has been used successfully in infants weighing as little as 1000 g.

Percutaneous balloon angioplasty has been used successfully as a palliative procedure to stabilize critically ill infants with coarctation of aorta syndrome. It is likely that surgical correction will be necessary after stabilization. Percutaneous balloon angioplasty is also being utilized to dilate recoarctations in postoperative patients.

Patients who do not require surgery early in life may be corrected electively at ages 3–5 years unless significant systemic hypertension develops.

Course & Prognosis

Children who survive the neonatal period without developing congestive heart failure do quite well throughout childhood and adolescence. Fatal complications (eg, hypertensive encephalopathy, intracranial bleeding) occur uncommonly. Subacute infective endocarditis is also rare before adolescence.

School-age children in whom coarctation was corrected during infancy are at significant risk for systemic hypertension and myocardial dysfunction. Careful exercise testing is mandatory prior to their participation in athletic activities.

Starting in the third decade of life, the patient may develop the onset of easy fatigability, dyspnea on exertion, cardiac enlargement, and left ventricular failure. Only one-fourth of these patients may be expected to live through the fourth decade. Death results from subacute infective endocarditis or hypertensive cardiovascular disease.

Hammon JW Jr et al: Operative repair of coarctation of the aorta in infancy: Results with and without ventricular septal defect. *Am J Cardiol* 1985;**55:**1555.

Moss AJ: Coarctation of the aorta: Current status. *J Pediatr* 1983;**102:**253.

Parker BP et al: Preoperative and postoperative renin levels in coarctation of the aorta. *Circulation* 1982;**66:**513.

Stafford MA, Griffiths SP, Gersony WM: Coarctation of the aorta: A study in delayed detection. *Pediatrics* 1982;**69:**159.

2. AORTIC STENOSIS

Essentials of Diagnosis

- Systolic ejection murmur at upper right sternal border.
- Thrill in carotid arteries.
- Systolic click at the apex.
- Dilatation of the ascending aorta on chest x-ray.

General Considerations

Aortic stenosis may be defined from the anatomic or physiologic point of view. Anatomically, it consists of an obstruction to the outflow from the left ventricle at or near the aortic valve. Physiologically, aortic stenosis may be defined as a condition in which a systolic pressure gradient of more than 10 mm Hg exists between the left ventricle and the aorta. Aortic stenosis accounts for approximately 5% of all cases of congenital heart disease. Anatomically, congenital aortic stenosis may be divided into 4 types:

A. Valvular Aortic Stenosis (75%): Critical aortic stenosis presenting in infancy usually consists of a unicuspid diaphragmlike structure without well-defined commissures. Preschool and school-age children more commonly present with a bicuspid valve. Teenagers and young adults characteristically present with tricuspid but partially fused leaflets. This lesion is more common in males than females.

B. Discrete Membranous Subvalvular Aortic Stenosis (20%): This consists of a membranous or fibrous ring just below the aortic valve. The ring forms a diaphragm with a hole in the middle and results in obstruction to left ventricular outflow. The aortic valve itself and the anterior leaflet of the mitral valve are often deformed.

C. Supravalvular Aortic Stenosis: In this variety, there is a constriction of the ascending aorta just above the coronary arteries. This condition is often associated with a family history, abnormal facies, and mental retardation (idiopathic hypercalcemia syndrome).

D. Idiopathic Hypertrophic Subaortic Stenosis (IHSS): In this case, there is a marked hypertrophy of the entire left ventricle and, predominantly, the ventricular septum. With contraction of the ventricle, the hypertrophic portion of the septum, together with the mitral valve, causes obstruction of left ventricular outflow. A family history is often present.

Obstruction to outflow from the left ventricle causes the left ventricle to work harder to maintain an adequate pressure and flow in the systemic arterial circuit, resulting in hypertrophy of the left ventricle and increased oxygen requirement. If the stenosis is severe, the oxygen requirements may exceed the capacity of the coronary arteries to supply oxygen, and relative coronary insufficiency may develop. In critical aortic stenosis, left ventricular failure may occur. The left ventricle is usually able to adapt to the increased pressure load for a considerable period of time before heart failure or coronary insufficiency develops.

Clinical Findings

A. Symptoms and Signs: Most patients with aortic stenosis have no cardiovascular symptoms. Except in the most severe cases, the patient may do well up until the third to fifth decade of life, although some patients have mild exercise intolerance and easy fatigability. A small percentage of patients have significant symptoms within the first decade, ie, dizziness and syncope. Sudden death, although uncommon, may occur in all forms of aortic stenosis, with the greatest risk being idiopathic hypertrophic subaortic stenosis.

Although isolated valvular aortic stenosis seldom causes symptoms in infancy, severe heart failure occasionally occurs when critical obstruction is present. The response to medical management is poor; therefore, an aggressive surgical approach is recommended.

The physical findings vary somewhat depending upon the anatomic type of lesion:

1. Valvular aortic stenosis—Affected patients are well developed and well nourished. The pulses are usually normal and equal throughout. If the stenosis is severe and there is a gradient of greater than 80 mm Hg, the pulses are small with a slow upstroke. Examination of the heart reveals a left ventricular thrust at the apex. A systolic thrill at the right base, the suprasternal notch, and both carotid arteries accompanies moderate disease. If only one carotid artery manifests a thrill, it is the right carotid (usually seen in milder disease).

The first heart sound is normal. A prominent aortic type ejection click or ejection sound is best heard at the apex. Very frequently, this click can be heard at the lower left sternal border and at the aortic area. It is separated from the first heart sound by a short but appreciable interval. It does not vary with respiration. The second heart sound at the pulmonary area is physiologically split. The aortic component of the second heart sound is of good intensity. There is a grade III–V/VI, rough, medium- to high-pitched ejection type systolic murmur, loudest at the first and second intercostal spaces, which radiates well into the suprasternal notch and along the carotids. The murmur also radiates fairly well down the lower left sternal border and can be heard at the apex. The murmur transmits to the neck, and its grade correlates roughly with the severity of the stenosis.

2. Discrete membranous subvalvular aortic stenosis—The findings are essentially the same as those of valvular aortic stenosis. Absence of an aortic ejection click is an important differentiating point, and the thrill and murmur are usually somewhat more intense at the left sternal border in the third and fourth intercostal spaces than at the aortic area. Frequently, however, the murmur is equally intense at both areas. A diastolic murmur of aortic insufficiency is commonly heard after 5 years of age.

3. Supravalvular aortic stenosis—Affected patients often have abnormal facies and are mentally retarded. The thrill and murmur are characteristically best heard in the suprasternal notch and along the carotids, although they are well transmitted over the aortic area and near the mid left sternal border. A difference in pulses and blood pressure between the right and left arms may be found, with the more prominent pulse and pressure in the right arm.

4. Asymmetric septal hypertrophy—The murmur in this case is ejection in quality, grade II–III/VI, and heard from the left sternal border toward the apex and sometimes associated with a murmur of mitral insufficiency. There is often an atrial fourth heart sound with a diastolic murmur. No ejection click is audible. The arterial pulse wave has a rapid upstroke and frequently a bisferious quality.

B. X-Ray Findings: In most cases, the heart is not enlarged. The left ventricle, however, is slightly prominent. In valvular and discrete subvalvular aortic stenosis, dilatation of the ascending aorta is frequently seen (more commonly in the former). The ascending aorta is usually normal in idiopathic hypertrophic subaortic stenosis and in supravalvular aortic stenosis.

C. Electrocardiography: There is some correlation between the severity of the obstruction and the ECG. Patients with mild aortic stenosis have normal ECGs. Patients with severe obstruction frequently demonstrate evidence of left ventricular hypertrophy and left ventricular strain, but many do not. In about 25% of severe cases, the ECG is normal. Progressive increase in left ventricular hypertrophy on serial ECGs indicates a significant degree of obstruction. Left ventricular strain is taken as a potential indication for operation.

D. Echocardiography: This has become a reliable noninvasive technique for the initial diagnosis and follow-up evaluation of idiopathic hypertrophic subaortic stenosis. It also provides clues to the progression of other forms of aortic stenosis. Cross-sectional echocardiography holds promise for a more precise noninvasive method for assessment of severity of valvular disease.

E. Cardiac Catheterization and Angiocardiography: Left heart catheterization demonstrates the pressure differential between the left ventricle and the aorta and the level at which the gradient exists. Patients with severe aortic stenosis may be asymptomatic and have normal ECGs and chest x-rays. Serial cardiac catheterization is frequently the only reliable guide to the progression and the severity of the lesion. In the case of valvular aortic stenosis, an asymptomatic patient with a resting gradient of

60–80 mm Hg is considered to require surgery. In the face of symptoms, patients with lesser gradients are surgical candidates. Cineangiocardiography is helpful in demonstrating the level of the obstruction.

Treatment

Because the results of surgery are too frequently unsatisfactory, surgical repair should only be considered in patients with symptoms or a large resting gradient (60–80 mm Hg). In many cases, the gradient can only be moderately to minimally relieved without producing aortic insufficiency (which is potentially more harmful than the lesion for which surgery was undertaken). Discrete subvalvular aortic stenosis requires a lesser gradient for surgical intervention, since continued trauma to the aortic valve by the subvalvular jet may destroy the valve. Unfortunately, simple resection is followed by recurrence in more than 25% of patients with subvalvular aortic stenosis. Asymmetric septal hypertrophy has even less satisfactory results than muscle resection; therefore, medical management with propranolol should be tried initially.

Patients for whom surgery is not strongly indicated should have close follow-up, and those over age 6 years should undergo yearly exercise testing. If exercise testing is normal, restriction of physical activity may not be necessary in patients with mild to moderate aortic stenosis; in many cases, these patients may participate in competitive sports.

Course & Prognosis

All forms of left ventricular outflow tract obstruction tend to be progressive diseases. However, regression of the obstruction has been documented in a few patients with supravalvular obstruction. Pediatric patients with left ventricular outflow tract obstruction—with the exception of those with critical aortic stenosis of infancy—are usually asymptomatic. Symptoms accompanying severe unoperated obstruction (angina, syncope, and congestive heart failure) are all rare currently because of detection and surgical intervention. The vast majority of children without asymmetric septal hypertrophy are not only asymptomatic but also tend to have the personality and capabilities to compete in sports. There is increasing evidence that pre- or postoperative children whose obstruction is mild to moderate have above-average oxygen consumption and maximum voluntary working capacity. Children in this category with normal findings on resting and exercising ECG and normal heart size may safely participate in vigorous physical activity, including nonisometric competitive sports.

Flaker G et al: Supravalvular stenosis. *Am J Cardiol* 1983;**51:**256.

Jones M, Barnhart GR, Morrow AG: Late results after operations for left ventricular outflow tract obstruction. *Am J Cardiol* 1982;**50:**569.

Waldman JD et al: The obstructive subaortic conus. *Circulation* 1984;**70:**339.

3. MITRAL VALVE PROLAPSE

Essentials of Diagnosis

- Midsystolic click best heard with patient in standing or squatting position.
- Occasional late systolic murmur.

General Considerations

Mitral valve prolapse is the most common entity to present with abnormal auscultatory findings in pediatric patients. It is secondary to redundant valve tissue or abnormal tissue comprising the mitral valve apparatus. The mitral valve prolapses, moving posteriorly or superiorly into the left atrium during ventricular systole. A systolic click occurs at the time of this movement and is the clinical hallmark of this entity. Mitral insufficiency may occur late in systole, causing an atypical, short, late systolic murmur with variable radiation. It is most commonly found in individuals with the following characteristics: over 6 years of age, female, slender habitus, and bony thoracic abnormalities. Its incidence is estimated to vary from 2 to 20%, with the higher part of the range representing incidence in slender teenage females.

Clinical Findings

A. Symptoms and Signs: The vast majority of patients with mitral valve prolapse are asymptomatic. Chest pain, palpitations, and dizziness are reported, but it is not clear whether or not these symptoms are more common in affected patients than in the normal population. Significant dysrhythmias are uncommon, and true exercise intolerance is rare. The standard approach to auscultation must be modified to diagnose mitral valve prolapse; ie, auscultation should be performed with the patient placed in various positions. Clicks with or without systolic murmur are more commonly elicited in the standing and squatting positions than in the supine and sitting positions. The systolic click occurs earlier in children than in adults; ie, it tends to be midsystolic rather than late systolic. Although it is usually heard at the apex, it may be audible at the left sternal border or even occasionally may be panthoracic. A midsystolic or systolic murmur following the click implies mitral insufficiency and is much less common than isolated prolapse. The murmur tends to be atypical for mitral insufficiency in that it is not pansystolic and radiates to the sternum rather than to the left axilla. A coexistent diastolic murmur of relative or real mitral stenosis is rare. Occasionally, a systolic "honk" is heard.

B. X-Ray Findings: In the rare case of significant mitral insufficiency, the left atrium may be enlarged; this is visualized best on lateral film x-ray. Most chest x-rays show normal findings, and their use is therefore largely unwarranted.

C. Electrocardiography: Despite the fact that flat or inverted T waves in precordial lead V_6 have been reported, almost all electrocardiographic findings are normal. Disabling chest pain is rare and should be assessed with ergometric electrocardiography.

D. Echocardiography: Significant posterior systolic movement of the posterior mitral valve leaflet is considered diagnostic. Many false-positive results are due to multiple leaflet images (chevroning) or to the presence of insignificant (small duration and amplitude) posterior systolic valve movement. False-negative results are also common, partly owing to performance of the procedure when the patient is in the supine position. If the physical findings are typical for isolated prolapse, echocardiography is not warranted.

E. Cardiac Catheterization and Angiography: Invasive procedures are very rarely indicated.

Treatment & Prognosis

Use of oral propranolol may be effective in rare cases of disabling chest pain. Prophylaxis for subacute infectious endocarditis is indicated only in individuals with associated mitral insufficiency.

The natural course of disease is largely unknown. Twenty years of observation indicate, however, that mitral valve prolapse in childhood is a largely benign entity. It merges with a common variation from normal in slender children and is associated with an asthenic body build that presumably results from altered geometry of the left ventricle and mitral valve.

Barlow JB, Pocock WA: Billowing, floppy, prolapsed or flail valves? *Am J Cardiol* 1985;**55:**501.

Barlow JB, Pocock WA, Obel IWP: Mitral valve prolapse: Primary, secondary, both or neither? *Am Heart J* 1981;**102:**140.

Worth DC et al: Prevalence of mitral valve prolapse in normal children. *J Am Coll Cardiol* 1985;**5:**1173.

4. OTHER CONGENITAL VALVULAR LESIONS

Congenital Mitral Stenosis

In this rare disorder, the valve leaflets are thickened and fused to produce a diaphragmlike or funnellike structure with an opening in the center. Frequent associated malformations include subaortic and aortic stenosis and coarctation of the aorta. This lesion complex is known as Shone's syndrome. Most patients develop symptoms early in life. Early symptoms include tachypnea, dyspnea, and severe failure to thrive. Physical examination reveals a regular sinus rhythm. The first heart sound is accentuated, and the pulmonary closure sound is loud. No opening snap can be heard. In most cases, a presystolic crescendo murmur is heard at the apex. Occasionally, only a middiastolic murmur can be heard. Rarely, no murmur at all is heard. Electrocardiography shows right axis deviation, biatrial enlargement, and right ventricular hypertrophy. X-ray reveals evidence of left atrial enlargement and, frequently, pulmonary venous congestion. Echocardiography shows abnormal valve structures with reduced excursion and left atrial enlargement. Cardiac catheterization reveals an elevated pulmonary capillary pressure and wedge pressure and pulmonary hypertension.

Surgical treatment, including valve replacement with a prosthetic mitral valve, has become possible even in infants weighing 3–5 kg.

Cor Triatriatum

This is an extremely rare abnormality in which the pulmonary veins enter a separate chamber rather than pass directly into the left atrium. The chamber communicates with the left atrium through an opening of variable size. The physiologic consequences of this condition are very similar to those of mitral stenosis. The clinical findings depend upon the size of the opening. If the opening is extremely small, symptoms develop very early in life. If the opening is large, patients may be asymptomatic for a considerable period of time. Echocardiography may reveal a hard shadow in the left atrium. Cardiac catheterization may be diagnostic. Finding a high pulmonary capillary pressure (high pulmonary venous pressure) and a low left atrial pressure (if the catheter can be passed through the foramen ovale into the true left atrial chamber) makes the diagnosis certain. Angiocardiographic studies may identify 2 "left atrial" chambers.

Surgical repair is usually successful.

Congenital Mitral Regurgitation

This is a relatively rare abnormality that is usually associated with other congenital heart lesions, including corrected transposition of the great vessels, endocardial cushion defect, and endocardial fibroelastosis. Uncomplicated congenital mitral regurgitation is very rare. It is sometimes present in patients with Marfan's syndrome. Occasionally, there is a congenital dilatation of the valve ring with an otherwise normal valve. In other cases, the chordae tendineae are malformed, resulting in mitral regurgitation.

Congenital Aortic Regurgitation

The most common causes of this disorder are bicuspid aortic valve, either uncomplicated or with coarctation of the aorta; ventricular septal defect and aortic insufficiency; and fenestration of the aortic valve cusp (one or more holes in the cusp).

Absence of the Pulmonary Valve

This rare abnormality is usually associated with ventricular septal defect. In about 50% of cases, severe infundibular pulmonary stenosis is present (tetralogy of Fallot).

Ebstein's Malformation of the Tricuspid Valve

This uncommon abnormality consists of downward displacement of the tricuspid valve such that the greater portion of the valve is attached to the ventricular wall rather than to the fibrous ring. As a result, the upper portion of the right ventricle is within the right atrium. The portion of the ventricle below the apex of the tricuspid valve is very small and represents the true functioning right ventricle. Clinically, there is a wide spectrum of abnormalities ranging from relative absence of symptoms to death in early infancy. The severity depends upon the degree of malattachment of the valve and the associated abnormalities. Echocardiography is useful in diagnosis.

Silver MA et al: Late clinical and hemodynamic results after either tricuspid valve replacement or annuloplasty for Ebstein's anomaly of the tricuspid valve. *Am J Cardiol* 1984;**54:**672.

Smith WM et al: The electrophysiologic basis and management of symptomatic recurrent tachycardia in patients with Ebstein's anomaly of the tricuspid valve. *Am J Cardiol* 1982;**49:**1223.

MYOCARDIAL DISEASES

Myocardial diseases are characterized by significant cardiac enlargement. Murmurs may or may not be present. Electrocardiographic changes include left ventricular hypertrophy, ST depression, and T wave inversion.

1. GLYCOGEN STORAGE DISEASE OF THE HEART

At least 10 types of glycogen storage disease are recognized. The type that primarily involves the heart is known as Pompe's disease. The deficient enzyme (acid maltase) is necessary for hydrolysis of the outer branches of glycogen, and its absence results in marked deposition of glycogen within the myocardium. Cardiac glycogenosis is a rare heritable (autosomal recessive) disorder.

Affected infants are usually normal at birth, but onset commonly begins by the sixth month of life. These children have a history of retardation of growth and development, feeding problems, poor weight gain, and then the findings of heart failure. Physical examination reveals generalized muscular weakness, a large tongue, cardiomegaly, no significant heart murmurs, and, occasionally, evidence of congestive heart failure. Chest x-rays reveal marked cardiomegaly with or without pulmonary venous congestion. The ECG shows a short PR interval with left ventricular hypertrophy and shows ST depression and T wave inversion over the left precordial leads. Echocardiography shows extremely thick ventricular wall structures.

Children with this disease usually die within the first year of life. Death may be sudden or due to progressive congestive heart failure.

2. ANOMALOUS ORIGIN OF THE LEFT CORONARY ARTERY

In this condition, the left coronary artery arises from the pulmonary artery rather than from the aorta. In the neonatal period, while the pulmonary arterial pressure is relatively high, blood is supplied to the left ventricle from the pulmonary artery. Accordingly, during this period the child is asymptomatic and does well. However, within the first 2 months of life, the pulmonary arterial pressure decreases to normal. This results in a marked decrease of flow to the left coronary artery. Infarction of the heart usually occurs. If the patient survives, collateral channels appear that join the peripheral branches of the right with the branches of the left coronary artery. As a result, the direction of blood flow in the left coronary artery changes. Whereas previously there was some flow from the pulmonary artery into the myocardium through the left coronary, flow now occurs from the right coronary artery through the collateral into the left coronary artery and then into the pulmonary artery. In essence, then, an arteriovenous fistula is formed that further removes blood from the myocardium. This results in further myocardial infarction and fibrosis. Death occurs eventually as a result of marked dilatation of the heart and congestive heart failure. At autopsy, the left ventricle is found to be markedly fibrosed and thin.

Clinical Findings

A. Symptoms and Signs: Patients appear to be normal at birth. Growth and development are relatively normal for a few months, although detailed questioning of the parents often discloses a history of intermittent episodes of severe abdominal pain, pallor, and sweating, especially during or after feeding. These episodes are thought to be secondary to "colic," and attacks are similar to anginal attacks in adults.

On physical examination, the patients are usually well developed and well nourished. The pulses are usually weak but equal throughout. The heart is enlarged but not very active. A murmur of mitral regurgitation is frequently present, although no murmur may be heard.

B. X-Ray Findings: Chest x-rays show significant cardiac enlargement with or without pulmonary venous congestion.

C. Electrocardiography: The ECG is usually diagnostic. There are T wave inversions in leads I and aVL. The precordial leads show T wave inversions from V_{4-7}. Deep Q waves are often seen in leads I, aVL, and V_{4-6}. These findings of myocardial infarction are similar to those in adults.

D. Echocardiography: The diagnosis can be made with 2-dimensional techniques by visualizing a single large right coronary artery arising from the aorta.

E. Cardiac Catheterization and Angiocardi-

ography: A small left-to-right shunt (a result of the flow of blood from the right through the left coronary artery into the pulmonary artery) can often be detected at the pulmonary artery level. Frequently, however, the shunt is very small and can be detected only by the most sensitive techniques, eg, by the use of a hydrogen electrode catheter. Cineangiocardiography following injection of contrast material into the root of the aorta shows absence of origin of the left coronary artery from the aorta. A huge right coronary artery fills directly from the aorta, and the contrast material will flow through the right coronary system into the left coronary arteries and finally into the pulmonary artery.

Treatment & Prognosis

Treatment remains controversial. Medical management with anticongestives and afterload reduction is advocated by some. Lengthy operations requiring cardiopulmonary bypass to effect 2 functional coronary arteries from the aorta have a high death rate in critically ill infants. Simple ligation of the left coronary artery or subclavian to coronary artery anastomosis (without cardiopulmonary bypass) should be considered for the most critically ill infants. More complex operations should only be considered for the more stable infants or older children.

The prognosis is guarded. No therapeutic modality has been shown to be superior in follow-up studies of survivors.

Midgley A et al: Repair of anomalous origin of the left coronary artery in the infant and small child. *J Am Coll Cardiol* 1984;**4:**1231.

3. ENDOCARDIAL FIBROELASTOSIS

The incidence of endocardial fibroelastosis has decreased dramatically over the past 2 decades, and this entity is now uncommon. The cause is not known, although intrauterine infection with mumps or coxsackievirus B has been suggested.

Pathologic examination discloses a marked milky white thickening of the endocardium, the subendocardial layers of the left ventricle, and, usually, the left atrium. The mitral valve is frequently involved also. The myocardial fibers themselves are fibrotic and disorganized, and associated hypervascularization is common. Serial sections often show coexistent evidence of myocarditis. Thus, endocardial fibroelastosis appears to be part of a continuum of primary endomyocardial diseases and may be a sequela to myocarditis.

Clinical Findings

A. Symptoms and Signs: Patients appear normal at birth, and growth and development during early infancy are normal. About half develop symptoms within the first 5 months of life, and most are symptomatic by age 1. An occasional patient may have no symptoms until age 5.

The symptoms and signs that do develop are associated with left ventricular heart failure. These include dyspnea, easy fatigability, feeding difficulties, and, eventually, findings of left and right heart failure.

On physical examination, these children are often small and undernourished. The heart is usually enlarged, and the heart tones are poor (when there is evidence of decompensation). A murmur of mitral regurgitation may be present.

B. X-Ray Findings: Chest x-rays show generalized cardiac enlargement with or without pulmonary venous congestion.

C. Electrocardiography: The ECG almost always shows evidence of left ventricular hypertrophy and, quite frequently, ST depression and T wave inversion. If there has been pulmonary hypertension secondary to left heart failure, right ventricular hypertrophy may be present. Right atrial hypertrophy is sometimes present. Complete heart block is occasionally seen.

D. Echocardiography: M mode and 2-dimensional techniques reveal dilatation of cardiac chambers and echo-dense endocardial images indicating decreased myocardial function.

E. Cardiac Catheterization and Angiocardiography: Catheterization reveals the absence of left-to-right shunts. Pulmonary hypertension may be present. Cineangiocardiography demonstrates diminished myocardial contractility.

Treatment & Prognosis

Treatment of endocardial fibroelastosis is medical and consists of adequate and prolonged use of digitalis and oral diuretics. If response to the usual dose is not satisfactory, the dosage of both digitalis and diuretics should be increased until a satisfactory response is noted or toxicity occurs. Afterload reduction would appear to be rational therapy for infants with this disease. Continue these agents for several years.

Some children appear to improve initially with treatment but then develop recurrent bouts of heart failure. Complete recovery in such patients is very infrequent, and most eventually die with intractable congestive heart failure. The prognosis is most favorable in patients who present between 6 months and 3 years of age and respond promptly to treatment.

Hutchins GM, Vie SA: The progression of interstitial myocarditis to idiopathic endocardial fibroelastosis. *Am J Pathol* 1972;**66:**483.

MUCOCUTANEOUS LYMPH NODE SYNDROME

Mucocutaneous lymph node syndrome, also known as Kawasaki disease, was first described in Japan in 1967. The acute illness is characterized by (1) prolonged fever (over 5 days) that is unresponsive to antibiotics; (2) conjunctivitis; (3) cracking and fissuring of the lips, with inflammation of mucous membranes; (4) cervical lymphadenopathy; (5) rash involving the trunk and extremities, with reddened palms and soles of the hands and feet and subsequent desquamation of tips of the toes and fingers; and (6) edema. Patients may also have associated arthritis. Thrombocytosis and increased sedimentation rate are seen on laboratory examination.

Cardiovascular complications during the acute illness include myocarditis, pericarditis, and arteritis that predisposes to aneurysm formation in the coronary arteries in approximately 20% of patients. Aneurysm formation may occur 7–45 days after the onset of illness. Acute myocardial infarction may occur during the acute illness secondary to thrombosis of these aneurysms. Death occurs in 1–2% of patients during this phase of the illness. Long-term follow-up of patients with aneurysms shows some resolution of aneurysms in half of those affected; the remainder may continue to have aneurysms, may develop stenosis, and, possibly later, may develop myocardial ischemia.

During the acute illness and for 2–3 months after, patients should be monitored closely by serial electrocardiography, chest x-ray, and M mode and 2-dimensional echocardiography. Selective coronary angiography is recommended in all patients to determine the extent of the disease.

Patients with acute illness are treated with moderate to high doses of aspirin until they become afebrile. Low doses of aspirin (3–5 mg/kg/d) are then used as antiplatelet therapy until the aneurysms are resolved or coronary arteries are demonstrated to be normal. Evidence of myocardial infarction warrants early cardiac catheterization and coronary bypass surgery if obstruction exists.

Burns JC et al: Coagulopathy and platelet activation in Kawasaki syndrome: Identification of patients at high risk for development of coronary artery aneurysms. *J Pediatr* 1984;**105:**206.

Kato H et al: Fate of coronary aneurysms in Kawasaki disease: Serial coronary angiography and long-term follow-up study. *Am J Cardiol* 1982;**49:**1758.

Melish ME, Hicks RV, Reddy V: Kawasaki syndrome: An update. *Hosp Pract* (March) 1982;**17:**99.

Multiple outbreaks of Kawasaki syndrome—United States. *MMWR* (Jan) 1985;**34:**33.

Satomi G et al: Systematic visualization of coronary arteries by two-dimensional echocardiography in children and infants: Evaluation in Kawasaki's disease and coronary arteriovenous fistulas. *Am Heart J* 1984;**107:**497.

CYANOTIC HEART DISEASE

TETRALOGY OF FALLOT

Essentials of Diagnosis

- Cyanosis after the neonatal period.
- Hypoxemic spells during infancy.
- Right-sided aortic arch in 25%.
- Systolic ejection murmur at upper left sternal border.

General Considerations

In Fallot's tetralogy, there is a ventricular septal defect and severe obstruction to right ventricular outflow such that the intracardiac shunt is predominantly from right to left. This is the most common type of cyanotic heart lesion, accounting for 10–15% of all cases of congenital heart disease. The ventricular defect is usually located in the membranous portion of the septum but may be totally surrounded by muscular tissue and is usually quite large. Obstruction to right ventricular outflow may be solely at the infundibular level (50–75%), at the valvular level alone (rarely), or at both levels (25% or more). The term tetralogy has been used to describe this combination of lesions, since there is always associated right ventricular hypertrophy and a varying degree of "overriding of the aorta." The overriding is present because of the position of the ventricular septal defect in relation to a dilated and often dextroposed aorta. These 2 factors (right ventricular hypertrophy and overriding aorta) plus the major lesions make up the tetralogy. A right-sided aortic arch is present in 25% of cases and an atrial septal defect in 15%.

Severe obstruction to right ventricular outflow plus a large ventricular septal defect results in a right-to-left shunt at the ventricular level and desaturation of the arterial blood. The degree of desaturation and the extent of cyanosis depend upon the size of the shunt. This in turn is dependent upon the resistance to outflow from the right ventricle, the size of the ventricular septal defect, and the systemic vascular resistance. The greater the obstruction, the larger the ventricular septal defect, and the lower the systemic vascular resistance, the greater the right-to-left shunt. Although the patient may be deeply cyanotic, the amount of pressure the right ventricle can develop is limited to that of the systemic (aortic) pressure. In other words, right ventricular pressure cannot exceed left ventricular pressure. The right ventricle is usually quite able to maintain this level of pressure without developing heart failure.

Clinical Findings

A. Symptoms and Signs: The clinical findings vary depending upon the degree of right ventricular outflow obstruction. Patients with a mild degree of obstruction are only minimally cyanotic or acyanotic and may even present initially with congestive heart failure. Those with maximal obstruction are deeply cyanotic from birth. However, few children are asymptomatic; most have cyanosis by 4 months of age; and the cyanosis usually is progressive. Growth and development are retarded, and easy fatigability and dyspnea on exertion are common. Squatting is seen when the children become old enough to walk.

Hypoxemic spells (cyanotic spells) are characterized by the following signs and symptoms: (1) sudden onset of cyanosis or deepening of cyanosis; (2) sudden onset of dyspnea; (3) alterations in consciousness, encompassing a spectrum from irritability to syncope; and (4) decrease in intensity or disappearance of the systolic murmur. These episodes may begin in the neonatal period and continue until nearly school age. It is unusual, however, for the initial episode to occur after 2 years of age. Acute treatment of cyanotic spells consists of giving oxygen and placing the patient in the knee-chest position. Acidosis, if present, should be corrected with intravenous sodium bicarbonate. Morphine sulfate should be administered cautiously by a parenteral route in a dosage of 0.1 mg/kg. Propranolol, 0.1–0.2 mg/kg intravenously, has been found to be useful. Chronic (daily) treatment of cyanotic spells with propranolol, 1 mg/kg orally every 4 hours while awake, remains controversial; however, in a significant number of patients, this regimen has prevented subsequent "spells" and made it possible to delay operation until total correction can be performed.

Patients with tetralogy are usually small and thin. The degree of cyanosis is variable. The fingers and toes show varying degrees of clubbing depending upon the age of the child and the severity of the cyanosis.

On examination of the heart, a right ventricular lift is palpable. No thrills are present. The first sound is normal; occasionally, there is an ejection click at the apex that is aortic in origin. The second sound is single and best heard at the lower left sternal border between the third and fourth intercostal spaces. The second heart sound at the pulmonary area is soft; however, aortic closure is loud and heard best in the third and fourth intercostal spaces at the left sternal border. There is a grade I–III/VI, rough, ejection type systolic murmur that is maximal at the left sternal border in the third intercostal space. This murmur radiates over the anterior and posterior lung fields. Diastolic murmurs are not present.

B. Laboratory Findings: The hemoglobin, hematocrit, and red blood count are usually mildly to markedly elevated, depending upon the degree of arterial oxygen desaturation.

C. X-Ray Findings: Chest x-rays reveal the overall heart size to be normal, and indeed the x-ray may sometimes be interpreted as being entirely normal. However, the right ventricle is hypertrophied, and this is often shown in the posteroanterior projection by an upturning of the apex (boot-shaped heart). The main pulmonary artery segment is usually concave, and the aorta in 25% of cases arches to the right. The pulmonary vascular markings are usually decreased.

D. Electrocardiography: The cardiac axis is to the right, ranging from +90 to +180 degrees. The P waves are usually normal, although there may be evidence of slight right atrial hypertrophy. Right ventricular hypertrophy is always present, but right ventricular strain patterns are rare.

E. Echocardiography: M mode and 2-dimensional techniques reveal thickening of the free right ventricular wall, with overriding of the aorta and a membranous ventricular septal defect. In addition, obstruction at the level of the infundibulum and pulmonary valve may be seen.

F. Cardiac Catheterization and Angiocardiography: Cardiac catheterization reveals the absence of a significant left-to-right shunt, although the hydrogen electrode curve may be positive in the right ventricle. There is arterial blood desaturation of varying degree. The right-to-left shunt exists at the ventricular level. The right ventricular pressure is at systemic levels, and the pressure contour in the right ventricle is almost identical with that of the left ventricle. The pulmonary artery pressure is extremely low (mean ranges of 5–10 mm Hg). The gradients and pressure may be noted at the valvular level, the infundibular level, or both. The catheter frequently is passed from the right ventricle into the overriding ascending aorta.

Cineangiocardiography is diagnostic. Injection of contrast material into the right ventricle reveals the right ventricular outflow obstruction and the right-to-left shunt at the ventricular level.

Treatment

A. Palliative Treatment: Palliative treatment is recommended for very small infants who are markedly symptomatic (severely cyanotic, frequent severe anoxic spells) and in whom complete correction would be difficult or impossible. It may be medical (chronic oral β-blocking agents) or, more often, surgical (creation of a systemic arterial to pulmonary arterial anastomosis).

The earliest procedure employed for this disease (Blalock-Taussig) consists of an anastomosis between the subclavian artery and the pulmonary artery. It is usually done on the side opposite the aortic arch. A synthetic anastomosis between the ascending aorta and the main pulmonary artery may be performed.

B. Total Correction: Total correction of tetralogy of Fallot is performed under the cardiopulmonary bypass. It involves opening the right ventricle, closing the ventricular septal defect, and removing the obstruction to right ventricular outflow. The surgical death rate varies from 2 to 15%. The major limiting anatomic feature of total correction is the size of the pulmonary artery and its branches. Children who survive the operation are markedly improved. There is complete disappearance of cyanosis, and clubbing disappears shortly thereafter. Growth and development improve markedly, and these patients often become asymptomatic within a short period of time. However, these patients remain at risk for sudden death due to dysrhythmias. Currently, major cardiovascular centers are performing total correction for virtually all infants with this condition, including newborns.

Course & Prognosis

Infants with the most severe form of the disease are usually deeply cyanotic at birth. Hypoxemic spells may occur during the neonatal period. Death is extremely rare during a severe hypoxemic spell. Many patients who survive the first year of life seem to improve. This may be due to the development of systemic-to-pulmonary collateral vessels. Although hypoxemic spells may decrease in severity, these children remain deeply cyanotic and markedly limited in their activity. They seldom survive the second decade of life without surgical treatment.

Infants with moderate obstruction to right ventricular outflow do fairly well. Although cyanosis is present in very early life, it is usually not severe. The cyanosis may progress in severity, and anoxic spells may occur. These patients do fairly well in later childhood, but their condition progressively deteriorates during the second and third decades of life. Death occurs by the third decade as a result of cerebrovascular accidents, brain abscess, subacute infective endocarditis, anoxia, or pulmonary hemorrhage.

Patients with the mildest form of the disease are said to have the "acyanotic" variety. The degree of obstruction is very mild, and the right-to-left shunt is small. Very frequently, there is a predominant left-to-right shunt. However, the degree of obstruction often increases as the patient gets older. This, combined with the increased activity, results in progressively worsening cyanosis. Many of these patients live relatively normal lives without severe symptoms. Life expectancy, however, is definitely decreased, and death usually occurs by the third to fourth decade.

In school-age children, complete repair usually results in fair to good function, although patients are occasionally subject to sudden death from dysrhythmias.

Edmonds LH, Stephenson LW, Gadzck JP: The Blalock-Taussig anastomosis in infants younger than 1 week of age. *Circulation* 1980;**62:**597.

Garson A Jr, Gillette PC, McNamara DG: Propranolol: The preferred palliation for tetralogy of Fallot. *Am J Cardiol* 1981;**47:**1098.

Garson A Jr et al: Prevention of sudden death after repair of tetralogy of Fallot. *J Am Coll Cardiol* 1985;**6:**221.

PULMONARY ATRESIA WITH VENTRICULAR SEPTAL DEFECT

This condition consists of complete atresia of the pulmonary valve in association with ventricular septal defect. Essentially it is an extreme form of tetralogy of Fallot. Since there is no flow outward from the right ventricle into the pulmonary artery, the pulmonary blood flow must be derived either from a patent ductus arteriosus or from collateral channels.

The clinical picture depends entirely upon the size of the ductus or the collateral channels (or both). If they are large, patients may do quite well and actually do better than those with severe tetralogy of Fallot. If effective pulmonary blood flow is small, death occurs secondary to severe anoxia early in life. This may occur suddenly with postnatal closure of a patent ductus arteriosus.

Echocardiography or cardiac catheterization and angiocardiography are diagnostic. If patent ductus arteriosus dependency is established, a prostaglandin E_1 infusion to dilate the patent ductus arteriosus may help stabilize the patient until surgery.

Infants who are severely hypoxemic require urgent systemic to pulmonary anastomosis in order to provide sufficient oxygenated blood to the body.

A corrective surgical procedure that has been successful in patients with adequate-sized pulmonary arteries consists of bypassing the obstructed right ventricular outflow and closing the ventricular septal defect.

Olin CL et al: Pulmonary atresia: Surgical considerations and results in 10 patients undergoing definitive repair. *Circulation* 1976;**54(Suppl 3):**35.

PULMONARY ATRESIA WITH INTACT VENTRICULAR SEPTUM

Essentials of Diagnosis

- Cyanosis at birth.
- Continuous murmur.
- Chest x-ray with concave pulmonary artery segment and apex tilted upward.

General Considerations

In this uncommon condition, the pulmonary valve is absent and is replaced by a small diaphragm consisting of the fused cusps. The ventricular septum is intact. The main pulmonary artery segment is somewhat hypoplastic but almost always patent. In the type 1 deformity (80%), the cavity volume of the right ventricle is extremely small and the wall is thickened and fibrotic. In type 2, the right ventricular cavity is frequently of normal size.

During intrauterine life, if the tricuspid valve is intact and normal, very little blood enters the right ventricle, since there is no outlet for this chamber. Almost all of the blood passes through the foramen ovale directly into the left side of the heart. In the type 2 deformity, there is usually an outlet for the right ventricle (tricuspid valve insufficiency), and the right ventricle receives a sufficient quantity of blood to permit it to develop in a relatively normal fashion.

Following birth, the pulmonary circulation is maintained primarily by a patent ductus arteriosus. Although a bronchial pulmonary collateral network is present, it is usually insufficient to maintain the pulmonary circulation. Accordingly, whether or not the patients live depends upon the patency of the ductus arteriosus. The ductus usually remains open for only a short period of time. As it closes, hypoxia becomes progressively more severe, and death eventually occurs.

Clinical Findings

A. Symptoms and Signs: Patients may be normal at birth, although they are usually cyanotic. Cyanosis becomes progressively more severe and is associated with severe dyspnea. A blowing systolic murmur due to the associated patent ductus arteriosus may be heard at the pulmonary area and under the left clavicle. In type 2 deformity, a loud pansystolic murmur due to the tricuspid insufficiency is heard at the lower left sternal border. Not infrequently, the liver is pulsating.

B. X-Ray Findings: Chest x-rays show a markedly enlarged heart with marked decrease in pulmonary vascular markings. With striking tricuspid insufficiency, right atrial enlargement may be massive and the cardiac silhouette may virtually fill the chest.

C. Electrocardiography: Electrocardiography reveals an axis that is usually normal in the frontal plane. Evidence for right atrial enlargement is usually striking. Voltage criteria for other chamber enlargement are variable.

D. Echocardiography: M mode or 2-dimensional echocardiography shows absence of the pulmonary valve, with varying degrees of hypoplasia of the right ventricular cavity.

E. Cardiac Catheterization and Angiocardiography: The diagnosis can be made on cardiac catheterization and cineangiocardiography. Right ventricular pressure is very high (greater than systemic). A cineangiocardiogram following injection of contrast material into the right ventricle reveals absence of filling of the pulmonary artery from the right ventricle. It also demonstrates the size of the right ventricular chamber and the presence or absence of tricuspid regurgitation, and right ventricular sinusoids that drain into the coronary arteries may fill.

Treatment & Prognosis

As in pulmonary atresia with ventricular septal defect, a prostaglandin E_1 infusion is useful in stabilizing the patient and maintaining patency of the ductus until surgery can be performed. Surgery should be undertaken as soon as the diagnosis is made by cardiac catheterization. A Rashkind atrial septostomy is performed to open up the communication across the atrial septum and permit adequate flow in both directions. Subsequent surgical approaches vary widely. In cases of type 1 deformity, it is necessary to immediately establish a surgical aorticopulmonary anastomosis (usually a Blalock-Taussig shunt). Later in infancy, a communication between the right ventricle and pulmonary artery should be created in an attempt to stimulate right ventricular cavity growth. In cases of type 2 deformity, a closed valvotomy may be all that is necessary initially, with a more definitive reconstruction of the right ventricular outflow tract accomplished at a later date.

The prognosis is unpredictable for patients with type 1 or type 2 deformity who survive the surgery. In type 1 patients, the dimensions of the right ventricle can increase significantly after the initial procedure.

de Leval M et al: Pulmonary atresia and intact ventricular septum: Surgical management based on a revised classification. *Circulation* 1982;**66:**272.

Lewis AB, Wells W, Lindesmith GG: Evaluation and surgical treatment of pulmonary atresia and intact ventricular septum in infancy. *Circulation* 1983;**67:**1318.

O'Connor WN et al: Pulmonary atresia with intact ventricular septum and ventriculocoronary communications. *Circulation* 1982;**65:**805.

TRICUSPID ATRESIA

Essentials of Diagnosis

- Marked cyanosis present from birth.
- ECG with left axis deviation, right atrial enlargement, and left ventricular hypertrophy.

General Considerations

This relatively rare condition (< 1% of cases of congenital heart disease) is characterized by complete atresia of the tricuspid valve. As a result, no direct communication exists between the right atrium and right ventricle.

Tricuspid atresia may be divided into 2 types depending upon the relationship of the great vessels:

Type 1. Without transposition of the great arteries: (a) No ventricular septal defect. Hypoplasia or atresia of the pulmonary artery. Patent ductus arteriosus. (b) Small ventricular septal defect. Pulmonary stenosis. Hypoplastic pulmonary artery. (c) Large ventricular septal defect and no pulmonary stenosis. Normal-sized pulmonary artery.

Type 2. With transposition of the great arteries: (a) With ventricular septal defect and pulmonary stenosis. (b) With ventricular septal defect but without pulmonary stenosis.

Since there is no direct communication between the right atrium and right ventricle, the entire systemic venous return must flow through the atrial septum (either an atrial septal defect or patent foramen ovale) into the left atrium. Accordingly, the left atrium receives both the systemic venous return and the pulmonary venous return. Complete mixing occurs in the left atrium, resulting in a greater or lesser degree of arterial desaturation.

As a result of this lack of direct communication, the development of the ventricle depends upon the presence of a left-to-right shunt at the ventricular level. Therefore, severe hypoplasia of the right ventricle occurs in those forms in which there is no ventricular septal defect or in which the ventricular septal defect is very small.

Clinical Findings

A. Symptoms and Signs: In the great majority of patients with tricuspid atresia, symptoms develop very early in infancy. Except in cases in which the pulmonary blood flow is great, cyanosis is present at birth. Growth and development are very poor, and there is usually easy fatigability on feeding, tachypnea, dyspnea, anoxic spells, and evidence of right heart failure. Patients with marked increase in pulmonary blood flow (types 1c and 2b) will develop evidence of left heart failure as well.

Clubbing is present if the child is old enough. On examination of the heart, a slight bulge on the right side of the sternum may occasionally be seen. The first heart sound is normal. The second heart sound is most often single (owing to aortic closure). A murmur is usually present, although it is variable. It ranges from grade I to grade III/VI in intensity and usually is a harsh blowing murmur heard best at the lower left sternal border.

B. X-Ray Findings: Chest x-rays are variable. The heart may be slightly to markedly enlarged. The main pulmonary artery segment is usually small or absent. The size of the right atrium varies from huge to only moderately enlarged, depending upon the size of the communication at the atrial level. The pulmonary vascular markings are usually decreased, although in types 1c and 2b they are increased.

C. Electrocardiography: The ECG is usually helpful. It often shows a left axis deviation with a counterclockwise loop in the frontal plane. The P waves are tall and peaked, indicative of right atrial hypertrophy. The size of the P wave depends upon the right atrial pressure, which in turn depends upon the size of the interatrial communication (the taller the P wave, the smaller the communication). Left ventricular hypertrophy or left ventricular preponderance is found in almost all cases. Voltage over the right precordium is usually low.

D. Echocardiography: M mode or 2-dimensional methods are diagnostic and show absence of the tricuspid valve.

E. Cardiac Catheterization and Angiocardiography: This reveals the marked right-to-left shunt at the atrial level and desaturation of the left atrial blood. Because of the complete mixing in the left atrial chambers, oxygen saturation in the left ventricle, right ventricle, pulmonary artery, and aorta is identical to that in the left atrium. The right atrial pressure is increased. Left ventricular and systemic pressures are normal. The catheter cannot be passed through the tricuspid valve from the right atrium to the right ventricle. The course of the catheter is always from right atrium into left atrium and from there into left ventricle.

Cineangiocardiography following injection of contrast material into the right atrium is diagnostic. It reveals the lack of communication of the right atrium with the right ventricle and the right-to-left shunt at the atrial level.

Treatment & Prognosis

In infants with high pulmonary artery flow, conventional anticongestive therapy should be given until the infant begins to outgrow the ventricular septal defect. At that point, a Fontan procedure (connection of right atrium to right ventricle or pulmonary artery) should be considered.

In infants with extremely low pulmonary artery flow, prostaglandin E_1 should be infused until an aorticopulmonary shunt can be performed. The Fontan procedure is rapidly gaining acceptance as the "corrective" procedure of choice. The optimal timing is controversial, but the procedure has been performed successfully in infants under 1 year of age at our institution.

The prognosis for all patients with tricuspid atresia depends on achieving a balance of pulmonary blood flow that permits adequate oxygenation of the tissues without producing intractable congestive heart failure. For children treated by the Fontan procedure, the prognosis is as yet undefined; initial results are moderately encouraging.

Disessa TG et al: Systemic venous and pulmonary arterial flow patterns after Fontan procedure for tricuspid atresia or single ventricle. *Circulation* 1984;**70:**898.

Nishioka K et al: Left ventricular volume characteristics in children with tricuspid atresia before and after surgery. *Am J Cardiol* 1981;**47:**1105.

Sanders SP et al: Clinical and hemodynamic results of Fontan operation for tricuspid atresia. *Am J Cardiol* 1982;**49:**1733.

HYPOPLASTIC LEFT HEART SYNDROME

Hypoplastic left heart syndrome includes a number of conditions in which there are either valvular or vascular lesions on the left side of the heart, resulting in hypoplasia of the left ventricle.

The lesions that make up this syndrome are mitral atresia, aortic atresia, or both. In all of these conditions, there is severe obstruction to either filling or emptying of the left ventricle. As a result, during intrauterine life, the quantity of blood filling the left ventricle is extremely small, resulting in hypoplasia of this chamber. Following birth, there is marked impairment of the circulation because of the very small size of the left ventricle and the presence of obstructing lesions. Congestive heart failure develops rapidly, in most cases within several days to 3 months of life.

Patients with aortic atresia develop congestive heart failure very early, usually within the first week. Death occurs earliest in this group. Patients with mitral atresia who have large atrial and ventricular communications may live longer. Some patients have lived beyond the first decade. Patients with involvement of the aortic arch usually die within 1 month or less.

The clinical picture depends upon the type of obstructing lesion. Cyanosis is usually present early in life and is usually generalized. Patients with hypoplasia or atresia of the aortic arch may show differential cyanosis. Murmurs may or may not be present and are usually nondiagnostic. Congestive heart failure develops early.

Chest x-rays usually are relatively normal at birth. Rapid and progressive cardiac enlargement then occurs, frequently associated with pulmonary venous congestion. These changes occur earliest in patients with aortic atresia.

The ECG usually demonstrates right axis deviation, right atrial hypertrophy, and right ventricular hypertrophy with relative paucity of left ventricular forces and absence of a Q wave in V_6.

Echocardiography is usually diagnostic and often eliminates the need for cardiac catheterization. A diminutive aorta and left ventricle with a poorly defined mitral valve in the presence of a normal and easily definable tricuspid valve are diagnostic.

During the past several years, a 2-stage complex surgical approach to palliation of aortic atresia has been advocated. Although not widely tried, this extremely high-risk approach offers some small hope for patients with aortic atresia.

Lang P, Norwood WI: Hemodynamic assessment after palliative surgery for hypoplastic left heart syndrome. *Circulation* 1983,68.104.

COMPLETE TRANSPOSITION OF THE GREAT ARTERIES

Essentials of Diagnosis

- Cyanotic newborn without respiratory distress.
- More common in males.

General Considerations

Complete transposition of the great vessels is the second most common variety of cyanotic congenital heart disease, accounting for about 16% of all cases. The male/female ratio is 3:1. It is due to an embryologic abnormality in the spiral division of the truncus arteriosus.

The aorta is located anterior to the pulmonary artery—either directly anterior or to the left or right. The pulmonary artery usually ascends parallel to the aorta rather than crosses it. In most cases, associated intracardiac abnormalities are present. These include ventricular septal defect, atrial septal defect, pulmonary stenosis, and patent ductus arteriosus. Obstructive changes within the pulmonary arteriolar bed are common in patients past infancy.

Transposition of the great vessels can be classified as follows:

Group 1. Transposition with intact ventricular septum: (a) Without pulmonary stenosis or (b) with pulmonary stenosis, subvalvular or valvular (or both).

Group 2. Transposition with ventricular septal defect: (a) With pulmonary tenosis, (b) with pulmonary vascular obstruction, or (c) without pulmonary vascular obstruction (normal pulmonary vascular resistance).

Since the aorta arises directly from the right ventricle, life would not be possible unless there were mixing between the systemic and pulmonary circulations; oxygenated blood from the pulmonary veins must in some way reach the systemic arterial circuit. In patients with intact ventricular septum (group 1), mixing occurs at the atrial and also at the ductal levels. However, in most patients, these communications are small, and the ductus arteriosus often closes shortly after birth. These patients are therefore severely cyanotic, and congestive heart failure occurs rapidly as a result of the marked increase in cardiac output. Patients with a ventricular septal defect show greater or lesser degrees of cyanosis depending upon the ratio of the pulmonary to systemic blood flow. Patients with ventricular septal defect and pulmonary stenosis (group 2a) are usually severely cyanotic because of the limited blood flow to the lungs. Patients with ventricular septal defect and pulmonary vascular obstruction (group 2b) show a moderate degree of cyanosis. Patients with ventricular septal defect and normal pulmonary vascular resistance (group 2c) show the least cyanosis but often develop heart failure very early because of the enormous pulmonary blood flow

Congestive heart failure develops not only because of the high cardiac output but also because of the poor oxygenation of the myocardium and the presence of systemic pressure in both ventricles.

Clinical Findings

A. Symptoms and Signs: Many of the neonates are quite large, some weighing 4 kg (9 lb) at birth, and most are cyanotic at birth, although cyanosis occasionally does not develop until later. Patients in groups 1 and 2a are most cyanotic; those in group 2c are least cyanotic. Retardation of growth and development after the neonatal period is common. Congestive heart failure occurs in patients in groups 1 and 2c. Patients in group 2a show no evidence of congestive heart failure but often have severe anoxic spells in early life; if they survive the first year of life, retardation of growth and development is common and cyanosis becomes progressively more severe. However, intellectual development may be unaffected.

Although these infants are usually large at birth, growth and development are retarded; thus, when they reach age 6 months to 1 year, they are usually below the third percentile in both height and weight. Cyanosis is marked. Clubbing is present in children over age 1. The findings on cardiovascular examination depend somewhat upon the intracardiac defects. Group 1a patients have only soft murmurs or none at all. The first heart sound is usually normal. The second heart sound is single and accentuated and is best heard at the lower left sternal border. Patients in group 1b have loud obstructive systolic murmurs that are maximal at the second and third intercostal spaces and the left sternal border, radiating well to the first and second intercostal spaces. Group 2a patients have a murmur of pulmonary stenosis (obstructive systolic murmur at the base of the heart, best heard to the right of the sternum). Those in group 2c have a systolic murmur along the lower sternal border and a mitral diastolic flow murmur at the apex.

B. X-Ray Findings: In the sick, blue newborn,

at a time when any diagnostic clues are greatly appreciated, the chest x-ray in transposition is often very nonspecific. In fact, at any age, the so-called characteristic findings may be lacking.

C. Electrocardiography and Echocardiography: Early in infancy, the ECG is usually of little positive help. It reveals the usual amount of right ventricular hypertrophy expected for age. The absence of positive findings of other lesions, such as left axis deviation of tricuspid atresia, provides some deductive information. Abnormal relationships of the great vessels by echo are suggestive of a lesion in the transposition group.

D. Cardiac Catheterization and Angiocardiography: Cardiac catheterization has a dual purpose in this malformation: diagnosis and therapy. The sequence is usually to enter the right ventricle and immediately record a contrast medium injection on videotape and ciné. As soon as the cardiologist has confidently demonstrated that complete transposition of the great arteries exists and that there are 2 well-developed ventricles, a Rashkind septostomy is performed.

Treatment

It has become increasingly apparent at many pediatric cardiology centers throughout the world that survival of patients with transposition of the great arteries depends on early, aggressive management.

A. Cardiac Catheterization: A routine for all types of transposition is as follows:

1. Newborn period—Diagnostic and therapeutic cardiac catheterization should be performed as soon as the patient achieves as much stability as the clinical course indicates is possible. The therapeutic part of the catheterization is, of course, the Rashkind balloon septostomy, which enlarges the atrial septal communication by repeatedly pulling a dye-filled balloon across the foramen ovale, tearing the septum. In patients with persistent significant hypoxia (P_{O2} < 20–25 mm Hg), administration of prostaglandin E_1 has been found to cause an immediate improvement in oxygenation, presumably owing to a decrease in pulmonary vascular resistance. We have found, however, that if the arterial pH remains constant, oxygenation virtually always improves spontaneously in several days.

2. At 4–6 months—Repeat the catheterization (with catheterization of the pulmonary artery to assess progression of pulmonary vascular obstruction), determine the presence or absence of left ventricle outflow obstruction, and repeat the Rashkind septostomy if indicated.

3. At 8–10 months—Repeat the catheterization if definitive surgery has not taken place before this time.

B. Complete Surgical Correction:

1. Elective surgery—All patients with favorable anatomic and hemodynamic criteria should be offered corrective surgery by 6 months of age. Surgery currently involves insertion of an intra-atrial baffle (by either a Mustard or a Senning operation) to redirect systemic and pulmonary venous blood to the appropriate pulmonary and aortic ventricles.

2. Early surgery—Certain patients, especially those with rapidly rising pulmonary artery pressures (with or without ventricular septal defect) and those with rapidly progressing left venticular outflow obstruction, may require surgical intervention as early as 1–2 weeks to 6 months of age (after the second cardiac catheterization). In patients with transposition, it is not uncommon for a ventricular septal defect to close spontaneously, depriving the patient of the necessary mixing of systemic and pulmonary circulations. A patent ductus arteriosus has not proved to be an asset in some cases and has inhibited atrial level mixing (despite an adequate atrial septostomy), necessitating ligation and early intra-atrial baffling.

3. Late surgery—Some patients, especially those in group 2a (ie, patients with ventricular septal defect and pulmonary stenosis), may have had early or relatively late development of severe left ventricular-pulmonary outflow obstruction. This is not ideally amenable to a Mustard correction but may be more suitable for a Rastelli operation (an aortic homograft from left ventricle to pulmonary arteries).

4. Palliative surgical correction—Open atrial septectomy and aorticopulmonary shunts may be used under special circumstances, but the trend is to perform early total correction whenever possible.

5. Anatomic correction—Since 1975, surgical techniques to "switch" the great vessels to their anatomically appropriate locations have undergone a painful and slow evolution. A key feature in the development of techniques has been careful patient selection. The left ventricular musculature in this entity rapidly loses its muscle mass and potential to meet systemic afterload unless a large ventricular septal defect or left ventricular outflow obstruction occurs; consequently, newborns with either of these conditions are appropriate candidates. The incidence of death from this type of surgery has fallen from 80% to approximately 25%. Although the death rate following an intra-atrial baffling procedure is considerably less, there is growing concern about the long-term ability of an anatomic right ventricle to function as a systemic circulation pump. During the next several years, many institutions will begin using anatomic correction techniques in selected patients.

Bical GR et al: Anatomic correction of transposition of the great arteries associated with ventricular septal defect. *Circulation* 1984;**70:**891.

Hurwitz RA et al: Radionuclide angiography in evaluation of patients after repair of transposition of the great arteries. *Am J Cardiol* 1982;**49:**761.

Park SC et al: Hemodynamic function after the Mustard operation for transposition of the great arteries. *Am J Cardiol* 1983;**51:**1514.

ORIGIN OF BOTH GREAT VESSELS FROM THE RIGHT VENTRICLE

In this rare malformation, the aorta is completely transposed, but the pulmonary artery occupies a relatively normal position. Accordingly, both great vessels arise from the right ventricle. Ventricular septal defect is present in all cases and provides the only outlet for the left ventricle.

This malformation may be divided into 5 types on the basis of the relationship of the ventricular septal defect to the great arteries and the presence or absence of pulmonary stenosis: (1) ventricular septal defect related to the aorta, (2) ventricular septal defect related to the pulmonary artery (Taussig-Bing type), (3) ventricular septal defect committed to both great vessels, (4) ventricular septal defect uncommitted to the great vessels, and (5) ventricular septal defect related to the aorta, with pulmonary stenosis (tetralogy of Fallot type).

The clinical and laboratory features depend on which of the 5 anatomic types occurs. Two-dimensional echocardiography has proved to be extremely important in the diagnosis and classification of this entity.

Surgical correction is most satisfactory in patients with ventricular septal defect related to the aorta and is effected by closing the defect and creating a tunnel from the left ventricle to the aorta via the patch. Correction of uncommitted defects or defects related to the pulmonary artery requires patch closure and directing the blood to the pulmonary artery, thereby creating a transposition of the great vessels and an associated interatrial rerouting procedure. The use of a valved external conduit may be necesssary in the complex varieties.

Pitlick P et al: Results of intraventricular baffle procedure for ventricular septal defect and double outlet right ventricle or d-transposition of the great arteries. *Am J Cardiol* 1981;**47:**307.

TOTAL ANOMALOUS PULMONARY VENOUS RETURN WITH OR WITHOUT OBSTRUCTION

Essentials of Diagnosis

- Mild cyanosis.
- Systolic ejection murmur with left sternal border flow rumble and accentuated P_2.
- Right atrial and right ventricular hypertrophy.

General Considerations

This malformation accounts for approximately 2% of all congenital heart lesions. The pulmonary venous blood does not drain into the left atrium but either directly or indirectly (via a systemic venous connection) into the right atrium. Thus, the entire venous drainage of the body drains into the right atrium.

This malformation may be classified according to the site of entry of the pulmonary veins into the right side of the heart.

Type 1 (55%): Entry into the left superior vena cava (persistent anterior cardinal vein) or right superior vena cava.

Type 2: Entry into the right atrium or into the coronary sinus.

Type 3: Entry below the diaphragm (usually into the portal vein).

Type 4: Multiple types of entry.

Since the entire venous drainage from the body drains into the right atrium, a right-to-left shunt is always present at the atrial level. This may take the form either of a large atrial septal defect or a patent foramen ovale. Relatively complete mixing of the systemic and pulmonary venous return occurs in the right atrium, so that the left atrial and hence the systemic arterial saturation levels approximately equal that of the right atrial saturation.

The degree of saturation of the blood (and thus the degree of cyanosis present) is determined by the ratio of the quantity of pulmonary blood flow to that of the systemic blood flow. If pulmonary vascular resistance is normal, the flow of blood into the pulmonary artery is much greater than that into the left side of the heart. In this case, there is much greater return from the pulmonary than from the systemic venous system, and the saturation within the right atrium is high. Affected patients function very well, with relatively normal pulmonary artery pressures, and at least physiologically are very similar to patients with very large atrial septal defects and normal pulmonary venous return.

If pulmonary vascular resistance is elevated, the ratio of pulmonary to systemic blood flow is much lower. When the pulmonary vascular resistance equals that of the systemic vascular resistance, equal amounts of blood flow in both directions. When this occurs, marked desaturation of the mixed blood develops and the patient is markedly cyanotic. Such patients do much less well and eventually develop severe right heart failure.

Clinical Findings

A. With Normal Pulmonary Vascular Resistance: The great majority of patients in this group have some elevation of the pulmonary artery pressure owing to the marked increase in pulmonary blood flow. In most cases, the pressure does not reach systemic levels.

1. Symptoms and signs—These patients may have a history of mild cyanosis in the neonatal period and during early infancy. Thereafter, they do relatively well except for frequent respiratory infections. They are usually rather small and thin and resemble patients with very large atrial septal defects.

Careful examination discloses duskiness of the nail beds and mucous membranes, but definite cyanosis and clubbing are usually not present. The arterial pulses are normal. The jugular venous pulses usually show a significant V wave. Examination of the heart shows left chest prominence. A right ventricular heaving impulse is palpable.

The pulmonary component of the second sound is usually increased in intensity. A grade II–IV/VI ejection type systolic murmur is heard at the pulmonary area. It radiates very well over the lung fields anteriorly and posteriorly. An early to middiastolic flow murmur is often heard at the lower left sternal border in the third and fourth intercostal spaces (tricuspid flow murmur).

2. X-ray findings—Chest x-ray reveals evidence of cardiac enlargement primarily involving the right atrium, right ventricle, and pulmonary artery. There is a marked increase in pulmonary vascular markings. There is often a characteristic contour called a "snowman" or "figure of 8," which is seen where the anomalous veins drain into a persistent left superior vena cava.

3. Electrocardiography—Electrocardiography reveals right axis deviation and varying degrees of right atrial and right ventricular hypertrophy. There is often a QR pattern over the right precordial leads.

4. Echocardiography—Demonstration by echocardiography of a chamber posterior to the left atrium is strongly suggestive of the diagnosis. However, echocardiographic discrimination between anomalies of pulmonary venous return and persistence of pulmonary fetal circulation is still difficult.

B. With Increased Pulmonary Vascular Resistance: This group includes patients in whom the pulmonary veins drain into a systemic venous structure below the diaphragm. It also includes a small number of patients in whom the venous drainage is into a systemic vein above the diaphragm.

1. Symptoms and signs—These infants are usually quite sick. Half die within the first 6 months; most are dead by age 1 year unless treated surgically. Cyanosis is common at birth and is quite evident by 1 week. Another common early symptom is severe tachypnea. Congestive heart failure develops later.

Cardiac examination discloses a striking right ventricular impulse. A shock of the second sound is palpable. The first heart sound is accentuated. The second heart sound is markedly accentuated and single. A grade I–II/VI ejection type systolic murmur is frequently heard over the pulmonary area with radiation over the lung fields. Diastolic murmurs are uncommon. In many cases, no murmur is heard at all.

2. X-ray findings—In the most severe and classic cases, the heart is small and pulmonary venous congestion is marked. In less severe cases, the heart may be slightly enlarged or normal in size, with only slight pulmonary venous congestion.

3. Electrocardiography—The ECG shows right axis deviation, right atrial hypertrophy, and right ventricular hypertrophy.

4. Echocardiography—Echocardiography may demonstrate the combination of a small left atrium and a vessel lying parallel and anterior to the descending aorta and to the left of the inferior vena cava. If this area remains echo-free with a contrast echocardiogram from below, the finding is diagnostic.

5. Cardiac catheterization and angiocardiography—These procedures are diagnostic. Cardiac catheterization demonstrates the presence of total anomalous pulmonary venous return and (usually) the site of entry of the anomalous veins. It also demonstrates the ratio of the pulmonary to systemic blood flow and the degree of pulmonary hypertension and pulmonary vascular resistance.

Cineangiocardiography following injection of contrast material into the right ventricle or pulmonary artery demonstrates the presence of anomalous pulmonary venous return and the site of entry of the anomalous veins. In cases of severe obstruction and a right-to-left patent ductus arteriosus, catheter balloon occlusion of the ductus may be necessary to achieve dense opacification of the pulmonary venous return.

Treatment

If immediate surgical intervention is not contemplated, atrial balloon septostomy should be performed during the initial diagnostic cardiac catheterization. This procedure coupled with vigorous medical management may sustain some infants for several months. Until recently, the surgical death rate in infants was greater than 90%. Within the past few years, however, certain centers have reported excellent results employing either cardiopulmonary bypass or deep hypothermia (cooling to 20 °C [68 °F]). A modification of the anastomosis allowing a larger communication has also greatly improved the surgical results. In such centers, the option of immediate surgical correction may be taken.

Course & Prognosis

Patients with normal pulmonary vascular resistance and only modest elevation of pulmonary artery pressures may do quite well through the second or third decade. Eventually, however, progressive increase in pulmonary vascular resistance and pulmonary hypertension does occur. Patients with increased pulmonary vascular resistance and pulmonary hypertension do poorly, and most die unless treated before age 1 year.

Clarke DR, Paton BC, Stewart JR: Surgical treatment of total anomalous pulmonary venous drainage. *Adv Cardiol* 1979;**26:**129.

Newfeld EA et al: Pulmonary vascular disease in total anomalous pulmonary venous drainage. *Circulation* 1980;**61:**103.

Snider AR et al: Evaluation of infradiaphragmatic total anomalous pulmonary venous connection with two-dimensional echocardiography. *Circulation* 1982;**66:**1129.

PERSISTENT TRUNCUS ARTERIOSUS

Essentials of Diagnosis

- Neonatal cyanosis.
- Systolic ejection click.

General Considerations

Persistent truncus arteriosus probably accounts for less than 1% of all congenital heart malformations. Only one (huge) great vessel arises from the heart and supplies both the systemic and pulmonary arterial beds. It develops embryologically as a result of complete lack of formation of the spiral ridges that divide the fetal truncus arteriosus into the aorta and pulmonary artery. A high ventricular septal defect is always present. The number of valve leaflets varies from 2 to 6, and the valve may be sufficient, insufficient, or stenotic.

The classification most commonly employed is divided into 4 types:

Type 1: One pulmonary artery that arises from the base of the trunk just above the semilunar valve and runs parallel with the ascending aorta (48%).

Type 2: Two pulmonary arteries that arise side by side from the posterior aspect of the truncus (29%).

Type 3: Two pulmonary arteries that arise independently from either side of the trunk (11%).

Type 4: No demonstrable pulmonary artery (12%). Pulmonary circulation is derived from bronchials arising from the descending thoracic aorta. (The existence of this variety of truncus is controversial. Many authorities consider it an extreme form of tetralogy of Fallot with an atretic main pulmonary artery.)

In this condition, blood leaves the heart through a single common exit. Therefore, the saturation of the blood in the pulmonary artery is the same as that in the systemic arteries. The degree of systemic arterial oxygen saturation depends upon the ratio of the pulmonary to systemic blood flow. If pulmonary vascular resistance is normal, the pulmonary blood flow is much greater than the systemic blood flow and the saturation is relatively high. If pulmonary vascular resistance is great, owing either to pulmonary vascular obstruction or to very small pulmonary arteries, pulmonary blood flow is reduced and oxygen saturation is low. The systolic pressures in both ventricles are identical to that in the aorta.

Clinical Findings

A. Symptoms and Signs: The clinical picture varies depending upon the degree of pulmonary blood flow.

1. Large pulmonary blood flow—Patients with large pulmonary blood flow do well and are usually acyanotic, though the nail beds are commonly dusky. They function similarly to patients with large ventricular septal defects and pulmonary hypertension. Examination of the heart reveals a hyperactive impulse, felt both at the apex and over the xiphoid process. A systolic thrill is common at the lower left sternal border. The first heart sound is normal. A loud early systolic ejection click is commonly heard. The second sound is single and accentuated. A grade IV/VI, completely pansystolic murmur is audible at the lower left sternal border. A diastolic flow murmur can often be heard at the apex (mitral flow murmur).

2. Decreased pulmonary blood flow—Patients with decreased pulmonary blood flow have marked cyanosis early and do very poorly. The most common manifestations include retardation of growth and development, easy fatigability, dyspnea on exertion, and congestive heart failure. The heart is not unduly active. The first and second heart sounds are loud. A systolic grade II–IV/VI murmur is heard at the lower left sternal border. No diastolic flow murmur is heard. A continuous heart murmur is very uncommon except in type 4, in which the continuous murmur is due to the large bronchial collateral vessels. A very loud systolic ejection click is commonly heard.

B. X-Ray Findings: Most common are a boot-shaped heart, absence of the main pulmonary artery segment, and a large aorta that frequently arches to the right. The pulmonary vascular markings vary depending upon the degree of pulmonary blood flow.

C. Electrocardiography: The axis is usually normal, though left axis deviation occurs rarely. Evidence of right ventricular hypertrophy or combined ventricular hypertrophy is commonly present. Left ventricular hypertrophy as an isolated finding is rare.

D. Echocardiography: A characteristic tracing would exhibit override of a single great artery (similar to tetralogy of Fallot) without a demonstrable right ventricular infundibulum.

E. Angiocardiography: This procedure is usually diagnostic. Injection of contrast material into the right ventricle demonstrates the presence of a ventricular septal defect and the single vessel arising from the heart. The exact type of truncus, however, may be somewhat difficult to determine even from angiocardiograms. It may occasionally also be difficult to differentiate this condition from pulmonary atresia and ventricular septal defect (pseudotruncus).

Treatment

Anticongestive measures and, in some cases, banding of the pulmonary artery are indicated for patients with high pulmonary blood flow and congestive failure. Aortic homografting for "total correction" of the truncus has been performed in selected patients. During the past several years, the number of severely symptomatic infants undergoing "total correction" in the first 6 months of life has increased.

Course & Prognosis

The outcome depends to a great extent upon the status of the pulmonary circulation. Patients with a low pulmonary blood flow usually do very poorly and die within 1 year. Those with increased pulmonary blood flow can survive for a variable period. A few cases of survival into the third decade have been reported. Death is usually due to congestive heart failure, hypoxia, subacute infective endocarditis, or brain abscess.

Juanida E, Haworth SG: Pulmonary vascular disease in children with truncus arteriosus. *Am J Cardiol* 1984;**54:**1315.

Spicer B et al: Repair of truncus arteriosus in neonates with the use of a valveless conduit. *Circulation* 1984;**70:**26.

DEXTROCARDIA

This lesion consists of right-sided heart with or without reversal of position of other organs (situs inversus). If there is no reversal of other organs, the heart usually has other severe defects. With complete situs inversus, the heart is usually normal.

Apical pulse and sounds are heard on the right side of the chest. X-ray shows the cardiac silhouette on the right side. On electrocardiography, the P waves are usually inverted in lead I; QRS is predominantly down in lead I; and lead II resembles normal lead III and vice versa. Two-dimensional echocardiography is extremely useful in defining the complex anatomy.

With situs inversus and no heart defects, the prognosis is excellent. If severe heart defects are present, definitive diagnosis is imperative, since corrective surgery is frequently beneficial.

Rao FS: Dextrocardia: Systematic approach to differential diagnosis. *Am J Cardiol* 1981;**102:**389.

Van Praagh R, Vlad P: Dextrocardia, mesocardia, and levocardia: The segmental approach to the diagnosis in congenital heart disease. Chap 36, pp 638–695, in: *Heart Disease in Infancy and Childhood,* 3rd ed. Keith JD, Rowe RD, Vlad P (editors). Macmillan, 1978.

ACQUIRED HEART DISEASE

RHEUMATIC FEVER

Rheumatic fever is a disease in transition. Although it is still an important disease in the USA, its frequency has diminished significantly over the past half century. Penicillin is largely responsible, but the decrease in frequency of rheumatic fever was already apparent before the antibiotic era. In the USA and other developed countries in the temperate zone, improvement in standards of living, general hygiene, and opportunities for medical care have greatly reduced the incidence of this disease.

The symptomatic presentation of the disease has also changed significantly in the USA within the past 2 decades. The frequency with which one encounters severe disabling carditis has greatly diminished, and the attack rate of acute rheumatic fever is considerably less than the original estimate of 0.3% in untreated children. Current manifestations of carditis are often mild and transient and require serial examinations by a skilled auscultator to confirm or rule out the diagnosis. One can only speculate on the reasons for these changes in the epidemiologic characteristics of the disease in different communities and on what role, if any, the liberal use of antibiotics may have played.

Group A β-hemolytic streptococcal infection of the respiratory tract is the essential environmental trigger that acts on predisposed individuals. The latest attempts to define host susceptibility implicate immune response (Ir) genes, which are present in approximately 15% of the population. The immune response triggered by colonization of the pharynx with group A streptococci consists of (1) sensitization of B lymphocytes by streptococcal antigens, (2) formation of antistreptococcal antibody, (3) formation of immune complexes that cross-react with cardiac sarcolemma antigens, and (4) myocardial and valvular inflammatory response.

The peak period of risk in the USA is age 5–15 years. The disease is slightly more common in girls and is now more common in blacks, perhaps reflecting socioeconomic factors. The average annual attack rate in the total North American population is less than one per 10,000, and the presence of rheumatic heart disease in the school-age population is less than one per 1000. The annual death rate from rheumatic heart disease in school-age children (whites and nonwhites) recorded a decade ago was less than one per 100,000.

Jones Criteria (Revised) for Diagnosis of Rheumatic Fever

- Major manifestations
  - Carditis
  - Polyarthritis
  - Sydenham's chorea
  - Erythema marginatum
  - Subcutaneous nodules
- Minor manifestations
  - Clinical
    - Previous rheumatic fever or rheumatic heart disease
    - Polyarthralgia
    - Fever
  - Laboratory
    - Acute phase reaction: elevated erythrocyte sedimentation rate, C-reactive protein, leukocytosis
    - Prolonged PR interval

Plus

Supporting evidence of preceding streptococcal infection, ie, increased titers of antistreptolysin O or other streptococcal antibodies, positive throat culture for group A *Streptococcus.*

Traditionally, 2 major or one major and 2 minor criteria (plus supporting evidence of streptococcal infection) justified the presumptive diagnosis of rheumatic fever. However, the major modern dilemma regarding diagnosis is that the physical findings may be so subtle and transient that the criteria are marginal. Since improper diagnosis has lifelong and serious consequences, it is justified to hospitalize patients with marginal findings so that serial clinical studies of the patient, including multiple examinations by a pediatric cardiologist, can be performed. If rheumatic fever appears likely on the basis of appropriate and careful evaluation but does not fully meet the Revised Jones Criteria, the diagnosis of suspect acute rheumatic fever is appropriate. This diagnosis mandates anti-infective prophylaxis but attempts to avoid the social and economic sequelae of the full diagnosis.

Major Manifestations of Rheumatic Fever

A. Active Carditis: Any one of the following—

1. A significant *new* murmur that is clearly mitral insufficiency (with or without a transient apical diastolic Carey-Coombs murmur) or aortic insufficiency. It should be remembered that mitral insufficiency, while commonly caused by rheumatic fever, has many other causes in childhood.

2. Pericarditis, manifested by a pericardial friction rub or evidence of pericardial effusion.

3. Evidence of congestive heart failure.

B. Polyarthritis: Two or more joints must be involved; involvement of one joint does not constitute a major manifestation. The joints may be involved simultaneously or (more diagnostically) in a migratory fashion. The most commonly involved joints are the ankles, knees, hips, wrists, elbows, and shoulders. Heat, redness, swelling, severe pain, and tenderness are usually all present. Arthralgia alone without the other signs of inflammation is not sufficient to meet the criterion of polyarthritis.

C. Subcutaneous Nodules: These are usually seen only in severe cases, and then most commonly over the joints, scalp, and spinal column. They vary from a few millimeters to 2 cm in diameter and are nontender and freely movable under the skin.

D. Erythema Marginatum: While this is a specific and major manifestation of acute rheumatic fever, many physicians fail to distinguish it from other skin lesions. It usually occurs only in severe cases and is rarely an essential diagnostic clue. It consists of a macular erythematous rash with a circinate border and appears primarily on the trunk and extremities. The face is usually not involved.

E. Sydenham's Chorea: Sydenham's chorea is characterized by emotional instability and involuntary movements. These findings become progressively more severe and are often followed by the development of ataxia and slurring of speech. Muscular weakness becomes apparent following the onset of the involuntary movements. The individual attack of chorea is self-limiting, although it may last up to 3 months. It is not uncommon to find involvement on only one side. Manifestations may not be apparent for months to years after the acute episode of rheumatic fever.

Minor Manifestations of Rheumatic Fever

A. Fever: The fever is usually low-grade, although occasionally it reaches 39.4–40 °C (103–104 °F).

B. Polyarthralgia: Pain in 2 or more joints without heat, swelling, and tenderness is a minor rather than a major manifestation.

C. Electrocardiographic Changes: Prolongation of the PR interval represents only a minor manifestation and does not qualify as active carditis.

D. Acute Phase Reaction: The sedimentation rate is accelerated and, more specifically, the C-reactive protein is elevated. Congestive heart failure does not influence the C-reactive protein and usually does not affect the sedimentation rate. Leukocytosis is the rule.

E. History: There is a prior history of acute rheumatic fever or the presence of inactive rheumatic heart disease.

Essential Manifestation

Except in cases of rheumatic fever presenting solely as Sydenham's chorea or long-standing carditis, there should be clear supporting evidence of a streptococcal infection such as scarlet fever, a positive throat culture for group A β-hemolytic *Streptococcus,* and increased antistreptolysin O or other streptococcal antibody titers. The antistreptolysin O titer is significantly higher in rheumatic fever than in uncomplicated streptococcal infections.

Other Manifestations

Associated findings may include erythema multiforme; abdominal, back, and precordial pain; and nontraumatic epistaxis, vomiting, malaise, weight loss, and anemia.

Treatment & Prophylaxis

A. Treatment of the Acute Episode:

1. Anti-infective therapy—Eradication of the streptococcal infection is essential. Benzathine penicillin G is the drug of choice. Depending on the age and weight of the patient, give a single intramuscular injection of 0.6–1.2 million units, or give 125–250 mg orally 4 times a day for 10 days. Erythromycin, 250 mg orally 4 times a day, may be substituted if the patient is allergic to penicillin.

2. Anti-inflammatory agents—

a. Aspirin—Patients with the contemporary form of the disease need significantly less aspirin than in the past. Currently, 30–60 mg/d is given in 4 divided doses; this dosage is often more than sufficient to effect dramatic relief of the arthritis and fever. In general, higher dosages carry a greater risk of side effects, and there are no proved short- or long-term benefits of giving high doses to effect salicylate blood levels of 20–30 mg/dL. The duration of therapy must be tailored to meet the needs of the patient, but use of aspirin for 2–6 weeks, with reduction in dosage toward the end of the course, is usually sufficient.

b. Corticosteroids—Corticosteroids are rarely indicated in current therapy. However, in the unusual patient with severe carditis and manifestations of congestive heart failure (as evidenced by radiographic findings of cardiomegaly or by cardiopulmonary symptoms or a gallop rhythm), therapy may not only be effective but lifesaving. Corticosteroid therapy may be given as follows: prednisone, 2 mg/kg/d orally for 2 weeks (or comparable doses of other corticosteroids); reduce prednisone to 1 mg/kg/d the third week, and begin aspirin, 50 mg/kg/d; stop prednisone at the end of 3 weeks, and continue aspirin for 8 weeks or until the C-reactive protein is negative and the sedimentation rate is falling.

3. Therapy of congestive heart failure—See Congestive Heart Failure, above.

4. Bed rest and ambulation—Strict bed rest is not required for patients with arthritis and mild carditis without congestive heart failure. It is preferable to maintain a regimen of bed-to-chair with bathroom privileges and meals at the table for patients who are relatively asymptomatic while on aspirin therapy. Asymptomatic patients can be kept in bed only under duress anyway. Patients with severe carditis (congestive heart failure) have no desire to get out of bed and should be at bed rest at least as long as corticosteroid therapy is required. *Gradual* indoor ambulation followed by modified outdoor activity may be ordered when symptoms have disappeared but there is still clinical and laboratory evidence of rheumatic activity. Modified bed rest for 2–6 weeks is generally adequate. Children should not return to school while there is clear evidence of rheumatic activity.

B. Treatment After the Acute Episode:

1. Prevention—The patient who has had rheumatic fever has a greatly increased risk of developing rheumatic fever following the next inadequately treated group A β-hemolytic streptococcal infection. *Prevention is thus the most important therapeutic course for the physician to emphasize.* The purpose of follow-up visits after the acute episode is not so much to evaluate the evolution of mitral insufficiency murmurs as to reinforce the physician's advice about the necessity for antibacterial prophylaxis with benzathine penicillin G. At such times, the physician should stress that greater protection is afforded by administration via the intramuscular route than via the oral route and that, in addition, failure to comply with regular oral medication programs increases the risk for recurrence of rheumatic fever. Thus, patients should be informed that the parenteral route will be favored until they are adults, at which time their internists may elect oral medication.

If myocardial or valvular disease persists, antibacterial prophylaxis is a lifelong commitment. More commonly with transient cardiac involvement, 3–5 years of therapy or discontinuance at adolescence is a practical and effective approach.

The following regimens are in current use:

a. Benzathine penicillin G, 1.2 million units intramuscularly every 28 days, is the drug of choice.

b. Sulfadiazine, 500 mg daily as a single oral dose for patients weighing over 27 kg (60 lb), is the drug of second choice. Blood dyscrasias and a lesser effectiveness in reducing streptococcal infections make this drug less satisfactory than benzathine penicillin G.

c. Penicillin G (buffered), 250,000 units orally twice daily, offers approximately the same protection afforded by sulfadiazine but is much less effective than intramuscular benzathine penicillin G (5.5 versus 0.4 streptococcal infections per 100 patient years).

d. Erythromycin, 250 mg orally twice a day, may be given to those patients who may be allergic to both penicillin and sulfonamides.

2. Residual valvular damage—Chronic congestive heart failure may follow a single severe episode of acute rheumatic carditis or, more commonly, may follow repeated episodes. In children in the USA, the usual manifestations of residual valvular damage are heart murmurs of mitral and aortic insufficiency; murmurs are not accompanied by congestive heart failure during most of the pediatric age period *as long as repeated attacks are prevented.*

Methods of managing congestive heart failure have been previously discussed. Children with severe valvular damage who cannot be adequately managed on a medical regimen must be considered for valve replacement—and considered before the myocardium is irreversibly damaged.

Markowitz M: The decline of rheumatic fever. *J Pediatr* 1985;**106:**545.

Zabriskie JB: Rheumatic fever: The interplay between host, genetics, and microbe. *Circulation* 1985;**71:**1077.

RHEUMATIC HEART DISEASE

Mitral Insufficiency

Mitral insufficiency, the most common valvular residual of acute rheumatic carditis, is characterized by a pansystolic murmur that localizes at the apex. In patients with mitral involvement, the murmur appears early in the course of rheumatic carditis, and—depending on the severity of the damage—may disappear over a period of days or months or may persist for life. Although rheumatic fever is a common cause of mitral insufficiency in pediatric patients, the mitral insufficiency murmur cannot be taken as diagnostic of a rheumatic episode.

Among the many other causes of mitral insufficiency, the most common is the mitral dysfunction syndrome, characterized by a mid to late apical systolic murmur introduced by a click.* Other causes are myocarditis, endocardial fibroelastosis, anomalous left coronary artery, and congenital anomalies of the mitral valve, which occur as isolated lesions or as part of a complex of anomalies (eg, endocardial cushion defects). It is thus essential to define the cause of mitral insufficiency in order to provide knowledgeable management—and not to prescribe a lifetime program of rheumatic fever prophylaxis for a patient who has only mitral dysfunction or to fail to provide appropriate surgical treatment if the mitral insufficiency is secondary to an anomalous left coronary artery.

Mitral Stenosis

There are murmurs of mitral stenosis which are secondary to structural stenosis of the valve; those which are due to relative excess of flow (in large volumes of regurgitation); and those which are present during acute valvulitis (Carey-Coombs murmur). Mitral stenosis due to structural stenosis is rarely encountered in the USA before 5–10 years following the first episode of acute rheumatic carditis and is much more commonly discovered in adults than in children. Early mitral stenosis murmurs, flow murmurs, and Carey-Coombs murmurs are short and heard in mid diastole. Established mitral stenosis murmurs become progressively longer in duration until they attain the classic crescendo, presystolic configuration.

Aortic Insufficiency

This early decrescendo diastolic murmur—heard maximally at the secondary aortic area—is not commonly encountered as the sole valvular involvement of rheumatic carditis, as is mitral insufficiency. It is the second most frequent valve affected in polyvalvular as well as in single valvular disease. It appears that the aortic valve is involved more often in males and in blacks. A short aortic systolic murmur due to excess flow may accompany the aortic insufficiency murmur.

Aortic Stenosis

Dominant aortic stenosis of rheumatic origin does not occur in pediatric patients. Aortic stenosis in children is congenital. In one large series, the shortest length of time observed for a patient to develop dominant aortic stenosis secondary to rheumatic heart disease was 20 years.

Vardi P et al: Clinical echocardiographic correlations in acute rheumatic fever. *Pediatrics* 1983;**71**:830.

* A word of caution about diagnosing the mitral dysfunction syndrome: The echocardiographic finding of prolapse (redundancy) of the mitral valve, which characterizes mitral dysfunction, may also be found in patients with acute rheumatic fever and recently acquired rheumatic heart disease.

MYOCARDITIS

In the great majority of cases, the cause of myocarditis is not determined. Coxsackievirus B is the commonest infectious agent isolated. Coxsackievirus A, rubella virus, cytomegalovirus, mumps virus, herpesvirus, adenovirus, and many other viral agents have been implicated. Virtually every other infectious agent, including bacteria, fungi, rickettsiae, chlamydiae, spirochetes, and parasites, has been suggested as a cause of myocarditis, but laboratory confirmation is seldom possible. It is important to emphasize that myocarditis is part of a spectrum of primary endomyocardial diseases and may be one of the causes of endocardial fibroelastosis.

Clinical Findings

A. Symptoms and Signs: The clinical picture usually falls into 2 separate patterns: (1) Onset of congestive heart failure is sudden in a newborn who has been in relatively good health 12–24 hours previously. This is a malignant form of the disease and is thought to be solely secondary to overwhelming viremia and tissue invasion of multiple organ systems, including the heart. (2) In the older child, the onset of cardiac findings tends to be much more gradual. There is often a history of an upper respiratory tract infection or gastroenteritis within the month prior to the development of cardiac findings. This is a more insidious form of the disease and may have a late postinfectious or autoimmune component. Recovery from the initial infection is followed by gradual and progressive development of easy fatigability, dyspnea on exertion, and malaise.

In the newborn infant, the signs of congestive heart failure are usually quite apparent. The skin is pale and gray, and peripheral cyanosis may be present. The pulses are rapid, weak, and thready. Edema of the face and extremities may be present. Significant cardiomegaly is present, and the left and right ventricular impulses are weak. On auscultation, the heart sounds may be poor, muffled, and distant. Third and fourth heart sounds are common, resulting in a gallop rhythm. Murmurs are usually absent, though a murmur of tricuspid or mitral insufficiency can occasionally be heard. Moist rales are usually present at both lung bases. The liver is enlarged and frequently tender. The level of the jugular venous pulse is elevated. In the latter group, the signs of congestive heart failure are often quite subtle.

B. X-Ray Findings: Generalized cardiomegaly involving all 4 chambers of the heart can be seen on x-ray. There is evidence of moderate to marked pulmonary venous congestion. Pneumonitis is commonly present.

C. Electrocardiography: The ECG is variable. Classically, there is evidence of low voltage of the QRS throughout all frontal and precordial leads and depression of the ST segment and inversion of the T waves in leads I, III, and aVF and in the left precordial leads during the acute malignant stage.

Dysrhythmias are common, and atrioventricular and intraventricular conduction disturbances may be present. With the more benign form—or during the recovery phase of the malignant form—high-voltage QRS complexes are commonly seen and are indicative of left ventricular hypertrophy.

Treatment

A. Digitalis: All patients with clinical findings of myocarditis should be started immediately on digitalis. Because the inflamed myocardium is markedly sensitive to digitalis, only about two-thirds of the usual total digitalizing dose should be employed. During the initial phase of therapy, frequent ECGs should be taken. If serious dysrhythmias or other evidence of digitalis intoxication develops, the drug should be stopped and not reinstituted until all evidence of digitalis toxicity has disappeared. If toxicity is not evident and there is no clinical response, digitalis doses should be increased until one or the other is noted.

B. Diuretics: Diuretics should be administered with caution, since they may potentiate digitalis toxicity.

C. Corticosteroids: The administration of corticosteroids is controversial but seems more rational when used in the treatment of the more benign postinfectious autoimmune cases. If the patient's condition continues to deteriorate despite anticongestive measures, corticosteroids are commonly employed.

Prognosis

The prognosis is related to the age at onset, the response to therapy, and the presence or absence of recurrences. If the patient is less than 6 months of age or older than 3 years, responds poorly to therapy, and manifests multiple recurrences of congestive heart failure, the prognosis is poor. Many patients recover clinically but have persistent cardiomegaly. It is possible that subclinical myocarditis in childhood is the pathophysiologic basis for some of the idiopathic myocardiopathies seen later in life.

Barson WJ et al: Survival following myocarditis and myocardial calcification associated with infection by coxsackievirus B-4. *Pediatrics* 1981;**68:**79.

Pulido S: Acute and subacute myocarditis. *Cardiovasc Rev Rep* 1984;**5:**912.

Ringel RE et al: Serologic evidence for *Chlamydia trachomatis* myocarditis. *Pediatrics* 1982;**70:**54.

INFECTIVE ENDOCARDITIS

Essentials of Diagnosis

- Preexisting organic heart murmur.
- Persistent fever.
- Increasing symptoms of heart disease (ranging from easy fatigability to heart failure).
- Splenomegaly (70%).
- Embolic phenomena (50%).
- Leukocytosis, elevated erythrocyte sedimentation rate, positive blood culture.

General Considerations

Bacterial infection of the endocardial surface of the heart or the intimal surface of certain arterial vessels (coarcted segment of aorta and ductus arteriosus) is a rare condition that usually occurs when an abnormality of the heart or great vessels exists. It may develop in a normal heart during the course of septicemia.

The incidence of infective endocarditis appears to be increasing owing to many factors, including (1) increased survival rates for children with congenital heart disease, (2) greater use of chronic central venous catheters, and (3) increased use of prosthetic material and valves. Pediatric patients without preexisting heart disease also are at increased risk for infective endocarditis owing to (1) increased survival rates for children with immune deficiencies, (2) greater use of chronic indwelling lines in critically ill newborns, and (3) increased incidence of intravenous drug abuse.

Patients at greatest risk include those with aorticopulmonary shunts, left-sided outflow obstruction, and ventricular septal defects. Predisposing factors can be identified approximately 30% of the time and include dental procedures, nonsterile surgical procedures, and cardiovascular surgery.

Organisms causing endocarditis include *Streptococcus viridans* (about 50% of cases), *Staphylococcus aureus* (about 30%), and fungal agents (about 10%).

Clinical Findings

A. History: Almost all patients have a history of heart disease. There may or may not be a history of infection or a surgical procedure (tooth extraction, tonsillectomy).

B. Symptoms, Signs, and Laboratory Findings: In one large study, the following symptoms, signs, and laboratory findings were reported (in order of decreasing frequency): changing murmurs, fever, positive blood culture, weight loss, cardiomegaly, elevated sedimentation rate, splenomegaly, petechiae, embolism, and leukocytosis. Other findings include hematuria, signs of congestive heart failure, clubbing, joint pains, and hepatomegaly. Echocardiography has become a valuable tool in diagnosing large vegetations.

Prevention

It is recommended that patients at risk for infective endocarditis be given appropriate antibiotics before any type of dental work (tooth extraction, cleaning) and before operations within the oropharynx, gastrointestinal tract, and genitourinary tract. Continuous antibiotic prophylaxis (as in the treatment of rheumatic fever) is *not* recommended in patients with congenital heart disease.

It is economically and logistically easier to give parents a supply of oral penicillin tablets to be used by their school-age children for dental procedures. The following schedule is sufficient for most patients: 500 mg of penicillin 1 hour prior to the procedure and 250 mg every 6 hours for the remainder of that day and for the 2 days following the procedure.

Treatment

In a patient with known heart disease, the presence of an otherwise unexplained fever should alert the physician to the possibility of infective endocarditis. A positive blood culture or other major findings of infective endocarditis confirm the diagnosis. If a positive blood culture is obtained and the organism is identified, specific treatment should be begun immediately. Even if blood cultures are negative after 48 hours, it is advisable to begin penicillin therapy (if there is other evidence of infective endocarditis), since most positive cultures are obtained within the first 48 hours. Penicillin is the drug choice in most cases. Other antibiotics may be added (see Chapter 38). If congestive heart failure occurs and progresses unremittingly in the face of adequate antibiotic therapy, surgical excision of the infected area and prosthetic valve replacement should be considered.

Course & Prognosis

The prognosis depends upon how early in the course of the infectious process treatment is instituted. The prognosis is better in patients in whom blood culture is positive. If congestive heart failure develops, the prognosis is usually poor.

Even though bacteriologic cure of the infectious process is achieved, death may occur as a result of congestive heart failure secondary to severe valvular destruction. Intractable congestive heart failure may occur weeks or months following bacteriologic cure. Embolization may occur following bacteriologic cure when vegetations tear off from the involved area.

The death rate for infective endocarditis is still about 20%.

Bisno AL et al: Treatment of infective endocarditis due to viridans streptococci. *Circulation* 1981;**63:**730A.

Brandenburg C et al: Infective endocarditis: A 25-year overview of diagnosis and therapy. *J Am Coll Cardiol* 1983;**1:**280.

Shulman ST: Prevention of bacterial endocarditis. *Pediatrics* 1985;**75:**603.

PERICARDITIS

Essentials of Diagnosis

- Retrosternal pain made worse by deep inspiration and decreased by leaning forward.
- Fever.
- Shortness of breath and grunting respirations are common.
- Pericardial friction rub.
- Tachycardia.
- Hepatomegaly and distention of the jugular veins.
- ECG with elevated ST segment.

General Considerations

Involvement of the pericardium rarely occurs as an isolated event. In the great majority of cases, pericardial disease occurs in association with a more generalized process. Important causes include rheumatic fever, viral pericarditis, purulent pericarditis, rheumatoid arthritis, uremia, and tuberculosis.

In the pediatric age group, pericardial disease usually takes the form of acute pericarditis. In most cases, there is effusion of fluid into the pericardial cavity. The consequences of such effusion depend upon the amount, type, and speed of fluid accumulation. Under certain circumstances, serious compression of the heart occurs. The direct compression and the body's attempt to correct it result in cardiac tamponade. Unless the pericardial fluid is evacuated, death occurs very rapidly.

Clinical Findings

A. Symptoms and Signs: The symptoms depend to a great extent upon the cause of the pericarditis. Pain is common. It is usually sharp and stabbing, located in the mid chest and in the shoulder and neck, made worse by deep inspiration, and considerably decreased by sitting up and leaning forward. Shortness of breath and grunting respirations are common findings in all patients.

The physical findings depend upon whether or not a significant amount of effusion is present: (1) In the absence of significant accumulation of fluid, the pulses are normal and the level of the jugular venous pulse is normal. On examination of the heart, a characteristic scratchy, high-pitched friction rub may be heard. It is often systolic and diastolic and can be located at any point between the apex and the left sternal border. The location and timing vary considerably from time to time. The heart sounds are usually normal, and the heart is not enlarged to percussion. (2) If there is a considerable accumulation of pericardial fluid, the cardiovascular findings are different. The heart is enlarged to percussion, but on inspection of the precordium, it seems to be very quiet. Auscultation reveals distant and muffled heart tones. Friction rub is usually not present. In the absence of cardiac tamponade, the peripheral, venous, and arterial pulses are normal.

Cardiac tamponade is characterized by distention of the jugular veins, tachycardia, enlargement of the liver, peripheral edema, and "paradoxic pulse," in which the systolic pressure drops by more than 10 mm Hg during inspiration. The term paradoxic pulse is a misnomer, since the drop is only an accentuation of a normal event. (Normally, the systolic pressure drops by no more than 5 mm Hg.) This finding is best determined with the use of a blood pressure cuff. At this point, the patient is critically ill and has all the symptoms and signs suggestive of right-sided congestive heart failure.

Not all patients with marked cardiac compression demonstrate all the findings listed above. If the patient appears critically ill and has evidence of pericarditis and effusion, treatment should be instituted even though all the clinical signs of cardiac tamponade are not present.

B. X-Ray Findings: In pericarditis without effusion, chest x-rays are normal. With pericardial effusion, the cardiac silhouette is enlarged, often in the shape of a water bottle, with blunting of the cardiodiaphragmatic borders. When there is evidence of cardiac tamponade, the lung fields are clear. This is in contrast to patients with myocardial dilatation, who show evidence of pulmonary congestion.

Cardiac fluoroscopy usually demonstrates absence of pulsations of the cardiac borders. This is helpful in differentiating this condition from myocarditis, in which the pulsations, although feeble, are present.

C. Electrocardiography: A number of electrocardiographic abnormalities occur in patients with pericarditis. Low voltage is commonly seen in patients with significant pericardial effusion, although the voltage may be normal. The ST segment is commonly elevated during the first week of involvement. The T wave is usually upright during this time. Following this, the ST segment is normal and the T wave becomes flattened. After about 2 weeks, the T wave inverts and remains inverted for several weeks or months. In contrast to findings in patients with myocardial infarction, there is no reciprocal relationship between the findings in lead I and lead III in the frontal plane and the right and left precordial leads.

D. Echocardiography: Echocardiography has become a most reliable form of noninvasive diagnosis of pericardial effusion. The results must be considered in the light of the clinical picture in deciding whether or not to remove the fluid.

Treatment

Treatment depends upon the cause of the pericarditis. Cardiac tamponade due to any cause must be treated by evacuation of the fluid. It is usually desirable to perform a wide resection of the pericardium through a surgical incision. However, needle insertion into the pericardial sac may be lifesaving in an emergency situation (see Chapter 35).

Prognosis

The prognosis depends to a great extent upon the cause of the pericardial disease. Cardiac tamponade due to any cause will result in death unless the fluid is evacuated.

See references below.

SPECIFIC DISEASES INVOLVING THE PERICARDIUM

Acute Rheumatic Fever

When pericarditis occurs during the course of acute rheumatic fever, it is almost always associated with involvement of the myocardium and endocardium (pancarditis). Thus, heart murmurs are almost always present. The pericarditis is usually of the serofibrinous variety and usually not associated with significant pericardial effusion.

Patients with acute rheumatic fever and pericarditis are usually very ill, with severe cardiac involvement. They respond extremely well to corticosteroid therapy. Pericarditis usually disappears rapidly (1 week) after corticosteroid therapy is started. Constrictive pericarditis almost never occurs secondary to this disease.

Viral Pericarditis

Viral pericarditis is uncommon in children and young adults. The most common cause is the coxsackievirus B4. Influenza virus has also been implicated. There is usually a history of a protracted upper respiratory tract infection.

The pericardial effusion usually lasts for several weeks. Cardiac tamponade is rare. Recurrences of pericardial effusion are quite common even months or years after the initial episode. Constrictive pericarditis has been reported in this disease.

Purulent Pericarditis

The most common causes of purulent pericarditis are pneumococci, streptococci, staphylococci, *Escherichia coli,* and *Haemophilus influenzae.* This is always secondary to infection elsewhere, although occasionally the primary site is not obvious. In addition to demonstrating signs of cardiac compression, patients are quite septic and run extremely high fevers. The purulent fluid accumulating within the pericardial sac is usually quite thick and filled with polymorphonuclear leukocytes. Although antibiotics will sterilize the pericardial fluid, pericardial tamponade commonly develops, and evacuation of the pericardial sac is usually necessary. Wide resection of the pericardium through a surgical incision performed in the operating room is most desirable, but pericardiocentesis is often dramatically effective and lifesaving. Drainage of the purulent fluid is followed by marked improvement of symptoms.

Postpericardiotomy Syndrome

Postpericardiotomy syndrome is characterized by fever, chest pain, friction rub, and elevation of ST segment noted on ECG 1–2 weeks after open heart surgery. It appears to be an autoimmune disease with high titers of antiheart antibody and with detectable evidence of fresh or reactivated viral illness. The syndrome is often self-limited and responds well to short courses of aspirin or corticosteroid therapy. Occasionally, it lasts for months to years and may require pericardiocentesis or pericardiectomy.

Clapp SK et al: Postoperative pericardial effusion and its relation to postpericardiotomy syndrome. *Pediatrics* 1980;**66:**585.

Engle MA et al: Viral illness and the postpericardiotomy syndrome. *Circulation* 1980;**62:**1151.

Fowler NO, Gabel M: The hemodynamic effects of cardiac tamponade. *Circulation* 1985;**71:**154.

Gersony WM, Hordof AJ: Infective endocarditis and diseases of the pericardium. *Pediatr Clin North Am* 1978;**25:**838.

HYPERTENSION*

Blood pressure determinations are being more routinely obtained in the examination of infants and children; as a result, systemic hypertension has become more widely recognized as a pediatric problem. Pediatric standards for blood pressure have been published, but the studies from which these standards were derived suffered from 3 methodologic problems. The first and most important is that the widest cuff that would fit between the axilla and antecubital fossa was not routinely used. The use of a wide cuff either has no effect on blood pressure or decreases blood pressure by a maximum of 5 mm Hg. Use of a narrow cuff, however, routinely increases blood pressure by 10–50 mm Hg. The second methodologic problem was lack of an ethnic cross section. Third, the fact that systemic blood pressure decreases with increasing altitude of residence was not taken into consideration.

These 3 problems were addressed in a recent study of a triracial population at sea level and at an altitude of 10,000 feet. The widest cuff that would fit between the axilla and antecubital fossa was used in each case. Most children from 10–11 years of age needed a standard adult-size cuff (bladder width of 12 cm), and many high school students needed a large adult-size cuff (width of 16 cm) or leg cuff (width of 18 cm). Results of the study are shown in Table 15–3. The 95th percentile value for blood pressure was similar for both sexes and all 3 ethnic groups. Blood pressure varied more with altitude and body weight than with sex or ethnic origin. If the blood pressure taken in a quiet atmosphere and sitting position exceeds the 95th percentile for systolic, diastolic muffle, or diastolic disappearance pressures, it should be repeated twice in 1- to 2-week intervals. If it is abnormal all 3 times, a pediatric hypertension diagnostic center should be consulted.

Essential hypertension is the most common form of pediatric hypertension. Coarctation of the thoracic or abdominal aorta, renal artery stenosis, renal disease, and pheochromocytoma should be ruled out.

Patients with essential hypertension often show improvement with reduction of obesity, reduction of excessive salt intake, institution of an exercise program, avoidance of cigarette smoking, and avoidance of use of oral contraceptives. The use of antihypertensive drugs in pediatric hypertension is controversial, but thiazide diuretics and propranolol are useful in selected cases.

* The diagnostic evaluation of renal hypertension and the treatment of hypertensive emergencies as well as the ambulatory treatment of chronic hypertension are discussed in Chapter 21.

Table 15–3. The 95th percentile value for blood pressure (mm Hg) taken in the sitting position.*

	Sea Level			10,000 Feet		
Age (yr)	**S**	**Dm**	**Dd**	**S**	**Dm**	**Dd**
5				92	72	62
6	106	64	60	96	74	66
7	108	72	66	98	76	70
8	110	76	70	104	80	70
9	114	80	76	106	80	70
10	118	82	76	108	80	70
11	124	82	78	108	80	72
12	128	84	78	108	80	72
13	132	84	80	116	84	76
14	136	86	80	120	84	76
15	140	88	80	120	84	80
16	140	90	80	120	84	80
17	140	92	80	122	84	80
18	140	92	80	130	84	80

* Blood pressures: S = systolic (Korotkoff's sound 1; onset of tapping); Dm = diastolic muffling (Korotkoff's sound 4); Dd = diastolic disappearance (Korotkoff's sound 5).

Fraser GE, Phillips RL, Harris R: Physical fitness and blood pressure in school children. *Circulation* 1983;**67:**405.

Jesse MJ: Essential hypertension in children. *Hosp Pract* (Nov) 1982;**17:**81.

Laird WP, Fixler DE: Left ventricular hypertrophy in adolescents with elevated blood pressure. *Pediatrics* 1981;**67:**255.

Loggie JM et al: Juvenile hypertension. *J Pediatr* 1984;**104:**657.

McCrory WW: Blood pressure in healthy children. *Pediatrics* 1982;**70:**143.

Steinfeld L et al: Sphygmomanometry in pediatric patients. *J Pediatr* 1978;**92:**934.

ATHEROSCLEROSIS AS A PEDIATRIC PROBLEM

Awareness of the importance of coronary artery risk factors in general—and atherosclerosis in particular—has risen dramatically in the general population during the past 25 years. In adults, the incidence of death from ischemic heart disease has been decreasing over the last decade, presumably as a result of modifying the diet or life-style to avoid known risks for heart disease. During this same decade, a large number of serum samples from the pediatric population have been collected and analyzed for lipids, and epidemiologic studies have been performed to determine the relationship of lipid levels to coronary heart disease. The level of serum lipids in childhood usually remains the same through adolescence. Biochemical abnormalities in the lipid profile appear early in childhood and correlate with higher risk for coronary artery disease in adulthood. High-density lipoprotein has been identified as an antiatherogenic agent through these studies.

The concept of pediatric screening for hyperlipidemia has been evaluated carefully. Currently, only children at high risk—ie, children with a family history of early myocardial infarction (prior to 50–55 years) in parents or grandparents or with known familial hyperlipidemia—are screened routinely. In addition, some researchers consider adolescents with total cholesterol levels of greater than 180 mg/dL or low-density lipoprotein levels of greater than 110 mg/dL to be at risk for coronary artery disease in adulthood.

In the majority of cases, treatment consists of dietary restrictions, exercise, abstinence from smoking, and avoidance of other ischemic heart disease risk factors. In patients with life-threatening familial hyperlipidemia, pharmacologic and surgical intervention (ileal bypass or portacaval shunt) may be considered.

Aristimuño GG et al: Influence of persistent obesity in children on cardiovascular risk factors: The Bogalusa Heart Study. *Circulation* 1984;**69:**895.

Glueck CJ: Detection of risk factors for coronary artery disease in children. *Pediatrics* 1980;**66:**834.

Moll PP et al: Total cholesterol and lipoproteins in school children. *Circulation* 1983;**67:**127.

Morrison JA, Glueck CJ: Pediatric risk factors for adult coronary heart disease: Primary atherosclerosis prevention. *Cardiovasc Rev Rep* 1981;**2:**1269.

Voller RD, Strong WB: Pediatric aspects of atherosclerosis. *Am Heart J* 1981;**101:**815.

DISORDERS OF RATE, RHYTHM, & ELECTROLYTE IMBALANCE

In normal cardiac conduction, depolarization occurs in the following sequence: sinoatrial node (depolarization cannot be seen on ECG), atria (P wave), atrioventricular node (PR segment), and bundles and ventricles (QRS). Repolarization (T wave) then occurs.

In evaluating cardiac dysrhythmia and abnormal findings on ECG, it is important to keep in mind the normal sequence of cardiac conduction as well as the normal intervals of conduction (PR, QRS, QT, etc) and the normal rates in children. A systematic approach to electrocardiography is essential.

SINUS DYSRHYTHMIA

It is normal to have phasic variation in heart rate (sinus dysrhythmia). Typically, dysrhythmia is associated with the respiratory cycle. Heart rate is accelerated on inspiration and decelerated on expiration. P–QRS–T intervals are normal.

SINUS BRADYCARDIA

Depending on the age of the patient, sinus bradycardia may be a normal finding, particularly when the patient is at rest or asleep. Sleeping infants and children commonly have sinus rates of 80/min or lower. In critically ill patients, common causes of bradycardia include hypoxia, use of medications, and central nervous system damage. Bradycardia is usually not a primary cardiac abnormality.

SINUS TACHYCARDIA

The heart rate normally accelerates in response to stress, eg, fever, hypovolemia, anemia, or congestive heart failure. Tachycardia with decreased cardiac output is more ominous and warrants evaluation for shock or tachyarrhythmia. Treatment may be indicated for correction of the underlying cause of tachycardia (transfusion for anemia, correction of hypovolemia or fever, etc).

PREMATURE ATRIAL CONTRACTIONS

Premature atrial contractions are triggered by an ectopic focus in the atrium. They are one of the most common premature beats seen in the pediatric population, particularly during the newborn period. They may be nonconducted (with associated QRS) (Fig 15–7A) or conducted (with premature P wave) (Fig 15–7B). There is usually some delay until the next normal sinus beat (compensatory pause). Depending on the ectopic focus of the premature contraction, the frontal plane vector of the P wave may be normal (+60 degrees) or abnormal. The PR interval may be short if the focus is close to the atrioventricular node.

As an isolated finding, premature atrial contractions are benign and require no treatment. They may occur more frequently in association with excessive caffeine ingestion. In patients with heart disease, premature atrial contractions are not treated unless they are associated with specific tachyarrhythmias or are frequent and cause decreased cardiac output.

PREMATURE JUNCTIONAL CONTRACTIONS

Premature junctional contractions occur high in the bundle of His and may or may not induce aberrant conduction (wide QRS configuration). Most often, they induce a narrow QRS complex (Fig 15–7C) with no preceding P wave and may have retrograde atrial depolarization (P wave seen on early portion of the T wave). When aberrantly conducted, premature junctional contractions cannot be distinguished from premature ventricular contractions except by invasive (electrophysiologic) study.

As an isolated finding, premature junctional contractions are usually benign and require no specific therapy. When associated with junctional tachycardia,

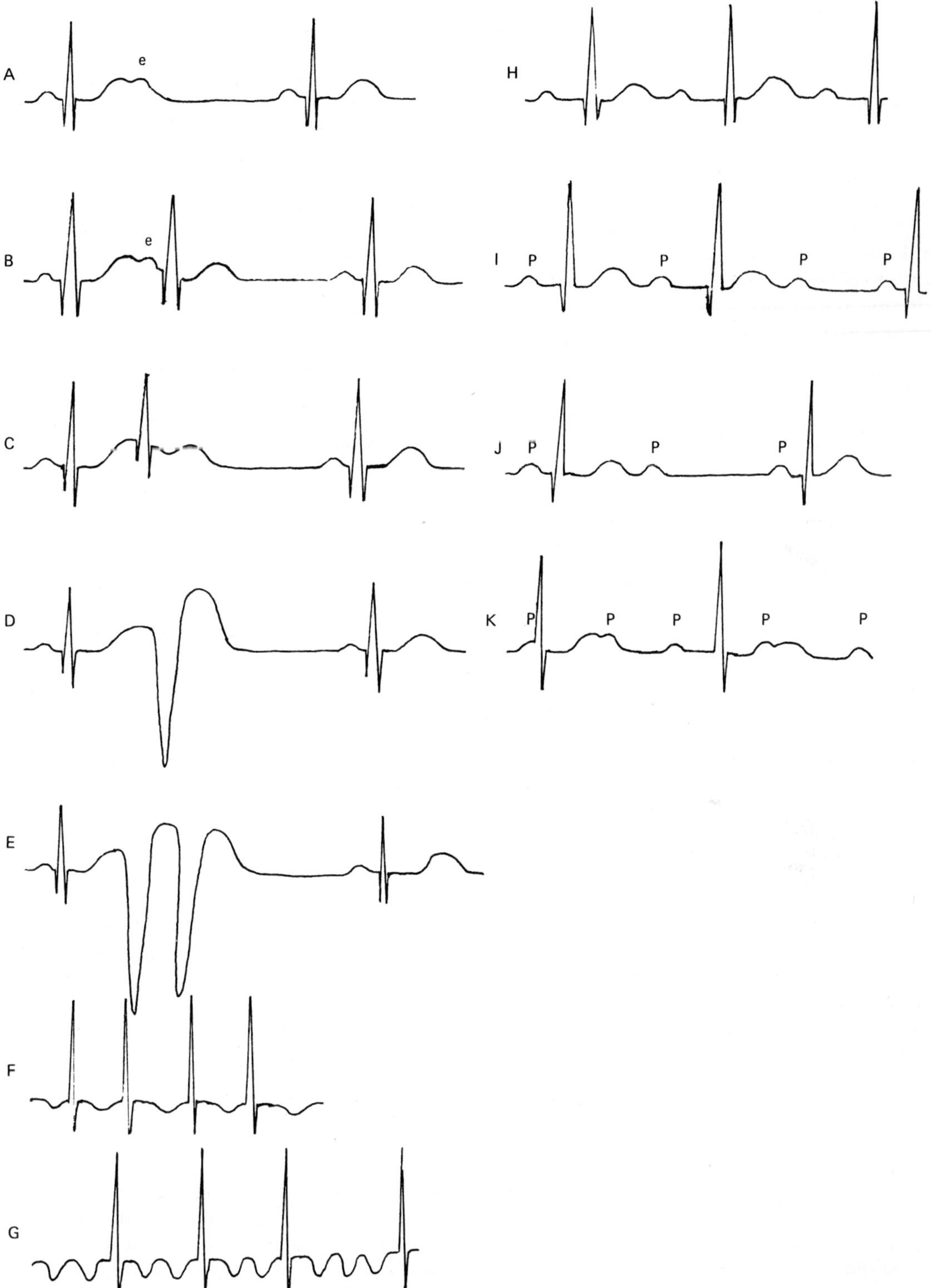

Figure 15–7. Dysrhythmias shown on ECG. *A:* Nonconducted premature atrial contraction. *B:* Conducted premature atrial contraction. *C:* Premature junctional contraction. *D:* Premature ventricular contraction. *E:* Premature ventricular contraction in couplet. *F:* Paroxysmal supraventricular tachycardia. *G:* Atrial flutter with variable conduction. *H:* First-degree atrioventricular heart block. *I:* Mobitz type I (Wenckebach type) second-degree atrioventricular heart block. *J:* Mobitz type II (2:1 type) second-degree atrioventricular heart block. *K:* Complete heart block. e = ectopic atrial premature beat; P = P wave.

they are one of the most difficult abnormalities to treat.

PREMATURE VENTRICULAR CONTRACTIONS

Premature ventricular contractions may originate in either ventricle and are characterized by a bizarre QRS of greater than 10 ms in duration, an abnormal T wave not preceded by a P wave (Fig 15–7D), and a compensatory pause (interval between 2 beats, including the premature contraction) equal to 2 normal cardiac cycles. Premature ventricular contractions originating from a single ectopic focus all have the same configuration; those of multifocal origin show varying configurations. The consecutive occurrence of more than one beat can result in coupling (Fig 15–7E) or ventricular tachycardia (3 or more consecutive ventricular beats).

Most unifocal premature ventricular contractions in otherwise normal patients are benign. The nature of contractions can be confirmed by having the patient exercise. As the heart rate increases, benign premature contractions disappear. If exercise results in an increase or coupling of contractions, there may be underlying disease. Multifocal premature ventricular contractions are always abnormal and are more dangerous. They may be associated with drug overdosages (cyclic antidepressant, digoxin toxicity, etc). When associated with organic heart disease, they must be thoroughly evaluated and treated if necessary. Phenytoin, propranolol, or quinidine is currently used for treatment.

PAROXYSMAL SUPRAVENTRICULAR TACHYCARDIA

Paroxysmal supraventricular tachycardia, the most common tachyarrhythmia of childhood, often presents in infancy. It is most often secondary to bypass tracts (accessory pathways between the atria and ventricles) whose conduction times differ from those of the atrioventricular node. With premature stimulation (preexcitation), these tracts can be activated and cause repetitive rapid stimulation of atria and ventricles (''circus phenomenon''). Only rarely is paroxysmal supraventricular tachycardia caused by ectopic foci.

Clinical Findings

A. Symptoms and Signs: Clinical presentation varies with the age of the patient. Infants tend to turn pale and mottled with onset of tachycardia and may become irritable. With long duration of tachycardia, symptoms of congestive heart failure develop. Heart rates can be from 240 to 300 beats per minute. Early diagnosis and prompt therapy are imperative in this group of patients. Older children may complain of dizziness, palpitations, fatigue, and chest pain. Heart rates usually range from 240 in the younger child to 150–180 in the teenager. Congestive heart failure is less common in children than in infants. Tachycardia may be associated with either congenital heart defects such as Ebstein's anomaly or acquired conditions such as cardiomyopathies and myocarditis. Complete noninvasive cardiovascular evaluation is indicated in all patients with a first episode of paroxysmal supraventricular tachycardia.

B. X-Ray Findings: Findings on chest x-ray are normal during the early course of dysrhythmia. If congestive heart failure is present, the heart is enlarged and there is evidence of pulmonary venous congestion.

C. Electrocardiography: Electrocardiography (Fig 15–7F) is the most important tool in the diagnosis of this condition.

1. The heart rate is very rapid, ranging from 160 to 320/min.
2. The rhythm is extremely regular. There is no variation in the PR interval throughout the entire tracing.
3. P waves may or may not be present. If they are present, there is no variation in the appearance of the P wave or in the PR interval. P waves may be difficult to find because they are superimposed upon the preceding T wave. Furthermore, if the abnormal focus is located within the atrioventricular node, the P waves will not be seen.
4. The QRS complex is usually the same as during normal sinus rhythm. However, the QRS complex is occasionally widened, in which case the condition may be difficult to differentiate from ventricular tachycardia (supraventricular tachycardia with aberrant ventricular conduction). Presence of a delta wave or slurring of the initial portion of the QRS, with a short PR interval during or after paroxysmal supraventricular tachycardia, is indicative of preexcitation.
5. Termination of the tachycardia is characterized by conversion to normal sinus rhythm. In contrast with atrial flutter, degrees of atrioventricular block do not develop.

Treatment

During initial episodes, all patients (particularly infants) require close monitoring of intravenous blood pressure. In severe failure, intra-atrial blood pressure should be monitored. Correction of acidosis or electrolyte abnormalities is also indicated.

A. Verapamil: The current drug of choice for acute conversion to normal sinus rhythm is verapamil, 0.1 mg/kg given intravenously as a slow push (1–2 minutes). Conversion usually occurs within 1–2 minutes. This dose may be repeated in 20 minutes. Transient hypotension may occur but usually does not require treatment.

B. Digitalis: Digitalis is still the drug of choice for long-term therapy (1–2 years). It can be used with or without verapamil, and conversion should be accomplished within 8–12 hours. Doses used are the same as those for congestive heart failure.

C. DC Cardioversion: DC cardioversion (1–2 J/kg) is also effective in more refractory cases of tachycardia and in critically ill infants. The procedure should be supervised by a cardiologist.

D. Other Drugs and Procedures: Other drugs such as propranolol, quinidine, or procainamide may be used when other measures fail.

The older child who has short episodes of tachycardia can learn Valsalva's maneuver to convert the dysrhythmia during reflex. Also very effective is placing a plastic bag full of ice cold water or crushed ice on the face. Ocular pressure or carotid massage is rarely of great benefit and is particularly dangerous in the infant.

Prognosis

Paroxysmal supraventricular tachycardia that presents during infancy has a low recurrence rate if the patient is treated with digitalis for 1–2 years. If it presents or recurs after infancy, long-term pharmacologic therapy is indicated. If pharmacologic intervention fails to control the tachycardia, surgical ablation should be considered.

ATRIAL FLUTTER & FIBRILLATION

Atrial flutter and fibrillation are quite rare in children and are most often associated with organic heart disease, particularly cardiomyopathies and myocarditis. Atrial flutter (Fig 15–7G) can present in infancy, and if 1:1 conduction of flutter occurs, it can mimic paroxysmal supraventricular tachycardia. Atrial rate is usually greater than 240 and is often 300. Ventricular rate depends on the degree of atrioventricular response and is usually slower. Atrial fibrillation is an irregular rhythm with variable rate.

DC cardioversion, followed by digitalization, is indicated for treatment of either of these entities. Either or both may require the addition of quinidine to the regimen for adequate control. Both forms of dysrhythmia are frequently difficult to control and should be managed under the supervision of a pediatric cardiologist.

VENTRICULAR TACHYCARDIA

Ventricular tachycardia, an uncommon dysrhythmia in children, is often associated with organic heart disease. It can be quite regular, although typically there is variation in the RR interval. All QRS complexes are widened and bizarre. The heart rate is usually 120–180 (less than that of paroxysmal supraventricular tachycardia). Intermittent runs of ventricular tachycardia frequently precede sustained tachycardia, which can develop into ventricular fibrillation.

The electrocardiographic pattern of ventricular tachycardia must be differentiated from that of hyperkalemia. Differentiation is accomplished by administering intravenous sodium bicarbonate or an intravenous flush of calcium chloride and continuously monitoring the ECG. If the QRS complexes narrow and T waves return to baseline, the diagnosis of hyperkalemia is suggested and can be confirmed by serum electrolyte evaluation.

Treatment for ventricular tachycardia is lidocaine, 1 mg/kg given as an intravenous bolus. If there is no response to lidocaine, DC cardioversion is indicated. Use of either of these modalities in patients with hyperkalemia can be fatal.

FIRST-DEGREE HEART BLOCK

First-degree heart block is an electrocardiographic diagnosis for prolongation of the PR interval (Fig 15–7H). The block does not in itself cause problems of heart function. However, it is commonly found in association with such congenital heart defects as ostium secundum type atrial septal defect and with such diseases as rheumatic carditis or viral myocarditis. The PR interval may also be prolonged as a result of digoxin therapy. This is a sign of digoxin effect, not toxicity.

SECOND-DEGREE HEART BLOCK

Mobitz type I (Wenckebach type) heart block is recognized by progressive prolongation of the PR interval until there is no QRS associated with a P wave (Fig 15–7I); then the cycle may repeat itself. In Mobitz type II (2:1 type) heart block, every other P wave has a dropped beat or nonconduction to the ventricles (Fig 15–7J).

Second-degree heart block of either type can occur in the normal heart but is usually associated with organic heart disease or drug intoxication. Treatment is correction of the underlying problem.

COMPLETE HEART BLOCK

In complete heart block, the atria and ventricles beat independently. The atrial rate is usually more rapid than the ventricular rate (Fig 15–7K). Ventricular rates can range from 40 to 80 beats per minute, while atrial rates may be 1½–3 times that rate.

Congenital complete heart block, the most common form of complete heart block, has a very high association with maternal systemic lupus erythematosus (80% at our institution). Serologic screening should be performed in the mother of an infant with complete heart block, even if she has no symptoms of systemic lupus erythematosus. Congenital complete heart block is also associated with corrected transposition of the great vessels, endocardial cushion defect, and endocardial fibroelastosis.

Acquired complete heart block can be secondary to acute myocarditis, digoxin toxicity, and open heart surgery.

Clinical Findings

Prenatal bradycardia is frequently noted in infants with congenital complete heart block. In the past, this finding occasionally indicated the need for emergency delivery of the infant; however, since the advent of fetal monitoring and fetal echocardiography, this is infrequently necessary. An overall assessment of postnatal adaptation to the heart block is important. Adaptation is largely dependent on the heart rate; infants with heart rates less than 60 are at significantly greater risk for low cardiac output and congestive heart failure. Wide QRS complexes and a rapid atrial rate are also poor prognostic signs. All patients have some heart murmur from increased stroke volume. In more symptomatic patients, the heart can be quite enlarged and pulmonary edema present. In older patients, Stokes-Adams syncope may be the presenting symptom, or heart block may be found on routine physical examination.

Full cardiac evaluation, including echocardiography, is indicated. Holter monitoring is used to assess the patient for evidence of ventricular ectopy and to document the slowest heart rate attained.

Treatment

In patients thought to be at risk for Stokes-Adams attacks or congestive heart failure, the treatment of choice is surgical insertion of a programmable permanent pacemaker. Until surgery is performed, patients can be temporarily assisted by intravenous drip of isoproterenol (Isuprel) or by transvenous pacemaker. Permanent transvenous pacemakers are increasingly used in pediatric patients.

ELECTROLYTE IMBALANCE

Potassium, calcium, and, to a lesser extent, magnesium imbalances are reflected on ECG. The electrolyte disturbances of potassium are of greatest concern to the pediatrician, and some familiarity with abnormal tracings found in hyperkalemia and hypokalemia is essential. In hyperkalemia (Fig 15–8), there is gradual progression from tall peaked T waves (5–7 meq/L) through widening of the QRS complex (8–9 meq/L) to a broad, almost sine wave configuration (>10 meq/

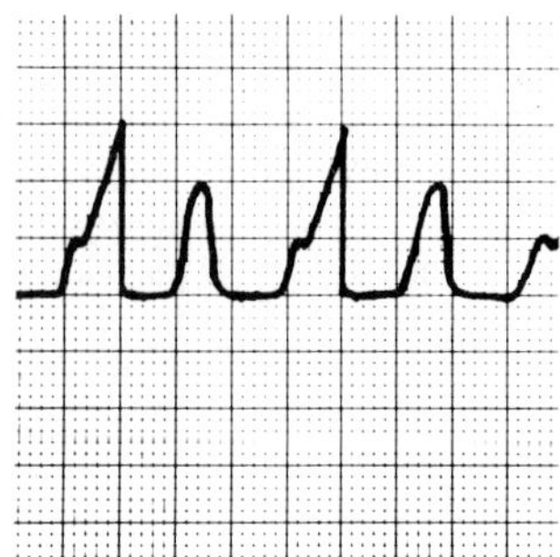
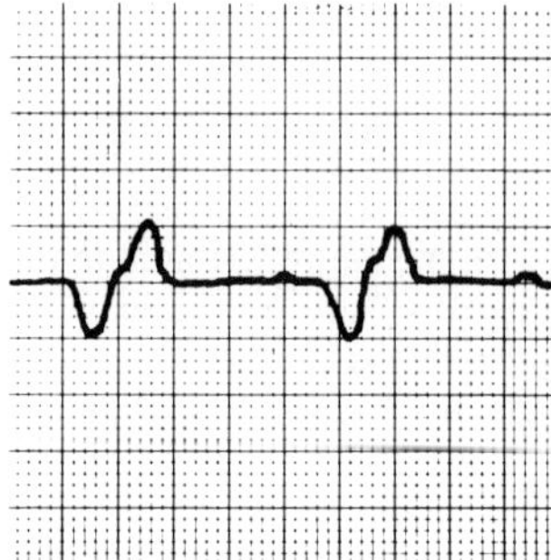

Figure 15–8. Hyperkalemia. *Left:* Serum K^+ of 8.5 meq/L. *Right:* Serum K^+ of 11 meq/L.

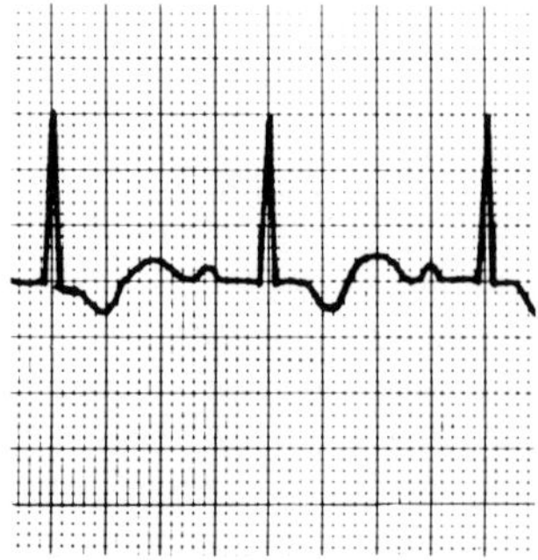
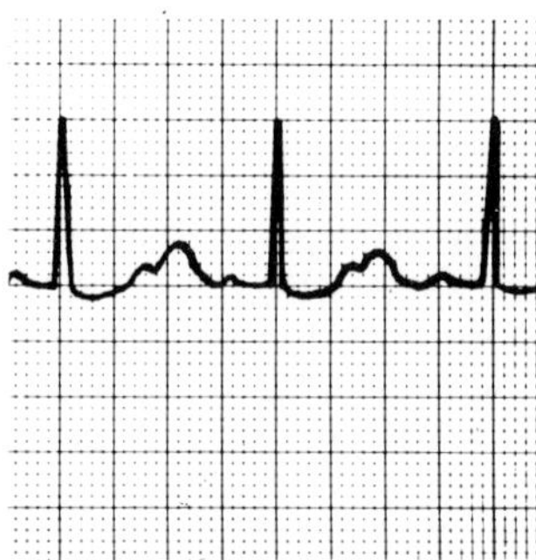

Figure 15–9. Hypokalemia. *Left:* Serum K^+ of 2.5 meq/L. *Right:* Serum K^+ of 3.5 meq/L.

L). Hypokalemia (Fig 15–9) is characterized by progressive prominence of the U wave and prolongation of the QT (really QU) interval with ST segment depression.

SELECTED REFERENCES

Garson A Jr, Gillette PC, McNamara DG: *A Guide to Cardiac Dysrhythmias in Children*. Grune & Stratton, 1980.

Gillette PC, Garson A Jr (editors): *Pediatric Cardiac Dysrhythmias*. Grune & Stratton, 1981.

Liebman J, Plonsey R, Gillette PC: *Pediatric Electrocardiography*. William & Wilkins, 1982.

Whittemore R, Hobbins JC, Engle MA: Pregnancy and its outcome in women with and without surgical treatment of congenital heart disease. *Am J Cardiol* 1982;**50:**641.

16 Hematologic Disorders

John H. Githens, MD, & William E. Hathaway, MD

Knowledge of the normal ranges by age is essential in the diagnosis of hematologic disorders of infancy and childhood. The normal values for bone marrow and peripheral blood are shown in Tables 16–1 and 16–2. They vary significantly with age.

The important changes shown in Table 16–2 include polycythemia in the neonatal period followed by physiologic anemia of infancy, which is maximal at 2½–3 months. Subsequently, there is a gradual rise of the hemoglobin, hematocrit, and red cell count through childhood. Adult levels are not reached until after puberty.

Screening for anemia should be done at birth, 9 months, 12 months, 18 months, 5 years, and 14 years of age. (See Chapter 6.)

The red blood cells of the newborn are macrocytic (8–9 μm in diameter). There is a gradual change to microcytosis at 3 months, with return to normal diameter (7.4 μm) by 8 months.

The white blood count may normally remain higher than in the adult throughout infancy and childhood. The differential white count shows a predominance of lymphocytes, which may normally comprise as much as 80% of the white blood cells through the first 6 years of life.

I. ANEMIAS

Anemia is always a manifestation of disease or nutritional deficiency. The cause should be determined by appropriate clinical and laboratory investigations or, if necessary, by therapeutic trial with specific replacement therapy. "Shotgun" treatment with multiple drugs is never indicated.

The cell indices that are most useful are the MCHC (mean corpuscular hemoglobin concentration), the MCH (mean corpuscular hemoglobin), and the MCV (mean corpuscular volume). The normal values are shown in Table 16–2.

The primary cause of anemia in infancy is nutritional iron deficiency. Anemias due to causes other than iron deficiency fall into 2 major groups: (1) those due to impaired red cell production, maturation, or release from the marrow; and (2) those due to acute blood loss or destruction (hemolysis). The studies needed to determine the exact cause are different for these 2 groups.

The essential test in differentiating anemias due to defective production from the hemolytic group is the reticulocyte count. This must be done prior to treatment with drugs or transfusion.

Diagnosis of Anemia

The following scheme for diagnosis of anemia is useful:

(1) Careful history: Duration of symptoms, diet, rate of growth, evidence of acute or chronic hemorrhage, jaundice, and a family history of anemia, jaundice, or gallbladder disease.

(2) Determination of hemoglobin, hematocrit, red blood cell count, MCH, MCV, MCHC, and examination of the smear. The blood smear often provides the clue for the final workup.

(a) If hypochromia is shown, the cause of iron deficiency should be sought and treated. Additional studies—serum iron and iron-binding capacity, serum proteins, examination of stools for blood, and bone marrow examination—may be indicated. Serum ferritin and free erythrocyte protoporphyrin can be useful in differentiating iron deficiency from other hypochromic anemias.

(b) If normochromia (or hyperchromia) is shown, the reticulocyte count is essential. If the reticulocyte count is low (due to defect in marrow production or

Table 16–1. Normal values of cellular elements in bone marrow in older infants and children.*

	Range (%)	Mean (%)
Myeloblasts	1–5	2
Myelocytes (including promyelocytes)	10–25	20
Nonsegmented polymorphonuclear cells (including metamyelocytes)	15–30	20
Segmented polymorphonuclear cells	5–30	25
Lymphocytes	5–25	13
Nucleated red cells (principally normoblasts)	15–30	20
Megakaryocytes	10–35/μL	
Total nucleated cell count	100,000–200,000/μL	

* From Smith CH: *Blood Diseases of Infancy and Childhood,* 2nd ed. Mosby, 1966.

Table 16–2. Normal peripheral blood values at various ages.*

	1st Day	2nd Day	6th Day	2 Weeks	1 Month	2 Months	3 Months	6 Months	1 Year	2 Years	5 Years	8–12 Years	Adults	
													Males	Females
Red blood cells (millions/μL)	5.9 (4.1–7.5)	6 (4.0–7.3)	5.4 (3.9–6.8)	5 (4.5–5.5)	4.7 (4.2–5.2)	4.1 (3.6–4.6)	4 (3.5–4.5)	4.5 (4–5)	4.6 (4.1–5.1)	4.7 (4.2–5.2)	4.7 (4.2–5.2)	5 (4.5–5.4)	5.4 (4.6–6.2)	4.8 (4.2–5.4)
Hemoglobin (g/dL)	19 (14–24)	19 (15–23)	18 (13–23)	16.5 (15–20)	14 (11–17)	12 (11–14)	11 (10–13)	11.5 (10.5–14.5)	12 (11–15)	13 (12–15)	13.5 (12.5–15)	14 (13–15.5)	16 (13–18)	14 (11–16)
White blood cells (per μL)	17,000 (8–38)		13,500 (6–17)	12,000 (5–16)	11,500 (5–15)	11,000 (5–15)	10,500 (5–15)	10,500 (5–15)	10,000 (5–15)	9,500 (5–14)	8,000 (5–13)	8,000 (5–12)	7,000 (5–10)	
PMNs† (%)	57	55	50	34	34	33	33	36	39	42	55	60	57–68	
Eosinophils (total) (per μL)	20–1000				150–1150		70–550	70–550					100–400	
Lymphocytes† (%)	20	20	37	55	56	56	57	55	53	49	36	31	25–33	
Monocytes† (%)	10	15	9	8	7	7	7	6	6	7	7	7	3–7	
Immature white cells (%)	10	5	0–1	0	0	0	0	0	0	0	0	0	0	
Platelets† (per μL)	350,000		325,000	300,000			260,000			250,000		260,000	260,000	
Nucleated red cells/ 100 white cells‡	0–10		0–0.3	0	0	0	0	0	0	0	0	0	0	
Reticulocytes (%)	3 (2–8)	3 (2–10)	1 (0.5–5)	0.4 (0–2)	0.2 (0–0.5)	0.5 (0.2–2)	2 (0.5–4)	0.8 (0.2–1.5)	1 (0.4–1.8)	1 (0.4–1.8)	1 (0.4–1.8)	1 (0.4–1.8)	1 (0.5–2)	
Mean diameter of red cells (μm)	8.6				8.1		5–7		7.4		7.4		7.5	
MCV§ (fL)	85–125		89–101	94–102	90		80	78	78	80	80	82	82–92	
MCHC§ (%)	36		35	34				33		32	34	34	34	
MCH§ (pg)	35–40		36	31	30		27	26	25	26	27	28	27–31	
Hematocrit (%)	54 ± 10		51	50	40		35	35	36	37	38	40	40–54	37–47

* Modified and reproduced, with permission, from Silver HK et al: *Handbook of Pediatrics,* 15th ed. Lange, 1986.
† Usual or average values; considerable individual variation may occur.
‡ Total nucleated red cells: first day, $< 1000/\mu L$.
§ MCV = mean corpuscular volume. MCHC = mean corpuscular hemoglobin concentration. MCH = mean corpuscular hemoglobin.

release), examine bone marrow (see Chapter 35); if high (due to hemolytic disease or acute hemorrhage), perform blood smear and Coombs test. If the Coombs is negative, perform red cell saline fragility test, autohemolysis test, hemoglobin electrophoresis, fetal hemoglobin determination, and Heinz body preparation. If spherocytosis or a hemoglobinopathy has not been identified, red cell enzyme studies are indicated.

ANEMIAS DUE TO DEFICIENT PRODUCTION

PHYSIOLOGIC "ANEMIA" OF THE NEWBORN & ANEMIA OF PREMATURITY

Essentials of Diagnosis

- Age 2–3 months.
- Normochromia or hyperchromia; microcytosis.

General Considerations

Physiologic "anemia" occurs in all full-term infants and reaches its low point (hemoglobin about 10–11 g/dL) at about age 2½ months. The exact mechanism is not known, although it is recognized that both erythropoietin release and bone marrow production cannot keep pace with somatic growth. At this age it is not due to iron deficiency. It is associated with the transition from production of fetal hemoglobin to adult hemoglobin. The increased O_2 release capacity of adult hemoglobin provides less stimulus for erythropoietin as it replaces fetal hemoglobin. The anemia may be more severe in premature infants, in whom the hemoglobin may drop to levels of 5–6 g/dL.

Clinical Findings

A. Symptoms and Signs: Slight pallor may be noted in full-term infants, but usually no other symptoms occur. If the anemia is severe in the premature infant, decreased activity and fatigue with feeding may occur.

B. Laboratory Findings:

1. Blood—Anemia is normochromic or hyperchromic, with microcytosis. Cell diameter may be as small as 5 μm. No other abnormalities are noted in the blood smear.

2. Bone marrow—The marrow appears relatively normal but shows slight erythroid hypoplasia; morphologic changes are not indicative of decreased production.

Differential Diagnosis

Iron deficiency anemia usually does not manifest itself until after the age of 2–3 months. Congenital hemolytic anemias that are associated with red cell membrane or red cell metabolic abnormalities (such as hereditary spherocytosis, pyruvate kinase deficiency, etc) are present from birth and should be considered. Congenital pure red cell hypoplastic anemia presents within the first few months of life; an extremely low reticulocyte count should suggest this diagnosis. Hemolysis associated with sepsis or following erythroblastosis fetalis should be considered. Chronic infection may increase the degree of anemia.

Treatment

Treatment should not be instituted unless the anemia is of sufficient severity to produce symptoms. Therefore, therapy is not indicated in the full-term infant. Treatment may be necessary in the premature infant if the hemoglobin drops below 7 or 8 g/dL and symptoms of lethargy and fatigue are noted.

The only effective treatment is blood transfusion, which should be given in the form of packed red cells in doses of 5–10 mL/kg. The anemia will not respond at this age to iron or folic acid or other hematinics.

Prognosis

Spontaneous recovery is apparent by about 12–14 weeks of age in all infants. Anemia that persists beyond 3 months usually has another cause.

Dallman PR: Anemia of prematurity. *Annu Rev Med* 1981; **32:**143.

O'Brien RT, Pearson HA: Physiologic anemia of the newborn infant. *J Pediatr* 1971;**79:**132.

Stockman JA III, Garcia JF, Oski FA: The anemia of prematurity: Factors governing the erythropoietin response. *N Engl J Med* 1977;**296:**647.

NUTRITIONAL ANEMIAS

Anemia is the most common manifestation of nutritional deficiency in children in the USA; it is even more frequent in other parts of the world. In the USA, iron deficiency is responsible for the majority of these nutritional anemias. Folic acid and vitamin B_{12} deficiencies are seen principally in economically underprivileged children. The need for exogenous iron is greatly increased during the first 2 years of life and again in adolescence because of the rapid growth of the child.

1. IRON DEFICIENCY ANEMIA

Essentials of Diagnosis

- Pallor, fatigue.
- Good weight gain, poor muscle tone.
- Delayed motor development.
- Poor dietary intake of iron.
- Age 6 months to 2 years.
- Hypochromic microcytic anemia.

General Considerations

The average diet contains 12–15 mg of iron (of which approximately 10% is absorbed), and the normal daily excretion of iron is less than 1 mg/d.

Iron deficiency on a nutritional basis generally occurs between 6 months and 2 years of age and is an extremely rare cause of anemia after age 3 except in adolescence. As infants rarely outgrow their iron stores prior to the age of 4 months, iron deficiency is almost never a cause of anemia in the first 3 months of life except with severe iron deficiency in the mother or following blood loss by hemorrhage in the infant. It has been demonstrated that iron deficiency is associated with abnormalities of the intestinal mucosa that allow for loss of serum proteins as well as chronic intestinal hemorrhage. In some cases, occult gastrointestinal blood loss may be a major factor. Thus, the exudative enteropathy that may occur secondary to dietary iron deficiency further aggravates the iron depletion in the body. Other primary conditions (eg, cow's milk intolerance) may cause exudative enteropathy and initiate the iron loss.

Iron deficiency is also seen in association with chronic hemorrhage or rapid growth. Infestation with hookworm or *Trichuris trichiura* should be considered as primary cause of chronic gastrointestinal blood loss in endemic areas.

The diagnosis depends largely on a history of a diet low in iron-containing solid foods with a high intake of milk (> 1 quart/d) and evidence of early rapid weight gain during the first 1–2 years of life. Hypochromia with microcytosis, decreased MCHC, and decreased serum iron with increased iron-binding capacity are characteristic.

Clinical Findings

A. Symptoms and Signs: Pallor, fatigue, irritability, and delayed motor development are common. The child is often fat and flabby, with poor muscle tone. Beeturia (red urine from the pigment of beets) occurs more frequently in iron-deficient children and may be a clue to the anemia. Nonhematologic manifestations of iron deficiency are caused in part by deficiencies in the cytochrome system. Irritability and decreased intellectual performance and perception have been demonstrated. Other symptoms include anorexia, koilonychia, atrophy of the tongue papillae, gastric achlorhydria, and the alterations in small bowel mucosa noted above. Pica is common in all age groups and includes geophagia (clay or dirt eating), pagophagia (ice eating), and amylophagia (starch eating).

B. Laboratory Findings: The hemoglobin is depressed and may be as low as 3–4 g/dL. The red cell count and hematocrit are proportionately higher, producing a significantly lowered MCHC (< 30%). The red cells on smear are microcytic and hypochromic, with a low MCV and low MCH for age. The reticulocyte count is usually normal, but it may be elevated in severe cases.

Serum iron need not be determined in childhood if the dietary and growth history readily explain the cause of the hypochromic anemia. If there is doubt regarding the diagnosis or the cause or if exudative enteropathy is suspected, this determination should be performed. Serum iron is low—usually below 30 μg/dL (normal, 90–150 μg/dL). Total iron-binding capacity is usually elevated to 350–500 μg/dL (normal, 250–350 μg/dL). Iron saturation is under 20% (normal, 30%), and serum ferritin is decreased to less than 10 ng/mL. Free erythrocyte protoporphyrin (FEP) is elevated. An FEP/hemoglobin ratio greater than 2.8 μg/g of hemoglobin usually indicates iron deficiency or lead poisoning. Values greater than 17.5 μg/g of hemoglobin, however, are usually caused by lead intoxication. Measurement of hemoglobin alone with a cutoff of 11 g/dL may be an effective screening test for iron deficiency during the first 2 years of life. If a trial of iron therapy results in a hemoglobin rise of at least 1 g/dL, mild iron deficiency is confirmed.

Bone marrow examination is usually not necessary in infants for the diagnosis of iron deficiency. Even normal children under 2 years of age deposit little or no iron in the form of hemosiderin in the marrow. In older children and adolescents, marrow examination with staining for iron may be helpful, since stainable iron should be present normally over the age of 2–3 years and will be absent in iron deficiency anemia.

The diagnosis is best confirmed by administration of an adequate dose of iron and the demonstration of a reticulocyte rise in 3–5 days and a hemoglobin rise in 7–14 days.

Differential Diagnosis

Iron deficiency anemia must be differentiated from several other hypochromic microcytic anemias caused by defective incorporation of iron into the hemoglobin molecule.

Thalassemia minor is the disorder that is most frequently confused with nutritional iron deficiency anemia, and it should be suspected in the child with an iron-resistant hypochromic anemia. Hypochromia and anemia may occur with any hemoglobinopathy involving the thalassemia gene. The serum iron will be elevated in these conditions, and the free erythrocyte protoporphyrin will be normal. Hemoglobin A_2 will be elevated in beta thalassemia minor.

Infection and inflammation interfere with erythropoiesis and utilization of iron. They produce hypochromic anemias that may be slightly microcytic. Although the serum iron and total iron-binding capacity are low, bone marrow hemosiderin will be present in the older child; search should be made for the presence of severe chronic infection or inflammatory disease. Other iron-resistant hypochromic anemias include anemia due to lead poisoning and vitamin B_6-dependent anemia.

Complications

Children with iron deficiency anemia are more susceptible than others to infection. In severe cases, heart failure may occur. Motor development is often delayed because of weakness. Anorexia and irritability cause additional feeding problems and further malnutrition. Severe iron deficiency interferes with the normal integrity of the gastrointestinal tract; exudative enteropathy associated with protein and additional iron loss may occur.

Prevention

Iron deficiency can be prevented in full-term infants by using iron-fortified infant formulas for 12 months or by the addition of iron-containing solid foods by 4 months of age. Breast-fed infants absorb up to 50% of the iron in the milk, but supplemental iron-fortified solid foods (such as infant cereals) are also recommended. Small preterm infants should receive iron-fortified formulas or supplemental iron medication by 2 months of age in a large prophylactic dose (2–4 mg/kg/d) of elemental iron.

Treatment

A. Oral Iron: The recommended oral dose of elemental iron is 1.5–2 mg/kg 3 times daily between meals (4.5–6 mg/kg/d). Although absorption is better if the medication is given between meals, it may cause gastrointestinal irritation; iron can be administered with food or even in milk. Various iron complexes and concentrates are available, but there is little evidence that any one is preferable to the others. Ferrous sulfate remains the drug of choice. Patients should be observed for a reticulocyte rise in 3–5 days and for a hemoglobin increase in 1–2 weeks. To replenish iron stores, therapy should be continued for 2 months after the hemoglobin has reached a normal level.

B. Intramuscular Iron: Iron dextran (Imferon) may be given intramuscularly if oral intolerance or malabsorption is present or if parental supervision is inadequate. The total dose can be calculated from the following formula:

$$\text{mg Iron} = \frac{\text{Desired hemoglobin} - \text{Initial hemoglobin}}{100} \times 80 \times \text{Weight in kg} \times 3.4$$

An additional 30% should be given to replace deficient iron stores. Daily doses should be limited to 1 mL (50 mg) in infants and 2 mL (100 mg) in very young children. When administering iron dextran, pull the skin to one side before injecting; this will prevent leakage to the skin. The response of the reticulocyte count and the hemoglobin to the intramuscular product is no more rapid than to oral administration of an adequate dose of ferrous sulfate.

C. Ascorbic Acid: Large doses of ascorbic acid increase absorption of iron from food but probably do not affect the efficacy of iron medication.

D. Blood Transfusions: Transfusion therapy is reserved for children with extremely low levels of hemoglobin who are bordering on congestive failure or who have serious acute infections. Packed red cells should be used and administered slowly in a dose not to exceed 10 mL/kg. In the severely ill child with impending or frank congestive failure, a partial exchange transfusion (isovolumetric) with packed red cells should be given.

E. Diet: Ultimate management of iron deficiency anemia requires improvement in the diet, with reduction of milk intake, use of iron-fortified formulas, and an increase in iron-containing foods such as meat, eggs, fortified infant cereals, and green vegetables.

Prognosis

Iron therapy will produce rapid and complete recovery within 2–4 weeks if the anemia is due to nutritional inadequacy. If the anemia persists, other causes must be found and treated.

Committee on Nutrition, American Academy of Pediatrics: Iron supplementation for infants. *Pediatrics* 1976;**58:**765.

Committee on Nutrition, American Academy of Pediatrics: Relationship between iron status and incidence of infection in infancy. *Pediatrics* 1978;**62:**246.

Dallman PR et al: Diagnosis of iron deficiency: The limitations of laboratory tests in predicting response to iron treatment in 1-year-old infants. *J Pediatr* 1981;**99:**376.

Dienard AS, Schwartz S, Yip R: Developmental changes in serum ferritin and erythrocyte protoporphyrin in normal (nonanemic) children. *Am J Clin Nutr* 1983;**38:**71.

Oski FA, Stockman JA III: Anemia due to inadequate iron sources or poor iron utilization. *Pediatr Clin North Am* 1980;**27:**237.

Siimes MA, Järvenpää AL: Prevention of anemia and iron deficiency in very low birth weight infants. *J Pediatr* 1982;**101:**277.

2. IRON-RESISTANT, MICROCYTIC HYPOCHROMIC ANEMIAS

Anemia of Infection & Inflammation

The hemoglobin usually ranges from 8 to 11 mg/dL, and the red cells may be slightly hypochromic. Serum iron and total iron-binding capacity are low. (See p 455 for details.) Free erythrocyte protoporphyrin and ferritin may be slightly elevated.

Thalassemia Minor

This is one of the more common forms of iron-resistant hypochromic anemia in children of black, Mediterranean, or Southeast Asian origin. The hemoglobin is usually in the range of 9–11 g/dL, and the red cells are significantly hypochromic. The blood smear may also show target cells and basophilic stippling. Serum iron, total iron-binding capacity, and ferritin are elevated. Free erythrocyte protoporphyrin is normal. A_2 hemoglobin is elevated in beta thalassemia minor, but normal in alpha thalassemia. (See p 474 for details.)

Anemia of Lead Poisoning

Microcytosis is common in children with severe

lead poisoning. It occurs in about 80% of patients with blood lead concentrations exceeding 70 μg/dL. Anemia is less common and is often due to associated iron deficiency. Lead poisoning can be suspected by the presence of basophilic stippling of erythrocytes. Moderate reticulocytosis occurs. A history of pica may be found in iron deficiency anemia but is particularly characteristic of the young child with lead ingestion. The serum iron may be low, normal, or elevated depending on the nutritional status, but sideroblasts are always present in the bone marrow. Free erythrocyte protoporphyrin is markedly elevated. Diagnostic studies for lead poisoning include long bone x-rays, serum lead levels, and urinary lead, coproporphyrin, and δ-aminolevulinic acid studies. Details of diagnosis and treatment are discussed in Chapter 30. Packed red cell transfusions may be indicated for correction of the anemia if it is severe.

Cohen AR, Trotsky MS, Pincus D: Reassessment of the microcytic anemia of lead poisoning. *Pediatrics* 1981;**67:**904.

Piomelli S et al: The FEP (free erythrocyte porphyrins) test: A screening micromethod for lead poisoning. *Pediatrics* 1973:**51:**254.

Pyridoxine-Responsive (Vitamin B_6-Responsive) Anemia

This rare condition is usually hereditary. It is characterized by severe microcytic hypochromic anemia. The onset may be early in infancy. Serum iron and ferritin are elevated. The bone marrow shows erythroid hyperplasia with large numbers of sideroblasts (nucleated normoblasts with iron inclusions). There is progressive hepatosplenomegaly. Abnormalities of tryptophan metabolism may be demonstrated by excessive excretion of xanthurenic acid, kynurenine, and kynurenic acid in urine after an oral loading dose of tryptophan. The diagnosis is proved by response of the anemia to parenterally administered pyridoxine. An adequate test dose is 100 mg, although most children will respond to 25 mg or less. The disorder is usually inherited as an X-linked recessive, and recovery is dependent upon continued administration of vitamin B_6. Phlebotomy has also been shown to be of value in older individuals in conjunction with vitamin B_6 therapy.

Acquired pyridoxine deficiency has been described in association with isoniazid therapy for tuberculosis. It responds readily to small oral doses of pyridoxine (2–5 mg/kg/d).

Hines JD: Effect of pyridoxine plus chronic phlebotomy on the function and morphology of bone marrow and liver in pyridoxine-responsive sideroblastic anemia. *Semin Hematol* 1976;**13:**133.

Sideroachrestic (Sideroblastic) Anemias

The sideroachrestic anemias comprise a group characterized by iron resistance, hypochromia, large iron stores, and high serum iron levels. The anemias are all due to a disturbance in hemoglobin biosynthesis, resulting in an increased number of sideroblasts—nucleated normoblasts with iron inclusions. The iron accumulates, since the cell is unable to incorporate iron into the hemoglobin molecule. Sideroblasts occur in low concentrations in normal persons but are markedly increased in this group of iron-refractory anemias. Siderocytes, which are erythrocytes with iron inclusions, are also markedly increased in number.

Most cases are familial, and some of them are apparently transmitted as an X-linked recessive disorder. Patients are occasionally anemic in early childhood, but the familial forms are more apt to express themselves fully in adult life.

The anemia is always hypochromic, with anisocytosis and poikilocytosis. It is refractory to parenteral iron therapy. The serum iron is increased, with almost complete saturation of the total iron-binding capacity.

Diagnosis is based on bone marrow examination, determination of the A_2 hemoglobin level by electrophoresis studies for lead intoxication, and a therapeutic trial with vitamin B_6 in order to differentiate the other iron-resistant hypochromic anemias.

Bottomley SS: Porphyrin and iron metabolism in sideroblastic anemia. *Semin Hematol* 1977;**14:**169.

Peto TEA, Pippard MJ, Weatherall DJ: Iron overload in mild sideroblastic anaemias. *Lancet* 1983;**1:**375.

3. MEGALOBLASTIC ANEMIAS

Megaloblastic anemias are characterized by oval macrocytes and hypersegmented polymorphonuclear neutrophils in the peripheral blood and megaloblasts in the bone marrow. They are due primarily to a deficiency of folic acid or vitamin B_{12} or a combination of both. These 2 substances function as coenzymes in the synthesis of nuclear protein.

Folic acid must be converted to folinic acid with the assistance of ascorbic acid. The gastric intrinsic factor is necessary for the absorption of vitamin B_{12}. Megaloblastic anemias develop in the absence of gastric intrinsic factor or as a result of dietary deficiencies of folic acid or, rarely, vitamin B_{12}, or they may appear in the presence of ascorbic acid deficiency if the folic acid intake is low.

Folic Acid Deficiency

Dietary deficiency of folic acid occurs most frequently in infancy. It appears in an acute form within the first few months of life and is almost always due to the combination of low folic acid intake and ascorbic acid deficiency. Whole cow's milk and human breast milk provide adequate folic acid. However, certain powdered milk products, unless supplemented, contain inadequate folate. Goat's milk is deficient in both folate and vitamin B_{12}, and its use is a major cause of nutritional megaloblastic anemia in infancy. Preterm infants and those with prolonged diarrhea are more likely to become deficient.

Folic acid-deficient megaloblastic anemia also occurs in older children with severe nutritional deficiency or with serious absorption problems such as celiac disease, intestinal bypass, or blind loops of the bowel.

Megaloblastic anemia may also result from infestation with the fish tapeworm *(Diphyllobothrium latum)*. The administration of certain anticonvulsant drugs (phenytoin, primidone, phenobarbital) and the use of isoniazid with cycloserine, phenylbutazone, nitrofurantoin, and methotrexate have been reported to cause megaloblastic anemia.

Folate deficiency also occurs secondary to increased utilization of folate in chronic hemolytic anemias such as sickle cell disease.

The characteristic findings are weakness, pallor, and anorexia in infancy. Glossitis and a beefy red tongue are occasionally noted, but the neurologic manifestations of pernicious anemia are not seen. The anemia is frequently severe, with hemoglobin levels below 4 g/dL. The red cell count is low and may be under 1 million/μL in severe cases. The blood smear shows macrocytes and significant anisocytosis and poikilocytosis. The red cells are usually normochromic but may be hypochromic if iron deficiency is also present. Leukopenia with neutropenia is usually present. Polymorphonuclear neutrophils are enlarged and hypersegmented. The platelets are usually moderately reduced. The reticulocyte count is low. Formiminoglutamic acid (FIGLU) is present in the urine in folic acid deficiency after histidine loading. The Schilling test will differentiate folic acid deficiency from defective vitamin B_{12} absorption. Erythrocyte transketolase activity is normal in folate deficiency but elevated in vitamin B_{12} deficiency.

The marrow examination is diagnostic. The smear is characterized by delayed maturation and the presence of the typical megaloblastic forms of the nucleated red cells. Giant metamyelocytes may be seen, and megakaryocyte nuclei may be hypersegmented.

Megaloblastic anemia due to folic acid deficiency responds rapidly to oral or parenteral administration of folic acid in a daily dosage of 5 mg. Two to 3 weeks of treatment are usually sufficient. A significant rise in the reticulocyte count will occur within a few days after therapy is started. Ascorbic acid in a dosage of about 200 mg/d orally should be given at the same time. In generalized malnutrition, vitamin B_{12} should also be given. Dietary changes should be instituted to prevent the recurrence of megaloblastic anemia.

Complete and permanent recovery will follow the administration of folic acid and ascorbic acid. Relapses occur only with dietary deficiencies.

Administration of folic acid in a dose of 25–50 μg/d is recommended for preterm infants under 1700 g during the first 3 months of life, since their absorption of folate is poor.

Chanarin I: Management of megaloblastic anaemia in the very young. *Br J Haematol* 1983;**53:**1.

Dallman PR: Iron, vitamin E, and folate in the preterm infant. *J Pediatr* 1974;**85:**742.

Kamel K et al: Folate requirements of children. 3. Response of children recovering from protein-calorie malnutrition to graded doses of parenterally administrered folic acid. *Am J Clin Nutr* 1972;**25:**152.

Taheri MR et al: The effect of folate analogues and vitamin B_{12} on provision of thymine nucleotides for DNA synthesis in megaloblastic anemia. *Blood* 1982;**59:**634.

Megaloblastic Anemia of Generalized Malnutrition

Megaloblastic anemia occurs among economically underprivileged children, particularly in tropical and subtropical countries, in association with poverty and poor dietary habits. It results from a low intake of both folic acid and vitamin B_{12} and often is associated with iron deficiency anemia. The bone marrow and other laboratory findings demonstrate the presence of megaloblastic changes in the marrow and iron deficiency. The peripheral blood usually shows both macrocytosis and hypochromia. The anemia of kwashiorkor, which occurs in severe nutritional deficiency associated with protein inadequacy, is usually normochromic and normocytic or, less commonly, macrocytic or megaloblastic.

Treatment should include folic acid, vitamin B_{12}, and iron, with dietary improvement for future prevention.

Cook JD et al: Nutritional deficiency and anemia in Latin America: A collaborative study. *Blood* 1971;**38:**591.

Congenital Megaloblastic Anemia

A few cases of megaloblastic anemia have been reported in infancy in association with a congenital metabolic block in nucleic acid formation. Large quantities of orotic acid appear in the urine because of the inborn error in pyrimidine metabolism. Patients respond well to treatment with uridine but are unresponsive to folic acid or vitamin B_{12}. Therapy must usually be continued throughout life.

Smith LH Jr: Pyrimidine metabolism in man. *N Engl J Med* 1973;**288:**764.

Vitamin B_{12} Deficiency & Juvenile Pernicious Anemia Syndromes

Vitamin B_{12} deficiency in childhood is usually due to dietary lack or malabsorption. Since the primary source of vitamin B_{12} is from meats, a deficiency can occur in families on a pure vegetarian diet and has been described in breast-fed infants of vegan mothers. Vitamin B_{12} malabsorption may occur in the presence of adequate intrinsic factor, with acquired intestinal lesions, with generalized intestinal malabsorption, and in a familial disease of infants characterized by selective malabsorption of B_{12}.

The pernicious anemia syndromes of childhood are all caused by impaired absorption of vitamin B_{12}.

Although pernicious anemia is rare in childhood, a number of different forms have been described. A congenital deficiency of intrinsic factor has been observed, with onset of symptoms in early infancy. Several forms of intrinsic factor defect have been differentiated with onset in the second decade—one type without antibodies, one type with antibodies to parietal cells and intrinsic factor (similar to the disease in adults), and pernicious anemia associated with various endocrinopathies.

The clinical picture is very similar to that in the adult, with anemia resulting in pallor, fatigue, and the development of anorexia and diarrhea. The presence of a beefy red, smooth, sore tongue and the development of neurologic manifestations differentiate this anemia from the other megaloblastic anemias of childhood. The central nervous system involvement includes ataxia, paresthesias of the hands and feet, impaired vibratory perception, a positive Babinski sign, and the absence of tendon reflexes.

Typical laboratory findings include a macrocytic anemia with anisocytosis and poikilocytosis. Neutropenia and thrombocytopenia are common, and the polymorphonuclear neutrophils are hypersegmented. Reticulocytes are within the normal range. The bone marrow is hyperplastic and shows characteristic megaloblastic abnormalities with a delay in maturation. Giant metamyelocytes and hypersegmented megakaryocytes are found.

The serum vitamin B_{12} concentration is usually less than 100 pg/mL (normal, 300–400 pg/mL).

Treatment consists of the administration of vitamin B_{12} (cyanocobalamin) by parenteral injection. In children, a dosage of 15–30 μg intramuscularly given 3–5 times per week for 2–4 weeks (or until blood values return to normal) is usually adequate. In large children or adolescents, the dose may be increased to 100 μg given at the same intervals. A maintenance dose of 100 μg should be administered by injection each month. This therapy usually produces an excellent remission, although it must be continued throughout life. Oral administration of vitamin B_{12}, liver injections, and folic acid therapy are not recommended. Treatment with folic acid alone will allow the neurologic manifestations to progress even though the anemia may be controlled.

Chanarin I: Management of megaloblastic anaemia in the very young. *Br J Haematol* 1983;**53:**1.

Higginbottom MC, Sweetman L, Nyhan WL: A syndrome of methylmalonic aciduria, homocystinuria, megaloblastic anemia, and neurologic abnormalities in a vitamin B_{12}-deficient breast-fed infant of a strict vegetarian. *N Engl J Med* 1978;**299:**317.

APLASTIC & HYPOPLASTIC ANEMIAS

CONGENITAL HYPOPLASTIC ANEMIA (Congenital Aregenerative Anemia, Congenital Pure Red Cell Anemia, Primary Erythroid Hypoplasia, Blackfan-Diamond Syndrome)

Essentials of Diagnosis

- Pallor, weakness, fatigue.
- Onset in first few months of life.
- Normochromic, macrocytic anemia.
- Very low reticulocyte count (often zero).
- Normal white blood cells and platelets.

General Considerations

Congenital pure red cell anemia usually manifests itself in the first 4 months of life—often immediately after birth—and should be suspected in an infant with severe normochromic anemia and a very low reticulocyte count in the presence of normal circulating white cells and platelets. The diagnosis is made by bone marrow examination; failure of erythropoiesis without equivalent depression of the white cells or platelets is characteristic. The disorder appears to be caused by a block in the maturation of the erythroid series at the stem cell or earliest erythroblast stage. However, recent studies suggest a possible autoimmune T cell mechanism. Thymoma is not present in the congenital childhood form. Although this is sometimes observed in adults with acquired pure red cell anemia, this form is very rare in childhood.

Clinical Findings

A. Symptoms and Signs: Pallor, fatigue, and weakness becoming progressively more severe from early infancy are produced by the anemia. Short stature and growth retardation are characteristic (in untreated cases). Occasionally, there are other associated anomalies, particularly of the kidneys.

B. Laboratory Findings:

1. Blood—The anemia is normochromic but macrocytic, with an MCV greater than 90 fL. The hemoglobin is often less than 5 g/dL. The reticulocyte count is characteristically very low and may be zero. The platelet count, white count, and differential count are normal.

2. Bone marrow—The bone marrow is characterized by a striking absence of nucleated red cell precursors without any depression of the granulocytic series or the megakaryocytes. Occasionally, very immature cells of the erythroid series may also be seen.

3. Other tests—Levels of erythropoietin are markedly elevated, and abnormalities of tryptophan metabolites have been described in the urine following a tryptophan loading test.

The erythrocytes have the characteristics of fetal red cells, with increased hemoglobin F, increased i antigen, and elevated levels of glycolytic enzymes. Activity of erythrocyte adenosine deaminase is increased.

Differential Diagnosis

Other conditions occurring in the neonatal period with depressed erythropoiesis in the presence of normal granulocytes and platelets include the anemia of prematurity and the anemia that often follows severe erythroblastosis fetalis. In both of these situations, reticulocytes should be present and the past history is suggestive.

Congenital pure red cell anemia may occasionally be confused with hemolytic anemia in the first few months of life, when physiologic processes inhibit the normal reticulocyte response to hemolysis.

A variant of pure red cell anemia has been described in infants with triphalangeal thumbs and neutropenia.

Transient erythroblastopenia of infancy may closely mimic congenital hypoplastic anemia. It can be differentiated by a later age of onset, normal MCV (< 80 fL), normal adenosine deaminase activity, and spontaneous recovery.

Complications

The principal complications are associated with therapy. Repeated blood transfusions have resulted in widespread hemosiderosis, at times progressing to hemochromatosis. Therapy with corticosteroids has resulted in marked impairment of physical growth and in osteoporosis.

Treatment

A. Corticosteroids: In many cases, the anemia responds dramatically to therapy with corticosteroids, particularly if therapy is begun before age 3. Oral prednisone is the most frequently used drug. The dosage ranges from 15 mg/d in infants up to 60 mg/d in older children. It should be given in divided doses. A significant response of the anemia will usually be seen within 3–4 weeks. Following this, the dosage should be reduced to determine the minimal level with which a remission can be obtained. Alternate-day therapy is often possible and may cause less interference with growth.

Other drugs such as testosterone and cobalt have no effect in this condition.

B. Blood Transfusions: Transfusions must be given in the presence of severe anemia and as a chronic supportive measure in the child who does not respond to corticosteroid therapy. Packed cells should be administered every 3–4 weeks to keep the hemoglobin above 11 g/dL.

C. Splenectomy: Splenectomy is occasionally of value but is never curative. Its effect is probably greatest in the child who has developed splenomegaly and has an extracorpuscular hemolytic component that is presumably in the spleen. This is confirmed by tagging normal donor red cells with radioactive chromium (^{51}Cr) and noting their shortened survival.

D. Iron Chelation Therapy: Deferoxamine has been used as a chelating agent in patients who require chronic transfusions. Administration by subcutaneous drip over 12 hours has been shown to be most effective. Ascorbic acid aids in mobilizing the iron stores for chelation. (See section on thalassemia.)

E. Bone Marrow Transplantation: This form of therapy has been attempted and may hold promise for the future.

Prognosis

Before the adrenocorticosteroids came into use, the course of congenital pure red cell anemia in many patients was one of chronic and progressive anemia with a fatal outcome. Repeated transfusions prolong life but cause hemosiderosis and hemochromatosis by the second decade.

The results of long-term corticosteroid therapy have not yet been evaluated. Many children have been maintained in remission throughout childhood. Markedly impaired growth appears to be the primary complication of corticosteroid treatment.

Occasionally, children have spontaneous remission during later childhood or at adolescence. The milder cases that show a few red cell precursors in the bone marrow are more apt to have remissions.

Alter BP: Childhood red cell aplasia. *Am J Pediatr Hematol Oncol* 1980;**2:**131.

Ambruso DR et al: Effect of subcutaneous deferoxamine and oral vitamin C on iron excretion in congenital hypoplastic anemia and refractory anemia associated with the 5q-syndrome. *Am J Pediatr Hematol Oncol* 1982;**4:**115.

Chan HS, Saunders EF, Freedman MH: Diamond-Blackfan syndrome. 1. Erythropoiesis in prednisone responsive and resistant disease. *Pediatr Res* 1982;**16:**474.

Glader BE, Backer K, Diamond LK: Elevated erythrocyte adenosine deaminase activity in congenital hypoplastic anemia. *N Engl J Med* 1983;**309:**1486.

TRANSIENT ERYTHROBLASTOPENIA OF INFANCY

This disorder is characterized by anemia, reticulocytopenia, and absence of erythroid precursors in an otherwise normal marrow. It appears acutely in infants and children, often preceded by an infection. Recovery usually occurs spontaneously within 1–2 weeks. It is differentiated from congenital hypoplastic anemia by the normal size of the red cells (MCV < 80 fL), normal hemoglobin F, and no increase in the i antigen. There is evidence in some cases to suggest an IgG-mediated autoimmune basis, and other cases may be due to viral suppression of erythroblastosis.

Labotka RJ, Maurer HS, Honig GR: Transient erythroblastopenia of childhood: Review of 17 cases, including a pair of identical twins. *Am J Dis Child* 1981;**135:**937.

Wang WC, Mentzer WC: Differentiation of transient erythroblastopenia of childhood from congenital hypoplastic anemia. *J Pediatr* 1976;**88:**784.

APLASTIC ANEMIA

Essentials of Diagnosis

- Weakness and pallor.
- Purpuras, petechiae, and bleeding.
- Frequent infections.
- Pancytopenia with empty bone marrow.

General Considerations

Aplastic anemia is characterized by a severe pancytopenia with an acellular marrow and normal-sized spleen.

In childhood, aplastic anemia may be of 3 general types.

A. Fanconi's Congenital Pancytopenia: See below.

B. Idiopathic Aplastic Anemia: In at least half of cases in childhood, no etiologic agent or specific congenital cause can be found. Recent studies suggest a possible T cell autoimmune mechanism.

C. Secondary (Acquired) Aplastic Anemia: Aplastic anemia may occur as a toxic reaction to various chemicals and drugs. Chloramphenicol accounts for the majority of cases in childhood. Other antibiotics, sulfonamides, benzene, acetone, toluene, phenylbutazone, mephenytoin, certain insecticides such as DDT, and heavy metals have all been incriminated. Glue sniffing has produced aplastic anemia and has also initiated aplastic crises in patients with sickle cell anemia. Large amounts of radiation and high doses of cytotoxic drugs such as mechlorethamine and the folic acid antagonists will also produce severe aplasia. Aplastic anemia has been observed as a complication of severe infectious hepatitis and may be caused by other viruses also.

Clinical Findings

A. Symptoms and Signs: Weakness, fatigue, and pallor are the result of the anemia; purpura and bleeding occur because of the thrombocytopenia; and severe generalized or localized infections are frequently due to neutropenia.

B. Laboratory Findings: Severe normochromic anemia is usually present, with some microcytosis. The reticulocyte count is usually very low, but in early cases with partial marrow destruction, it may be slightly elevated. The white count is usually less than 2000/μL, with a marked neutropenia. The platelet count is usually below 50,000/μL. Thrombocytopenia is often the earliest manifestation.

The bone marrow is practically devoid of normal marrow elements and is replaced with fat. A bone marrow section is indicated for absolute diagnosis.

The fetal hemoglobin level remains elevated in congenital aplastic anemia (Fanconi type) but may or may not rise in acquired forms.

Differential Diagnosis

Other causes of pancytopenia in childhood include infiltration with leukemia, Hodgkin's disease, Niemann-Pick disease, Gaucher's disease, Letterer-Siwe disease, osteopetrosis, myelofibrosis, and various toxic agents. Most of these conditions are associated with splenomegaly.

Complications

The disease is characteristically complicated by overwhelming infection and severe hemorrhage. With long-term transfusion therapy, problems may develop in association with leukoagglutinins, erythrocyte antibodies, and hemosiderosis.

A significant complication of prolonged testosterone therapy in childhood is the development of secondary sex characteristics in boys and evidence of masculinization and hirsutism in girls. Epiphyseal closure and stunting of growth have not been a problem in most cases, but patients should be checked periodically with bone x-rays for epiphyseal maturation.

Treatment

A. General Measures: Severely ill children should be protected from infection in their environment by being placed in "reverse isolation." Specific and appropriate antibiotics should be used for infection.

Transfusions are usually necessary. If bleeding is not present, packed red cells in a dose of 10–20 mL/kg should be used for treatment of the anemia when symptoms develop. For severe hemorrhage, platelet concentrates should be used. Buffy coat concentrate containing high numbers of white cells may be tried for severe antibiotic-resistant infections, although this will increase the incidence of future transfusion reactions due to the development of leukoagglutinins.

B. Drug Therapy:

1. Androgens—Androgens will produce remissions in a small proportion of both secondary and idiopathic cases of aplastic anemia in childhood. A patient who has a few residual marrow cells will respond more frequently than a patient with a totally empty bone marrow. The remission will frequently not occur until 1–2 months after treatment is started. Once a remission has been achieved, the lowest possible maintenance dose should be determined by gradual reduction of dosage. Temporary cessation of therapy may be indicated because of untoward drug side effects. Oxymetholone (2–4 mg/kg/d orally) has been used widely in the past. Hepatic toxicity and heptomas have been associated with long-term use. Nandrolone decanoate (1–1.5 mg/kg/wk intramuscularly) has proved effective in some cases and has not been associated with hepatic complications. Androgen therapy should probably be reserved for patients for whom a transplant donor is not available and who have not improved with antithymocyte globulin (ATG) therapy. Androgens may be given in conjunction with ATG.

2. Immunosuppressive therapy—Corticosteroids have generally not been effective in usual doses. However, up to 20% of patients respond to intravenous high-dose methylprednisolone, and up to 50% respond to therapy with antilymphocyte globulin (ALG) or antithymocyte globulin (ATG). Remissions have occasionally been observed following cyclophosphamide treatment. Data suggesting the presence of overactive suppressor thymocytes in some cases are confirmed by these responses. ATG with methylprednisolone is currently considered the therapy of choice for patients with no HLA-matched marrow donor. There is no good method for determining which patients will respond.

C. Bone Marrow Transplantation: Cure has been achieved in over 50% of patients with the use of homologous bone marrow transplantation using a sibling donor with the same tissue (HLA) type. Isogenic marrow grafting has been consistently successful when an identical twin with unaffected bone marrow is the donor. Early marrow transplantation is considered by many to be the treatment of choice when an HLA-matched sibling donor is available.

Prognosis

The prognosis for patients with either the secondary (acquired) or the idiopathic form of aplastic anemia is extremely poor when the bone marrow is totally empty and complete pancytopenia is present. In spite of supportive measures, these patients usually die of infection or hemorrhage within a period of a few months. Very few will respond to testosterone therapy. If some marrow elements remain, however, spontaneous remissions occasionally occur; remissions are sometimes induced with testosterone therapy. In the acquired form, a spontaneous remission may eventually occur 1–2 years after initiating treatment with testosterone or testosterone plus prednisone. Bone marrow transplantation with a histocompatible donor has provided a 50–60% cure rate (especially if done early in the disease), whereas the recovery with supportive therapy and androgens is only about 20%.

Camitta BM et al: A prospective study of androgens and bone marrow transplantation for treatment of severe aplastic anemia. *Blood* 1979;**53:**504.

Champlin R, Ho W, Gale RP: Antithymocyte globulin treatment in patients with aplastic anemia: A prospective randomized trial. *N Engl J Med* 1983;**308:**113.

Gordonsmith EC: Treatment of aplastic anemias. *Hosp Pract* (May) 1985;**20:**69.

Mangan KF: T-cell mediated suppression of hematopoiesis. (Editorial.) *N Engl J Med* 1985;**312:**306.

Najean Y, Girot R, Baumelou E: Prognostic factors and evolution of acquired aplastic anemia in childhood: A prospective analysis of 48 androgen-treated cases. *Am J Pediatr Hematol Oncol* 1982;**4:**273.

Sanders JE et al: Bone marrow transplantation in pediatric patients with aplastic anemia or acute leukemia. *Am J Pediatr Hematol Oncol* 1980;**2:**171.

Storb R et al: Graft-versus-host disease and survival in patients with aplastic anemia treated by marrow grafts from HLA-identical siblings. *N Engl J Med* 1983;**308:**302.

Workentin PI et al: Immunosuppressive therapy for severe aplastic anemia. *Am J Pediatr Hematol Oncol* 1980;**2:**327.

CONGENITAL APLASTIC ANEMIA WITH MULTIPLE CONGENITAL ANOMALIES (Fanconi's Anemia)

This is a familial aplastic anemia in which hypoplastic or aplastic bone marrow is associated with a number of other congenital anomalies. Occasionally, pancytopenia occurs in association with a hyperplastic marrow as a result of a delay in maturation. The most common defects are skeletal and include hypoplasia or absence or anomalies of the thumb, the thenar eminence, and the radius. Other skeletal anomalies may include syndactyly, congenital dislocation of the hips, and abnormalities of the long bones. Some affected children have patchy brown pigmentation of the skin, hypogenitalism, microcephaly, short stature, strabismus, ptosis of the eyelids, nystagmus, anomalies of the ears, and mental retardation. The condition may occur in siblings and is probably transmitted as an autosomal recessive trait. The hematologic manifestations rarely are manifested prior to age 1 and may appear at any time between ages 1 and 12. Thrombocytopenia is usually the first abnormality to be noted, followed later by neutropenia and anemia. Although the bone marrow in the typical patient is hypoplastic and progresses to aplasia, in rare cases it may be hyperplastic, with a delay in maturation of marrow elements.

The hematologic disorder is slowly progressive, and severe aplasia will develop in most cases. Death due to infection or bleeding will eventually occur if therapy is not instituted.

The clinical manifestations are principally those of the aplastic anemia (see above).

Fanconi's anemia is characterized by elevated fetal hemoglobin, an increased red cell MCV, and an increased number of chromosomal breaks. These findings are present prior to the onset of the pancytopenia and can aid in early diagnosis. The heterozygotes also have the chromosomal anomalies. Both the patients and the carriers have an increased risk of cancer, both for leukemia and for solid tumors. Prenatal diagnosis can be made by study of amniotic fluid fibroblasts for chromosomal breaks. For these studies, cell cultures must be stressed with alkylating agents such as diepoxybutane.

The majority of patients with Fanconi's anemia will respond to testosterone therapy or testosterone plus prednisone, although relapse will occur when drug therapy is discontinued. (See section on aplastic anemia for details of therapy.) Transfusion should be used in patients who do not respond to either testosterone or a combination of testosterone and prednisone. These children are especially prone to the development of hepatomas with long-term oxymetholone treatment; therefore, nandrolone decanoate treatment should be used instead.

The prognosis is much better since testosterone therapy came into use. However, long-term experience is beginning to suggest that many of these patients may eventually become resistant to testosterone therapy and die of the aplastic anemia in early adult life. Spontaneous recovery has occurred in a few cases during adolescence. Successful bone marrow transplantation using an unaffected histocompatible sibling donor has been reported in this disease.

Auerbach AD, Adler B, Chaganti RS: Prenatal and postnatal diagnosis and carrier detection of Fanconi anemia by a cytogenetic method. *Pediatrics* 1981;**67:**128.

Gözdaşoğlu S et al: Fanconi's aplastic anemia: Analysis of 18 cases. *Acta Haematol (Basel)* 1980;**64:**131.

McIntosh S, Breg WR, Lubiniecki AS: Fanconi's anemia: The preanemic phase. *Am J Pediatr Hematol Oncol* 1979;**1:**107.

CONGENITAL HYPOPLASTIC ANEMIA WITHOUT ASSOCIATED ANOMALIES

Several families have been reported with pancytopenia and hypoplastic or aplastic marrow without associated anomalies. This is probably a recessive hereditary disorder and closely related to Fanconi's anemia. Testosterone therapy may be effective.

ANEMIA OF RENAL FAILURE (Anemia of Uremia)

A severe normochromic anemia occurs in almost all forms of renal disease that have progressed to renal insufficiency. Although white cell production remains normal and platelet production may be normal, the bone marrow shows significant hypoplasia of the erythroid series.

The marrow hypoplasia is due to decreased circulating erythropoietin, which is normally produced principally in the kidney. Erythropoiesis is also suppressed (in vitro) by the serum of uremic patients. The only treatment available is blood transfusion, which should be given as packed cells in a dosage of 10–20 mL/kg when the hemoglobin drops below 7 g/dL or when symptoms occur. Drug therapy is not effective.

The anemia of renal disease is frequently complicated by an extracorpuscular hemolytic component that occurs in the presence of significant uremia. Hemolytic-uremic syndrome, a more severe form of hemolytic anemia that occurs occasionally in children in association with renal disease, is discussed in Chapter 21.

Wallner SF, Vautrin RM: Evidence that inhibition of erythropoiesis is important in the anemia of chronic renal failure. *J Lab Clin Med* 1981;**97:**170.

ANEMIA OF HYPOTHYROIDISM

Certain patients with hypothyroidism develop fairly severe normochromic anemias. The red cells frequently tend to be macrocytic. However, microcytic hypochromic anemia also has been described. The bone marrow shows hypocellularity of the erythroid series, with a normoblastic pattern.

Replacement therapy with thyroid hormone is effective in treating the anemia of the hypothyroid patient. Some of the hypochromic patients also respond partially to iron.

ANEMIA OF INFECTION & INFLAMMATION

Significant anemia usually develops in serious chronic infections or inflammatory diseases such as tuberculosis, chronic osteomyelitis, rheumatic fever, regional ileitis, and rheumatoid arthritis. It also may occur with acute inflammation. The anemia usually ranges between 8 and 11 g/dL of hemoglobin and is normochromic or slightly hypochromic. The reticulocyte count is usually normal or low. The mechanism is not clearly understood. However, the primary causes are a decrease in erythropoietin and a reticuloendothelial block in transfer of iron. In addition, there is a slight decrease in red cell survival time. The bone marrow appears normal and hemosiderin deposits are present, although the serum iron and the total iron-binding capacity are low. Ferritin and free erythrocyte protoporphyrin are elevated. Evidence of underlying infection or inflammatory disease is usually obvious.

There is no effective treatment except control of the infection and transfusions if the anemia is severe.

Abshire TC, Reeves JD: Anemia of acute inflammation in children. *J Pediatr* 1983;**103:**868.

Ward HP, Kurnick JE, Pisarczyk MJ: Serum level of erythropoietin in anemias associated with chronic infection, malignancy, and primary hematopoietic disease. *J Clin Invest* 1971;**50:**332.

ANEMIAS ASSOCIATED WITH MARROW REPLACEMENT (Myelophthisic Anemias)

Anemias resulting from bone marrow invasion or replacement are known as myelophthisic anemias.

The most common cause in childhood is invasion with leukemic cells or lymphosarcoma. The differentiation from aplastic anemia in the hypoplastic form of leukemia can only be made by bone marrow examination. Hodgkin's disease in its advanced form may also be associated with severe marrow involvement. Other malignant tumors (particularly neuroblastoma) may cause diffuse involvement of the marrow. The disseminated acute form of histiocytosis (Letterer-Siwe disease) may be associated with a diffuse involvement of the marrow. Some lipid storage diseases (eg, Gaucher's disease and Niemann-Pick disease) gradually invade the marrow. Osteopetrosis (Albers-Schönberg disease) in the acute infantile form is associated with severe encroachment on the marrow space by bone and usually presents initially as a myelophthisic anemia. True myelofibrosis with the development of classic agnogenic myeloid metaplasia is rarely seen in childhood.

All of these forms of myelophthisic anemia are characterized by the development of a normochromic anemia and associated thrombocytopenia. The presence of nucleated red cells and immature white cells with an elevated nucleated cell count in the peripheral blood suggests the existence of a myelophthisic process. Immature white and red cells are not always released, and they are probably related to the degree of extramedullary hematopoiesis. Splenomegaly is present in the majority of these conditions. The diagnosis is dependent upon finding the specific infiltrating process, osteopetrosis, or myelofibrosis in the bone marrow.

ANEMIAS DUE TO FAILURE OF RELEASE FROM THE MARROW

PRIMARY REFRACTORY ANEMIA (Refractory Normoblastic Anemia)

This condition is characterized by the paradoxic association of a hypercellular marrow and a moderate to severe chronic anemia, occasionally associated with neutropenia and thrombocytopenia. The reticulocyte count is low to normal. There are usually no other clinical findings, and the spleen is not enlarged. The marrow is markedly hypercellular, with normoblastic hyperplasia. Megaloblastic changes are usually present. Marrow hemosiderin is greatly increased.

The exact cause of this syndrome is not known, although many patients previously given this diagnosis may have had some type of dyserythropoietic anemia associated with intramedullary hemolysis (see next section). Treatment of the primary refractory anemias has been generally without success, and transfusion is usually the only treatment. In rare cases, splenectomy has been of slight value. Occasionally, congenital cases have responded to testosterone therapy. All patients should be given a trial of vitamin B, since the findings in pyridoxine-dependent anemias may be similar.

DYSERYTHROPOIETIC ANEMIAS

The dyserythropoietic anemias are characterized by maturation abnormalities in the bone marrow with associated intramedullary hemolysis. The clinical manifestations include the presence of intermittent scleral jaundice and splenomegaly. Anemia occasionally is not present. Some patients are well compensated, with hemoglobins and hematocrits within the normal range. The majority have a mild to moderate anemia of about 10 g/dL. Occasional patients show intermittent severe anemia associated with increased jaundice. They are frequently not recognized as having a hemolytic process, since the destruction takes place in the marrow and an excessive number of reticulocytes are not released. The reticulocyte count usually ranges from normal to a maximum of about 4%. In most of the reported familial cases, the mode of genetic transmission appears to be autosomal recessive. At least 4 different types have been described.

Additional laboratory findings include the presence of marked anisocytosis and poikilocytosis on the blood smear. There is usually an elevation of the indirect serum bilirubin to approximately 2 mg/dL. The haptoglobin is low or absent. Urobilin and urobilinogen are increased in the urine. The bone marrow pattern is diagnostic, with erythroid hyperplasia and characteristic erythroblasts showing several separate nuclei or with clover leaf-shaped nuclei.

Findings include elevated fetal hemoglobin and increased hemolysis in acidified serum (a positive Ham test) in the presence of a negative sugar water test in type II. A high proportion of cells are agglutinated by anti-i antibody. Osmotic fragility is normal or increased. The autohemolysis test and hemoglobin electrophoresis are normal. Iron stores are increased, and iron kinetics show a rapid plasma clearance.

The exact mechanism of the ineffective erythropoiesis and the intramedullary hemolysis has not been specifically explained.

The differential diagnosis includes Gilbert's disease, since patients with little or no anemia show primarily an elevated unconjugated (indirect reacting) serum bilirubin and intermittent scleral icterus. In patients with anemia, the differential diagnosis includes the other types of mild hemolytic disease.

Treatment is symptomatic.

Alloisio N et al: Alterations of globin chain synthesis and of red cell membrane proteins in congenital dyserythropoietic anemia I and II. *Pediatr Res* 1982;**16:**1016.

Lewis SM, Verwilghen RL: *Dyserythropoiesis*. Academic Press, 1977.

HEMOLYTIC ANEMIAS

The hemolytic anemias of childhood may be classified as hereditary or acquired. The hereditary group is of particular importance, since the manifestations usually present in infancy or childhood. They may be divided first into those associated with a defect of the red cell membrane, such as hereditary spherocytosis, and those due to abnormalities in red cell glycolysis. (This includes the majority of the nonspherocytic hemolytic anemias that are associated with specific red cell enzyme defects and the drug-induced hemolytic anemias.) Second, there is a large group of hemoglobinopathies that includes the anemias with abnormal hemoglobin chains, those with a genetically determined decrease in production of one of the hemoglobin chains, and those with unstable hemoglobin. The majority of the acquired hemolytic anemias are on an "autoimmune" basis; are secondary to drug or chemical poisoning; or are associated with sepsis from hemolytic organisms.

DISORDERS OF RED CELL MEMBRANE

1. HEREDITARY SPHEROCYTOSIS (Congenital Hemolytic Anemia, Congenital Hemolytic Jaundice)

Essentials of Diagnosis

- Anemia.
- Sudden weakness and jaundice.
- Splenomegaly.
- Spherocytosis, increased reticulocytes.
- Increased osmotic fragility, abnormal autohemolysis.
- Negative Coombs test.
- Positive family history of anemia, jaundice, or gallbladder disease.

General Considerations

Hereditary spherocytosis is a common inherited hemolytic anemia that occurs in about one in 5000 persons of Northern European ancestry. It is caused by an abnormal skeletal structure of the red cell membrane, probably due to a defect in spectrin. Instability of the membrane allows fragmentation and loss of surface area. There is also increased influx of water and sodium into the erythrocytes. Increased glycolysis is necessary to prevent the intracellular accumulation of sodium. Spherocytosis and decreased red cell survival occur when the cell is deprived of sufficient glucose. The cells are sequestered and destroyed in the spleen. Transfused cells from normal donors have a normal survival in the patient with spherocytosis, whereas spherocytic cells transfused into a normal recipient maintain their shortened survival rate. The disease may be mild to severe and is characterized by intermittent crises associated with rapid hemolysis and jaundice. Hypoplastic crises occasionally occur in association with decreased erythroid production in the bone marrow. In most instances, the disease is transmitted as an autosomal dominant, and abnormalities can usually be detected in one of the parents of the child even though they are asymptomatic. There have been occasional reports of families in which the abnormality cannot be found in other generations, suggesting that it can be transmitted as a recessive trait or occur as a mutation. Hereditary spherocytosis may be a cause of neonatal hyperbilirubinemia and may be confused with ABO incompatibility because of the presence of spherocytes in both conditions.

Clinical Findings

A. Symptoms and Signs: Jaundice usually occurs in the newborn period. Splenomegaly without other symptoms characterizes many of the cases in childhood. Chronic fatigue and malaise may be present, and abdominal pain is a frequent complaint. Gallbladder pain may occur in the adolescent.

Hemolytic or aplastic crises may develop and are associated with severe weakness, fatigue, fever, abdominal pain, and jaundice.

B. Laboratory Findings: Mild chronic anemia is characteristic. The hemoglobin usually varies from 9 to 11 g/dL, although a few cases may have almost normal levels of 12–13 g/dL. The red cells are microcytic and hyperchromic (MCV = 70–80 fL, and MCHC = 36–40%). Spherocytes characteristically are seen on the smear but may comprise no more than 10% of the cells prior to splenectomy. A persistently elevated reticulocyte count is characteristic. White cells and platelets are usually normal.

The bone marrow shows typical erythroid hyperplasia of hemolytic anemia (except during the hypoplastic crisis, when there may be marked reduction of erythropoiesis).

Osmotic fragility is increased, particularly after incubation at 37 °C for 24 hours. Autohemolysis of blood incubated for 48 hours is greatly increased. Incubation with glucose or ATP will decrease the hemolysis (usually to normal levels). Serum bilirubin may show elevation of the unconjugated portion. Stool urobilinogen is usually elevated. The Coombs test is negative, and hemoglobin electrophoresis reveals a normal pattern.

Complications

Severe jaundice may occur in the newborn period with the development of kernicterus if exchange transfusion is not performed. Splenectomy in the first 2 years of life is associated with increased susceptibility to overwhelming bacterial infections (particularly pneumococcal sepsis). Gallstones (composed principally of bile pigments) occur in up to 85% of young adults with this disease, and they may even develop during later childhood if splenectomy is not performed by the middle childhood years.

Treatment

There is no satisfactory medical treatment for this condition, but splenectomy is effective.

A. Exchange Transfusions: For hyperbilirubinemia in the neonatal period, exchange transfusion should be performed.

B. Surgical Treatment: Splenectomy is the treatment of choice in hereditary spherocytosis. Except in unusually severe cases, the procedure should be postponed until the child is at least 5 or 6 years of age, because of the increased risk of infection prior to this time. The operation is indicated in older children as soon as the diagnosis is confirmed, even though the degree of hemolysis may be mild. Cholecystectomy for cholelithiasis is rarely indicated in childhood, particularly if splenectomy is performed by 10 years of age.

C. Postoperative Anti-infective Prophylaxis: Prophylactic penicillin is recommended following splenectomy in all children. It should be continued throughout childhood and adolescence. Pneumococcal vaccine should be given before splenectomy.

D. Treatment of Hemolytic and Hypoplastic Crises: Crises associated with anemia are frequently precipitated by infection. Therapy should include antibiotics for bacterial infections and packed red cell transfusions for both hemolytic and hypoplastic crises.

Prognosis

Splenectomy will eliminate all signs and symptoms, and the red cell survival usually returns to normal following this procedure. The development of cholelithiasis will also be prevented if splenectomy is performed during childhood. The abnormal red cell morphology, increased osmotic fragility, and the abnormal findings on autohemolysis test persist following splenectomy but are of no clinical significance.

Agre P, Orringer EP, Bennett V: Deficient red-cell spectrin in severe, recessively inherited spherocytosis. *N Engl J Med* 1982;**306:**1155.

Kelleher JF et al: Human serum "parvovirus": A specific cause of aplastic crisis in children with hereditary spherocytosis. *J Pediatr* 1983;**102:**720.

Lux SE, Wolfe LC: Inherited disorders of the red cell membrane skeleton. *Pediatr Clin North Am* 1980;**27:**463.

Marchesi VT: The red cell membrane skeleton: Recent progress. *Blood* 1983;**61:**1.

2. OVALOCYTOSIS (Hereditary Elliptocytosis)

Hereditary elliptocytosis is characterized primarily by the presence of large numbers of oval and elliptic cells in the peripheral blood. It is usually discovered on routine examination, and the majority of patients are asymptomatic. The morphologic abnormality of the peripheral blood is transmitted as an autosomal dominant and occurs in both sexes. Approximately 12% of the heterozygous cases demonstrate evidence of mild hemolytic disease characterized by slight splenomegaly and reticulocytosis. There may be low-grade anemia, but even in these patients the hemoglobin is frequently within normal limits. Occasionally, neonatal jaundice is sufficiently severe to require exchange transfusions.

The nucleated precursors of the elliptic cells in the bone marrow are normal in shape, with the oval appearance occurring first at the reticulocyte stage or later. The mechanism of the abnormality is not known.

A few cases have been reported of children who are homozygous for the disease. These children have severe hemolytic anemia, with splenomegaly and hematologic evidence of hemolysis.

Treatment is not usually indicated except in severe cases, for which splenectomy is usually beneficial.

Lusher JM, Barnhart MI: The role of the spleen in the pathophysiology of hereditary spherocytosis and hereditary elliptocytosis. *Am J Pediatr Hematol Oncol* 1980;**2:**31.

Torlontano G et al: Hereditary elliptocytosis: Haemotological and metabolic findings. *Acta Haematol (Basel)* 1972;**48:**1.

3. STOMATOCYTOSIS

A rare form of hemolytic anemia has been described in which the red blood cells have a characteristic cup-shaped appearance. The anemia is mild, and the disease has the characteristics of a hemolytic process with elevated reticulocyte count. The red cells have increased osmotic fragility, increased autohemolysis, and reduced glutathione.

Splenectomy results in improvement.

4. ACANTHOCYTOSIS (Abetalipoproteinemia)

This rare autosomal recessive disorder is characterized by acanthocytes (thorny cells) in the blood, progressive ataxic neurologic disease, retinitis pigmentosa, malabsorption, and abetalipoproteinemia. Although the red cells are very abnormal, the degree of hemolysis is mild. (See also Chapter 33.)

Cooper RA, Gulbrandsen CL: The relationship between serum lipoproteins and red cell membranes in abetalipoproteinemia: Deficiency of lecithin:cholesterol acyltransferase. *J Lab Clin Med* 1971;**78:**323.

5. XEROCYTOSIS (Desiccytosis)

Xerocytosis is a rare autosomal dominant condition characterized by mild to moderate congenital hemolytic anemia. The number of reticulocytes is increased, and the blood smear usually shows shrunken, spicular cells in which hemoglobin is "puddled" on one side. Target cells, stomatocytes, and dense cells may also be present. This disorder is due to a membrane defect that causes loss of water and potassium but little change in intracellular sodium, and this results in intracellular dehydration. Diagnosis is made by measurement of red cell cations and isopyknic centrifugation. Osmotic fragility is usually decreased. Splenectomy has not been of value.

Glader BE et al: Desiccytosis associated with RBC potassium loss: A new congenital hemolytic syndrome. *Pediatr Res* 1973;**7**:350.

6. HYDROCYTOSIS

Hydrocytosis is a rare congenital hemolytic anemia in which the red cells have a primary defect in permeability that leads to cell swelling. Anemia varies from mild to severe, and the inheritance is usually autosomal dominant. The increase in cell water, which produces stomatocytes, can be demonstrated by either isopyknic centrifugation or osmotic gradient ectocytometry. Osmotic fragility is increased, and there is an increase in total red cell cation concentration due to increased intracellular sodium. Patients respond well to splenectomy.

Lande WM, Mentzer WC: Haemolytic anaemia associated with increased cation permeability. *Clin Haematol* 1985;**14**:89.

7. HEREDITARY PYROPOIKILOCYTOSIS

This is a rare disorder presenting in infancy with severe hemolytic anemia. It is characterized by extreme poikilocytosis with budding red cells, spherocytes, elliptocytes, and bizarrely shaped fragmented cells. The MCV is very low (25–55 fL), and osmotic fragility and autohemolysis are markedly increased. The red cells have unusual sensitivity to heat and will fragment at 45–46 °C (normally at 49 °C). Red cell membrane spectrin is abnormal and unusually heat-sensitive. Pyropoikilocytosis has been reported primarily in black families. Splenectomy results in marked improvement but not complete cure. Pyropoikilocytosis also has been reported to be transient in infancy in some families with mild hereditary elliptocytosis.

Castleberry RP et al: Hereditary pyropoikilocytosis: Ultrastructural and biochemical assessment. *Blood* 1979;**54**:25.

Prchal JT et al: Hereditary pyropoikilocytosis and elliptocytosis: Clinical, laboratory, and ultrastructural features in infants and children. *Pediatr Res* 1982;**16**:484.

8. ACQUIRED CELL MEMBRANE DEFECTS ASSOCIATED WITH HEMOLYSIS

Infantile Pyknocytosis

A transient hemolytic anemia has been described in newborn infants in association with a high degree of pyknocytosis of their red cells. Pyknocytes bear a close resemblance to burr cells or acanthocytes. They occur in small numbers in all newborn and premature infants, but in infants with hemolysis, as many as 50% of red cells may be pyknocytes. The exact cause remains unknown. The syndrome is characterized by hemolysis beginning during the first week of life, with jaundice, anemia, reticulocytosis, and splenomegaly. The anemia usually reaches its peak by 3 weeks of age, and recovery is spontaneous.

The diagnosis is based on the presence of large numbers of pyknocytes (> 6%) in association with a Coombs-negative hemolytic anemia.

Exchange transfusion may be necessary for the hyperbilirubinemia of pyknocytosis during the first week. Small transfusions are indicated for increasing anemia after that time.

Vitamin E Deficiency Hemolytic Anemia

Vitamin E deficiency may cause hemolysis and an increase in burr cells. It can be differentiated from pyknocytosis by demonstrating an increased hemolysis in hydrogen peroxide and a response to the administration of parenteral vitamin E.

The disorder occurs primarily in preterm infants after the fourth week of life and is due to poor absorption of vitamin E. It is aggravated by the oral administration of iron medication. A dosage of 25 units of vitamin E per day orally is adequate prophylaxis.

Lubin B, Chiu D: Properties of vitamin E-deficient erythrocytes following peroxidant injury. *Pediatr Res* 1982;**16**:928.

Melhorn DK, Gross S: Vitamin E-dependent anemia in the premature infant. 1. Effects of large doses of medicinal iron. *J Pediatr* 1971;**79**:569.

Liver Disease

Red cell membrane changes may occur in liver disease and can be associated with significant hemolytic anemia. The membrane abnormality is associated with changes in serum and membrane lipid involving the cholesterol-phospholipid ratio. The most severe form (usually seen in hepatocellular disease) is characterized by "spur" cells. The more common and milder form is characterized by target cells.

Cooper RA et al: An analysis of lipoproteins, bile acids, and red cell membranes associated with target cells and spur cells in patients with liver disease. *J Clin Invest* 1972; **51**:3182.

Renal Disease

A marked hemolytic anemia may occur secondary to the effect of elevated metabolites and urea in severe uremia. Burr cells are usually present. These changes are corrected by dialysis.

Hemolytic-Uremic Syndrome

Hemolytic anemia may be severe and often is the presenting complaint in this disorder. It is a microangiopathic anemia associated with destruction of red cells in small renal vessels and characterized by fragmented and burr-shaped cells. (See Chapter 21.)

Hemolysis With Disseminated Intravascular Coagulation

A microangiopathic hemolytic anemia with fragmented cells and burr cells is characteristic of this syndrome (see p 497).

DISORDERS OF RED CELL GLYCOLYSIS (The Hereditary Nonspherocytic Hemolytic Anemias)

Essentials of Diagnosis

- Moderate to severe anemia.
- Elevated reticulocyte count.
- Normal osmotic fragility test with abnormal autohemolysis.
- Splenomegaly.
- Present from birth, with neonatal jaundice.
- Negative Coombs test.

General Considerations

The hereditary nonspherocytic hemolytic anemias include a number of different defects in red cell metabolism. A number of specific enzymes necessary for erythrocyte glycolysis have been shown to be deficient in various forms of nonspherocytic hemolytic anemia. These enzyme deficiencies include glucose 6-phosphate dehydrogenase (G6PD), 6-phosphogluconate dehydrogenase, pyruvate kinase, triosephosphate isomerase, hexokinase, hexosephosphate isomerase, phosphoglycerate kinase, adenosinetriphosphatase (ATPase), 2,3-diphosphoglycerate mutase, phosphoglucose isomerase, phosphofructokinase, glyceraldehyde 3-phosphate dehydrogenase, lactate dehydrogenase, glutathione reductase, glutathione peroxidase, glutathione synthetase, and hereditary absence of glutathione. The most frequently encountered are those associated with G6PD or pyruvate kinase deficiency. These will be discussed in more detail in succeeding sections.

The hereditary pattern varies. Deficiency of G6PD is transmitted as an X-linked recessive, whereas pyruvate kinase deficiency and most of the other types occur as autosomal recessives.

Clinical Findings

A. Symptoms and Signs: Moderate to severe anemia is usually present and exists from early infancy. Neonatal hyperbilirubinemia is usually marked. In severe cases, symptoms of chronic anemia and jaundice persist. The spleen is enlarged.

B. Laboratory Findings: Anemia is moderate to severe, and the hemoglobin usually ranges from 5 to 9 g/dL. The red cells are normocytic and normochromic, although occasional microcytes are seen and, in pyruvate kinase deficiency, a few spherocytes. The reticulocyte count is markedly elevated; the white cell and platelet counts are normal. Bone marrow shows marked erythroid hyperplasia.

Red cell osmotic fragility is increased in pyruvate kinase deficiency and triosephosphate isomerase deficiency but is normal in other enzyme deficiencies.

The autohemolysis test is slightly increased in most types and is partially corrected by the addition of glucose and ATP. The test is markedly increased in pyruvate kinase deficiency; partial correction can be achieved with use of glucose and ATP. The test is also increased in triosephosphate isomerase deficiency; complete correction with glucose and ATP can be achieved in these cases.

Studies of red cell glycolysis with assays of specific enzymes are indicated in all cases that fall into this group, since the response to splenectomy may be dependent on the exact type of disease.

Differential Diagnosis

In the newborn period, hereditary nonspherocytic hemolytic anemia must be differentiated from erythroblastosis fetalis and ABO incompatibility by immunologic studies. It is differentiated from acquired hemolytic anemia by the early onset and the absence of a positive Coombs test. The differentiation from hereditary spherocytosis is based on the absence of spherocytes on the smear, the normal or only slightly increased red cell fragility, and the lack of complete correction with glucose in the autohemolysis test in the nonspherocytic hemolytic anemias.

Complications

The severe chronic anemia is usually associated with growth failure; hemosiderosis may occur in cases that require frequent transfusions. Cholelithiasis and cholecystitis may develop in later childhood.

Treatment

There is no specific therapy for most cases of nonspherocytic hemolytic anemia. Splenectomy is not as effective as in hereditary spherocytosis and is of no benefit in many cases. However, some patients (including those with pyruvate kinase deficiency) do show significant improvement following splenectomy; although no patients are completely cured and many do not respond at all, the operation is probably worth a trial. The possible value of splenectomy can be estimated by determining the red cell survival of cells from a patient with hereditary nonspherocytic hemolytic anemia after infusion into a normal individual who has undergone splenectomy for some other reason.

Prognosis

In the milder form of this disease, the prognosis is good; the patient can usually live with a mild chronic anemia. Cholelithiasis often develops in early adult life. The prognosis is similar with more severe forms that show improvement following splenectomy.

In the severe types that do not respond to splenectomy, frequent transfusions are required, physical growth is stunted, and hemochromatosis may develop from the iron administered by the frequent transfusions.

Beutler E: *Hemolytic Anemia in Disorders of Red Cell Metabolism.* Plenum Press, 1978.

Sullivan DW, Glader BE: Erythrocyte enzyme disorders in children. *Pediatr Clin North Am* 1980;**27**:449.

1. PYRUVATE KINASE DEFICIENCY HEMOLYTIC ANEMIA

A severe chornic hemolytic anemia is associated with erythrocyte pyruvate kinase deficiency. Although this is a rare disease, it is still one of the more frequently encountered specific entities in the group of nonspherocytic hereditary hemolytic anemias. It is transmitted as an autosomal recessive condition. It presents as a moderate or severe hemolytic anemia in the immediate neonatal period, with low hemoglobin levels even in cord blood. Jaundice in the newborn is a common complication, and exchange transfusion is usually required. Splenomegaly is the only consistent clinical finding. The reticulocytes in this disorder are particularly susceptible to splenic sequestration. Leg ulcers have been described in a family with a variant type of pyruvate kinase deficiency.

The anemia is normochromic, and there is a marked elevation of the reticulocyte count. The blood smear shows some microcytes and a few spherocytes. Differentiation from hereditary spherocytosis is not easy, because spherocytes may be seen in pyruvate kinase deficiency and red cell osmotic fragility may also be slightly increased; the autohemolysis test is markedly increased, as in spherocytosis. The most useful point of differentiation between thc 2 diseases is the fact that the red cell fragility is only slightly increased and the autohemolysis test is only partially corrected by glucose in pyruvate kinase deficiency, whereas the latter is markedly corrected in spherocytosis.

Family studies are also helpful in differentiating the 2 conditions, since pyruvate kinase deficiency is autosomal recessive whereas spherocytosis is usually dominant.

Red cell glycolysis and specific enzyme assays for pyruvate kinase are indicated if this condition is suspected. Several different mutant forms of the enzyme have been reported; recently, a mutant enzyme was described in patients with a similar disorder who appear to have adequate pyruvate kinase activity by the usual assay but who are found to have a pathologic isoenzyme that can be detected only by assays using low levels of substrate.

Treatment consists of splenectomy. Significant improvement usually follows this procedure, although complete cure is not achieved. Prior to splenectomy, repeated transfusions are usually necessary every few months. No drugs or other methods of management are effective.

The prognosis following splenectomy is fairly good, although the complications of cholelithiasis should be anticipated.

Glader BE, Nathan DG: Haemolysis due to pyruvate kinase deficiency and other glycolytic enzymopathies. *Clin Haematol* 1975;**4**:123.

Miwa S: Pyruvate kinase deficiency and other enzymopathies of the Embden-Meyerhof pathway. *Clin Haematol* 1981; **10**:57.

2. GLUCOSE 6-PHOSPHATE DEHYDROGENASE DEFICIENCY (Drug-Sensitive Hemolytic Anemia, Primaquine-Sensitive Hemolytic Anemia)

Drug-induced hemolytic anemia is most commonly associated with a red cell deficiency of glucose 6-phosphate dehydrogenase (G6PD). The deficiency is due to the presence of a labile G6PD enzyme that is present in young cells but rapidly disappears with cell aging. A large number of variant defective enzymes have been found in different racial groups. It is estimated that G6PD deficiency affects more than 125 million persons worldwide. Most persons with a G6PD defect have episodes of hemolysis only after exposure to certain oxidant drugs, although the more severe forms may be manifested by a chronic hereditary nonspherocytic hemolytic anemia.

The disease is transmitted as an X-linked recessive. Full expression occurs also in females who are homozygous for the gene; intermediate expression occurs in the heterozygous female carrier. In the USA, about 10% of black males manifest this enzyme deficiency, whereas only 1–2% of black females tend to be mildly symptomatic when challenged with drugs. This disease occurs also in Chinese people, Southeast Asians, and whites (particularly Greeks, Italians, Arabs, and Sephardic Jews). The exact mechanism of the enzyme defect is not quantitatively or qualitatively identical in all of these racial groups. The disorder is less severe in blacks than in other racial groups.

Symptoms usually occur only in association with oxidant drug exposure or infections. In the neonatal period, certain racial groups (Greek, Italian, and Chinese) may show increased hyperbilirubinemia, whereas full-term black infants do not. The most common offenders are the antimalarials, sulfonamides, sulfones, nitrofurans, antipyretics, analgesics, synthetic vitamin K, and uncooked fava beans. Hemolytic crises in patients with sickle cell anemia may be due in part to an associated G6PD deficiency.

The clinical picture is characterized by an acute hemolytic episode following exposure to one of these substances. The anemia is normochromic, and Heinz body formation is characteristic. An elevated reticulocyte count will appear within a few days.

Since only the older red cells are susceptible, the process becomes self-limited as a younger red cell population appears in response to the hemolytic process.

A specific laboratory diagnosis may be made by one of several tests, including the glutathione stability test, the dye reduction test using cresyl blue, the methemoglobin reduction test, and a commercially available dye reduction spot test. The G6PD levels and the screening test may be normal immediately after a hemolytic episode, because only young cells remain and these still may have normal enzyme activity.

Routine laboratory screening has been recommended for persons in the high-risk racial groups.

Treatment includes discontinuing exposure to the offending agent and transfusion of packed red cells.

Luzzatto L: Inherited haemolytic states: Glucose-6-phosphate dehydrogenase deficiency. *Clin Haematol* 1973;**4:**83.

Shannon K, Buchanan GR: Severe hemolytic anemia in black children with glucose-6-phosphate dehydrogenase deficiency. *Pediatrics* 1982;**70:**364.

SYNTHETIC VITAMIN K-INDUCED HEMOLYTIC ANEMIA OF THE NEWBORN

Another form of drug-induced hemolytic anemia occurs following the administration of synthetic vitamin K (Synkayvite) in large doses in the newborn period. Although the level of G6PD is not decreased in the newborn infant, the drug-induced hemolysis appears to be related to instability of reduced glutathione in the newborn red cells. This may be due in part to the low blood glucose levels that are characteristic of the neonatal period.

This complication can be prevented by limiting the dose of the synthetic vitamin K product to a total of 1 mg or by the use of vitamin K_1 (AquaMephyton, Mephyton, etc), which does not have the same chemical derivation.

Oski FA, Naiman JL: *Hematologic Problems in the Newborn,* 2nd ed. Saunders, 1972.

HEMOGLOBINOPATHIES: QUALITATIVE DEFECTS

1. SICKLE CELL ANEMIA

Essentials of Diagnosis

- Anemia, elevated reticulocyte count, jaundice.
- Positive sickling test, hemoglobin S and F.
- Splenomegaly in early childhood, with later disappearance.
- Crises with pain in the legs and abdomen.
- Usually black African ethnic origin.

General Considerations

Sickle hemoglobin is found primarily in black persons of African origin. However, it also occurs in other racial groups in Sicily, Italy, Greece, Turkey, Saudi Arabia, and India and occurs rarely in other Caucasians. Sickle cell anemia is seen in about one in 500 blacks in the USA. The incidence is much higher in some parts of Africa.

Sickle cell anemia occurs in individuals who are homozygous for the sickle cell gene. Sickle hemoglobin is characterized by a single amino acid substitution (valine for glutamic acid) at the 6 position in the beta globin chain of adult type (A_1) hemoglobin. The sickling trait is transmitted as a dominant; the carrier shows a combination of hemoglobin A_1 and sickle hemoglobin, whereas the patient with sickle cell anemia has only sickle, A_2, and fetal hemoglobins. The sickling process is often initiated by low oxygen tension and low pH. The sickled cells obstruct small vessels, and infarcts are frequent. Infarction accounts for the abdominal pain, bone pain, and gradual decrease in the size of the spleen (''autosplenectomy''). Functional hyposplenism occurs as early as 7 months of age.

Clinical Findings

A. Symptoms and Signs: The onset of symptoms is usually between 6 and 12 months of age, since high levels of fetal hemoglobin prevent sickling in the first few months of life. Functional hyposplenism (often associated with splenomegaly) occurs at this age and is associated with a high risk of sepsis and meningitis due to *Streptococcus pneumoniae* and *Haemophilus influenzae*. Acute splenic sequestration crises are common and result in life-threatening anemia. Pneumonia, urinary tract infections, and osteomyelitis (especially due to *Salmonella*) are also common, with the highest risk of infection occurring between the ages of 1 and 10 years. Moderately severe hemolytic anemia occurs by 1 year of age and causes mild scleral icterus. Hemolytic or hypoplastic crises may occur. Pain crises in the extremities and abdomen occur in varying degrees in most patients who develop the disease in early childhood. Strokes occur in about 10% of children and tend to be recurrent. Physical growth is often retarded; puberty may be delayed; and children are usually asthenic. Older children show enlargement of the facial and skull bones and may develop a ''tower skull.'' During adolescence, leg ulcers may develop and cholelithiasis often occurs. Pulmonary infarctions, priapism, hepatic dysfunction, cardiomegaly, systolic ejection murmur, and even heart failure may occur in older children and adolescents. Chronic sickling in the kidneys results in hyposthenuria (with dilute urine), occasional hematuria, and eventual renal function impairment. Repeated bone infarctions may result in aseptic necrosis (particularly in the hip or shoulder).

B. Laboratory Findings: The hemoglobin usually ranges between 7 and 10 g/dL. It may drop as low as 2–3 g/dL at the time of a sequestration or hypoplastic crisis. The reticulocyte count is markedly elevated. The anemia is normocytic or mildly macrocytic; the smear shows increased numbers of target cells and abnormalities of size and shape. Irreversible sickled cells (ISCs) may be seen on the ordinary blood smear and are common at the time of crisis. The sickling phenomenon can be demonstrated by reducing the oxygen tension in the finger with a small tourniquet prior to obtaining blood or by ringing the coverslip on a slide with petrolatum over a drop of blood. Fresh sodium metabisulfite, 2%, mixed on the slide with the drop of blood will bring out the sickling in a few minutes. The blood "solubility" tests are positive in the presence of sickle hemoglobin. Nucleated red cells are present and may equal the number of white cells. The total nucleated cell count is high. Serum bilirubin usually shows an elevation of unconjugated (indirect) bilirubin. The specific gravity of the urine becomes fixed at about 1.010 in later childhood, and both hemosiderinuria and hematuria may be seen.

The bone marrow shows marked erythroid hyperplasia. X-rays of the skull and spine reveal cortical thinning, enlargement of the marrow spaces, and increased trabecular markings.

Hemoglobin electrophoresis reveals only sickle (S), fetal (F), and A_2 hemoglobin. The fetal component usually varies between 5% and 20%, while A_2 is normal. Techniques for intrauterine diagnosis have been developed using cells from amniocentesis and restriction enzyme fragmentation of DNA.

Differential Diagnosis

The most important differentiation is from the other sickle hemoglobinopathies that are also common in the black population. The differentiation from sickle thalassemia and sickle hemoglobin C disease is made primarily by hemoglobin electrophoresis and determination of fetal and A_2 hemoglobin. The hematuria that occurs with sickle cell anemia must be differentiated from renal bleeding due to other causes. In crisis, the primary differentiation is from acute appendicitis in the presence of abdominal pain and tenderness and from rheumatic fever because of the frequent joint and bone pains and the systolic precordial murmur in sickle cell disease.

Hemoglobins D and G migrate electrophoretically on paper and cellulose acetate at pH 8.4 at the same rate as S and are indistinguishable by this method. They can be differentiated by the negative sickling test with hemoglobin D and G and by electrophoresis on citrate agar at pH 6.2. Study of the entire family is often of importance in determining the exact nature of the hemoglobinopathy.

Sickle cell trait associated with iron deficiency anemia can be differentiated by the presence of a low reticulocyte count, high red cell count, and hypochromia.

Complications

Repeated small vascular infarctions may result in damage to nearly every organ system. The early splenic involvement, with eventual splenic fibrosis, results in increased susceptibility to overwhelming infection. (See also Clinical Findings.)

Treatment

Treatment is instituted primarily for the crises. There is no known effective method for reducing the rate of chronic hemolysis or preventing crises. Both the splenic sequestration and hypoplastic crises should be treated with transfusion. Transfusions are also helpful in terminating prolonged "painful" crises. Packed red cells are usually used. A partial exchange with packed red cells is indicated in pulmonary and other severe crises and prior to surgery. Repeated transfusion every 3–4 weeks is being used with iron chelation therapy in patients with strokes and other severe complications. The use of oxygen, maintenance of good hydration, and correction of acidosis are the most important measures for management of the symptoms of crisis. Rest, analgesics, and sedatives may be sufficient in mild cases. Corticosteroids have been reported to be helpful in the management of painful swelling of the hands and feet. Clinical trials using testosterone to stimulate marrow production have been associated with an increased incidence of thrombosis. A number of antisickling drugs have been evaluated or are under investigation, but none have yet proved suitable for long-term clinical use. Urea and cyanate are effective but toxic. Hydroxyurea and 5-azacytidine (still under investigation) have been shown to cause moderate increases in fetal hemoglobin but are toxic. Bone marrow transplantation has been successful but would not be indicated in most patients because of the risk of the procedure.

In the young patient, early treatment of suspected sepsis with intravenous antibiotics is essential. Prevention of life-threatening pneumococcal disease may be accomplished by use of prophylactic penicillin throughout childhood. Pneumococcal and *H influenzae* vaccines should be administered to all children over 2 years of age with sickle cell disease. Folic acid, 1 mg/d, is given to prevent folate deficiency.

Prognosis

Overwhelming infection in early childhood has resulted in a mortality rate of more than 10% in the past. This can be reduced by early diagnosis of sickle cell anemia (by 6 months of age) and appropriate preventive and therapeutic measures. Diagnosis can be made by hemoglobin electrophoresis done at both alkaline and acid pH in the newborn or at age 4–6 months. Sickling or solubility tests will usually be normal during the first few months of life. Early diagnosis and parental counseling regarding complications such as sepsis and acute splenic sequestration can lead to improved medical care with reduced morbidity and mortality rates. In the future, relatively few patients should die in childhood of this disease. Many patients, however, die in early adult life. Progressive renal damage usually occurs, and death from uremia, heart failure, or pulmonary infarction is common. Some patients survive to over 60 years of age.

Ambruso DR et al: Urinary excretion of iron in response to subcutaneous deferoxamine in sickle cell anemia. *Am J Pediatr Hematol Oncol* 1980;**2:**111.

Ammann AJ: Current status of pneumococcal polysaccharide immunization in patients with sickle cell disease or impaired splenic function. *Am J Pediatr Hematol Oncol* 1982;**4:**301.

Castro OL et al: Managing sickle cell emergencies. *Patient Care* (Jan) 1985;**19:**92.

Powars DR: Natural history of sickle cell disease: The first ten years. *Semin Hematol* 1975;**12:**267.

Vichinsky EP, Johnson R, Lubin BH: Multidisciplinary approach to pain management in sickle cell disease. *Am J Pediatr Hematol Oncol* 1982;**4:**328.

Vichinsky EP, Lubin BH: Sickle cell anemia and related hemoglobinopathies. *Pediatr Clin North Am* 1980;**27:**429.

2. SICKLE CELL TRAIT

Sickle cell trait occurs in about 8–10% of blacks in the USA and in as much as 40% of the population in certain areas of Africa. The high incidence of the carrier state in African blacks has been attributed to the increased resistance to malaria in these individuals; this tends to selectively increase their representation in the population. It is generally asymptomatic, and anemia, reticulocytosis, and morphologic red cell changes are not observed. Hematuria is the principal complication and occurs in 3–4% of cases. Progressive impairment in the ability of the kidneys to concentrate urine is sometimes noted. Splenic infarction or sequestration may occur in the presence of low oxygen tension at extremely high altitudes—particularly with flying in unpressurized aircraft. Except for these unusual circumstances, the prognosis is excellent and the life expectancy is normal.

Heller P et al: Clinical implications of sickle-cell trait and glucose-6-phosphate dehydrogenase deficiency in hospitalized black male patients. *N Engl J Med* 1979;**300:**1001.

Knasel A: Is sickle cell trait a health hazard? Medical problems: A brief review. *Am J Pediatr Hematol Oncol* 1982;**4:**179.

Mahony BS, Githens JH: Sickling crises and altitude: Occurrence in the Colorado patient population. *Clin Pediatr* 1979;**18:**431.

Sears DA: The morbidity of sickle cell trait: A review of the literature. *Am J Med* 1978;**64:**1021.

3. HEMOGLOBIN S-C DISEASE

Hemoglobin S-C disease is caused by the double autosomal heterozygous state for both hemoglobin S and C. The incidence in the American black population is about one in 1500. Symptoms are similar to those of homozygous sickle cell disease but are much less marked. Persons with S-C disease are particularly prone to develop splenic sequestration crises at high altitudes or while flying in unpressurized aircraft. Some patients are prone to vaso-occlusive crises involving the lung, kidney, retina, and femoral head. Target cells are prominent, and a mild anemia with persistent reticulocytosis is usually present. The diagnosis is confirmed by hemoglobin electrophoresis and the sickling test, along with evaluation of other members of the family. The complications and general treatment are similar to those for sickle cell anemia, although most patients require no therapy. However, the retinopathy occurs in a high percentage of young adults and may result in blindness from retinal detachment or vitreous hemorrhage. These complications can be prevented by regular ophthalmologic examination and treatment of the characteristic neovascularization with laser beam coagulation or cryotherapy. Although the severity of the disease may vary, the prognosis is much better than in homozygous sickle disease, and the life span is usually not seriously affected.

Githens JH et al: Splenic sequestration syndrome at mountain altitudes in sickle/hemoglobin C disease. *J Pediatr* 1977; **90:**203.

Kim HC: Variants of sickle cell disease. Page 215 in: *Hemoglobinopathies in Children.* Schwartz E (editor). PSG Publishing Co., 1980.

Serjeant GR et al: The clinical features of haemoglobin SC disease in Jamaica. *Br J Haematol* 1973;**24:**491.

4. SICKLE BETA THALASSEMIA

This disease is due to the double autosomal heterozygous state for both hemoglobin S and beta thalassemia. In blacks with sickle beta$^+$ thalassemia, symptoms are similar to those of sickle cell anemia but are less marked. Painful vaso-occlusive crises may occur. Anemia is mild and microcytic—hemoglobin is in the range of 10–12 g/dL. Hemoglobin electrophoresis shows both A_1 and S hemoglobins but with S being over 50% (usually 60–80%). A_2 and fetal hemoglobins are also present and elevated.

Some patients with the Mediterranean beta thalassemia gene (sickle beta^0 thalassemia) have only S, F, and A_2 hemoglobins, making it difficult to differentiate them from patients with sickle cell anemia. The presence of a low MCV and elevated A_2 hemoglobin suggests this diagnosis. Family studies are needed to confirm the diagnosis. Symptomatic treatment may be required for crises. Life expectancy is probably normal in sickle beta$^+$ thalassemia but reduced in sickle beta^0 thalassemia.

Serjeant GR et al: The clinical features of sickle-cell-thalassaemia in Jamaica. *Br J Haematol* 1973;**24:**19.

5. HEMOGLOBIN C TRAIT & HEMOGLOBIN C DISEASE

Hemoglobin C trait occurs in approximately 2–3% of blacks in the USA. Individuals with the trait are heterozygous for the gene and are essentially asymptomatic; they have a normal life expectancy. The blood smear, however, reveals the presence of large numbers of target cells. Renal hematuria has occasionally been reported.

Hemoglobin C disease is rare and occurs in individuals who are homozygous for the gene. It occurs almost exclusively in blacks. Onset is at about 1 year of age, since the infant is protected by fetal hemoglobin. Patients usually demonstrate a mild hemolytic anemia with a persistently elevated reticulocyte count. Red cell morphology is characterized by many target cells, which are usually normocytic and normochromic. Tetragonal crystals of hemoglobin can be found in the erythrocyte. Osmotic fragility is decreased. The diagnosis is made by hemoglobin electrophoresis, which usually reveals 100% hemoglobin C. Fetal hemoglobin is usually not elevated. Moderate to marked splenomegaly is the only significant clinical finding. There are usually no symptoms, although abdominal pain, arthralgia, and jaundice may occur occasionally.

Treatment is usually not required, and transfusions are rarely needed. Splenectomy is occasionally indicated if anemia is severe.

6. HEMOGLOBIN M DISEASE

The designation M is given to several abnormal hemoglobins associated with methemoglobinemia. Affected individuals are heterozygous for the gene, and it is transmitted as an autosomal dominant. A number of different types have been described in which various abnormal amino acids are substituted in the poplypeptide chain, producing a hemoglobin molecule in which the iron remains in the ferric instead of the ferrous state and cannot combine with oxygen. The defect may be on either the alpha or the beta chain. Hemoglobin electrophoresis at the usual pH will not always demonstrate the abnormal hemoglobin, and special techniques are necessary to detect it by electrophoresis as well as spectroscopically.

The patient has marked and persistent cyanosis but is otherwise usually asymptomatic. Exercise tolerance may be normal, and life expectancy is not affected. When the abnormality is on the beta chain, the infant is unaffected for the first few months of life. Some persons with the M hemoglobinopathy of the beta chain may also have mild hemolysis.

This type of methemoglobinemia does not respond to any form of therapy.

Vichinsky EP, Lubin BH: Unstable hemoglobins, hemoglobins with altered oxygen affinity, and m-hemoglobins. *Pediatr Clin North Am* 1980;**27:**421.

7. HEMOGLOBIN E DISORDERS

Hemoglobin E is common in Southeast Asia and has been seen in the USA with increasing frequency. Hemoglobin E trait (heterozygous hemoglobin E) is totally asymptomatic, with no anemia. Occasional microcytes are seen on blood smear. Hemoglobin E disease (homozygous hemoglobin E) is a benign disorder. The blood smear shows many target cells and significant microcytosis, with a low MCV. There may be borderline anemia and mildly elevated reticulocyte levels. Slight splenomegaly occurs rarely.

The double heterozygous state of hemoglobin E and beta thalassemia results in moderate (beta$^+$ thalassemia-hemoglobin E) or severe (beta^0 thalassemia-hemoglobin E) anemia, with microcytosis, hypochromia, hemolysis, and splenomegaly. The more severe cases may be transfusion-dependent.

When hemoglobin E is submitted to electrophoresis at an alkaline pH, it migrates at the same rate as hemoglobin C, but it can be differentiated from hemoglobin C at an acid pH.

Frischer H, Bowman J: Hemoglobin E, an oxidatively unstable mutation. *J Lab Clin Med* 1975;**85:**531.

8. ABNORMAL D & G HEMOGLOBINS

Hemoglobins D and G are rare in the USA but occur with a higher incidence in other parts of the world. Hemoglobin D has been reported particularly from the Punjab area of India and in parts of Turkey and Africa, as well as occasionally in North American blacks and Indians. It is generally asymptomatic unless associated with another abnormal hemoglobin such as S. Hemoglobin G, even in the homozygous form, has not been associated with symptoms but has been described in combination with other abnormal hemoglobins as a cause of mild anemia.

The majority of the other abnormal hemoglobins that have been described occur only in the heterozygous form and are asymptomatic.

Ozsoylu S: Homozygous haemoglobin D Punjab. *Acta Haematol* 1976;**43:**353.

9. THERMOLABILE (UNSTABLE) HEMOGLOBINS

Since the first report in 1960, a number of families have now been described with a mild form of hemolytic anemia due to a hemoglobinopathy in which the hemoglobin is thermolabile. All of these patients with unstable hemoglobins have had mild anemia and scleral jaundice. They frequently report intermittent exacerbations of hemolysis, and in all cases a dark brown urine has been noted. Mild splenomegaly is usually present. The disorders appear to be transmitted as an autosomal dominant, with symptoms occurring in the heterozygous form.

The laboratory findings reveal a typical picture of a hemolytic anemia with a mild to moderate depression of the hemoglobin and hematocrit and a significant elevation of the reticulocyte count. The unconjugated (indirect reacting) serum bilirubin is often slightly elevated and haptoglobin levels are usually zero, confirming the evidence for hemolysis. The blood smear in some patients has demonstrated marked basophilic stippling. The osmotic fragility test may show both increased fragility and increased resistance. The autohemolysis test is normal. Specific diagnostic studies include the presence of Heinz bodies, particularly after incubation at 37 °C for 48 hours. Hemoglobin electrophoresis in some families has shown an abnormal hemoglobin on paper electrophoresis at pH 8.5. In all cases in which the abnormal hemoglobin was identified on electrophoresis, it has migrated more slowly than hemoglobin A_1 and frequently has been more readily identified on starch gel or agar gel. The percentage of abnormal hemoglobin identified has usually been low (in the range of 5–10%). The heat stability test is the best method for identification of the thermolabile hemoglobin. All of the reported hemoglobins precipitate with heating to 50 °C for 1 hour. The dark pigment in the urine has been identified as mesobilifuscin.

At least 50 different unstable hemoglobins have been identified to date. These include Scott, Zurich, Köln, Ubi 1, Summersmith, Dacie, Seattle, St. Mary's, Sydney, King's County, and others.

The differential diagnosis includes all of the hereditary hemolytic anemias such as spherocytosis and the nonspherocytic group as well as the other hemoglobinopathies. The autosomal dominant genetic transmission tends to exclude the majority of these except for spherocytosis. The diagnostic test is a demonstration of a thermolabile hemoglobin in the blood and the presence of mesobilifuscin in the urine.

The prognosis in most patients is probably good, since the anemia appears to be mild. There is no specific treatment.

Vichinsky EP, Lubin BH: Unstable hemoglobins, hemoglobins with altered oxygen affinity, and m-hemoglobins. *Pediatr Clin North Am* 1980;**27**:421.

10. HEMOGLOBINOPATHIES WITH ABNORMAL OXYGEN AFFINITY

Over 20 different hemoglobinopathies have been described in which the primary clinical sign is polycythemia. The individuals have been heterozygous for the abnormal hemoglobins (eg, hemoglobins Chesapeake, Malmö, Yakima, and Rainier), and the condition is usually transmitted as an autosomal dominant. These hemoglobins have an increased oxygen affinity that results in decreased tissue oxygenation and a compensatory erythrocytosis. Most affected individuals have been asymptomatic except for plethora.

At least 3 different hemoglobins have been described with low oxygen affinity. They may demonstrate cyanosis (hemoglobin Kansas) or anemia (hemoglobin Seattle).

THALASSEMIA SYNDROMES

1. BETA THALASSEMIA MINOR (Thalassemia Trait, Cooley's Carrier State)

Essentials of Diagnosis

- Mild hypochromic anemia.
- Unresponsiveness to iron.
- Elevated A_2 hemoglobin.
- Usually in Mediterranean, black, or Oriental persons.

General Considerations

Beta thalassemia is due to a genetic defect in the production of beta globin chains of hemoglobin. The patient with thalassemia minor is heterozygous for the gene.

Clinical Findings

A. Symptoms and Signs: There are usually no symptoms, and the only physical sign may be slight enlargement of the spleen.

B. Laboratory Findings: The anemia is usually mild; the hemoglobin is rarely under 9 g/dL and may be within normal limits. The red count and hematocrit are very slightly reduced. The red cells are small and hypochromic, and with low MCV and MCH. Target cells are often present, and stippled cells are seen occasionally. Variations in the size and shape of the cells are often noted. The reticulocyte count may be slightly elevated but is frequently within normal limits. Osmotic fragility is markedly decreased.

The diagnosis is confirmed by finding an elevation of the A_2 hemoglobin on electrophoresis in 90% of families; fetal hemoglobin is increased in 10% of families. (In alpha thalassemia—see below—the A_2 hemoglobin is normal.) The serum iron may be normal in infancy but becomes elevated. The bone marrow may show excessive iron deposition in the older child. Free erythrocyte protoporphyrin is normal.

Differential Diagnosis

The primary differentiation is from other mild hypochromic anemias. In childhood, nutritional iron deficiency presents the greatest problem but is readily differentiated by the finding of low serum iron levels and a response to iron therapy. In iron deficiency, free erythrocyte protoporphyrin is elevated, and the hemoglobin A_2 concentration is normal. Lead poisoning and pyridoxine-responsive anemia may present with a similar hematologic picture.

Several closely related thalassemialike carrier states have recently been described. One of these, the Lepore trait, is characterized by a mild hypochromic anemia and an abnormal hemoglobin on starch electrophoresis (but not on paper). It comprises approximately 10% of the hemoglobin.

Complications

There are no complications of thalassemia trait in childhood. In late adult life, excess accumulation of iron may lead to hemosiderosis.

Treatment

No therapy is indicated. Iron should definitely not be administered.

Ohene-Frempong K, Schwartz E: Clinical features of thalassemia. *Pediatr Clin North Am* 1980;**27:**403.

Stockman JA et al: The micromeasurement of free erythrocyte porphyrin (FEP) as a means of screening for β-thalassemia minor in subjects with microcytosis. *Blood* 1973;**42:**990.

2. BETA THALASSEMIA MAJOR (Cooley's Anemia, Mediterranean Anemia)

Essentials of Diagnosis

- Very severe anemia.
- Marked erythroblastemia.
- Splenomegaly and hepatomegaly.
- Elevated fetal hemoglobin.
- Usually in Mediterranean, black, or Oriental persons.

General Considerations

Thalassemia major appears in individuals who are homozygous for the thalassemia gene. Family studies show that both parents have thalassemia minor. Homozygous beta thalassemia is now believed to be due to a quantitative deficiency in production of beta chains of adult hemoglobin (hemoglobin A_1). This produces an intracorpuscular defect that is associated with marked hypochromia and a shortened red cell survival time. Ineffective erythropoiesis and increased intramedullary hemolysis contribute to the anemia. The gene is present in Africa, southern Europe, and Asia. It is believed that the selective increase in the gene in this area (which may reach an incidence of up to 50% in isolated communities) is due to the fact that the heterozygote has an increased resistance to malaria.

Clinical Findings

A. Symptoms and Signs: Severe anemia usually does not manifest itself clinically until about age 1, because of the protective effect of normal fetal hemoglobin. However, splenomegaly and mild anemia are often noted by 6 months. Massive splenomegaly and significant hepatomegaly are usually seen by age 2 and continue until the spleen extends into the pelvis. Physical growth and sexual development are markedly impaired, and there is increased susceptibility to infections. As the child approaches the school years, the widening of the flat bones of the face and skull in association with marrow hypertrophy gives all children with thalassemia major a characteristic facies: prominence of the malar eminences, depression of the bridge of the nose, a slightly oblique appearance of the eyes, and an enlargement of the superior maxilla with upward protrusion of the lip. The anemia is severe; after age 1, frequent transfusions are usually required. Jaundice may be present.

B. Laboratory Findings: The blood smear reveals a severe hypochromic microcytic anemia with marked anisocytosis and poikilocytosis. Target cells are prominent. Nucleated red cells are numerous and often exceed the circulating white blood cells. The hemoglobin is low (5–6 g/dL). The reticulocyte count is significantly elevated. Platelet and white cell counts are frequently high. Serum bilirubin is elevated. The diagnosis is confirmed by hemoglobin electrophoresis, which reveals no abnormal hemoglobin but a marked increase in fetal hemoglobin and in A_2 hemoglobin. The exact level of fetal hemoglobin should be determined by the alkali denaturation method. Osmotic fragility is markedly decreased. The bone marrow shows marked erythroid hyperplasia with increased iron deposition.

C. X-Ray Findings: Bone x-rays are very characteristic and reveal an increase in the medullary area with thinning of the cortex. The skull has a "hair-on-end" appearance.

Differential Diagnosis

There is usually no problem in the diagnosis of homozygous thalassemia, since essentially no other disease shows the characteristic peripheral blood and hemoglobin electrophoresis findings. The primary clinical differentiation is with the combinations of thalassemia and other abnormal hemoglobins as in thalassemia-hemoglobin S disease, thalassemia-hemoglobin E disease, etc. These have similar clinical pictures but are usually more mild. They are differentiated by the electrophoretic pattern.

Complications

Patients with thalassemia major have multiple complications. They have an increased susceptibility to infections, particularly following splenectomy. Acute benign nonspecific pericarditis is a common problem. Repeated fractures are associated with the thinning of cortical bone. The multiple transfusions that are required are ultimately associated with transfusion reactions and the development of leukocyte antibodies. Growth is impaired, and adolescent development of secondary sex characteristics is delayed. Cholelithiasis and cholecystitis are almost always present in the adolescent or young adult. The major complication, however, is the development of hemochromatosis secondary to excessive absorption and transfusion of iron in these patients. This results in cirrhosis and in heart failure. Cardiac complications are related primarily to the heavy deposition of iron in the myocardium, and death is usually due to heart failure.

Treatment

There is no specific treatment for thalassemia major. Infections should be treated promptly with antibiotics, and heart failure with digitalis and other appropriate therapy.

A. Transfusion: Blood transfusion is the primary therapeutic measure; packed red cells are indicated (in many cases, every 3–4 weeks) to maintain the hemoglobin level above 12 g/dL. This has been associated with increased vigor and well-being, improved growth, and fewer overall complications. Frequent transfusions reduce gastrointestinal absorption of iron. Hemochromatosis will still develop unless iron chelation is carried out. Life expectancy may be greater if the hemoglobin is maintained at a high level.

B. Chelation: The chelating agent deferoxamine (Desferal), when given by slow continuous infusion either intravenously or subcutaneously, has proved effective in removing iron. The subcutaneous route is most practical; the drug is administered by a small portable infusion pump in a dose of 2–4 g over a 12-hour period. Urinary excretion is enhanced by ascorbic acid given orally in a dose of 200–500 mg daily.

C. Folic Acid: A relative folic acid deficiency may develop because of the marked overproduction of bone marrow. Folic acid, 1 mg daily orally, is often of value.

D. Splenectomy: Splenectomy is usually of value in the older child and is definitely indicated if the transfusion requirements become progressively greater. It is also indicated for the abdominal discomfort and distention associated with massive enlargement of the organ. Although it does not change the basic rate of hemolysis, it will eliminate the hypersplenism, which further shortens survival of the patient's red cells and the transfused red cells. The hazard of severe and overwhelming infection following splenectomy is much greater in patients with thalassemia major than in any other group, and the use of prophylactic penicillin following this procedure is recommended. Pneumococcal and *Haemophilus influenzae* vaccines should also be administered.

E. Testosterone: Testosterone may stimulate bone marrow and enhance the patient's red cell production.

F. Bone Marrow Transplantation: This has been tried with success but is not recommended for most patients because of the risks of the procedure.

Prognosis

The prognosis has improved significantly in the past decades and should continue to improve with frequent transfusions to maintain a high level of hemoglobin and the use of chelating agents to remove iron and prevent hemosiderosis. Very few patients survived into adult life in the past, although the majority reached adolescence.

Cohen A, Martin M, Schwartz E: Response to long-term deferoxamine therapy in thalassemia. *J Pediatr* 1981;**99:**689.

Ohene-Frempong K, Schwartz E: Clinical features of thalassemia. *Pediatr Clin North Am* 1980;**27:**403.

Propper RD, Button LN, Nathan DG: New approaches to the transfusion management of thalassemia. *Blood* 1980;**55:**55.

Wolfe L et al: Prevention of cardiac disease by subcutaneous deferoxamine in patients with thalassemia major. *N Engl J Med* 1985;**312:**1600.

3. ALPHA THALASSEMIA

Defective production of alpha chains also results in anemia. Several different forms of alpha thalassemia have been described. The disorder has been recognized chiefly in Southeast Asia (especially Thailand) and in blacks. Recent evidence indicates that 4 alpha globin genes exist and that different degrees of severity of anemia are related to the number of gene deletions.

The alpha thalassemia carriers who lack one gene (''silent carriers'') are completely asymptomatic and have normal blood findings. Those with 2 deleted genes show mild hypochromia and microcytosis on the blood smear. No abnormal hemoglobin is demonstrated in older children with the 2-gene deletion, and there are no compensatory increases in hemoglobin A_2 or fetal hemoglobin. Bart's hemoglobin (4 gamma chains) is present in small amounts at birth. This mild form of alpha thalassemia has been found in 5–7% of blacks in the USA and is common in Southeast Asian and Arabian peoples.

The disorder previously called thalassemia-hemoglobin H disease is not recognized to be a form of alpha thalassemia in which 3 of the 4 genes are deleted. It has been described primarily in Southeast Asia (Philippines, southern China, and Thailand). The patient demonstrates a chronic microcytic anemia that is refractory to iron therapy and tends to resemble an intermediate form of beta thalassemia. Hemoglobin electrophoresis at pH 8.5 reveals a fast hemoglobin (hgb H) that migrates more rapidly than A_1. This hemoglobin is composed of 4 beta chains. Characteristic red cell inclusions are demonstrated by the reticulocyte stain upon incubation. There is no satisfactory treatment. Iron should not be administered to patients with any form of alpha thalassemia unless associated iron deficiency is present.

The most severe type of alpha thalassemia is caused by deletion of all 4 genes and is incompatible with life. These severely anemic and hydropic infants have only Bart's hemoglobin, since they are unable to produce any alpha hemoglobin chains. Intrauterine diagnosis of the alpha thalassemias is now possible.

Lie-Injo LE et al: Hb Bart's level in cord blood and deletions of alpha-globin genes. *Blood* 1982;**59:**370.

Orkin SH, Nathan DG: The thalassemias. *N Engl J Med* 1976;**295:**710.

Wong V et al: Diagnosis of homozygous alpha-thalassemia in cultured amniotic-fluid fibroblasts. *N Engl J Med* 1978; **298:**669.

4. THALASSEMIA VARIANTS

Double heterozygosity of thalassemia with other hemoglobinopathies such as C, S, and E is fairly common in certain parts of the world; these variants manifest themselves clinically as milder forms of thalassemia major. The diagnosis is made by hemoglobin electrophoresis, which shows a predominance of fetal hemoglobin and other abnormal hemoglobin. Family studies will reveal one parent to be a thalassemia carrier and the other a carrier of C, S, or E.

5. HEREDITARY PERSISTENCE OF FETAL HEMOGLOBIN

Hereditary persistence of fetal hemoglobin has been reported in both black and Greek families. It is usually found in the heterozygous form and is associated with no symptoms. The blood counts and blood smears are normal. The fetal hemoglobin level is approximately 20% after 2 years of age and higher than normal during infancy. The homozygous form is also asymptomatic. There is a deletion of both the beta globin gene and the gene that controls the switch from production of gamma to production of beta globin chains. The double heterozygous state with hemoglobin S is asymptomatic but can mimic homozygous (SS) disease on electrophoresis.

Wood WG, Clegg JB, Weatherall DJ: Hereditary persistence of fetal haemoglobin (HPFH) and delta beta thalassaemia. *Br J Haematol* 1979;**43:**509.

ACQUIRED HEMOLYTIC ANEMIAS

1. AUTOIMMUNE HEMOLYTIC ANEMIA

Essentials of Diagnosis

- Sudden pallor, fatigue, and jaundice.
- Splenomegaly.
- Positive Coombs test.
- Reticulocytosis and spherocytosis.

General Considerations

Acquired autoimmune hemolytic anemia is rare during the first 4 months of life but is one of the more common causes of acute acquired anemia after the first year. It is caused by antibodies that coat the red cells and are responsible for the positive direct Coombs test. Circulating antibodies are demonstrated by the indirect Coombs test. The "primary" (or idiopathic) cases may be associated with an unrecognized preceding infection. The possible importance of cytomegalovirus infection has recently been emphasized. The disease may be "symptomatic" and may occur in association with a known infection such as hepatitis, viral pneumonia, or infectious mononucleosis; or it may occur as a manifestation of a generalized autoimmune disease such as disseminated lupus erythematosus or with a type of cancer such as Hodgkin's disease or leukemia. The antibodies may be of the "cold-reacting" IgM type or "warm" antibodies of the IgG type.

Clinical Findings

A. Symptoms and Signs: The disease usually has an acute onset and is associated with weakness, pallor, and fatigue. Hemoglobinuria may be present. Jaundice and splenomegaly are often present. Occasional cases are chronic and insidious in onset. Clinical evidence of the underlying disease such as infection or lupus erythematosus may be present.

B. Laboratory Findings: The anemia is normochromic and normocytic and may be very severe, with hemoglobin levels as low as 3–4 g/dL. Occasionally, the secondary form of acquired hemolytic anemia may be very mild and may present with evidence of a positive Coombs test but with compensated anemia. Spherocytes are usually present, and within 24 hours nucleated red cells and reticulocytes are present in the peripheral blood. There is usually a significant leukocytosis, and the platelet count may be elevated. Bone marrow shows a marked erythroid hyperplasia. Both the direct and indirect Coombs tests are usually positive. Autoagglutination may be present, and because of this the patient may be incorrectly typed as AB, Rh-positive. The indirect serum bilirubin may be elevated, and the stool and urine urobilinogen are increased.

Differential Diagnosis

The principal condition to be differentiated in childhood is hereditary spherocytic anemia in crisis, since both diseases present with acute hemolysis and spherocytosis. The Coombs test differentiates the 2 anemias, since it is negative in hereditary spherocytosis. The Coombs test likewise differentiates autoimmune hemolytic anemia from essentially all other anemias except erythroblastosis.

Complications

The anemia may be very severe and result in shock, requiring emergency management. Thrombocytopenia may occur as an associated autoimmune condition. The complications of the underlying disease such as disseminated lupus erythematosus or lymphoma may be present in the symptomatic form.

Treatment

Medical management of the underlying disease is important in symptomatic cases.

A. Transfusion: Transfusion is necessary in the

acute disease and may be an emergency procedure. Difficulty in cross-matching will usually be encountered. A search should be made for blood that will provide the best major cross-match. Packed, washed cells are often more compatible. The IgG antibody is often type-specific (particularly to one of the Rh antigens), and cross-matching may be possible, whereas the IgM antibody is usually a panagglutinin (frequently anti-I). Transfusion occasionally must be given in spite of agglutination or a positive Coombs test in the major cross-match. Donor cells may be destroyed at a rapid rate, particularly if compatible blood cannot be found. Donor cells may be tagged with ^{51}Cr to determine their rate of survival in severe cases.

B. Immunosuppressive Therapy: Medical treatment to block the immune process or the reticuloendothelial system is indicated. Corticosteroid therapy in the form of hydrocortisone intravenously in large doses or prednisone, 2 mg/kg/d orally, should be tried initially. If a response is observed, the dose is decreased at weekly intervals until the lowest level that will maintain the patient in remission is reached. Other immunosuppressive drugs such as cyclophosphamide, mercaptopurine, or azathioprine may be tried alone or in conjunction with corticosteroid therapy.

C. Heparin: Heparin may be useful in the IgM type (which binds complement) because of its anticomplementary effect. It may also help prevent intravascular coagulation and the associated secondary renal disease.

D. Exchange Transfusion or Plasmapheresis: Plasma or whole blood exchange transfusion or plasmapheresis will temporarily wash out antibody and may be a lifesaving measure in severe cases.

E. Splenectomy: Splenectomy may be beneficial in cases in which all forms of medical treatment have failed. About 50% of cases may be expected to respond to this procedure, particularly those with an IgG antibody.

Prognosis

The disease is self-limited in most idiopathic cases in childhood, although hemolysis does not usually cease completely for months to years; the Coombs test often remains weakly positive for years. Most patients will show a response to corticosteroid therapy, and about 50% will improve with splenectomy. In the majority of chronic cases, there is a basic underlying disease or immunologic disorder.

Habibi B et al: Autoimmune hemolytic anemia in children: A review of 80 cases. *Am J Med* 1974;**56:**61.

Schreiber AD: Autoimmune hemolytic anemia. *Pediatr Clin North Am* 1980;**27:**253.

Taft EG, Propp RP, Sullivan SA: Plasma exchange for cold agglutinin hemolytic anemia. *Transfusion* 1977;**17:**173.

2. ACUTE "COOMBS-NEGATIVE" ACQUIRED HEMOLYTIC ANEMIA (Lederer's Anemia)

Severe episodes of hemolytic anemia that are not associated with a positive Coombs test are occasionally seen in children. The onset is acute and the duration short, with spontaneous recovery in a few weeks. The cause may be autoimmune, but the amount of cell-bound IgG is so small that the antibody cannot be detected by the Coombs test. Other more sensitive tests for antibody may be positive. An IgA antibody has been found in a few cases. An episode is often precipitated by an infectious process such as a urinary tract infection.

Transfusion is the treatment of choice; there is usually no problem with cross-matching the donor blood.

The prognosis is good, since most cases are self-limited.

Rosse WF: The detection of small amounts of antibody on the red cell in autoimmune hemolytic anemia. *Ser Haematol* 1974;**7:**358.

3. MISCELLANEOUS ACQUIRED (NONIMMUNE) HEMOLYTIC ANEMIAS

A wide variety of extracorpuscular mechanisms can produce hemolysis of a nonimmune type. Hemolysis in association with ingestion of oxidant drugs (eg, antimalarials, sulfonamides) or uncooked fava beans occurs primarily in individuals with a deficiency of G6PD. Certain other chemicals and drugs such as arsenic and benzene may produce hemolysis by their direct effect. Exposure to physical agents such as extreme heat or cold may cause hemolysis. Hemolytic anemia is a common complication of severe burns. Microangiopathic hemolytic anemia, characterized by fragmented cells (schistocytes), is often a major complication of disseminated intravascular coagulation and the hemolytic-uremic syndrome.

Many bacterial infections with hemolytic organisms such as *Bartonella bacilliformis* and *Clostridium perfringens* produce hemolysis. In the neonatal period, hemolytic anemia may be a complication of almost any infection, but it is seen most commonly with hemolytic staphylococcal and *Escherichia coli* infections. Malaria and some other parasitic diseases are characteristically associated with hemolysis. The venom of most poisonous snakes (in particular, the pit vipers of North America) contains a hemolysin, as do the venoms of certain spiders also. The management of the majority of the acquired toxic hemolytic anemias is dependent upon the removal of the offending agent or treatment of the toxic disorder. Transfusion may be important in the more severe cases.

Hemolysis in heart disease or after open heart

surgery has been reported. This has usually occurred in situations in which a jet of blood was driven against a Teflon prosthesis as well as in certain congenital valvular defects and with prosthetic valve replacement. The hemolysis is on a mechanical basis.

II. POLYCYTHEMIA & METHEMOGLOBINEMIA

PRIMARY ERYTHROCYTOSIS (Benign Familial Polycythemia)

This is the most common type of primary polycythemia of childhood. It differs from polycythemia vera in that it affects only the erythroid series; the white cell count and platelet count are normal. It frequently occurs on a familial basis as an autosomal dominant, although it may also occur as an autosomal recessive. There are usually no physical findings except for plethora and splenomegaly. The hemoglobin may be as high as 27 g/dL, with a hematocrit of 80% and a red cell count of 10 million/μL. There are usually no symptoms other than headache and lethargy. Recent studies in a number of families have revealed (1) an abnormal hemoglobin with increased oxygen affinity, (2) reduced red cell diphosphoglycerate, or (3) autonomous increase in erythropoietin production.

Treatment is not indicated unless symptoms are marked. Phlebotomy is the treatment of choice.

Adamson JW: Familial polycythemia. *Semin Hematol* 1975; **12:**383.

SECONDARY POLYCYTHEMIA (Compensatory Polycythemia)

Secondary polycthemia occurs in response to hypoxia in any condition that results in a lowered oxygen saturation of the blood. The most common cause of secondary polycythemia is cyanotic congenital heart disease. It also occurs in chronic pulmonary disease such as cystic fibrosis and in pulmonary arteriovenous shunts. Persons living at extremely high altitudes, as well as those with methemoglobinemia and sulfhemoglobinemia, develop polycythemia. It has on rare occasions been described without hypoxia in association with renal tumors, brain tumors, Cushing's disease, or hydronephrosis; in association with cobalt therapy; and in patients with certain unusual hemoglobinopathies.

Polycythemia occurs normally in the neonatal period; it is particularly exaggerated in preterm and small-for-gestational-age infants, in whom it is frequently associated with other symptoms. It may occur in infants of diabetic mothers, and it has recently been described as a manifestation of Down's syndrome in the newborn and as a complication of congenital adrenal hyperplasia.

Multiple coagulation and bleeding abnormalities have been described in severely polycythemic cardiac patients. These include thrombocytopenia, mild consumption coagulopathy, and increased anticoagulants with elevated fibrinolytic activity. Bleeding at surgery may be severe.

The ideal treatment of secondary polycythemia is correction of the underlying disorder. When this cannot be done, phlebotomy is often necessary to control the symptoms. Adequate hydration of the patient and phlebotomy with plasma replacement are indicated prior to major surgical procedures; these measures prevent the complications of thrombosis and hemorrhage. Isovolumetric exchange transfusion is the treatment of choice in severe cases.

Balcerzak SP, Bromberg PA: Secondary polycythemia. *Semin Hematol* 1975;**12:**353.

METHEMOGLOBINEMIA

Methemoglobin is formed when hemoglobin in a deoxygenated state is oxidized to the ferric form. Methemoglobin is being formed continuously in the red cells and is simultaneously reduced to hemoglobin by enzymes in the erythrocyte. Methemoglobin becomes unavailable for transport of oxygen and causes a shift in the dissociation curve of the residual oxyhemoglobin. Cyanosis is produced with methemoglobin levels of approximately 15% or greater. There are several mechanisms for the production of methemoglobinemia.

Congenital Methemoglobinemia Associated With Hemoglobin M

Congenital and familial methemoglobinemia associated with an abnormal hemoglobin molecule (hemoglobin M) is discussed under the hemoglobinopathies (see above). Affected patients are cyanotic but asymptomatic. They do not respond to any form of treatment.

Congenital Methemoglobinemia Due to Enzyme Deficiencies

Congenital methemoglobinemia is most frequently caused by congenital absence of a reducing factor in the erythrocyte that is responsible for the conversion of methemoglobin to hemoglobin in normal red cells. Most patients with this disease suffer from a deficiency of the reducing enzyme diaphorase I (coenzyme factor I). It is transmitted as an autosomal recessive trait. These patients may have as high as 40% methemoglobin but usually have no symptoms, although a mild compensatory polycythemia may be present.

Patients with methemoglobinemia associated with a deficiency of diaphorase I respond readily to treatment with ascorbic acid and with methylene blue (see below). However, treatment is not usually indicated.

Drug-Induced Methemoglobinemia

A number of compounds activate the oxidation of hemoglobin from the ferrous to the ferric state, forming methemoglobin. These include the nitrites and nitrates, chlorates, and quinones. Common drugs in this group are the aniline dyes, sulfonamides, acetanilid, phenacetin, bismuth subnitrate, and potassium chlorate. Poisoning with a drug or chemical containing one of these substances should be suspected in any infant or child who presents with sudden cyanosis. Methemoglobin levels in cases of poisoning may be extremely high and can produce severe anoxia and dyspnea with unconsciousness, circulatory failure, and death. Young infants and newborns are more susceptible to poisoning because their red cells have difficulty reducing hemoglobin, probably on the basis of a transient deficiency of DPNH-dependent hemoglobin reductase.

Patients with the acquired form of methemoglobinemia respond dramatically to methylene blue in a dosage of 2 mg/kg given intravenously. For infants and young children, a smaller dose (1–1.5 mg/kg) is recommended. Ascorbic acid administered orally or intravenously also reduces methemoglobin, but it acts more slowly.

Jaffé ER: Methaemoglobinaemia. *Clin Haematol* 1981;**10:**99.

III. DISORDERS OF LEUKOCYTES

NEUTROPENIA & AGRANULOCYTOSIS

Essentials of Diagnosis

- Increased frequency of infections.
- Ulceration of oral mucosa and throat.
- Normal red cells and platelets.

General Considerations

Neutropenia in infancy and childhood is usually defined as an absolute neutrophil (granulocyte) count of less than 1500/μL. However, in the first 2 years of life, normal infants may have absolute counts as low as 1000/μL. Most neutropenias in childhood are acquired and frequently caused by viral infections. A few are associated with other primary disorders, and some are congenital and hereditary. Many are physiologic in young children.

Neutropenias may result from absent or defective granulocyte stem cells, ineffective or suppressed myeloid maturation, decreased or absent monocyte production of granulopoietin (colony-stimulating factor), decreased marrow release, increased neutrophil destruction, or an increased neutrophil "marginating pool" (pseudoneutropenia).

Benign Neutropenias of Childhood

A. Physiologic Neutropenia: After the first few weeks of life, all infants and young children have neutropenic neutrophil levels in comparison with adult levels. The normal white blood cell count of infants and children may be as low as 5000–6000/μL, and the percentage of neutrophils may normally be as low as 18–20% during the first 3–4 years of life. A diagnosis of neutropenia should be considered in infancy and early childhood only if the absolute neutrophil count is below 1000/μL. (See Table 16–2 for normal values.)

B. Pseudoneutropenia: This term is used for neutropenia that is caused by excessive marginal pooling of neutrophils along vessel walls and in the spleen. Ordinarily, about 50% of neutrophils are in the marginal pool (which equals the circulating pool). Some children have excess margination, but these neutrophils are available when needed, and there is no increased susceptibility to infection. The diagnosis is made by administration of epinephrine, which causes release of marginal neutrophils into the circulation.

C. Chronic Benign Neutropenia of Childhood: Several series of cases have been described in which persistent neutropenia was noted throughout childhood. The bone marrow usually shows normal cellularity but abnormal maturation of granulocytes. In most cases, neutrophils represent about 10% of the circulating leukocytes, and infection is not a serious problem. Spontaneous remission may occur. The neutrophil count usually rises with bacterial infections and in response to administration of endotoxins or cortisone.

Acquired Neutrophils

A. Neutropenia Due to Infection: Most viral diseases cause neutropenia and are the most common cause in childhood. Although neutrophil depression is transient, it may last for up to 2 months. Absolute counts are usually in the range of 400–1000/μL but may be lower. The marrow shows maturation arrest. Overwhelming bacterial infection may cause neutropenia. In these cases, the marrow pool of more mature cells becomes depleted, and the neutrophils that are present are predominantly immature cells (bands and metamyelocytes).

B. Neutropenia Due to Drugs and Chemicals: Usage of drugs and chemicals should be investigated in all cases. In childhood, the more common drug-induced neutropenias occur with anticonvulsants, antimicrobial agents (chloramphenicol, sulfonamides, trimethoprim-sulfamethoxazole), antithyroid drugs, and phenylbutazone. Neutropenia is a common complication of exposure to large amounts of x-ray radiation and to cytotoxic drugs such as antimetabolites and nitrogen mustards.

C. Immune Neutropenia: Isoimmune neutropenia is occasionally seen in the newborn. It is caused by transplacental immunization of the mother to the leukocytes of her infant in a manner analogous to Rh immunization of the newborn. The granulocytopenia in these cases may be accompanied by temporary infection lasting up to 4 weeks. The diagnosis can be proved by demonstration of antibodies to the father's granulocytes in the maternal or infant serum. Neutropenia is due to peripheral destruction, and the marrow is usually normal. Maternal neutrophil antibodies may also cross the placenta in women with autoimmune neutropenias. Neutrophil antibodies may develop on an autoimmune basis in childhood. This commonly occurs in disseminated lupus erythematosus and has also been described in lymphomas and infectious mononucleosis.

Neutropenias Associated With Other Disorders

A. Neutropenia With Pure Red Cell Hypoplastic Anemia: A number of cases of pure red cell hypoplastic anemia have also been associated with neutropenia. Neutropenia is usually mild, and an increased incidence of infection has not been observed, although oral ulceration and staphylococcal infections of the skin have been reported in a few cases.

B. Pancreatic Insufficiency and Bone Marrow Dysfunction (Shwachman Syndrome): Neutropenia, anemia, and thrombocytopenia have been reported in association with pancreatic insufficiency in infancy and childhood. Although diarrhea, failure to thrive, short stature, and infections occur, the prognosis is better than in cystic fibrosis.

C. Neutropenia in Association With Immune Deficiency Syndromes: Neutropenia (constant or cyclic) may occur in agammaglobulinemia. It has also been seen in other immune deficiencies. The neutropenia rarely responds to immune globulin but may be controlled by fresh plasma infusions.

D. Neutropenia in Type IB Glycogen Storage Disease: Neutropenia and increased infections have recently been described in this disorder.

Congenital & Hereditary Neutropenias

Congenital neutropenias are usually present from birth and may range from very severe to relatively mild or cyclic. The milder forms may be transmitted as an autosomal dominant, and the parents should be evaluated. The severe agranulocytosis is often autosomal recessive.

The congenital neutropenias of infancy and childhood may be due to a basic stem cell defect, deficiencies in the colony-stimulating factor (granulopoietin) produced by the monocytes, a defect or inhibitor in the microenvironment in the marrow, or problems in release from the marrow that may be associated with defective chemotaxis.

A. Infantile Genetic Agranulocytosis (Kostman's Syndrome, Kostman's Hereditary Neutropenia): Several families have been described in which agranulocytosis occurred from infancy in several siblings without depression of other circulating cell elements. Agranulocytosis has been associated with either depression of the granulocytic series in the marrow or a delay in maturation. The course has been chronic, with a high mortality rate and no response to therapy. The genetic pattern suggests autosomal recessive transmission.

B. Chronic Hypoplastic Neutropenia: A few cases have been described of chronic neutropenia associated with hypoplasia of granulocytic precursors in the marrow. Complicating infections have been moderate to severe.

C. Periodic (Cyclic) Neutropenia: This is a rare condition that may occur at any age but usually begins in infancy and childhood. The disease is caused by fluctuating levels of granulopoietin. It is characterized by extreme granulocytopenia that occurs at approximately 3-week intervals, with recovery between attacks. The peripheral blood changes are reflected by a cyclic maturation arrest of the granulocytic series in the bone marrow. During the leukopenic episode, the white blood cell count is usually 2000–4000/μL, with granulocytes representing only 6–10% of the cells. The agranulocytic periods usually last about 10 days and are associated with the development of ulcers of the oral mucosa, fever, and sore throat. Various other infections may complicate the disease, and staphylococcal skin infections are common. Splenomegaly and lymphadenopathy have also been reported.

Clinical Findings

A. Symptoms and Signs: The symptoms are those of infection, with chills and fever. Sore throat and oral mucosa ulceration are common, and chronic or recurrent staphylococcal skin infection is frequent. In most cases, the spleen and liver are not enlarged. A complete history should be taken, and a physical examination should be performed to look for acquired or congenital causes of the disease. A family history should also be taken.

B. Laboratory Findings: Neutrophils are absent or markedly reduced in the peripheral blood. In the purer forms of neutropenia or agranulocytosis, the monocytes and lymphocytes will be normal and the red cells and platelets not affected. The bone marrow usually shows a normal erythroid series, with adequate megakaryocytes but a marked reduction in the myeloid cells or a significant delay in maturation of this series.

White blood cell counts should be taken for parents and siblings.

If there is no obvious acquired cause such as viral infection or drug ingestion and no other primary disease, tests should be performed as follows: White blood cell counts should be performed twice weekly for 2 months to diagnose cyclic neutropenia. An epinephrine stimulation test will diagnose pseudoneutropenia due to "marginal pooling." The absolute neutrophil count should more than double. Epinephrine, 0.1 mL (1:1000 solution), is given subcutaneously, and neutrophil counts are done at 5, 10, 20, 40, and 60 minutes. Bone marrow aspiration and biopsy are most important. If marrow is normally cellular, marrow release may be measured by stimulation with intravenous hydrocortisone, 50–100 mg, or typhoid vaccine, 0.5 mL subcutaneously. Neutrophil counts are recorded every 30 minutes for 4 hours. Measure immunoglobulins to detect associated dysgammaglobulinemias. Elevated urinary muramidase levels are found if increased neutrophil destruction is the cause. Other more specific tests to identify the mechanism of neutropenia include chemotactic studies and measurement of neutrophil antibodies if the marrow is highly cellular. Cultures of bone marrow and buffy coat are evaluated for colony-forming units and production of colony-stimulating factor (granulopoietin).

Differential Diagnosis

The isolated neutropenias should be differentiated from the pancytopenias such as aplastic anemia and the hypoplastic (aleukemic) form of childhood leukemia by bone marrow examination.

Complications

The complications are essentially those of infection. Septicemia and pneumonia are the most serious. Chronic infection with antibiotic-resistant staphylococci and *Pseudomonas* is frequent in severe cases.

Treatment

Removal of the toxic agent is essential if one can be identified. Otherwise, treatment consists of administering appropriate antibiotics. Prophylactic antimicrobial therapy is not indicated, and the patient should be managed with specific therapy directed toward the infecting organism.

Marrow stimulation with testosterone or with testosterone plus one of the corticosteroids (see Aplastic Anemia) may be tried in chronic cases, but there is little evidence that it is effective.

Fresh frozen plasma has produced remissions in a few cases with immune globulin deficiencies. Chloramphenicol has been reported to cause maturation of granulocytes in one type of congenital neutropenia.

Prognosis

The prognosis varies greatly with the cause and severity of the neutropenia. In severe cases with persistent agranulocytosis, the prognosis is very poor in spite of antibiotic therapy; in mild or cyclic forms of neutropenia, symptoms may be minimal and the prognosis for normal life expectancy excellent.

Adams GR, Pearson HA: Chloramphenicol-responsive chronic neutropenia. *N Engl J Med* 1983;**309:**1039.

Lange RD, Jones JB: Cyclic neutropenia: Review of clinical manifestations and management. *Am J Pediatr Hematol Oncol* 1981;**3:**363.

Priest JR et al: Transient autoimmune neutropenia due to anti-NA 1 antibody. *Am J Pediatr Hematol Oncol* 1980;**2:**195.

Weetman RM, Boxer LA: Childhood neutropenia. *Pediatr Clin North Am* 1980;**27:**361.

ACUTE INFECTIOUS LYMPHOCYTOSIS

Acute infectious lymphocytosis is a specific entity characterized hematologically by marked lymphocytosis that may range between 15,000 and 200,000 cells/μL. The predominant cell is a small mature lymphocyte. The disease is apparently infectious and tends to occur in epidemic form in institutions and families. The specific agent has not been determined, although a virus is suspected. An enterovirus similar to coxsackievirus A may be the cause.

In most cases, the condition is asymptomatic, and the diagnosis is made on the basis of a routine blood count. Epidemics have been reported in which symptoms were noted, including fever, upper respiratory tract manifestations, skin rashes, abdominal pain, diarrhea, and meningoencephalitis. Lymphadenopathy and splenomegaly are not present.

The bone marrow is normal except for a slight increase in mature lymphocytes. The disease can be readily differentiated from leukemia, since the lymphocytes of the peripheral blood are all mature and since chronic lymphatic leukemia does not occur in the pediatric age group. The blood smear is similar to that seen in pertussis.

There is no specific treatment. Symptomatic therapy is usually not needed.

The disease is self-limited, and the blood count usually returns to normal within a few weeks.

Horwitz MS, Moore GT: Acute infectious lymphocytosis: Etiology and epidemiologic study of outbreak. *N Engl J Med* 1968;**279:**399.

CHRONIC NONSPECIFIC INFECTIOUS LYMPHOCYTOSIS

This syndrome is characterized by moderate leukocytosis with a predominance of lymphocytes, low-grade fever, anorexia, pallor, irritability, increased fatigability, and abdominal pain. The peripheral blood usually shows a significant lymphocytosis, with total counts reaching 25,000/μL with as many as 80% lymphocytes. Most of the lymphocytes are of the small, mature type, although occasional larger cells may be seen. The cause is not known, but viral infection is suspected.

The symptoms and elevated lymphocyte count often persist for several months, and therapy is not helpful. Antibiotic therapy and restriction of physical activity are not indicated.

MYELOPROLIFERATIVE SYNDROMES

1. MYELOID METAPLASIA (Myelofibrosis, Myelosclerosis, Agnogenic Myeloid Metaplasia)

Myeloid metaplasia is a myeloproliferative condition associated with splenomegaly and a granulocytic leukemoid picture. In childhood, it occurs most frequently in the secondary form and is associated with replacement of the bone marrow by tumor, storage cells, or osteosclerosis (osteopetrosis, marble bone disease). The primary form, which is associated with idiopathic myelofibrosis (agnogenic myeloid metaplasia), is extremely rare in childhood.

The peripheral blood in this condition shows not only a marked increase in granulocytes, with many immature forms at all levels of maturation, but also a significant number of nucleated red cells and large immature platelets. The presence of immature hematopoietic cells in the peripheral blood is explained by the marked extramedullary hematopoiesis that occurs in the spleen and liver in this condition.

Treatment should be directed toward the primary disease if possible. The use of testosterone (see Aplastic Anemia) may be helpful in stimulating hematopoiesis in the bone marrow.

Boxer LA et al: Myelofibrosis-myeloid metaplasia in childhood. *Pediatrics* 1975;**55:**861.

2. FAMILIAL MYELOPROLIFERATIVE DISEASE

One family has been described with 9 children (related as first cousins) who developed a myeloproliferative disorder that appeared to be similar to either acute or subacute myelogenous leukemia. Hepatosplenomegaly, leukocytosis (with immature granulocytes), anemia, and thrombocytopenia were found. The liver and spleen showed extramedullary hematopoiesis. Six of the 9 children recovered in adolescence, and 3 died in infancy.

3. MYELOPROLIFERATIVE SYNDROME WITH ABSENT C GROUP CHROMOSOME

There have been several reports of myeloproliferative disorders associated with an absent chromosome of the C group. Massive hepatosplenomegaly (with extramedullary hematopoiesis), leukocytosis (with young granulocytes), anemia, and thrombocytopenia characterize this condition. The patients have usually progressed to an acute granulocytic leukemia, and the myeloproliferative phase should be considered preleukemic.

Humbert JR et al: Pre-leukemia in children with a missing bone marrow C chromosome and a myeloproliferative disorder. *Br J Haematol* 1971;**21:**705.

4. MYELOPROLIFERATIVE DISORDER OF DOWN'S SYNDROME

A severe myeloproliferative disorder affecting granulocytes, erythrocytes, platelets, or any combination of these cell lines may be present at birth in infants with Down's syndrome. The granulocytic hyperplasia with immature cells in the blood is the most common and has in the past been confused with acute or subacute myelogenous leukemia. It clears spontaneously and should not be treated with antileukemic therapy. There is a significant mortality rate from bleeding or infection in the first few weeks before the marrow recovers and matures.

Nix WL, Fernbach JD: Myeloproliferative diseases in childhood. *Am J Pediatr Hematol Oncol* 1981;**3:**397.

GRANULOCYTE FUNCTION DISORDERS

Disorders of neutrophil function include those related to cell movement, phagocytosis, and bacterial killing. Examples of primary defects in cell movement (chemotaxis) are **Chédiak-Higashi syndrome** (recurrent infections, decreased skin pigment, nystagmus, and giant granules in leukocytes and platelets) and **lazy leukocyte syndrome.** Acquired or transient defects in chemotaxis are associated with diabetes mellitus, burns, malnutrition, and corticosteroid therapy or may occur during the neonatal period. Disorders of phagocytosis are related to deficient opsonization of bacteria and are seen in patients with antibody deficiencies, lack of complement (C3), or primary cellular abnormality (actin dysfunction). The clinically important defects in microbial killing are related to intracellular oxygen-dependent mechanisms as seen in **chronic granulomatous disease** (X-linked disorder of chronic purulent infections of lymph nodes, skin, liver, lungs), severe G6PD deficiency, and myeloperoxidase deficiency.

Little specific therapy is available for patients with primary defects in granulocyte function. In general, treatment is directed toward management of infections and includes prompt antibiotic therapy with drugs that penetrate cell membranes (eg, chloramphenicol in chronic granulomatous disease), surgical drainage of suppurative lesions, and general supportive care. Ascorbate therapy has been used in Chédiak-Higashi syndrome; sulfisoxazole may help in chronic granulomatous disease. The prognosis is poor in severe disorders such as chronic granulomatous disease and Chédiak-Higashi syndrome. In cases of chemotaxic or opsonization defects, fresh plasma transfusions may be of benefit if a plasma component is deficient (antibody, complement).

Ambruso DR, Johnston RB: *Immunodeficiency Disorders*. Chandra RK (editor). Churchill Livingstone, 1981.

Gallin JI et al: Recent advances in chronic granulomatous disease. *Ann Intern Med* 1983;**99:**657.

Miller ME: Pathology of chemotaxis and random mobility. *Semin Hematol* 1975;**12:**59.

IV. BLEEDING DISORDERS

Bleeding disorders may be classified as (1) defects in small vessel hemostasis, which include (a) quantitative and qualitative abnormalities of platelets (thrombocytopenia, platelet function defects, and thrombocythemia) and (b) the vascular disorders; and (2) intravascular disorders (defects in blood coagulation).

The initial laboratory workup for screening patients with bleeding disorders should include a careful history and physical examination and all of the following laboratory investigations:

(1) Bleeding time to test small vessel integrity and platelet function.

(2) Platelet count or estimation of platelet number on blood smear.

(3) Partial thromboplastin time (PTT) to measure clotting activity of factors XII, IX, XI, VIII, X, II, V, and fibrinogen.

(4) One-stage prothrombin time (PT) to screen the tissue thromboplastin system of coagulation (factors II, V, VII, X, and fibrinogen).

(5) Thrombin time to measure antithrombin effect of fibrin split products or heparin as well as fibrinogen level and function.

(6) Fibrinogen determination.

With this battery of screening tests, it is usually possible to determine the general area of the defect and proceed with more specific tests in order to make an exact diagnosis.

Rapaport SI: Brief review: Preoperative hemostatic evaluation: Which tests, if any? *Blood* 1983;**61:**229.

ABNORMALITIES OF PLATELET NUMBER OR FUNCTION

IDIOPATHIC THROMBOCYTOPENIC PURPURA (Werlhof's Disease, Purpura Haemorrhagica)

Essentials of Diagnosis

- Petechiae, ecchymoses.
- Decreased platelet count.
- No splenomegaly.
- Normal bone marrow examination.

General Considerations

Acute idiopathic thrombocytopenic purpura is the most common bleeding disorder of childhood. It most frequently follows infections, particularly the common contagious diseases (rubella, varicella, and rubeola). As a rule, it is self-limited; this is particularly true of the postinfectious type, the majority of which cases recover spontaneously within a few months and approximately 90% within a year after onset. Chronic idiopathic thrombocytopenic purpura is rare in childhood.

Most cases of idiopathic thrombocytopenic purpura are felt to be an immunologic disorder, and platelet-associated IgG can usually be demonstrated. The spleen plays a major role by sequestering damaged platelets and by forming antibodies.

Clinical Findings

A. Symptoms and Signs: The onset is usually acute, with the appearance of multiple ecchymoses. Petechiae are often present, and epistaxis is common. There are no other physical findings, and the spleen is not palpable.

B. Laboratory Findings:

1. Blood—The platelet count is markedly reduced (usually $< 50{,}000/\mu L$), and platelets are decreased and frequently of larger size on peripheral blood smear. The white blood count and differential count are normal. Anemia is not present unless hemorrhage has occurred.

2. Bone marrow—The bone marrow usually shows increased numbers of megakaryocytes.

3. Other laboratory tests—The bleeding time is prolonged, and clot retraction is abnormal. PTT and PT are normal. Platelet-associated IgG may be demonstrated in the platelets or serum (platelet antibody testing).

Differential Diagnosis

The presence of a low platelet count immediately differentiates idiopathic thrombocytopenic purpura from all other bleeding disorders except those associated with thrombocytopenia. A normal white blood count and normal precursors in the bone marrow differentiate the idiopathic disease from leukemia and aplastic anemia. The bone marrow is important in making the differential diagnosis. The family history may be helpful in indicating hereditary or familial thrombocytopenia.

Complications

Severe exsanguinating hemorrhage and bleeding into vital organs are the primary complications of idiopathic thrombocytopenic purpura. Intracranial hemorrhage is the most serious. Complications of treatment include those associated with prolonged corticosteroid therapy. Splenectomy, particularly in children under age 2, may be associated with increased incidence of infection.

Treatment

A. General Measures: Avoidance of trauma is important, and in many postinfectious cases no other therapy may be required. In the presence of hemorrhage, blood transfusions may be necessary. Platelet transfusions are usually ineffective and should be reserved for life-threatening hemorrhage. The platelets (platelet concentrate or platelet pack) from 1 unit of blood per 6 kg of body weight are usually required to produce an observable rise in platelet count. Patients must avoid aspirin and aspirin-containing drugs.

B. Corticosteroids: Patients with a significant hemorrhagic tendency or with a platelet count less than 10,000/μL are treated with prednisone (2 mg/kg orally in divided daily doses) for a period of 2 weeks. The dosage is tapered and stopped during the third week. No further prednisone is given regardless of the level of the platelet count unless significant bleeding recurs, at which time the dosage of prednisone used is the smallest that will give symptomatic relief (usually 2.5–5 mg twice daily). The patient is then followed, using the general measures outlined above, until spontaneous remission occurs or until the patient is a candidate for splenectomy.

C. Splenectomy: Splenectomy produces permanent remission in most cases of idiopathic thrombocytopenic purpura; however, it is now usually reserved for children who have shown no evidence of spontaneous remission over a period of 6 months to 1 year, since about 90% of children with the disease will recover without surgical intervention within 1 year after onset. If symptoms are not controlled by medical management, splenectomy may be done prior to this time, and in most cases splenectomy is advised if symptoms persist beyond 1 year after onset. Fifty to 75% of chronic cases in childhood respond to the procedure.

Bleeding is rarely a complication of splenectomy, but platelet concentrates should be available during surgery. If the patient has been receiving corticosteroid therapy prior to surgery, the dose should be increased to the full therapeutic level during and after surgery.

Anticoagulant therapy is not indicated postoperatively even though the platelets may rise to levels of approximately 1 million.

The risk of overwhelming infection is low in the older child undergoing splenectomy. It does represent a significant risk in the young child, and the procedure should be postponed if possible until the child is older. Administration of pneumococcal vaccine and prophylactic penicillin following splenectomy is indicated.

D. Other Treatment Measures: In children who remain significantly thrombocytopenic after splenectomy or in young children in whom splenectomy may be of increased risk, therapy with intravenous immune globulin may be tried. A 5-day course of a special polyvalent intact immunoglobulin for intravenous use is frequently associated with a rise in platelets in refractory patients. This treatment appears to be more effective after splenectomy. Vincristine treatment may also be of benefit in selected patients, although other immunosuppressive agents (azathioprine, cyclophosphamide) have shown little benefit in children.

Prognosis

Spontaneous remission with permanent recovery occurs in almost 90% of cases of idiopathic thrombocytopenic purpura in childhood. (The incidence of spontaneous remission is much lower in adults.)

Ahn YS et al: The treatment of idiopathic thrombocytopenia with vinblastine-loaded platelets. *N Engl J Med* 1978;**298:**1101.

Andrew M, Barr RD: Increased platelet destruction in infancy and childhood. *Semin Thromb Hemostas* 1982;**8:**248.

Bussel JB et al: Intravenous gamma globulin treatment of chronic idiopathic thrombocytopenic purpura. *Blood* 1983;**62:**480.

Cheung N-K V et al: Platelet-associated immunoglobulin-G in childhood idiopathic thrombocytopenic purpura. *J Pediatr* 1983;**102:**366.

Sartorius JA: Steroid treatment of idiopathic thrombocytopenic purpura in children: Preliminary results of a randomized cooperative study. *Am J Pediatr Hematol Oncol* 1984;**6:**165.

THROMBOCYTOPENIA IN THE NEWBORN

Thrombocytopenia is one of the most common causes of purpura in the newborn and should be considered and investigated in any infant with petechiae or a significant bleeding tendency. A platelet count less than 150,000/μL establishes a diagnosis of thrombocytopenia in the neonatal period. A number of specific entities may be responsible (Table 16–3). Management is directed toward alleviation of the specific cause; special situations are discussed below.

Thrombocytopenia Associated With Platelet Alloimmunization

An uncommon cause of thrombocytopenia in the neonatal period is platelet alloimmunization, which

Table 16–3. Causes of neonatal thrombocytopenia.

Infection
Bacterial: Sepsis, congenital syphilis
Viral: Cytomegalic inclusion disease, disseminated herpes simplex, rubella syndrome, enteroviruses
Other: Toxoplasmosis
Immune disorders
Alloimmunization
Maternal antibody-induced disorders: Systemic lupus erythematosus, idiopathic thrombocytopenic purpura, drug-associated disorders
Bone marrow abnormality
Congenital megakaryocytic hypoplasia
Thrombocytopenia-absent radius syndrome
Fanconi's pancytopenia
Aplastic anemia
Myeloproliferative disease (Down's syndrome)
Osteopetrosis
Congenital leukemia
Maternal drugs
Tolbutamide
Thiazide diuretics
Infant drugs
Intravenous fat emulsion (eg, Intralipid)
Tolazoline
Intravascular coagulation syndromes
Disseminated intravascular coagulation
Large-vessel thrombosis (renal vein, aorta)
Necrotizing enterocolitis
Placental chorioangioma
Excessive peripheral utilization
Giant hemangioma
Hyperviscosity syndrome
Erythroblastosis fetalis
Other causes
Postexchange transfusion
Maternal hyperthyroidism
Metabolic disorders: Hyperglycinemia, cirrhosis, mucolipidosis
Thrombotic thrombocytopenic purpura
Postmature and small-for-gestational-age infants (often with maternal toxemia)
Neonatal neuroblastoma

is similar to the mechanism responsible for Rh blood group alloimmunization. Alloimmunization occurs when the platelet type of the infant differs from that of the mother and when a significant number of platelets cross from the fetal to the maternal circulation. Platelet antibodies can usually be demonstrated by platelet IgG-binding techniques. Petechiae are usually present shortly after birth, and a male may bleed from circumcision. The bone marrow usually shows normal to increased megakaryocytes. The disease is self-limited; platelets show a spontaneous rise within 2 weeks, with complete recovery by 4–6 weeks. Rarely, severe intracranial bleeding can occur.

Platelet transfusions may be used in an emergency. In very severe cases, exchange transfusion with fresh whole blood is effective in removing antibody and in replacing platelets temporarily; a platelet concentrate from the mother will be more effective in raising the platelet count.

Thrombocytopenia Associated With Idiopathic Thrombocytopenic Purpura in the Mother

Infants born to mothers with idiopathic thrombocytopenic purpura or systemic lupus erythematosus develop thrombocytopenia as a result of passive transfer of antibody from the mother to the infant. Evaluation of the maternal platelet count is indicated in any infant with thrombocytopenia. The persistence of antibodies in the infant's circulation is temporary, and spontaneous recovery is the rule. In severe cases (platelet count < 20,000/μL), which may be detected prior to delivery by careful sampling of the infant's scalp, cesarean section should be performed. Others have advocated the administration of corticosteroids to the mother for 10–14 days prior to vaginal delivery in order to increase the infant's platelet count. Severely thrombocytopenic infants (platelet count < 50,000/μL) can also be given a short course of corticosteroids.

Neonatal Thrombocytopenia Associated With Infections

Thrombocytopenia is commonly associated with severe generalized infections of the newborn period, particularly those which develop in utero. Megakaryocytes are decreased and immature, and splenomegaly is usually present. Other intrauterine infections such as syphilis, toxoplasmosis, and cytomegalic inclusion disease are almost invariably associated with thrombocytopenia, and thrombocytopenia is frequently present with bacterial sepsis and generalized infection with herpes simplex virus or other viruses.

In addition to specific treatment for the underlying disease if available, platelet transfusions may be indicated in severe cases. Platelet concentrate in a dosage of 10 mL/kg will raise the platelet count by about 75,000/μL.

Thrombocytopenia Associated With Giant Hemangiomas

A rare but important cause of thrombocytopenic purpura in the newborn is giant hemangioma. Platelet sequestration in the tumor results in peripheral depletion of platelets. The bone marrow usually shows marked hyperplasia of megakaryocytes. In the presence of massive hemangiomas, the thrombocytopenia may be associated with disseminated intravascular coagulation and result in fatal hemorrhage.

X-ray treatment of hemangiomas may be indicated. Heparinization is indicated if there is evidence of disseminated intravascular coagulation. Surgery is usually contraindicated because of the risk of hemorrhage. Prednisone therapy has been associated with marked regression of infantile hemangiomas.

Karpatkin M: Corticosteroid therapy in thrombocytopenic infants of women with autoimmune thrombocytopenia. *J Pediatr* 1984;**105:**623.

Karpatkin M, Porges RF, Karpatkin S: Platelet counts in infants of women with autoimmune thrombocytopenia: Effects of steroid administration to the mother. *N Engl J Med* 1981;**305:**936.

Kelton JG et al: The prenatal prediction of thrombocytopenia in infants of mothers with clinically diagnosed immune thrombocytopenia. *Am J Obstet Gynecol* 1982;**144:**449.

Pereyra R, Andrassy RJ, Mahour GH: Management of massive hepatic hemangiomas in infants and children: A review of 13 cases. *Pediatrics* 1982;**70:**254.

Scott JR et al: Fetal platelet counts in the obstetric management of immunologic thrombocytopenic purpura. *Am J Obstet Gynecol* 1980;**136:**495.

THROMBOCYTOPENIA ASSOCIATED WITH APLASTIC ANEMIA

Thrombocytopenia is frequently the first manifestation of aplastic anemia and may be present before neutropenia and anemia develop. The child who presents with amegakaryocytic thrombocytopenia in the first few years of life—particularly if there are associated skeletal anomalies—should be considered as a possible case of congenital pancytopenia of the Fanconi type.

THROMBOCYTOPENIA IN LEUKEMIA

Thrombocytopenia is almost invariably a major finding in acute leukemia of childhood. This is discussed in Chapter 31.

DRUG-INDUCED THROMBOCYTOPENIA

Drug-induced thrombocytopenia may be either amegakaryocytic or megakaryocytic. The myelosuppressive drugs and chemical toxins, as well as irradiation, tend to affect all marrow elements, including megakaryocytes. Thrombocytopenia thus is a primary presenting complication of the aplastic or hypoplastic anemias produced by these agents. They are discussed in detail in the section on aplastic anemia.

Megakaryocytic thrombocytopenia is an immune reaction resulting from sensitization of the patient by prior administration of drugs such as quinidine or quinine.

Once the cause of the purpura is understood, prevention is readily effected by removal of the sensitizing drug.

Hackett T, Kelton JG, Powers P: Drug-induced platelet destruction. *Semin Thromb Hemostas* 1982;**8:**116.

HEREDITARY THROMBOCYTOPENIAS

At least 3 types of hereditary thrombocytopenia can be recognized based on the mode of inheritance and characteristic clinical and laboratory findings: (1) Wiskott-Aldrich syndrome is characterized by X-linked thrombocytopenia, eczema, recurrent infections, and findings of low levels of IgA and IgM immunoglobulins, impaired delayed hypersensitivity and abnormal lymphocyte function, and decreased numbers of small, poorly functioning platelets with a short life span. Variants of this disorder without the severe immunologic difficulties may be confused with chronic idiopathic thrombocytopenic purpura, and patients with this disorder are at great risk of developing overwhelming infection if splenectomy is performed. (2) Bernard-Soulier giant platelet syndrome is a rare autosomal, incompletely recessive disorder characterized by giant, bizarre platelets of varying numbers but with normal in vitro function except for defective aggregation with ristocetin. (3) A heterogeneous group of thrombocytopenias with failure to release ADP (a release defect similar to that produced by aspirin) may be inherited by either the recessive or the dominant mode and can also be confused with chronic idiopathic thrombocytopenic purpura. Platelet function tests are usually abnormal. Occasionally, these disorders are seen in association with hereditary nephritis.

Bellucci S et al: Inherited platelet disorders. *Prog Hematol* 1983;**13:**223.

Lum LG et al: Splenectomy in the management of the thrombocytopenia of the Wiskott-Aldrich syndrome. *N Engl J Med* 1980;**302:**892.

SECONDARY HYPERSPLENISM

Thrombocytopenia is one of the earliest hematologic manifestations of secondary hypersplenism.

THROMBOTIC THROMBOCYTOPENIC PURPURA

Thrombotic thrombocytopenic purpura is a hemorrhagic disorder characterized by thrombocytopenia, purpura, fever, hemolytic anemia, transitory focal neurologic signs, and hepatic involvement. Hemolysis often precedes clinical purpura. The red blood cells show bizarre forms and fragmentation similar to that seen in the hemolytic-uremic syndrome. Other clinical signs and symptoms may occur in association with widespread intracapillary and intra-arteriolar thrombi that may affect not only the brain but also the kidneys, heart, and spleen. It has been suggested that the disorder is due to a deficiency of an inhibition to platelet aggregation induced by increased amounts of abnormal factor VIII-vWf.

The course is usually rapidly progressive and may terminate fatally within a few weeks, although chronic cases have been described.

Treatment, when effective, has included plasma infusions, plasmapheresis and replacement of plasma, and exchange transfusions. Platelet inhibitors (aspirin, dipyridamole, splenectomy, and corticosteroids) have also been successful.

Aster RH: Plasma therapy for thrombotic thrombocytopenic purpura: Sometimes it works, but why? *N Engl J Med* 1985;**312:**985.

Moake JL et al: Unusually large plasma factor VIII: von Willebrand factor multimers in chronic relapsing thrombotic thrombocytopenic purpura. *N Engl J Med* 1982;**307:**1432.

Myers TJ et al: Thrombotic thrombocytopenic purpura: Combined treatment with plasmapheresis and antiplatelet agents. *Ann Intern Med* 1980;**92:**149.

DISORDERS OF PLATELET FUNCTION

The hereditary disorders of platelet function are characterized by a bleeding diathesis, usually associated with a prolonged bleeding time in spite of normal numbers of platelets. The findings in these diseases are summarized in Table 16–4. Acquired disorders of platelet function include uremia, cirrhosis, disseminated intravascular coagulation, macroglobulinemias, systemic lupus erythematosus, vitamin B_{12} deficiency, myeloproliferative disorders, acyanotic congenital heart disease, and viral infections. Many pharmacologic agents decrease platelet function. Clinically, the most important of these include aspirin, dipyridamole, phenylbutazone, and synthetic penicillins.

Champion LA et al: The effects of four commonly used drugs on platelet function. *J Pediatr* 1976;**89:**653.

George JN et al: Molecular defects in interactions of platelets with the vessel wall. *N Engl J Med* 1984;**311:**1084.

Lusher JM, Barnhart MI (editors): *Acquired Bleeding Disorders in Children: Platelet Abnormalities and Laboratory Methods.* Masson, 1981.

Thompson CB et al: Size dependent platelet subpopulations: Relationship of platelet volume to ultrastructure, enzymatic activity, and function. *Br J Haematol* 1982;**50:**509.

VON WILLEBRAND'S DISEASE

Essentials of Diagnosis

- History of easy bruising and epistaxis from early childhood.
- Prolonged bleeding time with normal platelet count.
- Reduced levels of factor VIII complex.

General Considerations

Von Willebrand's disease is a familial bleeding disorder that is usually transmitted as a dominant trait and occurs in both sexes. It is associated both with a prolonged bleeding time and with a reduced level of factor VIII. The partial thromboplastin test is usually prolonged but may be normal.

Von Willebrand's disease and variants are due to abnormalities of the factor VIII molecule (VIII complex). In severe classic von Willebrand's disease, the factor VIII procoagulant activity (VIIIc), the portion of the molecule that corrects the bleeding time defect and supports ristocetin-induced aggregation of platelets (VIII-vWf), and the factor VIII measured by antibodies (VIII antigen) are reduced or absent. Variants of the disorder are seen in which combinations of the above attributes of the factor VIII molecule are defective.

Clinical Findings

A. Symptoms and Signs: There is usually a history of increased bruising and severe prolonged epistaxis. Increased bleeding will also occur with lacerations or at surgery. Excessive menstrual flow is a problem in the adolescent female. Petechiae are usually not observed, and hemarthrosis is rare.

B. Laboratory Findings: A prolonged bleeding time is present; platelet number and function are normal except for platelet retention in glass bead columns ("adhesiveness") and decreased platelet aggregation with the antibiotic ristocetin. These latter defects are

Table 16–4. Findings in hereditary platelet diseases.

Disease	Platelet Aggregations	Platelet Morphology	Mechanism	Genetic Transmission
Glanzmann's thrombasthenia	Decreased with ADP, collagen, thrombin, epinephrine.	Decreased adsorbed fibrinogen.	Absent membrane glycoprotein.	Autosomal recessive.
Storage pool disease	Absent release of ADP and serotonin; defective aggregation with collagen and epinephrine.	Decreased dense granules.	Decreased platelet storage pool of ADP, ATP, 5-hydroxytryptamine, Ca^{2+}.	Autosomal dominant (and recessive).
Defective release (aspirinlike)	Absent release; defective aggregation with collagen, epinephrine, and arachidonic acid.	Normal.	Cyclo-oxygenase deficiency.	Variable.
Bernard-Soulier syndrome	No aggregation with ristocetin; otherwise normal.	Giant platelets.	Absent membrane glycoprotein.	Autosomal recessive.

due to deficiency of the factor VIII-vWf portion of the VIII molecule. Factor VIIIc and VIII antigen are usually decreased but may be normal. Analysis of vWf multimers allows the disorder to be classified into types (I, IIa, IIb, III).

Treatment

The depressed levels of factor VIIIc can be easily corrected with freshly frozen plasma or cryoprecipitates. The VIIIc levels increase both after transfusion of VIIIc and as a result of endogenous production of VIIIc; therefore, VIIIc levels remain elevated longer than in classic hemophilia. In some patients, the platelet adhesiveness and bleeding time can be corrected by the use of freshly frozen, platelet-free plasma. Transfusions with cryoprecipitates are more effective than normal plasma in correcting the bleeding time. One bag of cryoprecipitate per 6 kg body weight given every 6–12 hours may be necessary to correct the bleeding time adequately. Infusions of desmopressin acetate (DDAVP) have been shown to be effective in raising the factor VIII complex levels in mild to moderate von Willebrand's disease (type I).

When dental extractions are necessary, management consists of systemic correction, local pressure, and use of aminocaproic acid (Amicar).

Prognosis

Patients with mild forms of the disease have a normal life expectancy, and bleeding can be controlled with the measures noted above or may cease spontaneously. In severe cases, it may be difficult to control hemorrhage, although recent methods of therapy with plasma and concentrates have greatly improved the outlook. Elective surgical procedures should be avoided.

Abildgaard CF et al: Serial studies in von Willebrand's disease: Variability versus "variants." *Blood* 1980;**56:**712.

Miller JL, Castella A: Platelet-type von Willebrand's disease: Characterization of a new bleeding disorder. *Blood* 1982; **60:**790.

Warrier AI, Lusher JM: DDAVP: A useful alternative to blood components in moderate hemophilia A and von Willebrand's disease. *J Pediatr* 1983;**102:**228.

Zimmerman TS, Ruggeri ZM: von Willebrand's disease. *Prog Hemost Thromb* 1982;**6:**202.

VASCULAR DEFECTS

ANAPHYLACTOID PURPURA (Schönlein-Henoch Purpura, Allergic Purpura)

Essentials of Diagnosis

- Purpuric cutaneous rash.
- Urticaria.
- Migratory polyarthritis.
- Gastrointestinal pain and hemorrhage.
- Hematuria.

General Considerations

Anaphylactoid purpura is characterized by a typical purpuric skin rash plus (in any combination) migratory arthritis, gastroenteritis, and nephritis. It is believed to be a vasculitis related to vessel damage by deposits of immune complexes (antigen-antibody). It is characterized by involvement of the small vessels, particularly in the skin, the gastrointestinal tract, and the kidneys. The cause of the allergic reaction is frequently not recognized, although in some parts of the world group A β-hemolytic streptococcal infection may precede the disease in some cases. Other inciting antigens such as drugs, other infections (viruses), food allergens, insect bites, and horse serum have been implicated.

Clinical Findings

A. Symptoms and Signs: Migratory polyarthritis very similar to that of rheumatic fever frequently precedes the onset of the skin rash. Gastrointestinal pain, diarrhea, and gastrointestinal bleeding are common. Nephritis occurs in about 50% of cases, either with symptomless proteinuria or hematuria or with nephrotic syndrome. The skin rash is diagnostic in appearance: It is characteristically distributed on the ankles, buttocks, and elbows; purpuric areas a few millimeters in diameter are present and may progress to form larger hemorrhages ("palpable purpura"). Petechial lesions occur, but the majority of skin or mucous membrane hemorrhages are slightly larger. The rash usually begins on the lower extremities, but the entire body may be involved. Erythematous and urticarial skin eruptions (which may become hemorrhagic) often accompany the hemorrhage. Cardiac involvement is rare.

B. Laboratory Findings: The platelet count, platelet function tests, bleeding time, and tourniquet test are usually negative. Blood coagulation is normal except for elevated factor VIII levels and an increase in fibrin split products. Urinalysis frequently reveals hematuria and proteinuria, but casts are unusual. Stool tests may be positive for occult blood, even though gross melena is not observed. The ASO titer is frequently elevated or the throat culture positive for group A β-hemolytic streptococci. Serum IgA globulins may be elevated.

Differential Diagnosis

The hemorrhagic rash of anaphylactoid purpura can be differentiated from thrombocytopenic purpura by the presence of raised skin lesions in the former and by the platelet count. The rash of septicemia (especially meningococcemia) may be very similar, although the distribution tends to be more generalized in sepsis. Blood culture may be necessary for final diagnosis.

Complications

Intussusception of the small bowel occurs in a significant number of patients with intestinal manifestations. The most important complications derive from the renal involvement. About 10% of patients develop renal failure as a result of advancing proliferative glomerulonephritis, and an equal number will have continuing hematuria, proteinuria, and hypertension after 2 years. About 25% have recurring hematuria, and in the remainder the renal disease clears completely. Clinical severity is proportionate to the extent of the lesion histologically; older children are more liable to severe involvement.

Treatment

There is no satisfactory treatment for anaphylactoid purpura. Corticosteroid therapy may be useful in patients with acute gastrointestinal manifestations. If the culture is positive for group A β-hemolytic streptococci or if the ASO titer is elevated, give penicillin in full therapeutic doses for 10 days. Aspirin is useful for the arthritis, and sedatives may benefit the patient with gastrointestinal pain. Immunosuppressive drugs such as cyclophosphamide and azathioprine are now contraindicated in the treatment of the nephritis.

Prognosis

The prognosis for recovery is good, although symptoms frequently recur over a period of several months. In patients who develop renal manifestations, approximately 50% may have persistent abnormal urinary findings. This occasionally progresses to significant impairment of renal function.

Kitchens CS: The anatomic basis of purpura. *Prog Hemost Thromb* 1980;**5:**211.

Saulsbury FT: Henoch-Schönlein purpura. *Pediatr Dermatol* 1984;**1:**195.

Weber TR et al: Massive gastric hemorrhage: An unusual complication of Henoch-Schönlein purpura. *J Pediatr Surg* 1983;**18:**576.

Yoshikawa N, White RH, Cameron AH: Prognostic significance of the glomerular changes in Henoch-Schönlein nephritis. *Clin Nephrol* 1981;**16:**223.

INTRAVASCULAR DEFECTS; COAGULATION FACTOR DEFICIENCIES

Essentials of Diagnosis

- Generalized bleeding tendency.
- Ecchymoses (not petechiae).
- Congenital (family history) or acquired (systemic illness).
- Abnormal partial thromboplastin time or prothrombin time (or both).

General Considerations

A congenital or acquired deficiency of one or more of the coagulation factors in the blood can result in a generalized bleeding diathesis. The bleeding tendency may be mild (bleeding only at time of severe traumas or surgical procedures), moderate, or severe (frequent spontaneous hemarthroses and ecchymoses) depending on the degree of the coagulation factor deficit. Fig 16–1 depicts the interaction of these factors in producing coagulation of the blood. Hemostasis in humans depends upon platelet and vascular factors as well as blood coagulation.

A specific hemorrhagic diathesis has been seen with a deficiency of each of the coagulation factors except Hageman factor (XII), calcium deficiency, prekallikrein, and high-molecular-weight kininogen. These disease entities are discussed below.

The diagnosis and classification of clinical coagulation factor deficiencies depend upon proper performance and interpretation of specific clotting tests that are briefly reviewed below.

Coagulation Tests

A. Whole Blood Coagulation Time (Lee-White): This test is too insensitive to be of value in diagnosis or treatment of patients with mild to moderate coagulation factor deficiencies. The clotting time is influenced by heparin and can therefore be used as a rough guide to heparinization. Although simple to perform, this procedure is not an adequate screening test and should be abandoned as a "routine" test. A more useful test is the activated whole blood clotting time (ACT), which is performed by addition of an activating agent (kaolin, silica) to the clotting tube.

B. One-Stage Prothrombin Time (Quick): This procedure consists of noting the clotting time of citrated plasma after addition of calcium and tissue thromboplastin. Normal adult values are between 11 and 13 seconds (100%). This is an adequate screening test for proconvertin (VII), proaccelerin (V), Stuart-Prower factor (X), and prothrombin (II). It does not measure the factors necessary for the earlier stages of coagulation or fibrinogen levels greater than 75 μg/dL.

C. Partial Thromboplastin Time (PTT): This test is performed much like the prothrombin time except that a phospholipid is added instead of tissue thromboplastin. In addition, a contact activator substance such as kaolin may be added to avert the influence of glass contact. The test is very sensitive, relatively easy to perform, and inexpensive. All coagulation factors except proconvertin are measured; therefore, it is the screening test of choice.

D. Thrombin Time: Bovine or human thrombin is added to plasma and the clotting time recorded. The normal adult range is 7–15 seconds or more, depending upon the amount of thrombin added. The test measures the conversion of fibrinogen to fibrin and is dependent upon the concentration of fibrinogen or inhibitors such as fibrin split products, antithrombins, and heparin.

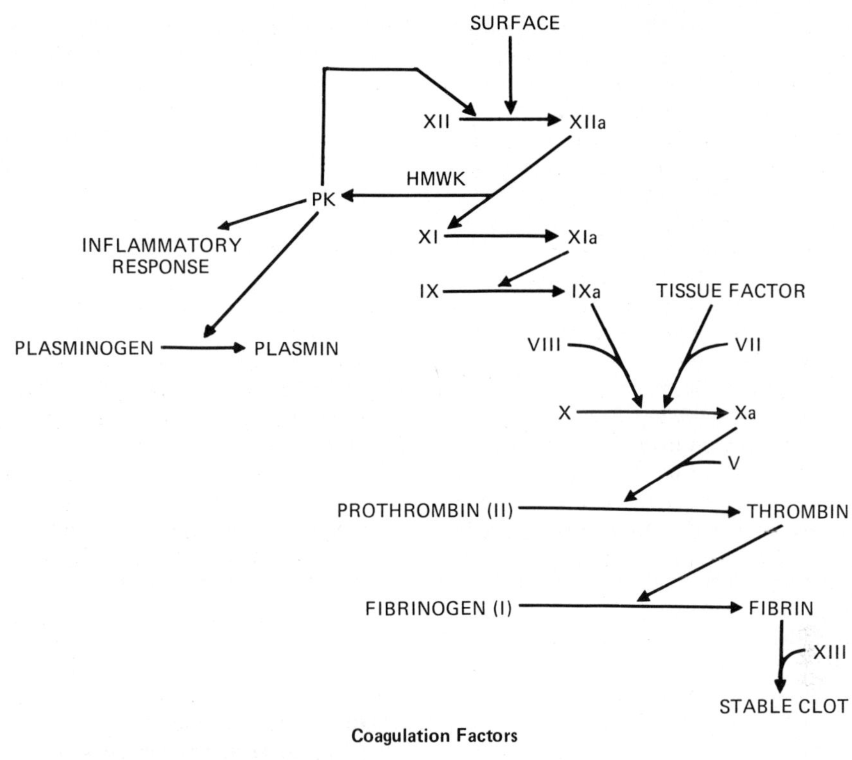

Coagulation Factors

I	Fibrinogen
II	Prothrombin
V	Ac-globulin, proaccelerin, labile factor
VII	Proconvertin, SPCA
VIII	Antihemophilic factor (AHF)
IX	Plasma thromboplastin component (PTC)
	IXa Activated form
X	Stuart-Prower factor
	Xa Activated form
XI	Plasma thromboplastin antecedent (PTA)
	XIa Activated form
XII	Hageman factor
	XIIa Activated form
XIII	Fibrin stabilizing factor, fibrinase
PK	Prekallikrein (Fletcher factor)
HMWK	High-molecular-weight kininogen

Figure 16–1. Blood coagulation scheme and terminology of coagulation factors.

E. Specific Factor Assays: Each of the coagulation factors can be assayed by an indirect clotting method using natural or synthetic factor-deficient substrates or chromogenic substrates and compared to the activity of normal plasma (100%).

F. Bleeding Time (Ivy or Template): Place a blood pressure cuff on the upper arm and inflate to 40 mm Hg. With an alcohol sponge, clean an area free of visible veins on the flexor surface of the forearm. In the Ivy method, using a sterile Bard-Parker No. 11 blade, make a puncture wound 5 mm deep and 2 mm wide. Note time of puncture; touch wound gently with sterile filter paper to absorb blood every 30 seconds until bleeding stops. Normal bleeding time is 1–7 minutes. A modification of this test using a template to make a cut 1 mm deep and 4 mm long is now frequently used (template bleeding time); the normal range is up to 9 minutes. A commercially available variation of this test (Simplate) is widely used.

G. Other Tests: Various other tests, available usually in research laboratories only, such as the thromboelastograph, thrombin generation time, euglobulin fibrinolysin time, and recalcification time, are sometimes helpful in identifying unusual circulating anticoagulants or hypercoagulability of the blood.

Triplett DA (editor): *Standardization of Coagulation Assays: An Overview.* College of American Pathologists, 1982.

AFIBRINOGENEMIA & DYSFIBRINOGENEMIA

There have been reports of several patients with a bleeding tendency and delayed clotting due to an abnormal molecule of fibrinogen (congenital dysfibrinogenemia). Immunologic determinations of fibrinogen are normal, but the thrombin and prothrombin times are often prolonged. Treatment is similar to that outlined for afibrinogenemia.

Congenital absence of fibrinogen produces a definite entity that resembles hemophilia clinically. However, the condition is inherited as an autosomal recessive and affects both sexes. The patients have persistent bleeding from small injuries, hematomas, ecchymoses, and hemarthroses. Although fatal bleeding from the umbilical cord has been reported, most cases are usually much less severe than classic hemophilia.

The principal laboratory finding in afibrinogenemia is complete absence of a fibrin clot by any of the usual clotting tests attempted. Whole blood and plasma are incoagulable even upon the addition of optimal amounts of calcium, thromboplastin, and thrombin. The erythrocyte sedimentation rate is zero. There is an absence of precipitable fibrinogen upon heating of plasma to 56 °C for 10 minutes. Specific assays for other coagulation factors are normal. Hypofibrinogenemia (fibrinogen level < 100 mg/dL) is also rarely seen.

Transfusion with whole blood, fresh plasma, or cryoprecipitate generally controls the acute bleeding episodes. The minimal hemostatic level of circulating fibrinogen is about 60 mg/dL (normal, 250–450 mg/dL). The half-life of transfused fibrinogen is about 4 days. Therefore, 10–20 mL of plasma per kilogram of body weight or one bag of cryoprecipitate per 6 kg should achieve hemostasis. This dose may need to be repeated daily depending upon the type and severity of bleeding and the rate of healing.

Mammen EF: Congenital coagulation disorders. *Semin Thromb Hemostas* 1983;**9:**1.

HEMOPHILIA A (Antihemophilic Factor [AHF, Factor VIIIc] Deficiency)

Classic hemophilia (hemophilia A) is a bleeding disorder characterized by decreased activity of circulating antihemophilic factor (AHF or factor VIIIc, the coagulant portion of the factor VIII complex molecule). The disease occurs in males and is inherited in an X-linked recessive manner. All degrees of severity of the disease have been reported.

Clinical Findings

A. Symptoms and Signs: Patients with severe hemophilia, characterized by frequent spontaneous bleeding epidodes involving skin, mucous membranes, joints, muscles, and viscera, have no circulating factor VIIIc activity. However, mild hemophilia is also recognized; these patients bleed only at times of severe trauma or surgery. They have 5–20% factor VIIIc activity. An intermediate group of patients with moderate symptoms (usually no severe joint involvement) have 1–5% factor VIIIc levels.

The most crippling aspect of hemophilia A is the tendency to develop chronic hemarthroses, especially of knees and elbows, which lead to fibrosis and joint contractures.

B. Laboratory Findings: In about 70% of families with this disease, the female carriers will have low levels of factor VIIIc (20–70%) and may occasionally be mildly symptomatic. Otherwise, low levels of factor VIIIc are not seen in a female unless the individual has von Willebrand's disease or a circulating anticoagulant or is the product of the union of a hemophiliac male and a carrier female. Carriers of hemophilia can be detected in most instances by determination of the ratio of factor VIIIc to factor VIII antigen.

Results of tests measuring intrinsic plasma thromboplastin formation (whole blood clotting time, plasma recalcification time, partial thromboplastin time [PTT], and thromboplastin generation test [TGT]) are all abnormal. The bleeding time and one-stage prothrombin time are usually normal. The specific diagnosis is made by showing failure of "correction" in a test system (PTT or TGT) by known factor VIIIc-deficient plasma. Coagulation assays have been developed to measure the actual percentage of factor VIIIc activity in a given biologic fluid. The whole blood clotting time can be normal in the presence of as little as 1–2% factor VIIIc and, therefore, is not a good test for diagnosis or guide to therapy. Factor VIII antigen and factor VIII-vWf levels are normal in classic hemophilia.

Complications

The principal complication of classic hemophilia is the development of an acquired circulating anticoagulant to factor VIIIc. Inhibitors or antibodies to factor VIIIc develop in about 15% of factor VIIIc-deficient hemophiliacs. Patients may have both mild and severe inhibitor states. Mild inhibitor or anticoagulant substances specific to factor VIIIc not uncommonly can be shown in factor VIIIc-deficient patients, but the development of a severe factor VIIIc inhibitor is a rare and dreaded complication. When this occurs, the patient is often resistant to all attempts at therapy. The inhibitor has been shown to be an antibody but is rarely amenable to immunosuppressive therapy. "Activated" prothrombin complex concentrates (Autoplex, Feiba Immuno) may be of help in stopping hemorrhage in these patients.

Other complications in hemophilia include chronic crippling arthritis due to repeated hemarthroses; development of pseudotumors as a result of multiple bleeding in one site; chronic hepatitis contracted through transfusion; and acquired immunodeficiency syndrome (AIDS), which may also be contracted through transfusion. The risk for developing AIDS may be significantly reduced by use of heat-treated concentrates.

Treatment

The basis of treatment of classic hemophilia is the administration of a factor VIIIc-containing substance in order to achieve adequate hemostasis. Factor VIIIc is temperature and storage labile in biologic fluids.

The in vitro half-life of infused factor VIIIc is about 12 hours.

The following substances can be used for therapy: (1) fresh frozen plasma or cryoprecipitates, stored at −30 °C for less than 12 months; and (2) lyophilized concentrates of factor VIIIc, reconstituted and given immediately.

Dosage and duration of therapy depend upon the type of bleeding seen clinically. Bleeding that occurs from lacerations of the skin or mucous membranes, tooth extractions, surgical wounds, or severe traumatic epistaxis usually requires more intense therapy than joint or soft tissue bleeding.

In order to achieve the desired in vivo level of factor VIIIc, use either of the following: (1) cryoprecipitated factor VIIIc, prepared from individual blood donors and supplied frozen in 10- to 20-mL amounts per plastic bag; or (2) commercially prepared factor VIIIc concentrates from large donor pools, supplied in lyophilized form in vials. Dosages can be calculated as follows:

$$\text{Units of factor VIIIc} = \text{Weight in kilograms} \times \text{Desired in vivo percentage level} \times 0.5$$

Cryoprecipitates usually contain 100 units* of factor VIIIc per bag; concentrate potency is designated on the vial. Fresh frozen plasma, 10 mL/kg, will produce an in vivo level of 15–20% factor VIIIc.

Treatment must be continued until adequate healing occurs—ie, 2–5 days for tooth extractions or epistaxis but 7–10 days for lacerations or surgical wounds. The principle of therapy is to rapidly achieve a hemostatic level of factor VIIIc (at least 20%) and to maintain this level until the lesion is adequately healed. For surgical procedures, levels of 30–40% are usually necessary for hemostasis. In mucous membrane bleeding or wounds (tongue, tooth socket), the duration of factor VIIIc therapy can often be reduced to 1–2 days if a fibrinolytic inhibitor, aminocaproic acid (Amicar), is given in a dosage of 100 mg/kg orally every 6 hours until healing is complete. Major surgical procedures and central nervous system bleeding usually require levels of 80–100% for adequate hemostasis.

Bleeding in joints or soft tissue areas can often be controlled by a single infusion of fresh frozen plasma, cryoprecipitates, or factor VIIIc concentrate to reach a single peak of 20%. If bleeding is severe, this dose should be repeated in 12 hours or a higher level achieved initially (ie, 40%). However, if the lesion is a dissecting hematoma that might threaten nerve function or endanger respiration or vision, a level of 20% should be maintained for at least 48 hours.

* A unit of factor VIIIc is the amount contained in 1 mL of fresh plasma at a 100% factor VIIIc activity level.

Corticosteroids may be helpful in instances of recurrent joint bleeding. Patients with renal bleeding have also benefited from corticosteroid therapy. Local hemostatic measures such as pressure or application of Gelfoam soaked in bovine thrombin are often helpful in cases of epistaxis. Patients with mild hemophilia should be treated with fresh frozen plasma, cryoprecipitates, or desmopressin acetate (DDAVP) in order to avoid complications of concentrate therapy.

Prognosis

With prophylaxis against injury, early treatment of bleeding episodes, careful orthopedic care of joint lesions, and attention to emotional, social, and educational adjustment, the prognosis for a useful normal life is good.

Brettler DB et al: A long-term study of hemophilic arthropathy of the knee on a program of factor VIII replacement given at the time of each hemarthrosis. *Am J Hematol* 1985;**18:**13.

Eyster ME et al: Development and early natural history of HTLV-III antibodies in persons with hemophilia. *JAMA* 1985;**253:**2219.

Kasper CK et al: Hematologic management of hemophilia A for surgery. *JAMA* 1985;**253:**1279.

Ratnoff OD, Jones PK: The laboratory diagnosis of the carrier state for classic hemophilia. *Ann Intern Med* 1977;**86:**521.

Wick MR et al: Non-A, non-B hepatitis associated with blood transfusion. *Transfusion* 1985;**25:**93.

HEMOPHILIA B
(PTC [Factor IX] Deficiency)

The mode of inheritance and clinical manifestations of hemophilia B (PTC deficiency, factor IX deficiency, Christmas disease) are the same as those of factor VIIIc deficiency (hemophilia A). Congenital PTC deficiency is 15–20% as prevalent as factor VIIIc deficiency. PTC is made in the liver and is vitamin K-dependent; therefore, acquired deficiencies of factor IX are fairly common.

In hereditary factor IX deficiency, the PTT is prolonged, but prothrombin time and thrombin time are normal. Diagnosis is confirmed by specific coagulation assay. Genetic variants of factor IX deficiency have been described; however, diagnosis and management are the same for all types.

Although factor IX is stable in storage and is not consumed during coagulation, the therapy of bleeding episodes differs little from that outlined above for classic hemophilia. The products that can be used include recently outdated blood bank plasma (approximately 3 weeks old) at 4 °C, plus fresh frozen plasma or factor IX concentrate. Unlike factor VIII, approximately half of the administered dose of factor IX diffuses into the extravascular space. Therefore, twice the calculated factor VIII dose (see above) should be given as plasma or factor IX concentrate (Konyne) initially. Subsequently, half of the initial dose can be given to achieve the desired in vivo level. (Factor IX has a half-life of 20–22 hours in vivo.) Cryoprecipitates and factor VIIIc concentrates do not contain sufficient PTC for use in this disease. The prognosis is good if the bleeding episodes are adequately controlled.

Pechet L et al: Relationship of factor IX antigen and coagulant in hemophilia B patients and carriers. *Thromb Haemost* 1979;**40:**465.

Raish RJ et al: Successful cardiac surgery following plasmapheresis in a patient with hemophilia B. *Transfusion* 1985; **25:**128.

HEMOPHILIA C (PTA [Factor XI] Deficiency)

PTA (factor XI) deficiency is a bleeding diathesis of mild to moderate severity. Inheritance is by the autosomal recessive mode. Heterozygotes rarely show a mild bleeding tendency at surgery or following severe trauma. Homozygous patients may have spontaneous hemorrhage (ecchymoses, epistaxis) in addition to bleeding due to trauma. Only rarely do patients with hemophilia C have spontaneous hemarthroses. Hemophilia C has been found mainly in Jews and comprises less than 5% of all hemophilioid diseases.

The defect may be very mild, and a sensitive coagulation test is required to identify the deficiency. Factor XI is a stable factor found in both serum and plasma and shows increased activity on contact with glass or after storage. Therefore, differentiation from PTC deficiency may be difficult unless tests are done with fresh plasma using known PTA-deficient plasma for assays. The prothrombin time and bleeding time (Ivy) are normal in PTA deficiency.

The bleeding defect is mild and requires treatment usually only at times of surgery (eg, tooth extractions) or trauma. PTA is a stable factor, and good levels are found in plasma stored for several weeks at 4 °C. Therefore, the principles of treatment outlined for PTC deficiency apply equally well to PTA deficiency.

The prognosis for an average life span is excellent.

Reese EA et al: Spontaneous factor XI inhibitors. *Arch Intern Med* 1984;**144:**525.

Seligsohn U, Modan M: Definition of the population at risk of bleeding due to factor XI deficiency in Ashkenazic Jews and the value of activated partial thromboplastin time in its detection. *Isr J Med Sci* 1981;**17:**413.

DEFICIENCIES OF LIVER-DEPENDENT COAGULATION FACTORS

The following clotting factors are known to be produced in the liver: fibrinogen (I), PTC (IX), prothrombin (II), proconvertin (VII), proaccelerin (V), Stuart-Prower factor (X), PTA (XI), and Hageman factor (XII). Vitamin K is necessary for the synthesis of II, VII, X, and IX. Hereditary bleeding diseases due to isolated deficiencies of prothrombin, proconvertin, proaccelerin, or Stuart-Prower factor are exceedingly rare. Congenital deficiencies of fibrinogen and PTC are discussed above.

Hereditary prothrombin deficiency, proconvertin deficiency, Stuart-Prower factor deficiency, and proaccelerin deficiency have been reported in both males and females and have a recessive mode of transmission. Mild to moderately severe bleeding manifestations can occur. The prothrombin time is uniformly prolonged in these disorders. The diagnosis is suspected when a patient is seen with a history of bleeding manifestations, a prolonged prothrombin time without liver disease, and no response to vitamin K therapy. The diagnosis must be confirmed by specific factor assays.

Treatment consists of transfusion of whole plasma in dosages sufficient to achieve at least 20–30% correction of the prothrombin time. Fresh plasma must be used for proaccelerin (V) deficiency, since this is a relatively unstable factor. Prothrombin complex concentrates (Konyne, Proplex) may be used for therapy of factor II, VII, and X when higher levels are desired.

Chiu HC et al: Heterogeneity of human factor V deficiency: Evidence for the existence of antigen-positive variants. *J Clin Invest* 1983;**72:**493.

Goldsmith GH Jr et al: Studies on a family with combined functional deficiencies of vitamin K-dependent coagulation factors. *J Clin Invest* 1982;**69:**1253.

Ragni MV et al: Factor VII deficiency. *Am J Hematol* 1981;**10:**79.

HAGEMAN FACTOR (FACTOR XII) DEFICIENCY; PREKALLIKREIN DEFICIENCY; HIGH-MOLECULAR-WEIGHT KININOGEN DEFICIENCY

Severe deficiencies of the ''contact'' factors (factor XII, or Hageman factor, prekallikrein, or Fletcher factor; and high-molecular-weight kininogen, or Fitzgerald factor) cause marked prolongation of the PTT but are not associated with a bleeding diathesis. Severe factor XII deficiency has been associated with thrombosis. Mild deficiencies of factor XII and high-molecular-weight kininogen also prolong the PTT and are frequently of clinical importance in the evaluation of a mildly prolonged PTT prior to surgical procedures.

Hathaway WE et al: Sensitivity of the activated partial thromboplastin time to mild factor deficiencies. Pages 131–136 in: *Standardization of Coagulation Assays: An Overview*. Triplett DA (editor). College of American Pathologists, 1982.

Hellstern P et al: Arterial and venous thrombosis and normal response to streptokinase treatment in a young patient with severe Hageman factor deficiency. *Acta Haematol (Basel)* 1983;**69:**123.

FIBRIN STABILIZING FACTOR (FACTOR XIII) DEFICIENCY; ALPHA$_2$ ANTIPLASMIN DEFICIENCY

Two separate but closely related coagulation factor deficiencies are associated with a severe bleeding diathesis characterized by mucous membrane, muscle, and joint hemorrhages. Fibrin stabilizing factor (factor XIII) deficiency and alpha$_2$ antiplasmin deficiency are autosomal recessive. Affected individuals may present with hemorrhage into the umbilical cord at birth. Factor XIII and alpha$_2$ antiplasmin are both necessary for stabilization and persistence of the fibrin clot; therefore, the usual screening tests of hemostasis (bleeding time, PTT, prothrombin time, thrombin time) are normal. Factor XIII deficiency is diagnosed by demonstration of plasma clot lysis in urea, 5 mol/L, and alpha$_2$ antiplasmin deficiency by increased lysis of whole blood and dilute plasma. Specific assays are available for both factors. Treatment consists of plasma transfusions, 10–15 mL/kg, to control acute bleeding episodes.

Kitchens CS, Newcomb TF: Factor XIII. *Medicine* 1979; **58:**413.

Miles LA et al: A bleeding disorder due to deficiency of alpha 2-antiplasmin. *Blood* 1982;**59:**1246.

ACQUIRED COAGULATION FACTOR DEFICIENCIES

1. HEMORRHAGIC DISEASE OF THE NEWBORN

A generalized bleeding diathesis can occur in newborn infants who are markedly deficient in vitamin K-dependent coagulation factors (factors II, VII, IX, and X). This clinical syndrome is called hemorrhagic disease of the newborn. It may be present at birth or may occur any time in the first 3 days of life. All newborn infants show a moderate deficiency of these vitamin K-dependent factors at a level of 25–60% of normal adult values. However, when the levels fall below 20% in infants who are vitamin K-deficient, a generalized bleeding tendency can ensue. Ecchymoses, gastrointestinal hemorrhage, hematuria, and cerebral hemorrhages may occur on the second to fourth days of life.

Hemorrhagic disease may also occur at 1–2 months of age in breast-fed infants who have not received prophylactic vitamin K at birth or who have malabsorption syndromes (see below). The prothrombin time is markedly prolonged to a level below 20% of normal. The PTT is also greatly prolonged. Platelet estimation and bleeding times are normal. In this age group, bleeding in association with a greatly prolonged prothrombin time is very suggestive of hemorrhagic disease of the newborn. The diagnosis is confirmed by the response to specific treatment and by demonstration of the precursor *p*rotein present *in v*itamin *K a*bsence (PIVKA) (abnormal prothrombin).

By definition, this disorder is due to severe vitamin K deficiency. Therefore, the disease can be prevented and treated adequately by a single intramuscular injection of 1 mg of vitamin K$_1$ (phytonadione). It is also recommended that this dose be given prophylactically to all newborn infants and to older breast-fed infants with protracted diarrhea. The prothrombin will become essentially normal within 12–24 hours, and the bleeding will stop within 6–12 hours after treatment with vitamin K. If life-threatening hemorrhage is present, a transfusion of fresh plasma (10 mL/kg) is indicated.

Infants of mothers receiving hydantoin or warfarin therapy are especially susceptible to vitamin K deficiency.

Lane PA, Hathaway WE: Vitamin K in infancy. *J Pediatr* 1985;**106:**351.

2. VITAMIN K DEFICIENCY IN OLDER CHILDREN

Older infants and children, especially if they were breast-fed, may develop vitamin K deficiency secondary to chronic diarrhea, malabsorption syndrome, obstructive jaundice, and defective synthesis associated with prolonged antibiotic therapy. The clinical and laboratory manifestations are similar to those seen in hemorrhagic disease of the newborn. Treatment is by administration of vitamin K$_1$ (phytonadione) in doses of 5–10 mg intravenously or intramuscularly.

Lane PA et al: Fatal intracranial hemorrhage in a normal infant secondary to vitamin K deficiency. *Pediatrics* 1983;**72:**562.

3. SECONDARY HEMORRHAGIC DIATHESIS OF THE NEWBORN

Premature and full-term infants frequently develop generalized bleeding tendencies associated with other illnesses such as respiratory distress syndrome, cyanotic congenital heart disease, cerebral anoxia, and severe sepsis. Factors often present and possibly related to this bleeding syndrome are "physiologic" depression of coagulation factors, hypoxia, acidosis, vascular fragility, defective platelet number and function, and increased fibrinolytic activity. Laboratory tests of bleeding and coagulation are difficult to interpret because results in affected patients overlap with those in normal infants. The values for these tests seen in "normal" full-term and premature infants are shown in Table 16–5. The pathophysiologic mechanisms of these secondary bleeding syndromes (cerebral hemorrhage, pulmonary hemorrhage, generalized bleeding tendency) are related to increased consumption (due to pathologic proteolysis) or decreased syn-

Table 16–5. Coagulation factor and test values in normal pregnant women and newborn infants.*

Category	Fibrinogen (mg/dL)	Factors									Platelet Count (per μL)	Euglobulin Lysis Time (minutes)	Partial Thromboplastin Time† (seconds)	Prothrombin Time (seconds)	Thrombin Time (seconds)
		II (%)	V (%)	VII (%)	VIII (%)	IX (%)	X (%)	XI (%)	XII (%)	XIII (titer)					
Normal adult or child	190–420	100	100	100	100	100	100	100	100	1/16	200,000–450,000	90–300	37–50	12–14	8–10
Term pregnancy	483	92	108	170	196	130	130	69	...	1/16	290,000	278	44	13	8
Premature infant (1500–2500 g), cord blood	233	25	67	37	100	34	29	30	33	1/8	220,000	214	90	17 (12–21)	14 (11–17)
Term infant, cord blood	216	41	92	56	100	27	55	36	47	1/8	190,000	84	71	13.5 (12–16)	12 (10–16)
Term infant, 48 hours	210	46	105	20	100	↓	45	39	25	...	200,000	105	65	16 (12–21)	13 (10–16)

Note: All levels expressed as means or ranges.

* Modified and reproduced, with permission, from Hathaway WE: Coagulation problems in the newborn infant. *Pediatr Clin North Am* 1970;**17**:929.

† Kaolin PTT.

thesis (due to functional impairment of the liver) of clotting factors and platelets.

Treatment consists of correcting the associated conditions and replacing clotting factors and platelets with doses of fresh frozen plasma, 10 mL/kg, or platelet concentrates, 10 mL/kg. Occasionally, exchange transfusion or heparinization is indicated.

Hathaway WE, Bonnar J: *Perinatal Coagulation.* Grune & Stratton, 1978.

4. DISSEMINATED INTRAVASCULAR COAGULATION

Essentials of Diagnosis

- Presence of disorder known to trigger disseminated intravascular coagulation.
- Evidence for activation of coagulation (prolonged PTT, prothrombin time, or thrombin time or decreased fibrinogen or platelets).
- Microangiopathic red cell changes.

General Considerations

Disseminated intravascular coagulation (DIC) is an acquired pathologic process characterized by activation of the coagulation system leading to thrombin generation, intravascular fibrin deposition, and platelet consumption. Microthrombi, composed of fibrin and platelets, may produce ischemic tissue damage as well as fragmentation of erythrocytes. The fibrinolytic system is also frequently activated, producing plasmin-mediated destruction of fibrin, fibrinogen, and other clotting factors (factor V, factor VIII). Degradation or split products of fibrin-fibrinogen are formed and function as anticoagulants and inhibitors of platelet function. Disseminated intravascular coagulation commonly accompanies disorders seen in critically ill infants and children. Conditions known to trigger disseminated intravascular coagulation include endothelial cell damage (endotoxin, virus), tissue destruction (necrosis, physical injuries), hypoxia (acidosis), ischemic and vascular changes (shock, hemangiomas), and release of tissue procoagulants (cancer, placental disorders).

Clinical Findings

Physical signs of the disorder include (1) evidence of a diffuse bleeding tendency (hematuria, melena, purpura, petechiae, persistent oozing from needle punctures or other invasive procedures); (2) circulatory collapse, poor skin perfusion, early ischemic changes; and (3) evidence of thrombotic lesions (major vessel thrombosis, gangrene, purpura fulminans).

The laboratory diagnosis of disseminated intravascular coagulation is outlined in Table 16–6. Tests that are most sensitive, easiest to perform, and best reflect the hemostatic capacity of the patient are the PTT, prothrombin time, platelet count, fibrinogen level, and a test for fibrin-fibrinogen split products (Thrombo-Wellco test for serum fibrin-fibrinogen split products; protamine precipitation test for plasma monomer-fibrin-fibrinogen split product complexes). If these tests are normal or only slightly abnormal, clinically significant disseminated intravascular coagulation is not present. When disseminated intravascular coagulation is present, varying degrees of abnormality may be seen with these screening tests, depending on the triggering event. Patients with infections may have primarily thrombocytopenia, only slight prolongation of PTT and prothrombin time, and mildly elevated fibrin-fibrinogen split products. Platelets may be consumed in bacterial sepsis without any other evidence of activated coagulation. Asphyxia (at any age) may produce significant consumption of fibrinogen and elevated fibrin-fibrinogen split products without depression of platelets. In the neonatal period, the PTT is often prolonged on a physiologic basis and is thus less useful as a screening test for disseminated intravascular coagulation.

Table 16–6. Laboratory tests that may be abnormal in disseminated intravascular coagulation.

Test	Mechanism of Abnormality
Prolonged partial thromboplastin time (PTT, APTT)	Decreased procoagulants, increased fibrin-fibrinogen split products.
Prolonged prothrombin time (PT)	Decreased fibrinogen, increased fibrin-fibrinogen split products.
Prolonged thrombin time (TT)	Decreased fibrinogen, increased fibrin-fibrinogen split products.
Prolonged reptilase time	Decreased fibrinogen, increased fibrin-fibrinogen split products.
Decreased platelet count	Platelet consumption.
Decreased fibrinogen level	Fibrinogen consumption.
Increased fibrin-fibrinogen split products	Plasmin degradation of fibrin and fibrinogen.
Prolonged bleeding time	Decreased platelets and decreased platelet function.
Decreased activity of coagulation factors XII, V, VII, VIII, II, and XIII and of prekallikrein, antithrombin III, and plasminogen	See text.

Differential Diagnosis

The differential diagnosis of a diffuse bleeding tendency in a critically ill patient must include other causes as well as disseminated intravascular coagulation. Uremic bleeding (due to a platelet function defect), severe hepatic coagulopathy (due to decreased synthesis of clotting factors), and vitamin K deficiency can all mimic disseminated intravascular coagulation or may be present along with it. Vitamin K deficiency can be easily diagnosed and treated, and uremia is not hard to recognize, but severe liver disease may be more difficult to diagnose. Patients with fulminant hepatitis or advanced cirrhosis often have evidence of both decreased production of liver factors and increased comsumption of platelets and fibrinogen.

Treatment

The most important aspects of therapy are identification and treatment of the triggering event. For bacterial sepsis, give antibiotic therapy and provide volume replacement and circulatory support. Relieve hypoxia, and correct acidosis in neonatal asphyxia and respiratory distress syndromes. Restore blood volume in hemorrhagic shock, and give antiviral agents in severe viral infections. If the precipitating event can be quickly treated (eg, hypoxia or shock), often no other therapy is needed. Serial determination with coagulation tests will help in deciding whether further therapy is indicated.

Replacement of depleted coagulation factors and platelets may be necessary in severe disseminated intravascular coagulation, especially with an associated bleeding diathesis or potential severe hemorrhage. Initial stabilization of children suspected of having disseminated intravascular coagulation should include use of fresh frozen plasma whenever volume expanders are indicated in order to replace depleted coagulation factors. Fibrinogen and other clotting factors can be replaced by use of fresh frozen plasma; 10–15 mL/kg will raise the clotting factor level by about 20%. Fibrinogen (and factor VIII) can be given in cryoprecipitates also; one bag of cryoprecipitate per 3 kg in infants or one bag of cryoprecipitate per 5 kg in older children will raise the fibrinogen level by about 75–100 mg/dL. Platelets are replaced by use of platelet concentrates; in the neonate, 10 mL of platelet concentrate per kilogram will raise the platelet count by about 75,000–100,000/μL. In older children, one bag of platelet concentrate per 5–6 kg is the usual dose. The minimal hemostatic levels of procoagulants are estimated by a platelet count of 30,000–50,000/μL, a prothrombin time of 18 seconds, and a fibrinogen level of 100 mg/dL.

In specific instances, interruption of the clotting process by heparin may be necessary when the triggering event cannot be quickly treated and consumptive coagulopathy or tissue necrosis is ongoing (eg, acute promyelocytic or monocytic leukemia, giant hemangioma, hemolytic-uremic syndrome in the patient with frank disseminated intravascular coagulation [infrequent], impending tissue necrosis or gangrene in septic shock, large vessel thrombosis, or purpura fulminans). In these instances, heparin will halt disseminated intravascular coagulation or allow for more effective replacement therapy while the primary disease is being specifically treated. The most effective and safest method of giving heparin is by continuous intravenous administration. A loading dose of 50 units/kg is followed by 10–15 units/kg/h by continuous intravenous infusion. Unless there is significant tissue necrosis, this dose is usually effective, and improvement on coagulation screening tests should occur in 12–24 hours or sooner.

In purpura fulminans, where heparin is absolutely indicated, a higher dose (20–25 units/kg/h) may be needed in order to halt the gangrenous process.

Feinstein DI: Diagnosis and management of disseminated intravascular coagulation: The role of heparin therapy. *Blood* 1982;**60**:284.

Miner ME et al: Disseminated intravascular coagulation fibrinolytic syndrome following head injury in children: Frequency and prognostic implications. *J Pediatr* 1982;**100**:687.

Silverman ED et al: Consumption coagulopathy associated with systemic juvenile rheumatoid arthritis. *J Pediatr* 1983; **103**:872.

5. CIRCULATING ANTICOAGULANTS

Acquired anticoagulants or coagulation inhibitors are of 2 types: (1) a blocking inhibitor such as the "lupus" anticoagulant, which prolongs the PTT and is not corrected by 1:1 mixing with normal plasma; and (2) specific coagulation factor inhibitors or antibodies, which progressively destroy a clotting factor (often factor VIII) on incubation with normal plasma at 37 °C. The lupus inhibitor is seen in disseminated lupus erythematosus and other collagen-vascular disorders, in postviral infections, and in patients who have been given certain drugs such as penicillin. Thrombosis rather than hemorrhage may be associated with the occurrence of the lupus anticoagulant. The second type is also found in patients with collagen-vascular disorders or may appear spontaneously postpartum and is associated with a bleeding tendency. Both types tend to disappear with time. Treatment with prednisone or immunosuppressive drugs may occasionally be indicated.

Heparin and dicumarol are potent anticoagulants when administered as drugs. Heparin affects the whole blood coagulation time or PTT primarily, whereas dicumarol affects the prothrombin time by inhibiting the utilization of vitamin K.

Mackay RJ et al: Deep vein thrombosis in association with a circulating endogenous anticoagulant. *J Pediatr* 1982; **101**:75.

Thiagarajan P, Shapiro SS: Lupus anticoagulants. In: *Disorders of Thrombin Formation.* Colman RW (editor). Churchill Livingstone, 1983.

6. HEREDITARY DEFICIENCIES OF ANTICOAGULANTS ASSOCIATED WITH THROMBOEMBOLIC DISEASE

Hereditary deficiencies of several physiologic anticoagulants are known to be associated with recurrent thromboembolic disease. Heterozygous deficiencies of antithrombin III-heparin cofactor, protein C, and protein S are expressed in an autosomal dominant fashion. Homozygous protein C deficiency is characterized by severe thrombosis or recurrent and often fatal purpura fulminans in newborn infants. Treatment of acute thrombosis is by systemic anticoagulation with or without replacement of the deficient factor.

Hereditary deficiencies in the amount and function of plasminogen as well as certain dysfibrinogenemias are associated with a lifelong thrombotic tendency.

Bertina RM et al: The use of a functional and immunologic assay for plasma protein C in the study of the heterogeneity of congenital protein C deficiency. *Thromb Haemost* 1984;**51**:1.

Comp PC, Esmon CT: Recurrent venous thromboembolism in patients with a partial deficiency of protein S. *N Engl J Med* 1984;**311**:1525.

Sills RH et al: Severe homozygous protein C deficiency. *J Pediatr* 1984;**105**:409.

Winter JH et al: Familial antithrombin-III deficiency. *Q J Med* 1982;**51**:373.

V. THE SPLEEN

SPLENOMEGALY

The child with a relatively isolated finding of splenomegaly frequently presents a puzzling diagnostic problem. In the diagnosis of chronic splenomegaly, the following categories of diseases should be considered: congestive splenomegaly, chronic infections, leukemia and lymphomas, hemolytic anemias, reticuloendothelioses, and storage diseases. The clinical findings in these entities and the recommended diagnostic procedures are summarized in Table 16–7.

DEVELOPMENTAL DEFECTS OF THE SPLEEN

Simultaneous injury, at about the 25th day of embryonic life, of the splenic anlage, atrioventricular cushions of the heart, and mesentery may account for the triad of situs inversus, congenital lesions of the heart, and asplenia. Fewer than 10% of cases of congenital absence of the spleen occur without serious heart lesions. Most infants with this triad die within a few weeks. The principal evidence of asplenia in

Table 16–7. Causes of chronic splenomegaly in children.

Cause	Associated Clinical Findings	Diagnostic Investigation
Congestive splenomegaly	History of umbilical vein catheter or neonatal omphalitis. Signs of portal hypertension (varices, hemorrhoids, dilated abdominal wall veins); pancytopenia, history of hepatitis or jaundice.	Complete blood count, platelet count, liver function tests, upper gastrointestinal x-rays.
Chronic infections	History of exposure to tuberculosis, histoplasmosis, coccidioidomycosis, other fungal disease; chronic sepsis (foreign body in bloodstream; subacute infective endocarditis).	Appropriate cultures and skin tests, ie, blood cultures, PPD, histoplasmin, coccidioidin skin tests; chest film.
Infectious mononucleosis	Fever, fatigue, pharyngitis, rash, adenopathy.	Heterophil antibodies.
Leukemia, lymphoma, Hodgkin's disease	Evidence of systemic involvement with fever, bleeding tendencies, and lymphadenopathy; pancytopenia.	Blood smear, bone marrow examination, spleen biopsy.
Hemolytic anemias	Anemia, jaundice; family history of anemia, jaundice, and gallbladder disease in young adults.	Reticulocyte count, Coombs test, spherocytosis (blood smear, osmotic fragility), autohemolysis test, gallium scan.
Reticuloendothelioses (histiocytosis X)	Chronic otitis media, seborrheic or petechial skin rashes, anemia, infections, lymphadenopathy.	Skeletal x-rays for bone lesions; biopsy of bone, liver, bone marrow, or lymph node.
Storage diseases	Family history of similar disorders, neurologic involvement, evidence of macular degeneration.	Biopsy of rectal mucosa, liver, bone marrow, spleen, or brain in search for storage cells.
Splenic cyst	Evidence of other infections (postinfectious cyst) or congenital anomalies; peculiar shape of spleen.	Radioisotope scans.

these infants consists of erythrocytic inclusions such as Howell-Jolly bodies, nucleated red cells, and Heinz bodies. A mild reticulocytosis and siderocytosis can be found. The discovery of these red cell inclusions in a patient with congenital heart disease is strong presumptive evidence of this syndrome.

No specific therapy is available.

Freedman RM et al: Development of splenic reticuloendothelial function in neonates. *J Pediatr* 1980;**96:**466.

Majeski JA, Upshur JK: Asplenia syndrome: A study of congenital anomalies in 16 cases. *JAMA* 1978;**240:**1508.

CONGESTIVE SPLENOMEGALY (Banti's Syndrome)

Banti's syndrome consists of an enlarged spleen, pancytopenia, and evidences of hepatic disease such as liver enlargement, decreased liver function as shown by appropriate tests, portal hypertension, and hepatic decompensation. Three separate entities are known to produce this syndrome: (1) vascular anomalies of the splenic and portal venous system; (2) thrombophlebitis of the portal and splenic veins, often secondary to infection following neonatal catheterization of the umbilical vein; and (3) cirrhosis of the liver. The age at onset and the presenting symptoms vary according to the cause.

Infections and neoplasms of the spleen are listed in Table 16–7 and discussed elsewhere in the text.

INFECTIONS FOLLOWING SPLENECTOMY

There is good evidence that infants and children who have undergone splenectomy are subsequently more susceptible to septicemia, meningitis, and pneumonia due to pneumococci, group A streptococci, *Haemophilus influenzae,* and enteric organisms. Children under 4 years of age and those with generalized disorders of the reticuloendothelial system are more frequently affected. The increased susceptibility to infection following splenectomy has not been explained, but it is probably related to the role of the spleen in antibody synthesis and phagocytic function. If possible, splenectomy should be delayed until after age 4, and prophylactic antibiotic therapy should be used after splenectomy in susceptible patients in addition to the administration of pneumococcal vaccine.

Krivit W: Overwhelming postsplenectomy infection. *Am J Hematol* 1977;**2:**193.

Kumpe DA et al: Partial splenic embolization in children with hypersplenism. *Radiology* 1985;**155:**357.

Linné T et al: Splenic function after nonsurgical management of splenic rupture. *J Pediatr* 1984;**105:**263.

Pearson HA: Splenectomy: Its risks and its roles. *Hosp Pract* (Aug) 1980;**15:**85.

TRANSFUSION REACTIONS

Essentials of Diagnosis

- Fever and chills during or after transfusion.
- Urticarial reaction with or without lymphadenopathy, joint pains, fever, hypotension, asthma.

General Considerations

The incidence of transfusion reactions is high—estimates range up to 20%. A common form is a febrile reaction which may be related to contamination with bacterial or other pyrogenic products or which may accompany hemolytic reactions or reactions in which transfused leukocytes are destroyed by antileukocyte antibodies present in the recipient. Urticarial reactions have been reported to occur in 1–3% of transfusions and are said to be more common in atopic individuals. Citrate toxicity, manifested largely as tetany and vascular collapse progressing at times to death, is an unusual complication of transfusion therapy. The transmission of serum hepatitis is also a potential problem, but careful screening of donors has helped to reduce the incidence of transmission.

Transfusion of mismatched blood may have any of the following adverse effects: symptoms and signs of intravascular or extravascular hemolysis; ischemia or bleeding; or a reaction involving antibodies formed to IgA, especially in IgA-deficient recipients. Allergic reactions to mismatched blood may result from passive sensitization of the recipient through blood from a donor sensitive to foods, drugs, inhalants or other allergens or from the infusion of allergen present in donor's plasma to which the recipient is sensitive. Hemolytic reactions are among the most severe transfusion reactions and have a high mortality rate.

Clinical Findings

A. Symptoms and Signs: Chills and fever are particularly common and may be associated with septicemia, hemolytic reactions, or reactions due to the presence of leukoagglutinins, especially if the patient has received multiple transfusions. Symptoms of hemolytic reactions may also include headache, nausea and vomiting, apprehension and anxiety, facial flushing, a feeling of warmth along the vein into which blood is being transfused, and abdominal or chest pains. Hypotension, oliguria, and frank renal failure with anuria may result.

Urticarial reactions with accompanying pruritus frequently occur without other symptoms but may also occur in conjunction with anaphylactic and hemolytic reactions. Anaphylactic reactions, which may include bronchial obstruction, hypotension, or laryngeal edema, are seen rarely. With allergic reactions, eosinophilia is sometimes noted.

B. Laboratory Findings: With hemolytic reactions, free hemoglobin is usually present in detectable amounts in the serum almost immediately and may also be found in the urine; serum bilirubin levels may become elevated within hours, as may methemoglobin levels also. The white blood count may be high or low. A Coombs test (direct and indirect) performed on posttransfusion recipient's blood should reveal the presence of antibody reactive with cells of the recipient or donor. In addition, red cell agglutinates can sometimes be seen in a sample of the recipient's blood. Agglutinins to other formed blood elements or antibody to donor immunoglobulins may be found.

Prevention

Antihistamines given 1 hour before the blood transfusion may be used prophylactically to decrease the incidence and severity of allergic reactions. Used prophylactically, *antihistamines do not completely eliminate the possibility of a severe transfusion reaction.* Febrile reactions to leukocytes can be avoided by using frozen washed red cells. Problems consequent to the administration of hemolyzed blood can largely be avoided with proper inspection of the blood and equipment prior to transfusion.

Treatment

Treatment consists chiefly of immediate discontinuation of the transfusion and maintenance of adequate blood volume and pressure with intravenous fluids and pressor amines. Other ancillary measures depend upon the degree and nature of the reaction.

Urticaria with pruritus unaccompanied by other signs or symptoms does not necessarily contraindicate continuing the transfusion, as is the case with mild febrile reactions.

The treatment of urticarial reactions, angioedema, laryngeal edema, asthma, serum sickness, and anaphylactic shock has been described elsewhere.

Epinephrine, 1:1000, 0.2–0.4 mL intramuscularly, remains the most important single drug early in the treatment of severe acute allergic reactions. Antihistamines may also be given intravenously. Corticosteroids have also been recommended for the treatment of allergic and hemolytic transfusion reactions, but their efficacy in acute reactions is questionable.

For citrate toxicity, treatment consists of discontinuation of the transfusion and *slow* administration of calcium chloride (5%) or calcium gluconate (10%), 5–20 mL intravenously.

With hemolytic reactions, recipient and donor blood should be retyped and cross-matched and recipient blood cross-matched against other possible donors. If the hemolytic reaction is severe—and in the absence of cardiac failure, severe dehydration, intracranial bleeding, or renal failure—a 20% solution of mannitol, 0.3 g/kg intravenously over 10–15 minutes, should be given in addition to intravenous fluids to ensure adequate urine flow. This may be repeated once in 2 hours if adequate urine flow is not attained.

Plasma expanders may be necessary to treat hypotension due to hypovolemia.

Corticosteroids—eg, hydrocortisone sodium succinate (Solu-Cortef), 4 mg/kg—should be added to intravenous fluids and infused in a 4- to 6-hour period.

Prognosis

The prognosis depends on the nature and degree of the reaction. Hemolytic reactions must be kept in mind, since they are associated with a high fatality rate.

Conrad ME (editor): Transfusion problems in hematology. *Semin Hematol* 1981;**18:**79. [Entire issue.]

Flaum MA et al: The hemostatic imbalance of plasma-exchange transfusion. *Blood* 1979;**54:**694.

Masouredis SP: Hazards of transfusion therapy. Pages 1314–1319 in *Hematology.* Williams WJ et al (editors). McGraw-Hill, 1972.

Mollison PL: Blood transfusion. In: *Clinical Medicine,* 7th ed. Blackwell, 1983.

SELECTED REFERENCES

Biggs R: *Human Coagulation, Haemostasis and Thrombosis,* 2nd ed. Blackwell, 1976.

Bloom AL, Thomas DP: *Haemostasis and Thrombosis.* Churchill Livingstone, 1981.

George JN, Nurden AT, Phillips DR: Molecular defects in interactions of platelets with the vessel wall. *N Engl J Med* 1984;**311:**1084.

Mollison PL: *Blood Transfusion in Clinical Medicine,* 7th ed. Blackwell, 1983.

Moncada S, Vane JR: Arachidonic acid metabolites and the interactions between platelets and blood-vessel walls. *N Engl J Med* 1979:**300:**1142.

Montgomery RR, Hathaway WE: Acute bleeding emergencies. *Pediatr Clin North Am* 1980;**27:**327.

Nathan DG, Oski FA: *Hematology of Infancy and Childhood,* 2nd ed. Saunders, 1981.

Oski FA, Naiman JL: *Hematologic Problems of the Newborn,* 2nd ed. Saunders, 1972.

Petz LD, Garratty G: *Acquired Immune Hemolytic Anemias.* Churchill Livingstone, 1980.

Sherwood WC, Cohen A (editors): *Transfusion Therapy: The Fetus, Infant, and Child.* Masson, 1980.

Smith CH: *Blood Diseases of Infancy and Childhood,* 4th ed. Mosby, 1978.

Stiehm ER, Fulginiti VA: *Immunologic Disorders in Infants and Children,* 2nd ed. Saunders, 1980.

Wintrobe MM et al: *Clinical Hematology,* 8th ed. Lea & Febiger, 1981.

17 Immunodeficiency

Anthony R. Hayward, MD, PhD, & Richard B. Johnston, Jr., MD

Resistance to infection is a complex phenomenon that depends upon a variety of factors, both nonspecific and specific. Since each of these factors has its special functional role, abnormalities in these factors (ie, immunodeficiency diseases) can result in different patterns of infection. Table 17–1 provides a summary of the major immunodeficiency diseases and a description of the typical patterns of infection that occur in the presence of these disorders.

NONSPECIFIC FACTORS IN RESISTANCE TO INFECTION

Specific immunity depends upon the formation of antibody and of increased numbers of lymphocytes primed to recognize specific antigens. This aspect of host defense will be discussed below. Nonspecific factors important in host defense against infection consist of physical and anatomic barriers (nonimmunologic systems), phagocyte function, and complement. Defects in those factors are discussed first.

Defects in Physical & Anatomic Barriers

Defects in the normal physical and anatomic barriers to microbial invasion are the most common predisposing cause of recurrent infections. As such, they should be systematically considered. Some typical diagnostic possibilities are presented in Table 17–1 according to their pathophysiologic mechanisms. Bacterial infections recurring in the same location should suggest one of the defects in this group. For example, localized infection may occur in the lung when vascular perfusion has been embarrassed by a sickle cell infarct, or infection may occur in areas of skin affected by the angiopathy of diabetes mellitus or the edema of nephrotic syndrome. Infection may localize behind obstruction to the normal outflow of air or of mucus, eg, from cystic fibrosis, foreign body, depression of the cough reflex by alcohol, or reflux from a tracheoesophageal fistula. Breaks in integument commonly predispose to infection, which may be localized or generalized. The frequency of enterobacterial pneumonia and septicemia in hospitalized patients receiving antibiotic therapy should remind physicians that normal commensal bacteria protect us from invasion by pathogens.

Defects of Phagocyte Function

The wider availability of assays of neutrophil and monocyte function has resulted in detection of an increasing number of abnormalities in this aspect of host defense. In most cases, the underlying molecular aberration is unknown or incompletely understood. The better substantiated disorders associated with an increased incidence of infection are listed in Table 17–2. Defects in more than one function may coexist; in these cases, categorization is based on the apparent relative severity of the defects.

Defects of chemotaxis may be due to abnormalities of the cell, either intrinsic or secondary; to a deficiency of complement-derived chemotactic factors; or to increased activity of cell-directed or chemotactic factor-directed inhibitors. Examples of primary cellular abnormalities are Chédiak-Higashi syndrome (see Chapter 16) and congenital deficiency of a family of plasma membrane glycoproteins that play an important role in adherence, chemotaxis, and phagocytosis. Patients with this latter disorder have delayed rejection of the umbilical stump after birth, severe periodontal disease, and recurrent infections of the skin and respiratory tract. Metabolic and nutritional disorders, including diabetes mellitus, the hypophosphatemia associated with hyperalimentation, and a wide variety of other conditions (Table 17–2), can be associated with depressed motility of phagocytic cells, presumably because the metabolic requirements for movement are not met. The association of depressed chemotaxis with hyperimmunoglobulinemia E, recurrent pyoderma, eczema, and otitis media appears to fit within this same category.

When the migration of neutrophils into sites of bacterial invasion is impaired, infections occur at these sites—namely, beneath the skin and in the mucous membranes of the respiratory tract. Thus, furunculosis, subcutaneous abscesses, oral ulcers, and pneumonia have been the most common infections in patients with defective cell motility. Staphylococci, which are common and energetic residents of the interface between the body and the outside world, have been the most frequent infecting organisms.

Deficient phagocytosis is most often due to a deficiency of opsonins, especially hypogammaglobulinemia. If there are insufficient numbers of wandering phagocytic cells (ie, neutropenia), the result is infection at peripheral sites of bacterial invasion; thus, the types of infections and the infecting organisms

Table 17–1. Typical patterns of infections seen in patients with immunodeficiency diseases.*

Physiologic Mechanism	Abnormality	Usual Pattern of Associated Infections: Organisms†	Usual Pattern of Associated Infections: Sites; Types‡
Nonimmunologic systems			
Vascular perfusion	Sickle cell disease, diabetes, edema (nephrotic syndrome, congestive heart failure).	Pyogenic and enteric bacteria.	Recurrent in same location.
Drainage	Urethral or ureteral stenosis; bronchial obstruction (cystic fibrosis, foreign body, drug-depressed cough, tracheoesophageal fistula, α_1-antitrypsin deficiency, ciliary dysfunction); auditory tube obstruction.		
Integumental barriers	Eczema, burns, skull fracture, sinus tract.		
Bacterial flora	Altered gut flora secondary to antibiotic therapy.	Pyogenic and enteric bacteria.	Diarrhea, bacteremia, pneumonia.
Phagocyte function			
Chemotaxis	Defective adherence (glycoprotein deficiency).	Staphylococci, enteric bacteria.	Skin and respiratory tract.
	Defects of neutrophil migration.	Staphylococci.	Skin and respiratory tract.
Phagocytosis	Opsonin deficiency.	(See Humoral systems, below.)	
	Neutropenia.	Staphylococci, enteric bacteria.	Skin and respiratory tract.
	Asplenia.	Pyogenic bacteria (pneumococci).	Septicemia, meningitis.
	Intrinsic cellular defects.	Staphylococci, enteric bacteria.	Skin and respiratory tract.
Killing	Chronic granulomatous disease.	Staphylococci, enteric bacteria, fungi.	Skin and RES§; abscesses.
Humoral systems			
Circulating antibody	Hypogammaglobulinemia.	Pyogenic bacteria.	Any site; localized and disseminated.
Mucosal antibody	IgA deficiency.	Pyogenic bacteria.	Respiratory tract.
Complement	Congenital deficiencies: C1q, C2, C3, factor I.	Pyogenic bacteria.	Bacteremia, meningitis, pyoderma.
	C5, C6, C7, C8, C9	*Neisseria meningitidis* or *Neisseria gonorrhoeae.*	Meningitis, pyogenic arthritis.
Cell-mediated immunity			
T lymphocytes	Deficiency in number or function.	Viruses, fungi, protozoa, bacteria.	Any site; localized and systemic.

* Reproduced, with permission, from Johnston RB Jr: Recurrent bacterial infections in children. *N Engl J Med* 1984;**310:**1237.

† Common infecting organisms are emphasized. Pyogenic bacteria include pneumococci, *Streptococcus pyogenes, Haemophilus influenzae,* meningococci, and staphylococci. Enteric bacteria include enterococci and the gram-negative bacilli common to the intestinal tract, especially *Escherichia coli, Pseudomonas* sp, *Klebsiella-Enterobacter* sp, and *Proteus* sp.

‡ Skin infections include furunculosis, subcutaneous abscesses, and cellulitis; respiratory tract infections include recurrent pneumonia, otitis media, and sinusitis.

§ RES denotes reticuloendothelial system (liver, lungs, lymph nodes, and spleen).

Table 17–2. Defects of phagocyte function.

Defects of cell movement (chemotaxis)
- Primary (intrinsic) cellular abnormalities
  - Chédiak-Higashi syndrome
  - Increased microtubule assembly and elevated cGMP
  - Lazy leukocyte syndrome
  - Absence of specific granules
  - Membrane glycoprotein deficiency
  - Kartagener's syndrome
  - Glycogenosis type Ib
- Secondary cellular abnormalities
  - Hyperimmunoglobulinemia E syndrome
  - Diabetes
  - Acrodermatitis enteropathica
  - Hypophosphatemia
  - Ethanol intoxication
  - Rheumatoid arthritis
  - Mannosidosis
  - Down's syndrome
  - Cancer
  - Severe infections
  - Burns
  - Malnutrition
  - Corticosteroid or immunosuppressive therapy
  - Bone marrow allotransplantation (graft-versus-host reaction)
  - Neonatal state
  - Influenza virus
  - Artificial blood substitutes
- Humoral deficiencies
  - Complement deficiencies
  - Absence of antagonist of chemotaxis inhibitor
- Humoral inhibitors
  - Chemotactic factor inhibitors (cancer, cirrhosis, sarcoidosis, leprosy)
  - Elevated IgA, circulating chemotactic factors (Wiskott-Aldrich syndrome, nephritis)
  - Autoantibody to neutrophil

Defects of phagocytosis
- Deficient opsonization (antibody or C3 deficiency)
- Neutropenia
- Hyposplenia
- Membrane glycoprotein deficiency
- Secondary cellular abnormalities
  - Hypophosphatemia
  - Diabetes
  - Corticosteroid therapy
  - Galactosemia
  - Viral infection
  - Circulating immune complexes
  - Macrophage "blockade," eg, with damaged erythrocytes

Defects of microbicidal activity
- Chronic granulomatous disease
- Glucose 6-phosphate dehydrogenase deficiency
- Myeloperoxidase deficiency
- Alkaline phosphastase deficiency
- Pyruvate kinase deficiency
- Malacoplakia
- Granule defects
  - Chédiak-Higashi syndrome
  - Absence of specific granules
  - Myelogenous or histiocytic leukemia
- Secondary cellular abnormalities
  - Leukemia
  - Viral infection
  - Felty's syndrome

are those seen in defects of chemotaxis. This pattern contrasts with that seen in individuals without spleens. Since neutrophils are present to protect the periphery, subcutaneous abscesses and pneumonia are not a problem in asplenic persons. Without the capacity of the spleen to filter the bloodstream, however, bacteremia can rapidly progress to fulminant septicemia, especially pneumococcal septicemia. Persons with sickle cell anemia have functional asplenia owing to engorgement of the spleen with sickled erythrocytes, which at least partially explains the predisposition of these individuals to serious pneumococcal infections.

It is clear that the killing of ingested microorganisms by phagocytes requires conversion of oxygen by the phagocytes to toxic metabolites, including superoxide anion and hydrogen peroxide. Neutrophils and macrophages that can phagocytose normally but cannot undergo this burst of oxidative metabolism cannot kill the ingested organisms. This oxidative defect of phagocytic cells is the basis for chronic granulomatous disease. This disorder is characterized by the formation of abscesses, both at sites of invasion beneath the skin and in the central phagocytic organs; liver, spleen, and lymph nodes. Marked lymphadenopathy, hepatosplenomegaly, pneumonia, and furunculosis are additional typical findings. Daily administration of sulfonamides or antibiotics has markedly reduced the severity of infections in many of these patients.

Marked deficiency of glucose 6-phosphate dehydrogenase in leukocytes results in a slightly milder form of chronic granulomatous disease. The other defects of microbial killing noted in Table 17–2, as tested in vitro, are generally much less pronounced than the defect of chronic granulomatous disease.

Anderson DC et al: Abnormalities of polymorphonuclear leukocyte function associated with a heritable deficiency of high molecular weight surface glycoproteins (GP138): Common relationship to diminished cell adherence. *J Clin Invest* 1984;**74:**536.

Gallin JI: Abnormal phagocyte chemotaxis: Pathophysiology, clinical manifestations, and management of patients. *Rev Infect Dis* 1981;**3:**1196.

Johnston RB: Defects of neutrophil function. *N Engl J Med* 1982;**307:**434.
Johnston RB, Newman SL: Chronic granulomatous disease. *Pediatr Clin North Am* 1977;**24:**365.

Defects of Complement

Complement is a system of serum proteins that interact in an orderly sequential fashion along 2 pathways. The classical pathway of complement activation is triggered by the interaction of antibody with an antigen or immune complex; the sequence of component activation is C1, 4, 2, 3, 5, 6, 7, 8, 9. During activation, factors that promote the vasodilatation which characterizes inflammation are split off from C3 and C5. The same C5 product (C5a) induces chemotaxis. Fixation of the major fragment of C3 (C3b) to invading microorganisms promotes their clearance by phagocytes. Fixation of all 9 components results in lysis of the organism or cell to which the components have attached. C3 can be activated and the biologic functions of chemotaxis, opsonization, and cytolysis can thereby be derived by activation of the alternative pathway, which bypasses C142. This system consists of properdin, C3b, and factors D and B.

Congenital deficiency of each of the 11 proteins of the classical pathway, properdin, and 4 control (inhibitor) proteins has been described, as set forth in Table 17–3. None of these deficiencies are common. As noted in the table, associated clinical disorders include nephritis, collagen-vascular disease, and recurrent infections. Complement hemolytic activity should be assayed in any patient with collagen-vascular disease, since in the presence of underlying complement deficiency the general pattern of disease often differs from the classic presentation and the threat of infections is greater. Complement activity should also be tested in all patients with a second episode of bacteremia (especially pneumococcal), a second episode of meningococcal meningitis, or disseminated gonococcal infection.

Recurrent angioedema without urticaria, usually beginning in late childhood, should lead one to suspect hereditary angioedema. Effective therapy exists for the disease in the form of danazol, a synthetic androgen that increases C1 inhibitor levels and prevents attacks. The diagnosis is suggested by decreased activity of whole complement, C4, and C2 and confirmed by direct assay of the C1 inhibitor.

Altenburger KM, Johnston RB: The complement system and its disorders in man. Pages 113–132 in: *Primary and Secondary Immunodeficiency Disorders.* Chandra RK (editor). Churchill Livingstone, 1984.
Smith TF, Johnston RB: The complement system: Implications for pediatrics. Pages 305–320 in: *Pediatrics Update: Reviews for Physicians, 1981.* Moss AJ, Stiehm ER (editors). Elsevier/North-Holland, 1981.

Table 17–3. Congenital deficiencies of the complement system.

Deficient Component	Associated Clinical Abnormalities
C1q	Bacterial and fungal infections, dermal vasculitis, systemic lupus erythematosus, discoid lupus erythematosus
C1r	Chronic glomerulonephritis, systemic lupus erythematosus, dermal vasculitis
C1s	Systemic lupus erythematosus
C2	Systemic lupus erythematosus, discoid lupus erythematosus, membranoproliferative glomerulonephritis, Henoch-Schönlein purpura, dermatomyositis, rheumatoid arthritis, pneumococcal septicemia
C3	Generalized pyogenic infections, systemic lupus erythematosus, chronic glomerulonephritis
C4	Systemic lupus erythematosus
C5	Systemic lupus erythermatosus, disseminated gonococcal infection
C5 (dysfunction)	Pyoderma, septicemia, Leiner's disease
C6	Gonococcal and meningococcal infections, systemic lupus erythematosus
C7	Systemic lupus erythematosus, ankylosing spondylitis, gonococcal and meningococcal infections
C8	Gonococcal and meningococcal infections, systemic lupus erythematosus
C9	Meningococcal meningitis
C1 inhibitor	Hereditary angioedema, systemic lupus erythematosus
Factor D	Recurrent sinusitis, bronchiectasis
Factor H	Hemolytic-uremic syndrome
Factor I	Generalized pyogenic infections
Properdin	Meningococcal meningitis

SPECIFIC FACTORS IN RESISTANCE TO INFECTION

Specific immunity is mediated by antibodies and by the specialized subsets of lymphocytes and monocytes that interact in cellular immunity. Since immunodeficiency may result from a failure of antibody immunity or cellular immunity (or both), these mechanisms are briefly summarized.

Antibodies are immunoglobulins and are composed of 2 types of polypeptide chains: H (heavy) and L (light) chains, according to their molecular weights. The L chains are of 2 varieties—kappa (κ) and lambda (λ)—and are the same in all immunoglobulin molecules. The H chains have regions that are distinctive for each of the immunoglobulin classes. These differences in amino acid sequences are responsible for the distinctive antigenic, physicochemical, and biologic properties of the 5 known members of the immunoglobulin family. The immunoglobulins

Table 17–4. Properties of immunoglobulins.*

	IgG (γG)	IgA (γA)	IgM (γM)	IgD (γD)	IgE (γE)
Molecular weight	150,000	$(180{,}000)_n$	900,000	150,000	200,000
Half-life (days)	25	6	5	2.8	...
Distribution	ECF	ECF, especially secretions	Plasma	...	ECF and fixed to target cells
Placental transfer	Yes	No	No	No	No
Subclasses	G1, G2, G3, G4	A1, A2	...	...	...
Complement fixation	Yes	No	Yes	No	No

* ECF = extracellular fluid.

recognized to date are IgG, IgA, IgM, IgD, and IgE. Some properties of the immunoglobulins are shown in Table 17–4. Immunoglobulins are secreted by plasma cells, which in turn are derived from B lymphocytes as a result of antigen stimulation. The B cell response to antigen generally requires help from specialized T cells and is also susceptible to T cell suppression.

Cellular immunity requires T lymphocytes and mononuclear phagocytes. In a skin test that is an example of delayed hypersensitivity, the skin lesions are infiltrated with lymphocytes and macrophages. The tuberculin reaction is a clinical example, and contact dermatitis is a disease mediated by this mechanism. Many features of delayed hypersensitivity result from the release, by antigen-activated T cells, of soluble factors (lymphokines) that act on macrophages, vascular endothelium, and other lymphocytes.

Other T cell-mediated responses include granulomatous tissue reactions, allograft rejection, and the killing of virus-infected cells. The T cell subsets that participate in different types of cellular immune response are distinguishable by commercially available monoclonal antibodies. Examples include the OKT 4 and Leu 3 antibodies, which bind to helper-amplifier T cells, and the OKT 8 and Leu 2 antibodies, which bind to suppressor and cytotoxic T cells. Helper and cytotoxic T cells also recognize antigen in association with different histocompatibility (HLA) antigens. OKT 4-positive T cells generally respond best to antigen present on monocytes and HLA-DR determinants, whereas cytotoxic T cells kill only cells with which they have HLA-A or -B antigens in common. These HLA restrictions are thought to account for some of the associations between certain HLA types and disease (eg, ankylosing spondylitis and juvenile diabetes). One practical consequence of the HLA restriction of T cell responses is that cellular immunity cannot be transferred between unrelated individuals by blood or lymphocyte transfusion unless the donor and recipient share HLA antigens. Antibodies, in contrast, are not HLA-restricted, so passive immunity is readily conferred by injection of immune serum globulin.

Natural killer (NK) cells are another type of blood mononuclear cell, but their origin is uncertain. They lyse tumor cells and virus-infected target cells without any requirement for HLA antigen sharing. NK cell activity is greatly increased by the γ interferon released by antigen-stimulated T lymphocytes. NK cells are relatively deficient in infants for the first months of life, and their activity is congenitally defective in the Chédiak-Higashi syndrome.

Marchalonis JJ: Cell interactions in immune responses. Chap 10, pp 115–128, in: *Basic & Clinical Immunology,* 3rd ed. Fudenberg HH et al (editors). Lange, 1980.

Roitt IR: *Essential Immunology,* 3rd ed. Blackwell, 1978.

CLASSIFICATION OF IMMUNODEFICIENCY

Immune responses are complex and can fail in many ways. Defects of specific immunity are broadly subdivided into those affecting predominantly antibody formation; those in which cellular immunity is mainly affected; and those in which both mechanisms are impaired. This classification, summarized in Table 17–5, is based on combinations of clinical and laboratory results. Family studies in which a mode of inheri-

Table 17–5. Classification of primary specific immunodeficiency.

Antibody deficiency disorders
- Congenital X-linked agammaglobulinemia
- X linked hypogammaglobulinemia with IgM
- Transient hypogammaglobulinemia
- Other varied hypogammaglobulinemia syndromes
- Selective IgA deficiency
- Other selective immunoglobulin deficiencies

Cellular immunodeficiency disorders
- Nucleoside phosphorylase deficiency
- Thymic hypoplasia
- Cartilage-hair hypoplasia

Combined immunodeficiency disorders
- Severe combined immunodeficiency syndromes
- Immunodeficiency with thymoma
- Lymphopenia with lymphocytotoxins

Other disorders associated with defects of specific immunity
- Wiskott-Aldrich syndrome
- Ataxia-telangiectasia
- Chronic mucocutaneous candidiasis

tance can be shown are the most secure basis for classification, and in a few instances the underlying single gene defect is known—eg, adenosine deaminase and purine nucleoside phosphorylase deficiencies. Occasionally, as in ataxia-telangiectasia, the phenotypic features are sufficiently characteristic to facilitate recognition. The fact that most cases of immunodeficiency are still reported as "varied immunodeficiency, largely unclassified" indicates that major advances remain to be made.

Ammann AJ, Fudenberg HH: Immunodeficiency diseases. Chap 25, pp 395–429, in: *Basic & Clinical Immunology*, 4th ed. Stites DP et al (editors). Lange, 1982.

Immunodeficiency. Technical Report Series No. 630. World Health Organization, 1978.

ANTIBODY DEFICIENCY

CONGENITAL X-LINKED AGAMMAGLOBULINEMIA

Antibody deficiency in this disorder is due to panhypogammaglobulinemia. Affected infants (males) lack plasma cells in bone marrow and lymph nodes and B lymphocytes in blood. The single gene inheritance points to a single protein defect, but it is not known which metabolic pathway is affected.

Clinical Findings

A. Symptoms and Signs: Affected boys are healthy for the first 3–6 months, during which time they are protected by maternal IgG. Symptoms are the result of infections: the upper and lower airways are most affected, with recurrent sinusitis, otitis media, bronchitis, and pneumonia. Septicemia and meningitis follow unless antibiotics are given. A few boys develop asymmetric arthritis, most often of the knee or ankle, which usually resolves after adequate IgG replacement is given. Tonsils and adenoids are small or absent.

B. Laboratory Findings: The blood count should be normal. Serum IgA and IgM are usually undetectable; during infancy, affected boys will have maternal IgG. Tests of cell-mediated immunity are usually normal at least initially, though reduced numbers of blood T cells, reduced lymphocyte response to mitogens, and increased T-suppressor activity have been found in some older boys, particularly in association with chronic viral infections.

Differential Diagnosis

This disorder must be differentiated from other types of antibody deficiency and severe combined immunodeficiency. Patients in the former group usually make at least some immunoglobulin—most commonly IgM—and children with transient hypogammaglobulinemia may have IgA in their saliva even when serum levels are low; moreover, they do not have X-linked transmission. A confident diagnosis of X-linked agammaglobulinemia requires an appropriate maternal family history—affected brothers are not enough. Sporadic cases and female carriers cannot be identified with any certainty at present, though absence of blood B cells in an affected boy would be suggestive, since children with most other types of immunodeficiency do have B cells.

Treatment

IgG may be replaced by (1) intramuscular injections of Red Cross or commercial concentrate (0.6–0.8 mL/kg every 4 weeks) or (2) intravenous infusions of specially prepared deaggregated IgG (100 mg/kg every 3 weeks). Intravenous treatment is inconvenient in young children, though high IgG levels can be achieved. Many patients manage well on intramuscular injections alone. The criterion for adequate treatment is freedom from infection, such as purulent sputum or conjunctivitis, until the next injection is given. Because the injection becomes bulky and painful as the child grows, the less painful intravenous route becomes increasingly attractive. However, the relatively expensive intravenous preparations must be used, since immunoglobulin prepared for intramuscular use contains aggregates that cause reactions (see below) if given intravenously. Plasma infusions are rarely used because of the risks of acquired immunodeficiency syndrome (AIDS) or hepatitis.

Reactions to immunoglobulin are more common in patients with varied immunodeficiency than in boys with congenital hypogammaglobulinemia. Their onset is generally within minutes of the injection. Symptoms include back and limb pain, anxiety, and tightness of the chest. Signs are tachycardia, shivering, fever, and, in severe cases, shock. Fatalities are very rare. Reactions are frequent in some patients and rare in others; their occurrence is sporadic and not generally due to hypersensitivity (anti-IgA reactions may be an exception). Skin tests are not helpful. Immunoglobulin replacement must be given, but if reactions are frequent, the possibility of changing to infusions of intravenous IgG preparations should be considered. Most patients can continue receiving intramuscular injections with the following precautions: (1) When the next injection is due, 1 mL of the concentrate is injected intramuscularly; if there are no adverse effects, the remainder is given after 30 minutes. (2) Resuscitation facilities and agents, including intravenous fluids and oxygen, should be present. Epinephrine subcutaneously, as for anaphylaxis, has been recommended.

Ammann AJ et al: Use of intravenous γ-globulin in antibody deficiency: Results of a multicenter controlled trial. *Clin Immunol Immunopathol* 1982;**22:**60.

X-LINKED HYPOGAMMAGLOBULINEMIA WITH IgM

Boys with this disorder have B lymphocytes and IgM-secreting plasma cells, but their B cell differentiation is inappropriately regulated, since they rarely make useful antibody responses. The nature of the defect and the reasons for failure of IgG and IgA production are not understood.

Clinical Findings

A. Symptoms and Signs: The spectrum of infections includes those found in agammaglobulinemic boys plus opportunists such as *Pneumocystis carinii* and *Candida*. Infections may be accompanied by lymphadenopathy and splenomegaly.

B. Laboratory Findings: IgG and IgA are low (after maternal IgG is lost); IgM levels vary greatly and may fall after IgG replacement is begun. Isohemagglutinin titers are low or absent, and responses to injected antigens usually fail. Many of the boys develop neutropenia or thrombocytopenia, either transient or persistent, which probably makes the prognosis worse. Lymphocyte reponse to mitogens may be low or may have an abnormal dose-response curve.

Differential Diagnosis

Persistently low IgG and IgA distinguish this type of antibody deficiency from transient hypogammaglobulinemia. The onset of infections in severe combined immunodeficiency is usually earlier, but this differentiation may have to be based on tests of T lymphocytes.

Treatment & Prognosis

Immunoglobulin replacement must be given as described above, with appropriate antibiotic treatment of infections.

There is an impression that these boys have more infections than those with agammaglobulinemia and that this results mainly from the neutropenia.

OTHER TYPES OF HYPOGAMMAGLOBULINEMIA

1. TRANSIENT HYPOGAMMAGLOBULINEMIA

Infants' IgG levels fall during the first 4–5 months of life while maternal IgG is diluted and catabolized. The physiologic trough that occurs before the infants' IgG production maintains adult levels is accentuated in premature and dysmature infants. IgG levels of 250–300 mg/dL lie within 2 standard deviations of the mean at 3–4 months of age, and the diagnosis of transient hypogammaglobulinemia is often made in infants with infections and levels in this range. The diagnosis should be made retrospectively, since the transitory nature of the hypogammaglobulinemia can only be established when immunoglobulin levels have returned to normal.

The only diagnostic laboratory findings are of low IgG, with or without low IgA and IgM, and subsequent return to normal levels. Salivary IgA is generally detectable, and, despite the low immunoglobulin levels, antibody activity (isohemagglutinin or anti-diphtheria or tetanus antibody) is present in serum. Tests for cellular immunity are normal.

No treatment is usually required other than appropriate antibiotics for bacterial infections. Infants with severe infections and hypogammaglobulinemia could rationally be given IgG injections, since maternal antibody to the infecting organism will be rapidly depleted, but this is rarely necessary. The prognosis for affected infants is (by definition) excellent provided they do not succumb to infection before normal immunity is achieved. There is, however, an association with severe combined immunodeficiency in siblings, so this is an indication for screening infants born later into the family.

2. VARIED HYPOGAMMAGLOBULINEMIA SYNDROMES

Antibody deficiency in patients with varied hypogammaglobulinemia syndromes may be congenital or acquired. A familial trend in some cases (including relatives with autoimmune disorders) and an excess of affected boys suggest that both multifactorial and single gene causes exist. Excessive suppression of B cell differentiation by T cells has been found in some patients, but this may be a secondary phenomenon. Patients with varied hypogammaglobulinemia outnumber patients with all other types of antibody deficiency except selective IgA deficiency.

Infections follow the patterns described for other types of antibody deficiency. Some patients have remarkably few infections despite long-standing, very low immunoglobulin levels.

The laboratory findings are heterogeneous. Low levels of one or more immunoglobulin classes are associated with varying degrees of impairment of cellular immunity. Autoantibody formation, raised IgE levels, and positive immediate hypersensitivity skin reactions occur.

Treatment is by IgG replacement and antibiotics as necessary. These syndromes are too heterogeneous for confident prognosis.

COMPLICATIONS OF HYPOGAMMAGLOBULINEMIA

About 10% of boys develop optic atrophy or ataxia, evolving slowly or rapidly into fatal encephalitis. Echoviruses have sometimes been isolated from their cerebrospinal fluid or brains at biopsy or necropsy. A smaller proportion develop a dermatomyositislike syndrome, with prominent peripheral cyanosis and myopathy but little heliotrope coloration. About 10% develop symptoms of diarrhea and malabsorption that resemble Crohn's disease and are generally unresponsive to dietary changes or antibiotics. A similar but treatable enteritis may be caused by *Giardia lamblia* infection: every effort should be made to make this diagnosis, since the response to metronidazole is good.

There are reports of an increased rate of cancer in patients with antibody deficiency. The association is predominantly with lymphoreticular proliferation, but—to judge from the natural history of the condition—proliferation is frequently not malignant.

Roord JJ et al: Echovirus infections of the CNS in congenital agammaglobulinemia. Page 449 in: *Progress in Immunodeficiency Research and Therapy*. Vol 1. Griscelli C, Vossen J (editors). Excerpta Medica, 1984.

SELECTIVE IMMUNOGLOBULIN DEFICIENCIES

1. IgA DEFICIENCY

With a prevalence of 1:500 in Caucasian populations, this is by far the most common defect of specific immunity. The proportion of IgA-deficient patients who ultimately develop symptoms is unknown, but it may be at most two-thirds. Most cases appear sporadically, but both dominant and recessive inheritance occurs, so the syndrome is heterogeneous. Postulated cellular mechanisms include an intrinsic defect of differentiation of B lymphocytes committed to IgA production and excessive suppression by T cells or monocytes.

Many patients have no symptoms, perhaps because they can adequately protect their mucosae with IgG and IgM. Failure of antibody responses in the IgG2 subclass is reported in symptomatic patients. When symptoms are present, they are predominantly due to upper respiratory tract infections or diarrhea. There are also strong associations with allergy (mainly respiratory and gut) and autoimmune disorders (thyroiditis, arthritis, vitiligo, etc).

Arbitrary criteria for diagnosis are serum IgA less than 5 mg/dL, absent salivary IgA, normal IgM and IgG, and normal cellular immunity. A search for anti-IgA antibodies may be important, as these can cause transfusion reactions. The selective lack of IgA responses and the presence of normal antibody responses in other immunoglobulin classes serve to distinguish IgA deficiency from varied immunodeficiency.

IgA replacement is impractical, though it is conceivable that colostrum feeding could modify severe gut symptoms. Treatment of symptomatic patients with IgG injections has been both advocated and condemned on theoretic grounds. Most IgA-deficient patients manage reasonably well with antibiotics only; atopic or autoimmune symptoms should be treated conventionally.

Buckley RH: Clinical and immunologic features of selective IgA deficiency. In: *Immunodeficiency in Man and Animals*. Bergsma D, Good RA, Finstad J (editors). Sinauer, 1975.

Oxelius V-A et al: IgG subclasses in selective IgA deficiency: Importance of IgG2-IgA deficiency. *N Engl J Med* 1981; **304:**1476.

2. SELECTIVE DEFICIENCIES OF OTHER CLASSES

Selective deficiencies of IgM, IgE, κ, and λ chains have been described but are rare. IgM deficiency has been associated with marked susceptibility to septicemia. Since replacement is impractical on a long-term basis, reliance is placed mainly on antibiotics.

SELECTIVE DEFECTS OF CELL-MEDIATED IMMUNITY

Purine nucleoside phosphorylase deficiency is the best defined; it results in increased intracellular levels of deoxyguanosine triphosphate (dGTP), which interfere with DNA synthesis, especially in T cells. T cell help to B cells is not prevented, probably because it is not dependent on cell division. The structural locus for purine nucleoside phosphorylase is on chromosome 14, and transmission is recessive. Presenting features have included progressive vaccinia, severe varicella, anemia, and failure to thrive; the age range is 6 months to 7 years. Investigations showed low normal blood lymphocyte counts, absent delayed hypersensitivity skin responses, and low or absent lymphocyte responses to mitogens. Serum immunoglobulins and antibody responses to injected antigens were normal. In many cases, an autoimmune hemolytic anemia was present. Diagnosis depends on enzyme measurement, and all patients with severely impaired cellular immunity who make immunoglobulin should probably be tested. Injections of deoxycytosine or thymosin and infusions of irradiated red cells are being evaluated as treatment measures.

Thymic hypoplasia (DiGeorge's syndrome) in its most severe form is associated with lack of parathyroid glands and with major vessel abnormalities such as truncus arteriosus, anomalous pulmonary venous drainage, or right-sided aortic arch. Other features include a small jaw, low-set ears, and a short philtrum. A positive family history is exceptional, and environmental damage to the fetus, probably between 5 and 7 weeks of gestation, seems the most likely cause. Clinical presentation usually results from cardiac failure or, after 24–48 hours, from hypocalcemia, and the diagnosis is sometimes made during the course of cardiac surgery, when no thymus is found in the mediastinum. Postoperative hypocalcemia can be severe and persistent, requiring both calcium and vitamin D supplements. Despite receiving fresh blood transfusions during cardiopulmonary bypass, patients do not usually develop graft-versus-host disease. Their susceptibility to infection is variable: a few have died with septicemia, and some have had chronic candidiasis; but many appear to respond normally. This may reflect the tendency for the number of T cells in the patients' blood to rise spontaneously over the course of several years.

Less severe degrees of thymic hypoplasia may be more common, though this diagnosis must be substantiated by evidence of cardiac, parathyroid, or thymic abnormality. Hypocalcemia and a small or absent thymus on chest x-ray may be secondary to infection. Grafting thymic hypoplasia patients with fetal thymus is often followed by rapid improvement in the lymphocyte response to mitogens. A graft of thymic epithelial cells has had similar effects. The improvement is so rapid that thymic humoral factors are thought to be responsible. Graft treatment is generally reserved for those who do not improve spontaneously.

Many patients with the American (but not Finnish) type of cartilage-hair hypoplasia have a moderate degree of lymphopenia, low lymphocyte responses to mitogens, and higher than normal morbidity and mortality rates from herpesvirus and poxvirus infections. There is no established treatment. Short-limbed dwarfs who are immunodeficient should probably be tested for adenosine deaminase deficiency, since this is treatable. Other types of immunodeficiency affecting predominantly cellular immunity exist but are poorly classified; currently, therefore, they are included in the "varied immunodeficiency" group. Their infections resemble those described above, with the frequent addition of chronic diarrhea and malabsorption and lung infections due to fungi and *Pneumocystis carinii*. Treatment is experimental and may include thymosin, transfer factor, and thymus grafts.

Ammann AJ, Sutliff W, Millinchick E: Antibody-mediated immunodeficiency in short-limbed dwarfism. *J Pediatr* 1974;**84**:200.

Conley ME et al: The spectrum of the DiGeorge syndrome. *J Pediatr* 1979;**94**:883.

Symposium: Enzyme defects and immune dysfunction. Ciba Foundation. Elsevier/North-Holland, 1979.

COMBINED IMMUNODEFICIENCY DISORDERS

SEVERE COMBINED IMMUNODEFICIENCY (SCID) (& Variants of SCID)

Essentials of Diagnosis

- Early onset of diarrhea, failure to thrive, and respiratory infections.
- Hypogammaglobulinemia.
- Severely impaired cellular immunity.

General Considerations

SCID comprises a heterogeneous group of conditions that have in common primary severe impairment of both antibody- and cell-mediated immunity. The term SCID is usually restricted to infants with congenital immunodeficiency, but equally severe defects can be caused by acquired immunodeficiency syndrome (AIDS) or lymphocyte loss. The heterogeneity of the congenital forms reflects the range of underlying metabolic defects that may interfere with lymphocyte development at different stages and the varying degrees of engraftment with maternal lymphocytes that can occur during gestation or at birth.

Clinical Findings

A. Symptoms and Signs: Diarrhea, vomiting, and cough are common symptoms. The diarrhea causes failure to thrive and, though it may briefly remit after dietary changes, recurs after a few days. The cough is usually persistent; it is often due to *Pneumocystis carinii* infection and can cause cyanosis. Skin rashes are common and frequently evanescent, except for rash following blood transfusion, which is due to graft-versus-host disease. A *Candida* diaper rash is usual. Findings initially include absence of tonsils or palpable lymph nodes; later, there is emaciation. The presence of a thymus shadow on chest x-ray speaks against the diagnosis.

B. Laboratory Findings: All patients with SCID have some degree of hypogammaglobulinemia and failure of antibody production (though maternal IgG will be present in infants). Lymphopenia is inconstant; in time, most patients become anemic. B lymphocytes (with surface IgM) are usually present in blood; T cells are absent. In vitro lymphocyte responses to mitogens and antigens are negative.

Variants of SCID

A. Adenosine Deaminase Deficiency: Adenosine deaminase converts adenosine and deoxyadenosine to inosine and deoxyinosine, respectively. Its structural locus is on chromosome 20, and individuals homozygous for a null gene account for about 20%

of cases of SCID. Raised deoxy-ATP levels inhibit ribonucleotide reductase, so that T lymphocytes are prevented from dividing. Affected infants may be near-normal at birth (presumably because their mothers keep deoxyadenosine levels down). Their cellular immunity fails first; they then become antibody-deficient, though they may continue to make small amounts of immunoglobulin for some time. Diagnosis is by assay of adenosine deaminase in red cell lysates. A bone marrow graft from a histocompatible sibling with normal red cell adenosine deaminase levels is the ideal treatment (see below), but others may benefit from infusions of irradiated normal red cells, since these contain adenosine deaminase.

B. SCID With Immunoglobulins: Affected patients have severely impaired cellular immunity, and although they may make small or large amounts of immunoglobulin (usually IgM), they do not make useful antibodies. Their clinical course is therefore similar to those with other types of SCID. The condition is heterogeneous in that both X-linked and autosomal recessive forms exist.

C. SCID With Reticuloendotheliosis: Skin rashes, lymphadenopathy, and splenomegaly are prominent, and biopsies show histiocytic infiltration and proliferation. Many of these cases probably resulted from partial engraftment with sufficient maternal T cells to cause graft-versus-host disease in the infant with SCID.

D. SCID With Leukopenia (Reticular Dysgenesis): Affected infants have severe neutropenia, often with reduced numbers of granulocyte precursors in the marrow. Only about 15 cases have been reported. There is a familial trend, but the severity of the neutropenia varies between affected siblings, so this may be a secondary feature.

E. SCID With Defective Expression of HLA Antigens: Affected patients are antibody-deficient, though they may make immunoglobulin and they have variable numbers of T and B cells in their blood. Their recognition requires functional tests rather than cell marker tests. Most cases have been found in North Africa.

Differential Diagnosis

Defects of cellular immunity should be suspected in infants (especially females) with antibody deficiency who continue to have diarrhea after IgG replacement. The main differential is between severe varied immunodeficiency and secondary immunodeficiency due to gastrointestinal disease, eg, long-standing gastroenteritis or intestinal lymphangiectasia. In secondary immunodeficiency, the blood lymphocyte response to phytohemagglutinin is usually not completely absent, and the serum albumin concentration may be low.

Treatment

Infants in whom the diagnosis is suspected should receive antibiotics for infection and IgG replacement if they are hypogammaglobulinemic. They should not be transfused with blood unless it has first been irradiated. With confirmation of the diagnosis, they may be started on trimethoprim-sulfamethoxazole for *Pneumocystis* prophylaxis. Bone marrow grafting offers the best hope for cure. If a histocompatible sibling is available, there is a high chance of success; the treatment can be given without depleting the marrow of T cells or immunosuppressing the recipient. Most SCID patients do not have histocompatible donors, and they are now treated with grafts of parental bone marrow from which the T cells are removed by lectins or monoclonal antibodies. Pregraft suppression may be required; reconstitution can take 4 months; and the overall success rate is about 60%.

OTHER DISORDERS ASSOCIATED WITH IMMUNODEFICIENCY

WISKOTT-ALDRICH SYNDROME

The clinical features of Wiskott-Aldrich syndrome are eczema, thrombocytopenia (see Chapter 16), and recurrent infections. The mode of inheritance is X-linked recessive, and presentation, with bloody diarrhea or cerebral hemorrhage, is usually in the first few years of life. The immunodeficiency tends to be progressive; early findings are a failure to make antibody to polysaccharide antigens, lack of isohemagglutinins, and hypercatabolism of immunoglobulins. Serum IgE is high in many cases, and impairment of cellular immunity is usually a late manifestation.

Splenectomy alleviates the thrombocytopenia; patients should be kept on antibiotics after this operation. A few patients have had successful marrow grafts. Survival through the teens is rare in untreated patients, though partial syndromes are sometimes diagnosed in adults.

ATAXIA-TELANGIECTASIA

Ataxia-telangiectasia is a recessively inherited disorder. Its neurologic manifestations (see Chapter 23) are its most crippling feature and are usually the first to attract attention. About 60% of patients lack serum IgE, and half lack IgA. The degree of impairment of cellular immunity is variable. The high frequency of epithelial and lymphoreticular cancers in these patients and their first-degree relatives may be due to a primary defect of DNA repair.

There is no treatment that is of established value.

CHRONIC MUCOCUTANEOUS CANDIDIASIS

The recurrent candidiasis—occasionally disfiguring—that these patients experience points to an underlying immunodeficiency, though the faulty mechanism has not been identified. Affected patients make anti-*Candida* antibodies, and their in vitro lymphocyte responses may be positive even when *Candida* skin tests are negative. Evidence for the complexity of this form of immunodeficiency includes the frequent association with endocrinopathy, sometimes autoimmune (affecting parathyroid, thyroid, pituitary, or gonads), and, less commonly, susceptibility to staphylococcal infections with defective neutrophil mobility. There is usually some control of the candidiasis with continuous ketoconazole treatment.

SECONDARY IMMUNODEFICIENCY

Secondary immunodeficiency is a common cause of pediatric illness. The mechanisms that may be impaired are summarized in Table 17–6, and the symptoms are generally those that would be anticipated from the combination of the primary disorder and the complicating immunodeficiency. Whenever possible, treatment should be of the primary disorder. Occasionally, immunologic methods may help, eg, zoster immune globulin may prevent varicella in patients with leukemia. IgG replacement is unlikely to help when loss (as in nephrotic syndrome) is responsible for hypogammaglobulinemia.

Table 17–6. Mechanisms of secondary immunodeficiency.

Failure of production of antibody or factors involved in cellular immunity	
Malnutrition: generalized; specific (protein, trace elements)	
Drugs interfering with lymphocyte function	
Measles and some other virus infections	
Loss	
Kidney:	Mostly immunoglobulin
Gut:	Affects immunoglobulin and lymphocytes; may cause malnutrition
Burns:	Loss is initially of immunoglobulin, with secondary effects on lymphocytes
Miscellaneous conditions	
Splenectomy	
Thymectomy	
Down's syndrome	
Infections:	
Protozoal	
Bacterial	
EB virus in X-linked lymphoproliferative syndrome	
Other lymphoproliferative syndromes	

Secondary immunodeficiency. In: *Immunodeficiency*. Technical Report Series No. 630. World Health Organization, 1978.

ACQUIRED IMMUNODEFICIENCY SYNDROME (AIDS)

Infection with human T leukemia virus III (HTLV-III) can result from blood transfusion or use of factor VIII concentrates or can be acquired from infected parents. The virus infects OKT 4-positive lymphocytes, and infants or children who develop the AIDS-related complex (ARC) have lymphadenopathy, hepatosplenomegaly, and high IgG levels. In an unknown proportion of cases, ARC progresses to AIDS, with failure to thrive, recurrent infections, and lymphopenia. Infections in pediatric cases are often bacterial and affect the respiratory tract, as in patients with antibody deficiency; symptomatic improvement following IgG replacement is reported. Conventional opportunistic infections (*Candida, Pneumocystis,* cytomegalovirus) follow as cell-mediated immunity fails.

Lapointe N et al: Twelve children with AIDS and their families. Page 345 in: *Progress in Immunodeficiency Research and Therapy*. Vol 1. Griscelli C, Vossen J (editors). Excerpta Medica, 1984.

INVESTIGATION OF IMMUNODEFICIENCY

Many children have a history of recurrent infections. Evaluation for a possible underlying anatomic anomaly or immune defect should begin with a thorough history, since this is the most useful diagnostic guide. Physical, environmental, and anatomic defects are, as a group, the commonest causes, and recurrent infections at a single site should prompt a search for a local abnormality. To recognize individual diagnostic possibilities within this group (Table 17–1), the physician must keep them in mind. The age at onset of infections may be an important clue. Infections associated with defects of phagocytes, C3, or cellular immunity commonly start within 2 months, whereas maternal antibody protects infants with hypogammaglobulinemia for 3–6 months. Antibody, complement, and phagocyte defects predispose mainly to bacterial infections; superficial candidiasis and severe herpesvirus and poxvirus infections are typical of cellular immunodeficiency. A simple protocol for testing these mechanisms is presented in Table 17–7.

Phagocyte Function

Evaluation of phagocyte function should begin

Table 17–7. A simple protocol for immunity testing.*

	Neutrophils	Complement	Antibody	Cell-Mediated Immunity
Simple clinical or laboratory test	Blood count and differential.		Isohemagglutinins, serum immunoglobulins.	Delayed hypersensitivity skin tests with *Candida, Trichophyton,* tetanus toxoid.
Special tests: first level	Neutrophil mobility, nitroblue tetrazolium reduction, Rebuck skin window.	Hemolytic complement, C3 level.	Antibodies to diphtheria or tetanus (IgG) or a range of viruses.	Whole blood phytohemagglutinin response.
Special tests: second level	Bacterial killing, chemiluminescence, leukocyte enzymes.	Measurement of individual components and inactivators.	Antibody responses to defined antigens: keyhole limpet hemocyanin, ΦX-174. Immunoglobulin subclasses.	Blood T cell numbers, T cell subpopulations, in vitro mediator production, response to antigens.

* For description of laboratory methods, see Rose NR, Friedman H: *Manual of Clinical Immunology.* American Society for Microbiology, 1980; and Thompson R: *Methods in Clinical Immunology.* Blackwell, 1980.

with white blood count, differential count, and blood smear in order to rule out neutropenia, to look for bizarrely shaped erythrocytes suggesting asplenia, and to ascertain the presence or absence of normal lysosomal granules in neutrophils. Chemotaxis can be evaluated by creating an area of inflammation in the skin through gentle abrasion and then noting the type and number of cells that migrate into the site and adhere to a sterile coverslip placed there. However, results with such an "inflammatory skin window" are not quantitative. In vitro systems for quantitating leukocyte motility are now available in many medical centers. Results with these must be interpreted cautiously, since secondary and transient defects in chemotaxis are common. Quantitation of ingestion and microbicidal activity requires special techniques available chiefly in research laboratories. However, the chemical reduction of nitroblue tetrazolium by phagocytic cells requires normal oxidative metabolism, and this test serves as a useful screening test for chronic granulomatous disease or leukocyte glucose 6-phosphate dehydrogenase deficiency. Myeloperoxidase can be detected within neutrophils and monocytes with a simple stain available in most oncology laboratories.

Complement

Deficiency of a classical pathway component can be excluded by a normal hemolytic complement titer. Any microbiology laboratory doing complement fixation assays can do this test, but it is essential that the patient's serum be separated within 30 minutes of collection and stored at −70 °C. There is little point in measuring individual complement component levels if the hemolytic titer is normal, unless it is to follow the activity of an immune complex-associated disease in which C4 and C3 may be low. Opsonizing defects can be due to classical or alternative pathway defects or, if yeast is used, to abnormal C5. Opsonizing tests are not widely available as screening tests.

Antibodies & Immunoglobulins

In patients who are not group AB, isohemagglutinins are the easiest naturally occurring antibodies to test for. They are of the IgM class; normally, they become detectable by 6 months of age and reach adult levels about a year later. Patients who have been immunized with typhoid-paratyphoid vaccine can be tested for anti-O antibodies. The importance of antibody tests is illustrated by the inverse correlation between isohemagglutinin titer and susceptibility to meningitis in patients with hypogammaglobulinemia, irrespective of their serum IgM levels. Lack of availability of Schick antigen means that in vitro methods are required to test for IgG antibodies. Many public health laboratories can measure antitetanus and antidiphtheria antibodies; antivirus antibodies are a possible alternative. In practice, it is often easier to measure serum immunoglobulins as a screening procedure than to test for antibodies, but it should be appreciated that some patients with varied immunodeficiency syndromes make immunoglobulin that does not have useful antibody activity. Properly performed immunoglobulin estimations are reproducible to ±10% for IgG and IgA and ±20% for IgM, so small changes are of no significance. Immunoglobulin concentrations are lower in infants than in adults (Table 17–8), and laboratories may erroneously report normal children's values as low. Comparisons of results from different laboratories may be difficult, because few commercial kit suppliers calibrate their control sera against the international standard. Simple protein electrophoresis is not sufficiently sensitive to make a confident diagnosis of hypogammaglobulinemia, though it is valuable for identifying the monoclonal excesses seen in multiple myeloma. Serum albumin should be measured at least once in patients with hypogammaglobulinemia to exclude secondary deficiencies due to loss. IgG or IgA subclass measurements may be abnormal in patients with varied immunodeficiency syndromes, but they are rarely helpful

Table 17–8. Relation of age to serum immunoglobulin (Ig) levels and isohemagglutinin activity (IHA).

	IgG (mg/dL) (Mean ±1 SD and Range)	IgA (mg/dL) (Mean ±1 SD and Range)	IgM (mg/dL) (Mean ±1 SD and Range)	IHA Titer (Mean and Range)
Cord blood	1086 ± 290 (740 – 1374)	2 ± 2 (0 – 15)	14 ± 6 (0 – 22)	0*
1–3 months	512 ± 152 (280 – 950)	16 ± 10 (4 – 36)	28 ± 14 (15 – 86)	1:5 0 – 1:10†
4–6 months	520 ± 180 (240 – 884)	22 ± 14 (11 – 52)	36 ± 18 (21 – 74)	1:10 0 – 1:160†
7–12 months	742 ± 226 (281 – 1280)	54 ± 17 (22 – 112)	76 ± 27 (36 – 150)	1:80 0 – 1:640‡
13–24 months	945 ± 270 (290 – 1300)	67 ± 19 (9 – 143)	88 ± 36 (18 – 210)	1:80 0 – 1:640‡
25–36 months	1030 ± 152 (546 – 1562)	89 ± 34 (21 – 196)	94 ± 23 (43 – 115)	1:160 1:10 – 1:640§
3–5 years	1150 ± 244 (546 – 1760)	126 ± 31 (56 – 284)	87 ± 24 (26 – 121)	1:80 1:5 – 1:640
6–8 years	1187 ± 289 (596 – 1744)	147 ± 35 (56 – 330)	108 ± 37 (54 – 260)	1:80 1:5 – 1:640
9–11 years	1217 ± 261 (744 – 1719)	146 ± 38 (44 – 208)	104 ± 46 (27 – 215)	1:160 1:20 – 1:640
12–16 years	1248 ± 221 (796 – 1647)	168 ± 54 (64 – 290)	96 ± 31 (60 – 140)	1:160 1:10 – 1:320

* IHA is rarely detectable in cord blood.
† 50% of normal infants have no isohemagglutinins at age 6 months.
‡ 10% of normal infants have no isohemagglutinins at age 1.
§ Beyond age 2, all normal individuals (except those with blood type AB) have isohemagglutinins.

clinically. Lymph node biopsies and marrow studies for architecture or plasma cells, and counts of blood B cells, are useful research tools but are not usually necessary for diagnosis.

Cellular Immunity

Cellular immunity can easily be evaluated by skin tests for delayed hypersensitivity, provided the patient is old enough to have become sensitized. Antigens that are suitable because sensitivity to them is widespread include candidin, trichophytin, streptokinase-streptodornase, and tetanus toxoid. In each case, 0.1 mL of an appropriate preparation is injected intradermally, and the site is inspected after 24 and 48 hours. A positive response consists of induration as well as erythema, which indicates that the patient's lymphocytes can both recognize and respond to antigen. Anergic patients and infants under 18 months, who are unlikely to respond to many of the test antigens, should have their lymphocyte response to phytohemagglutinin measured, preferably using a whole blood screening method. Causes of low response include lymphopenia, antilymphocyte antibodies, and intrinsic T cell defects, each of which can be further evaluated. Severe impairment of cellular immunity can be confirmed by failure of dinitrochlorobenzene sensitization, but this test should not be attempted until a negative phytohemagglutinin response has been confirmed, because dinitrochlorobenzene causes chemical burns. Purine pathway defects are best screened for by analysis of urine excretory products; the reliability of simple screening tests remains to be established. Enumerating T cells in blood with a pan-T monoclonal antibody is useful for the rapid diagnosis of thymic hypoplasia or severe combined immunodeficiency (SCID) and can be used for prenatal diagnosis in fetoscopy samples. Changes in T cell subsets occur with active immune responses: HTLV-III depletes OKT 4-positive cells, while many other viruses give increased proportions of OKT 8-positive cells.

Webster ADB: *The Assessment of Immunocompetence: Clinics in Immunology and Allergy.* Vol 1. Saunders, 1981.

HAZARDS OF IMMUNODEFICIENCY

IMMUNIZATIONS

Patients with severely impaired cell-mediated immunity are susceptible to progressive infections by attenuated strains of organisms used for immunization. Examples in which the outcome has been fatal include BCG bacilli and vaccinia virus. In general, antibody-deficient patients recover normally from virus infections, but there are exceptions—eg, adverse reactions have been attributed to polio and measles immunizations. Exposure of suspected immunodeficient patients to live immunogens should therefore be avoided until the patient's capacity to respond has been established. In practice, patients with defects of nonspecific immunity can usually be safely immunized with viruses and killed bacteria, but BCG should probably be avoided. Antibody-deficient patients would usually not profit from immunization anyway, and they will be protected from many endemic infections, such as measles, by their IgG replacement treatment.

Patients with transient or borderline immunodeficiency should not be given attenuated live virus vaccines until they have been shown to respond adequately to diphtheria or tetanus toxoids. These latter antigens are useful immunogens for testing the antibody responsiveness of patients. They are preferred in this respect to *Salmonella typhi* antigen (TAB), which may cause endotoxin shock in IgM-deficient patients.

GRAFT-VERSUS-HOST DISEASE (GVH)

Patients with severely impaired cellular immunity are unable to protect themselves from attack by foreign lymphocytes such as might be given in a blood transfusion or an incompletely matched graft. Delay in onset of symptoms depends mainly on the number of foreign cells given; the earliest is a rash after about a week, followed by diarrhea, hepatitis, pneumonitis, Coombs-positive anemia, thrombocytopenia, and leukopenia. Skin biopsy may provide tissue diagnosis. The cellular immunity of affected patients remains severely depressed, and this is accompanied by deficiency of OKT 4-positive or Leu 3-positive T cells in the blood. Mild cases of graft-versus-host disease may remit spontaneously or evolve into chronic disease. Severe cases are usually fatal. Treatment with adrenal corticosteroids and antilymphocyte globulin may improve the skin rash and hepatitis but is often followed by a fatal opportunistic infection. It is better to avoid giving blood transfusions to potentially immunodeficient patients—and this includes patients receiving heavy immunosuppression—without first irradiating the blood with 3000 rads.

CANCER

The overall cancer rate in immunodeficient patients of all ages is higher than in the general population, but this increase is less apparent in the pediatric age group. The principal concern of the oncologist should be to avoid mistaking the lymphoproliferation that accompanies some primary immunodeficiencies for lymphoma, since the methods of treatment are so different.

SELECTED REFERENCES

Asherson GL, Webster ADB: *Immunodeficiency Diseases*. Blackwell, 1980.

Bergsma D, Good RA, Finstad J (editors): *Immunodeficiency in Man and Animals*. Sinauer, 1975.

Seligmann M, Hitzig WH (editors): *Primary Immunodeficiencies*. Elsevier, 1980.

Soothill JF: Hayward AR, Wood CBS: *Pediatric Immunology*. Blackwell, 1983.

Stiehm ER, Fulginiti VA (editors): *Immunologic Disorders in Infants and Children*. Saunders, 1980.

Stites DP et al (editors): *Basic & Clinical Immunology*, 5th ed. Lange, 1984.

18 Rheumatic Diseases

J. Roger Hollister, MD

Rheumatic diseases have an autoimmune basis. Unknown factors in the environment act upon the immune system of patients who have inherited a predisposition to these diseases. Expression of disease is rarely seen in a familial pattern, although patients share common immunogenetic traits.

JUVENILE RHEUMATOID ARTHRITIS (Juvenile Chronic Arthritis)

Essentials of Diagnosis

- Nonmigratory monarticular or polyarticular arthropathy, with a tendency to involve large joints or proximal interphalangeal joints and lasting more than 3 months.
- Systemic manifestations with fever, erythematous rashes, nodules, leukocytosis, and, occasionally, iridocyclitis, pleuritis, pericarditis, and hepatitis.

General Considerations

Juvenile rheumatoid arthritis patients exhibit different immunogenetic traits from adult rheumatoid arthritis patients. In juvenile rheumatoid arthritis, HLA-DR5 is associated with iritis and the production of antinuclear antibodies, whereas HLA-DR4 is found in adult rheumatoid arthritis. These traits may be important in the formation of anti-suppressor cell antibodies, immune complex generation, and consequent chronic inflammatory disease.

Clinical Findings

A. Symptoms and Signs: There are 4 patterns of presentation in juvenile rheumatoid arthritis that provide clues to the prognosis and possible sequelae of the disease. In the acute febrile form, which is most common in children under age 4, an evanescent salmon-pink macular rash, arthritis, hepatosplenomegaly, leukocytosis, and polyserositis characterize the constellation described by George Still. These patients have episodic illness, and remission of the systemic features can be expected within 1 year. They do not develop iridocyclitis.

The polyarticular pattern resembles the adult disease, with chronic pain and swelling of many joints in a symmetric fashion. Both large and small joints are usually involved. Systemic features are less prominent, though low-grade fever, fatigue, rheumatoid nodules, and anemia may be present. These patients tend to have long-standing arthritis, although the disease may wax and wane. Iridocyclitis is occasionally seen in this group. Older children may have a positive latex fixation test.

The third pattern consists of pauciarticular disease characterized by chronic arthritis of a few joints, often the large weight-bearing joints, in an asymmetric distribution. The synovitis is usually mild and may be painless. Systemic features are uncommon, but there is serious extra-articular involvement with inflammation in the eye. Up to 30% of children with pauciarticular juvenile rheumatoid arthritis develop insidious, asymptomatic iridocyclitis that frequently causes blindness. The activity of the eye disease does not correlate with the activity of the arthritis. Therefore, routine ophthalmologic screening with slit lamp examination must be performed every 6 months until puberty.

The fourth pattern occurs in late childhood mainly in boys, of whom 75% have HLA-B27. The early clinical pattern is of pauciarticular disease involving the lower limbs; later, the sacroiliac joints may be involved, and ultimately the lumbar and thoracic spine.

B. Laboratory Findings: There is no diagnostic test for juvenile rheumatoid arthritis. Rheumatoid factor is positive by the latex fixation test in about 15% of cases, usually when onset of polyarticular disease occurs after age 8 years. Antinuclear antibodies are most often present in pauciarticular disease with iridocyclitis and may serve as an indication of this complication; they are also fairly common in the late-onset rheumatoid factor-positive group. A normal erythrocyte sedimentation rate does not exclude the diagnosis. Synovial fluid examination is rarely performed in childhood but will establish the presence of inflammation or infection, especially in monarticular cases.

C. X-Ray Findings: In the early stages of the disease, only soft tissue swelling and regional osteoporosis are seen. Cervical subluxation should be monitored by radiographs in patients with neck pain.

Differential Diagnosis

Monarticular arthritis is the most important differential disorder to establish. Pain in the hip or lower extremity is a frequent symptom with childhood cancer, especially leukemia, neuroblastoma, and rhabdomyosarcoma. Infiltration of bone by tumor and actual joint effusion may be seen. X-rays of the affected site and a careful examination of the blood smear for unusual cells and thrombocytopenia are necessary. In doubtful cases, bone marrow examination is indicated.

Bacterial arthritis is usually acute and monarticular except for arthritis associated with *Haemophilus influenzae* and gonorrhea, both of which are associated with a migratory pattern. Fever, leukocytosis, and increased sedimentation rate with an acute process in a single joint demand synovial fluid examination and culture to identify the pathogen. An elevated synovial fluid white count and low glucose (relative to plasma glucose) suggest sepsis.

The arthritis of rheumatic fever is migratory, transient, and often more painful than that of juvenile rheumatoid arthritis. Rheumatic fever is very rare under the age of 5 years. The murmur of rheumatic endocarditis should be carefully sought. Evidence of recent streptococcal infection is not specific for either condition. The fever pattern in rheumatic fever is low-grade and persistent in comparison to the intermittent fever in the systemic form of juvenile rheumatoid arthritis.

Articular involvement with inflammatory bowel disease, psoriasis, and Reiter's syndrome most often involves the lower extremities and frequently the heel. If there are associated abdominal complaints, weight loss, etc, contrast x-rays are indicated. Other forms of reactive arthritis are associated with various bacterial enteritis infections, the *Ixodes dammini* spirochete (Lyme disease), Henoch-Schönlein purpura, and Kawasaki syndrome (mucocutaneous lymph node syndrome). Gout has been reported very rarely in children. Chondromalacia patellae, which characteristically causes pain when the patient walks up and down stairs, may be confused with juvenile rheumatoid arthritis. There is patellar tenderness with this condition. Arthritis is the most frequent symptom of systemic lupus erythematosus; a careful history and investigation for multisystem disease will establish the diagnosis. Self-limited arthralgia and arthritis, usually involving the knee, can be associated with a number of viral infections and rubella immunization. A normal sedimentation rate may suggest the diagnosis.

Treatment

The objective of therapy is to restore function, relieve pain, and maintain joint motion. Salicylates are the treatment of choice at the outset. Aspirin, 75–100 mg/kg/d in 4 divided doses, will frequently relieve pain and inflammation and allow good physical therapy. A self-limited hepatotoxicity occurs with high-dose salicylate therapy, but most patients can continue to take aspirin. If the patient is exposed to chickenpox or Asian influenza, however, aspirin should be withheld to reduce the risk of Reye's syndrome. Range-of-motion exercises and muscle strengthening should be taught and supervised by a therapist, and a home program should be instituted. Bed rest is to be avoided except in the most acute stages. Joint casting is almost never indicated. In patients who fail to respond to aspirin, there are a number of alternatives. Corticosteroids are of value as a temporary measure during acute flare-ups and when there is acute systemic disease or iridocyclitis. Gold salts are of proved efficacy. The dose of gold salt (eg, gold sodium thiomalate) is 1 mg/kg/wk intramuscularly. As symptoms are controlled, the frequency of injection can be gradually decreased. White cell counts and urine testing for protein must be done on a regular basis. Auranofin, a recently licensed oral gold preparation, also appears to be safe and efficacious. The dose is 0.15 mg/kg/d. Diarrhea is the most common side effect. Blood counts and urinalysis should be monitored, as with parenteral gold. The newer nonsteriodal anti-inflammatory agents such as tolmetin, ibuprofen, and naproxen cause fewer gastric problems but otherwise appear to offer little advantage over aspirin. The use of penicillamine is currently under investigation. Its potency and toxicity are similar to those of gold. Immunosuppressive therapy with cytotoxic drugs such as methotrexate remains uncertain and should be reserved for patients who have failed to respond to other forms of therapy.

Iridocyclitis should be treated by an ophthalmologist. Orthopedic consultation on a regular basis is helpful, although surgery is seldom necessary.

Prognosis

In the primarily articular forms, disease activity progressively diminishes with age and ceases in about 95% of cases by puberty. In a few instances, this will persist into adult life. Problems after puberty therefore relate primarily to residual joint damage. Cases presenting in the teen years usually presage adult disease. The children most liable to be permanently handicapped are those with unremitting synovitis, hip involvement, or positive rheumatoid factor tests. Death may occur from persistent carditis or renal amyloidosis.

Ansell BM: *Rheumatic Disorders in Childhood.* Butterworth, 1980.

Baum J: Juvenile arthritis. *Am J Dis Child* 1981;**135:**557.

Giannini EH, Brewer EJ, Person DA: Auranofin in the treatment of juvenile rheumatoid arthritis. *J Pediatr* 1983;**102:**138.

Glass D et al: Early-onset pauciarticular juvenile rheumatoid arthritis associated with human leukocyte antigen-DRw5, iritis, and antinuclear antibody. *J Clin Invest* 1980;**66:**426.

Miller JJ III (editor): *Juvenile Rheumatoid Arthritis.* PSG, 1979.

Schaller J: Juvenile rheumatoid arthritis. *Pediatr in Rev* 1980;**2:**163.

SYSTEMIC LUPUS ERYTHEMATOSUS

Essentials of Diagnosis

- Multisystem inflammatory disease of joints, serous linings, skin, kidneys, and central nervous system.
- Antinuclear antibodies must be present in active, untreated disease.

General Considerations

Systemic lupus erythematosus is the prototype of immune complex diseases; its pathogenesis is related to deposition in the tissue of soluble immune complexes existing in the circulation. The spectrum of symptoms in systemic lupus erythematosus appears to be due not to tissue-specific autoantibodies but rather to damage to the tissue by lymphocytes, neutrophils, and complement evoked by the deposition of antigen-antibody complexes. In systemic lupus erythematosus, many such antigen-antibody systems are present, but the best correlation exists between DNA-anti-DNA complexes and the activity of the disease. Laboratory tests of these antibodies and complement components give an objective assessment of disease pathogenesis and response to therapy. The trigger for the formation of immune complexes in systemic lupus erythematosus has not been identified. Several studies indicate a suppressor cell defect that results in B lymphocyte hyperactivity, leading by implication to autoimmunity.

A drug-related syndrome resembling systemic lupus erythematosus may be produced by procainamide, hydantoin compounds, and isoniazid, among others. Affected patients recover on stopping the drug and do not manifest renal diease.

Clinical Findings

A. Symptoms and Signs: The onset is most common in females (8:1) between the ages of 9 and 15 years. The symptoms depend on what organ is involved with immune complex deposition.

1. Joint symptoms are the commonest presenting feature. Nondeforming arthritis may involve any joint, often in a symmetric manner. Myositis may also occur and is more painful than the inflammation in dermatomyositis.

2. Systemic manifestations include weakness, anorexia, fever, fatigue, and loss of weight.

3. Skin lesions include butterfly erythema and induration, small ulcerations in skin and mucous membranes, purpura, alopecia, and Raynaud's phenomenon. The sun sensitivity of the dermal lesions may be striking.

4. Polyserositis may include pleurisy with effusions, peritonitis, and pericarditis. Libman-Sacks endocarditis is rarely seen since corticosteriods became available for treatment.

5. Hepatosplenomegaly and lymphadenopathy may occur.

6. Renal systemic lupus erythematosus produces few symptoms at onset but is often progressive and is the leading cause of death. Renal biopsy is indicated in all patients with evidence of renal involvement, since the course of the renal disease varies with the lesion produced by immune complex deposition in the glomerular basement membrane. Late complications are nephrosis and uremia.

7. Central nervous system involvement produces a variety of symptoms such as seizures, coma, hemiplegia, focal neuropathies, and behavior disturbances, including psychosis. The psychosis may be impossible to distinguish from corticosteroid-induced psychosis. Neurologic disease is now the second leading cause of death in systemic lupus erythematosus.

B. Laboratory Findings: Leukopenia and anemia are frequently found with a high incidence of Coombs positivity. Thrombocytopenia and purpura may be early manifestations even in the absence of other organ involvement. The erythrocyte sedimentation rate is elevated, and hypergammaglobulinemia is often present. Renal involvement is indicated by the presence in the urine of red cells, white cells, red cell casts, and proteinuria.

The antinuclear antibody test is the most sensitive diagnostic test and has supplanted the LE preparation. The antinuclear antibody test is invariably positive in patients with active untreated systemic lupus erythematosus, and a negative antinuclear antibody test effectively excludes the diagnosis. Punch biopsy of involved and uninvolved skin in systemic lupus erythematosus shows deposits of immunoglobulin and complement at the dermal-epidermal junction. This rapid technique may be of aid in diagnostically difficult cases.

In managing the disease, elevated titers of anti-DNA antibody and depressed levels of serum complement (hemolytic, C3, or C4) accurately reflect active disease, especially renal, central nervous system, and skin disease. A CT scan demonstrating cerebral atrophy may be a unique finding in active central nervous system lupus.

Differential Diagnosis

Systemic lupus erythematosus may simulate many inflammatory diseases such as rheumatic fever, rheumatoid arthritis, and viral infections. It is essential to review all organ systems carefully to establish a clinical pattern. Renal and central nervous system involvement are unique to systemic lupus erythematosus. A negative antinuclear antibody test excludes the diagnosis of systemic lupus erythematosus. Commercial sera are now highly specific, and the test is generally reliable.

An overlap syndrome known as mixed connective tissue disease, with features of several collagen-vascular diseases, has recently been described in adults and children. The symptom complex is diverse and does not readily fit previous classifications. Arthritis, fever, skin tightening, Raynaud's phenomenon, muscle weakness, and rashes are most commonly present. Important factors in recognition of this disease entity are the relative infrequency of renal disease, which implies a better prognosis than systemic lupus erythematosus, and the corticosteroid responsiveness of symptoms, which distinguishes mixed connective tissue disease from scleroderma. The definition of the disease includes the presence of serum antibody to an extractable nuclear antigen. Patients are initially identified by a speckled pattern of immunofluorescence in the antinuclear antibody test. The specialized extractable nuclear antigen test demonstrates very high titers of up to 1:1,000,000 of the antibody. Pulmonary disease in childhood produces major morbidity.

Treatment

The treatment of systemic lupus erythematosus should be tailored to the organ system involved so that toxicities may be minimized. Prednisone, 0.5–1 mg/kg/d orally, has significantly lowered the mortality rate in systemic lupus erythematosus and should be used in all cases with renal, cardiac, or central nervous system involvement. The dose should be varied using clinical and laboratory parameters of disease activity, and the minimum amount of corticosteroid to control the disease should be used. Alternate-day regimens of corticosteroid are frequently possible. Skin manifestations may frequently be treated with antimalarials, eg, hydroxychloroquine, 4 mg/kg/d orally. Pleuritic pain or arthritis can often be managed with salicylates alone.

If disease control is inadequate with prednisone or if the dose required produces intolerable side effects, an immunosuppressant should be added. Either azathioprine, 2–3 mg/kg/d orally, or cyclophosphamide, 1–2 mg/kg/d orally, has been most widely used. These drugs are ineffective during acute crises such as seizures.

The toxicities of the regimens must be carefully considered. In life-threatening disease, the choices are easier. Growth failure, osteoporosis, Cushing's syndrome, adrenal suppression, and aseptic necrosis are serious side effects of chronic use of prednisone. When high doses of cortiocosteroids are used (> 2 mg/kg/d), the risk of sepsis is very real. Cyclophosphamide causes bladder epithelial dysplasia, hemorrhagic cystitis, and sterility. Azathioprine has been associated with liver damage and bone marrow suppression. Immunosuppressant treatment should be withheld if the total white count falls below 3000/μL or the neutrophil count below 1000/μL. Retinal damage from chloroquine derivatives has not been observed in the recommended dosage. Intravenous pulse steroid therapy and plasmapheresis are new treatments that may be useful in selected cases.

Amenorrhea may result from uncontrolled systemic lupus erythematosus but may also be a consequence of prednisone, cyclophosphamide, or azathioprine administration.

Course & Prognosis

The prognosis in systemic lupus erythematosus relates to the presence of renal or central nervous system involvement. With improved diagnosis, milder cases are now identified. Nonetheless, the survival rate has improved from 51% at 5 years in 1954 to 71% at 10 years in 1979. The disease has a natural waxing and waning cycle, and periods of complete remission are not unusual.

Abeles M et al: Systemic lupus erythematosus in the younger patient: Survival studies. *J Rheumatol* 1980;**7:**515.

Baron KS et al: Pulse methylprednisolone therapy in diffuse proliferative lupus nephritis. *J Pediatr* 1982;**101:**137.

Celermajer DS et al: Sex differences in childhood lupus nephritis. *Am J Dis Child* 1984;**138:**586.

Chudwin DS et al: Significance of a positive antinuclear antibody test in a pediatric population. *Am J Dis Child* 1983;**137:**1103.

Oetgen WJ, Boice JA, Lawless OJ: Mixed connective tissue disease in children and adolescents. *Pediatrics* 1981;**67:**333.

Singsen BH et al: Systemic lupus erythematosus in childhood: Correlations between changes in disease activity and serum complement levels. *J Pediatr* 1976;**89:**358.

DERMATOMYOSITIS (Polymyositis)

Essentials of Diagnosis

- Pathognomonic skin rash.
- Weakness of proximal muscles and occasionally of pharyngeal and laryngeal groups.
- Pathogenesis related to vasculitis.

General Considerations

Dermatomyositis, a rare inflammatory disease of muscle and skin in childhood, is uniquely responsive to corticosteroid treatment. The vasculitis observed in childhood dermatomyositis differs pathologically from the adult disease. Small arteries and veins are involved, with an exudate of neutrophils, lymphocytes, plasma cells, and histiocytes. The lesion progresses to intimal proliferation and thrombus formation. These vascular changes are found in the skin, muscle, kidney, retina, and gastrointestinal tract. Muscle regeneration is unusual in childhood disease. Postinflammatory calcinosis is frequent.

The autoimmune pathogenesis of dermatomyositis has been difficult to prove. Recent studies have shown that both cellular and humoral mechanisms may be involved. Lymphocytes from patients are stimulated to undergo blastogenesis in the presence of muscle tissue and will release lymphotoxin, which destroys cultured fetal muscle cells. Biopsies studied with immunofluorescence techniques demonstrate immunoglobulin and complement in a perivascular distribution. The putative antigen has not been identified. Suggestive data relating adult myositis to toxoplasmosis have not been found in children, and results of viral studies have been negative.

Clinical Findings

A. Symptoms and Signs: The predominant symptom is muscular weakness in a proximal distribution affecting pelvic and shoulder girdles. Tenderness, stiffness, and swelling may be found but are not striking. Neurologic findings such as absence of tendon reflexes are not seen until late in the disease. Pharyngeal and respiratory involvement can be life-threatening. Flexion contractures and muscle atrophy produce significant residual deformities. Calcinosis may follow the inflammation in muscle and skin. Vasculitis of the intestine causing hemorrhage or perforation is less frequently seen in recent years, perhaps owing to corticosteroid treatment.

The rash of dermatomyositis is very helpful in the diagnosis of unknown muscle disease. Characteristically, the rash involves the upper eyelids and extensor surfaces of the knuckles, elbows, and knees with a distinctive heliotrope color that progresses to a scaling and atrophic appearance. Periorbital edema is not uncommon. Late lesions include telangiectatic vessels on the face and extremities. None of the rashes associated with other childhood rheumatic diseases have these features of distribution. The activity of the rash frequently does not parallel the muscle disease.

B. Laboratory Findings: Determination of muscle enzyme levels is the most helpful tool in diagnosis and treatment. All enzymes, including serum aldolase, should be screened to detect an abnormality that reflects activity of the disease. The blood count, erythrocyte sedimentation rate, and acute phase reactants are frequently normal. No autoantibodies are found. Electromyography is useful to distinguish myopathic from neuropathic causes of muscle weakness. Muscle biopsy is indicated in doubtful cases of myositis without the pathognomonic rash.

Treatment

Prednisone in high doses (1–2 mg/kg/d orally) has been shown to speed recovery. The dose should be maintained or increased until muscle enzymes have returned to normal. Functional recovery will lag somewhat behind laboratory improvement. With improvement, the dose may be cut to that level which maintains disease control and normal muscle enzymes. Treatment must be continued for an average of 2 years. Immunosuppressant agents are rarely required in childhood dermatomyositis. Plasmapheresis may be tried in refractory cases but should be used early before irreversible muscle damage has occurred. Physical therapy is critical to prevent or allay contractures.

Course & Prognosis

Most children will recover and discontinue medications in 1–3 years. Relapses may occur. Functional ability is very good in most patients. Myositis in childhood is not associated with an increased risk of cancer.

Bowyer SL et al: Childhood dermatomyositis and factors predicting functional outcome and development of dystrophic calcification. *J Pediatr* 1983;**103:**882.

Miller G, Heckmatt JZ, Dubowitz V: Drug treatment of juvenile dermatomyositis. *Arch Dis Child* 1983;**58:**445.

Pachman LM, Cooke N: Juvenile dermatomyositis: A clinical and immunologic study. *J Pediatr* 1980;**96:**226.

Spencer CH et al: Course of treated juvenile dermatomyositis. *J Pediatr* 1984;**105:**399.

Spencer-Green G, Crowe WE, Levinson JE: Nailfold capillary abnormalities and clinical outcome in childhood dermatomyositis. *Arthritis Rheum* 1982;**25:**954.

POLYARTERITIS NODOSA

Polyarteritis nodosa is a rare disease, but a significant number of cases have been reported in childhood and infancy. No single cause has been found, but immune complex deposition as typified by hepatitis B antigen may mediate the inflammatory events.

Pathologically, the disease is a vasculitis of medium-sized arteries with fibrinoid degeneration in the media extending to the intima and adventitia. Neutrophils and eosinophils comprise the inflammatory reaction. Aneurysms may be palpated or seen radiographically. Thrombosis of diseased arteries may cause infarction in many organs. Fibrosis of vessels and surrounding tissues accompanies the healing stages.

Symptomatology involves many tissues, and diagnosis is difficult. In childhood, unexplained fever, conjunctivitis, central nervous system involvement, and cardiac disease are more prominent than is the case in adult disease. Many cases appear as acute myocarditis, and the peripheral neuropathy so common in the adult is unusual. Diagnosis depends on biopsy-proved vasculitis. Testicular biopsy may be helpful if accessible tissue is not available. The mucocutaneous lymph node syndrome is a recently described entity with many pathologic similarities to polyarteritis nodosa.

The mortality rate is high, especially with cardiac involvement. Treatment consists of prednisone, 1–1.5 mg/kg/d orally, and azathioprine, 1–2 mg/kg/d orally, but controlled studies of the efficacy of therapy of this rare disease are not yet available.

Bell DM et al: Kawasaki syndrome: Description of two outbreaks in the United States. *N Engl J Med* 1981;**304:**1568.

Fauci AS: Vasculitis. *J Allergy Clin Immunol* 1983;**72:**211.

Magilavy DB et al: A syndrome of childhood polyarteritis. *J Pediatr* 1977;**91:**25.

Reznik VM et al: Hepatitis B-associated vasculitis in an infant. *J Pediatr* 1981;**98:**252.

DIFFUSE SCLERODERMA (Progressive Systemic Sclerosis)

Scleroderma is a rare disease in childhood. Both the generalized systemic type and the more localized benign form (morphea) have been described. The diagnosis is made on a clinical basis with the finding of a skin disease that progresses from an edematous phase to an atrophic, taut, immobile dermis involving some or all of the skin. Systemic involvement may include Raynaud's phenomenon, arthralgias, pulmonary fibrosis, and renal disease. Involvement of the lungs and kidneys leads to rapid demise. Histologically, the diagnosis may not be specific but includes dermal atrophy with increased fibrosis and collagen content. The pathogenesis remains obscure, but recent studies indicate an increased synthesis of immature collagen by cultured scleroderma fibroblasts.

Penicillamine and newer antihypertensive agents may provide effective treatment in the future. Physical therapy is sometimes helpful in reducing debilitation from contractures and muscle wasting.

Dabich L, Sullivan DB, Cassidy JT: Scleroderma in the child. *J Pediatr* 1974;**85:**770.

Steen VD et al: Clinical and laboratory associations of anticentromere antibody in patients with progressive systemic sclerosis. *Arthritis Rheum* 1984;**27:**125.

MARFAN'S SYNDROME

First discovered by Marfan in 1896, this syndrome is now considered to be a diffuse abnormality of elastic tissue inherited as an autosomal dominant. The molecular defect is unknown, although the high urinary excretion of hydroxyproline indicates an increased rate of turnover of connective tissue fiber. Clinically, the impact of these changes is on the skeletal and cardiovascular systems and the eyes. Patients are characteristically tall and thin, and the upper body segment is proportionately shorter than the lower. In addition to arachnodactyly of the fingers—as indicated by a middle finger that is 1½ or more times the length of its metacarpal—bony defects include pectus carinatum or excavatum, a long narrow face and pointed head, high-arched palate, kyphoscoliosis, and an elongated great toe. The attendant laxity in the ligaments leads to pes planus, winging of the scapulas, genu recurvatum, and subluxation of the patellas, hips, elbows, and other joints. Femoral and diaphragmatic hernias are noted.

Weakening of the aortic media leads to aneurysms, usually of the ascending aorta, that may involve the valve. Lax chordae may lead to mitral as well as aortic incompetence. The pulmonary artery may be dilated. Dislocation of the lens due to weakness of the suspensory ligaments is characteristic but may be confused with homocystinuria. Blue scleras, myopia, retinal detachment, and megalocornea are other abnormalities of the eye, and glaucoma, iridocyclitis, and interstitial keratitis are complications of these disorders.

There is no specific treatment, although surgical correction of the cardiovascular complications may be appropriate. Prognosis is governed by the severity of these cardiovascular lesions. Homocystinuria should be excluded.

Murdoch JL et al: Life expectancy and causes of death in the Marfan syndrome. *N Engl J Med* 1972;**286:**804.

Siggers DC: Marfan syndrome treated with propranolol. *Birth Defects* 1975;**11:**332.

EHLERS-DANLOS SYNDROME

This is a rare heritable disorder of collagen that is probably transmitted as an autosomal dominant. Characteristically, the skin is pale, soft, and strikingly hyperextensible without being lax. Subcutaneous nodules develop over pressure points, and the skin in these areas is especially subject to trauma and the formation of shiny, parchmentlike, atrophic scars. The joints are hyperextensible, and there is a tendency to dislocation of hips, patellas, elbows, clavicles, and shoulders. Blue scleras, wide epicanthal folds, dislocation of the lens, and other eye signs occur.

A number of other congenital defects have been described in association with this syndrome, notably hiatal hernia, gastrointestinal diverticula, urinary tract anomalies, and aortic aneurysm and insufficiency, the latter being conspicuously difficult to repair because of tissue friability.

There is no specific treatment.

Lichtenstein JR et al: Defect in conversion of procollagen to collagen in a form of Ehlers-Danlos. *Science* 1973;**182:**298.

McKusick VA: Multiple forms of the Ehlers-Danlos syndrome. *Arch Surg* 1974;**109:**475.

LYME DISEASE (Lyme Arthritis)

Lyme disease (see also Chapter 27) is a form of arthritis that is often chronic. The first cases were reported in Lyme, Connecticut, in 1975, and subsequent cases have been observed in at least 15 other states. Lyme disease is thought to be due to a spirochete transmitted by a tick *(Ixodes dammini).*

The onset is commonly characterized by influenza-like symptoms (fever, malaise, headache, stiff neck). A target-shaped skin rash (erythema chronicum migrans) develops and may spread at the site of the tick bite. Lesions persist for 1 day to 3 weeks. About 90% of patients experience pain and arthritis, which mainly affects the large joints and may be present for many years (in some patients, since discovery of the disease in 1975). In 7–10% of patients, meningoencephalitis occurs, at times with facial paralysis and altered states of consciousness lasting from a few days to several weeks. No patient has died.

The eruption is arrested by use of either penicillin or tetracycline, but lesions may recur. Once arthritis has developed, antispirochetal therapy is of little value.

Bruhn FW: Lyme disease. *Am J Dis Child* 1984;**138:**467.

Steere AC et al: The spirochetal etiology of Lyme disease. *N Engl J Med* 1983;**308:**733.

19 Gastrointestinal Tract*

Arnold Silverman, MD, & Claude C. Roy, MD

VOMITING & REGURGITATION

Vomiting and regurgitation are especially common during infancy. Vomiting is the violent expulsion of gastric and sometimes intestinal contents. Regurgitation is expulsion of small amounts of esophageal or gastric contents without marked increase in intra-abdominal pressure. A number of disease conditions originating outside the gastrointestinal tract lead to vomiting. Table 19–1 lists the various causes of vomiting and regurgitation.

GASTROESOPHAGEAL REFLUX & HIATAL HERNIA

Hiatal hernias may be classified as follows: (1) paraesophageal hernia, in which the esophagus is normal up to the esophageal hiatus but the stomach is herniated into the thorax; and (2) sliding hernia, in which the esophagogastric junction is located above the esophageal hiatus. Sliding hernia is the most common type in children.

Clinical Findings

Paraesophageal hernias are rare and present with symptoms of complete esophageal obstruction. Symptoms of the sliding type of hiatal hernia may mimic chalasia. Hiatal hernia is found in some infants with rumination. Dysphagia, failure to thrive, anemia, vomiting, aspiration pneumonia, reactive airway disease, and neck contortions are common features. Pain occurs when esophagitis is present, and bleeding may occur with hematemesis and melena. Stricture formation gives rise to dysphagia and the vomiting of undigested food. Large hiatal hernias may remain completely asymptomatic but are commonly associated with reflux.

During the first few months of life, the cardiac sphincter is often functionally incompetent, and reflux can be observed. Continuous free reflux observed by cineradiography is abnormal and is often associated with the presence of a pouch of stomach above the diaphragm. Esophageal manometry will permit identification of the position of the lower esophageal sphincter and assessment of its activity. Around-the-clock monitoring of the pH in the lower esophagus is presently the best way to monitor gastroesophageal reflux. Both the number of episodes of reflux and the speed with which acid is cleared from the esophagus are good indicators of those hernias that are at risk of complications. Although reflux is often present with a hiatal hernia, this does not imply a causal relationship. Displacement of the sphincter into the chest does not necessarily lead to malfunction; consequently, hiatal hernias may be asymptomatic.

A barium swallow will identify larger hernias, but esophagoscopy should also be performed if bleeding occurs, if there are x-ray changes of esophagitis, and if pain is severe. Scintigraphy and extended pH monitoring of the area proximal to the lower esophageal sphincter give important information.

Complications

Gastroesophageal reflux is a well-known cause of disabling esophageal and respiratory complications and severe growth problems. Anemia, digital clubbing, and hypoproteinemia may also be found.

Treatment & Prognosis

In 85% of patients, conservative management is efficacious. Semi-upright positioning of the patient or, better, a 30-degree prone position around the clock may be necessary for at least 3 months after all symptoms have ceased. Small thickened feedings combined with antacids may also be of value. Pharmacologic agents (see Chalasia, below) may be tried if there is reflux.

Failure of medical management (15% of cases), malnutrition, anemia, recurrent pneumonia, esophagitis, and the presence of strictures are indications for surgical treatment. The Nissen fundoplication operation is an effective procedure.

CHALASIA

Clinically, 40% of newborn infants have a tendency to regurgitate. On fluoroscopy, regurgitation can be elicited in close to 50% of normal newborns. This is due to incompetence of the lower esophageal sphincter, often in combination with delayed gastric emptying.

In a small number of patients, vomiting is sufficient to cause failure to thrive. A significant degree of

*Esophageal atresia and tracheoesophageal fistula are discussed in Chapter 3.

Table 19–1. Causes of vomiting and regurgitation.

Gastrointestinal tract disorders	
Esophagus	**Intestine**
Chalasia	Atresia and stenosis
Achalasia	Meconium ileus
Diffuse esophageal spasm	Malrotation, volvulus
Hiatal hernia	Duplication
Peptic esophagitis	Intussusception
Atresia with or without fistula	Foreign body, polyposis
Congenital vascular or mucosal rings, webs	Soy or cow's milk protein intolerance
Stenosis	Gluten enteropathy
Duplication and diverticulum	Food allergy
Foreign body	Hirschsprung's disease
Periesophageal mass	Chronic pseudointestinal obstruction
Stomach	Appendicitis, perforations
Hypertrophic pyloric stenosis	Crohn's disease
Pylorospasm	Gastroenteritis, infestations
Diaphragmatic hernia	**Other abdominal organs**
Peptic disease and gastritis	Hepatitis
Gastric volvulus, diaphragm	Gallstones
Duodenum	Pancreatitis
Atresia, diaphragm	Peritonitis
Annular pancreas	
Duodenitis and ulcer	
Extra-gastrointestinal tract disorders	
Sepsis	Adrenal insufficiency
Pneumonia	Renal tubular acidosis
Otitis media	Inborn errors
Urinary tract infection	Urea cycle disorders
Meningitis	Phenylketonuria
Subdural effusion	Maple syrup urine disease
Hydrocephalus	Lactic acidosis
Brain tumor	Organic (propionic) aciduria
Reye's syndrome	Galactosemia
Cyclic vomiting	Fructose intolerance
Rumination	Tyrosinosis
Intoxications	Scleroderma
	Epidermolysis bullosa

esophagitis may occur. This can cause occult blood loss, iron deficiency anemia, hematemesis, strictures, and inflammatory esophageal polyps. Recurrent aspiration pneumonia, chronic cough, wheezing, and asthmalike attacks are reported. Apneic spells and sudden infant death syndrome or "near miss" episodes have been ascribed to gastroesophageal reflux. Gastroesophageal reflux is particularly frequent in neurologically impaired children.

Gastroesophageal reflux secondary to chalasia may mimic pyloric stenosis, outlet obstruction of the stomach, hiatal hernia, or esophageal stenosis.

Thickened feedings are helpful. The infant should be kept in a 30-degree prone position for 2–3 hours after each feeding, and it may be necessary to maintain this position 24 hours a day. Metoclopramide, 0.1–0.2 mg/kg given just prior to feeding, can be tried. Reflux may also be treated with bethanechol, 10 mg/m^2/d given every 8 hours in infants and 45 minutes before meals in children.

Chalasia is usually a mild transitory condition that normally disappears by 6–12 months of age. It is compatible with perfectly good health and a normal growth pattern.

Indications for surgery include (1) persistent vomiting with failure to thrive after 3 months of conservative treatment; (2) esophagitis refractory to medical treatment and the presence of strictures; (3) reflux proved to be the cause of a "near miss" episode, apneic spells, and chronic pulmonary problems; and (4) underlying central nervous system problems for which medical management is likely to fail.

Harnsberger JK et al: Long-term follow-up of surgery for gastroesophageal reflux in infants and children. *J Pediatr* 1983;**102:**505.

Herbst JJ: Gastroesophageal reflux. *J Pediatr* 1981;**98:**859.

Richter JE, Castell DO: Gastroesophageal reflux: Pathogenesis, diagnosis, and therapy. *Ann Intern Med* 1982;**97:**93.

Tunell WP et al: Gastroesophageal reflux in childhood: The dilemma of surgical success. *Ann Surg* 1983;**197:**560.

Werlin SL et al: Mechanisms of gastroesophageal reflux in children. *J Pediatr* 1980;**97:**244.

ACHALASIA OF THE ESOPHAGUS

Esophageal achalasia is characterized by failure of relaxation of the inferior esophageal sphincter (cardiospasm) and lack of propulsive peristalsis in the body of the esophagus.

Clinical Findings

A. Symptoms and Signs: Achalasia is seen in all age groups but is uncommon under the age of 5 years. The history of difficulty in swallowing solid food is intermittent at first and often goes back for many years. Typically, the dysphagia is manifested by retrosternal pain and frequent episodes of food "sticking" in the throat or upper chest. Affected children are described as slow eaters, consuming large amounts of fluids while eating. Familial cases have been described. The dysphagia is relieved by repeated swallowing movements (wet or dry) or by vomiting. Besides dysphagia and vomiting, bouts of coughing and wheezing are reported along with recurrent pneumonitis, anemia, and weight loss.

B. X-Ray and Manometric Studies: With delayed diagnosis, the barium swallow shows a grossly dilated esophagus (megaesophagus) with a narrowing at the distal end. The narrowed segment is usually very short. Cinefluoroscopic examination may show absence of normal peristalsis and failure of relaxation of the gastroesophageal sphincter.

The esophageal motility pattern confirms the abnormal propulsive peristalsis and malfunctioning of the lower esophageal sphincter. The pressure at rest in the lower esophageal sphincter may be normal or elevated and does not fall to the level of gastric pressure during swallowing.

Differential Diagnosis

Reflux esophagitis with or without hiatal hernia is the most common cause of organic esophageal stricture in childhood and must be ruled out by esophagoscopy, x-rays, pH probe, and manometric studies.

Treatment & Prognosis

Balloon (pneumatic) dilation is of value in most cases and can be repeated with recurrent symptoms. More definitive results can be achieved by means of a surgical procedure (Heller) consisting of longitudinal splitting of all the muscle coats down to the mucosa.

Because of the shorter duration of the illness in pediatric patients, the prognosis for return of the esophagus to normal caliber after surgical treatment is very good.

Berquist WE et al: Achalasia: Diagnosis, management and clinical course in 16 children. *Pediatrics* 1983;**71:**798.

Vantrappen G et al: Achalasia, diffuse esophageal spasm, and related motility disorders. *Gastroenterology* 1979;**76:**450.

CAUSTIC BURNS OF THE ESOPHAGUS

Stricture of the esophagus commonly follows ingestion of a caustic alkali, eg, lye, Clorox, Drano, ammonia. Lesions initially are of varying severity. Superficial esophagitis may be the only finding. On the other hand, ulceration and sometimes necrosis may lead to chemical mediastinitis and to peritonitis if the stomach is involved. The presence and extent of burning of the mouth do not correlate with the presence and degree of esophageal damage.

Children who have swallowed lye may present with oral lesions and shock. The usual clinical picture, however, is that of painful edematous lesions of the lips, mouth, and larynx. Over a period of a few hours or days, the initially extreme dysphagia subsides. If left untreated, the child remains asymptomatic for a few months until a stricture progressively develops. X-rays usually reveal more severe strictures in the areas of anatomic narrowing, eg, the cervical region and the point at which the left bronchus crosses the esophagus and cardia. Esophagoscopic findings are those of localized escharotic lesions. Severe morphologic stenosis occurs only if full-thickness necrosis of the deep muscle layers occurs. Single, dense, fairly localized strictures may occur, although in other cases the entire esophagus may become twisted and narrowed. Shortening of the esophagus may lead to a hiatal hernia.

The child with a history of alkali ingestion should have a careful examination of the lips and mouth and evaluation of the airway. Drooling is common. Oral lesions are frequent if solid agents have been ingested. Symptoms resulting from strictures may occur within 1 month following the accident, but more commonly the stricture formation does not lead to symptoms for many months or even years. Dysphagia is first manifest for solids and eventually for liquids.

The immediate home care should be familiar to all parents. Vomiting should not be induced. Hospitalization is recommended even if there is only a reasonable possibility of ingestion. Prednisone, 1–2 mg/kg/d (or its equivalent intravenously), is started immediately. Intravenous fluids may be necessary. Esophagoscopy should be done within 24–48 hours after ingestion. Treatment is stopped if there is no visible lesion or if only a first-degree burn is seen. Corticosteroids are continued and a program of bougienage started for more severe cases. In cases where x-rays show evidence of erosion into the mediastinum or peritoneum, antibiotics become mandatory. Intraluminal stenting may be beneficial.

Without early treatment, stricture formation is inevitable. Surgical replacement of the esophagus with a segment of colon may be necessary if dilation fails.

Benirschke K: Time bomb of lye ingestion. *Am J Dis Child* 1981;**135:**17.

Crain FC, Gershel JC, Mezey AP: Symptoms as predictors of esophageal injury. *Am J Dis Child* 1984;**138:**863.

Gaudreault P et al: Predictability of esophageal injury from signs and symptoms: A study of caustic ingestion in 378 children. *Pediatrics* 1983;**71:**767.

PYLORIC STENOSIS

Essentials of Diagnosis

- Vomiting, usually projectile.
- Constipation.
- Poor weight gain or weight loss.
- Dehydration.
- Palpable olive-sized tumor in the right upper quadrant.
- Typical hypoechoic mass of 1.5 cm or greater detected by ultrasonography.
- "String sign" and evidence of retained gastric contents on x-ray.

General Considerations

The cause of the increase in the size of the circular muscle of the pylorus is not known. Serum gastrin and secretin levels are normal. There is a coincidence of the disease in twins or fathers and sons. The disease occurs in one out of 500 births, and males are affected 3–4 times more commonly than females. The reported increased incidence in firstborns and in the spring and fall months is controversial.

Clinical Findings

A. Symptoms and Signs: Vomiting usually begins between 2 and 4 weeks of age and progresses to projectile vomiting after each feeding; in about 10% of cases, it may start at birth. In premature infants particularly, the onset of symptoms is often delayed. The vomitus does not contain bile but may be bloodstreaked. The infant is hungry and nurses avidly, but constipation and failure to thrive occur.

Dehydration, loss of skin turgor, fretfulness, and apathy may be present. The upper abdomen is distended, and gastric peristaltic waves from left to right may be seen. An olive-sized tumor can almost always be felt to the right of the umbilicus and is readily palpable immediately after the infant has vomited.

B. Laboratory Findings: Elevated levels of unconjugated bilirubin occur in 2–3% of cases. There is metabolic alkalosis with potassium depletion. Hemoconcentration is reflected by elevated hemoglobin and hematocrit values.

C. X-Ray and Ultrasonographic Findings: An upper gastrointestinal series reveals delay in gastric emptying and an elongated narrowed pyloric channel (''string sign''). There is invagination of the pylorus into the antrum. Ultrasonography shows a hypoechoic ring in front of the right kidney and medial to the gallbladder.

Differential Diagnosis

The absence of increased intracranial pressure, virilization, and hyperkalemia rules out intracranial lesions and congenital adrenal hyperplasia with adrenal insufficiency. In achalasia, the food is undigested; in annular pancreas, the vomitus contains bile. Sepsis and urinary tract infections can easily be ruled out. In simple cases of ''pylorospasm,'' there may be a delay in gastric emptying, but the elongated narrow pyloric canal is not seen and no tumor is present. Antral webs or diaphragms, duplications, cysts, and channel ulcers of the pyloric canal are rare causes of gastric outlet obstruction.

Treatment & Prognosis

Pyloromyotomy is the treatment of choice and consists of incision down to the mucosa and fully across the pyloric length. Surgery for pyloric stenosis is not an emergency procedure, and the necessary time should be taken to repair dehydration and electrolyte abnormalities and to assuage any gastritis by saline gastric irrigations.

Drug therapy is not widely recommended in the USA but has been used in other countries in patients whose symptoms begin late. However, surgery is eventually required in 30% of cases.

The outlook is excellent following surgery. Sometimes there is continued vomiting postoperatively in cases with a long preoperative history.

Benson CD: Infantile hypertrophic pyloric stenosis. Pages 890–895 in: *Pediatric Surgery,* 3rd ed. Ravitch MM et al (editors). Year Book, 1979.

Khamapirad T, Athey PA: Ultrasound diagnosis of hypertrophic pyloric stenosis. *J Pediatr* 1983;**102:**23.

Moazam F, Kolts BE, Rodgers B: In pursuit of the etiology of congenital hypertrophic pyloric stenosis. *J Pediatr Gastroenterol Nutr* 1982;**1:**97.

NEONATAL PERFORATIONS OF THE GASTROINTESTINAL TRACT

A number of gastrointestinal anomalies and diseases are responsible for intrauterine perforation and will give rise to sterile meconium peritonitis. X-ray evidence of calcifications indicates that the perforation occurred prenatally. Causes include perforation of the appendix, intestinal atresia or stenosis, malrotation with volvulus, meconium ileus, internal hernia, idiopathic perforation of the stomach and duodenum, intestinal duplication, intussusception, and Hirschsprung's disease. Postpartum perforation, usually in the first week of life, gives rise to a bacterial peritonitis. The most common cause is necrotizing enterocolitis. Other entities include perforated peptic ulcers, Hirschsprung's disease, intestinal atresia, gastroschisis, and malrotation with volvulus.

Stress ulcers and necrotizing enterocolitis of the newborn are manifestations of ischemic necrosis likely to be seen in neonates with asphyxia.

Prematurely born infants are more prone to develop perforation. The syndrome has been observed in identical twins. The affected newborns usually appear normal at birth; the average age at onset of symptoms is the third day of life. Refusal of feedings is followed by vomiting, sometimes bloody. The abdomen becomes rapidly distended; dyspnea and cyanosis frequently ensue and are followed by shock. X-ray findings may reveal free air under the diaphragm. The gastric air bubble is usually absent, especially when the perforation is large.

Fluid and electrolyte balance should be corrected while the abdomen is decompressed by nasogastric suction. Plasma volume maintenance and systemic antibiotics are indicated.

Surgery should be carried out as soon as the infant's condition will permit. The prognosis has not changed significantly over the last decade and is still poor.

Emanuel B et al: Perforation of the gastrointestinal tract in infancy and childhood. *Surg Gynecol Obstet* 1978;**146:**926.

Lloyd JR: Gastrointestinal perforation of the newborn. Pages 887–891 in: *Pediatric Surgery,* 3rd ed. Ravitch MM et al (editors). Year Book, 1979.

Roy CC et al: Gastrointestinal emergency problems in pediatric practice. *Clin Gastroenterol* 1981;**10:**225.

PEPTIC DISEASE

Essentials of Diagnosis

- Abdominal pain occurring late after meals or at night.
- Vomiting.

- Melena or hematemesis (or both).
- Unexplained anemia.
- Vague abdominal complaints in a patient with a strong family history.

General Considerations

A. Ulcerous Peptic Disease: The incidence of peptic ulcers in children is increasing, in part because of better diagnostic techniques. They may occur at any age but are more frequent in the age group from 12 to 18 years. Boys are affected twice as commonly as girls, and this preponderance is even greater beyond 12 years of age. Up to age 6, most ulcers are associated with an underlying illness, a drug, or a toxic substance. A positive family history is present in almost 50% of cases of duodenal ulcers.

Gastric ulcers are as common as duodenal ulcers up to age 6. In the 6- to 18-year-old group, duodenal ulcers are 5 times as common as gastric ulcers. The pathogenesis of gastric ulcers is not understood. There is a breakdown of the normal mucosal resistance to acid, bile, and bile acids. Furthermore, reflux of duodenal contents into the stomach occurs to a greater extent in patients with gastric ulcers. A number of factors favor back diffusion of hydrogen ions across the gastric mucosa, which causes extensive damage to the gastric mucosa. Aspirin is the only drug that has been proved to be ulcerogenic in humans. Hypoxia, hypotension, sepsis, and increased intracranial pressure are often responsible for secondary ulcers. Excess production of pepsin or acid is an important factor in the development of primary duodenal ulcers. The increased functional parietal mass could be inherited or acquired (islet cell adenoma, hypercalcemia). Patients with duodenal ulcers have normal fasting levels of gastrin but demonstrate increased gastrin release in response to feeding. The resultant hypersecretion of acid is neutralized by food. However, evacuation through the pylorus occurs more rapidly and is followed by a significantly higher rebound secretion of hydrochloric acid.

B. Nonulcerous Peptic Disease: Although the relationship between gastroduodenal inflammation and peptic ulcer is still unclear, studies in patients with dyspepsia suggest that nearly 60% have no ulcers but have evidence of gastroduodenitis, which is now considered a component of the peptic ulcer spectrum. One-third of patients with gastroduodenitis will eventually develop an ulcer, and a significant proportion have a previous history of a well-documented ulcer. Nonulcerous peptic disease warrants the same treatment as peptic ulcer disease.

Clinical Findings

A. Symptoms and Signs:

1. At 0–3 years of age—In infants past the neonatal period up to the age of 3, symptoms of primary ulcers include poor eating, vomiting, crying after meals, and melena or hematemesis. Secondary ulcers are more acute, and perforation may be the first sign.

2. At 3–6 years of age—Vomiting related to eating is always present. Gastric outlet obstruction may give rise to protracted vomiting. Periumbilical or generalized abdominal pain is common. The typical "ulcer pain" is rarely present. Melena, hematemesis, and perforation are the rule in cases of secondary ulcers.

3. At 6–18 years of age—Fewer than 50% of patients have the typical pain leading to an early diagnosis. Melena or hematemesis (or both) is noted in over 50%; occult bleeding and anemia without other symptoms are not uncommon. In addition to the acute illnesses responsible for secondary ulcers, certain chronic diseases such as chronic lung disease, Crohn's disease, cirrhosis of the liver, and rheumatoid arthritis are associated with an increased incidence of peptic disease.

B. Gastric Analysis: The chief value of gastric fluid analysis is to show that there is no hypersecretion such as would occur with the Zollinger-Ellison syndrome. Gastrin levels after a feeding are higher in children with duodenal ulcers. They should be obtained in cases of recurrent ulcers.

C. X-Ray Findings: Radiologic signs of ulceration or a deformity should be present. The frequency with which the radiologic sign of duodenal irritability is found makes the x-ray diagnosis often unreliable. In patients with severe degrees of duodenal irritability, a niche may not be demonstrated, since the barium is moved out of the bulb very rapidly.

D. Panendoscopy: Although a barium meal remains a useful diagnostic tool for 85% of active ulcers, endoscopy should be carried out if x-ray findings are negative or equivocal. In the case of a bleeding ulcer, endoscopy takes precedence over x-ray studies if it can be done within 48 hours of cessation of hematemesis or melena.

Differential Diagnosis

The diagnosis of acute secondary ulcers should be suspected in any child with a severe underlying disease who suddenly presents with abdominal distention, hematemesis, or melena. A wide spectrum of symptoms is associated with primary peptic ulcers. The differential diagnosis includes chronic idiopathic recurrent abdominal pain, irritable colon syndrome, esophagitis, chronic pancreatitis, cholelithiasis, and recurrent midgut volvulus. Suspicion is warranted when abdominal pain occurs at night or in the early morning hours, when recurrent vomiting is closely related to eating, and, finally, when there is a family history of duodenal ulcers even if gastrointestinal complaints are vague.

Treatment

Bed rest is unnecessary unless there are signs of duodenal obstruction, active bleeding, or perforation.

With outlet obstruction, gastric suction should be maintained for a few days before restarting oral intake. Foods that cause pain should be avoided. Beef broth, tea, coffee, spices, and carbonated beverages should be used sparingly, since they enhance gastric secretion. Three regular meals are advocated. Snacks are contraindicated, particularly at bedtime. Aspirin should be avoided. Antacids (15–30 mL) every 1–2 hours and at bedtime are given initially. Later, they should be given 1 and 3 hours after meals and at bedtime for 6 weeks. Anticholinergics should be given at bedtime only in exceptional cases of duodenal ulcers with significant hypersecretion.

Use of cimetidine, a histamine (H_2 receptor) antagonist, in a dosage of 25–40 mg/kg/d given with meals and at bedtime results in healing of 85% of duodenal ulcers within 6 weeks. It is not more effective than a large-dose antacid regimen. Maintenance therapy once or twice daily will prevent 80% of recurrences; ranitidine may prove to be longer-acting and to have fewer side effects. Combinations of antacids and cimetidine may be indicated for intractable peptic disease.

Surgical management is reserved for the complications, ie, perforation, hemorrhage, obstruction, or incapacitating and intractable pain.

Prognosis

Long-term studies show that up to 80% of children with duodenal ulcers have recurrent symptoms on long-term follow-up. The prognosis for recurrence is much lower in the younger group (0–6 years). Surgery for duodenal ulcers (pyloroplasty and vagotomy) gives excellent results.

Dunn S et al: Acute peptic ulcer in childhood. *Arch Surg* 1983;**118**:656.

Euler AR, Byrne WJ, Campbell MF: Basal and pentagastrin-stimulated gastric acid secretory rates in normal children and in those with peptic ulcer disease. *J Pediatr* 1983;**103**:766.

Greenlaw R et al: Gastroduodenitis: A broader concept of peptic ulcer disease. *Dig Dis Sci* 1980;**25**:660.

Nord KS, Lebenthal E: Peptic ulcer in children. *Am J Gastroenterol* 1980;**73**:75.

White A, Carachi R, Young DG: Duodenal ulceration presenting in childhood long-term follow-up. *J Pediatr Surg* 1984;**19**:6.

CONGENITAL DIAPHRAGMATIC HERNIA

Diaphragmatic hernia may be secondary to a posterolateral defect in the diaphragm (foramen of Bochdalek) or, in about 5% of cases, to a retrosternal defect (foramen of Morgagni). It represents failure of division of the thoracic and abdominal cavities at the eighth to tenth weeks of fetal life.

All degrees of protrusion of the abdominal viscera through the diaphragmatic opening into the thoracic cavity may occur. The extent of herniation determines the severity and the timing of the symptoms. In the posterolateral variety, more than 80% involve the left diaphragm.

Symptoms of mild to severe respiratory distress and cyanosis are usually present from birth, although some patients remain asymptomatic and the finding of a large diaphragmatic hernia with air-filled coils on x-ray is incidental to an x-ray examination. The abdomen is scaphoid. Breath sounds in the affected hemithorax are absent, with displacement of the point of maximal cardiac impulse.

Fatal cases (about 30%) have circulatory problems secondary to the mediastinal shift, giving rise to stretching and kinking of the great vessels. Pulmonary infections also constitute a major cause of death, along with prematurity, cardiac anomalies, and malrotation. The most frequent cause of death, however, is pulmonary insufficiency. The lung on the affected side is compressed and hypoplastic, with decreased numbers of generations of airways and pulmonary arteries throughout. The long-term follow-up of survivors shows that although hypoperfusion and a preemphysematous state can be identified, hypoplastic lungs remain asymptomatic at least until late in childhood.

In eventration of the diaphragm, a leaf of the diaphragm containing a diminution of muscular elements is ballooned into the chest and leads to identical but much milder symptoms.

Bloss RS, Aranda JV, Beardmore HE: Congenital diaphragmatic hernia: Pathophysiology and pharmacologic support. *Surgery* 1981;**89**:518.

Eichelberger MR et al: Agenesis of the left diaphragm: Surgical repair and physiologic consequences. *J Pediatr Surg* 1980;**15**:395.

Reid IS, Hutcherson RJ: Long-term follow-up of patients with congenital diaphragmatic hernia. *J Pediatr Surg* 1976;**11**:939.

CONGENITAL ATRESIAS & STENOSES OF THE GASTROINTESTINAL TRACT

The usual mode of presentation is neonatal intestinal obstruction. These conditions are sometimes diagnosed prenatally by ultrasonography when suggested by the presence of polyhydramnios. The triad of abdominal distention, bilious vomiting, and obstipation or failure to pass meconium constitutes the most important clue to diagnosis. Prematurity and the presence of other anomalies may also be useful. The localization and relative incidence of atresias and stenoses are given in Table 19–2.

CONGENITAL DUODENAL OBSTRUCTION

Extrinsic duodenal obstruction is usually due to congenital peritoneal bands with or without volvulus associated with midgut malrotation; to annular pancreas; or, more rarely, to duplication of the duodenum. An intrinsic type includes atresia, where only the

Table 19–2. Localization and incidence of gastrointestinal atresias and stenoses.

	Area Involved	Type of Lesion	Relative Frequency
Pylorus		Atresia Web or diaphragm (66%)	1%
Duodenum	Distal to the ampulla of Vater (80%)	Atresia Web or diaphragm (40%)	45%
Jejunoileal	Proximal jejunum and distal ileum (66%)	Atresia (multiple in 6–29%) Stenosis (20%)	50%
Colon	Left colon and rectum (50%)	Atresia (may be associated with atresias of the small bowel)	5–9%

lumen is obliterated by a membrane or where there is a complete gap between the 2 bowel ends. Atresia and stenosis may affect the duodenum proximal or distal to the ampulla of Vater. There is often a history of polyhydramnios.

Clinical Findings

A. Atresia: Vomiting (usually bile-stained) begins within a few hours after birth, with epigastric distention. Meconium may be normally passed. The association between duodenal atresia and severe congenital anomalies (30%), such as esophageal atresia, atresias elsewhere in the gastrointestinal tract, and cardiac and renal anomalies, is well described. Prematurity (25–50%) and Down's syndrome (20–30%) are other associated conditions.

B. Stenosis: Symptoms of duodenal obstruction are delayed for weeks, months, or years. Even though a postampullary location of the stenotic area is usual, the vomitus does not always contain bile. X-rays of the abdomen usually show gastric and duodenal gaseous distention proximal to the atretic site (''double bubble''). In cases of protracted vomiting and dehydration, there may be little air in the stomach; it is then advisable to instill 10 mL of air into the stomach to elicit the typical pattern. Total absence of gas in the intestinal tract distal to the obstruction suggests atresia or an extrinsic obstruction severe enough to completely occlude the lumen, while air scattered over the lower abdomen may indicate a partial duodenal obstruction of either the intrinsic or extrinsic variety. A barium enema may be helpful in determining the presence of a concomitant malrotation or of an area of atresia lower in the gastrointestinal tract.

Treatment & Prognosis

Thorough exploration is necessary at operation not only to find the cause of the obstruction but also to make sure that no additional pathologic anomalies are present lower in the gastrointestinal tract.

The mortality rate (35–40%) is significantly affected by prematurity, Down's syndrome, and associated congenital anomalies.

CONGENITAL JEJUNAL & ILEAL OBSTRUCTION

Bile-stained or fecal vomiting usually begins in the first 48 hours of life, and distention is frequent. Small amounts of meconium may be passed. Prematurity and severe congenital anomalies often coexist. Atresias, stenoses, and obstructing membranes may affect multiple sites. X-ray features include dilated loops of small bowel and absence of colonic gas. Barium enema will reveal a colon of restricted caliber (microcolon) if the atresia is in the lower small bowel. In over 10% of cases of jejunoileal atresia, there is absence of the mesentery, and the superior mesenteric artery cannot be identified beyond the origin of the right colic and ileocolic arteries. As a result, the ileum coils around one of these 2 arteries, giving rise to the ''Christmas tree'' deformity. The tenuous blood supply often leads to long areas of gangrenous bowel and compromises surgical anastomoses.

The differential diagnosis should include Hirschsprung's disease, paralytic ileus secondary to sepsis, gastroenteritis or pneumonia, midgut volvulus, and meconium ileus. In 10% of cases, this latter condition, the initial manifestation of cystic fibrosis, can be found in association with intestinal atresia.

Surgery is mandatory. The prognosis remains guarded.

Lynn HB: Duodenal obstruction: Atresia, stenosis and annular pancreas. Pages 902–911 in: *Pediatric Surgery,* 3rd ed. Ravitch MM et al (editors). Year Book, 1979.

Shigemoto H et al: Neonatal meconium obstruction in the ileum without mucoviscidosis. *J Pediatr Surg* 1978;**13:**475.

ANNULAR PANCREAS

The presence of an annular pancreas is usually associated with failure of segmental duodenal development. The symptoms are those of partial or complete duodenal obstruction. Down's syndrome and severe congenital anomalies of the gastrointestinal tract occur frequently. As with other gastrointestinal obstructive lesions of the neonate, polyhydramnios is commonly found. Clinical manifestations can occur late in childhood.

Treatment consists of duodenoduodenostomy or duodenojejunostomy without operative dissection or division of the pancreatic annulus.

Kiernan PD et al: Annular pancreas: Mayo Clinic experience from 1957 to 1976 with review of the literature. *Arch Surg* 1980;**115:**46.

Merrill JR, Raffensperger JG: Pediatric annular pancreas: Twenty years' experience. *J Pediatr Surg* 1976;**11:**921.

MIDGUT MALROTATION WITH OR WITHOUT VOLVULUS

Normally, the midgut (which extends from the duodenojejunal junction to the mid transverse colon and which is supplied by the superior mesenteric artery) returns to the intra-abdominal position during the tenth week of embryonic life, and the root of the mesentery rotates in a counterclockwise direction. This causes the colon to cross ventrally; the cecum moves from the left to the right lower quadrant, and the duodenum crosses dorsally to become partly retroperitoneal. When this rotation is incomplete, the posterior fixation of the mesentery is defective, so that the bowel from the ligament of Treitz to the mid transverse colon may twist, causing a volvulus around the pediclelike mesentery. Duodenal or ileal obstruction may later result through peritoneal bands from the mobile hepatic flexure or cecum. The majority of cases are asymptomatic.

Clinical Findings

A. Symptoms and Signs: Seventy-five percent of symptomatic cases show high intestinal obstruction within the first 3 weeks of life, with bile-stained vomitus, abdominal distention, and visible peristalsis. The first signs may occur later in life, with recurring symptoms of intermittent intestinal obstruction or, more rarely, with celiac syndrome or intermittent profuse watery diarrhea. Acute gastroenteritis may be an early symptom in infants under the age of 6 months. Severe associated congenital anomalies, especially cardiac, are said to occur in over 25% of symptomatic cases.

B. X-Ray Findings: In the newborn period, complete absence of air in the small bowel suggests duodenal atresia. An upper gastrointestinal series may show partial or complete obstruction. The diagnosis of malrotation can be further confirmed by barium enema, which shows a cecum that is mobile and abnormally located.

Treatment & Prognosis

Midgut volvulus is one of the most catastrophic diseases of the newborn period. The ischemia often involves the entire segment of the intestine in the region of the superior mesenteric artery (from the ligament of Treitz to the mid transverse colon). When necrosis is extensive, a second-look operation is recommended 48 hours after reducing the volvulus and dividing Ladd's bands. The prognosis in the newborn period is guarded in view of the incidence of perforation with peritonitis and of extensive intestinal necrosis.

Duke JH Jr, Yar MS: Primary small bowel volvulus. *Arch Surg* 1977;**112:**685.

Janik JS, Ein SH: Normal intestinal rotation with nonfixation: A cause of chronic abdominal pain. *J Pediatr Surg* 1979;**14:**670.

Stewart DR et al: Malrotation of the bowel in infants and children: A 15 year experience. *Surgery* 1976;**79:**716.

MAJOR ABDOMINAL WALL DEVELOPMENTAL DEFECTS

Omphalocele

This is a rare condition (1:10,000 births) associated with variable herniation of intestine and liver into the base of the umbilical cord. There is no defect of the abdominal wall, but cardiac anomalies (20%) and the midline syndromes are common. Primary closure of those less than 5 cm in diameter has a good prognosis. Attempts at primary repair of larger ones lead to respiratory failure or Budd-Chiari syndrome, which necessitates a staged enlargement of the abdominal cavity.

Gastroschisis

Herniation of bowel and other viscera through a defect in the abdominal wall is twice as frequent as omphalocele. There is no covering membrane, and the eviscerated bowel loops are dark red, edematous, and adherent. They are encased in a thick matrix of fibrinous material. Gangrene may be present. All patients have associated malrotation and some degree of congenital shortening of the small bowel. Associated intestinal atresias are common. Closure is by stages with a prosthetic abdominal wall. Prematurity (40%), the threat of sepsis, and malnutrition remain the long-term challenges of this entity. The postoperative course is usually difficult because of protracted intestinal obstruction and intestinal dysfunction. Total parenteral nutrition is often required for extended periods of time.

Congenital Deficiency of Abdominal Musculature

This disorder, known as the prune-belly syndrome, is apparent from the flaccid and wrinkled appearance of the abdominal wall. Almost all affected infants are males with undescended testes; 50% present with clubfoot. Between 20 and 25% also have cardiac and gastrointestinal anomalies. Urinary tract anomalies consist of urethral and functional bladder neck obstructions associated with a patent urachus. Corseting counteracts the abdominal wall weakness, but 60% die in infancy as a result of renal insufficiency or respiratory failure.

De Vries PA: The pathogenesis of gastroschisis and omphalocele. *J Pediatr Surg* 1980;**15:**245.

Stringel G, Filer RM: Prognostic factors in omphalocele and gastroschisis. *J Pediatr Surg* 1979;**14:**515.

Towne BH, Peters G, Chang JH: The problem of "giant" omphalocele. *J Pediatr Surg* 1980;**15:**543.

MECKEL'S DIVERTICULUM & OMPHALOMESENTERIC DUCT REMNANTS

Meckel's diverticulum is present in 1.5% of the population but rarely causes symptoms. Familial cases have been reported. Complications occur 3 times more frequently in males than in females, and in 50–60% of cases within the first 2 years of life. Heterotopic tissue (gastric mucosa mostly, but also pancreatic tissue and jejunal or colonic mucosa) is 10 times as likely to be present in symptomatic cases. Meckel's diverticulum is usually located within 100 cm of the ileocecal valve and runs antimesenterically, with its own blood supply.

Clinical Findings

A. Symptoms and Signs:

1. Hemorrhage–(40–60% of symptomatic cases.) Massive painless rectal bleeding or dark red stool is characteristic. Occult bleeding may lead to anemia. Shock may be present with low hemoglobin levels. Gastric mucosa and an ulcer of the ileal mucosa are found in the majority of cases presenting with hemorrhage.

2. Intestinal obstruction–(25% of symptomatic cases.)

a. Intussusception–Ileocolic intussusception occurs with early intestinal infarction. A mass is palpable.

b. Herniation or volvulus–Twisting of the bowel around a fibrous remnant of the vitelline duct extending from the tip of the diverticulum to the abdominal wall may occur with herniation around this cord or strangulation of the diverticulum in an inguinal hernia. In many cases, entrapment of a bowel loop under a band running between the diverticulum and the base of the mesentery has been associated with intestinal obstruction.

3. Diverticulitis–(10–20%.) Diverticulitis is clinically indistinguishable from acute appendicitis. Perforation and generalized peritonitis may occur in the young infant. There may be chronic recurrent abdominal pain, possibly due to the presence of an entrapped foreign body.

B. X-Ray Findings: An x-ray diagnosis of this condition is seldom made. Radionuclide imaging with ^{99m}Tc pertechnetate may be of value to demonstrate the diverticulum lined with heterotopic gastric mucosa. Stimulation of ^{99m}Tc pertechnetate uptake by both pentagastrin and cimetidine can reduce the number of false-negative results. Angiography may be useful when bleeding is brisk.

Treatment

A. Diverticulum: Treatment is surgical. At operation, close inspection of the ileum proximal and distal to the diverticulum may reveal ulcerations and heterotopic tissue adjacent to the neck of the diverticulum.

B. Other Remnants of the Omphalomesenteric Duct: Fecal discharge from the umbilicus is evidence of a patent omphalomesenteric duct. The duct may be completely closed, leading to persistence of a fibrous cord joining ileum and umbilicus and potentially the origin of a volvulus. In other instances, a mucoid discharge may be indicative of a mucocele, which can protrude through the umbilicus and be mistaken for an umbilical granuloma, since it is firm and bright red. In all cases, surgical excision of the omphalomesenteric remnant is indicated.

Prognosis

The prognosis for Meckel's diverticulum is good. Marked hemorrhage may occur but is rarely exsanguinating.

Benson CD: Surgical complications of Meckel's diverticulum. Pages 955–960 in: *Pediatric Surgery*, 3rd ed. Ravitch MM et al (editors). Year Book, 1979.

Hough JE, Konieczny KM: The sodium pertechnetate Tc 99m scan. *Pediatrics* 1975;**56**:34.

Mackey WC, Dineen P: A fifty-year experience with Meckel's diverticulum. *Surg Gynecol Obstet* 1983;**156**:56.

Pellerin D et al: Meckel's diverticulum: Review of 250 cases in children. *Ann Chir Infantile* 1976;**17**:157.

Treves S, Grand RJ, Eraklis AJ: Pentagastrin stimulation of technetium-99m uptake by ectopic gastric mucosa in Meckel's diverticulum. *Radiology* 1978;**128**:711.

DUPLICATIONS OF THE GASTROINTESTINAL TRACT

Duplications of the gastrointestinal tract are congenital malformations most often discovered during infancy. Duplications are spherical or tubular structures of various sizes and shapes that may occur anywhere along the gastrointestinal tract from the tongue to the anus. They usually contain fluid and sometimes blood if necrosis has taken place. Although most duplications are not communicating, they are intimately attached to the mesenteric side of the gut and share a common muscular coat. The intestinal epithelium is usually of the same type as that seen in the area of the gastrointestinal tract from which it originates; 20–30% contain ectopic gastric mucosa. Some duplications are attached to the spinal cord and are associated with the presence of hemivertebrae (neurenteric cysts). Abdominal duplications are much more common than the thoracic ones, which are usually attached to the esophagus.

Symptoms usually become manifest in infancy and consist of vomiting, abdominal distention, colicky pain, rectal bleeding, partial or total intestinal obstruction, or an abdominal mass. Physical examination reveals a rounded, smooth, freely movable mass, and x-rays of the abdomen show a noncalcified mass displacing the intestines or compressing the stomach. Scanning with ^{99m}Tc pertechnetate is useful in duplications containing gastric mucosa. Involvement of the terminal small bowel can give rise to an intussusception.

Prompt surgical treatment is indicated.

Favara B, Franciosi RA, Akers DR: Enteric duplications. Thirty-seven cases: A vascular theory of pathogenesis. *Am J Dis Child* 1971;**122**:501.

Pruksapong C et al: Gastric duplication. *J Pediatr Surg* 1979;**14**:83.

Silverman A, Roy CC: Duplications of the gastrointestinal tract. Page 75 in: *Pediatric Clinical Gastroenterology*, 3rd ed. Mosby, 1983.

NECROTIZING ENTEROCOLITIS

Essentials of Diagnosis

- The patient is likely to be a small premature (< 1600 g) and the product of an abnormal gestation and a complicated delivery.
- During the first weeks of life, regurgitation and vomiting are followed by abdominal distention, hematochezia, and signs of peritonitis.
- Lethargy, bradycardia, temperature instability, severe acidosis, apneic episodes, sepsis, and shock rapidly supervene.
- Plain film shows intramural gas bubbles (pneumatosis intestinalis).
- Late manifestations (strictures in the ileum or colon) usually occur within 3 months of the initial illness.

General Considerations

Necrotizing enterocolitis in the newborn infant is an acute fulminating disease associated with diffuse ulceration and necrosis of the gastrointestinal tract. The lower ileum is the most common site of the disease. In 75% of cases, there are also lesions in the colon. The stomach and upper small bowel are rarely affected. The disease affects 1–2% of all premature infants, the incidence being higher in the ones weighing less than 1600 grams. Necrotizing enterocolitis may occur as a complication of neonatal appendicitis, lower bowel obstruction (eg, meconium ileus, Hirschsprung's disease), or exchange transfusion in full-term newborns. Risk factors in premature infants include perinatal asphyxia, respiratory distress, congenital heart disease, and early or hyperosmolar feedings. Intolerance to soy and cow's milk protein has also been implicated. Breast feeding may offer some protection.

Clinical Findings

A. Symptoms and Signs: Symptoms may occur as early as the first day and as late as the fourth week. Feedings are poorly tolerated, and regurgitation and vomiting occur. This is followed by abdominal distention and bloody stools or obstipation. Signs of perforation and peritonitis may be the initial manifestations. Severe acidosis, sepsis, and shock rapidly supervene. In some cases, the course is not as fulminating, and the diagnosis may be more difficult or completely missed until the infant develops signs of progressive lower small bowel or colonic obstruction, the result of acquired strictures. These late manifestations of necrotizing enterocolitis occur usually within the first 3 months after the acute phase of the illness but may occur as late as age 1 year.

B. X-Ray Findings: A plain film may show, besides small bowel distention and evidence of obstruction, a feathered appearance indicative of ulceration and the accumulation of intramural gas bubbles (pneumatosis intestinalis). With progression of the disease, portal venous gas may be seen; with subsequent perforation, pneumoperitoneum is evident.

Treatment

Oral feedings should be withheld, nasogastric suction and intravenous fluids initiated, and diagnostic workup started. Parenteral antibiotics are indicated. Nonabsorbable oral antibiotics may also be given, since the intestinal flora is thought to be an important pathologic factor associated with the ischemic lesion. Plain films of the abdomen are done every 4–6 hours for the first few days to detect a perforation. Feedings are resumed cautiously when the nasogastric drainage is small and when pneumatosis and ileus have resolved for 72 hours. Any evidence of intestinal perforation or peritonitis is an indication for immediate operation.

After discharge, newborns who have had necrotizing enterocolitis must be followed closely for signs of partial obstruction, which usually occurs at 6–8 weeks but can occur as late as a year after the initial insult. The strictures more commonly affect the left colon (50–80%) and rarely the small bowel, other than the terminal ileum (10–20%).

Prevention

The following recommendations are made: (1) Delay oral feedings for 1–2 weeks in low-birth-weight neonates with a history of perinatal asphyxia. (2) Hyperosmolar formulas are not recommended in sick newborns. (3) In the presence of significant polycythemia (hematocrit > 75%), consider a small phlebotomy and exchange transfusion with plasma, using a peripheral vein. (4) Arterial umbilical catheters should lie in the aorta below the takeoff point of the renal arteries. (5) Venous umbilical catheters should not be positioned in the portal vein for an exchange transfusion.

Prognosis

The mortality rate is 25–30%. Prematurity and a history of asphyxia affect the prognosis adversely, as does onset before age 7 days. Much better results are seen in the full-term infant after exchange transfusion.

Abbasi S et al: Long-term assessment of growth, nutritional status, and gastrointestinal function in survivors of necrotizing enterocolitis. *J Pediatr* 1984;**104:**550.

Kliegman RM, Fanaroff AA: Necrotizing enterocolitis. *N Engl J Med* 1984;**310:**1093.

Kosloske AM, Burstein J, Bartow SA: Intestinal obstruction due to colonic stricture following neonatal necrotizing enterocolitis. *Ann Surg* 1980;**192:**202.

Stoll BJ et al: Epidemiology of necrotizing enterocolitis: A case control study. *J Pediatr* 1980;**96:**447.

Teasdale F et al: Neonatal necrotizing enterocolitis: The relation of age at the time of onset to prognosis. *Can Med Assoc J* 1980;**123:**387.

Wilson R et al: Risk factors for necrotizing enterocolitis in infants weighing more than 2000 grams at birth: A case control study. *Pediatrics* 1983;**71:**19.

PRIMARY PERITONITIS

The incidence of primary peritonitis has decreased with the availability of antibiotics. Most cases occur before the age of 5. In older children, the disease is 3–5 times more common in girls. The most common infecting organisms are *Escherichia coli* and hemolytic streptococci and pneumococci, although viruses have been implicated in a few cases. Especially at risk are infants who have undergone splenectomy. Peritonitis is a potential complication of nephrosis and cirrhosis in which ascites is present, and it may occur following a Kasai operation.

The onset is acute, with severe abdominal pain, fever, nausea, and vomiting. The abdomen is tender, with guarding, involuntary rigidity, and distention. Tenderness is present on rectal examination. The physical signs are identical to those associated with peritonitis secondary to, for example, a perforated appendix. However, the temperature is usually higher and the white blood cell count also higher (20,000–50,000/μL) than is usual in appendicitis. Diarrhea is not uncommonly seen in primary peritonitis and is much rarer in appendicitis.

Primary peritonitis must be distinguished from secondary peritonitis (see below).

A diagnostic paracentesis should be made and appropriate antibiotic therapy instituted. Surgical peritoneal drainage has been virtually abandoned except in cases of localized abscesses.

McDougal WS, Izant RJ Jr, Zollinger RM Jr: Primary peritonitis in infancy and childhood. *Ann Surg* 1975;**181:**310.

Weinstein MP et al: Spontaneous bacterial peritonitis. *Am J Med* 1978;**64:**592.

SECONDARY PERITONITIS

Secondary peritoneal infection commonly results from an abscessed or ruptured intra-abdominal viscus, usually the appendix. More rarely, peptic ulcer, cholecystitis, pancreatitis, regional enteritis, ulcerative colitis, midgut volvulus, intussusception, and strangulated hernia can cause secondary peritonitis. Abscesses may form in the pelvic, subhepatic, and subphrenic areas, but localization occurs less commonly in infants and young children than in adults.

Clinical Findings

A. Symptoms and Signs: Signs are often overshadowed by those of the underlying disorder. High fever is common except in newborn or debilitated infants, and shock may be present. Abdominal pain is diffuse and is exacerbated by movement. Vomiting is protracted and bilious. Constipation is marked unless there is localization, when small diarrheal stools may be passed. Restlessness, rapid pulse, and superficial grunting respirations are other common clinical features. Abdominal examination shows diffuse tenderness with muscular resistance and rebound tenderness. Peristalsis is usually absent. Irritation of the pelvic peritoneum is evidenced by pain on rectal examination. Abdominal paracentesis may help in establishing the diagnosis.

B. Laboratory Findings: A striking polymorphonuclear response is usual; later, the white blood cell count often drops to leukopenic levels.

Treatment & Prognosis

Preoperative hydration, correction of acid-base problems, antimicrobial therapy, gastric suction, and relief of pain significantly improve the mortality rate.

The operative management consists of removal or repair of the affected viscus, drainage of the localized abscess, and lavage of the peritoneal cavity with saline and antibiotics.

The mortality rate is probably around 1% in older children and 50% in newborns.

Bell MJ, Ternberg JL, Bower RJ: The microbial flora and antimicrobial therapy of neonatal peritonitis. *J Pediatr Surg* 1980;**15:**569.

Emanuel B, Zlotnik P, Raffensperger JG: Perforation of gastrointestinal tract in infancy and childhood. *Surg Gynecol Obstet* 1978;**146:**926.

Kosloske AM, Lilly JR: Paracentesis and lavage for diagnosis of intestinal gangrene in neonatal necrotizing enterocolitis. *J Pediatr Surg* 1978;**13:**315.

CONGENITAL AGANGLIONIC MEGACOLON (Hirschsprung's Disease)

Essentials of Diagnosis

- Partial or complete intestinal obstruction in the newborn period.
- Vomiting, diarrhea, abdominal distention, and shock in the newborn period.
- Obstinate constipation, abdominal enlargement, ribbonlike stools, and failure to thrive in infancy or childhood.
- Absence of fecal material on rectal examination.
- Narrowed colonic segment proximal to the anus on x-ray.
- Absence of ganglion cells in the narrowed segment.

General Considerations

Hirschsprung's disease is secondary to congenital absence of parasympathetic ganglion cells in one segment of the colon (a 4- to 25-cm rectal or rectosigmoid segment in 90% of cases), but it may involve the entire organ in 5%. Distal aganglionosis may also be acquired, presumably secondary to ischemia. **Zonal colonic aganglionosis** is exceedingly rare. The aperistaltic denervated segment is narrowed, with dilatation of the proximal uninvolved colon. In long-standing cases, the portion proximal to the narrowed segment may become thinned out, and ulcerations of the mucosa occur although perforations are rare. Protein-losing enteropathy may be present. A familial pattern has been described, particularly in total colonic aganglionosis. The disease is 4 times more common in boys than in girls, and 10–15% of patients have Down's syndrome.

Clinical Findings

A. Symptoms and Signs: Failure of the newborn to pass meconium—followed by vomiting, abdominal distention, and reluctance to feed—suggests a long aganglionic segment. The infant is irritable, and breathing may be rapid and grunting because of abdominal distention. In other cases, symptoms appear later and are those of partial intestinal obstruction. Stools may be infrequent and loose; vomiting may be bilious initially and fecal later. Abdominal distention is invariably present. Bouts of enterocolitis manifested by fever, explosive liquid diarrhea, and severe prostration are reported in about 50% of newborns with this disease. These episodes are serious and may lead to acute inflammatory and ischemic changes. Perforation (especially cecal) and sepsis are not unusual. In later infancy, alternating obstipation and diarrhea predominate. The older the child, the more likely to present with obstinate constipation. The stools are offensive and ribbonlike, the abdomen enlarged, and the veins prominent; peristaltic patterns are readily visible, and fecal masses are easily palpated. Intermittent bouts of intestinal obstruction due to fecal impaction, hypochromic anemia, hypoproteinemia, and failure to thrive are added features.

On digital rectal examination, the anal canal and rectum are devoid of fecal material and may feel narrow. If the involved segment is short, there may be a gush of flatus and of pale, liquid, offensive stool as the finger is withdrawn. The presence of fecal colonic impaction associated with an empty rectum is most suggestive of the disease. However, in cases of short segment aganglionosis, feces may be present in the rectal ampulla, and soiling may be a presenting symptom.

B. Laboratory Findings: The diagnosis is based on histologic evidence of aganglionosis and histochemical evidence of increased acetylcholinesterase activity. Rectal suction biopsies taken at 3, 4, and 5 cm readily establish the diagnosis, although some prefer a full-thickness rectal biopsy in order to have access to the ganglion cells between the muscular layers (Auerbach's plexus).

C. X-Ray Findings: X-ray examination of the abdomen may reveal dilated colonic loops and absence of gas from the pelvic colon on an erect lateral film. A barium enema, introducing a small amount of radiopaque material through a catheter with the tip inserted barely beyond the anal sphincter, will usually demonstrate the narrowed segment. A postevacuation film taken 12–48 hours later will show substantial residual barium and is more reliable because the narrowed segment can be absent, especially in patients up to 6 weeks of age.

D. Special Examinations: Manometric studies are sometimes useful in the diagnosis of aganglionosis and are essential in cases where the involvement is limited to a short segment, making histologic diagnosis difficult. Failure of the internal sphincter muscle to relax after balloon distention of the rectum is consistent with Hirschsprung's disease. Interpretation of acetylcholinesterase staining in newborns is sometimes difficult.

Differential Diagnosis

Congenital aganglionic megacolon accounts for 15–20% of cases of neonatal intestinal obstruction. Later in life, this disease must be differentiated from psychogenic megacolon. It can also be confused with celiac disease because of the striking abdominal distention and failure to thrive.

A number of disorders symptomatically similar to Hirschsprung's disease have been described: hypoganglionosis; immaturity of ganglion cells; and achalasia of the distal rectal segment and of segmental dilatation of the colon in the presence of a normal complement of ganglion cells.

Treatment

A colostomy should be performed in an area of the colon where ganglion cells have been demonstrated by frozen section. If the entire colon is involved, ileostomy is the procedure of choice. If enterocolitis is clinically present and radiologically demonstrated by the typical "sawtooth" appearance, saline irrigations should be repeatedly given through a rectal cannula. Plasma expanders and fluid and electrolyte homeostasis are essential before surgery. Resection of the aganglionic segment is delayed until the infant is at least 6 months of age. In healthy patients, staging is not necessary.

During operation, it is essential to ascertain from biopsies of the bowel that ganglion cells are present in the proximal portion of the resected bowel before the final anastomosis is made. The endorectal pull-through (Soave) procedure is the preferred surgical operation and leads to fewer long-term complications such as fecal and urinary incontinence.

Prognosis

Enterocolitis before or after surgery is associated with a 30% mortality rate; the rate appears to be higher in infants with a long aganglionic segment.

Hirschsprung's disease has recurred postoperatively in some cases because of the dropping out of ganglion cells secondary to vascular impairment and chronic inflammatory changes with stenosis.

Klein MD et al: Hirschsprung's disease in the newborn. *J Pediatr Surg* 1984;**19:**370.

Kleinhaus S et al: Hirschsprung's disease: A survey of the members of the Surgical Section of the American Academy of Pediatrics. *J Pediatr Surg* 1979;**14:**588.

Morikawa Y, Donahoe PK, Hendren WH: Manometry and histochemistry in the diagnosis of Hirschsprung's disease. *Pediatrics* 1979;**63:**865.
Soave F: Long-term results of operative treatment in Hirschsprung's disease. *Z Kinderchir* 1977;**22:**267.
Weinberg RJ et al: Acquired distal aganglionosis of the colon. *J Pediatr* 1982;**101:**406.

NEONATAL INTESTINAL OBSTRUCTION

Failure to pass meconium within the first 24 hours of life suggests intestinal obstruction. A diagnosis of obstruction is very likely if other symptoms such as distention or vomiting are present or if by 36 hours only a small amount of mucus or meconium has been passed. The evacuation of meconium may be quite normal in situations where the obstruction is high in the gastrointestinal tract.

In late pregnancy, the presence or suspicion of polyhydramnios is an indication for ultrasonography. It may show an echo-free sonolucent area and can demonstrate the presence of fetal intestinal obstruction, such as duodenal atresia, malrotation with jejunal atresia, gastroschisis, or Hirschsprung's disease.

The causes of neonatal intestinal obstruction can be listed as follows:

- Atresia
- Duplications, cysts, and bands
- Malrotation and midgut volvulus
- Gastrointestinal perforations
- Necrotizing enterocolitis
- Hirschsprung's disease
- Abnormal meconium
  - Meconium ileus
  - Meconium plug syndrome
- Functional obstruction
  - Neurologic immaturity in prematures
  - Small left colon syndrome
  - Sepsis
  - Respiratory distress syndrome
  - Maternal drugs
- Imperforate anus
- Incarcerated hernia
- Milk curds, lactobezoar

When the diagnosis is suspected, x-rays are in order. Air should reach the proximal small bowel during the first hour following delivery and the colon and rectum within 6 hours. Large amounts of air in the stomach may suggest a tracheoesophageal fistula, while the absence of air is evidence of esophageal atresia without a fistula or with a proximal fistula. A bubble of air to the right of the spine and adjacent to the stomach bubble ("double bubble") is diagnostic of duodenal atresia or annular pancreas. A few dilated loops beyond the stomach indicate atresia of the jejunum, whereas many air-filled loops usually suggest a lower small bowel or colonic obstruction.

Examination of the abdomen may not show much distention if vomiting is protracted or if nasogastric drainage is being carried out. An abdominal mass suggests meconium ileus, volvulus, or duplication. If crying is brought about by light palpation, acute abdomen is a likely diagnosis. Abdominal rigidity is rarely present even in the case of peritonitis. A gray cyanotic hue with distended veins is a common finding in cases of necrotic bowel with peritonitis. If rectal examination is followed by explosive passage of stool and gas, short-segment Hirschsprung's disease is likely to be present.

As soon as the diagnosis is suspected, nasogastric suction should be initiated. The infant should be kept in an incubator for maintenance of central temperature and oxygenation. Systemic antibiotics, vitamin K, salt-poor human albumin, water, and electrolytes should be given immediately. Improperly reconstituted or high-density calorie formulas may give rise to intestinal obstruction through the formation of milk-curd enteroliths or of lactobezoars.

Erenberg A, Shaw RD, Yousefzadah D: Lactobezoar in the low-birth-weight infant. *Pediatrics* 1979;**63:**642.
Roy CC, Morin CL, Weber AM: Gastrointestinal emergency problems in paediatric practice. *Clin Gastroenterol* 1981; **10:**225.
Stewart DR et al: Neonatal small left colon syndrome. *Ann Surg* 1977;**186:**741.
Thomas P: Incidence of some surgically correctable congenital abnormalities in South Australia. *J Pediatr Surg* 1977; **12:**693.

THE MECONIUM PLUG SYNDROME

Evidence of low intestinal obstruction becomes apparent on the second day of life. Little or no meconium is passed, and abdominal distention is followed by bile-stained vomiting and dehydration. On rectal examination, the anal canal may be abnormally small. Occasionally, the meconium plug may be passed, and large amounts of gas and meconium follow the rectal examination.

In addition to air distention seen on x-ray, fluid levels are observed in half of the patients. A barium enema performed under low pressure with a soft-tipped catheter is not only diagnostic, since it reveals a change in the caliber of the colon at the site of obstruction, but can also be therapeutic in dislodging the meconium plug. The finding of a microcolon distal to the plug makes the differentiation from Hirschsprung's disease impossible, especially since the meconium plug syndrome has been reported in Hirschsprung's disease.

Ruling out cystic fibrosis by a sweat test and Hirschsprung's disease by a rectal biopsy may be necessary if bowel function is not entirely normal after passage of the meconium.

Pochaczevsky R, Leonidas JC: The meconium plug syndrome: Roentgen evaluation and differentiation from Hirschsprung's disease and other pathological states. *Radium Ther Nucl Med* 1974;**120:**342.

Shigemoto H et al: Neonatal meconium obstruction in the ileum without mucoviscidosis. *J Pediatr Surg* 1978;**13:**475.

CHYLOUS ASCITES

Congenital chylous ascites may be observed in the newborn before feeding when there is an abnormality in the lymphatic system. If the thoracic duct is involved, chylothorax may be present. Later in life, the cause may be either a congenital lymphatic abnormality or secondary to tumors or peritoneal bands.

Clinical Findings

A. Symptoms and Signs: In both forms, a rapidly enlarging abdomen, diarrhea, and failure to thrive are noted, with a fluid wave and shifting dullness. Unilateral or generalized peripheral lymphedema may be present. In older children, the history is most important in that trauma, infection, tumor, and previous surgery may play an important role.

B. Laboratory Findings: Laboratory findings include hypoalbuminemia, hypogammaglobulinemia, and lymphopenia. Ascitic fluid obtained by paracentesis will have the composition of chyle if the patient has been fed; otherwise, it is indistinguishable from ascites secondary to cirrhosis.

Differential Diagnosis

Chylous ascites must be differentiated from ascites due to liver failure and, in the older child, from constrictive pericarditis and neoplastic, infectious, or inflammatory diseases causing lymphatic obstruction.

Complications & Sequelae

Severe chylous ascites can be fatal. Chronic loss of albumin and gamma globulin through the gastrointestinal tract may lead to edema and increase the risk of infection. Rapidly accumulating chylous ascites may cause respiratory complications.

Treatment & Prognosis

If there is a congenital abnormality due to hypoplasia, aplasia, or ectasia of the lymphatics, little can be done for the patient. Attempts to relieve the ascites by bringing the saphenous vein into the peritoneal cavity have had partial success. A fat-free diet supplemented with medium-chain triglycerides decreases the formation of chylous ascitic fluid. Total parenteral nutrition may be necessary.

The congenital form of chylous ascites may spontaneously disappear following paracentesis and a medium-chain triglyceride diet.

The prognosis is guarded, although spontaneous cures have been reported.

Cochran WJ et al: Chylous ascites in infants and children: A case report and literature review. *J Pediatr Gastroenterol Nutr* 1985;**4:**668.

Guttman FM, Montupet P, Bloss RS: Experience with peritoneovenous shunting for congenital chylous ascites in infants and children. *J Pediatr Surg* 1982;**17:**368.

CONGENITAL ANORECTAL ANOMALIES

Anorectal anomalies occur once in every 3000–4000 births, and most types are more common in males. Inspection of the perianal area is essential in all newborns.

Classification

A. Anterior Displacement of the Anal Opening: This condition is more common in girls than in boys. It may be associated with a posterior rectal shelf and usually is characterized by constipation that responds poorly to medical management.

B. Anal Stenosis: The anal aperture is very small and filled with a dot of meconium. Defecation is difficult, and there may be ribbonlike stools, fecal impaction, and abdominal distention. This malformation accounts for perhaps 10% of cases of anorectal anomalies.

C. Imperforate Anal Membrane: The infant fails to pass meconium, and a greenish bulging membrane is seen. After excision, bowel and sphincter function are normal.

D. Anal Agenesis: This results from defective development of the anus. The anal dimple is present, and stimulation of the perianal area leads to puckering indicative of the presence of the external sphincter. If there is no associated fistula, intestinal obstruction occurs. Fistulas may be perineal or vulvar in the female and perineal or urethral in the male. A perineal fistula presents as a streak of meconium buried in thickened perineal skin.

E. Rectal and Anal Agenesis: Rectal and anal agenesis accounts for 75% of total anorectal anomalies. Fistulas are almost invariably present. In the female, they may be vestibular or vaginal or may enter a urogenital sinus, which is a common passageway for the urethra and vagina. In the male, fistulas are rectovesical or rectourethral. Associated major congenital malformations are common. Sacral defects, prematurity, and hypoplastic internal and external sphincters significantly influence the prognosis for life and function.

F. Rectal Atresia: The anal canal and lower rectum form a blind pouch that is separated for a variable distance from the blind upper rectal pouch.

Clinical Findings

X-rays taken with the infant held upside down after the first 24 hours of life and with a radiopaque object held in place at the usual location of the anus will help determine the position of the terminal end of the bowel and the surgical approach.

Treatment & Prognosis

Dilation of the anus should be undertaken in cases

of anal stenosis. Treatment for imperforate anal membrane consists of excision of the membrane and dilation. Colostomy is advocated for all cases of rectal agenesis. In patients with anal agenesis and a visible fistula of sufficient size to pass meconium, treatment can be deferred. The male without a visible fistula may have a urethral fistula; therefore, colostomy is recommended.

Of the patients with "low" defects, 80–90% are continent after surgery; with "high" defects, only 30% achieve continence. Gracilis muscle transplants may improve continence. Levatorplasty may also be used as a secondary operation following surgery for anorectal agenesis.

The mortality rate is about 20%. The prognosis is worse in small premature infants and in infants with associated anomalies.

Brandesky G et al: Operations for the improvement of fecal incontinence. *Prog Pediatr Surg* 1976;**9:**105.

Kiesewetter WB et al: Imperforate anus. *Arch Surg* 1976; **111:**518

McGill CW et al: The clinical basis for a simplified classification of anorectal agenesis. *Surg Gynecol Obstet* 1978;**146:**177.

Nixon HH et al: The results of treatment of anorectal anomalies: A 13 to 20 year follow-up. *J Pediatr Surg* 1977;**12:**27.

Reisner SH et al: Determination of anterior displacement of the anus in newborn infants and children. *Pediatrics* 1984;**73:**216.

ACUTE ABDOMEN

Many disorders must be considered in the differential diagnosis of acute abdomen. Emergency surgery should not be considered until the differential diagnosis has been completed. The patient may be too young to describe symptoms, and the parent's description is a subjective interpretation of what he or she thinks is wrong. A partial etiologic classification of acute abdomen is shown in Table 19–3, with the most common causes noted.

History

A. Age of the Patient: The age of the patient significantly affects the history taking. Each age group requires a specific approach. A child younger than 2 years of age is unable to describe the symptoms, and the parent's belief that abdominal pain is present may not be accurate. The physician must consider other sources of pain, including referred pain. A child 2–5 years of age may not be able to give details about pain but will be able to point to its location. Children of this age rarely simulate pain or have psychogenic pain. Children 6 years of age or older are able to give a more reliable history and description of symptoms.

B. Sex of the Patient: Some entities are more frequently seen in males than in females (eg, intussusception and pyloric stenosis). The possibility of gynecologic disorders must not be overlooked in girls.

C. Patterns of Weight Loss and Growth: Chronic gastrointestinal diseases usually affect weight gain and growth rapidly. Information regarding weight and growth may help in differentiating benign from malignant disease and acute from chronic entities (eg, acute appendicitis from Crohn's ileitis).

D. Pain: The timing of pain in relation to meals and whether pain occurs during the night should be documented. Pain that awakens a child in the middle of the night is probably related to an organic lesion. Episodes of pain lasting longer than 1 hour are unusual in functional disorders.

Diagnosis is much easier when the child is old enough to point to the site of pain. Visceral pain generated by exaggerated physiologic motor activity (eg, as in gastroenteritis) will be felt in the midline of the abdomen owing to the bilateral sensitive innervation of the gastrointestinal tract. Visceral inflammation gives rise to more localized pain that is referred outside the periumbilical area. Its extension to the mesentery and peritoneum leads to pain sharply localized to the site of irritation.

Events occurring at the time of onset of abdominal

Table 19–3. Etiologic classification of acute abdomen.*

Mechanical Obstruction		Inflammatory Diseases and Infections			
Intraluminal Obstruction	**Extraluminal Obstruction**	**Gastrointestinal Disease**	**Paralytic Ileus**	**Blunt Trauma**	**Miscellaneous**
Foreign body Bezoar Fecalith Gallstone Parasites Meconium ileus equivalent Tumor Fecaloma	Hernia Intussusception Volvulus Duplication Stenosis Tumor Mesenteric cyst Superior mesenteric artery syndrome Pyloric stenosis	Appendicitis Crohn's disease Ulcerative colitis Henoch-Schönlein purpura and other causes of vasculitis Peptic ulcer Meckel's diverticulitis Acute gastroenteritis Pseudomembranous enterocolitis	Sepsis Pneumonia Pyelonephritis Peritonitis Pancreatitis Cholecystitis Renal and gallbladder stones Pelvic inflammation Lymphadenitis due to viral or bacterial infection	Accident Battered child syndrome	Lead poisoning Sickle cell crisis Familial Mediterranean fever Porphyria Diabetic acidosis Addisonian crisis Torsion of testis Torsion of ovarian pedicle

* Reproduced, with permission, from Roy CC, Morin CL, Weber AM: Gastrointestinal emergency problems in paediatric practice. *Clin Gastroenterol* 1981;**10:**225.

discomfort must be carefully recorded. Stressful situations in the family or at school are often associated with the onset of functional pain. Trauma is frequent in children and may go unnoticed during play. Child abuse must be considered when there are signs of trauma.

E. Family History: The family history and the psychosocial status of the family must be evaluated. A positive family history for acute intermittent porphyria, familial Mediterranean fever, or sickle cell anemia will suggest a diagnosis.

F. Psychologic History: Minimal behavioral disturbances should be looked for when functional pain or encopresis is suspected.

Clinical Findings

The physical examination of a child may be difficult to perform and interpret. Careful observation of an infant or preschool child prior to the physical examination will provide useful information. The physician might decide to keep the child under observation for a few hours if the examination is not satisfactory. Because palpation of the abdomen requires the cooperation of a relaxed patient, the physician may choose to examine an infant while the infant is sitting on the parent's lap. Quiet conversation or a toy will help to distract older children. When examination is impossible because of voluntary muscle contraction, use of diazepam (Valium), 0.1–0.2 mg/kg administered intramuscularly, is recommended. Spasm of the abdominal musculature may be missed and peritoneal irritation may be difficult to interpret in an uncooperative infant or child. Rebound tenderness is a more reliable sign, but involuntary muscle contraction can be absent even in cases of peritonitis, especially in infants.

A. Symptoms and Signs: Symptoms such as anorexia, vomiting, change in bowel habits, tenesmus, and bleeding should be noted. Symptoms not associated with gastrointestinal distress are also important. Child abuse is suggested by the presence of numerous ecchymoses far from a site of trauma, ocular lesions (eg, retinal hemorrhages), subdural hematomas, multiple fractures, or burns. Traumatic pancreatitis, perforation of a hollow viscus, rupture of a solid viscus, and intraparietal gastrointestinal hematoma have been described in the battered child syndrome. Infection-related symptoms are also important to recognize, especially in children 2–5 years of age, in whom infectious disease frequently occur. Henoch-Schönlein purpura also occurs in this age group. The presence of skin rash, especially with purpuric components, suggests the possibility of vasculitis involving the small bowel. Pica suggests the presence of a foreign body, parasites, or lead poisoning. Intussusception should be suspected in a 1-year-old child who is somnolent and has severe recurrent abdominal pain.

In each age group, different disease entities must be considered. In infants, the most common causes of acute abdomen are incarcerated inguinal hernia and intussusception. Gastrointestinal malformation, incarcerated umbilical hernia, and torsion of the testis or ovarian pedicle must also be considered. Intussusception typically occurs between 6 and 24 months of age. There is no justification for waiting for signs of severe abdominal distention, bile-stained vomitus, or bloody stool before considering the diagnosis. The sudden onset of severe abdominal pain in an otherwise healthy child or following viral infection is evidence for diagnosis, especially if the pain is episodic. In preschool children, acute abdomen is more often related to infection or an inflammatory process than to mechanical obstruction.

Causes of acute abdomen in older children include gastroenteritis, which may be confused with several disorders (eg, pneumonia with referred abdominal pain, which is not uncommon). Acute appendicitis is the condition most commonly requiring abdominal surgery during childhood. Urinary infection should always be ruled out. In children over 5 years of age, chronic recurrent abdominal pain is frequent (10% of cases presenting with abdominal discomfort), but experienced clinicians can easily differentiate this syndrome from acute abdomen according to symptoms and signs. In children 6 years of age or older, the differential diagnosis of acute abdomen is similar to that of adults. There is an increasing incidence of Crohn's disease among adolescents. There are several causes of intraluminal obstruction, and chronic constipation complicated by fecaloma and encopresis must not be confused with abdominal tumor with diarrhea. Intussusception or meconium ileus equivalent must be considered in an adolescent with cystic fibrosis who refuses to take pancreatic enzyme supplements.

B. Laboratory and X-Ray Findings:

1. Appendicitis—One of the most difficult diagnoses in children is that of acute appendicitis. Radiologic examination of the chest is mandatory, since referred pain due to pneumonia may be difficult to differentiate from pain due to appendicitis. Urinalysis rules out the possibility of urinary tract infection. Abdominal films may be helpful. Appendiceal fecaliths appear as laminated concretions in the right lower quadrant. Their identification in the presence of symptoms confirms the diagnosis. Areas devoid of bowel gas in the right lower quadrant are also signs, especially when air-fluid levels are present in the cecum or terminal ileum. This finding suggests localized ileus. Scoliosis with concavity oriented to the right lower quadrant and disappearance of the right psoas shadow are indirect signs of appendicitis. Eventually, the cecum is displaced by a significant periappendiceal abscess. Evaluation with barium enema or ultrasonography may be helpful in such cases. When tests and x-rays are inconclusive, the safest approach is to examine the patient several times over a period of a few hours. Sudden disappearance of severe pain may indicate perforation of the appendix. When findings of the history and physical examination do not disclose features incompatible with appendicitis, it is best not to wait for a definitive diagnosis but rather to perform surgery at once.

2. Intussusception—Abdominal x-rays are of particular importance when intussusception is suspected. In about one-third of cases, a plain film of the abdomen will be suggestive by showing absence of gas in one area, a mass effect or crescent shape indicating gas outlining the top of the invaginated bowel, or evidence of obstruction. Even if the film is normal, a barium enema must be given when there is severe recurrent colicky abdominal pain in a child 6 months to 2 years of age. Barium enema will not only provide the diagnosis but will cure the intussusception in about 75% of cases, since hydrostatic reduction by barium enema is the treatment of choice for this disorder.

Treatment

The child with acute abdomen rapidly becomes dehydrated. Adequate therapy, including correction of electrolyte imbalance, should be started immediately.

For management of specific entities, see the individual discussions below.

Roy CC, Morin CL, Weber AM: Gastrointestinal emergency problems in paediatric practice. *Clin Gastroenterol* 1981; **10:**225.

ACUTE APPENDICITIS

Essentials of Diagnosis

- Diffuse, crampy abdominal pain, followed by right lower quadrant pain.
- Vomiting and constipation.
- Anorexia.
- Low-grade fever (38–38.5 °C [100.4–101.3 °F]).
- Right lower quadrant tenderness with rebound tenderness and, eventually, guarding.
- White blood cell count < 15,000/μL, with raised neutrophil levels.

General Considerations

Acute appendicitis increases in frequency with age and is most frequent between ages 15 and 30. Luminal obstruction by fecaliths (25%) or parasites is a predisposing factor.

The incidence of perforation is very high (40%) in infants and children and appears to be increasing. In order to avoid delay in diagnosis, it is important to maintain close communication with parents, perform a thorough physical examination and sequential examinations of the abdomen over a period of several hours, and interpret correctly the evolving symptoms and signs. No patient with acute abdominal pain and fever should be sent home without appropriate laboratory and x-ray examinations.

Clinical Findings

A. Symptoms and Signs: The triad of persistent localized right lower quadrant pain, localized abdominal tenderness, and slight fever is strongly suggestive of appendicitis. Anorexia, vomiting, and constipation also occur. The clinical picture is often atypical, ie, generalized pain, tenderness around the umbilicus, and no leukocytosis. Diarrhea can substitute for constipation, and a subsiding upper respiratory tract infection may be found. Rectal examination should always be done. Since many infections give rise to symptoms mimicking appendicitis and since physical findings are often inconclusive, it is important to repeat examinations of the abdomen.

B. Laboratory Findings: White blood cell counts are seldom higher than 15,000/μL.

C. X-Ray Findings: A radiopaque fecalith is reportedly present in two-thirds of cases of ruptured appendix. The value of barium enema examination in atypical cases remains controversial.

Differential Diagnosis

The presence of intrathoracic infection (eg, pneumonia) or urinary tract infection should be kept in mind, along with other medical and surgical conditions leading to acute abdomen (see above).

Treatment & Prognosis

Appendectomy is indicated whenever the diagnosis of appendicitis cannot be ruled out after a period of close observation. Postoperative antibiotic therapy directed to the treatment of anaerobes and coliforms is reserved for cases with gangrenous or perforated appendix.

The mortality rate is less than 1% in patients during childhood, despite the high incidence of perforation.

Doraiswamy NV: Progress of acute appendicitis: A study in children. *Br J Surg* 1978;**65:**877.

Fedyshin P, Kelvin FM, Rice RP: Nonspecificity of barium enema findings in acute appendicitis. *AJR* 1984;**143:**99.

Puri P, O'Donwell B: Appendicitis in infancy. *J Pediatr Surg* 1978;**13:**173.

Savrin RA, Clatworthy HW: Appendiceal rupture: A continuing diagnostic problem. *Pediatrics* 1979;**63:**37.

FOREIGN BODIES IN THE ALIMENTARY TRACT

Most foreign bodies pass through the esophagus and the rest of the gastrointestinal tract without difficulty, although anything longer than 3–5 cm may have difficulty passing the duodenal loop at the region of the ligament of Treitz. Foreign bodies in the esophagus require immediate attention. Coins may remain in the stomach for 2–3 months before spontaneous passage. Gastric outlet obstruction should be considered. Camera batteries that contain 45% potassium hydroxide are especially hazardous and should be removed endoscopically if present in the esophagus or in the stomach after 24 hours.

A reasonable rule is that if a foreign body remains distal to the pylorus in one location for longer than 5 days, surgical removal should be considered, especially if symptoms occur. Close observation and, preferably, hospitalization are urged for children who have swallowed open safety pins and long sharp objects (eg, toothpicks).

Esophagogastroscopy will permit the removal of the majority of foreign bodies lodged in the esophagus and stomach. A Foley catheter introduced into the esophagus may obviate the need for endoscopy, especially for removal of coins.

Campbell JB, Foley LC: A safe alternative to endoscopic removal of blunt esophageal foreign bodies. *Arch Otolaryngol* 1983;**109:**323.

Litovitz TL: Battery ingestions: Product accessibility and clinical course. *Pediatrics* 1985;**75:**469.

Nandi P, Ong GB: Foreign body in the esophagus: Review of 2394 cases. *Br J Surg* 1978;**65:**5.

TRAUMATIC INJURIES OF THE GASTROINTESTINAL TRACT

Etiology

A. Neonatal Period: Severe intra-abdominal injuries are rare in the newborn period. Listlessness, rapid respirations in conjunction with fullness of the abdomen, an abdominal mass, and rapidly developing anemia are characteristic symptoms. The incidence of trauma increases in proportion to the size of the infant and is perhaps higher in breech deliveries. A ruptured spleen usually gives rise to immediate signs. Subcapsular hematomas of the liver secondary to laceration of the liver are quite common, especially if there have been manual attempts at resuscitation. Kidney injuries give rise to retroperitoneal hematomas. Peritoneal taps are helpful in making a diagnosis and deciding whether emergency surgery is indicated. If the peritoneal fluid is bloody, immediate surgery may be required.

B. Childhood: The peak age for abdominal trauma is between 6 and 8 years of age. Blunt trauma is by far the most common form of abdominal injury. Trauma isolated to the abdomen is the result of a fall in 80% of cases. In cases where multiple injuries are present, traffic accidents are the usual cause (60%).

C. Adolescence: In the teenage years, the peak incidence for abdominal trauma is between 15 and 18 years of age. Penetrating injuries outnumber blunt trauma injuries. Nearly 50% of cases are caused by automobile accidents. Sports accidents account for only 20% of all injuries in this age group.

Clinical Findings

Abdominal trauma is found in many children brought to the hospital following serious injury. Blunt trauma gives rise to little external evidence of internal injury, and multiple injuries may distract the examiner from the abdominal injury. Solid organs are more seriously and frequently injured than hollow viscera. Contusion of the pancreas may lead to acute pancreatitis or, later, a pseudocyst. Intramural hematomas in the duodenum or at the duodenojejunal junction are frequently seen in the battered child syndrome.

Treatment

All children suffering abdominal trauma or serious injuries that may have resulted in damage to abdominal structures and organs should be admitted to an intensive care unit. An airway should be provided when necessary. If shock is present or likely to occur, a large-caliber intravenous catheter should be promptly inserted along with a central venous pressure line. A nasogastric tube should be used for continuous suction. If the patient is unconscious, endotracheal intubation and a Foley catheter are necessary. Close observation and monitoring are in order during the workup, which may include x-rays, ultrasonography, CT scanning of the chest and abdomen, radionuclide imaging, intravenous urography, abdominal lavage, and abdominal arteriography.

Feins NR: Multiple trauma. *Pediatr Clin North Am* 1979; **26:**759.

Gornall P et al: Intra-abdominal injuries in battered baby syndrome. *Arch Dis Child* 1972;**47:**211.

Talbert JL, Rogers BM: Acute abdominal injuries in children. *Pediatr Ann* 1976;**5:**36.

ANAL FISSURE

Anal fissure consists of a slitlike tear in the anal canal, usually secondary to the passage of large, hard, dry fecal masses. Anal stenosis and trauma can be contributory factors, as can a crypt abscess following gastroenteritis.

The infant or child cries with defecation and will try to hold back stools. Sparse, bright red bleeding is seen on the outside of the stool or on the toilet tissue following defecation. The fissure can often be seen if the patient is held in a knee-chest position and the buttocks spread apart.

When a fissure cannot be identified, it is essential to rule out other causes of rectal bleeding. If there is no history of constipation, the physician should consider juvenile polyp, perianal inflammation (due to group A streptococcal infection), or inflammatory bowel disease.

Anal fissures should be treated promptly, especially in infancy, to break the constipation-fissure-constipation cycle. A stool softener should be given and is usually effective against constipation. If this does not prove sufficient, 30 mL of mineral oil administered rectally with an ear syringe is advocated. The introduction of a gloved, lubricated finger twice daily lessens sphincter spasm. Hot sitz baths after defecation may be helpful. In rare cases, silver nitrate cauterization may be necessary. In protracted cases, surgery is indicated.

Beck AR, Turell R: Pediatric proctology. *Surg Clin North Am* 1972;**52:**1055.

INTUSSUSCEPTION

Essentials of Diagnosis

- Paroxysmal, episodic abdominal pain and vomiting.
- Sausage-shaped mass in upper abdomen.
- Rectal passage of bloody material (mucus and stool).
- Barium enema evidence of intussusception.

General Considerations

Intussusception is the most frequent cause of intestinal obstruction in the first 2 years of life. It is 3 times more common in males than in females. In most cases (85%) the cause is not apparent, although polyps, Meckel's diverticulum, Henoch-Schönlein purpura, lymphomas, lipomas, constipation, parasites, foreign bodies, or adenovirus or rotavirus infections with hypertrophy of Peyer's patches are predisposing factors. Intussusception is relatively common in cystic fibrosis and usually relates to inspissated fecal material in the terminal ileum and colon. In children older than age 6 years, lymphoma is the most common lesion. Intermittent small bowel intussusception is a cause of recurrent abdominal pain in untreated patients with celiac disease.

The intussusception usually starts just proximal to the ileocecal valve, so that invagination is ileocolic. Other forms include ileoileal and colocolic. Swelling, hemorrhage, incarceration with necrosis, and eventual perforation and peritonitis occur as a result of impairment of venous return.

Clinical Findings

Characteristically, a thriving infant 3–12 months of age suddenly develops periodic abdominal pain with screaming and drawing up of the knees. Vomiting occurs soon afterward (90% of cases), and bloody bowel movements with mucus appear within the next 12 hours (50%). Severe prostration and fever supervene, and the abdomen is tender and becomes distended. On palpation, a sausage-shaped tumor may be found in the early stages. In rare cases, the onset may be painless or with diarrhea. Some patients show signs of altered consciousness (''knocked-out look'') or may have seizures.

The intussusception can persist for several days when obstruction is not complete, and such cases may present as separate attacks of enterocolitis. In older children, sudden attacks of abdominal pain may be related to chronic recurrent intussusception with spontaneous reduction.

Treatment

A. Conservative Measures: A barium enema is a safe procedure if the following recommendations are observed:

1. No attempt should be made at hydrostatic reduction if there are clinical signs of strangulated bowel, perforation, or severe toxicity.

2. The barium solution should be allowed to drip by gravity through a Foley bag catheter inserted in the rectum from a height not more than 1 meter (3½ feet) above the fluoroscopy table.

3. There should be no manipulation of the abdomen during hydrostatic reduction under fluoroscopic examination, since this may increase intraluminal pressure and thus the risk of perforation.

4. Upon reduction, there should be free reflux of barium into the ileum; this is better elicited in a post-evacuation film, which should be repeated in 24 hours.

B. Surgical Measures: For patients not suitable for hydrostatic reduction or in whom it is unsuccessful (25%), surgery is required. This has the advantages of demonstrating any lead point (such as Meckel's diverticulum) and of a lower recurrence rate.

Prognosis

Intussusception is almost uniformly fatal if untreated. The prognosis relates to the duration of the intussusception before reduction. The mortality rate is 1–2%. The patient should be hospitalized, since intussusception recurs in 3–4% of patients, usually within 24 hours after reduction.

Ein SH: Leading points in childhood intussusception. *J Pediatr Surg* 1977;**12**:367.

Ein SH, Stephens CA, Minor A: Painless intussusception. *J Pediatr Surg* 1976;**11**:563.

Hutchison IF: Intussusception in infancy and childhood. *Br J Surg* 1980;**67**:209.

Singer J: Altered consciousness as an early manifestation of intussusception. *Pediatrics* 1979;**64**:93.

INGUINAL HERNIA

A peritoneal sac precedes the testicle as it descends from the genital ridge to the scrotum. The lower portion of this sac envelops the testis to form the tunica vaginalis, and the remainder normally atrophies by the time of birth. Persistence of the processus vaginalis presents as a mass in the inguinal region when an abdominal structure or peritoneal fluid is forced into it. The persistent sac may be very short or may extend into the scrotum. In some cases, peritoneal fluid may become trapped in the tunica vaginalis of the testis (noncommunicating hydrocele). If the processus vaginalis remains open, peritoneal fluid or an abdominal structure may be forced into it (indirect inguinal hernia).

Most inguinal hernias are of the indirect type and occur much more frequently in boys than in girls (9:1). Hernias may be present at birth or may appear at any age thereafter. The incidence in premature infants is close to 5%. In those weighing 1000 g or less, inguinal hernia is reported in 30%. In this weight group, girls are more commonly affected than boys.

Clinical Findings

There are no symptoms associated with an empty hernial sac. In most cases, the hernia is a painless inguinal swelling varying in size. There may be a history of inguinal fullness associated with coughing or long periods of standing; or there may be a firm, globular, and tender swelling, sometimes associated with vomiting and abdominal distention.

Spontaneous reduction frequently occurs while sleeping or with mild external pressure. In some instances, a herniated loop of intestine may become partially obstructed, leading to pain, irritability, and incomplete intestinal obstruction. More rarely, the loop of bowel becomes incarcerated, and signs of complete intestinal obstruction are present. Gangrene of the testis may occur; in the female, the ovary may prolapse into the hernial sac.

Inspection of the 2 inguinal areas may reveal a characteristic bulging or mass. Infants should be observed for evidence of swelling after crying and older children after bearing down.

A suggestive history is often the only criterion for diagnosis, along with the "silk glove" feel of the rubbing together of the 2 walls of the empty hernial sac.

Differential Diagnosis

An inguinal mass may represent lymph nodes. They are usually multiple and more discrete. Hydrocele of the cord transilluminates. An undescended testis may be moved along the canal and is associated with absence of the testicle in the scrotum.

Treatment

Surgery is indicated. There is still controversy about exploring the opposite side. Herniography is helpful in determining the patency of the processus vaginalis, but patency does not necessarily lead to a hernia.

Incarcerated inguinal hernias occur most often in the first 10 months of life and are more common in girls than in boys. Manipulative reduction can be attempted after placing the sedated infant in the Trendelenburg position with an ice bag on the affected side. This is contraindicated if the incarcerated hernia has been present for more than 12 hours or if bloody stools are noted.

Harper RG, Garcia A, Sia C: Inguinal hernia: A common problem of premature infants weighing 1000 grams or less at birth. *Pediatrics* 1975;**56:**112.

McGregor DB et al: The unilateral pediatric inguinal hernia: Should the contralateral side be explored? *J Pediatr Surg* 1980;**15:**313.

Viidik T, Marshall DG: Direct inguinal hernias in infancy and early childhood. *J Pediatr Surg* 1980;**15:**646.

UMBILICAL HERNIA

Umbilical hernias are more common in premature than in full-term infants. This defect is also more common in black infants.

Excessive thinning of the skin distended by the hernia and progressive enlargement of the fascial defects are rarely reported unless there is increased intra-abdominal pressure due to organomegaly or ascites. Incarceration is the only dangerous problem and is limited to smaller hernias.

Most umbilical hernias heal spontaneously if the fascial defect has a diameter of less than 1 cm. Large defects may still disappear without treatment, but seldom before school age. Large defects and smaller hernias persisting up to school age should be treated surgically. Reducing the hernia and strapping the skin do not accelerate the healing process.

Hale DE et al: Umbilical hernia: What happens after age 5 years. *J Pediatr* 1981;**98:**415.

TUMORS OF THE GASTROINTESTINAL TRACT

1. JUVENILE POLYPS

Large juvenile polyps are nearly always pedunculated and solitary, with a stalk covered in part by colonic mucosa. The chorion is hyperplastic, vascular, and inflamed. The glandular portion shows branching, irregular proliferation, and cystic transformation. The polyps are always benign. Eighty percent are within reach of the sigmoidoscope and are solitary.

Rarely, colonic polyps are present in large numbers, with anemia, diarrhea, and severe protein loss. There are a few cases of generalized gastrointestinal juvenile polyposis involving the stomach and both the small and large bowel, and these cases are associated with a slightly increased risk of cancer. In patients with Canada-Cronkhite syndrome, the polyposis is accompanied by alopecia, onychodystrophy, hyperpigmentation, and malabsorption.

Polyps are rare before age 1, and their incidence reaches a maximum frequency between 3 and 5 years of age. They are uncommon after age 15 because of autoamputation. They are more frequent in boys. Small amounts of bright red blood in the stools, intermittent melena, and occult painless gastrointestinal bleeding with anemia in otherwise well children are the most frequent manifestations. Abdominal pain is infrequent, but a juvenile polyp can be the lead point for an intussusception. Low-lying polyps may prolapse during defecation. Rectal examination, sigmoidoscopy, and barium enema are essential to a full exploration for polyps.

All polyps are now accessible by flexible fiberoptic colonoscopy and can be safely removed by electrocautery. If histology confirms that the growth is a juvenile polyp, nothing further should be done.

Except in rare cases of generalized gastrointestinal juvenile polyposis, the prognosis is excellent.

Erbe RW: Inherited gastrointestinal polyposis syndromes. *N Engl J Med* 1976;**294:**1101.

Grotosky HW et al: Familial juvenile polyposis coli: A clinical

and pathologic study of a large kindred. *Gastroenterology* 1982;**82:**494.
Silverberg SG: "Juvenile" retention polyps of the colon and rectum. *Dig Dis Sci* 1970;**15:**617.

2. FAMILIAL POLYPOSIS

Familial polyposis is characterized by the presence in the colon of large numbers of adenomatous polyps varying in size from mucosal excrescences to large stalked polyps. A family history is obtained in roughly two-thirds of cases, and the entity is transmitted genetically as a dominant with reduced penetrance. Carcinoma of the colon usually develops before age 40, or approximately 15 years after onset of symptoms.

The disease has been identified in infants but is more likely to become symptomatic in the late teens. Diarrhea is usually the first symptom. Blood loss, anemia, and abdominal pain usually supervene. The initial symptoms may be those of carcinomatosis.

Sigmoidoscopy reveals great numbers of polyps of various sizes. Barium enema reveals a normal bowel wall but a great number of filling defects.

All members of the family should be carefully examined. Subtotal colectomy has been recommended, but many authors believe that keeping the rectal stump is dangerous, since carcinoma may develop despite frequent observation of the stump. Ileoanal pull-through or proctocolectomy with an ileostomy is the treatment of choice, since any individual with familial polyposis will eventually develop carcinoma of the colon if untreated.

Fazio VW: Polyposis coli and hereditary colon cancer. Pages 348–359 in: *Current Therapy in Gastroenterology and Liver Disease 1984–1985*. Bayless TM (editor). Mosby, 1984.
Jagelman DG: Familial polyposis coli. *Surg Clin North Am* 1983;**63:**117.

3. PEUTZ-JEGHERS SYNDROME

The polyps in this syndrome are classified as hamartomas. They may occur anywhere between the cardiac sphincter and the anus but are present most often in the small intestine. The presence of perioral, lip, and buccal mucosal pigmentation helps establish the diagnosis; it usually appears at birth or in infancy and has a tendency to lessen at puberty. The syndrome is inherited as an autosomal dominant trait.

Colicky abdominal pain, anemia, and gastrointestinal hemorrhage are common symptoms. Intussusception may occur when polyps are large.

Conservative treatment is advocated. Symptomatic and accessible lesions should be removed by colonoscopy or surgery. Carcinomatous change is reported but rare (2–3% of cases).

Howell J et al: Peutz-Jeghers polyps causing colocolic intussusception in infancy. *J Pediatr Surg* 1981;**16:**82.
Yosowitz P et al: Sporadic Peutz-Jeghers syndrome in early childhood. *Am J Dis Child* 1974;**128:**709.

4. GARDNER'S SYNDROME

This is a dominantly inherited condition consisting of soft tissue and bone tumors associated with multiple intestinal polyps predisposed to malignant change. The large bowel is the most common site of involvement. Management is similar to that described for familial polyposis.

Naylor EW, Lebenthal E: Early detection of adenomatous polyposis coli in Gardner's syndrome. *Pediatrics* 1979;**63:**222.

5. CANCER OF THE SMALL & LARGE INTESTINES

The most common small bowel cancer in children is lymphosarcoma. Intermittent abdominal pain, an abdominal mass, evidence of intussusception, or a celiaclike picture may be present. Long-term survivals are reported in patients without lymph node involvement at surgery.

Small carcinoid tumors of the appendix in children are not aggressive regardless of the degree of invasion. However, carcinoid tumors of the ileum may metastasize.

Adenocarcinoma of the colon is rare in the pediatric age group. The transverse colon and rectosigmoid are the 2 most commonly affected sites. The low 5-year survival rate has to do with the nonspecificity of presenting complaints and the large percentage of undifferentiated types. Children with a family history of cancer and chronic ulcerative colitis or familial polyposis are at greater risk but seldom develop cancer before age 15. Cancer of the colon usually develops in a previously intact colon.

Aiges HW et al: Adenocarcinoma of the colon in an adolescent with the family cancer syndrome. *J Pediatr* 1979;**94:**632.
Andersson A, Bergdahl L: Carcinoma of the colon in children: A report of six new cases and a review of the literature. *J Pediatr Surg* 1976;**11:**967.
Gray GM et al: Lymphomas involving the gastrointestinal tract. *Gastroenterology* 1982;**82:**143.
Katzka I et al: Assessment of colorectal cancer risk in patients with ulcerative colitis: Experience from a private practice. *Gastroenterology* 1983;**85:**22.

6. MESENTERIC CYSTS

These rare tumors may be small or large, single or multiloculated. Invariably thin-walled, they contain either serous, chylous, or hemorrhagic fluid. They are commonly located in the mesentery of the small intestine but may also be seen in the mesocolon.

The majority are asymptomatic. Traction on the mesentery eventually leads to colicky abdominal pain, which can be mild and recurrent but may present acutely with vomiting. Volvulus is reported, as is hemorrhage into the cyst. A rounded mass can occasionally be palpated or can be seen on x-ray to displace adjacent intestine. Abdominal ultrasonography is usually diagnostic.

Surgical removal is indicated.

Caropreso PR: Mesenteric cysts. *Arch Surg* 1974;**108**:242.

Christensen JA et al: Mesenteric cysts. *Am Surg* 1975;**41**:352.

7. INTESTINAL HEMANGIOMA

Hemangiomas of the bowel may be a source of acute or chronic blood loss and anemia. They may also cause intestinal obstruction by triggering intussusception, by local stricture, or by intramural hematoma formation. Thrombocytopenia and consumptive coagulopathy are occasional systemic complications. Some lesions are telangiectasias (Rendu-Osler-Weber syndrome), and others are capillary hemangiomas. However, the largest group consists of cavernous hemangiomas, which are large, thin-walled vessels arising from the submucosal vascular plexus. They may protrude into the lumen as polypoid lesions or may invade the intestine from mucosa to serosa.

Abrahamson J, Shandling B: Intestinal hemangiomata in childhood and a syndrome for diagnosis: A collective review. *J Pediatr Surg* 1973;**8**:487.

Mestre JR, Andres JM: Hereditary hemorrhagic telangiectasia causing hematemesis in an infant. *J Pediatr* 1982;**101**:577.

DIARRHEAL DISEASES*

Diarrhea may be defined as water and electrolyte malabsorption leading to accelerated excretion of intestinal contents. What constitutes diarrhea is sometimes difficult to define in terms of number or consistency of stools because there are wide variations in colonic function. Some infants may pass one firm stool every second to third day, whereas others may have 5–8 soft small stools daily. A gradual or sudden increase in the number of stools, a reduction in their consistency coupled with an increase in their fluid content (> 15g/kg/d), and a tendency for the stools to be green are more important factors.

Diarrhea may result from any of the following closely related pathogenetic mechanisms: (1) interruption of normal cell transport processes; (2) decrease in the surface area available for absorption, which may be due to shortening of the bowel or mucosal disease; (3) increase in intestinal motility; (4) presence in the intestine of large amounts of unabsorbable osmotically active molecules; and (5) abnormal increase in gastric or intestinal permeability, leading to increased secretion of water and electrolytes.

The physiologic consequences of diarrhea vary with its severity and duration, the age of the patient and state of nutrition prior to onset, and the presence or absence of associated symptoms. Acute diarrhea may lead to dehydration and acid-base disturbances (see Chapter 36), while chronic diarrhea is more likely to be associated with malnutrition as a consequence of malabsorption or insufficient intake of nutrients.

The differential diagnosis of chronic diarrhea is difficult, and the listing of causes in Table 19–4 is not necessarily complete. Note that a few microorganisms can cause subacute or chronic diarrhea.

* Epidemic diarrhea of the newborn is discussed in Chapter 3; diarrhea due to viral infections, in Chapter 26; diarrhea due to bacterial infections, in Chapter 27; and diarrhea due to parasitic infections, in Chapter 28.

Causes of Diarrhea Other Than Infectious

A. Antibiotic Therapy: Antibiotics such as ampicillin, neomycin, and tetracyclines commonly give rise to diarrhea. They lead to decreased glucose absorption and disaccharidase activity. In a clinical setting where a bacterial infection has been ruled out, they should be stopped and a lactose-free diet administered. At times, antibiotics may give rise to the overgrowth of a species of *Clostridium difficile* whose toxin is responsible for pseudomembranous colitis.

B. Parenteral Infections: Infections of the urinary tract and upper respiratory tract (especially otitis media) are at times associated with diarrhea, although the actual mechanism remains obscure. In the opinion of several investigators, a concomitant intestinal infection is likely.

C. Malnutrition: Malnutrition may lead to diarrhea because of an increased occurrence of enteral infections in malnourished children. Decreased disaccharidase activity, altered motility, or changes in the intestinal flora may be other factors.

D. Diet: Dietary causes of diarrhea are numerous. Overfeeding of a colicky infant is a common example. Introduction of new foods, such as fruit juices, egg yolk, vegetables, etc, can cause diarrhea. Intestinal irritants (spices and foods high in roughage) are also frequent offenders.

E. Allergic Diarrhea: Diarrhea caused by gastrointestinal allergy to dietary proteins is a frequently entertained diagnosis but a poorly documented clinical entity except in cases of milk sensitivity, which is discussed separately.

Irritable Colon Syndrome

Chronic nonspecific diarrhea of childhood is the most common type of diarrhea in the otherwise well and thriving child. The typical patient is a child 6–20 months of age who was a colicky baby and who starts having 3–6 loose mucoid stools per day during the waking hours. The child is active, looks healthy, has a good appetite, and is growing normally. The diarrhea worsens with a low-residue, low-fat, or high-carbohydrate diet and during periods of stress and infection. It clears spontaneously at about 3½ years of age. No organic disease is discoverable. The patho-

Table 19–4. Guide to differential diagnosis of chronic diarrhea in infants and children.

Disease	Age	Type of Diarrhea	Associated Clinical Features	Effects on Well-Being and Growth
Infections and infestations				
Salmonella, Yersinia, Campy-lobacter	Any age	Watery; may contain mucus, pus, and blood	Pain, vomiting, fever	Chronic foms are unusual but may lead to significant weight loss
Giardia lamblia	Any age	Bulky, pale, malodorous, often nocturnal	Abdominal distention, flatulence, anorexia	Failure to thrive, especially if associated immune defect
Parenteral infections				
Otitis media and urinary tract infection	< 2 yr	Usually mild	Symptoms of the underlying infection may be minimal	Vary with severity of infection
Postinfectious diarrhea (Carbohydrate intolerance, malnutrition)	< 2 yr	Can be severe if large carbohydrate intake or malnutrition	Clinical picture of carbohydrate intolerance or marasmus	Malnutrition often iatrogenic, ie, secondary to "starvation" diets
Dietary factors				
Overfeeding	< 6 mo	Watery	Colicky baby	None; baby is often fat
Milk protein allergy; soy protein allergy	< 2 mo	Watery to fatty; at times, mucus and blood	Vomiting, anemia; peripheral edema is rare	Mild (anemia) to severe (celiaclike)
Intolerance to certain foods	< 6 mo	Watery	Follows introduction of new foods	None
Acrodermatitis enteropathica	<12 mo	Severe in most	Alopecia, dermatitis, conjunctivitis, vomiting	Malnutrition
Primary bile acid malabsorption	< 1 mo	Intractable diarrhea	Dehydration, wasting	Failure to thrive
Irritable colon syndrome	6–36 mo	Watery, abundant; mucus, undigested foods	None; often follows a bout of acute diarrhea and vomiting	None unless iatrogenic
Toxic diarrhea (Antibiotics, iron preparations, chemotherapy, radiation)	Any age	Loose; may contain modest amount of fat	Vomiting, anorexia	In the case of radiation enterocolitis, malnutrition may be severe
Functional tumors (Neuroblastoma, Zollinger-Ellison syndrome, carcinoid, pancreatic cholera)	Any age	Severe, secretory diarrhea	Large spectrum of symptoms and signs; hypokalemia common	Variable
Carbohydrate malabsorption				
Congenital Sucrose-isomaltose	< 6 mo	Varies with sucrose intake	Abdominal distention and pain, flatulence	Poor growth common if early onset
Glucose-galactose	< 1 mo	Watery, intractable	Dehydration, acidosis	Failure to thrive
Acquired lactose intolerance	4–8 yr	Loose to watery	Abdominal pain, flatulence	Normal growth
Secondary Lactose	Any age	Watery	Follows intestinal infections	Variable
Glucose-galactose	< 2 yr	Severe, watery	After surgery, infections, stagnant loop syndrome	Dehydration, acidosis
Pancreatic disorders				
Cystic fibrosis	< 6 mo	Fatty	Repeated chest infections	Failure to thrive
Shwachman syndrome	< 2 yr	Fatty	Neutropenia, bone lesions	Variable degree of growth impairment
Chronic pancreatitis	Any age	Usually a late complication	Recurrent abdominal pain with vomiting	Variable degree of growth impairment
Celiac disease	< 2 yr	Mild to severe	Vomiting, anorexia, abdominal distention	Failure to thrive

Table 19–4 (cont'd). Guide to differential diagnosis of chronic diarrhea in infants and children.

Disease	Age	Type of Diarrhea	Associated Clinical Features	Effects on Well-Being and Growth
Intestinal lymphangiectasia	< 3 mo	Mild to severe with fatty stools	Infections, vomiting, lymphedema	Failure to thrive
Immune defects				
Acquired dysgammaglobulinemia and isolated IgA deficiency	Any age	Varying severity; often celiac syndrome	Recurrent sinopulmonary infections	Growth impairment
Defective cellular immunity	< 2 yr	Severe with fat malabsorption	Feeding difficulties, skin rash, stomatitis, repeated infections	Desperately ill with severe failure to thrive
Combined immune deficiency	< 1 mo			
Inborn errors				
Familial chloridorrhea	< 1 mo	Profuse, watery	Abdominal distention, alkalosis	Growth usually retarded
Abeta- and hypobetalipoproteinemia	< 3 mo	Fatty	Abdominal distention, CNS disease	Failure to thrive
Wolman's disease	< 1 mo	Severe, fatty	Vomiting, large liver	Severe malnutrition
Malabsorption of folic acid	< 1 mo	Watery	Severe anemia, stomatitis, seizures	Failure to thrive and mental retardation
Galactosemia, tyrosinosis	< 3 mo	Not invariably present	Vomiting, large liver, icterus, seizures	Failure to thrive
Anatomic abnormalities				
Congenital				
Malrotation, partial small or large bowel obstruction, short bowel	< 3 mo	Intractable diarrhea; may be celiaclike	Vomiting, abdominal distention	Failure to thrive
Acquired				
Blind or stagnant loop syndrome	Any age	Severe with carbohydrate and lipid malabsorption	History of surgery; vomiting, abdominal distention	Significant stunting of growth and malnutrition
Chronic intestinal pseudo-obstruction	Usually > 4 yr	Bouts of obstipation with chronic diarrhea	Recurrent bouts of intestinal obstruction	Progressive weight loss and growth impairment
Lymphosarcoma	> 4 yr	Loose and celiaclike	Crampy pain, intussusception	Weight loss and anemia
Familial polyposis	Teenagers	Loose, with blood	Abdominal pain, anemia	None unless cancer develops
Inflammatory bowel disease				
Crohn's disease	Usually > 10 yr	Loose stools, often nocturnal	Pain more severe in Crohn's; tenesmus more severe in chronic ulcerative colitis; anorexia, fever, extraintestinal manifestations often predominant in Crohn's	Growth retardation severe in Crohn's and less pronounced in chronic ulcerative colitis; delayed puberty.
Chronic ulcerative colitis	Usually > 10 yr	Diarrhea with blood; nocturnal		
Intractable diarrhea of early infancy (nonspecific enterocolitis)	< 3 mo	Explosive watery diarrhea	Vomiting and fever common at onset	Cachexia
Hirschsprung's enterocolitis	<1 yr	Pea soup and putrid	Abdominal distention, vomiting, fever, and periods of obstipation	Toxic, failure to thrive
Eosinophilic gastroenteritis	Any age	Watery and at times severe	Vomiting; eczema and asthma common	Failure to thrive common in infants
Malnutrition and maternal deprivation	< 1 yr	Loose stools	Apathy, lethargy; abnormal affect, signs of battering	Retarded growth and neuromotor development
Endocrinopathies				
Hyperthyroidism	Any age	Watery	Signs of hyperthyroidism	Accelerated bone age
Congenital adrenal hyperplasia	< 1 mo	Watery	Vomiting usually predominates	Failure to thrive

genesis of the disease remains obscure but may be related to infections. A high familial incidence of functional bowel disease is observed. Stool culture, assay for *C difficile* toxin, pH testing, and microscopy for *Giardia* should always be carried out.

The following measures are helpful: institution of a high-fat, low-carbohydrate, high-fiber diet; avoidance of between-meal snacks; and avoidance of chilled fluids, especially hyperosmolar fruit juices. Early toilet training is recommended. It may be helpful to give loperamide (Imodium), 0.1–0.2 mg/kg/d in 2–3 divided doses; cholestyramine (Questran), 2–4 g with breakfast; or psyllium agents, 1–2 tsp twice daily.

Greene HL, Ghishan FK: Excessive fluid intake as a cause of chronic diarrhea in young children. *J Pediatr* 1983;**102:**836.

Jonas A, Diver-Haber A: Stool output and composition in the chronic non-specific diarrhoea syndrome. *Arch Dis Child* 1982;**57:**35.

Lloyd-Still JD: Chronic diarrhoea of childhood and the misuse of elimination diets. *J Pediatr* 1979;**95:**10.

Intractable Diarrhea of Early Infancy

A. Symptoms and Signs: Onset is in the first 3–6 months of life. The initial phase is sometimes mistaken for a feeding problem. In most cases, however, it mimics infectious diarrhea with loose, greenish stools. The stools are rarely grossly bloody, but microscopic blood is often present. Vomiting and abdominal distention may suggest an underlying obstructive lesion. Dehydration, acidosis, and malnutrition rapidly supervene. After "resting the gastrointestinal tract" by means of intravenous therapy, resumption of oral feedings often precipitates a recurrence.

B. Diagnosis: Conditions such as enterocolitis associated with Hirschsprung's disease, cystic fibrosis, intestinal stenosis, malrotation, blind loop syndrome, short small bowel syndrome, allergic gastroenteropathy, celiac disease, disaccharidase deficiency, immunologic defects, vasoactive intestinal peptide, tumor, gastrinoma, lymphangiectasia, adrenogenital syndrome, neural crest tumors, glucose-galactose malabsorption, primary bile acid malabsorption, sepsis, urinary tract infections, and chloridorrhea may all lead to intractable diarrhea.

These diagnoses and infectious gastroenteritis can be verified or ruled out by the following emergency workup: (1) stool cultures (3 of them); (2) stool pH; (3) tests for fecal blood and reducing substances; (4) barium enema and upper gastrointestinal x-ray with small bowel follow-through; (5) blood count with small lymphocyte count; (6) blood pH and electrolytes; (7) sweat chloride test; (8) stool chymotrypsin; (9) protein electrophoresis and serum immunoglobulins; (10) rectosigmoidoscopy and rectal suction biopsy; and (11) small bowel biopsy.

If these conditions are ruled out in a young infant who still has diarrhea after 3 weeks and is steadily losing weight, a primary type of intractable diarrhea (nonspecific enterocolitis) becomes the most likely diagnosis.

C. Treatment: Fasting is recommended during the first few days while blood volume, electrolyte, and acid-base disturbances are repaired. A formula such as Pregestimil can be offered at a low concentration and in small volume while peripheral or central alimentation is continued. Continuous nasogastric feeding has distinct advantages as a means of providing a larger volume (200–250 mL/kg/d) at a lower osmolality (200–250 mosm/kg water). Breast milk has occasionally been used with some measure of success. Antidiarrheal medication, corticosteroids, and cholestyramine (Questran) have not been shown to be useful. Unfortunately, extended periods of parenteral nutrition are commonly necessary.

D. Prognosis: Although the outcome of this severe and challenging affliction has changed dramatically, morbidity rates are high, and the course is often unpredictable.

Larcher VF et al: Protracted diarrhoea in infancy: Analysis of 82 cases with particular reference to diagnosis and management. *Arch Dis Child* 1977;**52:**597.

Lo CW, Walker WA: Chronic protracted diarrhea of infancy: A nutritional disease. *Pediatrics* 1983;**72:**786.

MacLean WC Jr: Nutritional management of chronic diarrhea and malnutrition: Primary reliance on oral feeding. *J Pediatr* 1980;**97:**316.

Rossi TM et al: Extent and duration of small intestinal mucosal injury in intractable diarrhea of infancy. *Pediatrics* 1980;**66:**730.

CONSTIPATION

Constipation is the regular passage of firm or hard stools or of small, hard masses at long intervals. It may be accompanied by fecal soiling or encopresis. Familial, cultural, and social factors influence the genesis, development, and course. Psychologic factors, toilet-training techniques, diet (particularly excessive milk intake), overuse of laxatives, and enemas may also influence bowel habits. Neurologic (spinal cord lesions) and anatomic (anorectal) disorders, along with mental retardation, hypothyroidism, and hypercalcemia, are all well-known causes of constipation.

Clinical Findings

Many symptoms, such as fever, convulsions, nervousness, school failure, bad breath, and the like have been improperly attributed to constipation.

A. Simple Constipation: The infant often appears to be having difficulty passing a stool. The child's face may turn red and the legs are drawn up on the abdomen even when the stool passed is quite soft. This pattern may be erroneously considered to be an indication of constipation. Similarly, the infant 6–12 months of age may become flushed, withdraw the legs, and act as though there is a great deal of

Table 19–5. Causes of constipation.*

Idiopathic or constitutional causes	Abnormalities of myenteric ganglion cells
Dietary causes	Hirschsprung's disease
Undernutrition	Hypo- and hyperganglionosis
Protracted vomiting	Recklinghausen's disease
Excessive milk intake	Multiple endocrine neoplasia type IIB
Lack of bulk	Absence of abdominal musculature
Drug and cathartic abuse	Spinal cord defects
Structural defects of gastrointestinal tract	Metabolic and endocrine disorders
Anus and rectum	Hypothyroidism
Fissure, hemorrhoids, abscess	Hyperparathyroidism
Anterior location of anus	Renal tubular acidosis
Anal and rectal stenosis	Diabetes insipidus
Presacral teratoma	Vitamin D intoxication
Rectal prolapse	Idiopathic hypercalcemia
Small bowel and colon	Neurologic and psychiatric conditions
Tumor, stricture	Myotonic dystrophy
Chronic volvulus	Amyotonia congenita
Intussusception	Brain tumors
Internal hernia	Mental retardation
Smooth muscle diseases of gastrointestinal tract	Psychosis
Scleroderma and dermatomyositis	
Systemic lupus erythematosus	
Chronic intestinal pseudo-obstruction	

* Reproduced, with permission, from Silverman A, Roy CC: *Pediatric Clinical Gastroenterology,* 3rd ed. Mosby, 1983.

difficulty in passing a bowel movement when in fact the infant is attempting to withhold a stool. Failure to appreciate this normal developmental pattern may lead to the unwise use of laxatives or enemas. As children become ambulatory, many new and exciting activities interfere with the response to the "call to stool"; they may pass enough stool to relieve the pressure while continuing to play, or they may gradually develop an effective capacity to ignore the sensation of rectal fullness. In older children, school, games, social events, and factors such as inadequately cleaned toilets may all interfere with the development of any pattern of regularity.

B. Constipation With Encopresis: Psychogenic constipation is characterized by constant or intermittent "involuntary" seepage of feces when there is a mass of feces in the rectal ampulla and sigmoid colon. Children with psychogenic constipation prefer to soil themselves rather than pass large painful stools. In some cases, these children suffer from emotional problems that commonly disappear with relief of the constipation. In other cases, fecal soiling is a manifestation of an underlying emotional disturbance.

Differential Diagnosis

Constipation is prevalent among mentally retarded children with associated motor deficits and in those with hypothyroidism. Causes of constipation are listed in Table 19–5.

Distinguishing features from Hirschsprung's disease are summarized in Table 19–6. Rare cases of short-segment aganglionosis may present with symptoms and signs suggestive of chronic constipation with encopresis.

Treatment

A. Simple Constipation: A reduction of milk intake and increase of high-residue foods such as bran, whole wheat, fruits, and vegetables are usually curative. The use of a barley malt extract such as Maltsupex, 1–2 tsp added to feedings 2 or 3 times daily, is helpful in small infants. Stool softeners such as dioctyl sodium sulfosuccinate (Colace), 5–10 mg/kg/d, prevent excessive drying of the stool and are effective unless there is voluntary stool retention. Cathartics such as standardized extract of senna fruit (Senokot syrup), 1–2 tsp twice daily depending on age, can be used for short periods of time.

B. Constipation With Encopresis: Remove the fecal impaction by hypertonic phosphate enemas (Fleet enema) after overnight retention of 3–4 oz of mineral oil. A daily enema is advocated for the first week.

Mineral oil in orange juice should be given in amounts sufficient initially (15–60 mL twice daily)

Table 19–6. Differentiation of constipation and Hirschsprung's disease.

	Constipation	Hirschsprung's Disease
Onset	2–3 years	At birth
Abdominal distention	Rarely	Present
Nutritional growth	Normal	Poor
Soiling	Intermittent or constant	Never
Rectal examination	Ampulla full	Ampulla empty

to lead to incontinence; then reduce so that 2–3 loose stools are passed daily for a period of 6 months.

The prevention of stool holding and the establishment of a regular soft bowel movement pattern are accomplished by "toileting" the child at regular times each day and by the continued administration of mineral oil over a period of several months in a reduced dosage. A double dose of water-soluble vitamins is recommended while mineral oil is administered. After this initial phase, a stool softener (Colace, 5–10 mg/kg/24 h) should be administered on a chronic basis, but this should not begin until regular toilet habits have been acquired.

Psychiatric consultation may be indicated for patients with recurrent symptoms or overt, severe emotional disturbances.

Clayden GS, Lawson JO: Investigation and management of long-standing chronic constipation in childhood. *Arch Dis Child* 1976;**51:**918.

Fitzgerald JF: Difficulties with defecation and elimination in children. *Clin Gastroenterol* 1977;**6:**283.

Olness K, McParland FA, Piper J: Biofeedback: A new modality in the management of children with fecal soiling. *J Pediatr* 1980;**96:**505.

Schmitt BD: Encopresis. *Primary Care* 1984;**11:**497.

GASTROINTESTINAL BLEEDING

Vomiting or rectal evacuation of blood is an alarming symptom. The history should provide detailed answers to the following questions:

(1) *Is it really blood and is it coming from the gastrointestinal tract?* A number of substances may simulate hematochezia or melena; therefore, the presence of blood should be confirmed chemically (Hematest tablet). Information concerning genitourinary problems, coughing, or epistaxis may identify a source of bleeding elsewhere than in the gastrointestinal tract.

(2) *How much blood is there and what is its color and character?* Table 19–7 lists the sites of gastrointestinal bleeding in relationship to the amount and the appearance of the blood in the stools. Tables 19–8 and 19–9 list clinical causes of hematemesis and rectal bleeding.

(3) *Is the child acutely or chronically ill?* The physical examination should be thorough no matter how ill the patient is. Alertness to signs of portal hypertension, intestinal obstruction, or blood dyscrasia is particularly important. The nasal passages should be inspected for signs of recent epistaxis; the vagina for menstrual blood; and the anus for fissures and hemorrhoids.

A systolic blood pressure below 100 mm Hg and a pulse rate above 100/min in an older child suggest at least a 20% reduction of blood volume. A pulse rate increase of 20/min or a drop in systolic blood pressure greater than 10 mm Hg when the patient sits up is also a sensitive index of significant volume depletion.

Table 19–7. Identification of sites of gastrointestinal bleeding.

Symptom or Sign	Location of Bleeding Lesion
Effortless welling forth of bright red blood from the mouth	Esophageal varices; lacerations of gastric mucosa (Mallory-Weiss syndrome).
Vomiting of bright red blood or of "coffee grounds"	Lesion proximal to ligament of Treitz.
Melena	Lesion proximal to ligament of Treitz. Blood loss in excess of 50–100 mL/24 h.
Bright red or dark red blood in stools	Lesion in the ileum or colon. (Massive upper gastrointestinal bleeding may also be associated with bright red blood in stool.)
Streak of blood on outside of a stool	Lesion in the rectal ampulla or anal canal.

(4) *Is the child still bleeding?* A determination of vital signs every 15 minutes is essential to assess ongoing bleeding. Serial hematocrits are useful; remember, however, that plasma expansion subsequent to a loss of red cell mass may be delayed for hours and sometimes for days.

The most important maneuver for the assessment of the origin and severity of gastrointestinal bleeding is the introduction of a Levin tube in the stomach. Detection of blood in the gastric aspirate confirms a bleeding site proximal to the ligament of Treitz. However, its absence does not rule out the duodenum as the source.

Management

A hemorrhagic diathesis should be ruled out, and vitamin K should be given intravenously. In severe bleeding, needs for volume replacement are monitored by measurement of central venous pressure. In less severe cases, vital signs, serial hematocrits, and gastric aspirates are sufficient.

If blood is recovered from the gastric aspirate, gastric lavage with saline should be performed for 30–60 minutes, until only a blood-tinged return is obtained. Panendoscopy is then done and is particularly useful for identifying an active bleeding site; it is superior to barium contrast study for lesions such as esophageal varices, stress ulcers, and gastritis. In cases in which there has been no clinical evidence of ongoing bleeding during the 48 hours preceding admission, the upper gastrointestinal series is usually carried out as the initial diagnostic procedure. It is followed by the endoscopic procedure if the lesion is unidentified radiologically.

Except for Meckel's diverticulum and hemangiomas, most bleeding small bowel lesions also produce signs and symptoms suggesting intestinal obstruction.

Table 19–8. Causes of hematemesis in infants and children.*

Entity	Age	Amount of Blood	Clinical Features	Cause	Diagnostic Procedure
Swallowed maternal blood	Newborn	Variable	No other signs of illness	Delivery	Apt-Downey test
Stress ulcer	Any age	Large	Sickly appearance, pale; shock	CNS disease, sepsis, asphyxia	Endoscopy, nasogastric tube
Hemorrhagic gastritis	Newborn	Large	Sickly appearance, pale; shock	CNS disease, sepsis, asphyxia	Endoscopy, nasogastric tube
Hemorrhagic disease of newborn	Newborn	Variable	Melena, bleeding elsewhere	Vitamin K deficiency, liver disease, clotting defect	Clotting studies
Gastric volvulus	Newborn, infancy	Small	Intractable vomiting	Congenital defect, eventration of diaphragm	Upper gastrointestinal series
Peptic disease	Any age	Large	Relatively good health, vomiting, pain	Duodenal or antral ulcer	Endoscopy, upper gastrointestinal series
Esophageal varices	Any age	Large	Chronic illness or good health	Portal hypertension	Esophagoscopy
Peptic esophagitis	Any age	Small	Dysphagia, chronic vomiting	Incompetence of lower esophageal sphincter	pH monitoring
Foreign body	Infancy to later childhood	Small	Dysphagia	Large variety	Esophagoscopy and esophagography, plain films, endoscopy
Gastric outlet obstruction	Any age	Small	Vomiting, failure to thrive	Peptic disease, hypertrophic pyloric stenosis, malformations	Upper gastrointestinal series
Erosive gastritis or esophagitis	Any age	Small	Vomiting, pain, dysphagia	Ingestion of acids, alkali, iron, aspirin	Endoscopy
Gastritis	Any age	Small	Protracted vomiting	Infection, bile reflux	Endoscopy
Mallory-Weiss syndrome	Preschool to adolescence	Moderate to large	Retching, vomiting	Increased intraesophageal pressure	Esophagoscopy
Swallowed blood	Any age	Moderate to large	Nausea, epistaxis	Bleeding from mouth, gums, ears, nose, or throat	History taking

* Reproduced, with permission, from Silverman A, Roy CC: *Pediatric Clinical Gastroenterology,* 3rd ed. Mosby, 1983.

Table 19–9. Differential diagnosis and treatment of rectal bleeding in infants and children.

Cause	Usual Age Group	Additional Complaints	Amount of Blood	Color of Blood	Blood With Movement	Treatment
Swallowed foreign body	Any age	Usually none	Small	Dark	Yes	Surgery may be necessary
Systemic bleeding	Any age	Other evidence of bleeding	Variable	Dark or bright	Yes or no	As indicated
Hemorrhagic disease of the newborn	Newborn	Other evidence of bleeding	Variable	Dark or bright	Yes or no	Vitamin K_1, transfusion
Milk intolerance	Infants	Colicky abdominal pain	Moderate to large	Dark or bright	Yes	Eliminate allergen
Esophageal varices	> 4 years	Signs of portal hypertension	Variable	Usually dark	Yes	Medical initially; sometimes emergency surgery
Hemangioma or familial telangiectasia	Any age	Often telangiectasia elsewhere	Variable	Dark or bright	Yes or no	Usually none
Peptic ulcer	Any age	Abdominal pain	Usually small; can be massive	Dark	Yes	Bland diet
Duplication of bowel	Any age	Variable	Usually small	Usually dark	Yes	Surgery
Meckel's diverticulum	Young adult	None or anemia	Small to large; usually large	Dark or bright	Yes or no	Surgery
Volvulus	Infant or young child	Abdominal pain, intestinal obstruction	Small to large	Dark or bright	Yes or no	Surgery
Intussusception	< 18 months	Abdominal pain, mass	Small to large	Dark or bright	Yes	Surgery
Ulcerative colitis	> 4 years	Diarrhea, cramps	Small to large	Usually bright	Yes	Usually medical
Bacterial enteritis	Any age	Diarrhea, cramps	Small to large	Usually bright	Yes	Medical
Polyp	2–8 years	None	Small to large	Bright	No	Surgery
Inserted foreign body	Child	Pain	Small	Bright	No	Removal
Anal fissure or proctitis	< 2 years	Pain	Small	Bright	No	Soften stool, anal dilation, habit training
Swallowed maternal blood	Newborn	None	Variable	Dark	Yes	None
Hiatal hernia	Any age	Dysphagia, hematemesis	Usually small	Dark	Yes	Medical or surgical
Henoch-Schönlein purpura	3–10 years	Purpuric rash, arthritis, abdominal pain, hematuria	Variable	Dark	Yes	Medical or surgical
Lymphoid nodular hyperplasia	3–24 months	Loose stools	Small	Bright	Yes	None; corticosteroids by enema or systemically

A plain film of the abdomen and a barium enema should be done in such cases prior to laparotomy. If there is no obstruction and the bleeding seemingly comes from the colon or lower ileum, rectosigmoidoscopy and colonoscopy are done prior to barium enema. In the case of a nonobstructing small or large bowel lesion that bleeds actively and briskly (> 0.5 mL/min), angiography may be diagnostic. Scintigraphic scanning of the abdomen after injection of labeled red cells may be helpful.

The patient with upper gastrointestinal bleeding should be maintained in a semisitting position and a calm environment. Sedation is contraindicated. Ongoing bleeding is an indication for vasopressin, 20 units/1.73 m^2 intravenously over a 20-minute period. After that it may be necessary to sustain the infusion for 24 hours at a rate of 0.2–0.4 unit/1.73 m^2/min. It is rarely necessary to use a pediatric Sengstaken-Blakemore tube in cases of bleeding esophageal varices. Sclerotherapy of the varices is the treatment of choice.

The challenging patients are those with cirrhosis and abnormal clotting mechanisms. Emergency shunt operations are at times inevitable. Surgical treatment is also warranted in peptic disease and stress ulcers when severe ongoing bleeding continues over several days despite conservative management.

Hyams JS, Leichtner AM, Schwartz AN: Recent advances in diagnosis and treatment of gastrointestinal hemorrhage in infants and children. *J Pediatr* 1985;**106:**1.

McKusick KA et al: ^{99m}Tc red blood cells for detection of gastrointestinal bleeding. *AJR* 1981;**137:**1113.

Roy CC, Morin CL, Weber AM: Gastrointestinal emergency problems in paediatric practice. *Clin Gastroenterol* 1981; **10:**225.

RECURRENT ABDOMINAL PAIN

About 10% of unselected school children experience at least 3 attacks of recurrent abdominal pain severe enough to affect their activities. An organic cause can be found in fewer than 10% of cases, and there is usually evidence that the pain is a reaction to emotional stress. The age at onset is usually between 5 and 10 years.

Clinical Findings

A. Symptoms and Signs: Recurrent attacks of umbilical or periumbilical pain last less than 24 hours, usually only about an hour. There may be associated pallor, nausea, vomiting, and slight fever. The pain seldom radiates. An organic cause is suggested by a change in the pattern of the attack; a negative history of colic, diarrhea, and vomiting in infancy; and absence of associated emotional problems or a family history of migraine. The farther the pain is from the umbilicus, the more likely it is that an organic cause will be found. Emotional disturbances are common.

The pain usually bears little relationship to bowel habits and activity, although constipation is present in some. At times, pain may occur during meals or before the child leaves for school. A definite precipitating or particularly stressful situation in the child's life at the time the pains began can sometimes be elicited. A history of functional gastrointestinal complaints and migraine headaches is often found in family members.

A thorough physical examination is essential. Abdominal tenderness, if present, is diffuse and mild, although discomfort over the descending colon is common.

B. Laboratory and X-Ray Findings: Complete blood count, sedimentation rate, urinalysis, stool test for occult blood, and tuberculin testing usually suffice. If the syndrome is somewhat atypical, urine cultures, intravenous urography, voiding cystography, barium enema, and upper gastrointestinal x-rays should be done.

Differential Diagnosis

Organic causes relating to the urinary and gastrointestinal tracts, as well as extra-abdominal causes (Table 19–3), should be ruled out by appropriate studies. Oxyuriasis, "mesenteric lymphadenitis," and "chronic appendicitis" are improbable causes of recurrent abdominal pain. Milk intolerance due to lactose intolerance usually manifests itself by both pain and diarrhea. However, abdominal discomfort may at times be the only symptom. Abdominal migraine and abdominal epilepsy are truly rare conditions.

Treatment & Prognosis

Treatment consists of reassurance based on a thorough physical appraisal and a sympathetic explanation of the emotional basis. Therapy for emotional problems is sometimes required, but drugs should be avoided. The prognosis is good.

Appley J: *The Child With Abdominal Pain*, 2nd ed. Blackwell, 1975.

Liebman WM: Recurrent abdominal pain in children: A retrospective survey of 119 patients. *Clin Pediatr* 1978;**17:**149.

Silverman A, Roy CC: Psychophysiologic recurrent abdominal pain. Pages 418–430 in: *Pediatric Clinical Gastroenterology*, 3rd ed. Mosby, 1983.

THE MALABSORPTION SYNDROMES

Intestinal absorption is affected by the length of the small bowel and the amount of available surface area of the absorptive mucosa. Anatomic abnormalities and impaired motility of the small intestine interfere with normal propulsive movements and mixing of food with pancreatic and biliary secretions, and they can also lead to an altered bacterial flora. Impairment of portal venous return, anoxia, and lymphatic abnormalities also cause malabsorption, as can diseases interfering with pancreatic exocrine function and with the production and flow of biliary secretions. Other causes include disaccharidase deficiency, glucose-galactose malabsorption, abetalipoproteinemia, malnutrition, endocrine conditions, immune deficiencies, and emotional factors (maternal deprivation).

Clinical Findings

Gastrointestinal symptoms such as diarrhea, vomiting, anorexia, abdominal pain, and bloating are not always present, and the presenting complaints may not refer to the gastrointestinal tract. Certain physical features such as potbelly and wasted buttocks may indicate celiac disease. Personal observation of the stools for abnormal color, consistency, bulkiness, odor, mucus, and blood is important.

The following are the most helpful investigations:

A. Fat Absorption: Seventy-two-hour fecal fat excretion and coefficient of fat absorption, serum carotene and cholesterol, and prothrombin time.

B. Protein Absorption: Serum protein electrophoresis, fecal nitrogen, and fecal excretion of α_1-antitrypsin.

C. Carbohydrate Absorption: Glucose tolerance test, D-xylose absorption test, disaccharide absorption test, breath hydrogen analysis, and stool pH and reducing substances.

D. Absorption of Folic Acid and Vitamin B_{12}: Schilling test and serum folic acid and vitamin B_{12}.

E. Bacteriology and Parasitology: Assays of stool and duodenal juice.

F. X-Ray Studies: Upper gastrointestinal series with small bowel follow-through, barium enema, and bone age.

G. Sweat Test: Chloride determination.

H. Pancreatic Exocrine Function: Examination of duodenal aspirate (volume, viscosity, pH, and bicarbonate, trypsin, lipase, and amylase activity) and bentiromide excretion test.

I. Liver Function Tests: Bilirubin, transaminases, alkaline phosphatase, and sulfobromophthalein (BSP) excretion.

J. Miscellaneous: Peroral small bowel biopsy, rectosigmoidoscopy and rectal biopsy, immunoglobulin levels, lipoprotein electrophoresis, urine catecholamines, and endocrine function tests.

Differential Diagnosis

The pathophysiologic classification set forth in Table 19–10 may be helpful in view of the considerable variety of disorders giving rise to malabsorption.

Treatment & Prognosis

See specific syndromes (celiac disease, disaccharidase deficiency, etc).

Anderson CM: Malabsorption in children. *Clin Gastroenterol* 1977;**6:**355.

Friedman HI, Nylund B: Intestinal fat digestion, absorption, and transport: A review. *Am J Clin Nutr* 1980;**33:**1108.

Walker-Smith J: *Diseases of the Small Intestine in Childhood,* 2nd ed. Pitman, 1979.

PROTEIN-LOSING ENTEROPATHIES

Excessive loss of plasma proteins into the gastrointestinal tract occurs in association with a number of disorders, some of which are listed below.

Disorders Associated With Protein-Losing Enteropathy

A. Cardiac: Congestive heart failure, constrictive pericarditis, atrial septal defect, primary myocardial disease.

B. Gastric: Giant hypertrophic gastritis (Menetrier's disease), polyps.

C. Small Intestine: Celiac disease, intestinal lymphangiectasia, tropical sprue, regional enteritis, Whipple's disease, lymphosarcoma, acute gastrointestinal infection, allergic gastroenteropathy, blind loop syndrome, abetalipoproteinemia, chronic volvulus, malrotation with Ladd's bands.

D. Colon: Ulcerative colitis, Hirschsprung's disease, polyposis syndromes.

E. Other: Immunologic deficiency states.

Clinical Findings

The signs and symptoms include edema, chylous ascites, poor weight gain, deficiencies of fat-soluble vitamins, hypochromic anemia, and megaloblastic anemia secondary to vitamin B_{12} or folic acid malabsorption, with severe and long-standing gastrointestinal problems. Serum albumin is usually less than 2.5 g/dL. Normally, the gut plays only a minor role in albumin catabolism, and enhanced intestinal losses of protein are solely responsible for the hypoalbuminemia that occurs in most conditions leading to protein-losing enteropathies, except for an increased rate of catabolism or a decreased rate of synthesis in systemic diseases.

Differential Diagnosis

Hypoalbuminemia may be due to an increased catabolic rate or may be associated with cirrhosis, diseases in which there is mechanical or functional obstruction of lymph flow, or congenital malformations of lymphatics outside the gastrointestinal tract. It is especially important to rule out malnutrition and to make certain that no significant proteinuria is present. Lymphangiography is useful after age 2 years.

Treatment

Temporary benefits can be derived from albumin infusions in conjunction with intravenous furosemide. Treatment must be directed toward the primary underlying cause.

Hill RE et al: Fecal clearance of alpha 1-antitrypsin: A reliable measure of enteric protein loss in children. *J Pediatr* 1981;**99:**416.

Rothschild MA et al: Albumin synthesis. (2 parts.) *N Engl J Med* 1972;**286:**748, 816.

Waldman TA: Gastrointestinal protein loss in pediatrics. Page 442 in: *Pediatric Nuclear Medicine.* James AE, Wagner HN, Cooke RE (editors). Saunders, 1974.

CELIAC DISEASE (Gluten Enteropathy)

Essentials of Diagnosis

- Diarrhea and steatorrhea.
- Failure to thrive; loss of weight involving mostly the limbs and buttocks.
- Abdominal distention.
- Depressed rate of D-xylose absorption.
- Villous atrophy on small bowel biopsy.
- Improvement on gluten-free diet, and histologic relapse following reintroduction of gluten into the diet within a period of 2 years.
- Normal pancreatic and biliary secretions.

Table 19–10. Malabsorption syndromes.

- **Intraluminal phase abnormalities**
  - Acid hypersecretion; Zollinger-Ellison syndrome
  - Gastric resection
  - Inadequate lipolysis and proteolysis
  - Cystic fibrosis
  - Chronic pancreatitis
  - Pancreatic pseudocysts
  - Shwachman syndrome
  - Enterokinase deficiency
  - Lipase and colipase deficiency
  - Malnutrition
  - Decreased conjugated bile acids
    - Liver production and excretion
      - Neonatal hepatitis
      - Biliary atresia: intrahepatic and extrahepatic
      - Acute and chronic active hepatitis
      - Disease of the biliary tract
      - Cirrhosis
      - Fat malabsorption in the premature infant
    - Intestinal factors
    - Short bowel syndrome
    - Bacterial overgrowth
      - Blind loop
      - Fistula
      - Strictures, regional enteritis
      - Scleroderma, intestinal pseudo-obstruction
- **Intestinal phase abnormalities**
  - Mucosal diseases
    - Infection, bacterial or viral
    - Infestations
      - *Giardia lamblia*
      - Fish tapeworm
      - Hookworm
    - Malnutrition
      - Marasmus
      - Kwashiorkor
    - Dermatitis herpetiformis
    - Folic acid deficiency
    - Drugs: methotrexate, antibiotics
    - Crohn's disease
    - Chronic ulcerative disease
    - Cow's milk and soy protein intolerance
    - Secondary disaccharidase deficiency
    - Hirschsprung's disease with enterocolitis
    - Tropical sprue
    - Celiac disease
    - Radiation enteritis
    - Lymphoma
- **Intestinal phase abnormalities (cont'd)**
  - Circulatory disturbances
    - Cirrhosis
    - Congestive heart failure
  - Abnormal structure of gastrointestinal tract
    - Dumping syndrome after gastrectomy
    - Malrotation
    - Stenosis of jejunum or ileum
    - Small bowel resection; short bowel syndrome
    - Polyposis
  - Selective inborn absorptive defects
    - Congenital malabsorption of folic acid
    - Selective malabsorption of vitamin B_{12}
    - Cystinuria, methionine malabsorption
    - Hartnup disease, blue diaper syndrome
    - Glucose-galactose malabsorption
    - Primary disaccharidase deficiency
    - Acrodermatitis enteropathica
    - Abetalipoproteinemia
    - Congenital chloridorrhea
    - Primary hypomagnesemia
    - Hereditary fructose intolerance
    - Familial hypophosphatemic rickets
  - Endocrine diseases
    - Diabetes
    - Addison's disease
    - Hyperthyroidism
    - Hypoparathyroidism, pseudohypoparathyroidism
    - Neuroblastoma, ganglioneuroma
- **Delivery phase defects**
  - Whipple's disease
  - Intestinal lymphangiectasis
  - Congestive heart failure
  - Regional enteritis with lymphangiectasis
  - Lymphoma
  - Abetalipoproteinemia
- **Miscellaneous**
  - Renal insufficiency
  - Carcinoid, mastocytosis
  - Immunity defects
  - Familial dysautonomia
  - Maternal deprivation?
  - Collagen disease
  - Wolman's disease
  - Histiocytosis X
  - Intractable diarrhea of early infancy

General Considerations

Celiac disease is a specific disease entity associated with abnormal jejunal mucosa that improves with a strict gluten-free diet. It is a common but decreasing cause of malabsorption in infants. Most cases present during the second year of life, but the age at onset and the severity are both variable. The disease is more common in Europe and in Canada than in the USA and is uncommon in blacks and Orientals.

The underlying pathologic process is not yet clearly understood, but it is presently thought that the intestinal lesion is the result of a cell-mediated immune response in individuals susceptible to gluten—or, more specifically, to gliadin, the alcohol-soluble fraction of gluten.

Clinical Findings

A. Symptoms and Signs:

1. Diarrhea—Affected children present with a history of digestive disturbances starting at 6–12 months of age—the age at which wheat, rye, or oat glutens are first fed. Initially, the diarrhea may be intermittent and related to upper respiratory tract infections. Subsequently, it is continuous, with voluminous, bulky, pale, frothy, greasy, offensive floating stools. During celiac crises, dehydration, shock, and acidosis are commonly seen. Diarrhea is absent in 10% of cases.

2. Constipation, vomiting, and abdominal pain—This triad of symptoms may in a small number of cases dominate the clinical picture and suggest a diagnosis of intestinal obstruction.

3. Failure to thrive—The onset of diarrhea is usually accompanied by loss of appetite, failure to gain weight, and increased irritability.

4. Wasting and retardation of growth—In established cases, there is a loss of weight, which is most marked in the limbs and buttocks. The face remains plump, and the abdomen becomes distended secondary to a poor musculature and, more importantly, to accumulation of gas and fluid in the hypotonic intestinal tract with altered peristaltic activity. Growth failure may dominate the clinical picture.

5. Anemia and vitamin deficiencies—Anemia usually responds to iron and is rarely megaloblastic. Deficiencies in fat-soluble vitamins are common. Rickets can be seen when growth has not been completely halted by the disease; however, osteomalacia is more common, and pathologic fractures may occur. Hypoprothrombinemia can be severe, and some patients are known to present with severe intestinal hemorrhages.

B. Laboratory Findings:

1. Fat content of stools—A 3-day collection of stools usually reveals fecal fat levels over 4.5 g/d. However, steatorrhea may be absent in 10–25% of cases. It is important that a nonabsorbable marker, such as charcoal or carmine red, be given for accurate collection. A normal child will absorb 90–98% of ingested fats. The untreated celiac patient, on the other hand, will not absorb more than 65–85% of daily fat intake.

2. Impaired carbohydrate absorption—A low oral glucose tolerance curve is seen. Absorption of D-xylose is impaired, with blood levels lower than 20 mg/dL at 60 minutes.

3. Hypoproteinemia—Hypoalbuminemia can be severe enough to lead to edema. There is evidence of increased losses of protein in the gut lumen.

C. X-Ray Findings: A small bowel series can demonstrate a typical malabsorptive pattern characterized by segmentation, clumping of the barium column, and hypersecretion. These changes are nonspecific, and x-rays of the small bowel should therefore be taken to rule out structural defects that might cause malabsorption (Table 19–10).

D. Biopsy Findings: Peroral intestinal biopsy provides the only reliable evidence for the diagnosis of celiac disease. It is a safe and simple procedure even in infants.

Under the dissecting microscope, the jejunal mucosa presents a "crazy paving" appearance rather than the slender fingerlike projections that characterize normal villi. Under the light microscope, the celiac mucosa is readily recognized by amputation of the villi, by lengthening of the crypts of Lieberkühn, and by increased round cell infiltration of the lamina propria. Normal to nearly normal appearance of the lamina propria can be expected after withdrawal of gluten from the diet.

E. Serologic Tests: Measurements of gliadin antibody and reticulin antibody may be useful screening tests.

Differential Diagnosis

The differential diagnosis includes disorders that cause malabsorption. Strict adherence to 2 diagnostic criteria—ie, the characteristic small bowel microscopic changes and clinical improvement on a gluten-free diet—is essential. Whenever the mucosal lesion is not characteristic or the response to a gluten-free diet is not as good as expected, challenge with a gluten-containing diet is indicated. Biopsy should be performed as soon as the patient becomes symptomatic or after 6 months if the child remains healthy and is growing well on a normal diet.

Treatment

A. Diet: Treatment consists of dietary gluten restriction for life. Dietary supervision is essential. The diet (Table 19–11) should provide 25% more calories than calculated for expected weight plus protein amounts of 6–8 g/kg/d. Lactose is poorly tolerated in the acute stage, since the extensive mucosal damage leads to acquired disaccharidase deficiency. Normal amounts of fat are advisable.

In treating a severely affected child, the diet should be tailored to the child's appetite and capacity to absorb. A full gluten-free diet can usually be given after 2–3 weeks. Clinical improvement is usually evident within a week, and histologic repair is complete after 3–12 months.

B. Corticosteroids: Corticosteroid therapy can produce dramatic remissions. It is used only in celiac crises.

Table 19–11. Gluten-free diet.*

Foods allowed
Milk, cream, and cheese
Eggs
Meat, fish, and poultry (unless breaded or creamed)
Vegetables
Bread made from rice, corn, or gluten-free wheat flour
Cornflakes; cornmeal, puffed rice, or precooked gluten-free cereals
All clear soups
Fruit and fruit juices
Foods to be avoided
Bread, rolls, crackers, cakes, and cookies made from wheat or rye
Cereals, spaghetti, macaroni, and noodles made from wheat or rye
All canned soups except clear broth
Commercial ice cream
Prepared mixes and puddings
Commercial candies containing cereal products
Malted milk, beer, ale, and some instant coffees

* All possible sources of wheat, rye, and oats must be eliminated from the patient's diet.

Prognosis

Improvement and clinical recovery are the rule. However, disappearance of symptoms can be a protracted, intermittent process. Although good gastrointestinal tolerance for gluten may be eventually noted in a number of patients maintained on the gluten-free diet, most patients undergo a histologic relapse on reexposure. Malignant lymphoma of the small bowel is a long-term risk that is not averted by good dietary control.

Bullen AW, Losowsky MS: Cell-mediated immunity to gluten fraction III in adult celiac disease. *Gut* 1978;**19:**126.

Burgin-Wolff A et al: A reliable screening test for childhood celiac disease: Fluorescent immunosorbent test for gliadin antibodies. *J Pediatr* 1983;**102:**655.

Cacciari E et al: Short stature and celiac disease: A relationship to consider even in patients with no gastrointestinal tract symptoms. *J Pediatr* 1983;**103:**708.

Cooper BT et al: Celiac disease and malignancy. *Medicine* 1980;**59:**249.

Lebenthal E, Branski D: Childhood celiac disease: A reappraisal. *J Pediatr* 1981;**98:**681.

Packer SM et al: Gluten challenge in treated celiac disease. *Arch Dis Child* 1978;**53:**449.

DISACCHARIDASE DEFICIENCY

Essentials of Diagnosis

- Watery diarrhea, explosive and frothy.
- Stool pH < 5.5.
- Reducing substances present in stools and often in urine.
- Flat glucose tolerance test following disaccharide loading.
- A positive breath hydrogen test following an oral test dose of lactose or sucrose.

General Considerations

Carbohydrates account for a substantial proportion of the human diet. The polysaccharide starch and the disaccharides sucrose and lactose are quantitatively the most important and require hydrolysis before significant absorption can take place. Fig 19–1 summarizes the digestion sequence of the common polysaccharides and disaccharides.

Disaccharidases are localized in the brush border of the intestinal epithelial cells. Absolute levels are higher in the jejunum and in the proximal ileum than in the distal ileum and duodenum. Some substrates can be hydrolyzed by more than one enzyme, and, conversely, some enzymes act on more than one substrate.

In the primary form, the enzyme deficit is isolated, the disaccharide intolerance is likely to persist, intestinal histologic findings are normal, and a family history is common.

Since disaccharidases are confined to the outer cell layer of the intestinal epithelium, they are very susceptible to mucosal damage. A number of conditions are now known to give rise to the secondary type of disaccharidase deficiency, which is transient and involves a quantitative decrease in all enzymes, although lactose intolerance is by far the most common. Histologic examination reveals changes compatible with the underlying disorder. A familial incidence in these cases is uncommon.

Clinical Findings

A. Primary (Congenital):

1. Lactase deficiency—Congenital lactase deficiency is a rare condition leading to diarrhea after lactose is ingested. The stools are frothy and acid; their pH may fall below 4.5 owing to the presence of organic acids that stimulate peristalsis and hypersecretion. The osmotic action of unhydrolyzed lactose leads to catharsis. Vomiting is common. Severe malnutrition may occur. Reducing substances are usually present in the stools, and lactosuria may occur. Infants with lactosuria, aminoaciduria, proteinuria, acidosis, and elevated blood urea nitrogen have been described. An oral lactose tolerance test (2 g/kg) after dietary

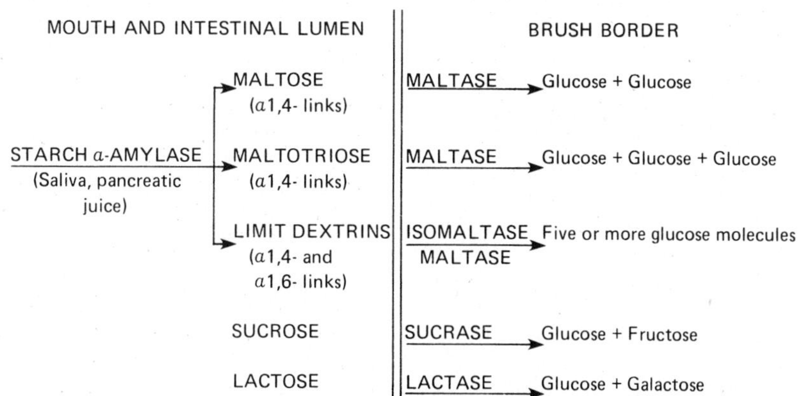

Figure 19–1. Digestion sequence of common polysaccharides and disaccharides.

lactose has been withdrawn is likely to result in symptoms of intolerance within 8 hours; the blood glucose levels show no appreciable rise. A better test is to measure the hydrogen in the expired air after an oral lactose load. If the milk does not give rise to symptoms initially, it is necessary to exclude small intestinal mucosal damage that may cause secondary lactase deficiency; this may be done by means of a small bowel biopsy, which also permits direct estimation of the disaccharidase.

Patients respond to the exclusion of lactose from their diets.

2. Sucrase and isomaltase deficiency—This is a combined defect that is inherited as an autosomal recessive trait. Diarrhea usually occurs only when sucrose is fed. Abdominal distention, failure to thrive, and toilet-training difficulties with chronic diarrhea may be the presenting symptoms. Since sucrase-isomaltase deficiencies have been found in siblings who had few or no symptoms, it is likely that a number of persons with this trait—particularly adults—remain unrecognized.

In making a diagnosis, it is important to remember that sucrose is not a reducing sugar. The usual 5 drops of stool and 10 drops of water added to a Clinitest tablet will not give a positive reaction unless 1 N HCl is substituted for the water and the mixture allowed to boil for a few seconds before adding the tablet. A sucrose tolerance test (2 g/kg) is likely to be flat and will lead to a positive breath test. Since many gastric and extraintestinal factors can account for very poor blood glucose rises, it is wise to check the stools for the presence of sucrose and to follow the sucrose tolerance test by the xylose absorption test. Shock may occur owing to osmotic water losses in some patients with lactase or sucrase-isomaltase deficiency with a standard dose of the disaccharide for the tolerance test. In sucrase-isomaltase deficiency, exclusion of sucrose is usually sufficient. Starch intolerance is rarely a problem, since the 1–6 linkages of starch hydrolyzed by isomaltase constitute only a small part of the molecule.

B. Secondary (Acquired):

1. Secondary lactase deficiency—Diarrhea may be produced in normal individuals if a large dose of lactose is ingested. The threshold for lactose tolerance is usually much lower than that for sucrose. Lactose intolerance develops spontaneously in a certain number of children and may cause abdominal pain without diarrhea. There is a high prevalence of lactose intolerance in certain racial groups (70% in North American blacks) after 3–5 years of age. Disaccharidase deficiency has been described in association with many different disorders. Neomycin and kanamycin administration have been shown to reduce lactase activity in adults. The list of conditions associated with secondary lactase deficiency includes celiac disease, giardiasis, malnutrition, viral or bacterial gastroenteritis, abetalipoproteinemia, cystic fibrosis, immunoglobulin deficiencies, extensive intestinal resections, and necrotizing enterocolitis.

2. Secondary sucrase deficiency—Intestinal mucosal damage tends to lower the levels of all disaccharidases. Signs of sucrose intolerance are usually masked by the more striking symptoms related to lactose. Infectious diarrhea is the most frequent cause of secondary sucrose intolerance.

Treatment

A. Lactose-Free Diet: Use a milk formula that does not contain lactose, eg, Nutramigen, Pregestimil, or soy formulas. Exclude foods containing whey, dry milk solids, and curds. It is important to see if labels indicate any lactose content, particularly with canned puréed baby foods. Cheeses (cottage, cheddar, cream), ice cream, sherbet, and chocolate milk powders also contain variable amounts of lactose, small amounts of which are tolerated.

B. Sucrose-Restricted Diet: See Table 19–12.

Prognosis

In the primary type, the enzyme deficiency is a lifelong defect. However, in both lactase and sucrase deficiencies, tolerance for the disaccharide tends to increase with age. The prognosis in the secondary or acquired forms of disaccharidase deficiency is that of the underlying illness. It is important to remember that normal tolerance for lactose may not be regained until many months after an acute mucosal injury.

Kilby A et al: Sucrase-isomaltase deficiency: A follow-up report. *Arch Dis Child* 1979;**53:**677.

Lebenthal E et al: Recurrent abdominal pain and lactose absorption in children. *Pediatrics* 1981;**67:**828.

Lifshitz F: Carbohydrate problems in paediatric gastroenterology. *Clin Gastroenterol* 1977;**6:**415.

Nose O et al: Breath hydrogen test for detecting lactose malabsorption in infants and children. *Arch Dis Child* 1979;**54:**436.

Table 19–12. Sucrose-restricted diet.*

Foods allowed
- Milk, cream, butter, cheese, and salad and cooking oils
- Eggs, meat, and fish
- Potatoes
- Asparagus, broccoli, brussels sprouts, cucumbers, spinach, tomatoes, and lettuce
- Grapes, cherries, strawberries, cranberries, and blackberries
- Homemade bread and pastries containing dextrose; homemade ice cream; and gelatin desserts
- Diet carbonated beverages, diet Kool-Aid, unsweetened cocoa, and vegetable juices

Foods to be avoided
- Fruits and vegetables not included in the above list, especially peas, beans, and lentils
- Breakfast cereals
- Commercial ice cream, pies, cookies, and cakes
- Jam, honey, jelly, candy, molasses, and maple syrup
- Kool-Aid and carbonated beverages
- Medicines made up in syrup

* The diet described here does contain small amounts of sucrose that are usually well tolerated.

Perman JA et al: Sucrose malabsorption in children: Noninvasive diagnosis by interval breath hydrogen determination. *J Pediatr* 1978;**93:**17.

GLUCOSE-GALACTOSE MALABSORPTION

Chronic diarrhea like that due to intestinal disaccharide deficiency may be due to the osmotic effect of monosaccharide malabsorption. A decreased rate of tubular reabsorption of glucose is often associated with the intestinal cell transport defect.

In the congenital form of the disease, severe diarrhea begins within a few days after birth. Small bowel histologic findings are normal. Glycosuria and aminoaciduria may occur. The glucose tolerance test is flat. Fructose is well tolerated. The diarrhea promptly subsides on withdrawal of glucose and galactose from the diet. The stool pH is not as acid as that reported in disaccharidase deficiencies; fecal reducing substances are consistently found. The clinical features associated with acquired disease are the same as those seen with disaccharidase deficiency states. The acquired form is mainly seen in the perinatal period but is also described in older infants. Both disaccharides and monosaccharides, including fructose, are malabsorbed. Necrotizing enterocolitis, intractable diarrhea of early infancy, postoperative phases of neonatal gastrointestinal surgery, and protein-calorie malnutrition are acquired forms of the entity that have been described in infants with extensive small bowel resections or during the course of a bout of gastroenteritis.

In the congenital form, total exclusion of glucose and galactose from the diet is manadatory. A satisfactory formula consists of fructose with a carbohydrate-free formula. The prognosis is good if the disease is diagnosed early, since tolerance for glucose and galactose improves with age.

Elsas LJ, Lambe DW: Familial glucose-galactose malabsorption: Remission of glucose intolerance. *J Pediatr* 1973; **83:**226.

Fairclough PD et al: Absorption of glucose and maltose in congenital glucose-galactose malabsorption. *Pediatr Res* 1978;**12:**1112.

Klish WJ et al: Intestinal surface area in infants with acquired monosaccharide intolerance. *J Pediatr* 1978;**92:**566.

INTESTINAL LYMPHANGIECTASIA

This form of protein-losing enteropathy results from a congenital abnormality of the lymphatic system and is often associated with lymphatic aberrations in the extremities. Obstruction to lymphatic drainage of the intestine leads to rupture of intestinal lacteals with leakage of lymph into the lumen of the bowel. Fat loss may be significant and lead to steatorrhea. Chronic loss of lymphocytes and of immunoglobulins is usual and increases the susceptibility to infections.

Clinical Findings

Peripheral edema, diarrhea, abdominal distention, lymphedematous extremities, chylous effusions, and repeated infections are common. Laboratory findings are low serum albumin, decreased immunoglobulin levels, lymphocytopenia, and anemia. Serum calcium is frequently depressed, and stool fat may be elevated. Lymphocytes may be seen in large numbers on a stool smear. Fecal α_1-antitrypsin studies confirm the gastrointestinal protein loss. X-ray studies reveal an edematous small bowel mucosal pattern, and biopsy reveals dilated lacteals in the villi and lamina propria. It should be noted that in certain cases where the disorder involves the submucosa, subserosa, mesentery, and omentum, the peroral biopsy may be normal, and laparotomy may be necessary to establish the diagnosis.

Differential Diagnosis

Other causes of protein-losing enteropathy must be considered, although an associated lymphedematous extremity strongly favors this diagnosis.

Complications & Sequelae

Failure to thrive, tetany, and frequent infections are the common complications of this disease. Lymphedema of an extremity may be disfiguring, since it leads to increased bone growth and hemihypertrophy.

Treatment & Prognosis

Surgery is needed when the lesion is localized to a small area of the bowel or in cases of constrictive pericarditis or obstructing tumors. This may include placement of a LeVeen or Denver shunt or construction of a saphenous vein-peritoneal anastomosis in intractable cases.

A low-fat diet reduces lymph flow. Medium-chain triglycerides as a fat source are effective only in the mucosal type of lymphangiectasia. Water-soluble vitamin and calcium supplements should be given. Antibiotics are used for specific infections. Total parenteral nutrition is helpful on a temporary basis.

The prognosis at present is not favorable, although there may be remission with age.

Tift WL, Lloyd JK: Intestinal lymphangiectasia: Long-term results with MCT diet. *Arch Dis Child* 1975;**50:**269.

Vardy PA, Lebenthal E, Shwachman H: Intestinal lymphangiectasia: A reappraisal. *Pediatrics* 1975;**55:**842.

COW'S MILK PROTEIN INTOLERANCE

Milk intolerance is more common in males and in children with a family history of allergy. The estimated incidence is 0.5–1%. There is a little evidence that breast feeding for a period of 3 months is protective even in infants from atopic families. The gastrointestinal features vary in severity and last from 6 weeks to 12 months of age. In some patients, severe colic is present. In others, vomiting is the predominant symptom, and diarrhea is chronic. In a third group, diarrhea is very severe and may lead to the syndrome called "intractable diarrhea of early infancy." Milk protein allergy commonly leads to the presence of occult blood in the stools. Gross blood can be seen and can be associated with "milk colitis." Pneumatosis intestinalis may suggest necrotizing enterocolitis. Eosinophilic gastroenteritis with a protein-losing enteropathy characterized by hypoalbuminemia and hypogammaglobulinemia is less commonly seen. It may involve the stomach or the small bowel. A celiaclike syndrome can occur secondary to milk sensitivity. Anaphylactic shock is a rare threat.

In most cases of milk sensitivity, milk protein elimination results in a rapid amelioration of symptoms. In evaluating the response of diarrhea suspected of being due to milk allergy, it is essential to remember that soy protein intolerance is reported with increasing frequency. Soy protein intolerance is clinically similar to cow's milk protein intolerance. It is best to use a casein hydrolysate formula as an elimination diet to prove the diagnosis. A normal 1-hour blood xylose level 4–12 weeks after clinical recovery, with a drop below 25 mg/dL 4 days after reintroduction of cow's milk protein, has been shown to be a reliable means of diagnosis.

Eastham EJ, Walker WA: Effect of cow's milk on gastrointestinal tract: A persistent dilemma for the pediatrician. *Pediatrics* 1977;**60**:477.

Gerrard JW, Shenassa M: Food allergy: Two common types as seen in breast and formula fed babies. *Ann Allergy* 1983;**50**:375.

Jenkins HR et al: Food allergy: The major cause of infantile colitis. *Arch Dis Child* 1984;**59**:326.

Kramer MS, Moroz B: Do breast-feeding and delayed introduction of solid foods protect against subsequent atopic eczema? *J Pediatr* 1981;**98**:546.

Lothe L, Lindberg T, Jakobsson I: Cow's milk formula as a cause of infantile colic: A double-blind study. *Pediatrics* 1982;**70**:7.

IMMUNOLOGIC DEFICIENCY STATES WITH DIARRHEA OR MALABSORPTION

It is now thought that both cellular and humoral immunity serve as a protective mechanism against pathogenic organisms by preventing the entry of foreign materials and regulating antigen absorption. Intestinal immunity plays an important role in various diseases of the gastrointestinal tract and in certain systemic disorders.

Intermittent diarrhea is a frequent finding in immunoglobulin deficiency states, but the cause is usually obscure. It is uncommon to find pathogenic bacteria in the stools, but giardiasis is common. Fifty to 60% of patients with idiopathic acquired hypogammaglobulinemia have steatorrhea and histologic changes consistent with the celiac syndrome. Lymphonodular hyperplasia is a common feature in this group of patients. Congenital or Bruton type agammaglobulinemics occasionally have abnormal intestinal morphology. Patients with isolated IgA deficiency have normal intestinal function but may also present with chronic diarrhea, a celiaclike picture, lymphoid nodular hyperplasia, and giardiasis. Patients with isolated cellular immunity defects or combined cellular and humoral immune incompetence all have severe chronic diarrhea leading to malnutrition. The cause is unknown, and mucosal biopsies are normal. A high incidence of disaccharidase deficiency is associated with immunologic deficits in children. Chronic granulomatous disease may be associated with intestinal symptoms suggestive of chronic inflammatory bowel disease. A rectal biopsy may reveal the presence of typical macrophages.

Treatment must be directed toward correction of the immunoglobulin defect. Gluten-free diets have been disappointing in most cases with villous atrophy. Dramatic improvement may follow the eradication of giardiasis. In patients exhibiting disaccharidase deficiencies, dietary manipulations are helpful.

Glassman M et al: High incidence of hypogammaglobulinemia in infants with diarrhea. *J Pediatr Gastroenterol Nutr* 1983;**2**:465.

Katz AJ, Rosen FS: Gastrointestinal complications of immunodeficiency syndromes. *Ciba Found Symp* 1977;**46**:243.

Ogra PL, Bienenstock J (editors): *The Mucosal Immune System in Health and Disease*. 81st Ross Conference on Pediatric Research. Columbus, Ohio, 1981.

CHRONIC ULCERATIVE COLITIS

Essentials of Diagnosis

- Rectal bleeding, bloody diarrhea, diarrhea with mucus or pus.
- Tenesmus and crampy abdominal pain.
- Extracolonic manifestations, fever, weight loss, retardation of growth, arthralgia, arthritis, mucocutaneous lesions, erythema nodosum, jaundice.
- Ragged mucosa with loss of haustral markings on barium enema.
- Acute inflammatory changes with crypt abscesses on rectal mucosal biopsy.

General Considerations

Ulcerative colitis is an acute, intermittent or chronic, relapsing disease of the mucosa and submucosa of varying lengths of the colon and rectum characterized by bloody stools, irregularly recurring fever, and many local or extracolonic signs and symptoms. Rectal involvement is seen in more than 90% of cases. It is not a rare disorder in children and has been reported in infants. Twenty percent of cases begin before age 20, with a peak between ages 10 and 19. Impairment of physical growth and delayed appearance of secondary sex characteristics are important complications, but studies indicate that the incidence of carcinoma is low.

An "autoimmune" basis for this disorder is suggested by the favorable response to corticosteroid treatment and by its close association with extraintestinal manifestations such as arthritis, erythema nodosum, uveitis, chronic active hepatitis, and autoimmune hemolytic anemia.

An increase in lymphocytotoxic antibody has been demonstrated in the serum of some patients with ulcerative colitis. Furthermore, leukocyte migration inhibition has been shown when lymphocytes from patients are exposed to antigens from normal human colon. An immune-mediated mechanism has also been supported by decreased IgE-containing lymphocytes and increased mast cells. Complement turnover studies have shown increased metabolism of C1q and C3. Cell-mediated immunity appears to be normal.

Although emotional stress can exacerbate the disease, studies have failed to identify psychosocial factors unique to these patients.

Clinical Findings

The diagnosis of ulcerative colitis is based upon a history of an acute onset of diarrhea or nonspecific gastroenteritis, the passage of bloody stools, abdominal cramping, tenesmus, fever, malaise, and anorexia. The onset may also be insidious, with a change in bowel habits from normal to constipation or continued constipation followed by the passage of blood, mucus, or pus. Less commonly, the course is fulminating, with high septic fever, extreme prostration, anorexia, vomiting, and an almost continuous bloody diarrhea. In such cases (toxic megacolon), the threat of colonic perforation is great and emergency surgery is mandatory.

The extracolonic manifestations may be the presenting symptoms and signs, especially with arthralgia or arthritis (15–20%). This is usually monarticular and involves the major joints. Joint symptoms wax and wane with the remissions and exacerbations of the primary disease. Rarely, they precede the signs of bowel involvement by months or years. Other extracolonic findings are erythema nodosum, pyoderma gangrenosum, and liver disease, either with hepatic enlargement or with abnormalities in liver function studies for which no cause is readily apparent.

The diagnosis of ulcerative colitis is established by sigmoidoscopic examination revealing a hyperemic, friable, bleeding mucosa. Early in the disease, special attention should be paid to discrete mucosal changes manifested by small indentations in the barium enema. Later, the ulcers are more easily identified. In advanced colitis, there is a loss of haustral markings, pseudopolyps, and narrowing and shortening of the colon. During the barium enema examination, it is important to fill the terminal ileum, since 10–15% of children with involvement of the entire colon have so-called backwash ileitis. Biopsy of the rectal mucosa reveals inflammatory cell infiltration and crypt abscesses and is particularly helpful in suggestive cases with negative sigmoidoscopic and radiologic findings.

A clinically milder form is usually associated with segmental disease affecting only the distal colon. In rare cases, the disease is limited to the rectum. Proctitis rarely progresses to involve other parts of the colon, and the risk of carcinoma is nil. Unfortunately, this form of the disease is rare in children, and 80% have pancolitis within a few years of onset.

Differential Diagnosis

Because ulcerative colitis is not a distinct histopathologic entity, it must be differentiated from acute infectious colitis that could be attributable to *Shigella, Salmonella, Yersinia, Campylobacter, Entamoeba histolytica,* invasive *Escherichia coli,* or *Aeromonas hydrophila.* A mild type of colitis may be mistaken for irritable colon; a severe form may suggest pseudomembranous colitis. In rare instances, connective tissue diseases have to be considered in the differential diagnosis. The most difficult entity to rule out is Crohn's colitis.

Complications

A. Local: With progression of the disease, ulcers within the mucosa may extend to the outer layers. The chronic course interspersed with acute exacerbations leads to extensive fibrosis and consequently to colonic or rectal stricture. Between areas of fibrosis, mucosa becomes "heaped up" and gives rise to pseudopolyps. Massive hemorrhage is uncommon, and toxic megacolon is rare in children. Perianal fissures, abscesses, and fistulas occur often.

B. Systemic: Arthritis, erythema nodosum, uveitis, and pyoderma gangrenosum may be seen. Retarded growth and chronic invalidism occur but are not as severe as in Crohn's disease. Fatty infiltration of the liver and, rarely, pericholangitis are seen in patients who have had the disease a long time. Sepsis and thromboembolic phenomena also occur.

The risk of carcinoma is about 2–3% after 10 years of the disease and increases to 25% after 20 years. The mortality rate from carcinoma is very high, so that prophylactic colectomy must always be considered in patients with long-standing disease, especially if the disease involves the entire colon and is continuous. It is advisable to have a surveillance plan to detect mucosal dysplasia.

Treatment

No method of management has proved uniformly successful. The effectiveness of the following measures must be individually determined and will further depend on the kind of relationship the physician has been able to establish with the patient, who is often apprehensive, emotionally immature, hostile, demanding, and depressed.

A. Diet: A high-protein, high-carbohydrate, high-vitamin, normal-fat diet is recommended. The main concern should be in serving attractive meals that the child will eat. Restrictive or bland diets are not necessary, although a milk-free and low-residue regimen may be tried.

B. Sulfasalazine: This drug is effective acutely and is useful in preventing relapses. Sulfapyridine is absorbed and excreted in the urine. The other component of the molecule, aminosalicylate, has anti-inflammatory effects on the mucosa. The response may be delayed for 1 week. Side effects are common and include headache, anorexia, and nausea. An exacerbation of diarrhea sometimes occurs. Systemic reactions include serum sickness and Heinz body hemolytic anemia. Pancreatitis is also reported.

1. Children under 10 years of age—Give 50 mg/kg/d as acute therapy in 3 divided doses with meals. Half this dosage is recommended to prevent relapses.

2. Children over 10 years of age—Give 2–3 g/d as acute therapy in 3 divided doses with meals. Give half this dosage to prevent an exacerbation.

C. Corticosteroids: These drugs are usually restricted to children with severe systemic manifestations and to those in whom sulfasalazine has not brought about any improvement.

1. Hydrocortisone—Hydrocortisone can be given intravenously in a dosage of 10 mg/kg/d for up to 10 days.

2. Oral prednisone and rectal corticosteroids—Give prednisone, 1–2 mg/kg orally daily for 6–8 weeks, followed by gradual weaning. Prednisone administered in a dose of 10–20 mg on an alternate-day basis minimizes side effects. There is no evidence that the corticosteroids may prevent relapses in patients who completely remit. Prednisone is often given on an alternate-day basis in conjunction with sulfasalazine.

Corticosteroid retention enemas, liquid or foam, given twice a day can be useful when the rectum is severely involved but are not effective when the disease extends beyond the sigmoid.

D. Azathioprine (Imuran): Azathioprine, 1.5–2 mg/kg/d orally, is used only when a high maintenance dose of corticosteroids is necessary to keep the disease under control and there are serious risks of corticosteroid-induced complications.

E. Symptomatic Therapy: Opiates are generally contraindicated because they contribute to the development of toxic megacolon. Anticholinergic agents can reduce hypermotility of the bowel. Sedatives and tranquilizers can be used as required.

F. Psychotherapy: The need for a formal psychiatric referral must be individualized.

G. Surgical Measures: Emergency surgery is lifesaving in fulminating disease with toxic megacolon or with severe hemorrhage, perforation, or obstruction. Because of the risk of carcinomatosis, endoscopy on an annual basis is recommended after 6 years of disease.

Proctocolectomy has been the traditional surgical procedure, but successful continent ileostomies have now been reported in children. An endorectal pull-through operation will prevent the need for an ileostomy, but few centers have had extensive experience with this procedure. Recent series show that almost 30% of children require surgery within 5 years of the onset of the disease.

H. Hyperalimentation: Total parenteral nutrition may be a valuable adjunct for the treatment of malnutrition but rarely produces remissions. Attempts at continuous enteral alimentation have generally been disappointing in ulcerative colitis—in contrast to the good results in Crohn's disease.

Prognosis

The overall prognosis for ulcerative colitis is good. In patients who from the onset have had pancolitis with anemia and hypoalbuminemia, the response to medical management may be initially good, but severe relapses may warrant early surgery. Rarely, the patient may expire during an acute fulminating attack of toxic ulcerative colitis (toxic megacolon). Many children (30–40%) respond favorably to medical management, doing well for months or years. These patients may have mild to moderate relapses, but on the whole they are able to have a normal life-style. A group of patients (20–45%) whose symptoms continue despite medical therapy require early surgery. The patient may die of carcinoma, acute exsanguinating hemorrhage, perforation of the colon, overwhelming sepsis, or sclerosing cholangitis and biliary cirrhosis.

Hamilton JR et al: Inflammatory bowel disease in children and adolescents. *Adv Pediatr* 1979;**26:**311.

Hyams JS et al: Course and prognosis after colectomy and ileostomy for inflammatory bowel disease in childhood and adolescence. *J Pediatr Surg* 1982;**17:**400.

Kirsner JB, Shorter RG: Recent developments in "nonspecific" inflammatory bowel disease. 2 parts. *N Engl J Med* 1982;**306:**775, 837.

CROHN'S DISEASE

Essentials of Diagnosis

- Fever, anemia, anorexia, weight loss.
- Crampy abdominal pain, diarrhea.
- Stunting of growth.
- Anal fistulas.
- X-ray evidence of segmental lesions characterized by thickened circular folds, cobblestoning, rigidity of the lumen, separation and fixation of loops, "string sign."
- Histologic demonstration of submucosal inflammation with fibrosis and of granulomatous lesions.

General Considerations

The terminal ileum and cecum are most commonly involved (80–90%), but any segment or combination of segments of the intestinal tract from stomach to anus may be affected. The tonsils and regional lymph nodes may also be involved. Nearly half of patients have ileocolitis. About 30% have disease limited to the small bowel. In children, the percentage of cases of Crohn's disease affecting only the large bowel (granulomatous colitis) or the anus is 25%. The wall is thickened and rigid, with longitudinal mucosal ulcerations and fissures, submucosal thickening, or cobblestone formation. Sinus tracts and fistulas may be present. Areas of disease may be separated by lengths of normal-appearing gut ("skip lesions"). Histologic features consist of a chronic granulomatous inflammatory reaction with edema and fibrosis involving all layers of the intestinal wall. The most useful diagnostic feature is the presence of noncaseating granulomas containing multinucleated giant cells and epithelioid cells. These focal lesions are found in 50% of cases; in another 25%, the inflammatory reaction is more diffuse. In cases where a nonspecific inflammatory process is reported, the diagnosis must be based on other criteria.

Crohn's disease is twice as frequent as chronic ulcerative colitis. Its cause remains unknown. Occurrence of the disease in members of the same family and a significantly higher incidence among Jews suggest a genetic factor. Psychiatric studies of the disease have not disclosed any specific emotional makeup or cause.

Clinical Findings

A. Symptoms and Signs: Teenagers and young adults are most often afflicted. Cases have been described within the first few months of life. In certain instances, extraintestinal symptoms such as arthritis, uveitis, stomatitis, erythema nodosum, unexplained fever, severe anorexia, or failure to grow may be the presenting symptoms. Anal lesions may antedate the intestinal manifestations by a few years. Crampy abdominal pain, often triggered by food, is usually the predominant symptom. In most instances it is periumbilical, but it may localize in the right lower quadrant. Thus, in one-third of patients the symptoms may mimic an attack of acute appendicitis. In such cases, the possibility of an acute ileitis that can be secondary to *Yersinia enterocolitica* infection should be considered, especially since only 10% of such cases become chronic. Diarrhea is the presenting complaint in one-third of cases. Bloody diarrhea is less frequent than in ulcerative colitis. Anorexia, weight loss, fever, and anemia are found in the majority of patients and often precede the gastrointestinal complaints.

Sigmoidoscopy may be normal or may show diffuse involvement, with lesions indistinguishable from those of ulcerative colitis.

B. Laboratory Findings: Routine laboratory studies contribute little to the diagnosis. Some degree of anemia is usually present. Megaloblastic anemia is rare but may occur as a consequence of vitamin B_{12} or folic acid malabsorption. Evidence for a protein-losing enteropathy can be documented by a decreased serum albumin concentration. Stool examination seldom reveals the presence of blood or pus, and cultures for infectious organisms are negative.

C. X-Ray Findings: X-ray examination should include both a small bowel series and a barium enema. When both ileum and colon are involved, the disease may resemble ulcerative colitis with backwash ileitis. However, the differentiation can usually be made on clinical, radiologic, pathologic, and therapeutic grounds.

Complications

Perforation and hemorrhage are rare. Intestinal obstruction, fistula, and abscess formation are frequent. Severe malnutrition is frequent and due to anorexia and fear of food-induced pain. It is a serious complication that may be compounded by malabsorption syndrome, protein-losing enteropathy, disaccharidase deficiency, and bile salt-induced diarrhea. Systemic complications include perianal disease, pyoderma gangrenosum, arthritis, amyloidosis, and a high incidence of severe growth retardation.

Treatment

Regional enteritis is not surgically curable, although 70% of patients will ultimately require surgery. The relapse rate 6 years after surgery exceeds 60%. The rate of recurrence in previously normal bowel is particularly high during the first 2 years after surgery. Recurrence at the site of anastomosis is most common; consequently, surgery is reserved for the intestinal complications of the disease such as obstruction, perforation, fistulas, and abscess formation. Studies suggest that when the granulomatous process is limited to the colon, the recurrence rate and the need for reoperation are substantially less than in cases of ileocolitis. Surgery should also be considered for those whose growth retardation fails to respond to an optional medical and nutritional program. To be effective, surgery must be performed before the pubertal growth spurt.

Evaluation of medical regimens is made difficult by the spontaneous exacerbations and remissions so characteristic of this disease. The medical management is that of a long-term chronic illness, with goals directed toward relieving disability rather than achieving a cure.

A. Nutrition: Dietary management should center around providing the anorexic patient with a diet high in calories and in proteins. Roughage should be eliminated if there is evidence of a stenotic bowel. Patients are advised to eliminate foods that seem to trigger symptoms. Supplemented calories in the form of liquid diets (Ensure, Isocal) are well tolerated. Vitamin and iron requirements should not be neglected. Total parenteral nutrition for periods of 4–6 weeks may not only improve the patient with severe malnutrition but may also induce a temporary remission. Both monomeric (Vivonex) and polymeric (Ensure) diets can be used to treat severe malnutrition rapidly and safely and will induce remissions of various duration by putting the distal bowel "at rest." These diets are preferably administered by tube on a continuous basis for periods of 3–4 weeks and make possible caloric ingestions of more than 80 kcal/kg in children and adolescents who may be taking less than 50%

of the recommended daily allowance for their age.

Parenteral nutrition is important in rehabilitation of the malnourished patient and is also effective in inducing remissions and healing enteral fistulas. Home total parenteral nutrition programs have been used with a considerable number of patients.

B. Symptomatic Treatment: Rest is important when the disease is active. Anxiety, depression, severe diarrhea, and pain can be treated with sedatives, tranquilizers, anticholinergic agents, and opiates, but they are seldom needed.

C. Antibiotics and Sulfasalazine: Broad-spectrum antibiotics may be helpful if there is evidence that malabsorption is partly due to significant upper small bowel bacterial contamination. Antibiotics are not generally effective in the treatment of perianal abscesses and fistulas. However, good results can be obtained with metronidazole (Flagyl), 1–1.5 g/1.73 m^2/d. There are also reports of satisfactory control of other forms of the disease with metronidazole, especially when sulfasalazine therapy proves ineffective. Sulfasalazine is not thought to be as effective in regional enteritis as in ulcerative colitis but is given to patients with Crohn's colitis and ileocolitis in the same dosage. It offers no protection against relapses but is effective in the acute stage of the disease.

D. Corticosteroids: Both short-term and chronic administration of corticosteroids are useful in the control of symptoms. Corticosteroids may alter the course of the disease and are particularly indicated in patients with systemic manifestations. However, there is no convincing evidence that they prevent relapses when given either pre- or postoperatively.

E. Immunosuppressive Therapy: Azathioprine (Imuran), 2 mg/kg/d orally, has been shown to prolong remissions, thus making it possible to maintain patients on smaller doses of corticosteroids. One study suggests that mercaptopurine, 1.5 mg/kg/d, may be more effective than azathioprine.

Prognosis

Although the mortality rate is low, the morbidity rate is high. The disease process is progressive in most cases, and its course is interspersed with both acute and chronic complications, leading to variable degrees of invalidism. Most patients experience symptoms that impose limits on the quality of their lifestyles. About 20% have severe disabling disease, whereas 20% have few symptoms and describe themselves as healthy.

Farmer RG, Whelan G, Fazio VW: Long-term follow-up of patients with Crohn's disease. *Gastroenterology* 1985;**88:**1818.

Fonkalsrud EW et al: Surgical management of Crohn's disease in children. *Am J Surg* 1979;**138:**15.

Gryboski JD: Crohn's disease in children. *Pediatr in Rev* 1981;**2:**239.

Motil KJ et al: The effect of disease, drug, and diet on whole body protein metabolism in adolescents with Crohn's disease and growth failure. *J Pediatr* 1982;**101:**345.

Rosenthal SR et al: Growth failure and inflammatory bowel disease: Approach to treatment of a complicated adolescent problem. *Pediatrics* 1983;**72:**481.

SELECTED REFERENCES

Davidson M (editor): Paediatric gastroenterology. *Clin Gastroenterol* 1977;**6:**251. [Entire issue.]

Lebenthal E: *Textbook of Gastroenterology and Nutrition in Infancy.* Raven Press, 1981.

Silverman A. Roy CC: *Pediatric Clinical Gastroenterology,* 3rd ed. Mosby, 1983.

Sleisenger MH, Fordtran JS: *Gastrointestinal Disease,* 3rd ed. Saunders, 1983.

Walker-Smith J: *Diseases of the Small Intestine in Childhood,* 2nd ed. Wiley, 1979.

Liver & Pancreas

20

Arnold Silverman, MD

LIVER

PROLONGED CHOLESTATIC NEONATAL JAUNDICE

The main clinical features of the group of disorders responsible for prolonged cholestatic neonatal jaundice are elevated direct-reacting bilirubin fraction (> 2 mg/dL), elevated serum bile acids (> 10 mmol/L), normal or partially or completely acholic stools, dark urine, and hepatomegaly.

Prolonged neonatal cholestasis may be due to intrahepatic or extrahepatic causes. Though many specific causes of intrahepatic cholestasis have been identified, only about 25% of all such cases are accounted for. With rare exceptions, extrahepatic cholestasis is due to anatomic defects that occur without specific known cause.

Attention to specific clinical clues will distinguish these 2 major categories of jaundice in 85% of cases. Histologic examination of tissue obtained by percutaneous liver biopsy will increase the accuracy of differentiation to over 95% (Table 20–1).

Table 20–1. Differentiating clinical and pathologic features of intra- and extrahepatic neonatal cholestasis.

	Intrahepatic	Extrahepatic
Clinical features	Preterm, small for gestational age, appears ill; hepatosplenomegaly, other organ or system involvement; incomplete cholestasis (stools with some color); associated cause identified (infections, metabolic, familial, etc).	Full-term, seems well, hepatomegaly (firm to hard), complete cholestasis (acholic stools > 10/d), polysplenia syndrome, equal right and left hepatic lobes.
Pathologic features	Cholestasis, lobular disarray, giant cells, portal inflammation, minimal fibrosis, rare neoductular formation, steatosis, extramedullary hematopoiesis.	Cholestasis, neoductular proliferation, portal fibrosis, bile lakes, normal lobular architecture, rare giant cells.

INTRAHEPATIC CHOLESTASIS

Intrahepatic cholestasis is characterized by patency of the extrahepatic biliary system, cholestasis, and abnormalities on liver function tests. A specific cause can be identified in about 25% of cases. Patency of the extrahepatic biliary tract can best be confirmed by nonsurgical means by hepatobiliary scintigraphy using ^{99m}Tc-diethyliminodiacetic acid (diethyl-IDA, DIDA) or ^{99m}Tc-*p*-isopropylacetanilidoiminodiacetic acid (PIPIDA). Radioactivity in the bowel within 4–14 hours is evidence of patency.

1. PERINATAL OR NEONATAL HEPATITIS DUE TO INFECTION

This diagnosis is justified in infants with jaundice, hepatomegaly, vomiting, lethargy, and other systemic signs if a perinatally acquired viral, bacterial, or protozoal infection can be established. Infection may occur by transplacental spread via the ascending route from vaginal or cervical structures into amniotic fluid, from swallowed contaminated products (maternal blood, urine) during delivery, or from breast milk, contaminated hands, etc. The infectious agents most apt to be associated with neonatal intrahepatic cholestasis include herpesvirus, varicella, coxsackievirus, cytomegalovirus, rubella virus, echoviruses 14 and 19, adenovirus, hepatitis B virus, *Treponema pallidum*, and *Toxoplasma gondii*. The degree of liver cell injury caused by these agents is variable, ranging from massive hepatic necrosis (herpesvirus) to focal necrosis and mild inflammation (cytomegalovirus, hepatitis B virus). Injury to critical hepatocyte organelles is usual, affecting bilirubin uptake, binding, conjugation, and excretion (mixed hyperbilirubinemia). Elevated bile acids are seen, and other liver function tests are likewise abnormal. Cholestasis results, with jaundice, and the infant generally appears ill.

Clinical Findings

A. Symptoms and Signs: Clinical symptoms usually appear in the first 2 weeks of life but may appear as late as 2–3 months. Jaundice may be noted in the first 24 hours or may develop later, after an anicteric period. Loss of appetite, poor sucking reflex, lethargy, and vomiting are frequent. Stools may be normal to pale in color but are seldom acholic. Dark urine stains the diaper. Hepatomegaly is present with a uniform, firm consistency. Splenomegaly is variable. Macular, papular, or petechial rashes may occur. In less severe cases, failure to thrive may be the major complaint. Unusual presentations include hypoproteinemia and anasarca (nonhemolytic hydrops) and hemorrhagic disease of the newborn.

B. Laboratory Findings: The blood count often shows neutropenia, thrombocytopenia, and signs of mild hemolysis. Mixed hyperbilirubinemia, elevated transaminases, prolongation of clotting studies, mild acidosis, and elevated cord serum IgM levels (over 60% of normal) suggest congenital infection. Nasopharyngeal washings, urine, stool, and cerebrospinal fluid should be cultured for virus. Specific serologic tests comparing infant and maternal levels are useful (TORCH titers), as are skull and long bone x-rays to determine the presence of intracranial calcifications or "celery stalking" in the metaphyseal regions of the humeri, femurs, and tibias.

Histologic examination of liver biopsy tissue obtained by the percutaneous route is a better way to distinguish intrahepatic from extrahepatic cholestasis than to identify a specific infectious agent within the liver tissue. Exceptions to this generalization include the finding of intracytoplasmic inclusions of cytomegalovirus in hepatocytes or bile duct epithelium cells and the finding of intranuclear acidophilic inclusions of herpesvirus. Variable degrees of lobular disarray characterized by focal necrosis, giant cell transformation, and ballooned pale hepatocytes with loss of cordlike arrangement of liver cells are usual. Portal changes are not striking, but modest neoductular proliferation and mild fibrosis may occur.

Differential Diagnosis

Great care must be taken to distinguish infectious causes of intrahepatic cholestasis from genetic or metabolic causes (inborn errors), since the clinical presentations are very similar. Galactosemia, congenital fructose intolerance, and tyrosinemia must be investigated promptly, because specific dietary therapy is available. Alpha$_1$-antitrypsin deficiency and cystic fibrosis must also be considered. Specific physical features may be helpful when considering Menkes' syndrome or Zellweger's syndrome.

Unless the diagnosis is spontaneous perforation of the bile ducts, infants with extrahepatic causes of cholestasis are seldom ill. Stools are usually completely acholic in appearance, and the liver is enlarged and firm—all helpful clinical clues.

Histologic examination is helpful in distinguishing most cases of intra- versus extrahepatic cholestasis (Table 20–1).

Treatment

Most forms of viral neonatal hepatitis are treated symptomatically. Fluids and adequate calories are encouraged. Vitamin K by injection, vitamins D and E orally, and calcium supplementation should be provided. Choleretics (cholestyramine, phenobarbital) are used if cholestasis persists. Corticosteroids are probably contraindicated. Use of specific antiviral agents (vidarabine, acyclovir) is recommended in herpesvirus disease. Penicillin for suspected syphilis or specific antibiotics for bacterial hepatitis need to be administered promptly. Infants born to women with hepatitis B should be given hepatitis B immune globulin and subsequently immunized with hepatitis B virus vaccine, as outlined in Chapter 5.

Prognosis

Multiple organ involvement is commonly associated with neonatal infectious hepatitis and has a poor outcome. Death from hepatic or cardiac failure, intractable acidosis, or intracranial hemorrhage is seen, especially in herpesvirus or echovirus infection and occasionally in cytomegalovirus or rubella infection. Hepatitis B virus may cause fulminant neonatal viral hepatitis. On the other hand, recovery with transplacental diseases may be complete or with sequelae, especially neurologic ones. Persistent liver disease results in mild chronic hepatitis, portal fibrosis, or cirrhosis. Chronic cholestasis may lead to dental enamel hypoplasia, biliary rickets, severe pruritus, and xanthoma.

Specific Infectious Agents

A. Neonatal Hepatitis Virus B Disease: Infection with hepatitis B (HB) virus may occur at any time during perinatal life, but the greatest risk to the newborn is when acute maternal disease with HB virus occurs during the last trimester of pregnancy or at the time of delivery. Hepatitis B virus has been found in most body fluids besides blood, including breast milk, but it does not seem to be present in feces. In chronic HBsAg carrier mothers, fetal and infant acquisition risk is greatest if the mother (1) is also HBeAg-positive and HBeAb-negative, (2) has detectable levels of serum-specific HB DNA polymerase, or (3) has high serum levels of HBcAb. These findings are markers of high infectivity.

Nomenclature for Hepatitis B Antigens and Antibodies

HBsAg = Hepatitis B surface antigen
HBsAb = Hepatitis B surface antibody
HBeAg = Hepatitis B e antigen
HBeAb = Hepatitis B e antibody
HBcAb = Hepatitis B core antibody

Neonatal liver disease due to HB virus is extremely variable. Fulminant hepatic necrosis has been reported, especially in association with intrapartum or postpartum transfusions of infected blood. However, it also can occur from maternally transmitted virus. In such cases, progressive jaundice, stupor, shrinking liver size, and coagulation abnormalities dominate the clinical picture. Respiratory and circulatory failure usually follow. Histologically, the liver shows massive hepatocyte necrosis, collapse of reticulum framework, minimal inflammation, and occasional pseudoacinar structures. Rare survivors are reported with reasonable restitution of liver architecture toward normal.

In less severe cases, focal hepatocyte necrosis is seen with a mild portal inflammatory response. Cholestasis is intracellular and canalicular. Chronic persistent hepatitis may be found for many years, with serologic evidence of persisting antigenemia (HBsAg) and mildly elevated serum transaminases. However, liver disease progressing to cirrhosis is fortunately very rare.

Mothers with markers for infectivity (HBsAg, HBeAg, DNA polymerase, HBcAb) may be chronic carriers, and their infants should receive hepatitis B immune globulin and hepatitis B virus vaccine (see Chapter 5).

B. Neonatal Bacterial Hepatitis: Most bacterial liver infections in newborns are acquired by transplacental invasion from amnionitis with ascending spread from maternal vaginal or cervical infection. Onset is abrupt, usually within 48–72 hours after delivery, with signs of sepsis and often shock. Jaundice, seen in less than 25% of cases, appears early and is of the mixed type. The liver enlarges rapidly, and the histologic picture is that of a diffuse hepatitis with or without micro- or macroabscess. The most common organisms are *Escherichia coli, Listeria monocytogenes,* and group B streptococci. Isolated neonatal liver abscess due to *E coli* or *Staphylococcus aureus* is often associated with omphalitis or umbilical vein catheterization. Bacterial hepatitis and neonatal liver abscesses require specific antibiotics in large doses and, rarely, surgical drainage. Deaths are common, but survivors show no long-term consequences of liver disease.

C. Neonatal Jaundice With Urinary Tract Infection: The typical appearance of jaundice in affected infants—usually males—is between the second and fourth weeks of life. The manifestations of this disorder are lethargy, fever, poor appetite, jaundice, and hepatomegaly. Except for mixed hyperbilirubinemia, other liver function tests are not remarkable. Leukocytosis is present, and pyuria is confirmed by culture techniques. The mechanism for the liver impairment is unknown, though toxic action of bacterial products (endotoxins) and the inflammatory response have been incriminated.

Treatment of the infection leads to prompt resolution of the cholestasis without hepatic sequelae.

Committee on Infectious Diseases, American Academy of Pediatrics: Prevention of hepatitis B virus infections. *Pediatrics* 1985;**75:**362.

Delaplane D et al: Fatal hepatitis B in early infancy: The importance of identifying HBsAg-positive pregnant women and providing immunoprophylaxis to their newborns. *Pediatrics* 1983;**72:**176.

Dupuy JM et al: Hepatitis B in children. 2. Study of children born to chronic HBsAg carrier mothers. *J Pediatr* 1978; **92:**200.

Majd M et al: Hepatobiliary scintigraphy with ^{99m}Tc-PIPIDA in the evaluation of neonatal jaundice. *Pediatrics* 1981; **67:**140.

2. INTRAHEPATIC CHOLESTASIS ASSOCIATED WITH INBORN ERRORS OF METABOLISM; FAMILIAL INTRAHEPATIC CHOLESTASIS; "TOXIC" & MISCELLANEOUS CAUSES OF INTRAHEPATIC CHOLESTASIS

These cholestatic syndromes are diagnosed by specific enzyme deficiencies or other inherited disorders; a positive history of certain precipitants associated with neonatal liver disease; and features of intrahepatic cholestasis—ie, jaundice, hepatomegaly, and normal to completely acholic stools. Some of the specific clinical conditions have characteristic clinical signs.

Neonatal Cholestasis Due to Enzyme Deficiencies or Other Inherited Disorders

Early specific diagnosis is important because dietary treatment may be available. Reversal of liver disease and clinical symptoms is prompt and permanent as long as the diet is maintained. As with other genetically inherited inborn errors of metabolism, proper counseling for parents of the affected infant should be done as soon as possible.

Cholestasis due to inborn errors of metabolism such as galactosemia, hereditary fructose intolerance, and tyrosinemia (see Chapter 33) appears as part of a distinct clinical presentation. Vomiting, lethargy, poor feeding, and irritability often precede jaundice. Firm hepatomegaly is a constant finding. The infants often appear septic, and gram-negative organisms can be cultured from the blood in 25–50% of cases, especially in patients with galactosemia.

Other inherited conditions occasionally presenting with features of intrahepatic cholestasis include Byler disease, cystic fibrosis, Niemann-Pick disease, cholestasis of North American Indian children, cerebrohepatorenal (Zellweger's) syndrome, and Menkes' kinky hair syndrome. A more common diagnostic problem of familial nature is α_1-antitrypsin deficiency (see below), especially when liver biopsy features in the presence of complete cholestasis (acholic stools) mimic those seen in histologic specimens from patients with extrahepatic causes of neonatal cholestasis.

"Toxic" Causes of Neonatal Cholestasis

A. Neonatal "Gut Shock" Conditions: Perinatal events that result in hypoperfusion of the gastrointestinal system are sometimes followed in 1–2 weeks by cholestasis. This is seen in premature infants with respiratory distress, severe hypoxia, hypoglycemia, shock, and acidosis. When these perinatal conditions develop in association with gastrointestinal lesions such as ruptured omphalocele, gastroschisis, or later necrotizing enterocolitis, a subsequent cholestatic picture is common (25–50% of cases).

Liver function studies reveal mixed hyperbilirubinemia, elevated alkaline phosphatase values, and variable elevation of the transaminases. Stools are seldom persistently acholic.

Choleretics (cholestyramine, phenobarbital) and nutritional support are the mainstays of treatment until the cholestasis resolves. In some cases, this may take 3–6 months. When total parenteral nutrition is required, an amino acid concentration of 2% or less is recommended.

Complete resolution of the hepatic abnormalities is the rule, but portal fibrosis with perilobular scarring is occasionally seen on follow-up biopsy.

B. Prolonged Parenteral Nutrition: Cholestasis may develop after 1–2 weeks in premature newborns receiving total parenteral nutrition.

The mechanism seems to result from both concentration of amino acids and duration of their use. Diminished stimulation to bile flow from prolonged absence of oral feedings, toxic additives in the solutions, and an improper ratio of neutral to aromatic amino acids have been considered as cholestatic "toxic" factors.

The prognosis is good. Rare cases of portal fibrosis or stable cirrhosis have been found on follow-up liver biopsy.

C. "Inspissated Bile Syndrome": This is the result of accumulation of bile in canaliculi and in the small and medium-sized bile ducts in hemolytic disease of the newborn (Rh, ABO). The same mechanisms may cause intrinsic obstruction of the common duct. In extreme hemolysis, the cholestasis may be seemingly complete with acholic stools. Levels of bilirubin may reach 40 mg/dL, primarily direct-reacting. If inspissation of bile occurs within the extrahepatic biliary tree, differentiation from biliary atresia may be difficult. A trial of choleretics (cholestyramine, phenobarbital, aluminum hydroxide gel, theophylline) is indicated. Once stools show a return to normal color, patency of the extrahepatic biliary tree is ensured. Small bile-colored plugs in the stools are sometimes reported by parents at the time stool color becomes normal. Though most cases slowly improve over 2–6 months, persistence of complete cholestasis for more than 6–8 weeks requires further studies (ultrasonography, ^{99m}Tc diethyl-IDA scanning, liver biopsy) with possible laparotomy for exploration of the extrahepatic biliary tree. Irrigation of the common duct is sometimes necessary to dislodge the obstructing inspissated biliary material.

Applebaum MN, Tholer MM: Reversibility of extensive liver damage in galactosemia. *Gastroenterology* 1975;**69:**496.

Dahms BB, Halpin TC Jr: Serial liver biopsies in parenteral nutrition-associated cholestasis of early infancy. *Gastroenterology* 1981;**81:**136.

Dosi PC et al: Perinatal factors underlying neonatal cholestasis. *J Pediatr* 1985;**106:**471.

Hardwick DF, Dimmick JE: Metabolic cirrhoses of infancy and early childhood. *Perspect Pediatr Pathol* 1976;**3:**103.

Odievre M et al: Hereditary fructose intolerance in childhood. *Am J Dis Child* 1978;**132:**605.

Riely CA: Familial intrahepatic cholestasis: An update. *Yale J Biol Med* 1979;**52:**89.

3. IDIOPATHIC NONFAMILIAL INTRAHEPATIC CHOLESTASIS (Giant Cell Hepatitis)

This type of cholestatic jaundice of unknown cause presents with the usual features of cholestasis and a typical appearance on histologic examination of biopsied liver tissue; it accounts for up to 75% of cases of neonatal intrahepatic cholestasis. The cholestasis may be mild to severe when clinically and biochemically it is indistinguishable from extrahepatic causes (10% of cases).

If the history includes smallness for gestational age or premature birth, poor feeding, emesis, or failure to thrive, that is consistent with intrahepatic cholestasis. Obviously, the presence of normal or intermittently normal color in stools is helpful information in ruling out an operable explanation for the cholestasis.

In cases of suspected "idiopathic" intrahepatic cholestasis, a trial of choleretics is indicated, with vitamin and nutritional support. Persistence of complete cholestasis after 4–6 weeks (acholic stools) warrants repeat liver biopsy and minilaparotomy with intraoperative cholangiography. A small but patent extrahepatic biliary tree is occasionally demonstrated (hypoplastic) and is probably the result rather than the cause of diminished bile flow. Cholecystostomy often results in improvement in cholestasis, but recurrences are possible when this form of drainage is discontinued.

Once a patent extrahepatic tree is confirmed, therapy should include choleretics (cholestyramine, phenobarbital), a special formula with medium-chain triglycerides (Pregestimil, Portagen), and supplemental fat-soluble vitamins in water-miscible form. These are continued as long as significant cholestasis remains.

Long-term consequences correlate best with the duration of the cholestasis. In general, failure to resolve the cholestatic picture is associated with progressive liver disease and evolving cirrhosis. This may occur either with normal numbers of interlobular bile ducts or when diminished numbers of ducts (paucity of interlobular ducts) result. Perilobular and intralobular fibrosis both progress, and portal hypertension eventually ensues, with splenomegaly and esophageal varices. Finally, ascites with rising bilirubin levels heralds the onset of hepatic failure.

This form of persistent neonatal cholestasis does not always lead to progressive liver disease, but severe pruritus and growth retardation are common (see below).

Balistreri WF: Neonatal cholestasis. *J Pediatr* 1985;**106:**171.
Ferry GD et al: Guide to early diagnosis of biliary obstruction in infancy. *Clin Pediatr* 1985;**24:**305.
Odievre M et al: Long-term prognosis for infants with intrahepatic cholestasis and patent extrahepatic biliary tract. *Arch Dis Child* 1981;**56:**373.

4. INTRAHEPATIC CHOLESTASIS WITH PAUCITY OF INTERLOBULAR BILE DUCTS (Anatomic Forms)

Anatomic forms of intrahepatic cholestasis may be classified according to whether or not they are associated with other malformations. One form (Alagille's syndrome [arteriohepatic dysplasia]) is sometimes recognized by identification of the characteristic facies, which in the newborn becomes more obvious with age. The forehead is prominent, as is the nasal bridge. The eyes are set deep and sometimes widely apart (hypertelorism). Often the chin is small and slightly pointed and projects forward. Cholestasis is usually incomplete, and stool color is normal. Pruritus begins by 3–4 months of age. Firm, smooth hepatomegaly is present, and cardiac murmurs are frequent. Xanthomas are rare early in the disease. Occasionally, early cholestasis is mild and not recognized.

Mild elevations of serum bilirubin are found (up to 2–8 mg/dL). Serum alkaline phosphatase is usually markedly elevated, as is the cholesterol level, especially early in life. Serum bile acids are always elevated. Transaminases are slightly increased, but clotting factors and other liver proteins are usually normal.

The cardiovascular abnormalities are variable; pulmonary stenosis is most common. Other lesions that may occur include atrial septal defect, coarctation of the aorta, and tetralogy of Fallot.

The vertebral arch defects include incomplete fusion of the vertebral body or anterior arch (butterfly deformity) and diminished interpedicle distance in the thoracolumbar spine.

Other abnormalities become manifest later in life. Growth retardation with normal growth hormone levels is commonly seen. A weak, high-pitched voice may be noted. Eye findings (posterior embryotoxon), renal abnormalities (dysplastic kidneys, tubular ectasia), and neurologic disorders due to vitamin E deficiency (areflexia, ataxia) eventually develop in some children.

In a second form, not often distinguishable on liver biopsy, there are no associated malformations. Biliary cirrhosis and liver failure usually occur before adolescence and are secondary to giant cell hepatitis or α_1-antitrypsin deficiency.

High doses (4–8 g/d) of cholestyramine are beneficial in controlling the pruritus and clearing xanthomas. Serum cholesterol levels fall to normal or near-normal by age 5 years. Phenobarbital is useful as adjuvant therapy to lower the bilirubin values. Good nutrition early in life, with supplemental water-miscible forms of fat-soluble vitamins, is important, especially to prevent rickets and the neurologic manifestations of vitamin E deficiency.

The prognosis is favorable in the syndromatic variety. Cholestasis disappears by age 2–3 years, and pruritus subsides before adolescence. Liver fibrosis is usually absent or minimal despite mild persistent biochemical abnormalities such as elevated serum bile acids, transaminases, and alkaline phosphatase, even after many years. Survival into adulthood is common in these cases. Though hypogonadism has been noted, fertility is not obviously affected. The cardiac, vertebral, ocular, or renal components seldom affect longevity.

Guggenheim MA et al: Progressive neuromuscular disease in children with chronic cholestasis and vitamin E deficiency: Diagnosis and treatment with alpha tocopherol. *J Pediatr* 1982;**100:**51.
Markowitz J et al: Arteriohepatic dysplasia. 1. Pitfalls in diagnosis and management. *Hepatology* 1983;**3:**74.
Riely CA et al: Arteriohepatic dysplasia: A benign syndrome of intrahepatic cholestasis with multiple organ involvement. *Ann Intern Med* 1979;**91:**520.

EXTRAHEPATIC NEONATAL CHOLESTASIS

Extrahepatic neonatal cholestasis is characterized by complete and persistent cholestasis (acholic stools) in the first 1–4 weeks of life, surgically proved lack of patency of the extrahepatic biliary tree (porta hepatis to ampulla of Vater) by intraoperative cholangiography, firm to hard hepatomegaly, and typical features on histologic examination of liver biopsy tissue. There are 4 conditions to consider as causative of extrahepatic cholestasis: biliary atresia, choledochal cyst, intrinsic obstruction of the common duct, and spontaneous perforation of the extrahepatic ducts.

Extrahepatic Biliary Atresia

In Caucasians, extrahepatic biliary atresia occurs in 1:8000–1:13,000 births, and the incidence in both sexes is equal. In Orientals, the incidence is higher, and the disorder is twice as common in girls. The abnormality found most commonly is complete atresia of all extrahepatic biliary structures, but there are variants. The specific cause is not known, although recent evidence supports an insult to the biliary structures in utero that progresses in postnatal life. Extrahepatic atresia has not been found in stillborn fetuses and is rarely seen in premature infants. Meconium and first-passed stools are usually normal in color, suggesting early patency of the ducts. Furthermore, the presence of patent intrahepatic bile ducts near the porta hepatis is not consistent with congenital absence of the primitive bile duct. Evidence obtained from surgically removed remnants of the extrahepatic biliary tree suggests an inflammatory or sclerosing cholangiopathy. Although an infectious cause seems reasonable, no agent has been consistently found in such cases. Though other congenital malformations, especially vascular ones, may occasionally be seen in extrahepatic biliary atresia, only polysplenia syndrome (situs inversus, levocardia, absence of the inferior vena cava) is consistently associated with extrahepatic biliary atresia.

Jaundice may be noted in the newborn period but is more often delayed until 2–3 weeks of age. The urine is dark and stains the diaper, and the stools are often pale yellow, buff-colored, gray, or acholic. Seepage of bilirubin products across the intestinal mucosa gives some yellow coloration to the stools. Hepatomegaly is common, and the liver may feel firm to hard; splenomegaly develops later. Pruritus, digital clubbing, xanthomas, and a rachitic rosary may be noted in slightly older patients. Murmurs reflecting increasing cardiovascular output or shunting through bronchial arteries may be heard over the entire precordium and back. By 2–3 months, the growth curves reveal poor weight gain, probably as a result of fat malabsorption, though vomiting and diarrhea are seldom reported. Late in the course, ascites and bleeding complications occur.

No single laboratory test will consistently differentiate this entity from other causes of "complete" obstructive jaundice. A ^{99m}Tc diethyl-IDA excretion study performed early in the course of disease and after pretreatment with phenobarbital (3–5 mg/kg/d for 5–7 days) may distinguish hepatocyte disease from small and large bile duct disease. Although biliary atresia is suggested by persistent elevation of serum γ-glutamyl transpeptidase or alkaline phosphatase levels, high cholesterol levels, and prolonged prothrombin times, these findings have also been reported in severe neonatal hepatitis. Furthermore, these tests will not differentiate the location of the obstruction within the extrahepatic system ("correctable" versus "noncorrectable" lesions). Generally, the transaminases are only modestly elevated in biliary atresia. Serum proteins and blood clotting factors are not affected early in the disease. Routine chest x-ray may reveal abnormalities suggestive of polysplenia syndrome. Ultrasonography of the biliary system should be performed to ascertain the presence of choledochal cyst. Biopsy specimens can differentiate intrahepatic causes of cholestasis from biliary atresia in over 90% of cases.

The major diagnostic dilemma is between this entity and "complete" intrahepatic cholestasis, choledochal cyst, or intrinsic bile duct obstruction (stones, bile plugs). Though spontaneous perforation of extrahepatic bile ducts leads to jaundice and acholic stools, the infants are usually quite ill with chemical peritonitis from biliary ascites, and hepatomegaly is not found.

Surgical exploration is necessary. Associated anomalies should be anticipated (malrotation, preduodenal portal vein, situs inversus). Preoperative attention to clotting studies is warranted, including partial thromboplastin time as well as prothrombin time. Laparotomy must always include liver biopsy and an operative cholangiogram if a gallbladder is present. The presence of bile in the gallbladder implies patency of the proximal extrahepatic duct system. Radiographic visualization of dye in the duodenum will exclude obstruction to the distal extrahepatic ducts. An absent gallbladder, the absence of bile within the lumen, or failure to visualize the duodenum on cholangiography dictates thorough exploration of the extrahepatic biliary tree to the porta hepatis.

In the absence of surgical correction, the following eventually develop: failure to thrive, marked pruritus, portal hypertension, hypersplenism, bleeding diathesis, rickets, ascites, and cyanosis. Bronchitis and pneumonia are common. Eventually, hepatic failure and death occur.

Except for the occasional example of "correctable" biliary atresia where choledocho- or cholecystojejunostomy is feasible, the standard procedure is hepatoportoenterostomy (Kasai procedure). Occasionally, portocholecystostomy may be performed if the gallbladder is present and the passage to the duodenum is patent. These procedures are best done in specialized centers where experienced surgical, pediatric, and nursing personnel are available. It is recommended that surgery be performed as early as possible (6–10 weeks); the Kasai procedure should not be undertaken in infants over 4 months of age, because the prognosis in these patients is hopeless.

Orthotopic liver transplantation is available, and the long-term prognosis seems to be improving in survivors.

Whether or not the Kasai procedure is performed, supportive medical treatment measures consist of vitamin and caloric support (using water-miscible forms of vitamins A, D, K, and E and formulas containing medium-chain triglycerides [Pregestimil]). Bacterial infections should be treated promptly and signs of bleeding tendency corrected with intramuscular vitamin K. Ascites can be managed with reduced sodium intake and spironolactone. Choleretics and bile acid-binding products (cholestyramine, aluminum hydroxide gel, phenobarbital) are of little value.

When bile flow is sustained, the 5-year survival rate is 35–50%. Complete surgical failures have the same outcome as nonoperated cases, but patients die sooner (age 8–15 months versus age 18–36 months). Death is usually due to liver failure, sepsis, acidosis, or respiratory failure secondary to intractable ascites. Surprisingly, terminal hemorrhage is unusual.

Barkin R, Lilly JR: Biliary atresia and the Kasai operation: Continuing care. *J Pediatr* 1980;**96:**1015.

Danks DM et al: Studies of the aetiology of neonatal hepatitis and biliary atresia. *Arch Dis Child* 1977;**52:**360.

Kobayashi A, Itabashi F, Ohbe Y: Long-term prognosis in biliary atresia after hepatic portoenterostomy: Analysis of 35 patients who survived beyond 5 years of age. *J Pediatr* 1984;**105:**243.

McClement JW, Howard ER, Mowat AP: Results of surgical treatment for extrahepatic biliary atresia in United Kingdom 1980–1982. *Br Med J* 1985;**290:**345.

Choledochal Cyst

Choledochal cyst is an unusual cause of extrahepatic neonatal cholestasis (2–5% of cases) that occurs with an increased incidence in Orientals. In most cases, the clinical manifestations, basic laboratory findings, and histopathologic features on liver biopsy are indistinguishable from those seen in biliary atresia. Neonatal symptomatic cysts are usually associated with atresia of the distal common duct—accounting for the diagnostic dilemma—and may simply be part of the spectrum of biliary atresia. However, a palpable subhepatic mass, positive ultrasound scan, or pressure deformity on the first and second portion of duodenum seen on upper gastrointestinal series promptly resolves the question. Immediate operation is indicated once abnormalities in clotting factors have been corrected. Discovery of such a mass eliminates the need for percutaneous liver biopsy or other extraneous studies.

Excision of the cyst and hepatojejunal anastomosis are recommended. In some cases, because of technical problems, only a cystojejunostomy can be performed.

The prognosis depends upon the presence or absence of associated evidence of atresia and the appearance of the intrahepatic ducts. If atresia is found, the prognosis is similar to that described for that disorder. If an isolated cyst is encountered, the outcome is generally excellent, with resolution of the jaundice and return to normal liver cellular architecture the rule. However, bouts of ascending cholangitis or obstruction of the anastomotic site may occur. The risk of biliary carcinoma developing within the cyst is about 1–3% at adulthood; therefore, cystectomy should be done whenever possible.

Harris VJ, Kahler J: Choledochal cyst: Delayed diagnosis in a jaundiced infant. *Pediatrics* 1978;**62:**235.

Kim SH: Choledochal cyst: Survey by the Surgical Section of the American Academy of Pediatrics. *J Pediatr Surg* 1981;**16:**402.

Spontaneous Perforation of the Extrahepatic Ducts

The sudden appearance of obstructive jaundice, acholic stools, and abdominal enlargment with ascites in a sick-appearing newborn is suggestive of this condition. The liver is usually normal in size, and a yellow-green discoloration can often be discerned under the umbilicus or in the scrotum. Aspiration of ascitic fluid reveals the bilious color and is best performed after intravenous injection of ^{99m}Tc diethyl-IDA. Radioisotope activity is present in the removed fluid, confirming the diagnosis.

Treatment is surgical. Simple drainage is sufficient in primary perforations. A diversion anastomosis is constructed in cases associated with choledochal cyst or stenosis.

The prognosis is generally good.

Howard ER et al: Spontaneous perforation of common bile duct in infants. *Arch Dis Child* 1976;**51:**883.

OTHER NEONATAL HYPERBILIRUBINEMIC CONDITIONS (NONCHOLESTATIC NONHEMOLYTIC)

This group of disorders associated with hyperbilirubinemia is of 2 types: (1) unconjugated hyperbilirubinemia, consisting of breast milk jaundice, Lucey-Driscoll syndrome, congenital hypothyroidism, upper intestinal obstruction, Gilbert's syndrome, Crigler-Najjar syndrome, and drug-induced hyperbilirubinemia; and (2) conjugated noncholestatic hyperbilirubinemia, consisting of Dubin-Johnson syndrome and Rotor's syndrome.

Persistent elevation of the indirect bilirubin fraction may occur in 1–3% of breast-fed infants. In some cases, it is due to an inhibitor of bilirubin conjugation appearing in mature breast milk. Pregnane-3α,20β-diol and nonesterified fatty acids have both been suggested as the inhibitor.

Hyperbilirubinemia does not usually exceed 10–15 mg/dL. The jaundice is noticeable by the fifth to seventh day of breast feeding and may accentuate the underlying physiologic jaundice. Physical examination is normal; urine does not stain the diaper; and the stools are golden-yellow.

The jaundice clears before 3 months in almost all infants, even when breast feedings are continued.

Kernicterus has never been reported in this condition. In special situations, breast feeding may be discontinued and replaced by formula feedings for 2–3 days until serum bilirubin decreases by 2–8 mg/dL. When breast feeding is reinstituted, the serum bilirubin may increase slightly but not to the previous level.

Some recommend heating the breast milk (56 °C [133 °F] for 15 minutes) before feedings for 4–5 consecutive days, as the inhibitor factor appears to be heat-labile. Lastly, phenobarbital (3–5 mg/kg/d) may be used to hasten maturation of the hepatocyte conjugating system. Blood levels of the drug should be monitored during therapy.

Poland RL: Breast-milk jaundice. *J Pediatr* 1981;**99:**86.

Congenital Hypothyroidism

Though the differential diagnosis should always include consideration of congenital hypothyroidism as a cause of indirect hyperbilirubinemia, the diagnosis may be obvious from other clinical and physical clues. The jaundice quickly clears with replacement thyroid hormone therapy, though the mechanism is unclear.

Smith DW et al: Congenital hypothyroidism: Signs and symptoms in the newborn period. *J Pediatr* 1975;**87:**958.

Upper Intestinal Obstruction

The association of indirect hyperbilirubinemia with high intestinal obstruction—eg, pyloric stenosis—in the newborn has been observed repeatedly, but the mechanism remains unproved. Diminished levels of hepatic glucuronyl transferase have been found on liver biopsy.

Treatment is that of the underlying obstructive condition (usually surgical), and jaundice disappears once adequate nutrition is achieved.

Wolley MM et al: Jaundice, hypertrophic pyloric stenosis and hepatic glucuronyl transferase. *J Pediatr Surg* 1974;**9:**359.

Gilbert's Syndrome

This is a common form of familial hyperbilirubinemia associated with a partial reduction of hepatic bilirubin uridine diphosphate glucuronyl transferase activity. Mild fluctuating jaundice, especially with illness, and vague constitutional symptoms are common. A shortened red cell survival has been shown in some patients. Subsidence of hyperbilirubinemia has been achieved in patients by administration of phenobarbital (5–8 mg/kg/d).

The disease is inherited as an autosomal dominant with incomplete penetrance. Males are affected more often than females (4:1). The findings on liver biopsy and most other liver function tests are normal except for prolonged BSP retention. An increase in the level of unconjugated bilirubin after a 2-day fast (300 kcal/d) of 1.4 mg/dL or more is consistent with the diagnosis of Gilbert's disease.

Gollan JL et al: Effect of dietary composition on the unconjugated hyperbilirubinemia of Gilbert's syndrome. *Gut* 1976; **17:**335.

Crigler-Najjar Syndrome

Patients with type I disease usually develop rapid severe elevation of unconjugated bilirubin, with neurologic consequences (kernicterus). Some survive without neurologic signs until adolescence and early adulthood, at which time deterioration may suddenly occur. The bile is colorless and contains only traces of unconjugated bilirubin. The glucuronyl transferase deficiency is inherited as an autosomal recessive. Phenobarbital is without effect, though phototherapy and cholestyramine may keep bilirubin levels below 25 mg/dL.

Occasionally, a milder autosomal dominant form (type II) without neurologic complications has been found. Hyperbilirubinemia is less severe, and the bile is pigmented and contains bilirubin diglucuronide. Patients with this form usually respond to phenobarbital.

Liver biopsy findings and liver function tests are consistently normal in both types.

Arrowsmith WA et al: Comparison of treatments for congenital non-obstructive non-hemolytic hyperbilirubinemia. *Arch Dis Child* 1975;**50:**197.
Wolkoff AW et al: Crigler-Najjar syndrome (type I) in an adult male. *Gastroenterology* 1979;**76:**840.

Drug-Induced Hyperbilirubinemia

Vitamin K and the sulfonamides may cause high levels of indirect bilirubin, either by reducing the available binding sites on albumin or by causing hemolysis in patients with hereditary deficiency of glucose 6-phosphate dehydrogenase.

Stern L: Drug interactions. 2. Drugs, the newborn infant and the binding of bilirubin to albumin. *Pediatrics* 1972;**49:**416.

Conjugated Noncholestatic Hyperbilirubinemia (Dubin-Johnson Syndrome & Rotor's Syndrome)

The diagnosis is aided by a positive family history and jaundice that persists or recurs.

The basic defect is impaired hepatocyte excretion of conjugated bilirubin, with a variable degree of impairment in uptake and conjugation complicating the picture. Bile acids are normally handled so that cholestasis does not occur. Bilirubin values range from 2 to 5 mg/dL, and other liver function tests are normal. In Rotor's syndrome, the liver is normal; in Dubin-Johnson syndrome, it is darkly pigmented on gross inspection. Microscopic examination reveals numerous dark-brown pigment granules, especially in the centrilobular regions. However, the amount of pigment varies within families, and some jaundiced members may have no demonstrable pigmentation in the liver. Otherwise, the liver is histologically normal. Oral cholecystography fails to visualize the gallbladder. Differences in the excretion patterns of BSP, in results of ^{99m}Tc-HIDA cholescintigraphy, and in urinary coproporphyrin I and III levels can help distinguish these conditions.

The prognosis is excellent, and no treatment is needed.

Bar-Meir S et al: ^{99m}Tc-HIDA cholescintigraphy in Dubin-Johnson and Rotor syndromes. *Radiology* 1982;**142:**743.
Kaplan MM: Case records of the Massachusetts General Hospital. *N Engl J Med* 1978;**299:**592.
Wolkoff AW et al: Rotor's syndrome: A distinct inheritable pathophysiologic entity. *Am J Med* 1976;**60:**173.

HEPATITIS A (Short-Incubation, MS-1, or Infectious Hepatitis)

Essentials of Diagnosis

- Gastrointestinal upset (anorexia, vomiting, diarrhea).
- Jaundice.
- Liver tenderness.
- Abnormal liver function tests.
- Positive liver biopsy.

- Local epidemic of the disease.
- Specific antibody rise.

General Considerations

This disease appears to be caused by a virus or strains of related viruses (27-nm particles) and tends to occur in both epidemic and sporadic fashion. Transmission by the fecal-oral route explains epidemic outbreaks from contaminated food or water supplies. Particles 27 nm in diameter have been found in stools during the acute phase of type A hepatitis and are similar in appearance to the enterovirus group. Sporadic cases usually result from contact with an affected individual. The overt form of the disease is easily recognized by the clinical manifestations, but a larger number of affected individuals have an anicteric and unrecognized form of the disease. This has been especially true in outbreaks of hepatitis A reported in day-care centers for children younger than 3 years of age. Both forms probably confer lifelong immunity to hepatitis A virus.

Antibody to this virus appears within 1–4 weeks of clinical symptoms. While the great majority of children with infectious hepatitis are asymptomatic or have mild disease and recover completely, some will develop a fulminating hepatitis, chronic hepatitis, or cirrhosis. Children who die during the initial attack of the disease do so from massive hepatic necrosis secondary to overwhelming viremia, an immunologic deficiency state, or perhaps exposure to a completely different strain of virus.

Clinical Findings

A. History: A history of direct exposure to a previously jaundiced individual or of eating seafood or drinking contaminated water in the recent past should be sought. Following an incubation period of 14–50 days, the initial symptoms of fever, anorexia, and vomiting usually precede the development of obvious jaundice by 5–10 days.

B. Symptoms and Signs: Fever, anorexia, vomiting, headache, and abdominal pain are the usual symptoms. Darkening of the urine, suggesting the presence of bile, precedes jaundice. Jaundice reaches a peak in 1–2 weeks and then begins to subside. The stools may become light or clay-colored during this time. Clinical improvement can be noted during the early phase of developing jaundice. Jaundice and liver tenderness are the most consistent physical findings. Splenomegaly may be present.

C. Laboratory Findings: An elevated serum bilirubin (both direct- and indirect-reacting) is common. The AST (SGOT) and ALT (SGPT) values are elevated, especially early in the course of the disease. A prolongation of BSP retention following disappearance of jaundice indicates severe residual damage. The sedimentation rate is elevated. Serum proteins are generally normal, but an elevation of the gamma globulin fraction (> 2.5 g/dL) can occur and indicates a worse prognosis. Hypoalbuminemia, hypoglycemia, and marked reduction in prothrombin time are serious prognostic findings. Urine bile and uribilinogen are increased. As the virus disappears, a specific serum IgM antibody rises. The IgG-specific antibody to hepatitis A virus can be detected by immune adherence test or complement fixation from 1 to 4 weeks after onset of the illness.

If the diagnosis is in doubt, a percutaneous liver biopsy may be safely performed in most children—provided the partial thromboplastin time, platelet count, and bleeding time are normal and the prothrombin time is greater than 50%. The presence of ascites may increase the risk of percutaneous liver biopsy. "Balloon cells" and acidophilic bodies are characteristic histologic findings. Liver cell necrosis may be diffuse or focal, with accompanying infiltration of inflammatory cells containing polymorphonuclear leukocytes, lymphocytes, macrophages, and plasma cells, particularly in portal areas. Some bile duct proliferation may be seen in the perilobular portal areas alongside areas of bile stasis. Regenerative liver cells and proliferation of reticuloendothelial cells are present. Occasionally, massive hepatocyte destruction is seen with scarcely a normal liver cell visible.

Differential Diagnosis

Before jaundice appears, the symptoms are those of a nonspecific viral enteritis. Other diseases with somewhat similar onset include pancreatitis, infectious mononucleosis, leptospirosis, drug-induced hepatitis, Wilson's disease, and, most often, type B hepatitis or non-A, non-B hepatitis. Acquired cytomegalovirus disease may also mimic hepatitis A.

Prevention

Some attempt at isolation of the patient is indicated, although the majority of patients with type A hepatitis are noninfectious by the time the disease becomes overt. Stool, urine, and blood-contaminated objects should be handled with extreme care for 1 month after the appearance of jaundice.

Passive-active immunization of exposed susceptibles can be achieved by giving standard immune globulin, 0.02–0.04 mL/kg intramuscularly, with casual contacts receiving approximately half this dose. Illness is prevented in 80–90% of individuals so treated if immune globulin is given within 1–2 weeks of exposure. Individuals traveling to endemic disease areas should receive 0.05 mL/kg as prophylaxis.

Treatment

There are no specific measures. Bed rest during the icteric phase appears to be helpful. Sedatives should be avoided. Do not use corticosteroids.

A. Diet: At the start of the illness, a light diet is preferable. Fruits, vegetables, and plenty of sugars are usually well tolerated. Adequate protein can be supplied by grilled meats or broiled fish with less than normal amounts of fat. B complex vitamins have been used on empiric grounds, but there is no good evidence to show that they alter the course of this disease.

B. Antibiotics: Antibiotics may be given to decrease the intestinal flora in anticipation of hepatic coma in fulminant cases (eg, neomycin, 20 mg/kg/d orally, or kanamycin or clindamycin in comparable doses). If signs of hepatic coma are noted, antibiotics must be discontinued so that lactulose solution, 15–60 mL every 6 hours orally, can be given, since antibiotics interfere with the action of this drug.

Prognosis

Ninety-five percent of children recover without sequelae. In rare cases of fulminating hepatitis, the patient may die in 5 days or may survive as long as 1–2 months. The prognosis is poor if the signs and symptoms of hepatic coma prevail, with deepening of jaundice and development of ascites. Incomplete resolution leads to prolonged hepatitis, chronic cholestatic hepatitis, or, rarely, chronic active hepatitis, which may have several expressions and clinical patterns. Rare cases of aplastic anemia following acute infectious hepatitis have also been reported. A benign relapse of symptoms may occur in 10–15% of cases after 6–10 weeks of apparent resolution.

Feinstone SM, Purcell RH: New methods for the serodiagnosis of hepatitis A. *Gastroenterology* 1980;**78:**1092.

Hadler SC et al: Risk factors for hepatitis A in day care centers. *J Infect Dis* 1982;**145:**255.

Hoofnagle JH: Type A and type B hepatitis. *Lab Med* 1983;**14:**705.

Tabor E et al: Asymptomatic viral hepatitis types A and B in an adolescent population. *Pediatrics* 1978;**62:**1026.

HEPATITIS B (Long-Incubation, MS-2, or Serum Hepatitis; Australia Antigen Hepatitis)

Essentials of Diagnosis

- Gastrointestinal upset, anorexia, vomiting, diarrhea.
- Jaundice, tender hepatomegaly, abnormal liver function tests.
- Serologic evidence of hepatitis B disease: HBsAg, HBeAg, HBcAb.
- History of parenteral exposure.

General Considerations

In contrast to infectious hepatitis, serum hepatitis has a slow onset with an incubation period of 21–135 days. The disease is due to a virus (42-nm Dane particle) that is usually acquired by the parenteral route, although person-to-person spread may occur with shared razors or toothbrushes as well as venereally. Breast milk, urine, and saliva have been shown to contain viral antigen. The identification of hepatitis virus B surface antigen (HBsAg) in 75–100% of patients with this type of hepatitis greatly assists the diagnosis of this entity. The incidence of this disease following blood transfusions varies directly with the number of units received. Data suggest that HBsAg may be present in 8.7% of blood donors.

The complete Dane particle is composed of a core (28-nm particle) that is found in the nucleus of infected liver cells and a double-shelled surface particle apparently formed in the cytoplasm where the completed virus particle is synthesized. The surface antigen in blood is termed HBsAg. This particle is found as a 22-nm spherical particle in the serum but occasionally occurs as a filamentous structure as well. The antibody to it is HBsAb. The core antigen is termed HBcAg and its antibody HBcAb. The core antigen also contains DNA polymerase, which can be measured in patients' blood during viremia. Another important antigen-antibody system associated with hepatitis B virus disease is the "e" antigen system. A soluble antigen, HBeAg, appears in the serum of infected patients early and correlates with active virus replication. Persistence of HBeAg is a marker of infectivity, while the appearance of HBeAb generally implies termination of the carrier state. Neonatal hepatitis B disease occurs in infants born of mothers with active disease in the last trimester and in those born of chronic carriers with markers of infectivity (HBsAg, HBeAg, DNA polymerase). (See p 564.)

Clinical Findings

A. Symptoms and Signs: The symptoms are nonspecific, consisting only of slight fever (which may be absent) and mild gastrointestinal upset. Visible jaundice is usually the first significant finding. It is accompanied by darkening of the urine and pale or clay-colored stools. Hepatomegaly is present. Occasionally, a symptom complex of macular rash, urticarial lesions, and arthritis antedates the appearance of icterus.

B. Laboratory Findings: The presence of HBsAg, HBcAb, or hepatitis B-specific DNA polymerase signifies acute hepatitis virus B disease. HBsAb may develop much later (months to years). Carriers of HBsAg also have detectable levels of HBcAb, and e antigen may also be present in the serum of patients with persistent antigenemia.

Liver function test results are similar to those discussed previously for infectious hepatitis (see above). Liver biopsy seldom differentiates hepatitis A and B disease.

Renal involvement may be suspected by urinary findings suggesting glomerulonephritis.

Differential Diagnosis

The differentiation between hepatitis A and hepatitis B disease is made easier by a history of parenteral exposure and an unusually long period of incubation. The history may suggest a drug-induced hepatitis, especially if a serum sickness prodrome is reported.

Prevention

Screening of blood donors to eliminate individuals who may have had hepatitis is the most dependable way of preventing serum hepatitis. The use of unsterilized hypodermic equipment is a danger that must be considered. Storing plasma at room temperature for 6 months or treating it with ultraviolet rays may decrease the risk of infection. Fibrinogen is as dangerous as plasma.

In individuals receiving numerous blood transfusions, passive immunization with immune globulin has met with variable success. Hepatitis B immune globulin, 0.04 mL/kg, may be of therapeutic value if given within 5–7 days of exposure. A repeat injection 1 month later is recommended.

Individuals in high-risk groups (hemophiliacs, renal dialysis patients, infants born of hepatitis B-infected mothers) can be actively immunized with hepatitis B virus vaccine (see Chapter 5).

Treatment

Supportive measures such as bed rest and a nutritious diet are used during the active stage of disease. Corticosteroids are contraindicated.

Prognosis

The prognosis is good, although fulminating hepatitis, chronic persistent hepatitis, or chronic active liver disease and cirrhosis may supervene. The course of the disease is variable, but jaundice seldom persists for more than 2 weeks. HBsAg disappears in 95% of cases at the time of clinical recovery. Persistent asymptomatic antigenemia may occur, particularly in children with Down's syndrome or leukemia and those undergoing chronic hemodialysis. Persistence of neonatally acquired HBsAg is common, and the presence of e antigen in the HBsAg carrier patient seems to convey a poorer prognosis.

Dupuy JM et al: Hepatitis B in children. 1. Analysis of 80 cases of acute and chronic hepatitis B. *J Pediatr* 1978,**92:**17.

Hoofnagle JH: Type A and type B hepatitis. *Lab Med* 1983;**14:**705.

Krugman S: The newly licensed hepatitis B vaccine. *JAMA* 1982;**247:**2012.

Trevisan A et al: Virologic features of chronic hepatitis B virus infection in childhood. *J Pediatr* 1982;**100:**366.

FULMINATING HEPATITIS (Acute Massive Hepatic Necrosis, Acute Yellow Atrophy)

Fulminating hepatitis has a mortality rate close to 95% in children. An unusual virulence of the infectious agent or peculiar host susceptibility is postulated in these cases. In the first few weeks of life, fulminant hepatic necrosis can be caused by herpesvirus, echovirus, or adenovirus. Metabolic disease may also be responsible. Later, hepatitis B virus and non-A, non-B hepatitis virus are sometimes causative. Hepatitis A virus rarely is responsible for this dreaded disease. Patients with immunologic deficiency diseases and those receiving immunosuppressive drugs are especially vulnerable.

Clinical Findings

In a number of patients, the disease proceeds in a rapidly fulminant course with deepening jaundice, deterioration of laboratory indices, ascites, a rapidly shrinking liver, and progressive coma. Terminally, some laboratory values, such as AST (SGOT) and ALT (SGPT), may improve at the time when the liver is getting smaller (massive necrosis and collapse). Another group of patients start with a course typical of "benign" hepatitis and then suddenly become ill once again during the second week of the disease. Fever, anorexia, vomiting, and abdominal pain may be noted, and worsening of liver function tests parallels changes in sensorium or impending coma. Hyperreflexia and upgoing toes are seen. A characteristic breath odor is present (fetor hepaticus). A generalized bleeding tendency occurs at this time. Impairment of renal function, manifested by either oliguria or anuria, is an ominous sign. The striking laboratory findings include elevated serum bilirubin levels (usually > 20 mg/dL), high AST and ALT (> 5000 IU/L) that may decrease terminally, low serum albumin, hypoglycemia, and prolonged prothrombin time. Blood ammonia levels may be elevated, whereas blood urea nitrogen is often very low initially. Hyperpnea is frequent, and a mixed respiratory alkalosis and metabolic acidosis is apparent from serum electrolyte values. A rise in the polymorphonuclear count often presages acute liver failure.

Differential Diagnosis

Other known causes of fulminating hepatitis such as drugs and other chemical poisons or naturally occurring plant toxins may be difficult to exclude. Patients with Reye's syndrome are typically anicteric. A liver biopsy may be helpful. Wilson's disease, acute leukemia, and Budd-Chiari syndrome should be considered.

Complications

Hepatic failure is soon followed by hepatic coma, the depth of which (stage I-IV) corresponds to the prognosis. Cirrhosis of the postnecrotic type is the usual sequela in the rare pediatric survivor, with some cases of chronic active hepatitis evolving from submassive hepatic necrosis. Cerebral edema may be the cause of death in 15–30% of patients. Complete restoration of normal histologic features is more likely in drug-induced hepatic encephalopathy. Sepsis, hemorrhage, renal failure, or cardiorespiratory arrest is a common terminal event.

Treatment

Many regimens have been tried, but controlled evaluation of therapy remains difficult. Exchange transfusion (with fresh heparinized blood) temporarily repairs both the chemical and hematologic abnormalities. Response may be delayed and repeated exchange transfusions necessary. Plasmapheresis with plasma exchange, total body washout, charcoal hemoperfusion, and hemodialysis using a special high-permeability membrane have been used in the treatment of fulminant hepatic failure. Removal of circulating toxins may be of greater benefit to extrahepatic organ function (brain) than to the liver itself. Reversal of hepatic encephalopathy may follow any of these therapeutic modalities but without improvement in the final prognosis. Survival in adults is not improved over the control group (about 20%). Organ transplantation has been tried in desperate situations.

Corticosteroids may actually be harmful. Sterilization of the colon with antibiotics such as clindamycin, neomycin, or kanamycin is recommended. Acidification of the colon with lactulose (Cephulac), 2–3 tablespoons 3 or 4 times daily, reduces blood ammonia levels and traps ammonia in the colon. Intravenous arginine and glutamine have been used to decrease blood ammonia levels, but their value is questionable. There is recent experimental evidence that insulin and glucagon given via the portal vein may be hepatotropic and of some help in fulminant hepatic necrosis. Growth hormone injections were also thought beneficial in isolated cases.

Close monitoring of fluid and electrolytes is mandatory and requires a central venous line. Maintenance of normal blood glucose levels is important. Diuretics, sedatives, and tranquilizers are to be avoided or used sparingly. Blood clotting factors may be provided by fresh frozen plasma or exchange transfusions. Early signs of cerebral edema are treated with dexamethasone (Decadron) and careful infusions of mannitol (0.5–1 g/kg).

Tracheostomy and mechanical support of ventilation in the comatose patient are indicated with respiratory failure. Antibiotics are indicated at this time. Controlled ventilation may be needed if signs of cerebral edema progress. Prophylactic immune globulin, 0.04 mL/kg intramuscularly, should be given to contacts of the patient.

Prognosis

The overall prognosis remains very grave. Exchange transfusions or other modes of heroic therapy do not improve survival figures. The presence of nests of liver cells seen on liver biopsy amounting to more than 25% of the total cells and rising levels of clotting factors V and VII coupled with rising levels of serum alpha-fetoprotein may signify a more favorable prognosis for early survival. Only the rare survivor escapes postnecrotic cirrhosis.

Hepatic encephalopathy today. *Lancet* 1984;**1:**489.

Mathiesen LR et al: Hepatitis type A, B, and non-A, non-B in fulminant hepatitis. *Gut* 1980;**21:**72.

Psacharopoulos HT et al: Fulminant hepatic failure in childhood. *Arch Dis Child* 1980;**55:**252.

CHRONIC ACTIVE HEPATITIS (Lupoid Hepatitis, Plasma Cell Hepatitis, Chronic Hepatitis)

Chronic active hepatitis is most common in teenage girls, though it does occur at all ages and in either sex. It may follow acute hepatitis B and perhaps hepatitis A or non-A, non-B hepatitis. Rarely, it evolves from drug-induced hepatitis or may develop in conjunction with such diseases as ulcerative colitis, Sjögren's syndrome, or autoimmune hemolytic anemia. Persistence of HBsAg has been noted in sera of patients, especially adults. Positive LE preparations, smooth muscle antibodies, antinuclear antibodies, and systemic manifestations, such as arthralgia, acne, and amenorrhea, suggest systemic lupus erythematosus with liver involvement. However, histologic findings in the liver are consistent with those described for chronic active hepatitis and not those of systemic lupus erythematosus. A genetic susceptibility to development of this entity is suggested by the increased incidence of the histocompatibility antigens HLA-A1 and HLA-B8. These histocompatibility antigens may code for the defect in suppressor T cell function also noted in patients with chronic active hepatitis. Increased autoimmune disease in families of patients and a high prevalence of seroimmunologic abnormalities in relatives have been noted.

Clinical Findings

Fever, malaise, recurrent or persistent jaundice, skin rash, arthritis, amenorrhea, gynecomastia, acne, pleurisy, pericarditis, or ulcerative colitis may be found in the history of these patients. Cutaneous signs of chronic liver disease may be noted (eg, spider angiomas, liver palms). Hepatosplenomegaly is frequently present. Digital clubbing may be found.

Liver function tests reveal smoldering disease with abnormal values for bilirubin, AST (SGOT), ALT (SGPT), BSP retention, and serum alkaline phosphatase. Serum albumin may be low. Serum gamma globulin levels are strikingly elevated (in the range of 2–6 g/dL), with reports of values as high as 11 g/dL. Low levels of C3 complement have been seen. Antibody to a liver-specific membrane lipoprotein has been found, corresponding to ongoing liver disease activity.

Histologic examination of liver biopsy specimens shows loss of the lobular limiting plate, "piecemeal" necrosis, portal fibrosis, an inflammatory reaction of lymphocytes and plasma cells in the portal areas as well as perivascularly, and some bile duct and Kupffer cell proliferation and pseudolobule formation.

Differential Diagnosis

Laboratory and histologic findings differentiate other types of chronic hepatitis (eg, Wilson's disease, chronic persistent hepatitis, α_1-antitrypsin disease, chronic pericholangitis, subacute hepatitis). Drug-induced (isoniazid, methyldopa) chronic active hepatitis should be ruled out. In acute, severe viral hepatitis, histologic examination may also show an "aggressive" lesion early in the disease (< 3 months).

Complications

Untreated disease that continues for months to years eventually results in postnecrotic cirrhosis. Persistent malaise, fatigue, and anorexia parallel disease activity. Bleeding from esophageal varices and development of ascites usually usher in hepatic failure.

Treatment

Corticosteroids (prednisone, 2 mg/kg/d) decrease the mortality rate during the early active phase of the disease. Azathioprine (Imuran), 1 mg/kg/d, is of value in decreasing the side effects of long-term corticosteroid therapy but should not be used alone during the "induction" phase of treatment. These therapeutic agents are now considered to be contraindicated in hepatitis B virus-caused disease. Remissions occur in 75–85% of cases. Treatment is continued for 1–2 years. Relapses are treated in a similar manner. In doubtful cases, a 3- to 6-month period of observation may be indicated prior to commencement of therapy.

Prognosis

The overall prognosis for chronic active hepatitis has been significantly improved by early therapy. Some report cures (normal histologic findings) in 15–20% of cases. Relapses (seen clinically and histologically) occur in 40–50% of cases after cessation of therapy; remissions follow re-treatment. Survival for 10 years is common despite residual cirrhosis. Progressive portal hypertension is seen, and complications (bleeding varices, ascites) require specific therapy.

Arasu TS et al: Treatment of chronic active hepatitis in children. *J Pediatr* 1979;**95:**514.

Czaja AJ et al: Corticosteroid-treated chronic active hepatitis in remission. *N Engl J Med* 1981;**304:**5.

Davis GL, Czaja AJ, Ludwig J: Development and prognosis of histologic cirrhosis in corticosteroid-treated hepatitis B surface antigen-negative chronic active hepatitis. *Gastroenterology* 1984;**87:**1222.

Fitzgerald JF: Chronic hepatitis. *J Pediatr* 1984;**104:**893.

Jensen MJ et al: Detection of antibodies directed against a liver-specific membrane lipoprotein in patients with acute and chronic active hepatitis. *N Engl J Med* 1978;**299:**1

Kayhan TN et al: Effect of corticosteroids on suppressor-cell activity in "autoimmune" and viral chronic active hepatitis. *N Engl J Med* 1982;**307:**1301.

Maggiore G et al: Treatment of autoimmune chronic active hepatitis in childhood. *J Pediatr* 1984;**104:**839.

POSTNECROTIC CIRRHOSIS

Many cases of postnecrotic cirrhosis occur without a prior episode of known hepatitis, but the disease may follow chronic liver disease (eg, neonatal hepatitis; viral hepatitis type A, B, or non-A, non-B; chronic active hepatitis; drug hepatitis) or certain inborn errors of metabolism. The course may be insidious, as in anicteric hepatitis, Wilson's disease, or α_1-antitrypsin deficiency, or the disease may progress with episodes of acute exacerbation of hepatitis. The underlying liver disease may be quiescent, and a stable cirrhosis may exist.

Clinical Findings

General malaise, loss of appetite, failure to thrive, and nausea are frequent complaints. The first indication of underlying liver disease may be ascites, gastrointestinal hemorrhage, or even hepatic coma, especially in the anicteric, insidious varieties. There may be variable hepatosplenomegaly, spider angiomas, and red and warm liver palms. A small shrunken liver may sometimes be detected by percussion over the right chest wall. Most often, the liver is slightly enlarged, especially in the subxiphoid region where it has a firm to hard quality. Gynecomastia may be noted in males. Digital clubbing is found in 10–15% of cases. Irregularities of menstruation and amenorrhea in adolescent girls may be early complaints.

Jaundice may or may not be present, and serum protein determinations often reveal a decreased level of albumin and increased level of gamma globulins. Prothrombin time is prolonged and usually unresponsive to vitamin K administration. "Burr" red cells may be noted on the peripheral blood smear. A mild anemia is present, and thrombocytopenia and leukopenia are present if hypersplenism exists.

Esophageal varices may be demonstrated by endoscopy or x-ray. Liver biopsy, preferably by laparoscopy or by surgical means, is necessary for confirmation of cirrhosis. Regenerating nodules and surrounding fibrosis are the hallmarks of cirrhosis.

Differential Diagnosis

The most important entities to be considered are Wilson's disease, chronic active hepatitis, and α_1-antitrypsin deficiency. Others might include glycogen storage disease (especially type IV), galactosemia, fructose intolerance, porphyria, infantile cirrhosis of India, and chronic passive congestion. (See Table 20–2.)

Complications

In addition to ascites and hepatic coma, complications of portal hypertension are frequent. On the other hand, some individuals with compensated postnecrotic cirrhosis may lead a relatively normal life. The young child often shows malnutrition as a result of fat malabsorption. Deficiencies of vitamin A, D, K, or E may be indicated by rickets, bleeding tendencies, hemolytic anemia, or mucous membrane lesions. Arteriovenous shunts lead to high-output murmurs, digital clubbing, and cyanosis.

Ascites accumulates because of low serum proteins and hyperaldosteronism. Initially, it responds to a low-salt diet but becomes refractory with time.

Hepatic encephalopathy is heralded by subtle per-

Table 20–2. Familial hepatic diseases associated with cirrhosis.

	Predominant Hepatic Pathology	Frequency of Hepatic Pathology	Diagnostic Procedure
Wilson's disease	Postnecrotic or macronodular cirrhosis	High	Biopsy, liver copper content, 24-hour urinary copper excretion, copper oxidase levels in serum
Cystic fibrosis	Macronodular biliary cirrhosis	Moderately high	Sweat chloride
Galactosemia	Postnecrotic cirrhosis	High	Galactose-1-phosphate uridyl transferase levels
Glycogen storage disease (type IV)	Macronodular	High	Amylo-1,4 → 1,6-transglucosidase (branching enzyme)
Fructose intolerance	Postnecrotic	Rare	Absence of fructose-1-phosphate aldolase
Infantile cirrhosis of India	Postnecrotic	Invariable	Clinical setting
Hepatic porphyrias	Postnecrotic	Low	Porphyrin excretion, liver biopsy
Rendu-Osler-Weber syndrome	Postnecrotic	Low	Skin lesion, biopsy
Tyrosinemia	Postnecrotic	High	Blood and urine amino acid screening tests
α_1-Antitrypsin deficiency	Postnecrotic	High	Blood α_1-antitrypsin levels
Byler disease	Postnecrotic	Invariable	Biopsy, serum cholesterol, family history, clinical setting
Cirrhosis of North American Indians	Postnecrotic	Invariable	Biopsy, serum cholesterol, family history, clinical setting

sonality changes and loss of memory. Later, tremors, dysarthria, and lethargy are seen prior to deep coma.

Treatment

Whenever possible, treatment of the underlying condition is indicated: corticosteroids and immunosuppressive drugs in chronic active hepatitis, copper-chelating agents for Wilson's disease, and specific dietary elimination for galactosemia or congenital fructose intolerance. Except in very young infants with metabolic cirrhotic changes, reversal of pathologic liver changes is incomplete. At best, stabilization of the cirrhosis is occasionally achieved. Severe hypersplenism may be treated by splenic embolization or splenectomy (half or total), and bleeding esophageal varices by endosclerosis. Surgical shunting procedures are seldom successful in children younger than 12 years of age. Ascites may be treated with a variety of diuretic agents such as chlorothiazide (Diuril) and spironolactone (Aldactone) in combination with a low-salt diet. More potent diuretic agents (eg, ethacrynic acid) must be used with care because of their tendency to produce potassium-deficient alkalosis. Peritoneovenous shunt (Le Veen shunt) may be tried in refractory cases. Nutrition can be improved with the use of medium-chain triglycerides with large doses of water-soluble vitamins. Portal encephalopathy can be treated by restricted protein intake, lactulose, and nonabsorbable antibiotics. Sedatives, diuretics, and gastrointestinal bleeding are frequent precipitants of the portal encephalopathy.

Prognosis

Postnecrotic cirrhosis follows an unpredictable pattern, with death occurring in the majority of patients within 10 years of diagnosis, usually from liver failure and hepatic coma. A rising bilirubin coupled with diuretic refractory ascites precedes by 6–12 months or less the final signs of hepatic decompensation. The terminal event may be generalized hemorrhage, sepsis, or cardiorespiratory arrest. Cerebral herniation occurs in 10–15% of cases as the major cause of death. Cirrhosis (especially cirrhosis due to hepatitis B disease) carries an increased risk of hepatocarcinoma.

Appleman HD: Cirrhosis: Morphologic dynamics for the nonmorphologist. *Am J Dig Dis* 1972;**17:**463.

Popper H et al: Hepatic fibrosis: Correlation of biochemical and morphological investigations. *Am J Med* 1970;**49:**701.

ALPHA$_1$-ANTITRYPSIN DEFICIENCY LIVER DISEASE

Essentials of Diagnosis

- Serum α_1-antitrypsin level less than 80 mg/dL.
- Identification of specific phenotype (Pi ZZ, SZ).
- Detection of diastase-resistant glycoprotein deposits in periportal hepatocytes.
- Histologic evidence of liver disease.
- Family history of early-onset pulmonary disease or liver disease.

General Considerations

The disease is due to a deficiency in the protease inhibitor system (Pi) predisposing patients to chronic liver disease and an early onset of pulmonary emphysema. It is most often associated with the Pi phenotype

ZZ. With the intermediate serum levels of α_1-antitrypsin present in the heterozygote phenotype (MZ), the incidence of liver disease is not greater than that in the general population despite the presence of glycoprotein deposits in hepatocytes and the rare reports of cirrhosis occurring in heterozygotes. The exact relationship between low levels of serum α_1-antitrypsin and the development of lung and liver disease is unclear. Inclusion bodies in the liver contain a protein component immunologically cross-reactive with serum α_1-antitrypsin, containing excess mannose but lacking sialic acid. This structural abnormality leads to aggregation in the endoplasmic reticulum and is resistant to sialization by sialyltransferase. Although all patients with the ZZ genotype have antitrypsin inclusions in hepatocytes, it may be the only histologic evidence of liver disease. However, the likelihood of developing severe liver disease in response to hepatic injury is definitely increased in patients homozygous for this condition. From 30 to 50% of adults with α_1-antitrypsin deficiency have been found to have cirrhosis. A few children will have only pulmonary or pulmonary and hepatic involvement.

Clinical Findings

A. Symptoms and Signs: α_1-Antitrypsin deficiency should be suspected in all small-for-gestational-age newborns with the "idiopathic" cholestatic syndrome. Poor appetite, lethargy, slight irritability, and jaundice suggest neonatal hepatitis but are not pathognomonic of any one cause. Hepatosplenomegaly is present.

In the older child, hepatomegaly or physical findings suggestive of cirrhosis (spider angiomas, pruritus, liver palms, digital clubbing, small liver size, splenomegaly), especially in the face of a negative history of liver disease, should always lead one to suspect α_1-antitrypsin deficiency. Recurrent pulmonary disease (bronchitis, pneumonia) may be present in a few children.

B. Laboratory Findings: Low levels (< 0.2 mg/dL) of the α_1-globulin fraction may be noted on serum protein fractionation. Specific quantitation of α_1-antitrypsin reveals levels of less than 80 mg/dL in homozygotes (ZZ) deficient in this glycoprotein. Specific Pi genotyping should be done to confirm the diagnosis. Liver function tests often reflect underlying hepatic pathologic changes. Bilirubin (mixed type), transaminases, and liver alkaline phosphatase are elevated in the acute stage, and low albumin and prolonged BSP retention occur in the cirrhotic stage. Hematologic assessment may reveal evidence of hypersplenism. The esophagogram frequently shows varices in advanced cases with portal hypertension.

Pathologic evidence of α_1-antitrypsin deficiency disease is seen in liver biopsy material, where diastase-fast eosinophilic intracellular granules and hyaline masses are noted, particularly in the periportal zones. This material can be definitively identified by immunofluorescence techniques and electron microscopy.

Differential Diagnosis

Other specific causes of neonatal cholestatic syndrome need to be considered (eg, giant cell hepatitis, cytomegalovirus disease, galactosemia, syphilis, fructose intolerance, choledochal cysts, biliary atresia), as well as causes of insidious cirrhosis in childhood (eg, anicteric viral hepatitis A or B, Wilson's disease, cystic fibrosis, glycogen storage disease). If pulmonary symptoms predominate, then cystic fibrosis, immune deficiency disease, tracheoesophageal anomalies, hiatal hernia, and hypoplastic pulmonary artery and lung disease should be considered.

Complications

Twenty-five to 60% of patients with α_1-antitrypsin deficiency may develop chronic liver disease with cirrhosis or decreased numbers of interlobular bile ducts. The infant may succumb in the first year.

Early-onset pulmonary emphysema occurs in young adults (age 30–40 years). An increased susceptibility to hepatocarcinoma has recently been noted in cirrhosis with α_1-antitrypsin deficiency.

Treatment

There is no specific treatment for the deficiency disorder. Replacement of the protein by transfusion therapy is handicapped by its short half-life (4–6 days). The neonatal cholestatic condition is treated with phenobarbital, 3–5 mg/kg/d orally; cholestyramine, 4–8 g/d orally; medium-chain triglyceride-containing formula; and water-miscible vitamins. Portal hypertension, esophageal bleeding, ascites, and other complications are treated as described elsewhere. Genetic counseling is indicated whenever the diagnosis is made. Diagnosis by prenatal screening is possible. Orthotopic liver transplantation has the potential of curing the disease.

Prognosis

With liver injury (due to viral infection, toxins, drugs, etc), 30–50% of these patients either die from progressive liver disease or develop cirrhosis. A correlation between histologic patterns and clinical course has been documented in the infantile form of the disease. Liver failure can be expected 5–15 years after development of cirrhosis.

Morse JO: Alpha$_1$-antitrypsin deficiency. (2 parts.) *N Engl J Med* 1978;**299:**1045, 1099.

Nebbia G et al: Early assessment of evolution of liver disease associated with alpha$_1$-antitrypsin deficiency in childhood. *J Pediatr* 1983;**102:**661.

Sveger T: Prospective study of children with alpha$_1$-antitrypsin deficiency: Eight-year-old follow-up. *J Pediatr* 1984;**104:**91.

BILIARY CIRRHOSIS

Congenital abnormalities of the bile ducts and cystic fibrosis account for most cases of biliary cirrhosis. Early biliary cirrhosis may be found in cases of unsuspected choledochal cyst, common duct stenosis, tumors of the bile duct, or Caroli's disease and in hypersensitivity reactions to certain drugs, eg, phenothiazines and phenytoin. Parasites *(Clonorchis sinensis, Fasciola, Ascaris)* may be causative. Sclerosing cholangitis leading to biliary cirrhosis occurs in some patients with chronic ulcerative colitis. If the extrahepatic biliary tree is atretic, the progress of disease is rapid. It is slow in cases of common duct stenosis or stricture, hypoplasia of the intrahepatic bile ducts, and cystic fibrosis. Patients who have had an ineffective hepatoportoenterostomy (Kasai procedure) progress to biliary cirrhosis with or without significant episodes of cholangitis.

Clinical Findings

The predominating signs and symptoms are those of persistent jaundice, marked pruritus, hepatosplenomegaly, spider nevi, palmar erythema, xanthomas, and gynecomastia in males. Failure to thrive and steatorrhea are frequent. Ascites may be present. Dark urine and pale stools are common.

Laboratory findings show the typical pattern of obstructive jaundice, with elevations of blood cholesterol, alkaline phosphatase, and bile acids. Serum albumin is often reduced, with the gamma globulin fraction elevated. Blood clotting tests are usually abnormal and corrected with vitamin K. Esophageal varices are common in severe biliary cirrhosis secondary to extrahepatic biliary atresia and cystic fibrosis.

Liver biopsy shows proliferation, dilatation, and plugging of bile ducts and fibrosis. Late in the course, there may be few functioning bile ducts. There may sometimes be confusion with congenital hepatic fibrosis. Radionuclide imaging with ^{99m}Tc conjugates in conjunction with ultrasonography, transhepatic cholangiography, and endoscopic or operative cholangiograms may be necessary.

Differential Diagnosis

During infancy, extrahepatic atresia, choledochal cyst, or paucity of the intrahepatic ducts must be considered as the most likely cause. Stricture or stenosis of the extrahepatic ducts may also cause biliary cirrhosis. Unrecognized intraductal tumor or cholelithiasis may lead to biliary cirrhosis. Cystic fibrosis can be ruled out by the sweat test. Ova and parasites should be sought in duodenal fluid and stool, especially in patients from Southeast Asia. Drug toxicity (phenytoin [Dilantin]) should be considered. Nonobstructive dilatation of the intrahepatic biliary tree (Caroli's syndrome) can lead to biliary cirrhosis. Rarely, sclerosing cholangitis may be seen in the adolescent with chronic ulcerative colitis.

Complications

Progressive deterioration and loss of liver cells with marked disruption of hepatic architecture is the common course. Hepatic decompensation, ascites, and coma eventually supervene. The consequences of portal hypertension, with bleeding esophageal varices and hypersplenism, are life-threatening. Early in the disease, severe pruritus may be disabling.

Treatment

Specific treatment is available only for surgically correctable lesions involving the extrahepatic biliary system, and surgery must be performed before the cirrhosis becomes well established. Early (age 2–3 months) surgery using the Kasai operation is currently a popular method of treatment for biliary atresia. Patients with other lesions are treated by supportive measures, including medium-chain triglycerides, water-miscible vitamins (A, D, E, and K), and cholestyramine (Questran) in large doses (8–15 g/d). Antibiotic therapy is indicated in cases where ascending cholangitis or pericholangitis is suspected. Anthelmintic drugs can be used where indicated. Liver transplantation may be considered for a curative procedure.

Prognosis

The prognosis is good only in surgically corrected lesions or in those amenable to specific measures. In the remainder, this is a progressive, ultimately fatal disease.

Starzl TE et al: Liver replacement for pediatric patients. *Pediatrics* 1979;**63:**825.

CHOLECYSTITIS, CHOLELITHIASIS, & ACUTE HYDROPS OF THE GALLBLADDER

Gallstones, often related to hemolytic anemias, are more common than cholecystitis in preadolescent children. Acute and chronic cholecystitis without gallstones is found in teenagers. This may be seen in association with a systemic disease (eg, typhoid fever, scarlet fever, measles) or secondary to anatomic obstruction, either congenital or acquired. Impairment of bile flow may be a consequence of external pressure from neoplasm, lymph node enlargement in the porta hepatis, or pancreatic pseudocyst. Bile flow is impaired by gallstones in the cystic duct, common duct, or ampulla of Vater, as well as by ductal anomalies and tumors.

Clinical Findings

A. History: Acute epigastric or right upper quadrant pain precipitated by eating fatty foods suggests biliary colic. Abdominal pain developing in a child with mucocutaneous lymph node syndrome (Kawasaki disease) is probably due to acute hydrops of the gallbladder. A careful inquiry may elicit evidence of congenital hemolytic anemia or sickle cell disease. The incidence of cholelithiasis increases sharply in the older teenager, especially in the face of obesity and pregnancy. There is also an increased risk of gallstones in children receiving total parenteral nutrition and in those with ileal disease.

B. Symptoms and Signs: Recurrent severe, steady upper abdominal pains with tenderness over the right upper quandrant and radiation of pain to the right shoulder are the most constant physical finding; jaundice and a palpable mass are much less frequent. Vomiting is quite common with acute hydrops.

C. Laboratory Findings: The white blood count may be normal or elevated. Serum bilirubin and alkaline phosphatase are usually variably elevated. Pancreatic amylase levels are elevated when there is obstruction at the ampulla.

D. X-Ray Findings: X-rays may visualize calculi, and an oral cholecystogram may show impairment or nonfunctioning of the gallbladder with or without calculi. Enlargement of the gallbladder and delayed or incomplete emptying following a fatty meal are definitely abnormal findings in children. Endoscopic cholangiography may be necessary if oral cholecystography is nondiagnostic or if better visualization of the common duct is desired. Ultrasonography in cases of acute hydrops or cholelithiasis has now replaced cholecystography.

Differential Diagnosis

The possibilities to be considered for recurrent epigastric and right upper quadrant pain include peptic disease, liver disease, pancreatic pseudocyst, intestinal or colonic inflammatory disease, and kidney disease. The association of abdominal pain in children with hematologic disorders and its postprandial occurrence after fatty foods is most helpful. The triad of pain, jaundice, and a mass should suggest choledochal cyst, but confirmation is best obtained by radiologic studies or even laparotomy. Acute hydrops is almost impossible to differentiate clinically from other inflammatory or obstructive bowel conditions.

Complications

The major concern in long-standing cases is biliary cirrhosis. Perforation of the gallbladder is extremely rare in children but does occur in acute cholecystitis. Obstructions at the level of the ampulla can result in pancreatitis.

Treatment

With the exception of acute hydrops, symptomatic gallbladder disease is best treated by removal of the gallbladder. Common duct patency should be verified by operative cholangiography. Acute hydrops has been treated by aspiration or drainage, but it may resolve spontaneously.

Prognosis

The prognosis in surgically treated patients is good. The postcholecystectomy syndrome is extremely rare in children.

Honoré LH: Cholesterol cholelithiasis in adolescent females. *Arch Surg* 1980;**115:**62.

Roslyn JJ et al: Increased risk of gallstones in children receiving total parenteral nutrition. *Pediatrics* 1983;**71:**784.

Sarnaik S et al: Incidence of cholelithiasis in sickle cell anemia using the ultrasonic gray-scale technique. *J Pediatr* 1980;**96:**1005.

Slovis TL et al: Sonography in the diagnosis and management of hydrops of the gallbladder in children with mucocutaneous lymph node syndrome. *Pediatrics* 1980;**65:**789.

PYOGENIC & AMEBIC LIVER ABSCESS

Pyogenic liver abscesses are usually secondary to bacterial seeding via the portal vein from infected viscera and occasionally from ascending cholangitis or gangrenous cholecystitis. The resulting lesion tends to be solitary and located in the right hepatic lobe. Bacterial seeding may also occur from infected burns, pyodermas, and osteomyelitis. Unusual causes include omphalitis, subacute infective endocarditis, pyelonephritis, and perinephric abscess. Multiple pyogenic liver abscesses are associated with severe sepsis. At particular risk are children receiving anti-inflammatory and immunosuppressive agents. Likewise, children with defects in white blood cell function (chronic granulomatous disease) are more prone to pyogenic hepatic abscesses, especially those due to *Staphylococcus aureus*. In adults there is a male preponderance, and the abscesses are usually solitary.

Although amebic liver abscess is still rare in children, a gradual increase in frequency has been noted, presumably as a result of increased travel through endemic areas (Mexico, Southeast Asia). *Entamoeba histolytica* invasion occurs via the large bowel, though a history of diarrhea (colitislike picture) is not always obtained.

Clinical Findings

With pyogenic liver abscess, nonspecific complaints of low-grade to septic fever, chills, malaise, and abdominal pain are frequent. Weight loss is very common, especially in delayed diagnosis. A few patients have shaking chills and jaundice. The dominant complaint is a constant dull pain over an enlarged liver that is tender to palpation. An elevated hemidiaphragm with reduced or absent respiratory excursion may be demonstrated on physical examination and confirmed by fluoroscopy. Laboratory studies show leukocytosis and at times anemia. Liver function tests reveal low-grade bilirubin elevation and an elevated alkaline phosphatase. Elevated vitamin B_{12} levels are reported. Amebic liver abscesses are usually heralded by an acute illness with high fever, chills, and leukocytosis. Early in the course, liver tests may suggest mild hepatitis. An occasional prodrome may include cough, dyspnea, and shoulder pain as rupture of the abscess into the right chest occurs. Consolidation of the right lower lobe is common (30%).

A radioisotope liver scan is the most useful diagnostic aid; its accuracy is around 80%. Hepatic arteriography, an ultrasonic liver scan, or hepatic angiography has likewise had success in demonstrating liver abscesses as small as 2 cm.

The distinction between pyogenic and amebic abscesses is best made by indirect hemagglutination test and the prompt response of the latter to antiamebic therapy (metronidazole). Examination of material obtained by needle aspiration of the abscess is often diagnostic.

Differential Diagnosis

Hepatitis, hepatoma, hydatid cyst, gallbladder disease, or biliary tract infections can mimic liver abscess. Subphrenic abscesses, empyema, and pneumonia may give a similar picture. Inflammatory disease of the intestines or of the biliary system may be complicated by liver abscess.

Complications

Spontaneous rupture of the abscess may occur with extension of infection into the subphrenic space, thorax, peritoneal cavity, and, occasionally, the pericardium. Bronchopleural fistula with large sputum production and hemoptysis can develop in severe cases. Simultaneously, the amebic liver abscess may be secondarily infected with bacteria (10–20% of cases). Metastatic hematogenous spread to the lungs and brain has been reported.

Treatment

When a solitary pyogenic liver abscess is localized, adequate surgical drainage should be performed. Cultures (aerobic and anaerobic) are taken and specific antibiotic therapy started. Both solitary and multiple pyogenic liver abscesses can also be treated by percutaneous needle aspiration and antibiotics.

Amebic abscesses should be treated promptly. Uncomplicated cases can be treated with oral metronidazole (Flagyl), 30–50 mg/kg/d in 3 divided doses for 10 days. Intravenous metronidazole can be used in patients unable to take oral medication. (***Caution:*** Metronidazole has been shown to be carcinogenic in rodents and mutagenic in bacteria; nevertheless, it is the best single drug currently available for treating invasive amebiasis.) In severe cases, give dehydroemetine, 1–1.5 mg/kg/d for 5–10 days, and cloroquine, 10–20 mg/kg/d in one or 2 divided doses for 21 days. Surgical drainage of the abscess is indicated when secondary bacterial infection exists. Failure to improve after 72 hours on drug therapy indicates superimposed bacterial infection or an incorrect diagnosis. The effect of treatment is best assessed by a liver scan, with resolution occurring over 3–6 months.

Prognosis

An unrecognized and untreated pyogenic liver abscess is universally fatal. The surgical cure rate is about 75%. Most amebic abscesses are cured with conservative medical management.

Chusid MJ: Pyogenic hepatic abscess in infancy and childhood. *Pediatrics* 1978;**62:**554.

Harrison HR, Crowe CP, Fulginiti VA: Amebic liver abscess in children: Clinical and epidemiologic features. *Pediatrics* 1979;**64:**923.

Herbert DA et al: Pyogenic liver abscesses: Successful nonsurgical therapy, *Lancet* 1982;**1:**134.

Rubin RH et al: Hepatic abscess: Changes in clinical, bacteriologic and therapeutic aspects. *Am J Med* 1974;**57:**601.

PREHEPATIC PORTAL HYPERTENSION

Essentials of Diagnosis

- Splenomegaly.
- Esophageal varices with hematemesis or melena.
- Elevated splenic pulp pressure.
- Normal wedge hepatic vein pressure.
- Normal liver histology.
- Impaired patency of splenic and portal veins shown by splenoportography and venous phase of superior mesenteric or splenic aortography.

General Considerations

Prehepatic portal hypertension from acquired abnormalities of the portal and splenic veins accounts for 5–8% of cases of gastrointestinal bleeding in children. A history of neonatal omphalitis, sepsis, dehydration, and umbilical vein catheterization is present in 30–50% of cases. Symptoms may occur before 1 year of age, but in most cases the diagnosis is not made until 3–5 years of age. Those with a positive neonatal history tend to become symptomatic earlier. Splenomegaly is often the first abnormal physical finding. Massive hematemesis or melena occurs within a few years.

A variety of portal or splenic vein malformations have been described, including valves, cavernous transformation, and atretic segments. The site of the venous obstruction may be anywhere from the hilum of the liver to the hilum of the spleen and may be suspected from abdominal ultrasound examination.

Clinical Findings

A. Symptoms and Signs: Splenomegaly in an otherwise well child is the most constant physical sign. Recurrent episodes of abdominal distention due to ascites may also be noted. The usual presenting symptoms are hematemesis and melena. An episode of bronchitis, tracheitis, or pneumonia with significant cough can precipitate esophageal bleeding. The presence of prehepatic portal hypertension is suggested by the following: (1) an episode of severe infection in the newborn period or early infancy—especially omphalitis, sepsis, gastroenteritis, severe dehydration, or prolonged or difficult umbilical vein catheterizations; (2) no previous evidence of liver disease; and (3) a history of well-being prior to onset or recognition of symptoms. In addition, transient ascites may occur following a bleeding episode.

B. Laboratory and X-Ray Findings: Most other

common causes of splenomegaly may be excluded by proper laboratory tests. Cultures, heterophil titer, blood smear examination, bone marrow studies, and liver function tests are necessary. Hypersplenism, mild leukopenia, and thrombocytopenia are present in most cases. Esophagography will reveal varices in over 80% of these patients, with the remainder discovered by fiberoptic esophagoscopy. In addition to normal liver function tests, confirmation of a normal liver is best obtained directly by liver biopsy or indirectly by measurement of wedge hepatic vein pressure (normal, 3–12 mm Hg). The finding of an elevated splenic pulp pressure (normal, 8–12 mm Hg) and demonstration of the block by simultaneous splenic portography confirm the diagnosis of prehepatic portal hypertension. Filling of collateral vessels to stomach and esophagus by the dye is frequently demonstrated. Selective arteriography using the superior mesenteric artery is recommended prior to definitive surgery to determine the patency of the superior mesenteric vein.

Differential Diagnosis

All causes of splenomegaly must be included in the differential diagnosis, the most common ones being infections, blood dyscrasias, lipidosis, reticuloendotheliosis, cirrhosis of the liver, and cysts or hemangiomas of the spleen. When hematemesis or melena occurs, other causes of gastrointestinal bleeding are possible, ie, gastric or duodenal ulcers, tumors, duplications, ulcerative bowel disease, and suprahepatic or hepatic venous obstructions.

Complications

The major manifestation and complication of this condition is bleeding esophageal varices. Fatal exsanguination appears to be uncommon, but hypovolemic shock or resulting anemia may require prompt treatment. Congestive splenomegaly with granulocytopenia and thrombocytopenia occurs. Rupture of the enlarged spleen due to trauma is always a threat. Leukopenia and thrombocytopenia seldom cause major symptoms. Unexplained fluctuating episodes of ascites may develop, and retroperitoneal edema has been reported (Clatworthy's sign).

Treatment

A. Surgical Measures: Except in specialized centers, the surgical treatment of this disease has been disappointing. Portacaval anastomosis would be the most satisfactory procedure, but the portal vein is often involved in the basic disease process, making it unsuitable for anastomosis except in rare cases. Children have previously been treated by means of simultaneous splenectomy and splenorenal shunts. Sustained patency of the shunt is unlikely in children under the age of 8–10 years except when placed by an experienced surgeon. Thrombosis of the shunt is soon followed by recurrent and often more severe hemorrhage from esophageal varices. Splenectomy increases the risk of overwhelming sepsis. More importantly, however, it removes a "safe" group of collateral vessels running from the splenic capsule to the azygos veins, thereby bypassing the esophageal and gastric drainage system.

Other surgical decompression procedures include anastomosis of the superior mesenteric vein to the inferior vena cava (mesocaval shunt), distal splenorenal shunt (Warren procedure), and the interposition mesocaval shunt using knitted Dacron or Teflon for the graft. Esophageal and gastric resection of the varices and transthoracic ligation of the varices have been used as more desperate measures.

B. Medical Treatment: Since a few children with this disease will die as a result of esophageal bleeding, every effort should be made to control the disease medically. The chances for successful surgical shunting procedures improve as the child gets older. The patient may spontaneously develop a decompressive shunt adequate to prevent major bleeding from the esophageal varices.

Spontaneous cessation of hemorrhage from esophageal varices occurs frequently. Shock must be treated with blood transfusions and anemia with iron. Gastric irrigation with iced 0.5% saline solution may help. A transient reduction of portal venous pressure may be achieved by the use of intravenous vasopressin (Pitressin). A dose of 0.1–0.3 unit/min given intravenously often stops the bleeding. The effect of vasopressin is constriction of the splanchnic and hepatic arterioles and consequent lowering of portal venous pressure. Hypertension, bradycardia, diminished cardiac output, water retention, and hyponatremia may occur with this form of treatment. Direct injection of the varices (sclerotherapy) is indicated when other measures fail and before surgery, especially in the child less than 10 years of age. Careful use of a pediatric Sengstaken-Blakemore tube can stop the bleeding.

Antacids, small feedings, and positioning may reduce gastric acidity or prevent esophageal reflux that may aggravate esophageal bleeding. Avoidance of contact sports in the presence of splenomegaly is advisable. Aspirin products should be avoided. Propranolol may reduce the risk of subsequent bleeding by lowering venous pressure in the portal drainage system.

Prognosis

The prognosis depends upon the site of the block, the effectiveness of sclerotherapy, the availability of suitable vessels for shunting procedures, and the experience of the surgeon. Each unsuccessful surgical procedure worsens the prognosis for life. Bleeding episodes, however, seem to diminish with adolescence.

The prognosis in patients managed by medical and supportive therapy may be better than in the surgically treated group, especially when surgery is performed at an early age. Portacaval encephalopathy is unusual in the postshunted child except when protein intake is excessive.

Altman RP, Krug J: Portal hypertension: American Academy of Pediatrics Surgical Section Survey, 1981. *J Pediatr Surg* 1982;**17**:567.

Alvarez F et al: Portal obstruction in children. (2 parts.) *J Pediatr* 1983;**103**:696, 703.

Bismuth H, Franco D: Portal diversion for portal hypertension in early childhood. *Ann Surg* 1976;**183**:439.

Stamatakis JD et al: Injection sclerotherapy for oesophageal varices in children. *Br J Surg* 1982;**69**:74.

SUPRAHEPATIC & INTRAHEPATIC (NONCIRRHOTIC) PORTAL HYPERTENSION

In the absence of cirrhosis, suprahepatic or intrahepatic causes of portal hypertension are rare. The following entities should be considered:

(1) Hepatic vein occlusion or thrombosis (Budd-Chiari syndrome): In most instances, no cause can be demonstrated. Endothelial injury to hepatic veins by bacterial endotoxins has been shown experimentally. The occasional association of hepatic vein thrombosis in inflammatory bowel disease (ulcerative colitis, regional enteritis, infectious diarrhea) favors the presence of endogenous toxins traversing the liver. Allergic vasculitis leading to endophlebitis of the hepatic veins has been occasionally described. In addition, hepatic vein obstruction may be secondary to tumor, abdominal trauma, hyperthermia, or sepsis, or it may occur following the repair of an omphalocele or gastroschisis. Vena caval bands, webs, or strictures above the hepatic veins are sometimes causative. Hepatic vein thrombosis may be a complication of oral contraceptive medications.

(2) Hepatic veno-occlusive disease (acute stage): This entity is often the result of ingestion of pyrrolizidine alkaloids (''bush tea''), which causes widespread occlusion of the small- and medium-sized hepatic veins, with congestion and necrosis of the neighboring parenchymal cells. It may develop after chemotherapy for acute leukemia or bone marrow transplantation. The acute form of the disease generally follows a nonspecific respiratory illness. The disease may be rapidly fatal, although about 50% of patients recover. A subacute and chronic form also exists. Increased use of herbal teas in the USA has been reponsible for several recently reported cases.

(3) Congenital hepatic fibrosis: This rare cause of intrahepatic presinusoidal portal hypertension is inherited as an autosomal recessive and usually requires liver biopsy for diagnosis. Splenoportography reveals patency of the portal venous system even though splenic pulp pressure is increased. The intrahepatic branches of the portal vein may be abnormal (duplicated). Renal abnormalities (microcystic disease) are often associated with the hepatic lesion; therefore, urography should be routinely performed.

(4) Hepatoportal sclerosis and schistosomal hepatic fibrosis: These are also rare causes of intrahepatic presinusoidal portal hypertension.

Clinical Findings

Patients with suprahepatic causes of portal hypertension have abdominal enlargement due to ascites as the presenting complaint in all but a few cases. Abdominal pain and tender hepatosplenomegaly are frequently found. Jaundice is present in about 25% of cases. Vomiting, hematemesis, and diarrhea are less common. The presence of distended superficial veins on the anterior abdomen along with dependent edema is usually seen with inferior vena cava obstruction. Absence of the hepatojugular reflex (jugular distention when pressure is applied to the liver) is a helpful clinical sign. Liver function tests are not usually helpful. Localization is difficult. An inferior venacavogram may reveal an intrinsic filling defect from an infiltrating tumor or from extrinsic pressure and obstruction of the inferior vena cava by an adjacent tumor or nodes. Care must be taken in interpreting extrinsic pressure defects of the subdiaphragmatic inferior vena cava in the face of ascites.

Simultaneous wedge hepatic vein pressure and hepatic venography are most useful procedures. Pressures should also be taken from the right heart and supradiaphragmatic portion of the inferior vena cava. These should eliminate cardiac (constrictive pericarditis) and pulmonary (primary pulmonary hypertension) disease from the differential diagnosis. Hepatic vein pressure and splenic pulp pressure are elevated. Obstruction to major hepatic vein ostia and smaller vessels may be demonstrated by this procedure. In the absence of obstruction, reflux across the sinusoids into the portal vein branches can be accomplished. In most instances, open liver biopsy should be undertaken. Marked central venous congestion and necrosis without fibrosis are striking. Endothelial thickening of hepatic veins may also be found.

Patients with congenital hepatic fibrosis present with hepatomegaly, abdominal pain (cholangitis), or prehepatic portal hypertension. Liver biopsy is diagnostic.

Differential Diagnosis

Cirrhosis of the liver due to any cause must be ruled out. Suprahepatic (cardiac and pulmonary) or infrahepatic causes of portal hypertension must also be excluded. Although ascites may occur in prehepatic portal hypertension, it is not common. Cutaneous signs of chronic liver disease are lacking, since this entity is usually acute. Noncirrhotic nodular transformation of the liver and hereditary telangiectasia should also be considered in the differential diagnosis of intrahepatic presinusoidal portal hypertension.

Complications

Without treatment, complete and persistent hepatic vein obstruction will lead to liver failure, coma, and death. A nonportal type of cirrhosis may develop in the chronic form of hepatic veno-occlusive disease in which small- and medium-sized hepatic veins are affected. Hematemesis due to bleeding esophageal varices is frequent in the few survivors. Death from renal failure may occur in rare cases of congenital hepatic fibrosis.

Treatment

Efforts to correct underlying causes must be undertaken promptly. Surgical removal of the occluding tumor or of the hepatic vein thrombi is possible when the large ostia are involved. Portacaval shunts and right atrial to inferior vena cava grafts have been attempted. Transcardiac membranotomy can be attempted when the obstruction lies in the inferior vena cava. Medical management with heparin, corticosteroids, and diuretics has had inconsistent results. Simple portacaval shunting is the treatment of choice in patients with congenital hepatic fibrosis and may be done prophylactically or after an esophageal bleed.

Prognosis

Hepatic vein obstruction carries a very high mortality rate (95%). In veno-occlusive disease, the prognosis is better, with complete recovery possible in 50% of acute forms and 5–10% of subacute forms.

Alvarez F et al: Congenital hepatic fibrosis in children. *J Pediatr* 1981;**99:**370.

Stillman AF et al: Hepatic veno-occlusive disease due to pyrrolizidine (Senecio) poisoning in Arizona. *Gastroenterology* 1977;**73:**349.

Taneja A et al: Budd-Chiari syndrome in childhood secondary to inferior vena caval obstruction. *Pediatrics* 1979;**63:**808.

Tang TT et al: Hepatomegaly and recurrent ascites in an 11-year-old boy. *J Pediatr* 1977;**91:**1015.

HEPATOMAS

Essentials of Diagnosis

- Abdominal enlargment and pain.
- Hepatomegaly with or without a definable mass.
- Weight loss.
- Anemia.
- Laparotomy and tissue biopsy.

General Considerations

Primary epithelial neoplasms of the liver represent 0.2–5.8% of all malignant conditions in the pediatric age group. The incidence is higher in Japan and China, where childhood cirrhosis is more commonly found. There are 2 basic morphologic types with certain clinical and prognostic differences. Hepatoblastoma predominates in male infants and children, with most cases appearing before age 3. The predominance of right-sided lesions has aroused interest, since the left lobe is supplied with oxygenated blood from the umbilical vein and the right lobe with portal vein blood, which has a lower oxygen saturation.

Hepatocarcinoma, the other major malignant tumor of the liver, occurs more frequently after age 3. This type of neoplasm carries a poorer prognosis than hepatoblastoma and for some reason causes more abdominal discomfort and pain. Hepatocarcinoma has been reported in children with postnecrotic cirrhosis or biliary cirrhosis, but these are the exceptions rather than the rule. The association of hepatocarcinoma with tyrosinemia and α_1-antitrypsin deficiency cirrhosis has also been reported. An interesting aspect of primary epithelial neoplasms of the liver has been the increased incidence of associated anomalies and unusual conditions found in these children. Virilization has been reported as a consequence of gonadotropin activity of the tumor. Leydig cell hyperplasia without spermatogenesis is found on testicular biopsy. Hemihypertrophy, congenital absence of the kidney, macroglossia, and Meckel's diverticulum have been found in association with hepatocarcinoma. The late development of hepatoma in patients treated with androgens must also be kept in mind.

Clinical Findings

A. History: Noticeable increase in abdominal girth with or without pain is the most constant feature of the history. Constitutional symptoms (anorexia, fatigue, fever, chills, etc) may be present.

B. Symptoms and Signs: Weight loss, pallor, and abdominal pain associated with a large abdomen are common. Physical examination reveals hepatomegaly with or without a definite tumor mass, usually to the right of the midline. Signs of chronic liver disease are usually absent.

C. Laboratory Findings: Normal to slightly distorted liver function tests are the rule. Anemia is frequently seen, especially in cases of hepatoblastoma. Final tissue diagnosis is best obtained at laparotomy. Cystathioninuria has been reported. Alpha-fetoprotein levels may be elevated, especially in hepatoblastoma.

D. X-Ray Findings: X-ray is at times helpful in demonstrating the tumor shadow or calcified foci in the neoplasm. An intravenous pyelogram will prove the intrahepatic origin of the mass. Specialized techniques such as radioactive liver scans and selective celiac axis or umbilical artery angiography are generally part of the preoperative workup. CT scanning and ultrasonography are useful both for diagnosis and for following tumor response to therapy.

Differential Diagnosis

In the absence of a palpable mass, the differential diagnosis is that of hepatomegaly with or without anemia. Hematologic and nutritional conditions should be ruled out, as well as lipid storage diseases, histiocytosis X, glycogen storage disease, congenital hepatic fibrosis, hepatic abscess (pyogenic or amebic), cysts, and hemangiomas. Parasitic infections, toxins, and drugs can cause identical symptoms. Veno-occlusive disease and thrombosis of the hepatic veins are also rare possibilities. Tumors in the left lobe may be mistaken for pancreatic pseudocysts.

Complications

Progressive enlargement of the tumor, abdominal discomfort, ascites, respiratory difficulty, and widespread metastases are the rule. Rupture of the neoplastic liver and intraperitoneal hemorrhage have been reported. Progressive anemia and emaciation predispose to an early septic death. Metastases are most frequently to the lungs and abdominal lymph nodes.

Treatment

An energetic surgical approach has brought forth the only long-term survivors. Complete resection of the lesion offers the only chance for a cure. It appears that every isolated lung metastasis should also be surgically resected. Radiotherapy and chemotherapy have been disappointing in the treatment of primary liver neoplasms, although new combinations of drugs are continually being evaluated.

Organ transplantation has been disappointing.

Prognosis

The survival rate if the tumor is completely removed is 60% for hepatoblastoma and 33% for hepatocellular carcinoma. Fibrolamellar oncocytic hepatocarcinoma has a more favorable prognosis. The overall survival and cure rate is less than 20%.

Clatworthy HW Jr, Schiller M, Grosfeld JL: Primary liver tumors in infancy and childhood. *Arch Surg* 1974;**109:**143.

Exelby PR et al: Liver tumors in children in the particular reference to hepatoblastoma and hepatocellular carcinoma. *J Pediatr Surg* 1975;**10:**329.

Farhi DC et al: Hepatocellular carcinoma in young people. *Cancer* 1983;**52:**1516.

WILSON'S DISEASE (Hepatolenticular Degeneration)

Essentials of Diagnosis

- Acute or chronic liver disease.
- Deteriorating neurologic status.
- Kayser-Fleischer rings.
- Elevated liver copper.
- Abnormalities in levels of ceruloplasmin and serum and urine copper.

General Considerations

In Wilson's disease, the increased hepatic copper may be due to an abnormal copper-binding protein or to a lysosomal defect that impairs the excretion of biliary copper. The disease should be considered in all children with evidence of liver disease or with suggestive neurologic signs. A family history is often present, and 25% of cases are identified by screening asymptomatic homozygous family members.

Clinical Findings

A. Symptoms and Signs: Hepatic involvement may be fulminant, may masquerade as chronic active liver disease, or may progress insidiously to postnecrotic cirrhosis. Findings include jaundice, hepatomegaly early in childhood, splenomegaly, Kayser-Fleischer rings, and neurologic manifestations such as tremor, dysarthria, and drooling beginning after 10 years of age. Deterioration in school performance is often the earliest neurologic expression of disease. The rings can sometimes be detected by unaided visual inspection as a brown band at the junction of the iris and cornea, but slit lamp examination is usually necessary.

B. Laboratory Findings: Early liver function tests are consistent with hepatocellular damage. Late in the course, only the BSP may be useful to assess the degree of liver damage.

The laboratory diagnosis of Wilson's disease is sometimes difficult. Serum ceruloplasmin levels are usually less than 20 mg/dL and are measured as copper oxidase rather than directly. (Normal values are 23–43 mg/dL.) Low values, however, are seen normally in infants under 3 months of age, and in 3–5% of homozygotes the levels may be normal. Serum copper levels are low, but the overlap with normal is too great for satisfactory discrimination. Urine copper levels in children over 3 years of age are normally less than 30 μg/d; in Wilson's disease, they are greater than 100 μg/d. Finally, the tissue content of copper from a liver biopsy, normally less than 20 μg/g wet tissue, is greater than 50 μg/g wet tissue in Wilson's disease.

Glycosuria, aminoaciduria, and elevated serum uric acid levels have been reported. Hemolysis and, on rare occasions, gallstones may be found on routine radiography; bone lesions simulating those of osteochondritis dissecans have also been found.

The coarse nodular cirrhosis and glycogen nuclei seen on liver biopsy may distinguish Wilson's disease from other types of cirrhosis. Early in the disease, vacuolation of liver cells, fatty degeneration, and lipofuscin granules can be seen, as well as Mallory bodies. The presence of the latter in a child is strongly suggestive of Wilson's disease.

Differential Diagnosis

During the icteric phase, acute viral hepatitis type A or B, α_1-antitrypsin deficiency, chronic active hepatitis, infantile cirrhosis of India, and drug-induced hepatitis are the usual diagnostic possibilities. Later, other causes of cirrhosis and portal hypertension need consideration. Laboratory testing for the specific factors listed above will differentiate Wilson's disease from the others. The radiocopper ceruloplasmin incorporation test is sometimes needed to differentiate Wilson's disease with a normal ceruloplasmin level from other liver disease with increased liver and urine copper values.

Complications

Progressive liver disease and hepatic coma and death are not uncommon. Recovery from the initial episode usually results in cirrhosis of the postnecrotic type. The complications of portal hypertension (variceal hemorrhage, ascites) are poorly tolerated by these patients. Progressive degenerating central nervous system disease and terminal aspiration pneumonia are common in untreated older people. Acute hemolytic disease may result in renal impairment.

Treatment

Penicillamine (Cuprimine), 900–1200 mg/d orally, is the drug of choice in all cases, whether symptomatic or not. It is best to begin with 250 mg/d and increase the dose weekly by 250-mg increments. Dietary restriction of copper intake is not practical. Supplementation with zinc sulfate may negate this problem. The dosage of penicillamine may be reduced after urinary copper levels return to normal. Vitamin B_6 is given to prevent optic neuritis. Levodopa may be helpful in cases where penicillamine is unsuccessful or results in toxicity.

General treatment measures for acute hepatitis are as outlined for infectious hepatitis. Portacaval shunting may be contraindicated in Wilson's disease. Orthotopic liver transplants can be curative if rejection can be controlled.

Prognosis

The prognosis of hepatitis due to Wilson's disease is not favorable, though reversal of the hepatic lesion following treatment has been reported in isolated cases. Eventual liver failure and coma often occur prior to brain death from neurologic complications. All siblings should be immediately screened and homozygotes treated even if asymptomatic.

McCullough AJ et al: Antemortem diagnosis and short-term survival of a patient with Wilson's disease presenting as fulminant hepatic failure. *Dig Dis Sci* 1984;**29:**862.

Perman JA et al: Laboratory measures of copper metabolism in the differentiation of chronic active hepatitis and Wilson's disease in children. *Pediatrics* 1979;**94:**564.

Spechler SJ, Loff RS: Wilson's disease: Diagnostic difficulties in the patient with chronic hepatitis and hypoceruloplasminemia. *Gastroenterology* 1980;**78:**803.

Werlin SL et al: Diagnostic dilemmas of Wilson's disease: Diagnosis and treatment. *Pediatrics* 1978;**62:**47.

REYE'S SYNDROME (Encephalopathy With Fatty Degeneration of the Viscera; White Liver Disease)

Essentials of Diagnosis

- Prodromal upper respiratory tract infection, influenza A or B illness, or chickenpox.
- Vomiting.
- Lethargy, drowsiness progressing to semicoma.
- Elevated AST (SGOT), hyperammonemia, normal or slightly elevated bilirubin, prolonged prothrombin time.
- Variable hypoglycemia.
- Microvesicular steatosis of liver, kidneys, brain, etc.

General Considerations

The number of reported cases of Reye's syndrome is decreasing, perhaps owing to a decline in the use of salicylates among younger children, who seem to be at greater risk. Vulnerability appears to be temporary, since the disease is rare in adults. Persistent attempts to implicate a single etiologic factor have failed. Varicella, influenza A and B, echovirus 2, coxsackie A virus, reovirus, and EB (Epstein-Barr) virus have been isolated from some patients. Epidemics of Reye's syndrome seem to cluster during influenza B epidemics. Toxic causes (insecticides, herbicides, aflatoxins), drugs (salicylates), and metabolic causes (defects in the urea cycle) have also been implicated. The mode of onset may lead to confusion with other causes of coma, particularly toxic encephalopathy and hepatic coma.

The mechanism is thought to be acute viral damage to mitochondria with consequent uncoupling of oxidative phosphorylation, although the encephalopathy may be largely due to a combination of the effect of elevated short-chain fatty acids and hyperammonemia.

Clinical Findings

A. Symptoms and Signs: Most cases give a history of minor upper respiratory tract illness of short duration preceding the development of vomiting, irrational behavior, progressive stupor, and coma. Resolving chickenpox may be present in 10–20% of cases. Restlessness and convulsions may also occur. Striking physical findings are hyperpnea, irregular respirations, and dilated, sluggishly reacting pupils. Jaundice is minimal or absent. The liver may be normal or slightly enlarged. If the prodrome has been prolonged, the liver may be reduced in size. Splenomegaly is not present. A positive Babinski sign and hyperreflexia in association with decorticate and decerebrate posturing are consistent with severe cerebral edema.

B. Laboratory Findings: Cerebrospinal fluid is acellular, and cerebrospinal fluid glucose may be low in younger patients. Cerebrospinal fluid pressure is variably elevated. The serum glucose is proportionately decreased. Moderate to severe elevations of AST (SGOT), ALT (SGPT), and lactate dehydrogenase are found. Serum bilirubin and alkaline phosphatase values are normal to slightly elevated. The prothrombin time is usually prolonged, and the blood ammonia is elevated (by definition). A mixed respiratory alkalosis and metabolic acidosis is seen. In a few cases, the blood urea nitrogen has been elevated. Hyperaminoacidemia (glutamine, alanine, lysine) and hypocitrullinemia are present.

Histopathologic changes in Reye's syndrome are most striking in the brain, liver, and kidneys; less commonly, changes in the heart and pancreas may be found. The brain shows gross cerebral edema, occasionally with evidence of herniation.

Histologically, loss of neurons and fatty vacuolation around small vessels have been noted. The liver shows diffuse microvesicular steatosis with minimal inflammatory changes. Glycogen is virtually absent from the hepatocytes in biopsies taken before giving hypertonic glucose. Ultrastructural changes are mitochondrial.

The kidney changes consist principally of swelling and fatty degeneration of the proximal lobules.

C. Electroencephalography: The EEG is diffusely abnormal, with marked slow-wave activity predominating.

Differential Diagnosis

Differentiation of Reye's syndrome from acute toxic encephalopathy or from hepatic coma or fulminating hepatitis can be made on clinical and laboratory grounds. A negative history and urine screen for ingestion of poisons and drugs, absence of cells in the cerebrospinal fluid, and absence of jaundice are significant. Fulminating hepatitis and hepatic coma in the absence of jaundice have been reported but are extremely rare. Liver biopsy and electromicroscopy can be diagnostic, and the procedure is indicated in atypical cases.

Complications

Aspiration pneumonitis and respiratory failure are common, as with any comatose patient. Most patients die of cerebral complications rather than hepatic or renal failure. Herniation of the brain stem due to cerebral edema is the most serious complication. Cardiac dysrhythmias may develop, as may inappropriate vasopressin excretion, diabetes insipidus, and acute pancreatitis.

Treatment

Treatment is supportive. A nasogastric tube, Foley catheter, and arterial and central venous pressure lines should be inserted immediately. Mechanical ventilation may become necessary if the patient reaches stage III coma (Lovejoy). Cerebral edema should be monitored directly, using an epidural transducer, subarachnoid bolt, or intraventricular tube. Intracranial pressures (ICP) should be kept below 15–20 mm Hg, and systemic blood pressure should be kept sufficiently high to maintain cerebral perfusion pressure (CPP) above 45–50 mm Hg. Respirator settings should keep the P_{CO_2} close to 25 mm Hg and the arterial pH at 7.5–7.6. Mannitol infusions (0.5–2 g/kg) can be given every 4 hours. At times, additional hyperosmolar agents are required to keep ICP below 25 mm Hg. Urea, 1 g/kg intravenously, or glycerol, 1.5 g/kg by nasogastric tube, may be tried, Maintenance fluids using 10% glucose should be given at a rate sufficient to produce a urine flow of 1–1.5 mL/kg/h. Careful attention to central venous pressure is needed when using hyperosmolar agents. Exchange transfusions have been used with success. Vitamin K, 3–5 mg intramuscularly, should be administered. Hypothermia (30–33 °C) and pharmacologic doses of pentobarbital (10–50 mg/kg/d) have been employed to decrease body (brain) metabolic needs during the period of uncontrolled intracranial pressure.

Prognosis

At least 70% of these patients survive. The prognosis is related to the depth of coma and the peak ammonia level on admission. Severe neurologic residuals are not uncommon in the younger children (< 2 years) who recover from prolonged stage III-IV coma. The prognosis is also worse for those children with a varicellar presentation. Relapses do occur after months to years of well-being, and patients with relapses should be screened for other metabolic defects.

Delong GR, Glick TH: Encephalopathy of Reye's syndrome: A review of pathogenetic hypotheses. *Pediatrics* 1982;**69:**53.

Rogers MF et al: National Reye syndrome surveillance, 1982. *Pediatrics* 1985;**75:**260.

Shaywitz BA, Rothstein P, Venes JL: Monitoring and management of increased intracranial pressure in Reye's syndrome: Results in 29 patients. *Pediatrics* 1980;**66:**198.

PANCREAS

ACUTE PANCREATITIS

Most cases of acute pancreatitis are due to drugs, viral infections, systemic diseases, or accidental or nonaccidental abdominal trauma, although 20% are idiopathic. Other cases resulting in obstruction to pancreatic flow include stones in the ampulla of Vater, choledochal cysts, tumors of the duodenum, pancreas divisum, and ascariasis. Acute pancreatitis has been seen with high-dosage corticosteroid therapy and administration of sulfasalazine, thiazides, valproic acid, and other drugs. It may also occur in cystic fibrosis, systemic lupus erythematosus, α_1-antitrypsin deficiency, diabetes, Crohn's disease, glycogen storage disease type I, hyperlipidemia types I and V and familial (hereditary) cases, hyperparathyroidism, Henoch-Schönlein purpura, Reye's syndrome, and malnutrition. Alcohol-induced pancreatitis should be considered in the teenage patient.

Clinical Findings

A. Symptoms and Signs: An acute onset of severe upper abdominal pain occasionally referred to the back, with vomiting and fever, is the common presenting picture. The abdomen is tender but not rigid, and bowel sounds are diminished. Jaundice may also be noted in less than one-third of cases. In cases due to trauma, an abdominal mass that is suggestive of pseudocyst may be felt. Ascites may be noted in such cases also.

B. Laboratory Findings: Leukocytosis and an elevated serum amylase and urine diastase should be expected early. Serum lipase is elevated and persists longer than serum amylase. The urinary amylase/creatinine ratio may be of value in less classic presentations. The immunoreactive trypsinogen test may also be of value. Serum calcium may be low and signifies a poor prognosis. Hyperglycemia and slightly elevated serum bilirubin values occur.

C. X-Ray Findings: Plain x-rays of the abdomen may show a localized ileus (sentinel loop). Ultrasonography shows decreased echodensity of the gland in comparison to the left lobe of the liver. Pseudocyst formation can also be seen early in the course. CT scanning is better for detecting pancreatic phlegmon or abscess formation. Endoscopic retrograde pancreatography may be useful in some cases.

Differential Diagnosis

Other causes of acute upper abdominal pain include lesions of the stomach, duodenum, liver, and biliary system; acute gastroenteritis or atypical appendicitis; pneumonia; volvulus; intussusception; and nonaccidental trauma.

Complications

Complications early in the disease include shock due to fluid and electrolyte disturbances, ileus, and hypocalcemic tetany. Later, there may be pseudocyst, phlegmon, or abscess formation (15% of cases), which may be associated with internal fistulas. Hypervolemia is seen between the third and fifth days, at which time renal tubular necrosis may occur. Impairment of oxygenation and respiratory distress may require assisted ventilation for some patients. Chronic pancreatitis, pancreatic insufficiency, and pancreatic lithiasis may occur as sequelae. Splenic vein thrombosis can also occur.

Treatment

Medical management includes rest, gastric suction, fluids, electrolyte replacement, and blood or plasma as needed. Peritoneal lavage is currently being evaluated in severe cases. Pain should be controlled with meperidine. Atropine may be used intramuscularly. Recurrence of pain after oral feedings may be prevented by giving pancreatic enzymes with the meal. Some (25–40%) pseudocysts will resolve spontaneously within 4–12 weeks.

Surgical treatment is reserved for stones, cysts, abscesses, and anatomic obstructive lesions. Drugs known to produce acute pancreatitis should be discontinued.

Prognosis

In the pediatric age group, the prognosis is surprisingly good with conservative management. The mortality rate is 5–10% in patients treated by operation and 1% in those treated medically. The morbidity rate is high in the surgical group as a result of fistula formation.

Cox KL et al: The ultrasonic and biochemical diagnosis of pancreatitis in children. *J Pediatr* 1980;**96:**407.

Forbes A, Leung JWC, Cotton PB: Relapsing acute and chronic pancreatitis. *Arch Dis Child* 1984;**59:**927.

Regan PT: Medical treatment of acute pancreatitis. *Mayo Clin Proc* 1979;**54:**432.

CHRONIC PANCREATITIS

Two forms of chronic pancreatitis have been reported: chronic fibrosing pancreatitis and the more common familial autosomal dominant chronic relapsing pancreatitis.

The causes include stenotic lesions of the ampulla of Vater, strictures of the pancreatic ducts, intraductal stones, pancreas divisum, and parasitic infestations or gallstones in the ampulla. Chronic intermittent disease may rarely follow mumps pancreatitis and may be a consequence of abdominal trauma with or without pseudocyst formation. Choledochal cyst may give rise to bouts of chronic relapsing pancreatitis. Hyperlipidemias (types I and V) and hyperparathyroidism should be considered.

Pancreatitis is rarely symptomatic in cystic fibrosis.

Clinical Findings

The diagnosis of the hereditary form is usually not made in childhood unless there is a similar history in other family members. The diagnosis of chronic fibrosing pancreatitis is made by surgical exploration demonstrating a normal duct system and typical histologic findings in the pancreatic biopsy.

A. Symptoms and Signs: There is usually a history of recurrent upper abdominal pain of variable severity but prolonged (1–6 days) duration. Radiation of the pain into the back is a frequent complaint. Fever and vomiting are not common in the chronic form. Abnormal stools and symptoms of diabetes may develop later in the course of this disease, and malnutrition due to failure of pancreatic exocrine secretions may also occur.

B. Laboratory Findings: The serum or urine amylase is usually elevated during the early acute attacks. Pancreatic insufficiency and reduced volume and bicarbonate response may be found at duodenal intubation after intravenous administration of synthetic cholecystokinin (0.2 μg/kg) and secretin (2 units/kg). A 3-fold increase of normal serum amylase values is considered a positive test for obstruction.

Blood lipids and urinary amino acids are elevated in familial forms of the disease associated with hyperlipoproteinemia and should be studied in all cases. Elevated blood glucose levels and glycosuria are frequently found in protracted disease. Sweat chloride should be checked for cystic fibrosis and serum calcium for hyperparathyroidism.

C. X-Ray Findings: X-rays of the abdomen may show pancreatic or gallbladder calcifications. Contrast studies may demonstrate other obstructive lesions in the region of the duodenum. Retrograde pancreatography may become a helpful tool in the nonsurgical diagnosis. Pancreatograms show ductal dilatation rather than obvious strictures or stenotic segments.

Differential Diagnosis

Other causes of recurrent abdominal pain must be considered. Specific causes such as hyperparathyroidism, systemic lupus erythematosus, infectious disease, and ductal obstruction by tumors, stones, or helminths must be excluded by appropriate tests.

Complications

Disabling abdominal pain, steatorrhea, nutritional deprivation, and diabetes are the most frequent complications. Pseudocyst formation is seen in 10–20% of cases. Pancreatic carcinoma occurs more frequently in hereditary pancreatitis, especially in patients with calcifications within the gland.

Treatment

When the hereditary form of chronic pancreatitis is suspected or proved, medical management of acute attacks is indicated (see Acute Pancreatitis, above). If ductal obstruction is strongly suspected, surgical exploration should be undertaken after endoscopic studies. Pancreatography and cholangiography can also be performed at laparotomy. Sphincterotomy and biopsy are recommended when obvious obstruction is not found. Relapses seem to occur in most patients. Pseudocysts may be marsupialized to the surface or drained into the stomach or into a loop of jejunum in those failing to regress spontaneously. Prophylactic total or subtotal pancreatic resection is advocated by some workers.

Prognosis

In the absence of a correctable lesion, the prognosis is not good. Disabling episodes of pain, pancreatic insufficiency, and diabetes may ensue. Narcotic addiction and suicide are risks in teenagers with disabling disease.

Ghishan FK et al: Chronic relapsing pancreatitis in childhood. *J Pediatr* 1983;**102:**514.

Niederau C, Glendell JH: Diagnosis of chronic pancreatitis. *Gastroenterology* 1985;**88:**1973.

ZOLLINGER-ELLISON SYNDROME

Zollinger-Ellison syndrome, consisting of non-B islet cell tumors of the pancreas, marked gastric hypersecretion, and severe atypical intractable peptic ulceration, is most common in males (4:1). When it occurs with multiple endocrine neoplasias, it is an autosomal dominant.

The ulcerogenic, gastrinlike hormone elaborated by these small pancreatic islet cell tumors and their metastases to liver or lymph nodes is responsible for the gastric hypersecretion and the intractable peptic disease. Intractable diarrhea of the secretory type may occur in the absence of peptic disease. Half of islet cell tumors in the pediatric age group have been malignant. To date, multiple adenomatosis has not been reported in children with Zollinger-Ellison syndrome.

Clinical Findings

Severe and intermittent abdominal pain, vomiting, hematemesis, melena, diarrhea, and steatorrhea are common. X-ray findings of hypertrophied gastric rugae, duodenal dilatation, and edematous small bowel mucosa all suggest gastric hypersecretion. Ulcers are found in the stomach, duodenum, or jejunum, singly or in multiples. Gastric analysis shows a marked increase in basal volume and titratable acidity after a 12-hour overnight collection. Gastric secretion volumes of 600–2000 mL have been reported during a 12-hour period. Measurement of circulating gastrin levels in the blood is usually diagnostic (> 300 pg/mL). A calcium infusion test or secretin suppression test may be needed to clarify "gray zone" gastrin levels. The histamine test rarely shows more than a 2-fold increase in acid output, since these patients are already secreting maximally.

Treatment

The use of histamine (H_2 receptor) antagonists is the treatment of choice. Primary and metastatic tumor tissue removal should be attempted; however, cures have been reported even when metastases have not been surgically removed and the primary tumor has not been found. Total gastrectomy is reserved for those whom medical therapy has failed.

Drake DP et al: Zollinger-Ellison syndrome in a child: Medical treatment with cimetidine. *Arch Dis Child* 1980;**55:**226.

Regan PT, Malagelada JR: A reappraisal of clinical, roentgenographic and endoscopic features of the Zollinger-Ellison syndrome. *Mayo Clin Proc* 1978;**53:**19.

Smith AL, Auldist AW: Successful surgical resection of an hepatic gastrinoma in a child. *J Pediatr Gastroenterol Nutr* 1984;**3:**801.

ISOLATED EXOCRINE PANCREATIC DEFECTS

Enterokinase (Enteropeptidase) Deficiency Disease (Formerly Trypsinogen Deficiency Disease)

In this rare genetic defect, absence of the enzyme enterokinase leads rapidly to severe protein malnutrition and hypoproteinemia. The key step in activating the proteolytic system within the duodenum is dependent upon the enzyme.

Trypsinogen is first converted to trypsin by enterokinase. Once formed, trypsin can replace enterokinase in the activation of the proenzyme. Trypsin is also needed to activate the conversion of chymotrypsinogen to chymotrypsin as well as procarboxypeptidase to carboxypeptidase. Consequently, the absence of enterokinase results in a complete loss of pancreatic proteolytic enzyme activity. Activation studies with exogenous trypsin and homogenates of normal duodenal mucosa have shown that trypsinogen, procarboxypeptidase, and chymotrypsinogen are present in samples of the patients' pancreatic juice and are qualitatively intact. The sweat chloride test is normal, and the diagnosis is made by duodenal intubation and analysis of pancreatic enzyme activity. Anemia has been associated with this entity but not neutropenia.

Treatment consists of feeding a formula containing a casein hydrolysate (eg, Nutramigen or Pregestimil) and adding pancreatic enzymes to the diet (Cotazym).

Ghishan FK et al: Isolated congenital enterokinase deficiency. *Gastroenterology* 1983;**85:**727.

Isolated Pancreatic Lipase Deficiency

Deficiencies related to malabsorption of the fat-soluble vitamins may be associated with fatty, offensive-smelling stools but no other findings. Neither pancreatic lipase nor a lipase inhibitor is present, and pancreatic trypsin and amylase activity are normal; however, the cofactor colipase is present. Nonpancreatic lipases remain active and prevent malnutrition. The sweat chloride iontophoresis test is normal. Direct assay of pancreatic juice for enzyme activity following intravenous stimulation with synthetic cholecystokinin (0.2 μg/kg) and secretin (2 units/kg) is required for diagnosis.

Improvement occurs with pancreatic enzymes. A low-fat diet or a formula containing medium-chain triglycerides is helpful.

Figarella C et al: Congenital pancreatic lipase deficiency. *J Pediatr* 1980;**96:**412.

PANCREATIC EXOCRINE HYPOPLASIA & CHRONIC NEUTROPENIA (Shwachman Syndrome)

This uncommon disease, characterized by diarrhea and failure to thrive, is due to pancreatic exocrine insufficiency. Pathologically, there is widespread fatty replacement of the gland acinar tissue. This is easily recognized on abdominal CT scan. There is no fibrosis or inflammation, and the pancreatic ducts appear to be normal. The islet cells are spared. The disease may be confused with cystic fibrosis, but the absence of elevated sweat chlorides distinguishes these entities. The association of immunoglobulin deficiencies is sometimes noted. There is evidence that the disease is genetically determined.

The history of failure to thrive, diarrhea, fatty stools, and, in most cases, freedom from respiratory infections should make one suspect this entity. Important laboratory findings include normal sweat electrolytes but absent or reduced pancreatic lipase, amylase, and trypsin on duodenal intubation. Leukopenia is often present, and the thrombocyte count is sometimes depressed. Small bowel is normal on histologic examination, and studies of absorption not dependent upon pancreatic enzymes yield normal results. The bone marrow is typically hypocellular, showing a "maturation arrest" of the granulocyte series. Metaphyseal dysostosis and an elevated fetal hemoglobin may occur. Hepatic dysfunction is also reported in some cases.

Normal sweat electrolytes and a negative history of repeated pulmonary infections differentiate this disease from cystic fibrosis. Small bowel biopsy supported by absorption tests, particularly with D-xylose, distinguishes the disorder from celiac disease. Cases of isolated lipase or enterokinase deficiency may be more difficult to distinguish. The association of exocrine pancreatic insufficiency with congenital anomalies (aplastic alae nasi, aplasia cutis, deafness) needs to be recognized. Consider cyclic neutropenia and neutropenia due to other causes.

The complications and sequelae of deficient pancreatic enzyme secretion are malnutrition, diarrhea, and growth failure. The degree of steatorrhea may lessen with age. The major sequela seems to be short stature, although long-term follow-up studies are not available. Increased numbers of infections may be the results of chronic neutropenia. Neutrophil mobility is also impaired in many patients and perhaps contributes to their susceptibility to infections.

Pancreatic enzyme replacement therapy has been fairly successful, although some patients get along without it. The prognosis appears to be good for those able to survive the increased number of bacterial infections early in life. However, an increased incidence of leukemia has been noted in these patients.

Aggett PJ: Shwachman's syndrome. *Arch Dis Child* 1980; **55:**331.

Hill RE et al: Steatorrhea and pancreatic insufficiency in Shwachman's syndrome. *Gastroenterology* 1982;**83:**22.

Woods WG et al: The occurrence of leukemia in patients with the Shwachman syndrome. *J Pediatr* 1981;**99:**425.

SELECTED REFERENCES

Alagille D, Odievre M: *Liver and Biliary Tract Disease in Children.* Wiley, 1978.

Grand RJ, Watkins JB (editors): Gastrointestinal and liver disease. *Pediatr Clin North Am* 1975;**22:**719. [Entire issue.]

Gryboski J, Walker A: *Gastrointestinal Problems in the Infant,* 2nd ed. Saunders, 1983.

Mowat A: *Liver Disorders in Childhood.* Butterworth, 1979.

Schiff L, Schiff ER: *Diseases of the liver,* 5th ed. Lippincott, 1982.

Silverberg M: *An Advanced Textbook of Pediatric Gastroenterology.* Medical Examination Publishing Co., 1983.

Silverman A, Roy CC: *Pediatric Clinical Gastroenterology,* 3rd ed. Mosby, 1983.

21 Kidney & Urinary Tract

Gary M. Lum, MD, James K. Todd, MD,
& Donough O'Brien, MD, FRCP

EVALUATION OF THE KIDNEY & URINARY TRACT

HISTORY

When renal disease is suspected, a careful history should elicit the following: (1) family history of cystic disease, hereditary nephritis, deafness, dialysis, or transplantation; (2) preceding acute or chronic illnesses (eg, urinary tract infection, pharyngitis, impetigo, or endocarditis); (3) rashes or joint pains; (4) growth delay or failure to thrive; (5) polyuria, polydipsia, enuresis, frequency, or dysuria; (6) hematuria or discolored urine; (7) pain (abdominal, costovertebral angle, or flank) or trauma; (8) sudden weight gain or periorbital swelling; and (9) exposure to drugs or toxins (especially nephrotoxins). In the newborn or small infant, additional information should be obtained regarding birth history, eg, Apgar scores, voiding, umbilical artery catheterization, and oligohydramnios. In patients with known chronic renal failure, the history should also elicit information on developing pallor, headache, lethargy, anorexia, or bone pain.

PHYSICAL EXAMINATION

Certain aspects of the physical examination deserve emphasis. General appearance is noted, with attention to the presence of low-set ears, skeletal deformity, and edema or pallor. Anomalies of the ears or eye defects may be associated with renal disease, as are anomalies of the external genitalia. The skin should be examined for lesions. The blood pressure should be carefully measured in a quiet setting. The cuff should cover two-thirds of the child's upper arm, and peripheral pulses should be noted. An ultrasonic device is useful for measurements in infants. Height and weight should be carefully recorded. The abdomen should be palpated, with careful attention to the kidneys or masses in the vicinity; note the presence of ascites.

LABORATORY EVALUATION OF RENAL FUNCTION

Urinalysis

Urinalysis is a rapid method for detection and evaluation of possible renal disease (see Chapter 35). Commercially available dipsticks can be used to detect blood and protein and to approximate the pH. Such detection, however, must be followed by a careful microscopic examination of the urinary sediment. The use of low illumination and a urine stain facilitates the examination. Casts should be sought at the periphery of the coverslip. Bacteria and cells are studied with the high-power objective. Crystals should be carefully described. The urine, if collected properly, can be sent for culture.

Serum Analysis

The standard indicators of renal function are serum levels of creatinine and urea nitrogen. The ratio of blood urea nitrogen to creatinine is normally about 10. In renal insufficiency, the levels rise. The ratio may increase in cases where renal perfusion or urine flow is decreased, since blood urea nitrogen levels are greatly affected by these and other factors (eg, nitrogen intake, catabolism, use of tetracyclines), whereas creatinine levels are affected much less. Therefore, the most reliable, easily assessed blood indicator of glomerular function is the serum level of creatinine.

Most laboratories report the "normal" range of serum creatinine as 0.8–1.2 mg/dL. However, many small children should have serum creatinine levels under 0.8 mg/dL, and only the larger adolescents should have levels exceeding 1 mg/dL. Thus, one must interpret with caution the "normal" creatinine levels reported.

Less precise but nonetheless important indicators of the presence of renal disease are abnormalities of serum electrolytes, pH, calcium, phosphorus, magnesium, or uric acid.

Measurement of Glomerular Filtration Rate (GFR)

The determination of GFR is of paramount importance in the evaluation of suspected renal disease or in the serial follow-up of the child with established renal insufficiency.

An estimate of GFR may be attained by measurements of the endogenous creatinine clearance (C_{Cr})

in milliliters per minute. A 24-hour urine collection is usually obtained; however, in small children when collection is difficult, a 12-hour daytime specimen, collected when urine flow rate is greatest, is acceptable. Careful explanation of the procedure for collecting a quantitative urine specimen should be made, so that the parent or patient understands fully the rationale of (1) first emptying the bladder (discarding that urine) and noting the time; and (2) putting all urine subsequently voided into the collection receptacle including the last void 12 or 24 hours later. Reliability of the 24-hour collection can be approximated by measurement of the total 24-hour creatinine excretion in the specimen. Total daily creatinine excretion in milligrams per kilogram of the patient's weight (creatinine index) should be in the range of 14–20. If the creatinine index of a 24-hour specimen is less than 12, inadequate collection should be suspected. Calculation by the following formula requires measurements of plasma creatinine (P_{Cr}) in milligrams per milliliter, urine creatinine (U_{Cr}) in milligrams per milliliter, and urine volume (V) expressed as milliliters per minute.

$$C_{Cr} = \frac{U_{Cr}V}{P_{Cr}}$$

Creatinine is a reflection of body muscle mass. Since accepted ranges of normal creatinine clearance are based on adult parameters, "correction" for size is needed to determine normal ranges in children. Clearance is "corrected" to a standard body surface area of 1.73 m^2, as shown in the following formula:

$$\text{“Corrected” } C_{Cr} = \frac{\text{Patient's } C_{Cr} \times 1.73 \text{ m}^2}{\text{Patient's body surface area}}$$

The normal range for creatinine clearance is 80–120 mL/min/1.73 m^2. A simple and tested formula for quick approximation of creatinine clearance incorporates the use of the plasma creatinine level and the child's length in centimeters:

$$C_{Cr} \text{ (mL/min/1.73 m}^2\text{)} = \frac{0.55 \times \text{Height in cm}}{P_{Cr} \text{ in mg/dL}}$$

Note: This formula takes into consideration an expression of body surface area; thus, further correction is not necessary. Use 0.45 × length in centimeters in newborns less than 1 year old. This method of calculation is not meant to detract from the importance of clearance determinations but is of great help to the clinician who desires a quick estimate of the appropriateness of a suspect level of plasma creatinine.

Counahan R et al: Estimation of glomerular filtration rate from plasma creatinine concentration. *Arch Dis Child* 1976; **51:**875.

Schwartz GJ et al: Plasma creatinine and urea concentration in children: Normal values for age and sex. *J Pediatr* 1976;**88:**828.

Urine Concentrating Ability

Inability to concentrate urine is often the first sign of chronic renal failure and is very often a factor responsible for severe dehydration seen in patients with chronic renal failure. Furthermore, a dilute urine in the presence of oliguria may be observed in acute tubular necrosis as well. Direct measurement of urine osmolality is easily obtained and may be more helpful in evaluating renal concentrating ability. Except under unusual circumstances, a first morning void would be expected to be concentrated and can be screened with a specific gravity analysis. Evaluation of severe abnormalities of urinary concentration or dilution is discussed under specific disease entities.

Evaluation of Hematuria & Proteinuria

Hematuria and proteinuria deserve special emphasis, since they are hallmarks of possibly significant glomerular alterations. In children with *asymptomatic* hematuria or proteinuria, the search for renal glomerular abnormalities will yield the most results. Careful microscopic urinalysis and laboratory analysis of renal function (see above) are included in the evaluation of hematuria and proteinuria.

Initial detection of hematuria, usually by dipstick but at times by the appearance of the urine, should be followed by confirmation with careful microscopic analysis. The presence of red cell casts supports the diagnosis of glomerulonephritis, but the absence of casts does not rule out the disease.

Poststreptococcal glomerulonephritis is the most commonly suspected entity in the differential diagnosis of childhood glomerulonephritis; therefore, associated streptococcal infections should be considered and ruled out on the basis of antistreptolysin, streptozyme, and serum complement tests.

Special serologic and immunologic studies, such as tests for antinuclear antibodies, anti-DNA antibodies, serum cryoglobulins, immune complexes, complement components, immunoglobulins, anti-glomerular basement membrane antibodies, and hepatitis-associated antigen, are useful in diagnosing various glomerulonephritides (see below) and may be appropriate in evaluating hematuria.

The diagnosis of benign hematuria therefore becomes one of exclusion. It is interesting to note that included in this group may be children who are found to have asymptomatic hypercalciuria as an explanation for their hematuria.

The association of proteinuria with hematuria is characteristic of more significant glomerular disease. Proteinuria alone, however, may indicate the presence of some benign as well as some more serious entities.

The dipstick test for proteinuria should be followed by quantitation of urinary protein excretion. The collection procedure is the same as described above for measurement of creatinine clearance. A 24-hour collection for protein excretion divided into "recumbent'' and ''upright'' collections is needed if orthostatic proteinuria is to be ruled out; otherwise, a 12-hour timed collection could suffice.

In the 24-hour collection used to determine the presence of orthostatic proteinuria, urine formed in the recumbent (sleeping) position must be separated from that formed in the upright position. This is easily accomplished by having the patient complete the upright collection with a void just before going to bed. Urine voided during the night or upon awakening in the morning, when the 24-hour collection is completed, constitutes the recumbent collection. The 2 quantities can then be used to calculate total protein excretion (and creatinine clearance if desired) and the amount of protein can be compared in upright versus recumbent specimens to determine an orthostatic component. Significant quantitative proteinuria exceeds 150 mg/24 h. If the proteinuria is orthostatic in nature, an abnormal quantity will be noted in the upright specimen and an acceptable quantity will be found in the recumbent specimen. Proteinuria exceeding 1.5 g should generally not be regarded as simply orthostatic.

In children under 6 years of age, proteinuria generally reflects anatomic abnormalities that require radiographic analysis (excretory urography or ultrasonography). The presence of proteinuria severe enough to cause hypoproteinemia (levels usually 2 g), edema, and hyperlipidemia may represent idiopathic nephrotic syndrome of childhood (ie, ''nil'' disease, minimal change disease, or lipoid nephrosis), especially in the absence of any other abnormalities. The presumptive diagnosis of idiopathic nephrotic syndrome of childhood is generally ''tested'' by response to corticosteroid therapy (see Proteinuria and Renal Disease, below). Renal biopsy may be indicated in cases of suspected idiopathic nephrotic syndrome of childhood with numerous relapses, severe corticosteroid side effects, or a dependency on or resistance to corticosteroid therapy. In older children, there is a greater likelihood of a more serious renal lesion causing nephrotic syndrome. Typical lesions that would not be expected to respond to corticosteroid therapy are focal glomerular sclerosis and membranous nephropathy (see Proteinuria and Renal Disease, below). A renal biopsy is required to confirm the diagnosis. Other indications for biopsy include proteinuria with hematuria (strongly suggestive of serious glomerular disease), decreased serum complement levels, decreasing renal function, and severe hypertension. Renal biopsy procedures are discussed below.

Abuelo JG: Proteinuria: Diagnostic principles and procedures. *Ann Intern Med* 1983;**98:**186.

Fairley KF et al: Hematuria: A simple method for identifying glomerular bleeding. *Kidney Int* 1982;**21:**105.

Stapleton FB et al: Hypercalciuria in children with hematuria. *N Engl J Med* 1984;**310:**1345.

West CD: Asymptomatic hematuria and proteinuria in children: Causes and appropriate diagnostic studies. *J Pediatr* 1976;**89:**173.

Special Tests of Renal Function

A. Acute Renal Failure: Measurements of urinary sodium osmolality, creatinine, and urea are useful in differentiating prerenal causes of renal insufficiency from true renal causes.

The physiologic response to decreased renal perfusion is an increase in urine concentration (osmolality usually $>$ 800 mosm/L), a rise in urinary solutes, and a decrease in urinary sodium (usually $<$ 20 meq/L). Therefore, when an increase in serum creatinine or blood urea nitrogen level or a decrease in urinary output suggests the possibility of renal failure, appropriate steps can be taken to assess the status of renal function by qualitative and quantitative urinalysis (see Acute Renal Failure, below).

B. Tubular Function: The detection of some substances in urine may reflect tubular dysfunction. For example, glucose should not be present in concentrations greater than 5 mg/dL. Hyperphosphaturia is generally seen in cases of significant tubular abnormalities (eg, Fanconi's syndrome). Measurement of the phosphate concentration of a 24-hour urine specimen and evaluation of tubular reabsorption of phosphorus (TRP) will help document renal tubular diseases as well as hyperparathyroid states.

TRP (expressed as percentage of reabsorption) is calculated as follows:

$$\text{TRP} = 100\left[1 - \frac{S_{Cr} \times U_{PO_4}}{S_{PO_4} \times U_{Cr}}\right]$$

where S_{Cr} = serum creatinine; U_{Cr} = urine creatinine; S_{PO_4} = serum phosphate; and U_{PO_4} = urine phosphate. All values for creatinine and phosphate are expressed in milligrams per deciliter for purposes of calculation. A TRP value of 80% or more is considered normal, although it depends somewhat on the S_{PO_4}.

The urinary excretion of amino acids in generalized tubular disease reflects a quantitative increase rather than a qualitative change. Aminoaciduria is usually assessed visually on a one-dimensional paper chromatograph of a sample containing a standard amount of creatinine.

The ability of the proximal tubule to reabsorb bicarbonate is affected in several disease states—including renal tubular acidosis, Fanconi's syndrome (which is present in diseases such as cystinosis), and chronic renal failure—and is discussed under specific entities, below.

LABORATORY EVALUATION OF IMMUNOLOGIC FUNCTION

Much of parenchymal renal disease is mediated by immune mechanisms, many of which are not well defined or known. Examples of mechanisms in the kidney include (1) deposition of circulating antigen-antibody complexes that are themselves injurious or incite injurious responses and (2) formation of antibody directed against the glomerular basement membrane itself (rare in children).

Complete immunologic assessment of a patient requires many studies that are not routinely performed in all laboratories. Nonetheless, some basic tests are generally available. Total serum complement (and components if possible) should be measured when immune-mediated renal injury is suspected. Serum immunoglobulins should be quantitated. Abnormal serum protein levels are often associated with immune complex deposition; in such cases, tests should be performed to detect antinuclear antibodies, hepatitis-associated antigen, rheumatoid factor, and cold-precipitable proteins (cryoglobulins).

Where indicated, special studies to measure circulating immune complexes, C3 ''nephritic'' factor, and anti-glomerular basement membrane (anti-GBM) antibody may be performed. Very often, the diagnosis rests on the description of renal histology.

Berger J et al: Immunochemistry of glomerulonephritis. In: *Advances in Nephrology*. Vol 1. Hamburger J, Crosnier J, Maxwell MH (editors). Year Book, 1971.

McIntosh RM et al: Cryoglobulins. 3. Further studies on the nature, incidence, clinical, diagnostic, prognostic, and immunopathologic significance of cryoproteins in renal disease. *Q J Med* 1975;**44:**285.

Wilson CB, Dixon FJ: Diagnosis of immunopathologic renal disease. *Kidney Int* 1974;**5:**389.

RADIOGRAPHIC EVALUATION

Although excretory urography remains a valuable procedure in assessing the anatomy and function of the kidney, collecting system, and bladder, renal ultrasonography is often the initial procedure in evaluation of a child's urinary tract. Such a noninvasive diagnostic method is especially helpful in evaluating small infants with renal insufficiency; abdominal masses (eg, Wilms' tumor, neuroblastoma); or renal enlargement due to obstructive uropathy, renal vein thrombosis, or cystic disease. Ultrasonography has also contributed greatly to the examination of the fetal kidneys in utero and has provided a means to demonstrate the prenatal presence of a normal urinary tract.

Radioisotope studies can provide valuable information concerning renal anatomy, blood flow, and glomerular, tubular, and collecting system function.

Evaluation of the lower urinary tract (voiding cystourethrography or cystoscopy) is indicated when vesicoureteral reflux or bladder outlet obstruction is suspected.

CT scanning may be valuable when the less costly procedures have failed to produce results, eg, in cases where subtle abnormalities cannot be detected by the above procedures.

More invasive studies such as renal venography or arteriography are rarely required in children. Their main indications include evaluation of renal vein or arterial thromboses, vascular masses, arteriovenous malformation, or renal artery stenosis.

Chevalier RL, Campbell F, Brenbridge AN: Nephrosonography and renal scintigraphy in evaluation of newborns with renomegaly. *Urology* 1984;**24:**96.

UROLOGIC STUDIES

Except for the evaluation of patients with suspected anatomic abnormalities, cystoscopy is rarely indicated in the evaluation of asymptomatic hematuria or proteinuria in children, since the yield is minimal.

Retrograde urography is rarely necessary but can be helpful for anatomic evaluation of of the collecting system in cases in which renal insufficiency or obstruction may interfere with assessment of the entire urinary tract.

Lebowitz RL: Urography in children: When should it be done? 2. Conditions other than infection. *Postgrad Med* (Nov) 1978;**64:**61.

RENAL BIOPSY

The ultimate diagnostic procedure in children with suspected renal parenchymal disease is renal biopsy. Histologic information valuable for diagnosis, treatment, and prognosis can be obtained from a well-performed renal biopsy followed by proper tissue preparation, examination, and interpretation of findings. Satisfactory evaluation of renal tissue requires examination by light microscopy, immunofluorescence microscopy, and electron microscopy.

When a biopsy is anticipated, a pediatric nephrologist should be consulted. In children, percutaneous renal biopsy with a Vim-Silverman needle is an acceptable, low-risk procedure when performed by an experienced physician; it avoids the risks of general anesthesia. An experienced surgeon should perform the biopsy if operative exposure of the kidney is necessary, if an increased risk factor (eg, bleeding disorder) is present, or if a wedge biopsy is preferred.

CONGENITAL ANOMALIES OF THE URINARY TRACT

RENAL PARENCHYMAL ANOMALIES

Congenital anomalies of the genitourinary tract are present in about 10% of children. Severity ranges from asymptomatic abnormalities, which may never cause problems even into adult years and are often found only at autopsy, to malformations incompatible with intrauterine or extrauterine life.

Although an anomaly may be inconsequential in and of itself, there may be associated abnormalities. For example, in patients with horseshoe kidney (ie, kidneys fused in their lower poles), there is a reported higher incidence of renal calculi. Unilateral agenesis can occur and is usually accompanied by compensatory hypertrophy of the contralateral kidney and thus should be compatible with normal renal function. Supernumerary and ectopic kidneys can also occur and are usually of no significance.

Bilateral Renal Agenesis

Bilateral renal agenesis is a rare malformation resulting in early death. Oligohydramnios is present and probably is the cause of the pulmonary hypoplasia and peculiar (Potter) facies of infants with this anomaly.

Renal Hypoplasia & Dysplasia

Renal hypoplasia and dysplasia represent a spectrum of anomalies. In simple hypoplasia, which may be unilateral or bilateral, histologic findings on renal biopsy are normal, but the affected organs are smaller than normal. In the various forms of dysplasia, immature, undifferentiated renal tissue persists. In some of the dysplasias, the number of normal nephrons is insufficient to sustain life once the child reaches a critical body size. Thus, these lesions are usually discovered when excretory urography is performed in a child who is noted to be uremic with no history of urinary tract disease or in a child with failure to thrive. Other forms include oligomeganephronia, which is characterized by the presence of only a few large glomeruli, and the cystic dysplasias, which are a broad group of malformations in the hypoplasia-dysplasia group and are characterized by the presence of renal cysts.

Simple Cysts

Simple cysts are usually single and may be of no clinical significance. However, they may be a site for development of renal stones or hematuria and thus require evaluation or removal.

Polycystic Kidney Disease

The infantile type of polycystic kidney disease (autosomal recessive) is characterized by large cystic kidneys, often associated with multiple organ systems affected by cystic malformations. Some children with this type die in the newborn period, but many will develop progressive deterioration toward end-stage renal failure. When the infantile type occurs at a later age, it may be predominantly manifested by liver rather than renal involvement. The adult type of polycystic kidney disease (autosomal dominant) may also be detected in the newborn period and depending on degree of severity could be fatal. Although renal insufficiency and hypertension usually occur late in this type, there are exceptions. Detailed discussion of this entity is beyond the scope of this text. Careful documentation (usually by ultrasonography), close monitoring and management of the complications of renal insufficiency, and genetic counseling are suggested.

Medullary Cystic Disease (Juvenile Nephronophthisis)

Medullary cystic disease is characterized by varying sizes of cysts in the medulla and is associated with tubular and interstitial nephritis. Children present with renal failure and signs of tubular dysfunction (decreased concentrating ability, Fanconi's syndrome). This lesion should not be confused with medullary sponge kidney (renal tubular ectasia), a frequently asymptomatic cystic disease usually found in adults.

Grantham JJ: Polycystic kidney disease: Hereditary and acquired. *Kidney* 1984;**17:**19.

Shokeir MHK: Expression of "adult" polycystic renal disease in the fetus and newborn. *Clin Genet* 1978;**14:**61.

Steele BT, Lirenman DS, Beattie CW: Nephronophthisis. *Am J Med* 1980;**68:**531.

DISTAL URINARY TRACT ANOMALIES

Obstruction of urine flow, infection, and stone formation, alone or in combination, are the hallmarks of distal urinary tract anomalies. Most of these anomalies will be suggested by excretory urography and cystourethrography. Some may be managed surgically; in others, therapy is limited to supportive treatment and prompt recognition and management of infection and chronic renal failure. Early recognition of reversible lesions is of the greatest importance. However, immediate postnatal detection and intervention may not be able to reverse the detrimental intrauterine effects.

Anomalies of the Ureter

Obstruction at the ureteropelvic junction is common and may be the result of intrinsic muscle abnormalities, aberrant vessels, or fibrous bands. The lesion can cause hydronephrosis and usually presents as an abdominal mass in the newborn. Obstruction can occur in other parts of the ureter, especially at its entrance into the bladder, with resulting proximal hydroureter and hydronephrosis. Obstruction or reflux may occur in ectopic ureters. Most often, these are associated with duplications of the collecting systems; the ectopic ureter generally drains the upper pole of the affected kidney. The need for repair of an ectopic ureter is assessed on the basis of its effect on the collecting system it drains and on the related kidney.

Anomalies of the Bladder & Urethra

Severe bladder malformations such as exstrophy are clinically obvious and provide a surgical challenge. More subtle—but urgent in terms of diagnosis—is obstruction of urine flow from aberrant posterior urethral valves. This anomaly, almost invariably confined to males, usually presents as anuria or a poor voiding stream in the newborn period; with severe obstruction of urine flow, ascites may occur and the kidneys and bladder may be easily palpable. As soon as the diagnosis is suspected, cystourethrography should be performed to confirm the diagnosis. Treatment consists of destruction of the valves, usually by transurethral fulguration. This procedure may be preceded by a period of vesical drainage. Other distal obstructions (bladder neck obstruction, distal urethral stenosis, and meatal stenosis) were once popular diagnoses but have now fallen into disrepute as specific entities.

Complex Anomalies

The prune-belly syndrome is an association of urinary tract anomalies with cryptorchidism and absent abdominal musculature. Although complex anomalies, especially renal dysplasia, usually cause early death or the need for dialysis or transplantation, some patients have lived into the third decade with varying degrees of renal insufficiency. Early urinary diversion is essential to sustain renal function. At the time of this surgery, a renal biopsy can be obtained and may suggest the likelihood of adequate function in the future.

Discussion of other complex malformations, as well as such external genitalia anomalies as hypospadias, is beyond the scope of this text.

Poole CA: Congenital obstructive uropathies. *Pediatr Nephrol* 1974;**1**:231.

GLOMERULAR DISEASE

ACUTE POSTINFECTIOUS GLOMERULONEPHRITIS

Clinical signs of acute glomerulonephritis include general malaise, anorexia, and headache, sometimes accompanied by fever, vomiting, and abdominal pain. Edema, especially periorbital edema, is usually noted; it is most often moderate but occasionally is severe and generalized. Hypertension is common and may be severe enough to be symptomatic even to the point of inducing heart failure or encephalopathy. The urine is described as "coffee-colored" or "smoky," with gross hematuria. The presence of red cell casts is suggestive of the diagnosis, but hematuria alone may be present and mild in subclinical cases. Proteinuria is common and is within "nephrotic range" only in the more serious forms of the disease. Mild elevations of the blood urea nitrogen and serum creatinine levels are expected, but occasionally acute renal failure occurs.

Acute Poststreptococcal Glomerulonephritis

Acute poststreptococcal glomerulonephritis is the most common form of postinfectious glomerulonephritis and the most frequently encountered in childhood. Although the cause is not certain, the condition is thought to be an immune-mediated disease. The epidemiologic relationship between certain strains of streptococci and glomerulonephritis is well recognized. Presumably, antigen-antibody complexes induced by the infection are formed in the bloodstream and deposited in the glomeruli. These deposited complexes may cause glomerular damage through activation of the complement system, or the decrease in serum C3 levels may simply be the result of induced inflammation.

The diagnosis of poststreptococcal disease may be supported by a recent history (7–14 days previously) of group A β-hemolytic streptococcal infection. Recent streptococcal infection can be demonstrated by an elevated antistreptolysin O titer or by elevation of one or more antibody titers in the streptozyme panel.

Gross histology shows enlargement of involved kidneys, with punctate cortical hemorrhages. Proliferation of glomerular cells and infiltration of the glomerulus with inflammatory cells are found on light microscopic examination. Immunofluorescence microscopy reveals characteristic deposition of complement and immunoglobulins; some investigators have demonstrated deposition of streptococcal antigens. Electron microscopy may further demonstrate the characteristic subendothelial electron-dense "lumps" or "bumps," presumably immune deposits.

There is no specific treatment for the nephritis. Appropriate antibiotic therapy is indicated for streptococcal infection, if still present. The disturbances in renal function and resulting hypertension may require dietary management, diuretics, or antihypertensive drugs. In severe cases with rapidly deteriorating renal function, renal biopsy and hemodialysis or peritoneal dialysis may be necessary and may be accompanied by attempts to influence the course by giving corticosteroids.

The acute abnormalities generally are resolved in 2–3 weeks. Serum complement may be normal as early as 3 days or as late as 30 days. Most children will recover completely, although microscopic hematuria may persist for 1–2 years. Although there are reports of significant chronic disease or abnormalities in adults, the outlook for children remains for the most part good, except in the rarest of instances. Typical resolution is expected. Nonetheless, persistent deterioration in renal function, urinary abnormalities beyond 18 months, persistent hypocomplementemia, and associated presence of nephrotic syndrome are ominous signs and are indications for renal biopsy.

Other Types of Postinfectious Glomerulonephritis

Glomerulonephritis has been associated with pneumococcal and staphylococcal infections and with various viral infections as well. These postinfectious diseases are also presumed to result from immune complex formation and glomerular deposition, and the clinical presentations may be indistinguishable. A chronic infectious nidus (as occurs, for example, in infective endocarditis) or a ventriculoatrial shunt infection can also elicit immune-mediated mechanisms and subsequent acute or chronic glomerulonephritis.

The treatment remains that of the underlying infection, with follow-up of effects on renal function and renal biopsy where the diagnosis is in question.

Baldwin DS: Poststreptococcal glomerulonephritis: A progressive disease? *Am J Med* 1977;**62:**1.

Baldwin DS et al: The long-term course of poststreptococcal glomerulonephritis. *Ann Intern Med* 1974;**80:**342.

MEMBRANOPROLIFERATIVE GLOMERULONEPHRITIS

Membranoproliferative glomerulonephritis, a chronic form of glomerulonephritis, is a specific disease entity with distinct histologic features, a more serious prognosis, and a variable response to suggested modes of therapy. There are several histologic classifications. Type I may be corticosteroid-sensitive. Type II is associated with evidence of persistent complement consumption and has been designated hypocomplemententemic membranoproliferative glomerulonephritis. Other types are less well known.

Clinical Findings

The development of this disease may be insidious, and it must be suspected in the course of evaluation of asymptomatic hematuria or proteinuria. Less commonly, the disease may present with gross hematuria, nephrotic syndrome, or renal insufficiency. This form of glomerulonephritis can mimic poststreptococcal glomerulonephritis, although the course may be more severe and associated with nephrosis or persistent hypocomplementemia. In such cases, definitive diagnosis requires renal biopsy.

Hypertension is often a severe problem and requires aggressive therapy. Nephrotic syndrome develops frequently.

Urinalysis nearly always reveals hematuria, although it may be exclusively microscopic. Proteinuria may be slight at first but increases as the disease progresses. The total hemolytic complement level in serum may be normal or depressed and may fluctuate in the course of the disease. The complement profile in this disease is characterized by activation of the alternative pathway of complement metabolism. The early components (C1, C2, C1q) may be normal, while C3 and C5–C9 are depressed. Progressive renal insufficiency, reflected in a progressively decreasing creatinine clearance, occurs frequently.

Some of the histologic findings of membranoproliferative glomerulonephritis occur in a number of other glomerular diseases, including systemic lupus erythematosus and conditions suggesting postinfectious glomerulonephritis. The diagnosis is established by the characteristic histologic appearance of the glomerular basement membrane under electron microscopic examination. The findings with immunofluorescence microscopy are variable; however, the presence of C3 proactivator and properdin and the absence of the first 3 components appear to be of some diagnostic value.

Treatment & Prognosis

At present, there is no universally accepted treatment to halt the progressive deterioration of renal function caused by this disease. There have been many encouraging reports about the response to corticosteroids; however, the use of these agents remains controversial. If corticosteroid therapy is attempted, severe hypertension can be a significant complication but must and can be vigorously controlled with medication. This approach and other approaches to therapy need further evaluation. Unfortunately, long-term effects are difficult to determine owing to the slow progression of the disease.

In the majority of patients, membranoproliferative glomerulonephritis progresses to end-stage disease. Deterioration generally occurs over a prolonged time (> 10 years). Type II disease frequently recurs in patients with transplanted organs.

Donadio JV: Membranoproliferative glomerulonephritis: A prospective clinical trial of platelet-inhibition therapy. *N Engl J Med* 1984;**310:**1421.

McAdams AJ, McEnery PT, West CD: Mesangiocapillary glomerulonephritis: Changes in glomerular morphology with long-term alternate-day prednisone therapy. *J Pediatr* 1975;**85:**23.

McEnery PT et al: Membranoproliferative glomerulonephritis: Improved survival with alternate-day prednisone therapy. *Clin Nephrol* 1980;**13:**117.

West CD, McAdams AJ: The chronic glomerulonephritides of childhood. (2 parts.) *J Pediatr* 1978;**93:**1, 167.

IgA NEPHROPATHY

IgA nephropathy is a syndrome recognized in children and characterized by asymptomatic microscopic hematuria and recurrent bouts of macroscopic hematuria, with no apparent deterioration in renal function. Histologically, the kidneys show changes ranging from normal morphology to segmental proliferation of a few of the glomeruli (focal glomerulonephritis). Many patients with IgA nephropathy have been shown to have deposits of immunoglobulins, mainly IgA, in the mesangial regions of the glomeruli. The significance of these deposits and their role in the clinical syndrome are not clear.

Clinical Findings

Between the episodes of gross hematuria, the patient's urine may either be clear or show microscopic hematuria. Proteinuria may also be present. Impairment of renal function rarely occurs, although there have been occasional reports of patients exhibiting progressive renal insufficiency. No consistent abnormalities in serum immunoglobulins have been reported, but serum IgA levels are thought to be elevated in approximately 50% of cases. The diagnosis is made on biopsy by demonstration of the characteristic immunoglobulin pattern. Similar histologic patterns may be found in other glomerular diseases, especially systemic lupus erythematosus and anaphylactoid purpura, which must be excluded before the diagnosis is confirmed. Many cases of benign hematuria reported in the past may be attributed to IgA nephropathy.

Treatment & Prognosis

No specific treatment is indicated. In the great majority of cases, the condition is benign and nonprogressive. Since renal insufficiency has been reported, however, children should be followed with serial determinations of renal function as long as hematuria persists. Recurrence of IgA deposition in transplanted kidneys has been reported.

Southwest Pediatric Nephrology Study Group: A multicenter study of IgA nephropathy in children. *Kidney Int* 1982; **22:**643.

Vernier RL: Recurrent hematuria and focal glomerulonephritis. *Kidney Int* 1975;**7:**224.

ANAPHYLACTOID PURPURA NEPHRITIS

Anaphylactoid purpura (Schönlein-Henoch purpura) is a vasculitis characterized by a purpuric rash, arthritis, and gastrointestinal symptoms. Renal involvement is common and ranges from asymptomatic hematuria to a less common, rapidly progressive, acute glomerulonephritis that may result in end-stage disease.

Clinical Findings

Symptoms and signs of anaphylactoid purpura, ie, typical cutaneous manifestations and arthritis, are usually the first to develop, often following an upper respiratory tract infection. Gastrointestinal pain occurs frequently, and bloody diarrhea may be a complaint. There are no characteristic serologic features, although there have been reports of elevated levels of serum complement. Significant renal involvement will produce the clinical findings of acute glomerulonephritis, and microscopic hematuria occurs in as many as 80% of cases. Severity of renal disease is not necessarily related to the extent of extrarenal manifestations. Occasionally, hematuria may precede the other findings, or significant renal disease may evolve after the resolution of other manifestations. Most severe disease is suggested by the presence of the nephrotic syndrome or persistent proteinuria and the continued reduction in renal function.

Renal biopsy demonstrates focal to proliferative glomerulonephritis and crescent formation in a large percentage of cases, especially those with progressive renal failure. Immunofluorescence reveals IgA and IgG in the mesangium. Although the presence of fibrin has been reported and has prompted the use of anticoagulants in isolated cases, the finding may be nonspecific.

Treatment & Prognosis

There is no universally accepted therapy for anaphylactoid purpura nephritis. In severe forms with relentless deterioration of renal function, use of corticosteroids, cytotoxic drugs, or anticoagulants has had varied effects, but no large-scale controlled studies have shown significant benefit from their use. Continued evaluation of approaches to the treatment of children with deteriorating function is warranted.

In general, the prognosis is good. However, chronic glomerular disease with renal failure progressing to end-stage disease can occur and is a major concern in patients with proteinuria exceeding 1 g/24 h or with crescent formation exceeding 50% on renal biopsy. In such cases, therapy may be initiated by an experienced nephrologist after the lesion and its severity are documented at biopsy.

HEREDITARY NEPHRITIS (Alport's Syndrome)

The genetics of hereditary nephritis are not established with certainty, but the disease appears to be transmitted as an autosomal dominant trait with variable penetrance and possible sex linkage. The sporadic occurrence is estimated to be about 18%. In its complete form, the hereditary nephritis described by Alport is characterized by renal parenchymal disease, sensorineural hearing loss, and abnormalities of the crystalline lens. In most cases encountered, the clinical expressions of ear and eye abnormalities occur less commonly than do renal manifestations.

Clinical Findings

Patients generally present with hematuria, but cases have been discovered through routine auditory examination or because of known family history. Hematuria is usually microscopic and may persist without deterioration of renal function. However, the renal lesion may progress, with an increase in severity of hematuria, proteinuria, hypertension, and other complications of renal insufficiency.

Renal morphology by light microscopy is variable, depending on the time of biopsy. Chronic inflammatory changes and scarring may be the only discernible evidence of disease. None of the findings are specific. There are no helpful findings on immunofluorescence examination. Electron microscopy reveals a characteristic lamination of the basement membrane, but this finding is not considered diagnostic.

Treatment & Prognosis

There is no treatment for the disease itself. Attention is directed toward the complications of chronic renal failure (eg, hypertension, hyperphosphatemia). In severely affected males (rarely, in females), hereditary nephritis will progress to end-stage disease and require dialysis, renal transplantation, or both. Because of the hereditary nature of the problem, donation of organs by family members should be discouraged. Genetic counseling should be offered.

Although females seem to have a higher incidence of the disease, Alport's syndrome in males is more likely to progress to end-stage kidney disease.

Ferguson AC, Rance CP: Hereditary nephropathy with nerve deafness (Alport's syndrome). *Am J Dis Child* 1972;**124:**84.

Gubler M et al: Alport's syndrome: A report of 58 cases and a review of the literature. *Am J Med* 1981;**70:**493.

Habib RH et al: Alport's syndrome: Experience at l'Hôpital Necker. *Kidney Int* 1982;**11:**S20.

LUPUS NEPHRITIS

Lupus nephritis is one of the most serious complications of systemic lupus erythematosus (see Chapter 18); if untreated, the severe renal involvement can progress to end-stage disease. Treatment of the renal lesion, as well as strict blood pressure control, can decrease the severity and death rate of systemic lupus erythematosus.

Clinical Findings

Manifestations of systemic lupus erythematosus are discussed in Chapter 18. Renal manifestations range from mild hematuria or proteinuria (or both) to acute glomerulonephritis. Unfortunately, mild presentations do not necessarily correlate with mild renal involvement. Renal abnormalities are occasionally the initial manifestations, and serologic analysis can confirm the diagnosis. Titers of anti-DNA antibody and levels of serum complement should be determined. A fall in total hemolytic complement and C3 or C4 levels and a rise in anti-DNA titers appear to reflect the activity of renal disease. Other findings may be similar to those encountered in acute glomerulonephritis.

On light microscopy, the renal histology varies from mild hypercellularity of the glomerular mesangium to diffuse glomerular proliferation and glomerular basement membrane abnormalities. Immunofluorescence reveals many immunoglobulins and complement. Electron microscopy demonstrates electron-dense deposits and other alterations of the glomerular basement membrane. Renal biopsy is extremely helpful in the classification and management of lupus nephritis, but a complete description of findings on biopsy is beyond the scope of this discussion.

Treatment & Prognosis

The use of corticosteroids has greatly affected the course of lupus nephritis. The approach to treatment is based on the severity of the renal lesion, as reflected by renal histology, serology, and activity of the urinary sediment. Concomitant use of other immunosuppressive agents (cyclophosphamide or azathioprine) is somewhat controversial, but recent analysis of experience with these agents is encouraging in cases of severe renal involvement and progressive deterioration. Plasmapheresis has been attempted, with variable results. Dialysis or transplantation may be indicated in patients with renal involvement progressing to end-stage disease.

Although the renal involvement is one of the more serious complications of systemic lupus erythematosus, the prognosis has improved with vigorous therapy directed at the renal lesion and with strict monitoring of associated hypertension.

Balow JE et al: Effect of treatment on the evolution of renal abnormalities in lupus nephritis. *N Engl J Med* 1984;**311:**491.

Dinant JH et al: Alternative modes of cyclophosphamide and azathioprine therapy in lupus nephritis. *Ann Intern Med* 1982;**96:**728.

ANTI-GLOMERULAR BASEMENT MEMBRANE DISEASE

Most immune-mediated glomerular diseases in children are probably caused by deposition of circulating antigen-antibody complexes in the glomerulus. Rarely, glomerulonephritis is mediated by antibodies directed against the glomerular basement membrane (anti-GBM antibodies). The association of a concomitant life-threatening pulmonary hemorrhage and antibody to pulmonary alveolar basement membrane is referred to as Goodpasture's syndrome.

Clinical Findings

The disease usually presents as acute glomerulonephritis that progresses quickly to renal failure. Pulmonary involvement is life-threatening. The severity of the clinical presentation usually prompts rapid intervention with dialysis and immediate histologic identification so that definitive therapy can be instituted.

Light microscopic findings are variable, depending upon the severity of epithelial cell proliferation in the glomeruli. Immunofluorescence reveals a characteristic linear staining pattern. Electron microscopy is nonspecific. The diagnosis is established by documentation of circulating anti-GBM antibody in the presence of the characteristic clinical and immunohistologic picture.

Treatment & Prognosis

A regimen of high doses of methylprednisolone plus concomitant use of immunosuppressive agents has been shown to be effective. Plasmapheresis is thought to be most effective for treatment and should be initiated whenever possible, especially if there is a threat of pulmonary hemorrhage. Dialysis may be indicated, and with the disappearance of anti-GBM antibody in the serum, a renal transplant may be feasible.

Early intervention (before the glomerular filtration rate is severely affected) can result in clinical remission. Relentless progression can, however, result in the need for continued dialysis or in death.

Briggs WA et al: Antiglomerular basement membrane antibody mediated glomerulonephritis and Goodpasture's syndrome. *Medicine* 1979;**58:**348.

Lockwood CM et al: Plasma exchange in nephritis. Page 383 in: *Year Book of Medicine, 1979*. Year Book, 1979.

IDIOPATHIC RAPIDLY PROGRESSIVE GLOMERULONEPHRITIS

Glomerulonephritis characterized by rapid progression to renal failure and perhaps end-stage disease is rarely seen in childhood. The cause is unknown, and association with other glomerulonephritides (some of which may also be rapidly progressive in nature) is obscure.

Clinical Findings

This disease clinically cannot be readily distinguished from other glomerulonephritides that may cause rapid deterioration in renal function (except by their exclusion).

Analysis by light microscopy reveals glomerular lesions characterized by severe and extensive epithelial cell proliferation. Many glomeruli will display epithelial crescents or fibrous scarring. Lesions may be focal in the acute stages, but they rapidly diffuse and involve the glomeruli. Findings on immunofluorescence and electron microscopy may support the histologic diagnosis.

Treatment & Prognosis

Therapy is controversial. Several investigators recommend early treatment with anticoagulants or corticosteroids. Others have recommended plasmapheresis. Regardless of treatment, the outcome has generally been discouraging. Treatment attempts should be initiated by an experienced nephrologist, and supportive measures such as dialysis should be available.

Responses to therapy are variable. Most patients fail to respond to treatment, and dialysis or transplantation is inevitable. Reports of efficacy of different therapeutic regimens continue to prompt aggressive therapeutic trials in light of the serious alternative.

Cole BR et al: "Pulse" methylprednisolone therapy in the treatment of severe glomerulonephritis. *J Pediatr* 1976; **88:**307.

Min KW et al: The morphogenesis of glomerular crescents in rapidly progressive glomerulonephritis. *Kidney Int* 1974; **5:**47.

Suc JM et al: The use of heparin in the treatment of idiopathic rapidly progressive glomerulonephritis. *Clin Nephrol* 1976; **5:**9.

PROTEINURIA & RENAL DISEASE

FUNCTIONAL PROTEINURIA

Urine is not normally completely protein-free, but the average excretion is well below 150 mg/24 h. Although isolated asymptomatic proteinuria may be secondary to renal disease or genitourinary tract abnormalities, proteinuria is not always associated with renal disease. The search for the cause of proteinuria should therefore include consideration of functional proteinuria.

Exertional proteinuria (the result of increased activity) is well recognized and may be accompanied by hematuria. Exertional proteinuria can be diagnosed by comparing urine specimens collected during or following activity with those collected at other times.

Febrile proteinuria can be seen in about 5% of febrile illnesses and is not necessarily due to the presence of underlying renal disease.

Orthostatic proteinuria is explained by hemodynamic adjustments leading to renal vein congestion. It has been suggested that lordosis may produce this proteinuria by increasing the convexity of the aorta, resulting in compression of the left renal vein. Documentation is accomplished by comparing the level of protein in urine produced in the upright position with that produced in the recumbent position (see Evaluation of Hematuria and Proteinuria, above).

Vehaskari VM et al: Isolated proteinuria: Analysis of a school-age population. *J Pediatr* 1972;**101:**661.

CONGENITAL NEPHROSIS

Congenital nephrosis is a rare, uniformly fatal renal disorder that is often observed in more than one sibling in a family. Autosomal recessive inheritance is suggested. The kidneys are pale and large and may show microcystic dilatations (microcystic disease) of the proximal tubules and glomerular changes. The latter consist of proliferation, crescent formation, and thickening of capillary walls.

The pathogenesis is unknown. A fundamental immunologic incompatibility between the mother and the infant is perhaps responsible, since mothers reject skin grafts of their nephrotic infants more rapidly than control mothers reject grafts of normal infants. The findings of gamma globulin and complement components of the glomerular loops are also evidence of immune-related injury to the kidneys.

Low birth weight (with an obstetric history of a large placenta), wide cranial sutures, delayed ossification, and mild edema are commonly noted at birth in infants with congenital nephrosis. The edema may become apparent after the first few weeks or months of life. Anasarca follows, and the abdomen can become greatly distended by ascites. Massive proteinuria associated with typically appearing nephrotic syndrome and hyperlipidemia is the rule. Hematuria is common. If the patient lives long enough, progressive renal failure occurs. Most affected infants succumb to infections at the age of a few months.

Treatment has little to offer. Prevention and effective management of urinary tract and other infections are important. Immunosuppressants and heparin have occasionally appeared to sustain renal function for a period, but their use is not widely recommended.

Criswold WR, McIntosh RM: Immunological studies in congenital nephrosis. *J Med Genet* 1972;**9**:245.

Marks MI et al: Proteinuria in children with febrile illnesses. *Arch Dis Child* 1970;**5**:250.

Thompson AL et al: Fixed and reproducible orthostatic proteinuria. *Ann Intern Med* 1970;**73**:235.

IDIOPATHIC NEPHROTIC SYNDROME OF CHILDHOOD ("Nil" Disease, Lipoid Nephrosis, Minimal Change Disease)

Nephrotic syndrome is characterized by proteinuria, hypoproteinemia, edema, and hyperlipidemia. It may occur as a result of any form of glomerular disease and may be associated with a variety of extrarenal conditions. In children under 5 years of age, the disease usually takes the form of idiopathic nephrotic syndrome of childhood ("nil" disease, lipoid nephrosis), which is characterized by certain clinical and laboratory findings. If necessary, examination of renal tissue may confirm the diagnosis. Light microscopy reveals no significant glomerular changes (or reveals "minimal changes"). The cause of the childhood syndrome is unknown. Most immunologic investigations have reported negative results; however, there have been recent suggestions of hormonal causes and of associated dysfunction of T lymphocytes.

Clinical Findings

Affected patients are generally under 5 years of age at the time of their first episode. Often following an influenzalike syndrome, the child is noted to have periorbital swelling and perhaps oliguria. Within a few days, increasing edema—even anasarca—becomes evident. Other than vague malaise and, occasionally, abdominal pain, complaints are few. Despite the impressive swelling and weight gain, the patient may show signs of intravascular volume depletion and may even present with shock. Hypertension is rarely present. With marked edema, there may also be dyspnea due to pleural effusions.

Despite heavy proteinuria, the urine sediment is usually normal. Although microscopic hematuria may rarely be found, its presence should raise the suspicion of other glomerular diseases, especially focal sclerosis. Serum chemistries reveal hypoalbuminemia and hyperlipidemia. Abnormal immunoglobulin levels such as high IgM and low IgG have also been reported. However, no other evidence of immunologic disorder is present (eg, complement is normal, and there is no cryoglobulinemia). Some azotemia may occur but is related to intravascular volume depletion rather than to impairment of function.

Glomerular morphology is unremarkable except for fusion of foot processes of the visceral epithelium of the glomerular basement membrane. This finding, however, is nonspecific and is seen in many proteinuric states. Another acceptable histologic description is one of "minimal changes" in the glomerular mesangium, with unremarkable findings on immunofluorescence and electron microscopic examination.

Complications

Infectious complications (eg, peritonitis) are occasionally encountered, and pneumococci are frequently responsible for these complications. Immunization with pneumococcal vaccine is helpful. Hypercoagulability may be present, and thromboembolic phenomena are commonly reported.

Treatment & Prognosis

As soon as the diagnosis of idiopathic nephrotic syndrome is made, therapy with corticosteroids should be initiated. Prednisone in a single dose of 2 mg/kg/d is the treatment of choice. When the urine becomes protein-free for 5 consecutive days, the dose of prednisone is reduced to 2 mg/kg every other day. Alternate-day corticosteroid therapy is continued for 2 months, after which the dosage is tapered downward over a period of 4 weeks and then discontinued. Striking corticosteroid dependency or partial resistance may suggest the existence of variants in the assumed diagnosis of minimal change disease. The 2 most often described entities are IgM nephropathy and diffuse mesangial hypercellularity. A similar course of corticosteroids is given if nephrosis recurs. If the rate of recurrence does not permit discontinuation of corticosteroids for at least 2 months at a time, confirmation of the lesion by renal biopsy and therapy with cytotoxic drugs should be considered.

Although chlorambucil is slow-acting, it is considered to be less toxic than cyclophosphamide. The dose is 0.1–0.2 mg/kg/d for 8 weeks. Prednisone is continued while chlorambucil is administered. Following the 8-week combined course, the prednisone is gradually tapered. White blood cell counts are followed weekly; if leukopenia occurs, it is mild and transient, resolving when the drug is temporarily stopped. The course can be resumed when leukopenia resolves in 1–2 days.

Renal biopsy is not essential in the child with typical idiopathic nephrotic syndrome. However, biopsy should be performed prior to institution of chlorambucil therapy or if the clinical picture is atypical. In the initial treatment course, failure of proteinuria to disappear after 8 weeks of daily corticosteroid therapy is another indication for biopsy.

Diuretics may be useful in the mobilization of symptomatic edema. However, they are not always effective and may lead to hypovolemia. Intravenous albumin and diuretics are useful if anasarca results in acute distress or if severe intravascular depletion occurs.

The prognosis of idiopathic nephrotic syndrome is often suggested by the initial response to corticosteroids. A prompt remission lasting for 3 years is almost always permanent. Failure to respond or early relapse usually heralds a prolonged series of relapses, which may indicate the presence of more serious nephropathy. Chlorambucil or other cytotoxic drug therapy is predictably successful only in children who respond to corticosteroids. As mentioned above, renal biopsy is recommended in atypical cases.

Childhood nephrotic syndrome associated with diffuse mesangial hypercellularity: A report of the Southwest Pediatric Nephrology Study Group. *Kidney Int* 1983;**23:**87.

International Study of Kidney Disease in Children: Early identification of frequent relapsers among children with minimal change nephrotic syndrome. *J Pediatr* 1982;**101:**514.

Oliver WJ, Kelsch RC: Nephrotic syndrome due to primary nephropathies. *Pediatr in Rev* 1981;**2:**311.

Sibley RK et al: A clinicopathologic study of forty-eight infants with nephrotic syndrome. *Kidney Int* 1985;**27:**544.

Williams SA et al: Long-term evaluation of chlorambucil plus prednisone in the idiopathic nephrotic syndrome of childhood. *N Engl J Med* 1980;**302:**929.

FOCAL GLOMERULAR SCLEROSIS

Focal glomerular sclerosis is characterized by the presence in renal biopsy specimens of normal-appearing glomeruli as well as some partially or completely sclerosed glomeruli. At presentation, the disease is often quite similar to idiopathic nephrotic syndrome; however, the response to corticosteroids is poor, and the clinical course is often one of progression to end-stage renal disease. Some of the confusion in the literature regarding focal glomerular sclerosis stems from the varied but similar terminology applied in its description. The histologic picture has been labeled focal sclerosing glomerulonephritis, focal and segmental glomerulosclerosis, and focal and segmental hyalinosis, to name a few. Since there may be 2 forms of the disease, Habib's classification of focal segmental and global glomerular fibrosis may be useful.

The glomerular abnormalities in this disease may be confined to the juxtamedullary glomeruli, especially early in the course. Therefore, care must be taken to obtain biopsy tissue that includes this area of the kidney.

Because some forms of the disease (eg, global glomerular fibrosis) are believed to be more responsive to corticosteroid therapy, histologic diagnosis is imperative. Renal biopsy is helpful in distinguishing this disorder from idiopathic nephrotic syndrome of childhood as well as for indicating the prognosis.

Arbus GS et al: Focal segmental glomerulosclerosis with idiopathic nephrotic syndrome: Three types of clinical response. *J Pediatr* 1982;**101:**40.

Bohle A et al: Minimal change lesion with nephrotic syndrome and focal glomerular sclerosis. *Clin Nephrol* 1974;**2:**52.

Habib R: Focal glomerular sclerosis. *Kidney Int* 1973;**4:**355.

Kohaut EC et al: The significance of focal glomerular sclerosis in children who have nephrotic syndrome. *Am J Clin Pathol* 1976;**66:**545.

Nash MA et al: Late development of chronic renal failure in steroid-responsive nephrotic syndrome. *J Pediatr* 1982; **101:**411.

MEMBRANOUS NEPHROPATHY (Membranous Glomerulonephritis)

Membranous nephropathy is occasionally seen in children and thus deserves mention. The usual presenting feature is proteinuria of variable degree. This lesion has been reported to occur in children of all ages, but the diagnosis is more frequently made in older children with "nephrotic range" proteinuria.

The lesion has been described in association with diseases such as hepatitis B antigenemia, systemic lupus erythematosus, congenital and secondary syphilis, and renal vein thrombosis; with immunologic disorders such as autoimmune thyroiditis; and with administration of drugs such as penicillamine. The pathogenesis is unknown, but it is thought that the glomerular lesion is the result of prolonged deposition of circulating antigen-antibody complexes.

The onset of membranous nephropathy is often insidious, but onset may be similar to that of idiopathic nephrotic syndrome of childhood (see above). Unlike with that entity, response to corticosteroids would not be expected in patients with membranous nephropathy. In these patients, the total serum complement and the C3 levels may be normal, but the C4 level is often depressed. Light microscopy reveals uniform, diffuse thickening of all glomerular capillary walls. Spikelike deposits are demonstrable along the epithelial side of the glomerular basement membrane. Immunofluorescence microscopy shows granular staining, primarily of IgG, along the capillary walls. Electron microscopy also demonstrates the deposits.

Treatment methods are controversial. Remissions have not been impressive; however, there is some long-term benefit in corticosteroid therapy. Generally, although the disease is chronic, the rate of progression to end-stage renal disease and death is low.

A controlled study of short-term prednisone treatment in adults with membranous nephropathy: Collaborative study of the adult idiopathic nephrotic syndrome. *N Engl J Med* 1979;**301:**1302.
Gaffney EF et al: Segmental membranous glomerulonephritis. *Arch Pathol Lab Med* 1982;**106:**409.
Latham P et al: Idiopathic membranous glomerulopathy in Canadian children: A clinicopathologic study. *J Pediatr* 1982; **101:**682.
Wagoner RD et al: Renal vein thrombosis in idiopathic membranous glomerulopathy and nephrotic syndrome: Incidence and significance. *Kidney Int* 1983;**23:**368.

ACUTE INTERSTITIAL NEPHRITIS

Acute interstitial nephritis, a relatively uncommon form of nephritis, is characterized by diffuse or focal inflammation and edema of the renal interstitium and secondary involvement of the tubules but little or no secondary glomerular damage unless a combined or chronic picture is encountered. It seems to be related most often to drugs (eg, antibiotics, especially methicillin).

Fever, rigor, abdominal or flank pain, and rashes may occur in drug-associated cases. In all cases, there is some degree of renal failure, with proteinuria and hematuria. The inflammation can be severe enough to cause rapid deterioration of renal function. Histologic demonstration of tubular and interstitial inflammation of the kidneys is helpful for diagnosis. Immediate identification and removal of the causative agent is imperative. A relentless course with progressive renal insufficiency or nephrotic syndrome may require supportive dialysis and treatment with corticosteroids.

Ellis D et al: Acute interstitial nephritis in children. *Pediatrics* 1981;**67:**862.

HEMOLYTIC-UREMIC SYNDROME

Because of the usual severe gastrointestinal involvement in hemolytic-uremic syndrome, severe fluid imbalance and thus prerenal causes are responsible for most cases of renal insufficiency in children with this syndrome. Although the glomerulonephritides as a group account for the majority of renal parenchymal causes of renal failure, the hemolytic-uremic syndrome is the most common single cause of renal failure in childhood.

The cause of this syndrome is not well established, but epidemiologic studies have suggested both a genetic and an infectious component. The primary lesion seems to be one of the endothelium of arterioles, especially in the kidney, with formation of platelet thrombi and resulting microangiopathic hemolysis.

Clinical Findings

Hemolytic-uremic syndrome is found most often in children under 2 years of age. It usually begins with a prodromal phase characterized by gastrointestinal symptoms, including abdominal pain, diarrhea, and vomiting. Oliguria, pallor, and bleeding manifestations, principally cutaneous and gastrointestinal, occur next. Hypertension and seizures develop in some infants, especially those who develop severe renal failure and fluid overload.

The triad of anemia, thrombocytopenia, and renal failure characterizes the syndrome. Anemia is profound and is associated with findings of red blood cell fragments on smear. A high reticulocyte count confirms the hemolytic nature of the anemia. The platelet count is almost invariably below 100,000/μL. Other coagulation abnormalities are less consistent. Serum fibrin split products are often present, but fulminant disseminated intravascular coagulation is rare. Renal failure is characterized by a high blood urea nitrogen level and, usually, severe oliguria. Macroscopic hematuria is often present; proteinuria and the nephrotic syndrome may also occur. Immunologic investigations are usually unrevealing. The serum complement level is normal.

Complications

The complications of hemolytic-uremic syndrome are usually those associated with acute renal failure. Neurologic problems, particularly seizures, may result from electrolyte abnormalities such as hyponatremia, hypertension, or central nervous system vascular disease. Severe bleeding and complicating infections must be anticipated.

Treatment

As with any case of acute renal failure, meticulous attention to fluid and electrolyte status as detailed in the discussion of acute renal failure (see below) is crucial. There is evidence that early dialysis improves the prognosis; the size of the patient and the bleeding tendency will usually dictate peritoneal dialysis as the technique of choice. Seizures usually respond to control of hyptertension and electrolyte abnormalities. It has been suggested that the plasma in these cases lacks a prostacyclin-stimulating factor, which is a potent inhibitor of platelet aggregation. Administration of plasma might therefore be helpful. Platelet inhibitors have also been tried, but the results have not been impressive, especially late in the disease. Aspirin can provide the same effect but at certain doses also undesirably inhibits prostacyclin synthesis. Red cell and platelet transfusions may be necessary; although the risk of volume overload is significant, it can be minimized by use of dialysis. While there is no universally accepted therapy for patients with this syndrome, the strict control of hypertension and nutrition and the use of dialysis appear to affect the long-term outcome.

Course & Prognosis

It has been suggested that geographic factors may determine the severity of hemolytic-uremic syndrome. Most commonly, children recover from the acute episode within a week, and follow-up examination reveals no residual renal insufficiency. However, some patients who recover from the acute episode have severe and occasionally progressive renal dysfunction. Thus, follow-up of children recovering from hemolytic-uremic syndrome should include serial determinations of renal function for 1–2 years and meticulous attention to blood pressure for 5 years. Although a very small group of patients die in the early phase from the complications of acute renal failure, most children—even those with renal failure requiring dialysis—recover completely.

Arenson EG, August CS: Preliminary report: Treatment of the hemolytic uremic syndrome with aspirin and dipyridamole. *J Pediatr* 1975;**86:**957.

Goldstein MH et al: Hemolytic-uremic syndrome. *Nephron* 1979;**23:**263.

Remuzzi G et al: Prostacyclin and thrombotic microangiopathy. *Semin Thromb Hemostas* 1980;**6:**391.

DISEASES OF THE RENAL VESSELS

RENAL VEIN THROMBOSIS

In the newborn period, renal vein thrombosis may suddenly complicate the course of sepsis or dehydration or be observed in an infant of a diabetic mother, or it may be the result of an umbilical vein indwelling line. In older children and adolescents, it may develop following trauma or without any apparent predisposing factors; in these cases, nephrotic syndrome may be associated with renal vein thrombosis. There may also be an underlying membranous glomerulonephropathy.

Clinical Findings

In the newborn, renal vein thrombosis generally presents with the sudden development of an abdominal mass. If the thrombosis is bilateral, oliguria may be present; urine output may be normal with a unilateral thrombus. In older children, flank pain, sometimes with a palpable mass, is a common presentation. In some children with proteinuria, however, the nephrotic syndrome may be the first sign of renal vein thrombosis.

No single laboratory test is diagnostic of renal vein thrombosis. Hematuria usually is present and occasionally is gross. Proteinuria is less constant. In the newborn, thrombocytopenia may be found; this is rare in older children. Delayed opacification of the involved kidney may be seen on excretory urography. If the collecting system shows a ''notching'' of the ureteral image, this may suggest collateral blood flow. Renal ultrasonography and radioisotope studies are noninvasive, helpful procedures. The definitive procedure, more invasive and not often necessary, is renal venography.

Treatment

Anticoagulation with heparin is the treatment of choice both in newborns and in older children. No clear-cut benefit from nephrectomy has been demonstrated, although this continues to be suggested. In the newborn, a course of heparin combined with treatment of the underlying problem is usually all that is required. Management in other cases is less straightforward. The tendency for recurrence and embolization has led some workers in this field to recommend long-term anticoagulation. If an underlying membranous glomerulonephritis is suspected, biopsy should be performed.

Course & Prognosis

The rate of deaths due to renal vein thrombosis in the newborn is usually related to the underlying cause. If the child survives the acute phase, the prognosis for adequate renal function is good. The entity is much less common in older children, but they may be expected to follow the course known to occur in adults. Renal vein thrombosis may recur in the same kidney or occur in the other kidney years after the original episode of thrombus formation. Extension into the vena cava, with fatal pulmonary emboli, is a known complication.

The nephrotic syndrome, often with membranous glomerulonephritis, is associated with renal vein thrombosis. In some cases, thrombosis may be a complication of nephrotic syndrome. There is also evidence that the thrombus itself may result in glomerulonephritis, possibly through the release of renal tubular antigens.

Mauer SM et al: Bilateral renal vein thrombosis in infancy: Report of a survivor following surgical intervention. *J Pediatr* 1971;**78:**509.

Moore HL et al: Unilateral renal vein thrombosis and the nephrotic syndrome. *Pediatrics* 1972;**50:**598.

RENAL ARTERIAL DISEASE

Children are susceptible to renovascular hypertension due to fibromuscular hyperplasia, congenital stenosis, or other renal arterial lesions. The proportion of hypertensive children with such demonstrable abnormalities, however, is quite small. Unfortunately, there are few clinical clues to underlying arterial lesions. Nonetheless, arterial lesions should be suspected in children whose hypertension is severe, beginning at 10 years of age or under, or associated with delayed visualization on excretory urogram. The diagnosis is established by renal arteriography with selective renal vein renin measurements. Some of these lesions may be repaired surgically (see Hypertension, below), but repair may be technically impossible in many small children. Although thrombosis of renal arteries is rare, it should be considered in a patient with acute onset of hypertension and hematuria in an appropriate setting (eg, in association with hyperviscosity or umbilical artery catheterization).

RENAL FAILURE

ACUTE RENAL FAILURE

Acute renal failure is a major complication of many conditions. It can be defined as the sudden inability to excrete urine of sufficient quantity or adequate composition to maintain normal body fluid homeostasis. It may be due to impaired renal perfusion, acute renal disease, renal ischemia, renal vascular compromise, or obstructive uropathy. Prerenal, renal, and postrenal causes are shown in Table 21–1.

Diminished circulating blood volume leads to lowered renal perfusion, and the decreased glomerular filtrate is further diminished by increased tubular reabsorption of sodium and water and by excessive amounts of circulating vasopressin (ADH) and aldosterone. Acute renal failure due to hypovolemia usually responds to volume replacement with isotonic saline solution, plasma, or blood, depending upon the cause of the deficit. If impaired renal perfusion is prolonged, renal damage may take days or weeks to resolve.

Table 21–1. Classification of causes of renal failure.

Prerenal
- Dehydration due to gastroenteritis, malnutrition, or diarrhea
- Hemorrhage, blood loss, aortic or renal vessel injury, trauma, surgery, cardiac surgery, renal arterial thrombosis
- Diabetic acidosis
- Pooling of interstitial fluid into local area of injury—burns, operative site, peritonitis
- Hypovolemia associated with nephrotic syndrome
- Shock
- Infusion of fluid with too little sodium

Renal
- Hemolytic-uremic syndrome
- Acute glomerulonephritis
- Extension of prerenal hypoperfusion
- Nephrotoxins
- Acute tubular necrosis or vascular nephropathy
- Renal (cortical) necrosis
- Intravascular coagulation—septic shock, hemorrhage
- Diseases of the kidney and vessels
- Iatrogenic disorders
- Severe infections
- Drowning, especially fresh water
- Treatment of neoplasms—hyperuricacidemia, hyperuricaciduria

Postrenal
- Obstruction due to tumor, hematoma, or the presence of posterior urethral valves or ureteropelvic junction stricture
- Sulfonamide crystals
- Uric acid crystals
- Stones
- Ureteroceles
- Trauma to a solitary kidney or collecting system
- Renal vein thrombosis

Clinical Findings

The hallmark of early renal failure is oliguria. The initial approach to an oliguric child should be aimed at classifying the problem in one of the categories outlined in Table 21–1. While an exact etiologic diagnosis is not necessary, accurate classification is helpful before initiating appropriate therapy.

If the cause of renal failure or oliguria is not clear, entities that can be treated (eg, volume depletion) should be considered first. After treatable problems are ruled out, a diagnosis of acute tubular necrosis (eg, vasomotor nephropathy, ischemic injury) may be entertained.

A. Postrenal Causes: Postrenal failure, which is quite rare in children, is found in newborns with anatomic abnormalities. If there is obstruction of the bladder outlet, it can be relieved by insertion of a urethral catheter; surgical correction follows. Occult postrenal obstruction must always be considered; if the diagnosis is made early enough, removal of the obstruction may prevent irreversible renal injury and the development of secondary chronic renal failure. Delayed voiding in the newborn period, anuria, or poor urinary stream usually suggests obstruction. The clinician must also consider lesions higher in the urinary system, such as ureteropelvic junctional obstruction, which usually presents as abdominal mass. Obstructive uropathy may or may not be accompanied by variable degrees of renal insufficiency.

B. Prerenal and Renal Causes: The differentiation of renal failure from oliguria secondary to prerenal factors is a crucial part of the diagnostic evaluation. Several factors are taken into consideration in making this decision. If the physical examination reveals dehydration and low blood pressure, then prerenal failure should be suspected. The child with edema, however, may be in either prerenal or renal failure. A patient with nephrotic syndrome, for example, may be grossly edematous but have a severely compromised intravascular volume and thus develop prerenal oliguria. Careful physical examination and laboratory evaluation will aid in distinguishing the entities. However, direct central venous measurement may be necessary.

If a central venous pressure of less than 3 cm of water is observed when a central venous line is inserted, a prerenal disturbance is likely. The presence of the central line will facilitate fluid expansion and the subsequent management of the child.

Table 21–2 lists additional factors in the differentiation of prerenal from renal failure.

Complications

Patients with acute renal failure due to acute tubular necrosis or other parenchymal renal disease are unable to excrete a water load. Hence, they easily develop hyponatremia, fluid overload, and hypertension or congestive heart failure and are at great risk of rapidly developing hyperkalemia and acidemia. Hypocalcemia and hypophosphatemia are expected abnormalities. Uremic symptoms may take hours or days to develop, but proper nutrition and fluid balance are immediate problems. Hemorrhage, anemia, and infection may also be problems.

Treatment

An indwelling catheter should be inserted and urine output monitored hourly. If insignificant quantities of urine are produced and renal failure is established, the catheter should be removed because it then represents more of a hazard than an aid.

A. Prerenal Factors: Exclude or rectify any prerenal factors. Hypovolemia should be corrected with blood, plasma, or isotonic saline solution until the blood pressure is normal. A fluid challenge of 20 mL/kg may be safely administered in most instances. If urine output does not rise above oliguric levels within 30–60 minutes, a central venous pressure line should be inserted, and additional blood, plasma, or saline should be infused until the central venous pressure has been restored to 3–6 mm Hg (or 4–8 cm of water).

If diuresis does not occur in response to the above measures, give furosemide (Lasix), 2.5 mg/kg as an intravenous push. Allow 1 hour for a response to occur. If the urine output remains low (< 200–250 mL/m^2/24 h), repeat and double the dose of furosemide (5 mg/kg). If no diuresis occurs, no further administration of diuretics will be helpful; institute the oliguric phase regimen given below. If diuresis does occur, continue furosemide if its use is necessary to sustain the diuresis. Acute tubular necrosis may be aborted in this manner. After several hours, the patient may at least convert to a phase of nonoliguric renal failure that may last for several days and occasionally requires no further diuretic therapy or dialysis. When this occurs, follow the nonoliguria phase regimen given below.

Table 21–2. Urine studies.

Prerenal Failure	Acute Renal Failure
Urine osmolality 50 mosm/kg greater than plasma osmolality	Urine osmolality equal to or less than plasma osmolality
Urine sodium < 10 meq/L	Urinary sodium > 20 meq/L
Ratio of urine creatinine to plasma creatinine > 14:1	Ratio of urine creatinine to plasma creatinine < 14:1
Specific gravity > 1.020	Specific gravity 1.012 – 1.018

B. Oliguric Phase: Once it has been determined that a prolonged oliguric phase is inevitable, an oliguric renal failure regimen should be instituted without delay. It is essential that the patient be monitored closely and that the following be done at least once a day: weigh the patient; record intake, output, and vital signs; and determine hematocrit, blood CO_2 content, blood urea nitrogen level, and serum levels of sodium, potassium, chloride, calcium, phosphorus, uric acid, and creatinine.

The principal complications of acute oliguric renal failure are (1) fluid overload, (2) hyperkalemia, (3) metabolic acidosis, (4) hypertension, and (5) uremia. Therapy is directed against each of these complications. However, keep in mind that dialysis greatly reduces morbidity and mortality due to acute renal failure.

The tendency to develop fluid overload requires a sharp reduction in fluid intake. This makes it difficult to provide enough calories to minimize tissue catabolism, metabolic acidosis, hyperkalemia, and uremia.

If able to retain oral feedings, the patient may be given carbohydrate- and fat-rich supplements that are very low in protein, potassium, and sodium (eg, Pedialyte). It is usually safer, however, to administer all calories intravenously by increasing the glucose concentration in the intravenous fluids to 15–20%.

Intravenous fluids are calculated as follows: (1) Give no allotment for urine as long as oliguria persists. (2) Give only about two-thirds of the patient's estimated sensible and insensible water loss requirements. (The rest will be provided by water from oxidation.) In dry air, patients usually require about 400 mL/m^2/d.

Hyperkalemia can be controlled by administration of an ion-exchange resin. An aqueous slurry containing 1 g of resin per kilogram of body weight is prepared and given as a retention enema every 4 hours. It is imperative that the cardiac effects be monitored by electrocardiography.

The presence of severe or persistent hyperkalemia, severe hypertension, congestive heart failure, or hemolytic-uremic syndrome justifies the use of peritoneal dialysis or hemodialysis. Early institution of dialysis (ie, before complications occur) is preferable and is helpful in fluid, electrolyte, and nutritional management.

C. Nonoliguric Phase: Some patients with acute renal failure may initially be nonoliguric; in others, this phase may follow almost immediately after a renal insult or may be entered by diuretic-induced conversion from an oliguric state or during recovery after a period of prolonged oliguria. In some patients, the nonoliguric phase is mild, lasts only a few days, and is characterized by slightly increased volumes of poorly concentrated urine. Other patients, however, may pass enormous volumes of isosthenuric, sodium-rich urine. Occasionally, this salt-wasting state may be accompanied by significant potassium wasting as well.

Patients in the nonoliguric phase require adequate quantities of water, sodium, and potassium to replace ongoing losses. Measurements of previous volumes and determinations of urinary electrolytes (Na^+, K^+, Cl^-) provide the best guide to therapy. Producing an adequate volume of urinary output usually averts the need for dialysis.

D. Indications for Dialysis: The need for dialysis in individual cases is determined on the basis of clinical findings. However, there are some definite indications for dialysis: (1) severe hyperkalemia unresponsive to usual medical therapy; (2) unrelenting metabolic acidosis (usually in a situation where fluid overload prevents sodium bicarbonate administration); (3) fluid overload with or without severe hypertension or congestive heart failure (a situation that would seriously compromise caloric or drug administration—a definite problem in the oliguric patient); and (4) symptoms of uremia, usually manifested in children by central nervous system depression.

The rate of rise of both blood urea nitrogen and serum creatinine levels may indicate the need for dialysis; it is generally accepted that the blood urea nitrogen level should not be allowed to exceed 100 mg/dL.

Early dialysis, when properly performed, can simplify management and reduce the death rate associated with renal failure.

E. Methods of Dialysis: The choice of peritoneal dialysis or hemodialysis depends on the availability of as well as the indications for these techniques. Peritoneal dialysis is generally preferred in children because of the relative ease of performance and good results. However, when the clinical situation calls for rapid correction of systemic abnormalities or removal of toxins from the blood, hemodialysis must be instituted, since the peritoneal process is quite slow. Peritoneal dialysis may be accomplished even in patients with recent abdominal surgery. However, patients with past surgery may have adhesions and be at significant risk for perforation of a viscus or mechanical problems with peritoneal dialysis. Ileus also impairs the process, as does poor mesenteric circulation.

It is beneficial to insert a chronic peritoneal dialysis catheter in cases in which repeated dialysis may become necessary. Since this procedure is not routinely performed except in specialized centers, it will not be fully discussed here.

F. Technique of Peritoneal Dialysis: The procedure should be performed by experienced persons.

1. Catheter insertion—

a. Appropriate sedative medication may be administered at the physician's discretion.

b. The bladder must be empty. The abdomen is surgically prepared (with special attention to the umbilicus, which is considered highly contaminated) and draped. Strict aseptic technique should be followed.

c. The site of insertion is approximately 2 cm below the umbilicus, in the midline. Alternate sites are lateral rectus to this site. The skin in the area is infiltrated with local anesthetic, and the infiltration is carried to the fascia of the rectus muscle. The site is then perforated with a 14-gauge Angiocath or similar device that allows "priming" of the peritoneal cavity with dialysate. This procedure aids in demonstrating peritoneal cavity access as well as providing a "cushion" against which the dialysis catheter may be inserted. If the dialysate flows freely and there is no patient discomfort, intraperitoneal positioning is correct. If this is not the case, stop the flow immediately, since preperitoneal instillation of dialysate will make subsequent insertion practically impossible.

d. The abdomen is thus "primed" with enough prewarmed (37 °C) dialysate to distend the abdomen (see Table 21–3 for amount; the presence of ascitic fluid may reduce the requirement), thus reducing the likelihood of viscus perforation and facilitating insertion of the dialysis catheter. After the abdomen is distended, the Angiocath is removed and the dialysis catheter inserted.

e. The commercially available acute dialysis catheter usually consists of (1) a stiff Teflon catheter with a curve in the perforated segment that enters the peritoneal cavity and (2) a straight, sharpened metal stylet. The stylet is inserted into the Teflon catheter to straighten it, and the sharp tip of the stylet then eases insertion. Another method employs a wire guide and a Teflon catheter.

f. Insertion of the dialysis catheter with stylet in place may be further aided by making a small incision (2–3 mm) through the skin at the chosen site. With slow, steady pressure and some twisting motions, the catheter is pushed first through the skin and subcutaneous tissue. Sudden absence of resistance suggests entrance into the peritoneal cavity. This will be evidenced by dialysate welling up into the catheter as it is advanced (without resistance) over the stylet and into the pelvic area.

g. Exact placement depends on which position

Table 21–3. Volumes of dialysate in peritoneal dialysis.

Weight	Initial*	Maximum Maintenance (as Tolerated)
< 10 kg	50 mL/kg	50–100 mL/kg
10–20 kg	250–500 mL	1000–1500 mL
20–40 kg	500–1000 mL	1000–2000 mL
> 40 kg	1000 mL	2000 mL

* Initial volumes may need to be reduced to 25–35% of the amounts shown in some critically ill patients and then more fluid added slowly as tolerated.

is observed to provide the best function. The entire perforated segment of the catheter must lie intraperitoneally (pediatric-sized catheters are small enough to be used in most infants and older children).

h. After sterile dressings are placed around the catheter, it may be held in the desired place with tape. Care should be taken to prevent catheter movement once it is in place. It is especially important to avoid inserting the catheter farther into the peritoneal cavity once the exterior portion is contaminated.

2. Instillation of dialysate—

a. Note the total amount of fluid used to test catheter function, and make certain that at least 75% of dialysate instilled is recovered. If ascites is present at the time of dialysis, the decision whether or not ascitic fluid should be freely removed from the peritoneal cavity should be based on the patient's intravascular volume status.

b. Fill the peritoneal cavity with volumes of dialysate as set forth in Table 21–3.

c. The dialysate is allowed to run in freely by gravity flow until the inflow volume is achieved. The fluid is allowed to remain in the peritoneal cavity for approximately 20 minutes. The outflow tubing is then unclamped, permitting the dialysate to drain by gravity into a receptacle. The usual regimen is 2 "exchanges" each hour. An accurate record is kept of the amount instilled and the amount removed, so that it can readily be determined whether the patient is losing appropriate amounts of fluid in the process. Variation of the glucose concentration of the fluid results in removal of fluid from the patient. Weight should be recorded pre- and postdialysis and whenever calculations show a net fluid balance. The process is usually continued for 48 hours at a time but can be continued for as long as necessary.

d. During dialysis, vital signs should be carefully monitored, and a sample of the dialysate removed from the patient should be cultured daily, especially if the fluid becomes turbid. The catheter is removed after 48 hours, since the risk of peritonitis increases with prolonged use of this type of catheter. A new catheter can be inserted if necessary.

e. Peritoneal dialysis may be repeated as necessary during the course of acute renal failure.

3. Choosing the proper dialysate—A typical commercially prepared peritoneal dialysate solution contains Na^+, 132 meq/L; Cl^-, 102 meq/L; lactate, 35 meq/L; Ca^{2+}, 3.5 meq/L; and Mg^{2+}, 1.5 meq/L. K^+ is usually omitted unless the serum K^+ level is less than 4 meq/L. Glucose is added in varying quantities depending upon the need to withdraw fluid from the patient. Glucose solutions are available in 1.5% or 4.25% concentration. The 1.5% glucose concentration is used to maintain a slight osmotic gradient between the patient's serum and the dialysate in order to prevent fluid absorption. The 4.25% glucose concentration may be used to remove fluid more avidly. Concentrations higher than 4.25% are no longer commercially available because they remove an excessive quantity of fluid, which tends to result in severe hypernatremia. Lactate, instead of bicarbonate, is used in the solutions to provide an adequate buffer base. (The effectiveness of such buffers in dialysate solutions depends upon their ability to metabolize to bicarbonate.) Any other additives can be specified at the time of dialysis and added to the dialysate as indicated. The only other commonly used additive is heparin; 500 units are added to each of the first 4–6 L of dialysate to prevent clotting in the catheter.

G. Complications of Dialysis: The complications of catheter insertion include bleeding (rarely major), bowel perforation, failure to obtain adequate return of fluid (usually requiring only repositioning of the patient or the catheter), respiratory distress (usually correctable by using smaller volumes of dialysate), and infection. Infection is by far the most common and one of the more serious complications of established peritoneal dialysis. However, if infection is detected early, treatment is relatively simple; ie, the appropriate antibiotics are added to the dialysate. Signs of peritonitis should be sought during the procedure but may not necessarily be present. If peritonitis is suspected, a sample of the dialysis solution recovered from the patient should be sent for culture and sensitivity testing, and a gram-stained smear should be examined to determine whether or not antibiotic treatment can be started while culture results are being determined.

Dysequilibrium syndrome, a complication more commonly seen with hemodialysis than with peritoneal dialysis, usually appears early (ie, shortly after the procedure is initiated). The symptoms range from nausea and vomiting to severe headache and seizures. Although the cause is not completely understood, the disorder is believed to be related to rapid removal of urea from the blood with delayed removal from brain tissue, resulting in cerebral edema. This complication is rare with peritoneal dialysis, probably because of the slower rate of change in solute removal.

Excessive water removal can readily be corrected by increasing intake. Mild anxiety or pain can be relieved with analgesics or sedatives, providing it is not related to a true malfunction of the catheter itself. The procedure should be painless; any undue discomfort should alert the physician to a serious intra-abdominal problem or to catheter malposition.

Course & Prognosis

The period of severe oliguria, if it occurs, usually lasts about 10 days. If oliguria lasts longer than 3 weeks or if there is complete anuria, a diagnosis of acute tubular necrosis is very unlikely; vascular injury, severe ischemia, or glomerulonephritis is more probable. The diuretic phase begins with progressive increases in urinary output, followed by the passage of large volumes of isosthenuric urine containing sodium levels of 80–150 meq/L. During the recovery phase, signs and symptoms subside rapidly, although polyuria may persist for several days or weeks. Urinary abnormalities usually disappear completely within a few months.

The prognosis is excellent in acute tubular necrosis (> 90% complete recovery) but poor in other forms of acute renal failure of renal origin such as vascular accident (< 10% recovery).

Dobrin RS et al: The critically ill child: Acute renal failure. *Pediatrics* 1971;**48**:286.
Kleinknecht D et al: Uremic and non-uremic complications in acute renal failure: Evaluation of early and frequent dialysis on prognosis. *Kidney Int* 1972;**1**:190.
Tenckhoff H: Peritoneal dialysis today: A new look. *Nephron* 1974;**12**:420.

CHRONIC RENAL FAILURE

In renal failure, kidney function is reduced to a level at which the kidneys are unable to maintain normal biochemical homeostasis. In acute renal failure, the nephrons are injured, often reversibly; in the chronic form, the nephrons are progressively destroyed, leading to gradually increasing uremia. Many kidney diseases lead to uremia, particularly obstructive or reflux nephropathy and glomerulonephritis of various types. Renal dysplasias and cystic disease of the kidney as well as cystinosis and oxalosis are less common causes of failure.

Pathophysiology

The kidney has a remarkable ability to compensate for the persistent loss of nephrons that occurs in chronic renal failure. However, by the time the glomerular filtration rate has dropped to 5–20 mL/min/1.73 m^2, this capacity begins to be exhausted. The resulting biochemical problems can be grouped according to the major substances handled by the kidney.

A. Water: Defects in urine concentrating ability appear early in most chronic renal diseases. Thus, the patient requires a larger than normal urine volume to excrete a given solute load. Clinically, this is reflected as polyuria with a urine of low specific gravity; the patient needs an increased water intake to meet the demands of this situation. In later stages, the ability to dilute the urine may be lost, and a urine of fixed specific gravity close to that of plasma will be excreted regardless of intake.

B. Nitrogenous Products: Blood urea nitrogen and serum creatinine and uric acid levels rise as the glomerular filtration rate (GFR) falls. However, the level of blood urea nitrogen is affected not only by GFR but also by dietary intake of protein and by urinary flow. Creatinine, on the other hand, is not reabsorbed by the tubules and is not influenced by dietary intake; for these reasons, serum creatinine has several advantages over urea as an index of renal failure.

C. Sodium and Potassium: Sodium loss is enhanced by osmotic diuresis and by a decreased capacity of the tubules to secrete hydrogen ions in exchange for sodium. Sodium retention is rare in chronic renal failure unless nephrotic syndrome is also present. Salt wasting can therefore be a serious problem and can be compounded by salt restriction or diuretics. Hyperkalemia is usually a very late problem in chronic renal failure, occurring in the oliguric phase.

D. Phosphorus and Calcium: A large percentage (85%) of the filtered phosphorus is normally reabsorbed; tubular rejection can therefore compensate for a decrease in GFR. However, retention of phosphorus occurs when the GFR drops. Serum phosphorus levels of 7–10 mg/dL are common, and calcium levels are correspondingly low. This phenomenon is related both to the fact that the transport of calcium across the bowel wall in uremia is unresponsive to normal amounts of vitamin D and to the reciprocal relationship of serum phosphorus and serum calcium. Hyperphosphatemia is detrimental to renal parenchyma and plays a role in the development of renal osteodystrophy.

E. Acid-Base Balance: Decreased ammonia production and retention of endogenous acid account for the metabolic acidosis seen in chronic renal failure.

F. Nutrition and Growth: A major problem in management of chronic renal failure is the effect of dietary manipulations on the child's growth and development. The clinician may be unavoidably accepting some compromise in growth and development in making the best of what remains of renal function. Dietary supplementation with essential amino acids or keto acids may improve the nutritional status of the child with chronic renal failure. Unfortunately, many children find the diet unacceptable. Early initiation of dialysis has been thought by many to be a possible solution to this problem, although nutritional status may still be a problem while the patient is undergoing dialysis. The decision is not an easy one, given the extreme nature of the therapy at a time when some degree of renal function still exists. However, an aggressive approach to the problem may still provide the best results regarding growth in these children.

Clinical Findings

Chronic renal failure must be thought of as a total body disease, with clinical and laboratory findings relating to nearly every organ system.

Anemia is a nearly constant finding in chronic renal failure. It is usually normochromic and normocytic and results from decreased production secondary to diminished renal erythropoietin synthesis. Nutritional deficiency also plays a role. Platelet dysfunction and other abnormalities of the coagulation system may be present. Bleeding phenomena, especially gastrointestinal bleeding, may be a problem.

Central nervous system manifestations of the condition may be subtle but are usually present. Confusion, apathy, and lethargy usually occur late in the course of disease; these may be unsuspected clinically until the patient is carefully evaluated. With advancing uremia, stupor and coma may be present. Associated electrolyte abnormalities (eg, hyponatremia) may precipitate seizures (more commonly, a result of untreated hypertension).

Cardiovascular manifestations may be life-threatening. Uremic pericarditis may develop. Congestive heart failure is seen more often, and hypertension is quite common. The hypertension may relate to volume overload, excessive renin excretion, or both.

The skeleton may be severely affected. The combination of hyperparathyroidism, vitamin D deficiency, and buffering of acids by the bone salts results in osteomalacia and rickets. Bone pain and severe deformities may result.

Anorexia is the primary gastrointestinal manifestation of this state. It is often a significant problem in that it may lead to dangerous nutritional deficiencies. Intractable vomiting may also occur with severe uremia.

Patients with chronic renal failure tend to be more susceptible to infections. Because of their generally debilitated state, they often handle infections poorly.

Treatment

A. General Measures: As with acute renal failure, the aim of treatment in chronic renal disease is the prevention of complications. The principles of management differ depending upon the degree of renal insufficiency. Serial determinations of serum creatinine and urea levels (and, when necessary, creatinine clearances or other measurements of GFR) are essential in monitoring and managing renal insufficiency.

1. GFR of 20–30 mL/min/1.73 m^2—With this degree of renal insufficiency, most homeostatic mechanisms are still operating effectively. The physician should be most concerned with maintaining existing function. However, at this time, a normal serum phosphorus level is likely the result of secondary hyperparathyroidism. Thus, surveillance on a regular basis is essential. Blood pressure is followed carefully and hypertension treated if detected. The degree of acidosis is also monitored, and acidosis can be treated if fluid retention is not a problem. Phosphate binders and vitamin D may be necessary. Good nutrition is important; severe dietary restrictions (except for phosphorus) are rarely necessary at this level of function. However, there is still concern over the role of dietary protein in progressive chronic renal failure.

2. GFR of 10–20 mL/min/1.73 m^2—The need for some dietary control usually becomes evident when further lowering of GFR occurs. A diet high in fats and carbohydrates and low in protein (< 1 g/kg) will provide adequate calories, with some reduction in nitrogenous waste products. The need for salt restriction depends upon the urine sodium excretion. In situations where salt losses are continuing (eg, medullary cystic disease), restriction may be unnecessary or even dangerous. Generally, modest sodium restriction (1 meq/kg/d) will be required; severe hypertension may necessitate further restriction. Patients in this category are usually hyperphosphatemic. Although dietary phosphate restriction is difficult to achieve, the use of phosphate binders in the form of calcium carbonate (eg, Titralac) decreases absorption of the anion. Hypocalcemia may respond to lowering the serum phosphate level, or additional measures such as vitamin D or calcium supplementation may be necessary.

3. GFR of 5–10 mL/min/1.73 m^2—When the GFR reaches this level, it is nearly inevitable that dialysis or transplantation will eventually be necessary. The best policy is to arrange for elective placement of a chronic peritoneal catheter or arteriovenous fistula when this stage is reached even if the child is clinically well. If hemodialysis is the therapeutic choice, early placement of an access for hemodialysis will permit the fistula time to mature so that it will be functioning well as soon as dialysis is required. Extremely careful follow-up is necessary at this point, with the physician's main role being early recognition of the need for initiating dialysis. Supplemental bicarbonate may be needed for acidosis. Anemia is likely to be present but may be well tolerated. Blood transfusions, however, should be kept to a minimum because of the danger of volume overload. There is some evidence that the anemia of renal failure may respond to androgens, but it will more likely improve with dialysis.

4. GFR under 5 mL/min/1.73 m^2—With this degree of function, end-stage renal failure is well established (although it may be symptomatic at a clearance somewhere under 10 mL/min), and dialysis is necessary to maintain homeostasis. Few small children will tolerate delaying dialysis to this level of function. Regardless, the child should have been followed carefully enough to this stage so that dialysis can be initiated electively rather than as an emergency procedure. (See Acute Renal Failure, above, for a discussion of dialysis.) Avoidance of such complications as pulmonary edema, hyperkalemia, and neurologic symptoms secondary to uremia is desirable. The alternative to dialysis is, of course, renal transplantation (see below).

B. Water and Calorie Conservation: Strict attention must be paid to water conservation, especially in patients with severe renal failure. In cases of complete anuria, water should be supplied to replace insensible loss minus water from oxidation (about 400 mL/m^2/24 h) plus water lost in stools, emesis, and urine. The amount to be given should be carefully calculated at least daily and checked against body weight.

Dietary restriction is difficult to organize for any child with a fickle appetite, and especially so when fluid must be restricted and calories must exceed 70% of the recommended dietary allowance. Flavored high calorie solutions and dietary supplements are useful.

In less severe cases, restriction of protein to 1 g/kg/24 h or less may help to lower blood urea levels. Many children with end-stage renal disease are undergoing dialysis, and continuing growth in these children is in part dependent on adequate dialysis and a high-calorie, high-protein intake. Supplements of essential amino acids (Amin-Aid, etc) can be helpful in decreasing catabolism and reducing blood urea levels. Various glucose polymers are available to increase caloric intake. Sodium and potassium regulation will also be important, except in those children who continue to elaborate generous volumes of urine. Water-soluble vitamins should be given in at least twice the recommended dietary allowance to children undergoing dialysis.

C. Electrolyte Homeostasis: The principles of fluid and electrolyte therapy are discussed in Chapter 36. Meticulous medical care can often sustain children in renal failure for many weeks without dialysis, but the cost may not be justified in light of current dialysis techniques. For example, elevated serum phosphorus levels can to some extent be controlled by a low-phosphorus diet in conjunction with phosphate binders. The use of calcium carbonate as the binder will also provide dietary calcium supplementation. Dihydrotachysterol and other vitamin D derivatives have been used to raise serum calcium levels; however, calcitriol (Rocaltrol) is most effective.

D. Blood Transfusions: Some children with renal failure become severely anemic and require transfusions, but it is remarkable how little they may be affected by hemoglobin levels as low as 6 g/dL. In general, if there is no cardiac failure and the patient is not overly fatigued, transfusions should be minimal. Since these patients may already have marginally high blood volumes, any increase may precipitate severe hypertension with convulsions or congestive heart failure. Packed cells should always be used and should be given very slowly and under the closest supervision, usually while the patient is receiving dialysis. Vascular accidents are frequent during and immediately after improperly supervised transfusions.

E. Management of Acidosis and Osteodystrophy: A low-protein diet will be helpful in decreasing metabolic acidosis, since proteins are the largest contributors of nonvolatile acids. The acidosis can be further alleviated by the administration of an alkalinizing solution. Unless renal failure is very advanced, attempts should be made to relieve bone pain and improve osteodystrophy by control of serum phosphorus, acidosis, and hyperparathyroidism and by the administration of calcitriol (Rocaltrol). Serum calcium, phosphorus, and alkaline phosphatase levels must be monitored. In evaluating the status of osteodystrophy, it is useful to periodically measure plasma parathyroid hormone even though alkaline phosphatase determinations are readily available.

F. Management of Hypertension: Hypertension in chronic renal failure is often a reflection of fluid overload. This possibility should always be considered first and treated if appropriate. (See Hypertension, below.)

G. Control of Infections: After appropriate cultures are obtained, antibiotics should be given. The dosage of certain antibiotics eliminated principally in the urine should be reduced in proportion to the decrease in renal function in order to prevent toxic effects. The effect of dialysis should also be taken into consideration.

H. Psychologic Support: As is true of most children with chronic illness, an important part of management is attention to the patient's and the family's emotional adaptation to the disease. Psychiatric counseling requires as much attention as the rather complicated medical management.

I. Dialysis and Transplantation: The best-tolerated method of treatment of end-stage renal disease is a successful and uncomplicated renal transplant. The idea of transplantation in a child at first seems ideal; however, despite the advances that have been made in organ transplantation procedures, there are some problems. Adequate growth and well-being are directly related to acceptance of the graft, the degree of normal function, and the side effects of medications employed.

Great advances have also been made in peritoneal dialysis and hemodialysis, both in technique and in our understanding of the specialized approach required by the treatments. Hemodialysis is now performed in major centers that devote their entire effort in dialysis toward the management of pediatric patients and is now being regarded as a reasonable long-range method of treatment of the child with end-stage renal disease. Treatment of terminal renal failure in children may thus consist of transplantation or dialysis as the situation warrants. The demonstrated feasibility of chronic peritoneal dialysis in children has made this treatment most often the initial choice of dialysis therapy for children. Peritoneal dialysis via an indwelling chronic catheter is well accepted by children and can be performed in the home.

The best measure of the success of chronic dialysis in children is the level of physical and psychosocial rehabilitation achieved. Patients continue to participate in day-to-day activities, attend school, and have even recorded reasonable growth. Although catch-up growth rarely occurs, patients can grow at an acceptable rate even though they remain in the third percentile. Even associated problems such as chronic anemia and bone disease are being better controlled.

Course & Prognosis

Severe chronic renal disease in childhood is all too often progressive and eventually fatal. The rates at which renal diseases progress are quite variable, however, and hard to predict. Intractable anemia and hypertension are bad signs, as are permanent electrolyte changes and neurologic symptoms. In the older child, there is an increasing tendency to initiate peritoneal dialysis or hemodialysis before a transplant, thus minimizing these complications.

Alliopoulous JC et al: Comparison of continuous cycling peritoneal dialysis with continuous ambulatory peritoneal dialysis in children. *J Pediatr* 1984;**105:**721.

Chesney RW et al: Increased growth after long-term oral 1 alpha,25-vitamin D_3 in childhood renal osteodystrophy. *N Engl J Med* 1978;**298:**238.

Fine RN et al: Long-term results of renal transplantation in children. *Pediatrics* 1978;**61:**641.

Grushkin CM, Korsch B, Fine RN: Hemodialysis in small children. *JAMA* 1972;**221:**869.

Mauer M et al: Long-term hemodialysis in the neonatal period. *Am J Dis Child* 1973;**125:**269.
Potter DE et al: Treatment of end-stage renal disease in children: A 15 year experience. *Kidney Int* 1980;**18:**103.
Rae A, Pendray M: Advantages of peritoneal dialysis in chronic renal failure. *JAMA* 1973;**225:**937.

HYPERTENSION

Hypertension in children is most commonly of renal origin. It is usually encountered as an anticipated complication of known renal parenchymal disease, but it may be found on routine physical examination in an otherwise normal child. Increased understanding of the roles of water and salt retention on the one hand and overactivity of the renin-angiotensin system on the other has done much to guide therapy; it is nevertheless clear that not all forms of hypertension are explicable by these 2 mechanisms.

Diagnosis

Confirmation of the diagnosis depends upon the repeated demonstration of a diastolic pressure 2 standard deviations above the mean (Table 21–4). The blood pressure cuff should be at least 20% wider than the diameter of the arm, since a narrow cuff will cause falsely high readings. It is also sometimes necessary to use a "leg" cuff for determinations in overweight adolescent children. Adolescent patients may have labile blood pressures; it is therefore important to check initial elevated readings again after a period of relaxation. It may be useful to have blood pressures recorded at home.

Table 21–4. Normal blood pressure for various ages (mm Hg).*

Ages	Mean Systolic ± 2 SD	Mean Diastolic ± 2 SD
1 month	80 ± 16	46 ± 16
6 months to 1 year	89 ± 29	60 ± 10†
1 year	96 ± 30	66 ± 25†
2 years	99 ± 25	64 ± 25†
3 years	100 ± 25	67 ± 23†
4 years	99 ± 20	65 ± 20†
5–6 years	94 ± 14	55 ± 9
6–7 years	100 ± 15	56 ± 8
7–8 years	102 ± 15	56 ± 8
8–9 years	105 ± 16	57 ± 9
9–10 years	107 ± 16	57 ± 9
10–11 years	111 ± 17	58 ± 10
11–12 years	113 ± 18	59 ± 10
12–13 years	115 ± 19	59 ± 10
13–14 years	118 ± 19	60 ± 10

* Reproduced, with permission, from Nadas A: *Pediatric Cardiology,* 2nd ed. Saunders, 1963.

† In this study the point of muffling was taken as the diastolic pressure.

Evaluation of renal hypertension in children is particularly directed toward the possibility of a unilateral lesion or other abnormality that might be susceptible to remedy by surgery. The evaluation of nonrenal possibilities suggested by the history or physical signs is detailed under these respective conditions.

Routine laboratory studies include a complete blood count, urinalysis, and urine culture and radiographic delineation of the urinary tract. A renal biopsy (which rarely reveals the cause of hypertension unless there is clinical evidence of renal disease) should always be undertaken with special care in the hypertensive patient and preferably after pressures have been controlled by therapy. Ureteric catheterization is not used now in lateralizing lesions; instead, the appropriate information is obtained from renal size, a rapid-sequence intravenous urogram, the renal scan, aortography with renal arteriography, and differential renal vein renin levels.

Treatment

A. Emergency Treatment of Acute Hypertension: A hypertensive emergency may be said to exist when central nervous system signs of hypertension appear, eg, papilledema or seizures. Retinal hemorrhages or exudates also indicate a need for prompt and effective control.

1. One of the most effective drugs for use in a true hypertensive emergency is diazoxide (Hyperstat IV), 5 mg/kg by a single, rapid intravenous injection.

2. Intravenous hydralazine can be effective in some cases. Dosage varies according to the severity of the hypertension and should begin at around 0.15 mg/kg.

3. Sodium nitroprusside is also effective in an intensive care setting for reducing severely elevated blood pressure. Intravenous administration of 0.5–10 μg/kg/min will reduce blood pressure in seconds, but the dose must be carefully monitored.

4. Furosemide, 1–5 mg/kg intravenously, will reduce blood volume and enhance the effectiveness of other drugs.

B. Ambulatory Treatment of Chronic Hypertension: The treatment of renoparenchymal hypertension is medical rather than surgical. Table 21–5 lists the drugs commonly used to treat hypertension on an ambulatory basis.

In general, treatment is started with a low dose, and the dose is raised at intervals (usually every few days) until control of blood pressure is achieved, postural hypotension becomes a problem, or undesirable side effects occur.

The order and combinations in which these drugs should be used are governed by the potency of the drugs, their freedom from side effects, and the severity of the hypertension. The mildest drug is probably hydrochlorothiazide used alone, followed by propranolol and hydralazine. Certain more recently introduced drugs promise much better control. These include minoxidil with propranolol; saralasin, an angiotensin II inhibitor; and captopril, an angiotensin I

Table 21–5. Antihypertensive drugs for ambulatory treatment.

Drug	Oral Dose	Major Side Effects*
Hydrochlorothiazide (Esidrix, HydroDiuril)	2–4 mg/kg/24 h as single dose or in 2 individual doses	Potassium depletion, hyperuricemia.
Furosemide (Lasix)	1–5 mg/kg/dose, 2–3 doses per day	Potassium and volume depletion.
Hydralazine (Apresoline)	0.75 mg/kg/24 h in 4–6 divided doses	Lupus erythematosus, tachycardia, headache.
Methyldopa (Aldomet)	10–40 mg/kg/24 h in 3 divided doses	False-positive Coombs test, hemolytic anemia, fever, leukopenia, abnormal liver function tests.
Propranolol (Inderal) with	0.2–5 mg/kg/dose, 2–3 doses per day	Syncope, cardiac failure, hypoglycemia.
Minoxidil (Loniten) (a piperidine-pyrimidine)	0.15 mg/kg/dose, 2–3 doses per day	Tachycardia, angina, fluid retention, hirsutism.
Captopril (Capoten)	0.3–2 mg/kg/dose, 2–3 doses per day	Rash, hyperkalemia, glomerulopathy.

* Many more side effects than those listed have been reported.

converting enzyme inhibitor. Clonidine in doses of 0.2–2.4 mg/d has been widely used in children. The use of calcium channel and receptor blockers has not been sufficiently evaluated in children.

It is advisable to teach capable parents how to take and record blood pressures at home.

Prognosis

The long-term effects of mild hypertension with onset during childhood are not well defined. However, studies indicate that serious hypertension, if not corrected, is associated with a very poor long-term prognosis. Approximately 50% of children with diastolic blood pressures persistently above 120 mm Hg will die within 10 years of diagnosis.

Dormois JC, Young JL, Nies AS: Minoxidil in severe hypertension: Value when conventional drugs have failed. *Am Heart J* 1975;**90:**360.

Friedman A: Effective use of captopril (angiotensin I converting enzyme inhibitor) in severe childhood hypertension. *J Pediatr* 1980;**97:**664.

Gill DG et al: Analysis of 100 children with severe and persistent hypertension. *Arch Dis Child* 1976;**51:**951.

Loggie JMH et al: Hypertension in the pediatric patient: A reappraisal. *J Pediatr* 1979;**94:**688.

Londe S, Goldring D: High blood pressure in children: Problems and guidelines for evaluation and treatment. *Am J Cardiol* 1976;**37:**650.

Rance CP et al: Persistent systemic hypertension in infants and children. *Pediatr Clin North Am* 1974;**21:**801.

Richard GA et al: A pathophysiologic basis for the diagnosis and treatment of the renal hypertensions. *Adv Pediatr* 1977;**24:**339.

INHERITED OR DEVELOPMENTAL DEFECTS OF THE URINARY TRACT

In recent years, there has been a substantial increase in the number of renal or urinary tract diseases that have been discovered to be hereditary or developmental in origin. Although many classification schemes have been proposed, no scheme is entirely adequate. The more important entities are listed below.

Cystic Diseases of Genetic Origin

A. Polycystic Disease:

- Polycystic disease of early infancy: Neonatal polycystic disease, Meckel's syndrome
- Polycystic disease of childhood: Medullary tubular ectasia, congenital hepatic fibrosis
- Adult polycystic disease

B. Cortical Cysts:

- Tuberous sclerosis complex
- Lindau's disease (cystic disease in syndromes of multiple malformations):
  - Cerebrohepatorenal syndrome of Zellweger
  - Autosomal trisomy syndromes D and E
  - Lissencephaly and oral-facial-digital syndromes
  - Schwartz-Jampel syndrome
- Asphyxiating thoracic dystrophy of Jeune
- Down's, Turner's, and Ehlers-Danlos syndromes

C. Medullary Cysts:

- Medullary sponge kidney
- Medullary cystic disease (nephronophthisis)

D. Hereditary and Familial Cystic Dysplasia

Dysplastic Renal Diseases

- Renal aplasia (unilateral, bilateral)
- Renal hypoplasia (unilateral, bilateral, total, segmental)
- Multicystic renal dysplasia (unilateral, bilateral, multilocular, postobstructive, etc)
- Familial and hereditary renal dysplasias
- Oligomeganephronia

Hereditary Diseases Associated With Nephritis

- Hereditary nephritis with deafness and ocular defects (Alport's syndrome)

Nail-patella syndrome
Familial hyperprolinemia
Hereditary nephrotic syndrome
Hereditary osteolysis with nephropathy
Hereditary nephritis with thoracic asphyxiant dystrophy syndrome

Hereditary Diseases Associated With Intrarenal Deposition of Metabolites

Angiokeratoma corporis diffusum (Fabry's disease)
Heredopathia atactica polyneuritiformis (Refsum's disease)
Various storage diseases (eg, G_{M1} monosialogangliosidosis, Hurler's syndrome, Niemann-Pick disease, familial metachromatic leukodystrophy, glycogenosis type I [von Gierke's disease], glycogenosis type II [Pompe's disease])
Hereditary amyloidosis (familial Mediterranean fever; heredofamilial urticaria with deafness and neuropathy; primary familial amyloidosis with polyneuropathy)

Hereditary Renal Diseases Associated With Tubular Transport Defects

Hartnup disease
Immunoglycinuria
Fanconi's syndrome
Oculocerebrorenal syndrome of Lowe
Cystinosis (infantile, adolescent, adult types)
Wilson's disease
Galactosemia
Hereditary fructose intolerance
Renal tubular acidosis (many types)
Hereditary tyrosinemia
Renal glycosuria
Vitamin D-resistant rickets
Pseudohypoparathyroidism
Vasopressin-resistant diabetes insipidus
Hypouricemia

Hereditary Diseases Associated With Lithiasis

Hyperoxaluria
L-Glyceric aciduria
Xanthinuria
Lesch-Nyhan syndrome and variants, gout
Nephropathy due to familial hyperparathyroidism
Cystinuria (types I, II, III)
Glycinuria

Miscellaneous

Hereditary intestinal vitamin B_{12} malabsorption
Total and partial lipodystrophy
Sickle cell anemia
Bartter's syndrome

Bernstein J: Heritable cystic disorders of the kidney: The mythology of polycystic disease. *Pediatr Clin North Am* 1971;**18**:435.

Bernstein J: The morphogenesis of renal parenchymal maldevelopment (renal dysplasia). *Pediatr Clin North Am* 1971; **18**:395.

Carter JE et al: Bilateral renal hypoplasia with oligomeganephronia. *Am J Dis Child* 1970;**120**:537.

Crocker JFS et al: Developmental defects of the kidney: A review of renal development and experimental studies of maldevelopment. *Pediatr Clin North Am* 1971;**18**:355.

Milne MD: Genetic aspects of renal disease. *Prog Med Genet* 1970;**7**:112.

DISORDERS OF THE RENAL TUBULES

Three subtypes of renal tubular acidosis are well recognized: (1) the "classic" form, called type I or distal renal tubular acidosis; (2) the bicarbonate "wasting" form, designated as type II or proximal renal tubular acidosis; and (3) type IV, or hyperkalemic renal tubular acidosis (rare in children), which is associated with hyporeninemic hypoaldosteronism. Type I and type II and their variants are encountered most frequently in children. Thus, discussion will focus on these 2 most commonly seen problems of urinary acidification.

The renal mechanisms controlling acid-base equilibrium are illustrated in Fig 21–1. Primary tubular disorders in childhood, such as glycinuria, hypouricemia, or renal glycosuria, may result from a defect in a single tubular transport pathway. In other conditions, especially secondary ones (eg, phosphaturia, aminoaciduria, and glycosuria in Fanconi's syndrome), multiple pathways may be involved. In some situations (eg, lysinuric protein intolerance, Hartnup disease, and cystinuria), the transport defect in the renal tubular epithelium may be reflected to a variable extent in the enteric lining cells.

Tubular dysfunction may also be secondary to other major metabolic disorders such as galactosemia, cystinosis, renal failure, hyperparathyroidism, mineralocorticoid deficiency, and Bartter's syndrome. Elaborate discussions of all these entities are beyond the scope of this text. A discussion of a few more frequently encountered entities follows.

DISTAL RENAL TUBULAR ACIDOSIS (TYPE I)

The most common form of distal renal tubular acidosis in childhood is the hereditary form. The clinical presentation is one of failure to thrive, anorexia, vomiting, and dehydration. Hyperchloremic metabolic acidosis occurs, with hypokalemia and a urinary pH exceeding 6.5. The severity of the acidosis depends usually on the presence of a bicarbonate "leak." (This variant of distal renal tubular acidosis with bicarbonate wasting has been called type III

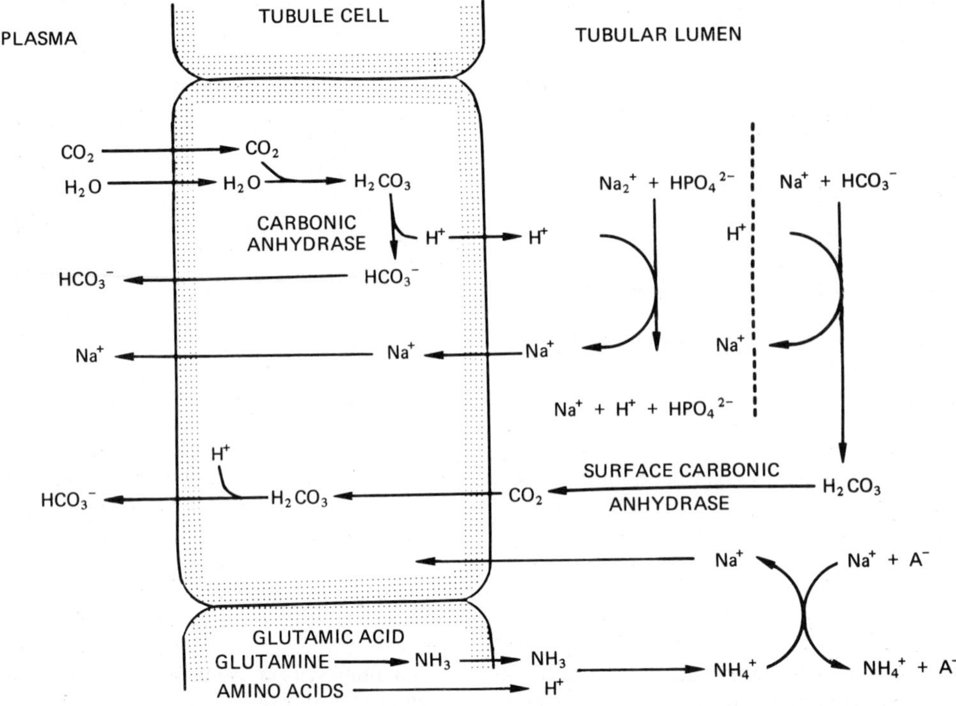

Figure 21–1. Tubular mechanisms for hydrogen ion excretion.

but for clinical purposes need not be considered as a distinct entity.) Concomitant hypercalciuria may lead to rickets, nephrocalcinosis, nephrolithiasis, and renal failure.

Other situations that may be responsible for distal renal tubular acidosis are malnutrition, hyperparathyroidism, vitamin D intoxication, Fabry's disease, various hypergammaglobulinemic states, amphotericin B intoxication, cirrhosis, sickle cell disease, hyperthyroidism, urinary tract obstruction, and genetic abnormalities such as Ehlers-Danlos syndrome or Marfan's syndrome.

The pathogenesis of distal renal tubular acidosis has not yet been clearly defined. Basically, there appears to be a defect in the distal nephron, in the tubular transport of hydrogen ion, or in the maintenance of a steep enough gradient for proper excretion of hydrogen ion. This defect can be accompanied by degrees of bicarbonate wasting, or the defect may not be severe enough to lead to frank acidosis. More studies are needed to clarify the role of a variety of abnormalities that may be associated with the distal defect.

The classic method for determining the ability to handle an acid load in suspected distal renal tubular acidosis is the administration of NH_4Cl. However, this approach has been challenged. Recent evidence has shown that during sodium bicarbonate loading, the CO_2 tension of the urine does not increase in patients with distal renal tubular acidosis as it does in normal controls; this reflects a problem with the dehydration of H_2CO_3 in these patients.

Since acid load testing can be somewhat cumbersome to perform and could produce severe acidosis, it is best to use a simplified method of bicarbonate titration (described in the next section) and alkali administration to rule out proximal (type II) renal tubular acidosis. The dose of alkali required to achieve a normal plasma HCO_3^- concentration in patients with distal renal tubular acidosis is low (seldom exceeds 2–3 meq/kg/24 h) in contrast to that required in proximal renal tubular acidosis. Higher doses are, however, needed if distal renal tubular acidosis is accompanied by bicarbonate wasting. Alkali therapy can result in reduced complications and improved growth.

Distal renal tubular acidosis is usually a permanent disorder, although it sometimes occurs as a secondary complication. If irreversible renal damage is prevented, the prognosis is good.

Chan CM: Renal tubular acidosis. *J Pediatr* 1982;**102:**327.

Quintanilla AP: Renal tubular acidosis. *Postgrad Med* (April) 1980;**67:**60.

Rodriguez-Soriano J et al: Natural history of primary distal renal tubular acidosis treated since infancy. *J Pediatr* 1982;**101:**669.

Sabastian A et al: Disorders of distal nephron function. *Am J Med* 1982;**72:**289.

Sabatini A et al: Disorders of acid-base balance. *Med Clin North Am* 1978;**62:**1223.

PROXIMAL RENAL TUBULAR ACIDOSIS (TYPE II)

In the proximal tubule, the dominant process in the control of acid-base balance is the exchange of tubule cell hydrogen ion for intraluminal sodium. Proximal renal tubular acidosis is characterized by an alkaline urine pH, loss of bicarbonate in the urine, and mildly reduced serum bicarbonate concentrations. About 85–90% of bicarbonate reabsorption occurs in the proximal tubules. The lesion in proximal renal tubular acidosis is a lowering of the renal bicarbonate threshold, ie, the concentration of serum bicarbonate above which bicarbonate appears in the urine. With more severe acidosis, the concentration of serum bicarbonate drops and bicarbonate disappears from the urine; this reflects normal distal tubular acidification.

The proximal type is the most common type of renal tubular acidosis encountered in children. It is often an isolated defect, and in the small or preterm infant, it can be considered to be a factor of renal immaturity. The onset in infants is accompanied by failure to thrive, hyperchloremic acidosis, hypokalemia, and, rarely, nephrocalcinosis. Secondary forms are the result of reflux or obstructive uropathy and are seen in association with other tubular disorders, eg, Fanconi's syndrome, cystinosis, Lowe's syndrome, Wilson's disease, galactosemia, hereditary fructose intolerance, tyrosinemia, and juvenile nephronophthisis (medullary cystic disease).

Bicarbonate titration can be used to demonstrate the lowered renal threshold for bicarbonate reabsorption in proximal renal tubular acidosis, thereby distinguishing the proximal defect from the distal defect. This procedure is rather cumbersome and requires strict adherence to a protocol of bicarbonate infusion and measurement of urine pH and bicarbonate levels. A practical differentiation can be made by oral administration of citrate or bicarbonate, gradually increasing the dose until the serum level of bicarbonate reaches 22 meq/L. Larger doses, usually exceeding 5 meq/kg/24 h, are generally required to achieve the described level of serum bicarbonate in proximal renal tubular acidosis.

The available forms of bicarbonate therapy that are somewhat more easily tolerated than sodium bicarbonate are the citrate solutions (eg, Bicitra, Polycitra). Shohl's solution is a standard solution of sodium citrate but requires mixing by a pharmacist. Generally, each milliliter of solution contains 1 meq of sodium citrate, which is metabolized to 1 meq of HCO_3^-. The required daily dosage is given in 3 divided doses. Potassium supplementation may be required, since the added sodium load presenting to the distal tubule may exaggerate potassium losses.

In cases of isolated defects, especially where the problem is related to renal immaturity, the prognosis is excellent. Alkali therapy can usually be discontinued after several months to 2 years. Growth should be normal, and the gradual increase in the serum bicarbonate level to above 22 meq/L heralds the presence of a raised bicarbonate threshold in the tubules. If the defect is part of a more complex tubular abnormality, the prognosis depends on the underlying disorder or syndrome.

Buckalew VM et al: Hereditary renal tubular acidosis. *Medicine* 1974;**53:**229.

McSherry E: Renal tubular acidosis in childhood. *Kidney Int* 1981;**20:**799.

Nash MA et al: Renal tubular acidosis. *J Pediatr* 1972;**80:**738.

Rodriguez-Soriano J, Vallo A, Garcia-Fuentes M: Distal renal tubular acidosis in infancy: A bicarbonate wasting state. *J Pediatr* 1975;**86:**524.

Vladuti A: Renal tubular acidosis: An autoimmune disease. *Lancet* 1973;**1:**265.

CONGENITAL HYPOKALEMIC ALKALOSIS (Bartter's Syndrome)

Bartter's syndrome is characterized by severe hypokalemic, hypochloremic metabolic alkalosis; extremely high levels of circulating renin and aldosterone; and a paradoxic absence of hypertension. On renal biopsy, there is striking juxtaglomerular hyperplasia. Most patients present in early infancy with severe failure to thrive.

The cause and pathogenesis are not known. The pathogenesis is thought to be related to sodium reabsorption defects in the proximal or distal tubule. Studies have associated elevated levels of prostaglandins with the syndrome, and treatment with inhibitors of prostaglandin (eg, indomethacin) has been advocated. A prostaglandin-independent chloride-reabsorptive defect has been proposed.

Treatment with prostaglandin inhibitors and potassium-conserving diuretics (eg, amiloride combined with magnesium supplements) may be beneficial. Although the prognosis is very poor, a few patients seem to have less severe forms of the disease that are compatible with longer survival.

Bartter's syndrome. (Editorial.) *Lancet* 1976;**2:**721.

Chan JCM: Bartter's syndrome. *Nephron* 1980;**26:**155.

Littlewood JM, Lee MR, Meadow SR: Treatment of Bartter's syndrome in early childhood with prostaglandin synthetase inhibitors. *Arch Dis Child* 1978;**53:**43.

Norby L et al: Prostaglandins and aspirin therapy in Bartter's syndrome. *Lancet* 1976;**2:**604.

Schwarz GJ, Cornfeld D: Propranolol in Bartter's syndrome. *N Engl J Med* 1974;**290:**966.

RENAL GLYCOSURIA

Renal glycosuria is a disorder that involves the proximal convoluted tubules of all nephrons. The basic mechanism does not seem to affect phosphorylation of glucose in the tubule but is assumed to interfere with the sodium- and energy-dependent steps of incorporation of glucose into the brush border. The degree to which this transport mechanism is inhibited can be determined by measuring the maximal tubular reabsorption of glucose (T_mG). The test is performed in conjunction with an inulin clearance test. The calculation is as follows:

$$T_mG \text{ in mg/min/1.73 m}^2 = (\text{Inulin clearance} \times \text{Plasma glucose concentration in mg/mL}) - \text{Glucose execretion in mg/min}$$

Normal values are 260–550 mg/min/1.73 m^2, whereas the range in renal glycosuria is 80–280 mg/min/1.73 m^2.

Structural alterations of the proximal convoluted tubules have been described; these changes seen on electron microscopy are degenerative and correlate well with the functional insufficiency of this area of the nephron.

In most patients, the total urinary glucose loss is insufficient to cause any symptoms or metabolic disturbance. Hyperglycemia does not occur. In some affected individuals, polyuria and polydipsia are present. During starvation and occasionally in pregnancy, the obligatory loss of carbohydrates may lead to acidosis.

No treatment is necessary. It is essential to rule out diabetes mellitus and renal tubular disorders, where glycosuria can be associated with aminoaciduria, phosphaturia, and acidification defects.

CYSTINOSIS

Three types of cystinosis have been identified: adult, adolescent, and infantile. The adult type is a relatively benign condition characterized by cystine deposition in the corneas, granulocytes, and fibroblasts but no renal disease. The adolescent type is also characterized by cystine deposition but is accompanied by the development of mild renal failure with Fanconi's syndrome during adolescence; growth is normal. The infantile type is both the most common and the most severe. Characteristically, children present in the first or second year of life with polyuria and on investigation are found to have renal rickets, generalized aminoaciduria, glycosuria, and a variable degree of renal tubular acidosis.

Cystinosis is an autosomal recessive condition that may be diagnosed in utero by obtaining fetal cells by amniocentesis, growing them in tissue culture, and measuring the avidity with which they incorporate ^{35}S-cystine.

The exact biochemical nature of the disease remains obscure. Cystine is stored in cellular lysosomes in virtually all tissues—the consequence of a now-recognized lysosomal cystine afflux transport system. Eventually, cystine accumulation results in cell damage and cell death, particularly in the renal tubules. Death from renal failure between ages 6 and 12 is the rule.

Whenever the diagnosis of cystinosis is suspected, a slit lamp examination of the corneas should be performed, as cystine crystal deposition causes an almost pathognomonic ground-glass "dazzle" appearance. Cystine crystals may also be readily observed in bone marrow aspirates (especially with phase microscopy) and in the thyroid. Thyroxine or thyroid-stimulating hormone levels should be obtained in order to check for hypothyroidism.

Cysteamine is under investigation for the treatment of cystinosis. Therapy with large doses of vitamin C yielded disappointing results. At present, the management of cystinosis is essentially that of chronic renal failure, with particular attention being paid to renal osteodystrophy. Renal homotransplantation shows significant promise in the palliation of cystinosis.

Girardin EP et al: Treatment of cystinosis with cysteamine. *J Pediatr* 1979;**94:**838.

Schneider JA et al: Cystinosis: A review. *Metabolism* 1977;**26:**817.

Schneider JA et al: Prenatal diagnosis of cystinosis. *N Engl J Med* 1974;**290:**878.

Segal S: Cystinosis and its treatment. *N Engl J Med* 1979;**300:**789.

PHOSPHATE-LOSING RENAL TUBULAR SYNDROMES & OTHER FORMS OF RICKETS

Recent investigation of the metabolic products of vitamin D_3 has done much to clarify the causes of various forms of rickets. Those forms due primarily to a lack of available calcium are described in Chapter 4. They include idiopathic hypercalciuria, in which there is low calcium intake or excessive urinary calcium loss; lack of vitamin D_3 because of low dietary intake or from steatorrhea; and vitamin D dependency and azotemic rickets. In vitamin D_3 dependency, there is an inborn or acquired inability to synthesize 1,25-dihydroxycholecalciferol (the calcium transport stimulating factor, type I), or there may be end-organ insensitivity to this factor (type II). Treatment consists of giving supplementary calcium or vitamin D in appropriate doses.

Diseases associated with decreased availability of phosphorus also cause rickets. Excessive use of aluminum hydroxide gels may be responsible, but this is very rare. Most commonly, the defect is an inherited or acquired one in which a defect of phosphorus reabsorption is variably associated with other transport defects (eg, defects in transporting amino acids, glucose, bicarbonate, hydrogen ion, or potassium). Certain generalized metabolic diseases—notably Wilson's disease, galactosemia, fructose intolerance, and cystinosis—may cause similar tubular damage. Treatment of the primary type is to give extra phosphorus. Treatment of the acquired forms is that of the basic disease.

Familial hypophosphatemic vitamin D-resistant rickets is an example of a tubular nephropathy in which only phosphorus transport is affected. The majority of cases present during the second year of life, but some have been reported to occur in the first 6 months.

Clinical features vary. Changes may be only biochemical, with a strikingly low serum phosphorus level and an elevated alkaline phosphatase level. Muscular hypotonia may be severe; growth failure, bowing of the legs, and enlargement of the wrists, knees, and costochondral junctions are often associated with spinal deformities. Craniosynostosis has been described in infants with this disease. Pathologic fractures may be seen on x-ray, as well as certain unique findings consisting of an irregular mosaic formation of the haversian system and trabecular "halos" of low-density bone.

In most cases, the serum phosphorus level is less than 2 mg/dL. The urinary calcium level is low, and the serum calcium level may be normal or slightly low. Serum levels of 1,25-dihydroxycholecalciferol are low, probably because high levels of phosphate in the tubule cell shut off the 1α-hydroxylase activity. Aminoaciduria is rare.

Treatment consists of giving 1–3 g of phosphorus daily either as a buffered monosodium and disodium hydrogen phosphate solution at pH 7.4 or as Fleet's Phospho-Soda. Magnesium oxide, 10–15 mg/kg/d by mouth, may also be of value. Supplementary calcitriol (Rocaltrol), up to 40 ng/kg/d, should be given if the serum calcium levels remain below normal.

Normal growth is never achieved unless every effort is made to keep the serum phosphorus level over 3 mg/dL both day and night.

Fraser D et al: Pathogenesis of hereditary vitamin D dependent rickets. *N Engl J Med* 1973;**289:**817.

Haussler MR, McCain TA: Basic and clinical concepts related to vitamin D metabolism and action. *N Engl J Med* 1977;**297:**974.

Reddy V et al: Magnesium-dependent vitamin-D-resistant rickets. *Lancet* 1974;**1:**963.

OCULOCEREBRORENAL SYNDROME (Lowe's Syndrome)

Lowe's syndrome has been described in males only and is therefore thought to be transmitted as an X-linked recessive gene leading to anomalies involving the eyes, brain, and kidneys. The physical stigmas and the degree of mental retardation are variable. In addition to congenital cataracts and buphthalmos, the typical facies includes prominent epicanthal folds, frontal prominence, and a tendency to scaphocephaly. Muscle hypotonia is a prominent finding. The incidence of hypophosphatemic rickets is variable; it is characterized by low serum phosphorus levels, low to normal serum calcium levels, and elevated serum alkaline phosphatase levels. Some degree of renal tubular acidosis is usually present, characterized by hyperchloremic acidosis, an alkaline urine, and a diminution in both titratable acidity and urinary ammonia in response to an ammonium chloride challenge. The aminoaciduria is usually generalized. Mothers of affected males have punctate lens opacities.

Alkaline therapy should be given to those presenting with tubular acidosis. Vitamin D requirements range from 10,000 to 20,000 IU daily.

Matin MA, Sylvester PE: Clinicopathological studies of the oculocerebrorenal syndrome of Lowe, Terrey and MacLachlen. *J Ment Defic Res* 1980;**24:**1.

DISORDERS OF THE COLLECTING DUCTS & RENAL PELVES

NEPHROGENIC DIABETES INSIPIDUS

In the normal kidney, the interstitial fluid of the papilla is hyperosmolar to the fluid in the collecting duct. The luminal cells have a specific receptor for antidiuretic hormone (ADH), which, acting via cAMP, permits water to move across the cell membrane in response to the osmotic gradient. In the common X-linked recessive form (type I) of nephrogenic diabetes insipidus, there is a disorder of the ADH:adenylate cyclase receptor, and urinary adenylate cyclase is not increased after administration of vasopressin. In the type II variety, cAMP is formed by ADH action but has no effect on water transport. There are probably many variants of this complex mechanism, which is also influenced by prostaglandin E_1 and by its inhibitor, indomethacin.

The symptoms are limited to polyuria, polydipsia, and failure to thrive. In some children, particularly if the solute intake is unrestricted, some acclimatization to an elevated serum osmolality may develop. However, these children are particularly liable to episodes of dehydration, fever, vomiting, and convulsions.

Clinically, the diagnosis can be made on the basis of a history of polydipsia and polyuria that are not sensitive to the administration of vasopressin, desmopressin acetate (DDAVP), or lypressin. It is wise to confirm this in all cases by performing a vasopressin test. Maximal water restriction, overnight if possible, does not increase the tubular reabsorption of water (T^cH_2O) to above 3 mL/min/m^2. If 5% dextrose is administered at the rate of 275 mL/m^2/h for 2 hours and vasopressin is given after 1 hour as an intravenous bolus of 0.005 unit/kg, the urine osmolality will not change during the period of infusion. The intravenous infusion of 2.5% saline at the rate of 0.25 mL/kg/min for not more than 45 minutes will result in only a small rise in urine osmolality in comparison to control infusion periods of normal saline. Theoretically, in psychogenic diabetes insipidus, vasopressin and hypertonic saline increase urine osmolality, but constant water loading seems to diminish renal response to ADH. Urine concentrating ability is impaired in a number of conditions—sickle cell anemia, pyelonephritis, potassium depletion, hypercalcemia, cystinosis and other renal tubular disorders, and obstructive uropathy—and as a result of nephrotoxic drugs.

In infants, it is usually best to allow water as demanded and to restrict salt. Serum sodium levels should be evaluated at intervals to ensure against hyperosmolality from inadvertent water restriction. In later childhood, sodium intake should continue to be restricted to 2–2.5 meq/kg/24 h. Studies have suggested that levels of C_{H_2O} are significantly decreased by use of chlorothiazide, 60 mg/m^2/24 h orally; ethacrynic acid (Edecrin), 120 mg/m^2/24 h orally; and indomethacin, 3 mg/kg/24 h. When ethacrynic acid is given, potassium chloride, 2–3 meq/kg/24 h orally, should also be given to prevent alkalosis due to excessive potassium loss.

Bell NH et al: Demonstration of a defect in the formation of 3′,5′-monophosphate in vasopressin-resistant diabetes insipidus. *Pediatr Res* 1974;**8:**223.

Schreiner RL et al: Congenital nephrogenic diabetes insipidus in a baby girl. *Arch Dis Child* 1978;**53:**906.

Usberti M et al: Renal prostaglandin E_2 in nephrogenic diabetes insipidus: Effects of inhibition of prostaglandin synthesis by indomethacin. *J Pediatr* 1980;**97:**476.

Verhoeven GFM, Wilson JD: The syndromes of primary hormone resistance. *Metabolism* 1979;**28:**253.

NEPHROLITHIASIS

Renal calculi in children may occur as a consequence of certain inborn errors of metabolism, eg, cystine in cystinosis, glycine in hyperglycinuria, urates in Lesch-Nyhan syndrome, and oxalates in oxalosis. Stones may occur secondary to hypercalciuria in distal tubular acidosis, and large stones are quite often seen in children with spina bifida who have paralyzed lower limbs. Treatment is limited to that of the primary condition, if possible. Surgical removal of stones should be considered only for obstruction, intractable severe pain, and chronic infection.

Cystinuria

Cystinuria, like Hartnup disease and a number of other disorders, is primarily an abnormality of amino acid transport across both the enteric and proximal renal tubular epithelium. There appear to be at least 3 biochemical types. In the first type, the bowel transport of basic amino acids and cystine is impaired, but transport of cysteine is not impaired. In the renal tubule, basic amino acids are again rejected by the tubule, but cystine absorption into kidney slices in vitro seems to be normal. The reasons for the cystinuria are, therefore, still obscure. Heterozygotes have no aminoaciduria. The second type is similar to the first, except that the heterozygotes excrete excess cystine and lysine in the urine, and cystine transport in the bowel is normal. In the third type, only the nephron is involved. The incidence of all types among institutionalized mentally retarded children is surprisingly high—about 0.2%.

The only clinical manifestations relate to stone formation. These include ureteral colic, dysuria, hematuria, proteinuria, and secondary urinary tract infection. The urinary excretion of cystine, lysine, arginine, and ornithine is increased.

The most reliable way to prevent stone formation is to maintain a constantly high free-water clearance. This involves a water intake of about 400 mL/m^2 every 4 hours night and day. If this is not effective, treatment with sodium bicarbonate, 6 g/m^2/d, should also be given. Such measures will certainly prevent increases in stone formation and very often lead to dissolution.

Operative removal of the stone may occasionally be required. Penicillamine (Cuprimine) in doses of 1000–1500 mg/m^2/d will also decrease cystine excretion and bring about partial or complete dissolution of stones. It is expensive, however, and may give rise to rashes that are just as objectionable as the problem of maintaining a high water intake.

Segal S: Disorders of renal amino acid transport. *N Engl J Med* 1976;**294:**1044.

Primary Hyperoxaluria

Oxalate production in humans is derived from the oxidative deamination of glycine to glyoxalate (about 40%), from the serine-glycolate pathway (about 50%), and from ascorbic acid. At least 2 enzymatic blocks have been described. Type 1 is a 2-oxo-glutarate; glyoxalate carboligase deficiency that inhibits the diversion of glyoxalate to γ-hydroxy-α-ketoglutarate. Type 2 is glyoxalate reductase deficiency.

Excess oxalate combines with calcium to form insoluble deposits in the kidneys, lungs, and other tissues. The onset is during childhood. The joints are occasionally involved, but the main impact is on the kidneys, where progressive oxalate deposition leads to fibrosis and eventual renal failure.

Pyridoxine supplementation and a low-oxalate diet have been tried as therapy, but the overall prognosis is poor, and most patients succumb to uremia by early adulthood. Renal transplantation is not very successful. Calcium carbimide, 1 mg/kg/24 h, has been tried as an inhibitor of the serine-glycolate pathway of oxalate production and was shown to substantially diminish oxalate excretion in type 1 oxalosis. The use of methylene blue has also been reported.

Hyperoxaluria may also occur secondary to ileal disease or after ileal resection.

Morgan JM et al: Successful renal transplantation in hyperoxaluria. *Arch Surg* 1974;**109:**430.

Vallman HB et al: Hyperoxaluria after resection of ileum in childhood. *Arch Dis Child* 1974;**49:**171.

Watts RWE: Oxaluria. *J R Coll Physicians Lond* 1973;**7:**161.

URINARY TRACT INFECTION

Infections of the urinary tract can range from asymptomatic bacteriuria to severe symptomatic pyelonephritis. As in the case of many pediatric diseases, signs and symptoms are less specific in younger children. Urinary tract infection is a common cause of fever in childhood, and even asymptomatic infections can result in significant renal damage, especially in infants. The clinician may be misled by erroneously interpreted clinical signs and laboratory data, resulting in either overdiagnosis (antibiotic side effects, cost, unnecessary procedures) or underdiagnosis (continued symptoms, progressive renal damage). Once the diagnosis of urinary tract infection is confirmed, an organized program of periodic follow-up should be established so that recurrences will be recognized. Most urinary tract infections can be managed by the primary physician without the need for specialized urologic procedures or surgery.

Predisposing Factors

A. Age and Sex: Approximately 1% of newborns develop urinary tract infection, sometimes associated with bacteremia. Males at this age are as likely to develop infection as females. After the newborn period, urinary tract infection is uncommon in males until later adult life. In boys with documented urinary tract infection, underlying urinary tract abnormalities should always be suspected.

The relatively high incidence of urinary tract infection in infants and preschool girls is due to excessive perineal fecal contamination, the short urethra, and infrequent and inadequate voiding. Infection in sexually active girls may be due to bacterial contamination of the bladder secondary to urethral trauma during intercourse.

B. Organisms: Although viruses are often excreted in urine, symptomatic urinary tract disease of viral origin (eg, hemorrhagic cystitis) is rare. Bacteria are by far the most common cause of urinary tract infection, the predominant organisms being *Escherichia coli, Klebsiella,* enteric streptococci, and *Staphylococcus epidermidis*—all common members of the normal rectal and perineal bacterial flora.

C. Route of Infection: Access of bacteria to the normally sterile bladder and kidneys appears to be retrourethral and may be enhanced by poor perineal hygiene, the short female urethra, pinworms, urethral instrumentation, or intercourse. In children with recurrent urinary tract infection, the bladder epithelial cells may show increased affinity for bacterial adherence.

Once bacteria are in the bladder, the urine serves as an excellent culture medium, but infection is usually avoided by the washout effect of voiding. Foreign bodies, urinary tract obstructions or anomalies, and infrequent or inadequate voiding may allow simple transient bacterial contamination of the bladder to progress to true persistent urinary tract infection. Vesicoureteral reflux, often seen in young children with urinary tract infection, can allow bacteria to gain access to the kidneys, with resulting pyelonephritis and renal damage.

Clinical Findings

A. Symptoms and Signs: Newborns may present with fever, hypothermia, poor feeding, jaundice, failure to thrive, or sepsis. Infants may have fever of unknown origin, poor feeding, failure to thrive, strong-smelling urine, and irritability. Preschool children may have abdominal pain, vomiting, strong-smelling urine, fever, enuresis, increased frequency of urination, dysuria, or urgency. School-age children may develop the "classic" signs of urinary tract infection, including enuresis, increased frequency of urination, dysuria, urgency, fever, and costovertebral angle tenderness (flank pain). Occasionally, children with bacterial urinary tract infection will present with hemorrhagic cystitis.

All age groups may suffer from asymptomatic infection that nonetheless can cause renal damage, predominantly in infants and young children, who have a greater propensity to develop vesicoureteral reflux. Those children who have urinary tract infection associated with fever, flank pain, severe abdominal pain, polymorphonuclear leukocytosis, an increased sedimentation rate, or increased C-reactive protein usually prove to have pyelonephritis. Asymptomatic children or those with "cystitis" symptoms (increased frequency of urination, burning on urination, dysuria, strong-smelling urine, recurrence of enuresis) may have infection of the lower tract that may asymptomatically involve the upper tract as well. It should be carefully noted that children with "classic" signs and symptoms of severe cystitis often do not have urinary tract infection but urethral irritation due to other causes (bubble bath, feminine hygiene sprays, vaginitis, pinworms, masturbation).

B. Laboratory Tests:

1. Obtaining a proper specimen—Bag urine specimens are frequently (30–60%) contaminated and not adequate for the definitive diagnosis of urinary tract infection. Clean-catch midstream specimens give a more accurate estimate of the bacteriologic state of the bladder urine but give false-positive results 10–20% of the time (again due to contamination) and may (if they are not first morning samples or if the patient has had a recent high fluid intake) yield colony counts under 10^5 colony-forming units per milliliter. Catheter-obtained urine (use a No. 5 feeding tube) is excellent for diagnosis as long as the first few milliliters are excluded from collection. The risk of introducing infection in most patients is very low. Suprapubic needle aspiration of urine is also an excellent way to avoid specimen contamination and confirm urinary tract infection, especially in patients with high fluid intake who may have colony counts under 10^5/mL.

2. Pyuria—The microscopic finding of more than 5 white blood cells per high-power field in a urine spun sediment is termed pyuria. Approximately 50% of patients with urinary tract infection (including pyelonephritis) *do not* have pyuria, and there are many causes of increased numbers of white cells in the urine (vaginal contamination, fever, appendicitis, viral illness) other than urinary tract infection. Thus, the presence of pyuria is a very poor basis for a diagnosis of urinary tract infection.

3. Microscopic bacteriuria—Microscopic observation of a urine spun sediment on high dry (40 ×) power does allow an accurate estimation of the presence of bacteria. A count of more than 100 bacteria per high-power field correlates well with actual colony counts exceeding 10^5/mL.

4. Urine cultures—The urine culture is the mainstay of urinary tract infection diagnosis. It can be performed in the office by the streak plate method or by commercial methods using agar-embedded dipslides. Colony counts exceeding 10^5/mL have in the past been considered indicative of true infection but are often associated with specimen (bag, clean-catch midstream) contamination; cases of infection with lower colony counts due to diuresis may be missed.

5. Nonculture detection of urinary tract infection—Two recently evaluated tests detect the chemical alterations on urine glucose and nitrite that are due to the modifying effects of bacteria in the overnight bladder urine. These methods (nitrite test, glucose test) only work on first morning overnight urine specimens but have the advantage that they give very few false-positive results, since contaminating organisms introduced during the collection process do not have time to chemically modify the urine prior to testing.

6. Proper diagnosis of urinary tract infection—In patients with serious symptoms of urinary tract infection, urine should be collected by catheterization or suprapubic needle aspiration to exclude contaminants that may be introduced in the clean-catch or bag collection process. If bacteria are seen on the spun sediment of a catheterized or suprapubically drawn specimen or if the patient grows more than 10^3 colony-forming units of any organism per milliliter (including *S epidermidis* or mixed organisms), the patient has a urinary tract infection.

If the patient is not severely symptomatic (or is being seen for follow-up of previous urinary tract infection), it is reasonable to postpone the visit until the next morning so that the patient can bring in a refrigerated first morning clean-catch specimen. This avoids the problem of falsely low colony counts and also allows testing by the nitrite test, which rarely gives false-positive results. If positive, a urine culture should be obtained and therapy initiated. If the nitrite test cannot be done or is negative, a spun sediment should be examined. If more than 100 bacteria are seen, a second clean-catch midstream specimen (or catheterized specimen) should be collected (to avoid the false-positive results of contaminated urine specimens) and examined. A count of more than 100 bacteria per high-power field on both specimens is diagnostic of urinary tract infection.

Treatment

A. Initial Treatment: Once urinary tract infection is confirmed, initial therapy should be based on the patient's history of antibiotic use, the location of the infection, and the cost of alternative antibiotics. Many drugs are available for treating urinary tract infection, but all of them will occasionally be ineffective because of inherent resistance of the organism.

For uncomplicated infection, a single oral antibiotic (eg, ampicillin, a sulfonamide, nitrofurantoin) that the patient has not used recently can be administered for 10 days. Single-dose therapy may also work, but its effectiveness must be confirmed by culture. For the patient with recurrent infection or suspected pyelonephritis (fever, vomiting, flank pain) or whose condition is unresponsive, antibiotic susceptibilities should be determined. A patient with suspected pyelonephritis need not always be admitted to the hospital but should be treated with 2 antibiotics (ampicillin, a sulfonamide, or a cephalosporin plus gentamicin or kanamycin). This regimen ensures adequate coverage until the patient improves and the results of antibiotic sensitivity tests are available, allowing selection of a single effective oral antibiotic. Therapy must be appropriately modified in patients with acute or chronic renal failure.

Most urinary tract infections can be successfully treated with inexpensive drugs given orally. Success requires confirmation by negative culture 2 days after the start of therapy if symptoms persist and 3–5 days after discontinuance of therapy in all cases.

B. Treatment of Refractory Infection: Persistent bacteriuria indicates superinfection with a different organism or with the same organism due to obstruction, the presence of a foreign body, or conversion of the organism to a variant form.

Intravenous urography should be considered with proved infection in newborns, boys, girls with symptoms of pyelonephritis, and girls with second urinary tract infections. Voiding cystourethrograms should be performed as above on boys and younger girls, but it is important to note that many young children have low-grade vesicoureteral reflux that does not require urologic intervention.

Obvious structural or obstructive anomalies necessitate referral to a urologist experienced in dealing with children. Conditions frequently diagnosed and treated as abnormalities (bladder outlet obstruction, meatal stenosis, distal urethral stenosis, duplication of the ureters) are also seen in otherwise normal children who do not require therapy. Repeated urethral dilation and cystoscopy are rarely if ever of value. Vesicoureteral reflux is common in younger children. If not severe, it will not result in renal damage and will disappear in time if repeated infections can be prevented. The presence of mild reflux does not ordinarily necessitate urologic consultation.

In patients without structural or functional urinary tract abnormalities, possible causes of recurrent infection are infrequent or incomplete voiding, poor perineal hygiene, pinworms, constipation, and bubble bath use. If attempts to deal with these problems are unsuccessful, single-dose prophylaxis at bedtime with agents such as nitrofurantoin or trimethoprim-sulfamethoxazole may be useful in combination with a program of frequent voiding.

C. Follow-Up of Patients With Urinary Tract Infection: All patients with urinary tract infection should be checked for recurrence every 1–2 months until they have remained free of infection for 1 year. Use of the nitrite test for home testing of first morning concentrated urine specimens may significantly reduce the cost of follow-up without compromising accuracy.

Prognosis

As long as urinary tract infections can be confined to the lower urinary tract (bladder and below), the prognosis is excellent. Once an infectious process has entered the kidney, the prognosis becomes more guarded. Hence, every diagnostic and therapeutic effort should be made to prevent recurrences.

American Academy of Pediatrics Section on Urology: Screening school children for urologic disease. *Pediatrics* 1977;**60:**239.

Kunin CM: *Detection, Prevention and Management of Urinary Tract Infections,* 3rd ed. Lea & Febiger, 1979.

Levitt SB: Medical versus surgical treatment of primary vesicoureteral reflux. *Pediatrics* 1981;**67:**392.

Stephens FD: Urologic aspects of recurrent urinary tract infection in children. *J Pediatr* 1972;**80:**725.

Todd JK: Diagnosis of urinary tract infections. *Pediatr Infect Dis* 1982;**1:**126.

Todd JK: Pediatrics: Urinary tract infections in children and adolescents. *Postgrad Med* (Nov) 1976;**60:**225.

ACUTE HEMORRHAGIC CYSTITIS

Acute hemorrhagic cystitis affects children of any race, age, or sex. It is usually of sudden onset and is characterized by gross total or terminal hematuria, dysuria, frequency, and urgency. It is sometimes associated with suprapubic pain, fever, and enuresis. Examination of urine usually shows only red cells and microscopic pyuria.

In 20–25% of cases, a viral cause can be found; the most common offender thus far identified has been adenovirus type 11. As adenovirus carriage is common, it is essential to document rises in viral neutralizing antibody titers as well as to recover the virus if it is desired to establish a viral cause.

A small proportion of cases appear to be caused by common bacterial pathogens. These should be identified and treated by means of systemic antibiotics.

Most cases are associated with sterile urine and remain idiopathic. Sterile hemorrhagic cystitis is not uncommon in patients receiving cyclophosphamide. Diagnostic studies should exclude other causes of hematuria.

Cases of viral and idiopathic acute hemorrhagic cystitis may be expected to resolve spontaneously in 10–14 days.

Mufson MA et al: Adenovirus infection in acute hemorrhagic cystitis. *Am J Dis Child* 1971;**121:**281.

SELECTED REFERENCES

Edelman CM (editor): *Pediatric Kidney Disease.* Vols 1 and 2. Little, Brown, 1978.

Fine RN, Gruskin A: *End Stage Renal Disease.* Saunders, 1984.

Heptinstall RH: *Pathology of the Kidney,* 3rd ed. Little, Brown, 1983.

Lieberman E (editor): *Clinical Pediatric Nephrology.* Lippincott, 1976.

Rubin MI, Barratt TM (editors): *Pediatric Nephrology.* Williams & Wilkins, 1975.

Strauss J (editor): *Pediatric Nephrology.* Vol 6. Stratton, 1981.

West CD, McAdams AJ: The chronic glomerulonephritides of childhood. (2 parts.) *J Pediatr* 1978;**93:**1, 167.

22 Orthopedics

Robert E. Eilert, MD

Orthopedics is the medical discipline that deals with disorders of neuromuscular and skeletal systems. Patients with orthopedic problems usually present with pain, loss of function, or deformity. Their symptoms must be considered not only in terms of the bones and joints but also in a more general sense relating to the anatomy, particularly of the extremities, and the blood vessels, skin, nerves, tendons, and muscles. As is true of most medical and surgical disorders, the diagnosis of orthopedic disorders can often be made on the basis of a carefully taken history. However, the physical examination is the most important feature of orthopedic diagnosis and depends upon an intimate knowledge of human anatomy.

DISTURBANCES OF PRENATAL ORIGIN

CONGENITAL AMPUTATIONS

Congenital amputations may be due to teratogens (eg, drugs or viruses), amniotic bands, or metabolic diseases (eg, diabetes in the mother) or, in rare cases, may be hereditary defects. Most are spontaneous and not genetically determined. The history of the pregnancy must be carefully reviewed in a search for possible teratogenic factors. According to the currently accepted international classification, amputations are either terminal or longitudinal. In terminal amputation, all parts are missing distal to the level of involvement—eg, absence of the forearm, wrist, and hand in the case of a terminal below-the-elbow amputation. A longitudinal amputation consists of partial absence of structures in the extremity along one side or the other. In radial clubhand, the entire radius is absent, but the thumb may be either hypoplastic or completely absent—ie, the effect on structures distal to the amputation may vary. Complex tissue defects are nearly always associated with longitudinal amputations in that the associated nerves and muscles are usually not completely represented when a bone is absent. Bones within the axial skeleton likewise may be absent. Congenital absence of the sacrum is often associated with diabetes in the mother.

Terminal amputations are treated by means of a prosthesis, eg, to compensate for shortness of one leg. With longitudinal deficiencies, constructive surgery may be feasible with the objective of reducing deformity and stabilizing joints. In certain types of severe anomalies, operative treatment is indicated to remove a portion of the malformed foot so that a prosthesis can be fitted early. This applies to such anomalies as congenital absence of the fibula, which is the lower extremity bone most commonly congenitally absent. Fortunately, there is rarely a problem with tenting of the skin by relative overgrowth of bone within the stump in congenital amputations.

Lower extremity prostheses are best fitted at about the time of normal walking (12–15 months of age). Lower extremity prostheses are consistently well accepted, as they are necessary for balancing and walking. Upper extremity prostheses are not as well accepted. Fitting the child with a dummy type prosthesis as early as 6 months of age has the advantage of instilling an accustomed pattern of proper length and bimanual manipulation. Children fitted later than age 2 years nearly always reject upper extremity prostheses.

Children quickly learn how to function with their prostheses and can lead active lives, participating in sports with peers.

Kruger LM: Recent advances in surgery of lower limb deficiencies. *Clin Orthop* 1980;**148:**97.

Shaperman J, Sumida CT: Recent advances in research in prosthetics for children. *Clin Orthop* 1980;**148:**26.

Swanson AB: A classification for congenital limb malformations. *J Hand Surg* 1976;**1:**8.

DEFORMITIES OF THE EXTREMITIES

1. METATARSUS VARUS

Metatarsus varus is characterized by adduction of the forefoot on the hindfoot, with the heel in normal position or slight valgus. The longitudinal arch is often creased vertically when the deformity is more rigid. The lateral border of the foot demonstrates sharp angulation at the level of the base of the fifth metatarsal, and this bone will be especially prominent. The deformity varies from flexible to rigid. Most flexible deformities are secondary to intrauterine posture and usually resolve spontaneously.

If the deformity is rigid and cannot be manipulated past the midline, it is worthwhile to use a plaster cast changed at weekly intervals to correct the deformity.

"Corrective" shoes do not live up to their name. Shoes are supportive, but shoe wedges have not been effective in correcting this type of deformity and are of more use for placating the parent than for any true therapeutic value. A few minutes spent explaining what can be achieved with shoes may avoid an unnecessary expense for the family. The prognosis for this common deformity of the foot is excellent, and few long-term problems are reported.

Bleck EE: Metatarsus adductus: Classification and relationship to outcomes of treatment. *J Pediatr Orthop* 1983;**3**:2.

Rushforth GF: The natural history of the hooked forefoot. *J Bone Joint Surg* [*Br*] 1978;**60**:530.

2. CLUBFOOT (Talipes Equinovarus)

When foot deformity consists of the following 3 elements, the diagnosis of classic talipes equinovarus, or clubfoot, is made: (1) equinus or plantar flexion of the foot at the ankle joint, (2) varus or inversion deformity of the heel, and (3) forefoot varus. The incidence of talipes equinovarus is approximately 1:1000 live births. Any infant with a clubfoot should be examined carefully for associated anomalies, especially of the spine. Clubfoot tends to follow a hereditary pattern in some families or may be part of a generalized neuromuscular syndrome such as arthrogryposis or myelodysplasia.

Treatment consists of massage and manipulation of the foot to stretch the contracted tissues on the medial and posterior aspects, followed by splinting to hold the correction. When this is instituted in the nursery shortly after birth, correction is achieved much more rapidly. When treatment is delayed, the foot tends to become more rigid within a matter of days. Treatment in the nursery by strapping and splinting is often effective. As the child gets older, casting following manipulation and stretching is necessary. The casts are applied sequentially, correcting first the forefoot adduction, then the inversion of the heel, and finally the equinus of the ankle. Treatment by means of casting requires patience and experience; if it is not done properly in sequence, iatrogenic deformities of the foot may result, such as rocker-bottom foot.

After full correction is obtained, a night brace is often prescribed for long-term maintenance of correction.

About half of children with clubfoot eventually need an operative procedure to lengthen the tightened structures about the foot.

A supple foot that is easily corrected by strapping and casting has a more favorable prognosis. If the foot is rigid and requires prolonged treatment to obtain correction, perhaps combined with surgery, the prognosis must be guarded.

Kite JH: Conservative treatment of the resistant recurrent clubfoot. *Clin Orthop* 1970;**70**:93.

Main BJ, Crider RJ: An analysis of residual deformity in clubfeet submitted to early operation. *J Bone Joint Surg* [*Br*] 1978;**60**:536.

3. CONGENITAL DYSPLASIA OF THE HIP JOINT (Congenital Dislocation of the Hip)

In a child with congenital dysplasia of the hip, the femoral head and the acetabulum may be in partial contact at birth. This condition is termed subluxation of the hip. A more severe defect is complete loss of contact between the femoral head and acetabulum, in which case there is frank dislocation of the hip, with the femoral head nearly always displaced laterally and superiorly due to muscle pull. At birth, there is lack of the development of both the acetabulum and the femur in cases of congenital hip dysplasia. The dysplasia becomes progressive with growth unless the dislocation is corrected. If the dislocation is corrected in the first few days or weeks of life, the dysplasia is completely reversible and a normal hip will develop. As the child becomes older and the dislocation or subluxation persists, the deformity will worsen to the point where it will not be completely reversible, especially after the walking age. For this reason, it is important to diagnose the deformity in the nursery or, at the latest, the 6-week checkup.

Clinical Findings

The diagnosis of congenital hip dislocation in the newborn depends upon demonstrating instability of the joint by placing the infant on its back and obtaining complete relaxation by feeding with a bottle if necessary. The examiner's long finger is then placed over the greater trochanter and the thumb over the inner side of the thigh. Both hips are flexed 90 degrees and then slowly abducted from the midline. With gentle pressure, an attempt is made to lift the greater trochanter forward. A feeling of slipping as the head goes into the acetabulum is a sign of instability (as first described by Ortolani). In other infants, the joint is more stable, and the deformity must be provoked by applying slight pressure with the thumb on the medial side of the thigh as the thigh is adducted, thus slipping the hip posteriorly and eliciting a jerk as the hip dislocates. This sign was first described by Barlow. The signs of instability are the most reliable criteria for diagnosing congenital dislocation of the hip in the newborn. X-rays of the pelvis are notoriously unreliable until about 6 weeks of age. Asymmetric skin folds are present in about 40% of newborns and therefore are not particularly helpful.

After the first month of life, the signs of instability as demonstrated by Ortolani's test or Barlow's test become less evident. Contractures begin to develop about the hip joint, causing limitation of abduction. Normally, the hip should abduct fully to 90 degrees on either side during the first few months of life. It is important that the pelvis be held level to detect asymmetry of abduction. When the hips and knees are flexed, the knees are at unequal heights, with the dislocated side lower (Allis's sign). After the first few weeks of life, x-ray examination becomes more valuable, with lateral displacement of the femoral head being the most reliable sign. In mild cases, the only abnormality may be increased steepness of acetabular alignment, so that the acetabular angle is greater than 35 degrees.

If congenital dislocation of the hip has not been diagnosed during the first year of life and the child begins to walk, there will be a painless limp and a lurch to the affected side, as first described by Trendelenburg. When the child stands on the affected leg, there is a dip of the pelvis on the opposite side owing to weakness of the gluteus medius muscle. This has been termed Trendelenburg's sign and accounts for the unusual swaying gait. In children with bilateral dislocations, the loss of abduction is almost symmetric and may be deceiving. Abduction, however, is never complete, and x-ray of the pelvis is indicated in children with incomplete abduction in the first few months of life. As a child with bilateral dislocation of the hips begins to walk, the gait is waddling. The perineum is widened as a result of lateral displacement of the hips, and there is flexion contracture as a result of posterior displacement of the hips. This flexion contracture contributes to marked lordosis, and the greater trochanters are easily palpable in their elevated position. Treatment is still possible in the first 2 years of life, but the results are not nearly as effective as in children treated in the nursery.

Treatment

Dislocation or dysplasia diagnosed in the first few weeks or months of life can easily be treated by splinting, with the hip maintained in flexion and abduction. Full abduction is contraindicated, as this often leads to avascular necrosis of the femoral head. The use of double or triple diapers is never indicated for medical reasons, since diapers are not adequate to obtain proper positioning of the hip. In cases of joint laxity without true dislocation, improvement will be spontaneous and diapers are excessive treatment.

Various splints to maintain flexion and abduction of the hip, such as the ones designed by Pavlik, Ilfeld, or von Rosen, are available. Treatment of children requiring splints is best supervised by an orthopedic surgeon with a special interest in the problem.

In the first 4 months of life, reduction can be obtained by simply flexing and abducting the hip; no other manipulation is usually necessary. If force is used to reduce the hip, the excessive pressure may cause avascular necrosis. In such cases, preoperative traction for 2–3 weeks is important to relax soft tissues about the hip. Following traction in which the femur is brought down opposite the acetabulum, reduction can be easily achieved without force under general anesthesia. It is then necessary to place the child in a plaster cast, which is used for approximately 6 months. The position in the cast should be carefully adjusted in order to avoid stretching of the delicate blood supply to the femoral head. The hip is flexed slightly more than 90 degrees and abducted only 45–60 degrees. Internal rotation is avoided, since this tends to "wring out" the blood vessels in the capsule of the joint. If the reduction is not stable within a reasonable range following closed reduction, open reduction may be necessary combined with plication of the lax capsule in order to maintain reduction.

If reduction is done at an older age, operations to correct the deformities of the acetabulum and femur may be necessary during growth.

Coleman SS: *Congenital Dysplasia and Dislocation of the Hip.* Mosby, 1978.

MacKenzie IG, Wilson JG: Problems encountered in the early diagnosis and management of congenital dislocation of the hip. *J Bone Joint Surg* [*Br*] 1981;**63:**38.

Weiner DS et al: Congenital dislocation of the hip: The relationship of premanipulation, traction and age to avascular necrosis of the femoral head. *J Bone Joint Surg* [*Am*] 1977;**59:**306.

4. TORTICOLLIS

Wryneck deformities in infancy may be due either to injury to the sternocleidomastoid muscle during delivery or to disease affecting the cervical spine. In the case of muscular deformity, the chin is rotated to the side opposite to the affected sternocleidomastoid muscle contracture, and the head is tilted toward the side of the contracture. A mass felt in the midportion of the sternocleidomastoid muscle does not represent a true tumor but fibrous transformation within the muscle.

In mild cases, passive stretching is usually effective. If the deformity has not been corrected by passive stretching within the first year of life, surgical division of the muscle will correct it. It is not necessary to excise the "tumor" of the sternocleidomastoid muscle, since this tends to resolve spontaneously. If the deformity is left untreated, an unsightly facial asymmetry will result.

Torticollis is occasionally associated with congenital deformities of the cervical spine, and x-rays of the spine are indicated in all cases.

Acute torticollis may follow upper respiratory infection or mild trauma in children. Rotatory subluxation of the upper cervical spine should be sought by appropriate x-ray views. Traction or a cervical collar usually results in resolution of the symptoms within 1 or 2 days.

Canale ST, Griffin DW, Hubbard CN: Congenital muscular torticollis: Long-term follow-up. *J Bone Joint Surg [Am]* 1982;**64:**810.

Dawson EG, Smith L: Atlantoaxial subluxation in children due to vertebral anomalies. *J Bone Joint Surg [Am]* 1979; **61:**582.

GENERALIZED AFFECTIONS OF SKELETON OR MESODERMAL TISSUES

1. ARTHROGRYPOSIS MULTIPLEX CONGENITA (Amyoplasia Congenita)

Arthrogryposis multiplex congenita consists of incomplete fibrous ankylosis (usually symmetric) of many or all of the joints of the body. There may be contractures either in flexion or extension. Upper extremity deformities usually consist of adduction of the shoulders, extension of the elbows, flexion of the wrists, and stiff, straight fingers with poor muscle control of the thumbs. In the lower extremities, common deformities are dislocation of the hips, extension of the knees, and severe clubfoot. The joints are fusiform and the joint capsules decreased in volume, producing contractures. Various investigations have attributed the basic defect to an abnormality of muscle or of the lower motor neuron. Muscular development is poor, and muscles may be represented only by fibrous bands. The joint deformities appear to be secondary to a lack of active motion during intrauterine development.

Passive mobilization of joints should be done early. Because of poor muscle control, however, joint mobility cannot be maintained by active motion. Prolonged casting for correction of deformities is contraindicated in these children, as further stiffness is often produced. Use of removable splints combined with vigorous therapy is the most effective conservative treatment. Surgical release of the affected joints is often necessary. The clubfoot associated with arthrogryposis is very stiff and nearly always requires an operation. Surgery about the knees, including capsulotomy, osteotomy, and tendon lengthening, is used to correct deformity. Dynamic correction by 2-pin skeletal traction may be effective in some knee contractures when combined with therapy to maintain motion while in traction. In the young child, a single vigorous attempt at reduction of the dislocated hip is worthwhile. Multiple operative procedures about the hip are contraindicated, as further stiffness may be produced with consequent impairment of motion. The dislocation of the hip that occurs in arthrogryposis is associated with severe dysplasia of the bones and does not respond to treatment as ordinary congenital hip dislocation does. Affected children are often able to walk with bilateral dislocation of the hips, and in cases of severe rigidity it is better to leave the hips out of joint. With lesser demands, the long-term disability is not as severe as it would be in a person with normal mobility and strength.

The long-term prognosis for physical and vocational independence is poor. Patients usually have normal intelligence, but they have such severe physical restrictions that gainful employment is hard to find.

Hahn G: Arthrogryposis: Pediatric review and habilitative aspects. *Clin Orthop* 1985;**194:**104.

2. MARFAN'S SYNDROME

Marfan's syndrome is characterized by unusually long fingers and toes (arachnodactyly); hypermobility of the joints; subluxation of the ocular lenses; other eye abnormalities including cataract, coloboma, megalocornea, strabismus, and nystagmus; a high-arched palate; a strong tendency to scoliosis; pectus carinatum; and thoracic aneurysms due to weakness of the media of the vessels. Serum mucoproteins may be decreased and urinary excretion of hydroxyproline increased. The condition is easily confused with homocystinuria, as the phenotypic presentation is identical. The 2 diseases may be differentiated by the presence of homocystine in the urine in homocystinuria.

Treatment is usually supportive for associated problems such as flatfeet. Scoliosis may involve more vigorous treatment by bracing or spine fusion. The long-term prognosis has improved for patients as better treatment for their aortic aneurysms has been devised.

Bornstein D, Byers DH: Collagen metabolism. In: *Current Concepts*. Upjohn, 1980.

3. CLEIDOCRANIAL DYSOSTOSIS

Cleidocranial dysostosis consists of absence of part or all of the clavicle and delay in ossification of the skull. The facial bones are often underdeveloped, with absence of the sinuses, a high-arched palate, and defective teeth. The skull is enlarged, especially in the parietal and frontal regions. Coxa vara deformity of the proximal femur is sometimes present but usually is not of sufficient magnitude to require surgery. Deficiency of ossification of the symphysis pubica may persist into adult life. The clavicular deformity allows affected patients to touch their shoulders in the midline but otherwise presents no difficulty. The pelvic deformities do not prevent normal pregnancy and childbirth. The syndrome has a strong hereditary tendency.

4. CRANIOFACIAL DYSOSTOSIS (Crouzon's Disease)

Craniofacial dysostosis is a syndrome consisting of acrocephaly, hypoplastic maxilla, beaked nose, protrusion of the lower lip, exophthalmos, exotropia, and hypertelorism. It is usually familial. No orthopedic treatment is necessary. Heroic efforts have been made by neurosurgeons and plastic surgeons to correct the grotesque deformity of patients, who generally have normal intelligence. These operative procedures are complicated and hazardous, involving multiple osteotomies of the skull and facial bones.

5. KLIPPEL-FEIL SYNDROME

Klippel-Feil syndrome is characterized by fusion of some or all of the cervical vertebrae. Multiple spinal anomalies may be present, with hemivertebrae and scoliosis. The neck is short and stiff, the hairline is low, and the ears are often low-set. Common associated defects include congenital scoliosis, cervical rib, spina bifida, torticollis, web neck, high scapula, renal anomalies, and deafness. Examination of the urinary tract by urinalysis, blood urea nitrogen, and intravenous urograms is indicated as well as a hearing test.

Scoliotic deformities, if progressive, may require treatment. Occasionally, it is necessary to correct the high scapula, also called **Sprengel's deformity** (see below).

Hensinger RN et al: Klippel-Feil syndrome. *J Bone Joint Surg [Am]* 1974;**56:**1246.

6. SPRENGEL'S DEFORMITY

Sprengel's deformity is a congenital condition in which one or both scapulas are elevated and small. The child cannot raise the arm completely on the affected side, and there may be torticollis. The deformity occurs alone or may be associated with Klippel-Feil syndrome.

If the deformity is functionally limiting, the scapula may be surgically relocated lower in the thorax. Excision of the upper portion of the scapula improves cosmetic appearance but has little effect on function.

Samilson RL: Congenital and development anomalies of the shoulder girdle. *Orthop Clin North Am* 1980;**11:**219.

7. OSTEOGENESIS IMPERFECTA

Osteogenesis imperfecta is a rare, mainly dominantly inherited connective tissue disease. The severe fetal type (osteogenesis imperfecta congenita) is characterized by multiple intrauterine or perinatal fractures. Affected children continue to have fractures and are dwarfed as a result of bony deformities and growth retardation. Intelligence is not affected. The shafts of the long bones are reduced in cortical thickness, and wormian bones are present in the skull. Other features include blue scleras, thin skin, hyperextensibility of ligaments, "otosclerosis" with significant hearing loss, and hypoplastic and deformed teeth. Recurrent epistaxis, easy bruisability, mild hyperpyrexia (which may increase significantly during anesthesia), and excessive diaphoresis are common. In the tarda type, fractures begin to occur at variable times after the perinatal period, resulting in relatively fewer fractures and deformities in these cases. The patients are sometimes suspected of having suffered induced fractures, and the condition should be ruled out in any case of nonaccidental trauma.

Metabolic defects include elevated serum pyrophosphate, increased neutrophil nitroblue tetrazolium (NBT), decreased platelet aggregation, and decreased incorporation of sulfate into acid mucopolysaccharides by skin fibroblasts. Normal parents can be counseled that the likelihood of a second affected child is negligible.

There is no effective treatment by medication. Surgical treatment involves correction of deformity of the long bones. Multiple intramedullary rods have been used to prevent deformity from poor healing of fractures.

The overall prognosis is poor, and patients are often confined to wheelchairs during adulthood.

Albright JA, Miller EA: Osteogenesis imperfecta. (Editorial.) *Clin Orthop* 1981;**159:**2.

Bauze RJ et al: A new look at osteogenesis imperfecta: A clinical, radiological and biochemical study of 42 patients. *J Bone Joint Surg [Br]* 1975;**57:**2.

8. IDIOPATHIC JUVENILE OSTEOPOROSIS

Idiopathic juvenile osteoporosis is an acute bone disease characterized by unexplained pathologic fractures of the spine and long bones. It affects boys and girls equally in the prepubertal years, and the degree of severity is variable. There is evidence of gross enteric malabsorption of calcium, which may reflect an abnormality of 1,25-dihydroxyergocalciferol synthesis.

9. OSTEOPETROSIS (Osteitis Condensans Generalisata; Marble Bone Disease; Albers-Schönberg Disease)

The clinical manifestations of osteopetrosis, a familial and hereditary syndrome, are bony deformities due to pathologic fractures, myelophthisic anemia, splenomegaly, visual and auditory disturbances, square head, facial paralysis, pigeon breast, and dwarfing. The findings may appear at any age. On x-ray examination, the bones show increased density, transverse bands in the shafts, clubbing of ends, and vertical striations of long bones. There is thickening about the cranial foramens, and there may be heterotopic calcification of soft tissues. Treatment with corticosteroids to ameliorate the hematologic abnormalities should be tried.

Yu AS et al: Osteopetrosis. *Arch Dis Child* 1971;**46**:257.

10. ACHONDROPLASIA (Classic Chondrodystrophy)

In achondroplasia, the arms and legs are short, with the upper arms and thighs proportionately shorter than the forearms and legs. Findings frequently include bowing of the extremities, a waddling gait, limitation of motion of major joints, relaxation of the ligaments, short stubby fingers of almost equal length, a prominent forehead, moderate hydrocephalus, depressed nasal bridge, and lumbar lordosis. Mentality and sexual function are normal. A family history is often present. X-rays demonstrate short, thick tubular bones and irregular epiphyseal plates. The ends of the bones are thick, with broadening and cupping. Epiphyseal ossification may be delayed.

Osteotomies of the long bones are occasionally necessary if deformities are severe.

The medullary canal is narrowed, so that herniated disk in adulthood may lead to acute paraplegia.

11. OSTEOCHONDRODYSTROPHY (Morquio's Disease)

Osteochondrodystrophy is characterized by shortening of the spine, kyphosis, scoliosis, moderate shortening of the extremities, pectus carinatum, protuberant abdomen, hepatosplenomegaly, and a waddling gait resulting from instability of the hips and laxity of the knee joints. The skull is minimally involved. The child may appear normal at birth but begins to develop deformities between 1 and 4 years of age as a result of abnormal deposition of mucopolysaccharides. The disorder is commonly familial. Inheritance appears to be on an autosomal recessive basis.

X-rays demonstrate wedge-shaped flattened vertebrae and irregular, malformed epiphyses. The ribs are broad and have been likened to canoe paddles. The lower extremities are more severely involved than the upper ones.

There is no treatment, and the prognosis is poor. Death may occur in childhood or adolescence. Progressive clouding of the cornea leads to increasing visual impairment.

Stanescu V, Stanescu R, Maroteaux P: Pathogenic mechanisms in osteochondrodysplasias. *J Bone Joint Surg* [*Am*] 1984;**66**:817.

12. CHONDROECTODERMAL DYSPLASIA (Ellis-van Creveld Syndrome)

Manifestations include ectodermal dysplasia, congenital heart disease, polydactyly, syndactyly, poorly formed teeth, and mental retardation. The disease is familial and inbred in certain ethnic groups such as the Amish people of Pennsylvania.

X-ray changes include chondrodystrophy; shortening and bowing of the tibias and fibulas; hyperplastic, eccentric proximal tibial metaphyses; and fusion of the carpal bones.

No treatment is available. The long-term prognosis depends on the severity of heart involvement.

Beals RK: Orthopaedic care for patients with skeletal dysplasia. In: *AAOS Symposium on Heritable Disorders of Connective Tissue*. Akeson WH, Bornstein P, Glimcher MJ (editors). Mosby, 1982.

McKusick VA: *Heritable Disorders of Connective Tissue*, 4th ed. Mosby, 1972.

Sillence DO, Rimoin DL: Chondroosseous morphology in the skeletal dysplasias. In: *AAOS Symposium on Heritable Disorders of Connective Tissue*. Akeson WH, Bornstein P, Glimcher MJ (editors). Mosby, 1982.

GROWTH DISTURBANCES OF THE MUSCULOSKELETAL SYSTEM

SCOLIOSIS

The term scoliosis denotes lateral curvature of the spine, which is always associated with some rotation of the involved vertebrae. Scoliosis is classified by its anatomic location, in either the thoracic or lumbar spine, with rare involvement of the cervical spine. The apex of the curve is designated right or left. Thus, a left thoracic scoliosis would denote a convex leftward curve in the thoracic region, and this is the most common type of idiopathic curve. Posterior curvature of the spine (kyphosis) is normal in the thoracic area, though excessive curvature may become pathologic. Anterior curvature is called lordosis and is normal in the lumbar spine. Idiopathic scoliosis generally begins at about 8 or 10 years of age and progresses during growth. In rare instances, infantile scoliosis may be seen in children 2 years of age or less.

Idiopathic scoliosis is about 4–5 times more common in girls than in boys. The disorder is usually asymptomatic in the adolescent years, but severe curvature may lead to impairment of pulmonary function or low back pain in later years. It is important to examine the back of any adolescent coming in for an incidental physical examination in order to identify scoliosis early. The examination is performed by having the patient bend forward 90 degrees with the hands joined in the midline. An abnormal finding consists of asymmetry of the height of the ribs or paravertebral muscles on one side, indicating rotation of the trunk associated with lateral curvature.

Diseases that may be associated with scoliosis include neurofibromatosis, Marfan's syndrome, cerebral palsy, muscular dystrophy, and poliomyelitis. Neurologic examination should be performed in all children with scoliosis to determine whether these disorders are present.

Five to 7% of cases of scoliosis are due to congenital vertebral anomalies such as a hemivertebral or unilateral vertebral bridge. These curves are more rigid than the more common idiopathic curve (see below) and will often increase with growth, especially during the rapid growth spurt during adolescence.

The most common type of scoliosis is so-called idiopathic scoliosis, which may be due to asymmetry of neuromuscular development. In 30% of cases, other family members are affected also; thus, a family survey is valuable for detecting the problem in siblings if one child has been found to have scoliosis.

Idiopathic infantile scoliosis, occurring in children 2–4 years of age, is quite uncommon in the USA; it is more common in Great Britain. If the curvature is less than 30 degrees, the prognosis is excellent, as 70% resolve spontaneously. If the curvature is more than 30 degrees, there may be progression, and the prognosis is therefore guarded.

Postural compensation of the spine may lead to lateral curvature from such causes as unequal length of the lower extremities. Antalgic scoliosis may result from pressure on the spinal cord or roots by infectious processes or herniation of the nucleus pulposus; the underlying cause must be sought. The curvature will resolve as the primary problem is treated.

Clinical Findings

A. Symptoms and Signs: Scoliosis in adolescents is classically asymptomatic. It is imperative to seek the underlying cause in any case where there is pain, since in these instances the scoliosis is almost always secondary to some other disorder such as a bone or spinal cord tumor. Deformity of the rib cage and asymmetry of the waistline are evident with curvatures of 30 degrees or more. A lesser curvature may be detected by the forward bending test as described above, which is designed to detect early abnormalities of rotation that are not apparent when the patient is standing erect.

B. X-Ray Findings: The most valuable x-rays are those taken of the entire spine in the standing position in both the anteroposterior and lateral planes. Usually, there is one primary curvature with a compensatory curvature that develops to balance the body. At times there may be 2 primary curvatures, usually in the left thoracic and right lumbar regions. Any right thoracic curvature should be suspected of being secondary to neurologic or muscular disease, prompting a more meticulous neurologic examination. If the curvatures of the spine are balanced (compensated), the head is centered over the center of the pelvis and the patient is "in balance." If the spinal alignment is uncompensated, the head will be displaced to one side, which produces an unsightly deformity. Rotation of the spine may be measured by use of spirit level as described by Bunnell (1984). This rotation is associated with a marked rib hump as the lateral curvature increases in severity. Deformity of the rib cage produces a decrease in the space available for the lung and is the cause of long-term problems.

Treatment

Curvatures of less than 20 degrees usually do not require treatment unless they show progression. Bracing is indicated for curvature of 20–40 degrees in a skeletally immature child. Treatment is indicated for any curvature that demonstrates progression on serial x-ray examination. Curvatures greater than 40 degrees are resistant to treatment by bracing. Thoracic curvatures greater than 60 degrees have been correlated with a poor pulmonary prognosis in adult life. Curvatures of such severity are an indication for surgical correction of the deformity and posterior spinal fusion to maintain the correction. Curvatures between 40 and 60 degrees may also require spinal fusion if they appear to be progressive or are causing decompensation of the spine or are cosmetically unacceptable.

Surgical fusion involves decortication of the bone over the laminas and spinous processes, with the addition of autogenous bone graft from the iliac crest. Postoperative correction is usually maintained by a Harrington or Luque rod, with activity restriction for several months until the fusion is solid.

Treatment is prolonged and difficult and is best done in centers where full support facilities are available.

Prognosis

Compensated small curvatures that do not progress may be well tolerated throughout life, with very little cosmetic concern. The patients should be counseled regarding the genetic transmission of scoliosis and cautioned that their children should be examined at regular intervals during growth. Large thoracic curvatures greater than 60 degrees are associated with shortened life span and may progress even during adult life. Large lumbar curvatures may lead to subluxation of the vertebrae and premature arthritic degeneration of the spine, producing disabling pain in adulthood. Early detection allows for simple brace treatment or surface electrical stimulation. In patients so treated, the long-term prognosis is excellent and surgery is not necessary. For this reason, school screening programs for scoliosis have gained popular support in many sections of the country.

Bunnell WP: An objective criterion for scoliosis screening. *J Bone Joint Surg* [*Am*] 1984;**66:**1381.

Lonstein JE, Carlson JM: The prediction of curve progression in untreated idiopathic scoliosis during growth. *J Bone Joint Surg* [*Am*] 1984; **66:**1061.

Luque ER: Segmental spinal instrumentation for correction of scoliosis. *Clin Orthop* 1982;**163:**192.

Moe JH et al: *Scoliosis and Other Spinal Deformities*. Saunders, 1978.

Weinstein SL, Favala DC, Ponseti IV: Idiopathic scoliosis: Long-term follow-up and prognosis of untreated patients. *J Bone Joint Surg* [*Am*] 1981;**63:**702.

EPIPHYSIOLYSIS (Slipped Capital Femoral Epiphysis)

Epiphysiolysis is the separation of the proximal femoral epiphysis through the growth plate. The head of the femur is usually displaced medially and posteriorly relative to the neck of the femur. The condition occurs in adolescence and is more common in overweight children. Slightly over 40% of the children so affected are of the obese, hypogenital body type. The cause is not clear, although some authorities have shown experimentally that the decreased strength of the perichondral ring stabilizing the epiphyseal area is sufficiently weakened by anatomic changes in adolescent years that the simple overload by excessive body weight can produce a pathologic fracture through the growth plate. Hormonal studies in these children have not demonstrated any abnormality. Anatomic study of the area of separation demonstrates a histologic picture identical to that seen with traumatic separation, and the condition occasionally occurs as an acute episode resulting from a fall or direct trauma to the hip.

More commonly, however, there are vague symptoms over a protracted period of time in an otherwise healthy child who presents with pain and limp. The pain is often referred into the thigh or the medial side of the knee. It is important to examine the hip joint in any child complaining of knee pain, particularly in adolescents. The consistent finding on physical examination is limitation of internal rotation of the hip. There usually is also an associated hip flexion contracture as well as local tenderness about the hip. X-rays should be taken in both the anteroposterior and lateral planes. These must be carefully examined in early cases in order to show an abnormality where displacement of the femoral head occurs posteriorly, which is usually most easily seen on the lateral view.

Treatment is based on the same principles that govern treatment of fracture of the femoral neck in adults in that the head of the femur is fixed to the neck of the femur and the fracture line allowed to heal. Unfortunately, the severe complication of avascular necrosis occurs in 30% of these patients. There has been a positive correlation between forceful reduction of the slip and avascular necrosis. In cases of acute slip, as evidenced by the absence of any callus formation about the growth plate, it may be possible to reduce the hip by gentle traction. In more chronic cases, a more expeditious procedure is to pin the slip in situ and perform correctional osteotomy later in order to realign the deformity. Remodeling of the fracture site often improves the position of the hip without further surgery. The pins used to maintain reduction should be removed once healing has occurred.

The long-term prognosis is guarded because most of these patients continue to be overweight and overstress their hip joints. Follow-up studies have shown a high incidence of premature degenerative arthritis in this group of patients—even those who do not develop avascular necrosis. The development of avascular necrosis almost guarantees a poor prognosis, since new bone does not replace the femoral head at this late stage of skeletal growth.

About 30% of patients have bilateral involvement, and patients should be followed for slipping of the opposite side, which may occur as long as 1 or 2 years after the primary episode.

Ratliff AHC: Slipped upper femoral epiphysis. In: *Hip Disorders in Children*. Lloyd-Roberts GC (editor). Butterworth, 1978.

GENU VARUM & GENU VALGUM

Genu varum (bowleg) is normal from infancy through 2 years of life. The alignment then changes to genu valgum (knock-knee) until about 8 years of age, at which time adult alignment is attained. Criteria for referral to an orthopedist include persistent bowing beyond age 2, bowing that is increasing rather than decreasing, bowing of one leg only, and knock-knee associated with short stature.

Bracing may be appropriate, or, rarely, an osteotomy is necessary for a severe problem such as Blount's disease (proximal tibial epiphyseal dysplasia).

Brighton CT: Structure and function of the growth plate. *Clin Orthop* 1978;**136:**22.

Staheli LT: Torsional deformity. *Pediatr Clin North Am* 1977;**24:**799.

Vankka E, Salenius P: Spontaneous correction of severe tibiofemoral deformity in growing children. *Acta Orthop Scand* 1982;**53:**567.

TIBIAL TORSION

The physician is often asked about "toeing in" in small children. The disorder is routinely asymptomatic. Tibial torsion is rotation of the leg between the knee and the ankle. Internal rotation amounts to about 20 degrees at birth but decreases to neutral rotation by 1 year of age. The deformity is sometimes accentuated by laxity of the knee ligaments, allowing excessive internal rotation of the leg in small children. In children who have a persistent internal rotation of the tibia beyond 1 year of age, it is often due to sleeping with feet turned in and can be reversed with an external rotation splint worn only at night.

FEMORAL ANTEVERSION

"Toeing in" beyond 2 or 3 years of age is usually based on femoral anteversion, which produces excessive internal rotation of the femur as compared to external rotation. This femoral alignment follows a natural history of progressive decrease toward neutral up to 8 years of age, with slower change to 16 years of age. Studies comparing the results of treatment with shoes or braces to the natural history have shown that little is gained by active treatment. Active external rotation exercises such as ballet, skating, or bicycle riding may be worthwhile. Osteotomy for rotational correction is rarely required. Refer those who have no external rotation of hip in extension.

Fabry G, MacEwen GD, Shands AR Jr: Torsion of the femur. *J Bone Joint Surg* [*Am*] 1973;**55:**1726.

COMMON FOOT PROBLEMS

When a child begins to stand and walk, the long arch of the foot is flat with a medial bulge over the inner border of the foot. The forefeet are mildly pronated or rotated inward, with a slight valgus alignment of the knees. As the child grows and muscle power improves, the long arch is better supported and more normal relationships occur in the lower extremities. (See also Metatarsus Varus and Talipes Equinovarus.)

1. FLATFOOT

Flatfoot is a normal condition in infants. Children presenting for examination should be checked to determine that the heel cord is of normal length when the heel is aligned in the neutral position, allowing complete dorsiflexion and plantar flexion. As long as the foot is supple and the presence of a longitudinal arch is noted when the child is sitting in a non-weight-bearing position, the parents can be assured that a normal arch will probably develop. There is usually a familial incidence of relaxed flatfeet in children who have prolonged malalignment of the foot. In any child with a shortened heel cord or stiffness of the foot, other causes of flatfoot such as tarsal coalition or vertical talus should be ruled out by a complete orthopedic examination and x-ray.

In the child with an ordinary relaxed flatfoot, no active treatment is indicated unless there is calf or leg pain. In children who have leg pains attributable to flatfeet, an orthopedic shoe with Thomas heel may relieve discomfort. An arch insert should not be prescribed unless passive correction of the arch is easily accomplished; otherwise, there will be irritation of the skin over the medial side of the foot.

Mosier KM, Asher M: Tarsal coalitions and peroneal spastic flatfoot: A review. *J Bone Joint Surg* [*Am*] 1984;**66:**976.

2. TALIPES CALCANEOVALGUS

Talipes calcaneovalgus is characterized by excessive dorsiflexion at the ankle and eversion of the foot. It is often present at birth and almost always corrects spontaneously. The deformity is the reverse of classic clubfoot (talipes equinovarus) and is due to intrauterine position.

Treatment consists of passive exercises by the mother, stretching the foot into plantar flexion. In rare instances, it may be necessary to use plaster casts to help with manipulation and positioning.

Complete correction is the rule.

3. CAVUS FOOT

In cavus foot, the deformity consists of an unusually high longitudinal arch of the foot. It may be hereditary or associated with neurologic conditions such as poliomyelitis, Charcot-Marie-Tooth disease, Friedreich's ataxia, or diastematomyelia. There is usually an associated contracture of the toe extensor, producing a claw toe deformity in which the metatarsal phalangeal joints are hyperextended and the interphalangeal joints acutely flexed. Any child presenting with cavus feet should have a careful neurologic examination including x-rays of the spine.

Stretching exercises for the heel cord and arch of the foot are indicated for conservative therapy. In resistant cases that do not respond to shoe adjustments (metatarsal bars and supports), operation may be necessary to lengthen the contracted extensor and flexor tendons. Arthrodesis of the foot may be necessary later. If these feet are left untreated, they are often painful and limit walking.

The overall prognosis is much poorer than with low arch or pes planus.

4. CLAW TOES

In patients with claw toes, there is a flexion deformity of either or both interphalangeal joints, which results in the "claw." The condition is usually congenital and may be seen in association with disorders of motor weakness, such as Charcot-Marie-Tooth disease or pes cavus. Surgical correction can alleviate symptoms if the toes are painful.

5. BUNIONS (Hallux Valgus)

Girls may present in adolescence with lateral deviation of the great toe associated with a prominence over the head of the first metatarsal. This deformity is painful only with shoe wear and almost always can be relieved by fitting shoes that are wide enough. Surgery should be avoided in the adolescent age group, as the results are much less successful than in adult patients with the same condition.

Coleman SS: *Complex Foot Deformities in Children.* Lea & Febiger, 1983.
Jones BS: Flatfoot. *J Bone Joint Surg [Br]* 1975;**57**:279.

EPIPHYSEAL GROWTH DISTURBANCES SECONDARY TO INFECTION OR TRAUMA

In the child under 1 year of age, there is direct vascular communication from the metaphysis to the epiphysis across the growth plate. For this reason, osteomyelitis occurring in the infant may produce permanent damage to the growth cartilage of the epiphysis with resulting angular deformity or decreased growth potential for the bone. Likewise, trauma, particularly of a compression variety, may damage part or all of the epiphysis. Once such damage occurs, deformity is progressive and may be severe, requiring osteotomy for angular deformity or epiphysiodesis for correction of leg length discrepancy.

ORTHOPEDIC ASPECTS OF ENDOCRINE DISEASES

Hormonal problems affecting the skeleton are discussed in Chapter 25. Only a brief orthopedic resume is presented here.

ADRENAL

Adrenocortical hyperfunction may lead to advanced skeletal age relative to chronologic age, with premature epiphyseal closure. In children receiving long-term high-dosage corticosteroid treatment, eg, in the treatment of asthma or nephrosis, there may be retardation of growth and delayed skeletal age.

THYROID

Hyperthyroidism or prolonged thyroid administration may lead to severe osteoporosis with secondary pathologic fracture.

Hypothyroidism is associated with retarded skeletal age and may result in a slipped capital femoral epiphysis in the adolescent. It is worthwhile to screen the patients with slipped capital femoral epiphysis for hypothyroidism.

PARATHYROID

1. HYPERPARATHYROIDISM

Parathyroid hormone exerts a direct effect upon bone, causing absorption of bone. Primary hyperparathyroidism is very rare in children. The skeletal effects of hyperparathyroidism in childhood are usually secondary to parathyroid stimulation by renal failure. X-ray changes associated with hyperparathyroidism are generalized osteoporosis and cortical atrophy that is most notable in the distal phalanges and about the necks of the metacarpals. It has been documented that slipped capital femoral epiphysis may occur as a result of the effect on the growth plate, with weakening in children with renal failure. The "brown tumors" of hyperparathyroidism are rare in childhood.

2. HYPOPARATHYROIDISM & PSEUDOHYPOPARATHYROIDISM

The signs and symptoms, laboratory findings, and x-ray findings in these 2 disorders are similar, and the distinction between them is difficult. The disease is commonly hereditary and associated with shortening of the fourth and fifth metacarpals and metatarsals. Formation of the growth plate is abnormal, and the epiphyseal ossification center may indent the metaphysis.

GONADS

In general, deficiency of gonadal hormones produces osteoporosis and delayed maturation of the skeleton. This is most commonly seen in association with Turner's syndrome in the child. Excessive amounts of estrogen such as occur in girls with Albright's syndrome produce not only sexual precocity but also premature closure of the growth centers, resulting in short stature.

DEGENERATIVE PROBLEMS (Arthritis, Bursitis, & Tenosynovitis)

Degenerative arthritis may follow childhood skeletal problems such as infection, slipped capital femoral epiphysis, avascular necrosis, or trauma or may occur in association with hemophilia. Early effective treatment of these disorders will prevent arthritis. Late treatment is often unsatisfactory.

Degenerative changes in the soft tissues around joints may occur as a result of overuse syndrome in adolescent athletes. Young boys throwing excessive numbers of pitches, especially curve balls, may develop "little leaguer's elbow," consisting of degenerative changes around the humeral condyles associated with pain, swelling, and limitation of motion. In order to enforce the rest necessary for healing, a plaster cast may be necessary. A more reasonable preventive measure is to limit the number of pitches thrown by children.

Acute bursitis is quite uncommon in childhood, and other causes should be ruled out before this diagnosis is accepted.

Tenosynovitis is most common in the region of the knees and feet. Children taking dancing lessons, particularly toe dancing, may have pain around the flexor tendon sheaths in the toes or ankles. Rest is effective treatment. At the knee level, there may be irritation of the patellar ligament, with associated swelling in the infrapatellar fat pad. Synovitis in this area is usually due to overuse and is also treated by rest. Corticosteroid injections are contraindicated.

TRAUMA

SOFT TISSUE TRAUMA (Sprains, Strains, & Contusions)

A sprain is the stretching of a ligament, and a strain is a stretch of a muscle or tendon. In either of these injuries, there may be some degree of tissue tearing. Contusions are generally due to tissue compression, with damage to blood vessels within the tissue and the formation of hematoma.

A severe sprain is one in which the ligament is completely divided, resulting in instability of the joint. A mild or moderate sprain is one in which incomplete tearing of the ligament occurs, but in which there is associated local pain and swelling.

Mild or moderate sprains are treated by rest of the affected joint, with ice and elevation to prevent prolonged symptoms. By definition, mild or moderate sprain is not associated with instability of the joint.

If there is more severe trauma resulting in tearing of a ligament, instability of the joint may be demonstrated by gross examination or by stress testing with x-ray documentation. Such deformity of the joint may cause persistent instability resulting from inaccurate apposition of the ligament ends during healing. If instability is evident, surgical repair of the torn ligament is indicated. If a muscle is torn, usually at its end, it should be repaired.

The initial treatment of any sprain consists of ice, compression, and elevation. The purpose of the treatment is to decrease local edema and residual stiffness resulting from gelling of blood proteins in the interstitial space. Splinting of the affected joint protects against further injury and relieves swelling and pain.

1. ANKLE SPRAINS

The history will indicate that the injury was by either forceful inversion or eversion. The more common inversion injury results in tearing or injury to the lateral ligaments, whereas an eversion injury will injure the medial ligaments of the ankle. The injured ligaments may be identified by means of careful palpation for point tenderness around the ankle. The joint should be supported or immobilized at a right angle, which is the functional position. Adhesive taping may be effective to maintain this position but should be applied by one skilled in the use of tape and changed frequently in order to prevent the formation of blisters and skin damage. A posterior plaster splint is more easily applied and gives good joint rest if the extremity is protected by using crutches for weight bearing. Prolonged use of a plaster cast is usually not necessary, but the sprained ankle should be rested sufficiently to allow complete healing. This may take 3–6 weeks. Because fractures usually receive more attention and adequate follow-up, the results are often better. A properly treated ankle sprain should not be the source of prolonged and repeated disability.

2. KNEE SPRAINS

Sprains of the collateral and cruciate ligaments are uncommon in children. These ligaments are so strong that it is more common to injure the epiphyseal growth plates, which are the weakest structures in the region of the knees of children. In adolescence, however, the joints and growth plates attain adult growth, and a rupture of the anterior cruciate ligament can result from a twisting injury that may avulse the anterior tibial spine. In such instances, the injury is apparent on physical examination and x-ray and requires anatomic reduction and immobilization for 6 weeks. In most instances, this means open operative correction.

Effusion of the knee after trauma deserves referral to an orthopedic specialist. The differential diagnosis includes torn ligament, torn meniscus, and osteochondral fracture. Nontraumatic effusion should be evaluated for inflammatory conditions (such as juvenile rheumatoid arthritis) or patellar malalignment.

3. INTERNAL DERANGEMENTS OF THE KNEE

Meniscal injuries are uncommon under age 12. Clicking or locking of the knee may occur in young children as a result of a discoid lateral meniscus, which is a rare type of congenital anomaly. As the child approaches adolescence, internal damage to the knee from a torsion weight-bearing injury may result in locking of the knee if tearing and displacement of the meniscus occur. Osteochondral fractures secondary to osteochondritis dissecans may also present as internal derangements of the knee in adolescence. Posttraumatic synovitis may mimic a meniscal lesion as well. In any severe injury to the knee, epiphyseal injury should be suspected; stress films will sometimes demonstrate separation of the distal femoral epiphysis in such cases. Epiphyseal injury should be suspected whenever there is tenderness on both sides of the metaphysis of the femur after injury.

Zaman M, Leonard MA: Meniscectomy in children: Results in 59 knees. *Injury* 1981;**12:**425.

4. BACK SPRAINS

Sprains of the ligaments and muscles of the back are unusual in children but may occur as a result of violent trauma from automobile accidents or athletic injuries. A child with back pain should not be presumed to have had trauma to the spine unless the history warrants that conclusion. The reason for back pain should be carefully sought by x-ray and physical examination. Inflammation, infection, and tumors are more common causes of back pain in children than sprains.

5. CONTUSIONS

Contusion of muscle with hematoma formation produces the familiar "charley horse" injury. Treatment of such injuries is by application of ice, compression, and rest. Exercise should be avoided for 5–7 days. Local heat may hasten healing once the acute phase of tenderness and swelling is past.

6. MYOSITIS OSSIFICANS

Ossification within muscle occurs when there is sufficient trauma to cause a hematoma that later heals in the manner of a fracture. The injury is usually a contusion and occurs most commonly in the quadriceps of the thigh or the triceps of the arm. When such a severe injury with hematoma is recognized, it is important to splint the extremity and avoid activity. If further activity is allowed, ossification may reach spectacular proportions and resemble an osteosarcoma.

Disability is great, with local swelling and heat and extreme pain upon the slightest motion of the adjacent joint. The limb should be rested, with the knee in extension or the elbow in 90 degrees of flexion, until the local reaction has subsided. Once local heat and tenderness have decreased, gentle active exercises may be initiated. Passive stretching exercises are not indicated, because they may stimulate the ossification reaction. It is occasionally necessary to excise excessive bony tissue if it interferes with muscle function once the reaction is mature. Surgery should not be attempted before 9 months to a year after injury, because it may restart the process and lead to an even more severe reaction.

TRAUMATIC SUBLUXATIONS & DISLOCATIONS

Dislocation of a joint is always associated with severe damage to the ligaments and joint capsule. In contrast to fracture treatment, which may be safely postponed, dislocations must be reduced immediately. Dislocations can usually be reduced by gentle sustained traction. It often happens that no anesthetic is necessary for several hours after the injury, because of the protective anesthesia produced by the injury. Following reduction, the joint should be splinted for transportation of the patient.

The dislocated joint should be treated by immobilization for at least 3 weeks, followed by graduated active exercises through a full range of motion. Physical therapy is usually not indicated for children with injuries. As a matter of fact, vigorous manipulation of the joint by a therapist may be harmful. The child should be permitted to perform therapy alone. No stretching should be permitted.

1. SUBLUXATION OF THE RADIAL HEAD (Nursemaid's Elbow)

Infants frequently sustain subluxation of the radial head as a result of being lifted or pulled by the hand. The child appears with the elbow fully pronated and painful. The usual complaint is that the child's elbow will not bend. X-rays are normal, but there is point tenderness over the radial head. When the elbow is placed in full supination and slowly moved from full flexion to full extension, a click may be palpated at the level of the radial head. The relief of pain is remarkable, as the child usually stops crying immediately. The elbow may be immobilized in a sling for comfort for a day.

Pulled elbow may be a clue to battering. This should be remembered during examination especially if the problem is recurrent.

2. RECURRENT DISLOCATION OF THE PATELLA

Recurrent dislocation of the patella is more common in loose-jointed individuals, especially adolescent girls. If the patella completely dislocates, it nearly always goes laterally. Pain is severe, and the patient is brought to the doctor with the knee slightly flexed and an obvious bony mass lateral to the knee joint and a flat area over the usual location of the patella anteriorly. X-rays confirm the diagnosis. The patella may be reduced by extending the knee and placing slight pressure on the patella while gentle traction is exerted on the leg. In subluxation of the patella, the symptoms may be more subtle, and the patient may say that the knee "gives out" or "jumps out of place."

In the case of complete dislocation, the knee should be immobilized for 3–4 weeks, followed by a physical therapy program for strengthening the quadriceps muscle. Operation may be necessary to tighten the knee joint capsule if dislocation or subluxation is recurrent. In such instances, if the patella is not stabilized, repeated dislocation produces damage to the articular cartilage of the patellofemoral joint and premature degenerative arthritis.

EPIPHYSEAL SEPARATIONS

In children, epiphyseal separations and fractures are more common than ligamentous injuries. This finding is based on the fact that the ligaments of the joints are generally stronger than the associated growth plates. In instances where dislocation is suspected, an x-ray should be taken in order to rule out epiphyseal fracture. Films of the opposite extremity, especially around the elbow, may be valuable for comparison. Reduction of a fractured epiphysis should be done under anesthesia in order to align the growth plate with the least amount of force necessary. Fractures across the growth plate may produce bony bridges that will cause premature cessation of growth or angular deformities in the growth plate. Epiphyseal fractures around the shoulder, wrist, and fingers can usually be treated by closed reduction, but fractures of the epiphyses around the elbow often require open reduction. In the lower extremity, accurate reduction of the epiphyseal plate is necessary to prevent joint deformity if a joint surface is involved. Unfortunately, some of the most severe injuries to the epiphyseal plate occur from compression injuries, where the amount of force is not immediately apparent. If angular deformities result, corrective osteotomy may be necessary.

TORUS FRACTURES

Torus fractures consist of "buckling" of the cortex as a result of minimal angular trauma. They usually occur in the distal radius or ulna. Alignment is satisfactory, and simple immobilization for 3–5 weeks is sufficient.

GREENSTICK FRACTURES

With greenstick fractures there is frank disruption of the cortex on one side of the bone but no discernible cleavage plane on the opposite side. These fractures are angulated but not displaced, as the bone ends are not separated. Reduction is achieved by straightening the arm into normal alignment, and reduction is maintained by a snugly fitting plaster cast. It is necessary to x-ray children with greenstick fractures again in a week to 10 days to make certain that the reduction has been maintained in plaster. A slight angular deformity will be corrected by remodeling of the bone. The farther the fracture is from the growing end of the bone, the longer the time required for healing. The fracture can be considered healed when there are no findings of tenderness and local swelling or heat and when adequate bony callus is seen on x-ray.

FRACTURE OF THE CLAVICLE

Clavicular fractures are very common injuries in infants and children. They can be immobilized by a figure-of-8 dressing that retracts the shoulders and brings the clavicle to normal length. The healing callus will be apparent when the fracture has consolidated, but this unsightly lump will generally resolve over a period of months to a year.

SUPRACONDYLAR FRACTURES OF THE HUMERUS

Supracondylar fractures tend to occur in the age group from 3 to 6 years and are potentially dangerous because of the proximity to the brachial artery in the distal arm. They are usually associated with a significant amount of trauma, so that swelling may be severe. **Volkmann's ischemic contracture** of muscle may occur as a result of vascular embarrassment. When severe swelling is present, the safest course is to place the arm in traction and carefully observe nerve function and the vascular supply to the hand. In these cases, the children should be hospitalized and followed carefully by experienced nurses. If the blood supply is compromised, exposure of the brachial artery may be necessary, although this is rarely needed when satisfactory reduction and traction are employed. Complications associated with supracondylar fractures also include a resultant cubitus valgus secondary to poor reduction. It is often difficult to ascertain adequacy of the reduction because a flexed position is necessary to maintain normal alignment. Such a "gunstock" deformity of the elbow may be somewhat unsightly but does not usually interfere with joint function.

Millis MB, Singer IJ, Hall JE: Supracondylar fracture of the humerus in children: Further experience with a study in orthopaedic decision-making. *Clin Orthop* 1984;**188:**90.

GENERAL COMMENTS ON OTHER FRACTURES IN CHILDREN

Reduction of fractures in children is usually accomplished by simple traction and manipulation; open reduction is rarely indicated. Remodeling of the fracture callus will usually produce an almost normal appearance of the bone over a matter of months. The younger the child, the more remodeling is possible. Angular deformities remodel with ease. Rotatory deformities do not remodel, and this produces the cubitus valgus deformity sometimes seen after supracondylar fractures.

The physician should be suspicious of child battering whenever the age of a fracture does not match the history given or when the severity of the injury is more than the alleged accident would have produced. In suspected cases of battering where no fracture is present on the initial x-ray, a repeat film 10 days later is in order. Bleeding beneath the periosteum will be calcified by 7–10 days, and the x-ray appearance is almost diagnostic of severe closed trauma characteristic of a battered child.

Cumming WA: Neonatal skeletal fractures: Birth trauma or child abuse? *J Can Assoc Radiol* 1979;**30:**30.

Ogden JA: *Skeletal Injury in the Child.* Lea & Febiger, 1982.

Rang M: *Children's Fractures,* 2nd ed. Lippincott, 1983.

Weber BG, Brunner C, Freuler F (editors): *Treatment of Fractures in Children and Adolescents.* Springer-Verlag, 1980.

INFECTIONS OF THE BONES & JOINTS

OSTEOMYELITIS

Osteomyelitis is an infectious process that usually starts in the spongy or medullary bone and then extends to involve compact or cortical bone. It is more common in boys than in girls or in adults of either sex. The lower extremities are most often affected, and there is commonly a history of trauma. Osteomyelitis may occur as a result of direct invasion from the outside through a penetrating wound (nail) or open fracture, but hematogenous spread of infection (eg, pyoderma or upper respiratory tract infection) from other infected areas is more common. The most common infecting organism is *Staphylococcus aureus,* which seems to have a special tendency to infect the metaphyses of growing bones. Anatomically, circulation in the long bones is such that the arterial supply to the metaphysis just below the growth plate is by end arteries, which turn sharply to end in venous sinusoids, causing a relative stasis. In the infant under 1 year of age, there is direct vascular communication with the epiphysis across the growth plate, so that direct spread may occur from the metaphysis to the epiphysis and subsequently into the joint. In the older child, the growth plate provides an effective barrier and the epiphysis is usually not involved, although the infection spreads retrograde from the metaphysis into the diaphysis and, by rupture through the cortical bone, down along the diaphysis beneath the periosteum.

1. EXOGENOUS OSTEOMYELITIS

In order to avoid osteomyelitis by direct extension, all wounds must be carefully examined and cleansed. Puncture wounds are especially liable to lead to osteomyelitis if not carefully debrided. Cultures of the wound made at the time of exploration and debridement may be useful if signs of inflammation and infection develop subsequently. Copious irrigation is necessary, and all nonviable skin, subcutaneous tissue, fascia, and muscle must be excised. In extensive or contaminated wounds, antibiotic coverage is indicated. Contaminated wounds should be left open and secondary closure performed 3–5 days later. If at the time of delayed closure further necrotic tissue is present, it should be excised. Leaving the wound open allows the infection to stay at the surface rather than extend inward to the bone.

Parenteral administration of antibiotics is satisfactory, and local irrigation is not needed. If the wound is acquired outside the hospital, penicillin is adequate for most wounds. After cultures have been read, an appropriate alternative antibiotic can be chosen if there is lingering inflammation. A tetanus toxoid booster is indicated for any questionable wound, but gas gangrene is better prevented by adequate debridement than by antitoxin.

Once exogenous osteomyelitis has become established, treatment becomes more complicated, requiring extensive surgical debridement and drainage followed by careful antibiotic management. These cases require hospitalization and the use of intravenous antibiotics.

2. HEMATOGENOUS OSTEOMYELITIS

Hematogenous osteomyelitis is usually caused by pyogenic bacteria; 85% of cases are due to staphylococci. Streptococci are rare causes of osteomyelitis today, but *Pseudomonas* organisms have often been documented in cases of nail puncture wounds. Children with sickle cell anemia are especially prone to osteomyelitis caused by salmonellae.

Clinical Findings

A. Symptoms and Signs: In infants, the manifestations of osteomyelitis may be quite subtle, presenting as irritability, diarrhea, or failure to feed properly; the temperature may be normal or slightly low; and the white blood count may be normal or only slightly elevated. In older children, the manifestations are more striking, with severe local tenderness and pain, high fever, rapid pulse, and elevated white blood count and sedimentation rate. Osteomyelitis of a lower extremity often presents around the knee in a child 7–10 years of age. Tenderness is most marked over the metaphysis of the bone where the process has its origin.

B. Laboratory Findings: Blood cultures are often positive early. The most significant test in infancy is the aspiration of pus when suspicion arises because of lack of movement in a painful extremity. It is useful to insert a needle to the bone in the area of suspected infection and aspirate any fluid present. This fluid can be smeared and stained for organisms as well as cultured. Even edema fluid may be useful for determining the causative organism. The white blood cell count is usually elevated, as is the sedimentation rate.

C. X-Ray Findings: The first manifestation to appear on x-ray is nonspecific local swelling. This is followed by elevation of the periosteum, with formation of new bone from the cambium layer of the periosteum occurring after 3–6 days. As the infection becomes chronic, areas of cortical bone are isolated by pus spreading down the medullary canal, causing rarefaction and demineralization of the bone. Such isolated pieces of cortex become ischemic and form sequestra (dead bone fragments). These x-ray findings are late, and osteomyelitis should be diagnosed clinically before significant x-ray findings are present. Bone scan is valuable in suspected cases before x-rays become positive.

Treatment

A. Specific Measures: Antibiotics should be started intravenously as soon as the diagnosis of osteomyelitis is made. Use of methicillin, another semisynthetic penicillin, or a cephalosporin that covers penicillinase-producing *Staphylococcus aureus* is recommended. Gentamicin can also be given to combat gram-negative organisms until the results of cultures are available. Antibiotics should be continued until swelling, tenderness, and local discharge have ceased and the white blood count and erythrocyte sedimentation rate are normal. Serial x-rays can also be used to follow bone healing. Antibiotic therapy by the intravenous route should be continued until all clinical signs are improved, including sedimentation rate. For a reliable family, oral medication may be started at that time (about 10 days), adjusting dosage by serum killing power and continued monitoring of erythrocyte sedimentation rate for at least 1 month after the rate has returned to normal.

B. General Measures: Splinting of the limb minimizes pain and decreases spread of the infection by lymphatic channels through the soft tissue. The splint should be removed periodically to allow active use of adjacent joints and prevent stiffening and muscle atrophy. In chronic osteomyelitis, splinting may be necessary to guard against fracture of the weakened bone.

C. Surgical Measures: Aspiration of the metaphysis is a useful diagnostic measure in any case of suspected osteomyelitis. Osteomyelitis represents a collection of pus under pressure within the body. In the first 24–72 hours, it may be possible to abort osteomyelitis by the use of antibiotics alone. However, if frank pus is aspirated from the bone, surgical drainage is indicated. If the infection has not shown a dramatic response within 24 hours in questionable cases, surgical drainage is also indicated. It is important that all devitalized soft tissue be removed and adequate exposure of the bone obtained in order to permit free drainage. Excessive amounts of bone should not be removed when draining acute osteomyelitis, since they may not be completely replaced by the normal healing process.

In questionable cases, little damage has been done by surgical drainage, but failure to drain the pus in acute cases may lead to more severe damage.

Prognosis

When osteomyelitis is diagnosed in the early clinical stages and prompt antibiotic therapy is begun, the prognosis is excellent. If the process has been unattended for a week to 10 days, there is almost always some permanent loss of bone structure, as well as the possibility of growth abnormality.

Jacobs RF et al: Management of *Pseudomonas* osteochondritis complicating puncture wounds of the foot. *Pediatrics* 1982;**69:**432.

Scoles PV, Aronoff SC: Antimicrobial therapy of childhood skeletal infections: Current concepts review. *J Bone Joint Surg* [*Am*] 1984;**66:**1487.

Treves S et al: Osteomyelitis: Early scintigraphic detection in children. *Pediatrics* 1976;**57:**183.

PYOGENIC ARTHRITIS

The source of pyogenic arthritis varies according to the age of the child. In the infant, pyogenic arthritis often develops by spread from adjacent osteomyelitis. In the older child, it presents as an isolated infection, usually without bony involvement. In teenagers with pyogenic arthritis, an underlying systemic disease is usually the cause, eg, an obvious generalized infection or an organism that has an affinity for joints, such as the gonococcus.

In infants, the most common cause of pyogenic arthritis is *Staphylococcus aureus,* although gram-negative organisms may be seen. In children between 4 months and 4 years of age, *Haemophilus influenzae* is a common causative organism.

The initial effusion of the joint rapidly becomes purulent. An effusion of the joint may accompany osteomyelitis in the adjacent bone. A white blood cell count exceeding 100,000/μL in the joint fluid indicates a definite purulent infection. Generally, spread of infection is from the bone into the joint, but unattended pyogenic arthritis may also affect adjacent bone. The sedimentation rate is elevated.

Clinical Findings

A. Symptoms and Signs: In older children, the signs are striking, with fever, malaise, vomiting, and restriction of motion. In infants, paralysis of the limb due to inflammatory neuritis may be evident. Infection of the hip joint in infants can be diagnosed if suspicion is aroused by decreased abduction of the hip in an infant who is irritable or feeding poorly. A history of umbilical catheter treatment in the newborn nursery should alert the physician to the possibility of pyogenic arthritis of the hip.

B. X-Ray Findings: Early distention of the joint capsule is nonspecific and difficult to measure by x-ray. In the infant with unrecognized pyogenic arthritis, dislocation of the joint may follow within a few days as a result of distention of the capsule by pus. Later changes include destruction of the joint space, resorption of epiphyseal cartilage, and erosion of the adjacent bone of the metaphysis.

Treatment

Diagnosis may be made by aspiration of the joint. In the hip joint, pyogenic arthritis is most easily treated by surgical drainage because the joint is deep and difficult to aspirate as well as being inaccessible to thorough cleaning through needle aspiration. In more superficial joints, such as the knee, aspiration of the joint at least twice daily may maintain adequate drainage. If fever and clinical symptoms do not subside within 24 hours after treatment is begun, open surgical drainage is indicated. Antibiotics can be specifically selected based on cultures of the aspirated pus. Before the results of cultures are available, treatment by methicillin and gentamicin will cover the usual etiologic organisms. It is not necessary to give intra-articular antibiotics, since good levels are achieved in the synovial fluid.

Prognosis

The prognosis is excellent if the joint is drained early, before damage to the articular cartilage has occurred. If infection is present for more than 24 hours, there is dissolution of the proteoglycans in the articular cartilage, with subsequent arthrosis and fibrosis of the joint. Damage to the growth plate may also occur, especially within the hip joint, where the epiphyseal plate is intracapsular.

Almquist EE: The changing epidemiology of septic arthritis in children. *Clin Orthop* 1980;**68:**96.

TUBERCULOUS ARTHRITIS

Tuberculous arthritis is now a rare disease in the USA. It must be considered, however, in children with resistant infections of the joints, especially if there is a history of tuberculosis in family members. Generally, the infection may be ruled out by skin testing. The joints most commonly affected in children are the intervertebral disks, resulting in gibbus or dorsal angular deformity at the site of the involvement.

Treatment is by local drainage of the "cold abscess," followed by antituberculosis therapy with isoniazid, rifampin, and ethambutol. Prolonged immobilization in a plaster bed is necessary in order to promote healing. Spinal fusion may be required to preserve stability of the vertebral column.

TRANSIENT SYNOVITIS OF THE HIP

The most common cause of limping and pain in the hip of children in the USA is transitory synovitis, an acute inflammatory reaction that often follows an upper respiratory infection and is generally self-limited. In questionable cases, aspiration of the hip yields only yellowish fluid, ruling out pyogenic arthritis. Generally, however, toxic synovitis of the hip is not associated with elevation of the white blood count or a temperature above 38.3 °C (101 °F). It classically affects children 3–10 years of age and is more common in boys. There is limitation of motion of the hip joint, particularly internal rotation, and x-ray changes are nonspecific, with some swelling apparent in the soft tissues around the joint.

Treatment consists of bed rest and the use of traction with slight flexion of the hip. Aspirin may shorten the course of the disease, although even with no treatment the disease usually is self-limited to a matter of days. It is important to maintain x-ray follow-up, since toxic synovitis may be the precursor of avascular necrosis of the femoral head (see next section) in a small percentage of patients. X-rays can be obtained at 1 month and 3 months, or earlier if there is persistent limp or pain.

Hardinge K: The etiology of transient synovitis of the hip. *J Bone Joint Surg* [*Br*] 1970;**52:**100.

VASCULAR LESIONS & AVASCULAR NECROSIS

AVASCULAR NECROSIS OF THE PROXIMAL FEMUR (Legg-Calvé-Perthes Disease)

The vascular supply of bone is generally precarious, and when it is interrupted, necrosis results. In contrast to other body tissues that undergo infarction, bone removes necrotic tissue and replaces it with living bone in a process called "creeping substitution." This replacement of necrotic bone may be so complete and so perfect that a completely normal bone results. Adequacy of replacement depends upon the age of the patient, the presence or absence of associated infection, congruity of the involved joint, and other physiologic and mechanical factors.

Because of their rapid growth in relation to their blood supply, the secondary ossification centers in the epiphyses are subject to avascular necrosis. The physicians who originally described the avascular lesions of the epiphyses and distinguished them from tuberculosis in the early 20th century were identified with the processes. Despite the number of different names referring to avascular necrosis of the epiphyses, the process is identical, ie, necrosis of bone followed by replacement.

Even though the pathologic and radiologic features of avascular necrosis of the epiphyses are well known, the cause is not generally agreed upon. Necrosis may follow known causes such as trauma or infection, but idiopathic lesions usually develop during periods of rapid growth of the epiphyses. Thus, the highest incidence of Legg-Calvé-Perthes disease is between 4 and 8 years of age.

Clinical Findings

A. Symptoms and Signs: Persistent pain is the most common symptom, and the patient may present with limp or limitation of motion.

B. Laboratory Findings: Laboratory findings, including studies of joint aspirates, are normal.

C. X-Ray Findings: X-ray findings correlate with the progression of the process and the extent of necrosis. The early finding is effusion of the joint associated with slight widening of the joint space and periarticular swelling. Decreased bone density in and around the joint is apparent after a few weeks. The necrotic ossification center appears more dense than the surrounding viable structures, and there is collapse or narrowing of the femoral head.

As replacement of the necrotic ossification center occurs, there is rarefaction of the bone in a patchwork fashion, producing alternating areas of rarefaction and relative density or "fragmentation" of the epiphysis.

In the hip, there may be widening of the femoral head associated with flattening, giving rise to the term **coxa plana.** If infarction has extended across the growth plate, there will be a radiolucent lesion within the metaphysis. If the growth center of the femoral head has been damaged so that normal growth does not occur, varus deformity of the femoral neck will occur as a result of overgrowth of the greater trochanteric apophysis.

Eventually, complete replacement of the epiphysis will become apparent as new bone replaces necrotic bone. The final shape of the head will depend upon the extent of the necrosis and collapse that has been allowed to occur.

Differential Diagnosis

Differential diagnosis must include inflammatory and infectious lesions of the joints or apophyses. Transient synovitis of the hip may be distinguished from Legg-Calvé-Perthes disease by serial x-rays.

Treatment

Treatment consists simply of protection of the joint. If the joint is deeply seated within the acetabulum and normal joint motion is maintained, a reasonably good result can be expected. The hip is held in abduction and internal rotation in order to fulfill this purpose. Braces are generally used. Surgery may be necessary for an uncooperative patient or one whose social or geographic circumstances do not allow use of a brace (living in a house trailer, in an unpaved rural area, etc).

Prognosis

The prognosis for complete replacement of the necrotic femoral head in a child is excellent, but the functional result will depend upon the amount of deformity that develops during the time the softened structure exists. In Legg-Calvé-Perthes disease, the prognosis depends upon the completeness of involvement of the epiphyseal center. In general, patients with metaphyseal defects, those in whom the disease develops late in childhood, and those who have more complete involvement of the femoral head have a poorer prognosis.

Osteochondrosis due to vascular lesion may affect various growth centers. Table 22–1 indicates the common sites and the typical ages at presentation.

Table 22–1. The osteochondroses.

Ossification Center	Eponym	Typical Age
Capital femoral	Legg-Calvé-Perthes disease	3–5
Tarsal navicular	Kohler's disease	6
Second metatarsal head	Freiberg's disease	12–14
Vertebral ring	Scheuermann's disease	13–16
Capitellum	Panner's disease	9–11
Tibial tubercle	Osgood-Schlatter disease	11–13
Calcaneus	Sever's disease	8–9

Calver R et al: Radionuclide scanning in the early diagnosis of Perthes' disease. *J Bone Joint Surg* [*Br*] 1981;**63:**379.
Catterall A: The natural history of Perthes disease. *J Bone Joint Surg* [*Br*] 1971;**53:**37.
McAndrew MP, Weinstein SL: A long-term follow-up of Legg-Calvé-Perthes disease. *J Bone Joint Surg* [*Am*] 1984;**66:**860.

OSTEOCHONDRITIS DISSECANS

In osteochondritis dissecans, there is a pie-shaped necrotic area of bone and cartilage adjacent to the articular surface. The fragment of bone may be broken off from the host bone and displaced into the joint as a loose body. If it remains attached, the necrotic fragment may be completely replaced by creeping substitution.

The pathologic process is precisely the same as that described above for avascular necrosing lesions of ossification centers. However, since these lesions are adjacent to articular cartilage, there may be joint damage.

The most common sites of these lesions are the knee (medial femoral condyle), the elbow joint (capitellum), and the talus (superior lateral dome).

Joint pain is the usual presenting complaint. However, local swelling or locking may be present, particularly if there is a fragment free in the joint. Laboratory studies are normal.

Treatment consists of protection of the involved area from mechanical damage. If there is a fragment free within the joint as a loose body, it must be surgically removed. For some marginal lesions, it may be worthwhile to drill the necrotic fragment in order to encourage more rapid vascular ingrowth and replacement. If large areas of a weight-bearing joint are involved, secondary degenerative arthritis may result.

Hughston JC, Hergenroeder PT, Courtenay BG: Osteochondritis dissecans of the femoral condyles. *J Bone Joint Surg* [*Am*] 1984;**66:**1340.

NEUROLOGIC DISORDERS INVOLVING THE MUSCULOSKELETAL SYSTEM

ORTHOPEDIC ASPECTS OF POLIOMYELITIS

Muscle Recovery

In paralytic poliomyelitis, it may not be possible for the complete pattern of anterior horn cell destruction to be determined in the initial stages, but some generalizations can be made:

(1) "Spotty" paralysis in a number of extremities has a good prognosis.

(2) A completely flail extremity will probably never show a significant functional recovery.

(3) Early muscle recovery is a good prognostic sign, with probable full functional recovery to be expected.

(4) Muscle recovery cannot be expected after 18 months from the time of onset.

(5) Muscle recovery must be steady and continuous. If a "plateau" is reached and maintained for 3 months, no further recovery of the muscle may be anticipated.

(6) Muscle "substitution" may produce functional improvement long after the first 18 months following the acute infection. Such muscle substitution may be functionally beneficial or may produce deformity due to unbalanced muscle power.

Reconstructive Procedures

Reconstructive orthopedic procedures may be directed at dividing restricting fascial contractures, transferring musculotendinous units for better balance of motor power, corrective osteotomies for bony angulation deformities, and various procedures to equalize leg length discrepancy. Procedures used to treat such lower motor neuron paralyses cover the entire range of operative orthopedics.

ORTHOPEDIC ASPECTS OF CEREBRAL PALSY

Early physical therapy to encourage completion of the normal developmental patterns may be of benefit in patients with cerebral palsy. The greatest gains from this type of therapy are obtained during the first few years of life, and therapy should not be continued with unrealistic goals when no improvement is apparent.

Bracing and splinting are of questionable benefit, although night splints may be useful in preventing equinus deformity of the feet or adduction contractures of the hips. Orthopedic surgery can offer procedures to weaken hyperactive spastic muscles, to transfer function of deforming spastic muscles, or to stabilize joints. In general, muscle transfers are unpredictable in cerebral palsy, and most orthopedic procedures are directed at weakening deforming forces or bony stabilization by osteotomy or arthrodesis.

Flexion and adduction of the hip due to hyperactivity of the adductors and flexors may produce a progressive paralytic dislocation of the hip. Congenital dislocation of the hip is unusual in cerebral palsy, but in more severely involved children, paralytic dislocation can lead to pain and dysfunction. Treatment of the dislocation once it has occurred is difficult and unsatisfactory. The principal preventive measure is abduction bracing, but this must often be supplemented by release of the adductors or hip flexors in order to prevent dislocation. In severe cases, osteotomy of the femur may also be necessary to correct the bony deformities of femoral anteversion and coxa valga that are invariably present.

Patients with predominantly an athetotic pattern are poor candidates for any surgical procedure or bracing. Neurosurgical procedures may be of some help.

Because it is difficult to predict the outcome of surgical procedures in cerebral palsy, the surgeon must examine patients on several occasions before any operative procedure is undertaken. Follow-up care by a physical therapist to maximize the anticipated long-term gains should be arranged before the operation.

Bleck EE: *Orthopaedic Management of Cerebral Palsy*. Saunders, 1979.

Eng GD, Koch B, Smokvina M: Brachial plexus palsy in neonates and children. *Arch Phys Med Rehabil* 1978;**59:**458.

Samilson RL: *Orthopaedic Aspects of Cerebral Palsy*. Lippincott, 1975.

ORTHOPEDIC ASPECTS OF MYELODYSPLASIA

Patients born with spina bifida cystica (aperta) should be examined early by an orthopedic surgeon. The level of neurologic involvement determines the imbalance of muscular force that will be present and apt to produce deformity with growth. The involvement is often asymmetric and tends to change during the first 12–18 months of life. Early closure of the sac is the rule, although there has been some hesitancy to treat all of these patients because of the extremely poor prognosis associated with congenital hydrocephalus, high levels of paralysis, and associated congenital anomalies. Associated musculoskeletal problems may include clubfoot, congenital dislocation of the hip, arthrogryposis type changes of the lower extremities, and congenital scoliosis, among others. The most common lesions are at the level of L3–4 and tend to affect the hip joint, with progressive dislocation occurring during growth. Foot deformities may be in any direction and are complicated by the fact that sensation is generally absent. Spinal deformities develop in a high percentage of these children, with scoliosis being present in approximately 40%. Ambulation is impossible without braces or splints, and careful urologic follow-up must be obtained to prevent complications from incontinence. A high percentage of these children have hydrocephalus, which may be evident at birth or shortly thereafter, requiring shunting. The shunts are sources of infection and may require frequent replacement.

In children who have a reasonable likelihood of walking, operative treatment consists of reduction of the hip and alignment of the feet in the weight-bearing position as well as stabilization of the vertebral scoliosis. In children who do not have extension power of the knee, ie, those who lack active quadriceps function, the likelihood of ambulation is greatly decreased. In such patients, aggressive surgery in the hip region may result in stiffening of the joints, thus preventing sitting. Multiple foot operations are also contraindicated in these children.

The overall management of the child with spina bifida should be coordinated in a multidiscipline clinic where all doctors working in cooperation with each other can work also with therapists, social workers, and teachers to provide the best possible care.

Lorber J: Spina bifida cystica: Results of 270 consecutive cases with criteria for selection for the future. *Arch Dis Child* 1972;**47:**854.

Menelaus MB: *The Orthopaedic Management of Spina Bifida Cystica,* 2nd ed. Churchill Livingstone, 1980.

Ramsey PL, Huff CW: Spina bifida: Ambulatory function and related hip problems. *J Bone Joint Surg* [*Am*] 1976;**58:**735.

NEOPLASIA OF THE MUSCULOSKELETAL SYSTEM

Neoplastic diseases of the mesodermal tissues constitute a very serious problem because of the poor prognosis of malignant tumors in these areas. Few of the benign lesions undergo malignant transformation, and it is important to establish a proper diagnosis and thus avoid undertreatment or overtreatment. The diagnosis depends upon correlation of the clinical, x-ray, and microscopic findings (Tables 22–2 to 22–6).

Table 22–2. Differentiating features of carcinoma and sarcoma.

	Carcinoma	Sarcoma
Tissue origin	Epithelial	Mesodermal
Age incidence	Middle age	Youth
Metastases	Regional nodes	Lungs
Radiation sensitivity	Sensitive. Some cures.	Resistant
Susceptibility to chemotherapeutic agents	Some specific drug sensitivities	More resistant
Prognosis	Variable	Poor

Table 22–3. Benign neoplasms: Osseous.

Disease	Clinical Features	X-Ray Features	Treatment	Prognosis
Osteocartilaginous exostosis (osteochondroma)	Pain-free mass. (Pain, if present, is due to super-imposed bursitis.) Single or multiple. Bone mass capped with cartilage. Masses enlarge during childhood and adolescence.	Metaphyseal position. Pedunculated or sessile. Cortex of host bone "turned out" into the lesion. Cartilage cap may be calcified. Long bones predominate.	Surgical excision if symptomatic, if lesion interferes with function, or enlarging mass in adult life.	Excellent. Malignant transformation is rare.
Osteoid osteoma	Pain with point tenderness. Night pain common. Pain often relieved by aspirin.	Radiolucent central nidus (about 1 cm in diameter) surrounded by spectacular osteosclerosis. Sclerosis may obscure nidus.	Surgical excision of nidus.	Excellent. No known malignant transformation.
Osteoblastoma (giant osteoid osteoma)	Pain similar to that of osteoid osteoma.	Nidus larger than 1 cm. Osteolytic phase may predominate.	Surgical excision.	Excellent.

Table 22–4. Benign neoplasms: Cartilaginous.

Disease	Clinical Features	X-Ray Features	Treatment	Prognosis
Chondroma	Usually silent lesions. Pain may be present. Pathologic fracture may occur.	Radiolucent lesions. Long bones predominate. Most common lesion of phalanges and metacarpals or metatarsals. Calcification may be present centrally. Little or no host reaction.	Surgical excision or curettage.	Excellent. Malignant transformation of chondromas of major bones occurs rarely in childhood.
Chondroblastoma (Codman's tumor)	Pain about a joint. Pathologic fracture may occur.	Radiolucent lesion of ossification center of child or adolescent. Occasionally perforates epiphyseal cartilage. Rarely calcification. Little or no reactive bone formation.	Surgical excision or curettage.	Excellent. No known malignant transformation.
Chondromyxofibroma	Usually silent lesion. Mass may be the presenting feature. Pathologic fracture may occur.	Long bones predominate (tibia, fibula, femur, humerus). Radiolucent lesion, may enlarge the host bone. Usually metaphyseal, linearly oriented. Usually well encapsulated.	Surgical excision or curettage.	Good. Lesion may recur after local excision.

In general, neoplasms of the mesodermal tissues are named according to the tissue produced (eg, osteosarcoma is one producing bone). However, because of the varied potentiality of mesodermal cells, several types of tissue may be present within the same tumor. This has resulted in confusion of nomenclature, with some tumors being given a bewildering combination of names. It has also resulted in a number of misdiagnoses, since a specimen from a single area may not represent tissue typical of the entire tumor. In addition, some of the tumors are so primitive that they rarely produce any recognizable type of adult tissue.

Biopsy is necessary for definitive diagnosis. Complications from biopsy are far outweighed by the advantages of correct diagnosis.

Ippolito E, Farsetti P, Tudisco C: Vertebra plana: Long-term follow-up in five patients. *J Bone Joint Surg* [*Am*] 1984;**66:**1364.

Jaffe N, Pochedly C, Miller D: *Bone Tumors in Children.* PSG, 1979.

Shapiro F, Simon F, Glimcher MJ: Hereditary multiple exostoses: Anthropometric, roentgenographic and clinical aspects. *J Bone Joint Surg* [*Am*] 1979;**61:**815.

Table 22–5. Benign neoplasms: Fibrous.

Disease	Clinical Features	X-Ray Features	Treatment	Prognosis
Nonossifying fibroma (benign cortical defect; benign metaphyseal defect)	Usually silent lesion. Rarely, pathologic fracture.	Radiolucent lesion. Metaphyseal location, linearly oriented. Eccentric position. Thin sclerotic border about lesion. May be multiple lesions.	No treatment needed. Lesions heal with time and growth.	Excellent.
Giant cell tumor	Extremely rare in children.	Radiolucent lesions.	Surgical excision or curettage.	Good. Malignant transformation rare. May undergo change to fibrosarcoma.

Table 22–6. Malignant neoplasms.

Disease	Clinical Features	X-Ray Features	Treatment	Prognosis
Osteosarcoma and chondrosarcoma	Pain the most common symptom. Mass, functional loss, limp occasionally present. Pathologic fracture common.	Destructive, expanding, invasive lesion. Minimal host reaction, but, if present, usually is a triangle between tumor, elevated periosteum, and cortex. Usually radiolucent, but lesional tissue may show ossification or calcification. Metaphyseal location common. Femur, tibia, humerus, and other long bones predominate.	Surgical excision or amputation. Radiation-resistant. Markedly improved prognosis (50–70%) results from use of surgery combined with doxorubicin and methotrexate in osteosarcoma. (See Chapter 31.)	Poor. Probably less than 5 or 10% cured. Metastases to lungs, occasionally to other bones. Life expectancy has been prolonged by use of chemotherapy.
Fibrosarcoma	Rare lesions in children.	Radiolucent, destructive, expanding, invasive lesion. Little or no host reaction. Long bones predominate.	Surgical excision or amputation.	Poor. Probably 10–15% cured. Metastases to lungs.
Ewing's tumor	Pain very common. Tenderness, fever, and leukocytosis also common. Frequent pathologic fracture. Frequently multicentric.	Radiolucent, destructive lesion, frequently in diaphyseal region of the bone. May be reactive bone formation about the lesion in successive layers—"onion skin" layering.	Radiation-sensitive but not curable. Surgical excision usually not desirable because of multiple areas of involvement. Chemotherapy by vincristine, doxorubicin, and cyclophosphamide.	Poor. Metastases to multiple organs.

MISCELLANEOUS DISEASES OF BONE

FIBROUS DYSPLASIA

Dysplastic fibrous tissue replacement of the medullary canal is accompanied by the formation of metaplastic bone in fibrous dysplasia. Three forms of the disease are recognized: monostotic, polyostotic, and polyostotic with endocrine disturbances (precocious puberty in females, hyperthyroidism, and hyperadrenalism, ie, Albright's syndrome).

Clinical Findings

A. Symptoms and Signs: The lesion or lesions may be asymptomatic. Pain, if present, is probably due to pathologic fractures. In females, endocrine disturbances may be present in the polyostotic variety and associated with café au lait spots.

B. Laboratory Findings: Laboratory findings are normal unless endocrine disturbances are present, in which case there may be increased secretion of gonadotropic, thyroid, or adrenal hormones.

C. X-Ray Findings: The lesion begins centrally within the medullary canal, usually of a long bone, and expands slowly. Pathologic fracture may occur. If metaplastic bone predominates, the contents of the lesion will be of the density of bone. Marked deformity of the bone may result, and a shepherd's crook deformity of the upper femur is a classic feature of the disease. The disease is often asymmetric, and limb length disturbances may occur as a result of stimulation of epiphyseal cartilage growth.

Differential Diagnosis

The differential diagnosis may include other fibrous lesions of bone as well as destructive lesions such as bone cyst, eosinophilic granuloma, aneurysmal bone cyst, nonossifying fibroma, enchondroma, and chondromyxoid fibroma.

Treatment

If the lesion is small and asymptomatic, no treatment is needed. If the lesion is large and produces or threatens pathologic fracture, curettage and bone grafting are indicated.

Prognosis

Unless the lesions impair epiphyseal growth, the prognosis is good. Lesions tend to enlarge during the growth period but are stable during adult life. Malignant transformation has not been recorded.

UNICAMERAL BONE CYST

Unicameral bone cyst appears in the metaphysis of a long bone, usually in the femur or humerus. It begins within the medullary canal adjacent to the epiphyseal cartilage. It probably results from some fault in enchondral ossification. The cyst is "active" as long as it abuts onto the metaphyseal side of the epiphyseal cartilage and "inactive" when a border of normal bone exists between the cyst and the epiphyseal cartilage. The lesion is usually identified when a pathologic fracture occurs, producing pain. Laboratory findings are normal. On x-rays, the cyst is identified centrally within the medullary canal, producing expansion of the cortex and thinning over the widest portion of the cyst.

Treatment consists of curettage of the cyst if it is producing pain. The cyst may heal after a fracture and not require treatment. Curettage should be delayed if surgery would risk damage to the adjacent growth plate. In such cases, methylprednisolone injection may be curative.

The prognosis is excellent. Many cysts will heal following pathologic fracture.

Scaglietti O: The effect of methylprednisolone acetate in the treatment of bone cysts. *J Bone Joint Surg* [*Br*] 1979;**61**:200.

ANEURYSMAL BONE CYST

Aneurysmal bone cyst is similar to unicameral bone cyst, but it contains blood rather than clear fluid. It usually occurs in a slightly eccentric position in the long bone, expanding the cortex of the bone but not breaking the cortex, although some extraosseous mass may be produced. On x-rays, the lesion appears somewhat larger than the width of the epiphyseal cartilage, and this feature distinguishes it from unicameral bone cyst.

The aneurysmal bone cyst is filled by large vascular lakes, and the stoma of the cyst contains fibrous tissue and areas of metaplastic ossification.

The lesion may appear quite aggressive histologically, and it is important to differentiate it from osteosarcoma or hemangioma. Treatment is by curettage and bone grafting, and the prognosis is excellent.

INFANTILE CORTICAL HYPEROSTOSIS (Caffey's Syndrome)

Infantile cortical hyperostosis is a benign disease of unknown cause that has its onset before 6 months of age and is characterized by irritability, fever, and nonsuppurating, tender, painful swellings. Swellings may involve almost any bone of the body and are frequently widespread. Classically, there are swellings of the mandible and clavicle in 50% of cases as well as of the ulna, humerus, and ribs. The disease is limited to the shafts of bones and does not involve subcutaneous tissues or joints. It is self-limited but may persist for weeks or months. Anemia, leukocytosis, an increased sedimentation rate, and elevation of the serum alkaline phosphatase are usually present. Cortical hyperostosis is demonstrable by a typical x-ray appearance and may be diagnosed on physical examination by an experienced pediatrician.

Fortunately, the disease appears to be decreasing in frequency. Corticosteroids are effective in severe cases.

The prognosis is good, and the disease usually terminates without deformity.

GANGLION

A ganglion is a smooth, small cystic mass connected by a pedicle to the joint capsule, usually on the dorsum of the wrist. It may also be seen in the tendon sheath over the flexor surfaces of the fingers. These ganglions can be excised if they interfere with function or cause persistent pain.

BAKER'S CYST

Baker's cyst is a herniation of the synovium in the knee joint into the popliteal region. In children, the diagnosis may be made by aspiration of mucinous fluid, but the cyst nearly always disappears with time. Whereas Baker's cysts may be indicative of intra-articular disease in the adult, they usually are of no clinical significance in children and rarely require excision.

Dinham JM: Popliteal cysts in children: The case against surgery. *J Bone Joint Surg* [*Br*] 1975;**57:**69.

SELECTED REFERENCES

Coleman SS: *Congenital Dysplasia and Dislocation of the Hip*. Mosby, 1978.

Drennan JC: *Orthopaedic Management of Neuromuscular Disorders*. Lippincott, 1983.

Lovell WW, Winter RB (editors): *Pediatric Orthopaedics*. Lippincott, 1978.

Menelaus M: *The Orthopaedic Management of Spina Bifida Cystica,* 2nd ed. Churchill Livingstone, 1980.

Ogden JA: *Skeletal Injury in the Child*. Lea & Febiger, 1982.

Rang M: *Children's Fractures,* 2nd ed. Lippincott, 1983.

Rockwood CA Jr, Wilkins KE, King RE (editors): *Fractures in Children*. Lippincott, 1984.

Sharrard WJW: *Paediatric Orthopaedics and Fractures,* 2nd ed. Blackwell, 1979.

Smith DW: *Recognizable Patterns of Human Malformation,* 3rd ed. Saunders, 1982.

Tachdjian MO: *The Child's Foot*. Saunders, 1985.

Tachdjian MO: *Pediatric Orthopedics*. Saunders, 1972.

Weber BG, Brunner CH, Freuler F (editors): *Treatment of Fractures in Children and Adolescents*. Springer-Verlag, 1980.

Winter RB: *Congenital Deformities of the Spine*. Thieme-Stratton, 1983.

Neurologic & Muscular Disorders

23

Gerhard Nellhaus, MD, David A. Stumpf, MD, PhD, & Paul G. Moe, MD

NEUROLOGIC ASSESSMENT & NEURODIAGNOSTIC PROCEDURES

NEUROLOGIC HISTORY & EXAMINATION

In obtaining the history of a neurologic disorder in an infant or child, much depends on the health care professional's expertise in interviewing and ability to communicate at the level and to the degree of sophistication of the patient and parents. Even the intelligent 3- to 4-year-old may provide helpful data if the health care professional is able to translate medical terminology into language the child understands.

The history should include information about perinatal events, with emphasis on the mother's health; nutrition; and use of medications, cigarettes, alcohol, or recreational drugs during pregnancy. A family history of genetic disorders should be elicited and additional information obtained from relatives if a genetic disorder is suspected. Available health records should be examined.

A systems review with emphasis on neuromuscular deficits may offer clues to the cause of the neurologic disorder. Aspects of the neurologic examination are described in Chapters 1, 2, and 7 and are outlined in detail by Paine and Oppe (see reference, below). Parts of the neurologic examination may need to be performed more than once to be certain of the accuracy of findings.

Considerable information about the behavior and neuromuscular function of an infant or child may be obtained during history taking by observing the child's alertness and curiosity, trust or apprehension, facial and eye movements, limb function, body posture and balance, etc. Frequent, gentle, casual touching of the infant or young child during the interview will help prepare the young patient for examination, as will letting the child play with the stethoscope, percussion hammer, or toys and items that may be used in developmental and neurologic testing. During examination, the infant or small child may be held in the parent's lap; this and the examiner's nearly constant eye contact with the child and soft measured pattern of talk will provide reassurance. To elicit the tendon reflexes of an infant or small child, the examiner's first and middle fingers can be used. A small cracker, jelly bean, or shiny penny may be used to test for reach, hand preference, and ability to maintain balance when picking up the object from a napkin on the floor. Much of the neurologic examination can be accomplished through play; it can and should be fun for the patient.

Although funduscopic examination is not always essential, it is frequently necessary in the neurologic evaluation. Mydriatic agents should generally *not* be used when pupillary reactions and size must be monitored closely (eg, in cases of possible brain swelling and herniation). If a mydriatic agent is used, pupillary reactions should be checked before it is instilled. The agent should be instilled at the beginning of the interview (to allow time for the patient to become calm while the evaluation proceeds) and the funduscopic evaluation deferred to the end of the neurologic examination. Adequate views of the fundi can often be obtained in semidarkness by having the child sit in someone's lap while another person directs the source of light and also makes a noise. Visual fields by confrontation or the threat maneuver, with the examiner's hand inside a puppet, may take repeated checking.

Depending on the child's age and ability to communicate, sensory testing may be limited to gross appreciation of touch, vibration, or a mildly painful, hidden stimulus (eg, a pin cupped in the examiner's hand).

Paine RS, Oppe TE: *Neurological Examination of Children.* Vols 20 and 21 of: *Clinics in Developmental Medicine.* Lippincott, 1966.

LUMBAR PUNCTURE

The principal purpose of lumbar puncture is to obtain an aliquot of cerebrospinal fluid for the diagnosis of infectious and inflammatory conditions of the central nervous system (Table 23–1). The uses of cerebrospinal fluid specimens in cytologic studies, bioassays of enzymes and neurotransmitters, and specific immunofluorescent staining tests for viruses are widening the clinical (and research) applicability of

Table 23–1. Characteristics of cerebrospinal fluid (CSF) in the normal child and in central nervous system infections and inflammatory conditions.

Condition	Initial Pressure (mm H_2O)	Appearance	Cells/μL	Protein (mg/dL)	Glucose (mg/dL)	Other Tests	Comments
Normal	< 180	Clear	0–5 lymphocytes. First 3 months, 1–3 PMNs. Neonates, up to 30 lymphocytes, 20–50 RBCs.	15–35 (lumbar). 5–15 (ventricular). Up to 150 (lumbar) for short time after birth; to 6 months, up to 65.	50–80 (two-thirds of blood glucose). May be increased after seizure.	CSF IgG index: < 0.7 units = CSF IgG/Serum IgG / CSF albumin/Serum albumin. Lactate dehydrogenase (LDH), 2–27 IU/L.	CSF protein in first month may be up to 170 mg/dL in small-for-dates or premature infants. No increase in WBCs due to seizure.
Bloody tap	Normal or low	Bloody (sometimes with clot)	One additional WBC/700 RBCs.	One additional mg/800 RBCs.	Normal		Spin down fluid; supernatant will be clear and colorless.
Bacterial meningitis, acute	200–750+	Opalescent to purulent	Up to 1000s, mostly PMNs. Early, few cells	Up to 100s.	Decreased; may be none.	Smear and culture mandatory. LDH > 24 IU/L.	Very early, glucose may be normal. Immunofluorescence tests.
Bacterial meningitis, partially treated	Usually increased	Clear or opalescent	Usually increased. PMNs usually predominate.	Elevated	Normal or decreased	LDH usually > 24 IU/L.	Smear and culture often negative.
Tuberculous meningitis	150–750+	Opalescent; fibrin web or pellicle	250–500, mostly lymphocytes. Early, more PMNs.	45–500; parallels cell count.	Decreased; may be none.	Smear for acid-fast organism; CSF culture and inoculation.	***Note:*** Bacterial meningitis may be superimposed.
Fungal meningitis	Increased	Variable; often clear	10–500. Early, more PMNs; then mostly lymphocytes.	Elevated and increasing.	Decreased	India ink preparations, culture inoculations, immunofluorescence tests.	Often superimposed in patients who are debilitated or on immunosuppressive or tumor therapy.
Aseptic meningoencephalitides	Normal or slightly increased	Clear unless cell count > 300	0 to few hundred, mostly lymphocytes; PMNs predominate early.	20–125	Normal; may be low in mumps.	CSF, stool, throat wash for viral cultures. LDH < 28 IU/L (90% < 24 IU/L).	Acute and convalescent antibody titers. In mumps, up to 1000 lymphocytes; serum amylase often elevated.
Neurosyphilis	Normal to 400	Clear unless protein is very high	10–100, mostly lymphocytes.	25–150; higher in meningitis.	Normal	Positive CSF serology. CSF IgG index increased.	Blood serology positive in untreated cases; *Treponema pallidum* immobilization test positive.
Parainfectious encephalomyelitis	80–450, usually increased	Usually clear	0–50, mostly lymphocytes.	15–75	Normal	CSF IgG index may be increased. Oligoclonal bands absent.	No organisms. Fulminant cases resemble bacterial meningitis.
Acute poliomyelitis	Usually normal	Clear or slightly opalescent	20–500+. Early, more PMNs; then mostly lymphocytes.	Normal to 150; often progressive increase.	Normal		Stool virus and serum antibody studies.
Polyneuritis Early	Normal and occasionally increased	Normal	Normal; occasionally slight increase.	Normal	Normal	Bacterial cultures negative; gamma globulin may be elevated.	Try to find cause (viral infections, toxins, lupus, infectious mononucleosis, diabetes, etc).
Late		Xanthochromic if protein high		45–1500			
Meningeal carcinomatosis	Often elevated	Clear to opalescent	Cytologic identification of tumor cells.	Often mildly to moderately elevated.	Often depressed		Seen with leukemia, medulloblastoma, meningeal melanosis, histiocytosis X. ***Note:*** May mimic meningitis.
Brain abscess	Normal or increased	Usually clear	5–500 in 80%; mostly PMNs.	Usually slightly increased.	Normal; occasionally decreased.		Cell count related to proximity to meninges; findings as in purulent meningitis if abscess perforates.

lumbar puncture. However, performing lumbar puncture for manometric determinations, cellular content, and protein levels in many conditions—including head injuries, brain and spinal cord tumors, and seizure disorders—has been superseded by the use of brain imaging and biochemical techniques that are far more specific.

Therapeutically, lumbar puncture may be employed for drainage of cerebrospinal fluid to reduce its hematotoxic effects in hemorrhagic conditions (eg, intraventricular hemorrhage in newborns, brain stem aneurysm) and to lower intracranial pressure in pseudotumor cerebri.

Lumbar puncture is usually performed with the patient in the lateral recumbent or decubitus position. Entry is at the level of the iliac crest or the L3–4 interspace, with the patient's head initially flexed and then extended. In small infants—especially premature infants and neonates in the first few months of life—lumbar puncture is more safely and satisfactorily performed with the infant in the sitting position and the head only slightly flexed or supported with a pillow propped between the outstretched arms and legs and resting against the infant's chest and abdomen. The wrists and ankles should be held by an assisting nurse, and the needle should be pointed slightly cephalad.

Note: Before lumbar puncture is performed, the fundi should always be checked for papilledema. Lumbar puncture is contraindicated in the presence of elevated intracranial pressure, especially when there are focal neurologic deficits, because of the risk of tentorial or tonsillar herniation. This risk is less likely when there is diffuse cerebral swelling than when elevated pressure is due to a mass lesion. Therefore, if equipment for CT brain scanning is readily available, lumbar puncture should usually be delayed until a scan can be done; it should not be delayed, however, if examination of cerebrospinal fluids is indispensable for diagnosis *and* vital therapeutic intervention.

Lumbar puncture must be performed promptly when a diffuse central nervous system infection (meningitis, meningoencephalitis, encephalitis, cerebritis) *is suspected.* Only a small-gauge needle should be used, and only enough fluid should be withdrawn to permit cell count, protein and glucose determination, and such stains and cultures (bacterial, fungal, viral) and other studies as may be helpful. A specimen of 2–3 mL is usually adequate for microchemical determinations.

It is important to obtain opening and closing cerebrospinal fluid pressures, if possible. To obtain valid pressure readings, the head, neck, and legs should gently be brought into a straight line. It may not be possible to obtain satisfactory pressures if the patient is sitting or if a small-gauge needle is used.

Craigmile TK, Welch K: Lumbar puncture and analysis of cerebrospinal fluid. Chapter 10 in: *Neurological Surgery.* Youmans J (editor). Saunders, 1973.

Cutler RWP, Spertel RB: Cerebrospinal fluid: A selective review. *Ann Neurol* 1982;**11:**1.

Gleason CA et al: Optimal position for a spinal tap in preterm infants. *Pediatrics* 1983;**71:**31.

ELECTROENCEPHALOGRAPHY

This widely used, noninvasive electrophysiologic method for recording cerebral activity has its most distinct clinical applicability in the study of seizure disorders. "Activation" techniques to accentuate abnormalities or disclose latent abnormalities include photic stimulation, well-sustained hyperventilation for 3 minutes, and depriving the patient of sleep from about midnight until after breakfast, at which time the EEG is recorded. The latter is an excellent though less widely employed "activation" method.

Electroencephalography is also used in the evaluation of tumors, cerebrovascular accidents, neurodegenerative diseases, and other neurologic disorders causing brain dysfunction; but, with some notable exceptions, it is nonspecific. Recordings over a 24-hour period or all-night recordings are invaluable in the diagnosis of sleep disturbances and narcolepsy. Electroencephalography with telemetry or simultaneous monitoring of behavior on videotape, although limited by cost to a relatively few laboratories, has great usefulness in selected cases. The EEG can be helpful in determining a possible cause or mechanism of coma and is frequently used to determine if coma is irreversible and brain death has occurred.

The limitations of electroencephalography are considerable, and results are often misinterpreted. In most cases, the duration of the actual tracing is only about 30 minutes, which is a very small fraction of the brain's overall activity. Many drugs—especially barbiturates, benzodiazepines, and most of those used in psychiatry—and "functional" disturbances have considerable effects on the EEG. About 15% of normal (nonepileptic) individuals, especially children, may show some paroxysmal activity on EEG. Electroencephalographic findings such as those seen in migraine, learning disabilities, or behavior disorders do not reflect permanent "brain damage." In fact, one of the very useful applications of the EEG is to show "normalization" as behavior disorders are relieved and certain seizure disorders are controlled by anticonvulsant drugs.

At present, use of CT scans, evoked potentials, positron emission tomography, regional cerebral blood flow studies, and magnetic resonance imaging has replaced the use of electroencephalography as a diagnostic and prognostic tool. The technique of brain electrical activity mapping has now become clinically practical. Using computerized "spectral" electroencephalographic analysis to objectify electroencephalographic readouts may enhance the clinical usefulness of the EEG.

Lewis DV, Freeman JM: The electroencephalogram in pediatric practice: Its use and abuse. *Pediatrics* 1977;**60:**324.

EVOKED POTENTIALS

Cortical auditory, visual, or somatosensory evoked potentials (evoked responses) may be recorded from the scalp surface over the temporal, occipital, or frontoparietal cortex after repetitive stimulation of the retina by light flashes, of the cochlea by sounds, or of the skin by galvanic stimuli of varying frequency and intensity, respectively. Computer averaging is used to recognize and enhance these responses while subtracting or suppressing the asynchronous background electroencephalographic activity. The presence or absence of evoked potential waves and their latencies (time from stimulus to wave peak or time between peaks) figure in the clinical interpretation.

The reproducible and quantifiable results obtained from brain stem auditory, pattern-shift visual, and short-latency somatosensory evoked potentials (see below) indicate the level of function of the relevant sensory pathway or system and indicate the site of anatomic disruption. While results of these tests alone are usually not diagnostic, the tests are noninvasive, sensitive, objective, and relatively inexpensive extensions of the clinical neurologic examination. Since the auditory and somatosensory tests and one type of visual test are totally passive, requiring only that the patient remain still, they are particularly useful in the evaluation of functions in neonates and small children as well as in patients unable to cooperate (eg, due to mental retardation, degenerative disorder, anesthesia, or coma). Knowledge of normal values and experience in testing of the applicable patient group are mandatory.

Brain Stem Auditory Evoked Potentials

A brief auditory stimulus (click) of varying intensity and frequency is delivered to the ear to activate the auditory nerve (nerve VIII) and sequentially activate the cochlear nucleus, tracts and nuclei of the lateral lemniscus, and inferior colliculus. Thus, this technique assesses hearing and function of the brain stem auditory tracts.

Hearing in the neonate or uncooperative (but sedated) patient can be objectively assessed, making the technique particularly useful in high-risk infants, especially those in intensive care nurseries, and in retarded and autistic patients. Brain stem auditory evoked potentials are used to judge brain stem dysfunction in sleep apnea and in "near miss" for sudden infant death syndrome. As high doses of anesthetic agents or barbiturates do not seriously affect results, the test is used to assess and monitor brain stem function of patients during surgery (in the operating room) and those in hypoxic-ischemic coma or coma following head injury. Absence of evoked potential waves beyond the first wave from the auditory nerve usually portends brain death. Brain stem auditory evoked potentials are also useful in the early evaluation of diseases affecting myelin—ie, the various leukodystrophies and multiple sclerosis (although auditory evoked potentials are less valuable than visual evoked potentials in the latter)—and in intrinsic brain stem gliomas. They are sometimes useful in evaluation of hereditary ataxias, Wilson's disease (hepatolenticular degeneration), and other degenerative disorders affecting the brain stem.

Pattern-Shift Visual Evoked Potentials

The preferred stimulus is a shift (reversal) of a checkerboard pattern, and the response is a single wave (called P100) generated in the striate and parastriate visual cortex. The absolute latency of P100 (time from stimulus to wave peak) and the difference in latency between the 2 eyes are sensitive indicators of disease. The amplitude of response is affected by any process resulting in poor fixation on the stimulus screen or affecting visual acuity. Ability to focus on a checkerboard pattern is thus necessary to evaluate visual acuity. (A bright flash visual evoked potential can be used in younger and uncooperative children, but the norms are less standardized.) Evoked potentials suggest that visual acuity may be 20/20 in infants by 6–7 months of age.

Clinical application of the test includes detection and monitoring of strabismus (ie, in amblyopia ex anopsia), optic neuritis, and lesions near the optic nerve and chiasm such as optic gliomas and craniopharyngiomas. Degenerative and immunologic diseases that affect visual transmission and may be detected early and followed by serial evaluations by this technique include adrenoleukodystrophy, Pelizaeus-Merzbacher disease, some spinocerebellar degenerations, sarcoidosis, and even multiple sclerosis. Flash visual evoked potentials are used to monitor function during surgery involving the eyes and optic nerve; to assess cortical or hysterical blindness; and to evaluate patients with photosensitive epilepsy, who may have exaggerated responses.

Short-Latency Somatosensory Evoked Potentials

Responses are commonly produced by electrical stimulation of peripheral sensory nerves, as this evokes potentials of greatest amplitude and clarity; finger tapping and muscle stretching may also be used. The function of this test is similar to that of the auditory test in closely correlating wave forms with function of the sensory pathways and permitting localization of conduction defects.

Short-latency somatosensory evoked potentials are used in the assessment of a wide variety of lesions of the peripheral nerve, root, spinal cord, and central nervous system following trauma, neuropathies (eg, in diabetes mellitus or Landry-Guillian-Barré syndrome), myelodysplasias, cerebral palsy, and many other disorders. The test procedure is often performed on an outpatient basis. One method is to stimulate the median nerve at the wrist with small (nonpainful) electrical shocks and record responses from the brachial plexus above the clavicle, the neck (cervical cord), and the opposite scalp area overlying the sensorimotor cortex. After stimulation from the knee (peroneal nerve) or ankle (tibial nerve), impulses are recorded from the lower lumbar spinal cord, cervical cord, and sensorimotor cortex. Such potentials are used to monitor spinal cord sensory functioning during surgery for disorders including scoliosis, myelodysplasias, and tumors and other lesions of the spinal cord or blood vessels supplying the cord. The technique is also used in leukodystrophies involving peripheral nerves, in multiple sclerosis, and in hysteria and malingering (anesthetic limbs). In the diagnosis of coma and brain death, somatosensory evoked potentials supplement the results of auditory evoked potentials.

Chiappa KH, Ropper AH: Evoked potentials in clinical medicine. (2 parts.) *N Engl J Med* 1982;**306:**1140, 1205.

Engler GL et al: Short-latency somatosensory evoked potentials during Harrington instrumentation for scoliosis. *J Bone Joint Surg [Am]* 1978;**60:**528.

Gupta PR, Dorfman LJ: Short-latency evoked potentials in diabetes. *Neurology* 1981;**31:**841.

Hecox KE, Cone B, Blaw ME: Brain stem auditory evoked response in the diagnosis of pediatric neurologic disease. *Neurology* 1981;**31:**832.

Rowe MJ III: The brain stem auditory evoked response in neurological disease: A review. *Ear Hear* 1981;**2:**41.

Shuhrocki F et al: Pattern-shift evoked responses: Two hundred patients with optic neuritis and/or multiple sclerosis. *Arch Neurol* 1978;**35:**65.

Sokol S: Infant visual development: Visual evoked potential estimates. *Ann NY Acad Sci* 1982;**388:**514.

Stockard J: Brain stem auditory evoked potentials in adult and infant sleep apnea syndromes, including sudden infant death syndrome, and near-miss for sudden infant death. *Ann NY Acad Sci* 1982;**388:**433.

Stockard J et al: Prognostic value of brain stem auditory evoked potentials in neonates. *Arch Neurol* 1983;**40:**360.

BRAIN ELECTRICAL ACTIVITY MAPPING (BEAM)

Brain electrical activity mapping is a relatively new technique in which electroencephalographic and evoked potential data recorded from multiple scalp electrodes are graphically displayed in color on a computer-driven video screen. Values between electrodes are obtained by interpolation. This procedure should increase the diagnostic accuracy of both anatomic and functional brain lesions.

Duffy FH: The BEAM method for neurophysiological diagnosis. *Ann NY Acad Sci* 1985;**457:**19.

PEDIATRIC NEURORADIOLOGIC PROCEDURES

Sedation for Procedures

Radiologic procedures in infants and children are usually performed by pediatric radiologists, but sedation for these procedures remains largely the responsibility of the physician caring for the child. The choice of sedation must take into account the patient's age and physical condition, the type of neurologic disorder, the effect and duration of the procedure, and whether immediate neurosurgery is anticipated. The prescribing physician should be familiar with the agent used.

In neonates and young infants, oral diphenhydramine may be sufficient. Morphine, 0.1 mg/kg intravenously, is also recommended, since its effects can be reversed with naloxone (Narcan), 0.01 mg/kg intravenously. Pentobarbital, 6 mg/kg for children weighing less than 15 kg and 5 mg/kg for larger children (up to a maximum of 200 mg) given intramuscularly at least 20 minutes before a procedure, has also been recommended. This usually achieves sedation for up to 2 hours. However, if sedation is inadequate 30 minutes after injection, and depending on the condition of the child, a second dose of pentobarbital, 2 mg/kg, is given. Pediatricians familiar with using a "cardiac cocktail," usually of intramuscularly administered meperidine, secobarbital, and promethazine or chlorpromazine, may employ this. General anesthesia may be indicated, especially if the child is to undergo surgery immediately on completion of a radiologic procedure.

Computerized Tomography (CT Scanning)

Computerized tomography (CT) consists of a series of cross-sectional ("axial") roentgenograms. The procedure is almost risk-free and can be performed on an outpatient basis. Radiation exposure is approximately the same as that from a skull roentgenogram series; shielded gonads receive less than 0.1 mrad. The images can be viewed on an oscilloscope as the scan is being done and later examined on printed-out films; both oscilloscope views and films record variations in tissue densities. CT scanning is of high sensitivity (88–96% of lesions over 1–2 cm can be seen) but low specificity (a tumor, focus of infection, or infarct may have the same appearance).

The CT scan is often repeated after intravenous injection of iodized contrast for "enhancement," which reflects the vascularity of a lesion or its surrounding tissues. Precautions should be taken to ensure that the patient is not hypersensitive to iodinated dyes and that allergic reactions can be managed promptly. Sufficient information is often obtained from a nonenhanced scan, reducing cost and risk.

Sedation may be required for CT scanning. For positioning the head of children up to 8 years of age, a specially shaped headrest may be needed. The indications for CT scanning and the findings in specific conditions are discussed below in the sections on specific disorders.

There have been rapid advances in the application of CT techniques to further refine brain imaging, eg, with magnetic resonance imaging and positron emission tomography, which are discussed below.

Coupling regional cerebral blood flow techniques with CT procedures in exploring physiologic processes is also under investigation.

Magnetic Resonance Imaging (MRI)

Magnetic or nuclear magnetic resonance (NMR) imaging is a noninvasive technique that uses the magnetic properties of certain nuclei to produce signals known as the proton spin-lattice relaxation time and the spin-spin relaxation time—signals that are based on the density of nuclei at a given point and on their immediate environment (lattice). Presently, the technique is based on detecting the response (resonance) of hydrogen proton nuclei to applied radiofrequency electromagnetic radiation; these nuclei are abundant in the body and more sensitive to magnetic resonance imaging than other nuclei. The strength of relaxation signals varies with the relationship of water to proteins and the amount of lipids present. The image displayed, which is made up of a mixture of signals and is similar to the CT film, provides high-resolution contrast of soft tissues. Magnetic resonance imaging can, in fact, provide information about the histologic, physiologic, and biochemical status of tissues, in addition to gross anatomic data.

Clinically, magnetic resonance imaging has been applied chiefly to the study of lesions in the head, but it can be used in examinations of the spine, body organs, and tissues such as muscles and nerves. It has been used to delineate brain tumors, edema, ischemic and hemorrhagic lesions, hydrocephalus, vascular disorders, inflammatory and infectious lesions, and degenerative processes. Magnetic resonance imaging can be used to study myelination and demyelination and, through the demonstration of changes in relaxation time, metabolic disorders of brain, muscles, and glands. Since bone causes no artifact in the images, the posterior fossa and its contents can be studied far better than with CT scans; even blood vessels and the cranial nerves can be imaged. On the other hand, the inability to detect calcification limits the detection of calcified lesions such as craniopharyngioma or leptomeningeal angiomatosis.

It is believed that the strong magnetic fields used in this procedure do not cause molecular or cellular damage. Work is progressing on imaging from nuclei other than hydrogen, such as phosphorus and sodium.

Positron Emission Tomography (PET)

Positron emission tomography is an imaging technique that measures the metabolic rate at a given site by CT scanning to detect positron (proton) emission. For measurement of local cerebral metabolism, the radiolabeled substrate most frequently used has been fluorodeoxyglucose ^{18}F by injection. Gray matter and white matter are clearly distinguishable; the skull and air- or fluid-filled cavities are least active metabolically.

Positron emission tomography has been used to study the cerebral metabolism of neonates and brain activation by visual or auditory stimuli. Pathologic states that have been studied include epilepsy (during and between seizures), brain infarcts and tumors, and dementias. In adult patients with schizophrenia, hypometabolism of the frontal lobes was detected by this technique.

Other radiolabeled substances sometimes used are ^{11}C-glucose, also by injection, and ^{11}CO by inhalation detectable subsequently in carboxyhemoglobin.

Clinical application is limited by the cost of the procedure and the need to have access to a nearby cyclotron where the radiopharmaceuticals can be prepared.

Ultrasonography

Ultrasonography offers a pictorial display (eg, echoencephalogram, echocardiogram) of the varying density of tissues in a given anatomic region or structure by recording the echoes of ultrasonic waves reflected from it. These waves, modulated by pulsations, are introduced into the tissue by means of a piezoelectric transducer. The many advantages of ultrasonography include the ability to make quick assessment of a structure and its positioning by means of portable equipment, without ionizing radiation and at about one-fourth of the cost of CT scanning. Sedation is usually not necessary, and ultrasonography can be repeated as often as indicated. In brain imaging, B mode and real-time sector scanners are usually employed, permitting excellent detail to be obtained in the coronal and sagittal planes. Contiguous structures can be studied by a continuous sweep and reviewed on videotape.

Ultrasonography has been used for in utero diagnosis of hydrocephalus and other anomalies. In neonates, the thin skull and the open anterior fontanelle have facilitated imaging of the brain, and ultrasonography is now used in many nurseries to screen and follow all infants of less than 32 weeks of gestation or under 1500 g for intracranial hemorrhage. Other uses in neonates include detection of hydrocephalus, major brain and spine malformations, and even calcifications from intrauterine infection with cytomegalovirus or *Toxoplasma*.

Cerebral Angiography

Arteriography remains a very useful procedure in the diagnosis of many cerebrovascular disorders, particularly vascular malformations, and is sometimes used when a potentially operable lesion is suspected. In some instances of brain tumor, arteriography may be necessary to define the precise location or vascular bed, to differentiate among tumors, or to distinguish tumor from abscess or infarction.

Air Encephalography

Brain examination by x-rays of the head after injection of air into the lumbar subarachnoid space (**pneumoencephalography**) or into a lateral ventricle (**ventriculography**) has largely been replaced by CT scanning. Air encephalography may on occasion still be necessary in the diagnosis of some brain tumors.

Metrizamide Ventriculography

A small amount (1 or 2 mL) of metrizamide, a water-soluble contrast material, may be injected into a lateral ventricle by direct puncture or via a preexisting shunt. Imaging is then carried out by standard x-ray or CT scanning. This permits visualization of the flow of cerebrospinal fluid (within the ventricle, between the ventricles, or between the ventricle and an intracerebral cyst) to determine the appropriate site of shunt placement or other surgical procedure.

Myelography

X-ray examination of the spine following injection of a dye, water-soluble contrast medium, or air into the subarachnoid space via the lumbar or, rarely, the cervical route may be indicated in cases of spinal cord tumors or various forms of spinal dysraphism and in rare instances of herniated disks in children. However, in most institutions, spine scanning or CT metrizamide myelography is now employed instead.

Bachman DS, Hodges FJ, Freeman JM: Computerized axial tomography in neurologic disorders of children. *Pediatrics* 1977;**59:**352.

Baker HL et al: Magnetic resonance imaging in a routine clinical setting. *Mayo Clin Proc* 1985;**60:**75.

Brant-Zawadzki M et al: Magnetic resonance of the brain: The optimal screening technique. *Radiology* 1984;**152:**71.

Creed L, Haber K: Ultrasonic evaluation of the infant head. *CRC Crit Rev Diagn Imaging* 1984;**21:**37.

Doyle LW et al: Regional cerebral glucose metabolism of newborn infants measured by positron emission tomography. *Dev Med Child Neurol* 1983;**25:**143.

Dykes FD, Abmann PA, Lazzara A: Cranial ultrasound in the detection of intracranial calcifications. *J Pediatr* 1982;**100:**406.

Harwood-Nash DC: Computed tomography and the abnormal brain in the neonate. *J Neuroradiol* 1981;**8:**125.

Harwood-Nash DC: Pediatric neuroradiological techniques. *J Neuroradiol* 1981;**8:**73.

Heller RM et al: Implications of nuclear magnetic resonance for the pediatrician. *Am J Dis Child* 1983;**136:**1045.

Hill ML, Breckle R, Gehrking WC: The prenatal detection of congenital malformations by ultrasonography. *Mayo Clin Proc* 1983;**58:**805.

Lenzi GL, Pantano P: Neurologic applications of positron emission tomography. *Neurol Clin* 1984;**2:**853.

Leonard JC et al: Nuclear magnetic resonance: An overview of its spectroscopic and imaging applications in pediatric patients. *J Pediatr* 1985;**106:**756.

Pinto RS, Becker MH: Computed tomography in pediatric diagnosis. *Am J Dis Child* 1977;**131:**583.

Rumack CM, Johnson ML: Role of computed tomography and ultrasound in neonatal brain imaging. *J Comput Tomogr* 1983;**7:**17.

Webster WE, Apert NM, Brownell GL: Radiation doses in pediatric nuclear medicine and diagnostic x-ray procedures. Pages 34–58 in: *Pediatric Nuclear Medicine*. James AE, Wagner HN Jr, Cooke RE (editors). Saunders, 1974.

DISORDERS AFFECTING THE NERVOUS SYSTEM IN INFANTS & CHILDREN

ALTERED STATES OF CONSCIOUSNESS

Essentials of Diagnosis

- Reduction or alteration in cognitive and affective mental functioning and in arousability or attentiveness.
- Acute onset.

General Considerations

Although altered states of consciousness are physiologically imprecisely defined, they denote rapidly evolving deviations of varying severity from the commonly accepted ranges of wakefulness and sleep and "reflected diffuse or bilateral impairment of cerebral functions or failure of the brain stem ascending reticular activating system or both" (Plum and Posner, 1980).

The following is a brief description of several types of altered states.

A. Clouding: Reduced attentiveness or awareness, with slowed thinking, sometimes unclear or disordered perceptions (especially visual ones), and disturbed sense of time; hyperirritability may alternate with drowsiness.

B. Confusion: Mental bewilderment, with variable disorientation for time, place, and other persons, consistent misinterpretation of stimuli, faulty memory, and often prolonged drowsiness during normal waking hours.

C. Delirium: Markedly abnormal mental state, with disorientation, hallucinations (especially visual ones), delusions, psychomotor overactivity, and, often, autonomic nervous system disturbances.

D. Obtundation: Mild to moderate reduction in alertness, with loss of interest in the environment, slow mental responsiveness, and, often, increased sleep.

E. Stupor: Unresponsiveness except to vigorous and repeated stimuli, with return to unresponsiveness when the stimulus ceases, and deep sleep.

F. Semicoma: Similar to stupor; often used to describe marked impairment of consciousness in which the patient responds with some purposeful movements to strong stimuli, especially pain.

G. Coma: Unresponsiveness to external stimuli and to inner needs.

Emergency Measures (See also Chapters 8 and 30.)

A. Airway: Perform endotracheal intubation or tracheostomy, if necessary. ***Caution:*** Stabilize the neck in trauma.

B. Breathing: Give oxygen and respiratory assistance by mechanical means.

C. Circulation: Insert an intravenous catheter, and give fluids. Administer dopamine, 5–20 μg/kg/min intravenously by continuous drip, for persistent hypotension.

D. Treatment of Reversible Causes: Stop seizures. Treat reversible causes as follows:

1. Opiate overdose—Give naloxone, 0.01 mg/kg intramuscularly or intravenously, to reverse effects of narcotics (larger doses to reverse effects of propoxyphene). Repeat every 15–30 minutes as needed.

2. Antidepressant overdose—Give physostigmine, 1 mg intravenously, to reverse effects of most antidepressants. This drug improves arousal.

3. Hypoglycemia—Give glucose as 50% dextrose solution (amount varies with size of the patient).

Causes of Altered States of Consciousness

A. Diffuse or Metabolic Dysfunctions:

1. Characteristics—The altered mental state precedes motor signs, which are usually symmetric. The pupils are usually reactive, and tremors and seizures are common. There may be hyper- or hypoventilation with acid-base imbalance.

2. Causes—These include poisons (eg, drugs in common use, household poisons, carbon monoxide); metabolic disorders (eg, hypoxemia and ischemia, Reye's syndrome, diabetic coma, uremia); cerebral infections (encephalitis); and intrinsic intracranial disorders (concussion, postictal state, subarachnoid hemorrhage, sudden increase in intracranial pressure secondary to a blocked shunt).

B. Supratentorial Mass Lesions Compromising the Diencephalon or Brain Stem:

1. Characteristics—Initial signs are often focal, with rostral to caudad progression of brain dysfunction. Motor signs are usually asymmetric.

2. Causes—Causes include intracranial hematomas (subdural, epidural, intracerebral), brain contusion, and infarction.

C. Subtentorial Mass or Destructive Lesions:

1. Characteristics—Brain stem signs precede or accompany the sudden onset of coma. Oculovestibular responses to ice-water lavage (caloric test) are always disturbed, and cranial nerve palsies are common. An unusual breathing pattern often marks the onset of coma.

2. Causes—The altered state may be due to a compressive lesion (posterior fossa hematoma, cerebellar mass lesion, basilar aneurysm) or to a destructive lesion (basilar migraine, brain stem or pontine hemorrhage).

D. Combined Causes: Intoxicant ingestion and head trauma may both be present.

Assessment of Impaired Consciousness & Coma

A relatively simple, generally applicable scheme of assessment, not requiring extensive neurologic competence, to follow a patient's course, predict outcome, promote understanding of the patient's state among physicians involved, and allow for comparisons between patients or the effects of treatment is the 15-point "Glasgow Coma Scale" (Fig 23–1), which rates both depth and duration of impaired consciousness and coma.

For purposes of assessment, the best motor response from the best limb is recorded. Limb injuries, immobilization, or paralysis may interfere with the assessment. A consistent stimulus should be used. Differences among limbs may reflect central or focal neurologic lesions. Abnormal flexion may be associ-

		Date				
		Time	Time	Time	Time	etc
	6 Obeying					
BEST	5 Localizes					
MOTOR	4 Withdraws					
RESPONSE	3 Abnormal flexing					
	2 Extensor response					
	1 None					
	5 Oriented					
BEST	4 Confused conversation					
VERBAL	3 Inappropriate words					
RESPONSE	2 Incomprehensible sounds					
	1 None					
	4 Spontaneous					
EYE	3 To speech					
OPENING	2 To pain					
	1 None					

Figure 23–1. "Glasgow Coma Scale" for recording assessment of consciousness. (After Teasdale and Jennett.) See text for adaptation of best verbal response for use in infants and toddlers.

ated with a slow assumption of the hemiplegic or decorticate posture with adduction of the shoulder. The extensor response includes "decerebrate" posturing and is associated in this scale with adduction and internal rotation of the shoulder and pronation of the forearm ("seal flipper posture").

Responses may be affected by conditions *not* related directly to the coma (eg, young age, mental retardation, hearing impairment). Thus, for infants and toddlers, the best verbal response on the "Glasgow Coma Scale" has been adapted as follows: 5 = fixes on, follows, and recognizes objects and persons; laughs. 4 = fixes on, follows, and recognizes objects inconstantly; recognition of persons uncertain. 3 = arousable only at times; does not drink. 2 = motor restlessness; unarousable. This adaptation is suitable for the profoundly retarded as well.

Examination & Clues to Causes of Coma

A. General Evaluation:

1. Vital signs—Status and possible causes are as follows:

a. Severe bradycardia—Increased intracranial pressure.

b. Hypertension—Raised intracranial pressure, intracerebral hemorrhage, hypertensive encephalopathy.

c. Hypotension—Shock (eg, from internal hemorrhage, gram-negative sepsis), alcohol intoxication, drug intoxication.

d. Fever—Acute infection, heat stroke, postictal state, toxic encephalopathies, intracranial bleeding.

e. Hypothermia—Barbiturates, alcohol, shock, exposure.

2. Breathing patterns—Patterns and associated causes are as follows:

a. Slow, deep breathing—Heavy sedation, postictal state, cerebral infections, increased intracranial pressure.

b. Slow, shallow breathing—Some sedatives, narcotics.

c. Hyperventilation or irregular breathing—Brain stem damage.

d. "Periodic" hyperpnea alternating with apnea (Cheyne-Stokes respiration)—Symmetric deep cerebral or diencephalic dysfunction.

e. Deep, rapid, gasping for breath (Kussmaul's respiration)—Acidosis.

f. Sustained, regular, rapid and deep breathing (central neurogenic hyperventilation)—Dysfunction between low midbrain and lower third of pons.

g. Blowing out of one cheek—Ipsilateral facial paralysis.

h. Odor of breath—Fruity odor of ketosis, foul odor of uremia, odor of alcohol.

3. Inspection and palpation—

a. Head—In infants, measure head circumference and note tension of anterior fontanelle. Examine the ears, mastoids, nose, and mouth for bleeding.

b. Skin—Examine for color (cyanotic in hypoxia; cherry red in carbon monoxide or atropine poisoning), signs of trauma, traces of toxic substances, needle marks, petechiae, ticks, and turgor.

c. Body—Check heart and lungs and palpate the abdomen. Check major vessels and pulses, noting bruits over eyes and neck.

B. Neurologic Evaluation:

1. Level of consciousness and coma—See above.

2. Neck flexion–(***Caution:*** Do *not* attempt if cervical injury is a possibility.) Nuchal rigidity suggests meningitis, subarachnoid hemorrhage, or herniation of cerebellar tonsils. ***Note:*** Nuchal rigidity may disappear in deep coma.

3. Eyes—See Pupils, below. Check the following:

a. Position at rest and eye movements.

b. Response to threat movements.

c. Status of fundi—(***Caution:*** Do *not* dilate pupils, since this obliterates critical signs.) Papilledema on funduscopic examination suggests increased intracranial pressure.

d. Response to doll's eye maneuver (oculocephalic reflex)—Movements may be conjugate, asymmetric, minimal, or absent.

e. Response to ice-water caloric testing (oculovestibular reflex)—This response *must* be checked in unconscious patients.

4. Pupils—Check size and reaction to light, using a hand lens if there is "no reaction." Status and possible causes are as follows:

a. Dilated, reactive pupils, sometimes on one side only—Postictal state.

b. Widely dilated, fixed pupils—Third nerve paralysis due to tentorial herniation or brain stem damage.

c. Pinpoint pupils—Narcotics, barbiturates, brain stem disorders.

5. Other cranial nerves—Check supraorbital pressure, corneal reflexes (nerve V), and gag reflex (nerve IX).

6. Motor function—Check the following:

a. Posture—Posture may appear decerebrate, decorticate, or hemiplegic.

b. Muscle tone—There may be signs of spasticity, paratonia, or flaccidity.

c. Symmetry of movement—Asymmetry of spontaneous movements or in response to pain suggests focal weakness.

d. Reflexes—Reflexes may be increased or diminished. Check for Babinski's sign and other primitive reflexes.

C. Laboratory Evaluation: The evaluation should be guided by the suspected cause.

1. Urinalysis—Urinalysis may be immediately helpful. Catheterize the patient if necessary. Perform a toxicology screen if indicated. Findings and their possible causes are as follows:

a. Glycosuria—Diabetes, salicylism, sometimes lead poisoning or cerebrovascular accidents.

b. Ketonuria—Starvation state.

c. Proteinuria—Renal disease, high fevers, lead and other poisonings.

d. Red to purple color on testing with ferric chloride or Phenistix—Salicylism, phenothiazines.

2. Blood—Blood tests include the following:

a. Typing and cross-matching for transfusion; toxicology studies.

b. Blood glucose, urea nitrogen, electrolyte, and arterial blood gas determinations.

c. Liver function studies. High enzyme levels and ammonia, with low bilirubin, are seen in Reye's syndrome.

d. Blood cultures if fever or septic shock is present.

e. Complete blood count and differential count. "Stippling" in small children suggests lead poisoning.

3. Gastric contents—Aspirate for diagnosis and therapeutic reasons.

4. Lumbar puncture—(See earlier section and also Chapter 35.) Lumbar puncture should *only* be performed *immediately* if bacterial meningitis is suspected or if the differential diagnosis includes other cerebral infections, subarachnoid hemorrhage, acute toxic encephalopathy (eg, Reye's syndrome), or acute necrotizing hemorrhagic encephalopathy.

D. Electroencephalography: Electroencephalography may be helpful (especially when it can be done promptly at the bedside) in directing attention to possible causes of coma before the biochemical laboratory can perform toxic or metabolic screens or in guiding the laboratory in what tests to run. Diffuse excessive fast (beta) activity is seen with many drugs, especially sedatives. Diffuse excessive slowing suggests infection and metabolic or "toxic" encephalopathies. Focal slowing points to a circumscribed area of brain tissue destruction, as seen in trauma, a cerebrovascular lesion, abscess, or focal encephalitis, eg, due to herpes simplex involving the temporal lobes.

E. X-Ray and Other Evaluation: X-rays should be taken when spinal cord injury or abdominal trauma is suspected. Nonessential x-ray studies should be deferred until the patient is not in a precarious state. CT brain scans should be performed in cases of severe head trauma, focal intracerebral infection, and suspected intracranial mass or destructive lesions. They should also be performed to evaluate increased intracranial pressure. Ultrasonography is indicated in infants with an open anterior fontanelle.

Treatment

The principle of treatment is to provide specific measures for specific problems. Emergency measures are outlined at the beginning of this section.

A. General Measures:

1. Above all, maintain vital functions. For hypotension, use dopamine.

2. Observe vital signs, the state of the pupils, and levels of consciousness closely. Monitor the ECG.

3. Turn the patient frequently to prevent hypostatic pneumonia.

4. Provide fluids by the intravenous route initially and by nasogastric feedings or gastrostomy if coma is prolonged. Monitor input and output.

5. Bladder care may require catheterization.

6. Avoid administration of sedatives. If the patient is very agitated and restlessness threatens to result in injuries, sedate the patient with diphenhydramine, chloral hydrate, or, occasionally, paraldehyde.

7. Prophylactic antibiotic therapy is rarely warranted.

8. Protect the patient's eyes.

B. Seizures: Seizures occur in about two-thirds of children with coma, with onset in 75% of cases. There is a high correlation between the cause of coma and both the occurrence and type of seizures: In about 80% of cases of coma with seizures at onset, the cause is an intracranial infection; with status epilepticus, it is either encephalitis or preexisting epilepsy. Focal seizures occur not only from a circumscribed brain lesion but often with meningitis, in which case seizures may be multifocal. Myoclonic seizures are seen most often in hypoxic-ischemic brain injury.

Seizures—especially status epilepticus—may complicate the treatment of the comatose child. Thus, it is not only important to treat seizures promptly; it may be highly advisable to treat prophylactically those children in whom there is a high degree of probability of developing seizures.

In the treatment or prevention of seizures in the comatose child, the following considerations are important:

1. The presence of antiepileptic drugs may be noted in the child, either because of prior treatment or accidental or intentional ingestion, with coma due to intoxication. Antiepileptic drug blood levels should be determined as soon as possible. (See Table 23–3.)

2. Intravenous diazepam (Valium) is useful in treating status epilepticus, but it may contribute to respiratory depression or arrest, especially in the presence of phenobarbital.

3. Phenytoin, administered intravenously as for status epilepticus, has the advantage of not depressing the level of consciousness, so that it does not mask the return of greater awareness or responsiveness. (Phenobarbital may mask responsiveness.)

4. Valproic acid is the drug of choice for myoclonic seizures and can be given rectally.

5. Anticonvulsant drug blood levels should be monitored.

6. If the child has had no seizures and is not known to have epilepsy, the antiepileptic drug given prophylactically may be withdrawn slowly upon recovery from coma. If, during withdrawal, a seizure should occur, the anticonvulsant should promptly be reinstituted at its effective dosage.

C. Increased Intracranial Pressure: Treat when elevated pressure is anticipated (as after significant hypoxia or head trauma) or present (as evidenced by papilledema or CT scan). Often a combination of approaches is necessary.

1. Physiologic program—

a. Restrict fluid to maintenance requirements, taking into consideration body temperature, tracheostomy, mist tent, and other factors. Maintain serum osmolality at about 300 mosm/L.

b. Induce hypothermia, since it reduces cerebral metabolism. Temperature should not fall below 32 °C (89.6 °F).

c. Keep head elevated at 30 degrees if possible.

d. Initiate controlled hyperventilation to maintain the arterial blood P_{aCO_2} at 25–28 mm Hg. Arterial blood gases, especially P_{CO_2}, should be monitored carefully.

e. Control systemic arterial pressure.

2. Corticosteroids—Corticosteroids are used prophylactically—especially preoperatively—and therapeutically.

a. Dexamethasone sodium phosphate, 0.15–0.25 mg/kg, is given intravenously initially, followed by 0.25 mg/kg/d intramuscularly in 3 or 4 doses; the dose is often tapered after 72 hours over a 3- to 4-day period.

b. Methylprednisolone sodium succinate is given in 4–5 times the dosage of dexamethasone (above).

3. Diuretics—These are most effective in acute cerebral edema while other therapy is being instituted. Serum electrolytes and osmolality should be monitored carefully.

a. Mannitol in 20% solution, 1–3 g/kg (often 1.5–2 g/kg), is given intravenously every 4–6 hours. The drug is often given repeatedly in smaller doses over several days.

b. Furosemide, 0.5–1 mg/kg, may be given.

4. Barbiturates—Pentobarbital, 5 mg/kg intravenously initially, followed by 2 mg/kg/h by intravenous infusion, is frequently used when intracranial pressure is being monitored. The blood level should be maintained at 25–35 μg/mL.

5. Withdrawal of cerebrospinal fluid—If an intraventricular cannula is in place, cerebrospinal fluid may be withdrawn.

6. Intracranial pressure monitoring—Techniques have been developed for the continuous monitoring of intracranial pressure to guide therapy for the reduction of increased pressure; these techniques provide more information than clinical observations alone. Ventricular fluid pressure is measured by means of tubing passed through a frontal bur hole into the lateral ventricle of the nondominant cerebral hemisphere. Subarachnoid pressure is also monitored. Pressures are displayed on a bedside monitor, often along with arterial pressure, ECG, and rectal temperature, and recorded by the nursing staff. Selection of patients for such monitoring may depend on the cause of increased pressure or may be guided by the "Glasgow Coma Scale" (Fig 23–1), particularly in trauma, where children with a score of 5 or better and a CT scan showing only diffuse brain swelling or no disease may not have to be monitored.

Handling of patients, especially those with seizures and episodes of tonic ("decorticate" or "decerebrate") posturing, produces sharp transient increases in pressure. Steep persistent rises may signify the evolution of a new process, such as an epidural hematoma.

The insertion of foreign bodies, and particularly of tubing into a ventricle, is not without the danger of producing bacterial intracranial infection or superimposing a new infection on a preexisting one.

Monitoring increased intracerebral pressure and treatment of increased pressure have led to significant increases in survival and improved neurologic status of survivors of severe head trauma and Reye's syndrome; children with hypoxic-ischemic encephalopathy, intracranial mass lesions, and multiple injuries do less well.

For a detailed description of the means and procedures employed, the reader is directed to the following references cited below: Bruce et al; Mayer and Walker; and Nussbaum and Galant.

"Brain Death"*

Statutory and other definitions of brain death vary in different jurisdictions. Many states have adopted the American Bar Association's "Uniform Brain Death Act." This states, "For legal purposes, a human body with irreversible cessation of brain function, according to usual and customary standards of medical practice, shall be considered dead." This statement deliberately avoids reference to *criteria* for establishing brain death. This approach is deemed wise because criteria are still evolving in response to each advancement in technology designed to assess brain function. Black (see reference below) provides a detailed discussion of many issues. At present, criteria for brain death are identical for pediatric and adult patients. A presidential commission developed useful guidelines as follows:

A. Prerequisite: Relevant diagnostic and therapeutic measures have been performed and have *excluded* reversible conditions (hypothermia, sedative drugs, neuromuscular blockade, metabolic coma, shock).

B. Criteria: *Clinical examination* has revealed the following:

1. Coma with cerebral unresponsiveness, ie, no purposeful vocal or motor responses. ***Note:*** Spinal reflexes persist after death.

2. Apnea, ie, no spontaneous respirations when checked periodically over a 10-minute interval.

3. Absent brain stem reflexes (pupillary, corneal, oculocephalic, oculovestibular, gag).

4. In the absence of confirmatory tests, the above criteria are found to be present for 12 hours. (In young children, longer periods of up to 72 hours have been recommended.)

C. Confirmation: The following confirmatory tests may be desirable: Electrocerebral silence—ie,

* ***Note:*** For "irreversible coma," see below.

a "flat" (isoelectric) EEG at maximal gains for 30 minutes—verifies brain death, except in cases of drug-induced coma and hypothermia and in young children. In young children, the EEG may show some activity, even though there is no blood flow to the child's brain and thus no hope for survival.

Absence of cerebral blood flow demonstrated by angiography or bedside brain flow study using an intravenously injected isotope is a safeguard when the diagnosis of brain death must be considered and other criteria have not been unequivocally met. This may include patients with small amounts of sedative drugs in their blood, those with small nonreactive pupils, those undergoing therapeutic procedures making examination of brain stem function impossible, or those being considered as organ donors.

In cases of brain death, the blood flow velocity in the common carotid artery (and the anterior cerebral artery in infants with an open fontanelle) may show a pattern of consistently marked reversal of blood flow in diastole and a single systolic peak.

Prognosis

Slightly over 50% of children with nontraumatic coma recover normally, about 30% die, and about 20% suffer mild to severe neurologic handicaps. Clinical variables that are assessable within 2–3 minutes of arrival at hospital and are useful in determining outcome include severity of coma, neuro-ophthalmologic signs, motor patterns, temperature, and seizure type. The risk of death is high if intracranial pressures are over 20 mm Hg and cerebral perfusion pressures are over 50 mm Hg on intracranial pressure monitoring.

In patients with brain death, apnea is accompanied by death of systemic tissues when respiratory support is discontinued. Patients with persistent vegetative states have **irreversible coma** with loss of all cerebral functions; however, in contrast to patients with brain death, these patients retain the vital functions of respiration, temperature, and blood pressure regulation. Occasionally, a minimal medullary activity is the only neurologic function retained, and standard tests may not detect this activity. In these rare patients, considered otherwise to have brain death, respirations may begin after termination of respiratory support. This emphasizes that, in practice, the ultimate test of brain death is disconnecting such support and observing the death of systemic organs.

Ashwal S, Schneider S: Failure of electroencephalography to diagnose brain death in comatose children. *Ann Neurol* 1979;**6:**512.

Black PM: Brain death: Medical progress. (2 parts.) *N Engl J Med* 1978;**229:**338, 393.

Bruce DA et al: Pathophysiology, treatment and outcome following severe head injury in children. *Childs Brain* 1979;**5:**177.

Gordon NS et al: The management of the comatose child: Consensus statement. *Neuropediatrics* 1983;**14:**3.

Guidelines for the determination of death: Report of the Medical Consultants on the Diagnosis of Death to the President's Commission for the Study of Ethical Problems in Medicine and Biomedical and Behavioral Research. (Special Communication.) *JAMA* 1981;**246:**2184.

Lütschg J et al: Brain-stem auditory evoked potentials and early somatosensory evoked potentials in neurointensively treated comatose children. *Am J Dis Child* 1983;**137:**421.

Mayer T, Walker ML: Emergency intracranial pressure monitoring in pediatrics: Management of the acute coma of brain insult. *Clin Pediatr* 1982;**21:**391.

McMenamin JB, Volpe JJ: Doppler ultrasonography in the determination of neonatal brain death. *Ann Neurol* 1983;**14:**302.

Nussbaum E, Galant SP: Intracranial pressure monitoring as a guide to prognosis in the nearly drowned, severely comatose child. *J Pediatr* 1983;**102:**215.

Plum F, Posner JB: *The Diagnosis of Stupor and Coma*, 3rd ed. Davis, 1980.

Rowland TW et al: Brain death in the pediatric intensive care unit: A clinical definition. *Am J Dis Child* 1983;**137:**547.

Seshia SS, Johnston R, Kasian G: Non-traumatic coma in childhood: Clinical variables in prediction of outcome. *Dev Med Child Neurol* 1983;**25:**493.

Teasdale G, Jennett B: Assessment of coma and impaired consciousness: A practical scale. *Lancet* 1974;**2:**81.

SEIZURE DISORDERS (Epilepsies)

Essentials of Diagnosis

- Recurrent nonfebrile seizures.
- Coincidental marked changes on EEG; interictal EEG also frequently abnormal.
- Family history of seizures in 30% of cases.

General Considerations

A seizure is a sudden, transient disturbance of brain function, manifested by involuntary motor, sensory, autonomic, or psychic phenomena, alone or in any combination, often accompanied by alteration or loss of consciousness. The incidence rate (new cases per 100,000 population) of seizures regardless of cause is 5–6% in newborns, including prematures; about 1% by 1 year of age; 0.5% by age 10; and 0.2% by age 15. While nearly 10% of children will have had one or more seizures by then, the prevalence of epilepsy is estimated at 1% in the total population.

Seizures recur following an initial unprovoked, nonfebrile generalized tonic-clonic (grand mal), simple focal, or complex partial (psychomotor) seizure in slightly over 50% of children, which is nearly twice the recurrence rate in adults. In children with a recurrent seizure, about 80% have more. Recurrence rates are highest in children with neurologic abnormalities, focal spikes on EEG, and complex partial seizures; they are lowest after a generalized convulsion in a neurologically intact child with a normal EEG.

Seizure disorders are often divided into 2 classes: the "symptomatic" (acquired or secondary) epilepsies, in which a cause is identified or strongly suspected; and "idiopathic" (essential or primary) epilepsy, defined by exclusion, in which no cause is known, but a significant genetic component is presumed. Some degree of genetic predisposition is thought to play a role even in many seizure disorders of known cause.

For clinical reasons, most if not all seizures in children up to 18 months or 2 years of age are held to be "symptomatic." Causes include pre- and perinatal insults and congenital malformations; after delivery, systemic and central nervous system infections "provoke" most seizures in children, with trauma, metabolic and electrolyte disturbances, toxins, vascular disorders, and degenerative diseases responsible for only a few percent. Primary or secondary neoplastic lesions account for fewer than 1% of "symptomatic" seizures in children, compared with 25% in adults.

Seizures are subject to modifying conditions and interacting factors. Some patients have generalized tonic-clonic or focal motor seizures chiefly during sleep—sometimes just after falling asleep and sometimes in the early morning hours. "Absence" or petit mal, akinetic, and myoclonic spells—often loosely referred to collectively as minor motor seizures—tend to occur in clusters in the morning around breakfast time and again in the afternoon or around supper time. Lack of sleep, emotional stress or excitement, intercurrent infections, alcohol, and some drugs may play a "triggering" role; there may be an "upsurge" at the start of the school year. Seizure frequency and the need for medication may be decreased by changes in environment or lessened stress, as during vacations, visits with relatives, or even in the hospital.

Mixed seizure patterns occur frequently in children. Patterns may also change with maturation, and the treatment of one kind of seizure may unmask another.

Clinical Findings

A. Seizure Types: Based on both clinical manifestations and age at onset, the more common seizure disorders encountered in infancy, childhood, and adolescence are presented in Table 23–2, along with pathogenic factors, commonly encountered electroencephalographic findings, and preferred modes of treatment. It must be emphasized that there have been many diverse attempts at seizure classification, principally on the basis of clinical patterns and pathophysiology (including electroencephalographic patterns), but almost all have proved either too cumbersome or too simple. It must also be stressed that, in many of the more difficult to manage chronic epilepsies of early life, so-called partial or focal seizures or those of the "minor motor" variety (as in Lennox-Gastaut syndrome and with absences) may appear sooner or later mixed with focal seizures of the complex partial type or with generalized (grand mal) convulsions.

B. Status Epilepticus: Any true seizure of at least 30 minutes or more, or a series of seizures extending over such a period, constitutes status epilepticus. The term is usually applied to (1) convulsive status epilepticus or a series of tonic-clonic seizures occurring in rapid succession without recovery of the normal alert state between spells, and (2) nonconvulsive status epilepticus, such as focal (motor, complex partial) and myoclonic status, as well as absence status or "spike-wave stupor" during which consciousness is impaired but not lost.

In treating status epilepticus, vigorous initial therapy is more likely to control seizures than the repeated administration of small doses of various anticonvulsants, whose cumulative effect may produce respiratory depression or marked central nervous system depression.

C. Breath-Holding Spells (Reflex Hypoxic Crisis): Although not a true epileptic disorder, the typical breath-holding spell is characterized by violent crying and breath-holding precipitated by slight injury, anger, frustration, fear, or the desire for attention in a young child (usually between 6 months and 4 years of age). The child becomes hypoxic and cyanotic, loses consciousness, may be opisthotonic, and may have a brief generalized seizure. In about 10% of cases, such spells are ushered in by pallor.

Unless the child sustains a head injury, these spells are benign. The description usually establishes the diagnosis. It is helpful to remember that cyanosis or pallor almost always precedes loss of consciousness, whereas in grand mal epilepsy consciousness is lost first. Neurologic examination and EEG are normal, although reflex slowing produced on the EEG by ocular compression is diagnostically helpful.

Breath-holding spells almost always disappear between 4 and 6 years of age. Anticonvulsant therapy usually is of no benefit; in the spells ushered in by pallor, atropine may be useful (0.01 mg/kg/d in divided doses; maximum, 0.4 mg).

D. Febrile Convulsions: Recommended criteria for febrile convulsions are fever of at least 38 °C (100.5 °F); age less than 6 years; no previous nonfebrile convulsion (even with recurrent febrile convulsion); and no primary neurologic illness or acute systemic metabolic disorder. Febrile convulsions are considered separately here because of their high incidence and the continuing concern over treatment.

The cumulative incidence of febrile convulsions by the criteria above is about 2.5%, but they constitute about 40% of all first seizures in children. Pharyngotonsillitis and otitis media are the most common associated illnesses; most febrile convulsions occur with temperatures over 39 °C (102.2 °F). Immunizations do not play a role per se except for associated fever. Many authorities exclude from this entity seizures associated with roseola infantum and acute *Salmonella* or *Shigella* infections.

The family history is positive for febrile convulsions in over 40% of cases and for nonfebrile seizures in 15%. A significantly increased prevalence of dermatoglyphic abnormalities has been reported in children with febrile convulsions and in their parents and suggests a polygenic mode of inheritance. Boys appear to be slightly more susceptible than girls. Risk

Table 23–2. Seizures by age at onset, pattern, and preferred treatment.

Age Group and Seizure Type	Age at Onset	Clinical Manifestations	Causative Factors	Electroencephalographic Pattern	Other Diagnostic Studies	Treatment and Comments* (Anticonvulsants by Order of Choice)
Neonatal seizures	Birth to 2 weeks	Often "atypical": sudden limpness or tonic posturing, brief apnea and cyanosis; odd cry; eyes "rolling up," "blinking" or "mouthing" or "chewing" movements; nystagmus; twitchiness or clonic movements—focal, multifocal, or generalized.	Neurologic insults (hypoxia/ischemia; intracranial hemorrhage) present more in first 3 days or after eighth day; metabolic disturbances alone between third and eighth days; hypoglycemia, hypocalcemia, hypophosphatemia, hyper- and hyponatremia. Drug withdrawal. Pyridoxine deficiency and other metabolic causes. CNS infections and structural abnormalities.	Highly variable; often rhythmic slowing; independent abnormalities may shift.	Lumbar puncture; serum Ca^{2+}, PO_4^{3-}, glucose, Mg^{2+}; BUN, amino acid screen, blood ammonia, organic acid screen, TORCHES screen.† Ultrasound and/or CT scan for suspected intracranial hemorrhage and structural abnormalities.	Phenobarbital, IV or IM; if seizures not controlled, add phenytoin IV (loading dose 20 mg/kg each). Diazepam, approximately 0.2 mg/kg. Treat underlying disorder. Seizures due to brain damage often resistant to anticonvulsants. When cause in doubt, stop protein feedings until enzyme deficiencies of urea cycle or amino metabolism ruled out.
West's syndrome: "infantile spasms." (See also Lennox-Gastaut syndrome, below.)	3–18 months; occasionally up to 4 years	Sudden, usually symmetric adduction and flexion of limbs with concomitant flexion of head and trunk; also abduction and extensor movements like Moro reflex. Tendency for spasms to occur in clusters, on waking or falling asleep, or when fatigued, or may be noted particularly when the infant is being handled, is ill, or is otherwise irritable. Tendency for each patient to have own stereotyped pattern.	Pre- or perinatal brain damage or malformation in approximately one-third; biochemical, infectious, degenerative causes in approximately one-third; unknown in approximately one-third. With early onset, pyridoxine deficiency, amino- or organic aciduria. Tuberous sclerosis in 5–10%. Chronic inflammatory disease and toxoplasmosis. Aicardi syndrome (females with mental retardation, agenesis of corpus callosum, ocular and vertebral anomalies).	Hypsarrhythmia: chaotic high-voltage slow waves, random spikes, all leads (90%); other abnormalities in rest. Rarely "normal." EEG normalization usually correlates with reduction of seizures; not helpful prognostically regarding mental development.	Funduscopic and skin examination; trial of pyridoxine. Amino- and organic acid screen. Chronic inflammatory disease. TORCHES screen.† CT scan may be justified to (1) establish definite diagnosis, (2) aid in genetic counseling.	Corticotropin preferred (5–8 units/kg/d IM divided in 2 doses for 14–21 days, then slow withdrawal). Some prefer oral corticosteroids. Diazepam, clonazepam, valproic acid. In resistant cases, ketogenic or medium-chain triglyceride (MCT) diet (see text). Retardation of varying degree in approximately 90% of cases.
Febrile convulsions	3 months to 5 years	Usually generalized seizures, less than 15 minutes; rarely focal in onset. May lead to status epilepticus.	Nonneurologic febrile illness (temperature rise to 40 °C [104 °F] or higher); family history frequently positive for febrile convulsions.	Normal interictal EEG, especially when obtained 8–10 days after seizure.	In infants or whenever suspicion of meningitis exists, perform lumbar puncture.	Treat underlying illness, fever. Prophylaxis with phenobarbital or valproic acid if phenobarbital not tolerated, with neurologic deficits, prolonged seizure, family history of epilepsy.
Myoclonic-astatic (akinetic, atonic) seizures, formerly "petit mal variant." With mental retardation, Lennox-Gastaut syndrome.	Any time in childhood; normally 2–7 years	Shocklike violent contractions of one or more muscle groups, singly or irregularly repetitive; may fling patient suddenly to side, forward, or backward. Usually no or only brief loss of consciousness. Half of patients or more also have generalized grand mal seizures.	Multiple causes, usually resulting in diffuse neuronal damage. History of West's syndrome; pre- or perinatal brain damage; viral meningoencephalitides; subacute sclerosing panencephalitis; CNS degenerative disorders; lead or other encephalopathies; structural cerebral abnormalities, eg, porencephaly.	Atypical slow (1–2.5 Hz) spike-wave complexes ("petit mal variant") and bursts of high-voltage generalized spikes, often with diffusely slow background frequencies. See text.	As dictated by index of suspicion. Lumbar puncture with measles antibody titer and CSF IgG index. Nerve conduction studies. Urine for lead, arylsulfatase A, etc. Skin biopsy for electron microscopy and enzyme studies. CT scan and brain biopsy may be justified.	Difficult to treat. "Cocktail" of carbamazepine and valproic acid, clonazepam, or methsuximide plus acetazolamide. Imipramine alone or as adjunct. Diazepam. Consider phenacemide, mephenytoin. Ketogenic or medium-chain triglyceride (MCT) diet. ACTH or corticosteroids as in West's syndrome. Protect head with helmet and chin padding.

Absence ("petit mal"). Also juvenile and myoclonic absence.	3–15 years	Lapses of consciousness or vacant stares, lasting about 10 seconds; often in "clusters." Automatisms of face and hands; clonic activity in 30–45%. Often confused with complex partial seizures but no aura or postictal confusion.	Unknown. Genetic component: probably an autosomal dominant gene. Rarely may usher in childhood form of CNS lipidosis.	Three-second bilaterally synchronous, symmetric, high-voltage spikes and waves. EEG "normalization" correlates closely with control of seizures.	Hyperventilation when patient on inadequate or no medication often provokes attacks. Studies for CNS degenerative diseases. CT scan is rarely of value.	Valproic acid or ethosuximide; with latter, add phenobarbital if EEG suggests other abnormalities (grand mal). Acetazolamide. In resistant cases, ketogenic or MCT diet. Also, in resistant cases, valproic acid and ethosuximide together.
Simple partial or focal seizures (motor/sensory/jacksonian). (Complex partial or psychomotor seizures, below.)	Any age	Seizure may involve any part of body; may spread in fixed pattern (jacksonian march), becoming generalized. In children, epileptogenic focus often "shifts," and epileptic manifestations may change concomitantly.	Often secondary to birth trauma, inflammatory process, vascular accidents, meningoencephalitis, etc. If seizures are coupled with new or progressive neurologic deficits, a structural lesion (eg, brain tumor) is likely.	Focal spikes or slow waves in appropriate cortical region; sometimes diffusely abnormal or even normal.	If seizures are difficult to control or progressive deficits occur, neuroradiodiagnostic studies, particularly CT brain scan, imperative (see text).	Carbamazepine, phenytoin, phenobarbital, or primidone. Valproic acid useful adjunct.
Complex partial seizures (psychomotor, temporal lobe, or limbic seizures).	Any age‡	Aura may be a sensation of fear, epigastric discomfort, odd smell or taste (usually unpleasant), visual or auditory hallucination (either vague and "unformed" or well-formed image, words, music). Aura and seizure *stereotyped* for each patient. Seizure may consist of vague stare; facial, tongue, or swallowing movements and throaty sounds; or various complex automatisms. Unlike absences, complex partial seizures tend not to occur in clusters but singly and to last longer (1 minute or more), followed by confusion. History of aura (or child running to adult from "vague fear") and of automatisms involving more than face and hands establishes diagnosis. About 60% also develop generalized grand mal seizures.	As above. Temporal lobes especially sensitive to hypoxia; thus, this seizure type may be sequela of birth trauma, febrile convulsions, etc. Also especially vulnerable to certain viral infections, especially herpes simplex. Remediable other causes are small cryptic tumors or vascular malformations.	As above, but occurring in temporal lobe and its connections, eg, frontotemporal, temporoparietal, temporo-occipital regions.	CT scan when structural lesion suspected. Temporal lobe biopsy when herpes simplex encephalitis suspected (see text). Carotid amobarbital injection when lateralization of speech dominance in question.	Carbamazepine, phenytoin, phenobarbital, or primidone. More than one drug often necessary. Methsuximide or valproic acid may be useful. Phenacemide or mephenytoin in difficult-to-control seizures. In cases uncontrolled by drugs and where a primary epileptogenic focus is identifiable, excision of anterior third of temporal lobe. Adjunctive psychotherapy required frequently.

* ***Note:*** When using anticonvulsants, continue treatment for at least a 2- to 4-year seizure-free period.
† TORCHES is a mnemonic formula for *to*xoplasmosis, *r*ubella, *c*ytomegalovirus, *he*rpes simplex, and *s*yphilis.
‡ May be difficult to recognize in younger children.

Table 23–2 (cont'd). Seizures by age at onset, pattern, and preferred treatment.

Age Group and Seizure Type	Age at Onset	Clinical Manifestations	Causative Factors	Electroencephalographic Pattern	Other Diagnostic Studies	Treatment and Comments* (Anticonvulsants by Order of Choice)
"Convulsive equivalents"; also called "abdominal," "autonomic," "diencephalic," "thalamic-hypothalamic" epilepsy, or "vegetative" seizure disorder	Any age‡	Variety of episodic visceral or sensory disturbances for which no other cause may be found, eg, recurrent abdominal pain, cyclic vomiting, headaches, dizzy spells, episodes of profuse sweating, laughing or crying jags, other paroxysmal alterations of mood or behavior, occasionally incontinence.	Unknown. The episodes may have a "migrainous" quality, and there is often a family history of epilepsy or migraine. Diagnosis depends on (1) paroxysmal, repetitive nature of attacks; (2) absence of explanatory pathologic findings; (3) positive response to therapeutic trial of phenytoin or phenobarbital. Abnormal epileptiform EEG.	Variety of EEG abnormalities in about 70% of cases, sometimes only during attack. One-fourth of children eventually have generalized or psychomotor seizures. May go on to regular migraine.	As indicated by symptomatology.	Phenytoin, about 7 mg/kg preferred. Phenobarbital, 5 mg/kg; occasionally Donnatal in very young child. Careful diagnosis important to avoid confusion with migraine.
"Benign epilepsy of childhood" (with "centrotemporal" or "rolandic" foci)	5–16 years	Partial motor or generalized seizures. Similar seizure patterns may be observed in patients with focal cortical lesions.	Seizure history or abnormal EEG findings in relatives of 40% of affected probands and 18–20% of parents and siblings, suggesting transmission by a single autosomal dominant gene, possibly with age-dependent penetrance.	Centrotemporal spikes or sharp waves ("rolandic discharges") appearing paroxysmally against a normal EEG background.	Serum Ca^{2+} and glucose, BUN, urinalysis. Seldom need CT scan.	Phenobarbital or phenytoin (or both). Primidone.
Juvenile myoclonic epilepsy (of Janz)	Late childhood and adolescence, peaking at 13 years.	Mild myoclonic jerks of neck and shoulder flexor muscles after waking up ("awakening" grand mal seizures). Intelligence usually normal.	40% of relatives have myoclonias, especially in females; 15% have the abnormal EEG pattern without clinical attacks.	Interictal EEG shows fast variety of spike-and-wave sequences or 4- to 6-Hz multispike-and-wave complexes.	Differentiate from progressive myoclonic encephalopathy of Unverricht-Lafora and other degenerative disorders by appropriate biopsies (muscle, liver, etc).	Valproic acid.
Generalized tonic-clonic seizures (grand mal)	Any age	Loss of consciousness; tonic-clonic movements, often preceded by vague aura or cry. Bladder and bowel incontinence in approximately 15%. Postictal confusion; sleep. Often mixed with or masking other seizure patterns.	Often unknown. Genetic component. May be seen with metabolic disturbances, trauma, infection, intoxication, degenerative disorders, brain tumors, etc.	Bilaterally synchronous, symmetric multiple high-voltage spikes, spikes and waves, mixed patterns. Often normal under age 4.	As above.	Phenobarbital in first 12 months; carbamazepine or valproic acid; phenytoin; primidone. Combinations may be necessary. Acetazolamide as adjunct.

* ***Note:*** When using anticonvulsants, continue treatment for at least a 2- to 4-year seizure-free period.

† TORCHES is a mnemonic formula for *to*xoplasmosis, *r*ubella, *c*ytomegalovirus, *he*rpes simplex, and *s*yphilis.

‡ May be difficult to recognize in younger children.

factors such as intrauterine insults, low birth weight, or perinatal complications appear to be similar in febrile convulsions and epilepsy.

Febrile convulsions are "simple" when generalized, less than 15 minutes long, or not in series totaling more than 30 minutes; they are "complex" when focal, prolonged, or multiple ("clustered") in a 24-hour period.

Meningitis must be ruled out. Meningitis may present as a febrile convulsion in 13% of cases, especially in a child under age 2; in 35% of cases, meningeal signs are lacking. Lumbar puncture should be performed in children (1) with any suspicion of meningitis, (2) under 2 years of age, (3) with a first febrile convulsion, and (4) when recovery from a febrile convulsion is slow. Because meningitis may present as a recurrent febrile convulsion, the physician's index of suspicion must remain high, and repeat lumbar punctures are often warranted. Other studies, such as complete blood count, CT scans, and measurements of serum electrolyte, calcium, and blood glucose levels, are rarely useful in uncomplicated febrile seizures. Electroencephalography should be done if the febrile convulsion was complex or if there are abnormal neurologic findings; if possible, it is best to wait a week, since by then only 5% or less of EEGs will be abnormal. However, abnormalities do not predict recurrent febrile convulsions or even the development of epilepsy. The child should be hospitalized when febrile convulsions are severe or multiple, when meningitis or other serious illness is suspected, or when the parents or caretakers are for any reason unable to take care of the child.

Recurrent febrile convulsions occur in about 30–40% of untreated cases. Half of recurrent febrile convulsions occur within 6 months after the initial seizure, and 90% within 30 months. A family history of nonfebrile seizures, complex or multiple initial febrile convulsions, and especially abnormal developmental and neurologic status correlate positively with recurrences.

Epilepsy (ie, recurrent nonfebrile convulsions) develops in a relatively small percentage of children with febrile seizures followed for 15 years. Children at high risk, in whom up to 13% may develop epilepsy, are those with at least 2 of 3 risk factors: family history of nonfebrile seizures, abnormal neurologic or developmental status prior to the initial febrile convulsion, or a complex febrile seizure. (Occurrence of the initial febrile convulsion before 6 months of age may be a fourth factor.) Children with only one or none of these factors are considered at low risk, with only 2–3% developing epilepsy.

The risk of recurrent febrile convulsions can be greatly reduced by daily long-term use of phenobarbital, with the single daily dose sufficient to maintain blood levels between 15 and 20 μg/dL. If phenobarbital is not tolerated, valproic acid is as effective but must be monitored more closely. Rectal diazepam (as a suppository or liquid squirted from a small tube; not yet available in the USA), administered promptly at the onset of an acute febrile illness, is absorbed rapidly enough to provide a high degree of protection.

"Simple" febrile convulsions, even when recurrent, usually do not result in any neurologic or mental impairment. Any deficit found may have either antedated the seizure or resulted from the underlying but unrecognized cause of the febrile seizure, such as roseola infantum, encephalitis, or severe hypernatremia at the time of fever. Effective anticonvulsant prophylaxis of febrile convulsions does not prevent subsequent epilepsy or significant neurologic impairment.

The consensus now is that children at low risk (see above) should not be treated, since the side effects of phenobarbital and valproic acid (Table 23–3) are significant. Prophylaxis should be considered for those at high risk and particularly for any child with neurologic sequelae after a febrile seizure, even if sequelae are transient. Prophylaxis should be continued for at least 2 years or for one seizure-free year after the last seizure, whichever is the longer period. Some may wish to treat after 2 or 3 febrile convulsions.

In counseling the parents and involving them in the decision of whether or not to treat their child, the physician should indicate that most febrile convulsions are benign; continuous treatment for 1 or 2 years poses distinct problems, and intermittent therapy—except with rectal diazepam (not yet available in the USA)—is ineffective; and successful prophylaxis does not lessen the risk of epilepsy. How to manage fever and seizures is, of course, part of the counsel given. The decision of whether to treat will also be based on the physician's consideration of several factors: (1) the possibility that the "simple," brief, generalized, single seizure (with its 2–3% risk of subsequent epilepsy) may have started as a focal one, may have lasted more than 15 minutes, or may have been one of several, carrying a risk of epilepsy 4 times greater; (2) the possibility that any seizure in a small child may lead to hospitalization, which is costly both in emotional and financial terms; and (3) the fact that the seizure itself may be upsetting to the family. Although febrile convulsions occur commonly enough in early childhood, the best approach to the problem is an individualized and flexible one.

E. Laboratory Findings: *Note:* The diagnostic workup should be guided by the age and immediate condition of the child and the demands of the situation. (See also Table 23–2.)

1. Blood—Glucose, calcium, phosphorus, and blood urea nitrogen or nonprotein nitrogen levels should be determined. Measurements of sodium, chloride, and, possibly, magnesium are indicated for most first nonfebrile convulsions. Screening for TORCHES (Table 23–2) and tests for lead and for sickle cell anemia may be warranted.

2. Urine—Reducing substances should be measured. Ferric chloride or Phenistix test, urinalysis, and chromatography for amino acids and organic acids are performed when indicated.

3. Lumbar puncture—Although not a routine procedure, spinal tap should usually be done in infants and young children up to about 2 years of age following the first convulsion, especially if the child is febrile, as discussed above.

Lumbar puncture (see earlier section and also Chapter 35) is not warranted in clear-cut breath-holding spells, recurrent febrile convulsions when the cause of the fever is unequivocally extracranial, or when there is a definite risk of brain herniation from increased intracranial pressure due to a mass. If a mass lesion is suspected, CT brain scanning should precede lumbar puncture in all but desperate situations thought to be due to bacterial infection.

4. Subdural tap—Subdural tap should be considered in an infant with an open anterior fontanelle if there is any possibility of trauma or postmeningitic effusion.

F. Radiologic Findings: Skull x-rays yield little diagnostic information in children with seizures and are not cost-effective. CT brain scanning, on the other hand, is highly informative in selected cases; even in unselected series of epileptic children, abnormalities in the range of 25%, albeit often of atrophic lesions, will be found. Indications for CT scanning and the percentages of abnormalities found are as follows: infantile spasms (60%), Lennox-Gastaut syndrome (35%), persistent unilateral or focal seizures (50%), partial complex (psychomotor) seizures (15%), and difficult-to-control generalized convulsions (15%).

Other clear indications for CT evaluation include persistent seizures despite adequate anticonvulsant treatment; progressive neurologic deficits, especially in the presence of localized slowing on EEG; status epilepticus, especially if focal; suspicion of increased intracranial pressure; and, of course, any child considered for surgical treatment of intractable seizures.

Unexpected CT findings in children, totaling between 2% and 6% of studies, have included tumors, cerebrovascular lesions or malformations, tuberous sclerosis, intracranial calcifications due to infectious processes, and other anomalies. After status epilepticus, severe brain edema was demonstrated to be followed by cerebral atrophy.

Thus, in children with seizures, CT brain scans may be well worth their cost in providing diagnostic information, therapeutic guidance, and a data base for prognosis and in some cases for genetic counseling.

X-rays of long bones or a skeletal survey should be ordered when there is a suspicion of lead poisoning, trauma (''battered child''), or occult tumor.

G. Electroencephalography: The limitations of electroencephalography, even in epilepsy where it is most useful, are considerable. *A seizure is a clinical phenomenon;* an EEG showing epileptiform activity may confirm and even extend the clinical diagnosis, but it cannot make it.

The EEG need not be abnormal in the presence of a definite seizure disorder. Normal EEGs are seen following a first generalized seizure in one-third of children under 4 years of age; the initial EEG is normal in about 20% of older epileptic children and in around 10% of adults with epilepsy. These percentages are reduced when serial tracings are obtained, but never completely eliminated. On the other hand, various grades of ''dysrhythmias'' are frequently observed in children; focal spikes and generalized spike-wave discharges are seen in 30% of close nonepileptic relatives of patients with centrencephalic epilepsy.

1. Diagnostic value—The greatest value of the EEG in convulsive disorders is in helping to classify seizure types and thus to select appropriate therapy (Tables 23–2 and 23–3). Petit mal absences and partial complex or psychomotor seizures are sometimes difficult to distinguish, especially when the physician must rely on the history and cannot observe one; their differing electroencephalographic patterns will then prove most helpful. Another rather frequent illustration of the role of the EEG in guiding therapy is the finding of mixed seizure patterns in a child who clinically has only grand mal or only petit mal absences, since some anticonvulsants efficacious for one seizure type may provoke the other. The EEG may often help in diagnosing neonatal seizures with minimal and ''atypical'' clinical manifestations; it may show ''hypsarrhythmia'' in infantile spasms or the pattern associated with the Lennox-Gastaut syndrome, both expressions of diffuse brain dysfunctioning of multiple causes and generally of grave significance. The EEG may help differentiate ''convulsive equivalents'' from somatic complaints of psychogenic origin.

The EEG may show focal slowing that, if constant—particularly when there are corresponding focal seizure manifestations and abnormal neurologic findings—will alert the physician to the presence of a structural lesion, in which case brain imaging may establish the cause and help determine further investigation and treatment.

2. Prognostic value—A normal EEG following a first convulsion suggests (but does not guarantee) a favorable prognosis. Markedly abnormal EEGs may become normal with treatment (1) immediately following intravenous injection of 50 mg vitamin B_6 in pyridoxine dependency or deficiency; (2) in infantile spasms and sometimes the Lennox-Gastaut syndrome (corticotropin or corticosteroids); (3) in petit mal absences (anticonvulsants); and (4) in petit mal and other minor motor seizures, including the Lennox-Gastaut syndrome (ketogenic diet). If so, it is likely that seizure control will be achieved (although this offers no clues to the mental status of the patient).

Electroencephalography should be repeated when there is an increase in the severity and frequency of seizures despite exhaustive and adequate anticonvulsant therapy; when there is a significant change in the clinical seizure pattern; or when there are progressive neurologic deficits. Focal or diffuse slowing may indicate a progressive lesion.

The EEG may be quite helpful in determining when to discontinue anticonvulsant therapy. The presence or absence of epileptiform activity on the EEG prior to withdrawal of anticonvulsants after a seizure-free period of several years on the medications has been shown to be correlated with the degree of risk of recurrence of seizures.

3. Interpretation—The techniques of recording and interpreting the EEG constitute a separate area of specialization. The most typical patterns are mentioned in Table 23–2.

Note: The 14- and 6-per-second positive spike pattern observed most frequently in adolescents, particularly during light sleep, has been claimed to be associated with convulsive equivalents and dissocial or asocial behavior; it is now considered a normal finding.

H. Additional Investigations: In patients with difficult-to-control partial seizures of complex symptomatology, particularly when these may be difficult to differentiate from pseudoseizures, an EEG with simultaneous audiovisual monitoring may be extremely helpful in directing proper treatment.

In patients with difficult-to-control seizures whose EEGs as ordinarily recorded are not informative, all-night or 24-hour tracings may be desirable. In considering surgery, EEG activation with methohexital (Brevital), under an anesthesiologist's supervision, may be used to provide information about the primary epileptic focus. Other special diagnostic techniques of value in selected patients include videotape monitoring, telemetry, positron emission tomography, brain electrical activity mapping, and (if surgery is contemplated) implantation of depth electrodes.

Differential Diagnosis

A. Fainting: In syncope, as cerebral blood flow drops, the patient usually reports that "things went black" before "sinking to the ground." Tonic-clonic movements rarely occur. As blood flow to the brain increases (when the patient lies recumbent or sits with head hanging between the legs), consciousness returns. There are no postictal phenomena, and usually there is no retrograde amnesia.

B. Conversion Hysteria ("Hysteroepilepsy"): The differentiation from epilepsy may be extremely difficult, particularly if the patient has true seizures but also mimics attacks. This is most often observed in immature adolescents. The character of the spells (pseudoseizures) may be quite convincing, depending on how much the patient knows about epilepsy and whether seizures were ever observed by the patient. Self-injury or urination is a possibility if there is a strong sadomasochistic component to the patient's conversion reaction. In less sophisticated patients, the attacks tend to be "bizarre." During the attack, the patient is often resistive. Even when the patient mimics postictal stupor, the pupillary dilatation and Babinski responses so often seen immediately after a true seizure are usually not present. The EEG during an attack simply shows muscle artifact, but no preceding "buildup," paroxysmal activity, or postseizure slowing is seen, and "interictal" EEGs are repeatedly normal; however, a "provocative" EEG (ie, with suggestion that a seizure will occur) can be immensely helpful.

C. Narcolepsy: See Sleep Disorders, below.

Complications

Emotional disturbances—notably anxiety, depression, anger, feelings of guilt and inadequacy—often occur as a reaction to the seizures in the parents of the affected child as well as in the child old enough to understand. The seizures—and particularly the hallucinatory auras and psychomotor attacks—frequently set off in the prepubescent and adolescent youngster fantasies (and sometimes obsessive ruminations) about dying and death that may become so strong as to lead to suicidal behavior and suicidal attempts. The limitations many school systems place on epileptic children add to the problem. Commonly, the child expresses feelings by "acting out."

Pseudoretardation may occur in poorly controlled epileptic children because their seizures—or the subclinical paroxysms sustained—may interfere with their learning ability. Anticonvulsants are less likely to "slow the child down" but may do so when given in toxic amounts; phenobarbital is particularly implicated.

True mental retardation is most commonly part of the same pathologic process that causes the seizures but may occasionally occur when seizures are frequent, prolonged, and accompanied by hypoxia.

Physical injuries, especially lacerations of the forehead and chin, are frequent in astatic or akinetic seizures (drop attacks). In all other seizure disorders in childhood, injuries as a direct result of an attack are impressively rare.

Treatment

The ideal treatment of seizures is the correction of specific causes. However, even when a biochemical disorder (eg, leucine hypoglycemia), a tumor, or septic meningitis is being treated, anticonvulsant drugs are often still required.

A. Precautionary Management of Individual Brief Seizures: Protect the patient against self-injury and aspiration of vomitus. Beyond that, no specific therapy is necessary. The less done to the patient during a relatively brief seizure (up to 10 or 15 minutes), the better. Thrusting a spoon handle or tongue depressor into the clenched mouth of a convulsing patient or trying to restrain tonic-clonic movements may cause worse injuries than a bitten tongue or bruised limb. Mouth-to-mouth resuscitation is rarely (if ever) necessary.

B. General Management of the Young Epileptic:

1. Education—The patient and the parents must be helped to understand the problem of seizures and their management. Many children—some even as young as 3 years of age—are capable of cooperating with the physician in problems of seizure control.

All bottles containing antiepileptic drugs should bear a contents label. The parents should know the names and dosage of the anticonvulsants being administered.

Materials on epilepsy—including pamphlets (some in Spanish), monographs, films, and videotapes suitable for children and teenagers, parents, teachers, and medical professionals—may be purchased through the Epilepsy Foundation of America, Materials Service Center, 4351 Garden City Drive, Landover, MD 20785. The Foundation's local chapter and other community organizations are eager to provide guidance and other services. In many cities, there are support groups for older children and adolescents and for their parents and others concerned.

2. Privileges and precautions in daily life—Encourage normal living within reasonable bounds. Children should engage in physical activities appropriate to their age and social group. After seizure control is established, swimming is generally permissible with a "buddy system" or adequate lifeguard coverage. High diving and high climbing should not be permitted. Physical training and sports (other than "contact" sports) are usually to be welcomed rather than restricted. Driving is discussed below.

Loss of sleep should be avoided. Emotional disturbances may need therapy. Alcoholic intake, a serious problem usually beginning in adolescence, should be avoided, as it may precipitate seizures. Prompt attention should be given to infections. Further neurologic disturbances should be brought to the physician's attention promptly.

Although every effort should be made to control seizures, this must not interfere with a child's ability to function. Sometimes a child is better off having an occasional mild seizure than being so heavily sedated as to impair function at home, in school, or at play. This often requires much art and fortitude on the part of the physician. Indeed, some pediatricians and pediatric neurologists, after discussion with the parents, are now *not* instituting anticonvulsant therapy after up to 3 nonfebrile convulsions in an otherwise neurologically intact child.

3. Driving—Driving becomes important to most youngsters at age 15 or 16. Restrictions vary from state to state; in most, a learner's permit or driver's license will be issued if the patient has been under a physician's care and free of seizures for at least 2 years, provided the treatment or basic neurologic problem does not interfere with the ability to drive. A guide to this and other legal matters pertaining to persons with epilepsy is published by the Epilepsy Foundation of America, whose Legal Advocacy Department may be able to provide additional information (see reference below).

4. Pregnancy—In the pregnant teenager with epilepsy, the possibility of teratogenic effects of anticonvulsants, such as facial clefts (about 5%), must be weighed against the risks from seizures. Such malformations occur in the infants of about 2.5% of untreated epileptic mothers.

C. Principles of Anticonvulsant Therapy:

1. Treat with the drug appropriate to the clinical situation, as outlined in Tables 23–2, 23–3, and 23–4.

2. Start with one drug in conventional dosage, and increase the dosage until seizures are controlled. If seizures are not controlled on the tolerated maximal dosage of one major anticonvulsant, gradually switch over to another before adding a second anticonvulsant. The dosages and usually effective blood levels listed in Table 23–3 are guides. Individual variations must be expected. The "therapeutic range" may also vary somewhat with the method used to determine levels. ***Note:*** Blood levels of antiepileptic drugs are discussed below.

3. Advise the parents and the patient that the prolonged use of anticonvulsant drugs will not produce significant or permanent "mental slowing" (although the underlying cause of the seizures might) and that prevention of seizures for 3–4 years or so substantially reduces the chances of recurrence. Advise them also that anticonvulsants are given to prevent further seizures and that they should be taken as prescribed. Changes in medications or dosages should not be made without the physician's knowledge. Unsupervised sudden withdrawal of anticonvulsant drugs may precipitate severe seizures or even status epilepticus.

Anticonvulsants must be kept where they cannot be ingested by small children or suicidal patients.

4. Check the patient at intervals, depending on the underlying cause of the seizures, the degree of control, and the toxic properties of the anticonvulsant drug or drugs used. Blood counts, urinalyses, and liver function or other biologic tests must be obtained periodically in the case of some anticonvulsants, as indicated in Table 23–3.

Periodic neurologic reevaluation is important. CT scanning may be indicated, as discussed under radiologic findings, above. Repeat EEGs are not needed to achieve seizure control. Indications for repeat EEGs are discussed above.

5. Continue anticonvulsant treatment until the patient is free of seizures for 2 or more years or, in some cases, through adolescence. In about 75% of cases, seizures may not recur. Such variables as younger age at onset, normal EEG, and ease of controlling seizures carry a favorable prognosis, while later onset, slowing or spikes on EEG, a history of atypical febrile convulsions, and possibly an abnormal neurologic examination carry a higher risk of recurrence.

6. In general, there is no need to withdraw anticonvulsants before taking an EEG.

7. Discontinue anticonvulsants gradually. If it becomes necessary to withdraw anticonvulsants abruptly, the patient should be under close medical surveillance. If seizures recur during or after with-

drawal, anticonvulsant therapy should be reinstituted and again maintained for at least 2 or more years.

D. Blood Levels of Antiepileptic Drugs:

1. General comments—Most anticonvulsants take 5–6 times the length of their half-life to reach the "steady state" indicated in Table 23–3. This must be considered when blood levels are assessed after anticonvulsants are started or dosages are changed.

Individuals vary in their metabolism and their particular pharmacokinetic characteristics. These and external factors, including, for example, food intake or illness, also affect the blood level. Thus, the level reached on a milligram per kilogram or surface area basis varies among patients.

Experience and clinical research in the determination of antiepileptic blood levels have shown that there is *some* correlation between (1) drug dose and blood level, (2) blood level and therapeutic effect, and (3) blood level and *some* toxic effects.

2. Effective levels—The ranges given in Table 23–3 are those within which seizure control without toxicity will be achieved in most patients. The level for any given individual will vary not only with metabolic makeup (including biochemical defects) but also with the nature and severity of the seizures and their underlying cause, with other medications being taken, and other factors. Seizure control may be achieved at lower levels in some; and higher levels may be reached without toxicity in others. When control is achieved at a lower level, the dose should *not* be increased merely to get the level into the "therapeutic range." Likewise, toxic side effects will be experienced at different levels even *within* the "therapeutic range"; lowering the dose will usually resolve the problem, but sometimes the drug must be withdrawn or another added (or both). Some serious toxic effects, including allergic reactions, LE phenomenon, and bone marrow or liver toxicity, are independent of dosage; liver toxicity especially may be the effect not just of a particular drug but also of its use in a patient who is or has been on several—and often a whole gamut—of other drugs.

3. Interaction of antiepileptic drugs—Blood levels of anticonvulsants may be affected by other drugs used. Examples are shown in Table 23–5. Individual variations occur; adjustment of doses may be required.

4. Indications for blood levels—Drug blood levels should be measured in a new patient or after a new drug is introduced and seizure control without toxicity is achieved to determine the "effective level" for that patient. Blood level monitoring is useful also when expected control on a "usual" dosage has not been achieved, either with a single drug or after adding another; when seizures recur in a previously well-controlled patient; or when control is poor in a patient on anticonvulsants seen for the first time. A low level may indicate inadequate dosage, drug interaction, or—quite frequently—noncompliance with the therapeutic regimen prescribed. A high level may indicate refractoriness, drug interaction, or a worsening neurologic process. ***Note:*** Brief and limited "breakthroughs" are common in children (particularly younger ones) with intercurrent infections or significant excitement or other stresses, and they do *not* necessitate blood levels.

Blood levels are mandatory when there are signs and symptoms of toxicity—particularly where there is polydrug therapy, the dosage of a drug has been raised, or another drug has been added. Blood levels may be the only means of detecting intoxication in a comatose patient or very young child. Toxic levels also occur with drug abuse or liver disease.

Finally, when the patient is well controlled (or is controlled as well as one may hope for in a patient refractory to antiepileptics or one with difficult-to-control seizures) and free of toxic signs, blood levels are desirable once or twice a year.

E. Side Effects of Antiepileptic Drugs: (See also Table 23–3.)

1. Serious allergic reactions usually necessitate discontinuance of a drug. However, not every rash in a child receiving an anticonvulsant is due to the drug. If a useful antiepileptic drug is discontinued for this reason and the rash disappears, restarting the drug in a smaller dosage is often warranted to see if the reaction recurs.

2. Signs of drug toxicity will often disappear when the daily dosage is reduced by 25–30%.

3. The sedative effect of many of the anticonvulsants is often easily counteracted by the judicious use of coffee or dextroamphetamine sulfate, 2.5–5 mg at breakfast and 2.5 mg at noon.

4. Gingival hyperplasia secondary to phenytoin is best minimized through good dental hygiene but occasionally requires gingivectomy. This condition (but not hypertrichosis) usually disappears within about 6 months after the drug is discontinued.

F. Guides to Therapy of Specific Seizure Disorders: See Tables 23–2, 23–3, and 23–4.

G. Management of Status Epilepticus: Diazepam (Valium) is the drug of choice. In general, 0.2 ± 0.05 mg/kg or 6 mg/m^2 administered intravenously over 1–3 minutes will achieve control; if necessary, half the initial amount should be given again. Pulse and blood pressure should be monitored during the injection; if these drop markedly, the injection should be temporarily halted until cardiovascular function returns to normal. In recurrent status epilepticus, intravenous diazepam may be repeated every 3–4 hours.

Lorazepam is also proving highly effective, with longer action than diazepam and little or no respiratory depression.

Phenytoin, 10–20 mg/kg slowly intravenously, is often useful in status epilepticus, especially where it is desirable to avoid depressing the level of consciousness. Lidocaine (Xylocaine) is very useful for rapid (though brief) control of focal motor seizures.

For further details on drug use in status epilepticus, see Table 23–3.

Table 23–3. Guide to pediatric anticonvulsant drug therapy.

Drug	Average Total (mg/kg/d)	in	Divided Doses	Steady State: Days	Effective Blood Levels (μg/mL)*	Side Effects and Precautions†	Usage and Remarks
Primary anticonvulsant							
Carbamazepine (Tegretol)	15–25	:	3–4	3–6	4–12 (> 15)	Thrombocytopenia, leukopenia, rash. Rare: hepatoxicity; bone marrow depression; dystonia; inappropriate ADH secretion; bizarre behaviors; tics.	Monitor CBC, platelet count, liver functions first 6 months closely; then periodically. Blood effects usually early and transient. May cause mild hypocalcemia.
Valproic acid (Depakene, Depakote)	15–60	:	2–3	2–4	50–120 (> 200)	Few side effects. Occasional gastric discomfort. Rare: hepatotoxicity; hyperammonemia.	For prophylaxis in febrile convulsion, see text. Monitor CBC, platelets, liver functions (especially split fibrinogen) first 6 months closely; then periodically. Can be given rectally.
Phenytoin (Dilantin)	5–10	:	2	5–10	5–20 (> 25)	Gum hypertrophy, hirsutism, ataxia, nystagmus, diplopia, rash, anorexia, nausea, osteomalacia. Severe toxicity may cause pseudodementia and liver damage. Rare: macrocytic anemia, lymph node involvement, exfoliative dermatitis, peripheral neuropathy.	Generally very effective and safe. No effect on behavior. Good dental hygiene reduces gum hyperplasia. May aggravate absence and myoclonic seizures. Check linear growth periodically; obtain Ca^{2+} and bone films as indicated: consider supplemental vitamin D. Poorly absorbed by neonatal gut. Absorption after intramuscular injection erratic. Useful in neonatal seizures and status epilepticus. ***Note:*** Suspension not recommended.
Phenobarbital	3–8	:	1	10–21	15–40 (> 45)	Irritability and overactivity in many children; sedative effects in others. Mild ataxia, nystagmus, skin rash. Osteomalacia. May interfere with learning.	Safest overall drug. Bitter taste. Higher blood levels sometimes required and tolerated in severe chronic epileptics. Check linear growth periodically; obtain Ca^{2+} and bone films as indicated; consider supplemental vitamin D. Useful in neonatal seizures and status epilepticus.
Primidone (Mysoline)	10–25	:	3–4	1–5	4–12 (> 15)	Drowsiness, ataxia, vertigo, anorexia, nausea, vomiting, rash.	Start slowly with 25–35% of expected maintenance dose; increase every 2 days until full dose reached. Most useful when phenobarbital not tolerated. Suspension pleasant.
Ethosuximide (Zarontin)	10–40	:	1–2	5–6	40–100 (> 150)	Nausea, gastric discomfort. Rare: bone marrow depression; hepatotoxicity.	May aggravate generalized seizures. Combine with valproic acid in refractory absence seizures.
Clonazepam (Clonopin)	0.1–0.2	:	2–3	5–10	15–80 ng/mL (≥ 80)	Drowsiness(> 50%): soporific effects greatest drawback. Behavior problems (25%). Slurred speech, ataxia, salivation.	Start slowly with 10–25% of expected maintenance dose; increase every 2–3 days. Very useful with difficult to treat minor motor seizures (astatic, myoclonic, infantile spasms; absences). Tolerance often occurs after a few months, but drug may be restarted after period of withdrawal. May aggravate generalized seizures.
Adjunctive or secondary drug							
Acetazolamide (Diamox)	5–20	:	2–3	(Not known)	. . .	Anorexia; numbness and tingling. Increase in urinary frequency; hence, do not give in evening.	Supplement to other medications, especially in absences and complex partial seizures. Also in females 4 days prior to and in the first 2–3 days of menstrual periods.

Methsuximide (Celontin)	15–30	:	3–4	(Not known)	10–40 (normethsuxi-mide)	Drowsiness, ataxia, headache, diplopia. Skin rash (15%).	Useful in complex partial and myoclonic-astatic seizures.
Clorazepate (Tranxene)	0.3–1	:	2–3	(Not known)	0.2–1.5 (> 2)	Lethargy.	May be useful adjunct in generalized tonic-clonic, partial, and astatic seizures.
Mephenytoin (Mesantoin)	4–15	:	2	(Not known)	5–25 (as ethylphenyl-hydantoin)	Mild: Rash, drowsiness, ataxia. ***Warning:*** Aplastic anemia, agranulocytosis.	A good anticonvulsant, especially in difficult to control complex partial, and possibly myoclonic-astatic, seizures. Fear of bone marrow depression limits use. Monthly CBC.
Phenacemide (Phenurone)	25–50	:	2–4	(Not known)	. . .	Rash, anorexia, nausea. ***Warning:*** Hepatitis, psychosis, blood dyscrasias.	Especially effective in complex partial seizures when all other drugs fail. Frequent CBC, liver function tests initial 3–4 months, then 2–4/yr.
Diazepam (Valium)	0.20 ± 0.05	:	3	(Not known)	. . .	Somnolence.	Useful in myoclonic-astatic and absence seizures and infantile spasms. Often ineffective after a few months. First choice in status epilepticus, below.
Dextroamphetamine (Dexedrine)	0.25–0.75	:	Breakfast and noon	(Not known)	. . .	Nervousness, palpitations, anorexia, insomnia.	To counteract sedative effect of other drugs. Narcolepsy. In behavior disorders of younger children. Growth retardation with chronic use reversible.
Trimethadione (Tridione)	20–50	:	3–4	(Not known)	470–1200 (dimethadione)	Rash, photophobia, irritability. ***Warning:*** Leukopenia, agranulocytosis, nephrosis. LE phenomenon.	Useful primarily in absences if ethosuximide and valproic acid fail. May aggravate generalized seizures; if so, add phenobarbital. Monthly CBC, urinalysis.
Mephobarbital (Mebaral)	4–10	:	1–2	(Not known)	15–40 (phenobarbital)	As with phenobarbital.	Twice the quantity of phenobarbital required for comparable effect.
Treatment of status epilepticus							
Diazepam (Valium)	0.2 ± 0.05 mg/kg IV initially. Repeat dose 0.1 mg/kg.					Administer slowly IV. Monitor pulse and blood pressure. May cause respiratory depression in presence of phenobarbital.	May need to be repeated every 3–4 hours. Follow with phenytoin or phenobarbital for long-range control. ***Note:*** Administration IM for status epilepticus ineffective.
Lorazepam	0.05–0.2 mg/kg IV. May repeat.					Mild respiratory depression.	May be more effective than diazepam.
Phenobarbital	5–20 mg/kg IV initially. Repeat dose 5 mg/kg IV.					See above.	Rule out pyridoxine deficiency. In neonatal seizures, load with 15–30 mg/kg IV (IM if IV impossible).
Phenytoin (Dilantin)	10–20 mg/kg IV initially. Repeat dose every 6–8 hours 2 or 3 times.					Administer IV over a 5-minute period. IM absorption uncertain. Monitor blood levels.	Adjunct in neonatal seizures (20 mg/kg IV) if phenobarbital alone fails; oral maintenance dose is 10–25 mg/kg/d.
Paraldehyde	0.1–0.15 mL/kg IV; 0.2–0.3 mL/kg rectally.					Administer slowly IV mixed in saline; rectal dose in vegetable oil, 1:1. Avoid in patient with pulmonary disease or in croupette.	Avoid IM administration if possible: may cause fat necrosis. Do not use plastic syringes.
Lidocaine (Xylocaine)	2 mg/kg IV.					Administer slowly.	Useful especially when reluctant to give more diazepam, barbiturates, or paraldehyde. Effect brief (about 30 min).
General anesthesia if other measures fail.							
Treatment of infantile spasms							
See text regarding use of corticotropin or corticosteroids and of ketogenic diet. Also, clonazepam, diazepam, or valproic acid, especially with recurrences.							

* In monotherapy. (Level at which clinical toxicity usually becomes manifest.)
† The interaction of antiepileptic drugs is outlined in Table 23–5.

Table 23–4. Anticonvulsants in monotherapy.

Seizures With Generalized Onset			Focal Onset (Partial)
Tonic-clonic	**Absence**	**Myoclonic-astatic**	**Simple *and* complex**
Carbamazepine	Valproic acid	Valproic acid	Carbamazepine
Valproic acid	Ethosuximide	Clonazepam	Phenytoin
Phenytoin*	Clonazepam	Ethosuximide	Primidone
Phenobarbital†			Phenobarbital

* Drug of second choice in neonatal seizures and in children under 1 year of age.
† Drug of first choice in neonatal seizures and often in children under 1 year of age.

Table 23–5. Interaction of antiepileptic drugs.*

Level of	Increased by	Decreased by	Variable or Unchanged by
Carbamazepine†	Acetazolamide Isoniazid	Phenobarbital Phenytoin Primidone	Clonazepam
Clonazepam	Little interaction	Little interaction	
Ethosuximide	Little interaction	Little interaction	
Phenobarbital	Amphetamine Methylphenidate Valproic acid		Clonazepam Phenytoin
Phenytoin	Amphetamine Isoniazid Methsuximide	Primidone Salicylates	Carbamazepine Clonazepam Phenobarbital Valproic acid
Primidone	Amphetamine Isoniazid Methylphenidate Valproic acid	Acetazolamide Carbamazepine	Phenytoin
Valproic acid†		Phenobarbital Phenytoin Primidone	

* Interactions vary in individuals. Reports on interactions not always consistent.
† Carbamazepine and valproic acid may decrease each other.

Note: General anesthesia may have to be used to control status epilepticus if the usual measures fail.

Once seizure control and an effective blood level are achieved, phenobarbital, 3–5 mg/kg, or phenytoin, 5–7 mg/kg, should be administered (the route depending on the situation) for long-term control.

H. Corticotropin and Corticosteroids:

1. Indications—These drugs are indicated for infantile spasms not due to causes amenable to specific therapy and in the Lennox-Gastaut syndrome, which cannot be controlled by anticonvulsant drugs.

The duration of therapy is guided by cessation of clinical seizures and "normalization" of the EEG. Corticotropin or the oral corticosteroids are usually continued in full doses for 2–3 weeks and then, if seizures have ceased, are tapered by about 25% every 2 weeks for a total treatment period of about 2 months. If seizures recur, increase the dosage to the last effective level and maintain the patient for up to 6 months on this dosage before again attempting withdrawal.

2. Dosages—

a. Corticotropin gel (Acthar Gel), starting with 5–8 units/kg/d intramuscularly in 2 divided doses. Parents can be taught to give the injections.

b. Cortisone, starting with 6–8 mg/kg/d orally in 3 divided doses.

c. Prednisone, starting with 2–4 mg/kg/d orally in 3 divided doses.

d. In astatic and myoclonic seizures, give another major anticonvulsant also.

3. Precautions—Give additional potassium, guard against infections, and discuss the cushingoid appearance and its disappearance. Do not withdraw oral corticosteroids suddenly.

I. Ketogenic or Medium-Chain Triglyceride Diet in Treatment of Epilepsy: A ketogenic diet should be recommended in astatic and myoclonic seizures and absence seizures not responsive to drug therapy; it is occasionally recommended for infantile spasms that do not respond to corticotropin or the corticosteroids. Ketosis is induced by a diet high in fats and very limited in carbohydrates with sufficient protein for body maintenance and growth; by the feeding of medium-chain triglycerides (MCT); or by a combination of these methods. The MCT diet induces ketosis more readily than does a high level of dietary fats and hence requires less carbohydrate restriction. The mechanism for the anticonvulsant action of the ketogenic diet is not yet understood, although various hypotheses have been put forth. However, it is the ketosis, not the acidosis, that raises the seizure threshold. It is usually most effective in young children (ie, those under the age of 8 years), but when all other measures fail, it should be tried even in adolescents.

As ketosis is achieved, a repeat EEG may be helpful; seizure control by the diet is more likely to occur if the EEG shows improvement.

The ketogenic diet is difficult and expensive, tends to be monotonous, and depends upon the ability of the mother to weigh out the foods as well as upon absolute adherence to the diet prescribed. Whether the ketosis is achieved by high fat meals or an MCT diet is often a matter of the physician's, the dietitian's, or the patient's preference. The result may also depend on which form of the diet is better tolerated. Full cooperation of *all* family members is required, including the patient if old enough. However, when seizure control is achieved by this method, the child is alert, often needs no anticonvulsants or only small amounts, and parental and patient satisfaction is most gratifying.

J. Surgery: In seizure disorders intractable to anticonvulsant therapy and primarily of focal origin, neurosurgery should be considered. Useful procedures, depending on the lesion, include corticectomy, hemispherectomy, anterior temporal lobectomy (for complex partial seizures), callosotomy (or commissurotomy), and stereotactic ablation.

Aicardi J, Chevrie JJ: Convulsive status epilepticus in infants and children. A study of 239 cases. *Epilepsia* 1970;**11:**187.

Camfield PR et al: Epilepsy after a first unprovoked seizure in childhood. *Neurology* 1985;**35:**1657.

Committee on Drugs, American Academy of Pediatrics: Behavioral and cognitive effects of anticonvulsant therapy. *Pediatrics* 1985;**76:**644.

Consensus statement: Febrile seizures: Long-term management of children with fever-associated seizures. *Pediatrics* 1980; **66:**1009.

Delgado-Escueta AV, Treiman DM, Walsh GO: Medical progress: The treatable epilepsies. (2 parts.) *N Engl J Med* 1983;**308:**1508, 1576.

Ellison PH: Management of seizures in the high-risk infant. *Clin Perinatol* 1984;**11:**175.

Epilepsy Foundation of America: *The Legal Rights of Persons With Epilepsy: An Overview of Legal Issues, Federal Laws, and State Laws Affecting Persons With Epilepsy,* 5th ed. Epilepsy Foundation of America, 1985.

Finlayson RE, Lucas AR: Pseudoepileptic seizures in children and adolescents. *Mayo Clin Proc* 1979;**54:**83.

Gomez MR, Klass DW: Neurological progress: Epilepsies of infancy and childhood. *Ann Neurol* 1983;**13:**113.

Green JR: Surgical treatment of epilepsy during childhood and adolescence: Percival Bailey Oration. *Surg Neurol* 1977; **8:**71.

Holmes GL: Partial seizures in children. *Pediatrics* 1986; **77:**725.

Homan RW, Walker JE: Clinical studies of lorazepam in status epilepticus. Chap 51, pp 493–498, in: *Advances in Neurology.* Vol 34: *Status Epilepticus.* Delgado-Escueta AV et al (editors). Raven, 1983.

Hurst DL: The use of imipramine in minor motor seizures. *Pediatr Neurol* 1986;**2:**13.

Huttenlocher PR: Ketonemia and seizures: Metabolic and anticonvulsant effects of two ketogenic diets in childhood epilepsy. *Pediatr Res* 1976;**10:**536.

Kutt H: Interactions between anticonvulsants and other commonly prescribed drugs. *Epilepsia* 1984;**25(Suppl 2):**S118.

Meldrum B: Physiological changes during prolonged seizures and epileptic brain damage. *Neuropaediatrie* 1978;**9:**203.

Mitchell WG, Greenwood RS, Messenheimer JA: Abdominal epilepsy: Cyclic vomiting as the major symptom of simple partial seizures. *Arch Neurol* 1983;**40:**251.

Morselli PL, Pippenger CE, Penry JK (editors): *Antiepileptic Drug Therapy in Pediatrics.* Raven Press, 1983.

Painter MJ, Bergman I, Crumrine P: Neonatal seizures. *Pediatr Clin North Am* 1986;**33:**91.

Riikonen R: Infantile spasms: Modern practical aspects. *Acta Paediatr Scand* 1984;**73:**1.

Shinnar S et al: Discontinuing antiepileptic medication in children with epilepsy after two years without seizures: A prospective study. *N Engl J Med* 1985;**313:**976.

Taylor DC, McKinlay I: When not to treat epilepsy with drugs: Annotations. *Dev Med Child Neurol* 1984;**26:**822.

Vajda FJE, Aicardi J: Reassessment of the concept of a therapeutic range of anticonvulsant plasma levels. *Dev Med Child Neurol* 1983;**25:**660.

HEADACHES

Headache is not usually a psychosomatic symptom in very young children, whereas this is more often the case—even in association with vomiting—in older children and adolescents. Headaches occur in 37% and migraine in 2.7% of children by 7 years of age; by 14 years, the rates are 69% and 10.9%, respectively. A careful description of the headaches, associated circumstances, and other neurologic and systemic symptoms should be obtained. The family history and emotional problems should be discussed in detail. Systemic and neurologic examination, including blood pressure, ophthalmoscopic examination, and urinalysis, will usually distinguish organic from psychogenic headaches. Differential features are given in Table 23–6.

If there is evidence of a specific intracranial cause or systemic disorder (eg, renal disease), diagnosis and treatment should be directed at the primary disorder.

Table 23–6. Differential features of headaches in children.

	Muscule Contraction (Tension/Psychogenic)	Vascular (Migraine)	Traction and Inflammatory (Increased Intracranial Pressure)
Time course	Chronic, recurrent.	Acute, paroxysmal, recurrent.	Chronic or intermittent but increasingly frequent; *progressive severity.*
Prodromes	No.	Yes.	No.
Description	Diffuse, bandlike, tight.	Intense, pulsatile, unilateral in older child (70%).	Diffuse; more occipital with infratentorial mass, more frontal with supratentorial mass.
Characteristic findings	Feelings of inadequacy, depression, or anxiety.	Neurologic symptoms and signs usually transient.	Positive neurologic signs, especially papilledema.
Predisposing factors	Problems at home or school or socially (sexually).	Positive family history (75%); head trauma.	No.

Muscle Contraction (Tension) Headaches

Often described as "dull" or "like a tight band," of slow onset, diffuse, occipital and sometimes nuchal in location, lasting for hours, and rarely disabling, tension headaches are a frequent complaint in school-age and especially adolescent children.

Salicylates are often successful in relieving the discomfort. Antianxiety drugs such as chlordiazepoxide (Librium), 5–10 mg 2–3 times daily, are occasionally indicated, along with supportive therapy. Primary attention should be directed at the precipitating and chronic causes of the emotional strain.

Vascular Headaches (Migraine)

Migraine attacks are usually paroxysmal, throbbing, pulsating, or pounding in character (initial vasoconstriction of intracranial vessels followed by vasodilatation of extracranial vessels). The pain in children is as often bilateral as unilateral, frontal or retro-orbital as hemicranial. Between attacks, the child is asymptomatic. Migraine in children is associated (in order of frequency) with nausea, gastric discomfort, or vomiting; dizziness or vertigo; photophobia, visual auras, and, less frequently, visual loss; sensory and motor disturbances, especially involving face and arm; speech disturbances; and, occasionally, hemiplegia (sometimes alternating), acute confusional states, or impairment of space, time, and body image perceptions (termed the "Alice-in-Wonderland syndrome"). The child frequently seeks rest in a dark, quiet room.

Migraine of varying severity may occur in up to 6.6% of children between 7 and 14 years of age. Onset by age 4 is not uncommon. After 10 years of age, it is twice as common in girls as in boys. The family history is positive for migraine in up to 75% of patients and not infrequently also for epilepsy. School stresses (headache often occurs after school) and foods occasionally precipitate migraine. Head trauma may precipitate onset. In most instances, the migraine attack is brief (hours, not days), and sleep gives relief. Motion sickness is an associated feature in 45% of cases.

EEG may be abnormally slow to mildly or moderately dysrhythmic in up to 80% of patients (emphasizing the relationship between migraine and epilepsy). Neuroradiologic studies, such as CT scanning, are usually not warranted unless there are definite neurologic or progressive abnormalities; in rare instances, an arteriovenous malformation may present as migraine.

Salicylates are often effective in children. The patient should be allowed to remain quiet in a darkened room. In children over 12 years of age, severe migraine may often be controlled by Fiorinal,* Lanorinal,* or Fioricet,† 1 capsule every 4 hours. If these measures are ineffective, especially in the older child, and when anxiety and nausea are prominent symptoms, Cafergot P-B,‡ ½–1 tablet at the first sign of an attack and ½–1 additional tablet every 30 minutes for a total of 2–4 tablets, is often useful. Cafergot P-B suppositories may be used when vomiting precludes oral medication.

In the prevention of severe, frequent, and disabling migraine—especially in children too young to alert an adult to their symptoms or to follow the above regimen—prophylaxis is recommended as follows: propranolol (Inderal), 10–40 mg 3 times daily depending on weight (contraindications are respiratory and cardiac disorders); cyproheptadine (Periactin), 0.2–0.4 mg/kg/d in 2–3 divided doses; or phenytoin (Dilantin) or phenobarbital (used in patients with or without abnormal findings on EEG or family history of seizures). Antidepressants such as imipramine (Tofranil) or amitriptyline (Elavil) may be useful (10–25 mg 2–3 times daily). In children, methysergide maleate (Sansert) is not recommended.

Cluster Headaches (Horton's Headaches)

Also known as histaminic cephalalgia, this presumably allergic disorder is uncommon in children. It is characterized by intense unilateral pain in the orbital area and often radiating to part or all of the face on the affected side. Other manifestations include conjunctival congestion, tearing, and flushing. Attacks may be relieved by inhalation of 100% oxygen, 5–7 L/min for 10 minutes; sublingual ergotamine, 1–2 mg; or, if there is no response, oral prednisone in a single dose (10–40 mg) or as a short course. In chronic cluster headaches, lithium carbonate to a level of about 1 mg/L may be prophylactic.

Headaches Due to Refractive Error

In school-age children, more headaches are blamed on eye problems than can be substantiated by ophthalmologic examination. Attention should be directed to underlying emotional disturbances.

Headache as an Epileptic Phenomenon

Headaches, when associated with epilepsy, may occur as an aura (usually in complex partial seizures) or in postictal states. Occasionally, headaches occur as a "convulsive equivalent" with some alteration of consciousness and paroxysmal activity in the EEG (Table 23–2).

Diamond S, Dalessio DJ: *The Practicing Physician's Approach to Headache,* 3rd ed. Williams & Wilkins, 1982.

* One capsule of Fiorinal or Lanorinal contains butalbital, 50 mg; aspirin, 325 mg; and caffeine, 40 mg.

† One capsule of Fioricet contains butalbital, 50 mg; acetaminophen, 325 mg; and caffeine, 40 mg.

‡ Cafergot P-B contains ergotamine tartrate, 1 mg; caffeine, 100 mg; Bellafoline (alkaloids of belladonna, as malates), 0.125 mg; and pentobarbital sodium, 30 mg.

Fenichel GM: Migraine in children. *Neurol Clin* 1985;**3:**77.
Gascon GG: Chronic and recurrent headaches in children and adolescents. *Pediatr Clin North Am* 1984;**31:**1027.
Waters WE: Headache and the eye. *Lancet* 1970;**2:**1.

SLEEP DISORDERS

Sleep Apnea Syndrome in Older Children

Sleep apnea syndrome should be considered if there is a history of restless sleep with snoring or respiratory noise during sleep and frequent awakenings from sleep in an older child who shows poor school performance associated with excessive daytime sleepiness or irritability and hyperactivity. Children with these problems frequently have hypertrophied tonsils or adenoids, causing partial airway obstruction; occasionally, they have facial dysmorphism, neuromuscular disorders with muscle hypotonia and poor pharyngeal muscle control, and hyperplastic tissues, as seen in myxedema, Hodgkin's disease, or pickwickian syndrome. Evaluation includes soft tissue x-rays of the lateral neck; chest x-ray; electrocardiography to rule out cardiomegaly, sinus dysrhythmias, and incipient or actual right-sided heart failure; arterial blood gas determinations while awake and during sleep; and polysomnography. Therapy is generally surgical, ranging from tonsillectomy and adenoidectomy when appropriate to tracheostomy when medical measures fail.

Narcolepsy

Narcolepsy, a primary disorder of sleep and wakefulness, is characterized by chronic, excessive daytime sleeping that occurs regardless of activity or surroundings and is not relieved by increased sleep at night. Onset occurs as early as 3 years of age and has been reported before 10 years of age in about 18% of patients and between puberty and the late teens in 60%. Narcolepsy usually interferes severely with normal living. Often months to years after onset, there may also be cataplexy (transient partial or total loss of muscle tone, often triggered by laughter, anger, or other emotional upsurge), hypnagogic hallucinations (visual or auditory), and the sensation of paralysis on falling asleep. Studies have shown that rapid eye movement (REM) sleep, with loss of muscle tone and an electroencephalographic low-amplitude mixed frequency pattern, occurs within 15 minutes of sleep onset in patients with narcolepsy, while normal subjects experience 80–100 minutes or longer of non-REM (NREM) sleep before the initial REM period.

Narcolepsy is treated with a central nervous system stimulant (dextroamphetamine or long-acting methylphenidate is preferred); occasionally, a tricyclic antidepressant, in low dosages titrated to the need of the patient, is added to the treatment regimen. The condition persists throughout life.

Somnambulism

Somnambulism has been assigned to a group of sleep disturbances known as disorders of arousal. It is characterized by abrupt onset early in the night of an episode of veiled consciousness and coordinated activity (eg, walking, sometimes moving objects without seeming purpose). The episode is of relatively brief duration and ceases spontaneously. There is poor recall of the event on waking in the morning. Somnambulism may be related to mental activities occurring in stages 3 and 4 of NREM sleep. The incidence has been estimated at only 2–3%, but up to 15% of cases are reported in children 6–16 years of age, with boys affected more often than girls and many youngsters having recurrent episodes. No psychopathologic features can usually be demonstrated, but a strong association (30%) between childhood migraine and somnambulism has been noted, and episodes of somnambulism may be triggered in predisposed children by stresses, including febrile illnesses.

No treatment of somnambulism is required, and it is not necessary to seek psychiatric counsel.

Night Terrors

Night terrors (pavor nocturnus) is a disorder of arousal from NREM sleep. It usually occurs in children 3–8 years of age and rarely occurs after adolescence. The disorder is characterized by sudden (but only partial) waking, with the severely frightened child unable to be fully roused or comforted. Concomitant autonomic symptoms include rapid breathing, tachycardia, and perspiring. The next morning, the child has no recall of any nightmare. Psychopathologic mechanisms are unclear, but falling asleep after watching scenes of violence on television or hearing frightening stories may play a role. Elimination of such causes and administration of a mild antianxiety agent such as chlordiazepoxide (Librium) may be helpful. It is important to differentiate these episodes from complex partial (psychomotor) seizures.

Barabas G, Ferrari M, Matthews WS: Childhood migraine and somnambulism. *Neurology* 1983;**33:**948.
Ferber R: Sleep, sleeplessness, and sleep disruptions in infants and young children. *Ann Clin Res* 1985;**17:**227.
Frank Y et al: Obstructive sleep apnea and its therapy: Clinical and polysomnographic manifestations. *Pediatrics* 1983;**71:**737.
Guilleminault C, Korobkin R, Winkle R: A review of 50 children with obstructive sleep apnea syndrome. *Lung* 1981;**159:**275.
Klackenberg G: Somnambulism in childhood: Prevalence, course and behavioral correlations. *Acta Paediatr Scand* 1982;**71:**495.
Regestein QR, Reich P, Mufson MJ: Narcolepsy: An initial clinical approach. *J Clin Psychiatry* 1983;**44:**166.
Willig R et al: Narcolepsy in a 7-year-old child. *J Pediatr* 1983;**102:**725.

HEAD INJURIES

Postnatal head trauma is a common problem in pediatrics and has important medical, psychologic, epidemiologic, and, often, legal aspects. Accidents, particularly those involving motor vehicles, are by far the leading cause of death in toddlers, children, and adolescents in the western world, and craniocerebral injury is a leading cause of hospitalization of children. The nature and severity of brain damage primarily determine the patient's neurologic status, course, and prognosis rather than the presence and extent of soft tissue injuries or of skull fractures per se. Brain damage may be due to sudden **deceleration** of the moving head, as when a falling child hits its head on the ground; or to **acceleration** of the relatively stationary head, as when it is struck by a ball or thrown against a windshield in a vehicular accident—as well as the shearing effects of torsional or rotational forces. Intracranial injuries are thus secondary to the relative inertia of the soft brain and its covering membranes and vessels compared to the momentum of the bony cranium, as well as to actual deformation of the cranial vault.

Perinatal brain injuries, etiologically and clinically unique, are dealt with in a separate section below.

Immediate Assessment

Uncertainty and justifiable concern are created by the knowledge that some patients who appear to have sustained only minor head trauma may, sooner or later, develop major sequelae. Most children present with **concussion syndrome:** Immediately after the head injury, there is brief disturbance or loss of conciousness, often with a focal or tonic-clonic seizure, irritability, drowsiness, retching or vomiting, and unsteadiness. The decision whether to hospitalize for observation or not is often based on social considerations as well as medical ones.

The initial examination will include a search for many of the symptoms and signs discussed in the section on altered states of consciousness, where particular findings and their significance are dealt with in detail. Some additional observations are as follows:

A. Vital Signs: Hyperventilation is common in excited, irritable children, as is a rapid pulse. Though the child may look pale or flushed or feel clammy, a normal blood pressure will be reassuring. Initial mild hypothermia may be followed by low-grade fever for 1 or 2 days.

Hypotension often suggests bleeding into the viscera, with splenic or hepatic rupture, especially after an automobile or bicycle accident.

B. Ocular Signs: Pupillary size and reactivity should be noted and followed closely. Abnormal findings have been detailed previously. Orbital ecchymosis (raccoon sign) suggests basilar skull fracture. Retinal flame-shaped or preretinal subhyaloid hemorrhages are seen with subdural or subarachnoid hemorrhages. Dilated, nonpulsating retinal veins are the first sign of papilledema, which may develop within a few hours after onset of increased intracranial pressure.

C. Inspection and Palpation:

1. Skull—Note signs of trauma, especially puncture wounds and deep scalp lacerations. Linear fractures, like widely separated sutures, may result in a "cracked pot sound" on percussion. Depressed fractures are usually palpable. If the anterior fontanelle is still patent, its size and tension should be noted. Head circumference should be measured.

2. Neck—Great caution must be exercised in checking the cervical spine and, if injury is suspected, in moving the patient. Nuchal rigidity may be due to injury or to subarachnoid bleeding.

3. Ears and nose—The tympanic membranes and nasal passages should be checked for blood or cerebrospinal fluid leakage. If mucous discharges are glucose-positive, they must be analyzed chemically and microscopically to identify them as cerebrospinal fluid. Bleeding from one or both ears or ecchymosis over the mastoid region (Battle's sign) suggests basilar skull fracture but may be due to other mechanisms.

4. Extremities, abdomen, and back—These should be inspected rapidly for fractures and signs of recent as well as old trauma (never forgetting that the child may have been physically abused in multiple ways). The abdomen should be examined carefully to rule out visceral bleeding.

D. Neurologic Examination: The extent of neurologic examination depends not only on the state of consciousness but also on the degree of irritability or, more positively, the degree of cooperation of the patient. For a short time after concussion or convulsion, there may be transient and alternating findings, such as paresis or positive Babinski responses. Of ultimate concern are persistent and, more importantly, progressive findings, signifying focal contusion and laceration, intracranial bleeding, and swelling. Paralysis may be on the same side as the lesion in uncal herniation (Kernohan's syndrome). While unsteadiness and generalized clumsiness are common in children after head trauma, nystagmus and progressive ataxia, especially in association with vertigo and vomiting, suggest posterior fossa hematoma (a curable lesion).

The limitations of the reflex examination were mentioned in the section on altered states of consciousness. Likewise, the sensory examination is usually of little value, but it must be done to the extent possible if spinal cord injury is suspected.

Radiologic Evaluation

A. Skull X-Rays: "Routine" skull x-rays are of little help, especially when CT head scanning is available. When skull x-rays were taken for medicolegal reasons only, fractures were found in fewer than 0.5% of cases; and when taken because there had been head trauma, only about 7% showed fractures. Even then, the findings rarely affect management. In closed head injuries, there is no correlation between fractures and complications, prognosis, or sequelae.

Skull x-rays may be indicated (but only if CT scanning cannot be performed) in the following situations: (1) obvious moderate to severe and all open head injuries; (2) possible depressed, compound, or basilar fracture; (3) possible foreign body: (4) hypocoagulable hematologic states; (5) cases in which the parent, guardian, or patient is clearly litigious or the patient is a ward of a governmental body; and (6) cases in which there is no history or external signs of head trauma but it is suspected and evidence is needed, as may be the case in an abused child. X-rays should be postponed in a restless, uncooperative child.

B. Other Plain Films: Whenever spinal cord injury is suspected, spine films must be obtained as soon as feasible; the patient must be moved with utmost care. X-rays of the extremities, chest, and abdomen should be taken when injury to these parts is thought likely. One strong indication is suspected child abuse.

C. CT Scanning: When severe head trauma occurs and neurosurgical intervention is contemplated, a nonenhanced CT brain scan should be obtained immediately. This obviates the need for plain skull films, as the scan will disclose depressed fractures, bony fragments, and foreign particles and will localize and differentiate between high-density acute hematomas, lower density edema and contusion, and evolving hydrocephalus. Epidural hematomas may have a dense convex lens configuration; subdural hematomas, a crescent-shaped one; and contusion, a "salt-and-pepper" appearance owing to blood scattered in areas of edema. If the patient's condition permits, contrast-enhanced CT scanning may be performed to define underlying pathologic conditions, especially of a vascular nature.

D. Cerebral Angiography: This may be used where CT scanning is not available or for further definition of a suspected lesion such as arterial dissection or thrombosis of a major vessel.

Classification

Head injuries are often categorized clinically on the basis of the skull injury, the degree of severity, and the suspected or actually defined underlying intracranial damage.

In **closed** head injuries, the skull is intact or the injury is limited to undisplaced skull fractures. **Open** head injuries include those with fairly deep and large scalp lacerations requiring suturing; compound, comminuted, or depressed skull fractures; and varying degrees of brain tissue damage.

In **mild** head injuries, neurologic functioning, including the state of consciousness, is either not disturbed at all or only for seconds or a few minutes, and there are no or only very transient neurologic changes. The presentation may be as in the **concussion syndrome** described above, but such symptoms, including headache, are mild and usually last only a few hours or at most 1 or 2 days. This picture may, however, also be seen with mild brain contusion and even with limited subarachnoid bleeding.

With **moderate** head injuries, presenting also as **concussion syndrome,** consciousness is lost or disturbed for several minutes to perhaps an hour. Abnormal neurologic signs are frequent though often relatively transient, but the posttraumatic period is characterized by more severe headache, irritability, drowsiness, and, sometimes, confusion. Vomiting for 12–36 hours and mild to moderate fever are common. The overall picture, however, is one of resolution of symptoms within 1 or 2 days. This state is usually associated with some cerebral edema, contusion, or laceration.

Severe head injuries may result in immediate unconsciousness lasting an hour or more or in sudden or progressive deterioration of the level of consciousness after an initial lucid period. This state may be best and most uniformly assessed by the "Glasgow Coma Scale," described in the section on altered states of consciousness. If consciousness is preserved, the posttraumatic period may be characterized by unremitting headache, marked fluctuations in levels of orientation and states of behavior, and vomiting. This state is usually associated with extensive brain swelling, cerebral contusion and laceration, intracranial bleeding, or brain stem damage, with abnormal neurologic signs that persist for hours or days or permanently.

Criteria for Home Care or Hospitalization

A. Home Management: Most children with mild to moderate concussion syndromes can be cared for at home if parents or caretakers are considered reliable, telephone contact can be maintained, and the home is within a reasonable distance from a treatment center. Since the course of epidural hematoma may be atypical in children, with signs and symptoms often not apparent until more than 24 hours following the head injury, even overnight admission of a child lucid on initial examination does not ensure early diagnosis of this serious complication.

Instructions for home care should include the following: (1) checking level of awareness or ease of arousal from sleep every 2–4 hours; (2) size and equality of pupils, and especially their reactivity to light; (3) double vision or eyes "looking straight or askew"; (4) ability to move all extremities; (5) telephone contact with the physician at least once in the first 24–48 hours, and especially when there is the least question of any abnormality, deterioration, or failure to return to normal.

It is usually neither possible nor necessary to warn the parents of all the possible sequelae of head trauma, thereby increasing their anxiety, but it is essential to stress their responsibility for obtaining medical attention promptly whenever any somatic or behavioral changes in the child cause concern. Specific emphasis should be given to persistent unusual behavior, headaches, vomiting, visual complaints, motor dysfunctioning, or otherwise unexplained fever—not only in the first 48 hours after the head injury but even a few weeks later. Only prompt reevaluation will ensure early diagnosis of posttraumatic complications.

General management of common sequelae of head trauma, such as headache, restlessness, and fluid accumulation, are discussed below in the section on treatment.

B. Hospitalization: Children should be hospitalized in the following circumstances: (1) when the social situation makes it doubtful that the child will be observed carefully and that physician contact will be maintained; (2) when there are significant neurologic deficits or injuries, including compound or depressed skull fracture or clinical or x-ray evidence of a basilar fracture; (3) when loss of consciousness lasted more than a few minutes; (4) when there is failure of neurologic functions to return rapidly to normal or during an hour or so while the child can be observed in the physician's office or clinic; and (5) when there are signs of deterioration.

Nonradiologic Evaluations (Chiefly in the Hospitalized Patient)

A. Lumbar Puncture: (See the discussions at the beginning of this chapter and in Chapter 35.) There are virtually *no* indications and many contraindications to spinal taps following head trauma. Cerebrospinal fluid examination is indicated *only* when intracranial infection or toxic encephalopathy is suspected. Many children become unsteady and fall or suffer a convulsion at the beginning of these processes; these processes, not the fall, require the tap.

B. Subdural Taps: A prerequisite to subdural taps is that the anterior fontanelle is still open or the coronal sutures are sufficiently patent to allow a subdural needle (20- or 22-gauge with short bevel) to pass. Subdural taps may be indicated if, following the intial posttraumatic period, the infant or toddler continues to do poorly, has convulsions, develops fever, has a falling hemoglobin level, or shows progressive neurologic signs or abnormally enlarging head circumference. Up to 18 months of age, transillumination of the head is usually positive in chronic *(but not acute)* subdural hematomas.

A small amount of air (10–15 mL) may be injected after removal of an equal amount of fluid; brow-up, brow-down, and lateral skull films may then disclose the extent of the subdural space and of the brain compression or atrophy.

C. Exploratory Bur Holes: These should not be performed for diagnostic purposes, especially when CT scanning or cerebral angiography is available.

Indications for trephination in an emergency are noted under surgical measures, below.

D. Electroencephalography: The EEG is frequently abnormal in the immediate posttraumatic period; findings are often out of proportion to clinical symptoms and are of doubtful significance.

Electroencephalography may be indicated when posttraumatic lethargy persists longer than expected clinically; when there are progressive neurologic deficits or when seizures occur beyond the immediate posttraumatic period; and, occasionally, when there are posttraumatic paroxysmal outbursts of behavioral disturbances, which may reflect seizures.

Differential Diagnosis

Head trauma due to an accident reported by a reliable historian, whether that is the patient or a witness, would appear to be an obvious diagnosis. But the injury is often not observed; the history given may be false or misleading, as when the accident is really an instance of child abuse; or a fall may be due to some neurologic disorder, a seizure, intoxication, or other causes discussed in the section on altered states of consciousness (above).

Complications & Sequelae

A. Posttraumatic Seizures: Such seizures may be focal or generalized, varying with age, site, and severity of injury. Seizures in the first 24 hours occur in 6–15% of children with head injuries of all types; they are more common in younger children and following brain lacerations. They may be very brief, or there may even be status epilepticus.

Seizures with onset about 1 week after the acute incident carry a higher risk of recurrence. Chronic posttraumatic epilepsy occurs in only about 2% of the total group but in 5–10% of children who suffered brain lacerations or initial unconsciousness of an hour or more. Over 50% of these seizures occur within the first 6 months; over 80% within 2 years.

A prudent approach is a 6-month treatment plan for any child who had seizures in the first week after the head injury; for any child in whom posttraumatic seizures emerged later, treatment should continue for 3–4 seizure-free years.

B. Space-Occupying Lesions: Up to 3% of children with head injuries seen at major hospitals have space-occupying lesions.

1. Epidural hematoma—The classic picture of a hemispheric extradural (epidural) hematoma is transient disturbance or loss of consciousness followed by a symptom-free ("lucid") interval of a few hours to a day, and then progressive clouding of consciousness and evolution of a dilated fixed pupil and hemiparesis. The usual cause is bleeding from a torn middle meningeal artery or vein.

In children, this classic sequence is rare. A history of impairment or loss of consciousness is frequently lacking. The symptom-free interval is often atypical because of nonspecific irritability, headache, vomiting, and other complaints; in about one-half of children, the lucid interval is longer than 48 hours' duration, and the course may be fluctuating rather than progressive, without loss of consciousness. As in adults, the site of injury is usually temporal, but skull fractures overlying the middle meningeal artery are often *not* present and the source of bleeding may be from its smaller branches or from torn diploic veins or bridging vessels. Extradural hematomas of clinical significance are uncommon under the age of 4 years.

Extradural hematomas of the posterior fossa may be difficult to diagnose clinically in children. The presenting symptoms and signs may relate chiefly to the obstruction of cerebrospinal fluid flow and consequent development of increased intracranial pressure. Cerebellar signs and cranial nerve palsies should suggest this diagnosis.

Close observation over several days is necessary to detect early signs of epidural hematoma so that neurosurgical consultation and neuroradiodiagnostic studies can be requested promptly.

With CT scanning, an increasing number of children with neurologic symptoms likely to resolve and no signs of brain herniation are found to have subacute or chronic extradural hematomas, which can be followed by scanning and which (like many chronic subdural hematomas) resorb spontaneously.

2. Subdural hematoma—Subdural hematoma is most common in children with a history of head trauma, but the history is often lacking. The male/female incidence is 2:1. Acute subdural hematoma may occur in association with contusion or laceration. Chronic subdural hematoma is more common. The clinical course is highly variable, depending primarily on the underlying damage to the cerebral substance and the age of the child. In infants and young children with open fontanelles and sutures, there may be considerable delay before symptoms develop. The most common presenting features in children are seizures (about 75% of cases), vomiting (60%), drowsiness, irritability, or other personality changes (50%), developmental retardation (20%), and failure to thrive (10%). The presenting signs consist of increased head size and bulging fontanelles (80%), retinal hemorrhages (40–65%), anemia (50–70%), extraocular (especially sixth nerve) palsies (40%), hemiparesis (35%), quadriplegia (10%), and fever (10%). There is a high associated incidence of scars and long bone or rib fractures due to "battering."

3. Intracerebral hematoma—Intracerebral hematoma is less common than epidural or subdural hematoma. When it does occur, multiple small areas of hemorrhage are more common; larger hematomas may develop beneath a depressed skull fracture. The symptoms and signs vary greatly with the size and location of the hematoma. The frontal and temporal lobes are most frequently involved.

C. Subarachnoid Hemorrhage: In children, traumatic subarachnoid hemorrhage is often relatively asymptomatic and therefore infrequently diagnosed. Nuchal rigidity, disturbance or loss of consciousness, and seizures are the nonspecific presenting symptoms. (For details, see Cerebrovascular Disorders, below.)

D. Cerebrospinal Fluid Rhinorrhea and Otorrhea: These disorders are infrequent in children. Cerebrospinal fluid leakage from the nose occurs with fracture of the frontal bone and associated dural and arachnoid tearing. The flow of fluid is increased by erect posture, coughing, and straining. Cerebrospinal fluid otorrhea with basilar fracture may be of serious prognostic significance.

Infections, particularly meningitis, are a potential threat in cerebrospinal fluid leakage. Most cerebrospinal fluid leaks heal within 2 weeks in children kept at rest; chronic leaks require surgical repair of the dural tear.

E. Cerebral Edema: Diffuse brain swelling is a common problem in severe head trauma. It produces lethargy, altered mentation, and signs of increased intracranial pressure but no focal signs. Increased pressure with midbrain dysfunction from central herniation may be fatal. Treatment is discussed on p 654.

F. Posttraumatic Central Nervous System Structural Complications:

1. Posttraumatic hydrocephalus The incidence of this complication is not known. It is seen most often in infants and toddlers and is most commonly due to aqueductal gliosis or basilar arachnoiditis. Congenital anomalies of the cerebrospinal fluid pathways may play a role.

2. Posttraumatic focal deficits—Cranial nerve palsies (most commonly abducens or facial palsy), optic atrophy, anosmia, motor deficits, diabetes insipidus, or aphasia may occur.

3. Leptomeningeal cyst—Infants and younger children (usually under age 3) with linear fracture or diastatic suture separation may develop a leptomeningeal cyst—also referred to as cephalhydrocele, spurious cranial meningocele, or "growing skull fracture." This is due to a tear of the dura and arachnoid or entrapment of the arachnoid between the separated bony parts. Cerebrospinal fluid then accumulates under the scalp, resulting in a fluctuant, often pulsatile swelling that can usually be transilluminated. It should not be aspirated, because there is a risk of infection. In some cases, the continued pulsatile effect of the cerebral tissue or loculated fluid causes progressive separation of the bony parts and further damage to the underlying brain. Skull x-rays 2–3 months following the initial trauma usually establish the diagnosis. Early surgical repair of the defect is indicated.

G. Postconcussion Syndrome: The manifestations of the postconcussion syndrome in children vary markedly from those seen in adults. The symptoms also vary with age (preschool, elementary school, older child). The chief complaints usually center around disturbances of behavior (aggressiveness, regression, withdrawal, antisocial acts) and sleep, and they may include enuresis, tension phenomena (irritability, emotional lability), phobias (fear of cars, fear of going out alone), and deterioration in school performance. Somatic complaints such as headache, vertigo or dizziness, tinnitus, and neck pains are more common in later childhood.

Compensation neurosis in children is usually induced by the parents and may cause secondary emotional problems. Repeated questioning by adults concerning somatic symptoms and repeated physical, neurologic, or psychologic examinations may, through suggestion and arousal of anxiety, provoke multiple complaints and behavioral and emotional difficulties in the child.

H. Posttraumatic Mental Retardation: Pseudoretardation (secondary to emotional problems) is not uncommon, but true intellectual loss usually occurs only with very severe injuries. The presence of microcephaly with a head circumference more than 2 SD below the mean for the age at which the accident occurred suggests that mental deficiency antedated the trauma. Psychologic testing may be useful.

Treatment

A. Emergency Measures:

1. Maintain airway and treat shock—See Altered States of Consciousness, above.

2. Anticonvulsants—For status epilepticus, give diazepam (Valium) followed by phenytoin (Dilantin); the latter does not depress the level of consciousness. (See Seizure Disorders.)

B. General Measures:

1. Observation—Criteria for home care or hospitalization are discussed above. Specific attention must be paid to level of consciousness or ease of arousal from sleep, pupillary reactions, and vital signs. In the child hospitalized for severe head trauma, the "Glasgow Coma Scale" is an excellent guide in recording recovery or warning of deterioration.

2. Restlessness—Diphenhydramine (Benadryl) is often an effective and safe sedative in very young children. Chloral hydrate and paraldehyde may also be used. Opiates or similar compounds such as pentazocine (Talwin) should not be used.

3. Headache—Give aspirin or acetaminophen (Tylenol) in appropriate doses.

4. Fluids—If the child is able to take fluids by mouth, maintain on clear fluids (noncarbonated soft drinks, sweetened tea, etc) until it is reasonably certain that vomiting will not occur. Intravenous fluids, if indicated, should be on the low side of maintenance requirements; a slight deficit in the first 3–4 days will counteract cerebral edema and minimize the possibility of water intoxication due to inappropriate ADH secretion.

5. Tetanus prophylaxis—Tetanus toxoid (or tetanus toxoid plus diphtheria toxoid), 0.5 mL, should be given for scalp wounds, particularly if "dirty," and if the child has not had a booster within 4 years.

6. Antibiotics—These should be given only on specific indications. With major "dirty" wounds—especially if there is dural tearing and extensive cerebral tissue damage—give antibiotics in therapeutic dosages as for purulent meningitis of unknown cause (see Chapter 38).

Prophylactic antibiotics are not advised in basilar skull fractures or cerebrospinal fluid leaks from the nose or ear. However, at the first sign of fever or meningeal involvement, lumbar puncture must be performed, cerebrospinal fluid analyzed, and the most appropriate antibiotics chosen.

7. Treatment of cerebral edema—See Increased Intracranial Pressure, p 654.

8. Maintenance of normal body temperature—Hypothermia by physical means may be instituted as part of the treatment of increased intracranial pressure. The use of chlorpromazine in the immediate posttraumatic period is not recommended.

9. Battering—If clinical and x-ray evidence suggests that the child has been abused, appropriate measures must be taken to ensure social service and psychiatric follow-up (see Chapter 24).

C. Surgical Measures: The chief obligation of the physician caring for the child is early recognition of complications that require prompt diagnostic studies and neurosurgical intervention.

Note: If there are compelling clinical reasons to suspect epidural hematoma and the patient is deteriorating rapidly, it is better to relieve pressure by trephination immediately than to risk serious delay in treatment by transporting the patient a long distance to a medical center. Relief of pressure may be lifesaving. Major lacerations are best dealt with by the surgeon.

1. Fractures—"Ping-pong ball" skull fractures in very young infants usually correct themselves within a few weeks and require no treatment. This is also true of slightly depressed skull fractures. Depressed fractures involving the inner table of the skull and their accompanying dural and cerebral defects require surgical therapy.

2. Cranioplasty—Repair of major skull defects can often be deferred in young children until they reach school age, when the skull attains over 90% of adult growth.

Prognosis

The outlook in children who have suffered head injuries is far better than in adults. Well over 90% of those who sustain concussions and simple linear fractures are free of symptoms after the initial period.

Even in severe head trauma, over 80% of children make a good recovery, 2–7% sustain moderate to severe disabilities, 3% are irreparably damaged, and 8–9% die. The improved outcome in recent years is due to advances in immediate care (eg, paramedical services, helicopter transport, trauma center services); the use of CT brain scanning for early recognition of neurosurgical problems; and advances in intensive care (eg, the monitoring and control of increased intracranial pressure).

Behavioral and emotional problems constitute the bulk of posttraumatic difficulties in children but normally disappear within a few months or a year.

Bruce DA et al: Pathophysiology, treatment and outcome following severe head injury in children. *Childs Brain* 1979;**5:**174.

Einhorn A, Mizrahi EM: Basilar skull fractures in children: The incidence of CNS infection and the use of antibiotics. *Am J Dis Child* 1978;**132:**1121.

Levin HS et al: Memory and intellectual ability after head injury in children and adolescents. *Neurosurgery* 1982;**11:**668.

Mahoney WJ et al: Long-term outcome of children with severe head trauma and prolonged coma. *Pediatrics* 1983;**71:**756.

Porta M et al: Surgical treatment of chronic subdural hematomas in infants. *Surg Neurol* 1979;**11**:107.

Singer HS, Freeman JM: Head trauma for the pediatrician. *Pediatrics* 1978;**62**:819.

Stuart GG et al: Severe head injury managed without intracranial pressure monitoring. *J Neurosurg* 1983;**59**:601.

PERINATAL HEAD INJURIES

The incidence of head injuries during birth is not known. Such injuries, notably intracranial hemorrhage, are estimated to account for 3–5 deaths per 1000 live births, or 10–20% of all neonatal deaths. Unlike the violent impact responsible for postnatal head trauma, most perinatal injuries are produced by prolonged gradual pressure on the head. A negative pressure gradient as the head goes through the birth canal may play a role. Predisposing or contributing factors include premature birth, cephalopelvic disproportion, shoulder dystocia, breech and precipitate delivery, prolonged labor, and misapplication of forceps or vacuum extractors.

Clinical Findings

A. Symptoms and Signs:

1. Soft tissue injuries—There may be erythema, abrasions, and necrosis of the face and scalp, caput succedaneum, scalpel injuries following cesarean section, or cephalhematoma. The latter usually does not appear until several hours after birth and does not transilluminate; occasionally, this subperiosteal hematoma grows so large as to cause symptoms due to hypovolemia and anemia.

2. Fractures—Linear skull fractures are often asymptomatic and not recognized unless accompanied by other findings. About 25% of cephalhematomas are associated with fractures. In occipital fractures with separation of the basal and squamous portions due to undue traction on the hyperextended spine while the head is still fixed in the maternal pelvis during breech delivery, there usually is massive and almost invariably fatal hemorrhage.

3. Intracranial hemorrhage—Extradural hemorrhage due to birth trauma is rare; it is always associated with skull fracture, often a depressed one. Subarachnoid bleeding is estimated to occur in over 10% of newborns; its major consequence is arachnoiditis and subsequent "communicating hydrocephalus." Subdural hematomas are uncommon owing to improved obstetric techniques, with subacute and chronic forms seen more often than acute forms. Intracerebral hemorrhage is seen with both trauma and hypoxia; it may be massive, as with tentorial laceration, especially at the juncture with the falx, with tearing of sinuses and veins, including the great vein of Galen.

Clinical manifestations vary with the cause, site, and extent of the hemorrhage; none are specific. Very limited bleeding may be asymptomatic; when more extensive, the triad of apneic spells and cyanosis, depressed consciousness, and convulsions is common. There may be irritability or listlessness, floppiness or hypertonicity, jitteriness, or a paucity of spontaneous motor activity. The cry may become shrill ("cerebral cry"); the fontanelles may be full and tense; and the sutures may widen. Focal signs are relatively uncommon and usually appear late; these include asymmetry of posture, tone, and reflexes. Because retinal hemorrhages are frequent even in well newborns, their presence is nondiagnostic. Transillumination of the head is usually negative early, as any subdural hematoma is still clotted. The most dependable findings pointing to neurologic damage are persistent asymmetry or absence of the Moro response, virtual absence of head control when the infant is pulled gently from the supine into the sitting position (traction response), and poor or absent sucking.

Intracranial hemorrhage seen chiefly in small premature infants may be intracerebellar (which is infrequently diagnosed during life and hence of uncertain clinical significance in survivors) and periventricular (which is clinically the most important and affects 40–50% of small premature infants). Periventricular-intraventricular hemorrhage, with bleeding from capillaries and less often from capillary-venule junctions, affects the premature infant primarily because the persistent subependymal matrix offers inadequate support to these small vessels. Bleeding initially is commonly at the level of the foramen of Monro and the head of the caudate, extending in about 80% or more of cases into the ventricles.

Periventricular-intraventricular hemorrhage may present in a variety of ways. In the "catastrophic," often fatal form, there is sudden development over minutes to a few hours of respiratory difficulties, hypotension, acidosis, hypothermia, depressed consciousness or coma, fixed pupils, absent oculovestibular responses, hypotonia, or sometimes opisthotonos, and seizures. In the "saltatory" form, running a waxing and waning course, there evolve over several hours more subtle alterations of consciousness, increases or decreases in spontaneous motor activity, abnormal eye movements or position, autonomic dysfunctions, and seizures; transient cessation of such symptoms may alternate with their recurrence over many hours or days. Premature infants may have asymptomatic periventricular-intraventricular hemorrhages.

B. Laboratory Findings:

1. Blood—Rapid decreases in the hematocrit or hemoglobin level occur with massive bleeding, whether into the subperiosteum or intracranially. Coagulation tests may be abnormal. Hypocalcemia occurs commonly in infants following a traumatic birth, but blood glucose, phosphorus, magnesium, sodium, pH, total CO_2, and P_{CO_2} levels should also be determined. The percentage of serum creatine kinase (CK) due to brain isoenzyme (CK-BB) may be elevated in term infants with hypoxic brain injury.

2. Cerebrospinal fluid—Cerebrospinal fluid xanthochromia, a high red cell count that does not diminish from the first tube or aliquot to the third or fourth, and a protein level over 150 mg/dL are characteristic findings. A low cerebrospinal fluid glucose level in the absence of infection is most apt to be due to hypoglycemia, but it also occurs 5–8 days after subarachnoid hemorrhage.

3. CT scanning and ultrasonography—See Intracranial Tumors (below).

Prevention

Administration of phenobarbital to prevent periventricular-intraventricular hemorrhages in infants at risk continues to be debated, but it has been reported to reduce the severity of bleeding. Intramuscular vitamin E (15 mg/kg on day 1 and 10 mg/kg on days 2, 4, and 6) has been found to reduce both the incidence and the severity of these hemorrhages in very low birth weight infants.

Treatment

Treatment is largely symptomatic. Specific treatment is directed at metabolic and electrolyte disturbances, infections, and seizures.

Vitamin K_1 (phytonadione), 1 mg intramuscularly (if not previously administered to the mother), may be given to the infant with intracranial hemorrhage to reduce the possibility of bleeding associated with vitamin K deficiency.

Repeated subdural taps are required in the presence of effusions. Shunting (subdural-peritoneal or subdural-pleural) is occasionally necessary.

Different forms of therapy for intraventricular hemorrhage have been suggested, but their exact value has not been determined. Treatments proposed include efforts to reduce pressure by removing cerebrospinal fluid (by daily lumbar puncture) or decreasing its production (with acetazolamide, furosemide). Hydrocephalus is a frequent complication, but shunting may have to be delayed until the clot liquefies.

Prognosis

The prognosis in infants with uncomplicated scalp injuries, linear fractures, "ping-pong ball" depressions, and cephalhematomas is good.

In infants with subacute and chronic subdural hematomas secondary to birth trauma, the prognosis is reasonably good if effusions are evacuated by tapping or by surgical means. However, the incidence of neurologic complications—particularly hydrocephalus, microcephaly, and seizures due to the underlying cortical damage—remains fairly high.

Newborns who survive major intracranial bleeding frequently have focal neurologic deficits, mental retardation, and seizures. The problem may be compounded by the hypoxia that often accompanies bleeding. The overall prognosis for life of the small newborn (< 2500 g) with repetitive seizures due to intraventricular hemorrhage is extremely guarded.

Focal seizures, especially of the complex partial type (or "mesial temporal lobe" epilepsy) have been related to the squeezing of the head during the birth process even when there is no significant clinical evidence of birth trauma. Onset of these seizures may be delayed for many years. Lesser degrees of head trauma may cause attention deficit disorder or minimal brain dysfunction.

Allan WC, Volpe JJ: Periventricular-intraventricular hemorrhage. *Pediatr Clin North Am* 1986;**33:**47.

Bada HS, Salmon JH, Pearson DH: Early surgical intervention in posthemorrhagic hydrocephalus. *Childs Brain* 1979; **5:**109.

Partridge JC et al: Optimal timing for diagnostic cranial ultrasound in low-birth-weight infants: Detection of intracranial hemorrhage and ventricular dilation. *J Pediatr* 1983; **102:**281.

Rayburn WF et al: Obstetric care and intraventricular hemorrhage in the low-birth-weight infant. *Obstet Gynecol* 1983; **62:**408.

Volpe JJ et al: Positron emission tomography in the newborn: Extensive impairment of regional cerebral blood flow with intraventricular hemorrhage and hemorrhagic intracerebral involvement. *Pediatrics* 1983;**72:**589.

TUMORS OF THE CENTRAL NERVOUS SYSTEM

1. INTRACRANIAL TUMORS

Essentials of Diagnosis

- Focal neurologic deficits, usually slowly progressive.
- Increased intracranial pressure with unremitting headache, vomiting, and papilledema.
- Lesion demonstrated neuroradiologically.

General Considerations

Cancer is (after accidents) the second most frequent cause of death in children over 1 year of age, with central nervous system tumors second only to the leukemias. The incidence of brain tumors in children under 15 years of age is about 24 per million per year. Familial cases occur; environmental causes have been implicated. For various reasons, specific diagnosis may be delayed for 6 months or more.

The sites, incidence, findings, and histologic types of brain tumors in children are shown in Table 23–7.

Meningiomas, acoustic neurinomas, and pituitary adenomas are rare in children. With the exception of leukemic infiltration, tumors metastatic to the brain are also uncommon; they include neuroblastoma, Wilms' tumor, and Ewing's sarcoma. Since the survival period for children with brain tumors is longer now than in the past, extraneural metastases are seen more frequently.

Clinical Findings

A. Symptoms and Signs: See Table 23–7.

1. Increased intracranial pressure—Signs of increased pressure may be due either to obstruction of cerebrospinal fluid flow with resulting hydrocephalus or to the tumor mass itself. Headaches may be constant and grow more severe, or they may be intermittent but increasingly frequent; they tend to be frontal in supratentorial tumors and occipital in infratentorial tumors. In infants and young children, irritability, lethargy, or banging the head or the fists against the head may be signs of headache.

2. Disturbances of higher functions and of sensory perception—These tend to be neglected by many patients and are not noted by young children.

3. Disturbances of vision—Especially in the very young, disturbances of vision are often not appreciated. Hemianopia may be demonstrated by opticokinetic testing or by playing with the child, bringing targets into the peripheral field while having the child fix on another object in front.

4. Progressive speech disturbances—These point to involvement of the language-dominant (usually the left) hemisphere.

5. Skin lesions—Skin lesions (eg, café au lait spots, hypopigmented patches, angiomas) point to neurocutaneous dysplasia, in which there is a high incidence of brain tumors of all types.

B. Laboratory Findings: Endocrine status should be assessed if pituitary and hypothalamic involvement is suspected or evident. ***Note:*** Lumbar puncture for cerebrospinal fluid examination is rarely justified—*and usually contraindicated*—when brain tumor is suspected. If cerebrospinal fluid is obtained at the time of operation or diagnostic examination, it should be cultured, evaluated by cell count and protein and glucose levels, and examined by cytologic techniques for tumor cells to rule out other treatable disorders (Table 23–1).

C. Radiologic Findings:

1. Skull x-rays—X-rays offer little not seen better by CT scanning. In long-standing increased intracranial pressure in older children, erosion of the posterior clinoids and thinning of sphenoid ridges are seen. Increased digital markings are an unreliable finding.

2. CT brain scanning—This is the procedure of choice for the evaluation of suspected intracranial tumors and for the selection of patients for whom further study may still be indicated. CT scanning will show the site of the tumor, associated edema, and hydrocephalus and will frequently suggest the histologic nature of the tumor by its density. Contrast enhancement is a further refinement. Intrinsic calcifications of the tumor, as in craniopharyngioma, oligodendroglioma, and even in minute amounts in optic and in brain stem gliomas, can be visualized. Cysticercosis may show "candle-guttering" of the ventricular walls.

3. Cerebral angiography—Angiography may offer additional information by demonstrating the abnormal vasculature around the tumor bed preoperatively, or in occasional vascular tumors.

4. Air encephalography—Air encephalography via the ventricular route when there is increased intracranial pressure, and via the lumbar route when not, is now infrequently used where CT scanning is available. Metrizamide (Amipaque) is often used instead of air with CT scanning. These modes are used to diagnose craniopharyngioma or other lesions in the sellar area (eg, optic gliomas) and, occasionally, posterior fossa tumors.

5. Magnetic resonance imaging—This procedure is becoming increasingly available and is especially useful in demonstrating posterior fossa tumors.

D. Electroencephalography: The EEG may show focal slowing and is of localizing value in about 70% of supratentorial tumors. False localization may occur. In infratentorial tumors, the EEG may merely show generalized slowing in the occipital and temporal regions or bifrontal slowing.

Differential Diagnosis

A clinical picture similar to that of brain tumor, with a history of insidious onset and progressive, unremitting course, headache, vomiting, seizures, and focal neurologic deficits, may be produced by any of the following disorders: subdural hematoma, toxic encephalopathies (eg, lead, uremia), "pseudotumor cerebri" of varying causes, brain abscess, tuberculoma or other granuloma, encephalitides (eg, herpes simplex), cerebral cysticercosis, degenerative central nervous system diseases, and slowly expanding or "leaking" cerebrovascular malformations. These can usually be differentiated by appropriate diagnostic studies.

Treatment

A. Surgical Treatment: Total extirpation is the procedure of choice if the location and type of tumor permit. Other types of treatment are partial removal or biopsy, surgical decompression, and shunting procedures for relief of cerebrospinal fluid obstruction.

B. Radiation Therapy: Radiation therapy is indicated in conjunction with surgery in many tumors. It is of particular importance to give radiation therapy along the entire neuraxis in medulloblastoma after the diagnosis has been confirmed by biopsy. Radiation therapy is given alone for intrinsic tumors of the brain stem and those around the pineal gland and quadrigeminal plate. In the latter instances, shunting for relief of obstructive hydrocephalus may first be necessary.

C. Antitumor Chemotherapy: In progressive or recurrent brain tumors following surgery and irradiation, high response rates are reported with combination chemotherapy, including *m*echlorethamine, vincristine (*O*ncovin), *p*rocarbazine, and *p*rednisone (MOPP). Lomustine (CCNU) may be useful. Chemotherapy for medulloblastoma is controversial. Methotrexate has been used for meningeal sarcoma and leukemia and in seeding of medulloblastoma both intrathecally and for intraventricular perfusion with removal of the perfusate from the lumbar subarachnoid space.

D. Replacement Hormone Therapy: This is usually required in craniopharyngiomas and pituitary and hypothalamic tumors. Corticosteroids (especially

Table 23–7. Brain tumors.

Site	Symptoms and Signs	Radiologic Findings	Tumor Type and Characteristics	Treatment and Prognosis
Cerebellum and fourth ventricle (50% of cases)	Evidence of increased intracranial pressure.* Cerebellar signs.† Signs due to pressure on adjacent structures.‡ Personality and behavioral changes. Occasionally emaciation.	1. CT scan of posterior fossa shows displacement or obliteration of fourth ventricle and resultant hydrocephalus; mural nodule of cystic astrocytoma usually identified. Contrast-enhanced CT scan demonstrates even better the differing densities of tumors common to this region, and their calcification. 2. Angiography may be needed to visualize tumors in cerebellopontine angle or cerebellar hemangioblastoma. 3. Air or metrizamide encephalography also used to demonstrate cerebellopontine or low vermis lesions.	1. Astrocytoma (17%): slow growth 3/5–4/5 cystic. Prognosis depends on histology of tumor. 2. Medulloblastoma (20%): rapid growth, seen mostly at age 2–6 years, about 60% in boys; seeds along CSF pathways. 3. Less common: ependymoma (5%), hemangioblastoma, choroid plexus papilloma.	Surgical removal. Follow by intensive x-ray therapy if removal is incomplete. Prognosis is good if removal is complete. Gross surgical excision, and x-ray therapy to site, cerebrum, and spinal canal. Shunt to relieve CSF obstruction. Prognosis improved: 80% survive 5 or more years. Surgical cure possible with hemangioblastoma and choroid plexus papilloma.
Brain stem (10% of cases)	1. Cranial nerve palsies (IX–X, VII, VI, V–chiefly sensory root), pyramidal tract signs (hemiparesis), and cerebellar ataxia. 2. Rarely, signs of increased intracranial pressure* or emaciation.	Demonstration of posterior fossa and displacement of cerebral aqueduct and fourth ventricle by CT scan; calcifications may be present.	Astrocytoma (10% varying grades, frequently malignant; polar spongioblastoma): usually rapid growth and recurrence. More common at age 3–8 years. Affects sexes equally.	X-ray therapy to site: remission rate for short periods. Prognosis grave: average survival 1 year, particularly when medulla is involved. 25% survive 5 years. Posterior fossa craniotomy only for aspiration of cystic intrinsic stem tumors or resection of juxtastem and cervicomedullary tumors. Chemotherapy has given variable results. Shunt for relief of CSF obstruction.
Midbrain and third ventricle (1% of cases)	1. Personality and behavioral changes, often early. 2. Evidence of increased intracranial pressure.* 3. Pyramidal tract signs and cerebellar signs.† 4. Inability to rotate eyes upward. 5. Sudden loss of consciousness; seizures rare.	CT scan shows displacement or obliteration of third ventricle and resultant hydrocephalus. Pineal rarely calcified in childhood.	Astrocytomas, teratomas including pinealoma (2% with macrogenitosomia praecox in boys), ependymoma. Choroid plexus papilloma (0.5–2%) and colloid cyst (rare).	Shunt procedure (ventriculocisternal, etc) for relief of CSF obstruction, and intensive x-ray therapy. Prognosis poor. With total surgical removal, prognosis good.
Diencephalon (1% of cases)	1. Emaciated; good intake. 2. Often very active, euphoric. 3. Few neurologic findings: occasional vertical nystagmus, tremor, ataxia. 4. Pale; without anemia. 5. Frequently: eosinophilia, decreased T_4 and pituitary reserve.	CT scan shows defect in floor of third ventricle and other midline findings.	Usually astrocytomas; less common: oligodendroglioma, glioma, ependymoma, glioblastoma.	X-ray treatment. Shunt for relief of CSF obstruction. Prognosis variable; generally poor.
Suprasellar region (13% of cases)	1. Visual disorders (visual field defects, optic atrophy). 2. Hypothalamic disorders (including diabetes insipidus, adiposity). 3. Pituitary disorders (growth arrest, hypothyroidism, delayed sexual maturation). 4. Evidence of increased intracranial pressure.*	1. Skull films: suprasellar calcification in about 90%. Deformities of sella turcica frequent. Optic foramens $\geqslant$ 8 mm in optic gliomas. 2. CT scan shows deformity, obliteration of suprasellar cistern; hydrocephalus if foramens of Monro blocked. Optic nerves thickened in optic glioma, may show calcification. CT scan may miss cystic craniopharyngioma, isodense with brain. 3. Encephalography if craniopharyngioma suspected clinically, not shown by CT.	Optic glioma (5%): high incidence of café au lait spots. The feet and hands may be large in infants and young children if the diencephalon is involved. Craniopharyngioma (8%): often dormant for years; over half intrasellar and suprasellar. Males predominate.	X-ray if optic chiasm is involved. Surgical removal if only one optic nerve is involved. Prognosis is fair to good. Conservative approach advised. Complete excision of craniopharyngioma with hormone replacement is now often feasible; or drainage of cyst and irradiation. Prognosis with complete removal is good. Repeated surgery often necessary if complete removal cannot be achieved.

* Evidence of increased intracranial pressure includes headache, vomiting (often without nausea, and before breakfast), diplopia, blurred vision, papilledema; personality changes, including irritability, apathy, disturbances in sleep and eating patterns, are frequent. Bulging of open anterior fontanelle. Sudden enlargement of the head if head circumferences have been plotted is detectable when sutures are still open or after sutures have split. Alterations of consciousness. Stiff neck with tonsillar herniation.

† Cerebellar signs; ataxia, dysmetria, nystagmus. Truncal ataxia in absence of lateralizing signs most common in vermis tumors.

‡ Signs due to pressure on adjacent structures: for posterior fossa, may include head tilting, cranial nerve signs, pyramidal tract signs, suboccipital tenderness, stiff neck.

Table 23–7 (cont'd). Brain tumors.

Site	Symptoms and Signs	Radiologic Findings	Tumor Type and Characteristics	Treatment and Prognosis
Cerebral hemispheres and lateral ventricles (25% of cases)	1. Evidence of increased intracranial pressure.* 2. Seizures (generalized, psychomotor, focal) in about 40%. 3. Neurologic deficits include hemiparesis (40%), visual field defects, ataxia, personality changes.	CT scan highly diagnostic (near 100%). Edema, ventricular deformation, shift; increased density with contrast enhancement correlates with vascularity of lesion. Tumors as small as 0.5 cm in diameter may be detected.	Gliomas; primary astrocytomas in 10%; glioblastomas in 10%. Meningiomas (up to 2%). Leptomeningeal sarcoma. Ependymoma (2%) and choroid plexus papilloma (0.5–2%).	Surgical biopsy or excision where possible. X-ray treatment. Prognosis varies with tumor type. Chemotherapy gaining in trial and usage. Surgical excision of choroid plexus papilloma; occasionally, hydrocephalus persists and requires shunt procedure.

* Evidence of increased intracranial pressure includes headache, vomiting (often without nausea, and before breakfast), diplopia, blurred vision, papilledema; personality changes, including irritability, apathy, disturbances in sleep and eating patterns, are frequent. Bulging of open anterior fontanelle. Sudden enlargement of the head if head circumferences have been plotted is detectable when sutures are still open or after sutures have split. Alterations of consciousness. Stiff neck with tonsillar herniation.

dexamethasone) may be given prior to and for a few days following surgery to reduce cerebral edema. (See Increased Intracranial Pressure, p 654.)

E. Anticonvulsants: Anticonvulsants are given as outlined in the section on seizure disorders. In general, phenobarbital, phenytoin, carbamazepine, and primidone (singly or in combination) are the drugs of choice for seizures due to brain tumors.

F. Treatment for Increased Intracranial Pressure: See discussion on p 654.

Prognosis

The overall operative mortality rate is about 5%. The older the child and the less malignant the tumor, the better the outlook. (See Table 23–7.)

A. Benign Tumors: (About 47% of cases.) Total excision is essentially curative. In suprasellar tumors, a normal life span but with neurologic and endocrine impairment is common following surgery or irradiation (or both).

B. Malignant Tumors: (About 53% of cases.) Advances in radiologic diagnosis, surgery, radiation therapy, and chemotherapy are improving the outlook. In medulloblastoma, CT scanning and more extensive surgical removal were reported to result in relapse-free survival for 4 years and overall survival for 10 years in 80% of cases. In brain stem glioma and in most ependymomas, death within 1–5 years of diagnosis is the usual outcome.

Berger MS et al: Pediatric brain stem tumors: Radiographic, pathological, and clinical correlations. *Neurosurgery* 1983;**12:**298.

Cohen ME, Duffner PK: *Brain Tumors in Children: Principles of Diagnosis and Treatment.* Raven, 1984.

Gunneson-Nordin V et al: Gliomas of the anterior visual pathway in children: Tumor behaviour and effect of treatment. *Neuropediatrics* 1982;**13:**82.

Jooma R, Hayward RD, Grant DN: Intracranial neoplasms during the first year of life: Analysis of one hundred consecutive cases. *Neurosurgery* 1984;**14:**31.

Kun LE et al: Quality of life in children treated for brain tumors: Intellectual, emotional, and academic function. *J Neurosurg* 1983;**58:**1.

Norris DG et al: Improved relapse-free survival in medulloblastoma utilizing modern techniques. *Neurosurgery* 1981; **9:**661.

Schott LH, Naidich TP, Gan J: Common pediatric brain tumors: Typical computed tomographic appearances. *J Comput Tomogr* 1983;**7:**3.

Shalet SM: Growth and hormonal status of children treated for brain tumors. *Childs Brain* 1982;**9:**284.

Zuniga OF et al: Hamartoma of CNS associated with precocious puberty. *Am J Dis Child* 1983;**137:**127.

2. PSEUDOTUMOR CEREBRI (Benign Intracranial Hypertension, Serous Meningitis, Meningeal Hydrops, Otitic Hydrocephalus, Toxic Hydrocephalus)

Essentials of Diagnosis

- Symptoms and signs of increased intracranial pressure.
- Normal or small but undisplaced ventricles.

General Considerations

The diagnosis of pseudotumor cerebri can be made only by excluding intracranial disorders that result in significant distortion, displacement, or enlargement of the ventricular system.

Pseudotumor cerebri, as reflected in its many synonyms, may be due to or associated with any of the following: (1) Inflammatory processes such as mastoiditis and lateral sinus obstruction (more often on the right than the left), poliomyelitis, Landry-Guillain-Barré syndrome, Lyme disease, head trauma, Schilder's diffuse sclerosis, and other demyelinating disorders. (2) Encephalopathies such as lead poisoning, hypo- or hypervitaminosis A, or toxicity due to insecticides, tetracyclines, or nalidixic acid; cystic fibrosis and other chronic lung disorders. (3) Endocrinopathies such as hypocalcemia, Addison's disease, functional hyperpituitarism (perhaps); menstrual dysfunctions, including menarche, pregnancy, and galactorrhea. (4) Prolonged corticosteroid therapy, especially with triamcinolone, usually during withdrawal. (5) Enzyme deficiency such as galactokinase. (6)

Catch-up brain growth, as with refeeding after psychosocial or nutritional deprivation. (7) Immune disorders, including systemic lupus erythematosus, periarteritis nodosa, and serum sickness.

Familial cases have been reported.

Clinical Findings

A. Symptoms and Signs: The presenting symptoms are nonspecific and nonlocalizing: headache, vomiting, blurred vision, photophobia, diplopia, dizziness, tinnitus, incoordination, drowsiness and stupor, and, rarely, convulsions.

On physical examination, signs of the causative or associated disorder may be present. Neurologic findings, in order of frequency, are papilledema, abducens nerve palsies, nystagmus, ataxia, pyramidal tract signs, and central or peripheral facial weakness. Visual acuity and visual fields should be evaluated in any child able to cooperate whose intelligence and age (often as early as 3–4 years) permit reliable testing.

B. Laboratory Findings: Studies should be guided by the clinical suspicion of the causes previously mentioned.

C. Lumbar Puncture: Lumbar puncture should not be performed until after the demonstration of normal or small but undisplaced ventricles. Cerebrospinal fluid is under increased pressure. It is generally acellular, with normal to low protein levels and normal glucose levels. In Landry-Guillain-Barré syndrome or immune disorders, protein levels may be elevated.

D. Radiologic Findings: CT scanning is the procedure of choice to demonstrate the presence of normal-sized or small ventricles. X-rays of the skull, mastoid sinuses, chest, and abdomen and a skeletal survey may help in diagnosis. The author has seen 2 instances where pseudotumor resulted from compression of the confluens of the sinuses by a metastatic neuroblastoma with a pinpoint lucency in the occipital skull and a lateral sinus obstruction due to unsuspected metastatic involvement of a mastoid by Ewing's sarcoma.

E. Electroencephalography: The EEG is often normal or diffusely slow and adds little diagnostically.

Treatment

Specific associated conditions are treated appropriately.

In patients receiving corticosteroids, a temporary increase in dosage may succeed in alleviating symptoms, to be followed by gradual withdrawal.

Measures aimed at reducing cerebrospinal fluid pressure, though of transient value, may relieve symptoms until remission occurs. In a child with intractable headache, vomiting, and other somatic complaints, lumbar puncture with removal of sufficient cerebrospinal fluid to lower initial pressure by 50% may be of benefit. Glycerol or furosemide may also be of value.

Visual acuity should be determined at frequent intervals. If there is loss of acuity or if the disorder is present in a young child (in whom visual acuity is difficult to measure) with long-standing increased intracranial pressure, a lumboperitoneal shunt or subtemporal decompression should be considered.

Prognosis

Pseudotumor cerebri is usually a self-limited condition with no residua. Careful follow-up is recommended, since some cases recur or a brain tumor eventually becomes manifest.

Corbett JJ: Problems in the diagnosis and treatment of pseudotumor cerebri: The 1982 Silversides Lecture. *Can J Neurol Sci* 1983;**10:**221.

Couch R, Camfield PR, Tibbles JAR: The changing picture of pseudotumor cerebri in children. *Can J Neurol Sci* 1985;**12:**48.

3. SPINAL CORD TUMORS

The relatively low incidence of spinal cord tumors in children often results in serious delay in diagnosis or in a misdiagnosis of "progressive cerebral palsy," a degenerative disorder, or even an emotional disorder.

Such tumors may be extra- or intramedullary and include dermoid cysts, teratomas, neuroblastomas, astrocytomas, ependymomas, and other types.

Symptoms and signs usually progress more slowly than in transverse myelitis or other causes of acute flaccid paralysis (Table 23–12) and include disturbances of gait, pain in the back and legs (more common in extramedullary tumors), weakness and disturbances of sensation in the legs, and loss of acquired sphincter control.

Neurologic findings—often symmetric with intramedullary and asymmetric with extramedullary tumors and varying with their site and extent—include curvature of the spine and localized tenderness; weakness, spasms, sensory deficits, and pathologic reflexes of the lower extremities; and dribbling of urine and loss of anal sphincter tone. Café au lait spots suggest neurofibromatosis. Some forms of spinal dysraphism (see below) may behave like spinal cord tumors.

The diagnosis is made roentgenographically. In 70% of patients, spine films show destructive changes of the vertebrae involved. If cord tumor is strongly suspected, spinal puncture or manometry testing for block may worsen the patient's status. The initial spinal tap should be for a myelogram. A neurosurgeon should be involved in case the patient's condition deteriorates and immediate surgery is needed.

Myelography, using CT scanning enhanced by intrathecal metrizamide, outlines intra- and paraspinal lesions far better than conventional myelography. Occasionally, the cisternal route must be employed. Where the history extends over only hours or 1–2 days, transverse myelitis is more likely; this may be aggravated by myelography. The cerebrospinal fluid may be xanthochromic, with a high protein content, and may contain tumor cells on cytologic examination.

With benign tumors, total excision and cure are often possible. In malignant tumors, decompressive laminectomy, partial excision, irradiation, and chemotherapy are employed, but the prognosis is poor regardless of treatment.

DiLorenzo N, Giuffre R, Fortuna A: Primary spinal neoplasms in childhood. Analysis of 1234 publishesd cases (including 56 personal cases) by pathology, sex, age and site: Differences from the situation in adults. *Neurochirurgia* 1982;**25:**153.

Kiwak KJ, Deray MJ, Shields WD: Torticollis in three children with syringomyelia and spinal cord tumor. *Neurology* 1983;**33:**946.

Resjo IM et al: CT metrizamide myelography for intraspinal and paraspinal neoplasms in infants and children. *AJR* 1979;**132:**367.

CEREBROVASCULAR DISORDERS

About 1–1.5% of all admissions to teaching hospitals (or 5% of pediatric neurologic disorders) are due to cerebrovascular disorders. Intracerebral vascular disease accounts for 17% of pediatric necropsies. Congenital heart disease is the commonest condition predisposing to ischemic stroke.

The deficits in children tend to be more often global or multifocal than strokes in adults.

The syndrome of **acute hemiplegias in childhood,** which is often termed acute infantile hemiplegia as if it were a single pathologic entity, requires additional description. The essential feature is the relatively rapid acquisition of hemiplegia in a previously neurologically intact child. The hemiplegia appears most often between 1 month and 6 years of age (usually under 3 years). The onset may be sudden or may evolve over a period of minutes to 1 or 2 days, frequently with an intermittent ("stuttering") progression. Cerebral vasculitis with resultant intravascular thrombosis is considered the principal cause, but it may be difficult to demonstrate angiographically. The syndrome occurs most often in association with infections of the upper respiratory tract and, next most commonly, with head trauma and with blunt injuries to the internal carotid artery or its surrounding tissues. Almost any of the conditions underlying cerebrovascular disorders in childhood (Table 23–8) may be responsible. Frequently, however, no cause can be identified; this has led to the term idiopathic infantile hemiplegia.

Clinical Findings

A. Symptoms and Signs: These vary with the nature, site, and extent of the lesion. Factors that may make it difficult to pinpoint the lesions clinically include alterations in level of consciousness; disturbances of sensorium, mood, behavior, and cognitive and perceptual functions; the frequency of seizures; and the more widespread nature of the deficits in younger children (Table 23–8).

Fever is observed frequently and may be part of an underlying or associated systemic disorder or may be of central origin. Vasomotor disturbances of involved extremities may be observed.

Retinal hemorrhages may occur with sudden increases in intracranial pressure, as in subarachnoid hemorrhage or from acute subdural hematomas, but should raise the suspicion of head trauma—especially child battering.

Seizures, which may be focal but frequently become generalized, occur in 50% or more of patients. They may precede, accompany, or follow the onset of other neurologic (especially motor) deficits.

In **acute hemiplegia,** the hemiplegia may be flaccid initially. Spasticity usually appears within a few days to 2 weeks. Hemianopia and hemisensory deficits are also often present. The seizures may remain entirely confined to the involved side, resulting in the "hemiplegia-hemiepilepsy" syndrome.

B. Laboratory Findings: Blood count, sedimentation rate, urinalysis, and electrolyte levels are usually normal; when grossly abnormal, they tend to reflect an underlying systemic disease.

Special studies as suggested by clinical indices may include screening for blood dyscrasias, including coagulation and cysteine screening tests, antinuclear antibody test (ANA), LE cell preparations, and renal function studies. Bacterial, serologic, and virologic studies should be performed in all cases associated with an inflammatory process.

Lumbar puncture should be performed in the presence of fever and meningeal signs to rule out treatable forms of intracranial infections. Except when these findings dominate the clinical picture, lumbar puncture should be deferred until CT brain scanning has shown that tentorial or tonsillar herniation is unlikely. The cerebrospinal fluid findings in cerebrovascular disorders are variable (Table 23–8).

C. Radiologic Findings: CT brain scanning with enhancement provides valuable information about the site and nature of the pathologic process.

Cerebral angiography following CT scanning is the definitive diagnostic procedure in cerebrovascular disorders *when a surgically remediable lesion is suspected,* as in small hematomas encasing an arteriovenous malformation. Arteriography via femoral catheterization will permit a "4-vessel" study of the carotid and vertebral arteries. In children with congenital heart disease who have had a stroke, cerebral angiography may be done at the time of cardiac catheterization by advancing the catheter into the aortic arch and then injecting dye.

D. Other Neurodiagnostic Studies: Isotopic scanning may be useful when CT scanning does not explain the clinical picture, particularly in demonstrating small telangiectatic lesions not detectable on a CT scan; for such lesions in the brain stem, auditory evoked potentials may also be useful. Isotopic scanning may be necessary when allergy to the contrast material precludes obtaining an enhanced CT scan.

Electroencephalography may be used as an adjunct

Table 23–8. Cerebrovascular disorders in childhood.

	Dural Sinus and Cerebral Venous Thrombosis	Arterial Thrombosis	Cerebral Embolism	Intracranial Hemorrhage (Primary Intracerebral and Subarachnoid)
Onset	Usually less sudden and clear-cut than in arterial occlusive disease. Usually unrelated to activity.	Sudden, but prodromal episodes may occur. Unrelated to activity.	Sudden onset; no prodrome. Unrelated to activity.	Sudden onset; severe headache, vomiting, loss of consciousness. Related to activity.
Underlying conditions	Pyogenic infections of leptomeninges and cranial structures (ear, face, sinuses). Marasmic states and severe dehydration. Congenital heart disease. Blood dyscrasias (sickle cell disease, polycythemia, thrombotic thrombocytopenia). Lead and other toxic encephalopathies. Trauma. Metastatic tumor. Sturge-Weber disease. Use of birth control pills.	"Idiopathic" (hemiplegia in infancy). Cyanotic congenital heart disease. Inflammatory disease of arteries: "collagen" diseases, granulomatous (Takayasu's arteritis), acute infections, syphilis. Trauma or extrinsic compression. Dissecting aneurysm. Arteriosclerosis (progeria). Thrombotic phenomenon: homocystinuria. Rarely: diabetes mellitus. Delayed effect by 2–22 years of large-dose radiation treatment. Amphetamine abuse, both IV and orally.	Atrial fibrillation and other "arrhythmias": congenital heart disease (R → L shunt), rheumatic heart disease. Acute or subacute infective endocarditis. Air: complications of heart, neck, or chest surgery. Fat: complications of fractures of bone, heart surgery. Septic: pneumonia or lung abscess (especially in congenital heart disease). Newborn: infarcted necrotic placental tissue. Tumor. Coronary.	Trauma: birth (intraventricular), subdural hemorrhage, epidural hemorrhage, cavernous sinus fistula. Vascular malformations: arteriovenous, angiomas, aneurysms. Hemorrhagic disorders (leukemia, aplastic anemia, hemophilia, sickle cell anemia, thrombocytopenic/anaphylactoid purpura, liver disease, vitamin deficiencies [K, C, B_1], anticonvulsants). Hypertensive encephalopathy (renal disease, pheochromocytoma). Toxic or infectious encephalopathy. Intracranial tumors.
Neurologic findings	Altered state of consciousness. Increased intracranial pressure. Focal neurologic deficits (leg, arm). Seizures, focal and generalized.	Seizures, frequently focal. Focal neurologic deficits. Behavioral and intellectual changes. Rapid improvement at times.	Transient loss of consciousness common. Seizures, often focal. Focal neurologic deficits (sometimes multiple). Rapid improvement at times.	Consciousness commonly lost; may be regained quickly. Marked meningeal signs (**not** seen in neonate). Focal neurologic deficits. Seizures, generalized and focal.
Special clinical clues	Lateral dural sinus: mastoiditis. Superior sagittal sinus: caput medusae. Cavernous sinus: homolateral exophthalmos, periorbital edema, palsies of cranial nerves III, IV, VI, and V.	Inflammatory disease: multifocal involvement common. Takayasu's arteritis: pulseless upper limbs. Moyamoya syndrome (progressive alternating hemiplegia with basal arterial stenosis and diencephalic telangiectasia). Somatic constitution (progeria, arachnodactyly). Signs of trauma. "Needle marks" in drug abuse.	Emboli to other organs (spleen, kidneys, lungs). Air embolism: transient blindness. Fat embolism: respiratory distress, blood-tinged sputum in postoperative period, fat droplets in urine, retinal vessels.	Trauma (hemorrhage, subhyaloid hemorrhages, bruises, fractures on x-rays). Malformations: bruit, heart failure, hydrocephalus, cutaneous stigmas. Previous seizures/neurologic deficit. Coarctation/polycystic kidney. Hemorrhagic diathesis: skin, joints, gastrointestinal tract, newborn. Hypertensive encephalopathy: blood pressure elevated, uremia.
CSF (Lumbar puncture usually follows CT brain scan.)	Findings vary with primary process. Protein often elevated. Sometimes bloody. If PMNs are present, suspect infection.	Early: usually normal. Later: slight monocytic pleocytosis and protein elevation.	Usually normal. Some pleocytosis and protein elevation in infective endocarditis.	Bloody CSF all tubes, xanthochromic supernatant. Protein elevated. Sugar may be decreased. Fluid may be clear if hemorrhage is intracerebral only.
Cerebral angiography*	Angiogram on venous phase or sinogram may show obstruction site. Sinogram may be dangerous.	Angiography early may show occlusion or narrowing. (Later studies usually negative.)	Angiography usually normal, as emboli commonly lodge in small peripheral vessels.	Angiography usually able to identify subdural and epidural hematoma, site and type of malformation, intracerebral tumor, clot.
CT brain scan* (usually precedes angiography)	In the first week, intra- and extracranial hematomas show greater density than brain tissue on CT scan. Blood with AV malformations and large aneurysms are seen as localized areas of increased radioabsorption, usually related to dilated draining veins; enhancement may be needed. Ischemic infarcts intially appear as areas of homogeneous lucency with edema, after about a week as irregularly marginated lucencies without "mass effect" but markedly enhanced by contrast material owing to altered capillary permeability, and in the chronic phase as an area of radiolucency without enhancement associated with focal or diffuse cerebral atrophy. Small infants may require serial CT scans.			

* In many instances and where readily available, CT brain scan should precede and may even obviate cerebral angiography. See x-ray findings, below.

in assessing associated seizures and depressed levels of consciousness.

For subdural taps, see p 674.

E. Electrocardiography: Electrocardiography is indicated if there is clinical evidence of heart disease, hypertension, or an arteriovenous malformation that may cause a work overload of the heart.

Differential Diagnosis

A. Postictal (Todd's) Paralysis: Focal motor paralysis lasting 2–3 days may follow seizures that are entirely focal or of focal onset.

B. "Cerebral Palsy" With Hemiplegia: Parents sometimes become aware of the presence of hemiplegia or other neurologic deficits only when the child is ill or has the first seizure. The findings of early spasticity—and particularly of atrophy of affected limbs—favor an old deficit, often congenital or of perinatal onset.

C. Other Causes: Focal neurologic deficits, including hemiplegia, may appear suddenly with a variety of inflammatory conditions of the brain, including meningitis, encephalitis, and brain abscess. With central nervous system tumors, degenerative processes (eg, Schilder's diffuse sclerosis or multiple sclerosis), or "slow virus" infections, the deficits are usually slower to evolve than in cerebrovascular disorders but may be apoplectic in onset. In the case of neoplasm, neurologic deficits of acute onset are usually due to hemorrhage.

Complications

The complications may be those of the underlying disease process. Frequent complications include seizures (particularly generalized status epilepticus), pneumonia, coma, decubiti, contractures, and hydrocephalus.

Treatment

A. Medical Measures: Great care must be given to airway, fluid and electrolyte balance, and infections. (See Altered States of Consciousness, p 654.)

Systemic hypertension should be lowered with caution. Too sudden a drop in arterial pressure may precipitate further cerebral hypoxia.

Specific therapies depend on the underlying condition and may include heparinization for multiple embolic phenomena or consumption coagulopathies, antibiotics for bacterial infections, and multiple tapping of a subdural hematoma.

B. Neurosurgical Measures: In addition to drainage of subdural hematomas (often performed by pediatricians), specific neurosurgical measures include removal of a large intracerebral clot; endarterectomy of a stenosed carotid artery and removal of thrombus; clipping, trapping, coating, or "embolization" of an aneurysm; extirpation of an accessible arteriovenous malformation; excision or biopsy of a tumor; drainage of a brain abscess; and shunting for hydrocephalus.

C. Long-Term Management: In addition to anticonvulsant treatment, educational, psychologic, physical, and speech therapy are often required.

Prognosis

The course may be brief, with complete recovery. Death may occur, depending on the precipitating cause or complications.

Residual motor and sensory deficits are common, especially with hemiplegias that occur at an early age. The upper extremity tends to be more involved than the lower. Visual field and parietal lobe defects contribute to the learning disabilities.

Seizures—mostly focal, but also other types—persist in affected children.

Impairment of mental abilities roughly parallels the frequency and severity of seizure disorders. In about three-fourths of cases, there are learning disabilities, hyperactivity, disturbances of behavior, and other signs of "maturational lag."

Children, as a group, recover more language function than adults with similar lesions; however, recovery is less complete than previously supposed.

Gold AP, Carter S: Acute hemiplegia of infancy and childhood. *Pediatr Clin North Am* 1976;**23:**413.

Golden GS: Stroke syndromes in childhood. *Neurol Clin* 1985;**3:**59.

Imai WK, Everhart R, Sanders JM: Cerebral venous sinus thrombois: Report of a case and review of the literature. *Pediatrics* 1982;**70:**965.

Ladurner G et al: Computed tomography in children with strokes. *Eur Neurol* 1982;**21:**235.

Mori K et al: Basilar artery occlusion in childhood. *Arch Neurol* 1979;**36:**100.

Sarnaik SA, Lusher JM: Neurological complications of sickle cell anemia. *Am J Pediatr Hematol Oncol* 1982;**4:**386.

Schauseil-Zips U et al: Intracranial arteriovenous malformations and aneurysms in childhood and adolescence. *Eur J Pediatr* 1983;**140:**260.

Schoenberg BS, Mellinger JF, Schoenberg DG: Cerebrovascular disease in infants and children: A study of incidence, clinical features, and survival. *Neurology* 1978;**28:**763.

Wilkins RH: Natural history of intracranial vascular malformations: A review. *Neurosurgery* 1985;**16:**421.

Woods BT, Carey S: Language deficits after apparent clinical recovery from childhood aphasia. *Ann Neurol* 1979;**6:**405.

Yamashiro Y, Takahashi H, Takahashi K: Cerebrovascular moyamoya disease. *Eur J Pediatr* 1984;**142:**44.

MALFORMATIONS OF THE CENTRAL NERVOUS SYSTEM

In about 3% of newborns, structural anomalies of prenatal origin are recognizable at birth and affect their well-being and viability. One-third of these "major" malformations involve the central nervous system, resulting in up to 75% of fetal and 40% of infant deaths. Causes are numerous and may be multifactorial: They may be genetic; due to maternal age, infections, or illnesses; or due to the effects of drugs or other substances ingested by the mother or to which she was exposed. Most often, the cause is not known. This section deals with some of the more common neurologic malformations due to disturbed induction at 3–6 weeks of gestation or neuronal migration, proliferation, and organization in the second to sixth fetal months.

Icenogle DA, Kaplan MA: A review of congenital neurologic malformations. *Clin Pediatr* 1981;**20:**565.

Kalter H, Warkany J: Congenital malformations: Etiologic factors and their role in prevention. (2 parts.) *N Engl J Med* 1983;**308:**424, 491.

1. SPINAL DYSRAPHISM

Essentials of Diagnosis

- Any defect of fusion in the dorsal midline.
- May be cutaneous, vertebral, meningeal, or neural.

General Considerations

Developmental anomalies involving the spinal

cord and its coverings are extremely common. The incidence of those forms of neural clefts without meningeal protrusion is not known. Vestigial or primarily superficial manifestations, such as dermal dimples and sinuses, vascular nevi, and abnormal tufts of hair, are extremely common. Spina bifida occulta, often an incidental x-ray finding, is estimated to occur in up to 25% of younger children in whom the posterior vertebral arches will eventually fuse; it is seen in about 5% or more of all individuals. Spina bifida cystica occurs in about 2 per 1000 births, with one meningomyelocele per 700–800 births. The incidence of neural tube defects has, however, been declining in recent years, more rapidly in females. Many environmental causes, including viral and irradiation injuries to the embryo, have been implicated epidemiologically and experimentally. Genetic factors may play a role; eg, in spina bifida cystica, the family history is positive in about 8% of cases.

As a matter of considerable clinical practicality, the various forms of spinal dysraphism can be grouped into (1) noncystic forms, in which there is no hernial protrusion of the meninges of the cord; and (2) cystic forms, with herniation of the meninges through a defect of the neural arch in which the hernial sac contains cerebrospinal fluid (meningocele) and often also nervous tissue (meningomyelocele).

Clinical Findings

A. Symptoms and Signs:

1. Cutaneous manifestations—

a. Noncystic—In noncystic forms of spinal dysraphism, a skin depression or dermal dimple may mark the outlet of a fistulous or fibrous tract extending to the meninges and representing a dermal sinus. On close inspection, a tiny pore may be seen. There may be chronic or intermittent drainage of a whitish secretion from such a sinus; this may lead to cystic dilatation if the sinus is partially obliterated. Commonly seen also in the midline as evidence of dysraphism are port wine angiomatous nevi; tufts or patches or even tails of hair, which may be long and coarse, sometimes silky, and often dark in blond children; and subcutaneous diffuse, soft lipomatous lesions. Such superficial stigmas may be absent, may appear singly or in close but variable association, or may even ''split'' on each side of the midline.

b. Cystic—Cystic defects are usually detected at birth, but occasionally the overlying skin is so thick that detection is delayed. A large vascular nevus, lipoma, or abnormal growth of hair may be an associated superficial finding. The differentiation between meningocele and meningomyelocele is usually made by noting the absence (meningocele) or presence of neurologic deficits, observing the presence of neural elements on transillumination of the sac, or eliciting reflex responses upon tapping the sac gently; however, in some instances, a definite diagnosis can only be established by surgical exploration. Pressure on the sac may cause the anterior fontanelle to bulge. An exception to these statements must be made for the rare neurenteric cysts (see below), in which no superficial lesions are usually present.

2. Orthopedic manifestations—Plainly visible or palpable anomalies of the spinal column may include scoliosis, anomalies associated with Klippel-Feil syndrome, and, occasionally, bifid vertebrae; in many instances, however, the abnormalities are seen only on x-ray (see below). Deformities of the feet or legs are the most common (and may be the only) evidence of noncystic spinal dysraphism. They may be highly variable in extent and kind and stationary or progressive depending upon the degree of neurologic deficit. There may be a marked difference in size between the 2 legs or feet, inversion (clubfoot) or eversion, and pes cavus or pes cavovarus. Dislocation of the hips may be present. As expected from the low incidence of dysraphism involving primarily the cervical cord, the upper extremities are far less commonly involved.

3. Motor disturbances—The orthopedic manifestations are often accompanied by muscle weakness and disturbances of reflexes. The nature and extent depend entirely on the lesion in the spinal cord and roots and help to identify the anatomic site. Particularly in such noncystic forms as diastematomyelia—and in symptomatic spina bifida occulta and ''tethering'' of the cord—the first signs may appear between 2 and 8 years of age in the form of progressive leg weakness and gait disturbance. In meningomyelocele, the legs may be partially, asymmetrically, or totally paralyzed and areflexic from birth.

4. Urinary and rectal disturbances—Atonic bladder (with dribbling) and poor anal sphincter tone are commonly present at birth in lumbosacral meningomyeloceles. In noncystic forms of dysraphism, urinary incontinence usually appears after the disturbances of gait and reflects pressure on or traction of the lower cord (or both) by an adherent lipoma or other connective tissue; loss of voluntary control of the anal sphincter in these types is less common but may occur in time. When urinary incontinence is present, intravenous urography may disclose the presence of various upper genitourinary anomalies.

5. Cerebral malformations—Disturbances of brain growth with noncystic forms are relatively infrequent but may occur. With cystic forms, encephalic anomalies are far more common; hydrocephalus occurs in 65% of cases with meningomyelocele, almost invariably in association with one of the forms of Arnold-Chiari malformation, and in 10% of meningoceles. Encephalocele, schizencephaly, cyclopia, and, often, microcephaly also represent aspects of dysraphism of the neuraxis; indeed, it is not unusual to find a hydrocephalic brain that after shunting or on postmortem examination turns out to be microcephalic.

6. Sensory deficits—Disturbances of sensation commonly parallel the motor deficits in meningomyelocele, where the upper level of the defect may be demonstrated by pricking the infant's skin; wrinkling or corrugation denotes an intact dermatome. In noncystic forms of dysraphism, sensory disturbances are much less common; where there is pressure or traction on the cord, there may be loss of pain leading to neurogenic arthropathies (Charcot joints). Trophic disturbances of the skin may also be seen.

B. Laboratory Findings: Abnormal findings relate principally to the 2 major complications of spinal dysraphism: meningitis and urinary tract disease (see below). In meningitis, the infection is frequently mixed, with both skin (*Staphylococcus epidermidis* and others) and gram-negative organisms present. When there is dribbling or other clinical or x-ray evidence of genitourinary tract disturbance, urinalysis, urine cultures, blood urea nitrogen, and creatinine clearance should be obtained and followed.

C. Radiologic Findings:

1. Plain x-rays of the spine—In overt spinal dysraphism, spine x-rays usually disclose the extent of the neural arch defect. In diastematomyelia, a ridge may protrude from the body of one or more vertebrae which splits or fixes the spinal cord or cauda equina and which may consist of bone, cartilage, and fibrous tissue. The radiopacity of the lesion depends on the degree of calcification of this spur; nonvisualization on plain spine films does not rule out this diagnosis. CT spine scanning is more informative.

2. Ultrasonography—This technique screens patients for a variety of dysraphisms, including meningomyeloceles, tethering of the cord, and sacrococcygeal teratomas.

3. Myelography—Myelography should be performed in cases of progressively more symptomatic noncystic forms of dysraphism, particularly if there is a possibility of diastematomyelia, tethering of the cord, or a neurenteric cyst—which may behave clinically like spinal cord tumors. Myelography is usually done with metrizamide, followed by CT scanning.

4. CT scanning—In meningomyelocele, CT brain scanning shortly after birth provides 2 extremely important pieces of information: (1) the presence of hydrocephalus (irrespective of occipitofrontal head circumference) and (2) the approximate thickness of the cortical mantle or pallium. CT spine scanning will define the nature of soft-tissue masses and of the underlying bony anomalies. It can detect small amounts of calcification in a diastematomyelic spur.

5. Air encephalography—Ventriculography is employed if CT scanning is not available to determine the presence and extent of hydrocephalus.

6. Urologic studies—Cystometrograms and intravenous urograms are indicated in all children with obvious or suspected urinary tract involvement secondary to spinal cord involvement.

Differential Diagnosis

Meningomyelocele usually presents little diagnostic difficulty. Meningocele is not infrequently confused with a subcutaneous lipoma, and indeed the 2 may be associated. The differentiation between meningocele and meningomyelocele is sometimes only made during operation. Because of traction or pressure on the cord (or a combination of both), considerable diagnostic difficulty may be encountered in those forms of dysraphism which give rise to symptoms not unlike those of spinal cord tumors or even syringomyelia. Such may be the case (as the child grows) with fibrolipomas, tethering of the cord or cauda equina by fibrous bands to the bone or skin directly or through meningeal attachment, a tight filum terminale, or a spur that partially or completely bisects the cord (diastematomyelia). Primarily orthopedic findings such as pes cavus or Charcot joints involve consideration of Friedreich's ataxia, diabetes mellitus, congenital insensitivity to pain, familial dysautonomia, and even congenital syphilis. Occasionally, cystic forms of dysraphism are placed anteriorly, causing symptoms of a space-occupying lesion in the thoracic, abdominal, or pelvic cavity or of a spinal cord tumor. (See also Spinal Cord Tumors, above.) Neurenteric cysts are anteriorly placed, usually in the lower cervical or upper thoracic area.

Complications

Meningitis occurs in nearly 15% of cases of spina bifida cystica if the sac ruptures. It occurs far less frequently with congenital dermal sinus, but when it does, it may give rise to recurrent episodes of bacterial meningitis until the sinus is discovered. If the sinus is not readily located in the back or at the nose, shaving the back of the head or a pneumoencephalogram may be required. Infections are often due to *Escherichia coli, Pseudomonas aeruginosa,* or *S epidermidis.*

Urinary tract infections, bladder atony, vesicoureteral reflux, hydronephrosis, and, eventually, renal failure are frequent complications, particularly in spina bifida cystica.

Spine and limb orthopedic complications are frequently minimized by early intervention.

Hydrocephalus is an early and frequent problem with spina bifida cystica, and its complications (discussed in the next section) adversely affect the prognosis.

Skin problems may occur owing to breakdown in the saddle area from bladder and bowel incontinence or in association with trophic disturbances.

Treatment

A. Neurosurgical Considerations:

1. Noncystic forms of spinal dysraphism—These may require neurosurgical intervention to relieve pressure or traction on the spinal cord, removal of a diastematomyelic spur, or excision of a dermal fistula and exploration for any connected tumor. It must be emphasized that *a dermal sinus should never be probed, as this may result in infection, especially of the central nervous system.*

2. Spina bifida cystica—Approaches to this complex problem vary. Decisions about treatment must be based on the extent of neurologic and systemic involvement, the consequent morbidity, the prognosis for physical and mental function, and the emotional, social, and financial impact on the family.

a. Meningoceles—Meningoceles should be repaired early if there is danger of rupture of the sac.

b. Meningomyeloceles—Newborn infants with meningomyeloceles are selected for immediate treatment in many centers today on the basis of the absence of major adverse criteria (Fig 23–2). Many physicians require the presence of 2 or more adverse criteria before withholding treatment. It is increasingly clear that there is no urgency in surgical intervention, since survival rates of over 90% at 10 months are similar for those with early, delayed, and late surgery and since there is no significant association between time of surgery and development of ventriculitis, worsening paralysis, or developmental delay.

c. Hydrocephalus—Hydrocephalus may be arrested by administration of isosorbide only, isosorbide followed by a shunt, or by shunt alone. Occasionally, with reduction of cerebrospinal fluid pressure, the meningocele collapses, followed by epithelialization of the sac.

B. Care of the Sac When Neurosurgical Repair Is Delayed: Application of silver nitrate to the thin membrane covering a sac is advocated by some to encourage epithelialization. To protect the sac, a "doughnut" of foam rubber or other spongy material, covered by plastic, wide and high enough to wall in the sac, and secured around the abdomen, is useful. It may be roofed by sterile gauze, but contact of the gauze with the sac—whether "dry" or covered with petrolatum—should be avoided.

C. Orthopedic Considerations: Surgery and braces are recommended to the extent that these measures will aid ambulation. Scoliosis is a frequent and serious complication. Correction of foot deformities and dislocation of the hips should not be undertaken if there is little hope that the child will ever walk.

In a child with neurogenic arthropathy, behavioral modification to reduce the frequency of trauma to the joints as well as physically protecting the joints (as by padding) is helpful.

D. Urologic Considerations: The renal status should be assessed early and watched closely. Measures for reducing the incidence of pyuria and renal complications include suprapubic manual expression of urine from the bladder, the use of an indwelling catheter, and ureteroileostomy.

"Prophylactic" antibiotic therapy is not advisable, but specific infections must be treated. Methenamine mandelate (Mandelamine) or cranberry juice to acidify the urine to pH 5.0 or less may reduce the frequency of infections.

E. Fecal Incontinence: Constipating foods and drugs may be of help. Colostomy is sometimes advisable for social reasons in older children who are otherwise able to function.

F. Skin Care: Skin hygiene should be maintained, particularly around the anus, vulva, and pressure areas, if these are involved.

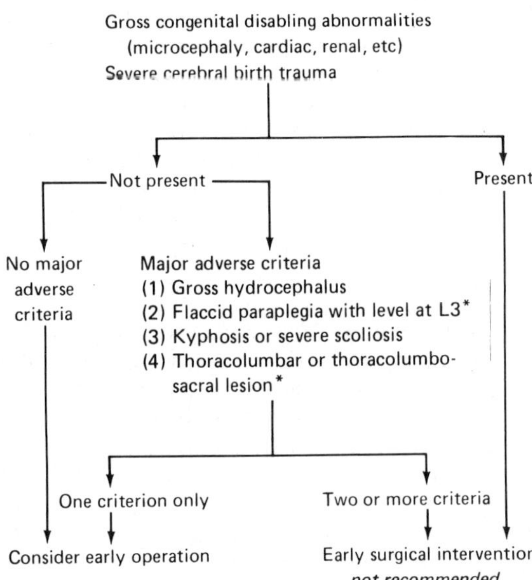

Figure 23–2. Proposed criteria for neurosurgical intervention in newborns with open meningomyeloceles. (After Stein et al.) *These often occur together.

Prognosis

In noncystic forms of spinal dysraphism, the prognosis for life and function is excellent if proper treatment is carried out. The degree of residual neurologic, orthopedic, and genitourinary deficit is often minimal but depends on the extent of involvement. With "release" of a tethered cord, urinary incontinence and gait disturbances, even when present for several years, may resolve.

Complete cures can be achieved by excision of neurenteric cysts. With meningoceles, the prognosis is that of the complications.

Of the infants with meningomyeloceles who are treated, about 15% die in early childhood, the most common causes being meningitis and ventriculitis, hydrocephalus, and other major malformations. Most of those with 2 or more major adverse criteria (Fig 23–2) die, over 90% within the first 6 months.

Among long-term survivors, a few have no handicaps or only arrested hydrocephalus; 30–60% are reported as "educationally" normal (IQ > 80), although many have multiple handicaps. The features most significantly related to low intelligence are central nervous system infection (with or without shunt) and thin pallium (< 2.5 cm). Impairment of renal function with uremia is the most serious long-term threat.

Women with a child or first-degree relative with a neural tube defect—and with advanced maternal age—should be monitored between the 14th and 16th weeks of pregnancy for elevated amniotic levels of alpha-fetoprotein (or possibly acetylcholinesterase) and between the 19th and 20th weeks with serial ultrasound studies of the fetus and sometimes amniography for the presence of such a defect. Since the predictive value of positive tests is 99.9%, a rational decision concerning continuation of such a pregnancy may be made. To prevent neural tube defects, some physicians recommend that such tests be performed in all women with a previous pregnancy complicated by multiple congenital malformations (or a family history of this), maternal viral or fungal infection, the presence of poly- or oligohydramnios, or first-trimester hemorrhage; some advocate such tests in all women.

Charney EB et al: Management of the newborn with myelomeningocele: Time for a decision-making process. *Pediatrics* 1985;**75:**58.

Frerepau PH et al: Diastematomyelia: Report of 21 cases surgically treated by a neurosurgical and orthopedic team. *Childs Brain* 1983;**10:**328.

Lorber J, Salfield SAW: Results of selective treatment of spina bifida cystica. *Arch Dis Child* 1981;**56:**822.

McLaughlin JF et al: Influence of prognosis on decisions regarding the care of newborns with myelodysplasia. *N Engl J Med* 1985;**312:**1589.

McLone DG et al: Central nervous system infections as a limiting factor in the intelligence of children with myelomeningocele. *Pediatrics* 1982;**70:**338.

Naidich TP et al: Sonography of the caudal spine and back: Congenital anomalies in children. *AJNR* 1984;**5:**221.

Park TS et al: Experience with surgical decompression of the Arnold-Chiari malformation in young infants with myelomeningocele. *Neurosurgery* 1983;**13:**147.

Sheffield LJ et al: A clinical approach to the use of predictive values in the prenatal diagnosis of neural tube defects. *Am J Obstet Gynecol* 1983;**145:**319.

Stein SC, Schut L, Ames MD: Selection for early treatment of myelomeningocele: A retrospective analysis of selection procedures. *Dev Med Child Neurol* 1975;**17:**311.

Windham GC, Edmonds LD: Current trends in the incidence of neural tube defects. *Pediatrics* 1982;**70:**333.

2. HYDROCEPHALUS

Essentials of Diagnosis

- Abnormal enlargement of the cerebral ventricles due to an increased pressure gradient between the intraventricular fluid and the brain.
- In infants and children, hydrocephalus is usually accompanied by macrocephaly.

General Considerations

Most cases of hydrocephalus in infancy and childhood are due to obstruction of cerebrospinal fluid flow, the aqueduct between the third and fourth ventricle being the most common site of blockage. Developmental causes include aqueductal stenosis (including X-linked cases) or aqueductal atresia; absence or atresia of the foramens of Luschka and Magendie (Dandy-Walker syndrome); Arnold-Chiari malformation (3 types are described; myelomeningocele is frequently, but not necessarily, associated); arteriovenous malformation of the great vein of Galen, compressing the aqueduct; and other anomalies, including block of the interventricular foramens (of Monro). Intrauterine and postnatally acquired causes include inflammatory states, whether from infection or hemorrhage, with resulting gliosis of the aqueduct, and arachnoiditis (''communicating hydrocephalus''). Intracranial mass lesions such as tumor, abscess, and hematoma also may cause obstruction to cerebrospinal fluid flow.

A nonobstructive or oversecretion type of hydrocephalus is due to choroid plexus papilloma.

Clinical Findings

A. Symptoms and Signs: Manifestations vary with age at onset, the underlying cause, and the rapidity with which hydrocephalus develops.

In infants with an open anterior fontanelle and patent sutures, symptoms of increased intracranial pressure are often delayed or minimal. The anterior fontanelle may be full and tense and the sutures palpably separated; there may be frontal bossing and a ''setting sun'' sign, in which the eyes appear to be depressed, with more sclera than normal showing above the iris. The head may transilluminate abnormally and percuss like a watermelon.

Abducens palsies with increased intracranial pressure are common in all age groups. When hydrocephalus is due to more acute obstruction, there may be vomiting, irritability, and listlessness.

The findings in older infants and children may include Macewen's cracked pot sign of sprung sutures, papilledema, difficulties in walking, disturbances of muscle tone and reflexes, and incoordination. An unusual form of presentation is the pendular, or side-to-side, movement that gives rise to the ''bobble-head doll syndrome.'' Cranial bruits are common in children, especially with increased intracranial pressure, but may suggest a vascular malformation.

B. Laboratory Findings: The composition of the ventricular or spinal fluid may offer some clues to the cause of hydrocephalus. Markedly elevated cerebrospinal fluid protein is often seen in choroid plexus papilloma and occasionally after a central nervous system infection or hemorrhage. Low cerebrospinal fluid glucose without evidence of current infection is seen in postinfectious, and sometimes in posthemorrhagic, hydrocephalus or in meningeal invasion by tumor (eg, leukemia, medulloblastoma). Increased 5-hydroxyindoleacetic acid is found in the cerebrospinal fluid in obstructive hydrocephalus. Cytologic examination of cerebrospinal fluid may show the presence of tumor cells.

C. Radiologic Findings: Plain skull films may show the cranium to be disproportionately large with respect to the face; there may be signs of increased intracranial pressure, lytic lesions, or a large, flat occipital shelf suggestive of Dandy-Walker syndrome.

CT brain scanning or ultrasonography will determine the size of the ventricles, the site of cerebrospinal fluid block, and the most likely cause. Ventriculography, especially if done with metrizamide and combined with CT scanning, may give additional information.

Magnetic resonance imaging is of particular value in demonstrating Arnold-Chiari malformations.

Differential Diagnosis

Hydrocephalus, remediable by surgical intervention, should be considered in the differential diagnosis of the enlarged head (macrocranium), discussed in a subsequent section (see Abnormal Head Growth, below).

Hydranencephaly consists of replacement of the cerebral hemispheres by a fluid-filled sac, usually due either to profound schizencephaly and bilateral porencephaly or to a massive encephalomalacic process that reduces the cerebral mantle to a thin membrane. The appearance of the newborn may be grossly normal. The head is usually not enlarged. If the diencephalon and midbrain are intact, as is usually the case, no difficulties occur with feeding, respiration, and other vegetative functions in the first months of life. Diagnosis may be delayed until the parents note slow development or defective vision. Some spasticity and persistence of primitive postural reflexes are usually evident. Hydranencephaly may be diagnosed by transillumination of the head, ultrasonography, or CT scanning.

Complications

In untreated cases, continuing increased intracranial pressure may lead to neurologic deterioration. Rarely, hydrocephalus may rupture.

In ''shunted'' cases, complications include (1) sudden rise in intracranial pressure, due either to blockage or other malfunction of the shunt (the site varies with the type of assembly); (2) infections (most frequently due to coagulase-positive *Staphylococcus epidermidis*), including septicemia, meningitis, and ventriculitis, with the shunt itself often the nidus of infection, possibly because of its interference with host defenses; (3) electrolyte imbalances; and (4) subdural hematoma following abrupt collapse of enlarged ventricles.

Prevention

Early recognition of hydrocephalus is best accomplished by periodic physical and neurologic examinations, including serial head measurements.

Fetal hydrocephalus, diagnosed by ultrasonography, may be treated with a ventriculoamniotic shunt, replaced after birth by a ventriculoperitoneal shunt.

Treatment

A. Observations and Evaluation: Careful observation over a short period may be indicated before deciding to operate. It is usually best not to operate if the patient is clinically well and the rate of enlargement does not exceed that indicated on a standard head circumference chart or appears to be arresting. In moderate cases, a clinical trial of isosorbide or furosemide may be warranted.

B. Medical Treatment: If the rate of head enlargement is slow to moderate or if more time is needed for observation and evaluation, isosorbide (Ismotic) may be used in an effort to halt progression. It is given in a 50% solution, 8 mg/kg/d (up to 12 mg/kg/d) in 4 divided doses, orally or by nasogastric tube, until a response is achieved or until it is necessary to proceed with surgery.

C. Surgical Treatment: The neurosurgical approach is dictated by the underlying condition and the surgeon's preference. Associated meningomyelocele or other anomalies must be dealt with also.

1. ''Shunting techniques'' involve a variety of systems that route cerebrospinal fluid from a lateral ventricle (usually the right) to the peritoneum or atrium. Other routes are now used rarely. In comparison with ventriculoatrial shunts, ventriculoperitoneal shunts are easier to insert and revise, have fewer and less serious complications, and are associated with lower death rates; the need for revision may also be less.

2. ''Direct'' nonshunting operations consist of third ventriculostomy and choroid plexectomy (imperative in choroid plexus papilloma).

3. The Rickham reservoir with catheter is used as a temporary measure.

D. Prophylactic Care of Shunts: Prophylactic antibiotic therapy (eg, oxacillin, gentamicin, or both) at the time a shunt is inserted is recommended to reduce infection. It is often given systemically as well as intraventricularly.

The shunt systems are usually fitted with a device (valve, tubing, etc) that permits ''pumping'' or flushing through of cerebrospinal fluid to reduce stasis, fibrin clot formation, and infection. How often a shunt should be pumped will vary with the system. Serial head circumference measurements will indicate when the hydrocephalic process ''arrests'' and head growth resumes a normal pattern. A repeat CT scan may demonstrate the reduction in ventricular size within hours after shunting; it is part of the preoperative evalution of the child with shunt failure. Shunt functioning and dependency may be evaluated by measuring pressure in the shunt reservoir and imaging the shunt system after injecting a radionuclide. Cerebrospinal fluid should be obtained when the reservoir is tapped for cell count, culture, and protein and glucose measurements.

Prognosis

In general, if progressive hydrocephalus can be arrested, the prognosis for function is improved. Even if the child is severely retarded and has other handicaps that do not threaten life, ''social shunts'' are justifiable, since the difficulties of caring for the child are markedly eased and the cost of care considerably lowered by reducing the necessity for institutionalization.

The width of the cerebral mantle may not be a reliable prognostic finding.

A. Nonoperated Group: The survival rate at

10 years is about 25%. Of the survivors, about one-fifth can function "competitively," and the remainder require supervision and maintenance.

B. Operated Group: The survival rate at 10 years is about 60%, with over half of the surviving children able to care for themselves. (About 25% of survivors have normal or higher than normal IQs.)

C. Shunt Dependency: The question of shunt dependency is unsettled. At some point in ventricular enlargement, the ependymal surface may be sufficiently large to absorb the net amount of cerebrospinal fluid not handled by the usual pathways. Such "spontaneous arrests" may occur in 40–50% of children surviving the first 1–2 years.

Ehle A, Sklar F: Visual evoked potentials in infants with hydrocephalus. *Neurology* 1979;**29:**1541.

Fitz CR, Harwood-Nash DC: Computed tomography in hydrocephalus. *J Comput Tomogr* 1978;**2:**91.

Freeman JM, D'Souza B: Obstruction of CSF shunts. (Editorial.) *Pediatrics* 1979;**64:**111.

Gardner P, Leipzig T, Phillips P: Infections of central nervous system shunts. *Med Clin North Am* 1985;**69:**297.

Lorber J: The family history of uncomplicated congenital hydrocephalus: An epidemiological study based on 270 probands. *Br Med J* 1984;**289:**281.

Lorber J, Salfield J, Lonton T: Isosorbide in the management of infantile hydrocephalus. *Dev Med Child Neurol* 1983;**25:**502.

Pretorius DH et al: Clinical course of fetal hydrocephalus: 40 cases. *AJNR* 1985;**6:**23.

Renier D et al: Factors causing acute shunt infection: Computer analysis of 1174 operations. *J Neurosurg* 1984;**61:**1072.

Shurtleff DB, Stuntz JT, Hayden PW: Experience with 1201 cerebrospinal fluid shunt procedures. *Pediatr Neurosci* 1985/86;**12:**49.

Tomasovic JJ, Nellhaus G, Moe P: The bobble-head doll syndrome: An early sign of hydrocephalus. *Dev Med Child Neurol* 1975;**17:**777.

3. CRANIOSYNOSTOSIS

Primary craniosynostosis is a developmental disorder of the membranous bones of the skull that results in closure of one or more cranial sutures in utero, beginning with dysostosis of the several bones of the cranial base. Diagnosis at birth is possible by inspection and palpation of the bony ridges along the suture lines, confirmed by radiologic imaging. Occasionally, there is a genetic basis for the defect. Associated anomalies are found in nearly one-third of cases.

Classification

(1) Sagittal sutures only are involved in over 50% of cases, resulting in dolichocephaly (scaphocephaly) with elongation and narrowing of the skull. It is much more common in boys. It may occur as a dominant trait.

(2) Coronal suture involvement accounts for almost 20% of cases, predominantly in girls. When bilateral, as it is in about half of these cases, the result is brachycephaly with a broad, shortened skull.

(3) Metopic suture involvement (10%) results in a pointed, ridged forehead, or trigonocephaly.

(4) Involvement of all the sutures (about 8%) results in a "turret" skull (oxycephaly, acrocephaly).

(5) Other combinations occur occasionally, such as fusion of the sagittal and coronal, lambdoidal, or metopic sutures, or of the lambdoidal and squamous sutures. Unilateral lambdoidal or coronal synostosis is called plagiocephaly.

(6) Allied entities (singly or in combination) are acrocephaly with syndactyly (acrocephalosyndactyly, or Apert's disease, craniofacial dysostosis (Crouzon's disease), and hydrocephalus.

Clinical Findings

In synostosis of a single suture, there are usually no symptoms other than the skull deformity. Signs and symptoms of increased intracranial pressure, strabismus, visual loss, optic atrophy, mental retardation, and, occasionally, seizures occur with brain compression if multiple sutures are involved or if there is hydrocephalus; in the latter case, the head circumference may be abnormally large.

Except where multiple sutures are involved, the normal head circumference and neurologic examination clearly differentiate primary from secondary craniosynostosis, which is usually accompanied by microcephaly.

The suture involvement is defined better by CT scanning than by standard x-rays. The entire suture need not be involved. Radionuclides with a predilection for areas of osteoblastic activity will delineate the fusing—but not the fused—sutures. Symmetric involvement of sutures and craniofacial disproportion are seen in microcephaly. CT scanning will also disclose possible hydrocephalus.

Treatment

If multiple sutures are involved, early neurosurgical intervention with excision of sutures in the first weeks of life is recommended. If there is a deformity of the orbits, orbital decompression is required. The principal reason for sagittal synostosis surgery is cosmetic.

About 13% of patients, chiefly those with bilateral coronal or multiple suture involvement, require reoperation because of recurrent increased intracranial pressure or evidence of fusion after craniectomy.

Prognosis

Cosmetic improvement occurs in about 75% of patients, with those operated on early and having only one or 2 sutures involved showing the best results, ie, an essentially normal-looking head.

Three to 5% with primary craniosynostosis exhibit varying degrees of mental retardation; it occurs most often in trigonocephaly and less often in sagittal synostosis.

Cohen MM: Genetic perspectives on craniosynostosis and syndromes with craniosynostosis. *J Neurosurg* 1977;**47:**886.

Furuya Y et al: Computerized tomography of cranial sutures. 2. Abnormalities of sutures and skull deformity in craniosynostosis. *J Neurosurg* 1984;**61:**59.

Jane JA et al: Immediate correction of sagittal synostosis. *J Neurosurg* 1978;**49:**705.

ABNORMAL HEAD SIZE

Essentials of Diagnosis

- Serial head circumference measurements that cross percentile curves on a growth graph.
- A single head circumference measurement 3 SD or more above or below the mean.
- A single head circumference measurement between 2 and 3 SD above or below the mean, depending on the clinical situation, and followed up by deviating serial measurements.

General Considerations

Abnormal head growth, resulting in micro- or macrocephaly, is often not due to congenital malformations. These malformations, however, may enter into the differential diagnosis. Normally, the maximal occipitofrontal circumference is an indirect measure of intracranial capacity and of brain size. Head circumference is about 65% of adult size at term birth, nearly 80% at 6 months, and slightly over 90% at 2 years, reflecting a brain about 25%, 50%, and 75% of adult size at these ages.

The variables governing head growth are many. The average head circumference in males is about 1 cm larger than in females from term birth on, except during girls' earlier pubertal spurt. Generally, taller people have larger heads and parental head sizes influence the child's head size, but there is no direct ratio between head circumference and other somatic measures. Worldwide, significant undernutrition is reflected by head circumference curves as much as 1 SD below those in well-fed populations. Within the range of normal, head size and degree of intelligence cannot be correlated.

Head circumference should be measured at each well child care visit and oftener on indications, as when the child—or even the adolescent—is seen for a possible disorder of growth and development or for a neurologic problem or when the head circumference falls 2 SD below or above the mean or crosses percentiles.

A thin, flexible, nonexpandable measuring tape should be used and the maximal occipitofrontal circumference checked at least twice. Variances of 0.5 cm in measurement are common and are about equal to the difference between a "full" or close-cut hair style. The measurement should then be plotted on a graph of standard head circumference based on sex.

1. MICROCEPHALY

A head circumference 3 SD or more below the mean for age and sex or increasing too slowly or not at all denotes microcephaly. A head circumference of near 2 SD below the mean *and falling off* is equally significant.

Etiology

The causes of microcephaly with irreparable interference with brain development are as follows:

(1) Defects of the primordium (anlage) of the brain are present in a variety of chromosomal and dysmorphic syndromes and in disorders of brain cell migration. Associated anomalies are common.

(2) Intrauterine brain injuries occur with fetal exposure to chemical agents (alcohol is the commonest, but anticonvulsants are also implicated); with TORCHES infections (*to*xoplasmosis, *r*ubella, *c*ytomegalovirus, *he*rpes simplex, *s*yphilis) or exposure to ionizing radiation in the first 2 trimesters; or with placental insufficiency from other causes.

(3) Brain insults in the last trimester, at birth, and postnatally occur with infections, toxins, metabolic disorders, severe hypoxia and prolonged acidosis, head trauma, cerebrovascular accidents, and degenerative central nervous system disorders. The brain may stop growing or there may be areas of focal destruction, depending upon the cause.

Clinical Findings

A. Symptoms and Signs: Microcephaly may be suspected in the full-term newborn and in infants up to 6 months of age whose chest circumference, unless the child is very obese, exceeds the head circumference. It may be discovered when the child is examined because of delayed developmental milestones or neurologic problems such as seizures or spasticity. There may be a marked backward slope of the forehead, as in familial microcephaly, with narrowing of the temporal diameter; and there is occipital flattening, which is not positional. Skull asymmetries are seen in many dysmorphic and chromosomal disorders; when the cranium is small but has a normal configuration, the brain may be more diffusely retarded in its growth, or a midline defect may be present. The palate may be high-arched and the teeth dysplastic.

B. Laboratory Findings: These vary with the cause. Abnormal dermatoglyphics may be present when the injury occurred before the 19th week of gestation. Screening for TORCHES and amino acid abnormalities should usually be done. Karyotyping should be considered.

C. Radiologic Findings: Skull films are indicated if craniosynostosis involves multiple sutures and is surgically remediable. They are also indicated in dysmorphic syndromes. Ordinarily, microcephaly causes secondary craniosynostosis. CT brain scanning may aid in diagnosis (eg, of intracranial calcifications, malformations, atrophy), prognosis, and genetic counseling. Spine films may occasionally show bony dysraphism.

Differential Diagnosis

Primary craniosynostosis involving multiple sutures is easily differentiated by inspection, the finding of bony ridges along suture lines, and radiologic studies. Treatable undergrowth of the brain due to hypopituitarism or severe protein-calorie undernutrition is recognized by the history and clinical findings.

Treatment & Prognosis

Except for the treatable disorders noted above, treatment is usually supportive and directed at the multiple neurologic and sensory deficits and any endocrine disturbances (eg, diabetes insipidus) encountered. About 90% of children with head circumferences more than 2 SD below the mean show variable degrees of mental retardation, the notable exceptions occurring either when there is "catch-up" head growth in the first 3 years of life or in cases of hypopituitarism. The rates of death and disability vary with underlying causes and complications.

2. MACROCEPHALY (Megalencephaly)

A head circumference more than 3 SD above the mean for age and sex or increasing too rapidly denotes macrocephaly and suggests an abnormally large brain (megalencephaly). A head circumference of 2 SD above the mean, followed by accelerating growth, is equally significant *but may not be pathologic.*

Clinical Findings

Clinical and laboratory findings vary with the underlying process. In infants, transillumination of the skull with an intensely bright flashlight or "Chun's gun" in a completely darkened room may disclose chronic subdural effusions, hydrocephalus, hydranencephaly, and large cystic defects.

A surgically or medically treatable condition must be ruled out; thus, the first major decison is whether and when to perform a CT scan.

A. CT Scan Not Indicated:

1. "Catch-up growth," as in the thriving, neurologically intact premature infant whose rapid head enlargement is most marked in the first weeks of life, or the infant in the early phase of recovery from deprivation dwarfism. As the expected "normal" is reached, head circumference growth slows down, then follows the percentile curve normal for the child.

2. Familial megalencephaly, where another family member may have an unusually large head and there are no signs or symptoms referable to such disorders as neurocutaneous dysplasias (especially neurofibromatosis) or cerebral gigantism (Sotos' syndrome), nor significant mental or neurologic abnormalities in the child.

3. Biochemical disorders involving brain substance (see Central Nervous System Degenerative Disorders of Infancy and Childhood, below), such as the mucopolysaccharidoses and reticuloendothelioses, which are best defined by biochemical techniques.

4. The older infant or child who is either so relatively intact or so profoundly neurologically damaged that serial head circumference measurements about 2–4 weeks apart for a few weeks or months, with equally close attention to neurologic status, may obviate the need for a CT scan.

B. CT Scan Indicated: CT (and in some centers, magnetic resonance) brain imaging—or ultrasonography, if the anterior fontanelle is open—is used to define any structural cause of macrocephaly and to determine an operable disorder. Even when the condition is nontreatable (or benign), the information gained may permit more accurate diagnosis and prognosis, guide management and genetic counseling, and serve as a basis for comparison should future abnormal cranial growth or neurologic changes necessitate a repeat CT scan.

Classification

Macrocephaly may be classified according to treatment options as follows:

A. Operable or Medically Treatable Primary Disorder:

1. Hydrocephalus, as discussed above.

2. Extracerebral lesions without hydrocephalus, such as subdural effusions, epidermoidoma, and some of the dysplasias, as they affect the skull and may cause increased intracranial pressure.

3. Cerebral disorders or malformations without increased intracranial pressure, as may be seen with porencephalic cysts or very slowly growing tumors (especially in infants and very young children); or with increased intracranial pressure, as in toxic encephalopathies, brain tumors, or pseudotumor cerebri.

B. Primary Disorder Not Treatable by Operation or Otherwise:

1. Hydrocephalus with cortical mantle less than 0.5 cm thick (some say 1 cm).

2. Cranioskeletal dysplasias, most notably neurofibromatosis, where there may be hemihypertrophy. It must be remembered that in some neurocutaneous dysplasias, brain tumors may arise at any time.

3. Cerebral gigantism (Sotos' syndrome), a dysmorphic syndrome characterized by large neonatal size or excessive growth in the first 4 years, with advanced bone age, macrocranium with high forehead, frontal bossing, hypertelorism, antimongoloid slant of the palpebral fissures, prominent jaw, and high-arched palate. Developmental delays and some degree of mental retardation are common. The syndrome may be familial.

4. Hydranencephaly (though the head is usually large only relative to a small body).

C. Nonpathologic Macrocephaly:

1. Constitutional gigantism, where the child and other family members are unsually tall but lack all

other stigmas of a neurocutaneous syndrome or cerebral gigantism.

2. Sporadic benign megalencephaly, where no other family member is unusually large or has an unusually large head size, and the child is developmentally and neurologically intact. The child may be excessively tall. In some of these cases, CT ventricular measurements (bifrontal and bicaudate distances) may be slightly enlarged. These children should be followed with serial head circumference measurements and neurologic examinations.

Dodge PR, Holmes SJ, Sotos JF: Cerebral gigantism. *Dev Med Child Neurol* 1983;**25**:248.

Ellison PH: Re-evaluation of the approach to an enlarging head in infancy. *Dev Med Child Neurol* 1978;**20**:738.

Lorber J, Priestley BL: Children with large heads: A practical approach to diagnosis in 557 children, with special reference to 109 children with megalencephaly. *Dev Med Child Neurol* 1981;**23**:494.

Nellhaus G: Head circumference from birth to eighteen years: Practical composite international and interracial graphs. *Pediatrics* 1968;**41**:106.

Stoch MB et al: Psychosocial outcome and CT findings after gross undernourishment during infancy: A 20-year developmental study. *Dev Med Child Neurol* 1982;**24**:419.

NEUROCUTANEOUS DYSPLASIAS

The neurocutaneous dysplasias are a large group of hamartomatous disorders in which tissues of neuroectodermal origin are chiefly involved; tissues arising from meso- and endoderm are often also affected. Visible manifestations may be present as birthmarks or may show up later. Many of the disorders are genetically determined; mutation rates are high in some, and others are wholly sporadic.

Classically cited are neurofibromatosis and tuberous sclerosis, both genetically determined and common; encephalofacial angiomatosis, less common and sporadic; and Hippel-Lindau disease, relatively rare but hereditary.

1. NEUROFIBROMATOSIS (Recklinghausen's Disease)

Neurofibromatosis is so protean in its manifestations that no single one defines it. Five or more café au lait spots at least 0.5 cm in diameter are the hallmark of the disorder but are not essential to the diagnosis. It is quite common (as common as muscular dystrophy; twice as common as cystic fibrosis). It may be transmitted as an autosomal dominant with variable penetrance (occurring in one out of 3000 births) or in sporadic fashion, with a mutation rate as high as 50%.

Clinical Findings

A. Symptoms and Signs:

1. Dermatologic features—In addition to 5 or more café au lait spots (fewer than 1% of individuals without Recklinghausen's disease have more than 2), axillary freckles and subcutaneous neurofibroma are virtually diagnostic. Freckles in the perineum and on the neck and lipomas are common; hemangiomas and lymphangiomas are less common.

2. Neurologic features—These include neuromas of cranial, peripheral, or autonomic nerves or of the spinal cord; optic nerve gliomas (involving either one nerve or the optic chiasm), not infrequent in childhood; acoustic (eighth nerve) neurinoma, usually bilateral in childhood; intracranial tumors, especially astrocytomas of varying degrees of malignancy; seizures (often indicative of intracranial tumors, but sometimes unrelated); asymptomatic megalencephaly; nonspecifically abnormal EEGs without other neurologic deficit; and central nervous system malformations, including meningocele and syringomyelia.

3. Mental functioning—Mild to moderate retardation occurs in nearly 10% of patients.

4. Skeletal involvement—There is a high incidence of kyphoscoliosis, defects of vertebral bodies and of the skull, elephantiasic hypertrophy, and rarefaction and cystlike destruction of bone. Recklinghausen's disease is occasionally associated with vitamin D-resistant rickets.

5. Other systems—Findings include delayed or precocious sex development, diabetes mellitus, thyroid and parathyroid disorders, pheochromocytomas, melanoblastosis, congenital glaucoma, soft tissue tumors (eg, retroperitoneal fibrosarcomas), leukemia, and vascular lesions, especially of the cerebrum or kidneys.

B. Laboratory, Radiologic, and Other Findings: None are specific. Radiologic studies, electroencephalography, and tests of endocrine function may be indicated on the basis of suspected involvement. Levels of neuronal growth factor have given mixed results as a discriminant for neurofibromatosis.

Differential Diagnosis

The light brown (café au lait) spots in neurofibromatosis are smooth-bordered, while the spots in polyostotic fibrous dysplasia are jagged-edged ("coast of Maine"); the distinction is not absolute.

Treatment & Prognosis

Treatment is directed toward specific problems, eg, neurosurgical removal or radiation therapy for tumors, orthopedic correction of scoliosis. The heritable nature of the disorder should be made clear.

The prognosis depends entirely on the manifestations: excellent where there are only skin or bone lesions, poor with malignant tumors. Overall, survival rates are somewhat impaired in relatives with neurofibromatosis, worse in probands, and worst in female probands.

Riccardi VM: Von Recklinghausen neurofibromatosis. *N Engl J Med* 1981;**305**:1617.

Riopelle RJ: Serum neuronal growth factor levels in von Reck-

linghausen's neurofibromatosis. *Ann Neurol* 1984;**16:**54.
Sorensen SA, Mulvihill JJ, Nielsen A: Long-term follow-up of von Recklinghausen neurofibromatosis: Survival and malignant neoplasms. *N Engl J Med* 1986;**314:**1010.

2. TUBEROUS SCLEROSIS (Bourneville's Disease)

Tuberous sclerosis is a neurocutaneous dysplasia characterized by the triad of mental retardation, pathognomonic facial fibroangiomas or poorly pigmented spots of skin or hair (or both), and epilepsy. It is transmitted as an autosomal dominant, possibly modified by a second unlinked dominant gene, and the mutation rate may be as high as 80%.

Clinical Findings

A. Symptoms and Signs:

1. Dermatologic features—Virtually diagnostic are the hypomelanotic "ash leaf" spots on the skin (mistakenly called "vitiligo"), which may be present at birth or appear in the first 2 years of life; these are often best demonstrated with Wood's light. Equally characteristic are Pringle's spots (erroneously labeled "adenoma sebaceum" by Pringle), usually appearing by the fourth year of life, and of 2 types: reddish angiofibromatous seedlike growths, and yellowish to brown, mostly fibromatous small nodules. Also seen are other angiomas; café au lait spots with smooth borders; shagreen patches of grayish-green or brown rough leathery skin; patches of poorly pigmented scalp hair; and subungual fibromas of fingers and toes found at adolescence and more often in girls.

2. Neurologic features—Seizures occur in over 85% of cases and may be the only manifestation in some family members. About 2–5% of patients with infantile spasms with hypsarrhythmia and mental retardation have tuberous sclerosis. Formation of nodules ("tubers") containing atypical large glial cells results in subependymal calcifications or irregularities of the ventricular walls; these are seen earliest and best on a CT scan. The cerebellum, brain stem, and spinal cord are rarely if ever involved. Mass lesions include gliomas, gangliogliomas, and cystic lesions. The EEG is often nonspecifically abnormal even in asymptomatic family members.

3. Mental retardation—Mental retardation is frequent and may be the sole manifestation in a member of an affected family. Tuberous sclerosis patients account for 0.3–0.6% of the institutionalized mentally retarded.

4. Ocular involvement—Retinal phakomas or "mulberry lesions" at the edge of the optic disk are found in 8% of affected individuals; other eye defects include optic atrophy, nystagmus, and even blindness.

5. Skeletal involvement—Findings include periosteal thickening and central cystic rarefactions of fingers and toes, hyperostosis of cranium, poly- and syndactyly, and vertebral defects.

6. Visceral manifestations—Renal hamartomas, cardiac rhabdomyomas, pulmonary vascular fibrosis, and various mixed tumors of other viscera are seen.

7. Other manifestations—Endocrinopathies, cleft lip and palate, branchial cleft cysts, congenital heart disease, and genital dysplasias may be present.

B. Radiologic Findings: Ultrasonography and CT scanning may show the diagnostic subependymal nodules and calcifications, even in very young patients. A renal echogram may show cysts.

Differential Diagnosis

The triad of seizures, typical skin lesions, and mental retardation present in any combination in a family suggests tuberous sclerosis. The diagnosis, sometimes difficult in the early stages or incomplete forms, may be facilitated by Wood's lamp examination of the skin, a CT brain scan, and possibly a renal echogram. These studies may also detect lesions in apparently unaffected parents and siblings.

Treatment & Prognosis

Treatment is nonspecific except as required for seizures, brain tumors, or visceral lesions. The heritable nature of the disorder should be made clear.

The most severely affected patients have a shortened life span, with death occurring at variable times as a result of status epilepticus, brain or visceral tumors, or intercurrent infections. In mild or atypical cases, life span may be normal.

Cassidy SB et al: Family studies in tuberous sclerosis: Evaluation of apparently unaffected parents. *JAMA* 1983;**249:**1302.
Gomez MR, Kuntz NL, Westmoreland BF: Tuberous sclerosis, early onset of seizures, and mental subnormality: Study of discordant homozygous twins. *Neurology* 1982;**32:**604.
Hunt A: Tuberous sclerosis: A survey of 97 cases. (3 parts.) *Dev Med Child Neurol* 1983;**25:**346, 350, 353.

3. ENCEPHALOFACIAL ANGIOMATOSIS (Sturge-Weber Disease)

Sturge-Weber disease consists of a port wine nevus on the upper part of the face and leptomeningeal angiomatosis of the cerebral cortex on the same side. It occurs sporadically. The facial lesions are present at birth, but other manifestations may not become evident for a year or more.

Clinical Findings

A. Symptoms and Signs: A purplish cutaneous nevus covers at least the upper eyelid or supraorbital region of the face (hence also called "trigeminal" angiomatosis) and scalp and may involve both sides of the face and other parts of the body. Seizures, both focal and generalized, occur in up to 90% of cases, often in the first year of life. Hemiparesis on the side contralateral to the face lesion is found in about one-third of cases and is frequently associated with hemiatrophy. Mental retardation of varying degree is present in about half of cases.

Buphthalmos (congenital glaucoma) occurs in about one-third of cases; hemianopia is common.

Angiomatous involvement of the oropharynx and viscera and hypertrophy of extremities covered by angiomatous skin may be present.

B. Radiologic Findings: CT brain scanning identifies the diagnostic double-contoured calcifications corresponding to cerebral gyri before they can be seen on skull x-rays. With enhancement, a CT scan may show the leptomeningeal angiomatosis. Skull films may show bony enlargement with large vascular channels over the involved side. Angiography should be reserved for children in whom cerebrovascular complications arise or who are being considered for hemispherectomy.

C. Electroencephalography: The EEG usually shows nonspecific abnormalities over the involved hemisphere early in the disease.

Differential Diagnosis

The diagnosis can be made on the basis of the facial lesion, especially when contralateral seizures and neurologic deficits are present. The diagnosis is confirmed by the typical intracranial calcifications seen on CT scan; rarely, calcification may occur even in the absence of the facial stain.

Complications

Intracranial bleeding may occur into the subdural or subarachnoid space, with worsening of the neurologic status. Focal status epilepticus may occur.

Treatment & Prognosis

For the treatment of seizures, see Seizure Disorders. Physical therapy may be indicated for hemiplegia. Glaucoma should be treated as outlined in Chapter 11. In cases with unilateral seizures, early hemispherectomy to prevent neurologic deterioration should be considered. Argon laser treatment of the port wine stains lightens them in over 70% of cases.

The prognosis varies with the extent of the leptomeningeal angiomatosis, the severity of the seizure disorder, and the occurrence of cerebrovascular accidents.

Di Trapani G et al: Light microscopy and ultrastructural studies of Sturge-Weber disease. *Childs Brain* 1982;**9:**23.

Hoffman HJ et al: Hemispherectomy for Sturge-Weber syndrome. *Childs Brain* 1974;**5:**233.

Nellhaus G, Haberland C, Hill BJ: Sturge-Weber disease with bilateral intracranial calcifications at birth and unusual pathologic findings. *Acta Neurol Scand* 1967;**43:**314.

4. HIPPEL-LINDAU DISEASE (Retinocerebellar Angiomatosis)

Hippel-Lindau disease is an unusual, dominantly transmitted condition characterized by hemangioblastomas of the retina and cerebellum. Brain stem and spinal angiomatosis, benign and malignant cystic tumors of the abdominal organs, and tumors of the sympathetic chain are often associated. Cutaneous hemangiomas occur rarely. Morbidity and deaths are usually due to the ocular and nervous system vascular lesions, pheochromocytoma, and renal cell carcinoma; pancreatic insufficiency has been reported. Polycythemia is frequently present.

The diagnosis may be confirmed by the family history and by a CT scan of the posterior fossa, spinal cord, or abdominal organs as indicated. Angiography is indicated when surgery is contemplated.

Retinal lesions may be dealt with by photo- or diathermy coagulation. Other tumors may require surgical removal.

Feldberg MAM, van Waes PFGM, Schonfeld DHW: Hippel-Lindau disease. *Radiol Clin* 1978;**47:**91.

CENTRAL NERVOUS SYSTEM DEGENERATIVE DISORDERS OF INFANCY & CHILDHOOD

Essentials of Diagnosis

- Arrest of psychomotor development.
- Loss, usually progressive but at variable rates, of mental and motor functioning and often vision.
- Seizures are common in some disorders.
- Symptoms and signs vary with age at onset and primary sites of involvement of specific types.

General Considerations

The central nervous system degenerative disorders of infancy and childhood are fortunately rare. An early clinical pattern of decline often follows normal early development. Referral for sophisticated biochemical testing is usually necessary before definitive diagnosis can be made.

Clinical Findings

A. Symptoms:

1. Where white matter is primarily involved, motor disturbances usually appear first. Hypotonia or flaccidity in infants may precede the eventual spasticity, or if the child has begun to walk, incoordination (ataxia or dystonia) may be noted first, accompanied or followed by derangements of swallowing and of vocalization or speech. Vision is disturbed early. Convulsions usually appear late in the course if at all.

2. Where gray matter is primarily involved, convulsions often precede disturbances of mental and motor functions.

3. Where the disorder is diffuse, the clinical picture may be mixed or may present predominantly with the features of a white or gray matter disturbance.

B. Signs: (See also Tables 23–9 and 23–10.) Certain signs, though rarely specific, together with data regarding age at onset and family history, will help in selecting the biochemical or other definitive studies for the diagnosis of a neurodegenerative disorder.

1. Eye signs—"Cherry-red" maculas often suggest Tay-Sachs and G_{M2} gangliosidosis variants; they sometimes point to generalized (G_{M1}) gangliosidoses, Niemann-Pick disease, and infantile Gaucher's disease. Other signs and their suggested disorders are as follows: "salt and pepper" maculas, neuronal ceroid lipofuscinosis; optic atrophy, leukodystrophies; retinitis pigmentosa, Bassen-Kornzweig syndrome and Refsum's disease; Kayser-Fleischer rings, Wilson's disease; and corneal clouding, some mucopolysaccharidoses.

2. Hepatosplenomegaly—This variable finding may suggest Niemann-Pick disease, infantile Gaucher's disease, gangliosidoses, mucopolysaccharidoses, some glycogen storage diseases, and carnitine deficiency. (See also Table 23–13.)

3. Areflexia—Areflexia may suggest globoid and metachromatic leukodystrophies.

C. Laboratory Findings: (See also Tables 23–9, 23–10, and 33–12.)

1. Specific enzyme deficiencies are known to cause many of these degenerative diseases. Assays are often available to test for enzyme abnormalities in leukocytes or cultured fibroblasts, including those from amniotic fluid.

2. Cerebrospinal fluid protein is usually increased in leukodystrophies. Gamma globulin and, more specifically, measles or rubella antibodies are increased in subacute sclerosing panencephalitis (SSPE).

3. Nerve conduction velocities are reduced in some leukodystrophies. Occasionally, biopsy of specific tissues may provide diagnostic information.

Differential Diagnosis

A period of observation may be necessary before it becomes clear that one is dealing with a degenerative process. Pseudodegeneration may occur as a result of a severe seizure disorder or other illness, or a child may regress because of gross emotional neglect or stress. Acquired deafness sometimes produces regression in cognitive function mimicking a degenerative course. Retarded children with static brain damage are often thought by their parents to be regressing when in actuality a younger sibling or other child is noted to be outstripping the older one. Thus, the differential diagnosis of central nervous system degenerative disorders must include "cerebral palsy," seizure disorders, space-occupying lesions (including subdural hematomas or brain tumors), neurocutaneous dysplasias, chromosomal defects, disorders of glucose or protein and amino or organic acid metabolism, and chronic central nervous system infections.

Tables 23–9 and 23–10 summarize the differential aspects of many of the degenerative central nervous system disorders of infancy and childhood.

Complications

Pneumonia, usually due to aspiration, is the most common complication and the usual cause of death.

Prevention

The heritable nature of specific disorders should be made clear. Enzymatic or electron microscopic techniques involving studies of leukocytes, skin fibroblasts, and amniotic cells identify the carriers, affected fetuses, or presymptomatic cases.

Treatment

Specific effective treatment (chelators in Wilson's disease, low phytanic acid diet in Refsum's syndrome, vitamin E in abetalipoproteinemia) may arrest or reverse neurologic symptoms.

In most degenerative central nervous system diseases, treatment is purely symptomatic, consisting of control of seizures, maintenance of nutrition (often via feeding gastrostomy), and treatment of infections. In acute attacks of "multiple sclerosis" and possibly in "Schilder's disease," corticotropin (4 mg/kg/d intramuscularly initially, with rapidly decreasing doses if there is a good response)—or prednisone—may shorten the duration of the attack without altering the frequency of exacerbations or the ultimate outcome. In subacute sclerosing panencephalitis, prolonged remissions may occur with continuous treatment with inosiplex (Isoprinosine; a drug still investigational in the USA), 100 mg/kg/d in divided doses.

Prognosis

By definition, the degenerative central nervous system diseases lead to progressive loss of function and premature death within months or a few years.

Arsenio-Nunes ML, Goutières F, Aicardi J: An ultramicroscopic study of skin and conjunctival biopsies in neurological disorders of childhood. *Ann Neurol* 1981;**9:**163.

Bye AME, Kendall B, Wilson J: Multiple sclerosis in childhood: A new look. *Dev Med Child Neurol* 1985; **27:**215.

Dyken PR: Subacute sclerosing panencephalitis: Current status. *Neurol Clin* 1985;**3:**179.

Dyken PR, Krawiecki N: Neurodegenerative diseases of infancy and childhood. *Ann Neurol* 1983;**13:**351.

Johnson WG: The clinical spectrum of hexosaminidase deficiency diseases. *Neurology* 1981;**31:**1453.

MacFaul R et al: Metachromatic leukodystrophy: Review of 38 cases. *Arch Dis Child* 1982;**57:**168.

Markland ON et al: Brain stem auditory, visual, and somatosensory evoked potentials in leukodystrophies. *Electroencephalogr Clin Neurophysiol* 1982;**54:**39.

O'Neil BP, Moser HW: Adrenoleukodystrophy. *Can J Neurol Sci* 1982;**9:**449.

Poser CM et al: Schilder's myelinoclastic diffuse sclerosis. *Pediatrics* 1986;**77:**107.

Prick MJJ et al: Progressive infantile poliodystrophy (Alper's disease) with a defect in citric acid cycle activity in liver and fibroblasts. *Neuropediatrics* 1982;**13:**108.

Rosenberg RN: Biochemical genetics of neurologic disease. *N Engl J Med* 1981;**305:**1181.

Sorbi S, Blass JP: Abnormal activation of pyruvate dehydrogenase in Leigh disease fibroblasts. *Neurology* 1982;**32:**555.

Walter GL: Myoencephalopathies with abnormal mitochondria: A review. *Clin Neuropathol* 1983;**2:**101.

Table 23–9. Central nervous system degenerative disorders of infancy.

Disease	Enzyme Defect and Genetics	Onset	Early Manifestations	Vision and Hearing	Somatic Findings	Motor System	Seizures	Laboratory and Tissue Studies	Course
WHITE MATTER									
Globoid (Krabbe's) leukodystrophy	Recessive. Galactocerebrosidase and lactosylceramidase I deficiency.	First 6 months; "late-onset forms."	Feeding difficulties. Shrill cry. Irritability. Arching of back.	Optic atrophy, mid-course to late. Hyperacusis occasionally.	Head often small. Often underweight.	Early spasticity, occasionally preceded by hypotonia. Prolonged nerve conduction.	Early. Myoclonic and generalized.	CSF protein elevated; usually normal in late-onset forms. Sural nerve: nonspecific myelin breakdown. Enzyme deficiency in leukocytes, cultured skin fibroblasts.	Rapid. Death usually by 1½–2 years. Late-onset cases may live 5–10 years.
Metachromatic leukodystrophy	Recessive. Arylsulfatase A deficiency.	Second year. Less often, later in childhood.	Incoordination, especially gait disturbance; then general regression. Reverse in juveniles.	Optic atrophy, usually late. Hearing normal.	Head enlarged late. None in juvenile form.	Combined upper and lower motor neuron signs. Ataxia. Prolonged nerve conduction.	Infrequent, usually late and generalized.	Metachromatic cells in urine; negative sulfatase A test. CSF protein elevated; occasionally normal early. Sural nerve biopsy: metachromasia. Enzyme deficiency in leukocytes, cultured skin fibroblasts.	Moderately slow. Death in infantile form by 3–8 years, in "juvenile" form by 10–15 years.
Adrenoleukodystrophy and variants	X-linked recessive.	5–10 years.	Impaired intellect, behavioral problems.	"Cortical blindness and deafness."		Ataxia, spasticity. Motor deficits may be asymmetric, or one-sided initially.	Occasionally.	Hyperpigmentation and adrenocortical insufficiency.* ACTH elevated. Accumulation of very long chain fatty acids.	Fairly rapid, death usually within 2–3 years after onset.
Pelizaeus-Merzbacher disease	X-linked recessive; rare female.	(?) Birth to 2 years.	"Eye rolling" often shortly after birth. Head bobbing. Slow loss of intellect.	Slowly developing optic atrophy. Hearing normal.	Head and body normal.	Cerebellar signs early, hyperactive deep reflexes. Spasticity usually only very late.	Usually only late.	None specific. Brain biopsy: extensive demyelination with small perivascular islands of intact myelin.	Exceedingly slow, often seemingly stationary. Many survive well into adult life.
DIFFUSE, BUT PRIMARILY GRAY MATTER									
Poliodystrophy (Alpers' disease)	Occasionally familial, recessive. Possibly viral. Metabolic forms.	Infancy to adolescence.	Variable: loss of intellect, seizures, incoordination.	"Cortical blindness and deafness."	Head normal initially; may fail to grow.	Variable: incoordination, spasticity.	Often initial manifestation: myoclonic, akinetic, and generalized.	Non specific. CSF protein normal or slightly elevated. Extensive neuronal loss in cortex: may occur very late. Citric acid cycle defects. ?Increased serum pyruvate, lactate.	Usually rapid, with death within 1–3 years after onset.
Tay-Sachs disease and G_{M2} gangliosidosis variants: Sandhoff disease; juvenile; chronic-adult.	Recessive. Hexosaminidase deficiencies. Tay-Sachs 93% East European Jewish, hexosaminidase A and S. Others panethnic. Sandhoff hexosaminidase A and B.	Tay-Sachs, Sandhoff similar: 3–6 months. Others 2–6 years or later. Juvenile-partial hexosaminidase A.	Variable: shrill cry, loss of vision, infantile spasms, arrest of development. In juvenile and chronic forms: motor difficulties; later, mental difficulties.	Cherry-red macula, early blindness. Hyperacusis early. Strabismus in juvenile form, blindness late.	Head enlarged late. Liver occasionally enlarged. None in juvenile or chronic forms.	Initially floppy. Eventual decerebrate rigidity. In juvenile and chronic forms: dysarthria, ataxia, spasticity.	Frequent, in mid-course and late. Infantile spasms and generalized.	Blood smears: vacuolated lymphocytes; basophilic hypergranulation. Enzyme deficiencies in serum, leukocytes, or cultured skin fibroblasts.	Moderately rapid. Death usually by 2–5 years. In juvenile form, 5–15 years.

Niemann-Pick disease and variants	50% Jewish. Recessive. Sphingomyelinase deficiency. In variants, enzyme defects unknown.	First 6 months. In variants, later onset; often non-Jewish.	Slow development. Protruding belly.	Cherry-red macula in 35–50%. Blindness late. Deafness occasionally.	Head usually normal. Spleen enlarged more than liver. Occasional xanthomas of skin.	Initially floppy. Eventually spastic. Occasionally extrapyramidal signs.	Rare and late.	Blood: vacuolated lymphocytes; increased lipids. X-rays: "mottled" lungs, decalcified bones. "Foam cells" in bone marrow, spleen, lymph nodes; lipid analysis of nodes.	Moderately slow. Death usually by 3–5 years.
Infantile Gaucher's disease (glucosyl ceramide lipidosis)	Recessive. Glucocerebrosidase deficiency.	First 6 months; rarely, late infancy.	Stridor or hoarse cry. Retraction. Feeding difficulties.	Occasional cherry-red macula. Convergent squint. Deafness occasionally.	Head usually normal. Liver and spleen equally enlarged.	Opisthotonos early, followed rapidly by decerebrate rigidity.	Rare and late	Anemia. Increased acid phosphatase. X-rays: thinned cortex, trabeculation of bones. "Gaucher cells" in bone marrow, spleen. Enzyme deficiency in leukocytes or cultured skin fibroblasts.	Very rapid.
Lipogranulomatosis (Farber's disease)	Ceramidase deficiency.	Early in infancy.	Hoarseness, irritability, restricted joint movements.	Usually normal.	Painful nodular swelling of joints; subcutaneous nodules.	Psychomotor retardation and progressive paralysis.	Usually none.	Chest x-rays may show pulmonary infiltrates. Nodules: granulomatous lesions, resembling those in reticuloendotheliosis.	Rapid: death usually in 1–2 years.
Generalized gangliosidosis and juvenile type (G_{M1} gangliosidoses)	Recessive. Beta-galactosidase deficiency.	First year; less often, second year.	Arrest of development. Protruding belly. Coarse facies in infantile (generalized) form.	50% "cherry-red spot." Hearing usually normal. In juvenile type, occasionallyretinitis pigmentosa.	Head enlarged early. Liver enlarged more than spleen.	Initially floppy, eventually spastic.	Usually late.	Blood: vacuolated lymphocytes. X-rays: dorsolumbar kyphosis, "beaking" of vertebrae. "Foam cells" similar to those in Niemann-Pick disease.	Very rapid. Death within a few years. Slower in juvenile type.
Subacute necrotizing encephalomyelopathy (Leigh's disease)	Recessive. Variable: thiamine triphosphate "inhibitor." Also deficiency of pyruvate carboxylase, pyruvate dehydrogenase.	Infancy to late childhood.	Difficulties in feeding. Feeble or absent cry. Floppiness.	Optic atrophy, often early. Roving eye movements.	Head usually normal, occasionally small. Cardiac and renal tubular dysfunction occasionally.	Flaccid and immobile; may become spastic. Spinocerebellar forms.	Rare and late.	Increased blood lactate and pyruvate. CSF, urine for "inhibitor." "Inhibitor" in brain, liver, heart, skeletal muscle.	Usually rapid in infants, but may be slow with death after several years. Central hypoventilation a frequent cause of death.
"Steel wool," or "kinky hair," disease (Menkes')	X-linked recessive. Defect in copper absorption.	Infancy.	Peculiar facies. Secondary hair white, twisted, split. Hypothermia.	May show optic disk pallor and microcysts of pigment epithelium.	Normal to small.	Variable: floppy to spastic.	Myoclonic, infantile spasms, status epilepticus.	Defective absorption of copper. Cerebralangiographyshowselongated arteries. Hair shows pili torti, split shafts. CT scan may show diffuse multifocal areas of low density.	Moderately rapid. Death usually by 3–4 years.
Huntington's disease.	Dominant. Genetic marker on chromosome 4.	10% childhood onset.	Rigidity, dementia.	Ophthalmoplegia late.	None.	Rigidity. Chorea frequently absent in children.	50% with major motor seizures.	CT scan may show "butterfly" atrophy of caudate and putamen.	Moderately rapid with death in 5–15 years.
Bassen-Kornzweig disease	Recessive. Primary defect unknown.	Early childhood.	Diarrhea in infancy.	Retinitis pigmentosa; late ophthalmoplegia.	None.	Ataxia, late extrapyramidal movement disorder.	None.	Abetalipoproteinemia; acanthocytosis, low serum vitamin E.	Progression arrested with vitamin E.

* CSF gamma globulin (IgG) is considered elevated in children when above 9% of total protein (possibly even > 8.3%); definitively elevated when > 14%.

Table 23–10. Central nervous system degenerative disorders of childhood.*

Disease	Enzyme Defect and Genetics	Onset	Early Manifestations	Vision and Hearing	Motor System	Seizures	Laboratory and Tissue Studies	Course
Neuroaxonal degeneration (Seitelberger's disease). Same as, or resembling, Hallervorden-Spatz disease	Familial, (?) recessive. Girls more frequent than boys. Defect unknown.	1–3 years.	Arrest of development and dementia. Loss of motor functions. Occasionally hypesthesia over trunk and legs.	Nystagmus frequent; optic atrophy, hearing impairment.	Combined upper and lower motor neuron lesions. Early, may lie in "frog" position.	Variable, but usually not a prominent feature.	Denervation on EMG; elevated serum LDH and transaminase. Increased iron uptake in region of basal ganglia by scintillation counter probes over the temples. Brain and sural nerve: axonal swellings or "spheroids." Iron deposition in globus pallidus.	Very slowly progressive, with death early in second decade or earlier.
Neuronal ceroid lipofuscinosis (cerebromacular degenerations): Late infantile cerebral sphingolipidosis (Bielschowsky-Jansky disease)	Recessive. Defect unknown.	2–4 years.	Ataxia. Visual difficulties. Arrested intellectual development.	Pigmentary degeneration of macula. Optic atrophy. Hearing may be impaired.	Ataxia, spasticity progressing to decerebrate rigidity.	Often early: myoclonic and later generalized; difficult to control.	Blood: vacuolated lymphocytes, azurophilic dispersed hypergranulation of polymorphonuclear cells. Electroretinography helpful. Bone marrow: sea-blue histiocytes. In skin, skeletal muscle, peripheral nerves, brain: "curvilinear bodies" and "fingerprint profiles"; autofluorescent lipopigments.	Moderately slow. Death in 3–8 years.
Subacute sclerosing panencephalitis (Dawson's disease, SSPE)	None. Relatively common. Measles "slow virus" infection. Also reported as result of rubella.	3–22 years. Rarely earlier or later.	Impaired intellect, emotional lability, incoordination.	Occasionally chorioretinitis or optic atrophy. Hearing normal.	Ataxia, slurred speech, occasionally involuntary movements, spasticity progressing to decerebrate rigidity.	Myoclonic and akinetic seizures relatively early; later, focal and generalized.	CSF protein normal to moderately elevated. High CSF gamma globulin;† oligoclonal bands. Elevated CSF and serum measles (or rubella) antibody titers. Characteristic EEG. Brain biopsy: inclusion body encephalitis; culturing of measles virus, possibly rubella virus.	Variable, from death in months to years. Remissions of variable duration may occur. Isoprinosine produces long-term remissions.
Multiple sclerosis (See also Transverse Myelitis and Neuromyelitis Optica, Table 23–12.)	None. Diagnosis difficult in childhood. Defect unknown. ?Slow virus infection.	2 years on.	Highly variable: may strike one or more sites of CNS. Paresthesias common.	Optic neuritis; diplopia, nystagmus at some time. Vestibulocochlear nerves occasionally affected.	Motor weakness, spasticity, ataxia, sphincter disturbances, slurred speech, mental difficulties.	Rare: focal or generalized.	CSF may show slight pleocytosis, elevation of protein and gamma globulin;† oligoclonal bands present. CT scan may show areas of demyelination. Auditory, visual, and somatosensory evoked responses often show lesions in respective pathways. Changes in T cell subsets.	Variable: complete remission possible. Recurrent attacks and involvement of multiple sites are prerequisites for diagnosis.
Cerebrotendinous xanthomatosis	?Recessive. Abnormal accumulation of cholesterol.	Late childhood to adolescence.	Xanthomas in tendons. Mental deterioration.	Cataracts; xanthelasma.	Cerebellar deficits. Late: bulbar paralysis.	Myoclonus.	Xanthomas may appear in lungs. Xanthomas in tendons (especially Achilles).	Very slowly progressive into middle life. Replace deficient bile acid.
Wilson's disease (hepatolenticular degeneration)	Recessive. Accumulation of copper.	Adolescence.	Ataxia, dysarthria, mental changes.	Normal. Kayser-Fleischer rings.	Spasticity and incoordination.	Rare.	Liver copper, 24-hour urine copper increased.	Reversed with chelators.
Refsum's disease	Recessive. Phytanic acid oxidase deficiency.	5–10 years.	Ataxia, ichthyosis, cardiomyopathy.	Retinitis pigmentosa.	Ataxia.	None.	Serum phytanic acid elevated; slow nerve conduction velocity, elevated CSF protein.	Treat with low phytanic acid diet.

* For late infantile metachromatic leukodystrophy, Pelizaeus-Merzbacher disease, poliodystrophy, Gaucher's disease of later onset, and subacute necrotizing encephalomyelopathy, see Table 23–9.

† CSF gamma globulin (IgG) is considered elevated in children when > 9% of total protein (possibly even > 8.3%); definitively elevated when > 14%.

ATAXIAS OF CHILDHOOD

1. ACUTE CEREBELLAR ATAXIA

Acute cerebellar ataxia occurs most commonly in children 2–6 years of age. The onset is abrupt, and the evolution of symptoms is rapid. In about half of cases, there is a prodromal illness with fever, respiratory or gastrointestinal symptoms, or an exanthem within 3 weeks of onset. Associated viral infections include varicella, rubeola, mumps, rubella, echovirus infections, poliomyelitis, infectious mononucleosis, and influenza. Bacterial infections such as scarlet fever and salmonellosis have also been incriminated.

Clinical Findings

A. Symptoms and Signs: Ataxia of the trunk and extremities may be severe, so that the child exhibits a staggering, reeling gait and inability to sit without support or to reach for objects; or there may be only mild unsteadiness. Hypotonia, tremor of the extremities, and horizontal nystagmus may be present. Speech may be slurred. The child frequently is irritable, and vomiting may occur.

There are no clinical signs of increased intracranial pressure. Sensory and reflex testing usually shows no abnormalities.

B. Laboratory Findings: Cerebrospinal fluid pressure and protein and glucose levels are normal; slight lymphocytosis (up to about 30/μL) may be present. Attempts should be made to identify the etiologic viral agent by appropriate studies of spinal fluid, stool, throat washings, and paired sera.

C. Radiologic and Other Findings: CT scans and x-rays of long bones are normal. The EEG may be normal or may show nonspecific slowing.

Differential Diagnosis

Acute cerebellar ataxia must be differentiated from acute cerebellar syndromes due to phenytoin, phenobarbital, primidone, or lead intoxication. For phenytoin, the toxic level in serum is usually above 25 μg/mL; for phenobarbital, above 50 μg/mL; for primidone, above 14 μg/mL. (See Seizure Disorders.) With lead intoxication, papilledema, anemia, basophilic stippling of erythrocytes, proteinuria, typical x-rays, and elevated cerebrospinal fluid protein are clinical clues, confirmed by serum, urine, or hair lead levels. An occult neuroblastoma, usually seen with the polymyoclonia-opsoclonus syndrome (see below) that once was included in acute cerebellar ataxia, must also be ruled out.

In rare cases, acute cerebellar ataxia may be the presenting sign of acute bacterial meningitis or may be mimicked by corticosteroid withdrawal, vasculitides such as in polyarteritis nodosa, trauma, the first attack of ataxia in a metabolic disorder such as Hartnup disease, or the onset of acute disseminated encephalomyelitis or of multiple sclerosis. The history and physical findings may differentiate these disturbances, but appropriate laboratory studies are often necessary. For ataxias with more chronic onset and course, see the sections on spinocerebellar degeneration (below) and the other degenerative disorders.

Treatment & Prognosis

Treatment is supportive. The use of corticosteroids has no rational justification.

Between 80 and 90% of children with acute cerebellar ataxia not secondary to drugs recover without sequelae within 6–8 weeks. In the remainder, neurologic disturbances, including disorders of behavior and of learning, ataxia, abnormal eye movements, and speech impairment, may persist for months or years, and recovery may remain incomplete.

French JH, Familusi JB: Cerebellar disorders in childhood. *Pediatr Ann* 1983;**12:**825.

2. POLYMYOCLONIA-OPSOCLONUS SYNDROME OF CHILDHOOD (Infantile Myoclonic Encephalopathy, "Dancing Eyes-Dancing Feet" Syndrome)

The symptoms and signs of this syndrome are at first similar to those of "acute cerebellar ataxia." Often of sudden onset, there is severe incoordination of the trunk and extremities with lightninglike jerking or flinging movements of a group of muscles, causing the child to be in constant motion while awake. Extraocular muscle involvement results in sudden irregular eye movements (opsoclonus). Irritability and vomiting are present often, but there is no depression of level of consciousness. This syndrome occurs in association with viral infections, tumors of neural crest origin, and many other disorders. Immunologic mechanisms have been postulated to be responsible. There are usually no signs of increased intracranial pressure. Cerebrospinal fluid may show normal or mildly increased protein levels. Special techniques show increased cerebrospinal fluid levels of plasmocytes and abnormal immunoglobulins. The EEG may be slightly slow, but when performed together with electromyography, it shows no evidence of association between cortical discharges and the muscle movements. An assiduous search must be made to rule out tumor of neural crest origin by x-rays of the chest and abdomen, skeletal survey, and intravenous urography as well as by assays of urinary catecholamine metabolites (vanilmandelic acid, etc) and cystathionine.

The symptoms respond (often dramatically) to large doses of corticotropin. Otherwise, treatment is as for specific entities. When a neural crest (or possibly other) tumor is found, surgical excision should be followed by irradiation and chemotherapy. Life span is determined by the biologic behavior of the tumor.

The syndrome is usually self-limited but may be

characterized by exacerbations and remissions. However, even after removal of a neural crest tumor and without other evidence of its recurrence, symptoms may reappear. A high incidence of mild mental retardation has also been recorded.

Boltshauser E, Deonna TH, Hirt HR: Myoclonic encephalopathy of infants or "dancing eyes syndrome": Report of 7 cases with long-term follow-up and review of the literature (cases with and without neuroblastoma). *Helv Paediatr Acta* 1979;**34:**119.

Rivner MH et al: Opsoclonus in *Hemophilus influenzae* meningitis. *Neurology* 1982;**32:**661.

3. SPINOCEREBELLAR DEGENERATION DISORDERS

Spinocerebellar degeneration disorders may be hereditary or may occur in sporadic distribution. Hereditary disorders include Friedreich's ataxia, dominant hereditary ataxia, and a group of miscellaneous diseases.

Friedreich's Ataxia

This is a recessive disorder characterized by onset of gait ataxia or scoliosis before puberty, becoming progressively worse in the first 2 years and later. Reflexes, light touch, and position sensation are reduced. Dysarthria becomes progressively more severe. Cardiomyopathy usually develops, and diabetes mellitus is found in 40% of patients, with half of these requiring insulin. Pes cavus typically is found.

Patients with Friedreich's ataxia have a deficiency of the mitochondrial malic enzyme in fibroblasts and muscle. However, it may not be the primary defect, or there may be more than one gene coding for the subunits of this enzyme.

Treatment includes surgery for scoliosis and intervention as needed for cardiac disease and diabetes. Patients are usually confined to a wheelchair after age 20 years. Death occurs, usually from heart failure or dysrhythmias, in the third or fourth decade; some patients survive longer.

Dominant Ataxia

This disease (also known as olivopontocerebellar atrophy, Holmes's ataxia, Marie's ataxia, etc) occurs with varying manifestations, even among members of the same family. Ataxia occurs at onset, and progression continues with ophthalmoplegias, extrapyramidal tract and motor neuron degeneration, and later dementia. Levodopa may ameliorate rigidity and bradykinesia, but no other therapy is available. Only 10% have onset in childhood, and their course is often more rapid.

Miscellaneous Hereditary Ataxias

Associated findings permit identification of these recessive disorders. These include ataxia-telangiectasia (telangiectasia, immune defects; see below), Wilson's disease (Kayser-Fleischer rings), Refsum's disease (ichthyosis, cardiomyopathy, retinitis pigmentosa, large nerves), Rett's syndrome (regression to autism at 7–18 months in girls, loss of use of hands, progressive failure of brain growth), and abetalipoproteinemia (infantile diarrhea, acanthocytosis, retinitis pigmentosa). Patients with juvenile and chronic gangliosidoses and some hemolytic anemias and long-term survivors of Chédiak-Higashi disease may develop a spinocerebellar degeneration. Idiopathic familial ataxia is called Behr's syndrome. Neuropathies such as Charcot-Marie-Tooth disease produce ataxia.

Bird T, Crill W: Visual evoked responses in hereditary ataxias and spinal degenerations. *Ann Neurol* 1981;**9:**243.

Hagberg B et al: A progressive syndrome of autism, dementia, ataxia, and loss of purposeful hand use in girls: Rett's syndrome. Report of 35 cases. *Ann Neurol* 1983;**14:**471.

Stumpf DA: The inherited ataxias. *Neurol Clin* 1985;**3:**47.

ATAXIA-TELANGIECTASIA (Louis-Bar Syndrome)

Ataxia-telangiectasia is a multisystemic disorder, inherited as an autosomal recessive trait. It is characterized by progressive ataxia; telangiectasia of the bulbar conjunctiva, external ears, nares, and (later) other body surfaces, appearing in the third to sixth year; and recurrent respiratory, sinus, and ear infections. Ocular dyspraxia, slurred speech, choreoathetosis, hypotonia and areflexia, and psychomotor and growth retardation may be present. Endocrinopathies are common. Nerve conduction velocities may be reduced. The entire nervous system may be affected in late stages of the disease. A spectrum of involvement may be seen in the same family. Immunodeficiencies of IgA and IgE are common (see Chapter 17), and the incidence of certain cancers is high.

Ataxia-telangiectasia: A multisystem hereditary disease with immunodeficiency, impaired organ maturation, x-ray hypersensitivity, and a high incidence of neoplasia. (NIH Conference.) *Ann Intern Med* 1983;**99:**367.

EXTRAPYRAMIDAL DISORDERS

Extrapyramidal disorders are characterized by the presence in the waking state of one or more of the following features: dyskinesias, athetosis, ballismus, tremors, rigidity, and dystonias. (These terms are explained below.)

For the most part, precise pathologic and anatomic localization is not completely understood. Motor pathways synapsing in the striatum (putamen and caudate nucleus), globus pallidus, red nucleus, substantia nigra, and the body of Luys are involved; this "system" is modulated by pathways originating in the thalamus, cerebellum, and reticular formation.

Symptoms

A. Chorea: Involuntary, purposeless, sudden jerky and irregular movements involving the face, trunk, and extremities are usually provoked and increased by voluntary activity and tension, are decreased by relaxation, and disappear in sleep. Gait is markedly disturbed; the legs are flung out or may suddenly flex, and the arms flail about. Hypotonia is frequent. There is waxing and waning of the grip ("milkmaid's grip"). The tongue darts in and out. Feeding and other activities requiring fine muscular coordination are impaired. There is facial grimacing. Speech is irregular and indistinct. The knee jerk may be "hung up"; ie, following stimulation, the lower leg may be slow to return to the prestimulus position or even the extended position for several seconds. The arm and leg are usually affected equally; however, the 2 sides of the body may be unequally involved, with only one side seemingly affected (hemichorea).

B. Athetosis: There is a recurring series of slow, writhing movements, including vermicular movements in the fingers and waves of grimaces. Muscular hypertonia is frequent; the muscles may become hypertrophied from the constant activity. Swallowing and speech may be severely impaired. Tendon reflexes may be difficult to obtain.

C. Choreoathetosis: A combination of chorea and athetosis occurs rather frequently.

D. Ballismus: Ballismus is characterized by violent flinging about of the limbs, with movements of large amplitude, usually related to contractions of the proximal musculature and usually unilateral (hemiballismus).

E. Dystonia: Disturbed muscle tone leads to abnormal postures and slow, sustained, and nonpatterned movements involving chiefly the trunk, neck, and proximal muscles of the extremities. Dystonia is worsened by voluntary activity and emotional tension. The spine is commonly twisted and the feet held in the equinus position and inverted; the hands are less affected. Occasionally, only the neck is involved (spasmodic torticolis or retrocollis). In addition to muscle spasm, hypertonia is common. Tendon reflexes are difficult to elicit. Ultimately, there may be paucity of movements because of the marked rigidity and contractures.

F. Tremors: These are fine to coarse, oscillatory movements. Resting tremors, which are best demonstrated with the patient's arms outstretched and fingers spread, are inhibited by volitional movements. In intention or action tremor, oscillations increase at the end of a movement.

G. Rigidity: Increased muscle tone with fairly constant contraction of the flexors and extensors results in increased resistance through the full range of passive motion. Deep tendon reflexes are normal or only slightly increased.

H. "Parkinsonian" Syndrome: There is a combination of abnormal posture, resting tremor, and rigidity. The "pill-rolling" tremor is increased by emotional tension and inhibited by volitional actions. Rigidity is of the "cogwheel" type because of a regularly jerky "give" in resistance when a flexed extremity is extended passively. Voluntary movements are slow; gait is shuffling, with lack of arm swing. Paucity of spontaneous movements is common. In children, there may be a frozen open-mouthed facies. Speech is slow and monotonous. Coordination and tendon reflexes are usually normal. In many instances, patients can run better than walk.

Hagberg B, Kyllerman M, Steen G: Dyskinesia and dystonia in neurometabolic disorders. *Neuropaediatrie* 1980;**10:**305.

Nellhaus G: Abnormal head movements of young children: A review. *Dev Med Child Neurol* 1983;**25:**384.

Rondot P: Involuntary movements and neurotransmitters. *Neuropediatrics* 1983;**14:**59.

1. POSTNATALLY ACQUIRED EXTRAPYRAMIDAL DISORDERS

DRUG-INDUCED EXTRAPYRAMIDAL SYNDROMES

Essentials of Diagnosis

- Chorea, dystonia, dyskinesia, tetanuslike syndrome, meningismus, myoclonic jerks, bizarre posturing, or generalized seizures.
- Autonomic disturbances.
- Ingestion of phenothiazines, butyrophenone, methylphenidate, or other neuroleptics; phenytoin, carbamazepine.

General Considerations

The diagnosis may be suspected in children who have received a phenothiazine derivative or butyrophenone (Haldol) within the preceding 48 hours. Severe bradykinesia due to anticonvulsants has been reported.

The clinical picture may be complicated by the signs and symptoms of the illness that led to the administration of the offending drug. Phenothiazine intoxication should be suspected first in the presence of extrapyramidal symptoms of acute onset.

Clinical Findings

A. Symptoms and Signs: Frequently seen are cogwheel rigidity, tremors, severe speech and swallowing disturbances, masked facies, dystonias, and dyskinesias. Constant or intermittent spasms of the neck and back muscles, jaws, face, tongue, and limbs, as well as a "sardonic smile," may suggest tetanus. Opisthotonos and spasms of the legs on straight leg raising may suggest meningismus. Oculogyric crisis may occur. Some patients have myoclonic jerks or generalized seizures, including status epilepticus. Bradykinesia may be the chief finding. Autonomic disturbances such as tachycardia, hypotension, salivation, blurred vision, and bladder paralysis may occur. Movements are not present during sleep.

B. Laboratory Findings: Testing the urine with Phenistix or ferric chloride up to 18–24 hours after the last dose of phenothiazine often gives a reddish-purple reaction. A toxicology screen may be required. If antiepileptic drugs are suspected, anticonvulsant (especially phenytoin) levels should be measured.

Differential Diagnosis

Common misdiagnoses, as may be suspected from the symptoms, are hysteria, meningitis (especially with an underlying febrile illness accompanied by vomiting), tetanus, and Sydenham's chorea.

The differential diagnosis should also include neuroleptic malignant syndrome, an uncommon idiosyncratic reaction to antipsychotics, characterized by pronounced muscular rigidity, fever, autonomic dysfunctions, and altered states of consciousness.

Treatment

In severe cases, give one of the following: (1) diazepam (Valium), 5–10 mg slowly intravenously (may need to repeat in smaller dose or oral dose); (2) diphenhydramine (Benadryl), 2 mg/kg slowly intravenously, and repeat cautiously if necessary for a total of 5 mg/kg/d; (3) caffeine and sodium benzoate, 10 mg/kg intravenously or intramuscularly (may repeat); (4) promethazine (Phenergan), 0.5 mg/kg intramuscularly; (5) benztropine (Cogentin), 0.5 mg intravenously, intramuscularly, or orally (may repeat); or (6) trihexyphenidyl (Artane), 0.5 mg orally (may repeat). Phenobarbital and atropine have also been used. With bradykinesia due to phenytoin, that drug should be reduced or withdrawn.

Gualtieri CT et al: Tardive dyskinesia and other clinical consequences of neuroleptic treatment in children and adolescents. *Am J Psychiatry* 1984;**141**:20.

Klein SK, Levinsohn MW, Blumer JL: Accidental chlorpromazine ingestion as a cause of neuroleptic malignant syndrome in children. *J Pediatr* 1985;**107**:970.

Rainier-Pope CR: Treatment with diazepam of children with drug-induced extrapyramidal symptoms. *S Afr Med J* 1979;**55**:328.

Weiner WJ, Nausieda PA, Klawans HL: Methylphenidate-induced chorea: Case report and pharmacologic implications. *Neurology* 1978;**28**:1041.

SYDENHAM'S POSTRHEUMATIC CHOREA

Sydenham's chorea is characterized by an acute onset of choreiform movements and variable degrees of psychologic disturbance. It is frequently associated with endocarditis and arthritis. Although the disorder follows infections with β-hemolytic streptococci, the interval between infection and chorea may be greatly delayed; throat cultures and antistreptolysin O (ASO) titers may therefore be negative. Psychic predisposition may also play a role. Chorea has also been associated with hypocalcemia and with vascular lupus erythematosus, toxic, viral, infectious and parainfectious, and degenerative encephalopathies.

Clinical Findings

A. Symptoms and Signs: See description of chorea in the introduction to this section. In addition to the jerky incoordinate movements, the following are noted: emotional lability, waxing and waning ("milkmaid's") grip, darting tongue, "spooning" of the extended hands and their tendency to pronate, and knee jerks slow to return from the extended to their prestimulus position ("hung up"). Seizures, while uncommon, may be masked by choreic jerks.

B. Laboratory Findings: Anemia, leukocytosis, and an increased erythrocyte sedimentation rate may be present. The ASO titer may be elevated and C-reactive protein present. Throat culture is sometimes positive for β-hemolytic streptococci.

Electrocardiography may occasionally show cardiac involvement. Electroencephalography may show nonspecific slowing or seizure activity.

Differential Diagnosis

The diagnosis is usually not difficult. Tics, drug-induced extrapyramidal syndromes, Huntington's chorea, and hepatolenticular degeneration (Wilson's disease), as well as other rare movement disorders, can usually be ruled out on historical and clinical grounds.

Treatment

There is no specific treatment. Sodium valproate in a dosage of 20 mg plus 5 mg/kg may suppress the involuntary movements in a few days, or one of the following may be used for sedation: (1) chlorpromazine (Thorazine), 15–25 mg 3 times daily initially and increased slowly until the involuntary movements are markedly reduced or cease or until the patient is overly drowsy; or (2) phenobarbital, 2–3 mg/kg orally 3 times daily. Corticosteroids have also been used.

All patients should be given antistreptococcal prophylaxis with penicillin G (200,000 units twice daily) or sulfonamide drugs.

Prognosis

Sydenham's chorea is a self-limiting disease that may last from a few weeks to about 2 years. Two-thirds of patients relapse one or more times, but the ultimate outcome does not appear to be worse in those with recurrences. Valvular heart disease occurs in about one-third of patients, particularly if other rheumatic manifestations appear. Psychoneurotic disturbances, if not already present at the onset of illness, occur in a significant percentage of patients.

Dhanaraj M et al: Sodium valproate in Sydenham's chorea. *Neurology* 1985;**35**:114.

Nausieda PA et al: Sydenham chorea: An update. *Neurology* 1980;**30**:331.

Peters ACB et al: ECHO 25 focal encephalitis and subacute hemichorea. *Neurology* 1979;**29**:676.

TICS (Habit Spasms)

Tics, or habit spasms, are quick repetitive but irregular movements, often stereotyped, and briefly suppressible. Coordination and muscle tone are not affected. A psychogenic basis is seldom discernible.

Transient tics of childhood (12–24% incidence in school-age children) last from 1 month to 1 year and seldom need treatment. Many children with tics have a history of encephalopathic past events, "soft signs" on neurologic examination, and school problems.

Facial tics such as grimaces, twitches, and blinking predominate, but the trunk and extremities are often involved and there are twisting or flinging movements. Vocal tics are less common.

Gilles de la Tourette's syndrome is a chronic disorder of multiple fluctuating motor tics and involuntary vocalizations. Tics evolve slowly, new ones being added to or replacing old ones. Coprolalia and echolalia are relatively infrequent. Partial forms are common. The usual age at onset is 2–15 years, and familial incidence is 35–50%; the disorder is now reported in almost all ethnic groups. Gilles de la Tourette's syndrome may be triggered by stimulants or other chemical agents; one of the authors has observed similar findings in 2 retardates receiving long-term neuroleptic drug therapy for aggressivity. Thus, the syndrome may have multiple causes. An imbalance of neurotransmitters, especially dopamine and serotonin, has been hypothesized.

In relatively mild cases, tics are self-limited and, when disregarded, disappear. When attention is paid to one tic, it may disappear only to be replaced by another that is often worse. If the tic and its underlying anxiety or compulsive neurosis are severe, psychiatric evaluation and treatment are needed. Drug therapy has little place in the treatment of tics except in Gilles de la Tourette's syndrome, for which haloperidol (Haldol), 1–5 mg/d, is the best-established treatment, benefiting 80% of patients. Because of side effects, including tardive dyskinesia, its usefulness may be limited. Use of clonidine, 0.125–0.3 mg/d, results in significant improvement in at least half of cases, without serious side effects or the development of tolerance to the drug. Attention to speech, academic, and behavior problems is at least as important as medication.

Caine ED: Gilles de la Tourette's syndrome: A review of clinical and research studies and consideration of future directions for investigation. *Arch Neurol* 1985;**42:**393.

Leckman JF et al: Short- and long-term treatment of Tourette's syndrome with clonidine: A clinical perspective. *Neurology* 1985;**35:**343.

2. CONGENITAL CHOREOATHETOSIS & RIGIDITY

Congenital chorea, athetosis, and rigidity, in varying combinations and degrees of severity, may present in infancy, childhood, or adolescence. Various familial forms have been identified.

About 15% of all children with cerebral palsy (see below) have choreoathetosis (dyskinesias). Patients may be divided into those exhibiting chiefly (1) double chorea, (2) double athetosis, (3) rigidity without movement disorder, (4) atypical movement disorders, (5) transitional types between any of the aforementioned 4 groups (the majority), and (6) those in whom the disorder is complicated by paralysis, spasticity, and other symptoms. The more severe the degree of involvement, the earlier the onset. Other neurologic disorders such as seizures, visual and hearing deficits, and mental retardation may be present.

Laboratory studies include CT brain scanning and x-rays of the hips (for dislocation); electroencephalograpy, if seizures are evident; amino acid chromatography (aminoacidurias are present in rare cases); tests of vision and hearing; and psychometrics.

Treatment is largely confined to physical and educational therapy. In selected cases, thalamotomies have been successful. Diazepam (Valium) may reduce the rigidity, but drug therapy to date has generally been of little avail. Levodopa alone or in combination with diazepam has occasionally been effective. Orthopedic correction of deformities is indicated in some cases.

Hanson RA, Berenberg W, Byers RK: Changing motor patterns in cerebral palsy. *Dev Med Child Neurol* 1970;**12:**309.

Lance JW: Familial paroxysmal dystonic choreoathetosis and its differentiation from related syndromes. *Ann Neurol* 1977;**2:**285.

3. PROGRESSIVE EXTRAPYRAMIDAL DISORDERS*

HUNTINGTON'S CHOREA

Huntington's chorea is rare in the first decade of life. The childhood picture has given rise to the term "striatocortical degeneration." It varies from the adult form in several respects: (1) Dementia occurs early and progresses rapidly. (2) A "striatal" syndrome with rigidity and akinesia predominates over choreoathetoid features. (3) Dysarthria is common and occurs early. (4) Cerebellar dysfunctions (tremors and ataxia) may be presenting features. (5) Seizures, often difficult to control, occur sooner or later in most (rare in adults). (6) Average duration of illness after onset is a little over 9 years (compared to over 13 years in adults).

* Wilson's disease is discussed in Chapter 20.

The disease is transmitted in autosomal dominant fashion, but a family history is frequently denied or unobtainable.

The biochemical defect is not yet defined; the deficiency most constantly found is a marked decrease of gamma-aminobutyric acid (GABA) and its synthesizing enzyme, glutamic acid decarboxylase, in the basal ganglia. A CT scan may show caudate and cortical atrophy; it may thus be most helpful in the differential diagnosis of Huntington's chorea and tardive dyskinesia. The EEG is frequently but nonspecifically abnormal, showing fast, low-voltage activity as well as asymmetry and disorganization.

The initial diagnosis may include the other conditions discussed in this section as well as cerebral palsy.

There is no treatment. The disease is fatal within a few years to about 15 years after onset. Diazepam, haloperidol, phenothiazines, and reserpine may afford some—if only temporary—relief. Seizures are treated in the manner discussed under seizure disorders. Genetic counseling is of paramount importance. Chromosomal identification of the carrier state may become available in the near future, while positron emission tomography may identify an afflicted individual at a very early stage.

Osborne JP, Munson P, Burman D: Huntington's chorea: Report of 3 cases and review of the literature. *Arch Dis Child* 1982;**57:**99.

DYSTONIA MUSCULORUM DEFORMANS

Dystonia musculorum deformans is an extrapyramidal disorder characterized by dystonic postures and fairly slow involuntary movements of uncertain cause.

In about two-thirds of cases, the disorder begins with hypertonia of calf muscles, producing plantar flexion and inversion and adduction of the foot, but it may also start in the wrist or neck. The face, organs of speech, and fingers are usually spared. The disease soon progresses along the extremity to the trunk, resulting eventually in severe lordosis; slow, powerful, widespread movements, which may succeed each other in waves; and bizarre postures due to spasm of some muscle groups and relaxation of others.

This disorder is inherited (1) as an automosal recessive, predominantly in Jewish children, with onset between 4 and 16 years of age and a rapid course; and (2) as a dominant, more variable in onset and with a slower course, with no ethnic predilection.

Symptoms and signs vary with the stage of the disease. The involuntary movements, accentuated by emotional upsets and activity (especially walking or running), are often bizarre and complex. They disappear in sleep. Strength, coordination, and reflexes are intact on examination if proper relaxation can be achieved. Intelligence is not affected, but many emotional problems develop.

Increased levels of dopamine β-hydroxylase in plasma may be found in the dominant form.

This condition must be differentiated from the other progressive extrapyramidal disorders discussed in this section and from toxic encephalopathies and hysteria.

Therapeutic responses to levodopa, carbamazepine, and diazepam are reported; sedation may be needed for sleep. Some cases of severe axial dystonias in children have responded to combined therapy with tetrabenazine, pimozide, and trihexyphenidyl (Artane). Pallidectomy and thalamotomy have afforded relief for several years in some patients.

The course is usually very slowly progressive, and the disease may be arrested for several years. Children involved earliest have the most rapid course.

Garg BP: Dystonia musculorum deformans: Implications of therapeutic response to levodopa and carbamazepine. *Arch Neurol* 1982;**39:**376.

Marsden CD, Marion MH, Quinn N: The treatment of severe dystonia in children and adults. *J Neurol Neurosurg Psychiatry* 1984;**47:**1166.

Ziegler DK: Prolonged relief of dystonic movements with diazepam. *Neurology* 1981;**31:**1457.

OTHER PROGRESSIVE EXTRAPYRAMIDAL DISORDERS

Hallervorden-Spatz disease and progressive pallidal degeneration are rare, slowly progressive extrapyramidal disorders whose diagnoses usually depend on the family history or autopsy findings. In familial calcification of the basal ganglia, the diagnosis is made on CT scan. Juvenile parkinsonism is a familial disorder due to impaired ability to synthesize dopamine; it may result in clinical symptoms first (or only) when major tranquilizers are used, but it responds to treatment with levodopa and carbidopa. Delayed-onset parkinsonism or dystonia may occur as a consequence of a variety of cerebral insults.

Burke RE, Fahn S, Gold AP: Delayed-onset dystonia in patients with "static" encephalopathy. *J Neurol Neurosurg Psychiatry* 1980;**43:**789.

Carlier G, Dubru JM: Familial juvenile parkinsonism. *Acta Paediatr Belg* 1979;**32:**123.

INFECTIONS & INFLAMMATIONS OF THE CENTRAL NERVOUS SYSTEM

One of the most significant clinical attributes of any infection of the central nervous system is its anatomic distribution, ie, meninges, cerebrum, cerebellum, bulb, or spinal cord. Most central nervous system infections in infants and young children are meningoencephalitides, although one or the other aspect (meningitis or encephalitis) may be more marked.

Specific infections are discussed in Chapters 26–29.

Laboratory Findings

A. Cerebrospinal Fluid: (See Table 23–1.) The diagnosis usually, though not always, depends on the cerebrospinal fluid findings. Cerebrospinal fluid examination should include total and differential cell count, levels of protein and glucose (with concomitant blood glucose levels), and Gram's stain and cultures (including special studies for acid-fast organisms, viruses, and fungi). Enzymatic and fluorescent antibody studies and tests for syphilis may be indicated.

Note: The techniques and risks of lumbar puncture are discussed on p 645.

B. Other Means of Identification of Etiologic Agent: The blood, nose, throat, urine, stools, stomach, lungs, and aspirates from petechiae, vesicles, or pus pockets may all provide material for direct isolation of the responsible infective agent. When the child does not clearly have a bacterial infection, serum should be set aside at the time of admission for serologic studies about 3 weeks later with a paired convalescent serum. Heterophil studies, febrile agglutinins, and skin tests (eg, tuberculosis, trichinosis, histoplasmosis) should be performed as indicated.

C. Neurodiagnostic Studies: Special neurodiagnostic studies, particularly CT scanning, may occasionally be necessary to differentiate nonsurgical from specifically surgical lesions and infections (eg, encephalitis with marked focal features from brain abscess; tuberculoma from brain tumor).

ACUTE PURULENT MENINGITIS

Purulent meningitis in infants and children remains a serious threat to life and neurologic competence in the survivors, despite the availability and use of potent specific and broad-spectrum antibiotics and a wide array of supportive measures. The more immature the child, the greater the susceptibility and the less specific the symptoms. Early diagnosis depends upon a high index of suspicion. Prompt treatment, which may prevent or minimize permanent central nervous system damage, may have to be initiated before the infectious organism is identified and specific antimicrobial therapy instituted.

Clinical Findings

A. Symptoms and Signs: Meningeal irritation is manifested by resistance to neck flexion. Kernig's sign (difficulty in extending the leg at the knee when the thigh is flexed at the hip in a patient in supine position) and Brudzinski's sign (passive flexion of the neck followed by flexion of the knees and hips) are often seen. However, neck stiffness and other symptoms (Table 23–11) may take several hours to develop and may vary with age. In addition, note the presence of extracranial infections, petechiae, alterations in the state of consciousness, head circumference in the younger age group, cranial nerve palsies, and other focal neurologic deficits.

Many of these symptoms and signs may, however, also be present with meningismus. Meningismus refers to meningeal irritation, especially nuchal rigidity, *not* due to central nervous system infection; it may accompany a variety of other disorders, including pneumonia, severe pharyngitis and cervical adenopathy, subarachnoid hemorrhage, acute phenothiazine intoxication, rheumatoid arthritis with cervical spine involvement, tetanus, and even dysentery and urinary tract infection. Lumbar puncture may be necessary for diagnosis.

B. Laboratory Findings: (See Table 23–1.) Cerebrospinal fluid usually shows pleocytosis, low glucose levels, elevated protein levels, and positive Gram's stain and cultures, unless the meningitis has been partially treated. Repeat lumbar punctures in suspect cases may be most helpful.

The most common etiologic agents, in order of frequency, are as follows: (1) in newborns, *Escherichia coli* and other gram-negative organisms; group B streptococci and *Listeria monocytogenes;* and (far less frequently) hemolytic staphylococci and other organisms; and (2) in older infants and children, *Haemophilus influenzae* (especially in children 2–7 years of age), more prevalent in fall and early winter; pneumococci; and meningococci (epidemics every 8–10 years), more prevalent in early spring.

Complications & Sequelae

A. Seizures: There is a high incidence of convulsions in infants up to about 18 months of age. Prophylactic anticonvulsant treatment with valproic acid or phenobarbital is often recommended in this age group.

B. Water Intoxication: Hypothalamic irritation from inflammation in the basal meninges may cause

Table 23–11. Symptoms and signs of purulent meningitis.

Symptoms and Signs	Newborn	Up to 2 Years	Over 2 Years
Irregular respirations/ cyanosis	+		
Fever	+	+	+
Hypothermia	+		
Vomiting	+	+	+
Diarrhea	+		
Jaundice	+		
Drowsiness	+	+	+
Jitteriness	+	+	
Bulging fontanelle	+	+	
Convulsions	Early	Early	Late
Stiff neck	Very late	Late	+
Headache			+
Ataxia			Early

inappropriate antidiuretic hormone secretion. The resulting hyponatremia is best treated by fluid restriction.

C. Subdural Effusions: The incidence of subdural effusion in infants with meningitis approaches 50%; it is less common after 18 months. Symptoms include prolongation or recurrence of fever, irritability, listlessness, poor appetite, vomiting, seizures, and focal neurologic deficits.

Important clues to the presence of a subdural effusion are abnormal increase in head circumference, bulging or tenseness of a previously flat anterior fontanelle, and positive transillumination in infants up to about 18 months. CT scanning may define the extent and loculation. The diagnosis is made by finding 2 mL or more of subdural fluid with a high protein content on subdural tap if the fontanelle is open, or through a bur hole or suture if the fontanelle is closed.

Most small effusions resolve spontaneously. If treatment is necessary, subdural taps should be done, if possible. Neurosurgical consultation is indicated if significant subdural effusions (ie, those causing symptoms or persistently infected) cannot be "dried up" after 4–5 weeks and especially if increased intracranial pressure persists.

D. Hydrocephalus: Hydrocephalus (discussed in an earlier section) is most prevalent in newborns and very young infants as a result of inflammatory obstruction of cerebrospinal fluid pathways.

E. Other Neurologic Sequelae: Neurologic sequelae of meningitis in childhood occur in 10–20% of survivors, most often in the youngest and in those in whom diagnosis and adequate therapy were delayed. The finding of significant subdural effusions per se has no prognostic significance. Severe seizures, prolonged depression of consciousness, and other evidence of major cerebral injury during the acute phase of meningitis are the indices of major sequelae. In order of frequency, they are "minimal brain dysfunction" syndrome and mild to severe mental retardation, recurrent seizures, hearing loss and ataxia, hydrocephalus, and motor deficits, including hemiparesis.

Treatment & Prognosis

Antibiotic, fluid and electrolyte, and anticonvulsant therapy are discussed in separate sections. Corticosteroids are not indicated except possibly when there is massive cerebral edema. Treatment of complications is discussed above.

Among interacting factors determining outcome—and assuming good medical management once the diagnosis is made—the 3 most important are age, causative agent, and time of diagnosis. In pediatric practice, the highest mortality rate (30–50%) occurs in newborns and young infants with meningitides due to gram-negative organisms and in those already in coma or near coma at diagnosis.

Bolan G, Barza M: Acute bacterial meningitis in children and adults: A perspective. *Med Clin North Am* 1985;**69:**231.

Brien H: Comparison between cerebral spinal fluid concentrations of glucose, total protein, chloride, lactate, and total amino acids for the differential diagnosis of meningitis. *Scand J Infect Dis* 1983;**15:**277.

Meade RH: Bacterial meningitis in the neonatal infant. *Med Clin North Am* 1985;**69:**257.

CIRCUMSCRIBED PYOGENIC INTRACRANIAL INFECTIONS (Brain Abscesses)

Brain abscesses are usually secondary to a suppurative infection elsewhere; occasionally, they are introduced directly, as after a compound skull fracture or penetrating foreign body (eg, pencil points). The source of infection is unknown in 5–15% of cases. Sources of direct extension are chronic otitis media and mastoiditis, the nasal cavity and accessory sinuses (frontal, sphenoid), and meningitis (via venous thrombosis). Metastatic spread occurs from the lungs and pleura or from subacute infective endocarditis. ***Note:*** Brain abscesses occur in nearly 5% of patients with cyanotic congenital heart disease.

The causative agents are often mixed and tend to be the same organisms responsible for middle ear and sinus infections. In metastatic abscesses, organisms may be even more diversified and include mycotic and parasitic organisms and *Salmonella typhi.*

Clinical Findings

A. Symptoms and Signs: Manifestations often evolve rapidly and include localized severe headache, fever and malaise, drowsiness progressing to confusion and stupor, nausea and vomiting, focal and generalized seizures, and focal motor, sensory, and speech deficits varying with the site and size of the pyogenic collection, degree of cerebral edema, and age of the child. (***Note:*** Focal signs may be obscured by depressed level of consciousness and seizures.) Stiff neck is seen with meningeal involvement, cerebellar abscess, and tonsillar herniation. Point tenderness to pressure on the cranium over the abscess area may be present. Papilledema may be a late finding.

B. Laboratory Findings:

1. Blood—Leukocytosis, with shift to the left and elevated sedimentation rate, is common.

2. Cerebrospinal fluid—(See Table 23–1.) Increased pressure is frequent; pleocytosis is variable. Protein levels may be normal to moderately elevated; glucose levels are often normal. Counterimmunoelectrophoresis often promptly identifies the causative organism, even when routine cultures are negative owing to prior antibiotic treatment.

C. Radiologic Findings: CT brain scanning is the procedure of choice in suspected subdural empyema or brain abscess. It often demonstrates the size of the abscess, its location, the thickness of its capsule, and any effects on the ventricular system. As pus may be isodense with brain tissue, it may be difficult to visualize without enhancing the CT scan with contrast material, after which a typical thin white ring shadow is seen. CT scanning is also used to monitor the disappearance of the abscess and will demonstrate any of its complications, such as hydrocephalus or ependymal adhesions.

Paranasal sinus, mastoid, and chest films should be taken to seek a possible source of infection.

D. Electroencephalography: An EEG should be taken if seizures complicate the intracranial infection. With an abscess, there may initially be diffuse high-voltage slow activity; as the abscess becomes circumscribed, this evolves into a slow wave focus.

Differential Diagnosis

On clinical grounds, the differential diagnosis between brain abscess and other pyogenic intracranial infections cannot be made with certainty. In extradural abscess, the course may be slow and relatively benign; in subdural empyema, often a complication of sinusitis or osteomyelitis, symptoms may evolve rapidly. CT brain scanning provides definitive information.

Treatment & Prognosis

Antibiotics should be given intravenously in large amounts with broad coverage. Surgical evacuation of pus and excision of the abscess are often indicated.

The death rate is high and is directly related to delay in diagnosis and treatment. With multiple abscesses, the death rate is very high. In about 50% of cases, the duration of illness from first symptoms to death is 5–14 days. Early diagnosis and prompt treatment offer an excellent chance of complete recovery if the underlying disease process is cured.

Jadavji T, Humphreys RP, Prober CG: Brain abscesses in infants and children. *Pediatr Infect Dis* 1985;**4**:394.

Kaplan K: Brain abscess. *Med Clin North Am* 1985;**69**:345.

Silverberg AL, DiNubile MJ: Subdural empyema and cranial epidural abscess. *Med Clin North Am* 1985;**69**:361.

SUBACUTE MENINGOENCEPHALITIS

Subacute meningoencephalitis may occur as a complication of primary tuberculosis or may be due to fungal infection or sarcoidosis. These infections involve the meninges of the base of the brain and panarteritis of the pial vessels.

Clinical Findings

A. Symptoms and Signs: Manifestations often evolve gradually and include fever, malaise, and irritability; headache, vomiting, and photophobia; drowsiness, stupor, and coma; focal and generalized seizures; focal motor deficits, including hemiparesis, paresis of the extraocular muscles, and Bell's palsy; and deafness. Meningeal signs may be absent or minimal, but increased intracranial pressure is common.

B. Laboratory Findings:

1. Blood—The erythrocyte sedimentation rate may be elevated.

2. Cerebrospinal fluid—(See Table 23–1.) In both tuberculous and mycotic meningitis, cell counts may range from just above 10 to about 500/μL, initially mostly polymorphonuclear cells but soon predominantly lymphocytes. Cerebrospinal fluid protein levels are mildly to moderately elevated ("pellicle" in tuberculous meningitis). Cerebrospinal fluid glucose levels may be normal initially and fall rapidly. Special smears for tubercle bacilli (acid-fast) and fungi (India ink) should be prepared and appropriate cultures started. Antibodies to *Cryptococcus* may be demonstrated.

C. Diagnosis of Specific Types: Disorders with a similar initial clinical course and gross cerebrospinal fluid findings include the following:

1. Tuberculous meningitis—Two-thirds of cases occur in the first decade, most between 6 and 24 months of age. A positive tuberculin skin test and chest x-ray strongly favor the diagnosis. Without treatment, the course is unremitting.

2. Mycotic meningitides—The course is usually slowly progressive, but prolonged remissions occur. Definitive diagnosis depends on cultural identification of the etiologic agent. Skin tests are often positive.

a. Cryptococcal meningitis (torulosis) is usually associated with chronic debilitating disorders such as tuberculosis, leukemia, and Hodgkin's disease or occurs in renal or liver transplant recipients.

b. Nocardiosis and aspergillosis are rare but again are more common in patients who have undergone transplants or are receiving immunosuppressive drugs.

c. Actinomycosis may spread to the central nervous system from a primary site in the face, neck, or cecum.

d. Mucormycosis may produce systemic infection with orbital cellulitis or thrombosis of the internal carotid artery.

3. Central nervous system sarcoidosis—Recurrent cranial neuropathies are frequent. Eosinophilia is present in about 35% of cases and hypergammaglobulinemia in about 50%. Hypercalcemia with normal serum phosphate levels is common. Lymph node and tongue biopsies and the Kveim test may establish the diagnosis.

D. Radiologic Findings: Chest films should be taken for signs of pulmonary tuberculosis, sarcoidosis, or other infections. CT brain scanning will demonstrate cerebritis, intracranial calcifications, brain abscess, and hydrocephalus. Vasculitis may be suspected from focal or diffuse ischemic changes.

Differential Diagnosis

Brain abscess may resemble subacute meningoencephalitis early, but focal headache and neurologic findings usually point to the diagnosis. Meningeal carcinomatosis, as in leukemia, sarcoma, pinealoma, etc, may be diagnosed by cytologic studies of the cerebrospinal fluid. CT scanning will demonstrate intracranial calcifications, as with a tuberculoma, but mycotic aneurysm can usually be seen only with arteriography.

Treatment & Prognosis

For appropriate antibiotic and anticonvulsant therapy, see under those sections. Observe carefully for toxic reactions to the anti-infective agents.

Neurosurgical evacuation of brain abscess may be required (eg, in actinomycosis) as well as neurosurgical relief of hydrocephalus by "shunting."

The prognosis varies with the disease process and its extent and severity. Many fungal infections, especially histoplasmosis, mucormycosis, nocardiosis, and aspergillosis, respond poorly if at all to the best available treatment.

Molavi A, LeFrock JL: Tuberculous meningitis. *Med Clin North Am* 1985;**69:**315.

Salaki JS, Louria DB, Chmel H: Fungal and yeast infections of the central nervous system: A clinical review. *Medicine* 1984;**63:**108.

Sodeman TM, Dock N: Laboratory diagnosis of parasitic and fungal diseases of the central nervous system. *Ann Clin Lab Sci* 1976;**6:**47.

"ASEPTIC" MENINGITIS, ENCEPHALITIS, & MENINGOENCEPHALITIS*

This clinical grouping encompasses those acute and subacute inflammatory conditions of the meninges or encephalon and often, but to a variable extent, both, in which (1) no flaccid paralysis is present; ie, there is no clinical involvement of the spinal cord or peripheral nerves (see below); and (2) no bacterial or fungal organisms are found on smear or cultures of the cerebrospinal fluid, which otherwise may show such changes as pleocytosis and increased protein. The diagnosis is often presumptive, and the diagnostic category (and even the specific entity) may be suggested by the patient's history. Clinical differentiation between entities is often difficult, since the signs and symptoms overlap considerably because of the nonspecificity of pathologic involvement. Definitive diagnosis can often be established only by laboratory studies, but even this is limited by the laboratory's ability to perform viral cultures or serodiagnostic investigations.

Herpes simplex (inclusion body) encephalitis deserves special consideration. In the newborn, it presents as a diffuse meningoencephalitis and is due to maternal genital infection with herpes simplex virus type 2. In the older child, adolescent, or adult, it occurs at any season and is due to herpes simplex virus type 1. Indicative of inferior frontal and temporal lobe involvement are behavioral changes, speech disturbances, seizures of various degree, and other localizing deficits. The EEG shows slowing or periodic slow-wave complexes in 80% of cases. Radionuclide scanning may show increased uptake, and CT scanning (especially with contrast enhancement) or magnetic resonance imaging may demonstrate the areas of involvement in a very high percentage of cases. *Brain biopsy is requisite* for fluorescent antibody staining and viral isolation, as well as for identification of other treatable causes (present in 20% of cases). Early diagnosis is essential. Acyclovir, 30 mg/kg/d intravenously for at least 10 days, is currently the antiviral treatment of choice in biopsy-proved cases of herpes simplex encephalitis. In children and adolescents—especially those with a score of at least 10 in the "Glasgow Coma Scale" (Fig 23–1) at onset of therapy—acyclovir treatment offers a favorable prognosis in terms of decreased rates of mortality and long-term sequelae.

* For consideration of specific clinical and laboratory features of the individual etiologic syndromes of aseptic meningitis, consult the chapters on viral, bacterial, and fungal diseases. Specific and supportive therapy is discussed in those chapters. Anti-infective therapy is discussed in Chapter 38.

Weiner LP, Fleming OJ: Viral infections of the nervous system. *J Neurosurg* 1984;**61:**207.

Whitley RJ et al and the NIAID collaborative antiviral study group: Vidarabine versus acyclovir therapy in herpes simplex encephalitis. *N Engl J Med* 1986;**314:**144.

ENCEPHALOPATHIES IN IMMUNOCOMPROMISED PATIENTS

About 45–75% of patients who are immunologically compromised, whether due to acquired immunodeficiency syndrome (AIDS) (see Chapter 17) or to long-term immunosuppressive therapy following organ transplantation or lymphoma, may develop and die from a clinically indistinct syndrome that encompasses elements of central nervous system degeneration, mass lesions, and infections and inflammations of the nervous system as described above. Treatment is for the specific problem, but the prognosis is extremely poor.

Belman AL et al: Neurological complications in infants and children with acquired immune deficiency syndrome. *Ann Neurol* 1985;**18:**560.

Epstein LG et al: Progressive encephalopathy in children with acquired immune deficiency syndrome. *Ann Neurol* 1985; **17:**488.

Rubin RH, Hooper DC: Central nervous system infection in the compromised host. *Med Clin North Am* 1985;**69:**281.

PYOGENIC SPINAL CORD INFECTIONS

Pyogenic infections of the spinal cord, although relatively uncommon in children, must be considered in the differential diagnosis of cord lesions, as prompt treatment is required. *Staphylococcus aureus* is the most common pathogen. Infection occurs by direct extension or metastasis from a focus of infection such as a skin furuncle, osteomyelitis, empyema, perinephric abscess, infected wound, or other septic process.

The onset of spinal cord infection, which is more rapid than that of spinal cord tumor, mimics that of noninfectious transverse myelitis.(See Table 23–12.)

Clinical Findings

A. Symptoms and Signs: The principal symptom, sometimes obscured for a while by the underlying illness, is severe localized back pain followed by root pain in the trunk or legs. Flaccid paralysis of the legs, accompanied by sensory loss, develops rapidly. Urinary retention is common. Headache, high fever, a stiff back, and vomiting are present in acute cases but often minimal in chronic ones.

Findings include rigidity of the spine, localized exquisite spine tenderness, lost tendon reflexes, and bilateral plantar extensor signs. Sensory loss, loss of urinary sphincter function, and, less commonly, fecal incontinence may occur.

B. Laboratory Findings:

1. Blood—Leukocytosis and elevation of the erythrocyte sedimentation rate are the rule. Blood cultures are often positive.

2. Cerebrospinal fluid—If epidural spinal abscess is suspected, spinal puncture is contraindicated.

Cerebrospinal fluid examination can be deferred and cervical puncture performed later during myelography. Spinal fluid xanthochromia and pleocytosis are often present; protein levels are usually moderately increased; glucose levels are normal. Cerebrospinal fluid cultures, however, often are negative.

C. Radiologic Findings: In spinal epidural abscess, evidence of osteomyelitis or an adjacent soft tissue mass is evident on spine x-rays in about 50% of cases.

Myelography is best performed in conjunction with diagnostic spinal puncture or via cisternal puncture or as CT metrizamide myelography.

Differential Diagnosis

The differential diagnosis involves principally 2 conditions:(1) transverse myelitis (Table 23–12) and other forms of acute flaccid paralysis, and (2) spinal cord tumors (see p 682).

Treatment & Prognosis

Treatment must be instituted promptly and consists of appropriate antibiotics in massive doses, neurosurgical decompression, and evacuation of the abscess or removal of granuloma.

The prognosis is good if cord compression is relieved early and infection is controlled.

Enberg RN, Kaplan RJ: Spinal epidural abscess in children. *Clin Pediatr* 1974;**13:**247.

Verner EF, Musher DM: Spinal epidural abscess. *Med Clin North Am* 1985;**69:**375.

SYNDROMES PRESENTING AS ACUTE FLACCID PARALYSIS

Flaccid paralysis evolving over hours or over a few days suggests, in the early clinical stages, the following: paralytic spinal poliomyelitis and encephalomyelitis, Landry-Guillain-Barré syndrome, secondary acute myelopathies and polyneuropathies, tick-bite paralysis, botulism (especially in infancy), and transverse myelitis.

Intercurrent nonspecific infections with predominantly flulike respiratory and gastrointestinal symptoms are so common in children as to suggest the diagnosis of Landry-Guillain-Barré syndrome ("acute idiopathic polyneuritis") almost too readily, diverting the physician's attention from the search for more specific causes.

While the sensory examination is important in these syndromes, it is often of dubious accuracy and hence of limited usefulness in the younger age group. Diagnosis (Table 23–12) is based on the clinical features of the illness, viral isolation, and serologic studies.

Differential Diagnosis

Abrupt onset of paralysis is usually from vascular causes that are uncommon in childhood, as from bleeding of an arteriovenous malformation, hemorrhage within a tumor or within or outside the spinal cord due to trauma, or thrombosis of the anterior spinal artery. A more gradual progression of weakness, often associated with pain over the spine and radiating in root distribution, may be due to spinal cord tumors, pyogenic infections, or traumatic hematomas. When performing a diagnostic lumbar puncture, the physician should be aware of compressive lesions, be ready to instill a nonionic dye for myelography, and have neurosurgical consultation available. Paralysis due to a conversion reaction, especially in a girl who may have been sexually assaulted or abused, can usually be diagnosed by careful history and repeated neurologic examinations. Wound botulism may mimic Landry-Guillain-Barré syndrome.

Complications

A. Respiratory Paralysis: Early and careful attention to oxygenation is essential and may require administration of oxygen, intubation, mechanical respiratory assistance, and careful suctioning of secretions.

Early signs of hypoxia are increasing anxiety and a rise in diastolic and systolic blood pressures. Cyanosis is a late sign. Deteriorating spirometric findings (FEV_1 and total vital capacity) may require controlled intubation and respiratory support.

B. Infections: Pneumonia is common, especially with respiratory paralysis. Prophylactic antibiotic administration is generally contraindicated. Antibiotic therapy is best guided by results of cultures.

Bladder infections are most common when an in-

Table 23–12. Acute flaccid paralyses in children.

	Poliomyelitis (Paralytic, Spinal, and Bulbar), With or Without Encephalitis	Landry-Guillain-Barré Syndrome ("Acute Idiopathic Polyneuritis")	Secondary Acute Myelopathies and Polyneuropathies*	Tick-Bite Paralysis	Transverse Myelitis and Neuromyelitis Optica
Etiology	Poliovirus types I, II, and III; occasionally mimicked by mumps.	Unknown. Possibly an autosensitivity phenomenon. Mycoplasmal and viral infections (including infectious mononucleosis) and various systemic or toxic disorders may be underlying cause.	Associated with infections (especially exanthems, diphtheria, etc), vaccination, metabolic and endocrine disturbances, allergic and immune disorders, intoxicants, neoplasms, other miscellaneous conditions.	Probable interference with transmission of nerve impulse caused by toxin in tick saliva.	Usually unknown; immunodeficiency state (?)
History	None, or inadequate polio immunization. Upper respiratory or gastrointestinal symptoms followed by brief respite. Bulbar paralysis more frequent after tonsillectomy. Often in epidemics, in summer and early fall.	Nonspecific respiratory or gastrointestinal symptoms in preceding 5–14 days common. Any season, though slightly lower incidence in summer.	Varies with etiology. Parainfectious paralyses may occur with or after primary illness. Paralyses due to allergic or immune disorders and neoplasms are usually of slow onset; rapid with IV heroin. Irradiation of spinal column for tumor.	Exposure to ticks (dog tick in eastern USA; wood ticks). Irritability 12–24 hours before onset of a rapidly progressive ascending paralysis.	Occasionally, symptoms compatible with multiple sclerosis or optic neuritis. Progression from onset to paraplegia very rapid, usually without a history of bacterial infection.
Presenting complaints	Febrile usually. Meningeal signs, muscle tenderness, and spasm. Weakness widespread or segmental (cervical, thoracic, lumbar). Bulbar symptoms early or before extremity weakness. Anxiety. Delirium.	Symmetric weakness of lower extremities, which may ascend rapidly to arms, trunk, and face. Muscle tenderness and spinal root pains frequent. Verbal child may complain of paresthesias. Fever uncommon. Facial weakness early. Miller-Fisher variant presents as ataxia and ophthalmoplegia.	Symptomatology similar to Landry-Guillain-Barré syndrome, but may be masked by primary disease. In parainfectious and postvaccinal myelitides, initial complaints include low-grade fever, severe back pain, and sensory loss as well as those characteristics of encephalitis.	Rapid onset and progression of ascending flaccid paralysis; often accompanied by pain and paresthesias. Paralysis of upper extremities usually occurs on second day after onset.	Root and back pain in about one-third to one-half of cases. Sensory loss below level of lesion accompanying rapidly developing paralysis. Sphincter difficulties common.
Findings†	Flaccid weakness, usually asymmetric. Lumbar: legs, lower abdomen. Cervical: shoulder, arm, neck, diaphragm. Thoracic: intercostals, spine, upper abdomen. Bulbar: respiratory, lower cranial, upper cranial nerves. Occasionally papilledema, encephalitic syndrome, ataxia. Fever in first days. Autonomic disturbances common.	Flaccid weakness, symmetric, usually greater proximally, but may be more distal or equal in distribution. Facial diplegia in about 85%, then IX–X, XI, III–VI. Bulbar involvement may occur. Slight distal impairment of position, vibration, touch; difficult to assess in young children.	Findings similar to those in Landry-Guillain-Barré syndrome. Sensory loss may be greater. Level of spinal cord involvement may be better defined. Findings may be masked or distorted by those of the associated primary disorder or encephalitic component.	Flaccid, symmetric paralysis. Cranial nerve and bulbar (respiratory) paralysis, ataxia, sphincter disturbances, and sensory deficits may occur. Some fever. Diagnosis rests on finding tick, which is especially likely to be on occipital scalp.	Paraplegia with areflexia below level of lesion early; later, may have hyperreflexia. Sensory loss below and hyperesthesia or normal sensation above level of lesion. Paralysis of bladder and rectum. Optic atrophy or neuritis may be present.
CSF	Pleocytosis (20–500+ cells) with PMN predominance in first few days, followed by rapid decrease and monocytic preponderance. Glucose normal. Protein frequently elevated (50–150 mg/dL).	Cytoalbuminologic dissociation: 10 or fewer mononuclear cells with high protein after first week. Normal glucose. Gamma globulin may be elevated.	CSF as for Landry-Guillain-Barré syndrome. In parainfectious and postvaccinal cases, mild pleocytosis (15–250 cells, principally monocytes) and protein elevation up to 150 mg/dL common.	Normal.	Usually no manometric block; CSF may show increased protein, pleocytosis with predominantly monocytes, increased gamma globulin.
EMG	Denervation after 10–21 days. Nerve conduction may be slowed slightly.	Denervation after 10–21 days. Nerve conduction velocities markedly decreased.	Denervation after 10–21 days. Nerve conduction slowed only in neuropathies.	Nerve conduction slowed; returns rapidly to normal after removal of tick.	Normal early. Denervation at level of lesion after 10–21 days.
Other studies	Initially, leukocytosis. Virus in stool and throat. Serologic titers.	Search for specific cause such as infection, intoxication, metabolic or endocrine disease, allergic phenomena, neoplasm. Lymphocyte transformation demonstrated. *Mycoplasma pneumoniae* implicated.	EEG diffusely slow, with focal or generalized seizure potentials when an encephalitic component is present. Appropriate studies to define associated primary disorder.	Leukocytosis, often with moderate eosinophilia.	Normal spine x-rays speak against spinal epidural abscess. Myelography may be irritative and should be employed cautiously; false positives occur, secondary to swelling of the cord.

* See Infant Botulism on p 723.

† ***Note:*** In flaccid paralysis, the deep reflexes are depressed or absent.

Table 23–12 (cont'd). Acute flaccid paralyses in children.

	Poliomyelitis (Paralytic, Spinal, and Bulbar), With or Without Encephalitis	Landry-Guillain-Barré Syndrome ("Acute Idiopathic Polyneuritis")	Secondary Acute Myelopathies and Polyneuropathies	Tick-Bite Paralysis	Transverse Myelitis and Neuromyelitis Optica
Course and prognosis	Paralysis usually maximal 3–5 days after onset. Transient bladder paralysis may occur. Outlook varies with extent and severity of involvement. ***Note:*** Threat greatest from respiratory failure and superinfection. Early muscle atrophy common.	Course progressive over a few days to about 2 weeks. Transient bladder paralysis may occur. ***Note:*** Threat greatest from respiratory failure and superinfection. Majority recover completely; residual weakness in up to one-fifth of cases.	Course and prognosis vary greatly with underlying disease process, extent of the paralytic and encephalitic involvement, presence of bladder and bowel paralysis, and respiratory complications.	Total removal of tick is followed by rapid improvement and recovery. Otherwise, mortality rate due to respiratory paralysis is very high.	Large degree of functional recovery possible. Corticosteroids are of benefit in shortening duration of acute attack (especially the first) but not in preventing recurrences or altering the overall course.

dwelling catheter is required for bladder paralysis. Prophylactic administration of methenamine mandelate (Mandelamine), 30 mg/kg orally, or the use of bladder irrigations with antibiotics is recommended. Recovery from myelitis may be delayed by urinary tract infection.

Treatment

There is no specific treatment except removal of ticks in tick-bite paralysis, erythromycin in *Mycoplasma* infection, and botulism equine antitoxin in wound botulism. Recognized associated disorders (eg, endocrine, neoplastic, toxic) should be treated by appropriate means. Supportive care also involves "pulmonary toilette," adequate fluids and nutrition, bladder and bowel care, prevention of decubiti, and, often, psychiatric support. For treatment of seizures with encephalitic components, see Seizure Disorders, above.

A. Corticosteroids: These agents are believed by most to be of no benefit in Landry-Guillain-Barré syndrome. Autonomic symptoms (eg, hypertension) may require treatment in polyneuritis.

B. Plasmapheresis: Plasma exchange has been beneficial in severe cases of Landry-Guillain-Barré syndrome.

C. Physical Therapy: Rehabilitative measures are best instituted when acute symptoms have subsided and the patient is stable.

Prognosis

The prognosis varies greatly with the extent of involvement, duration of the inflammatory process, complications, and other factors. See Table 23–12.

Freeman JM: Diagnosis and evaluation of acute paraplegia. *Pediatr in Rev* 1983;**4:**328.

Gamstorp I: Encephalomyelo-radiculoneuropathy: Involvement of the CNS in children with the Guillain-Barré-Strohl syndrome. *Dev Med Child Neurol* 1974;**16:**654.

Keller MA et al: Wound botulism in pediatrics. *Am J Dis Child* 1982;**136:**320.

McCarthy JT, Amer J: Postvaricella acute transverse myelitis: A case presentation and review of the literature. *Pediatrics* 1978;**62:**202.

Novak RW, Jones G, Ch'ien LT: Acute transverse myelopathy in childhood: A study of four cases. *Clin Pediatr* 1978; **17:**894.

Yoshioka M, Kuroki S, Mizue H: Plasmapheresis in the treatment of Guillain-Barré syndrome in childhood. *Pediatr Neurol* 1985;**1:**329.

DISORDERS OF CHILDHOOD AFFECTING MUSCLES

This section is concerned with specific muscle and neuromuscular disorders, including the muscular dystrophies, myasthenia gravis, and miscellaneous congenital neuromuscular disorders. (See Table 23–13.)

Certain studies that are commonly used in the diagnosis of muscle diseases merit special consideration.

Serum Enzymes

Among muscle enzymes—creatine kinase (CK), aldolase, glutamic-oxaloacetic transaminase (GOT), and lactic dehydrogenase—helpful in the diagnosis and in following the course of some muscle disorders, usually only CK is now followed. Normal CK values in males are up to 190 IU/L (and slightly higher during mid adolescence); values in females are usually slightly lower than those in males. Blood should be drawn before muscle biopsy, which may lead to release of the enzyme. Corticosteroids may suppress levels despite very active muscle disease.

Muscle Imaging

Ultrasonography, CT scanning, and magnetic resonance imaging (MRI) are now employed in the diagnosis and assessment of muscular dystrophies, congenital myopathies and myotonias, spinal muscular atrophies, and some neuropathies. MRI in particular may diagnose muscle diseases due to enzymopathies, such as McArdle's phosphorylase deficiency, and MRI and CT scanning are useful in carrier detection.

Table 23–13. Muscular dystrophies and myotonias of childhood.

Disease	Genetic Pattern	Age at Onset	Early Manifestations	Involved Muscles
Muscular dystrophies				
Duchenne's muscular dystrophy (pseudohypertrophic, infantile)	X-linked recessive; autosomal recessive unusual. Thirty to 50% have no family history.	2–6 years; rarer in infancy or at birth (congenital muscular dystrophy).	Clumsiness, easy fatigability on walking, on running and climbing stairs. Walking on toes; waddling gait. Lordosis. (Climbing up on legs rising from supine position—Gowers' maneuver.) Severe delay in motor development in congenital form.	Axial and proximal before distal. Pelvic girdle; pseudohypertrophy of gastrocnemius (90%), triceps brachii, and vastus lateralis. Shoulder girdle usually later; also articulation difficulties. Eventually, cardiomyopathy (50%).
Becker's muscular dystrophy (late onset)	X-linked recessive.	Childhood (usually later than in Duchenne's).	Similar to Duchenne's.	Similar to Duchenne's.
Limb-girdle muscular dystrophy A. Pelvifemoral (Leyden-Möbius) B. Scapulohumeral (Erb's juvenile)	Autosomal recessive in 60%; high sporadic incidence. A. Relatively common. B. Rare.	Variable: early childhood to adulthood.	Weakness, with distribution according to type. Waddling gait, difficulty climbing stairs. Lordosis.	A. Pelvic girdle usually involved first and to greater extent. B. Shoulder girdle often asymmetric. Quadriceps and hamstrings may be weakest. Pseudohypertrophy of calves uncommon.
Facioscapulohumeral muscular dystrophy (Landouzy-Déjérine) Scapuloperoneal variant	Autosomal dominant; sporadic cases not uncommon.	Usually late childhood and adolescence; rare in infancy; not uncommon in twenties.	Diminished facial movements with inability to close eyes, smile, or whistle. Face may be flat, unlined. Difficulty in raising arms over head. Lordosis. Tripping in scapuloperoneal type.	Facial muscles followed by shoulder girdle, with occasional spread to hips or distal legs (scapuloperoneal variant).
Distal myopathies A. Gowers' type B. Welander's	Autosomal dominant.	A. Gowers': some early; usually adult. B. Welander's: usually adult; occasionally adolescence.	Gowers': wasting of cranial musculature. Welander's: weakness of hands and feet; rarely, muscles of face and tongue.	Distal muscle weakness, especially small muscles of hands and feet.
"Oculocraniosomatic syndrome" (ophthalmoplegia and "ragged reds"; progressive external ophthalmoplegia)	(?)Acquired; 80% female; other hereditary neurologic disorders may be found in patient or family.	Variable: from infancy to adult life; most at about 10 years of age.	Ptosis and limitation of eye movements; hearing and visual loss (retinitis pigmentosa); intellectual loss; cerebellar disturbances (ataxia).	Extraocular muscles, often asymmetric. Variable involvement of axial muscles; cardiac muscles, with conduction defect.
Congenital myopathies:				
Central core	Generally, autosomal dominance with variable penetrance.	Onset generally prenatal.	Infantile hypotonia, delay in attaining motor milestones. Mild weakness.	Often diffuse and variable, mainly proximal, legs more than arms.
Nemaline (rodbody) Myotubular (centronuclear) Congenital fiber type disproportion	Autosomal recessive also reported. Genetics unclear.	Onset usually in infancy, occasionally later childhood.	Nemaline: associated dysmorphism (face, spine, feet, pigeon chest). Myotubular: may show ptosis, facial weakness.	Nemaline: some diffuse muscle wasting. May include extraocular muscles.
Myotonias				
Myotonia congenita (Thomsen)	Autosomal dominant (autosomal recessive cases reported).	Early infancy to late childhood.	Difficulty in relaxing muscles after contracting them, especially after sleep; aggravated by cold, excitement.	Hands especially; muscles may be diffusely enlarged, giving patient Herculean appearance.
Myotonic dystrophy (Steinert)	Autosomal dominant.	Late childhood to adolescence; neonatal and infantile forms increasingly recognized.	Myotonia of grasp, tongue; worsened by cold, emotions. "Hatchet-face." In infancy, floppiness with facial diplegia; arthrogryposis multiplex. Nasal voice. Weakness and easy fatigability. Thin ribs on chest x-ray. Mild to moderate mental retardation in about 80% may precede muscular symptoms.	Wasting and weakness of facial muscles, including muscles of mastication; sternocleidomastoids, hands. Myotonic phenomena: "bunching up" of muscles of tongue, thenar eminence, finger extensors after tapping with percussion hammer.
Carnitine deficiency (Lipid storage myopathy)	Genetics not known.	Early childhood to adolescence.	Intermittent attacks of metabolic acidosis; fluctuating hepatomegaly. Weakness similar to Duchenne's.	Progressive weakness, including voice, muscles of mastication and swallowing, ptosis; diffuse involvement of neck muscles, pectoral and pelvic girdle.

Electromyography

Electromyography is often helpful in grossly differentiating ''myopathic'' from ''neurogenic'' processes. Fibrillations occur in both. In the myopathies, very low spikes are more typical, and the motor unit action potentials seen during contraction characteristically are of short duration, polyphasic, and increased in number for the strength of the contraction (increased interference pattern). ''Neurogenic'' findings include decreased numbers of motor units, which may be polyphasic, larger than normal, or both. The interference pattern is decreased.

In myotonic dystrophy, the EMG is characterized by prolonged discharge of electrical activity on movement of the probing needle (''dive bomber'' sound), though these discharges may be found to a lesser

Table 23–13 (cont'd). Muscular dystrophies and myotonias of childhood.

Reflexes	Muscle Biopsy Findings	Other Diagnostic Studies	Treatment	Prognosis
Knee jerks ± or 0; ankle jerks + to + +, occasionally, extensor plantar response (Babinski sign).	Degeneration and variation in fiber size; proliferation of connective tissue. Basophilia, phagocytosis. Poor differentiation of fiber types on ATPase reaction; deficiency of type 2B fibers.	EMG myopathic. CK (4000–5000 IU) very high with decrease toward normal over the years. ECG. Chest x-ray.	Physical therapy, braces, wheelchair eventually, weight control.	Ten percent show nonprogressive mental retardation. Death from pneumonia 10–15 years after diagnosis with 75% of patients dead by age 20.
Similar to Duchenne's.	Similar to above, except type 2B fibers present.	Similar to above, although muscle enzymes may not be as elevated.	As above. Wheelchair in late childhood or early adult life.	Slower progression than Duchenne's, with death usually in adulthood.
Usually present.	Variation in muscle fiber size with many very large fibers. Fiber splitting and internal nuclei common. Many "moth-eaten" whorled fibers.	EMG myopathic. CK variable: often normal but may be elevated. ECG.	Physical therapy, weight control.	Mildly progressive: spread from lower to upper limbs may take 15–20 years. Life expectancy mid to late adulthood.
Present.	Predominantly large fibers with scattered tiny atrophic fibers, "moth-eaten" and whorled fibers. Inflammatory response. Little or no fiber splitting, fibrosis, or type 1 fiber predominance.	EMG myopathic. Muscle enzymes usually normal.	Physical therapy where indicated. Wheelchair in old age.	Very slowly progressive, often with plateaus, except in infantile form where there may be difficulties in walking by adolescence. Usually normal life span.
Present.	Nonspecifically myopathic.	EMG myopathic. Muscle enzymes may be mildly elevated.	None.	Normal life expectancy.
Depressed to ± or 0.	Mitochondrial abnormalities. "Ragged red" fibers. Changes in fiber size, usually due to type 2 fiber atrophy.	CK usually normal. ECG with conduction block. CSF protein elevated. Nerve conduction slowed. CT brain scan and brain stem auditory evoked response may be abnormal.	Plastic retraction of eyelids. Cardiac support. Corticosteroids of benefit where denervation present.	Dysphagia may develop (50%) as well as generalized muscle weakness. Prognosis fair if disease is confined to ocular muscles. In severe cases, spongy vacuolization of brain and brain stem.
Normal to ± or 0.	Specific histochemical findings determine diagnosis. Central core: amorphous areas in fiber devoid of oxidative enzymes. Nemaline: red rods with trichrome stain. Myotubular: central nuclei in areas devoid of myofibrils; type 2B fibers hypertrophy.	Muscle enzymes usually normal. CK may be slightly elevated.	Physical therapy to prevent contractures and strengthen existing muscles. Correction of dislocated hips or other deformities.	Usually very slowly progressive or nonprogressive, with plateaus and improvements possible, depending on type. Weakness occasionally increases in adolescence.
Normal.	Nonspecific and minor changes; type 2B fibers may be absent.	EMG "myotonic."	Usually none. Phenytoin, especially in cold weather, may improve muscle functioning.	Normal life expectancy, with only mild disability.
In infantile form, marked hyporeflexia.	Type I fiber atrophy, type 2 hypertrophy, sarcoplasmic masses, internal nuclei, phagocytosis, fibrosis, and cellular reaction.	EMG markedly "myotonic." Motor nerve conduction velocities slow. Hormonal studies, especially testosterone, glucose tolerance test, thyroid tests. ECG. Chest x-ray and pulmonary function tests. Immunoglobulins.	Procainamide, 250 mg 3 times daily orally, increased to tolerance; phenytoin, 5–7 mg/kg/d orally. Carbamazepine, 15–25 mg/kg/d orally, emerging as treatment of choice.	Frontal baldness, cataracts (85%), gonadal atrophy (85% of males), thyroid dysfunction, diabetes mellitus (20%). Cardiac conduction defects; impaired pulmonary function. Low IgG. Life expectancy normal to slightly decreased, though severely handicapped in late adult life.
Normal initially, progressively less active.	Lipid droplets separating myofibrils and distending intermyofibrillar space. Type 1 fibers contain most lipid droplets.	Marked deficiency of muscle carnitine (normal: 7.5–28 nmol/mg noncollagen protein). Liver biopsy: excessive lipid hepatocytes.	Combined carnitine and prednisone treatment may be of benefit.	Untreated, fatal within a very few years.

degree also in other conditions. In myotonic dystrophy during attempted relaxation after a contraction, electrical activity persists parallel with the protracted relaxation of muscle.

Muscle Biopsy

Properly executed (by "open" biopsy or by using the Bergstrom muscle biopsy needle), this is usually most helpful. Histochemical techniques, histogram analysis of muscle fiber types, and electron microscopy are offering new classifications of the myopathies. Findings common to the myopathies include variation in the size and shape of muscle fibers, increase in connective tissue, interstitial infiltration of fatty tissue, degenerative changes in muscle fibers, and central location of nuclei.

Findings more characteristic of certain myopathies include the sarcoplasmic masses and striking chains of central nuclei in myotonic dystrophy; the cysts in trichinosis and toxoplasmosis; the vacuoles in the periodic paralyses, thyrotoxicosis, chloroquine myopathy, and lupus erythematosus; the patterns of special stains in central core disease and nemaline myopathy; and the electron microscopic findings in giant mitochondrial myopathy.

Brooke MH: *A Clinician's View of Neuromuscular Diseases*, 2nd ed. Williams & Wilkins, 1985.

Coulter DL, Allen RJ: Abrupt neurological deterioration in children with Kearns-Sayre syndrome. *Arch Neurol* 1981; **38:**247.

Furukawa T, Peter JB: The muscular dystrophies and related disorders. (2 parts.) *JAMA* 1978;**239:**1537, 1654.

Heckman JZ, Leeman S, Dubowitz V: Ultrasound imaging in the diagnosis of muscle disease. *J Pediatr* 1982;**101:**656.

Lanzi G et al: Myotonic dystrophy in childhood. *Acta Neurol Belg* 1982;**82:**150.

McMenamin JB, Becker LE, Murphy EG: Congenital muscular dystrophy: A clinicopathologic report of 24 cases. *J Pediatr* 1982:**100:**692.

Miller RG et al: Emery-Dreifuss muscular dystrophy with autosomal dominant transmission. *Neurology* 1985;**35:**1230.

Parker D et al: Encephalopathy and fatal myopathy in two siblings: Their association with partial deficiency of muscle carnitine. *Am J Dis Child* 1982;**136:**598.

Scott JA, Rosenthal DI, Brady TJ: The evaluation of musculoskeletal disease with magnetic resonance imaging. *Radiol Clin North Am* 1984;**22:**917.

Sechi GP et al: Carbamazepine versus diphenylhydantoin in the treatment of myotonia. *Eur Neurol* 1983;**22:**113.

Stern LM et al: Carrier detection in Duchenne muscular dystrophy using computed tomography. *Clin Genet* 1985;**27:**392.

BENIGN ACUTE CHILDHOOD MYOSITIS

Benign acute childhood myositis (myalgia cruris epidemica) is characterized by transient severe muscle pain and weakness affecting mainly the calves and occurring 1–2 days following an upper respiratory tract infection. Though symptoms involve mainly the gastrocnemius muscles, all skeletal muscles appear to be invaded directly by virus; recurrent episodes are due to different viral types. By demonstration of seroconversion or by isolation of the virus, acute myositis has been shown to be largely due to influenza types B and A and occasionally due to parainfluenza and adenovirus.

Ruff RL, Secrist D: Viral studies in benign acute childhood myositis. *Arch Neurol* 1982;**39:**261.

THE PERIODIC PARALYSES

Hypokalemic Periodic Paralysis

This condition is inherited as a dominant trait, with decreased occurrence in females, but it may appear sporadically. A family history of migraine is often present. Onset is usually about the end of the first decade of life. The proximal muscles are affected first. The muscles innervated by the cranial nerves are spared—eg, the extraocular muscles, the muscles of facial expression, mastication, and swallowing, and the tongue muscles. The diaphragm, which is usually spared, has its embryonic origin in bulbar territory. Attacks of weakness may be precipitated by rest after exercise, exposure to cold, emotional stress, and high dietary intake of carbohydrate and sodium.

Attacks may last for days but may be aborted by mild exercise. The disease may progress to a chronic form of weakness and atrophy, but in general, attacks are less frequent after middle age. Permanent muscular weakness sometimes occurs.

The serum potassium level is low during an attack.

Provocative tests that induce weakness and thus confirm the diagnosis include (1) exercise and (2) giving insulin, 0.25 unit/kg subcutaneously, simultaneously with glucose, 0.8 g/kg orally.

Hyperthyroidism, particularly in Japanese persons, may produce similar periodic weakness.

Acetazolamide, 5–30 mg/kg/d orally, is usually effective in preventing attacks. Alternative treatment consists of giving potassium chloride, 2–10 g orally, to terminate an attack, and 2–10 g at bedtime between attacks. The patient should be encouraged to eat a low-carbohydrate, low-sodium diet. Thiamine may abort the effects of carbohydrates. Unnecessary exposure to cold should be avoided.

The disorder is consistent with a normal life span.

Hyperkalemic Periodic Paralysis

This form of periodic paralysis has its onset in the first decade of life and is usually detected in infancy because of "staring" eyes (myotonic form of lid lag) or a very feeble cry (especially on waking). It is inherited as an autosomal dominant. Pseudohypertrophy of the calves is often present. There is an increased incidence of diabetes mellitus. The attacks are relatively short, lasting 30 minutes to 2 hours, and may be precipitated by rest after exercise, cold, and fatigue. Attacks usually occur in children of school age and then abate, though permanent muscle weakness may develop.

The serum potassium level rises during attacks. The EMG may show myotonia of the external ocular and facial muscles.

Treatment is with hydrochlorothiazide, 50 mg/d orally, or acetazolamide, 250 mg/d orally. Dichlorphenamide (Daranide), 50 mg/d orally, has also been recommended. The dose must be adjusted for each case.

The disorder is consistent with a normal life span.

Normokalemic Periodic Paralysis

In this disorder, the onset is in the first decade of life. It is inherited as an autosomal dominant. Attacks come on during rest after exercise, with cold, following ingestion of foods high in potassium (eg, many fruit juices), and following ingestion of alcohol. The attacks may last for days.

In normokalemic paralysis, serum electrolyte levels do not change during attacks. Muscle biopsy may show vacuolar myopathy.

Treatment consists of increased salt intake; acetazolamide, 250 mg/d orally, with dosage adjusted for each case; and fludrocortisone, 0.1 mg/d orally.

The prognosis is good.

Pearson CM: The periodic paralyses: Differential features and pathological observations in permanent myopathic weakness. *Brain* 1964;**87:**341.

MYASTHENIA GRAVIS

Essentials of Diagnosis

- Weakness, chiefly of muscles innervated by the brain stem, usually coming on or increasing with use (fatigue).
- Positive response to neostigmine and edrophonium.
- Acetylcholine receptor antibodies in serum (except in congenital form).

General Considerations

Myasthenia gravis is characterized by easy fatigability of muscles, particularly the extraocular muscles and those of mastication, swallowing, and respiration. However, in the neonatal period or early infancy, the weakness may be so constant and general that an affected infant may present nonspecifically as a "floppy infant." Girls are involved more frequently than boys. The age at onset is over 10 years in 75% of cases, often shortly after menarche. If diagnosed before age 10, congenital myasthenia should be considered in retrospect. Thyrotoxicosis is found in almost 10% of affected female patients. The essential abnormality is a circulating antibody that binds to the acetylcholine receptor protein and thus reduces the number of motor end plates for binding by acetylcholine.

Clinical Findings

A. Symptoms and Signs:

1. Neonatal (transient) myasthenia gravis—This occurs in 12% of infants born to myasthenic mothers and, rarely, in those born to asymptomatic thymectomized mothers. The condition is due to maternal acetylcholine receptor antibody transferred across the placenta; a thymic factor in the infant may also be involved. A sibling may have died in the neonatal period with similar symptoms and nondiagnostic autopsy. The infant is "floppy," with a weak Moro reflex but normal knee jerks. Most striking are ineffective sucking, difficulty in swallowing, pooling of secretions, and a weak cry despite lack of evidence of other neurologic damage. In contrast to other forms of myasthenia gravis, in this neonatal form the eyes are usually wide open and extraocular muscle palsies are usually not present, but facial weakness is obvious.

2. Congenital (persistent) myasthenia gravis—In this form of the disease, the mothers of affected infants rarely have myasthenia gravis but other relatives may. Sex distribution is equal. Extraocular muscle palsies and ptosis are often prominent; there may be a weak cry, fatigue with sucking, and hypotonia. Symptoms are often subtle and not recognized initially. Differential diagnosis includes many other causes of the "floppy infant" syndrome (see p 722), such as infant botulism, ocular myopathy, congenital ptosis, and Möbius' syndrome (facial nuclear aplasia and other anomalies). This condition is *not* caused by receptor antibodies and often responds poorly to therapy. It may result from a genetic abnormality of the acetylcholine receptor protein.

3. Juvenile myasthenia gravis—In this autoimmune form, the symptoms and signs are like those in adults. Receptor antibodies are usually present. The patient may be first seen by an otolaryngologist or psychiatrist. The more prominent signs are difficulty in chewing, dysphagia, a nasal voice, ptosis, and ophthalmoplegia. Pathologic fatigability of limbs, chiefly involving the proximal limb and neck muscles, may be more prominent than the bulbar signs and may lead to an initial diagnosis of conversion hysteria, muscular dystrophy, or polymyositis. Associated disorders include seizures, neoplasia, diabetes mellitus, hyperthyroidism, asthma, rheumatoid arthritis, and other autoimmune conditions.

An acute fulminant form of myasthenia gravis has been reported in children age 2–10 years and presents with rapidly progressive respiratory difficulties. Bulbar paralysis may evolve within 24 hours. There is no history of myasthenia. The differential diagnosis includes Landry-Guillain-Barré syndrome and bulbar poliomyelitis. Administration of anticholinesterase agents establishes the diagnosis and is lifesaving.

B. Laboratory Findings:

1. Neostigmine test—In newborns and very

young infants, the neostigmine (Prostigmin) test is preferable to the edrophonium (Tensilon) test because the longer duration of its response permits better observation, especially of sucking and swallowing movements. The test dose of neostigmine is 0.02 mg/kg subcutaneously, usually given with atropine, 0.01 mg/kg subcutaneously. There is a delay of about 10 minutes before the effect may be manifest. The physician should be prepared to suction secretions.

2. Edrophonium test—Testing with edrophonium is used in older children who are capable of cooperating in certain tasks, such as raising and lowering their eyelids and squeezing a sphygmomanometer bulb or the examiner's hands. The test dose is 0.1–1 mL intravenously, depending on the size of the child. Maximum improvement occurs within 2 minutes.

3. Other laboratory tests—Serum acetylcholine receptor antibodies are found in the neonatal and juvenile forms. Lancaster red-green tests of ocular motility with edrophonium are often positive in patients able to cooperate. In juveniles, an EEG and thyroid and other endocrine and immunologic studies are appropriate.

C. Electrical Studies of Muscle: Repetitive stimulation of a motor nerve at slow rates (3/s) with recording over the appropriate muscle reveals a progressive fall in amplitude of the muscle potential in myasthenic patients. A maximal stimulus must be given. At higher rates of stimulation (50/s), there may be a transient repair of this defect before the progressive decline is seen.

If this study is negative, single fiber electromyography is now employed to determine if "mean jitter" exceeds normal.

D. Radiologic Findings: Chest x-ray and laminagraphy in older children may disclose thymus enlargement.

Treatment

A. General and Supportive Care: In the newborn or in a child in myasthenic or cholinergic crisis (see below), suctioning of secretions is essential. Respiratory assistance may be required.

Treatment should be carried out by physicians with experience in this disorder. In older children, some of the responsibility for adjustment of drug dosage may be left to the patient.

B. Anticholinesterase Drug Therapy: *Note:* There is increasing concern that anticholinesterase drugs may eventually damage the motor end plates.

1. Pyridostigmine (Mestinon)—The dose must be adjusted for each patient. A frequent starting dose is 15–30 mg orally every 6 hours.

2. Neostigmine (Prostigmin)—Fifteen milligrams of neostigmine are roughly equivalent to 60 mg of pyridostigmine. Neostigmine often causes gastric hypermobility with diarrhea, but it is the drug of choice in newborns, in whom prompt treatment may be lifesaving.

3. Atropine—Atropine may be added on a maintenance basis to control mild cholinergic side effects such as hypersecretion, abdominal cramps, and nausea and vomiting.

4. Immunologic intervention—This is primarily by use of prednisone; advisability of use in younger children is not definitely determined. Plasmapheresis is effective in removing acetylcholine receptor antibody in severely affected patients.

5. Myasthenic crisis—Relatively sudden difficulties in swallowing and respiration may be observed in myasthenic patients. Edrophonium will result in dramatic but brief improvement; this may make it difficult to evaluate the condition of the small child. Suctioning, tracheostomy, respiratory assistance, and fluid and electrolyte maintenance may be required.

6. Cholinergic crisis—Cholinergic crisis may result from overdosage of anticholinesterase drugs. The resulting weakness may be similar to that of myasthenia, and the muscarinic effects (diarrhea, sweating, lacrimation, miosis, bradycardia, hypotension) are often absent or difficult to evaluate. The edrophonium test may help to determine whether the patient is receiving too little of the drug or is manifesting toxic symptoms due to overdosage. Improvement after the drugs are withdrawn suggests cholinergic crisis. Respirator facilities should be available. The patient may require atropine and tracheostomy.

C. Surgical Measures: Early thymectomy is beneficial in many patients whose disease is not confined to ocular symptoms; the effects may be delayed. Experienced surgical and postsurgical care are prerequisites.

Prognosis

Neonatal (transient) myasthenia presents a great threat to life, primarily due to aspiration of secretions. With proper treatment, the symptoms usually begin to disappear within a few days to 2–3 weeks, after which the child usually requires no further treatment.

In the congenital (persistent) form, the symptoms may initially be as acute as in the transient variety; more commonly, however, they are relatively benign and constant, with gradual worsening as the child grows older. Life span is not usually affected.

In the juvenile form, patients may become resistant or unresponsive to anticholinesterase compounds and require corticosteroids or treatment in a hospital, where respiratory assistance can be given as needed. The overall prognosis for survival and for remission and improvement after therapy with prednisone and thymectomy is now considered to be favorable.

Death in myasthenic or cholinergic crisis may occur unless prompt treatment is given.

Engel AG: Myasthenia gravis and myasthenic syndromes: Neurological progress. *Ann Neurol* 1984;**16:**519.

Lefvert AK, Osterman PO: Newborn infants to myasthenic mothers: A clinical study and investigation of acetylcholine receptor antibodies in 17 children. *Neurology* 1983;**33:**133.

Pascuzzi RM, Coslett HB, Johns TR: Long-term corticosteroid treatment of myasthenia gravis: Report of 116 patients. *Ann Neurol* 1984;**15:**291.

Rodriguez M et al: Myasthenia gravis in children: Long-term follow-up. *Ann Neurol* 1983;**13**:504.
Snead OC et al: Juvenile myasthenia gravis. *Neurology* 1980;**30**:732.

CONGENITAL ABSENCE OF MUSCLES*

Congenital absence (sometimes only partial) of one or more muscles, usually unilateral, and particularly of the pectoralis (sternal portion), trapezius, serratus anterior, quadratus femoris, or omohyoid, is not unusual. Heredofamilial cases have been reported. Other deformities, eg, syndactyly, microdactyly, and muscular dystrophy, may be present. Absence of muscles of the abdominal wall (prune belly) may be associated with anomalies of the gastrointestinal tract, urinary tract (Eagle's syndrome), or extremities or with cryptorchidism. Treatment is determined by the specific abnormalities present.

PERIPHERAL NERVE PALSIES

1. THE ASYMMETRIC FACE

Facial asymmetry may be present at birth or develop later, either suddenly or gradually, unilaterally or bilaterally. Nuclear or peripheral involvement of the facial nerves results in sagging or drooping of the mouth and inability to close one or both eyes, particularly with crying in newborns and infants. Inability to wrinkle the forehead may be demonstrated in infants and young children by getting them to follow an object (light) moved vertically above the forehead. Loss of taste of the anterior two-thirds of the tongue on the involved side may be demonstrated in intelligent, cooperative children by age 4 or 5; playing with a younger child and the judicious use of a tongue blade may enable the physician to note if the child's face puckers up when something sour (eg, lemon juice) is applied with a swab to the anterior tongue. Ability to wrinkle the forehead is preserved, owing to bilateral innervation, in supranuclear or central facial paralysis.

Injuries to the facial nerve at birth occur in 0.25–6.5% of consecutive live births. Forceps delivery is the cause in some cases; in others, the side of the face affected may have abutted in utero against the sacral prominence. Often, no cause can be established.

Facial weakness in early life may be due to agenesis of the affected muscles or to supranuclear causes (part of Möbius' syndrome) or may even be familial. Myasthenia gravis, polyneuritis, and myotonic dystrophy must be considered. Facial asymmetry due to hypoplasia of one side of the cranium associated with contralateral hemiatrophy and spastic hemiparesis (due, in most instances, to an intrauterine cerebrovascular accident affecting one hemisphere) is usually differentiated easily, as is the hemiatrophy of one side of the body seen in Silver's syndrome.

Acquired peripheral facial weakness (Bell's palsy) of sudden onset and unknown cause is common in children. It may be a presenting sign of a disorder such as tumor, hypertension, infectious mononucleosis, or Landry-Guillain-Barré syndrome, usually diagnosable by the history, physical examination, and appropriate laboratory tests.

In the vast majority of cases of isolated peripheral facial palsy—both those present at birth and those acquired later—improvement begins within 1–2 weeks, and near or total recovery of function is observed within 2 months. Methylcellulose drops, 1%, should be instilled into the eyes to protect the cornea during the day; at night, the lid should be taped down with cellophane tape. Upward massage of the face for 5–10 minutes 3–4 times a day may help maintain muscle tone. Prednisone therapy reduces the pain of Bell's palsy and promotes recovery of facial strength and reduction of motor synkinesis ("crocodile tears").

Faradic or galvanic stimulation of facial muscles is not advised.

In the few children with permanent and cosmetically disfiguring facial weakness, plastic surgical intervention at 6 years of age or older may be of benefit. New procedures, such as attachment of facial muscles to the temporal muscle, are being developed.

Adour KK: Current concepts in neurology: Diagnosis and management of facial paralysis. *N Engl J Med* 1982;**307**:348.
Sudarshan A, Goldie WD: The spectrum of congenital facial diplegia (Moëbius syndrome). *Pediatr Neurol* 1985;**1**:180.

2. BRACHIAL PLEXUS INJURIES (Erb's Palsy, Klumpke's Paralysis)

Traction injuries of the brachial plexus are most common in newborns, occurring in 0.1% of spontaneous, 1.2% of breech, 1.3% of forceps, and 0.25% of all deliveries. The complexity of the brachial plexus precludes any absolute classification, but injuries are usually divided into those affecting the upper plexus (Erb's palsy) and those affecting the lower plexus (Klumpke's paralysis).

Erb's palsy, involving chiefly the fifth and sixth cervical roots, is seen in 99% of cases. It is usually associated with difficult breech delivery, forceps delivery (especially in brow and face presentations), or misapplication of the vacuum extractor. The arm is maintained in adduction and internal rotation at the shoulder, with the lower arm pronated, assuming

* Arthrogryposis multiplex, or contractures and fixation about multiple joints, is discussed briefly in a later section on the floppy infant. Clubfoot, Sprengel's deformity, and torticollis are discussed in Chapter 22.

the "waiter's tip" position. Loss of sensation may be difficult to assess in newborns.

In Klumpke's paralysis, involving chiefly the lower brachial plexus (eighth cervical and first thoracic roots), the small muscles of the hand and wrist flexors are affected, causing a "claw hand." Horner's syndrome may also be present. The injury, usually caused by manipulation during delivery, results in hyperabduction of the arm at the shoulder.

Swinging a child by one arm or jerking the arm may also cause lower plexus injuries ("nursemaid's palsy").

The palsies observed are usually due to avulsion of the plexus, with contusion, edema, and some hemorrhage. X-ray studies of the shoulder will rule out fractures of the clavicle or cervical spine as well as dislocations.

In most instances, recovery occurs spontaneously within a few days or weeks. However, contractures of the shoulder and especially the elbow joints and atrophy of the affected muscles may occur; positioning in the so-called Statue of Liberty or airplane wing position, formerly advised, has been said to contribute to these problems. Passive range-of-motion exercises, which can be taught to the parents, are most helpful in preventing contractures. Electromyography and CT metrizamide myelography can delineate the extent of injury and aid in prognosis, as well as determine the patients in whom surgical exploration and reparative procedures may be justified.

Greenwald AG, Schute PC, Shiveley JL: Brachial plexus birth palsy: A 10-year report on the incidence and prognosis. *J Pediatr Orthop* 1984;**4:**689.

Painter MJ, Bergman I: Obstetrical trauma to the neonatal central and peripheral nervous system. *Semin Perinatol* 1982; **6:**89.

3. OTHER PERIPHERAL NERVE INJURIES

Injuries to the radial and ulnar nerves occur with fractures of the humerus; ulnar and median nerve injuries may result from deep wrist lacerations; and fracture of the fibula may cause peroneal palsy. These usually require neurosurgery. Femoral nerve palsies occasionally occur with diabetes mellitus in teenagers.

"Shoulder strap" or "pack" paralysis of the long thoracic nerve, resulting in winging of the scapula, occurs in youngsters who carry heavy rucksacks with poorly padded straps.

An avoidable paralysis is that of the sciatic nerve following injections into the buttock. Penicillin and tetracycline injected into newborns or small thin children are the most common offenders. The resulting fibrosis, chiefly around the outer portion of the sciatic nerve, comprising elements making up the common peroneal nerve, causes footdrop and adduction and inversion of the foot. Sensory loss over the outer side of the lower leg and dorsum of the foot may be demonstrated by electrical and other studies. In most cases, at least partial recovery occurs over the course of a few weeks to 6 months. Occasionally, surgical exploration of the buttock with neurolysis is justified. Postinjection sciatic neuropathy can be prevented by giving injections into the anterior lateral aspect of the thigh.

Gilles FH, Matson DD: Sciatic nerve injury following misplaced gluteal injection. *J Pediatr* 1970;**76:**247.

CHRONIC POLYNEUROPATHY

Polyneuropathy, usually insidious in onset and slowly progressive, occurs in children of any age. The presenting complaints are chiefly disturbances of gait and easy fatigability in walking or running and, slightly less often, weakness or clumsiness of the hands. Pain, tenderness, or paresthesias are less frequently mentioned. Neurologic examination discloses muscular weakness, greatest in the distal portions of the extremities, with steppage gait and depressed or absent deep tendon reflexes. Cranial nerves are sometimes affected. Sensory deficits (difficult to demonstrate in fearful children or those under 5 years of age) cover a stocking and glove distribution. The muscles may be tender, and trophic changes such as a glossy or "parchment" skin and absent sweating may occur. Thickening of the ulnar and peroneal nerves may be felt. Pure sensory neuropathies show up as chronic trauma.

Known causes include (1) toxins, eg, lead, arsenic, mercurials, vincristine, and benzene; (2) systemic disorders, eg, diabetes mellitus, chronic uremia, recurrent hypoglycemia, porphyria, polyarteritis nodosa, and lupus erythematosus; (3) "inflammatory" states, eg, "chronic or recurrent Landry-Guillain-Barré syndrome" and neuritis associated with mumps or diphtheria; (4) hereditary, often degenerative conditions, which in some classifications include certain storage diseases, leukodystrophies, spinocerebellar degenerations with neurogenic components, and Bassen-Kornzweig disease (Table 23–9); and (5) the hereditary sensory or combined motor and sensory neuropathies. Polyneuropathies associated with carcinomas, beriberi or other vitamin deficiencies, or excessive vitamin B_6 intake are not reported or are exceedingly rare in children.

Of the 4 defined hereditary sensory neuropathies, the prototype is **familial dysautonomia,** also called Riley-Day syndrome and hereditary sensory neuropathy type III. Transmitted as an autosomal recessive trait and seen mostly in Jewish children, this disorder has its onset in infancy. It is characterized by vomiting and difficulties in feeding, which are due to abnormal esophageal motility; pulmonary infections; decreased or absent tearing; indifference to pain; diminished or absent tendon reflexes; absence of fungiform papillae of the tongue; emotional lability; abnormal temperature control, with excessive sweating; labile blood pressure; abnormal intradermal histidine responses; and other evidences of autonomic dysfunctioning. Mental retardation may be present. Neurologic findings include a marked decrease in unmyelinated fibers of cutaneous nerves and decreased myelinization in dorsal root fibers and the posterior columns of the spinal cord.

There are 5 hereditary conditions with combined motor and sensory neuropathies. Type I, **peroneal muscular atrophy,** is the classic hypertrophic de- and remyelinating form of Charcot-Marie-Tooth disease. It is usually inherited as an autosomal dominant trait, often linked to the Duffy blood group, but also appears as a recessive trait or sporadically. Beginning in the first or, less often, the second decade of life, there is progressive weakness and atrophy of the intrinsic muscles of the feet (causing pes cavus and hammer toe), then affecting the anterolateral calves and thighs ("stork legs"), and eventually involving the hands. Tendon reflexes are diminished or lost. Nerve conduction velocities are severely reduced owing to extensive segmental demyelinization and axonal loss. Peripheral nerves may be hypertrophic owing to remyelinization. Cerebrospinal fluid protein levels are generally elevated. Ataxia, tremor, distal weakness, sensory loss, and rate of progression are more prominent in this type than in the other 4 types. Type II, sometimes called the **neuronal-axonal form of Charcot-Marie-Tooth disease,** is inherited as an autosomal dominant, has its onset in the second decade of life or later, and often presents with complaints of leg cramps, numbness and tingling, and gait difficulties. Findings are similar to though much less severe than those in type I, with tendon reflexes preserved and much slower progression. Nerve conduction velocities may be normal or only modestly reduced. Nerve biopsy shows axonal loss with prominent demyelinization. Cerebrospinal fluid protein levels are usually normal. Type III, **hypertrophic interstitial neuritis,** is frequently equated with Déjérine-Sottas disease and is inherited as an autosomal recessive. The onset is often in infancy, and patients present with delayed motor development; weakness is slowly progressive. Findings may include clubfoot, kyphoscoliosis, pupillary abnormalities, deafness, absent tendon reflexes, ataxia, and sensory loss except for pain and temperature. Peripheral nerves are hypertrophic, and nerve conduction velocities are reduced. Cerebrospinal fluid protein levels are usually elevated. Type IV, **Refsum's disease,** is described in Table 23–10. Type V, **familial spastic paraplegia,** is inherited as an autosomal dominant, usually has its onset in the second decade or later, and is characterized by progressive spasticity and hyperreflexia. Motor conduction velocities in the lower extremities may be normal or diminished. Sensations are usually intact; however, with increasing age, sensory deficits reflect a decrease in myelinated peripheral sensory neurons.

Laboratory diagnosis of chronic polyneuropathy is made by measurement of motor and sensory nerve conduction velocities; electromyography may show a neurogenic polyphasic pattern. Cerebrospinal protein levels are often elevated, with IgG index sometimes increased as well. Nerve biopsy, with teasing of the fibers as well as staining for metachromasia, is advised to demonstrate loss of myelin and (to a lesser degree) loss of axons and increased connective tissue or concentric lamellas ("onion skin appearance") around the nerve fiber. Muscle biopsy may show the pattern associated with denervation. Other laboratory studies, directed toward specific causes mentioned above, include screening for heavy metals and for metabolic, renal, or vascular disorders. Chronic lead intoxication, which rarely causes neuropathy in childhood, may escape detection until the child is given edetate calcium disodium (EDTA) and lead levels are determined in timed urines. Three- and 4-fold rises then are diagnostic.

Therapy is directed at specific disorders whenever possible. Occasionally, the weakness is profound and involves bulbar nerves, in which case tracheostomy and respiratory assistance are required. Corticosteroid therapy may be of considerable benefit in cases in which the cause is unknown or neuropathy is considered to be due to "chronic inflammation" (as is not the case in acute Landry-Guillain-Barré syndrome). Prednisone, 1–2.5 mg/kg/d orally, with tapering to the least effective dose—discontinued if the process seems to be arresting and reinstituted when symptoms recur—is recommended. Prednisone should probably not be used for treatment of peroneal muscular atrophy. In all cases considered for corticosteroid, the risks and benefits should be carefully weighed. When treatable, symptoms regress and may disappear altogether over a period of months.

Long-term prognosis varies with the cause and the ability to offer specific therapy. In the "corticosteroid-dependent" group, residual deficits and deaths within a few years are more frequent.

Axelrod FB, Pearson J: Congenital sensory neuropathies: Diagnostic distinction from familial dysautonomia. *Am J Dis Child* 1984;**138:**947.

Dyck PJ et al: Prednisone improves chronic inflammatory demyelinating polyradiculoneuropathy more than no treatment. *Ann Neurol* 1982;**11:**136.

Dyck PJ et al: Prednisone-responsive hereditary motor and sensory neuropathy. *Mayo Clin Proc* 1982;**57:**239.

Evans OB: Polyneuropathy in childhood. *Pediatrics* 1979; **64:**96.

Hagberg B, Westerberg B: The nosology of genetic peripheral neuropathies in Swedish children. *Dev Med Child Neurol* 1983;**25:**3.

Prensky AL, Dodson WE: The steroid treatment of hereditary motor and sensory neuropathy. *Neuropediatrics* 1984; **15:**203.

MISCELLANEOUS NEUROMUSCULAR DISORDERS

FLOPPY INFANT SYNDROME

Essentials of Diagnosis

- In early infancy, decreased muscular activity, both spontaneous and in response to postural reflex testing and to passive motion.
- In young infants, "frog posture" or other unusual positions at rest.
- In older infants, delay in motor milestones.

General Considerations

In the young infant, ventral suspension, ie, supporting the infant with a hand under the chest, normally results in the infant's holding its head slightly up (45 degrees or less), the back straight or nearly so, the arms flexed at the elbows and slightly abducted, and the knees partly flexed. The floppy infant droops over the hand like an inverted U. Even the normal newborn attempts to keep the head in the same plane as the body when pulled up from supine to sitting by the hands ("traction response"). Marked head lag is characteristic of the floppy infant. Hyperextensibility of the joints is not a dependable criterion.

The usual reasons for seeking medical evaluation in older infants are delays in walking, running, or climbing stairs or difficulties and lack of endurance in motor activities.

Hypotonia or decreased motor activity is a frequent presenting complaint in neuromuscular disorders but may also accompany a variety of systemic conditions or may be due to certain disorders of connective tissue.

Clinical Types

A. Paralytic Group: There is significant lack of movement against gravity (eg, failure to kick the legs, hold up the arms, or attempt to stand when held) or in response to stimuli such as tickling or slight pain.

B. Nonparalytic Group: There is floppiness without significant paralysis.

Note: Deep tendon reflexes may be depressed or absent in the nonparalytic group also. Brisk reflexes with hypotonia point to suprasegmental or general cerebral dysfunction.

1. PARALYTIC GROUP

Hereditary Progressive Spinal Muscular Atrophies

These disorders are inherited as autosomal recessives, but rare instances of dominant transmission occur. Intrauterine diagnosis is not yet possible. Treatment is supportive and consists of minimizing respiratory infections, preventing contractures, and enabling those who can do so to use crutches or a wheelchair.

A. Infantile Form (Werdnig-Hoffmann Disease): This is the commonest of the paralytic forms of floppy infant syndrome. Onset may be in utero, with loss of fetal movements, or paralysis may appear gradually or fairly abruptly in the early weeks or months of life. The infant usually lies in the frog position, breathing diaphragmatically, exhibiting sternal retraction due to paralysis of intercostal muscles, and moving the legs only slightly if at all. The facies is alert. The cry may be weak, and secretions tend to pool in the pharynx owing to bulbar involvement. Fasciculation of the tongue is seen frequently. Fasciculations of the muscles of the extremities are usually hidden by baby fat. Tremors of the fingers may be seen, usually in slightly older and less severely involved children. Deep tendon reflexes are lost early—first in the lower extremities—as the paralysis proceeds cephalad. Sensation is normal.

The diagnosis is based on a "neurogenic" electromyographic pattern and muscle biopsy, which shows a neuropathic pattern of large bundles of atrophied fibers interspersed with bundles of normal or hypertrophied fibers. Soft tissue x-rays show marked muscle atrophy, and this may help in gauging needed depth for muscle biopsy. Muscle enzymes are usually normal but may be slightly elevated in milder variants.

Pneumonia, often due to aspiration, is the commonest complication, and most of the afflicted infants die within 2–3 years.

B. Variants: Less rapidly progressive forms may represent a continuum of the disorder, but—pending biochemical definition—not specific entities.

1. Weakness appearing late—Muscle weakness, chiefly of the legs, may not be recognized until the time when infants might be expected to sit up by themselves or to be walking; there may be other signs of retarded motor development as well. Intelligence is not affected. Muscles of respiration may be relatively spared, and the upper extremities may be strong enough so that the child can learn to walk with crutches, the legs and lower trunk being braced, or to use a wheelchair. Hence, maximum physical rehabilitation is indicated. In general, the more insidious and the later the onset of weakness and the more limited its extent, the better the prognosis. Some patients may live a normal life span.

2. Juvenile spinal muscular atrophy of Kugelberg-Welander—Onset is between 2 years of age and the late teens. The larger proximal muscles, especially of the pelvic girdle, are affected first; the lower legs and arms are involved relatively late. The muscles of the trunk and those supplied by the cranial nerves are usually spared. Muscle enzymes are usually normal, the EMG is "neurogenic," and muscle biopsy is more "myopathic" than in Werdnig-Hoffmann disease. Progression is usually slow. Males may be affected more severely. Every effort should be made to permit the patient to lead as independent a life as possible.

Myopathies

The congenital, relatively nonprogressive myopathies, muscular dystrophy, myotonic dystrophy, polymyositis, and periodic paralysis are discussed elsewhere. Most cases of congenital or early infantile muscular dystrophy reported in the past probably represented congenital myopathies (Table 23–13). Congenital muscular dystrophy, diagnosed by muscle biopsy, occurs in 2 forms: (1) a benign form, with gradual improvement in strength; and (2) a severe form, in which there is either rapid progression of weakness and death in the first months or year of life or severe disability with little or no progression but lifelong marked limitation of activity.

Glycogenosis With Muscle Involvement

Glycogen storage diseases are described in Chapter 33. Patients with type II (Pompe's disease, due to a deficiency of acid maltase) are most likely to present as floppy infants. The weakness in type III (limit dextrinosis) is less marked than in type II, while the rare instances of type IV (amylopectinosis) are severely hypotonic. Muscle cramps on exertion or easy fatigability, rather than floppiness in infancy, is the presenting complaint in type V (McArdle's phosphorylase deficiency) or the glycogenosis due to phosphofructokinase deficiency or phosphohexose isomerase inhibition.

Myasthenia Gravis

Neonatal transient and congenital persistent myasthenia gravis, presenting as "paralytic" floppy infants, is described elsewhere in this chapter.

Infant Botulism

A syndrome of generalized weakness, caused by neurotoxin from the germination of ingested spores of *Clostridium botulinum,* has now been recognized worldwide in hundreds of infants under 1 year of age (most commonly younger than 6 months). In the USA, the incidence in infants at risk ranges from 10 in 100,000 in California to 29 in 100,000 in Hawaii. A high incidence is also reported in Australia.

Infant botulism, as initially described in 1976, has a wide spectrum: In its mild form, infants present with a history of poor feeding and failure to thrive, have mild hypotonia, and are otherwise asymptomatic carriers of *C botulinum,* with or without toxin detected in stool; they do not require hospitalization. In its most virulent form, the condition is said to be indistinguishable by history or general autopsy from the sudden infant death syndrome, the diagnosis resting solely on the stool findings.

In the "classic" form, which requires hospitalization, infants develop the following over the course of hours to 4–5 days: increasing feeding difficulties, floppiness, constipation, weak cry, lethargy, irritability, droopy eyelids, loss of facial expression, respiratory difficulties including apneic spells, and aspiration pneumonitis. Findings corresponding to bulbar and skeletal involvement include loss of head and limb control; loss of sucking, gag, and stretch reflexes; dilated pupils; and ptosis and paralysis of the extraocular muscles. Electromyography shows brief, low-amplitude motor unit action potentials that are overabundant for the amount of power extended or stimulus used.

Stool (obtained by enema if necessary) is positive for *C botulinum* and either toxin type A or B; in one case, toxin was found in the serum. Illness has not been reported in any other members of families with affected infants. Worldwide, honey containing *C botulinum* organisms, used as a sweetener or laxative, has been responsible for about one-third of cases; thus, honey should not be fed to young infants. Other sources of the organism include soil, house dust, and dust-laden water. Since *C botulinum* is present ubiquitously and exposure to spores is nearly universal, some special condition (as yet undefined) of the intestine in infants contributes significantly to infant botulism.

Treatment requires supportive care, including gavage feeding and, in 40%, mechanically assisted ventilation. Botulism antitoxin has not been required. Aminoglycosides potentiate neuromuscular blockade of botulinus toxin and should not be used in treating associated pulmonary infections. The illness may persist for several weeks, but complete recovery is the rule. The overall death rate is 3%.

The differential diagnosis includes many of the other causes of floppy infant syndrome, particularly myasthenia gravis, in which there is a response to neostigmine, and infantile polyneuritis, especially of the "corticosteriod-responsive" type. The latter condition is characterized by (1) prolonged nerve conduction time and denervation on electromyographic examination; (2) usually marked elevation of cerebrospinal fluid protein levels for age; and (3) lack of progressive cerebral involvement, as in metachromatic and globoid leukodystrophies. Nerve biopsy may be justified. Diagnosis of this polyneuropathy may require a therapeutic trial of corticosteroids, resulting in improvement.

Arthrogryposis Multiplex (Congenital Deformities About Multiple Joints)

This symptom complex, sometimes associated with hypotonia, may be of "neurogenic" or "myopathic" origin (or both) and may be associated with a wide variety of other anomalies. Orthopedic aspects are discussed in Chapter 22.

Spinal Cord Lesions

Severe limpness in newborns following breech extraction with stretching or actual tearing of the lower cervical to upper thoracic spinal cord is rarely seen today, owing to improved obstetric delivery. Klumpke's lower brachial plexus paralysis may be present; the abdomen is usually exceedingly soft, and the lower extremities are flaccid. Urinary retention is present initially; later, the bladder may function autonomously. Myelography, but not spine films, may define the lesion. After a few weeks, spasticity of the lower limbs becomes obvious. Treatment is symptomatic and consists of bladder and skin care and eventual mobilization on crutches or in a wheelchair.

2. NONPARALYTIC GROUP

In infants in the "floppy" state without paralysis, tendon reflexes, though depressed, may be elicited. Creatine kinase and electromyogram are usually normal. Prolonged nerve conduction velocities point to polyneuritis or leukodystrophy. Muscle biopsies, utilizing special stains and histographic analysis, often show a remarkable reduction in size of type II fibers associated with decreased voluntary motor activity.

Central Nervous System Lesions (Above Spinal Cord)

Limpness in the neonatal period and early infancy and subsequent delay in achieving motor milestones are the presenting features in a large number of children with a variety of central nervous system disorders, including mental retardation, as in trisomy 21. In many such cases, no specific diagnosis can be made. Close observation and scoring of motor patterns and adaptive behavior, as by the Denver Developmental Screening Test, are most helpful. Several categories deserve specific attention.

A. "Prespastic (Atonic) Diplegia": Various forms of pre- or perinatal encephalopathy can be categorized as "prespastic diplegia." Findings include profound limpness at or shortly after birth, depressed or absent deep tendon reflexes initially, poor sucking and feeding, weak or shrill cry, poor Moro responses, weak or absent grasp responses, and visual and auditory inattention. Tendon reflexes usually become hyperactive within a few weeks. When the affected infant is held up, supported under the armpits by the examiner's hands, the legs are flexed at the hips and knees and, instead of going limp, the infant exhibits increased tone (Foerster's sign). Because of their initially floppy state, these infants are often classified as atonic or hypotonic diplegics; however, most, if not all, eventually exhibit hypertonicity, thus justifying a diagnosis of "prespastic diplegia." (See also Cerebral Palsy.)

B. Hypotonic, Hypokinetic Forms of "Minimal Brain Dysfunction": Floppiness may occur in infants who eventually exhibit attention deficit disorder, usually without hyperactivity. The diagnosis rests on close follow-up.

C. Degenerative Central Nervous System Disorders: Degenerative diseases of infancy presenting with hypotonia include globoid and metachromatic leukodystrophy, subacute necrotizing encephalomyelopathy, G_{M2} gangliosidosis, and generalized gangliosidosis (Table 23–9).

D. Other Disorders: Congenital choreoathetosis, discussed earlier, often presents as hypotonia; involuntary movements of the limbs and facial grimacing are not noted until the second half of the first year or later. Delays in motor milestones are the rule.

Children with congenital cerebellar ataxia and, even more rarely, those with exceedingly early forms of Friedreich's ataxia show hypotonia and subsequent incoordination when they begin to reach, sit, stand, or walk. CT brain scanning may disclose cerebellar dysplasia.

"Systemic" Causes

Limpness without motor paralysis is a presenting or accompanying feature of many other disorders seen in children. These include the following:

A. Malnutrition: Nutritional deprivation, cystic fibrosis, celiac disease, scurvy, rickets, etc.

B. Debilitating Diseases: Severe infections; congenital heart, lung, and renal diseases; etc.

C. Metabolic Disorders: Infantile hypercalcemia, hypophosphatasia, etc.

D. Endocrinopathies: Hypothyroidism, adrenocortical hyperfunction, gonadal dysgenesis (Turner's syndrome), hypotonia-hypogonadal-obesity syndrome of Prader-Willi, etc.

E. Other Disorders: Familial dysautonomia (of Riley-Day).

Heritable Disorders of Connective Tissue

Children with osteogenesis imperfecta, Marfan's syndrome, Ehlers-Danlos syndrome, and congenital laxity of ligaments, besides being floppy, are often "double-jointed" or "rubber-jointed." The first 3 disorders present characteristic pictures discussed elsewhere. The last condition is entirely benign.

Essential Hypotonia

Floppy infants who do not fall into the previously mentioned categories are often classified as having "essential" or, less properly, "benign congenital" hypotonia. This is a diagnosis of exclusion, made less and less frequently as diagnostic techniques improve. In essential hypotonia, the family history is usually negative. The muscles show no atrophy or fasciculations; tendon reflexes may be present, diminished, or absent. Respiratory difficulties are encountered occasionally. "Immaturity" of the motor end plates has been offered as a possible cause of the condition. Muscle biopsy, which should include special stains and electron microscopy, may show either no pathologic features or universally small fibers without histochemical or connective tissue changes. The outlook is for partial to full recovery in well over 50% of children so reported.

Dubowitz V: *The Floppy Infant*, 2nd ed. Clinics in Developmental Medicine, No. 76. Heinemann, 1980.
Gamstorp I, Sarnat HG (editors): *Progressive Spinal Muscular Atrophies*. Raven Press, 1984.
Long SS: Botulism in infancy. *Pediatr Infect Dis* 1984;**3**:266.
Zellweger H: The floppy infant: A practical approach. *Helv Paediatr Acta* 1983;**38**:301.

CEREBRAL PALSY

Essentials of Diagnosis

- Impairment of movement and posture since birth or early infancy.
- Nonprogressive and nonhereditary.

General Considerations

Cerebral palsy is a term of clinical convenience for disorders of impaired motor functioning and posture with onset before or at birth or during the first year of life, basically nonprogressive, and varying widely in their causes, manifestations, and prognosis. The most obvious manifestation is impaired ability of voluntary muscles. In the USA, cerebral palsy affects about 0.2% of neonatal survivors.

Classification

Classification is commonly based on the predominant motor deficit.

A. Spastic Forms: About 75% of cases. Often associated with other forms.

1. Quadriplegia (tetraplegia)—The 4 extremities may be involved about equally, or upper limbs may show more severe involvement. The main lesion is in the cerebral white matter. Quadriplegia due to perinatal damage often shows symptoms earlier than that due to fetal undernutrition or prematurity. Nearly 90% of patients are profoundly retarded.

2. Diplegia—Legs involved more than arms.

3. Hemiplegia—One side involved primarily.

4. Paraplegia—Legs only involved.

5. Monoplegia—One extremity only involved.

6. Triplegia—Three extremities involved.

B. Ataxia: About 15% of cases. Pure and in combination with other forms.

C. Dyskinesia (Choreoathetosis): (See Extrapyramidal Disorders.) About 5% of cases. Often associated with rigidity or spastic quadri- or diplegia.

D. Hypotonic Form: Fewer than 1% of cases. Persistent hypotonia with variable degrees of weakness.

Etiology

The cause is often obscure or multiple. No definite etiologic diagnosis is possible in over one-third of cases. The incidence is high among infants small for gestational age. Intrauterine hypoxia is a frequent cause. Other known causes are intrauterine bleeding, infections, toxins, congenital malformations, obstetric complications (including birth hypoxia), neonatal infections, kernicterus, neonatal hypoglycemia, acidosis, and a small number of genetic syndromes (about 2%).

Associated Deficits

A. Seizures: Seizures afflict about 50% of all children with cerebral palsy and are more prevalent in those with severe involvement.

B. Mental Retardation: Mild to moderate retardation is seen in 26% of patients and profound retardation in 27%. The incidence highly correlates with the severity of cerebral palsy.

C. Sensory and Speech Deficits: Impairment of speech, vision, hearing, and perceptual functions is found often in varying degrees and combinations.

Clinical Findings

A. Symptoms and Signs: The typical spastic child exhibits muscular hypertonicity of the clasp knife type that may eventually end in contractures. In the limb or limbs involved, tendon reflexes, if sufficient muscle relaxation can be achieved, are hyperactive; clonus may be present, and the plantar responses are often extensor. While voluntary control, especially of fine movements, is decreased, there is spread or overflow of associated movements. In extreme cases, the child may lie with elbows flexed and fists clenched (straphanger's posture) and legs crossed or scissored. In early infancy, the child may appear floppy, although tendon jerks are abnormally increased (hypotonic, atonic, or prespastic diplegia). Rigidity often accompanies cerebral palsy.

Ataxia may be difficult to delineate in the presence of spasticity or hyperkinetic movements.

Microcephaly (head circumference < 2 SD below the mean for age and sex and decreasing) is present in about 25% of spastic quadri- and diplegics.

Partial atrophy of the cranium on the involved side or of involved extremities is observed frequently, but dependable statistics are not available.

A smaller hand or foot, when coupled with mild weakness on muscle testing or hyperreflexia, often justifies a diagnosis of mild cerebral palsy of which the patient or the family may not even have been aware.

B. Laboratory and Other Findings: No routine workup can be outlined. The clinical findings, the presence or absence of seizures, and the overall outlook for the child—particularly with respect to intelligence and the ability to carry on activities of daily living—determine what studies, if any, should be performed. Hip films in abduction are indicated to rule out dislocations secondary to spasticity. Electroencephalography is indicated when seizures are present or suspected. In some cases, CT scanning may aid in determining the prognosis.

Urine screening tests for aminoacidurias (and in choreoathetosis with self-abuse, serum uric acid determinations) should be considered to rule out Lesch-Nyhan syndrome.

Differential Diagnosis

The diagnosis is usually not difficult. Progressive deterioration in the first 3 months is more likely to denote a metabolic disorder; subsequently, it denotes one of the central nervous system degenerative disorders (Tables 23–9 and 23–10). In the ataxic form, cerebellar dysgenesis (sometimes familial) or a spinocerebellar degeneration may have to be ruled out.

Prevention

Obstetric advances involving late third-trimester management and delivery have resulted in signficant gains. Much more needs to be done in prenatal care, especially during the second and early third trimester. The number of cases in which cerebral palsy is associated with aggressive efforts to salvage premature infants has decreased as a result of advances in neonatal care.

Treatment

Realistically, a child with cerebral palsy should be helped to achieve maximum potential rather than "normality." Special educational programming depends on the physical and mental potential of the child. The degree of improvement with physical therapy correlates positively with better intelligence. Treat seizures as in other children. The orthopedic aspects of cerebral palsy are discussed in Chapter 22.

Spasticity occasionally is reduced by diazepam (Valium), dantrolene (Dantrium), or baclofen (Lioresal). Optimal doses vary with degree of spasticity, size and age of the child, and other medications taken. Surgical amelioration of moderate to severe spasticity in cerebral palsy has been attempted by various procedures over many years.

Management of "hyperactivity" is dealt with below in connection with attention deficit disorder.

Psychologic counseling and support of the child and family are of paramount importance.

Prognosis

In patients with severe cerebral palsy, especially spastics with profound retardation and seizures that are difficult to control, death due to intercurrent infections is not uncommon; nearly half die by 10 years of age. In nearly 30% of patients, chiefly in those with mild involvement, motor deficits resolve by the seventh birthday. Many children with cerebral palsy and average or near-average intelligence lead fairly normal, satisfying, and productive lives.

Broggi G et al: Long-term results of stereotactic thalamotomy for cerebral palsy. *Neurosurgery* 1983;**12:**195.

Davidoff RA: Antispasticity drugs: Mechanisms of action. *Ann Neurol* 1985;**17:**107.

Kudrjavcev T et al: Cerebral palsy—Survival rates, associated handicaps, and distribution by clinical subtype: Rochester, MN, 1950–1976. *Neurology* 1985;**35:**900.

Marquis P et al: Extrapyramidal cerebral palsy: A changing view. *Dev Behav Pediatr* 1982;**3:**65.

Milner-Brown HS, Penn RD: Pathophysiological mechanisms in cerebral palsy. *J Neurol Neurosurg Psychiatry* 1979; **42:**606.

ATTENTION DEFICIT DISORDER (Minimal Brain Dysfunction)

Essentials of Diagnosis

- Developmentally inappropriate inattention and impulsivity.
- Hyperactivity a frequent, but not invariable, component.

General Considerations

The term attention deficit disorder was adopted in 1980 by the American Psychiatric Association in its *Diagnostic and Statistical Manual of Mental Disorders (DSM-III)* to describe the syndrome of childhood and adolescence previously most widely known as minimal brain dysfunction, a term still much in use. Other terms previously used include minimal or minor cerebral dysfunction, minimal brain damage, hyperactive child syndrome, and hyperkinetic reaction of childhood.

Minimal brain dysfunction is used to describe "children of near average, average, or above average general intelligence with certain learning or behavioral disabilities ranging from mild to severe, which are associated with deviations of function of the central nervous system. These deviations may manifest themselves by various conbinations of impairment in perception, conceptualization, language, memory, and control of attention, impulse, or motor function."*

The present *DSM-III* designation focuses on "attentional difficulties" that "are prominent and virtually always present among children with these diagnoses." The presence or absence of hyperactivity categorizes 2 subtypes, though whether these represent 2 aspects of the same disorder or represent distinct entities is not known. A third ("residual") subtype categorizes "individuals once diagnosed as having attentional deficit disorder with hyperactivity in which hyperactivity is no longer present, but other signs of the disorder persist."

The term attention deficit disorder may even cover dysfunctions in children referred to in the professional literature as developmental or learning disabilities, developmental dyslexia, perceptual handicaps, or perceptual motor dysfunction. *DSM-III* recognizes this by stating that "specific developmental disorders"—language, reading, writing, arithmetic, etc—"are common"; these are coded in *DSM-III* on a "second axis." Attention deficit may, with some frequency, be a part of learning disability.

* Clements SD: Minimal brain dysfunction in children. Pages 9–10 in: NINDB Monograph No. 3. US Department of Health, Education, and Welfare, 1966.

Etiology

Attention deficit disorder is common; it has been estimated to occur in 3% of prepubertal (school-age) children in the USA, with boys affected 3–10 times more often than girls. Presumed causes include virtually any illness or trauma occurring before, during, or after birth and affecting the brain either obviously or by implication. Genetic factors may play a role; familial incidence is not uncommon.

Artificial food colors and preservatives have recently been implicated as specific precipitants of "hyperactivity"; though that claim has many enthusiastic supporters, it may be valid in some instances only. A claim has been made that chronic low-level lead exposure may cause attention deficit disorder in some cases. Support for this claim comes from experimental evidence that newborn rats suckled on milk that was high in lead content became "hyperactive" and had high levels of lead and a 20% decrease in dopamine levels in brain tissue.

Clinical Findings

A. Symptoms and Signs: Attentional problems may be evident during early childhood, as demonstrated by the child's persistent failure to carry through on instructions at home or in nursery school or inability to continue in play and other activities for periods of time appropriate to the child's age. Attentional problems may become particularly evident when the child is in a group and must compete for attention, eg, at home when guests are present or in groups at church or school. Children with attention deficit disorder are described as unable to sit still, fidgety, easily distractible, "stimulus-bound," "organically driven," and "constantly on the go." The hyperactivity so common to children with the disorder is thought to reflect a lack of focus or of organization of activity, so that activity appears to be haphazard and not "goal-oriented." It is also evident that the child may not lack attentiveness or be hyperactive in every setting or situation.

Associated behavioral features, varying somewhat with age, include low frustration tolerance, temper outbursts, increased mood lability, lack of response to discipline, negativism, and a lack of flexibility, with reluctance to try something new (reluctance to risk failure). Frequently, the child is impaired academically as well as socially, and because the child experiences many frustrations and failures, there is often a high level of anxiety and depression. This, in turn, is expressed in "acting out," aggressiveness, and progressively increasing hyperactivity.

Disturbances of feeding and sleeping patterns were often noted in early infancy, with frequent formula changes and delays in sleeping through the night. Motor milestones were usually attained at normal ages, but the child was noted to be clumsy, with trouble in learning to dress, button clothes, and tie shoes. Language development was often "a little slow."

On neurologic examination, the physician is apt to be less impressed than the parents or teachers by the child's "hyperactivity." The chief findings are "maladroitness," or nonspecific incoordination; overflow "choreiform" as well as mirror movements or synkinesis (observed best by having the child wiggle the fingers of one outstretched hand and noting extraneous movements of the other hand or the feet); and difficulties in sequencing, as in clapping the hands in a rhythmic pattern. In comparison with children of the same age, the affected child may show a "maturational lag" in abilities involving motor skills, postural stability, right-left orientation, higher motor-sensory integration, or eye-hand coordination. Together with mild disturbances of muscle tone (especially slight spasticity in the lower extremities), hyperreflexia, and occasional Babinski responses, these findings are said to constitute "neurologic soft signs" indicative of brain dysfunctioning. Neither eye nor hand dominance nor "mixed laterality" have proved to be related to the learning problems. On serial examination, the "soft signs" are often difficult to reduplicate.

Minor somatic anomalies, which may be more common than in "normal" children, include abnormalities in the shape of the head, facies, pinnas of the ears, palate, and hands; mild deviations in head circumference may be present. In only about 5% of children with attention deficit disorder can a recognized neurologic disorder be diagnosed. In the author's experience, the most frequent association has been with neurofibromatosis, partial tuberous sclerosis, and arrested hydrocephalus, often manifested by the "cocktail party syndrome" of meaningless chatter. Attention deficit disorder occurs more frequently in children born prematurely and may reflect the fact that premature infants who die at birth show more lipid-laden cells both in superficial cortical and in deep basal brain areas, compatible with hypoxic-ischemic brain damage.

B. Electroencephalogic, Radiologic, and Other Findings: Abnormal findings on EEG are reported in 27–88% of cases, but there is no clear correlation between electroencephalographic findings and any of the functional disturbances; indeed, on follow-up studies, children labeled as hyperkinetic who had abnormal EEGs had normal ones later, while those with initially normal studies later had dysrhythmic EEGs.

In about one-third of involved children, CT brain scanning shows mild cerebral atrophy, reversal of the usual right-left asymmetry, or other anomalies.

On psychologic evaluation, the child with attention deficit disorder may do least well on tests involving short-term memory. On the Wechsler Intelligence Scale for Children, the profile for attentional deficits shows arithmetic, digit span, and coding scores to be low relative to the other subtest scores. Especially useful in some cases are such instruments as the Luria-Nebraska Children's Battery or the Halstead-Reitan Neuropsychological Test Batteries for Children.

Technologic advances in assessing dynamic brain

function promise to offer better neurophysiologic correlates of attentional deficits and of hyperactivity. Abnormalities in evoked potentials on visual, auditory, and somatosensory stimulation are reported. Complex computer-assisted analyses of EEG and evoked potentials—eg, with neurometrics and with brain electrical activity mapping, which provides a visual display of brain functioning—are being used. Regional cerebral blood flow studies (coupled with CT brain scan techniques) and positron emission tomography are other methods.

Pharmacologic investigations have demonstrated diminished catecholamine activity, particularly as related to brain dopamine levels, in some "hyperkinetic" children whose "paradoxic" response to stimulant drugs suggests that they are, in fact, "underaroused."

Treatment

A. General and Supportive Care: The physician's task is not only to rule out severe and possibly progressive neurologic or emotional disorders but to act as "ombudsman" for the child and to guide parents and teachers. The diagnosis must be as accurate as possible, and the physician should keep in mind that the reported complaints and disabilities, as well as the neurologic, electroencephalographic, and even psychometric findings, may be observed in children with different organic, emotional, and social problems, and that these may be present together to a greater or lesser extent. In discussing the problems, the author has often described the child as being "dyssynchronous," ie, "out of phase" in developmental, behavioral, and educational progression and maturation. Parents quickly appreciate the term "dyssynchronous" when it is explained in terms of such analogies as the automatic shift of an automobile synchronized to changes in speed. Lack of synchronization (or letting the clutch out at the wrong time when using a standard shift) results in grinding the gears or the car bucking like a bronco. The "dyssynchronous child" may be likened in effect to an orchestra whose instruments are all playing slightly out of tune and off the beat or whose conductor is not in complete command, so that what is heard is somewhat chaotic and cacophonous. For the more visually oriented parent, the "dyssynchronous child" may be likened to a television image in which the horizontal and vertical components are not aligned or where there is a great deal of "snow," offering a recognizable but distorted picture.

The term dyssynchronous may be taken to reflect an imbalance between central excitation and inhibition, the complex feedback mechanisms thought to produce the synchronized discharges essential to the arousal state and attentiveness, fine coordinated movements, and rhythmic electrical brain activity. The term dyssynchronous, while emphasizing the functional aspects of the disorder, also suggests something of its neurophysiologic basis as inferred from clinical findings: a disturbance, possibly synaptic in character, of the timing and orderliness of neuronal interplay. This appellation avoids the implication of demonstrable and irreversible anatomic injury contained in the term brain damage; rather, it offers the hope—founded on clinical experience—of adjustment and "synchronization," with maturation aided by education. Thus, this term carries within it the challenge for investigative and therapeutic efforts.

The physician can be supportive to parents, teachers, and other professionals. Behavior modification, with emphasis on and rewarding of acceptable behavior, instead of the common tendency to pay greatest attention to the child who is misbehaving or failing, is often of benefit. Parents, siblings, teachers, and peers can all be involved in behavior modification programs, preferably under the guidance of a clinical psychologist. However, such techniques as "contingent ignoring" and "time out" for unacceptable behavior must be used with scrupulous restraint, since their potential for harm is great. "Cognitive behavior modification" is a technique for dealing with attentional deficits and learning disabilities.

Remedial tutoring is best done not by the parents but by an intelligent, calm, patient, and kind high school or college student for 20- to 30-minute periods several days a week. A wide variety of inexpensive methods to help improve coordination and overcome specific learning disabilities may be devised. While a common concern of teachers and parents is that the child cannot read or write, raising the specter of "developmental dyslexia," it must be recognized that an ever-decreasing number of parents read to their children or are seen reading by their children; that television is a deterrent to reading; and that dyslexia may be familial.

There is little rationale for "patterning" as a form of therapy except to channel parental anxieties into exhaustive, compulsive, and ritualistic activities. While some "hyperkinetic" children may show some response to the "elimination diet" free of synthetic food additives, most studies do not substantiate this.

B. Drug Therapy: Drug therapy, especially stimulant medications to reduce hyperactivity, must be used judiciously, sparingly, and only as an adjunct to behavior modification. Dextroamphetamine (5–20 mg in the morning and 2.5–10 mg at noon) has proved useful in diverting the nondirected behavior into more goal-oriented activity. Methylphenidate (Ritalin), used widely in dosages varying from 0.3 to 1 mg/kg/d, is now available in a 20-mg sustained-release tablet, so that the need for twice-daily administration is avoided. The toxic effects of these agents (including initial suppression of growth) and their potential for abuse must be carefully considered. Pemoline (Cylert), 37.5 mg/d orally at first and increasing at 1-week intervals by 18.75 mg until the desired clinical response is obtained, is not recommended for children under age 6. The mean daily effective dose ranges from 56.25 to 75 mg. One of the main advantages of this drug may be its more sustained, smoother action. Side effects, especially anorexia and insomnia, often subside with continued administration or reduction of dosage.

In prescribing dextroamphetamine, methylphenidate, or pemoline, the physician needs to monitor the child's growth; "drug holidays" on weekends and during school vacations may minimize the risk of growth retardation. That effect appears to be dose-related yet temporary, with no effect on adult size.

The author's preference is for dextroamphetamine as more predictable and more easily adjustable than the other stimulants. In proper dosages, it does not have the potential for psychosis or extrapyramidal side effects reported for methylphenidate. Dextroamphetamine also has some anticonvulsant properties, useful when the child has seizures.

Other drugs used are thioridazine (Mellaril), chlorpromazine (Thorazine), chlordiazepoxide (Librium), imipramine (Tofranil), and in younger children, diphenhydramine (Benadryl). Whatever drug is used, its potential for harm must be understood. Coffee has proved useful.

Prognosis

As time goes by, the restless hyperactive child tends to remain very active but in a more organized and less disturbing fashion. Distractibility continues to be a major handicap, resulting in significantly poorer performance in school or on jobs. Emotional immaturity continues to be characteristic of the child's behavior. Not infrequently, more serious emotional disorders, including delinquency and substance abuse, result from the failures and disapproval experienced by the child.

Obviously, with the large number of children involved, major educational and preventive psychologic efforts are required.

American Psychiatric Association: *Diagnostic and Statistical Manual of Mental Disorders,* 3rd ed. American Psychiatric Association, 1980.

Berry CA, Shaywitz SE, Shaywitz BA: Girls with attention deficit disorder: A silent minority? A report on behavioral and cognitive characteristics. *Pediatrics* 1985;**76:**801.

Fuller PW, Guthrie RD, Alvord EC Jr: A proposed neuropathological basis for learning disabilities in children born prematurely. *Dev Med Child Neurol* 1983;**25:**214.

Howell DC, Huessy HR, Hassuk B: Fifteen-year follow-up of a behavioral history of attention deficit disorder. *Pediatrics* 1985;**76:**185.

Lou HC, Henriksen L, Bruhn P: Focal cerebral hypoperfusion in children with dysphasia and/or attention deficit disorder. *Arch Neurol* 1984;**41:**825.

Ottinger DR et al: Evaluating drug effectiveness in an office setting for children with attention deficit disorders. *Clin Pediatr* 1985;**24:**245.

Rappaport L et al: Children's descriptions of their developmental dysfunctions: Field testing of a self-administered student profile. *Am J Dis Child* 1983;**137:**369.

Snyder RD: The right not to read. *Pediatrics* 1979;**63:**791.

Sparrow S, Zigler E: Evaluation of patterning treatment for retarded children. *Pediatrics* 1978;**62:**137.

Steinhausen HC, Romahn G, Göbel D: Computer analyzed EEG in methylphenidate-responsive hyperactive children. *Neuropediatrics* 1984;**15:**28.

Symposium on learning disorders. *Pediatr Clin North Am* 1984;**31:**279. [Entire issue.]

Wender EH: The food additive-free diet in the treatment of behavior disorders: A review. *J Dev Behav Pediatr* 1986;**7:**35.

SELECTED REFERENCES

American Society of Pediatric Neurosurgeons: *Concepts in Pediatric Neurosurgery.* Vols 1–4. Karger, 1981–1983.

Chusid JG: *Correlative Neuroanatomy & Functional Neurology,* 19th ed. Lange, 1985.

Dubowitz V: *Muscle Disorders in Childhood.* Saunders, 1978.

Menkes JH: *Textbook of Child Neurology,* 3rd ed. Lea & Febiger, 1985.

Swaiman KF, Wright FS (editors): *The Practice of Pediatric Neurology,* 2nd ed. Mosby, 1982.

Volpe JJ: *Neurology of the Newborn.* Saunders, 1981.

24 Psychosocial Aspects of Pediatrics & Psychiatric Disorders

Dane G. Prugh, MD, & Anthony J. Kisley, MD

GENERAL PRINCIPLES OF PSYCHIATRIC EXAMINATION & TREATMENT

THE APPROACH TO INTERVIEWING

Most physicians find that the traditional question-and-answer or "checklist" method of taking a history is not flexible enough to elicit significant psychosocial material. The "open-ended question" allows parents or patients to take the lead and to respond with material they are most concerned about. Physicians should feel comfortable with their own interviewing techniques and not attempt to imitate others.

In addition to what the patient says, the physician can learn much from observation of the patient and from noting how the relationship is developing. The quality of this relationship will affect not only the accuracy of the data obtained but response to recommended therapeutic measures as well. A warm, friendly, and nonjudgmental attitude will make it easier for the patient and his or her parents to talk freely. The doctor's skill in "listening actively" will facilitate discovery of the multiple determinants underlying what the patient actually says. Quick advice should be avoided, as well as premature promises about the success of treatment; both can promote overdependency or lead to disappointment.

Adequate time should be permitted for interviews. A good deal can be learned in 20–30 minutes, and longer interviews can be scheduled if necessary. The appointment schedule should be adhered to.

Interviewing the Parents

At the initial contact with the family, both parents should be seen together. Valuable impressions can be gained about the marital relationship, attitudes about parenthood, and attitudes toward the child, the illness, and the adjustment problem imposed by the illness.

In most cases, the physician can simply begin by asking, "What seems to be the matter?" The parents should be encouraged to tell the story in their own way, guided as necessary by comments and questions. The ostensible chief complaint may turn out not to be the parents' greatest concern. Patience is required, and intrusive (or leading) questioning early in the interview only delays the flow of significant material.

Observing the parents' attitudes and feelings will help direct the physician's inquiries to fill in gaps in the history. Repeating an emotion-laden word or phrase may enable a parent who temporarily blocks to continue. A note to oneself about things the parent does not say may lead to important clues at a later time.

It is important to note how the parents seem to feel about the physician and what they expect will be achieved by going forward with the relationship. A sympathetic, tolerant, and respectful attitude will help convince them that the physician is interested in helping them with their problem.

Other people should be accorded the respect and dignity they deserve. Women should not be called "mother" as a device for saving the time necessary to learn their names. Some parents really are "troublesome" and "impossible to please," but the physician who encounters too many problems of this sort must consider whether the fault is all on that side and should seek psychiatric advice if it seems likely to help. It is sometimes necessary to suggest to parents that they might be better satisfied with another doctor.

Parental demands for quick advice and easy solutions are usually symptoms of the parents' own anxieties. The parents will soon lose confidence in a physician who jumps to conclusions based on insufficient facts. No parent loses respect for a physician who admits not knowing what is wrong or what to do and states that further investigation and thought are necessary.

Certain historical data carry an emotional charge, and some revelations are painful and difficult. This is particularly true of familial or hereditary illnesses and of emotional disturbances in children and parents. For example, parents of children with seizure disorders may at first withhold information about epilepsy in close relatives. Parents also recognize that their feelings about a child may help to explain behavioral disturbances. In asking questions about behavior problems, it is important not to adopt an approach the anxious parent may misinterpret as a critical attack: "Did you want this child?" "Does your son masturbate?" "Was your little girl jealous of the new baby?" In the initial interview, such questions provoke conventional replies or defensive indignation. Such information must be gathered by inference or by the use of indirect questioning. Nonverbal behavior such as blushing, nail biting, or neuromuscular tension may give important clues.

The history should elicit relevant details about the family's circumstances—eg, their position as members of a minority group, unsatisfying work experiences leading to depression in the father, and part-time employment that keeps the mother away from home at the child's bedtime. It is important to identify family illnesses relevant to the child's problem without compulsively reading out lists of all the possibilities.

Parents may have difficulty remembering details of the child's birth, growth and development, past illnesses, and their child-rearing practices. Confirmation from other sources may be required.

The most significant emotional data often do not emerge during the first interview. Parents can rarely discuss their deep feelings until a basic sense of trust in the doctor has been allowed to develop. The parents must be allowed to talk at their own pace. The act of talking helps to discharge initial tensions and overcome anxiety. Expectant waiting is vital even if the parent appears to be on the verge of tears. Rather than interrupt the expression of strong emotions the physician should encourage a tense and troubled mother to cry. The release of such feelings in a sympathetic atmosphere may help the parent and strengthen the relationship with the physician.

In terminating the initial interview, it is wise to return to the area of the parents' major concern. The physician can then ask questions prompted by leads gathered to this point. This indicates to the parents that the doctor fully comprehends their concern and intends to deal with it therapeutically.

Interviewing the Child

Infants and young preschool children are usually seen with the mother. The physician may give the child a toy, tongue depressor, or other object to play with. If the parent talks too freely in the child's presence, the child may play in the waiting room while the pediatrician and the parent talk alone.

The physician may learn a good deal by observing the child at play during the interview. The child's level of development can be roughly assessed by observing the degree of complexity and organization of play, the duration of the child's attention span, and other clues. The child's attitude toward the physician, which often reflects parental anxiety, may also be apparent in drawings, play with dolls, and the child's general demeanor.

With older children and adolescents, the initial interview may be handled in different ways under different circumstances. If the parents are concerned about what they think is an emotional problem, it may be wise to see them together without the child the first time so that they can talk freely. If it is clear when the appointment is made that the parents and an adolescent child are in bitter conflict, seeing the child first may help to allay the suspicion that doctors and parents are allied in opposition to the needs and desires of teenagers. With anxious, suspicious children, one or both parents and the child should be seen together at the first interview so the child will know that "secret information" is not being disclosed. Later, the parents and the child can be seen separately.

At the end of an evaluation, it may help to see the parents and the child together.

At some point, the physician should see the child alone. This is best done in an office rather than an examining room. The parents should tell the child that the doctor is interested in the problems that make boys and girls worried or unhappy.

With an older child, verbal data may be more accurate and voluminous after a positive relationship has been established. At the first contact, school-age children or adolescents may be inhibited and withdrawn. The physician should avoid making premature judgments of the child's mental status or capacities under these circumstances.

The physician, by being unaggressive and friendly and keeping the conversation at the child's level (without condescension), can easily secure the child's cooperation and confidence. Toys may be given to the child, who is encouraged to talk while playing. Once engrossed, the child may begin talking spontaneously, or the physician may comment on the play activities.

A great deal can be learned about conflicts or anxieties by observing the child at play. A 4-year-old boy who creates a toy drama in which a smaller boy doll "beats up" a larger boy doll before "throwing it off a cliff" reveals much about his feelings toward his 6-year-old brother. It is wise not to make immediate interpretations of the child's feelings, however, to avoid causing anxiety. Later (in this example), the physician can bring up the child's feelings about his siblings, referring to the play incident and suggesting that maybe he feels "like that boy." Firm but kindly limits should be set on aggressive or destructive play.

With the child who can talk fairly freely, one can evaluate how well the patient understands the symptoms or disability in terms of its effect upon school performance, adjustment within the peer group, and the home situation. With frightened or withdrawn children, data of this sort may have to be sought indirectly by asking what they want to do when they grow up. If a school-age child cannot offer at least one possibility, it can be inferred that there are fears about "growing up." The child can be asked to make 3 wishes; a significantly depressed child may not be able to think of one. If an ill child does not include "getting well" as one of the wishes, there are usually conflicts about returning to school or other (perhaps unconscious) fears.

Sick children can be asked what they would do if they were well, or children who cannot talk easily about themselves can be asked what a hypothetical child ("Let's pretend we know a boy who . . .") should wish for or do in a particular situation. Most children cannot talk easily at first about their feelings toward their parents. With such an approach, most children from late preschool age onward can be helped to understand their symptoms or behavior as a problem or a worry that can be remedied.

Preadolescent and adolescent children are usually capable of understanding the reason for the interview and, if adequately prepared by the parents, may openly express a desire for help. If the parents have used the visit to the physician as a threat or punishment or if the child is present at the recommendation of school or judicial authorities, the physician should quickly clarify the situation with the youngster so that a therapeutic alliance can be established. Authoritarian strictures, lectures, and unsought advice are detrimental to such a relationship. Frightened adolescents should be put at ease. Hostile or defensive young people usually have reasons for their behavior, and a physician who can accept these attitudes nonjudgmentally is likely to discover the reasons. An open and neutral position and an evident desire to help will in time convince even the most cynical adolescent that the physician is sincere. (See also Chapter 9.)

A formal mental status examination is difficult in children and often insulting to adolescents. Clinical observations, questions about school, and asking the child to write his or her name or to draw a picture will usually provide sufficiently accurate impressions of attention span, orientation in time and place, and perceptual and motor functions. School-age children, when asked to draw a picture of a person, will usually draw a person of the same sex.

A rough estimate of intelligence may be obtained in a similar way. Pediatricians have demonstrated their capacity, in a controlled study, to make a surprisingly accurate evaluation of the developmental quotient of infants and young children. Their main errors lie in underestimating the capacities of sick children and overestimating the abilities of mentally retarded ones.

Most available tests of reading ability are complicated and lengthy. The physician should be familiar with first, second, and third grade readers and should have one of each available in case a reading problem is suspected. For adequate evaluation in the cognitive area, a clinical child psychologist is needed.

Observation of Child & Parent

From the moment the parent enters the office, valuable clinical impressions are available to the physician or to an alert nurse or secretary. Some parents cannot permit the child to answer a question independently, manifesting a need to dominate the child or the situation. Other parents constantly correct their child or demand conformity to impossibly high standards of conduct and behavior.

If the father and mother are interviewed together, they may disclose disagreements in child-rearing practices. Some parents pay little attention to their children, such as the mother who does not stand close to protect the infant from falling off the examining table. Parents with unconscious needs to deny the extent or seriousness of a child's obvious illness may take a belittling or bantering attitude toward its symptomatic expression and urge the child to run and play like other children do.

The physician should record such observations and test them against later impressions. Observations of this sort are most readily available to the physician who visits the home and enjoys continuity of contact with the parents and the child. The parents' standards of care and the patterns of family living are often more evident on a home visit than in the office.

Call JD: Psychiatric evaluation of the infant and child. Chap 33, pp 1615–1624, in: *Comprehensive Textbook of Psychiatry,* 4th ed. Kaplan HI, Sadock BJ (editors). Williams & Wilkins, 1985.

Gardner RA: *Therapeutic Communication With Children: The Mutual Storytelling Technique.* Jason Aronson, 1971.

Korsch BM: Pediatrician-patient relations. In: *Ambulatory Pediatrics,* 2nd ed. Green M, Haggerty RJ (editors). Saunders, 1976.

Prugh DG: General principles of clinical examination. In: *The Psychosocial Aspects of Pediatrics.* Lea & Febiger, 1983.

THE APPROACH TO PHYSICAL EXAMINATION OF THE CHILD

Preparation for the Examination

The physician can anticipate active participation by the child in the physical examination but must be prepared for resigned submission, passive resistance, or even active refusal and violent battle. The degree of rapport already established with the parent and child may determine the diagnostic success of the examination. If the child is seriously ill, the physical examination may be done while the latter portion of the history is being taken to save time and to decrease the suspense of the anxious child and the parent.

Refusal by preschool children to remove certain items of clothing may indicate anxiety over being so completely exposed rather than sexual modesty. This initial apprehension should be respected, and it is soon overcome. Older children may retain their underpants, which can be dropped for genital examination when they are more at ease.

A relaxed and unhurried approach is vital. A few moments spent in conversation, using the child's first name or nickname, may save time and struggle. Some explanation of each step, as in examining the throat or darkening the room for ophthalmoscopic examination, can be given quietly, using terms the child can understand.

Permitting young children to handle certain instruments such as the stethoscope before they are used (eg, listening to their own heartbeat) may overcome tension. "Blowing out" the light of the otoscope is a time-honored pediatric method of distracting toddlers from their apprehension about the examination.

Variations in Handling at Different Ages

A. Very Young Infants: With the very young infant, little difficulty is encountered if the parent is relaxed and trusting. Pacifiers may be used if the infant is crying or restless. Much of the examination may be performed while the parent holds and feeds the infant, affording the physician an opportunity to observe the feeding approach and the parent a chance to talk about the infant's clinical status or developmental progress.

B. Older Infants Up to 1½ Years of Age: In the second half of the first year, stranger or separation anxiety causes most infants to show some fear of the physician even if health examinations have been on a regular basis. The physician may hand the parent a tongue depressor or similar object to give to the infant sitting in the parent's lap, permitting the infant to appraise the physician from a safe vantage point. The infant who can crawl or toddle may later approach the physician and make friendly overtures.

The infant often resists being examined while supine or on the examining table, and it may be best to have the infant sitting on the parent's lap. The infant's head is then held against the parent's shoulder for examination of the ears and throat. The nurse may be able to obtain a more positive initial response from an older infant than the physician can.

C. Children 1½–3 Years of Age: During the normal period of negativism in the latter part of the second and early part of the third year, the child may refuse to cooperate with some parts of the examination such as "opening wide" for examination of the throat. Patience is required. A stubbornly negativistic child, diverted at this point to some other activity, may later abandon a rebellious stand. Physical battles inevitably result in the child's loss of trust in the physician.

D. Preschool Children: The preschool child can usually be examined on a table. Most children at this age are frightened when they are compelled to lie down and feel less anxious when they are sitting.

E. School-Age Children: Older preschool and school-age children will disclose much about how they feel about themselves and their bodies during the physical examination, including fears or misconceptions about the body and how it works and grows and concerns about minor blemishes. The child may raise these issues with a trusted physician, or the parents may ask about such matters if the examination is conducted in an unhurried and confiding manner.

F. Adolescents: With adolescents, feelings of modesty may become apparent during the examination. Such feelings should be respected, and these young people should be handled in the same way as adults. Fears may emerge in boys concerning growth lags or other real or imaginary deviations; in girls, concerning the onset of menses and the development of secondary sex characteristics. During the examination of girls of this age by a male physician, a female nurse should always be present. (See also Chapter 9.)

Parent Attendance

Some physicians prefer to exclude an anxious mother from the physical examination, recognizing that the child often submits more passively in her absence. This approach carries with it not only the pain of separation but also the implication of punishment by the physician. The parent may react with feelings of guilt or resentment, surmising that the physician thinks she is a poor parent. It is almost always best to permit the parent to remain with the infant or young child.

An apprehensive parent who asks to leave during the examination should usually be permitted to do so, but it is better that she leave before rather than during the examination. If the mother leaves the room, the child should be told where she will be and when she will return. If restraint is indicated, it should be carried out promptly, with a brief explanation of its need.

Precautions in Examination

The physician's hands and instruments should be warm, since any coldness to the touch may add to the child's fear or resistance. With younger children, examination of the ears and throat should be done last. Rectal temperatures may be resisted, in which case an axillary temperature reading will suffice. For children beyond infancy, rectal examinations should be performed with great care and gentleness and with adequate explanation. A "blowing" game may aid in securing cooperation during examination of the chest. Time spent in putting the child at ease will provide sufficient relaxation of the abdominal musculature for an accurate examination of the abdomen. Caution should be observed in the vaginal inspection of preadolescent or adolescent girls.

After the examination, the child should be given time to ask questions about procedures or instruments used or about any other phase of the examination. Plans for preparation of the child for further laboratory procedures, other medical or surgical experiences, or hospitalization should be considered.

The physician should always terminate the interview with a friendly and personal farewell to the child.

SPECIAL TESTS

Psychologic Tests

When properly administered by trained personnel, psychologic tests can be of great diagnostic assistance. Like laboratory tests, they must be interpreted in the light of the clinical findings. A single psychologic test, like a single laboratory test, may not be accurate, especially if the child is tired, sick, or anxious.

Intelligence testing is discussed in Chapter 7.

Electroencephalography

Although the older literature indicates that a large percentage of patients with emotional illnesses have abnormal EEGs, recent investigators have found a strikingly high incidence of so-called abnormal waves in normally developing children. For example, it was once thought that 14- and 6-per-second spikes were associated with behavioral disorders, but these wave patterns have also been found in normal children and adolescents. In one large study, well over half of children without symptoms showed these abnormalities, especially children 4–9 years of age. Many so-called abnormal waves may be better described as transient phenomena occurring during critical periods of integrative development in the central nervous system.

The EEG should be interpreted only as one of many factors in the clinical evaluation of the patient.

Preparation of the child for electroencephalographic testing is important, as the wires and machine may arouse fears of "electricity." The child may also need to be told that the machine is not a mind reader.

Metcalf DR, Jordan K: EEG ontogenesis in normal children. In: *Drugs, Development, and Cerebral Function*. Smith WL (editor). Thomas, 1971.

Osselton JW, Kiloh LG: *Clinical Electroencephalography*. Butterworth, 1961.

Prugh DG: Special methods of evaluation. In: *The Psychosocial Aspects of Pediatrics*. Lea & Febiger, 1983.

IMPLEMENTATION OF RESULTS OF THE CLINICAL EXAMINATION

After the physician has made a satisfactory appraisal of the child and the family, a plan of therapy or program of well child care should be set forth. In making recommendations for therapy, the physician's duty is to be confident and strong but at the same time appropriately humble, patient, and understanding of the parents' anguish or uncertainty. Explanations should be conveyed in language appropriate to the parents' sophistication and level of education, and detailed or complicated instructions should be in writing.

In discussing a child's emotional problem with the parents, the physician should not imply that they have "caused" it. The parents may suspect that the problem is an emotional one. If they initially thought the problem was a physical one, the physician can begin by reassuring them that there are no serious physical abnormalities. The doctor's opinion that the symptoms can be caused or aggravated by "emotional tension" can then be offered, and the parents can be asked whether they have noticed evidence of any such tension. The physician can indicate that such problems are "nobody's fault" and can suggest that there are ways of helping the child to overcome the difficulties. With help, the parents can be encouraged to think of things that should be done or things that they might, in retrospect, want to change about their ways of handling the child. Most parents will respond positively, after some initial defensiveness, to such an approach.

The child should also be given an explanation—in age-appropriate terms—of the clinical problems and the plans for management. Whether the parents should be present at this time depends on the child's age and other circumstances individually considered.

INDICATIONS FOR PSYCHIATRIC REFERRAL

The decision about which cases the pediatrician can treat and which should be referred to a child psychiatrist or child guidance clinic depends to a large extent on the pediatrician's interests and training. Of all health professionals, the pediatrician is in the best position to educate parents about the special problems of childhood and to help them handle ordinary behavior problems. However, some problems are simply not within the pediatrician's competence. In doubtful cases, consultation with a child psychiatrist is the best and safest course.

Criteria for Referral

The following criteria should be considered as guidelines for referral.

A. Home Environment: A severely handicapping home environment or seriously disturbed parents will generally warrant a prolonged relationship with mental health professionals.

B. Age Discrepancy: At certain ages, most children have outgrown particular habits or behavior. If they do not, psychiatric study may be indicated.

C. Intensity or Frequency of Symptoms: Under emotional or physical stress, most children may regress, but persistent regressive behavior may indicate psychologic fixations.

D. Degree of Social Disadvantage or Impairment: Certain modes of behavior tend to be self-perpetuating. For example, the aggressive child who makes many enemies has no choice but to continue to fight.

E. The Child's Inner Suffering: This is frequently overlooked by parents, teachers, and physicians, as with the well-behaved student who is not achieving.

F. Intractable Behavior: The persistence of symptoms despite the efforts of the child and others to change them is a cardinal clue to intrapsychic conflicts.

Preparation for Referral

Once it is decided that referral is necessary, the pediatrician can help to ensure a successful outcome by preparing the child and the parents for it. Parents may be afraid of the word psychiatry; may feel that they have failed as parents; or may fear that they will be lectured or condemned.

The physician must explain to the parents why the child needs help. It is best to discuss the symptoms in terms of the child's discomfort, as indications of ''lack of confidence'' or of being ''mixed up.''

The second step involves dealing with the parents' possible objections to psychiatric aid. Some parents need to be told that normal children can have emotional problems and that they need not fear that the child will be stigmatized. Parents need reassurance about the confidentiality of such matters. A sense of guilt may prevent them from accepting help or recognizing their own involvement. The physician must not argue with the parents and should explain that there are undoubtedly many important reasons for their child's difficulties.

The last step involves conveying a realistic understanding of what psychiatric therapy can accomplish. The physician should not make extravagant promises or concrete predictions but should convince the parents that help is both needed and available.

In talking with children, openness and honesty are essential. Children should be told where they are going, why, and what the basic problems are along the way.

Freud A: Assessment of childhood disturbances. *Psychoanal Study Child* 1962;**17:**149.

Moskowitz JA: The pediatrician calls for psychiatric referral: Notes on achieving a successful consultation. *Clin Pediatr* 1968;**7:**733.

Rae-Grant Q: The primary care and referrals of children with emotional and behavior disorders. Chap 30, pp 664–677, in: *Psychological Problems of the Child in His Family,* 2nd ed. Steinhauer PD, Rae-Grant Q (editors). Basic Books, 1983.

PSYCHOTHERAPY

There are several different schools of psychotherapy based on different frames of references, but the aims and methods of treatment tend to be similar in all. In some types of emotional problems, a supportive or directive approach is indicated; in others, the patient's defenses and life experiences need to be explored; and in still others, the therapeutic effect of allowing the patient to talk about (ventilate) disturbing feelings is of dominant importance. Psychotherapy may also be classified as interpretive, suggestive, persuasive, or educative or be characterized in terms of its depth, duration, and intensity. Isolating a single therapeutic element as a basis for classification is an artificial approach, since each of the factors listed is present in some degree in every psychotherapeutic relationship. The dimensions of psychotherapy are best described as a continuum extending from the supportive end, where little uncovering of deeper conflicts occur, to the insight-promoting end, in which ''operative'' or interpretative activity is predominant. (See also Chapter 9.)

Adams PL: *A Primer of Child Psychotherapy.* Little, Brown, 1974.

Harrison SI, Carek DJ: *A Guide to Psychotherapy.* Little, Brown, 1966.

Lord JP: *A Guide to Individual Psychotherapy With School-Age Children and Adolescents.* Thomas, 1985.

Prugh DG: The psychotherapeutic aspects of the role of the pediatrician. In: *The Psychosocial Aspects of Pediatrics.* Lea & Febiger, 1983.

Schaefer CE: *Therapeutic Use of Child's Play.* Jason Aronson, 1976.

Schaefer CE, Breismeister JM, Fitton MF (editors): *Family Therapy Techniques for Problem Behaviors of Children and Teenagers.* Jossey-Bass, 1984.

Swanson FL: *Psychotherapists and Children: A Procedural Guide.* Pitman, 1970.

PSYCHOPHARMACOLOGIC AGENTS

Psychoactive drugs play a significant role in the treatment of emotional disorders of childhood. They cannot replace the interpersonal relationship, which is the main tool of the physician, but they can be effective in reducing anxiety and overactivity. Reduction of impulsiveness and irritability is usually accompanied by less anxiety and improved attention span. On occasion, drug therapy can increase spontaneous activity and responsiveness in states of apathy and depression. The effects on complex behavior patterns, on the other hand, are much more difficult to predict during drug therapy.

There is no evidence that psychoactive drugs can improve intellectual functioning directly. Although it is possible to modify a child's responses to current experiences with drugs, they cannot undo previously learned behavior or alter neurotic patterns. Much information is still needed on the effects of specific drugs and their mode of action, as our knowledge remains largely empiric.

Principles of Drug Treatment

A. Drug and Diagnosis Must Be Matched: The condition of a disturbed child must be accurately diagnosed before the effective treatment can be given. An appropriate drug—eg, an antipsychotic tranquilizer—can help control behavior even in severe psychoses. With appropriate drug administration, some severely disturbed children may become amenable to psychotherapy. Although neurotic disorders rarely respond lastingly to drugs, some children with intrapsychic conflicts suffering from persistent anxiety, inhibitions, and phobias become more spontaneous and increase their adaptive functioning when given tranquilizing drugs.

Personality disorders and mental retardation are generally not benefited by drugs. Hyperkinesia may benefit from stimulant drugs. Reactive disorders rarely justify drug use except as sedation is necessary for cases of acute anxiety.

B. Benefit Should Exceed Toxicity: The physician who uses drugs should have a thorough knowledge of their pharmacologic properties, including their side effects and potential toxicity. The severity of the child's disorder and the potential for improvement must justify the possible impact of side effects and toxicity.

C. Use Special Precautions in Young Patients: Data cannot always be extrapolated from adult medicine to pediatrics. A child's response to a psychoactive drug may be quite different from that of an adult.

Special clinical testing of drugs potentially valuable for disturbed children is essential, as a drug's action may be other than predicted because of the immature and developing qualities of the child.

Dosage must be individualized for each patient, since undertreatment as well as overtreatment may result from metabolic differences at different ages. Dosage must be carefully regulated so as not to impair a child's intellectual acuity and maturation.

D. Use Familiar Drugs: A well-tested and familiar drug should be employed until a newer or unfamiliar one establishes its superiority. Unexpected toxicity from a less well known agent may not become apparent until it has been in general use for a long period.

E. Use Drugs Sparingly: Drugs should not be used any longer than necessary. Dosage should be reduced periodically to rate improvement or worsening of symptoms.

F. Seek Other Forms of Therapy: Since pharmacotherapy of emotional disorders affects symptoms rather than the underlying disease, the physician must continue attempts to identify and eliminate the physical, psychologic, and social factors causing the disturbance.

MAJOR TRANQUILIZERS

The major (''antipsychotic'') tranquilizers have been of greatest use in treating hospitalized, severely disturbed, or psychotic children because they exert a calming effect on agitated, impulsive, or excited states without causing paradoxic excitement or anesthesia. They can also reduce or eliminate delusions, hallucinations, and some schizophrenic ideation and thus make these children more communicative.

The dosage is increased at intervals of several days until a satisfactory response is obtained or until side effects limit further increases in dosage or force discontinuance of therapy. In acute situations, an initial parenteral dose may be given.

These agents should not be used to alleviate neurotic anxiety.

The major tranquilizers can be classified according to their chemical structure or pharmacologic properties.

Phenothiazine Derivatives & Similar Potent Drugs

The tranquilizers most commonly used are phenothiazine derivatives. Chlorprothixene (Taractan) is chemically and pharmacologically similar. Haloperidol (Haldol) is a butyrophenone comparable to the stimulant tranquilizers listed below but is not approved for use in patients under 12.

The phenothiazines can be further classified according to the degree of sedation induced and the likelihood of extrapyramidal side effects.

A. Sedation Prominent: The only important example is promethazine (Phenergan).

B. Standard Agents: Included are chlorpromazine (Thorazine) and thioridazine (Mellaril).

C. Stimulant Tranquilizers: These agents cause comparatively less sedation for the same therapeutic effect but are also more likely to cause extrapyramidal side effects. Trifluoperazine (Stelazine) and prochlorperazine (Compazine) are the important drugs in this group. Children are especially susceptible to side effects and may manifest violent dystonias or choreiform movements as well as tremors, rigidity, and akathisia. Parenteral administration should be avoided.

Other side effects are atropinelike or anticholinergic responses (constipation, blurred vision, dryness of the mouth, difficult micturition), postural hypotension, and lethargy or drowsiness. Endocrine abnormalities, skin changes (dermatitis, photosensitivity), and lowered body temperature are less common.

Rare cases of aplastic anemia and agranulocytosis have been reported. Cholangiolitic jaundice (intrahepatic obstruction) was once a common side effect of chlorpromazine administration but is now rare. Convulsions may occur when very high dosages are used or when epilepsy or other predisposition to convulsions is present. The ''seizures'' seen after accidental ingestion of stimulant tranquilizers are usually dystonias.

Toxicity or troublesome side effects can be managed by decreasing the dosage or changing to another drug. Extrapyramidal signs can usually be relieved by antiparkinsonism drugs.

Rauwolfia Alkaloids (Reserpine)

Reserpine has been replaced as a major tranquilizer by the phenothiazines, and its use is now limited to the treatment of hypertension. In addition to the side effects mentioned above, it causes nasal congestion, gastric hypersecretion, and diarrhea.

MINOR TRANQUILIZERS & SEDATIVES

This group of drugs is mainly employed as antianxiety agents, but they may have additional roles as sedatives and anticonvulsants. They have the following characteristics in common:

(1) A dose-related depressant effect on the central nervous system. Small doses will achieve sedation, relief of anxiety, and encouragement of normal sleep. Increasing doses lead to disinhibition and—commonly in children, especially in the presence of pain, anxiety, or restraint—to a paradoxic excitement. Even larger doses lead to general anesthesia and ultimately to medullary depression and death.

(2) Habituation and withdrawal. This occurs rarely in children, although misuse of secobarbital and other sedatives involves younger age groups each year.

Classification

These drugs can be classified according to their chemical structure, but it is more useful to classify them according to rapidity of action and duration of effect. Those with a rapid onset of action have a short effect, and those with a longer latent period have a correspondingly prolonged effect.

A. Short-Acting: Pentobarbital, secobarbital, chloral hydrate, paraldehyde, diphenhydramine.

B. Intermediate-Acting: Amobarbital; the benzodiazepines such as diazepam (Valium), chlordiazepoxide (Librium), and flurazepam (Dalmane); a propanediol carbamate such as meprobamate (Equanil, Miltown); and the piperidinediones such as glutethimide (Doriden).

C. Long-Acting: Phenobarbital, mephobarbital (Mebaral), oxazepam (Serax).

Actions

Barbiturates mimic the effects of alcohol. They suppress the higher control centers and may have a mild euphoriant or depressant effect as well as adversely affecting psychomotor coordination. The barbiturates are addicting and are often used as a means of suicide. Tolerance develops easily, so that increasing doses are required to procure equivalent effects.

In terms of drug management, compared to the propanediol family of drugs and the barbiturates, the benzodiazepines are less depressing to the central nervous system vital center and therefore have less potential for use in suicide attempts. An additional advantage of the benzodiazepines over the barbiturates is that the margin between the therapeutic and sedative doses is wider, allowing greater latitude in establishing optimal therapeutic doses.

STIMULANTS

Stimulants have been found to be effective in the treatment of children who are hyperactive. There is a syndrome in young children that is characterized by a chronic history of short attention span, emotional lability, impulsiveness, and moderate to severe hyperactivity. "Soft" neurologic signs, abnormal EEG, and learning problems may also be present. Drugs are not indicated for all such children, and least of all for those whose symptoms are related to environmental factors. Although some hyperactive children with chronic or acute anxiety may respond to stimulants, care should be taken not to regard drug therapy as the only resource that can be offered. The decision to prescribe medication will depend upon an assessment of the chronicity and severity of the symptoms.

Treatment of school-age children with either dextroamphetamine or methylphenidate (Ritalin) is initiated with 5 mg at breakfast and lunch, increasing by 5-mg increments every several days until improvement occurs or side effects (anorexia or insomnia) appear. Daily dosages of up to 30 mg of dextroamphetamine and 40 mg of methylphenidate may be needed. Frequent consultations with the classroom teacher will help determine the drug's effectiveness and permit dosage adjustments. If after 2 weeks no noticeable improvement has occurred, the drug should be discontinued.

Caution should be exercised in the use of stimulants with children under 6 years of age.

If effective, these drugs can be employed until puberty, when they are usually no longer necessary and when abuse can more readily occur.

Alexandris A, Lundell F: Effect of thioridazine, amphetamine, and placebo on hyperkinetic syndrome and cognitive area in mentally deficient children. *Can Med Assoc J* 1968;**98:**92.

Charlton MH: Use of Ritalin in hyperactive children. *NY State J Med* 1972;**2:**2058.

Connors CK, Eisenberg L, Barcai A: Effect of dextroamphetamine on children: Studies on subjects with learning disabilities and school behavior problems. *Arch Gen Psychiatry* 1967;**17:**478.

ANTIDEPRESSANTS & LITHIUM

Whether the antidepressant drugs (tricyclics, monoamine oxidase inhibitors) will find a place in pediatric practice has not been established. The types of depression treated successfully with these drugs in adults do not occur as clearly in children and adolescents. Imipramine and other drugs in this group can have serious toxic effects.

On the other hand, there is some evidence in the literature that lithium has been effective in the treatment of bipolar type (manic-depressive) disorders, which do occur, though rarely, in adolescence. Lithium is useful for the acute manic phase as well as serving as a modulator for the highs and lows characteristic of the bipolar patient. Lithium can be lethal if given without careful patient selection, adequate clinical control, and frequent determination of serum lithium levels.

Herreno FA: Lithium carbonate toxicity. *JAMA* 1973;**266:**1109.

Prugh DG: Psychopharmacologic treatment. In: *The Psychosocial Aspects of Pediatrics.* Lea & Febiger, 1983.

Stallone F et al: The use of lithium in affective disorders. 3. A double-blind study of prophylaxis in bipolar illness. *Am J Psychiatry* 1973;**130:**1006.

Werry JS: An overview of pediatric psychopharmacology. *J Am Acad Child Psychiatry* 1982;**21:**3.

Wiener J (editor): *Diagnosis and Psychopharmacology of Childhood and Adolescent Disorders.* Wiley, 1985.

THE PEDIATRICIAN & OTHER SERVICES IN THE COMMUNITY

The pediatrician can contribute to the early treatment and in some cases prevention of some major current social issues. Such problems as adoption, disturbed families, delinquency, child battering, illegitimate pregnancies, and homicide can be partially solved or prevented by the kind of early intervention the pediatrician is in a position to offer. Physicians responsible for the care of children should be familiar with the mental health, family service, and other agencies in their communities and should use them when necessary.

Pediatricians may act as coordinators of the contributions of other professionals in the health team, as in a comprehensive approach to the management of children in a hospital ward. In the community, they may act as consultants to nursery schools, public schools, courts, camps, social agencies, or child guidance clinics. They can also use their influence to promote the development of needed mental health resources, which may aid them and other health professionals in preventing emotional disorders and other types of unhealthy adaptation and personality development. (See also Chapter 9.)

PSYCHOTHERAPEUTIC ASPECTS OF THE ROLE OF THE PEDIATRICIAN

Various aspects of the psychotherapeutic role of the pediatrician in dealing with children and their parents include, among others, emotionally supportive contacts during the prenatal period; later, helping the parents to promote the child's healthy personality development; and preparation of the child and parents for potentially stressful experiences such as hospitalization or surgery.

Some aspects of supportive psychotherapy the pediatrician can use in dealing with parents, older children, and adolescents have already been mentioned. In working with parents of children with mild psychologic disorders or with chronic illnesses or handicaps, the pediatrician can provide emotional support. Parents can more easily ventilate their feelings and develop spontaneous insights if they are offered help in clarifying conflicting feelings or gently confronted with apparent inconsistencies in their attitudes.

The pediatrician may reflect feelings back to the parents by repeating emotion-laden words, offering them an opportunity to explore conflicts further, at times verbalizing for them certain feelings or thoughts. Advice, counseling, or help in working through feelings already recognized should be made available, particularly in the case of serious illness. Suggestion and persuasion can be used to foster constructive changes in the parents' attitudes and behavior.

The use of toys and play interviews can help younger children to clarify their fears, confusion, or conflicts, offering them a chance to discharge tension or master anxieties through "playing out" their feelings.

Verbal discussion and counseling can be helpful for older children and adolescents if they can talk easily, but improvement may often occur on a nonverbal level as a result of patients' perceptions of the pediatrician's attitudes toward them and their parents.

Confidentiality of the older child's or adolescent's intimate revelations should be maintained and explained to the parents. Exceptions should be made only with the young person's knowledge and only when obviously necessary, such as a potential suicide attempt or serious delinquency.

Young patients may transfer attitudes or feelings toward key figures from past experience onto the pediatrician. Being aware of the origin of these transferences should enable the pediatrician to deal with them without taking any of it personally. If the pediatrician commonly responds with anger or frustration to certain types of behavior, those responses should be examined critically in the light of the physician's own experiences to determine whether a countertransference phenomenon is operating.

The pediatrician may sometimes employ family interviews, especially if communication between parents and child or adolescent seems blocked. An active, directive approach is needed in such situations to help the family maintain control and avoid explosive releases of hostile feelings. Group discussions, often with the aid of a social worker or other mental health professional, may be of value for parents of chronically ill children or for adolescents with hemophilia, diabetes, or other chronic disorders. They also may be employed with groups of parents of well children in a kind of "child study" approach.

Bolian GC: Diagnosis and treatment: Psychosocial aspects of well child care. *Pediatrics* 1967;**39:**280.

Coddington RD: The use of brief psychotherapy in a pediatric practice. *J Pediatr* 1962;**60:**259.

Prugh DG: The psychotherapeutic aspects of the role of the pediatrician. In: *The Psychosocial Aspects of Pediatrics.* Lea & Febiger, 1983.

Prugh DG, Eckhardt LO: Guidance by physicians and nurses: A developmental approach. In: *Helping Parents Help Their Children.* Arnold LE (editor). Brunner/Mazel, 1978.
Shulman JL: The management of the irate parent. *J Pediatr* 1970;**77**:338.

SPECIFIC CLINICAL DISORDERS

Although the definition of normality in development and behavior has a certain relativity because of individual variations and different cultural settings, an assessment of healthy behavioral responses can be made.

Appropriateness of behavior to the age of the child or stage of development is a basic consideration, and the same is true of the balance of progressive versus regressive forces and the general "smoothness" of development. The latter includes the clinician's assessment of the child's adaptation in the present as well as mastery of stresses in the past. Such considerations may be modified in accordance with the child's endowment and current developmental level, the nature of the stresses in the particular family and social setting, and other factors.

The following classification is that offered in the *Diagnostic and Statistical Manual of Mental Disorders (DSM-III),* the official classification adopted in 1980 by the American Psychiatric Association. In previous editions, the classification of emotional and mental disorders offered by the Committee on Child Psychiatry of the Group for Advancement of Psychiatry (GAP) has been used. In the material to follow, the major headings are retained from the GAP classification, but the diagnoses are drawn from *DSM-III,* which is the first official classification to contain a section on "Disorders Usually First Seen in Infancy, Childhood, or Adolescence." Healthy responses do not appear in the *DSM-III* classification. In *DSM-III,* a new principle of evaluation requires that every case be assessed on several axes, each of which refers to a different class of information. Specific criteria for diagnoses are spelled out in *DSM-III,* and a number of symptoms, such as those of substance abuse and kleptomania, are included among the diagnostic categories. If the physician uses *DSM-III* to make a diagnosis for insurance purposes, it is wise to consult with a child psychiatrist.

HEALTHY RESPONSES

1. DEVELOPMENTAL CRISES

Developmental crises are brief and transient upheavals that are related to a particular developmental stage and involve attempts to resolve appropriate psychosocial tasks. The child appears normal except for the manifestations of the developmental crisis.

Examples include "stranger" and "separation" anxieties of the second half of the first year, related to the capacity of the infant to distinguish between the mother and others. Anxiety, oppositional behavior, and other manifestations are most marked when developmental tasks are normally most demanding, as when the young child is first separated from the parent.

Treatment consists of a supportive counseling approach to help the child master the crisis and move on to the next stage of development. Anticipatory counseling of the parents is helpful so that they will not handle the child too permissively or too punitively at such times. Inappropriately handled, a developmental crisis may become a reactive disorder (see below) or may crystallize into a psychoneurotic or personality disorder. If a developmental crisis comes too early or too late, it may represent a developmental deviation.

2. SITUATIONAL CRISES

Situational crises are usually transient and brief and are related to situations in the family or environment that represent acutely stressful circumstances for a particular child. The resulting behavioral problems appear to be normal adaptive responses to crisis situations and not deeply disturbed behavior. The child appears normal on examination except for the behavioral response to the crisis situation.

Examples of situational crises include the death of a parent or other serious family crisis and the mild regression that may occur upon return from the hospital after a tonsillectomy. Depression may be apparent in grief reactions. Depressive equivalents may be manifested by temporary loss of appetite, sleep disturbances, or change in activity level. Regression is often characterized by a transient refusal to speak in infants or loss of bowel and bladder control in toddlers.

Treatment is primarily supportive, since the crises are self-limited. Anticipatory guidance of the parents and preventive measures such as preparation of the child and parents for hospitalization can be vital.

Prolonged stressful circumstances with inadequate parental response can lead to reactive disorders or more structured psychopathologic disorders.

Erikson EH: *Childhood and Society,* 2nd ed. Norton, 1963.
Friedman SB: Management of death in a parent or sibling. In: *Ambulatory Pediatrics,* 2nd ed. Green M, Haggerty RJ (editors). Saunders, 1976.
Lewis M: *Clinical Aspects of Child Development,* 2nd ed. Lea & Febiger, 1982.
Prugh DG: Healthy responses. In: *The Psychosocial Aspects of Pediatrics.* Lea & Febiger, 1983.
Sugar M: Children of divorce. *Pediatrics* 1970;**46**:588.

REACTIVE DISORDERS

In *DSM-III*, the term "reactive disorders" is not used. Instead, some disorders of this type are included in the childhood section of the classification under the headings of "reactive attachment disorder of infancy," "separation anxiety disorder," "avoidant disorder of childhood or adolescence," "overanxious disorder," and "atypical eating disorder." The childhood section also includes diagnoses for "other disorders with physical manifestations" (such as encopresis, enuresis, and sleep terrors), "conduct disorder," "attention deficit disorder" (with or without hyperactivity), and "identity disorder." In the adult section, diagnoses can be found for "posttraumatic stress disorder" and "adjustment disorder" (with depressed or anxious mood, disturbance of conduct, mixed emotional features, work or academic inhibition, withdrawal, and atypical features). Open depressive disorders of a reactive nature can only be diagnosed in the adult section under "major affective disorders" as "major depression" (single episode or recurrent). Categories such as "academic problem," "childhood or adolescent antisocial behavior," "parent-child problem" (which includes child abuse), "other specified family circumstances," and "other interpersonal problem" are categorized in *DSM-III* under "Codes for Conditions Not Attributable to a Mental Disorder That Are a Focus of Attention or Treatment."

Pathologic behavior or symptoms may occur in response to disturbing events or situations. They are usually transient but may develop into more severe and chronic problems. Such responses are most common in preschool and early school-age children. The child is usually normal on examination but may have had previous adaptive difficulties.

The reactive disorders differ from situational crises in the matter of degree. A disturbing situation arising acutely may have a profound effect. Examples include illness and hospitalization, accidents, loss of a parent, school pressures, and parental behavior problems. The important consideration is not the strength of the stimulus but the intensity of the child's reaction, which is a function of ego development, adaptive capacity, past experience, and original endowment. Psychophysiologic disorders such as peptic ulcer or ulcerative colitis may be precipitated in the predisposed youngster. Depression or regressive behavior may include withdrawal, thumb-sucking, wetting or soiling, or excessive daydreaming and preoccupation with fantasy. Acting-out behavior may occur.

Treatment is similar to that of situational crisis: supportive counseling for the parents, with anticipatory guidance and clarification of misconceptions, and emotional support for the child. "Replacement" therapy in the hospital, with the use of parent substitutes or liberalized visiting hours, will help to compensate for emotional deprivation. In some cases, a reactive disorder may be superimposed upon a psychoneurosis, a personality disorder, or even a chronic psychosis of moderate severity. Such disorders involving temporary arrest in development may evolve into a developmental deviation or psychoneurosis, and formal intensive psychotherapy may be necessary.

Reactive disorders in preschool children involving anxiety, regressive behavior, and mild depression or regressive enuresis, encopresis, and thumb-sucking may occur following hospitalization and surgery. These disorders can be prevented by telling parents and children what to expect during hospitalization, by daily visits and overnight stays by parents once the child is hospitalized, and by the use of outpatient treatment facilities or motel facilities by parents. Education of parents and frequent parental visits can also prevent reactive attachment disorders of infancy. Some milder cases of regressive encopresis and enuresis, atypical eating disorders, conduct disorders, posttraumatic stress disorders, and adjustment disorders will respond to counseling of the child and parents by the pediatrician. More severe cases and marked reactive depressions will respond only to psychotherapy. Attention deficit disorders with hyperactivity will often respond to stimulant drugs as part of a comprehensive approach; special remedial education is indicated for those with or without hyperactivity.

Kaplan DM: Study and treatment of an acute emotional disorder. *Am J Orthopsychiatry* 1965;**35:**69.

Prugh DG: Reactive disorders. In: *The Psychosocial Aspects of Pediatrics.* Lea & Febiger, 1983.

DEVELOPMENTAL DEVIATIONS

In the Group for Advancement of Psychiatry (GAP) classification, developmental deviations are regarded as becoming manifest over a period of months or years as innate characteristics of the child's development. Single dimensions of development may be involved (eg, motor, sensory, speech, or cognitive functions; social development; psychosexual development; affective or emotional development; and integrative development), or deviations may be characterized by lags, unevenness, or precocities in maturational steps. Deviations in maturational patterns such as the capacity for control of rhythmic integration in bodily functions are also included. In the childhood section of *DSM-III,* only "specific developmental disorders," such as reading, arithmetic, language, and articulation disorders, can be diagnosed. "Separation anxiety disorder" and "identity disorder" (including "gender identity disorder") in the childhood section of *DSM-III* may also be regarded as developmental deviations, as may certain cases of "psychosexual disorder" included in the adult section.

Types of Developmental Deviations

A. Motor Development: Examples are hyperactivity, hypoactivity, incoordination, and handedness, along with other predominantly motor capacities, where brain damage is not involved.

B. Sensory Development: Difficulty in monitoring stimuli from tactile to social in nature. Affected children may overreact or be apathetic to stimuli.

C. Speech Development: Significant delays other than those due to deafness, oppositional behavior, elective mutism, brain damage, or early childhood psychosis. Disorders of articulation, rhythm, or phonation or an infantile type of speech comprehension may be evident. Normal word repetition by a healthy child in the preschool phase and stuttering as a conversion symptom are not included in this group.

D. Cognitive Function: Problems of symbolic or abstract thinking such as reading, writing, and arithmetic. "Pseudoretarded" and significantly precocious youngsters are in this category.

E. Social Development: Examples are delayed tolerance for separation from the mother, marked shyness, dependence, inhibitions, and immaturely aggressive behavior.

F. Psychosexual Development: Examples are timing of sexual curiosity, persistence of infantile autoerotic patterns, and markedly precocious or delayed heterosexual interests.

G. Affective (Emotional) Development: The child may show moderate anxiety, emotional lability not appropriate to age, marked overcontrol of emotions, mild depression or apathy, and cyclothymic behavior.

H. Integrative Development: Lack of impulse control or frustration tolerance and uneven use or overuse of defense mechanisms (eg, projection or denial).

Treatment

In many developmental deviations, no formal treatment is necessary. Explanation to the parents of the nature of the deviation may suffice, and anticipatory guidance for the parents and counseling for the child are often helpful. Psychotherapy may be necessary in cases involving sweeping lags in maturational patterns or developing personality disturbances. It may also be necessary for marked separation anxiety disorders, identity disorders, or disorders in psychosexual development.

Stimulant drugs may be useful for a child with marked hyperactivity enhanced by overcontrolling parental responses; psychotherapy may be necessary in addition. Special remedial education is indicated for developmental reading and arithmetic disorders and other cognitive lags, as is speech therapy for language and articulation disorders and lags in speech development.

Baker L, Cantwell DP: Developmental articulation disorder. In: *Comprehensive Textbook of Psychiatry,* 4th ed. Kaplan HI, Sadock BJ (editors). Williams & Wilkins, 1985.

Baker L, Cantwell DP: Developmental language disorder. In: *Comprehensive Textbook of Psychiatry,* 4th ed. Kaplan HI, Sadock BJ (editors). Williams & Wilkins, 1985.

Cantwell DP: Developmental arithmetic disorder. In: *Comprehensive Textbook of Psychiatry,* 4th ed. Kaplan HI, Sadock BJ (editors). Williams & Wilkins, 1985.

Chess S: Individuality in children: Its importance to the pediatrician. *J Pediatr* 1966;**69**:676.

Jansky JJ: Developmental reading disorder. In: *Comprehensive Textbook of Psychiatry,* 4th ed. Kaplan HI, Sadock BJ (editors). Williams & Wilkins, 1985.

Malone C: Developmental deviations considered in the light of environmental factors. In: *The Drifters.* Pavenstedt E (editor). Little, Brown, 1967.

Prugh DG: Developmental deviations. In: *The Psychosocial Aspects of Pediatrics.* Lea & Febiger, 1983.

Thomas A, Chess S: *Temperament and Development.* Brunner/Mazel, 1977.

PSYCHONEUROTIC DISORDERS

Psychoneurotic disorders are ordinarily chronic and structured in nature, pervading the whole personality. They are characterized by psychologic symptoms (free-floating anxiety, obsessive thoughts, and phobias) that can be crippling. They arise from the child's internalized unconscious conflicts, often with apparent reference to current family situations.

Psychoneuroses in flagrant form are not common before early school age. No gross disturbances in reality testing are observed in spite of the apparent irrationality of the child's fears or other symptoms. As indicated in *DSM-III,* diagnoses of neurotic disorders are included in the adult section under "affective," "anxiety," "somatoform," "dissociative," and "psychosexual disorders" (the latter including homosexuality, transsexualism, and gender identity disorder of childhood).

Types of Psychoneuroses in the Pediatric Age Group

A. Anxiety Type: These disorders are included under "anxiety disorders" in the adult section of *DSM-III.* The conflict breaks into awareness as an intense and diffuse feeling of apprehension or impending disaster—in contrast to normal apprehensions, conscious fears, or content-specific phobias. The physiologic concomitants of anxiety, in contrast to psychophysiologic disorders, do not lead to structural changes in involved organ systems.

B. Phobic Type: These disorders are categorized under "anxiety disorders" in the adult section of *DSM-III.* There is unconscious displacement onto an object or situation in the external environment that has symbolic significance for the child. Examples are fear of animals, school, dirt, disease, or elevators. Phobias, with their internalized and structured character, should be distinguished from developmental crises involving separation anxiety and the mild fears and transient phobias associated with stressful experiences in reactive disorders. School phobias are discussed below.

C. Conversion Type: These disorders are included under "somatoform disorders" in the adult section of *DSM-III.* Tics, which are ordinarily considered to be conversion disorders, are included in the childhood section under "stereotyped movement disorders" (transient, chronic, and atypical tic disorders). Tourette's disorder and "atypical stereotyped movement disorder" are also included in this category. The original conflict is expressed as a somatic dysfunction of organs supplied by the voluntary portion of the central nervous system—usually the striated musculature or somatosensory apparatus. Included are disturbances of motor function, as in paralysis or motor tics; alterations in sensory perception, as in cases of blindness or deafness; disturbances in awareness, as in conversion syncope or convulsivelike phenomena; and disturbances in the total body image, as in psychologic invalidism associated with extreme weakness or bizarre paralyses. The following may also be conversion expressions: dysfunctions of the upper and lower ends of the gastrointestinal tract, as in certain types of vomiting or encopresis; of the voluntary components of respiration, as in hyperventilation and respiration (coughing or barking); and of the genitourinary organs, as in certain types of enuresis or bladder atony. Electroencephalographic changes are nonspecific, and local structural abnormalities have not been demonstrated except those secondary to long-standing conversions. Personality disorders and borderline psychoses may be associated and may justify multiple diagnoses.

D. Dissociative Type: These disorders are included in the adult section of *DSM-III* as "dissociative disorders." Included in this category are fugue states, cataplexy, transient catatonic states without underlying psychosis, and conditions with aimless motor discharge or "freezing." Disturbances in consciousness may occur with hypnagogic or hypnopompic or so-called twilight states, marked somnambulism, and pseudodelirious and stuporous states. Depersonalization, dissociated or multiple personalities (in late adolescence), amnesia, Ganser's syndrome (in adolescence), and pseudopsychotic states or "hysterical psychoses" may be present episodically. Although a hysterical personality may be involved, other psychopathologic disorders may be present also. Panic states (usually reactive disorders), acute brain syndromes, psychotic conditions, and epileptic equivalents must be differentiated.

E. Obsessive-Compulsive Type: These disorders are included under "anxiety disorders" in the adult section of *DSM-III*. They are characterized by various rituals such as excessive orderliness and washing compulsions, with marked anxiety if there is interference by the parents or others. Disorders must be distinguished from the normal ritualism in early childhood associated with bedtime or toilet training or pseudocompulsive rituals in the early school years.

F. Depressive Type: In *DSM-III*, these disorders are included in the adult section under "major affective disorders" in the category of "major depression" (single episode or recurrent). They are often expressed differently in children than in adults. Symptoms include eating and sleeping disturbances and hyperactivity. Chronic depressive disorders are modified by the child's stage of development and must be distinguished from the more acute reactive disorders in which depression may be involved (eg, the anaclitic type). Depression may be a component of any clinical problem from developmental crisis to psychosis. (See also Chapter 9.)

Treatment

Treatment may be minimal (eg, supportive counseling), since some mild psychoneurotic disorders resolve spontaneously. However, intensive psychotherapy for parents and child is often required and is usually successful, especially in the anxiety, phobic, conversion, and depressive types. Severe obsessive-compulsive and dissociative disorders often require child analysis.

Tranquilizing agents are of limited value but may be used to control free-floating anxiety.

Adams PL: Family characteristics of obsessive children. *Am J Psychiatry* 1972;**128:**1414.

Enzer NB, Walker PA: Hyperventilation syndrome in childhood. *J Pediatr* 1967;**70:**521.

Friedman SB: Conversion symptoms in adolescents. *Pediatr Clin North Am* 1973;**20:**873.

Goodwin DW et al: Follow-up studies in obsessional neurosis. *Arch Gen Psychiatry* 1969;**20:**182.

Lucas AR: Gilles de la Tourette's disease: An overview. *NY State J Med* 1970;**70:**2197.

Malmquist CP: Depression in childhood and adolescence. *N Engl J Med* 1971;**284:**955.

Poznanski EO, Krahenbuhl V, Zrull JP: Childhood depression: A longitudinal perspective. *J Am Acad Child Psychiatry* 1976;**15:**491.

Prugh DG: Psychoneurotic disorders. In: *The Psychosocial Aspects of Pediatrics*. Lea & Febiger, 1983.

Rachman S, Costello CG: The etiology and treatment of children's phobias: A review. In: *Childhood Psychopathology: An Anthology of Basic Readings*. Harrison S, McDermott J (editors). Internat Univ Press, 1972.

Rock NL: Conversion reactions in childhood. *J Am Acad Child Psychiatry* 1971;**10:**65.

Werkman SL: Anxiety disorders. In: *Comprehensive Textbook of Psychiatry*, 4th ed. Kaplan HI, Sadock BJ (editors). Williams & Wilkins, 1985.

PERSONALITY DISORDERS

This category is retained in *DSM-III* in the adult portion of the classification. The subcategories include "paranoid"; "schizoid"; "schizotypal"; "histrionic" (hysterical); "narcissistic"; "antisocial"; "borderline"; "avoidant"; "dependent"; "compulsive"; "passive-aggressive"; and "atypical, mixed or other personality disorder."

In children and adolescents, personality disorders do not assume the full-blown character seen in adults; thus, the terms "compulsive," "hysterical," "anxious," "overly dependent," "overly independent," "oppositional," "overly inhibited," "isolated," "mistrustful," "tension discharge," "sociosyntonic," and "sexual deviation" are more characteristic. Personality disorders involving fixed sexual deviation may properly be regarded as "psychosexual disorders," a category in the adult section of *DSM-III*. Borderline psychotic personality disorders are also seen in childhood.

Personality disorders in childhood (not commonly seen in flagrant form before late school age) are usually chronic and structured in nature, pervading the child's entire personality. They are manifested as chronic or fixed pathologic behavioral characteristics derived from responses to earlier conflicts that have become ingrained in the personality structure rather than psychologic symptom formation. No gross distortion in reality testing is observed in spite of the apparent irrationality of the child's behavior.

In discussing these disorders, the concept of a continuum is useful. At one end are the relatively well organized personalities with, for example, constructively compulsive traits or somewhat overdependent features, representing mild to moderate exaggerations of healthy personality trends. These may blend into the environment and may pass almost unnoticed unless the interpersonal network of relationships suddenly or radically changes. At the other end are markedly impulsive, sometimes poorly organized personalities that dramatically come into conflict with society as a result of their sexual or social patterns of behavior.

Symptom formation of a psychoneurotic nature is rarely seen, and in most cases the traits are not perceived by the child as a source of anxiety. Premonitory patterns are often seen during infancy and early childhood as fixations in early psychosexual and psychosocial development.

Treatment & Prognosis

Treatment and prognosis vary according to severity. In its milder forms, the disorder may offer sublimatory outlets (eg, compulsiveness may make for good work habits). More severe forms are more crippling and interfere with effective academic or social functions (eg, delinquency, poor impulse control) or conflict with a new social setting (eg, transfer to new school in large city).

While counseling of children and parents may be sufficient in cases of mild disorders of the obsessive, hysterical, anxious, overly dependent, oppositional, or overly inhibited types, intensive psychotherapy on an outpatient basis is usually necessary for more severe disorders, including the true sexual deviations. Day hospitalization programs with a psychoeducational approach or special classes are indicated if associated learning difficulties are present.

Children with moderate to severe isolated, mistrustful, or impulse-ridden personality types generally require intensive treatment on a residential basis. This is particularly the case when delinquency and drug or alcohol problems are involved. A residential setting, whether it be a hospital, cottage type group living setting, group foster home, or treatment-oriented correctional institution, should provide warmth, structure, consistent limits, and positive psychotherapeutic relationships with a well-trained staff who have adequate mental health consultation services available. (See also Chapter 9.)

Lewis DO: Conduct disorder and juvenile delinquency. In: *Comprehensive Textbook of Psychiatry,* 4th ed. Kaplan HI, Sadock BJ (editors). Williams & Wilkins, 1985.

Prugh DG: Personality disorders. In: *The Psychosocial Aspects of Pediatrics*. Lea & Febiger, 1983.

Vaillant GE, Perry JC: Personality disorders. Chap 21, pp 958–986, in: *Comprehensive Textbook of Psychiatry,* 4th ed. Kaplan HI, Sadock BJ (editors). Williams & Wilkins, 1985.

Zuger B: Effeminate behavior present in boys from early childhood. 1. The clinical syndrome and follow-up studies. *J Pediatr* 1966;**69:**1098.

PSYCHOTIC DISORDERS

In *DSM-III,* a category of "pervasive developmental disorders" is included in the childhood section, with subcategories for "infantile autism," "childhood-onset pervasive developmental disorder," and "atypical" types. Interactional psychotic disorders are not included. "Schizophreniform disorder," encountered in school-age children, is listed under "Psychotic Disorders Not Elsewhere Classified" in the adult section. "Schizophrenic disorders," seen in adolescence, are also listed in the adult section. "Brief reactive psychosis" and "atypical psychosis," seen also in adolescence, are included in the adult section. Acute confusional states do not appear in *DSM-III*. Manic-depressive ("bipolar disorder, mixed") and paranoid psychotic disorders, seen only in late adolescence, can be diagnosed in the adult section.

Psychoses may be of sudden or gradual onset in infancy, childhood, or adolescence, with differences in the clinical picture in relation to developmental level. The essential features are failure to develop awareness of or withdrawal from reality, with preoccupation with inner fantasy life; failure to develop emotional relationships with human figures, or retreat from established relationships; inability to express emotions appropriately or to use speech communicatively; and bizarre, stereotyped, or otherwise seriously inappropriate behavior.

Hallucinations and delusions, as well as other classic characteristics of adult psychoses, are rarely encountered until late school age or early adolescence.

Obsessions, compulsions, phobias, and other psychologic or behavioral symptoms may occur in psychotic children. They are markedly intense and tenacious, and the child usually has no awareness of their lack of logic or appropriateness. Biologic predisposing factors are involved.

Type of Psychoses in the Pediatric Age Group

A. Psychoses of Early Childhood:

1. Early infantile autism—This must be distinguished from autism secondary to brain damage or mental retardation. The onset is within the first year of life, and the child remains aloof from all human contact, being preoccupied with inanimate objects. The child resists any change with outbursts of temper or anxiety when routines are altered. Speech is delayed or absent, and sleep and feeding problems are severe. Intellectual functioning is restricted or uneven, probably related to perceptual and communication problems.

2. Pervasive developmental disorder, childhood onset—These disorders of infancy and early childhood include the so-called symbiotic psychoses. The problem revolves around the failure of the youngster to master the step of separation and individuation, often because of the mother's inability to allow the child to separate from her. The psychotic disorder is often precipitated in the second to fourth years by some shift in the mother-child relationship such as the birth of a sibling or a family crisis. The overdependent child then shows intense separation anxiety and clinging, with regressive manifestations. The picture is one of gradual withdrawal, emotional aloofness, autistic behavior, and distorted perception of reality.

3. Atypical psychotic disorders—Other psychoses of early childhood include "atypical" or fragmented ego development in children who exhibit some autistic behavior and emotional aloofness.

B. Psychoses of Later Childhood: Schizophreniform psychotic disorders occur in the school-age period and are characterized by a gradual onset of neurotic symptoms followed by concrete thinking, loose associations, hypochondriacal tendencies, and intense temper outbursts. Later developments may include a breakdown in reality testing, autism, anxiety, and uncontrollable phobias. Bizarre behavior and stereotyped motor patterns, such as whirling, are often observed. Other children may have sudden and wild outbursts of aggressive or self-mutilating behavior, inappropriate mood swings, and suicide threats or attempts. Organic brain syndromes and severe panic states with a temporary thought disorder due to anxiety require careful differential assessment.

C. Psychoses of Adolescence:

1. Acute confusional state—This is a "psychosis" of adolescence with an abrupt onset of acute and intense anxiety, depressive trends, confusion in thinking, and feelings of depersonalization. The crisis of identity is very common, but evidence of a true thought disorder or marked breakdown in reality testing is usually lacking. While rapid recovery is the rule, a deep-seated personality disorder may underlie the psychotic picture. Differential considerations include neurotic panic states and the severe upsets seen in normal adolescents.

2. Adult types of schizophrenia—These occur in late adolescence, with minor differences related to the developmental level. Manifestations include the myriad symptoms seen in adults.

3. Other psychotic disorders—These include brief reactive psychoses, often characterized by sweeping regression in a number of dimensions of personality functioning but without true thought disorders. Such disorders have an excellent prognosis in terms of response to hospitalization and treatment. Atypical psychoses include Ganser's syndrome (syndrome of "approximate answers"), which also has a very good prognosis when seen in adolescence.

Treatment & Prognosis

Treatment and prognosis vary considerably. The psychotic disorders of early childhood have a more guarded prognosis.

A. Young Children: Patients with early infantile autism have a guarded prognosis and often require long-term hospital care. Interactional psychotic disorders fare somewhat better and may respond to outpatient treatment of the child and the parents. Such treatment can often clarify the child's basic intellectual endowment and help the parents to accept, when necessary, later placement for treatment. In the management of these young children, play therapy as a restitutional experience for emotional deprivation—and simultaneous therapy for the parents—may be usefully combined with the contributions of a therapeutic nursery school. Operant conditioning (positive reinforcement by praise, affection, or reward for healthy behavior) has been helpful in teaching these youngsters speech and socialization. Placement in a nursery school requires preceding treatment to alleviate the separation anxiety of the child and the parents.

Family conjoint therapy and tranquilizing agents have limited value, the latter being useful when the child is very anxious, hyperactive, or destructive.

B. School-Age Children: For the school-age child with a schizophreniform psychosis, short-term psychiatric hospitalization with several weeks to several months of milieu therapy and individual psychotherapy for the child and parents often assists the youngster with an acute onset to recompensate so that further therapy can be continued on an outpatient basis. This may include family conjoint therapy (wherein the family is treated together and separately). The chronically psychotic child may require long-term residential treatment or long-term placement in small cottage-type group living quarters or professional group foster homes.

The psychoactive drugs are useful mainly in controlling outbursts of panic or aggressive behavior.

C. Older Children: The adolescent or postadolescent psychotic disorders often respond well to brief psychiatric hospitalization of only a few days or weeks. This is particularly true of the acute confusional state. Patients with sweeping regressive states may require several months of hospitalization. Very few adolescents, even with adult type schizophrenic disorders, require long-term hospitalization, and only a small proportion have further episodes or become chronically schizophrenic.

Psychoactive drugs are more effective in adolescents than in children and are used adjunctively with psychotherapeutic measures.

Campbell M: Biological intervention in psychoses of childhood. *J Autism Child Schizo* 1973;**3:**347.

Campbell M, Green WH: Pervasive developmental disorders of childhood. Chap 35, pp 1672–1683, in: *Comprehensive Textbook of Psychiatry,* 4th ed. Kaplan HI, Sadock BJ (editors). Williams & Wilkins, 1985.

Jordan K, Prugh D: Schizophreniform psychosis in childhood. *Am J Psychiatry* 1971;**128:**323.

Mahler MS: On early infantile psychosis: The symbiotic and autistic syndromes. *J Am Acad Child Psychiatry* 1965;**4:**554.

Prugh DG: Psychotic disorders. In: *The Psychosocial Aspects of Pediatrics.* Lea & Febiger, 1983.

Rutter M: Infantile autism and other child psychoses. In: *Child and Adolescent Psychiatry: Modern Approaches,* 2nd ed. Rutter M, Hersov L (editors). Blackwell, 1984.

PSYCHOPHYSIOLOGIC DISORDERS

In *DSM-III,* these are referred to as psychologic disorders affecting physical conditions. Such disorders involve organs or organ systems innervated by the autonomic nervous system—in contrast to conversion disorders, which involve the striated musculature and somatosensory apparatus. Biologic predisposing factors appear to be involved, with probable latent biochemical defects. Psychologic and social factors act as additional predisposing, precipitating, and perpetuating influences. More than one organ system may be involved.

Anxiety is not alleviated by these disorders—in contrast to conversion disorders, where anxiety is repressed and "bound" in the symbolic symptom.

No type-specific personality profile, parent-child relationship, or family pattern has as yet been associated with individual psychophysiologic disorders, although some may occur in conjunction with personality disorders.

These disorders may be mild or severe and transient or chronic. A continuum probably exists ranging from cases with milder biologic predisposition and greater psychologic involvement to those that are more heavily "loaded" biologically, requiring less psychologic influence for their appearance and perpetuation.

A brief summary of the various organ systems affected and the clinical manifestations follows. Treatment and prognosis are then discussed at the end of this section.

Skin

Psychophysiologic skin disorders include certain cases of neurodermatitis, seborrheic dermatitis, psoriasis, pruritus, alopecia, eczema, urticaria, angioneurotic edema, and acne. Atopic eczema may persist into childhood or may disappear and recur in late childhood and adolescence, with patches of dermatitis becoming widespread and severe during early adolescence. Affected children are generally rigid, tense, and at times compulsive, with a tendency to repress strong emotions, particularly toward an overcontrolling mother. Exacerbations during adolescence are usually related to increased conflicts over independence and sexuality. The latter considerations are also involved in urticaria patients, who are often shy, passive, and immature, with feelings of inadequacy, unconscious exhibitionistic trends, and overdependency upon the mother.

Kremer MM: Psychological impact of acne in adolescents. *J Am Med Wom Assoc* 1969;**24:**309.

Musculoskeletal System

Psychophysiologic musculoskeletal disorders include certain cases of low back pain, rheumatoid arthritis, "tension" headaches and other myalgias, muscle cramps, bruxism, and specific types of malocclusion (the latter may involve some conversion components). Children with rheumatoid arthritis often exhibit conflicts over the handling of aggression and dependency, and exacerbations are often related to shifts in family balance.

Cleveland SE, Reitmann EE, Brewer EJ: Psychological factors in juvenile rheumatoid arthritis. *Arthritis Rheum* 1965; **8:**1152.

McAnarney EG, Freedman SB: Psychological problems of children with chronic juvenile arthritis. *Pediatrics* 1974;**5:**523.

Respiratory System

Psychophysiologic respiratory disorders may include certain cases of bronchial asthma, allergic rhinitis, chronic sinusitis, hiccup, breath-holding spells, and hyperventilation. Psychologic factors contributing to asthmatic attacks include threatened separation from the parents and parental marital conflicts.

Creer TL, Renne CM, Chai H: The application of behavioral techniques to childhood asthma. In: *Behavioral Pediatrics: Research and Practice.* Russo D, Varni J (editors). Plenum Press, 1982.

Enzer NB, Walker PA: Hyperventilation syndrome in childhood. *J Pediatr* 1967;**70:**521.

Mattson A: Psychological aspects of childhood asthma. *Pediatr Clin North Am* 1975;**22:**77.

Cardiovascular System

Psychophysiologic cardiovascular disorders may overlap with respiratory disorders and include some cases of paroxysmal tachycardia, peripheral vascular spasm (eg, Raynaud's disease and central angiospastic retinopathy), migraine, erythromelalgia, causalgia, vasodepressor syncope, epistaxis, essential hypertension, hypotension, and eclampsia in adolescents. Intense autonomic responses to emotional trauma can trigger paroxysmal tachycardia, which may lead to syncope. Children with orthostatic hypotension often appear to be tense, anxious, emotionally restricted, and "not sure where they stand" in their families. Similar characteristics occur in children or adolescents with vasodepressor syncope, often precipitated by sudden fright or pain anticipation. This syncope should be distinguished from conversion syncope, which often occurs in hysterical girls who have other conversion phenomena but no vascular changes. Migraine presents during the school-age period (headache is rare in preschool children) and is often triggered by emotional crises. The patients tend to be rather rigid, sometimes compulsive individuals in tense families.

Falstein EI, Rosenblum AH: Juvenile paroxysmal supraventricular tachycardia: Psychosomatic and psychodynamic aspects. *J Am Acad Child Psychiatry* 1962;**1**:246.

Green M: Fainting. In: *Ambulatory Pediatrics,* 2nd ed. Green M, Haggerty RJ (editors). Saunders, 1976.

Holguin J, Fenichel E: Migraine. *J Pediatr* 1967;**70**:290.

Katcher AL: Hypertension in adolescent children. *Med Clin North Am* 1964;**48:**1467.

Gastrointestinal System

The psychophysiologic gastrointestinal disorders comprise a large category of varied clinical disorders. Since the gastrointestinal tract is so responsive to emotional factors, it is unusual to find gastrointestinal disorders that are not affected by the psychic adjustment of the individual. Some of the more common problems include pylorospasm, gastric hyperacidity, pseudo-peptic ulcer syndrome, idiopathic celiac disease, nontropical sprue in adolescents, megacolon (aganglionic type), constipation, diarrhea, and cyclic vomiting in tense, overprotected children in families with these tendencies. The following syndromes are usually included under this category; however, in *DSM-III,* anorexia nervosa and bulimia are classified separately as eating disorders.

A. Rumination: Rumination is the voluntary regurgitation of previously swallowed food in infants 3–12 months of age; the food may be vomited or retained in the mouth, chewed, and reswallowed. The infant induces regurgitation by backward movements of the head and neck, by intense sucking, and occasionally by also sucking on the fingers. Regurgitation is accompanied by an appearance of great satisfaction, in contrast to the apathy or irritability often seen between episodes.

The cause is not clear, but there is some evidence of reduced mother-infant contact. Improvement with intensive maternal caretaking is the most promising development. Rumination has rarely been seen to begin during nonorganic failure to thrive, and its relationship to this diagnosis and to chalasia is not clear. Untreated, it can lead to severe malnutrition, which is occasionally fatal.

B. Pica: Pica is the continued eating of nonnutritive substances, often unpleasant or dangerous, usually during the second or third year of life. Retardation, neglect, and iron or zinc deficiency may be implicated. Prevention of poisoning or bezoar formation and provision of additional supervision and companionship for the child may be important.

C. Recurrent Abdominal Pain: There is usually no organic basis for pain; however, the differential diagnosis should include lactose intolerance. In most cases, symptoms are epigastric or periumbilical and are usually related to some emotional crisis in tense, apprehensive, timid, and often overly conscientious children who have experienced parental overprotection. Fourteen- and 6-per-second electroencephalographic spikes are not diagnostic; they occur in many normal children in the early school-age period. School phobia or identification with a family member with abdominal pain is sometimes reported.

D. Peptic Ulcer: Peptic ulcers in school-age children and adolescents are different from those in adults and probably more common. Abdominal pain is not well localized, nausea and vomiting are common, and symptoms are not closely related to meals. Individuals who develop peptic ulcer have high blood pepsinogen levels from infancy, reflecting tendencies toward gastric hypersecretion. Children who have difficulty in handling hostile feelings, are demanding of affection, and are passive and dependent are apt to develop peptic ulcers in stressful situations.

E. Ulcerative Colitis: Children with ulcerative colitis are often overdependent, passive, inhibited, and compulsive, and frequently manipulate the parents. Precipitation of fulminant cases usually takes place in a situation with actual or threatened loss of emotional support from a key figure. Exacerbations are frequently related to family crises. Other psychologic factors include familial patterns of autonomic response to stress, involving the lower gastrointestinal tract in "bowel oriented" families, conditioning of the defecation reflex to emotional conflict in coercive toilet training, and maternal overprotection and overdominance in early childhood. These factors lead to overdependence and resentment by the child.

F. Regional Ileitis: Patients with regional ileitis have psychosocial similarities to those with ulcerative colitis and mucous colitis, the latter being generally less disturbed.

G. Obesity: Obesity results basically from an excess of intake over output of calories as a result of hyperphagia, usually in families with a tendency toward overeating and obesity. From a psychosocial view, there are 2 major groups: the **reactive** type, responding to an emotionally traumatic experience (eg, the death of a parent or a school failure); and the **developmental** type, where the origins are principally in the disturbed family's tendencies toward overeating, with probably some biologic predisposition also involved. The child is often overvalued by the family, sometimes because of the loss of a previous child. Obesity occurs as a result of overfeeding and continues from infancy on. The mother usually dominates and protects the child, and after an early period of demanding behavior, the child becomes passive, overdependent, and immature. In such children, feelings of helplessness, despair, and withdrawal from social interaction are associated with more overeating, and food is used as a solace to ward off depression or hostile feelings. The "wall of weight" is a way of hiding from social problems and is often used to ward off sexual conflicts with feelings of ugliness.

H. Anorexia Nervosa: This syndrome occurs in late school age to postadolescence, usually in females. It consists of loss of appetite; denial of physical hunger; aversion to food; severe weight loss; emaciation and pallor; amenorrhea; lowered body temperature; decreased metabolism, pulse rate, and blood pressure; flat or occasionally diabetic blood glucose curves; dry skin; brittle nails; cold intolerance; and, in severe and protracted cases, other symptoms and signs such as gastric hypoacidity and diarrhea. Activity levels remain high even with marked emaciation. Patients are often preoccupied or irritable and have difficulty in verbalizing their feelings. The onset is often related to menarche or traumatic incidents with serious dieting that continues out of control. The parents are frequently in the food business. The mother and daughter often have an ambivalent (hostile-dependent) relationship, and the involvement with the father often has had a seductive quality. During preadolescence, such patients are often overconscientious, energetic, high achievers, but they remain strongly dependent upon the parents.

Three main groups of patients are seen: (1) those with psychoneurotic disorders (mixed hysterical and phobic trends) with sexual implications and symbolic meanings attributed to eating and body weight; (2) those with obsessive-compulsive personality disorders; and (3) schizophrenic or near-psychotic individuals with massive projection tendencies and fears of poisoning. A few show the syndrome as a severe reactive disorder, at times with strongly depressive trends. (See also Chapter 9.)

I. Bulimia: This disorder, with onset usually in adolescence or early adult life, is characterized by episodes of "binge" eating—gorging of very large quantities of foods in a short time—usually foods that are high-carbohydrate and soft in texture (easy to swallow). The episode is usually terminated by self-induced vomiting, often followed by excessive use of cathartics or diuretics or occasionally by fasting. Depressed mood and self-deprecation are common following binges.

Bulimia may be more difficult to diagnose than anorexia nervosa, because weight may fluctuate but never reach extremes. Most patients are women with concerns about maintaining a slim figure but who also have difficulty controlling impulses in behaviors other than appetite.

Various forms of treatment have been tried with no predictable success thus far. Behavior modification therapy in a hospital setting combined with psychotherapy may, over a protracted interval, give the best hope of cure. Depression, occasionally leading to suicide, must be taken seriously in these patients. (See also Chapter 9.)

Bruch H: *Eating Disorders*. Basic Books, 1973.

Davidson M: The irritable colon of children (chronic nonspecific diarrhea syndrome). *J Pediatr* 1966;**69:**1027.

Green M: Psychogenic recurrent abdominal pain: Diagnosis and treatment. *Pediatrics* 1967;**40:**84.

Halmi KA: Eating disorders. In: *Comprehensive Textbook of Psychiatry,* 4th ed. Kaplan HI, Sadock BJ (editors). Williams & Wilkins, 1985.

Heald F: Obesity in the adolescent. In: *Symposium on Adolescence*. Meiks LT, Green M (editors). Saunders, 1960.

Leiken SJ, Caplan H: Psychogenic polydipsia. *Am J Psychiatry* 1967;**123:**1563.

Lesser LI et al: Anorexia nervosa in children. *Am J Orthopsychiatry* 1960;**30:**572.

Liebman R, Honig P, Berger H: A family therapy process for the treatment of psychogenic abdominal pain. In: *Family Therapy Techniques for Problem Behaviors of Children and Teenagers*. Schaefer CE, Briesmeister JM, Fitton MF (editors). Jossey-Bass, 1984.

Lowe CU, Coursin DB, Heald FP: Obesity in childhood. *Pediatrics* 1967;**40:**455.

Menking M et al: Rumination: A near-fatal psychiatric disease of infancy. *N Engl J Med* 1969;**280:**802.

Millar TP: Peptic ulcers in children. In: *Modern Perspectives in International Child Psychiatry*. Howells J (editor). Oliver & Boyd, 1969.

Prugh DG, Jordan K: The management of ulcerative colitis in childhood. In: *Modern Perspectives in International Child Psychiatry*. Howells J (editor). Oliver & Boyd, 1969.

Reinhart JB, Succop RA: Regional enteritis in pediatric patients: Psychiatric aspects. *J Am Acad Child Psychiatry* 1968;**7:**252.

Genital & Urinary Systems

Psychophysiologic genitourinary disorders include certain cases of menstrual disturbances, functional uterine bleeding, leukorrhea, polyuria and dysuria, vesical paralysis, urethral and vaginal discharges, and persistent glycosuria without diabetes. Disturbances of sexual function (eg, vaginismus, frigidity, frequent erections, dyspareunia, and priapism) are often conversion reactions but may include psychophysiologic components. Menstrual problems are the rule in early adolescence, but they may be intensified or perpetuated by emotional conflicts. Dysmenorrhea has an incidence of up to 12% in high school girls and may be influenced by attitudes of inconvenience or disgust, particularly in middle-class girls. Persistence of the symptom indicates difficulty in accepting the feminine role and the responsibilities of womanhood. Premenstrual tension is often intensified by sexual or identity conflicts. Habitual abortion occurs with significant conflicts over sexuality and motherhood. Impotence in adolescent boys is rare, but it may cause problems in teenage marriages—as may frigidity in girls.

Heald FP, Masland RP, Sturgis SH: Dysmenorrhea in adolescence. *Pediatrics* 1957;**20:**121.

Heiman H: The role of stress situations and psychological factors in functional uterine bleeding. *J Mt Sinai Hosp* 1956;**23:**755.

Endocrine System

Psychophysiologic endocrine disorders include certain cases of hyperinsulinism, growth disturbance, diabetes, hyperthyroidism, and, in adolescents, pseudocyesis and disorders of lactation. Emotional conflicts about "growing up" are related to some cases of delayed puberty or delayed onset of menarche. In pseudocyesis, enlargement of the abdomen is a conversion phenomenon, but the physiologic changes of pregnancy derive from obscure psychologic influences on endocrine function. It usually occurs in hysterical personalities with underlying conflicts over feminine identity and motherhood. In more seriously disturbed adolescents, it may occur after the first experience of kissing or petting. Diabetes is significantly influenced by psychologic mechanisms. It is often precipitated or exacerbated in a setting of increased conflict, most often involving a real or threatened loss of a key relationship. Although most juvenile diabetics show increased symptoms in adolescence, those more disturbed may have an exceptionally "stormy course," with coma precipitated by emotional conflict, rebellious overeating, or inattention to insulin requirements. Children and adolescents with thyrotoxicosis often experience the onset in gradually intensifying stressful situations, particularly those involving emotional relationships.

Evans SL, Reinhart JB, Succop RA: Failure to thrive: A study of 45 children and their families. *J Am Acad Child Psychiatry* 1972;**11:**440.

Greaves D, Green PE, West LJ: Psychodynamic and psychophysiological aspects of pseudocyesis. *Psychosom Med* 1960;**22:**24.

Silver HK, Finkelstein M: Deprivation dwarfism. *J Pediatr* 1967;**70:**317.

Nervous System

Psychophysiologic nervous system disorders include idiopathic epilepsy (grand mal, petit mal, psychomotor epilepsy, and epileptic equivalents), narcolepsy, certain types of sleep disturbance, dizziness, vertigo, hyperactivity, motion sickness, and some recurrent fevers of psychologic origin.

A. Epilepsy: Epilepsy, with its unfortunate stigma, frequently produces psychic trauma, although a personality disorder may antedate its onset. The youngster may have feelings of inferiority and shyness and feel different from others. Irritability, temper outbursts, or aggressive behavior may be exhibited prior to a seizure. These children tend to experience fears of death before a seizure and may fear they have said or done something "bad" during the interval of postictal amnesia. The anxious parents are frequently overly restrictive about activity. They often blame themselves for the hereditary factor and often equate the seizures with death or "craziness."

Few children deteriorate, intellectually or otherwise, if adequate seizure control is achieved. Seizures often are more frequent or precipitated initially during periods of emotional conflict or family crises. Some children learn to inhibit or touch off seizures, the latter sometimes being used in a manipulative way.

The diagnosis of "epileptic equivalent" on the basis of exaggerated fears, repeated tantrums, aggressive behavior, marked withdrawal, or sleepwalking in association with an abnormal EEG is often inappropriate. Most children suspected of such equivalents show disturbances in behavior related to family conflicts.

Conditions formerly thought to bear some relationship to idiopathic epilepsy include migraine, recurrent abdominal pain, cyclic vomiting, and narcolepsy.

B. Narcolepsy: Narcolepsy is uncommon in childhood and more frequent in boys. It is characterized by paroxysmal and recurrent attacks of irresistible sleep, often precipitated by a sudden alteration in emotional state related to conflict situations. Attacks may come on suddenly, occurring 1–2 times a day or many times a day. They may be associated with cataplexy and hypnagogic hallucinations. The sleep during attacks is light, and the patient is easily awakened. Nocturnal sleep is usually normal, although an earlier appearance of REM sleep has been reported. The major factors are usually psychopathologic, often related to conflicts over competition or the expression of unacceptable aggressive influences. The EEG is normal between attacks, and there is no significant relationship to epilepsy. Narcolepsy is to be differentiated from the pickwickian syndrome, in which sudden attacks of somnolence occur in markedly obese children.

C. Motion Sickness: Motion sickness in cars, trains, elevators, swings, etc, is more common in children than in adults; seasickness and airplane sickness are less frequent in children. Psychologic factors are involved to varying degrees in different children. Tense, apprehensive, or phobic children are most often affected, and family arguments during driving are frequent precipitating factors. Most children improve markedly by adolescence.

D. Hyperactivity: This picture occurs in many children without signs of brain damage. Anxious children who are active from birth may show this symptom, with impulsiveness and distractibility in response to overrestrictiveness or other family tensions.

Friedman AP, Harms E: *Headaches in Children.* Thomas, 1967.

Reinhart JB, Evans SL, McFadden DJ: Cyclic vomiting: Seen through the psychiatrist's eye. *Pediatrics* 1977;**59:**371.

Yoss RE, Daly DD: Narcolepsy in children. *Pediatrics* 1960;**25:**1025.

Fever

Fever of psychophysiologic origin may occur in children who show excitement or continued emotional tension in the absence of physical overactivity. Chronic low-grade fever may occur in infants with "hospitalism" or in school-age children who are anxious or tense. In the latter case, the mother is often overanxious and continues to take the child's temperature every day long after the subsidence of a mild infection. The fever usually disappears upon discontinuation of the daily measurements. Discussion of the parents' apprehension related to guilt or other feelings rather than simple reassurance may be helpful.

Renbourn ET: Body temperature and pulse rate in boys and young men prior to sporting contests: A study of emotional hyperthermia with a review of the literature. *J Psychosom Res* 1960;**4:**149.

Organs of Special Sense

Psychophysiologic disorders of organs of special

sense include certain cases of glaucoma, blepharospasm, amblyopia, Meniere's syndrome, and certain types of tinnitus and hyperacusis.

General Principles of Treatment & Prognosis in Pediatric Psychophysiologic Disorders

Treatment and prognosis are related to the multiple interactive factors involved in these disorders. Included are the nature of the biologic predisposition, the degree of personality disturbance and family disruption, the extent of the contribution of psychosocial factors to the perpetuation of the disorder, and the likelihood of its response to psychotherapeutic treatment and medical measures.

The basic approach to treatment should be founded upon an adequate diagnostic evaluation with due consideration of the relative importance of somatic and psychologic factors.

In some disorders, only treatment of the basic emotional deprivation, with "replacement measures" offered by parent substitutes, together with parental treatment, offers any chance of amelioration. In others with mild psychologic components, as in some cases of asthma, medical measures alone will suffice. In some mildly disturbed children—eg, in cases of obesity, menstrual problems, and recurrent abdominal pain—the pediatrician may use a supportive psychotherapeutic approach to the child and parents, with psychiatric consultation initially and as needed. If the patient is hospitalized, brief visits at the beginning or end of each day may be more effective than 1–2 hours a week, with the encouragement of an initially dependent relationship upon the pediatrician and, later, gradual "weaning." Long-term follow-up may be indicated, particularly for children with ulcerative colitis (even those treated surgically), who may have later exacerbations at times of emotional trauma.

In more seriously disturbed children with severe conditions of tension headache, asthma, menstrual problems, narcolepsy, quiescent ulcerative colitis, and management problems of diabetes, intensive psychotherapy for the child and parents may have to be conducted by a child psychiatrist or other mental health professional. In most such disorders, supportive psychotherapeutic measures should be undertaken at the beginning, with later use of more intensive measures if necessary. In potentially serious and life-threatening disorders such as acute ulcerative colitis or diabetes, psychotherapeutic treatment should never be undertaken without concomitant medical treatment and follow-up.

In some instances, notably anorexia nervosa, psychiatric hospitalization may be required. Under these circumstances, the psychiatrist may act as a coordinator, drawing upon the contribution of the pediatrician and other consultants regarding the medical or surgical aspects of treatment.

Certain basic principles in the handling of children with psychophysiologic (and many other) illnesses can be listed briefly as follows: **continuity** of the relationship with the child and parents by a single physician (usually the pediatrician); **communication** among professionals, in order to bring about true and respectful **collaboration** among disciplines and **consistency** in management; **consultation** with child psychiatrists and other specialists; and **coordination** of all such activities into a unified plan of therapy with the most appropriate balance of physical, psychologic, and social measures.

Kavanaugh JG Jr, Mattson A: Psychophysiologic disorders. In: *Basic Handbook of Child Psychiatry*. Noshpitz JD (editor). Basic Books, 1979.

Mattson A, Kim SP: Psychological factors affecting physical conditions (psychosomatic disorders). In: *Comprehensive Textbook of Psychiatry*, 4th ed. Kaplan HI, Sadock BJ (editors). Williams & Wilkins, 1985.

Prugh DG: Psychophysiologic disorders. In: *The Psychosocial Aspects of Pediatrics*. Lea & Febiger, 1983.

Prugh DG, Eckhardt LO: Special consideration in the treatment of psychophysical disorders in children. In: *Basic Handbook of Child Psychiatry*. Noshpitz JD (editor). Basic Books, 1979.

See also Selected References at end of chapter.

BRAIN SYNDROMES

Essentials of Diagnosis

- Impairment of orientation, judgment, discrimination, learning, memory, other cognitive functions; emotional liability.
- Evidence of cerebral dysfunction, including (1) abnormal neurologic findings, (2) definitively abnormal EEG, (3) perceptual-motor disturbances on psychologic testing, and (4) a history of insult to the central nervous system. (Three out of 4 should be present to establish the diagnosis.)
- Psychologic disturbances, either preexisting or secondary to brain damage. There is no "pure" cerebral dysfunction without accompanying psychologic reactions.

General Considerations

In *DSM-III*, these are referred to as "Organic Mental Disorders" (with delirium, delusions, or depression, or uncomplicated). Brain syndromes result from localized or diffuse damage to brain tissue, particularly the cerebral cortex, due to any cause. The severity of the associated psychotic, neurotic, or behavioral disorders is not necessarily proportionate to the degree of brain damage. The psychologic accompaniment of brain damage is determined by predisposing personality patterns, current emotional conflicts, the child's level of development, family interpersonal relationships, and the nature of the brain disorder and its meaning to the child and the parents. As in adults, such associated disorders are often regarded as having been released by the brain disorder or superimposed on or intertwined with it. In infants and young children, however, later personality development may be influenced by such disorders, whose manifestations may be quite different from those in older children and adults. The young child appears to be able to a great extent to compensate for insults to the central nervous system as maturation proceeds. Functions most recently developed may be most vulnerable to such insults, whereas those developed earlier may be less affected. On the other hand, functions not yet developed may be interfered with, particularly those relating to the cognitive aspects of learning and impulse control. It is thus much harder in children than in adults to correlate the severity of cognitive impairment with the severity of the brain lesion.

Children affected by localized rather than diffuse brain lesions may react in various ways depending only in part upon the brain functions that are interfered with.

Brain syndromes of diffuse nature are classified as acute (reversible) or chronic (permanent). The emphasis in the following paragraphs is on the psychologic and social consequences of brain damage in children.

Clinical Findings

A. Acute Brain Syndrome: Acute brain disorders may be due to intracranial infection, systemic infection, drug or poison (including alcohol) intoxication, trauma, circulatory disturbances, certain types of convulsive disorders, metabolic disturbances such as chronic renal problems, and certain disorders of unknown cause (eg, multiple sclerosis).

The principal manifestation in children (as in adults) is delirium, a disturbance in awareness resulting from alterations of cerebral metabolism. The clinical picture may be gross and easily identifiable, characterized by wildly agitated or confused behavior and hallucinatory experiences arising from distorted perception or interpretation of stimuli. A subclinical form, however, may present with subtle disturbances in awareness or mildly stuporous states, withdrawn or ''difficult'' behavior, or irrational fears. In such cases, a rough mental status examination adapted to the child's level of development will often reveal disorientation and misinterpretation of external stimuli. An EEG may aid in diagnosis, revealing large slow waves and disorganization that disappear upon correction of the disturbance in cerebral metabolism. Perceptual-motor difficulties may persist for some time and may lead to learning difficulties upon return to school even though the brain lesion has completely healed.

Recognition of subclinical forms may be difficult, and the clinician must keep the possibility in mind to avoid overlooking the delirium or to prevent misdiagnosis as psychotic behavior on a psychosocial basis.

Preexisting or underlying psychotic, psychoneurotic, or personality disorders may become more manifest after such insults to the central nervous system, and reactive disorders or later developmental deviations in cognitive or other areas may result.

B. Chronic Brain Syndrome: These disorders result from relatively permanent, more or less irreversible, diffuse impairment of cerebral tissue function. They may be due to congenital cranial anomalies, cerebral palsy, and other disorders arising from prenatal or perinatal damage to the brain; central nervous system syphilis; intoxications of various types; brain trauma; convulsive disorders; disturbances of metabolism, growth, or nutrition; intracranial neoplasm; or heredodegenerative factors such as Schilder's encephalopathy and Heller's infantile dementia. Some disturbances in memory, judgment, orientation, comprehension, affect, and learning capacity may persist permanently, accompanied at times by remarkable compensations in individual children during the course of development.

There appears to be no specific type of personality disorder in children with chronic brain syndromes. Many children become overly dependent, with frequent developmental lags in personality organization and other developmental deviations. These psychologic factors appear in varying admixtures with the effects upon behavior of the underlying brain damage, and some of the psychologic features may be reactions to the child's obvious limitations in personal performance and ability.

One particular syndrome often seen in young children with diffuse cerebrocortical damage is frequently but not invariably characterized by hyperactivity, distractibility, impulsiveness, and electroencephalographic and electromyographic abnormalities. Difficulties in perceptual-motor functions, spatial orientation, and cerebral integration lead to problems in employing symbols (eg, reading and writing) and in abstract concept formation. Specific neurologic lesions are rarely demonstrable, and the diagnosis must be based on the history and clinical findings. However, children with significant psychologic disturbances may also exhibit difficulties in impulse control, distractibility, and hyperactivity, together with delayed perceptual-motor development and dysrhythmic electroencephalographic patterns. Signs of cerebral dysfunction are not always due to organic lesions alone; therefore, diagnoses of ''organicity'' or ''minimal brain damage'' based principally on behavioral manifestations seem open to much question.

Many children with chronic brain syndrome are not significantly retarded in intellectual development. They often show significant learning difficulties, however, due to perceptual-motor handicaps, and may function at a mentally retarded level with psychologic and social factors playing a contributory role. If mental retardation is present, this should be specified by means of appropriate tests. In each instance, the predominant personality picture associated with the brain syndrome should be noted, eg, developmental deviations of affective nature, or personality, psychoneurotic, or psychotic disorders.

Cerebral palsy. (See also Chapter 23.) Children with cerebral palsy exhibit motor disabilities of a predominantly extrapyramidal type characterized by choreiform and athetoid movements and frequent sensory and perceptual defects, all of which predispose to learning difficulties and poor achievement on intelligence tests. Speech problems are often present. The physical defects, combined with the child's inability to discharge tensions through physical activity and play, produce anxiety, emotional conflicts, and feelings of difference from others and a negative self-image. Some parents feel guilty and handle the child overprotectively, whereas others may feel ashamed, resentful, or hopeless. Insufficient stimulation or a pessimistic appraisal of the child's prospects by parents, physicians, and teachers may lead to inadequate education in addition to the inherent learning problems.

Children with cerebral palsy are often emotionally immature, introverted, overly dependent, fearful, irritable, and egocentric. Emotional conflicts are commonly most severe during adolescence, although children with athetosis or ataxia may be surprisingly cheerful and outgoing (often with lack of insight into their limitations).

An important and encouraging characteristic of cerebral palsy is its stationary, nonprogressive course.

Treatment

A. Acute Brain Syndrome: The essential problem in the psychologic management of acute brain syndrome is the control of delirium while the underlying cause is being sought and treated. The child must be helped to deal with misperceptions of stimuli in the environment. Shadows may be seen as "witches" or "ghosts," or medical instruments as the weapons of "killers," ie, the doctors and nurses. A school-age child whose parents are not present may feel abandoned or even orphaned. Instead of darkening the room to cut down on stimuli, it is important to keep the child's room adequately lighted, especially at night, when such misperceptions are most severe and frightening. A special nurse, relative, or foster grandparent should be in the room at all times during the day and should be available at night to serve as an external "auxiliary ego" who can help the child correct misperceptions and misinterpretations.

Chloral hydrate is probably the best-tolerated sedative in childhood delirium, and large doses may be required. Paraldehyde given orally or rectally is the ideal sedative in adolescents, although the odor may be offensive. Barbiturates tend to cause confusion and should be avoided.

It is essential to maintain the tie with the parents, the only truly familiar figures in the delirious child's confused world, through daily visiting or overnight stay by one or the other, even for school-age children. If the parent is ill or far away and cannot visit regularly, substitute parenting becomes all the more vital. A familiar blanket or toy from home or postcards that can be read to the child will be of some help.

The anxieties and guilt of the parents must also be dealt with, especially in cases involving accidents or poisonings.

B. Chronic Brain Syndrome: Treatment measures, in addition to those directed toward the basic cause of brain dysfunction, include remedial education in small "ungraded" classes from which the child should move to normal classes as soon as possible. Individual tutoring may help to retain the child in the age-appropriate classroom. Special remedial teaching techniques using auditory, tactile, and kinesthetic stimuli may be of value.

Children with brain damage and significant emotional problems, including anxiety over performance, problems in impulse control, a negative self-image, and resistance to learning, often respond to psychotherapy for themselves and their parents. Such therapy may at first be largely supportive. Educational components, including some tutoring, may be included.

Cerebral palsy. (See also Chapter 23.) Whereas some parents of children with cerebral palsy may simply give up, others go to great lengths to push the child toward normality with "gimmicks" or cure-alls such as the Doman-Delacato approach, which involves a great deal of effort and money. This has been shown by a controlled study to be of no more value than other training methods and may cause emotional problems as a result of the pressure it places on the child.

In addition to physical therapy, speech therapy, and drug therapy (including tranquilizers) as indicated, special educational measures, sheltered workshops, and group therapy or discussions for the parents of such children may be helpful, as may individual psychotherapy for the more seriously disturbed. There is no substitute for the physician's continuing supportive relationship with the child and the parents, working with representatives of other disciplines. Children with cerebral palsy, many of whom are not inherently retarded, may make surprisingly adequate emotional and vocational adjustments in spite of continuing problems.

Psychoactive drugs may be of some value. Hyperactivity, impulsiveness, and distractibility may be controlled by the judicious use of amphetamines. Phenothiazines may help control anxiety or destructive behavior. Residential treatment may be necessary for children with severe emotional disturbances.

Prognosis

A. Acute Brain Syndrome: The prognosis for children with acute brain syndrome depends upon the degree of structural brain damage and upon host resistance factors. With appropriate antibiotic therapy, the various types of bacterial meningitis may resolve with little residual damage. The viral encephalitides cannot be controlled so well, but children who have been in coma even for several months may regain complete function, gradually "relearning" lost skills from walking to reading. In all of these disorders—particularly head trauma—the response of the child is influenced by parental reactions. A minor concussion may provoke overprotective patterns of parental behavior with psychologic difficulties during convalescence in spite of complete recovery.

If the child recovers completely, the possibility of persistence of perceptual-motor deficits for some weeks should be explained to the parents and teachers in order to permit gradual return to optimal academic performance.

B. Chronic Brain Syndrome: Infants and children show a remarkable tendency to compensate for diffuse damage to the cerebral cortex, especially if attention is paid to the psychosocial needs of the child and the parents.

Prugh DG: Brain syndromes. In: *The Psychosocial Aspects of Pediatrics*. Lea & Febiger, 1983.

Prugh DG et al: A clinical study of delirium in children and adolescents. *Psychosom Med* 1980;**42(Part 2, Suppl):**177.

Rourke BP et al: *Child Neuropsychology: An Introduction to Theory, Research, and Clinical Practice*. Guilford, 1983.

Schmitt BD: The minimal brain dysfunction myth. *Am J Dis Child* 1975;**129:**1313.

MENTAL RETARDATION

This category is discussed in Chapter 7.

COMMON PROBLEMS IN PEDIATRIC PRACTICE

COLIC

Colic or paroxysmal fussing is a common problem in young infants. It is most common in the evening. It may build up in a crescendo, with the baby drawing its legs up onto the abdomen, and is frequently relieved by the passage of flatus. This stage usually begins at age 2–3 weeks and disappears by 10–12 weeks—the so-called "3-months' colic." The course is not clear, but "developmental colic" may be related to overready response to stimulation, irregular gastrointestinal peristalsis, and other as yet unintegrated autonomic functions characteristic of the first 2–3 months. The evening hours in the home often involve more stimulation from the father, anxiety about the infant's sleep on the part of a tired young mother, and perhaps concerns about the reactions of relatives or neighbors to continued crying.

Observations suggest that prolonged and severe colic, often persisting until the latter part of the first year, occurs most commonly in infants who are overactive and tense from birth (the so-called hypertonic infant, with a "lean and hungry look"). There may be some relationship to greater activity of the infant in utero and higher levels of maternal anxiety during pregnancy. Maternal and family tensions, as well as possible allergic tendencies, have been implicated.

Management of Colic

Anticipatory guidance about avoiding overstimulation (particularly of more active infants) during the first 3 months may be helpful in minimizing developmental colic, as is the knowledge that it ordinarily disappears by 3 months. A pacifier can be soothing and does no harm unless used too frely by an overly anxious parent to prevent any crying or unless employed as a substitute for tactile, rhythmic, and other forms of soothing. If colic is prolonged and severe, more sucking time during feeding may be required for emotional satisfaction.

Counseling is important, giving the parent an opportunity to "think out loud," with the nonjudgmental help of the physician, about family tensions centering around living arrangements, overstimulation of the infant by the father when he comes home in the evening, arguments over handling the infant, criticisms of in-laws in the home, or other matters.

Brazelton TB: Crying in infancy. *Pediatrics* 1962;**29:**579.

Hyams JS, Liebman WM, Prugh DG: The fussy infant: Dealing with colic: *Patient Care* 1985;**19:**93.

SCHOOL PHOBIA

A special type of inability to attend school called school phobia is a syndrome involving a morbid or irrational dread of some aspect of the school situation. Somatic complaints include abdominal pain, nausea, vomiting, diarrhea, headache, pallor, faintness, feelings of weakness, and low-grade fever. These symptoms appear in the morning before school, usually disappear by the time school is out or before, and do not appear on weekends or school holidays.

The basic fear is not of going to school but of leaving home or of separation from the family. Such fears occur in mild form, often with abdominal pain, in many normal children going off to full day school for the first time. With reassurance and firm support from the parents, they usually disappear within a few days, although they may recur during the first several years of school attendance, after vacations, or during convalescence from illness. Some young school-age children with more intense fears are undergoing prolonged separation anxiety or experiencing a developmental crisis.

The classic picture of psychoneurotic school phobia involves an overly dependent, shy, and anxious child with a very solicitous or controlling mother and a passive father. The mother often has a strong need for closeness with the child, fears the child is growing away from her, and communicates to the child her anxiety about what might happen during periods of separation. There is usually a precipitating factor such as an unpleasant experience at school, illness or a new baby at home, or an increase in marital friction. The child's fear of separation is displaced onto the school as a "dangerous" place, and unconscious feelings of resentment over parental domination are projected onto the school in the form of fears of punishment or attack. The mother takes the child's fears too seriously and becomes concerned about accidents, attacks by strangers or other children at school, etc. The child in turn, if permitted to remain at home, becomes more guilty and socially isolated, clings more closely to the mother, and may provoke feelings of frustration and anger in her by continuing to do what she seemed to want before (stay home from school).

In young children in the early grades, the school phobia syndrome usually involves marked separation anxiety, a developmental crisis, or a mild form of phobic neurosis. In junior and senior high school students, it is usually a manifestation of a more severe personality disorder, occasionally a borderline psychosis. (See also Chapter 9.)

Management of School Phobia

The pediatrician plays an important role in the management of this pediatric-psychiatric emergency. The emergency situation represents the first phase of treatment, which may be handled by the pediatrician who is willing to work with the parents, the child, and the school authorities and who understands the background of the difficulty.

Early return to school is the immediate goal. The pediatrician should first do a thorough physical appraisal; if abdominal pain or other gastrointestinal symptoms have been present for weeks or months, barium x-ray examination is necessary to rule out peptic ulcer (often of the acute type), which occasionally coexists with school phobia. If the physical findings are within normal limits, the pediatrician should reassure the parents that no physical abnormalities are present and explain that "emotional tension" can be responsible for all of the symptoms, adding—in a noncritical, nonjudgmental way—that the child seems to be easily frightened by "new experiences," of which school is the most typical. Rather than interpreting their role in the problem, the pediatrician should ask the parents what they feel might be involved.

With this approach, many parents can begin to recognize, without too much defensiveness or guilt, that they have kept the child "too close" to them. The pediatrician can then suggest that they "think out loud" about ways to help the child become more independent. The importance of the child's early return to school should be emphasized—pointing out, if necessary, that every day at home will only make it harder for the child to have a successful school experience.

The pediatrician should talk with the principal or, with the principal's permission, with the teacher, school social worker, or psychologist in order to learn how they interpret the problem. If the school authorities agree, the mother should be instructed to take the child to school and, if necessary, to the classroom, even remaining there briefly. If the mother is too anxious, the father may accompany her or may take the child to school himself. If neither parent feels able to accompany the child, it may be possible for an adult relative, another adult (such as the school nurse), or even an older child to see that the child gets to school. Once in the classroom, the younger school-age child usually settles in and does well academically. In some cases, it may be necessary to arrange for return to school at first on a part-time basis or to one class only. It may sometimes be necessary to change teachers or even arrange a transfer to another school.

Certain children may be unable to remain for long in the classroom and may ask to go home because of abdominal pain or other symptoms. The child should be sent to the school nurse, allowed to lie down briefly, and should then return, with reassurance and encouragement, to the classroom. If the child is permitted to call home, the parents may not be able to resist pleas for rescue. No matter how worried the parents are, the physician should not give a medical certificate for home teaching, since psychologic invalidism and other psychopathologic disorders may result.

If these emergency measures are not effective, early referral to a psychiatric clinic is warranted. In a few cases, threats of legal action may be necessary to spur dilatory parents into responsible efforts to secure for the child the education they are required by statute to provide.

Even if early return to school is achieved, referral for psychotherapy is usually indicated to work out underlying conflicts and prevent recurrences. If the parents are reluctant to take this step, the pediatrician can take comfort from follow-up studies showing that most such children are able to remain in school and to perform adequately without crippling neurotic symptoms.

With children in junior high or high school, who are usually more severely disturbed, the "first aid" approach should be tried and may be successful. Often it is not, however, and many adolescents with school phobia require long-term intensive psychotherapy and even psychiatric hospitalization. With some mildly disturbed adolescents, brief pediatric hospitalization, drawing upon psychiatric consultation, may be all that is required.

Schmitt B: School phobia, the great imitator: A pediatric viewpoint. *Pediatrics* 1971;**48:**433.

Williams HR, Prugh DG: School phobia. In: *Ambulatory Pediatrics,* 2nd ed. Green M, Haggerty RJ (editors). Saunders, 1976.

Volden S: School phobia and other childhood neuroses: A systematic study of the children and their families. *Am J Psychiatry* 1975;**132:**8.

ENURESIS & ENCOPRESIS

Two major challenges for the pediatrician are offered by enuresis and encopresis. These symptoms are not necessarily associated with any specific personality picture. Both represent normal patterns until the expected age of training. Thereafter, they may represent a regressive component of a reactive disorder (in late preschool children), a developmental deviation in control mechanisms, a conversion symptom as part of a psychoneurotic disorder, or one of a constellation of symptoms in a chronic personality disorder or psychosis.

1. ENURESIS

Continuing enuresis (beyond about age 5) may be diurnal or nocturnal. Both types are often associated with coercive toilet training in infancy. Other causes are parental neglect or permissiveness; and some children with an apparent developmental lag in bladder control mechanisms not associated with other disturbances continue to be picked up at night when they wet the bedclothes. A familial tendency toward enuresis has been reported in some cases.

Diurnal enuresis is constant dribbling during the day beyond the point of occasional accidents caused by anxiety or momentary "forgetting" to empty a full bladder, as often happens in late preschool children. It may become a problem if the child enters nursery school, or it may remain mild and relatively unnoticed until kindergarten. It may or may not be associated with nocturnal enuresis and is associated with a higher incidence of encopresis.

Diurnal wetting may be influenced by shyness about asking to go to the toilet, fear of strange toilets, negativistic tendencies, or chronic anxiety. In older school-age children, diurnal enuresis is encountered most often in chronically anxious children, those with personality disorders of the anxiety type, and those with oppositional personality traits. In general, it is more difficult to treat with the usual methods (described below) than the nocturnal type. A supportive relationship with the pediatrician and counseling for the child and the parents may be of help. Psychiatric consultation should usually be obtained, however, and many of these children require referral for intensive psychotherapy.

Children with **nocturnal enuresis** seem to experience greater than normal urgency in response to bladder distention during sleep. Their bladder capacity is not strikingly diminished, however, and at least as measured by electroencephalographic studies, their sleep is not deeper. There appears to be no association with epilepsy (most epileptic children do not have enuresis). Most have no neurologic disorders related to true incontinence or structural abnormalities of the bladder or proximal urethra. The problem seems to be one of external sphincter control, and abnormalities higher in the urinary tract appear to play no significant role.

Diagnostic studies should usually be restricted to urinalysis to rule out cystitis (which might cause urinary urgency) or, at most, an intravenous urogram if abnormalities are suspected. Retrograde cystoscopy in children with normal urine specimens should be avoided, as it can provoke severe anxiety in young school-age children, who still have fears of bodily (especially genital) mutilation. If done without general anesthesia in neurotic adolescents, the experience can become paradoxically pleasurable, particularly in girls with hysterical trends and masochistic needs.

Classification of Causes

Children with nocturnal enuresis fall into several groups from a psychosocial point of view, which may account for the conflicting findings in the literature regarding personality pictures and parent-child relationships.

A. Developmental Lag: One group shows a continuing struggle for control with the parents in this area, often arising from an apparent developmental lag in control mechanisms that upsets the parents. These are not usually seriously disturbed children, although they may be timid, anxious, and immature. The symptom is more or less "encapsulated" and may represent a failure to achieve conditioned nighttime control.

B. Psychoneurotic Disorders: Boys with nocturnal enuresis are usually passive, inhibited, and often overly dependent or have phobic tendencies. They may identify with a dominant mother or be fearful of a punitive father. The symptoms appear to be of a conversion nature, involving relaxation of the external sphincter in relation to unconscious sexual conflicts, often expressed in terrifying nightmares during which loss of control occurs.

Girls with this symptom seem to be more active, sometimes overly independent, and competitive toward boys, with a tendency toward more masculine identification in an attempt to handle sexual fears. The content of the conversion symptom seems to carry an unconsciously hostile component toward their mothers or toward men who could injure them.

C. Tension Discharge Disorders: Children (usually boys) with tension discharge disorders, frequently of the impulse-ridden type, show problems in control in a number of areas. They often have dysrhythmic EEGs, although these seem to be related to immaturity in central nervous system development rather than to other causes. In some children with previously repressed neurotic conflicts, fire setting is encountered, together with dreams of firemen or of firehoses putting out fires. In many cases, the fathers have been overly punitive and the mothers unaffectionate. Broken homes are a frequent historical component, and most of these children have experienced considerable emotional deprivation.

D. Other Disorders: A few disturbed children with much resentment underlying passive-aggressive behavior demonstrate a "revenge" type of enuresis—ie, bed-wetting represents a volitional act. Psychotic children may have enuresis because of negativism or an inability to comprehend the significance of toilet training.

Treatment

Treatment should be related to the type of personality and family picture. For children whose enuresis represents a developmental lag in bladder control mechanisms, often with a related struggle for control, various methods can be employed successfully, eg, the gold star chart, drugs such as atropine or imipramine (Tofranil), and conditioning approaches such as the Eneurtone apparatus. Probably the most important ingredient in all these approaches is a positive doctor-patient relationship.

In the context of such a relationship, the physician should explain to the parents that the child cannot help the enuresis. They should be assured that the problem is not "their fault" and encouraged to stop pressuring or punishing the child in favor of the prescription, whatever it may be. By developing a positive relationship with the child, the pediatrician can help allay feelings of guilt, shame, or resentment and develop motivation for independent control with the help of the prescribed method. In some instances, control has been achieved during the evaluation process even before the prescription has been written.

Maxwell MD, Seldrup J: Imipramine in the treatment of childhood enuresis. *Practitioner* 1971;**207:**809.

Oppel WC, Harper PA, Rider RV: Social, psychological, and neurological factors associated with nocturnal enuresis. *Pediatrics* 1968;**42:**627.

Parker L, Whitehead W: Treatment of urinary and fecal incontinence in children. In: *Behavioral Pediatrics: Research and Practice.* Russo D, Varni J (editors). Plenum Press, 1982.

Pierce CM: Enuresis. In: *Comprehensive Textbook of Psychiatry,* 4th ed. Kaplan HI, Sadock BJ (editors). Williams & Wilkins, 1985.

Stanfield B: Enuresis: Its pathogenesis and management. *Clin Pediatr* 1972;**11:**343.

Werry JS, Cohrssen J: Enuresis: An etiologic and therapeutic study. *J Pediatr* 1965;**67:**423.

2. ENCOPRESIS

Children with encopresis fall into 3 different groups. In many cases, the symptom begins as stool withholding in late infancy, and the majority of these children have experienced coercive toilet training.

Classification of Causes

A. Developmental Failure: In one group, failure to develop conditioned control of the external anal sphincter results in continual soiling from infancy. Affected children generally have a relaxed anal sphincter. "Paradoxic diarrhea" often occurs, with a flow of mucoid material around a central fecal mass. These children frequently show strong oppositional behavior tendencies, with negativism in response to parental pressure or restrictions. Nonaganglionic megacolon of psychophysiologic origin may be present.

B. Inhibited, Dependent Children: Another group of children with encopresis often exhibit inhibited, dependent, compulsive tendencies and may show much concern about cleanliness in other areas. The symptom, often of regressive onset, seems to be a type of conversion reaction, representing the expression of unconscious hostility and resistance toward the parents—usually a dominating, overcontrolling, compulsive mother with strong unconscious interests in bowel functions and a passive, retiring, uninterested father. Soiling occurs rarely at school but is common on the way home, as the child returns to the area of conflict. "Hiding" the stool, wrapped in underwear, in a bureau drawer where the mother will find it frequently underlines the hostile significance of the soiling. In these children, the stool is often soft and formed, without paradoxic diarrhea.

C. Seriously Disturbed Children: Still another group of children with encopresis are much more seriously disturbed. They may manifest deep personality disorders, of mistrustful or isolated nature, with defects in reality testing of near-psychotic proportions, and some have shown "revenge" encopresis. Some may have been frankly psychotic since infancy, failing to comprehend control, whereas in others encopresis may have developed as one of a group of bizarre symptoms involved in a schizophreniform psychotic disorder. Paradoxic diarrhea may or may not be present. A few children have psychotic parents who have made no attempt to offer training. The parents of most are themselves disturbed, and they may occasionally interfere with treatment because of their fears or suspicions.

Treatment

Treatment should be geared to the personality and family patterns. If fecal impaction is present, hypertonic phosphate or oil retention enemas can be used in the hospital. Later, a mild laxative can be prescribed. Mineral oil is effective, but many children and parents are upset by the "leaking" that occurs. A regular evacuation each day may help reestablish bowel habits.

The support of the pediatrician, helping the parents to understand that the symptom is not their fault or the child's fault and encouraging them not to use pressure or punishment in controlling it, is fundamental to any therapeutic approach. The child usually feels embarrassed and guilty and can rarely talk about it easily but can be encouraged to participate in the reestablishment of bowel routines and control.

The above approach is surprisingly effective in the group who have resisted control by overly rigid parents and to some extent in school-age children who develop regressive encopresis with conversion mechanisms.

Psychiatric consultation may be necessary, and some children and parents may require intensive long-term psychotherapy.

"Cleaning out" procedures and establishment of bowel routines may be resisted by the child or the parents out of fear of harm.

Parker L, Whitehead W: Treatment of urinary and fecal incontinence in children. In: *Behavioral Pediatrics: Research and Practice*. Russo D, Varni J (editors). Plenum Press, 1982.

Pierce CM: Encopresis: In: *Comprehensive Textbook of Psychiatry*, 4th ed. Kaplan HI, Sadock BJ (editors). Williams & Wilkins, 1985.

Silver D: Encopresis: Discussion of etiology and management. *Clin Pediatr* 1969;**8:**225.

SUICIDE ATTEMPTS

Depression in adolescents, as in younger children, often takes different forms from depression in adults. Overt depression, with feelings of worthlessness, psychomotor retardation, and other physical changes, is much less common than in adults. Withdrawal, excessive daydreaming, anorexia, mood swings, sleep disturbances (inability to fall asleep or inability to get up in the morning), hyperactivity or hypoactivity, feelings of helplessness or hopelessness, and even hostility, temper outbursts, or aggressive behavior (warding off depression) are common depressive equivalents of which the adolescent may not be consciously aware.

Threats of suicide are common in children and often represent attempts to punish the parents. ("You'll be sorry if I die.") Children are unable to comprehend the reality of death until age 9 or 10 years. Suicide attempts are rare and usually do not reflect serious wishes to die but rather a desire for self-punishment or retaliation against the parents; however, they may accidentally be successful or may be carried out more efficiently than intended. The incidence of attempts rises rapidly after age 14. Although accurate reporting is rare, suicide is the fourth most frequent cause of death in late adolescence and the second most frequent cause in college students of high economic status.

Adolescent suicide rates vary from country to country (highest in Japan, Switzerland, and Finland) and from region to region (highest in the Rocky Mountain and Pacific Coast states in the USA). They appear to be higher in middle-class groups and in urban areas, and they show some seasonal incidence in temperate countries (highest in the spring) and some variation in relation to historical epochs and social crises. The adolescent (and young adult) suicide rate has increased dramatically in the recent past, and this increase may be due in part to more honest reporting of suicides previously recorded as accidental deaths. The rate among boys, particularly, may be even higher than reported if automobile accidents are considered, since self-destructive or suicidal motives may be involved in deaths due to vehicle accidents.

In the USA, the suicide rate was formerly higher among adolescent girls than boys. The rate of successful suicide in boys is now at least double that of girls, although girls make more attempts. Boys employ firearms and explosives most commonly, with hanging or strangulation next most common. Girls most frequently have employed poison or drugs, although firearms and explosives have recently become more common.

In addition to social, economic, or historical factors and a greater acceptance of suicide as a method of protest or problem solving, it may be that child-rearing attitudes related to shame, guilt, or achievement and individual and family or situational factors are involved in most suicide attempts. A small proportion of adolescents who attempt suicide are psychotic, and these episodes may be bizarre attempts at self-mutilation rather than actual suicide. Some have chronic personality disorders (hysterical and others), and their attempts may be clearly manipulative of parents or peers. Immature, sensitive, shy, anxious, emotionally labile adolescents with low self-esteem who come from disorganized or disturbed families are vulnerable to stressful events and may regard suicide as a solution. Others are reasonably healthy adolescents reacting to some specific situation such as chronic illness, pressure for school achievement, or sudden loss of another person or of self-esteem, as with a broken love affair or a bitter fight with a parent. Factors involved include one or more of the following: depression; feelings of unworthiness; internalized anger at another (with guilt and depression); boredom; attempts to gain affection and esteem or to punish a parent, boyfriend, or girlfriend; a desire to join a dead relative; or even the acting out of an unconscious wish of a parent or identification with a parent who has committed suicide. Many adolescents do not really wish to die, and the attempt is a cry for help. Even a true wish to die is more short-lived in adolescents than in adults. The adolescent often tells the parents about the attempt or leaves a note or a pill bottle where it can easily be found. During the course of a suicide attempt, the child may have a change of heart when it is too late or may want to draw back but feels compelled to carry out the threat so as not to look foolish or feel weak and silly.

Many parents feel ashamed and guilty when an adolescent son or daughter attempts suicide, and the doctor may unconsciously conspire with them to forget it or "sweep it under the rug." Every attempt at suicide or threat of suicide should be taken seriously. If an attempt is made that produces no response from the parents, the adolescent may try again with more determination and tragic results.

Signs of depression or depressive equivalents are a serious indication that a suicide attempt may be made. Although emotional lability is one of the characteristics of adolescence, true depression should never be dealt with by a "pat on the back" or a "buck up" approach. An opportunity to ventilate feelings to an understanding adult may be of great help, or more formal therapy may be necessary.

If an adolescent asks for a chance to talk with a physician or other adult, an interview should be arranged promptly. It is hard enough to encourage teenagers to talk to adults at most times; if a request for an opportunity to talk is made, granting it may help to prevent impulsive suicide attempts.

If a suicide attempt has been made, pediatric hospitalization can provide the time, with the help of a psychiatrist and social worker, to convince the parents of the seriousness of the adolescent's plea for help. Supportive counseling or environmental manipulation may suffice, or more intensive psychotherapy can be started at once if indicated.

It is unwise to send home from the emergency room an adolescent who has made even a patently superficial and manipulative suicidal attempt such as the ingestion of a small amount of an innocuous drug or a quantity of barbiturates that can easily be dealt with by gastric lavage. The family will often not return for follow-up therapy, and more serious attempts may occur. If the adolescent appears seriously disturbed, emergency psychiatric hospitalization is necessary. (See also Chapter 9.)

Lewis M, Solnit A: The adolescent in a suicidal crisis: Collaborative care on a pediatric ward. In: *Modern Perspectives in Child Development*. Solnit A, Provence S (editors). Internat Univ Press, 1963.

Mattsson A, Seese LR, Hawkins JW: Suicidal behavior as a child psychiatric emergency: Clinical characteristics and follow-up results. *Arch Gen Psychiatry* 1969:**20:**100.

Pfeffer CR: Suicidal behavior of children: A review with implications for research and practice. *Am J Psychiatry* 1981;**138:**154.

Prugh DG: Suicidal attempts. In: *The Psychosocial Aspects of Pediatrics*. Lea & Febiger, 1983.

DRUG ABUSE

Drug addiction and the use of drugs by adolescents are some of the most controversial topics of our times. Physicians should keep informed about what drugs are being abused in their geographic areas and be prepared to give appropriate counseling to parents and teenagers as well as to treat overdoses and side effects. (See also Chapter 9.)

LSD & Other Hallucinogens

The biologic effects of LSD and related compounds have been carefully studied; they resemble sympathomimetic agents and produce such changes as increased pulse and heart rate, rise in blood pressure, mydriasis, tremors of extremities, cold sweaty palms, flushing, chills and shivering, increased salivation, nausea, and anorexia. The psychologic effects may last from 1–2 hours to more than a day. The LSD effect usually lasts 4–8 hours.

The effects depend on the person taking the drug, the expectation of what will happen, the setting in which it is taken, the other people in the setting, previous experiences with the drug, the physiologic and psychologic states of the subject, and other variables.

Changes in perception (especially visual) are often experienced by nonpsychotic subjects who take oral doses of LSD as small as 30 μg. They include enhancement of colors, alterations in the perception of one's own body, vivid hallucinations, and synesthesias. Mood changes include depression, euphoria, and lability of mood; anxiety is frequent, sometimes to the point of panic. Feelings of depersonalization and estrangement are often reported. Changes in thinking may include flights of ideas, perseveration, a feeling of insight into universal and transcendental phenomena (the "psychedelic experience"), and intense preoccupation with one's own thought and bodily processes. Other cognitive changes consist of difficulty in concentration on reality-oriented tasks, distractibility, abandonment of logical and causal thinking, and changes in time sense.

Untoward psychologic effects ("bad trips") include the appearance of a serious schizophreniform psychotic illness (usually precipitated by the drug experience in borderline psychotic individuals); prolonged depressive reaction (including a number of reported suicides); continuing anxiety (panic), depersonalization, and recurrent catatonia, with intermittent return ("flashback") of hallucinatory experiences; and serious injury or death in a few cases.

Some reports have indicated that persons who take LSD have an increased number of "breaks" in chromosomes, lasting at least 6 months, and that the offspring of women who have taken LSD early in pregnancy also exhibit such chromosomal alterations (continuing up to 5 years of age). Similar findings have been reported in animals. These results need to be carefully validated, but caution in the use of LSD, especially by pregnant women, seems justified on this basis.

Because the manufacture and sale of many of the compounds used as hallucinogens is a federal offense, the extent of their abuse is difficult to determine. Statements regarding large numbers of young people who have experimented with or used these drugs are often exaggerated and inflammatory. Various surveys report that up to 15% of college students in selected colleges have admitted trying LSD. Undoubtedly, a number have tried the experience once only for "kicks" or out of curiosity; some anxious persons with conflicts have continued the practice; and others with "an empty feeling," alienation and isolation (anomie), may continue to seek stimulation of any kind by the use of these drugs. Some openly report the experience as frightening; others describe it in rapturous terms.

Although feelings of universal insight seem to occur in some individuals, there is no evidence that LSD changes personality for the better. In addition, those who experience such insights rarely can describe them clearly to others, and there is little evidence that the experiences have resulted in any personal or social benefit. The use of LSD as an adjunct to psychotherapy in chronically psychotic children has been reported, but no carefully controlled studies are available.

LSD is relatively easy to manufacture and easily available from illegal sources, and there is no way to detect its presence in the body. Thus, in spite of realistic concerns about adverse psychologic and biologic effects of LSD (and presumably other psychedelic drugs also), there is no easy way to control its distribution. The largest group of users appears to be teenagers and young adults who characteristically are "looking for answers" and are only too ready to rebel against the established order and break its rules. To make laws against use or possession of these drugs is more likely to encourage experimentation with them than the reverse. Such legislation also means that large numbers of young people who will soon outgrow their rebelliousness in the course of development will be socially hampered by a police record.

At present, the incidence of experimentation with these drugs seems to be decreasing. Young people are aware of the information about chromosomal damage and appear to respect that type of data more than rules or laws.

Marihuana

Marihuana is more widely used today than the psychedelic (hallucinogenic, psychotomimetic) drugs, with estimates of up to 50% or more in some reported studies of college students. Its effects are not well studied because of the illegal status of the substance in many areas. They appear to involve relaxation of inhibitions in some individuals, although most users describe an introspective attitude under the influence of marihuana even in a group. The drug does not appear to be significantly involved in episodes of antisocial, destructive, or criminal behavior. It is not addictive and does not predispose to other addictions. The furor among adults over its use seems unjustified, as most young people control its use or eventually give it up.

Heroin

Heroin does seem to have some addictive qualities, although physical dependence on it or other "addictive" drugs (with great desire and increasing tolerance) also involves certain psychologic needs for escape from reality conflicts, fear of withdrawal symptoms, or a conditioning process. Deaths have occurred from overdosage, and tetanus, malaria, hepatitis, syphilis, and other infections have resulted from the use of unsterile needles.

The Hydrocarbons

Inhalation of hydrocarbons (glue or plastic cement, lighter fluid, or gasoline fumes) seems to produce a state resembling alcoholic intoxication, ie, an initial "jag" with pleasant exhilaration, euphoria, and excitement. Ataxia, slurred speech, and (at times) diplopia and tinnitus follow, with drowsiness, stupor, and brief coma appearing later. As tolerance develops, large amounts of inhalant become necessary for a reaction. Nausea, anorexia, weight loss, irritability, inattentiveness, somnolence, excessive salivation, and fetor oris may result from glue sniffing, but serious physiologic effects do not occur. Gasoline sniffing, which has been reported in children as young as age 18 months, has caused occasional accidental deaths.

Although not addictive, the hydrocarbons offer easy habituation. They are used—particularly glue—principally by boys who usually have significant psychosocial problems. The same is true of individuals who become habituated to the amphetamines, barbiturates, alcohol, or tobacco in childhood or early adolescence.

Management of Drug Abuse

The approach to the use of drugs should be medical, psychologic, and social rather than restrictive or punitive. This is true of serious addictive problems as well; even alcoholism has been recognized recently by the courts as an illness requiring treatment and not primarily an offense against society. Indeed, recent indications are that alcohol is becoming the drug most widely abused by young people.

An understanding approach by the parents to guidance and discipline, with some limits but with some flexibility, will prevent many young people from resorting to the habitual use of drugs of any kind.

For those who have experienced "bad trips" or other untoward effects of drug abuse or for those in higher-income families who engage in chronic drug abuse because of emotional disturbance or rebellion, psychiatric treatment is usually indicated. Younger adolescents who have indulged in glue sniffing because of psychologic problems may often be successfully treated by the pediatrician with the help of psychiatric consultation and therapy for the parents by a social worker or other mental health professional. Other social and economic measures are necessary to deal with the fundamental problems of poverty and discrimination, which favor the use of drugs by adolescents in disadvantaged neighborhoods.

Deisher RW et al: Drug abuse in adolescence: The use of harmful drugs—a pediatric concern. *Pediatrics* 1969;**44:**131.

Levine S, Korenblum M, Golombek H: Substance abuse. In: *Psychological Problems of the Child in His Family,* 2nd ed. Steinhauer PD, Rae-Grant Q (editors). Basic Books, 1983.

Litt IF, Cohen MI: The drug-using adolescent and pediatric patient. *J Pediatr* 1970;**77:**195.

Proskauer S, Rolland RS: Youth who use drugs: Psychodynamic diagnosis and treatment planning. *J Am Acad Child Psychiatry* 1973;**12:**32.

Prugh DG: Drug abuse. In: *The Psychosocial Aspects of Pediatrics.* Lea & Febiger, 1983.

MANAGEMENT OF PSYCHOLOGIC ASPECTS OF ILLNESS & INJURY

ACUTE ILLNESS OR INJURY

The child's response to acute illness or injury depends upon the particular organ system affected, the level of psychosocial development, the meaning of the illness to the child and family, the nature of necessary treatment, and other factors. In general, there are broad patterns of responses characteristic of children at different developmental levels, with variations due to individual differences.

The direct effects of acute illness on behavior may include listlessness, prostration, irritability, and disturbances in sleep and appetite. Restlessness and hyperactivity often complicate the management of milder illnesses, especially in preschool children. In biologically predisposed youngsters, physiologic concomitants of anxiety may appear, including tachycardia, palpitation, hyperventilation, and diarrhea—at times leading to diagnostic confusion with hyperthyroidism, rheumatic fever, etc. A young child's efforts to resist parental control may lead to eating and sleeping problems that may persist long after recovery.

Emotional and behavioral regression in response to illness is common in older infants and young children and occurs to some degree in school-age children and adolescents as well. Depression may also occur with return of primitive fears and feelings of helplessness and hopelessness. In more severe reactions, compulsive or ritualized, stereotyped behavior may occur and may subside rapidly or continue as a reactive disorder.

Misinterpretations of the meaning of the illness or accident as punishment are common in preschool children and may occur in school-age children as well. Late preschool and early school-age children may have fears of bodily mutilation, especially when sensitive areas such as the genitalia, eyes, or mouth are involved. In older school-age children, conversion and dissociative reactions may be encountered, often associated with subclinical delirium in response to drug administration or high fever or during convalescence.

The potentially deleterious effects of bed rest too strenuously enforced must be borne in mind and balanced against the sometimes doubtful advantages.

Prugh DG: Acute illness and injury. In: *The Psychosocial Aspects of Pediatrics*. Lea & Febiger, 1983.

CHRONIC ILLNESS & SERIOUS INJURY

Chronic illness or handicapping injuries may have serious consequences for the child's personality development and family functioning. The child's previous adaptive capacity and the parent-child family balance appear to be the most important prognostic factors. These children's personalities appear to fall along a continuum ranging from overdependent, overanxious, and passive or withdrawn to overly independent, with strong tendencies to deny illness. A number of these youngsters become realistically dependent and accept their limitations, developing adequate social roles and methods and sublimating their energies in constructive ways. Parental patterns range from overanxiousness, overprotectiveness, and overindulgence, often with difficulties in setting limits on the child's demands, to refusal to accept the severity of the child's disability, projection of personal guilt onto others (including the doctor), reluctance to cooperate with treatment programs, and, occasionally, rejection or isolation of the child.

Many parents ultimately learn to accept an unwell child's limitations without discomfort so that they can permit an appropriate degree of dependency while still helping the child to find and reach his or her full potential. (See also Chapter 9.)

Child's Reaction

Many children with chronic illnesses or handicaps have difficulties in maintaining a sound body image. Adolescents especially may show marked reactions to disfigurement or physical handicap.

In reaction to catastrophic illness or injury, school-age children and adolescents show a phasic response consisting initially of an **impact phase** involving realistic fears of death, soon followed by marked regression, strong denial of long-term damage, and the use of primitive fantasy (eg, daydreams of being a great athlete). After days or weeks, the **phase of recoil** is characterized by dawning recognition of the seriousness of the situation and by grief, or "mourning for the loss of the self"; this represents a constructive process, but it may be masked by demanding behavior. Severe depression may be present during this phase. The **phase of restitution** is characterized by the reemergence of premorbid personality traits such as overdependence or unrealistic overindependence. Management must be geared to the patient's progress through these phases.

Parents' Reactions

Parents show a parallel phasic response. A phase of "denial and disbelief" may persist for days, weeks, or months, sometimes accompanied by "shopping" for other opinions. During the succeeding phase of "fear and frustration," the parents may be depressed and guilty and may project blame onto each other or onto other persons. Marital crises may occur during this time. After weeks or months, the parents usually arrive at the phase of "intelligent inquiry and planning," in which they are able to handle their feelings and to live fairly comfortably although with some ambiguity.

Attempts to force either the parents or the child to face the reality of the situation before they are ready only increase the denial. Indeed, some denial—within limits—may be necessary to maintain hope.

Management of Reactions

During the management of chronic illness or handicap, the child and parents can be helped to focus on small, day-to-day steps as well as to ventilate feelings of frustration, anxiety, or guilt. Other supportive measures include occupational therapy in the home, gradual resumption of activity, and redirection of the child's energies into new activities as a substitute for those that are now restricted by the disability.

Home teachers may make it possible for the child to keep up with school. The child should attend school, even on a part-time basis, either in a special class or, ideally, a regular class. Vocational training compatible with the adolescent's intellectual and physical capacities can be arranged with the help of community resources. For the child too disabled to leave home, service agencies can often build a social club in the home. Group discussions among parents of children with similar problems may be of value in offering emotional support, as may similar approaches with handicapped adolescents.

Paradoxic Responses to Treatment

Children with deep-seated emotional conflicts who have adapted to the role of an invalid in families with unhealthy interpersonal relationships may find it difficult to respond to treatment in a positive way and may instead decompensate or develop a variety of symptomatic reactions. A gradual rehabilitative approach is necessary for such children and parents, and psychiatric consultation or formal psychotherapy is often required.

Prognosis

Emotional factors such as depression over actual or symbolic loss of key figures or lack of motivation to recover may adversely influence the course of serious illnesses such as carcinoma, leukemia, lymphoma, and especially infectious hepatitis, which seems to exert a specific depressive effect upon the psyche. Supportive psychologic measures should be part of the total treatment plan for children and adolescents with many of these disorders. Psychiatric consultation is often helpful and should be sought whenever the physician feels inadequate in treating an emotional component that is menacing the patient's total mental and physical well-being.

Downey JA, Low NL: *The Child With Disabling Illness: Principles of Rehabilitation.* Saunders, 1974.

Eisenberg MG, Sutkin LC, Jansen MA: *Chronic Illness and Disability Through the Life Span: Effects on Self and Family.* Springer, 1984.

Green M, Solnit AJ: Reactions to the threatened loss of a child: A vulnerable child syndrome. *Pediatrics* 1964;**34:**58.

Mattsson A: Long-term physical illness in children: A challenge to psychosocial adaptation. *Pediatrics* 1972;**50:**801.

Prugh DG: Chronic illness and handicap in children. In: *The Psychosocial Aspects of Pediatrics.* Lea & Febiger, 1983.

Prugh DG: Stages and phases in the response of children and adolescents to illness or injury. In: *Advances in Behavioral Pediatrics.* Vol 1. Camp BW (editor). JAI Press, 1980.

Prugh DG: Toward an understanding of psychosomatic concepts in relation to illness in children. In: *Modern Perspectives in Child Development.* Solnit AJ, Provence S (editors). Internat Univ Press, 1963.

Prugh DG, Eckhardt LO: Children's reactions to illness, hospitalization, and surgery. In: *Modern Synopsis of Comprehensive Textbook of Psychiatry,* 3rd ed. Freedman AM, Kaplan HI (editors). Williams & Wilkins, 1980.

HOSPITALIZATION

The management of children before, during, and after hospitalization is an important part of pediatric treatment, since most children have this experience at some time or other (3.5 million a year under age 15). Hospitalization, with its separation from home and the various treatment procedures encountered, may cause a variety of reactions depending upon the child's level of psychosocial development, the family's response, the meaning of the illness and hospitalization, the type of treatment required, and other factors. As children become older, they develop a realistic understanding of the usefulness of hospitals and become less likely to harbor painful fantasies about the need for hospitalization during periods of acute illness.

Child's Reaction

A. Infants Under 6 Months of Age: Young infants usually show temporary "global responses" to unfamiliar methods of feeding and handling, which may confuse mothers on return home.

B. Older Infants: Beginning in the second half of the first year, infants experience stranger anxiety and fears of separation, with regression and depression.

C. Young Children: Children up to age 4 appear most vulnerable to separation from the mother. Children of this age often experience a sequence of protest, despair, and detachment, the latter often associated with withdrawal and depression if separation without adequate mother-substitute relationships continues beyond a few days or 1–2 weeks.

D. Children From Age 4 to Early School Age: Children in this age group may experience separation anxiety but are usually more acutely preoccupied with fears of mutilation.

E. Older School-Age Children: Older children are usually able to comprehend the reality of the hospital experience more objectively but may still show signs of mild regression and anxiety over bodily functioning, etc. Fears of genital inadequacy, muscular weakness, and loss of body control or helplessness during anesthesia may enhance the feelings of anxiety and inferiority that are characteristic of this stage of development. The same trends may be seen in adolescents but in a muted form. They may have difficulty in accepting the authority of the medical staff.

Parents' Reactions

The parents' anxiety over a child's illness may be worsened if the child is hospitalized. They may fear criticism from the hospital staff regarding their role in the illness itself or their effectiveness as parents and thus may adopt a rival attitude toward nurses or physicians in an attempt to disarm the implied criticism of their own parental abilities. Feeling left out or unwanted is also common among parents. A few parents project their own guilt onto the hospital staff and blame them for the child's difficulties. Some parents with excessive anxiety are themselves unable to separate comfortably from the child; a few, with intense guilt, may be unable to visit.

Preparation for Hospitalization

All children should be told simply and truthfully why they are going to the hospital, what being in a hospital is like, and what will be done to make them comfortable. They must be assured that their parents will remain in contact with them. When the physician decides that hospitalization is necessary, the parents should be told what to tell the child. The parents' apprehension, guilt feelings, or conflicts can be dealt with as necessary at this time.

Preschool children should not be prepared for elective hospitalization more than a week or so in advance—enough time for questions but not too much for anxiety to build up. In some instances, a group session with the physician, parents, and child may be helpful in order to support anxious parents or to give the child the feeling of being involved in the planning.

Thorough exposition of the medical or surgical implications and procedures is not necessary for most children, although adolescents may wish to know more details. Practical discussions about mealtimes, use of a bedpan, etc, may be of value for older preschool children. "Playing out" situations in the hospital with a toy doctor's or nurse's kit may help to prevent anxiety. Visits to the hospital may be useful for school-age children. Booklets about "going to the hospital" may be of value if an opportunity for questions is offered, but they should not convey the impression that being in hospital is like "being at a party," with entertainment, treats, etc.

Reactions to Painful Procedures

Procedures such as venipunctures, injections, and lumbar punctures are frightening to young children, and very young children cannot be expected to cooperate unassisted. Older children can sometimes be made interested in the doctor's instruments and their purpose, so that they can cooperate to some extent in controlling their response to pain. The doctor should always explain that some pain will occur, without minimizing or exaggerating it. Children should be told when and where it will hurt and encouraged to cry if they feel like it. Firm but kindly restraint should be used as necessary, with the explanation that it is being done to help the child hold still so that "it won't hurt so much." The main thought to be conveyed is that the young patient, the doctor, and the nurse have an alliance that will help get the task done with as little discomfort as possible.

Posthospitalization

Most children manifest at least mildly disturbed behavior for a few days or several weeks after returning home. This posthospitalization reaction may persist if reinforced by parental anxiety or guilt. Anticipatory guidance and support for the parents in gradually "weaning" the child from regressive behavior can be of valuable preventive significance.

During convalescence, some children find it hard to relinquish the greater dependency involved in the acute phase of the illness and may dread the imminent return to competitive school responsibilities. Flexibility in matters of bed rest, meals, and treatment routines may be appropriate—eg, rest on the living room couch, in contact with other members of the family, may be more therapeutic than in the bedroom, where the relative isolation can lead to further regression.

The child should return to an integrated family life and to school as soon as possible.

The Child in the Hospital

Hospitalization is not necessarily a traumatic experience for a child, although it should be used as sparingly as possible. Preschool or previously disturbed children are most vulnerable to adverse reactions. In addition to improvement in physical health as a result of hospitalization, some older children benefit from the opportunity to relate to other children and adults outside the home, especially if the family has been disturbed or isolated.

Previously unrecognized psychologic problems in a child with physical illness may become obvious as a result of a comprehensive evaluation in a hospital setting, where one may observe at greater length the behavior of the child and the interaction between the child and the parents.

During hospitalization, the child's "life space" and ties with reality should be maintained. The teacher is a familiar nonmedical figure, and schooling should be available even during brief periods of hospitalization. Recreational therapists, social group workers, and occupational therapists can provide valuable emotional support and opportunities for "playing out" feelings about the hospital staff and procedures while at the same time offering age-appropriate recreational outlets.

Early ambulation (in carts if necessary) and family style eating arrangements offer social experiences that may facilitate convalescence and improve appetite.

It is sometimes difficult to coordinate the activities of physicians, consultants, nurses, social workers, teachers, recreational staff, "foster grandparents," and other persons involved. A weekly or biweekly ward management conference chaired by a senior pediatrician or clinical director will facilitate communication and increase the effectiveness of the total effort.

The most vital mental health need while the child is in the hospital is maintenance of the tie with the family. The "therapeutic alliance" between the parents and the hospital staff is a concept of great importance. The hospital should be organized to provide a balance between the advantages of the parents' presence and the treatment obligations of the staff, with separate visiting and treatment areas if possible. Flexible daily visiting schedules are directly correlated with less disturbed behavior on the part of the older preschool and school-age child, and cross-infection has been shown to be minimal. Some facilities permit unrestricted visiting and overnight stay by parents. For preschool children, who are more anxious over separation and whose understanding is limited, overnight stay or "living in" by the parent is the most effective preventive measure. Individualized planning about visiting is necessary, since some parents will not be able to take advantage of such opportunities for a variety of reasons.

Alternatives to hospitalization should be considered. For example, motel facilities adjacent to a child's hospital have been developed where the parents of a child who is being studied diagnostically can stay. Day care can be planned for children with chronic illnesses or diagnostic problems who do not require hospitalization. Greater use can be made of home care if a "family team" can be organized for this purpose.

Asarnoff P, Hardgrove C (editors): *The Family in Child Health Care.* Wiley, 1981.

Glaser HD: Group discussions with mothers and hospitalized children. *Pediatrics* 1960;**26:**132.

Prugh DG: Reactions of children and families to hospitalization and medical and surgical procedures. In: *The Psychosocial Aspects of Pediatrics.* Lea & Febiger, 1983.

Prugh DG: *Respect for the Cultural Heritage of the Hospitalized Child: First Elizabeth M. Staub Memorial Lecture.* Bulletin of the Association for Child Care in Hospitals, Fall, 1975.

Shore MF (editor): *Red Is the Color of Hurting: Planning for Children in the Hospital.* US Department of Health, Education, and Welfare, 1966.

Solnit AJ: Hospitalization: An aid to physical and psychological health in childhood. *Am J Dis Child* 1960;**99:**155.

SURGERY

The child who requires an operation needs special preparation if psychologic problems are to be avoided. For school-age children, the explanation should be simple and brief, without many details, and the child should be permitted to ask questions freely both before and after surgery. Most children can talk more easily and understand more fully if a simple drawing is used to explain the procedure. Even early adolescent boys may fear, for example, that a colectomy for ulcerative colitis may somehow interfere with their capacity for "becoming a man." The pediatrician should make sure that preparation takes place, no matter who does it. Preparation of the parents is equally important, as they too may have significant misconceptions. If possible, elective operations should be avoided in children 4–6 years of age, since fears of bodily mutilation are greatest at this time.

Anesthesia

Anesthesia may evoke fears of death or of loss of self-control in school-age children. They may have fears they will say or do "something bad" and may also be concerned about what might be done to their bodily organs while they are helpless. Induction and recovery states should be explained in appropriate terms. Some children need to be reassured they will not wake up before the operation is over. Others may mistake the onset of unconsciousness for impending death and need to be told that "going to sleep" will be temporary and will be followed by complete awakening. Preliminary "playing out" of the induction process by the anesthetist or other personnel aids in the child's mastery of the situation. If possible, the child should be spared the experience of seeing instruments, the operating room, etc.

Since oral barbiturates may have a stimulant effect on preschool children unless given in large doses, administration of a basal anesthetic (eg, thiopental) in the child's room (with the parent present) may help relax an overly anxious child and prevent resistance on the way to the operating room. When the child awakes, the parent should be there; this is especially important for young children. School-age children can be helped to adjust to the ward setting and staff by being admitted a day in advance of an operation. (This is not ordinarily helpful for preschool children.)

Principles of this kind have also been shown to be effective in cutting down on the amount of anesthetic necessary and in reducing the incidence and severity of postoperative reactions.

Mutilating Operations

Special problems may arise in regard to operations with unavoidably mutilating results, such as amputations. The child who misinterprets the procedure as a punishment for a past misdeed may become aggressive (in fantasied self-defense) or withdrawn (feeling helpless and hopeless).

Occasionally, persistent denial of loss of a body part, such as a limb, can lead to difficulties in planning for prosthetic devices. Psychiatric consultation should be freely used.

Burns

A severely burned child who feels guilty about the accident and fearful of the loss of the parents' love may become seriously depressed, respond poorly to surgical procedures, and fail to heal adequately. The presence of a foster grandparent may literally save the life of a severely burned preschool child who is regressive and depressed about not being held any more by the parents—not comprehending that the burns prevent the parents from holding the child. Hypnosis may be helpful in minimizing pain during dressing changes; drugs are not as helpful in children as in adults. Most children with extensive burns have emotional problems even following successful surgical treatment. Psychotherapy has been shown to ameliorate or prevent such problems.

Bernstein NR: Observations on the use of hypnosis with burned children on a pediatric ward. *Int J Clin Exp Hypn* 1965;**13:**1.

Cytryn L, Cytryn E: Psychological implications of cryptorchidism. *J Am Acad Child Psychiatry* 1967;**6:**131.

Eckhardt LO, Prugh DG: Preparing children psychologically for painful medical and surgical procedures. In: *Psychosocial Aspects of Pediatric Care.* Gellert E (editor). Grune & Stratton, 1978.

Fine RN et al: Renal homotransplantation in children. *J Pediatr* 1970;**76:**347.

Gardner GG: The uses of hypnotherapy in pediatrics: A review. *Pediatrics* 1978;**62:**228.

Jessner L, Blom GE, Waldfogel S: Emotional implications of tonsillectomy and adenoidectomy in children. *Psychoanal Study Child* 1952;**7:**126.

Melamed BG, Robbins RL, Graves S: Preparation for surgery and medical procedures. In: *Behavioral Pediatrics: Research and Practice.* Russo D, Varni J (editors). Plenum Press, 1982.

TERMINAL ILLNESS

Recent advances in medical and surgical care have brought about a change in the composition of the patient population in many children's hospitals. The pediatric practitioner is spending more and more time in caring for children with chronic and sometimes fatal illnesses. The physician must be able to deal constructively with parents and children in these tragic circumstances. The management of dying children is perhaps one of the most difficult tasks the pediatrician faces today.

Explaining a fatal illness is a complicated task often attended by some risk. However, not to interpret the fatal illness at some level is a disservice to the patient and the patient's family. Knowing the child and family and understanding the child's concept of death may help provide answers in specific situations.

The Young Child

The chief concerns of a young child who is dying are fear of separation from the parents and a desire to be spared pain. When death comes acutely, the child's awareness is often blunted by delirium, stupor, or coma. In a more gradual terminal experience, there is often evidence of depression, withdrawal, fearfulness, and apprehension. Although most children with a fatal illness do not ask explicitly if they are going to die, children over the age of 4 or 5 may do so. Parents and others may have different ideas about how to respond to such questions. The physician should not answer without the parents' permission, since they may prefer to do it themselves or with the help of a religious counselor. When the physician does answer, it is important to find out why the child thinks dying is a possibility. It may be that the concealed purpose of the question is simply to make certain that someone will be there at the time and that there will be no pain.

The Older Child

Older children and adolescents have more understanding about impending death than the parents or hospital staff may realize.

Staff members often maintain an unconscious "conspiracy of silence" and may even stay away from these children to avoid the topic. In some cases, everyone involved may feel more comfortable if the topic is brought into the open. Young people can be told that they might die but that everything possible will be done to help them get well. They should be assured that pain relief will be available and that they will not be left alone if they become seriously ill.

When a child dies, other children on the ward inevitably sense that something serious has happened and may need to be reassured that their condition is different.

Parents' Reactions

Parental reactions include the entire continuum from complete withdrawal from the child, through "mourning in advance" and an early detachment, to the extreme of denial and unrealistic expectations accompanied by poor reality testing. The reaction of the parents also depends on the circumstances of the illness or injury, the degree of their guilt, and the nature of the prior family relationship.

The physician must keep in mind the nature of the disease, the age of the child, and the family concept of death. When the diagnosis and prognosis are certain, the parents should be told, frankly but gently, even though they may be overwhelmed and may want to go elsewhere for further medical care. The possibility of a fatal illnesss should never be mentioned to parents as part of a differential diagnosis, since some parents may continue to treat the child as a doomed creature even after the possibility has been ruled out.

If the parents are able to help care for the child in the hospital during the terminal phase, they should be encouraged to do so. Some parents cannot bring themselves to help, however, and they should not be made to feel guilty if this is so. The physician must be ready to accept whatever feelings the parents display, even permitting them to bring other family members in to mourn with the child or to take the child home to die if that is their cultural tradition. Parents should be allowed to vent their feelings and perhaps even be encouraged to engage in the normal mourning process if there is an obvious lack of expression in an overly inhibited family. In the hospital, parents may gain much emotional support from other parents or social workers. Other community resources may be available also, so that the parents can have someone to whom they can express their feelings outside the hospital. Religious counselors, other family members, or psychiatric consultants may be helpful in understanding such situations and in working out a plan for some sort of help.

Parents frequently require a continuing supportive relationship with the pediatrician after the child's death. An appointment should be made to see them within several weeks, as their guilt and anxiety may lead them to repeat questions already asked. Such an opportunity for "working through" their feelings may help them to avoid conceiving another child right away to take the place of the lost one, with obvious difficulties ahead.

Easson WM: *The Dying Child: Management of the Child or Adolescent Who Is Dying*. Thomas, 1970.

Friedman SB: Management of fatal illness in children. In: *Ambulatory Pediatrics,* 2nd ed. Green M, Haggerty RJ (editors). Saunders, 1976.

Koocher GP, O'Malley JE: *The Damocles Syndrome: Psychological Consequences of Surviving Childhood Cancer*. McGraw-Hill, 1984.

Prugh DG: Psychosocial aspects of the management of fatal illness. In: *The Psychosocial Aspects of Pediatrics*. Lea & Febiger, 1983.

Vernick J, Karon M: Who's afraid of death on a leukemia ward? *Am J Dis Child* 1965;**109:**393.

CHILD ABUSE & NEGLECT*

In the USA, over 80% of cases of abuse and neglect causing physical or developmental trauma in children and adolescents are the result of harmful actions of parents or other caretakers, with the vast majority attributable to the parents themselves. At least 10% of major injuries in children under 4 years of age are due to nonaccidental trauma. The number of sexual abuse cases that are reported is increasing rapidly, probably because of increased professional and public awareness and detection of the problem. Survey studies indicate that as many as 40% of women and 20% of men have been sexually molested at some time and that only a small percentage of these incidents had been reported. Currently, only 8% of reports of child abuse fall into the category of sexual abuse, but in light of the above survey statistics, it appears that this figure is not an accurate reflection of the number of cases that actually occur. The offender in sexual abuse cases is usually a relative (the parent or stepparent in 50% of cases), neighbor, baby-sitter, or trusted family friend. Occasionally, several members of a family are involved in an incestuous relationship.

Physicians and nurses (and other specified classes of child care professionals) are legally required to report suspected child abuse or neglect. Remaining alert to the possibility of abuse or neglect in children with injuries, developmental and emotional problems, and vague symptoms of illness will help make the diagnosis in more subtle cases.

* Contributed by Ruth S. Kempe, MD.

Classification

A. Physical Abuse: This category includes injuries caused by undue physical punishment, violence, or poisoning.

B. Neglect: Neglect is the primary diagnosis in over 45% of cases of child maltreatment and is a concomitant of many other forms of abuse. Neglect is not always willful; lack of knowledge, financial hardship, and other factors may prevent parents from providing adequately for their children. Types of neglect include (1) lack of nurturance, leading to growth failure (formerly called nonorganic failure to thrive), attachment difficulties and other psychologic disturbances, and developmental delays associated with failure to respond appropriately to the needs of a developing infant or child; (2) lack of supervision, which exposes the child to increased risks of injury and emotional trauma; (3) medical neglect, including failure to provide for well child care (eg, immunizations) and failure to seek medical attention for illness, which may result in exacerbation of an easily treated problem (eg, untreated recurrent otitis media resulting in hearing loss); and (4) educational neglect, including failure to teach the child the minimal information necessary to cope with his or her environment and failure to send the school-age child to school on a regular schedule.

C. Emotional Abuse: This is usually manifested as verbal criticism and demeaning and overt rejection of the child. It may progress to completely ignoring the child, isolating him or her from all social contact, or scapegoating of one child in the family. Emotional abuse almost always accompanies other forms of neglect and abuse.

D. Sexual Abuse: Sexual abuse may be confined to fondling or may involve seduction with oral, anal, and vaginal intercourse or rape. Children of any age may be sexually abused, but the offender is usually at least 5 years older than the victim. At least one-third of sexually abused children are physically abused or neglected as well.

E. "Munchausen-by-Proxy" Syndrome: Munchausen's syndrome involves seeking medical help for fictitious illnesses and providing a false history to support the claims. In the "by-proxy" form of the syndrome, the parent or caretaker (usually the mother) reports fictitious illnesses in the child or even induces illness (eg, by giving the child drugs or noxious substances) to obtain medical attention. The disturbed adult is very persistent and usually goes from one doctor to the next to obtain medical and surgical care and is sometimes successful in having the child hospitalized repeatedly.

Diagnosis

A multidisciplinary approach to diagnosis and treatment of child abuse and neglect involves physicians, nurses, social workers, and other medical and community professionals, often forming a special child protection team in larger communities or hospitals. Expertise is directed toward protecting the abused child and siblings but also preventing wrongful accusations of parents or caretakers by investigating whether injuries could have been accidental or self-inflicted.

A. History and Physical Examination:

1. Physical abuse—Details of the circumstances leading to injury should be elicited, and the child's medical history should be taken as described elsewhere in the text. Findings should be carefully recorded and photographs taken if appropriate.

In cases due to violence or excessive punishment, there may be obvious signs of injury, such as bruises, swelling, abrasions, lacerations, or cuts; marks made by slapping, tying, choking, or striking with a belt and belt buckle; or stocking and glove burns on an extremity, often due to immersion in hot water. With dislocations or fractures, commonly of the long bones and ribs, there may be tenderness or pain and resistance to movement. Skull fractures may be present even if there are no signs of intracranial injury. Retinal hemorrhages, an early sign of subdural hematoma, usually appear within 2 hours of injury. Subdural hematoma may be caused by direct trauma or shaking of an infant. Alterations in mental status may be due to head injury, drug ingestion, or poisoning.

2. Neglect—Signs of neglect include malnutrition, cradle cap (in infants) or dental caries (in children), evidence of chronic lack of personal cleanliness, and inadequate or dirty clothing. The parents may show lack of concern and support for the child, and the child may exhibit poor attachment to the parents, delayed development, and inappropriate social responses to parents and others.

3. Sexual abuse—Specific or generalized fears, social withdrawal, psychosomatic symptoms, school failure, or sexual preoccupation (often evidenced in overt masturbation or sexually seductive behavior with adults or other children) may alert teachers, parents, or physicians to the possibility of recent or past sexual abuse in a child or adolescent. In most cases, however, the diagnosis usually depends on the ability of the child to tell someone who will respond by enlisting medical or social service help.

The adequacy of the initial interview of the child is particularly important, and law enforcement personnel and the medical specialist may wish to arrange for a joint meeting or a videotaped interview performed by someone skilled in the field of interviewing children who are sexually abused. The child's comfort in the interviewing situation is of primary importance. The child should be encouraged to talk freely and provide details about who was involved and where, how, when, and how often the sexual encounters occurred. Questions should be nonleading, specific, and appropriate to the child's developmental age, so that there is confidence in the reliability of the child's report. Children under 3 years of age may only be able to indicate who was involved and how they were handled. Observing the young child's behavior in a play situation or the child's ability to demonstrate sexual experience by use of dolls may be helpful if these techniques are accompanied by appropriate questioning.

Perineal examination, performed in the presence of another person, should be done only after a good relationship has been established with the child so that there is a minimum of anxiety. The sex of the examiner may depend on the sex and age of the child and of the sex offender. Inspection of the genitalia may reveal hymenal tears or scars, or there may be irritation and redness of the vaginal or anal area. Some investigators believe that a vaginal opening exceeding 4 mm in a prepubertal girl is indicative of sexual abuse, but this requires further studies. The absence of specific findings on perineal examination does not rule out sexual abuse.

B. Laboratory, Radiologic, and Other Studies:

1. Physical abuse or neglect—If caretakers attribute bruises and similar marks to the child's easy bruisability, a bleeding screen (see Chapter 16) should be performed. If poisoning or ingestion of drugs or other noxious substances (eg, salt added to an infant formula) is suspected, a blood and urine screen and determination of electrolyte values should be performed. Ultrasonography can be useful in diagnosing some visceral injuries. X-rays should be taken in cases in which physical abuse is suspected in infants under 3 years of age and in older children with physical findings or with siblings who have been abused. Fractures in different stages of healing are usually diagnostic of nonaccidental trauma unless there is documented bone disease. Radionuclide bone scanning may be especially useful in detecting recent fractures, and CT scanning is helpful in the diagnosis of intracranial injuries.

In cases in which sudden death occurs in a child and abuse or neglect is suspected, a thorough postmortem examination should be performed to detect signs of bone or visceral injury, poisoning, and other indications of abuse, especially if the child is over the usual age for sudden infant death syndrome (see Chapter 14).

2. Sexual abuse—Rape kits for collecting appropriate specimens should be available for those who treat sexual abuse regularly. A serologic test for syphilis should be performed, and specimens from oral, anal, and vaginal orifices should be cultured for gonococci. Swabs should also be analyzed for prostatic acid phosphatase, spermatozoa, and ABO antigen if sexual abuse has occurred within 48 hours; however, only about 20–30% of these will yield positive results. Rape kits also include equipment to collect and analyze pubic hair.

C. Psychosocial Evaluation: An evaluation of the family should be undertaken if any form of abuse (physical, sexual, emotional, etc) or neglect is suspected. This should include a thorough evaluation of (1) the family's current environmental and socioeconomic status, including housing and financial problems; (2) the parents' marital situation, including the quality and status of the marriage (discord, stress, separation); (3) psychologic support systems (help from relatives and friends, isolation of the family, inability to trust or use outside support) and family responses to crises; (4) health problems of the parents, eg, physical illness, mental retardation, emotional problems, psychiatric disorders, or drug or alcohol abuse; (5) social problems of the parents, eg, history of violence or law breaking; (6) parent-child interactions, including attachment, ability to perceive and respond to the needs of the child, expectations of the child (realistic or unrealistic), and specific methods of discipline and how frequently they are employed; (7) the parents' perceptions of their child's behavior and, if perceived as unacceptable, examples of this; and (8) the parents' own experience during childhood. The majority of abusive and neglectful parents were themselves abused and neglected during childhood.

Management

A. Acute Medical Care: The acute medical needs of the child are addressed while the diagnostic process is under way. Treatment and follow-up for fractures, malnutrition, and other injuries and disorders are discussed elsewhere in the text. In cases of sexual abuse, the reader should consult Chapter 9 for discussions of sexually transmitted disease and pregnancy. Studies indicate that the risk of pregnancy is low, with incidence rates varying from 1 to 10% in several reports.

B. Immediate Protection of the Child: Hospitalization is often indicated because of the child's medical condition. In other cases, hospitalization or placement in a crisis care facility may be indicated for the child's protection while the home environment is evaluated.

High-risk factors that mitigate against an early return to the home include any injury in a young infant, since injuries tend to escalate in severity in cases of recurrent abuse; present serious or life-threatening injuries; a history of repeated injuries requiring treatment in the child or a sibling; fatal injury in a sibling; injuries resulting from sadistic behavior; abuse or neglect of a child who is particularly vulnerable, eg, physically handicapped, mentally retarded, or suffering from a severe behavior disorder; and cases in which a parent is mentally retarded, violent, emotionally disturbed, or addicted to drugs or alcohol. In the latter category, psychiatric evaluation of the parent is indicated to determine if parenting skills are adequate, and careful follow-up is needed to ensure that the parent is functioning well.

C. Long-Term Planning for the Family: Planning for protection of the child and treatment of the parents and child may require the expertise of various medical, social, and law enforcement personnel. In about 25% of substantiated reports of child abuse or neglect, the courts become involved in determining placement of the child.

While foster care placement is sometimes indicated, it should be considered a temporary measure to ensure the child's safety during the early stages of treatment for the parents and child.

1. Services to aid the parents—Onc or more of the following may be recommended: individual psychotherapy or individual counseling; self-help groups, such as Parents Anonymous; parenting classes or parent-child interaction sessions with a developmental specialist; respite care (ie, use of day-care centers, crisis nurseries, or voluntary temporary placement at times of major stress); and family or marriage counseling. The latter is considered most effective in coping with incest but should be considered in all cases of abuse or neglect when the family is to be reunited. In some cases, drug dependency programs or job training or rehabilitation services may be indicated.

2. Services to aid the child—For young children with developmental delays or emotional disturbances, therapeutic or specialized day-care services or preschool sessions may be indicated. Issues to be addressed in individual or group therapy for older children who show emotional disturbances subsequent to abuse or neglect include difficulties with relationships, expressed by lack of basic trust and by feelings of deprivation, dependency, sadness, and anger; behavioral difficulties, such as poor control of impulses and poor socialization skills; and negative self-image, with lack of self-confidence and poorly developed sense of identity. A few children will require psychiatric hospitalization or residential treatment because of the extensive nature of their emotional difficulties (eg, severe depression with suicidal tendencies, severe behavior disorders). Chapter 9 discusses treatment of problems that may develop or reach serious proportions in adolescence (eg, school truancy or failure, drug or alcohol abuse, depression, and suicidal behavior).

Prognosis & Prevention

Early diagnosis and treatment in cases of child abuse and neglect are essential to prevent future episodes of maltreatment and reduce the severity of physical, developmental, and psychologic effects on the victimized children. Parents who have themselves been severely neglected or abused in childhood are often the offenders in these cases and may respond slowly to counseling or therapy, whereas the children usually respond quickly to a safe and supportive environment. This poses the dilemma of how much time to allow parents to change their behavior while the child is without a permanent home (eg, in a foster home). If it appears that the parents will never achieve adequate parenting skills (as occurs in about 10% of those in treatment), it may be advantageous to the child to seek early court involvement to terminate parental rights and place the child in a permanent home.

Because of the generational repetition of abuse and neglect, as well as the difficulties in treating parents quickly, prevention of this problem is an urgent and major social concern. Measures to heighten social awareness and prevent abuse and neglect could include incorporation of concepts of human development (both physical and psychologic) into the school curriculum at all levels, educational programs for future parents, and support programs for all new parents.

Finkelhor D: *Child Sexual Abuse: New Theory and Research.* Free Press, 1984.

Fraiberg S: *Clinical Studies in Infant Mental Health.* Basic Books, 1980.

Helfer RE, Kempe RS: *The Battered Child.* Chicago Univ Press, 1986.

Mrazek PB, Kempe CH (editors): *Sexually Abused Children and Their Families.* Pergamon Press, 1981.

Schmitt BD: *The Child Protection Team Handbook.* Garland STPM Press, 1978.

SELECTED REFERENCES

Ackerman N: *Treating the Troubled Family.* Basic Books, 1966.

Apley J, McKeith R: *The Child and His Symptoms.* Davis, 1968.

Arnold LE (editor): *Helping Parents Help Their Children.* Brunner/Mazel, 1978.

Bakwin H, Bakwin RM: *Clinical Management of Behavior Disorders in Children,* rev ed. Saunders, 1967.

Berlin IN (editor): *Bibliography of Child Psychiatry and Child Mental Health,* 2nd ed. Human Sciences Press, 1976.

Birch HG: *Brain Damage in Children.* Williams & Wilkins, 1964.

Call JD, Galenson E, Tyson RL (editors): *Frontiers in Infant Psychiatry.* Vol 1. Basic Books, 1983.

Camp BW (editor): *Advances in Behavioral Pediatrics.* JAI Press, 1980–present. [Annual.]

Chess S, Hassibi M: *Principles and Practice of Child Psychiatry.* Plenum Press, 1978.

Chess S, Thomas A: *Annual Progress in Child Psychiatry and Child Development.* Brunner/Mazel, 1967–present. [Annual.]

Christopherson ER, Abernathy JE: Research in ambulatory pediatrics. In: *Behavioral Pediatrics: Research and Practice.* Russo DC, Varni JW (editors). Plenum Press, 1982.

Committee on Child Psychiatry: *Psychopathological Disorders in Childhood: Theoretical Considerations and a Proposed Classification.* GAP Report No. 62. Group for the Advancement of Psychiatry, 1968.

Diagnostic and Statistical Manual of Mental Disorders (DSM-III), 3rd ed. American Psychiatric Association, 1980.

Erikson EH: *Childhood and Society,* 2nd ed. Norton, 1963.

Farley GK, Eckhardt LO, Hebert FB: *Handbook of Child and Adolescent Psychiatric Emergencies,* 2nd ed. Medical Examination Publishing Co., 1986.

Freud A: *Normality and Pathology in Childhood: Assessment of Development.* Internat Univ Press, 1965.

Gellert E (editor): *Psychosocial Aspects of Pediatric Care.* Grune & Stratton, 1978.

Green M, Haggerty RJ (editors): *Ambulatory Pediatrics,* 2nd ed. Saunders, 1976.

Grossman HJ et al (editors): *Assessing Development and Treating Disorders Within a Family Context.* American Medical Association, 1979.

Harrison SI, Carek DJ: *A Guide to Psychotherapy.* Little, Brown, 1966.

Helfer RE, Kempe RS: *The Battered Child,* 4th ed. Univ of Chicago Press. [In press.]

Hill O (editor): *Modern Trends in Psychosomatic Medicine.* Butterworth, 1970.

Hoffman L, Hoffman M (editors): *Review of Child Development Research.* Vol 5. Russell Sage Foundation, 1975.

Howells JO (editor): *Modern Perspectives in International Child Psychiatry.* Oliver & Boyd, 1969.

Kanner L: *Child Psychiatry.* Thomas, 1962.

Kaplan HI, Sadock RJ (editors): *Comprehensive Textbook of Psychiatry,* 4th ed. Williams & Wilkins, 1985.

Lewis M: *Clinical Aspects of Child Development,* 2nd ed. Lea & Febiger, 1982.

Noshpitz JD (editor): *Basic Handbook of Child Psychiatry.* Basic Books, 1979.

Ollendich TH, Hersen M (editors): *Handbook of Child Psychopathology.* Plenum, 1983.

Patton RG, Gardner LI: *Growth Failure and Maternal Deprivation.* Thomas, 1963.

Pearson GHJ (editor): *A Handbook of Child Psychoanalysis.* Basic Books, 1968.

Prugh DG: *The Psychosocial Aspects of Pediatrics.* Lea & Febiger, 1983.

Psychoanalytic Study of the Child. Internat Univ Press, 1945–present. [Annual. Various editors.]

Rourke BP et al: *Child Neuropsychology: An Introduction to Theory, Research, and Clinical Practice.* Guilford, 1983.

Russo DC, Varni JW (editors): *Behavioral Pediatrics: Research and Practice.* Plenum Press, 1982.

Rutter M, Hersov L: *Child and Adolescent Psychiatry: Modern Approaches,* 2nd ed. Blackwell, 1984.

Schulman JI: *Management of Emotional Disorders in Pediatric Practice: With a Focus on Techniques of Interviewing.* Year Book, 1967.

Sex and the College Student. GAP Report No. 60. Group for the Advancement of Psychiatry, 1965.

Shaw CR (editor): *The Psychiatric Disorders of Childhood.* Appleton-Century-Crofts, 1966.

Shirley HF: *Pediatric Psychiatry.* Harvard Univ Press, 1963.

Simmons J: *Psychiatric Examination of the Child,* 2nd ed. Lea & Febiger, 1983.

Solnit AJ, Provence S (editors): *Modern Perspectives in Child Development.* Internat Univ Press, 1963.

Steinhauer PD, Rae-Grant Q (editors): *Psychological Problems of the Child in His Family,* 2nd ed. Basic Books, 1983.

Stuart HP, Prugh DG (editors): *The Healthy Child: His Physical, Psychological and Social Characteristics.* Harvard Univ Press, 1960.

Verville E: *Behavior Problems of Children.* Saunders, 1967.

Weiner HJ: *Psychobiology and Human Disease.* Elsevier, 1977.

25 Endocrine Disorders

Henry K. Silver, MD, Ronald W. Gotlin, MD, & Georgeanna J. Klingensmith, MD

Endocrine disorders are relatively infrequent in childhood, but a knowledge of the endocrine system is essential in order to differentiate its disorders from congenital malformations and from normal variations in the timing and pattern of development (ie, ''constitutional'' deviations from average). One should attempt to understand the pathogenesis of endocrine abnormalities so that the physiologic and chemical evidences of specific hormonal dysfunctions can be correlated with structural abnormalities, particularly as they affect growth and development.

DISTURBANCES OF GROWTH & DEVELOPMENT

Disturbances of growth and development are the most common presenting complaints in the pediatric endocrine clinic. It is estimated that over 1 million children in the USA have abnormal short stature and that there are at least 10 million children whose growth is potentially abnormal.

Failure to thrive is a term usually reserved for infants who fail to gain weight and is most often due to undernutrition (see below).

Tall stature is a much less frequent presenting complaint than short stature and is usually a matter of concern to adolescent girls. The recent trend toward acceptance of tall stature in women has decreased the number of young people evaluated and treated for tall stature in our clinics.

SHORT STATURE

Abnormally short stature in relation to age is a common finding in childhood. In most instances, it is due to a normal variation from the usual pattern of growth. The possible roles of such factors as sex, race, size of parents and other family members, nutrition, pubertal maturation, and emotional status must all be evaluated in the total assessment of the child.

The causes of unusually short stature are listed in Table 25–1. In most instances, the causes can be differentiated on the basis of the history, significant findings on physical examination, and stage of skeletal maturation as assessed by radiography.

1. CONSTITUTIONAL SHORT STATURE

Many children have a constitutional delay in growth and skeletal maturation. In all other respects, they appear entirely normal. There is often a history of a similar pattern of growth in one of the parents or other members of the family. Although puberty is delayed, normal puberty eventually occurs. These children usually reach normal adult height although at a later than average age.

In many children with constitutional short stature, birth weight and length are not affected, but the rate of growth is decreased during infancy and just prior to puberty. At other times, the infant is small at birth and growth velocity is normal, with the growth curve paralleling the fifth percentile.

With the exception of severe cases, no treatment for the short stature is indicated. The child and the parents should be helped to understand the normality of the situation. In severe cases, short controlled courses of anabolic and androgenic corticosteroids may be efficacious.

2. GROWTH HORMONE DEFICIENCY

When rigid diagnostic criteria are employed, instances of growth hormone (GH) deficiency are found in approximately one in 4000 children. About half of the cases are idiopathic (rarely familial); the remainder are secondary to pituitary or hypothalamic disease. In the majority of instances, a deficiency or impairment in hypothalamic secretion of GH-releasing hormone is suspected. Major causes are infection, trauma, reticuloendotheliosis, and craniopharyngioma or other tumors such as gliomas. GH deficiency may be an isolated defect or may occur in combination with other pituitary hormone deficiencies. Idiopathic GH deficiency affects both sexes equally.

At birth, affected children are of normal weight, but length may be reduced. The most characteristic clinical feature of the child with GH deficiency is a linear growth rate as little as one-half that of the normal child. Growth retardation may begin during infancy or may be delayed until later childhood. Other

Table 25–1. Causes of short stature.

Familial, racial, or genetic

Constitutional retarded growth and delayed adolescence

Endocrine disturbances
- Hypopituitarism
  - Isolated somatotropin or somatotropin-releasing hormone deficiency
  - Somatotropin deficiency with other pituitary hormone deficiencies
- Hypothyroidism
- Adrenal insufficiency
- Cushing's disease and Cushing's syndrome (including iatrogenic causes)
- Sexual precocity (androgen or estrogen excess)
- Diabetes mellitus (poorly controlled)
- Diabetes insipidus
- Hyperaldosteronism

Primordial short stature
- Intrauterine growth retardation
  - Placental insufficiency
  - Intrauterine infection
- Primordial dwarfism with premature aging
  - Progeria (Hutchinson-Gilford syndrome)
  - Progeroid syndrome
    - Werner's syndrome
    - Cachectic (Cockayne's syndrome)
- Short stature without associated anomalies
- Short stature with associated anomalies (eg, Seckel's bird-headed dwarfism, leprechaunism, Silver's syndrome, Bloom's syndrome, Cornelia de Lange syndrome, Hallerman-Streiff syndrome)

Inborn errors of metabolism
- Altered metabolism of calcium or phosphorus (eg, hypophosphatemic rickets, hypophosphatasia, infantile hypercalcemia, pseudohypoparathyroidism)
- Storage diseases
  - Mucopolysaccharidoses (eg, Hurler's syndrome, Hunter's syndrome)
  - Mucolipidoses (eg, generalized gangliosidosis, fucosidosis, mannosidosis)
  - Sphingolipidoses (eg, Tay-Sachs disease, Niemann-Pick disease, Gaucher's disease)
  - Miscellaneous (eg, cystinosis)
- Aminoacidemias and aminoacidurias

Inborn errors of metabolism (cont'd)
- Epithelial transport disorders (eg, renal tubular acidosis, cystic fibrosis, Bartter's syndrome, vasopressin-resistant diabetes insipidus, pseudohypoparathyroidism)
- Organic acidemias and acidurias (eg, methylmalonic aciduria, orotic aciduria, maple syrup urine disease, isovaleric acidemia)
- Metabolic anemias (eg, sickle cell disease, thalassemia, pyruvate kinase deficiency)
- Disorders of mineral metabolism (eg, Wilson's disease, magnesium malabsorption syndrome)
- Body defense disorders (eg, Bruton's agammaglobulinemia, thymic aplasia, chronic granulomatous disease)

Constitutional (intrinsic) diseases of bone
- Defects of growth of tubular bones or spine (eg, achondroplasia, metatropic dwarfism, diastrophic dwarfism, metaphyseal chondrodysplasia)
- Disorganized development of cartilage and fibrous components of the skeleton (eg, multiple cartilaginous exostoses, fibrous dysplasia with skin pigmentation, precocious puberty of McCune-Albright)
- Abnormalities of density of cortical diaphyseal structure or metaphyseal modeling (eg, osteogenesis imperfecta congenita, osteopetrosis, tubular stenosis)

Short stature associated with chromosomal defects
- Autosomal (eg, Down's syndrome, cri du chat syndrome, trisomy 18)
- Sex chromosomal (eg, Turner's syndrome-XO, penta X, XXXY)

Chronic systemic diseases, congenital defects, and cancers (eg, chronic infection and infestation, inflammatory bowel disease, hepatic disease, cardiovascular disease, hematologic disease, central nervous system disease, pulmonary disease, renal disease, malnutrition, cancers, collagen vascular disease)

Psychosocial dwarfism (deprivation dwarfism)

Miscellaneous syndromes (eg, arthrogryposis multiplex congenita, cerebrohepatorenal syndrome, Noonan's syndrome, Prader-Willi syndrome, Riley-Day syndrome)

findings include infantile fat distribution, youthful facial features, midfacial hypoplasia, and delayed sexual maturation. Epiphyseal maturation (''bone age'') is delayed. Headaches, visual field defects, abnormalities on funduscopic examination, polyuria, and polydipsia may precede or accompany the onset of growth failure in cases resulting from central nervous system disease. Abnormal skull radiographs or CT scans are common in organic hypopituitarism.

GH deficiency is associated with low levels of GH in the serum and with the failure of GH levels to increase appreciably during normal physiologic sleep, after exercise, or in response to arginine, glucagon, levodopa, clonidine, or insulin. Spontaneous hypoglycemia, augmented insulin sensitivity, and various findings due to other pituitary hormone deficiencies may be present.

Human pituitary GH has recently been implicated in deaths resulting from a degenerative neurologic disease. Therefore, the treatment of choice is synthetic human GH alone or in conjunction with other hormones. Results of clinical trials with GH-releasing hormone (somatotropin-releasing hormone) have been encouraging, and this agent may be employed in the future in patients with hypothalamic GH-releasing hormone deficiency. Protein anabolic agents may be effective in promoting linear growth but may cause undue acceleration of epiphyseal closure with a resultant lessening of adult height. Anabolic agents should ideally be used at the time of puberty and in combination with GH.

The greatest controversy surrounding GH therapy is its usefulness in a normal short child and in short-stature syndromes not associated with GH deficiency. At this time, the treatment of the normal short child with GH must be considered an experimental practice.

3. HYPOTHYROIDISM

Hypothyroidism in childhood (discussed in a subsequent section) is invariably associated with poor growth and delayed osseous maturation. In occasional cases, short stature may be the principal finding.

4. PRIMORDIAL SHORT STATURE (Intrauterine Growth Retardation)

Primordial short stature may occur in a number of disorders, including craniofacial disproportion (eg, Seckel's bird-headed dwarfism), Silver's syndrome, some cases of progeric and cachectic dwarfism (eg, Hutchinson-Gilford dwarfism), or may occur in individuals with no accompanying significant physical abnormalities. Children with these conditions are small at birth; both birth weight and length are below normal for gestational age. They grow parallel to but below the fifth percentile. Plasma GH levels are usually normal but may be elevated. In most instances, skeletal maturation (''bone age'') corresponds to chronologic age or is only mildly retarded, in contrast to the striking delay often present in children with GH and thyroid deficiency.

There is no satisfactory long-term treatment for primordial short stature, although growth hormone in large doses may be efficacious.

5. SHORT STATURE DUE TO EMOTIONAL FACTORS (Psychosocial Short Stature, Deprivation Dwarfism)

Psychologic deprivation with disturbances in motor and personality development may be associated with short stature. Although the growth retardation in some affected individuals is the result of undernutrition, in others undernutrition does not seem to be the major factor. In some instances, in addition to being small, the child may have increased (often voracious) appetite and a marked delay in skeletal maturation. Polydipsia and polyuria are sometimes present. These children are of normal size at birth and grow normally for a variable period of time before growth slows. A history of feeding problems in early infancy is common. Sleep is often restless. Emotional disturbances in the family are the rule. Plasma GH levels during sleep or in response to pharmacologic stimulation may be diminished.

Foster home placement or a significant change in the psychologic and emotional environment at home usually results in significantly improved growth and personality and decreased appetite and dietary intake.

DIFFERENTIAL DIAGNOSIS OF SHORT STATURE

Short stature may accompany or be caused by a large number of conditions (Table 25–1). When the etiologic diagnosis is not apparent from the history and physical examination, the following laboratory studies, in addition to bone age, are useful in detecting or categorizing the common causes of short stature:

(1) Complete blood count (to detect chronic anemia, infection, cancer).

(2) Erythrocyte sedimentation rate (often elevated in collagen vascular disease, cancer, chronic infection, inflammatory bowel disease).

(3) Urinalysis and microscopic examination (occult pyelonephritis, glomerulonephritis, renal tubular disease, etc).

(4) Stool examination for occult blood, parasites, and parasite ova (inflammatory bowel disease, overwhelming parasitism).

(5) Serum electroyltes and phosphorus (mild adrenal insufficiency, renal tubular diseases, parathyroid disease, rickets, etc).

(6) Blood urea nitrogen (occult renal insufficiency).

(7) Buccal smear and karyotyping (should be performed in all short girls with delayed sexual maturation with or without clinical features of Turner's syndrome).

(8) Thyroid function assessment: thyroxine (T_4) and thyroid-stimulating hormone (TSH) assay (short stature may be the only sign of hypothyroidism).

(9) GH evaluation. Blood samples for GH determination should be obtained following 20 minutes of exercise, during normal sleep, or after administration of one of the conventional provocative agents (arginine, glucagon, levodopa, clonidine, or insulin). Samples obtained during the first 90 minutes of sleep are preferable, since they demonstrate both the presence and the physiologic release of GH.

Chappel SC, Ulloa-Aguirre A, Coutifaris C: Biosynthesis and secretion of follicle-stimulating hormone. *Endocr Rev* 1983;**4:**179.

Craft WH et al: High incidence of perinatal insult in children with idiopathic hypopituitarism. *J Pediatr* 1980;**96:**397.

Delitala G et al: Cholinergic receptor control mechanisms for

L-dopa, apomorphine, and clonidine-induced growth hormone secretion in man. *J Clin Endocrinol Metab* 1983;**54:**1145.
Frasier SD: Human pituitary growth hormone (hGH) therapy in growth hormone deficiency. *Endocr Rev* 1983;**4:**155.
Gotlin RW: Assessing normal growth. Chap 11, pp 549–566, in: *Primary Care*. Poole SR (editor). Saunders, 1984.
Gotlin RW, Mace JW: Diagnosis and management of short stature in childhood and adolescence. (2 parts.) *Curr Probl Pediatr* (Feb) 1972;**2:**3; (March) 1972;**2:**3.
Greenhill LL et al: Growth disturbances in hyperkinetic children. (Letter.) *Pediatrics,* 1980;**66:**152.
Hopwood NJ et al: The effect of synthetic androgens on the hypothalamic-pituitary-gonadal axis in boys with constitutionally delayed growth. *J Pediatr* 1979;**94:**657.
Plotnick LP et al: Human growth hormone treatment of children with growth failure and normal growth hormone levels by immunoassay: Lack of correlation with somatomedin generation. *Pediatrics* 1983;**71:**324.
Powell GF, Hopwood NJ, Barrett ES: Growth hormone studies before and during catch-up growth in a child with emotional deprivation and short stature. *J Clin Endocrinol Metab* 1973;**37:**674.
Russo L, Moore WV: Comparison of subcutaneous and intramuscular administration of human growth hormone in the therapy of growth hormone deficiency. *J Clin Endocrinol Metab* 1982;**55:**1003.
Siegel SF et al: Comparison of physiologic and pharmacologic assessment of growth hormone secretion. *Am J Dis Child* 1984;**138:**540.
Silver HK, Finkelstein M: Deprivation dwarfism. *J Pediatr* 1967;**70:**317.
Tanner JM, Whitehouse RH: Clinical longitudinal standards for height, weight, height velocity, weight velocity, and stages of puberty. *Arch Dis Child* 1976;**51:**170.
Thomsett MJ et al: Endocrine and neurologic outcome in childhood craniopharyngioma: Review of effect of treatment in 42 patients. *J Pediatr* 1980;**97:**728.
Thorner MO et al: Acceleration of growth in two children treated with human growth hormone-releasing factor. *N Engl J Med* 1985;**312:**4.
Underwood LE et al: Degenerative neurologic disease in patients formerly treated with human growth hormone. *J Pediatr* 1985;**107:**10.
Van Wyk JJ, Underwood LE: Growth hormone, somatomedins, and growth failure. *Hosp Pract* (Aug) 1978;**13:**57.
Zachmann M et al: Anthropometric measurements in patients with growth hormone deficiency before treatment with human growth hormone. *Eur J Pediatr* 1980;**133:**277.

FAILURE TO THRIVE

Failure to thrive is present when there is a perceptible declination of growth from an established pattern or when the patient's height and weight plot consistently below the third percentile. (The term is usually reserved for infants who for various reasons fail to gain weight.) Linear growth and head circumference may also be affected; when this occurs, the underlying condition is generally more severe. There are many reasons for failure to thrive (see below and Table 25–1), although a specific cause often cannot be established. Nonaccidental trauma may be an important cause of failure to thrive.

Classification & Etiologic Diagnosis

The diagnosis of failure to thrive is usually apparent on the basis of the history and physical examination. When it is not, it is helpful to compare the patient's chronologic age with the height age (median age for the patient's height), weight age, and head circumference. On the basis of these measurements, 3 principal patterns can be defined that provide a starting point in the diagnostic approach.

Group 1. (Most common type.) Normal head circumference; weight reduced out of proportion to height: In the majority of cases of failure to thrive, malnutrition is present as a result of either deficient caloric intake or malabsorption.

Group 2. Normal or enlarged head circumference for age; weight only moderately reduced, usually in proportion to height: Structural dystrophies, constitutional dwarfism, endocrinopathies.

Group 3. Subnormal head circumference; weight reduced in proportion to height: Primary central nervous system deficit; intrauterine growth retardation.

An initial period of observed nutritional rehabilitation, usually in a hospital setting, is often helpful in the diagnosis. The child should be placed on a regular diet for age, and intake and weight should be carefully plotted for 1–2 weeks. During this period, the presence of lactose intolerance is determined by checking pH and the presence of reducing substances in the stools. If stools are abnormal, the child should be further observed on a lactose-free diet. Caloric intake should be increased if weight gain does not occur but intake is well tolerated. The following 3 patterns are often noted during rehabilitation. Pattern 1 is by far the most common.

Pattern 1. (Most common type.) Intake adequate; weight gain satisfactory: Feeding technique at fault. Disturbed infant-mother relationship leading to decreased caloric intake.

Pattern 2. Intake adequate; no weight gain: If weight gain is unsatisfactory after increasing the calories to an adequate level (based on the infant's ideal weight for height), malabsorption is a likely diagnosis.

If malabsorption is present, it is usually necessary to differentiate pancreatic exocrine insufficiency (cystic fibrosis) from abnormalities of intestinal mucosa (celiac disease). In cystic fibrosis, growth velocity commonly declines from the time of birth, and appetite usually is voracious. In celiac disease, growth velocity is usually not reduced until 6–12 months of age, and inadequate caloric intake may be a prominent feature.

Pattern 3. Intake inadequate:

(1) Sucking or swallowing difficulties: Central nervous system or neuromuscular disease;

esophageal or oropharyngeal malformations.

(2) Inability to eat large amounts is common in patients with cardiopulmonary disease or in anorexic children suffering from chronic infections, inflammatory bowel disease, and endocrine problems (eg, hypothyroidism). Patients with celiac disease often have inadequate caloric intake in addition to malabsorption.

(3) Vomiting, spitting up, or rumination: Upper intestinal obstruction (eg, pyloric stenosis, hiatal hernia, chalasia), chronic metabolic aberrations and acidosis (eg, renal insufficiency, diabetes mellitus and insipidus, methylmalonic acidemia), aldosterone insufficiency, increased intracranial pressure, psychosocial abnormalities.

Laboratory Aids to Diagnosis

The laboratory may provide adjunctive information helpful in the differential diagnosis.

A. Initial: Initial laboratory investigations at the time of admission might be limited to the following:

1. Blood—Complete blood count, sedimentation rate.
2. Urine—Urinalysis (including microscopic examination of sediment) and culture and colony count.
3. Stool—Culture, pH, reducing substances, and occult blood test (Hematest).
4. Tuberculin test.
5. Other tests as specifically indicated.

B. Definitive: The following laboratory investigations are recommended after the period of nutritional rehabilitation, when the patient has been classified in one of the 3 categories listed above.

1. Pattern 1—No further diagnostic laboratory tests are indicated. Maternal (and family) psychologic evaluation may be indicated.

2. Pattern 2—Evaluation of malabsorption.

a. Stool fat (72-hour specimen) on a diet with normal fat content.

b. Stool trypsin on *fresh* specimen.

c. Sweat chloride test.

d. Serum vitamin E, zinc, and D-xylose levels after an oral xylose load.

e. Peroral small bowel biopsy with histologic studies, analysis of intestinal disaccharidase activity, duodenal aspiration for pancreatic enzyme activity, culture and examination for *Giardia lamblia.*

f. Liver function tests (eg, serum alkaline phosphatase, bilirubin).

3. Pattern 3—

a. With vomiting—

(1) Serum electrolytes, pH, total CO_2, glucose, blood urea nitrogen, serum and urine osmolarities, serum and urine organic and amino acids.

(2) Upper gastrointestinal series and cineesophageography.

(3) Skull x-rays or CT scans for increased intracranial pressure, subdural hematoma, or fracture.

b. Without vomiting—

(1) Sigmoidoscopy, rectal biopsy (ulcerative or granulomatous colitis).

(2) Barium enema (ulcerative colitis or Hirschsprung's disease).

(3) Upper gastrointestinal series and follow-through (regional enteritis, malrotations).

(4) Thyroid function tests.

C. Other Tests: Further testing (adrenal function tests, intravenous urograms, etc) may be indicated.

Treatment & Prognosis

Treatment will vary according to the underlying disorder. Most patients will gain weight and thrive on an adequate caloric intake. Maternal counseling and support are often required over a prolonged period. In some cases, foster home placement may be required.

The outcome is dependent on the underlying disorder. In general, infants whose length and, particularly, head circumference are affected along with weight have a less favorable prognosis.

Gardner LI: The nosology of failure to thrive: Why is psychosocial deprivation, its major cause, undiagnosed? *Am J Dis Child* 1978;**132:**961.

Gross SJ et al: Head growth and developmental outcome in very low birth weight infants. *Pediatrics* 1983;**71:**70.

Hufton IW, Oates RK: Nonorganic failure to thrive: A long-term follow-up. *Pediatrics* 1977;**59:**73.

TALL STATURE

Tall stature is usually of concern only to adolescent and preadolescent girls. The upper limit of acceptable height of both sexes appears to be increasing, but there are occasions when the patient and her parents desire to influence the pattern of growth.

On the basis of family history, previous pattern of growth, stage of physiologic development, assessment of epiphyseal development ("bone age"), and standard growth data, the physician should make a tentative estimate of the patient's eventual height. Although there are several conditions (Table 25–2) that may produce tall stature, by far the most common cause is a constitutional variation from the average.

Reassurance and counseling should be tried first and are usually the only forms of therapy required. If the predicted height appears to be excessive, hormonal therapy with estrogen (eg, ethinyl estradiol, 0.2–0.3 mg daily), cycled with a progestational agent 7 days out of 28 days, has been suggested. Estrogens are of less value when the physiologic age (as determined by stage of sexual maturity and epiphyseal development) has reached the 12-year-old level and may be of little value even when administered at earlier ages. Estrogens act to accelerate epiphyseal closure and may be continued until fusion occurs.

Table 25–2. Causes of tall stature.

Constitutional (familial, genetic)
Endocrine causes
Somatotropin excess (pituitary gigantism)
Androgen excess (tall as children, short as adults)
True sexual precocity
Pseudosexual precocity
Androgen deficiency (normal height as children, tall as adults)
Klinefelter's syndrome
Anorchia (infection, trauma, idiopathic)
Hyperthyroidism
Genetic causes
Klinefelter's syndrome
Syndromes of XYY, XXYY (tall as adults)
Miscellaneous syndromes and entities
Marfan's syndrome
Cerebral gigantism (Sotos' syndrome)
Total lipodystrophy
Diencephalic syndrome
Homocystinuria

Because of the unknown long-term effects of hormone administration to children, these agents should be used with great caution.

Andersen H et al: Treatment of girls with excessive height prediction: Follow-up of forty girls treated with intramuscular estradiol and progesterone. *Acta Paediatr Scand* 1980; **69:**293.

Colle ML, Alperin H, Greenblatt RB: The tall girl: Prediction of mature height and management. *Arch Dis Child* 1977; **52:**118.

Wettenhall HNB, Cahill C, Roche AF: Tall girls: A survey of 15 years of management and treatment. *J Pediatr* 1975; **86:**602.

Whitehead EM et al: Pituitary gigantism: A disabling condition. *Clin Endocrinol* 1982;**17:**271.

THYROID

FETAL DEVELOPMENT OF THE THYROID

By the seventh week of intrauterine development, the thyroid gland has migrated to its definitive location and the thyroglossal duct has atrophied. Cell differentiation and function progress over the next 7 weeks, and by the 14th week the thyroid is capable of hormone synthesis. At this stage, TSH is detectable in the fetal serum and pituitary gland.

Under normal conditions, neither TSH nor thyroid hormones cross the placenta in appreciable amounts, and the fetal pituitary-thyroid axis functions independently of the maternal pituitary-thyroid axis.

Antithyroid drugs, including radioactive iodine, freely cross the placenta, and goitrous hypothyroid newborns may be born to hyperthyroid mothers who undergo treatment during pregnancy.

Although maternal TSH does not reach the fetus, pregnant hyperthyroid mothers may transmit human-specific thyroid stimulator immunoglobulin (HTSI) transplacentally, resulting in thyrotoxic newborns who may exhibit exophthalmos. Since HTSI may be present in the serum of "controlled," previously hyperthyroid mothers, the possible transmission of HTSI should be considered in all mothers in whom hyperthyroidism is or has been present.

Physiology

Under the stimulation of pituitary TSH, the thyroid gland traps, concentrates, and organifies iodine, synthesizes and couples mono- and diiodotyrosine, and releases active thyroid hormones into the circulation (Fig 25–1).

The quantity released is proportionate to the needs of the organism and is maintained by a negative feedback mechanism involving pituitary TSH and "free" thyroid hormone (Fig 25–2).

Active hormone produced in excess of physiologic needs is stored within the thyroid follicles as colloid. Upon release into the circulation, T_4 and T_3 are bound to thyroid hormone-binding globulin (TBG), albumin, and prealbumin. The binding affinity of TBG for T_4 is approximately 20 times greater than for T_3. A small percentage ($< 1\%$) of T_3 and T_4 is not bound but is "free" and exists in equilibrium with the "bound" form. In the peripheral tissues, T_4 is deiodinated to T_3, and the physiologic activity of thyroid hormone depends primarily on the amount of free T_3 presented to the cells.

Causes of Thyroid Disturbances

Physiologic disturbances of the thyroid gland may be due to the following causes:

(1) Decreased thyroid tissue: Hypofunction may result from congenital aplasia or hypoplasia, destruction due to inflammatory disease (thyroiditis), neoplasm, thyroidectomy, or irradiation.

(2) Inborn errors in the synthesis of thyroid hormone: Defects may occur in any of the metabolic steps shown in Fig 25–1 as well as in the binding and release of T_4 and T_3 from thyroglobulin.

(3) Iodine deficiency.

(4) Inhibition of thyroidal iodide uptake and concentration by drugs (eg, thiocyanates, perchlorates, nitrates).

(5) Interference with thyroid enzyme activity by antithyroid compounds. Antithyroid compounds include thiourea, thiouracil and its derivatives, cobalt, large doses of iodides, and certain foods such as cabbage, turnips, and soybeans. Iodides also interfere with the release of thyroid hormone.

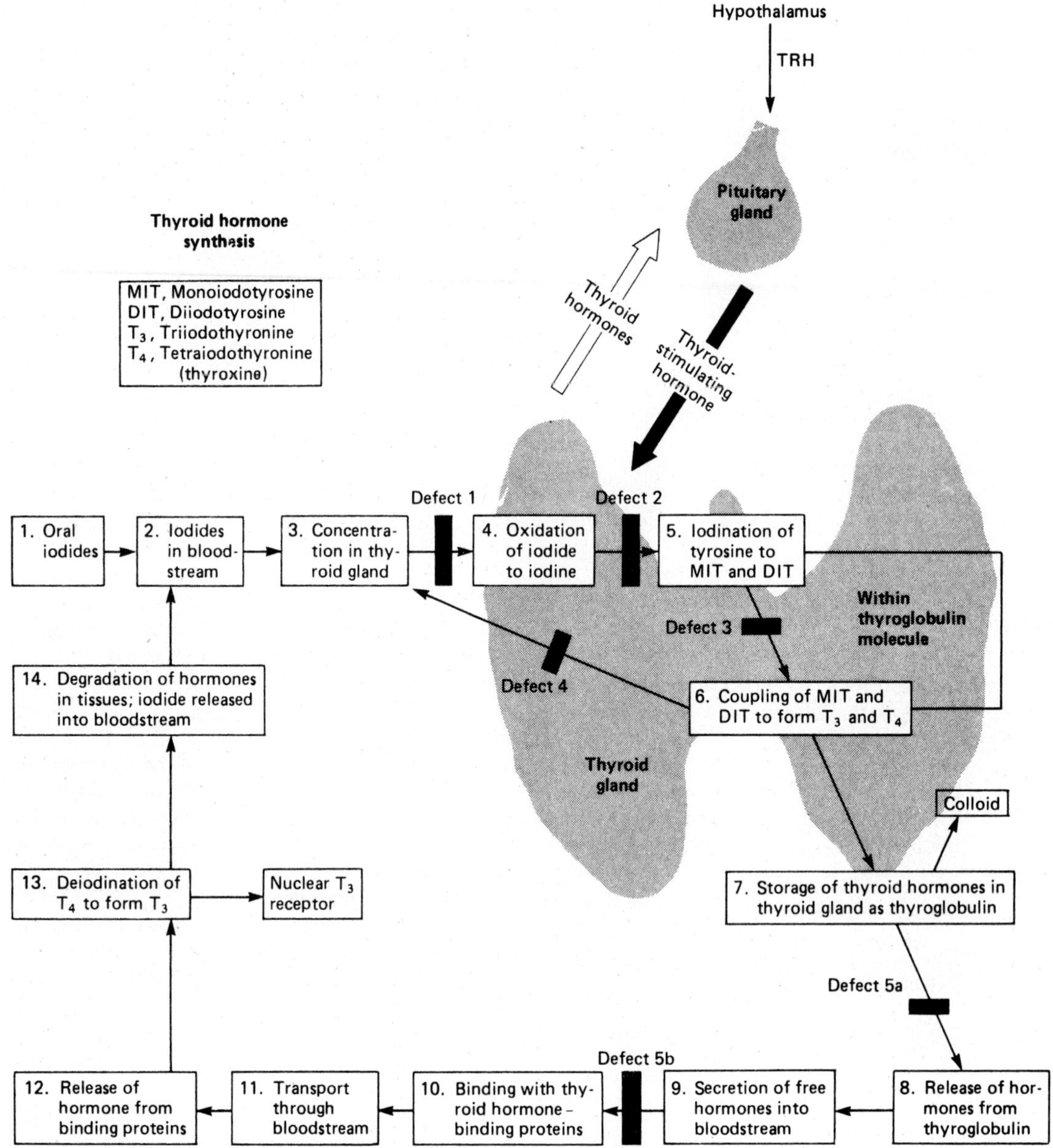

Figure 25–1. Synthesis of thyroxine (T_4) and triiodothyronine (T_3). (Adapted, with permission, from: Current Concepts of Thyroid Disease. [Programmed instruction course in *Spectrum.*] Pfizer Laboratories Division, Chas Pfizer & Co, Inc, 1965.) (See Table 25–3 for causes of defects.)

(6) Disorders of the hypothalamus and pituitary gland that result in impairment of either thyrotropin-releasing hormone (TRH) or thyrotropin secretion.

(7) Defects in the peripheral tissue conversion of T_4 to T_3.

Release of Thyroid Hormone & Its Function

The principal functions of the thyroid gland are to synthesize and store T_4 and T_3 and to release them in response to bodily need. A number of chemical reactions are involved in thyroid hormone formation. The thyroid gland is regulated and stimulated by TSH; HTSI is important only in hyperthyroid states. TSH production may be inhibited by either endogenous or exogenous thyroid hormone. At birth, the T_4 approximates that of the mother. There is a rapid increase of T_4 during the second to fifth days of life in response to a TSH surge resulting from umbilical cord clamping and then a gradual decrease over several weeks or months.

The total T_4 is low in various forms of hypothyroid-

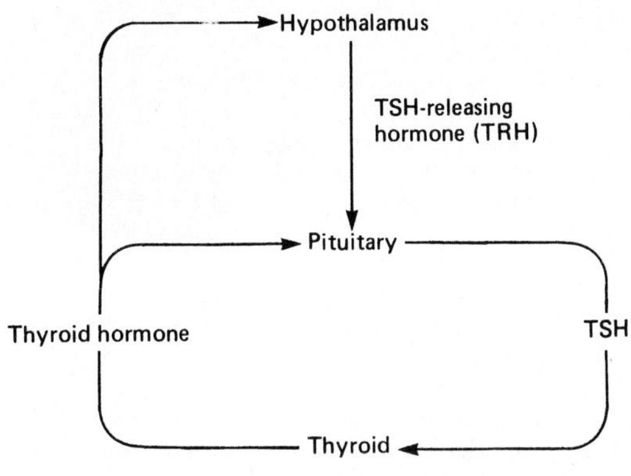

Figure 25–2. Pituitary-thyroid control.

ism and may be reduced in premature infants, particularly with respiratory distress, subacute and chronic thyroiditis, hypopituitarism, nephrosis, cirrhosis, hypoproteinemia, malnutrition, and following therapy with T_3. Prolonged administration of high doses of adrenocorticosteroids as well as sulfonamides, testosterone, phenytoin (Dilantin), and salicylates may also produce a decrease in T_4.

The total T_3 and T_4 are high in hyperthyroidism amd may be elevated in the acute forms of thyroiditis and acute hepatitis; in some types of inborn errors in the synthesis, release, or binding of thyroid hormone; following the administration of estrogens or during pregnancy; and following the administration of various iodine-containing globulins.

TBG is increased in pregnancy, after estrogen therapy (including oral contraceptives), occasionally as a genetic variation, in certain hepatic disorders, following administration of phenothiazines, and occasionally from unknown cause. TBG is decreased in familial TBG deficiency; following the administration of glucocorticoids, androgens, or anabolic steroids; in nephrotic syndrome with marked hypoproteinemia; in some forms of hepatic disease; in patients receiving phenytoin; and as an idiopathic finding. T_3, which appears to be the active thyroid hormone, acts fairly rapidly but has a shorter duration of action. Receptors for T_3 are present on the cell membrane, mitochondria, and nucleus and within the cytosol; the physiologic action of thyroid hormone is complex.

Engler D, Burger AG: The deiodination of the iodothyronines and of their derivatives in man. *Endocr Rev* 1984;**5:**151.

Larsen PR, Silva JE, Kaplan MM: Relationship between circulating and intracellular thyroid hormones: Physiological and clinical implications. *Endocr Rev* 1981;**2:**87.

Lenzen S, Bailey CJ: Thyroid hormones, gonadal and adrenocortical steroids and the function of the islets of Langerhans. *Endocr Rev* 1984;**5:**411.

Sterling K: Thyroid hormone action at the cellular level. (2 parts.) *N Engl J Med* 1979;**300:**117, 173.

HYPOTHYROIDISM (Congenital & Acquired [Juvenile] Hypothyroidism)

Essentials of Diagnosis

- Growth retardation, diminished physical activity, sluggish circulation, constipation, thick tongue, poor muscle tone, hoarseness, intellectual retardation.
- Delayed dental and skeletal maturation. Rarely, "stippling" of epiphyses.
- Thyroid function studies low (T_4 and T_3 resin uptake); TSH levels elevated in primary hypothyroidism.

General Considerations

Thyroid hormone deficiency may be either congenital (with or without the physical features of cretinism) or acquired (juvenile hypothyroidism) and may be due to many causes.

Various types of enzymatic defects have been described (Table 25–3 and Fig 25–1) that result from inborn errors of metabolism. With the exception of that group associated with congenital nerve deafness (Pendred's syndrome), there are no distinguishing clinical features among the various types. In children who have enzymatic defects, thyroid enlargement may not be present in the newborn period but generally occurs within the first 2 decades of life. Enzymatic defects have a familial autosomal recessive inheritance pattern.

Under the influence of increased TSH stimulation, rapid uptake occurs and reaches peak levels in about 2 hours. In patients with the very rare iodide-trapping defect, the goiter is small and the uptake of radioactive iodine is negligible. Patients with a defect in iodide organification rapidly release labeled iodine from the gland; this release may be significantly and abnormally augmented by the administration of potassium thiocyanate or perchlorate. Comparison of the levels of protein-bound iodine (PBI) and T_4 may be helpful in coupling and deiodinase defects, revealing a greater than normal discrepancy in the blood levels of these substances that reflects impaired thyroglobulin proteolysis, abnormal plasma binding, or the presence of abnormal circulating iodoproteins. Further clarification of the defect generally requires chromatographic fractionation of iodinated compounds in the serum, urine, and thyroid tissue.

A number of drugs and goitrogens taken during pregnancy (eg, cabbage, soybeans, aminosalicylic acid, thiourea derivatives, resorcinol, phenylbutazone, cobalt, and iodides in therapeutic doses for asthma—particularly in individuals who have also received adrenocortical steroids) have been reported to cause goiter and in some instances hypothyroidism also. Since many of these agents cross the placental barrier freely, they should be used with great caution during pregnancy. If these agents are taken by a pregnant woman, the goiter and decreased thyroid function

Table 25–3. Causes of hypothyroidism.*

A. Congenital (Cretinism):
1. Aplasia, hypoplasia, or associated with maldescent of thyroid–
   a. Embryonic defect of development.
   b. Autoimmune disease (?).
2. Familial iodine-induced goiter secondary to metabolic inborn errors–
   a. Iodide transport defect (defect 1).
   b. Organification defect (defect 2)–
      (1) Lack of iodine peroxidase.
      (2) Lack of iodine transferase; Pendred's syndrome, associated with congenital nerve deafness.
   c. Coupling defect (defect 3).
   d. Iodotyrosine deiodinase defect (defect 4).
   e. Abnormal iodinated polypeptide (defects 5a and 5b)–
      (1) Resulting from defect in intrathyroidal proteolysis of thyroglobulin.
      (2) Abnormal plasma binding preventing use of T_4 by peripheral cells.
   f. Inability of tissues to convert T_4 to T_3.
3. Maternal ingestion of medications during pregnancy–
   a. Maternal radioiodine.
   b. Goitrogens (propylthiouracil, methimazole).
   c. Iodides.
4. Iodide deficiency (endemic cretinism).
5. Idiopathic.

B. Acquired (Juvenile Hypothyroidism):
1. Thyroidectomy or radioiodine therapy for–
   a. Thyrotoxicosis.
   b. Cancer.
   c. Lingual thyroid.
   d. Isolated midline thyroid.
2. Destruction by x-ray.
3. Thyrotropin deficiency–
   a. Isolated.
   b. Associated with other pituitary tropic hormone deficiencies.
4. TRH deficiency due to hypothalamic injury or disease.
5. Autoimmune disease (lymphocytic thyroiditis).
6. Chronic infections.
7. Medications–
   a. Iodides–
      (1) Prolonged, excessive ingestion.
      (2) Deficiency.
   b. Cobalt.
8. Idiopathic.

* Information in parentheses (defect 1, etc) refers to specific defects in Fig 25–1.

that are produced in the newborn are generally transient and seldom a problem.

The majority of cases in childhood, particularly in the presence of a history of goiter, appear to be the result of previously unsuspected lymphocytic thyroiditis (see Thyroiditis, below).

Clinical Findings

The severity of the findings in cases of thyroid deficiency depends on the age at onset and the degree of interference with production of thyroid hormone.

A. Symptoms and Signs:

1. Functional changes—Even with congenital absence of the thyroid gland, the first finding may not appear for several days or weeks. Findings include physical and mental sluggishness; pale, gray, cool or mottled skin; nonpitting myxedema; decreased intestinal activity (constipation); large tongue; poor muscle tone, giving rise to a protuberant abdomen, umbilical hernia, and lumbar lordosis; hypothermia; bradycardia; diminished sweating (variable); decreased pulse pressure; hoarse voice or cry; delayed transient deafness; and slow relaxation after elicitation of deep tendon reflexes. Nasal obstruction and discharge and persistent jaundice may be present in the neonatal period.

The skin may be dry, thick, scaly, and coarse, with a yellowish tinge due to excessive deposition of carotene. The hair is dry, coarse, and brittle (variable) and may be excessive. Lateral thinning of the eyebrows may occur. The axillary and supraclavicular fat pads may be prominent in infants. Muscular hypertrophy (Debré-Sémélaigne syndrome) occasionally is present.

2. Retardation of growth and development—Findings include shortness of stature; infantile skeletal proportions with relatively short extremities; infantile naso-orbital configuration (bridge of nose flat, broad, and underdeveloped; eyes seem to be widely spaced); delayed osseous development (retarded "bone age"); delayed closure of the fontanelles; and retarded dental development. In hypothyroidism resulting from enzymatic defects, ingestion of goitrogens, or chronic lymphocytic thyroiditis, the thyroid gland may be enlarged. Thyroid enlargement in children is usually symmetric and the gland is moderately firm without nodularity, but in chronic lymphocytic thyroiditis, a cobblestone surface is present. Size and shape are often apparent on inspection in children. Slowing of mental responsiveness and retardation of development of the brain may occur, and in many cases a coincidental congenital malformation of the brain is present also.

3. Alterations in sexual development (usually retardation, sometimes precocity)—Menometrorrhagia may be seen in older girls; galactorrhea is occasionally found.

B. X-Ray Findings: Epiphyseal development ("bone age") is delayed. Centers of ossification, especially of the hip, may show multiple small centers or a single, stippled, porous or fragmented center (epiphyseal dysgenesis). Vertebrae may show anterior beaking. The cardiac shadow is increased. Coxa vara and coxa plana may occur.

C. Laboratory Findings: T_4 is decreased. Radioiodine uptake is below 10% (normal: 10–50%).* (Both may be normal or elevated in goitrous cretinism and in some cases of thyroiditis.) The binding of T_3 by erythrocytes or resin in vitro (T_3 test) is lowered. With primary hypothyroidism, the plasma TSH is elevated. Serum cholesterol and carotene are usually elevated in childhood but may be low or normal in infants. Cessation of therapy in previously treated hypothyroid patients produces a marked rise in serum cholesterol levels in 6–8 weeks. Urinary creatine excretion is decreased and creatinine increased. Serum alkaline phosphatase is occasionally reduced, and urinary hydroxyproline is low. Circulating autoantibodies to thyroid constituents may be present. Erythrocyte glucose 6-phosphate dehydrogenase activity is decreased. Plasma growth hormone may be decreased, with subnormal response to insulin-induced hypoglycemia and arginine stimulation.

Screening Programs for Neonatal Hypothyroidism

Congenital hypothyroidism may be recognized during the first month of life but may be so mild as to go unrecognized for months. Every effort should be made to establish the diagnosis of hypothyroidism as early as possible, since untreated hypothyroidism may be associated with irreversible damage to the central nervous system. Adequate treatment initiated prior to the first or second month of life is associated with a favorable prognosis. Mandatory newborn infant screening programs facilitate prompt diagnosis (within 30–60 days after birth) and therapy of congenital hypothyroidism. Screening programs utilize either T_4 or TSH. TSH may be a more sensitive index of thyroid hypofunction.

Differential Diagnosis

The various causes of primary hypothyroidism due to intrinsic defects of the thyroid gland must be differentiated from pituitary and hypothalamic failure with secondary thyroid insufficiency. TSH measurements before and after, TRH administration and radioactive iodide uptake studies before and after exogenous TSH administration (5–10 units daily for 3 days) are useful in differentiation. Since pituitary insufficiency may be associated with both secondary hypoadrenocorticism and secondary hypothyroidism, treatment of the latter alone may precipitate an adrenal crisis.

Down's syndrome, chondrodystrophy, generalized gangliosidosis, I-cell disease, Hurler's and Hunter's syndromes, and certain other causes of short stature as well as macroglossia due to abnormalities of the lymphatics of the tongue can all be readily distinguished by the clinical manifestations and by appropriate laboratory studies. Although other individual findings of the hypothyroid child may suggest exogenous obesity, congenital heart disease, or some type of anemia as the primary diagnosis, a careful appraisal of the entire clinical and laboratory picture should permit establishment of the proper diagnosis.

* The presence of iodides in bread in recent years has resulted in a significant decrease in normal values of radioiodine uptake. The normal levels for any particular area should be ascertained.

Treatment

Levothyroxine is the drug of choice in a dose of 100 $\mu g/m^2$ once daily. In newborns and infants, use 0.025 mg of levothyroxine initially and increase the dosage by 0.025–0.05 mg every 1–2 weeks until the required level is reached. Serum T_4 and TSH levels should be used as a guide to adequate therapy.

The hypothyroid patient may be quite responsive to thyroid, usually shows improvement 7–21 days after starting therapy, and may be sensitive to slight excesses of thyroid hormone.

Triiodothyronine (liothyronine sodium; Cytomel) may be employed when a more rapid and short-lived effect is desired (eg, in the TSH suppression test) but probably is not as effective for maintenance therapy as levothyroxine. In the treatment of neonatal goiter with or without hypothyroidism resulting from drugs and goitrogens taken by the pregnant woman, temporary use of levothyroxine is sufficient to bring about rapid disappearance of the enlargement.

Dop CV et al: Pseudotumor cerebri associated with initiation of levothyroxine therapy for juvenile hypothyroidism. *N Engl J Med* 1983;**308:**1076.

Fisher DA et al: Screening for congenital hypothyroidism: Results of screening one million North American infants. *J Pediatr* 1979;**94:**700.

Hollingsworth DR, Alexander NM: Amniotic fluid concentrations of iodothyronines and thyrotropin do not reliably predict fetal thyroid status in pregnancies complicated by maternal thyroid disorders or anencephaly. *J Clin Endocrinol Metab* 1983;**54:**349.

Iseki M et al: Sequential serum measurements of thyrotropin-binding inhibitor immunoglobulin G in transient familial neonatal hypothyroidism. *J Clin Endocrinol Metab* 1983; **57:**384.

Klein AH et al: Thyroid hormone and thyrotropin responses to parturition in premature infants with and without the respiratory distress syndrome. *Pediatrics* 1979;**63:**380.

Letarte J et al: Lack of protective effect of breast-feeding in congenital hypothyroidism: Report of 12 cases. *Pediatrics* 1980;**65:**703.

Melmed S et al: Comparison of methods for assessing thyroid function in nonthyroidal illness. *J Clin Endocrinol Metab* 1982;**54:**307.

Tachman ML, Guthrie GP Jr: Hypothyroidism: Diversity of presentation. *Endocr Rev* 1984;**5:**456.

THYROIDITIS

With the exception of chronic lymphocytic thyroiditis (Hashimoto's disease), the forms of thyroiditis listed in Table 25–4 are uncommon in childhood. In contrast, Hashimoto's disease is perhaps the most common endocrine condition in pediatric patients, particularly in female adolescents.

Table 25–4. Causes of thyroiditis.

I. Thyroiditis due to infectious agents.
  A. Acute bacterial thyroiditis (acute suppurative thyroiditis).
  B. Subacute viral thyroiditis (nonsuppurative, or De Quervain's, thyroiditis).
  C. Chronic or recurring thyroiditis.
II. Thyroiditis due to autoimmunity (chronic lymphocytic, or Hashimoto's, thyroiditis).
III. Thyroiditis due to physical agents.
  A. Radiation.
  B. Trauma.
IV. Thyroiditis of unknown etiology.
  A. Riedel's thyroiditis.

1. ACUTE SUPPURATIVE THYROIDITIS

Acute thyroiditis is rare but may occur after various bacterial infections, including those of the skin, pharynx, or larynx. The most common pathogens are streptococci, pneumococci, staphylococci, and anaerobic agents. The patient is invariably toxic, and the thyroid gland is exquisitely tender. There may be radiation of pain to the ear or chest. There is usually no consistently associated endocrine disturbance. Specific antibiotic therapy should be administered.

2. SUBACUTE NONSUPPURATIVE THYROIDITIS

Subacute thyroiditis (De Quervain's thyroiditis) is rare in the USA. In most cases, the cause is a virus (mumps virus, influenza virus, adenovirus, echovirus, coxsackievirus, infectious mononucleosis virus). Subacute thyroiditis is characterized by an insidious onset, fever, malaise, sore throat, dysphagia, pain in the thyroid gland that may radiate to the ears, and mild and transient manifestations of hypermetabolism. The thyroid gland is firm, and the enlargement may be confined to one lobe. Radioiodine uptake is usually reduced, but thyroid hormone levels in the blood are typically elevated.

3. CHRONIC LYMPHOCYTIC THYROIDITIS (Chronic Autoimmune Thyroiditis, Hashimoto's Thyroiditis, Lymphadenoid Goiter)

Essentials of Diagnosis

- Firm, freely movable, and diffusely enlarged goiter.
- T_4 normal, elevated, or decreased depending on stage of disease.
- Antibodies to various thyroid gland fractions.

General Considerations

Chronic lymphocytic thyroiditis is being seen with increasing frequency in all age groups and currently is the most common cause of goiter and hypothyroidism in childhood. In children and adolescents, it has a peak incidence between the age of 8 and 15 years and occurs most commonly in females. The disease is the result of a defect in immunoregulation (probably involving suppressor T cells) that allows the persistence of a clone of T cells, which induces a cell-mediated immune response (autoimmunity). The defect is probably inherited and is often associated with other autoimmune disorders (eg, Graves' disease, Addison's disease, hypoparathyroidism, type I diabetes mellitus, pernicious anemia). The defect can be located on histocompatibility loci of chromosome 6, most frequently at HLA-Dw3.

Clinical Findings

A. Symptoms and Signs: The goiter is characteristically firm, freely movable, nontender, "pebbly" in consistency, and diffusely enlarged, although it may be asymmetric. In long-standing cases, nodules and, rarely, malignant changes have been described. The onset is usually insidious. Most cases occur without clinical manifestations and are completely painless. The symptoms consist mainly of moderate tracheal compression with a sense of fullness, hoarseness, and dysphagia. There are no local signs of inflammation and no evidence of systemic infection.

B. Laboratory Findings: Laboratory findings are variable. Levels of T_4 and reverse T_3 (rT_3) may be normal, elevated (2%), or depressed. TSH levels may be slightly elevated. A variety of abnormalities in radioactive iodide uptake studies have been described; thyroid scans usually show a diffuse or patchy pattern, and cold nodules have been reported. Thyroid antibodies are usually present, though sometimes at low levels. Surgical or needle biopsy is diagnostic but seldom indicated.

Treatment

The treatment of choice for autoimmune thyroiditis is thyroid hormone in full therapeutic doses (levothyroxine, 100 $\mu g/m^3$). Approximately two-thirds of patients will have a decrease in the size of the goiter. Hypothyroidism is believed to be a common end result of autoimmune thyroiditis.

4. RIEDEL'S STRUMA (Chronic Fibrous Thyroiditis, Woody Thyroiditis, Invasive Thyroiditis)

Riedel's struma is rare in the USA, particularly in children. The cause is not known, but the disease may represent a late stage of chronic lymphocytic thyroiditis. The disease is characterized by marked and invasive fibrosis that extends beyond the thyroid gland to involve the trachea, esophagus, blood vessels, nerves, and muscles of the neck, so that the gland becomes fixed to these tissues. Since differentiation from carcinoma of the thyroid is usually impossible by clinical means alone, the diagnosis is usually made by surgical biopsy.

Adrenocorticosteroids may be helpful, but surgery is frequently necessary to relieve fibrotic obstruction or constriction of neighboring structures.

Czernichow P et al: Plasma thyroglobulin measurements help determine the type of thyroid defect in congenital hypothyroidism. *J Clin Endocrinol Metab* 1983;**56**:242.

Fisher DA et al: The diagnosis of Hashimoto's thyroiditis. *J Clin Endocrinol Metab* 1975;**40**:795.

Greene JN: Subacute thyroiditis. *Am J Med* 1971;**51**:97.

How J et al: T lymphocyte sensitization and suppressor T lymphocyte defect in patients long after treatment for Graves' disease. *Clin Endocrinol* 1983;**18**:61.

Hurley JR: Thyroiditis. *DM* (Dec) 1977;**24**:1.

Iwatani Y et al: T lymphocyte subsets in autoimmune thyroid diseases and subacute thyroiditis detected with monoclonal antibodies. *J Clin Endocrinol Metab* 1983;**56**:251.

Kidd A et al: Immunologic aspects of Graves' and Hashimoto's diseases. *Metabolism* 1980;**29**:80.

Kirkland RT et al: Solitary thyroid nodules in 30 children and report of a child with a thyroid abscess. *Pediatrics* 1973; **51**:85.

Reiter EO et al: Childhood thyromegaly: Recent developments. *J Pediatr* 1981;**99**:507.

Strakosch CR et al: Immunology of autoimmune thyroid diseases. *N Engl J Med* 1982;**307**:1499.

Weetman AP, McGregor AM: Autoimmune thyroid disease: Developments in our understanding. *Endocr Rev* 1984; **5**:309.

HYPERTHYROIDISM

Essentials of Diagnosis

- Nervousness, irritability, emotional lability, tremor, excessive appetite, weight loss, smooth warm skin, perspiration, and heat intolerance.
- Goiter, exophthalmos, tachycardia, increased pulse pressure.
- Thyroid function studies elevated (eg, T_4, T_3, rT_3, radioiodine uptake).

General Considerations

The cause of hyperthyroidism has not been precisely determined. Nevertheless, it is evident that abnormalities in the immune system are operative in the pathogenesis. Moreover, the association of hyperthyroidism and certain additional diseases that have an autoimmune basis and a familial pattern with a predilection for females supports a heritable and autoimmune basis. In addition, psychic trauma, psychologic maladjustments, disturbances in pituitary function, and infectious diseases may play a part in triggering the thyrotoxic state. Recently, an IgG antibody to thyroid, human-specific thyroid stimulator immunoglobulin (HTSI), has been implicated in the pathogenesis of hyperthyroidism. Since HTSI is an IgG, it may cross the placenta from a thyrotoxic mother and affect the fetus and neonate. Transient congenital hyperthyroidism may occur in infants of thyrotoxic mothers. Hyperthyroidism may be found with tumors of the thyroid, with other tumors producing thyrotropinlike substances, and with exogenous thyroid hormone excess.

Clinical Findings

A. Symptoms and Signs: Hyperthyroidism is 5 times as common in females as in males. The disease is most likely to appear in childhood at age 12–14 years, with only 20% of cases present before 10 years of age. The course of hyperthyroidism tends to be cyclic, with spontaneous remissions and exacerbations, but it tends to progress rapidly. Findings include weakness, dyspnea, emotional instability, "nervousness" (inability to sit still), marked variability in mood, tremors and movements that may simulate chorea, personality disturbances, warm and moist skin, flushed face, palpitation, tachycardia, systolic hypertension with increased pulse pressure, and dysphagia. Proptosis and exophthalmos are common in hyperthyroid children. Goiter is present in more than 80% of cases and is characteristically diffuse and usually firm. A bruit and thrill may be present. Variable degrees of accelerated growth and development occur, and loss of weight is common in spite of polyphagia. (An occasional adolescent may gain weight.) Amenorrhea may occur in adolescent girls.

B. Laboratory Findings: The T_4 and free T_4 are elevated except in rare cases in which only the blood T_3 level is elevated ("T_3 thyrotoxicosis"). There is increased binding of radioactive T_3 to shed blood or resin in the T_3 test. Radioiodine uptake is above 35–40% at 24 hours and suppressed less than 40% after administration of T_3 (25 μg 3–4 times daily for 7 days). The basal metabolic rate is elevated, but testing for this is frequently unreliable and is seldom used. Serum cholesterol is low; glycosuria may occur. Agglutinating antibodies to thyroglobulin are found in most patients. Circulating THS is usually depressed, and HTSI is often present in plasma. Erythrocyte glucose 6-phosphate dehydrogenase activity is increased. Urinary hydroxyproline is increased, and urinary creatine may be elevated.

C. X-Ray Findings: Rarely, abnormal skull x-rays are found in some patients with primary pituitary disease. Skeletal maturation assessed radiographically is advanced in younger children. In newborns, accelerated maturation may be associated with subsequent premature closure of the cranial sutures.

Differential Diagnosis

Although the well-established case of hyperthyroidism seldom presents a problem in diagnosis, the findings in the early stage of the disease may be confused with chorea or, more commonly, with findings seen in the euthyroid child with a goiter (usually an adolescent girl who is nervous, emotionally labile, and manifests a rapid pulse and increased perspiration). Careful and sometimes repeated clinical and laboratory evaluation may be required before the proper diagnosis can be established. Moreover, it should be recognized that thyrotoxic symptoms may occur with thyroiditis and rarely with thyroid cancer.

Various states with signs of hypermetabolism (severe anemia, leukemia, chronic infections, pheochromocytoma, as well as muscle-wasting disease) may occasionally be confused with hyperthyroidism, but differentiation can usually be readily made by the clinical manifestations and by appropriate laboratory studies.

Treatment

The course of hyperthyroidism may exhibit fluctuations of improvement and remission. In some mild cases, therapy may not be required.

Both surgical and medical methods are available for treating the manifestations of hyperthyroidism.

A. General Measures: Rest in bed is advisable only in severe cases, in preparation for surgery, or at the beginning of a medical regimen. The diet should be high in calories, carbohydrates, and vitamins (particularly vitamin B_1).

Propranolol (Inderal), a β-adrenergic blocking agent, may be useful in controlling symptoms of nervous instability and tachycardia. Propranolol may also be helpful in controlling life-threatening cardiac complications that may occur in thyroid storm (severe thyrotoxicosis, fever, and altered consciousness). The drug is particularly useful preoperatively in doses of 20–100 mg every 6 hours.

B. Medical Treatment: With medical treatment, clinical response may be noted in 2–3 weeks and adequate control in 2–3 months. The thyroid frequently increases in size after initiation of treatment but usually will decrease in size within several months.

1. Propylthiouracil—This drug interferes with the intrathyroidal hormonogenesis and the peripheral conversion of T_4 to T_3. The correct dose must always be individually assessed. Propylthiouracil may be used in the initial treatment of the patient with hyperthyroidism, but if the T_4 fails to return to a normal range—or if it rises rapidly with reduction in drug dosage after 18–24 months of therapy—continued or alternative therapy may be necessary. Relapses occur in 10–30% of cases, and severe cases may not respond. Short-term therapy is occasionally successful, but treatment usually must be continued for at least 2–3 years with the smallest drug dosage that will produce a euthyroid state. The safety of prolonged treatment has not been evaluated.

a. Initial dosage—Give 75–300 mg/d in 3–4 divided doses 6–8 hours apart until tests of thyroid function are normal and all signs and symptoms have subsided. Larger doses may be necessary.

b. Maintenance—Give 50–100 mg/d in 2–3 divided doses. Some authors recommend continuing the drug at higher levels until the euthyroid state is approached or reached and then giving oral thyroid. Thyroid may also be given if the gland enlarges significantly or remains enlarged after 2–3 months with propylthiouracil therapy.

c. Toxicity—Granulocytopenia, fever, and rash may occur. Discontinue the drug and consider giving antibiotics and a short course of one of the adrenocorticosteroids.

2. Methimazole (Tapazole)—This drug may be used in one-fifteenth to one-tenth the dosage of propylthiouracil. However, toxic reactions may be more common with methimazole than with propylthiouracil.

3. Iodide—Medical treatment with continuous iodide administration alone usually produces a rapid but brief response. Since the effectiveness of iodide is short-lived, it is generally recommended only for acute management. A progressive increase in dosage is often required for satisfactory control, and toxic reactions to iodide are not uncommon.

C. Radiation Therapy: Radioactive iodide (^{131}I) may be used as alternative therapy for children and adolescents who fail to respond to medical treatment or who are unable to complete a course of medical treatment. Reports do not support the fear of an increased incidence of thyroid cancer, particularly when an ablative dose of ^{131}I is employed. Therapy with thyroid hormone is necessary after thyroid ablation.

D. Surgical Measures: Subtotal thyroidectomy is considered by many to be the treatment of choice, especially when a close follow-up of the patient is difficult or impossible. In childhood, surgery should be employed in patients when medical treatment is impossible or has been unsuccessful. The patient should be prepared first with bed rest, diet, and propranolol (as above) and with iodide and propylthiouracil as follows: Propylthiouracil (as above) should be given for 2–4 weeks. Iodide (as saturated solution of potassium iodide) is added 10–21 days before surgery is scheduled. Iodides act by blocking the effect of TSH on the thyroid, with resultant decrease in iodine trapping (with reduction of vascularity), and by inhibiting the release of hormone, thus reducing the possibility of thyroid storm. Give 1–10 drops daily for 10–21 days. Continue the drug for 1 week after surgery.

Progressive exophthalmos following surgery is uncommon in childhood.

E. Management of Congenital (Transient) Hyperthyroidism: Temporary treatment of congenital hyperthyroidism may be necessary, in which case iodides appear to be the drugs of choice. Reserpine or propranolol may be necessary to control cardiac dysrhythmias. Transection of an enlarged thyroid isthmus may be of value if respiratory distress is present.

Course & Prognosis

Improvement may occur without therapy in as many as one-third of cases, but partial remissions and exacerbations may continue for several years. With medical treatment alone, prolonged remissions may be expected in one-half to two-thirds of cases. Surgical therapy probably yields about the same number of satisfactory results. Postoperative hypothyroidism is not uncommon, and hypoparathyroidism and other complications may occur after surgery. Because of the comparatively high incidence of carcinoma in nodular goiters of childhood, such glands should be removed routinely once the thyrotoxicosis is in remission.

Congenital hyperthyroidism has a significant death rate in the neonatal period, but the eventual prognosis in surviving infants is excellent.

Becker DV: Choice of therapy for Graves' hyperthyroidism. (Editorial.) *N Engl J Med* 1984;**311:**464.

Buckingham BA et al: Hyperthyroidism in children: A reevaluation of treatment. *Am J Dis Child* 1981;**135:**112.

Collen RJ et al: Remission rates of children and adolescents with thyrotoxicosis treated with antithyroid drugs. *Pediatrics* 1980;**65:**550.

Daneman D, Howard NJ: Neonatal thyrotoxicosis: Intellectual impairment and craniosynostosis in later years. *J Pediatr* 1980;**97:**257.

Hamburger JI: Management of hyperthyroidism in children and adolescents. *J Clin Endocrinol Metab* 1985;**60:**1019.

Hollingsworth DR, Mabry CC, Eckerd JM: Hereditary aspects of Graves' disease in infancy and childhood. *J Pediatr* 1972;**81:**446.

How J et al: T lymphocyte sensitization and suppressor T lymphocyte defect in patients long after treatment for Graves' disease. *Clin Endocrinol* 1983;**18:**61.

Larsen PR: Thyroid-pituitary interaction: Feedback regulation of thyrotropin secretion by thyroid hormones. *N Engl J Med* 1982;**306:**23.

Mitsuma T et al: T_3 toxicosis in childhood: Hyperthyroidism due to isolated hypersecretion of triiodothyronine. *J Pediatr* 1972;**81:**982.

Sridama V et al: Long-term follow-up study of compensated low-dose ^{131}I therapy for Graves' disease. *N Engl J Med* 1984;**311:**426.

Sugrue D et al: Hyperthyroidism in the land of Graves: Results of treatment by surgery, radio-iodine and carbimazole in 837 cases. *Q J Med* 1980;**49:**51.

CARCINOMA OF THE THYROID

Carcinoma of the thyroid is uncommon in childhood. The presentation is usually asymptomatic, asymmetric thyroid enlargement. Neck discomfort, dysphagia, voice changes, and respiratory difficulty are unusual but may be noted. Fifty percent of children will have metastatic disease at the time of presentation. The most common site of metastasis is to regional lymph nodes; thus, careful examination of the neck may demonstrate enlarged nodes. Pulmonary metastasis occurs in 5% of cases.

Thyroid function tests are normal. Thyroid carcinoma may elaborate thyroglobulin; if present, it is a useful tumor marker. A technetium or iodine scan of the thyroid is the most definitive diagnostic test. A chest radiograph may be useful to exclude pulmonary metastasis.

Papillary carcinoma is the most common form in childhood, and the prognosis with treatment is relatively good, with a survival rate greater than 80% after 10–20 years. The treatment of choice is surgical extirpation of the entire gland and removal of all involved lymph nodes. Radical neck dissection is usually not indicated. If metastatic disease is not identified at surgery, replacement thyroid hormone is generally the only further therapy required. Follow-up thyroid scans every 2–5 years are recommended.

Other less common malignant tumors of the thyroid include follicular, medullary, and undifferentiated carcinomas, lymphomas, and sarcomas. Medullary carcinoma of the thyroid may be familial (autosomal dominant), usually occurs as a component of type II multiple endocrine neoplasia, and has been associated with excessive elaboration of gastrin and calcitonin and with pheochromocytoma, parathyroid hyperplasia, and mucosal neuromas. The treatment and prognosis depend upon the cell type present.

Joppich I et al: Thyroid carcinoma in childhood. *Prog Pediatr Surg* 1983;**16:**23.

Kaplan MM et al: Risk factors for thyroid abnormalities after neck irradiation for childhood cancer. *Am J Med* 1983; **74:**272.

Panza N et al: ^{131}I total body scan and serum thyroglobulin assay in the follow-up of surgically treated patients affected by differentiated thyroid carcinoma. *J Nucl Med Allied Sci* 1984;**28:**9.

Schimke RN: Genetic aspects of multiple endocrine neoplasia. *Annu Rev Med* 1984;**35:**25.

DISORDERS OF CALCIUM HOMEOSTASIS

Parathyroid hormone (PTH) and vitamin D are the principal hormonal factors in the human that maintain calcium homeostasis. These agents exert their action primarily in bone, small intestine, and kidney.

The integrated action of PTH and vitamin D maintains the serum calcium level within a narrow normal range and contributes to normal bone mineralization. Deficiencies and excesses of these agents—as well as abnormalities in their receptors or in the metabolic transformation of vitamin D—lead to the clinical disturbances described below and shown in Tables 25–5 and 25–6. Less important calciotropic factors (eg, calcitonin, magnesium, and phosphorus) also influence calcium homeostasis.

HYPOPARATHYROIDISM

Essentials of Diagnosis

- Tetany with numbness, tingling, cramps, carpopedal spasm, positive Trousseau and Chvostek signs, loss of consciousness, convulsions, photophobia, diarrhea, and laryngospasm.

Table 25–5. Parathyroid deficiency states.

Disease or Condition	Synonym	Inheritance Pattern	Major Clinical Features	Metabolic Features							
				Serum Concentration				Urinary Excretion			
								Basal Conditions		Response to Parathyroid Hormone	
				Ca^{2+}	P	Alk Ptase	PTH	Ca^{2+}	P	P	Cyclic AMP
"Idiopathic" (spontaneous), surgical, or "autoimmune" hypoparathyroidism	Autoimmune polyendocrinopathy. Thyroiditis and hypoparathyroidism (Schmidt's syndrome). Absence of parathyroid glands and thymic aplasia (DiGeorge's syndrome)	X-linked or autosomal recessive in autoimmune type	Tetany, seizures, photophobia, diarrhea, positive Chvostek and Trousseau signs, candidiasis. In autoimmune type, other autoimmune diseases (eg, adrenal insufficiency, thyroiditis, pernicious anemia, diabetes mellitus).	↓ (N)	↑	↓ (N)	↓	↓ (N)	↓	N	N
Pseudohypoparathyroidism and pseudopseudohypoparathyroidism	Albright's syndrome	X-linked dominant	Brachymetacarpal and metatarsal short stature; mental subnormality; ectopic calcification of lenses, basal ganglia, and subcutaneous tissue.	↓ (N)	↑ (N)	↓ ↑ (N)	↑	↓ (N)	↓	↓	↓
Pseudohypoparathyroidism type II	PTH unresponsiveness	Unknown	Seizures. Phenotype normal.	↓	↑		↑	↓	↓	↓	N
Pseudohypohyperparathyroidism with osteitis fibrosa	Renal resistance to parathyroid hormone with osteitis fibrosa*	Probably familial	Clinical features of hypocalcemia. Phenotype normal.	↓	↑	↑	↑	N (↑)	↓ (N)	↓	↓
Pseudoidiopathic hypoparathyroidism†			Clinical features of hypoparathyroidism. Phenotype normal.	↓	↓		↑†	↓	↓	N	N

* The opposite (ie, skeletal unresponsiveness to PTH with normal renal responsiveness) has been described.
† Molecular anomaly of PTH proposed.

Table 25–6. Rickets and disorders of calcium metabolism.*

Disease or Condition	Synonym	Inheritance Pattern	Clinical Features	Metabolic Features: Serum Concentration Ca^{2+}	Serum Concentration P	Serum Concentration Alk Ptase	Serum Concentration PTH	Urinary Excretion Ca^{2+}	Urinary Excretion P	Treatment
Hypoparathyroid states	See Table 25–5.									Vitamin D and calcium
Transient tetany of the newborn			Tetany, focal seizures. More common in prematures and infants of diabetic mothers. Rarely described in association with maternal hyperparathyroidism.	↓	↓ (N)	↓ (N)	↓ (N)	↓ (N)	↑ (N)	Diet high in calcium, low in phosphate. Vitamin D may be necessary.
Malabsorption syndrome	Disease entities associated with malabsorption include cystic fibrosis, celiac disease, sprue, Shwachman syndrome; hypoplasia of cartilage and hair.	Generally familial with mode of inheritance related to specific disease	Steatorrhea, failure to thrive. Some forms associated with neutropenia, skeletal anomalies, immunologic deficiencies, and abnormalities of cartilage and hair.	↓ (N)	(N) ↓	↑ (N)	↑ (N)	↓	N (↑ ↓)	Vitamin D, calcium, and magnesium (hypomagnesemic states)
Chronic renal insufficiency			Growth failure, undernutrition, skeletal changes.	↓ (N)	↑	↑ (N)	↑	↓ (N)	↓	Diet high in calcium, low in phosphorus; vitamin D
Vitamin D-deficient rickets	Infantile rickets		Rickets.	↓ (N)	↓	↑	↑	↑	↑	Vitamin D and calcium
Familial hypophosphatemic vitamin D-resistant rickets†	(1) Hereditary vitamin D-resistant rickets (2) Phosphate diabetes (3) X-linked hypophosphatemia	X-linked dominant (occasionally autosomal dominant or sporadic)	Skeletal deformities, growth retardation.	N (↓)	↓	N	N (↑)	N	↑	Oral phosphate and vitamin D
Hereditary vitamin D-refractory rickets‡ Type I Type II	(1) Hypophosphatemic vitamin D-refractory rickets (2) Pseudo-vitamin D-deficiency rickets	Autosomal recessive	Severe rachitic bone changes; generalized aminoaciduria.	↓	↓ (N)	↑	↑		↑	Vitamin D (calciferol) in large doses or approximately physiologic doses of 1,25-dihydroxycholecalciferol

* Normal tubular reabsorption of phosphate (TRP) is 83–98%; the lower values are associated with higher serum levels of phosphorus. In hypoparathyroidism, TRP varies from 40 to 70%. Low values for TRP are also found in some forms of inherited renal tubular disease, eg, vitamin D-resistant rickets.

† A variety of diseases (cystinosis, galactosemia, tyrosinosis, Wilson's disease, hereditary fructose intolerance) are associated with renal tubular defects and should be considered in the differential diagnosis.

‡ Type I has been shown to be the result of defective renal 1α-hydroxylation of 25-hydroxycholecalciferol; type II is due to tissue unresponsiveness to normal levels of 1,25-dihydroxycholecalciferol.

- Candidal infections, defective nails and teeth, cataracts, and calcific bodies in the subcutaneous tissues and basal ganglia.
- Serum and urine calcium normal or low; serum phosphorus high; urine phosphorus low; alkaline phosphatase normal or low; azotemia absent. Inappropriately low parathyroid hormone:ionized calcium ratio.

General Considerations

Bone and kidney are the target organs of PTH, and most of the hormonal effects are mediated by interaction with a plasma membrane-bound receptor and activation of the adenylate cyclase complex—a complex consisting of at least 3 distinct proteins. Manifestations of PTH deficiency (Table 25–5) result either from an absolute deficiency in the hormone or from "resistant states" related to abnormalities of the receptor complex of the PTH molecule. Hypoparathyroidism may be idiopathic (possibly as the result of autoimmune phenomenon) or may result from parathyroidectomy. Hypoparathyroidism may develop following thyroidectomy, with either acute or insidious onset, and may be transient or permanent. Parathyroid deficiency has been reported following x-ray irradiation of the neck or the administration of therapeutic doses of radioactive iodine for carcinoma of the thyroid. Two types of transient hypoparathyroidism may be present in the newborn, both of which are due to a relative deficiency of PTH or hormone action. An early form occurs within the first 2 weeks of life in newborns with a history of birth asphyxia or those born to mothers with diabetes mellitus or hyperparathyroidism. Hypomagnesemia may also be seen in the early type and augments the severity of hypocalcemia. The more common later form occurs almost exclusively in infants fed a milk formula with a high phosphate:calcium ratio.

Autoimmune hypoparathyroidism with demonstrable antibodies to parathyroid tissue may be associated with candidal infection, Addison's disease, diabetes mellitus, pernicious anemia, alopecia, thyroiditis, hypogonadism, and steatorrhea. This form of hypoparathyroidism is often familial (autosomal recessive) and is associated with certain human leukocyte antigen (HLA) types. Infections resulting from lack of immune reaction to *Candida* (in spite of normal generalized T cell function) may lead to severe intractable candidiasis of the nails, skin, and gastrointestinal mucous membranes. Because of the frequent association of adrenocortical insufficiency with parathyroid insufficiency, adrenocortical function should be tested repeatedly.

Congenital absence of the parathyroids may occur in association with congenital absence of the thymus (with resultant thymic dependent immunologic deficiency) and cardiovascular, cerebral, and ocular defects (eg, DiGeorge's syndrome).

Clinical Findings

A. Symptoms and Signs: Prolonged hypocalcemia causes tetany (see below), photophobia, blepharospasm, and diarrhea and may be associated with chronic conjunctivitis, cataracts, numbness of the extremities, poor dentition, skin rashes, alopecia, ectodermal dysplasias, candidal infections, "idiopathic" epilepsy, or symmetric punctate calcifications of basal ganglia. In early infancy, respiratory distress may be the presenting finding.

Tetany is manifested by numbness, cramps, and twitchings of the extremities; carpopedal spasm and laryngospasm; positive Chvostek sign (tapping of the face in front of the ear produces spasm of the facial muscles); positive peroneal sign (tapping the fibular side of the leg over the peroneal nerve produces abduction and dorsiflexion of the foot); positive Trousseau sign (compression of the upper arm with an inflated blood pressure cuff for 2–4 minutes to a pressure above systolic blood pressure produces carpopedal spasm); positive Erb sign (use of a galvanic current to determine hyperexcitability); unexplained bizarre behavior; irritability; loss of consciousness; convulsions; and retarded physical and mental development. Headache, vomiting, diarrhea, increased intracranial pressure, papilledema, and pseudopapilledema may occur.

B. Laboratory Findings: (Table 25–5.) Serum calcium is decreased, serum phosphorus increased, and serum alkaline phosphatase usually normal. Urinary excretion of calcium and phosphorus is decreased. The Ellsworth-Howard test is positive; ie, there is a markedly increased excretion of urinary phosphorus and cyclic AMP following a single intravenous injection (200–500 units) of parathyroid extract. False-negative results are common. Alternatively, there is a rise in serum calcium, a fall in serum phosphorus, and an increase in urine phosphorus following the intramuscular injection of parathyroid extract, 400–1000 units in divided doses daily for 3–4 days. Renal clearance of phosphorus is decreased, and the maximum tubular reabsorption of phosphate falls by 12–30%.

C. X-Ray Findings: Soft tissue and cerebral (basal ganglia) calcification may occur in idiopathic hypoparathyroidism but is less common than in pseudohypoparathyroidism.

Differential Diagnosis

The differential diagnosis of hypoparathyroid states is outlined in Table 25–5. Convulsions suggest epilepsy and other chronic disorders of the central nervous system, while the group of findings referable to the central nervous system (headache, vomiting, increased intracranial pressure, and convulsions) may make differentiation from brain tumor difficult.

Treatment

The objective of treatment is to maintain the serum calcium and phosphate at an approximately normal level.

A. Acute or Severe Tetany: Correct hypocalcemia immediately with calcium intravenously and orally. Thiazide diuretics (eg, chlorthalidone) are also useful in acute management.

Because calcium chloride may cause necrosis and abscess formation at the site of injection, calcium gluconate, 0.1–0.2 g/kg as a 10% solution added to a 5% glucose solution and injected slowly intravenously with careful monitoring of the heart, is generally preferred. Subsequent control may be obtained with calcium orally, although intravenous calcium may be repeated. For short-term therapy, calcium chloride as a dilute solution orally is useful because it produces systemic acidosis and an increase of ionized calcium; calcium lactate or carbonate is the treatment of choice for prolonged oral therapy for both the raising of calcium and lowering of phosphate in the serum.

B. Maintenance Management of Hypoparathyroidism and Chronic Hypocalcemia:

1. Drugs—Give ergocalciferol, dihydrotachysterol, or calcitriol. Ergocalciferol may not reach its peak effect for 3–7 days, but activity of all vitamin D preparations persists for weeks or months. Careful control of dosage with frequent determinations of serum and urine calcium and urine concentrating ability is essential to avoid hypercalcemia, with resultant nephrocalcinosis and renal damage.

2. Diet—Give a high-calcium diet, with added calcium lactate or carbonate. The dose is 300–1200 mg of calcium lactate or carbonate 3–4 times daily with meals. Because calcium is efficiently absorbed, large doses of vitamin D are rarely necessary.

Course & Prognosis

Abnormal mineral concentrations in extracellular fluid are easily corrected with conventional dietary and drug treatments, and most signs and symptoms can be ameliorated. Central nervous system manifestations are usually reversible, and the prognosis for intellectual development is excellent. A major goal of therapy is avoidance of hypercalcemia and resultant renal damage; therefore, high doses of long-acting vitamin D preparations must be carefully monitored. Difficult therapeutic problems arise when manifestations are referable to other autoimmune diseases or when the immune defect gives rise to overgrowth of *Candida*.

Aarskog D, Aksnes L, Markestad T: Effect of parathyroid hormone on cAMP and 1,25-dihydroxyvitamin D formation and renal handling of phosphate in vitamin D-dependent rickets. *Pediatrics* 1983;**71**:59.

Adams JS et al: Vitamin-D synthesis and metabolism after ultraviolet irradiation of normal and vitamin-D-deficient subjects. *N Engl J Med* 1982;**306**:722.

Arulanantham K, Dwyer JM, Genel M: Evidence for defective immunoregulation in the syndrome of familial candidiasis endocrinopathy. *N Engl J Med* 1979;**300**:164.

Birkbeck JA, Scott HF: 25-Hydroxycholecalciferol serum levels in breast-fed infants. *Arch Dis Child* 1908;**55**:691.

Bosley AR, Verrier-Jones ER, Campbell MJ: Aetiological factors in rickets of prematurity. *Arch Dis Child* 1980;**55**:683.

Canalis E: The hormonal and local regulation of bone formation. *Endocr Rev* 1983;**4**:62.

Chesney RW et al: Long-term influence of calcitriol (1,25-dihydroxyvitamin D) and supplemental phosphate in X-linked hypophosphatemic rickets. *Pediatrics* 1983;**71**:559.

Chudley AE et al: Nutritional rickets in 2 very low birthweight infants with chronic lung disease. *Arch Dis Child* 1980; **55**:687.

Drezner MK et al: Evaluation of a role for 1,25-dihydroxyvitamin D_3 in the pathogenesis and treatment of X-linked hypophosphatemic rickets and osteomalacia. *J Clin Invest* 1980;**66**:1020.

Glorieux FH et al: Bone response to phosphate salts, ergocalciferol, and calcitriol in hypophosphatemic vitamin D-resistant rickets. *N Engl J Med* 1980;**303**:1023.

Nash MA et al: Hyperphosphatemia with insufficient parathyroid response in renal failure. *J Pediatr* 1981;**98**:247.

Raisz LG, Kream BE: Regulation of bone formation. *N Engl J Med* 1983;**309**:83.

Rasmussen H et al. Long-term treatment of familial hypophosphatemic rickets with oral phosphate and 1α-hydroxyvitamin D_3. *J Pediatr* 1981;**99**:16.

Salle BL et al: Early oral administration of vitamin D and its metabolites in premature neonates: Effect on mineral homeostasis. *Pediatr Res* 1982;**16**:75.

Schneider AB, Sherwood LM: Pathogenesis and management of hypoparathyroidism and other hypocalcemic disorders. *Metabolism* 1975;**24**:871.

Spiegel AM, Marx SJ: Parathyroid hormone and vitamin D receptors. *Clin Endocrinol Metab* 1983;**12**:221.

PSEUDOHYPOPARATHYROIDISM (Albright's Syndrome & Pseudopseudohypoparathyroidism)

Pseudohypoparathyroidism is a familial hereditary X-linked disease with a female to male ratio of approximately 2:1. It is characterized by adequate parathyroid hormone but a failure of response of the end-organ (the renal tubule, bone, or both) to the hormone. The failure of response is the result of an abnormality in the adenylate cyclase complex, a complex consisting of at least 3 distinct proteins. The specific abnormality is related to a diminution in the quantity of one of these units (the G unit), which is also low in other tissues. Hence, resistance to other hormones acting through the adenylate cyclase complex has been described in pseudohypoparathyroidism.

Patients with pseudohypoparathyroidism may have the same signs and symptoms seen in hypocalcemia and the same chemical findings seen in idiopathic hypoparathyroidism (Table 25–5). In addition, these patients have round, full faces; irregularly shortened digits (with the index and third digits often longer than the first, fourth, and fifth digits); a short, thickset body; delayed and defective dentition; and mental retardation. The hair is dry and coarse, and nails and skin are thickened. Candidiasis has not been reported. X-rays may show thickness of the long bones with limitation of growth at the metaphyseal ends. There may be chondrodysplastic changes in the bones of the hands, demineralization of the bones, thickening of the cortices, and exostoses. Ectopic calcification of the basal ganglia and subcutaneous tissues may occur with or without abnormal serum calcium levels. Corneal and lenticular opacities may be present.

Treatment is the same as for hypoparathyroidism.

Similar phenotypic findings may be found in **pseudopseudohypoparathyroidism,** which is a variant of pseudohypoparathyroidism in which the blood chemistry findings are normal. No treatment is necessary.

In both pseudo- and pseudopseudohypoparathyroidism, the parathyroid glands are hyperplastic, serum levels of PTH are elevated, and the kidneys are relatively unresponsive to PTH. Elevated calcitonin concentration is the consequence rather than the cause of hypocalcemia.

Morimoto S et al: Differentiation of pseudo- and idiopathic hypoparathyroidism by measuring urinary calcitonin. *J Clin Endocrinol Metab* 1983;**57:**1216.

Schneider AB, Sherwood LM: Pathogenesis and management of hypoparathyroidism and other hypocalcemic disorders. *Metabolism* 1975;**24:**871.

Spiegel AM, Marx SJ: Parathyroid hormone and vitamin D receptors. *Clin Endocrinol Metab* 1983;**12:**221.

HYPERPARATHYROIDISM & HYPERCALCEMIC STATES

Essentials of Diagnosis

- Elevated blood levels of PTH.
- Serum (and urine) ionized calcium elevated; urine phosphate high with low or normal serum phosphate; alkaline phosphatase normal or elevated.
- Abdominal pain, polyuria, polydipsia, hypertension, nephrocalcinosis, uremia, intractable peptic ulcer, constipation, renal stones, and pancreatitis.
- Bone pain and, rarely, pathologic fractures. X-ray shows subperiosteal resorption, loss of lamina dura of teeth, renal parenchymal calcification or stones, and bone cysts or "brown tumors."
- Unusual behavior and mood swings.

General Considerations

Hyperparathyroidism is rare in childhood and may be primary or secondary (Table 25–7). The most common cause of primary hyperparathyroidism is adenoma of the gland. Diffuse parathyroid hyperplasia or multiple adenoma has also been described in families. The most common causes of the secondary form are chronic renal disease (glomerulonephritis, pyelonephritis), rickets, and congenital anomalies of the genitourinary tract. Rarely, hyperparathyroidism may be found in osteogenesis imperfecta and cancers with bony metastases. Familial hyperparathyroidism may be an isolated disease or associated with other endocrine adenomas of type I and, less commonly, type II multiple endocrine neoplasia (MEN) syndromes.

Table 25–7. Hypercalcemic states.

I. Primary hyperparathyroidism:
  A. Hyperplasia.
  B. Adenoma.
  C. Familial, including multiple endocrine neoplasia types I and II.
  D. Ectopic parathyroid hormone secretion.

II. Hypercalcemic states other than hyperparathyroidism associated with increased intestinal or renal absorption of calcium:
  A. Hypervitaminosis D (including idiopathic hypercalcemia of infancy).
  B. Milk-alkali syndrome.
  C. Thiazide administration.
  D. Sarcoidosis.
  E. Phosphate depletion.

III. Hypercalcemic states other than hyperparathyroidism associated with increased immobilization of bone mineral:
  A. Hyperthyroidism.
  B. Immobilization.
  C. Malignant neoplasms:
    1. Ectopic parathyroid hormone secretion.
    2. Prostaglandin-secreting tumor and perhaps prostaglandin release from subcutaneous fat necrosis.
    3. Tumors metastatic to bone.
    4. Myeloma.

Clinical Findings

A. Symptoms and Signs:

1. Due to hypercalcemia—Findings include hypotonicity and weakness of muscles; apathy, mood swings, and bizarre behavior; nausea, vomiting, abdominal pain, constipation, and loss of weight; hyperextensibility of joints; and hypertension, cardiac irregularities, bradycardia, and shortening of the QT interval. Calcium deposits may occur in the cornea or conjunctiva ("band keratopathy"). Detection of this important finding may require slit lamp examination of the eye. Coma occurs rarely. Intractable peptic ulcer and pancreatitis occur in adults and rarely in children.

2. Due to increased calcium and phosphorus excretion—Findings include loss of renal concentrating ability, polyuria, polydipsia, precipitation of calcium phosphate in the renal parenchyma or as urinary calculi, and progressive renal damage.

3. Related to changes in the skeleton—There may be bone pain, osteitis fibrosa, subperiosteal absorption of phalanges, absence of lamina dura around the teeth, spontaneous fractures, and a "moth-eaten" appearance of the skull.

B. X-Ray Findings: Bone changes may be subtle in children, even when radiography shows nephrocalcinosis. When bone changes occur, the distal clavicle and middle phalanges are initially affected. Later, there is a generalized demineralization with a predilection for subperiosteal cortical bone.

Treatment

Treatment consists of complete removal of the tumor or subtotal removal of hyperplastic parathyroid glands. Preoperatively, intake of dietary calcium should be restricted and hypercalcemia controlled with normal saline infusion and nonthiazide diuretics. Postoperatively, observe carefully for evidence of hypocalcemic tetany; this may occur with total serum calcium within normal limits if a precipitous drop in calcium has occurred. The diet should be high in calcium and vitamin D.

Treatment of secondary hyperparathyroidism is directed at the underlying disease. Diminution in the absorption of phosphate with aluminum hydroxide orally is helpful. The hypocalcemia of severe renal disease (creatinine clearance < 15 mL/min) results from impaired renal activation of vitamin D. Treatment with calcitriol has been useful in this disorder.

Course & Prognosis

The prognosis following removal of a single adenoma is excellent. The prognosis following subtotal parathyroidectomy and removal of multiple adenomas and diffuse hyperplasia or removal of an adenoma is usually good and depends on correction of the underlying defect. In patients with multiple sites of parathyroid adenoma or hyperplasia, the possibility of a familial disease (eg, multiple endocrine neoplasia) must be considered. Since this may be either a sporadic or autosomal dominant condition, other family members are at risk and genetic counseling is indicated.

Goldsmith RE et al: Familial hyperparathyroidism: Description of a large family kindred with physiologic observations and a review of the literature. *Ann Intern Med* 1976;**84:**36.

Mundy GR, Martin TJ: The hypercalcemia of malignancy: Pathogenesis and management. *Metabolism* 1982;**31:**1247.

Scholz DA et al: Primary hyperparathyroidism with multiple parathyroid gland enlargement: Review of 53 cases. *Mayo Clin Proc* 1978;**53:**792.

HYPERVITAMINOSIS D

Exposure to sunlight and ingestion of vitamin D in a normal diet do not result in hypervitaminosis D and hypercalcemia, except possibly in sarcoidosis. Vitamin D intoxication is the result of ingestion of excessive amounts of vitamin D, some forms of which may be stored for months in adipose tissue.

Signs and symptoms of vitamin D-induced hypercalcemia are the same as with other hypercalcemic states and include abdominal, renal, central nervous system, and bone findings. Renal insufficiency may be irreversible and is the result of renovascular effects of hypercalcemia and precipitation of calcium phosphate in the renal interstitial tissue. Ectopic calcification can occur in many other tissues, including the cornea and the gastric mucosa.

Treatment depends on the stage of hypercalcemic toxicity. Because of adipose tissue storage of vitamin D, several months of treatment may be necessary. Dietary intake of foods fortified with vitamin D (eg, milk) and calcium should be reduced or eliminated, if possible. Hypercalcemia can be treated with intravenous fluids and nonthiazide diuretics. Adrenocorticosteroids, salmon calcitonin, and the antibiotic mithramycin have also been employed with some success.

The central nervous system manifestations may be dramatic, and deaths have occurred during acute crises. Chronic brain damage in young infants has been reported. The insidious nature of the renal insult may result in renal insufficiency and failure by the time diagnosis is established.

IDIOPATHIC HYPERCALCEMIA

Idiopathic hypercalcemia (Williams's syndrome) is an uncommon disorder characterized in its severe form by peculiar ("elfin") facies (receding mandible, depressed bridge of nose, relatively large mouth, prominent lips, hanging jowls, large low-set ears, prominent eyes, occasional esotropia, and hypertelorism), failure to thrive, mental and motor retardation, irritability, purposeless movements, constipation, hypotonia, polyuria, polydipsia, hypertension, and cardiac defects (ie, supravalvular aortic stenosis or peripheral pulmonic stenosis). Generalized osteosclerosis is common, and there may be premature craniosynostosis and nephrocalcinosis with evidence of urinary tract disease. In addition to the hypercalcemia, there may be hypophosphatemia, hypercholesterolemia, azotemia, and elevation of serum carotene and vitamin A.

Clinical manifestations may not appear for several months. The disease may be due to the increased intake of vitamin D during pregnancy, a defect in the metabolism of or responsiveness to vitamin D, abnormal sterol synthesis, or some as yet unrecognized mechanism.

Treatment is by rigid restriction of dietary calcium and vitamin D.

IMMOBILIZATION HYPERCALCEMIA

Abrupt immobilization of a rapidly growing adolescent following an injury may lead to a rapid decrease in bond deposition with continued bone resorption, calcium mobilization, and hypercalcemia. For reasons that are not completely understood, immobilization may be associated with elevated parathyroid hormone levels in spite of elevated levels of ionized calcium.

Hyman LR et al: Immobilization hypercalcemia. *Am J Dis Child* 1972;**124:**723.

Lerman S, Canterbury JM, Reiss E: Parathyroid hormone and the hypercalcemia of immobilization. *J Clin Endocrinol Metab* 1977;**45:**425.

HYPOPHOSPHATASIA & PSEUDOHYPOPHOSPHATASIA

Hypophosphatasia is an uncommon inherited (autosomal recessive) condition characterized by a specific deficiency of alkaline phosphatase activity in serum, bone, and tissues. Radiographically, there is inadequate mineralization of epiphyseal cartilage and osteoid, with localized areas of radiolucency. The disease is radiographically and histologically similar to bone lesions of other types of rickets, although in hypophosphatasia the lesions are not more severe in sites of rapid growth. The earlier the age at onset, the more severe the condition. Failure to thrive, feeding problems, dwarfing, hyperpyrexia, premature loss of teeth, widening of the sutures, bulging fontanelles, convulsions, bony deformities, hyperpigmentation, conjunctival calcification, band keratopathy, and renal lesions have been reported in some cases. Premature closure of cranial sutures may occur. Calcium and phosphate concentrations in the extracellular fluid are usually normal, although calcium levels may be elevated. When this occurs, signs and symptoms may be similar to those of idiopathic hypercalcemia; late features include osteoporosis, pseudofractures, and rachitic deformities. The plasma and urine of patients and heterozygote carriers contain phosphoethanolamine in excessive amounts. In some cases, marked metaphyseal irregularities may occur. A condition known as **pseudohypophosphatasia** has been described in which the clinical features of hypophosphatasia are seen in association with normal levels of alkaline phosphatase.

No specific treatment is available, but adrenocorticosteroids may be of value. The mortality rate is high in infancy. Adults are usually asymptomatic.

Whyte MP et al: Enzyme replacement therapy for infantile hypophosphatasia attempted by intravenous infusions of alkaline phosphatase-rich Paget plasma: Results in three additional patients. *J Pediatr* 1984;**105:**926.

ADRENAL CORTEX

The adrenal cortex develops from the dorsal coelomic mesothelium between the fourth and sixth weeks of fetal life. By 8–9 weeks of gestation, the fetal adrenal cortex contains the enzymes necessary to produce cortisol from progesterone. At 7–9 weeks of gestation, the fetal pituitary seems capable of producing and releasing adrenocorticotropic hormone (ACTH) to provide regulation of adrenal hormone production.

The adult adrenal cortex is composed of 3 distinct zones. The glomerulosa is the outermost zone and seems to be the exclusive source of aldosterone, the major mineralocorticoid in humans. The zona fasciculata is the largest cortical zone and is the source of cortisol, the major glucocorticoid. The zona reticularis is the innermost zone (adjacent to the adrenal medulla) and appears to produce mainly adrenal androgens and estrogens.

During fetal life, these 3 zones comprise only a minor portion of the adrenal cortex. The predominant portion is the fetal zone, or provisional cortex, which is capable of producing glucocorticoids, mineralocorticoids, androgens, and estrogens but is relatively deficient in production of 3β-hydroxydehydrogenase and Δ^5-Δ^4 isomerase (Fig 25–3). Therefore, placentally produced progesterone serves as the major precursor for fetal adrenal production of cortisol and aldosterone.

The adrenal cortex produces cortisol under the control of pituitary ACTH. The quantity of cortisol produced is regulated by a negative-feedback mechanism involving the pituitary and hypothalamus (Fig 25–4). This negative-feedback control is superimposed on a diurnal pattern of ACTH release. ACTH release is greatest during early morning hours and least in late afternoon.

The action of glucocorticoids (cortisol and cortisone) are myriad and incompletely understood. Glucocorticoids are catabolic and antianabolic; ie, they promote release of amino acids from muscle and increase gluconeogenesis while decreasing incorporation of amino acids into muscle protein. They also antagonize insulin action and permit lipogenesis. Glucocorticoids may influence blood pressure by affecting sodium and, therefore, water retention. A further influence on vascular volume is the glucocorticoid effect on arterioles, resulting in increased peripheral vascular resistance.

Mineralocorticoids (primarily aldosterone in humans) promote sodium retention and permit potassium excretion. While ACTH can affect aldosterone production, the usual regulators of aldosterone secretion are mediated via the renin-aldosterone system in response to changes in intravascular volume and serum sodium concentrations. Serum potassium concentrations may directly influence aldosterone release.

ADRENOCORTICAL INSUFFICIENCY (Adrenal Crisis, Addison's Disease)

Essentials of Diagnosis

Acute form (adrenal crisis):

- Vomiting, dehydration, hypotension, circulatory collapse.
- Serum sodium low; serum potassium high.
- Blood and urine adrenocorticosteroids low.
- A definite precipitating factor usually present (eg, acute illness, trauma).

Chronic form (Addison's disease):

- Weakness, fatigue, pallor; episodes of nausea, vomiting, and diarrhea; increased appetite for salt.
- Increased pigmentation, hypotension; small heart.

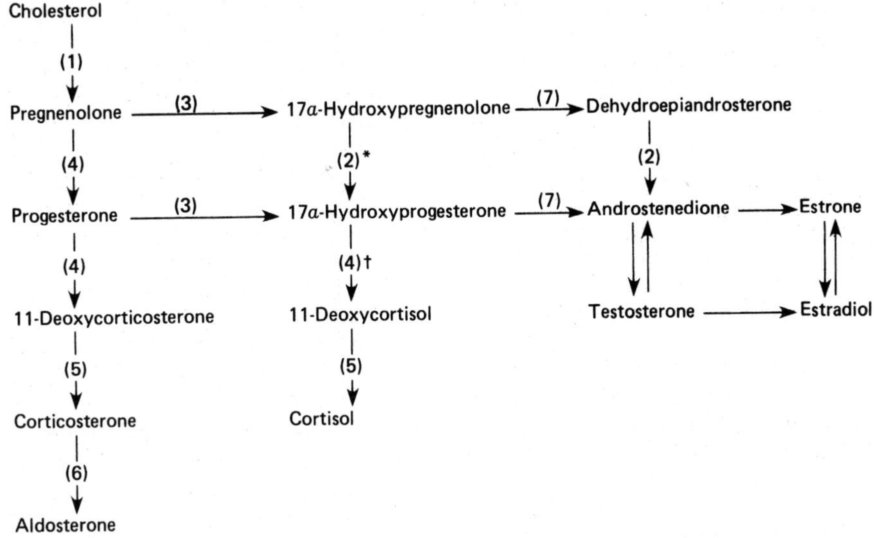

Figure 25–3. Synthesis of cortisol, aldosterone, testosterone, and estrogen in the adrenal gland.

- Serum sodium low, serum potassium high; blood and urine adrenocorticosteroids decreased; eosinophilia.

General Considerations

Adrenocortical hypofunction may be due to congenital absence or atrophy (toxic factors, autoimmune phenomena) of the adrenal; an enzymatic defect leading to decreased production of cortisol; infection (eg, tuberculosis); or destruction of the gland by tumor or hemorrhage (Waterhouse-Friderichsen syndrome) and calcification. In some cases, it occurs as a consequence of inadequate secretion of corticotropin (ACTH) due to anterior pituitary or hypothalamic disease. In the latter condition, hyperpigmentation does not occur. Any acute illness, surgery, trauma, or exposure to excessive heat may precipitate an adrenal crisis. A temporary salt-losing disorder, possibly due to either mineralocorticoid deficiency or renal tubular insensitivity to mineralocorticoid, may occur during infancy.

Fractional types of adrenocortical insuffiency, including forms with deficiency of glucocorticoid, aldosterone, or other mineral-regulating steroids but with normal production of other hormones of the adrenal, have been described.

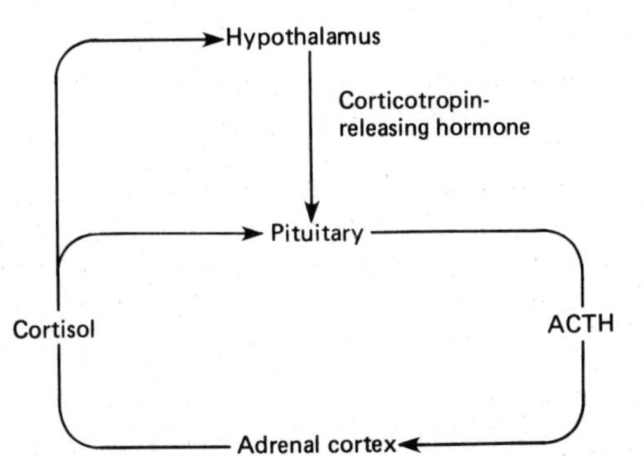

Figure 25–4. Pituitary-adrenal cortex control.

Clinical Findings

A. Symptoms and Signs:

1. Acute form (adrenal crisis)—Manifestations include nausea and vomiting, diarrhea, abdominal pain, dehydration, fever (which may be followed by hypothermia), hypotension, circulatory collapse, and confusion or coma.

2. Chronic form (Addison's disease)—The leading causes of adrenal insufficiency today are hereditary enzymatic defects with congenital adrenal hyperplasia and idiopathic loss of adrenal function, the latter thought to be due to autoimmune mechanisms. Adrenal destruction may also occur secondary to infectious processes (eg, tuberculosis) and neoplasms. A rare form of familial Addison's disease may be seen in association with cerebral sclerosis and spastic paraplegia. Idiopathic Addison's disease may be familial and has been described in association with hypoparathyroidism, candidiasis, hypothyroidism, pernicious anemia, hypogonadism, and diabetes mellitus. The finding of circulating antibodies to adrenal tissue and other tissues involved in these conditions suggests that an autoimmune mechanism, probably related to a defect in immunoregulation involving suppressor T cell function, is the cause.

Signs and symptoms include fatigue, hypotension, weakness, failure to gain or loss of weight, increased appetite for salt, diarrhea, vomiting (which may become forceful and sometimes projectile), and dehydration. Diffuse tanning with increased pigmentation over pressure points, scars, and mucous membranes may be present. A small heart may be seen on x-ray.

B. Laboratory Findings:

1. Suggestive of adrenal insufficiency—Serum sodium, chloride, and bicarbonate, P_{CO_2}, and blood pH and blood volume are decreased. Serum potassium and blood urea nitrogen are increased. Urinary sodium is elevated, and the sodium:potassium ratio is high despite low serum sodium.

Eosinophilia* and moderate neutropenia may be present.

2. Confirmatory tests—The following tests measure the functional capacity of the adrenal cortex:

a. The corticotropin (ACTH) stimulation test is the most definitive test.

b. Plasma ACTH levels are elevated while cortisol and urinary 17-hydroxycorticosteroid levels are low and fail to rise with ACTH stimulation.

c. Urinary 17-hydroxycorticosteroid excretion is decreased.

d. Urinary 17-ketosteroid output is lower except in cases due to congenital adrenal hyperplasia or adrenal cortex tumor. This test is of little value in younger children, who normally excrete less than 1 mg/d.

e. The metyrapone (Metopirone) test is useful in demonstrating normal pituitary function and in the diagnosis of adrenal insufficiency secondary to pituitary insufficiency. This test may provoke acute adrenal insufficiency in an individual with compromised adrenal function.

Differential Diagnosis

Acute adrenal insufficiency must be differentiated from severe acute infections, diabetic coma, various disturbances of the central nervous system, and acute poisoning. In the neonatal period, adrenal insufficiency may be clinically indistinguishable from respiratory distress, intracranial hemorrhage, or sepsis.

Chronic adrenocortical insufficiency must be differentiated from anorexia nervosa, certain muscular disorders (myasthenia gravis, etc), salt-losing nephritis, chronic debilitating infections (tuberculosis, etc), and recurrent spontaneous hypoglycemia.

Treatment

A. Acute Form (Adrenal Crisis):

1. Replacement therapy—

a. Hydrocortisone sodium succinate (Solu-Cortef), 2 mg/kg diluted in 2–10 mL of water intravenously, is given over 2–5 minutes. Follow this with an infusion of normal saline and 5–10% glucose, 100 mL/kg/24 h intravenously. Then give hydrocortisone sodium succinate, 1.5 mg/kg (12.5 mg/m^2), intravenously every 4–6 hours until stabilization is achieved and oral therapy tolerated.

b. Desoxycorticosterone acetate (DOCA), 1–2 mg/d intramuscularly, is given as part of initial therapy. This is repeated every 12–24 hours depending on the state of hydration, electrolyte status, and blood pressure.

c. Ten percent glucose in normal saline, 20 mL/kg intravenously in the first 2 hours, may be of value, particularly in infants with adrenal crisis who have congenital adrenal hyperplasia. Avoid overtreatment.

2. Hypotension—Specific treatment includes volume expansion (eg, hydrocortisone sodium succinate, normal saline solution, albumin). Plasma or blood transfusion, 22 mL/kg, should be used also as necessary to maintain blood pressure. Rarely, one of the following additions is necessary:

a. Isoproterenol, 2.5–5 mg in 500 mL of 5% dextrose and 0.45% saline solution infused over a period of 2–8 hours to maintain blood pressure.

b. Norepinephrine bitartrate, 4 mL (1 mg/mL) added to 1000 mL of electrolyte solution for use by intravenous drip. Determine response to an initial dose of 0.25–0.5 mL of dilute solution per 10 kilograms, and then stabilize flow at a rate sufficient to maintain blood pressure (usual rate: 0.5–1 mL/min). This drug is very potent, and great care must be employed in its use.

3. Infections—Treat infections with large doses of appropriate antibiotic or chemotherapeutic agents.

4. Waterhouse-Friderichsen syndrome with fulminant infections—The use of adrenocorticosteroids and norepinephrine in the treatment or "prophylaxis" of fulminant infections is felt by some not to be justified, since it may augment the generalized Shwartzman reaction seen in the renal cortices of fatal cases of meningococcemia. However, corticosteroids should be used in the presence of adrenal insufficiency, particularly with hypotension and circulatory collapse.

5. Fluids and electrolytes—Give 10% glucose in saline, 20 mL/kg intravenously. ***Caution:*** Avoid overtreatment. Total parenteral fluid in the first 8

* A normal number of eosinophils during stress (eg, the day after operation or in the presence of a severe infection) is also suggestive of insufficiency.

hours should not exceed the maintenance fluid requirement of the normal child (see Chapter 36). Fruit juices, ginger ale, milk, and soft foods should be given as soon as possible.

B. Maintenance Therapy of Chronic Form (Addison's Disease): Following initial stabilization, the most effective substitution therapy is generally hydrocortisone or cortisone given with supplementary desoxycorticosterone or fludrocortisone. Overtreatment should be avoided, since it may result in obesity, growth retardation, or other cushingoid features.

Additional hydrocortisone, desoxycorticosterone, or sodium chloride, singly or in combination, may be necessary with acute illness, surgery, trauma, or other stress reactions.

Supportive adrenocortical therapy should be given whenever surgical operations are performed on patients who have at some time received prolonged therapy with adrenocorticosteroids. (See below.)

1. Glucocorticoids (hydrocortisone or equivalent)—Increase the dosage of all glucocorticoids to 2–4 times the usual dosage during intercurrent illness or times of stress.

a. Hydrocortisone—Give 15–20 mg/m^2/d orally in 3–4 divided doses. For adrenal enzyme defects with excess ACTH, 25% of the dose is given in the morning and afternoon and 50% at night. For all other causes of adrenocortical insufficiency, 50% of the daily dose is given in the morning.

b. Cortisone acetate—Give 25–30 mg/m^2/d orally divided in 3 daily doses as hydrocortisone; or 12.5 mg/m^2/d intramuscularly given as 37.5 mg/m^2 intramuscularly every 3 days.

c. Prednisone—Give 5–6 mg/m^2/d orally in 2–3 divided doses. Its potency may preclude necessary minor modulations in dosage. More potent glucocorticoids should not be used.

2. Mineralocorticoids (desoxycorticosterone acetate [DOCA] and related drugs)—The dosage should be gradually increased or decreased to maintain normal serum sodium levels and blood volume and avoid hypertension. Increases with stress are not necessary.

a. Fludrocortisone (Florinef)—Give 0.05–0.2 mg orally once a day.

b. DOCA in oil—Give 1 mg/d intramuscularly.

c. Pellets containing DOCA may be implanted subcutaneously in the subscapular area. In general, two 125-mg pellets provide adequate therapy. Reimplantation is necessary every 6–9 months.

3. Salt—The child should be given ready access to table salt; an infant should be offered salted food or formula several times a day. Frequent blood pressure determinations in the recumbent position should be made to be certain that hypertension is avoided.

C. Corticosteroids in Patients With Adrenocortical Insufficiency Who Undergo Surgery:

1. Preoperatively—Give cortisone acetate intramuscularly as follows (single dose):

a. 48 hours before surgery, 15 mg/m^2.

b. 24 hours before surgery, 15 mg/m^2.

c. 12 hours before surgery, 15 mg/m^2.

d. 1 hour before surgery, 15 mg/m^2.

In addition, give hydrocortisone sodium succinate (Solu-Cortef), 15 mg/m^2, 1 hour before surgery.

2. During operation—Administer hydrocortisone sodium succinate, 25–100 mg intravenously, with 5–10% glucose in saline throughout surgery.

3. During recovery—Hydrocortisone sodium succinate, 12.5 mg/m^2 intravenously, is given every 4–6 hours until oral doses are tolerated. The oral dose of 3–5 times maintenance is gradually tapered to the maintenance dose as the patient recovers.

Course & Prognosis

A. Acute: The course of acute adrenal insufficiency is rapid, and death may occur within a few hours unless adequate treatment is given. Spontaneous recovery is unlikely. Newborn infants with severe adrenal hemorrhages seldom respond even to vigorous therapy. Patients who have received treatment with adrenocorticosteroids may exhibit adrenal collapse if they undergo surgery or other acute stress for as long as 6–24 months after corticosteroids are discontinued.

In all forms of acute adrenal insufficiency, once the crisis has passed, the patient should be observed carefully and evaluated with laboratory tests to assess the degree of permanent adrenal insufficiency.

B. Chronic: Adequately treated chronic adrenocortical insufficiency is consistent with a relatively normal life. Since patients may become dehydrated quickly during minor infections, they must be observed carefully and receive prompt treatment under such circumstances.

Gutai JP, Migeon CJ: Adrenal insufficiency during the neonatal period. *Clin Perinatol* 1975;**2:**163.

Khalid BA et al: Steroid replacement in Addison's disease and in subjects adrenalectomized for Cushing's disease: Comparison of various glucocorticoids. *J Clin Endocrinol Metab* 1982;**55:**551.

Pakravan P et al: Familial congenital absence of adrenal glands: Evaluation of glucocorticoid, mineralocorticoid, and estrogen metabolism in the perinatal period. *J Pediatr* 1974;**84:**74.

Riley WJ, Maclaren NK, Neufeld M: Adrenal autoantibodies and Addison disease in insulin-dependent diabetes mellitus. *J Pediatr* 1980;**97:**191.

Scott RS, Donald RA, Espiner EA: Plasma ACTH and cortisol profiles in Addisonian patients receiving conventional substitution therapy. *Clin Endocrinol* 1978;**9:**571.

Thistlethwaite D et al: Familial glucocorticoid deficiency: Studies of diagnosis and pathogenesis. *Arch Dis Child* 1975; **50:**291.

ADRENOCORTICAL HYPERFUNCTION

1. CUSHING'S SYNDROME

Essentials of Diagnosis

- "Truncal type" adiposity with thin extremities, moon face, weakness, plethora, easy bruisability, purplish striae, growth retardation.
- Hypertension, osteoporosis, glycosuria.
- Elevated serum and urine adrenocorticosteroids with loss of normal diurnal variation; low serum potassium; eosinopenia.
- Early in the disease process, few of the classic features may be present.

General Considerations

The principal findings in Cushing's syndrome in childhood result from excessive secretion of glucocorticoids and androgens. Depletion of body protein stores and abnormal carbohydrate and fat metabolism are typical. There may also be lesser degrees of overproduction of the mineralocorticoids. It has been suggested that in Cushing's syndrome with bilateral adrenal hyperplasia there is decreased responsiveness of the hypothalamic-pituitary "feedback" mechanism that regulates the release or production of ACTH. This may then result in a constant but only slightly excessive elevation in the secretion of ACTH or lead to qualitative or quantitative change in the diurnal variation.

Cushing's syndrome is more common in females. In children under 12, it is usually iatrogenic (secondary to therapeutic doses of corticotropin or one of the corticosteroids). It may rarely be due to an adrenal tumor or associated with a basophilic adenoma of the pituitary gland, adrenocortical hyperplasia, or an extrapituitary ACTH-producing tumor.

Clinical Findings

A. Symptoms and Signs:

1. Due to excessive secretion of the glucocorticoid hormones—Findings include "buffalo type" adiposity, most marked on the face, neck, and trunk (a fat pad in the interscapular area is characteristic); easy fatigability and weakness; plethoric facies; purplish striae; easy bruisability; ecchymoses; hirsutism; osteoporosis; hypertension; diabetes mellitus (usually latent), pain in the back; muscle wasting and weakness; and marked retardation of growth.

2. Due to excessive secretion of mineralocorticoids—Hypernatremia, increased blood volume, edema, and hypertension may be found.

3. Due to excessive secretion of androgens—Manifestation include hirsutism, acne, and varying degrees of excessive masculinization.

4. Menstrual irregularities—Menstrual irregularities occur during puberty in older girls.

B. Laboratory Findings:

1. Blood—

a. Serum cortisol levels are elevated. There may be a loss of the normal diurnal variation.

b. Serum chloride and potassium may be lowered.

c. Serum sodium and HCO_3^- content may be elevated (metabolic alkalosis).

d. Plasma ACTH concentrations are slightly elevated with adrenal hyperplasia; decreased in cases of adrenal tumor; and greatly increased with ACTH-producing pituitary or extrapituitary tumors. The white count shows polymorphonuclear leukocytosis with lymphopenia, and the eosinophil count is low ($< 50/\mu L$). The red cell count may be elevated.

2. Urine—

a. Urinary free cortisol excretion is elevated. This may be the most useful diagnostic test.

b. Urinary 17-hydroxycorticosteroid levels are elevated.

c. Urinary 17-ketosteroids may be normal but are usually elevated in association with adrenal tumor.

d. Glycosuria may be present.

3. Response to corticotropin (ACTH) and corticosteroids—The response to corticotropin (ACTH) stimulation is excessive in patients with adrenal hyperplasia; a poor response is usually found in those with tumor. There is a diminished adrenal response to small doses (0.5 mg) of dexamethasone in the dexamethasone suppression test; larger doses will cause suppression of adrenal activity when the disease is due to adrenal hyperplasia. Adenomas and adrenal carcinomas may rarely be suppressed by large doses of dexamethasone (4–16 mg/d in 4 divided doses).

C. Radiologic Findings: A CT scan of the pituitary may demonstrate a pituitary adenoma. A CT scan of the adrenals will demonstrate an adenoma and may demonstrate bilateral hyperplasia. Radionuclide studies of the adrenals may be useful in complex cases. Urograms may be abnormal. Adrenal calcification may be present. Osteoporosis (evident first in the spine and pelvis) with compression fractures may be seen in advanced cases.

Differential Diagnosis

Children with obesity, particularly in the presence of striae and hypertension, are frequently suspected of having Cushing's syndrome. The growth rate may be helpful in differentiating the two. Children with Cushing's syndrome have a poor growth rate, while those with exogenous obesity usually have a normal or slightly increased growth rate. In addition, the color of the striae (purplish in Cushing's syndrome, pink in obesity) and the distribution of the obesity assist in the differentiation. The urinary free cortisol excretion is always normal in obesity. The urinary excretion of corticosteroids may not be helpful, since they may be elevated in obesity (usually in proportion to the weight and surface area).

Treatment

In all cases of primary adrenal hyperfunction due

to tumor, surgical removal, if possible, is indicated. Corticotropin (ACTH) should be given preoperatively and postoperatively to stimulate the nontumorous adrenal cortex, which is generally atrophied. Adrenocorticosteroids should be administered for 1–2 days before surgery and continued during and after operation. Supplemental potassium, salt, and mineralocorticoids may be necessary. (See above outline of corticosteroid administration in surgical patients.)

Adrenal hyperplasia resulting from a pituitary microadenoma may respond to pituitary irradiation or microadrenalectomy. Total adrenalectomy may be necessary. Pituitary irradiation, radioactive implantation, electrocoagulation, or ablation has sometimes been of value in adults. Substitution therapy may be necessary after these measures.

The use of mitotane (Lysodren), a DDT derivative toxic to the adrenal cortex, and aminoglutethimide, an inhibitor of steroid synthesis, has been suggested, but their usefulness in children with adrenal tumors has not been determined.

Prognosis

If the tumor is malignant, the prognosis is poor; if benign, cure is to be expected following proper preparation and surgery.

Pituitary enlargement has been reported in some cases of Cushing's syndrome following both partial and complete adrenalectomy.

Cushing's syndrome (perhaps due to pituitary adenoma) may occasionally undergo spontaneous remission.

Although most of the changes resulting from adrenocorticosteroid excess disappear, hypertension, diabetes mellitus, and osteoporosis may persist, and the rate of growth may continue to be poor.

Aron DC et al: Cushing's syndrome: Problems in management. *Endocr Rev* 1982;**3:**229.

Giombetti R et al: Cushing's syndrome in infants: A case complicated by monilial endocarditis. *Am J Dis Child* 1971; **122:**264.

Jennings AS, Liddle GW, Orth DN: Results of treating childhood Cushing's disease with pituitary irradiation. *N Engl J Med* 1977;**297:**957.

Krieger DT: Physiopathology of Cushing's disease. *Endocr Rev* 1983;**4:**22.

Krieger DT et al: Cyproheptadine-induced remission of Cushing's disease. *N Engl J Med* 1975;**293:**893.

Lee PA, Weldon VV, Migeon CJ: Short stature as the only clinical sign of Cushing's syndrome. *J Pediatr* 1975;**86:**89.

McArthur RG et al: Cushing's disease in children: Findings in 13 cases. *Mayo Clin Proc* 1972;**47:**318.

Streeten DH et al: Hypercortisolism in childhood: Shortcomings of conventional diagnostic criteria. *Pediatrics* 1975;**56:**797.

Streeten DH et al: Normal and abnormal function of the hypothalamic-pituitary-adrenocortical system in man. *Endocr Rev* 1984;**5:**371.

2. ADRENOGENITAL SYNDROME

Essentials of Diagnosis

- Pseudohermaphroditism in females, with urogenital sinus, enlargement of clitoris, and other evidence of virilization.
- Isosexual precocity in males with infantile testes.
- Excessive growth; early development of sexual hair.
- Urinary 17-ketosteroids elevated; plasma 17α-hydroxyprogesterone and urinary pregnanetriol increased in the commonest form.
- May be associated with electrolyte and water disturbances, particularly in the newborn period.

General Considerations

The adrenogenital syndrome occurs when adrenal androgens or estrogens or both are produced in excessive amounts for the age of the child, resulting in precocious and sometimes heterosexual development of the genitalia. The most common form of this syndrome is the congenital familial (autosomal recessive) form, also known as congenital adrenal hyperplasia. This form, which affects males and females equally, is due to an inborn error of metabolism with a deficiency of one of the adrenocortical enzymes required for cortisol or sex hormone synthesis (Fig 25–3). Enzyme deficiencies that cause defects in cortisol and aldosterone synthesis have been described.

Over 80% of cases are caused by a 21-hydroxylase enzyme deficiency, approximately 10% by an 11-hydroxylase enzyme deficiency, and the remainder by deficiencies of the other 5 enzymes (Fig 25–3). In some forms, the infant may appear normal at birth, with symptoms occurring later. In all forms except 17,20-desmolase deficiency, there is diminished secretion of cortisol resulting in excessive secretion of ACTH, which causes adrenal hyperplasia with increased production of various adrenal hormone precursors and increased urinary excretion of their metabolites. Increased pigmentation, especially of the scrotum, labia majora, and nipples, frequently results from excessive ACTH secretion.

Studies in patients with 21-hydroxylase deficiency indicate that the clinical type (salt-wasting versus non-salt-wasting) is usually consistent within a family and that there is a close genetic linkage of the 21-hydroxylase gene to the HLA complex on chromosome 6. The latter finding has allowed more precise heterozygote detection and prenatal diagnosis. Population studies indicate that the defective gene is present in one out of 50–100 people and that the incidence of the disorder is one per 5000–15,000 people. Hormonal evaluation of unaffected family members following ACTH stimulation allows detection of the heterozygote with an 80–90% certainty, and a combination of hormonal and HLA studies can increase the number of cases detected. HLA typing in combination with measurement of 17α-hydroxyprogesterone and androstenedione in amniotic fluid has been used in the prenatal diagnosis of 21-hydroxylase deficiency. The potential for mass screening with a microfilter paper technique to evaluate 17α-hydroxyprogesterone is under investigation.

Nonclassic presentations of 21-hydroxylase deficiency have been reported with increasing frequency. Affected individuals have a normal phenotype at birth and develop evidence of virilization during later childhood, adolescence, or early adulthood. In these cases, previously referred to as late-onset or acquired enzyme deficiencies, results of hormonal studies are characteristic of 21-hydroxylase deficiency. An asymptomatic form has also been identified in which individuals have none of the phenotypic features of the disorder but have hormonal study results identical to those in patients with nonclassic 21-hydroxylase deficiency. The nonclassic form appears to be less severe than the classic form, and the fact that members of the same family may have classic, nonclassic, and asymptomatic forms suggests that the disorders are due to allelic variations of the same enzyme. Proof for this awaits gene mapping of the 21-hydroxylase gene and its variants.

Pseudohermaphroditism can be caused by factors other than enzyme deficiencies. In females, these include virilizing maternal tumors or androgens or related hormones taken by the mother during the first trimester of pregnancy. In these cases, the condition does not progress after birth, and cortisol deficiency with abnormal steroidogenesis is not present. Pseudohermaphroditism occurs rarely with gonadal dysgenesis.

Adrenogenital syndrome may also result from tumors of the adrenal, ovary, or testis or from idiopathic adrenal hyperplasia later in life. Symptoms begin after birth and progress until treated.

Clinical Findings

A. Symptoms and Signs:

1. Adrenogenital syndrome in females—In females with potentially normal ovaries and uterus, masculinization occurs and sexual development is along heterosexual lines.

a. Congenital bilateral hyperplasia of the adrenal cortex secondary to enzyme deficiency (pseudohermaphroditism)—The abnormality of the external genitalia may vary from mild enlargement of the clitoris to complete fusion of the labioscrotal folds, forming a penile urethra, and enlargement of the clitoris to form a normal-sized phallus. If left untreated, growth in height and skeletal maturation are excessive, and patients become muscular. Pubic hair appears early (often before the second birthday); acne may be excessive; and the voice may be deep. Excessive pigmentation may develop. Dentition is normal or only slightly advanced for the chronologic age. Similar abnormalities may be present in siblings and cousins. Signs of associated adrenal insufficiency may be present during the first days of life or later.

b. Postnatal adrenogenital syndrome (virilism)—This disorder may be due to adrenal hyperplasia or tumor or to arrhenoblastoma (extremely rare). Enlargement of the clitoris occurs, but other changes of the genitalia are not found. The family history is negative for similar abnormalities. If a tumor is present, it may be palpably enlarged. Other findings are similar to those of pseudohermaphroditism.

2. Adrenogenital syndrome in males (macrogenitosomia praecox)—In males, sexual development is along isosexual lines.

a. Congenital bilateral hyperplasia of the adrenal cortex due to enzyme deficiency—The infant may appear normal at birth, but during the first few months of life enlargement of the penis will be noted. There may be increased pigmentation resulting from excessive secretion of ACTH. Other symptoms and signs are similar to those of the congenital form in females. The testes are soft and not enlarged except in the rare male in whom aberrant adrenal cells may be present in the testes and produce unilateral or bilateral symmetric or asymmetric enlargement. Signs of adrenal glucocorticoid insufficiency may be present. In the complete form of the 21-hydroxylase deficiency, mineralocorticoid deficiency may lead to hyponatremia, hyperkalemia, anorexia, vomiting, decreased blood volume, circulatory collapse, and death.

b. Tumor—The findings may be identical with those of congenital bilateral hyperplasia of the adrenal cortex except that they appear at a later age. The tumor may be palpably enlarged. Rarely, an adrenal tumor in a male may produce feminization with gynecomastia.

B. Laboratory Findings:

1. Blood and urine—Hormonal studies are essential for accurate diagnosis. Findings characteristic of the enzyme deficiencies are shown in Table 25–8. With adrenal tumor, production and excretion of dehydroepiandrosterone are greatly elevated.

2. Genetic studies—When available, rapid chromosomal diagnosis is the diagnostic test of choice. In any newborn with ambiguous genitalia, a buccal smear interpreted by an experienced individual should be done as soon as possible. Ideally, fluorescent staining for the Y chromosome should be performed if the buccal smear is interpreted as chromatin-negative. In female pseudohermaphrodites, the nuclear chromatin pattern is positive.

3. Dexamethasone suppression test—If dexamethasone, 2–4 mg/d in 4 divided doses for 7 days, reduces 17-ketosteroids to normal, hyperplasia rather than adenoma is the probable diagnosis.

C. X-Ray Findings: Vaginograms using contrast material may indicate the presence of a urogenital sinus. Displacement of the kidney and calcification in the area of the adrenal may be seen on x-rays of patients with tumors. Bone age is advanced with 21- and 11-hydroxylase defects but may not be evident in the first year. Adrenal ultra-sonography may be useful in localizing an adrenal tumor.

Table 25–8. Laboratory and clinical findings in adrenal enzyme defects resulting in adrenogenital syndrome.

Enzyme Deficiency*	Urinary 17-Ketosteroids	Elevated Plasma Metabolite	Plasma Androgens	Aldosterone	Hypertension/ Salt Loss	External Genitalia†
20,22-Desmolase (1)	↓↓↓		↓↓↓	↓↓↓	−/+	M: feminized F: normal
3β-Hydroxydehydrogenase (2)	↑↑(DHEA)	Pregnenolone	↑(DHEA)	↓↓↓	−/+	M: feminized F: masculinized
17-Hydroxylase (3)	↓↓↓	Progesterone	↓↓	↓↓(↑Deoxycorticosterone)	+/−	M: feminized F: normal
21-Hydroxylase (simple) (4)	↑↑↑	17α-Hydroxyprogesterone	↑↑	↑	−/−	M: normal F: masculinized
21-Hydroxylase (salt-wasting) (4)	↑↑↑	17α-Hydroxyprogesterone	↑↑	↓↓	−/+	M: normal F: masculinized
11-Hydroxylase (5)	↑↑	11-Deoxycortisol	↑↑	↓↓(↑Deoxycorticosterone)	+/−	M: normal F: masculinized
17,20-Desmolase (7)	↓↓↓		↓↓	Normal	−/−	M: feminized F: normal

* The numbers refer to the position of enzyme action as shown in Fig 25–3.
† M = male, F = female.

Treatment

A. Congenital Hyperplasia of the Cortex:

1. Initially, cortisone acetate, given in a dosage of 10–25 mg/d orally or 10–25 mg intramuscularly every 3 days to infants or 25–100 mg/d orally to older children, will suppress abnormal adrenal steroidogenesis within 2 weeks. The maintenance dose is the same as that given on p 791. In congenital hyperplasia, if oral medication is given, 50% of the daily dose should be given in the late evening to suppress the early morning ACTH rise. Dosage is regulated to maintain a normal growth rate, a normal rate of osseous maturation, and the normal range of urinary 17-ketosteroid excretion; in cases of 21-hydroxylase deficiency, the plasma 17α-hydroxyprogesterone and dehydroepiandrosterone sulfate levels should also be kept within the normal range. In adolescent females, menses are a sensitive index of adequacy of therapy. Therapy should be continued throughout life in both males and females because of the possibility of malignant degeneration of the hyperplastic adrenal.

2. Other aspects of treatment are as for Addison's disease (eg, mineralocorticoid therapy and glucocorticoid increases with stress; see pp 789–791). Occasionally, inadequate mineralocorticoid therapy will lead to increased renin levels and elevated 17-ketosteroid production in the face of adequate or excessive glucocorticoid therapy.

3. Clitororecession is often indicated in the first year of life. Vaginoplasty for labial fusion should be performed in early childhood; it may be indicated during infancy if vaginal-urinary reflux and genitourinary tract infections occur. Partial clitoridectomy is occasionally indicated if the clitoris is abnormally large or sensitive.

B. Tumor: Because the malignant lesions cannot be distinguished clinically from the benign ones, surgical removal is indicated whenever a tumor has been diagnosed. Preoperative and postoperative treatment is as for Cushing's syndrome due to tumor.

Course & Prognosis

When therapy for enzyme deficiency is started in early infancy, abnormal metabolic effects are not observed and masculinization does not progress.

Unless adequately controlled, uncomplicated congenital adrenal hyperplasia causes sexual precocity and masculinization throughout childhood. Affected individuals will be tall as children but short as adults. Treatment with the corticosteroids permits normal growth, development, and sexual maturation. If started when somatic development is over 12–14 years (as determined by bone age), true sexual precocity may supervene, with thelarche and often menses in females and testicular androgen production in males.

Patient education stressing lifelong therapy is important for compliance in adolescence and later life.

Female pseudohermaphrodites mistakenly raised as males for more than 3 years may have serious psychologic disturbances if their sex is "changed" after that time. Extensive psychologic evaluation is mandatory in determining the course of action.

When adrenogenital syndrome is caused by a tumor, progression of signs and symptoms will cease after surgical removal; however, evidences of masculinization, particularly deepening of the voice, may persist.

Duck SC: Acceptable linear growth in congenital adrenal hyperplasia. *J Pediatr* 1980;**97:**93.

Gutai J et al: The detection of the heterozygous carrier for congenital virilizing adrenal hyperplasia. *J Pediatr* 1977;**90:**924.

Holcombe JH et al: Neonatal salt loss in the hypertensive form of congenital adrenal hyperplasia. *Pediatrics* 1980;**65:**777.

Hughes IA, Winter JS: Serum 17 OH-progesterone in the diagnosis and management of congenital adrenal hyperplasia. *J Pediatr* 1976;**88:**766.

Klingensmith GJ et al: Glucocorticoid treatment of girls with congenital adrenal hyperplasia: Effects on height, sexual maturation and fertility. *J Pediatr* 1977;**90:**996.

Kohn B et al: Late onset steroid 21-hydroxylase deficiency: A variant of classical congenital adrenal hyperplasia. *J Clin Endocrinol Metab* 1982;**55:**817.

Migeon CJ: Diagnosis and management of congenital adrenal hyperplasia. *Hosp Pract* (March) 1977;**12:**75.

New MI et al: Congenital adrenal hyperplasia and related conditions. Chapter 47 in: *The Metabolic Basis of Inherited Disease,* 5th ed. Stanbury JB et al (editors). McGraw-Hill, 1983.

Pang S et al: Amniotic fluid concentrations of delta 5 and delta 4 steroids in fetuses with congenital adrenal hyperplasia due to 21-hydroxylase deficiency and in anencephalic fetuses. *J Clin Endocrinol Metab* 1980;**51:**223.

Schnakenburg K, Bidlingmaier F, Knorr D: 17-Hydroxyprogesterone, androstenedione, and testosterone in normal children and in prepubertal patients in congenital adrenal hyperplasia. *Eur J Pediatr* 1980;**133:**259.

Villee DB, Crigler JF Jr: The adrenogenital syndrome. *Clin Perinatol* 1976;**3:**211.

Wentz AC et al: Gonadotropin output and response to LRH administration in congenital virilizing adrenal hyperplasia. *J Clin Endocrinol Metab* 1976;**42:**239.

3. PRIMARY HYPERALDOSTERONISM

Primary hyperaldosteronism may be caused by a benign adrenal tumor or by adrenal hyperplasia. It is characterized by paresthesias, tetany, weakness, periodic "paralysis," low serum potassium, elevated serum sodium, hypertension, metabolic alkalosis, and production of a large volume of alkaline urine with elevated protein content and low fixed specific gravity; the latter does not respond to vasopressin (Pitressin). The glucose tolerance test is frequently abnormal. Plasma and urinary aldosterone are elevated, but other steroid levels are variable. Edema is absent. Plasma renin levels are decreased (in contrast to increased levels in secondary hyperaldosteronism, eg, that due to renal vascular disease and Bartter's syndrome). In patients with tumor, the administration of ACTH may further increase the excretion of aldosterone. Marked decrease of aldosterone-induced hypokalemia, alkalosis, hypochloremia, or hypernatremia after the administration of a glucocorticoid or an aldosterone antagonist such as spironolactone (Aldactone), which blocks the action of aldosterone upon the renal tubule, may be of diagnostic value.

Treatment is with glucocorticoid administration, surgical removal of the tumor, or subtotal or total adrenalectomy for hyperplasia.

Baehler RW: Studies on the pathogenesis of Bartter's syndrome. *Am J Med* 1980;**69:**933.

Milla PJ et al: Salt-losing syndrome in 2 infants with defective 18-dehydrogenation in aldosterone biosynthesis. *Arch Dis Child* 1977;**52:**580.

Vaughan NJ et al: The diagnosis of primary hyperaldosteronism. *Lancet* 1981;**1:**120.

White EA et al: Use of computed tomography in diagnosing the cause of primary aldosteronism. *N Engl J Med* 1980;**303:**1503.

Wilson JX: The renin-angiotensin system in nonmammalian vertebrates. *Endocr Rev* 1984;**5:**45.

ADRENOCORTICOSTEROIDS & CORTICOTROPIN (ACTH)

Under the regulation of adrenocorticotropic hormone (ACTH, corticotropin), the intact adrenal elaborates adrenocorticosteroids having glucocorticoid activity and a minimal but significant amount of mineralocorticoid effect. The latter is complemented by adrenocorticosteroids that possess primarily mineralocorticoid activity and in addition to ACTH are under the regulatory control of vascular compartment volume and electrolyte concentration (ie, sodium). Adrenal androgens are also elaborated, but in the normal subject the quantity is insignificant before puberty.

Numerous synthetic preparations possessing variable ratios of glucocorticoid and mineralocorticoid activity are available (Table 25–9) and are employed widely in a variety of clinical conditions. With the exception of the deficiency states, these agents are not curative and may have many undesirable side effects. Moreover, prolonged use of these agents orally, parenterally, or topically may result in suppression of ACTH with ultimate adrenal atrophy and insufficiency.

Actions

The adrenocorticosteroids exert a direct or permissive effect on virtually every tissue of the body; major known effects include the following:

(1) Gluconeogenesis and glycogen synthesis in the liver.

(2) Stimulation of fat synthesis and redistribution of body fat.

(3) Catabolism of protein with an increase in nitrogen and phosphorus excretion.

(4) Decrease in lymphoid and thymic tissue, resulting in a decreased cellular response to inflammation and hypersensitivity.

(5) Alteration of central nervous system excitation.

(6) Retardation of connective tissue mitosis and migration, decreasing wound healing.

(7) Improved capillary tone and increased vascular compartment volume and pressure.

(8) In the case of mineralocorticoids, control of cation flux across membranes, with sodium retention and potassium excretion.

Uses

The adrenocorticosteroids and corticotropin are commonly employed in the following conditions in childhood:

Table 25–9. Adrenocorticosteroids.

	Trade Names	Potency/mg Compared to Cortisol* (Glucocorticoid Effect)	Potency/mg Compared to Cortisol (Sodium-Retaining Effect)
Glucocorticoids			
Hydrocortisone (cortisol)	Cortef, Cortril, Hydrocortone, Solu-Cortef	1	1
Cortisone	Cortone	4/5	1
Prednisone	Deltasone, Meticorten	4–5	2/5
Methylpredinisolone	Medrol	5–6	Minimal effect
Triamcinolone	Aristocort, Kenacort, Kenalog	5–6	Minimal effect
Paramethasone	Haldrone	10–12	
Dexamethasone	Decadron, Hexadrol	25–30	Minimal effect
Betamethasone	Celestone	25	
Mineralocorticoids			
Fludrocortisone (9α-fluorocortisol)	Florinef	15–20	300–400
Desoxycorticosterone acetate	DOCA, Percorten Acetate	No effect	15
Desoxycorticosterone pivalate (trimethylacetate)	Percorten Pivalate	No effect	
Aldosterone	Not available commercially	30	500

* To convert hydrocortisone dosage to equivalent dosage in any of the other preparations listed in this table, divide by the potency factors shown.

(1) Adrenogenital syndrome, adrenal insufficiency. (Corticotropin is not effective in these disorders.)

(2) Nephrotic syndrome.

(3) Ulcerative colitis and ileitis.

(4) Allergic disorders: Bronchial asthma (including status asthmaticus), intractable hay fever (pollinosis), urticaria, angioneurotic edema, serum sickness, atopic dermatitis, atopic eczema, exfoliative dermatitis.

(5) Inflammatory eye disease: Uveitis, chorioretinitis, sympathetic ophthalmia, iritis, iridocyclitis, retinitis centralis, herpes zoster (not herpes simplex) ophthalmicus, optic neuritis, retrobulbar neuritis.

(6) Collagen diseases: Rheumatoid arthritis, acute rheumatic fever, disseminated lupus erythematosus, scleroderma, dermatomyositis.

(7) Neoplastic diseases (temporary remission): Pulmonary granulomatosis, lymphoma, Hodgkin's disease, acute leukemia.

(8) Blood dyscrasias: Idiopathic thrombocytopenic purpura, allergic purpura, aplastic anemia, acquired hemolytic anemia.

(9) Miscellaneous conditions: Idiopathic hypoglycemia, infantile cortical hyperostosis, reticuloendotheliosis, thymic enlargement, sarcoidosis, pulmonary fibrosis, transfusion reactions, contact dermatitis (including poison oak), drug reactions, neurodermatitis.

Contraindications

A. Absolute Contraindications: Use is contraindicated in active, questionably healed, or suspected tuberculosis (unless treated concomitantly with specific antituberculosis agents).

B. Relative Contraindications: These drugs should be used with extreme caution in herpes simplex of the eye, osteoporosis, peptic ulcer and other active diseases of the gastrointestinal tract (except ileitis and ulcerative colitis), active infections, marked emotional instability, and thrombophlebitis.

Untoward Reactions of Therapy

With high dosage or prolonged use, adrenocorticosteroids may lead to any or all of the clinical manifestations of Cushing's syndrome. These side effects may result either from synthetic and exogenous agents (by any route, including topical) or from the use of corticotropin, which stimulates excess production of endogenous adrenocorticosteroids. Use of a large single dose given once every 48 hours (alternate-day therapy) lessens the incidence and severity of side effects.

A. Endocrine Disorders:

1. Hyperglycemia and glycosuria (of particular significance in early chemical diabetes).
2. Cushing's syndrome.
3. Persistent suppression of pituitary-adrenal re-

sponsiveness to stress with resultant hypoadrenocorticism.

B. Electrolyte and Mineral Disorders:

1. Marked retention of sodium and water, producing edema, increased blood volume, and hypertension (more common in endogenous hyperadrenal states).

2. Potassium loss with symptoms of hypokalemia.

3. Hypocalcemia, tetany.

C. Protein and Skeletal Disorders:

1. Negative nitrogen balance, with loss of body protein and bone protein, resulting in osteoporosis, pathologic fractures, and aseptic bone necrosis.

2. Suppression of growth, retarded skeletal maturation.

3. Muscular weakness and wasting.

D. Effect on Gastrointestinal Tract:

1. Excessive appetite and intake of food.

2. Activation or production of peptic ulcer.

3. Gastrointestinal bleeding from ulceration or from unknown cause (particularly in children with hepatic disease).

4. Fatty liver with embolism, pancreatitis, nodular panniculitis.

E. Lowering of Resistance to Infectious Agents; Silent Infection; Decreased Inflammatory Reaction:

1. Susceptibility to acute pulmonary or disseminated fungal infections; intestinal parasitic infections.

2. Activation of tuberculosis; false-negative tuberculin reaction.

3. Stimulation of activity of herpes simplex virus.

F. Neuropsychiatric Disorders:

1. Euphoria, excitability, psychotic behavior, and status epilepticus with electroencephalographic changes.

2. Increased intracranial pressure with ''pseudotumor cerebri'' syndrome.

G. Hemorrhagic Disorders:

1. Bleeding into the skin as a result of increased capillary fragility.

2. Thrombosis, thrombophlebitis, cerebral hemorrhage.

H. Miscellaneous:

1. Myocarditis, pleuritis, and arteritis following abrupt cessation of therapy.

2. Cardiomegaly.

3. Nephrosclerosis proteinuria.

4. Acne (in older children), hirsutism, amenorrhea.

5. Posterior subcapsular cataracts; glaucoma.

Axelrod L: Glucocorticoid therapy. *Medicine* 1976;**55:**39.

Chamberlain P, Meyer WJ: Management of pituitary-adrenal suppression secondary to corticosteroid therapy. *Pediatrics* 1981;**67:**245.

Khalid BA et al: Steroid replacement in Addison's disease and in subjects adrenalectomized for Cushing's disease: Comparison of various glucocorticords. *J Clin Endocrinol Metab* 1982;**55:**551.

Lee SS: Topical steroids. *Int J Dermatol* 1981;**20:**632.

Messer J et al: Association of adrenocorticosteroid therapy and peptic ulcer disease. *N Engl J Med* 1983;**309:**21.

Nelson AM, Conn DL: Series on pharmacology in practice. 9. Glucocorticoids in rheumatic diseases. *Mayo Clin Proc* 1980;**55:**758.

Rimsza ME: Complications of corticosteroid therapy. *Am J Dis Child* 1978;**132:**806.

Slocumb CH, Polley HF: Adrenocortical steroids—then and now. (Editorial.) *Mayo Clin Proc* 1980;**55:**774.

ADRENAL MEDULLA

PHEOCHROMOCYTOMA (Chromaffinoma)

Pheochromocytoma is an uncommon tumor, with approximately 10% of the total number of cases occurring in childhood. The tumor may be located wherever there is any chromaffin tissue (adrenal medulla, sympathetic ganglia, carotid body, etc). It may be multiple, familial (autosomal dominant, in which case a high prevalence of multiple endocrine neoplasia exists), recurrent, and (sometimes) malignant.

Although clinical manifestations of pheochromocytoma may result from physical expansion of lesions into surrounding tissue (eg, spinal cord), generally manifestations are due to excessive secretion of epinephrine or norepinephrine. Attacks of anxiety and headaches should arouse suspicion. Other findings are palpitation and tachycardia, dizziness, weakness, nausea and vomiting, diarrhea, dilated pupils with blurring of vision, abdominal and precordial pain, hypertension (usually persistent), postural hypotension, discomfort from heat, and vasomotor and sweating episodes. The symptoms may be sustained, producing all of the above findings plus papilledema, retinopathy, and enlargement of the heart. There is an increased incidence of pheochromocytomas in patients and families with the pheochromatoses, neurofibromatosis, and type II multiple endocrine neoplasia (see carcinoma of the thyroid, above). Neuroblastomas, neurogangliomas, and other neural tumors may cause increased secretion of pressor amines and occasionally simulate the findings of a pheochromocytoma. Carcinoid tumors may produce cardiovascular changes similar to those associated with pheochromocytoma.

Laboratory diagnosis is possible in over 90% of cases. Serum catecholamines are elevated, particularly while the patient is symptomatic, and urinary excretion of catecholamines parallels this elevation. (Elevated levels may be limited to the period of a paroxysm.) The 24-hour urine collection shows increased excretion of metanephrines and vanilmandelic acid (VMA, 3-methoxy-4-hydroxymandelic acid). Provocative tests employing histamine, tyramine, or glucagon and the phentolamine (Regitine) test may be abnormal; however, the former are dangerous and these agents are rarely necessary. Displacement of the kidney may be shown by routine x-ray and the tumor identified by CT scanning. Angiocatheterization and measurement of blood levels of catecholamines may be helpful in localizing the tumor prior to surgery.

Surgical removal of the tumor is the treatment of choice; this is a dangerous procedure and may produce sudden paroxysm and death. Oral phenoxybenzamine (Dibenzyline) or intravenous phentolamine is used preoperatively. Profound hypotension may occur as the tumor is removed; this may be controlled with an infusion of norepinephrine, which may have to be continued for 1–2 days.

Complete relief of symptoms is to be expected after recovery from removal of the nonmalignant tumor unless irreversible secondary vascular changes have occurred. If untreated, severe cardiac, renal, and cerebral damage may result.

Bravo EB, Gifford RW Jr: Pheochromocytoma: Diagnosis, localization and management. *N Engl J Med* 1984;**311:**1298.

Cryer PE: Physiology and pathophysiology of the human sympathoadrenal neuroendocrine system. *N Engl J Med* 1980; **303:**436.

Motulsky HJ, Insel PA: Adrenergic receptors in man. *N Engl J Med* 1982;**307:**18.

Weinshilbaum RM: Biochemical genetics of catecholamines in humans. *Mayo Clin Proc* 1983;**58:**319.

PITUITARY

DIABETES INSIPIDUS

Essentials of Diagnosis

- Polydipsia (4–40 L/d); excessive polyuria.
- Urine specific gravity < 1.010; osmolality < 280 mosm/kg.
- Inability to concentrate urine on fluid restriction.
- Hyperosmolality of plasma.
- Responsive to vasopressin.

General Considerations

Diabetes insipidus with inability to elaborate a concentrated urine may result from deficient secretion of vasopressin (ADH), lack of response of the kidney to ADH, or failure of osmoreceptors and pressor receptors to respond to elevations of osmolality and decreased intravascular volume.

Hypofunction of the hypothalamus or posterior pituitary with deficiency of ADH (neurogenic diabetes insipidus) may be idiopathic or may be associated with lesions of the posterior pituitary or hypothalamus (trauma, infections, suprasellar cysts, tumors, reticuloendotheliosis, or some developmental abnormality). Familial ADH deficiency may be transmitted as an autosomal dominant or X-linked recessive trait. In nephrogenic diabetes insipidus, the renal tubules fail to respond to physiologic or pharmacologic doses of vasopressin, and no lesion of the pituitary or hypothalamus can be demonstrated; this disease is believed to be X-linked with variable degrees of penetrance, with a milder variant in carrier females (see Chapter 21). When no specific cause for neurogenic diabetes insipidus can be determined, the search for an underlying lesion should be continued for many years.

Clinical Findings

The onset is often sudden, with polyuria, intense thirst, constipation, and evidences of dehydration. The child who awakens at night to urinate is very thirsty and drinks copiously. In young infants on an ordinary feeding regimen, polyuria may not be obvious and the infant may present with severe dehydration manifested by a high fever, circulatory collapse, and convulsions. In long-standing cases, growth retardation, lack of sexual maturation, and central nervous system damage may occur. The inability to concentrate urine is reflected by serum osmolalities that may be elevated to 305 mosm/kg (occasionally higher), but urine osmolality remains below this level (usually < 280 mosm/kg). Familial diabetes insipidus may have an insidious onset and a progressive course.

In cases of ADH deficiency and associated damage to the hypothalamic thirst center or hypothalamic-pituitary centers controlling ACTH production, the clinical features may be "masked" and polydipsia may not occur. The administration of corticotropin (ACTH) or adrenocorticosteroids may "unmask" the ADH deficiency by increasing the glomerular filtration rate and distal tubule perfusion.

Differential Diagnosis

Diabetes insipidus may be differentiated from psychogenic polydipsia (compulsive water drinking, potomania) and polyuria by permitting the usual intake of fluid and then withholding water for 7 hours. The test should be terminated if distress is clinically notable and associated with a weight loss exceeding 3% of body weight. Patients with long-standing psychogenic polydipsia may be unable to concentrate urine initially, and the test may have to be repeated after several days of water restriction. Eventually, in these patients, dehydration will increase urine osmolality well above plasma osmolality. With neurogenic and nephrogenic diabetes insipidus, the urine osmolality usually does not increase above 280 mosm/kg (specific gravity 1.010) even after the period of dehydration. Normal children and those with psychogenic polydipsia will respond to the dehydration with a urinary osmolality above 450 mosm/kg (specific gravity > 1.020). The vasopressin (Pitressin) and hypertonic saline tests may be employed to distinguish between the various forms of diabetes insipidus.

Decreased urinary concentrating ability may also occur with hypokalemia and with various forms of hypercalcemia (including hypervitaminosis D) and renal tubular abnormalities (eg, Fanconi's syndrome).

Treatment

A. Medical Treatment: The treatment of choice for total diabetes insipidus is desmopressin acetate (1-deamino-8-D-arginine vasopressin; DDAVP) administered intranasally. The dosage must be adjusted, but the duration of action is generally at least 12 hours and eliminates troublesome nocturia. Replacement with lypressin (8-lysine vasopressin; Diapid) is of less value because of short duration of action.

The use of one of the thiazide diuretics, ethacrynic acid, or even salt restriction may be of value for short periods in both the neurogenic and nephrogenic types. Moreover, the treatment of nephrogenic diabetes insipidus appears to be enhanced by the administration of abundant quantities of water at short intervals, low-sodium diet, and minimum but nutritionally adequate amounts of protein.

Chlorpropamide (Diabinese) has been found to have an antidiuretic effect through its augmentation of endogenous ADH effect. Chlorpropamide, clofibrate, and carbamazepine all stimulate the release of ADH. Their use in the treatment of diabetes insipidus is less satisfactory than the use of desmopressin acetate; hypotension and hypoglycemia are uncommon side effects.

B. Other Therapy: X-ray therapy, surgery, antitumor chemotherapy, or a combination of these may be used for some cases of tumor (eg, reticuloendotheliosis).

Prognosis

In the absence of associated defects, life expectancy should be normal (if severe dehydration in infancy is avoided). Hydronephrosis and hydroureter are not uncommon sequelae of prolonged polyuria; patients should also be observed carefully for urinary tract infection.

Gold PW et al: Abnormalities in plasma and cerebrospinal-fluid arginine vasopressin in patients with anorexia nervosa. *N Engl J Med* 1983;**308:**1117.

Hendricks SA et al: Differential diagnosis of diabetes insipidus: Use of DDAVP to terminate the seven-hour water deprivation test. *J Pediatr* 1981;**98:**224.

Lee WP et al: Vasopressin analog DDAVP in the treatment of diabetes insipidus. *Am J Dis Child* 1976;**130:**166.

Zerbe RL, Robertson GL: A comparison of plasma vasopressin measurements with a standard indirect test in the differential diagnosis of polyuria. *N Engl J Med* 1981;**305:**1539.

PINEAL

The pineal gland is made up of parenchymal cells (pinealocytes) and is often assigned an endocrine function (eg, regulation of somatic growth, sexual maturation, body pigmentation, blood glucose regulation, and a day/night-sensitive neuroendocrine regulatory function). Pineal tumors are rarely associated with sexual precocity in the male. Cases of gonadotropin-secreting choriocarcinomas of the pineal with secondary Leydig cell activation and resultant sexual precocity have been reported.

Preslock JP: The pineal gland: Basic implications and clinical correlations. *Endocr Rev* 1984;**5:**282.

Reiter RJ et al: The pineal and its hormones in the control of reproduction in mammals. *Endocr Rev* 1980;**1:**109.

Wurtman RJ, Moskowitz MA: The pineal organ. (2 parts.) *N Engl J Med* 1977;**296:**1329, 1383.

OVARIES & TESTES

DEVELOPMENT & PHYSIOLOGY

The gonads develop from a bipotential anlage in the genital ridge of the coelomic cavity. The primordial germ cells, which will become the oocytes and spermatocytes, arise in the yolk sac and migrate to the genital ridge by the fourth week after conception, when the gonad is identifiable. Between the fourth and eighth weeks of gestation, differentiation into an ovary or testis occurs; by 7–9 weeks, the fetal testis begins to produce androgens, and granulosa cells can be identified in the ovary. Testicular androgen production at this time occurs in response to placental human chorionic gonadotropin (hCG) and is necessary for male sexual differentiation. Between 9 and 12 weeks of gestational age, the fetal pituitary starts to produce luteinizing hormone (LH) and follicle-stimulating hormone (FSH); these fetal pituitary hormones are important for gonadal development. In response to fetal gonadotropins, ovarian follicular development can progress to the graafian follicle stage. In the testes, Leydig cell production of testosterone continues until several months after birth.

Throughout childhood, pulsatile secretion of FSH and LH occurs at 60- to 90-minute intervals and affects the output of gonadal hormones (Fig 25–5). As puberty approaches, the amplitude of the peaks increases, at first during the night and later during the day as well. As the basal LH levels rise, estrogen production from the ovaries or testosterone production from the testes increases toward adult levels.

Chappel SC et al: Biosynthesis and secretion of follicle-stimulating hormone. *Endocr Rev* 1983;**4:**179.

Marut EL, Huang SC, Hodgen GD: Distinguishing the steroidogenic roles of granulosa and theca cells of the dominant ovarian follicle and corpus luteum. *J Clin Endocrinol Metab* 1983;**57:**925.

Reiter EO, Grumbach MM: Neuroendocrine control mecha-

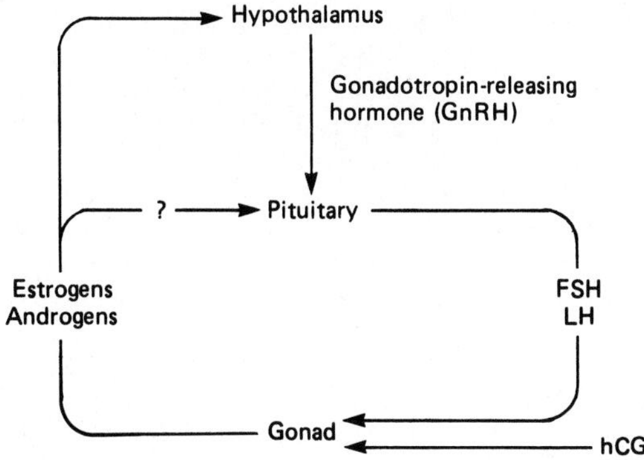

Figure 25–5. Hormonal regulation of gonadal function.

nisms and the onset of puberty. *Annu Rev Physiol* 1982; **44:**595.

Winters SJ, Troen P: Reexamination of pulsatile luteinizing hormone secretion in primary testicular failure. *J Clin Endocrinol Metab* 1983;**57:**432.

SEXUAL DIFFERENTIATION

Normal Sexual Differentiation

For normal sexual differentiation to occur, a specific sequence of events must take place. The bipotential gonad requires at least two X chromosomes to develop into an ovary; in the absence of a second X chromosome, a fibrous streak develops along the genital ridge. If a Y chromosome is present, a testis develops. The Y chromosome allows the production of H-Y antigen, a protein that appears to program the organization of the undifferentiated gonad into a testis. Between the seventh and 14th weeks of gestation, testosterone (produced by the fetal testis in response to placental hCG) acts locally to induce the formation and growth of the internal male accessory sex structures and acts peripherally to induce masculinization of the external genitalia, eg, fusion of the labioscrotal folds and formation of a penile urethra. Growth of the penis occurs mainly in the late second and third trimesters, requiring stimulation of the testis by fetal pituitary gonadotropins. In the absence of androgens, the external genitalia feminize and a vagina is formed. Müllerian duct *N* inhibiting factor, a glycoprotein produced by the testis, causes regression of the internal female duct structures; in the absence of this factor, the uterus and uterine (fallopian) tubes develop and mature.

Abnormal Sexual Differentiation

Abnormalities of sexual differentiation frequently result in ambiguous external genitalia. The causes for abnormal sexual differentiation may be divided into 4 major categories:

A. Abnormalities in Normal Gonadal Differentiation: These usually result from an identifiable abnormality of the sex chromosomes. Klinefelter's syndrome (see Chapter 33) with an XXY karyotype usually has a male phenotype. Turner's syndrome (see Chapter 33) usually has a female phenotype. Mosaic forms of gonadal dysgenesis that contain a Y-bearing cell line have an ambiguous and variable external phenotype. Idiopathic testicular failure prior to completion of sexual differentiation will result in ambiguous genitalia. True hermaphroditism, with the presence of both spermatocytes and oocytes, is rare and produces external genitalia that range in type from almost fully masculine to almost completely feminine.

B. Abnormalities in Testosterone Synthesis or Action: These disorders cause male pseudohermaphroditism, frequently with ambiguous genitalia. Enzyme defects in testosterone synthesis may affect only testosterone synthesis, or they may also affect the synthesis of cortisol, as in variants of the adrenogenital syndrome. Defects in testosterone action result from either absent or defective end-organ receptors or a defect in peripheral testosterone metabolism to dihydrotestosterone due to 5α-reductase deficiency. The androgen receptor defect may be complete (testicular feminization) or incomplete (Reifenstein's syndrome and its variants).

C. Presence of Excessive Androgens in a Female Fetus: These disorders cause female pseudohermaphroditism and usually result in ambiguous genitalia. Excessive adrenal androgen production secondary to an adrenal enzyme defect in cortisol synthesis (ie, adrenogenital syndrome) is seen in 95% of patients with female pseudohermaphroditism and approximately half of all patients with ambiguous genitalia. Occasionally, maternally derived androgens may cause masculinization of the female fetus.

D. Miscellaneous Syndromes: These are usually associated with multiple congenital anomalies, especially of the urinary tract and intestine. Occasionally, teratogenic agents may result in anomalous sexual development.

Amrhein JA et al: Partial androgen insensitivity: The Reifenstein syndrome revisited. *N Engl J Med* 1977;**297:**350.

Baker SW: Psychosexual differentiation in the human. *Biol Reprod* 1980:**22:**61.

Donahoe PK et al: Mixed gonadal dysgenesis: Pathogenesis and management. *J Pediatr Surg* 1979;**14:**287.

Griffen JE, Wilson JD: The syndrome of androgen resistance. *N Engl J Med* 1980;**302:**198.

Haseltine FP, Ohno S: Mechanisms of gonadal differentiation. *Science* 1981;**211:**1272.

Josso N, Briad M: Embryonic testicular regression syndrome: Variable phenotypic expression in siblings. *J Pediatr* 1980;**97:**200.

Kaufman FR et al: Male pseudohermaphroditism due to 17,20-desmolase deficiency. *J Clin Endocrinol Metab* 1983;**57:**32.

Kwan M et al: The nature of androgen action on male sexuality: A combined laboratory-self-report study on hypogonadal men. *J Clin Endocrinol Metab* 1983;**57:**557.

Pandridge WM: Androgens and sexual behavior. *Ann Intern Med* 1982;**96**:488.
Saengen P: Abnormal sexual differentiation. *J Pediatr* 1984; **104**:1.
van Niekerk WA: True hermaphroditism: An analytic review with a report of 3 new cases. *Am J Obstet Gynecol* 1976; **126**:890.
Wilson ID, George FW, Griffin JE: The hormonal control of sexual development. *Science* 1981;**211**:1278.

ABNORMALITIES IN OVARIAN FUNCTION

The ovary is composed of follicles (germ cells surrounded by granulosa cells), theca cells immediately surrounding the follicle, and stromal or supporting tissue. The ovary produces several types of hormones, the most important of which are estrogens and progesterone. At least 3 natural estrogens have been identified: estrone, 17β-estradiol (the most potent), and estriol. Production of the major ovarian estrogen, estradiol, is stimulated by LH secretion (Fig 25–5). Significant quantities of estrogen are not produced until the onset of puberty. Estrogens stimulate the growth of the uterus, vagina, and breasts. They also appear to be essential for the adolescent growth spurt occurring in girls.

Most patients with significant ovarian abnormalities in childhood exhibit precocious puberty, delayed puberty (or primary amenorrhea), or secondary amenorrhea.

1. PRECOCIOUS PUBERTY IN GIRLS

Puberty is considered precocious if the onset of secondary sexual characteristics occurs prior to 8 years of age. Precocious puberty is 9 times more common in girls than in boys. It may have its onset at any age. True (complete) precocious puberty refers to sexual maturation in which hypothalamic-pituitary maturation initiates the sexual development; in pseudoprecocity, the process is initiated elsewhere. True precocious puberty is always isosexual and may progress to the production of mature ova. In pseudoprecocity, sexual characteristics may be isosexual or heterosexual; secondary sexual characteristics develop, but the hypothalamic-pituitary-gonadal axis (Fig 25–5) does not mature and oocyte maturation does not occur.

Clinical Findings

A. Symptoms and Signs: Although the first sign of sexual development in girls is usually breast development, followed by pubic hair growth and vaginal bleeding, the pattern of development may be variable. The interval between breast development and menstruation (normally about 2 years) may be less than 1 year or more than 6 years. On careful abdominal examination of girls with ovarian or adrenal tumors, a mass may be palpated. The information gained from a rectoabdominal or pelvic examination must be weighed carefully against the discomfort and trauma this may cause to a young child; ultrasonography may be a desirable substitute. A growth spurt may precede or accompany the development of secondary sexual characteristics. Children with precocious puberty have accelerated growth during childhood but are often short as adults, since osseous maturation (bone age) advances at a more rapid rate than linear growth (height age) during the period of accelerated growth. A history of excessive mood changes and emotional lability frequently is obtained.

B. Laboratory Findings: In true precocious puberty, radioimmunoassays generally reveal that levels of serum or plasma gonadotropins are in the pubertal range. Early in the course of the disorder, random determinations may be within the prepubertal range. In these cases, further evaluation of serum LH and FSH levels after stimulation with gonadotropin-releasing hormone (GnRH) is necessary. In cases of true precocious puberty, a rise in LH and FSH levels will occur 30 and 60 minutes after intravenous stimulation with 100 μg of GnRH.

Estrogen levels can be determined as estradiol or as total serum estrogens. Adrenal androgen levels measured as androstenedione or dehydroepiandrosterone (DHEA) may be in the pubertal range. In pseudoprecocity, measurements of urinary 17-ketosteroid and pregnanetriol levels will identify adrenal tumors or enzyme defects (see Adrenogenital Syndrome, above).

C. X-Ray Findings: A bone age determination at the onset and every 6–12 months is helpful in predicting the effect of the precocity on adult height.

Abdominal and pelvic ultrasonography performed by a skilled radiologist can usually identify an ovarian mass, demonstrate an adrenal mass greater than 5 cm, and reveal follicular ovarian cysts if present. Serial examinations are useful in demonstrating significant changes. A cranial CT scan with special attention to the hypothalamic and pituitary regions will identify mass lesions and other structural abnormalities of the central nervous system. Some cases of precocious puberty due to organic brain lesions may produce no clinical manifestations for prolonged periods. When these conditions are suspected, examinations for central nervous system lesions should be performed periodically.

Differential Diagnosis

The causes of true precocious and pseudoprecocious puberty are outlined in Table 25–10. Precocious and pseudoprecocious puberty should be differentiated from premature thelarche and premature adrenarche, which are both benign. The most important differential diagnosis is between true precocious and pseudoprecocious puberty. Helpful laboratory and x-ray findings to differentiate between these are discussed above. Most (80–90%) girls with precocious puberty have true precocious puberty. Prior to the advent of sophis-

Table 25–10. Causes of isosexual precocious development.

True (complete) precocious puberty Constitutional (functional, idiopathic) Tumors producing destruction of the pineal (principally in males) Polyostotic fibrous dysplasia (McCune-Albright syndrome) (principally in females; often incomplete; usually infertile) Hypothalamic lesions (hamartomas, hyperplasia, congenital malformations, tumors) Tumors in vicinity of the third ventricle Internal hydrocephalus Cerebral and meningocerebral infections (postencephalitis, postmeningitis) Degenerative, possibly congenital encephalopathy Tuberous sclerosis Recklinghausen's disease Cystic arachnoiditis Therapeutic administration of gonadotropin Exogenous obesity **Pseudoprecocious (incomplete) puberty** Adrenal abnormalities Adrenocortical hyperplasia (males) Adrenocortical tumors Hyperplastic ectopic adrenal tissue Cushing's syndrome (males)	Gonadal tumors Tumors of the ovary—Granulosa cell tumor (most common), theca cell tumor, teratoma, choriocarcinoma, dysgerminoma, luteoma Tumors of the testes—Interstitial (Leydig) cell tumor, teratoma Premature pubarche (premature adrenarche) (both sexes) Without cerebral disease (constitutional?) With cerebral disease Premature thelarche (premature gynarche) (females) Without cerebral disease (constitutional?) With cerebral disease Drug-induced **Unclassified causes** With elevated gonadotropins Associated with hypothyroidism Presacral teratoma Primary liver cell tumors (hepatoma) (males only) Choriocarcinoma and seminoma of the testes Others Hyperinsulinism Primordial dwarfism Silver's syndrome (short stature, congenital asymmetry, and variations in the pattern of sexual development) Thyrotropin-releasing hormone excess

ticated CT scanners, 75–95% of these cases were considered idiopathic. CT scanning now demonstrates that many of them are due to static (presumably congenital) mass lesions in the hypothalamus.

Treatment

Treatment of the underlying cause of pseudoprecocious puberty (removal of the tumor or correction of the adrenal enzyme disorder) usually results in cessation of abnormal pubertal development.

Successful medical intervention in true precocious puberty has only recently been available. Because long-term safety has not been established, therapy is limited to children with rapidly progressive bone maturation, significant menstrual bleeding, or both. The most successful therapy employs analogs of gonadotropin-releasing hormone. The analogs block pituitary LH synthesis and release, and this results in the return of estrogen levels to prepubertal values. In most cases, menses cease, secondary sexual development stabilizes or regresses, and linear growth and bone maturation slow to prepubertal rates.

In patients with McCune-Albright syndrome, analogs of gonadotropin-releasing hormone may not be helpful. Therapy with antiandrogens, agents that block steroid synthesis (eg, ketoconazole), or both may be useful.

Regardless of the cause of precocious puberty or the medical therapy selected, the psychologic management of the patient and family is essential.

Cacciari E et al: How many cases of true precocious puberty in girls are idiopathic? *J Pediatr* 1983;**102:**357.

Comite F et al: Cyclical ovarian function resistant to treatment with an analogue of luteinizing hormone-releasing hormone in McCune-Albright syndrome. *N Engl J Med* 1984; **311:**1032.

Comite F et al: Short-term treatment of idiopathic precocious puberty with a long-acting analogue of LHRH. *N Engl J Med* 1981;**305:**1546.

D'Armiento M et al: McCune-Albright syndrome: Evidence for autonomous multiendocrine hyperfunction. *J Pediatr* 1983;**102:**584.

Harlan WR, Harlan EA, Grillo GP: Secondary sex characteristics of girls 12 to 17 years of age: The U.S. Health Examination Survey. *J Pediatr* 1980;**96:**1074.

Lippe BM, Sample WF: Pelvic ultrasonography in pediatric and adolescent endocrine disorders. *J Pediatr* 1978;**92:**897.

Mills JL et al: Premature thelarche: Natural history and etiologic investigation. *Am J Dis Child* 1981;**135:**743.

Wollner N et al: Malignant ovarian tumors in childhood: Prognosis in relation to initial therapy. *Cancer* 1976;**37:**1953.

2. AMENORRHEA

Primary amenorrhea is failure of menarche to occur in a girl who is 14 years of age or older and whose sexual development has not progressed beyond Tanner stage I or in a girl of any age who is over 2½–3 years postpubarche and has not yet menstruated. Secondary amenorrhea is cessation of menses after an interval of time equal to at least 6 months postmenarche or 3 menstrual cycles. A careful history and physical examination (with pelvic examination) are necessary to determine possible causes of amenorrhea (Table 25–11) to indicate the degree of evaluation required.

Primary Amenorrhea

Common causes of primary amenorrhea include physiologic or constitutional delay, Mayer-Rokitansky-Küster-Hauser syndrome, Turner's syndrome, chronic illness, and pseudoamenorrhea.

In pseudoamenorrhea, the patient is menstruating but has a genital tract obstruction that prevents release of menstrual blood. Sexual development is usually at Tanner stage IV or V, and cyclic abdominal pain without menstruation is noted. Pelvic examination may reveal an imperforate hymen, transverse vaginal ridge, or other obstruction. Treatment is surgical.

Mayer-Rokitansky-Küster-Hauser syndrome is characterized by congenital müllerian agenesis with normal ovaries, normal ovarian function, and normal breast development. Pelvic examination reveals an absent vagina and various uterine abnormalities with or without additional renal and skeletal anomalies. Full evaluation is necessary, including karyotyping, intravenous pyelography, and laparoscopy. Therapy for this syndrome is surgical vaginoplasty.

Turner's syndrome (XO syndrome, gonadal dysgenesis) should be considered in patients with short stature and sexual infantilism. This is a form of hypergonadotropic hypogonadism in which the estrogen level is low (or absent), FSH and LH levels are elevated, bone maturation is usually delayed, buccal smear is sometimes chromatin-negative, and karyotype is abnormal. The stigmas of Turner's syndrome are described in Chapter 33. Current treatment for the short stature includes low doses of estrogens, anabolic steroids, and human growth hormone separately or in combination. At the time of adolescence, a combination of estrogen and progesterone in physiologic doses is indicated.

Table 25–11. Causes of secondary amenorrhea.*

With Normal Ovarian Function
- A. Congenital
  - 1. Cryptomenorrhea
  - 2. Absence of uterus
- B. Acquired
  - 1. Intrauterine synechia (Asherman's syndrome)
  - 2. Hysterectomy
  - 3. After abortion, infection, or cesarean section

With Decreased Ovarian Secretion of Estrogen, Progestogen, or Androgen
- A. With high gonadotropins (primary ovarian failure)
  - 1. Congenital
    - a. Ovarian agenesis
    - b. Gonadal dysgenesis
    - c. Gonadotropin-resistant ovary syndrome
  - 2. Acquired
    - a. Premature menopause
    - b. Surgical oophorectomy
    - c. Radiation castration
    - d. Ovarian destruction by infection (rarely)
    - e. Following chemotherapy (cyclophosphamide [Cytoxan])
- B. With low or normal gonadotropins (secondary ovarian failure)
  - 1. Feminizing ovarian tumor
  - 2. Hypothalamic-pituitary dysfunction
    - a. Congenital deficiency of gonadotropin secretion
    - b. Acquired
      - i. Organic CNS disease
      - ii. Functional aberration of hypothalamic-pituitary axis
        - Psychogenic
        - Starvation (eg, anorexia nervosa)
        - Physical exertion (eg, marathon runners, ballet dancers)
        - Intercurrent disease
        - Extragenital endocrine disorders
        - Pharmacologic (eg, with tranquilizers or after prolonged use of antifertility hormones)
        - Unknown

With Increased Ovarian Androgen Secretion
- A. Masculinizing ovarian tumor
- B. Continuous estrus syndrome (polycystic ovary syndrome)

* Modified and reproduced, with permission, from Ross G, Vande Wiele R: Ovaries. In: *Textbook of Endocrinology*, 6th ed. Williams RH (editor). Saunders, 1981.

Secondary Amenorrhea

Common causes of secondary amenorrhea include stress, pregnancy, major weight loss, polycystic ovary syndrome, and prolactin excess. Stress-induced amenorrhea is often noted in teenagers, but it should be diagnosed only after a careful evaluation. Pregnancy and pregnancy complications are the most frequent causes of secondary amenorrhea in sexually active teenagers.

Irregular menses (oligomenorrhea) or amenorrhea may result from severe weight loss secondary to dieting, vigorous exercise (eg, in marathon runners), depression, anorexia nervosa, or chronic illness. In the normal ovulating female, it is believed that a major source of estrogen is from aromatization of androgens in peripheral adipose tissue. When the proportion of body weight as fat falls below a critical level (< 15–25%), there is less estrogen and eventual hypothalamic dysfunction. This hypothesis has been advanced to explain amenorrhea in athletes and patients with anorexia nervosa.

In polycystic ovary syndrome (Stein-Leventhal syndrome), secondary amenorrhea is the result of chronic anovulation. Occasionally, dysfunctional uterine bleeding is the only finding; the full syndrome consists of obesity, hirsutism, secondary amenorrhea, bilaterally enlarged ovaries, and, in some cases, clitoromegaly. The results of tests of endocrine function reveal normal FSH concentrations, elevated LH levels, and borderline to elevated adrenal or ovarian androgen levels. Polycystic ovary syndrome may be idiopathic or secondary to adrenocortical hyperplasia or an adrenocortical neoplasm. Laparoscopy, ovarian biopsy, endometrial biopsy, or a combination of these procedures may be necessary for final diagnosis. Treatment consists of correction of the estrogen: androgen ratio and induction of ovulation in patients who wish to become pregnant.

Other causes of amenorrhea are shown in Table 25–11. Chronic illness and central nervous system disorders should always be considered. When galactorrhea and amenorrhea occur together, hyperprolactinemia, drug ingestion, hypothyroidism, stress, and hypothalamic injury should be considered.

Approximately 2% of women taking birth control pills will note a delay (> 6 months) in the return of spontaneous menstruation after cessation of therapy.

Bachmann GA, Kemmann E: Prevalence of oligomenorrhea and amenorrhea in a college population. *Am J Obstet Gynecol* 1982;**144:**98.

Dewhurst J: Secondary amenorrhea. *Pediatr Ann* 1981;**10:**38.

Emans SJ, Grace E, Goldstein DP: Oligomenorrhea in adolescent girls. *J Pediatr* 1980;**97:**815.

Frisch RE, McArthur JW: Menstrual cycles: Fatness as a determinant of minimal weight for height necessary for their maintenance or onset. *Science* 1974;**185:**949.

Hall JG et al: Turner's syndrome. *West J Med* 1982;**137:**32.

Hurley DM et al: Induction of ovulation and fertility in amenorrheic women by pulsatile low-dose gonadotropin-releasing hormone. *N Engl J Med* 1984;**310:**1069.

Molitch ME, Reichlin S: Hyperprolactinemic disorders. *DM* (Sept) 1982;**28:**1.

Odell WD: Symposium on Adolescent Gynecology and Endocrinology. 1. Physiology of sexual maturation and primary amenorrhea. *West J Med* 1979;**131:**401.

Patton ML, Woolf PD: Hyperprolactinemia and delayed puberty: A report of three cases and their response to therapy. *Pediatrics* 1983;**71:**572.

Root AW, Reiter EO: Evaluation and management of the child with delayed pubertal development. *Fertil Steril* 1976; **27:**745.

Smith NJ: Excessive weight loss and food aversion in athletes simulating anorexia nervosa. *Pediatrics* 1980;**66:**139.

Yen SS: The polycystic ovary syndrome. *Clin Endocrinol* 1980;**12:**177.

ABNORMALITIES IN TESTICULAR FUNCTION

The major testicular hormone, testosterone, is produced by the Leydig (interstitial) cells. Production of testicular androgens is stimulated by LH secretion (Fig 25–5). Appreciable amounts of androgen usually begin to appear in boys at 12 years of age and are responsible, wholly or in part, for growth of internal and external genitalia and development of secondary sexual characteristics, including pubic, axillary, and facial hair. Androgens induce nitrogen retention, accelerate bone growth, and determine the closure of the epiphyseal junctions.

The seminiferous tubules are composed of germinal epithelium and Sertoli cells. Testicular androgens in combination with pituitary FSH stimulate the development and maturation of the germinal epithelium and thus promote spermatogenesis. The Sertoli cells activate the germinal epithelium and may produce inhibin, a hormone that inhibits secretion of FSH from the anterior pituitary. In addition, the Sertoli cells provide mechanical support for the germinal epithelium.

Abnormalities in testicular function may present as delayed or precocious sexual development, as cryptorchidism, or as gynecomastia.

1. PRECOCIOUS PUBERTY IN BOYS

Puberty is considered precocious in boys if secondary sexual characteristics appear prior to 9 years of age. Precocious puberty is much less common in boys than in girls. In boys presenting with sexual precocity, pseudoprecocious puberty is as common as true precocious puberty. In addition, boys with true precocious puberty are more likely to have an identifiable pathologic process rather than idiopathic precocious puberty.

Recent descriptions of gonadotropin-independent precocious puberty suggest this as the cause of familial male precocious puberty. In affected males, testicular production of testosterone occurs without the known stimulatory mechanisms. The biochemical basis for this remains obscure.

Clinical Findings

A. Symptoms and Signs: In precocious development, increases in somatic growth and pubic hair growth are the common presenting complaints. Testicular size may differentiate between true precocity, in which the testicles usually enlarge, and pseudoprecocity (most commonly due to andrenocortical hyperplasia), in which the testicles usually remain small. There are some exceptions: In advanced cases of pseudoprecocity, some testicular enlargement may occur, since seminiferous tubule elements may be stimulated by prolonged elevated androgen levels. In the very young child with early true precocity, minimal increases of testosterone may result in dramatic increases in penis size and pubic hair growth, with very little testicular enlargement. Tumors of the testis will present with asymmetric testicular enlargement.

B. Laboratory Findings: LH and FSH levels are elevated in boys with true sexual precocity. Sexual precocity caused by the adrenogenital syndrome is associated with abnormal levels of plasma 17α-hydroxyprogesterone, plasma 11-deoxycortisol, urinary 17-ketosteroids, or a combination of these findings. The level of serum or plasma testosterone aids in the differentiation of true precocity and pseudoprecocity. Determination of hCG levels to evaluate for hepatoma may be necessary in boys with true sexual precocity.

C. X-Ray Findings: Diagnostic studies are similar to those used to evaluate sexual precocity in girls (see above). Ultrasonography may be useful in detection of testicular tumors.

Differential Diagnosis

The causes of sexual precocity are outlined in Table 25–10. In boys, it is of particular importance to differentiate between pseudoprecocity and true sexual precocity.

Treatment

Specific therapy should be utilized in cases in which the cause is known and amenable to therapy. Treatment of idiopathic true precocious puberty in boys is similar to that in girls (see above).

Treatment of gonadotropin-independent precocious puberty (testitoxicosis) with agents that block steroid synthesis (eg, ketoconazole), with antiandrogens (eg, spironolactone), or with a combination of both has been reported to be successful.

2. SEXUAL INFANTILISM (Primary & Secondary Testicular Failure)

Lack of development of secondary sexual characteristics after the age of 17 years suggests abnormal testicular maturation. While delay of puberty until 17 years of age may be physiologically normal, it is generally of concern to a boy if pubertal changes do not occur by 14–15 years of age, and evaluation should be initiated at that time.

Sexual infantilism may be difficult to differentiate from benign constitutionally delayed adolescence. Although the latter may be associated with a delay in testicular function, normal puberty occurs at a later date.

The differentiation of primary and secondary testicular failure is based on the cause of the disorder. In general, primary failure results from absence, malfunction, or destruction of testicular tissue; secondary failure results from pituitary or hypothalamic insufficiency.

Primary testicular failure may be due to anorchia, surgical castration, Klinefelter's syndrome or other sex chromosomal abnormalities, a genetic defect in testosterone synthesis or action, inflammation and destruction of the testes following infection or toxic agents (mumps, irradiation, autoimmune disorders, syphilis, gonorrhea), trauma, or tumor.

Causes of secondary testicular failure resulting from central nervous system or hypothalamic-pituitary dysfunction include panhypopituitarism, isolated LH deficiency, Kallmann's syndrome, and isolated FSH deficiency. Destructive lesions in or near the anterior pituitary, especially craniopharyngiomas and gliomas, may result in hypothalamic or pituitary dysfunction. Prader-Willi syndrome and Laurence-Moon-Biedl syndrome are associated with LH and FSH deficiency. Miscellaneous causes include chronic debilitating disease and hypothyroidism.

Clinical Findings

A. Symptoms and Signs: Physical examination may not be helpful in differentiating primary from secondary gonadal insufficiency. While cryptorchidism suggests primary testicular failure, failure of testicular descent may occur with pituitary insufficiency.

B. Laboratory Findings: In primary testicular failure, the serum testosterone level will be low, while LH and FSH values will be elevated into the castrate range. In secondary testicular failure, levels of all 3 hormones will be below the normal adult range. To establish the ability of the testes to respond to stimulation, hCG may be given; a dose of 2000 mg/m^2 given every other day for 3 doses should result in a rise in the serum testosterone level to above 200 mg/dL. Determination of LH and FSH responses to exogenous GnRH may be useful.

Chromosomal karyotype should be determined in primary testicular failure of unknown cause.

C. X-Ray Findings: Skeletal maturation is usually delayed. A cranial CT scan should be performed in secondary testicular failure.

Treatment

Specific therapy is indicated when the cause of testicular failure is known. Treatment with testosterone enanthate, 200 mg every 3–4 weeks intramuscularly, may be given until sexual maturity is reached. In patients with primary testicular failure, replacement therapy with testosterone, 300–400 mg every 3–4 weeks, may be continued indefinitely. Specific therapy may be followed by fertility in patients with hypothalamic-pituitary insufficiency.

Bourguignon JP et al: Hypopituitarism and idiopathic delayed puberty: A longitudinal study in an attempt to diagnose gonadotropin deficiency before puberty. *J Clin Endocrinol Metab* 1982;**54:**733.

Guthrie RD, Smith DW, Graham CB: Testosterone treatment for micropenis during early childhood. *J Pediatr* 1973; **83:**247.

Hoffman AR et al: Induction of puberty in men by long-term pulsatile administration of low-dose gonadotropin-releasing hormone. *N Engl J Med* 1982;**307:**1237.

Parker MW et al: Effect of testosterone on somatomedin-C concentrations in prepubertal boys. *J Clin Endocrinol Metab* 1984;**58:**87.

Ratcliffe SG et al: Klinefelter's syndrome in adolescence. *Arch Dis Child* 1982;**57:**6.

Spitz IM et al: The prolactin response to thyrotropin-releasing hormone differentiates isolated gonadotropin deficiency from delayed puberty. *N Engl J Med* 1983;**308:**575.

3. CRYPTORCHIDISM

Cryptorchidism (undescended testes) is a common disorder in children. It may be unilateral or bilateral and may be classified as ectopic cryptorchidism or true cryptorchidism.

Approximately 3% of term male newborns and 30% of premature males have undescended testes at birth. In over half of these cases, the testes will descend by the second month; by age 1 year, 80% of all undescended testes are in the scrotum. Further descent may occur through puberty, the latter perhaps stimulated by endogenous gonadotropin. If cryptorchidism persists into adult life, failure of spermatogenesis occurs but testicular androgen production usually remains intact. The incidence of malignant neoplasm (usually seminoma) is appreciably greater in those testes which remain in the abdomen after puberty.

Ectopic testes are presumed to develop normally but are diverted as they descend through the inguinal canal. They are subclassified on the basis of their location; surgery is indicated once the diagnosis is established.

True cryptorchidism in most cases is thought to be the result of an abnormality in testicular development (dysgenesis). Cryptorchid testes frequently have a short spermatic artery, poor blood supply, or both. While early scrotal positioning of these testes will obviate further damage related to intra-abdominal location, the testes generally remain abnormal, spermatogenesis is rare, and the risk of malignant neoplasm is increased. These testes should probably be removed if spermatogenesis does not occur after a reasonable period of observation.

Bilateral cryptorchidism is a common feature in prepubertal castrate syndrome, Noonan's syndrome, and disorders of androgen synthesis or action; it is seen less commonly with Klinefelter's syndrome, Sertoli-cell-only syndrome, and hypogonadotropin states.

Clinical Findings

Testosterone levels may be obtained after hCG stimulation to confirm the presence or absence of abdominal testes. The child with bilaterally undescended testes should be evaluated for sex chromosome abnormalities and genetic sex determined by buccal smear or chromosome analysis in the newborn period.

Differential Diagnosis

In palpating for the testes, the cremasteric reflex may be elicited, with a resultant ascent of the testes into the inguinal canal or abdomen **(pseudocryptorchidism).** To prevent this, the fingers first should be placed across the upper portion of the inguinal canal, obstructing ascent. Examination while the child is in a warm bath is also helpful. No treatment is necessary, and the prognosis for testicular descent and competence is excellent.

Treatment

The best age for medical or surgical treatment has not been determined, but there is a trend toward operation in infancy or early childhood. Surgical repair is indicated for cryptorchidism persisting beyond puberty.

Gonadotropin therapy (chorionic gonadotropin, 4000–5000 units intramuscularly 3–5 times a week for 2–3 weeks) is recommended by some before surgery.

Androgen treatment (ie, testosterone enanthate) is indicated only as replacement therapy in the male beyond the normal age of puberty who has been shown to lack functional testes.

Garagorri JM et al: Results of early treatment of cryptorchidism with human chorionic gonadotropin. *J Pediatr* 1981; **101:**923.

Gendrel D et al: Correlation of pituitary and testicular responses to stimulation tests in cryptorchid children. *Acta Endocrinol* 1977;**86:**641.

4. GYNECOMASTIA

See Chapter 9.

TESTICULAR TUMORS

The primary malignant tumors of the testis are seminomas and teratomas. Seminomas are rare in childhood; they may be hormone-producing. The major hormone-producing tumor of the testis is the Leydig cell tumor. It is frequently associated with sexual precocity. Other testicular tumors (choriocarcinomas and dysgerminomas) have been reported in association with sexual precocity.

Treatment of testicular tumors is by surgical removal. The prognosis in patients with Leydig cell tumors is generally good.

Murphy GP: Testicular cancer. *CA* 1983;**33:**100.

OVARIAN TUMORS

Ovarian tumors are not rare in children and account for approximately 1% of cases of female sexual precocity. They may occur at any age; are usually large, benign, and unilateral; and may be estrogen-producing. The most common estrogen-producing tumor is the granulosa cell tumor, but thecomas, luteomas, mixed types, and theca-lutein and follicular cysts have all been described in association with sexual precocity. In most instances, an ovarian tumor is palpable abdominally or rectally by the time sexual development has occurred. Exceptions to this rule, although rare, are notable.

Other ovarian tumors (teratomas, choriocarcinomas, and dysgerminomas) have been reported in association with sexual precocity.

Treatment is surgical removal. Recurrences are uncommon.

DIABETES MELLITUS *

Essentials of Diagnosis

- Hyperglycemia and glycosuria, with or without ketonuria.
- Weight loss, polyuria, polydipsia, and abdominal or leg cramps.
- Enuresis, mild appetite loss, emotional disturbances, lassitude.
- Fewer than 5% of cases present in coma or precoma.
- Diminished glucose tolerance.

General Considerations

In individuals under 18 years of age, the incidence of diabetes mellitus is between 1 and 3.5 per 1000, depending on the population surveyed.

In most cases of juvenile diabetes—or insulin-dependent diabetes mellitus (IDDM; type I diabetes mellitus) as it is now more commonly called—the pathologic process is thought to have been taking place for several months before there is actual evidence of clinical insulin deficiency. The cause remains unknown. In part it is genetic, possibly due to polymorphism of one of the HLA-DR antigens. Genetic markers on chromosome 6 are associated with a considerably increased risk of disease. The risk in DR3 heterozygotes compared to the population at large is 3.7; in DR4 heterozygotes, 9.7; and in DR3/DR4 mixed heterozygotes, 45.8. The actual trigger of the inflammatory response in genetically susceptible individuals is unknown, but enteroviruses have been implicated.

The disease can now be detected in its earliest stages in siblings by the presence of islet cell cytoplasmic antibodies associated with a progressing impairment of insulin response to an intravenous glucose load. If effective treatment with immunosuppressive agents or by other means at this early stage could be achieved, this would clearly be an advance; the possibility is currently being explored.

With the progressive destruction of islet cells, insulin no longer stimulates protein synthesis at the ribosomal level or effectively binds hexokinase to the electron transport chain on the mitochondrial surface. The latter leads to diminished availability of oxaloacetate. To replace these lessened energy resources from glucose, increased breakdown of fat and protein to acetylcoenzyme A occurs. Peripheral utilization of fatty acids and amino acids, however, is incomplete, and both are converted to ketone bodies in the liver.

Clinical Findings

A. Symptoms and Signs:

1. Severe diabetes—In most affected children, diabetes is first recognized at the point when insulin production begins to fall below physiologic needs. Nowadays, fewer than 5% of patients are actually in or near coma when first seen. The characteristic symptoms of loss of weight, polyuria, polydipsia, and abdominal or leg cramps are recognized largely in retrospect. Dehydration is sometimes severe.

2. Mild diabetes—With increasing frequency, patients are presenting with more benign cases of diabetes. A few are detected accidentally by urinalysis before overt symptoms appear. Others present with enuresis associated with polyuria, moderate weight loss, or mild problems of poor appetite and lassitude or emotional disturbances. Very rarely, diabetes presents with delayed insulin release following a glucose load, with hypoglycemia 3 hours or so after a glucose load, or as nonketotic (hyperosmolar) coma. Maturity-onset diabetes (MODY) is occasionally seen in an obese teenager. This can usually be managed by diet restriction. By extending screening programs to young people, more such cases could be identified.

In most juvenile diabetics, a "honeymoon" period occurs shortly after initial stabilization, when insulin requirements are often small; but in nearly every case, the insulin dose must be raised to conventional levels in a few weeks. Very occasionally, this phase will last over a year, and it can sometimes be contained by the use of sulfonylureas.

Well-controlled diabetics show no abnormal physical signs.

3. Pseudodiabetes—Pseudodiabetes is a transient diabetic state occurring in the newborn or occasionally in older children with infections. It is primarily due to hyperglucagonemia and may require a short course of treatment with regular insulin.

4. Hyperosmolar nonketotic coma—This is characterized by severe hyperglycemia, hyperosmolality, and dehydration without ketoacidosis. It is usually seen in adult-onset diabetes; it is uncommon in children. Restoration of extracellular water with isotonic fluids is a primary goal of treatment.

B. Laboratory Findings:

1. Glycosuria—Glycosuria may be identified by glucose oxidase tapes, eg, Tes-Tape and Clinistix. Clinitest tablets are less sensitive.

2. Hyperglycemia—A fasting blood glucose value exceeding 120 mg/dL is almost certainly due to diabetes mellitus. The use of Chemstrip bG strips or a reflectometer in the home or office is now essential to monitor treatment.

3. Glucose tolerance tests—Glucose tolerance tests (Fig 25–6) are not usually necessary in childhood.

4. Serum insulin levels—Serum insulin levels may be normal or moderately elevated at the onset of juvenile diabetes. A delayed insulin response to glucose is indicative of prediabetes.

5. Other laboratory measurements—A number of additional laboratory parameters are coming to be used in the appraisal of long-term control. Stable hemoglobin A_{1c} levels are 11 ± 2% of total hemoglobin in children with reasonably well controlled diabetes and are 6.3 ± 2% in normal children. A level

* This section is contributed by Donough O'Brien, MD, FRCP.

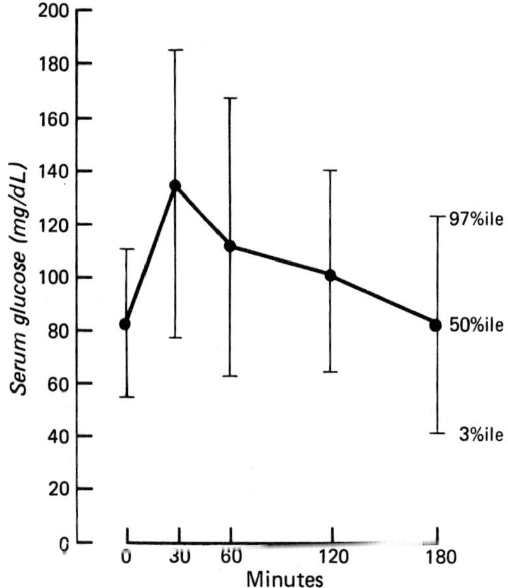

Figure 25–6. Serum glucose percentile levels after administration of glucose, 1.75 g/kg orally.

below 10% is indicative of excellent control. Fasting plasma cholesterol and HDL levels should be monitored.

Conventional (ICA-IgG) and complement-fixing (CF-ICA) islet cell antibodies are usually found in serum many months before the disease is clinically overt. Presence of these antibodies in siblings of patients or in susceptible HLA types may one day be an indication for intervention to prevent B cell destruction.

At the onset of type I diabetes, there is an increase in T cells positive for Ia antigen. Beyond indicating an immunologic response, the significance of this finding is not known.

Differential Diagnosis

The differential diagnosis of diabetes mellitus is not difficult, since this is virtually the only condition that gives rise to glycosuria and hyperglycemia with ketosis.

Abnormal glucose tolerance tests with glycosuria may be encountered in a variety of conditions in which there is an increased production of glucocorticoids or catecholamines. These include certain hypothalamic and pituitary tumors, adrenal tumors or hyperplasia, and pheochromocytomas. Since the hyperglycemia in these states is a reflection of increased gluconeogenesis and glycogenolysis and not of insulin insufficiency, there is no ketosis. Renal glycosuria is not associated with hyperglycemia.

Treatment

A. Management of Ketosis and Coma:

1. General management—The treatment of severe diabetic acidosis is based on fundamental principles. Insulin is given to restore normal carbohydrate utilization and triglyceride and protein synthesis. Extracellular fluid volume must be restored to compensate for losses due to vomiting and to the osmotic diuresis caused by unmetabolized glucose in the urine. Serum hyperosmolality must be gradually normalized and intracellular stores of potassium replenished. The serum phosphorus level must be raised in some cases in order to maintain normal erythrocyte 2,3-diphosphoglycerate levels and tissue oxygenation. Severe acid-base distortions may have to be corrected both for homeostatic reasons and to ensure optimal insulin action. Diabetic ketoacidosis, except as an initial presentation, is nowadays almost always due to poor compliance with treatment.

2. Initial laboratory studies—The laboratory routine should include a complete blood count; examination of the urine for blood cells, protein, ketone bodies, and glucose; and appropriate cultures as required for the investigation of suspected infectious disease.

The acid-base status should be estimated by measuring blood pH and P_{CO_2} or serum bicarbonate and anion gap. Baseline serum (or plasma) ketones, glucose, sodium, potassium, and chloride levels should be recorded, as well as blood urea nitrogen, serum phosphate, and serum osmolality in severe cases. Serum acetoacetic acid should be measured by Acetest tablet dilution. (More specific tests are too time-consuming for routine use.)

3. Initial management—The following protocol is for children with diabetic ketoacidosis who have been hospitalized because they are new diabetics; because they have severe acidosis, central nervous system symptoms, or repeated vomiting; because they are unable to take oral fluids; or because they have not responded to home or outpatient management.

a. General clinical management—

(1) Take a routine history and perform a physical examination, with special attention to the possibility of precipitating causes such as infection, emotional stress, or failure to take insulin.

(2) Reassure the patient, who should be kept warm. Antiemetics (eg, promethazine, 0.5 mg/kg intramuscularly) may be helpful if the child is vomiting but not comatose. Promethazine suppositories are likewise helpful.

(3) If there is vomiting or abdominal distention with a risk of aspiration due to coma or precoma, start continuous gastric suction. Unconscious patients must be catheterized.

(4) Start a flow sheet for medications, fluids, insulin, and laboratory values. Record all intake and output meticulously. Keep all records in a format that anyone can easily and accurately grasp.

(5) In severe cases, assess the degree of shock and the need for blood or other volume expanders. Also attach an electrocardiographic monitoring line for K^+ changes. Plasma volume expansion with col-

loid should be used with caution in the child whose lean body mass has been depleted, because of the risk of cardiac failure. This is indirectly but more safely achieved by rapid replacement of extracellular fluid losses using near isotonic fluids.

b. Insulin—No insulin should be given until a baseline serum glucose level has been determined. Insulin is then given by continuous intravenous infusion. This achieves a relatively constant serum insulin level without the hazard of hypoglycemia and a smoother and more predictable fall in serum glucose and ketones. The normal priming dose is 0.2 unit/kg intravenously. Subsequently, the dose is 0.1–0.15 unit/kg/h intravenously until the serum acetoacetic acid is only moderately elevated when tested by Acetest tablet in 1:2 dilution. During this period, serum acetoacetic acid by Acetest tablet should be measured every 2 hours before the insulin dose. Blood glucose by Dextrostix should be measured hourly as a screening measure to detect hypoglycemia early if it occurs. If the serum glucose has fallen below 250 mg/dL and serum acetoacetic acid is still elevated, the intravenous insulin regimen should be continued until serum ketones are normal, and glucose should be administered intravenously. In the interval before daily long-acting insulin is started and after serum ketones are normal and the blood glucose is less than 250 mg/dL, the intravenous insulin can be continued or one or more doses of regular insulin, 0.1–0.2 unit/kg/h, can be given subcutaneously.

The first dose of long-acting insulin should be started on the first or second morning after admission provided vomiting has stopped. A tentative starting total dose of 0.3–0.5 unit/kg/24 h is advised in new patients.

c. Fluid and electrolyte management—

(1) Initial volume expansion—If the patient is in a severely dehydrated or borderline shock state, give physiologic solution (isotonic saline or lactated Ringer's injection), 20 mL/kg (600 mL/m^2) or more over the first hour. If the serum glucose is high (> 250 mg/dL), there is no reason to add glucose until the serum glucose falls below this level. Blood glucose levels should be determined at hourly intervals to be certain that hypoglycemia does not occur—or the Dextrostix method can be used. If the patient is severely acidotic or has not voided, it is appropriate to wait to add potassium until after the initial fluid volume reexpansion in the first hour of therapy.

(2) Twenty-four-hour fluid volume—

(a) Replacement—Most children with mild diabetic ketoacidosis can be treated at home with additional regular insulin, fluids such as apple or grape juice, and promethazine (Phenergan) suppositories, 12.5 or 25 mg, if there is vomiting. Somewhat more serious cases can usually be managed with a few hours of outpatient fluid therapy. It is unusual to need inpatient therapy except in cases in which insulin has been deliberately withheld.

A convenient rule is to give 0.5 normal saline in a dosage of 600 mL/m^2 for the first 1–2 hours. Insulin is added as soon as the blood glucose level is known, and glucose, potassium, phosphate, and bicarbonate may be added as detailed below. Depending on the hydration needs, intravenous fluids can be slowed to twice the maintenance dose (see Table 36–3) after 2–3 hours. Most young patients can be sent home after 6 hours.

(b) Potassium—Potassium is a special problem because high urinary losses occur in association with normal serum levels due to the inability of K^+ to be retained intracellularly in the presence of acidosis. As acidosis is corrected, it is not unusual to see serum potassium levels fall in spite of large potassium replacements. In general, all intravenous fluids should contain 20–30 meq of K^+ per liter once voiding is established. Electrocardiographic strips (lead II) may give the best indication of total body potassium deficit or change. Supplements may be in the form of potassium chloride or phosphate.

(c) Phosphorus—Serum phosphorus, like potassium, may be initially elevated in diabetic acidosis only to fall rapidly during therapy. It is still not clear that low serum phosphorus causes clinical problems, but there is some evidence that neurologic disturbances may respond to raising the serum phosphorus. On theoretic grounds, a low serum phosphorus may be reflected in a low red cell 2,3-diphosphoglycerate, causing a leftward shift of the O_2 dissociation curve. This in turn may cause peripheral anoxia, especially with restoration of normal blood pH. In replacing phosphate, give half of all potassium requirements as potassium phosphate and check serum phosphate levels.

(d) Osmolarity—Measurement of serum osmolarity may be helpful in severely comatose patients. If the serum osmolality is very high (> 350 mmol/L), the blood glucose and dehydration should be corrected less rapidly, because of the danger of the dysequilibrium syndrome. All of the above considerations apply in treating hyperosmolar coma, but special attention must be given to the slow amelioration of serum hyperosmolality.

(e) Acid-base management—Specific acid-base correction with alkali is usually not necessary unless the blood pH is under 7.15. The acidosis appears to be of 2 kinds. When plasma and extracellular volume sustain normal renal perfusion, the urine contains large amounts of sodium salts of keto acids, the tubules have difficulty excreting hydrogen ion (urine pH is acid), and there is a hyperchloremic acidosis. If renal perfusion is diminished, however, keto acids are not excreted and there is a high anion gap acidosis. There is evidence that hyperchloremic acidosis is slower to resolve, so that bicarbonate therapy should be more readily used in these instances according to the conventional formula below:

$$\text{meq Bicarbonate required} = \text{Base excess in meq/L} \times 0.3 \times \text{Body weight in kg}$$

4. Continuing management of the ketotic patient—After the first period of adjustment, there is seldom any need to give insulin more than once or twice a day. The particular long-term regimen to be selected depends initially on the age of the child. Most young children dislike injections, especially at the beginning, so that it is always worthwhile to try to achieve satisfactory control with one injection a day. Semilente and ultralente in equal parts, totaling 0.3–0.5 unit/kg/d, may work very well; or one part of regular insulin to 3 or more parts of NPH or lente insulin may also be effective. After the patient reaches about 12 years of age, it is usually best to start right away with one part of regular pure pork insulin to 2 or more parts of pure pork lente or NPH insulin given 20–30 minutes before breakfast and dinner; the total insulin dose in the morning should be approximately twice that in the evening, although individual needs are quite variable.

The duration of action of various insulin preparations is shown in Table 25–12.

Synthetic human insulin is now widely available but does not seem to offer any particular advantage over pure pork insulin.

In the following days, the patient should be encouraged to return to full activity and a normal diet, while the insulin dosage is adjusted on the basis of serum and urine glucose levels and urine acetone along the lines suggested below for long-term management. At this stage, education of the patient and family must begin. After the nature and prospects of the disease have been explained, they must be shown the techniques of giving insulin, testing the urine for acetone and glucose, and home blood glucose monitoring. It is important to go over these routines repeatedly, especially in the early months of the disease. A good clinic nurse, especially one who can make home visits, can be invaluable in helping families to understand and manage diabetes in a child.

B. Management of Less Severe Acidosis: Most cases of juvenile diabetes now present without severe acidosis. The initial phases of management and education can usually be conducted on an outpatient basis if the family and physician can assign sufficient time for the purpose. Recurring acidosis in established cases is usually linked to infection or to stress; sometimes it is due to insulin overdose (the Somogyi effect).

Table 25–12. Duration of action of various insulins.

Insulin	Duration of Maximum Effect (hours)	End of Effect (hours)
Human	1–4	6
Pure pork regular	2–5	8
NPH	4–12	24
Semilente	5–10	16
Lente (30% semi, 70% ultra)	7–15	22
Ultralente	10–30	36

Patients with mild acidosis should be started with an insulin dosage of 0.3–0.5 unit/kg/d. The insulin is gradually increased until hyperglycemia and glycosuria are controlled.

It is probably not necessary to contrive an episode of hypoglycemia, even under controlled conditions. However, patients or their parents must be warned of the characteristic symptoms of headache, abdominal pain, and shakiness and instructed to control it with a snack, orange juice, lump of sugar, etc.

C. Long-Term Management of All Patients: The objective of long-term management is to achieve "control." In children, this can be defined as a high level of physical and emotional health; continuing normal growth with freedom from hypoglycemic reactions; no acetone in the urine; glycosuria that seldom exceeds 1% in early morning, pre-lunch, pre-supper, or late evening urine specimens; and blood glucose levels that are usually between 80 and 180 mg/dL. The hemoglobin A_{1c}, depending on methodology, should be less than 10%. The following are important in achieving this:

1. Patient follow-up and continuing education—Continued observation of the child with diabetes is most important. Initially, this should be weekly or at any time the need should arise; telephone contacts should be encouraged. During this period, if patients will keep careful records of either blood glucose levels 2 or 3 times a day or of urine glucose and acetone, it is usually possible to anticipate the fluctuations in insulin need that are characteristic of the early years of juvenile-onset diabetes. Later on, supervision can be much less close and will depend primarily on the patient's and the family's confidence in managing diet and insulin dosage. Puberty is often a period of instability in carbohydrate metabolism, but more frequently the problems at this age are, again, the emotional ones that may stem from feelings of being different or depressed or angry as a result of the diabetes. The patient must be encouraged to participate in all activities. Vigorous exercise is especially helpful in controlling diabetes, although hypoglycemia must be avoided. It is important, particularly in the early months, to constantly renew and augment the patient's and family's understanding of diabetes both in general terms and in the specific practical matters of giving the injections, diet management, activity, and immediate treatment of infections. Many families need emotional support and counseling. Special counseling to control stress is often of great help.

2. Insulin—Patterns of insulin administration have changed in recent years. Mixtures of equal parts of semilente and ultralente insulin or 1:3 or 1:4 mixtures of regular insulin and either lente or NPH insulin are still useful in the young child for injection once a day. In older children, however, the trend is toward the newer, highly purified pork insulins. These are usually given twice daily, 20–30 minutes before breakfast or dinner in the proportion of one part of regular insulin to 3 or more parts of NPH or lente insulin, with twice as much insulin given in the morning as in the evening. The total dose of insulin is usually around 0.8–1 unit/kg/d; but in adolescents, in children who exercise a lot and have a high caloric intake, and in obese patients, doses may reach around 1.8 units/kg/d. If these levels are encountered, insulin overdose must always be considered also. The pattern of insulin administration varies according to the needs and preferences of the child.

Human insulin is now available but seems to offer no special advantages; it is more rapidly absorbed and should be used in a 1:3 or higher ratio with NPH insulin and given at least 30 minutes before mealtime.

The new insulins are less likely to provoke subcutaneous reactions (especially atrophy) and can usually be injected into the same site each time. It is not necessary to sterilize the skin before the injection if it is already "clean," and disposable syringes may be recapped after use and kept in the refrigerator for up to 7 injections.

Insulin dosage should be readjusted from time to time on the basis of routine urine tests for glucose and acetone as well as occasional 24-hour urine glucose determinations or home blood glucose determinations by reflectometer or glucose oxidase strip. Parents and patients should be encouraged to acquire confidence in making small adjustments in insulin dosage in response to gradual changes with growth and short-term increases with infection.

3. Diet—The essence of dietary control of diabetes is to have a normal diet and to eat the same kinds of foods at the same time and in the same amounts each day. Snacks in midmorning, afternoon, and evening serve to avert hypoglycemia and spread the carbohydrate load. Weighing is seldom necessary, but a simple understanding of nutrition is important. In small children, good dietary discipline should not be pressed to the point of causing emotional problems; but beyond adolescence, every effort should be made to obtain compliance in the interest of good control and a diminished prospect of complications.

In most cases, it is sufficient to establish, with the help of a nutritionist, that the family diet offers a conventional assembly of calories (100 kcal × age in years + 1000), about 15–20% from proteins, 35–40% from fat, and 45–55% from carbohydrates, as well as other nutrients.

Understanding the dietary exchange system may be helpful in achieving control. This is outlined in the pamphlet *Exchange Lists for Meal Planning*, published by the American Diabetes Association, 600 Fifth Avenue, New York, NY 10020. In general, the idea of the exchange diet is to develop "equivalents" in each food group that are similar to each other in quantity and in calories. Instructions concerning the diet should be given by a dietitian or nutritionist.

In establishing the dietary pattern, it is important to consider the hypoglycemic effect of exercise. Adjusting snack times to cover exercise and, in some cases, reducing insulin dosage may be necessary. Another consideration is the use of protein and fat in the bedtime snack, which helps to prevent low blood glucose levels during the prolonged nighttime fast.

Young people with diabetes are vulnerable to hypertriglyceridemia and hypercholesterolemia. The long-term significance of these abnormalities is still debated; but until the controversy is resolved, it may be prudent to measure triglycerides and cholesterol annually and to institute dietary measures that are likely to maintain homeostasis of blood lipids. The use of 2% milk, polyunsaturated vegetable oil margarines (instead of butter), and polyunsaturated cooking oils is recommended on these grounds. Special dietetic foods, with the possible exception of artificial sweeteners, should not be encouraged for young diabetics; not only are such foods expensive and unnecessary, but above all they differentiate the affected child from the rest of the family.

In a setting where "fad diets" are so much a part of the social scene, it is not surprising that diabetes has been the focus of enthusiasts proposing diets with varying degrees of scientific basis. Brewer's yeast as a source of "glucose tolerance factor" and guar gum to delay absorption of glucose have been advocated but have not been demonstrated to be effective in young diabetic patients. The use of alternative sweeteners such as saccharin and aspartame in drinks and other products makes life much easier for the child with diabetes. Sorbitol and fructose are sugars that can be metabolized without forming glucose if sufficient insulin is present and the child is in good diabetic control. A high-fiber, low-fat diet in which carbohydrate is given as complex carbohydrate may be helpful but has found less favor among young diabetics than among adult diabetics. Perhaps as the different functions and properties of fibers and carbohydrates become known, more progress will be made in that area. Obesity in a young diabetic deserves the same attention and presents the same problems as in the nondiabetic, but with the added burden of insulin resistance in the diabetic. In the small subset of diabetic adolescents with maturity-onset diabetes of the young (MODY) and obesity (more often seen in girls than boys), the diabetes can usually be controlled by weight reduction and refined carbohydrate restriction.

Alcohol and drug intake can be considerable problems in teenagers with diabetes. Initially, use of alcoholic beverages usually results in increased blood glucose levels. Later, low blood glucose levels will be more likely, owing to sleeping late the next day, missed snacks, and a reduction of gluconeogenesis. The role of diet in control of diabetes is still rigidly fixed in the public mind, so that parents, relatives, and friends of diabetics often place exaggerated importance on the diet.

4. Managing hypoglycemia—It is wise for the patient to carry hard candy in case hypoglycemic symptoms are experienced. This is especially likely following unanticipated strenuous physical exertion. In certain cases, it is also advisable for the parents to be instructed in the use of glucagon to counteract hypoglycemia by giving 1 mg intramuscularly. If glucagon is used, the child must be given some easily absorbed carbohydrate as soon as possible to restore the liver glycogen. "Instant glucose" is a very viscous glucose solution obtainable in tubes from the local Diabetes Association. It can be squeezed into the cheeks of a semiconscious child and absorbed without danger of aspiration.

5. Urine testing—Because of the variability in the renal clearance of glucose, routine urine testing for glucose in type I diabetes has largely been replaced by home blood glucose monitoring. It is nevertheless important to measure urine ketones during episodes of acute illness.

6. Blood glucose estimations—Isolated and occasional blood glucose estimations are of little value except during acute illness. From later childhood on, however, home blood glucose monitoring has become the standard for assessing control. If the patient is ill, frequent testing is helpful; in normal times, 4–6 tests a week are sufficient. Half of these tests should be in the morning before breakfast, and the others should be in late afternoon, before dinner, or before bed.

7. Recent advances—There have been a number of advances recently in addition to the availability of new insulins and the practice of home blood glucose monitoring (discussed above). These now include a number of individually programmable pocket calculators that will indicate insulin dose; the physician, of course, must enter the algorithm. The use of insulin pumps is already declining. For the occasional highly motivated and technically gifted young adult, they can offer excellent control. However, for most adolescents, they are still too cumbersome and do not offer better control than injections twice daily; there is also some evidence that they lead to sustained hyperinsulinism, which possibly may hasten microvascular changes.

Human islet cell transplantation has been achieved and offers promise in the future. Increased knowledge about the immunologic nature of the primary lesion is leading to some interesting but equivocally successful trials of immunosuppressive therapy in the early stages of the disease.

Complications

Complications during the course of diabetes in children are not common. During presenting coma, extensive neurologic signs may develop, but the outlook is good. Hypoglycemia, which is also rarely a presenting symptom, may be frequent and severe enough to cause brain damage. Limited joint mobility, especially of the fifth proximal interphalangeal joint, seems to be a rather common problem and an index of later degenerative vascular disease. Peripheral neuritis and exudative retinopathy may occasionally be seen in childhood. Poorly controlled diabetes in young children over a long period may lead to a syndrome of hepatomegaly, delayed puberty, and dwarfism (Mauriac's syndrome). Emotional disturbances are common, especially in the early teen years. Vaginal candidiasis is seen occasionally.

Some children become very readily ketotic during episodes of stress. In some instances, they may be helped by small doses of propranolol.

One of the commonest causes of poor control is the Somogyi effect, which occurs as a result of sequential overdosage of insulin in response to occult hypoglycemia, followed by pressor amine-induced hyperglycemia spuriously interpreted as due to insufficient insulin. Treatment in this instance consists of reduction of the insulin dosage.

Both atrophy and hypertrophy of subcutaneous fat occur around injection sites but are much less common with the increased use of pure pork insulins.

Prognosis

Parents will want to know in what ways the overall life expectancy may be altered for their diabetic children. In this respect, there is now a mean expectancy of some 20 years after the onset of the disease before the onset of major complications. However, the prepubertal years do not contribute to the anticipated time of onset of these complications.

Baum JD et al: Immediate metabolic response to a low dose of insulin in children presenting with diabetes. *Arch Dis Child* 1975;**50:**373.

Cahill GF, McDevitt HO: Insulin-dependent diabetes mellitus: The initial lesion. *N Engl J Med* 1981;**304:**1454.

Chase HP et al: *Understanding Juvenile Diabetes,* 5th ed. Univ of Colo Med Ctr Press, 1983.

Jackson RA et al: Increased circulating Ia-antigen bearing T cells in type I diabetes mellitus. *N Engl J Med* 1982;**306:**785.

Rosenbloom AL et al: Limited joint mobility in childhood diabetes mellitus indicates increased risk for microvascular disease. *N Engl J Med* 1981;**305:**191.

Rotter JI, Rimoin DL: The genetics of glucose intolerance disorders. *Am J Med* 1981;**70:**116.

Skyler JS: Human insulin of recombinant DNA origin. *Diabetes Care* 1982;**5:**1.

Stiller CR et al: Effects of cyclosporine immunosuppression in insulin-dependent diabetes mellitus of recent onset. *Science* 1984;**223:**1362.

PRADER-WILLI SYNDROME

Children with Prader-Willi syndrome show obesity, short stature, and mental retardation with hypotonia in the newborn period. The males show hypogonadism. There is a tendency to develop diabetes in later childhood. Their appetites may be very hard to control, and this leads in turn to behavior problems and sometimes to the pickwickian syndrome.

Crinic KA et al: Preventing mental retardation associated with gross obesity in the Prader-Willi syndrome. *Pediatrics* 1980;**66:**787.

Ledbetter DH et al: Deletions of chromosome 15 as a cause of the Prader-Willi syndrome. *Am J Med* 1981;**70:**116.

Merritt RJ et al: Consequences of modified fasting in obese pediatric and adolescent patients. 1. Protein-sparing modified fast. *J Pediatr* 1980;**96:**13.

Tolis G et al: Anterior pituitary function in the Prader-Labhart-Willi syndrome. *J Clin Endocrinol Metab* 1974;**39:**1061.

SELECTED REFERENCES

Alsever RN, Gotlin RW: *Handbook of Endocrine Tests in Adults and Children,* 2nd ed. Year Book, 1978.

Gardner LI: *Endocrine and Genetic Diseases of Childhood and Adolescence,* 2nd ed. Saunders, 1975.

Harrison HE, Harrison HC: Disorders of calcium and phosphate metabolism in childhood and adolescence. *Major Probl Clin Pediatr* 1979;**20:**1.

Stanbury JB et al (editors): *The Metabolic Basis of Inherited Disease,* 5th ed. McGraw-Hill, 1983.

Villee DB: *Human Endocrinology: A Developmental Approach.* Saunders, 1975.

Williams RH: *Textbook of Endocrinology,* 7th ed. Saunders, 1985.

Infections: Viral & Rickettsial 26

Vincent A. Fulginiti, MD

I. VIRAL INFECTIONS*

The proper collection, shipping, and identification of specimens are essential to adequate diagnosis. In the discussions of specific viral diseases that follow are listed the specimens to be submitted, special procedures in handling and shipping such specimens (where applicable), and what information the physician can expect from the viral diagnostic laboratory.

In the past, diagnostic tests for viruses were of limited value because the results were reported long after clinical decisions had to be made. Rapid diagnosis can now be made with modern techniques employing fluorescent antibody staining of cells taken directly from the patient (eg, identification of respiratory syncytial virus in pharyngeal cells) or staining of cell cultures 1 or 2 days after they are inoculated with specimens from the patient (eg, identification of herpesvirus in tissue culture). Newer methods of antigen detection, such as the enzyme-linked immunosorbent assay (ELISA), also provide rapid results enabling clinicians to choose the appropriate drugs for treatment and determine the prognosis. In some cases, the more traditional methods of isolating or identifying the causative organism are used to supplement the rapid tests. Clinicians should contact the nearest viral diagnostic laboratory for assistance in obtaining and shipping specimens for testing.

General considerations that apply to the diagnosis of viral diseases are as follows:

(1) Viral diagnosis usually depends upon isolation of the offending agent or demonstration of the host response on the basis of a rising titer of specific serum antibody (or both).

(2) The rapid diagnostic tests usually employ specimens obtained by swabbing mucosal surfaces and skin lesions (especially vesicular fluid). The specimens must contain cells, since the cells are examined for the presence of viral antigens. In special circumstances (eg, if herpetic encephalitis is suspected), organ biopsy specimens can be submitted for direct examination.

(3) The more traditional diagnostic tests commonly employ specimens of body fluids, secretions, or tissue. An adequate sample can usually be obtained by swabbing the appropriate orifice or mucous membrane and immersing the swab immediately in a medium designed to protect the agent during shipping and handling—usually a mixture of salts and protein, which can be supplied by the laboratory. (Veal infusion broth with 0.5% albumin or Hanks' balanced salt solution is adequate.) It is almost always necessary to freeze the specimen immediately and keep it frozen until it reaches the laboratory. (Respiratory syncytial virus and cytomegalovirus may be destroyed by freezing and must be kept on ordinary ice during transport.)

(4) Viral antibody titration depends upon the collection of paired sera—a first ("acute") specimen collected as early as possible in the course of the illness and a second ("convalescent") serum collected usually 2–4 weeks later. Accurate serologic diagnosis depends upon aseptic direct venipuncture, careful separation of serum to avoid hemolysis, and maintenance in the frozen state until receipt in the laboratory.

Richman D et al: Immunoenzymatic staining of viral and chlamydial antigens in cell culture. *Diagn Microbiol Infect Dis* 1985;**3**:353.

Richman D et al: Summary of a workshop on new and useful methods in rapid viral diagnosis. *J Infect Dis* 1984;**150**:941.

MYXOVIRUSES

INFLUENZA

Influenza viruses cause sporadic clinical illness in infants and children in nonepidemic infections that account for 5–10% of all serious respiratory infections. Most frequent is the upper respiratory infection syndrome, although croup, bronchiolitis, and pneumonia also occur. During epidemics, a sudden onset of fever and "toxic" symptoms may accompany respiratory manifestations.

Except in major epidemics, clinical identification of influenza infection may be impossible. Influenza is mimicked by other respiratory viral infections. "Flu" syndrome seen in adults is uncommon in children.

Rapid identification of influenza virus can be accomplished by fluorescent antibody staining of pharyngeal and nasal epithelial cells. Attempts should

* For prevention, see Chapter 5.

be made to isolate the virus in order to determine its antigenic type. Serum antibody obtained early and late in the course of infection can aid in identification of viruses and control of epidemics.

Current isolates of influenza viruses are identified in regional reference laboratories and aid in the preparation of vaccines for the prevention of influenza, either in the upcoming season or in the future. In addition, the identification of influenza virus activity alerts the clinician to avoid the use of salicylates and thereby avoid the risk of Reye's syndrome.

Reye's syndrome (encephalopathy with fatty degeneration of the viscera) has recently occurred in epidemic fashion closely paralleling influenza type B epidemics. Other viruses—notably varicella—had previously been implicated as etiologic agents of this syndrome. The exact relationship between influenza virus and Reye's syndrome is unclear. Use of aspirin during acute illness has been associated with Reye's syndrome in 4 epidemiologic studies. Most authorities recommend avoidance of salicylates during acute influenza infections in children. If an upper respiratory infection is followed by excessive vomiting and convulsions, the physician should consider this diagnosis. Coma, hypoglycemia, and liver dysfunction are later confirmatory findings. (See Chapter 20 for details of the diagnosis and treatment of Reye's syndrome.)

Clinical Findings

A. History: The history is compatible with various types of respiratory infections of "viral" nature. A history of the same illness in other members of the family or school group or of more severe illness in younger siblings can often be obtained.

B. Symptoms and Signs: There are no distinguishing clinical characteristics except the abrupt onset of high fever and "toxic" symptoms that are in contrast to most other respiratory viruses. Influenza type C virus has been associated with the croup syndrome in infants.

C. Laboratory Findings: The usual laboratory tests are of little help. Epithelial cells (pharyngeal, nasal) can be examined with fluorescein-labeled antibody for rapid identification of influenza virus. A swab of the secretions should be sent in an appropriate medium to the laboratory. Paired sera obtained early in the course of the illness and after 2–3 weeks are of value in retrospective diagnosis.

D. X-Ray Findings: Chest x-rays may reveal extensive bronchial pneumonia or simply hyperaeration.

Differential Diagnosis

This is primarily an etiologic differential diagnosis, since many viruses produce the same syndrome. With croup, it is important to differentiate from *Haemophilus influenzae* epiglottitis (cherry-red epiglottis, severe systemic illness, positive throat and blood cultures); spasmodic or allergic croup (history of early respiratory symptoms or fever); and obstructive croup (history of choking or gagging on food, x-ray demonstration of foreign body or its effects).

Complications & Sequelae

Pneumonia may be followed by bacterial superinfections (particularly staphylococcal), with empyema, pyopneumothorax, etc. Croup may be associated with drying of the tracheal mucous membranes (with subsequent encrustation and obstruction), cardiac arrest, subcutaneous or mediastinal emphysema, and pneumothorax. Reye's syndrome has been associated with prior influenza virus infection, particularly type B infection.

Prevention

Amantadine (Symmetrel) is useful in preventing influenza type A infection. In highly susceptible individuals (such as children with chronic illnesses or immunodeficiency) in whom influenza infection could cause serious morbidity or death, prophylaxis with amantadine during the season of prevalence should be considered. The dosage is 4.4–8.8 mg/kg/d for children under 10 years of age (with a maximum of 150 mg/d) or 200 mg/d for those over 10 years of age; administer as a single daily dose or in 2 divided doses within a 24-hour period. Amantadine does not interfere with vaccine-induced immunity and can be administered concomitantly with influenza vaccine (see Chapter 5).

Treatment & Prognosis

Supportive measures are critical, especially in croup. Support of the airway, judicial tracheostomy, and attention to hydration and nutrition and to peripheral cardiovascular integrity may be lifesaving. (Croup is discussed further in Chapter 14.)

Amantadine (Symmetrel) can ameliorate influenza type A illness if begun within 24–48 hours of onset and continued for 5–7 days. The dosage is as indicated above. Experimental trials of ribavirin indicate that it has some effect in ameliorating established disease in adults, but there is little information on its effectiveness in children.

In general, complete recovery is the rule. Children—particularly young infants with croup—may die from cardiac arrest or other complications. Tracheostomy may prolong convalescence and require care beyond the period of acute infection.

Connor E, Powell K: Fulminant pneumonia caused by concomitant infection with influenza B virus and *Staphylococcus aureus*. *J Pediatr* 1985;**106:**447.

Glezen WP: Serious morbidity and mortality associated with influenza epidemics. *Epidemiol Rev* 1982;**4:**25.

Glezen WP, Couch RB, Six HR: The influenzae herald wave. *Am J Epidemiol* 1982;**116:**589.

Mullooly JP, Barker WH: Impact of type A influenza on children: A retrospective study. *Am J Public Health* 1982;**72:**1008.

Puck JM et al: Protection of infants from infection with influenza A virus by transplacentally acquired antibody. *J Infect Dis* 1980;**142:**844.

Wilson SZ et al: Treatment of influenza A (H1N1) virus infection with ribavirin aerosol. *Antimicrob Agents Chemother* 1984;**26:**200.

Wright P: Influenza in children: Prepared for this year's peak? *J Respir Dis* 1984;**10:**56.

PARAINFLUENZA

The parainfluenza viruses are among the more important respiratory viruses in childhood because they cause croup and upper respiratory illness.* Parainfluenza type 3 is most important very early in life, as most 1-year-old infants have been infected. The history, differential diagnosis, complications, and treatment are as for influenza (see above).

Although it is difficult to distinguish parainfluenza infections from other respiratory viral illnesses, the presence of hoarseness suggests this cause. This is particularly true if one member of the family has croup and the others upper respiratory infection with hoarseness. Rapid viral diagnosis is feasible, and identification of group and type is possible by laboratory examination of secretions and by antibody titration. Corticosteroid therapy of croup is controversial and not recommended by the author.

Recovery is the rule. Reinfection is common, but second infections tend to be less severe and produce less fever. Prolonged infections can occur in immunodeficient children.

Glezen WP et al: Parainfluenza virus type 3: Seasonality and risk of infection and reinfection in young children. *J Infect Dis* 1984;**150:**851.

Welliver R et al: Natural history of parainfluenza virus infection in childhood. *J Pediatr* 1982;**101:**180.

MUMPS

Essentials of Diagnosis

- History of exposure 14–21 days previously.
- Unilateral or bilateral parotid gland swelling.
- Aseptic meningitis with or without parotitis.
- Pancreatitis, orchitis, oophoritis (or combination).

General Considerations

Mumps is a common childhood infection that is asymptomatic in 30–40% of cases. Most children are infected, and lifetime immunity results. A few remain susceptible throughout adolescence and adult life, when parotitis with orchitis may occur. T cell-associated immunity may be the critical determinant of recovery and resistance.

Clinical Findings

A. History: Contact results in infection 14–21 days later. Only 60–70% of patients develop symptoms, and bilateral (or unilateral) painful swelling of the parotid glands is usually the only manifestation of the disease. Parotitis may be accompanied by mild respiratory symptoms. Occasionally, central nervous system symptoms appear prior to or in the absence of parotid gland involvement. Abdominal pain is a frequent complaint and may represent pancreatic involvement.

Recently, mumps virus pancreatitis has been suggested as a precursor of juvenile diabetes mellitus. Most of the evidence is epidemiologic, ie, a correlation between the incidence of mumps and of diabetes in children within 2–4 years. Specific data linking mumps virus infection of the pancreas and subsequent diabetes mellitus are lacking.

B. Symptoms and Signs:

1. Parotitis or salivary gland form—Smooth, tender enlargement of the affected salivary gland or glands is the most common finding. Lymphedema of the face is frequently present also and makes the swelling indistinct at its margins. Obliteration of the angle of the mandible is a useful diagnostic sign, as is the alignment of the fusiform swelling with the line formed by the long axis of the ear and the ramus of the mandible. Upward and lateral displacement of the earlobe is noted. The opening of Stensen's duct may be pointed and reddened.

Involvement of the submaxillary and sublingual glands produces swelling in the lateral and anterior aspects of the neck, respectively. Both are palpated just beneath the mandible and may appear to be fused with it as a result of surrounding lymphedema.

Systemic symptoms may consist of high fever and headache or mild respiratory symptoms or may be absent.

2. Meningoencephalitis—Mumps virus is the most common cause of aseptic meningitis in childhood. Cerebrospinal fluid pleocytosis is said to occur in 10–50% of all cases of mumps, although overt clinical symptoms are less common.

Aseptic meningitis may be accompanied by, may precede, or may occur in the absence of parotitis. Fever and headache increase, nuchal rigidity is noted, and gastrointestinal symptoms (nausea and vomiting) may occur. Central nervous system irritability is uncommon, and convulsions are rare. Recovery is rapid, with symptoms subsiding in 3–10 days, almost always without sequelae.

3. Pancreatitis—Mild to moderate abdominal pain may be present in the parotitic form of mumps. When severe epigastric pain occurs in association with nausea, persistent vomiting, high fever, chills, and severe prostration, pancreatitis should be suspected.

4. Orchitis or oophoritis—The gonads may be involved in postpubertal individuals with sudden onset of fever, chills, systemic symptoms, and testicular pain (males) or lower abdominal pain (females). Testicular swelling and extreme pain occur. Symptoms subside in 3–14 days, with abdominal tenderness being most persistent.

5. Other glandular involvement—Rarely, overt inflammation of the thyroid, Bartholin's glands, and breasts may be seen.

6. Endocardial fibroelastosis and subacute thyroiditis—These have recently been said to be due

* See Index for discussions of these diseases in other chapters.

to mumps virus infection, but the association has not been proved.

7. Other findings—Other possible manifestations include nephritis (rare), unilateral nerve deafness (1:15,000 cases of mumps), ophthalmologic disorders (optic neuritis, dacryoadenitis, uveokeratitis and scleritis, and central retinal vein thrombosis), arthritis, and postmumps thrombophlebitis.

C. Laboratory Findings: In almost 75% of patients, serum amylase levels rise in proportion to the glandular swelling. Return to normal values occurs in 2–3 weeks. Cerebrospinal fluid pleocytosis with lymphocytosis (often 500–1000 cells/μL) is associated with elevated cerebrospinal fluid protein and normal cerebrospinal fluid glucose values.

Mumps virus may be isolated from saliva, the pharynx, or urine and, in cases of aseptic meningitis, from the cerebrospinal fluid. A 4-fold rise in serum antibody titer is diagnostic and is particularly useful in the diagnosis of nonsalivary gland forms of the disease. Serum should be collected as early as possible in the clinical course and again in 2 weeks. Antibody can now be assayed by the enzyme-linked immunosorbent assay (ELISA).

The mumps virus skin test is no longer available.

Differential Diagnosis

The glandular forms of the disease must be distinguished from other acute causes of swelling in the neck: cervical lymphadenitis (location; coexistence of pharyngeal, tonsillar, or skin infection; leukocytosis with shift to the left; discreteness; absence of serum amylase elevation), acute suppurative parotitis (local inflammation, unilateral involvement, leukocytosis, purulent secretion from salivary duct), acute obstructive parotitis (visualization of calculus in the duct, history of previous episodes), other viral parotitides (coxsackievirus and lymphocytic choriomeningitis virus infections, distinguishable by virologic methods), acute lymphoma or lymphosarcoma (painless enlargement, involvement of lymph nodes, bone marrow findings), and acute episodes of recurrent parotitis (history of previous episodes, sialography reveals sialectasia).

Pancreatitis and oophoritis may be confused with other causes of acute abdominal pain, such as a ruptured viscus, acute appendicitis (especially in females with right-sided oophoritis), and peptic ulcer. A history of exposure to mumps, a high degree of suspicion, and serum amylase elevation all contribute to diagnosis.

Meningoencephalitis occurring in the absence of parotitis must be distinguished from all other causes. This can usually be done by laboratory evaluation.

Complications

Rare sequelae of meningoencephalitis include deafness (auditory nerve damage), postinfectious encephalitis syndrome or myelitis, facial neuritis, and myocarditis.

Contrary to common belief, mumps orchitis and oophoritis do not result in sterility. Most often it is unilateral, and even with bilateral infection total atrophy of the gonads is unlikely.

Mumps virus infection has been implicated as a cause of diabetes mellitus in some children.

Treatment & Prognosis

Control of fever, pain, and discomfort is occasionally necessary. Orchitis is best treated by conservative management, with rest, testicular support, and analgesics, although some physicians favor systemic corticosteroid therapy, which may result in more rapid subsidence of testicular swelling. Hydrocortisone, 10 mg/kg/24 h orally for 2–4 days, is the preferred treatment. Surgical intervention and hormonal therapy appear to offer no advantages.

Mumps is usually a self-limited infection lasting approximately 1 week in all forms. Recovery is spontaneous and complete, and sequelae are rare. Immunity is lifelong. Episodes of parotitis after mumps infection are due to other causes.

Brown NJ, Richmond ST: Fatal mumps myocarditis in an 8-month-old child. *Br Med J* 1980;**2:**356.

Hayden GF et al: Current status of mumps and mumps vaccine in the United States. *Pediatrics* 1978;**62:**965.

Helmke K et al: Islet cell antibodies in children with mumps infection. *Lancet* 1980;**2:**211.

Koskiniemi M et al: Clinical appearance on outcome in mumps encephalitis in children. *Acta Paediatr Scand* 1983;**72:**603.

Peig M et al: Post-mumps diabetes mellitus. (Letter.) *Lancet* 1981;**1:**1007.

Tsutsumi H et al: T-cell mediated cytotoxic response to mumps virus in humans. *Infect Immun* 1980;**30:**129.

Westmore GA et al: Isolation of mumps virus from the inner ear after sudden deafness. *Br Med J* 1979;**1:**14.

RESPIRATORY SYNCYTIAL VIRUS (RSV) DISEASE

Essentials of Diagnosis

- Bronchiolitis in very young infants is probably due to RSV.
- Illnesses are indistinguishable from other respiratory viral diseases (see Influenza).

General Considerations

RSV is the single most important cause of viral respiratory disease in infants and children, accounting for nearly 40% of all serious respiratory illnesses and for almost 70% of all cases of bronchiolitis. Children are infected early in life, and by age 1 most have acquired antibody. RSV infection appears to occur even when serum neutralizing antibody is present, and reinfection is common.

Clinical Findings

A. History: (See also Influenza.) A history of preceding upper respiratory symptoms is frequent in RSV infections, which then progress to lower tract disease. Fever is a more frequent finding in RSV infection than in other myxovirus diseases. Apneic episodes have been described in the course of RSV infections in premature and young infants.

B. Symptoms and Signs:

1. Upper respiratory infections—Nonspecific symptoms of rhinitis, nasal stuffiness, and bronchitis are seen. Cough and fever may be more frequent with RSV infections.

2. Bronchiolitis—Dyspnea and, frequently, severe respiratory distress, usually associated with copious, occasionally thick nasal and pharyngeal secretions, are the principal manifestations. Hyperaeration of lungs occurs, with fine rales and marked expiratory wheezing. Fever may be high. Retractions may be evident, and severe respiratory effort is a frequent finding. There is evidence suggesting that the term "bronchiolitis" as used here is too restrictive. Some children will have milder episodes of wheezing with the same pathophysiologic basis. Such children are seen in the physician's office and should be regarded as having the same airway events as the more classic cases in which the child requires hospitalization.

3. Bronchial pneumonia—Dyspnea and tachypnea are evident. Rales may or may not be present. Expiratory wheezing is not part of the picture of bronchial pneumonia.

4. Sudden death—A small proportion of sudden infant deaths may be due to overwhelming RSV infection, particularly in very young infants.

5. Nosocomial infections—Nosocomial infections with RSV among hospitalized infants and hospital staff have been noted. Spread is primarily by hand contact; thorough hand washing is imperative.

C. Laboratory Findings: Virologic diagnosis depends upon isolation of RSV or demonstration of a 4-fold antibody rise in paired sera. Throat or nasopharyngeal swabs placed in an appropriate medium and kept cold but not frozen are essential. Freezing may destroy the virus. Rapid diagnosis is possible by fluorescent antibody identification of RSV in upper respiratory cells.

D. X-Ray Findings: In bronchiolitis, generalized hyperaeration is often quite marked, with depression of the diaphragm, precardiac and retrosternal hyperaerated lungs, and diminished respiratory excursion on fluoroscopy. Pneumonia results in a similar pattern to a less marked degree. Patchy, diffuse peripheral infiltrates may be seen with both but are more prominent in pneumonia.

Differential Diagnosis

The differentiation between RSV and other respiratory viral infections can only be made by laboratory identification of the virus. Clues to RSV infection include wheezing, fever, and cough, which are prominent in RSV infection but may occur with other types of infection also. Bronchiolitis must be distinguished from pneumonia (lack of expiratory wheezing, prominence of pulmonary infiltrates) and allergic asthma (history of recurrence, family history, other signs or symptoms of atopy). Aspiration of a foreign body is characterized by a history of unilateral emphysema and diagnosed by endoscopic visualization; cystic fibrosis is diagnosed on the basis of sweat chloride determination, family history, and a history of meconium ileus or gastrointestinal symptoms.

Complications

Secondary bacterial infection may occur. Cardiac failure is a rare combination. Accumulating evidence suggests that RSV infections of the lung at a young age may be associated with restrictive airway dysfunction later in life.

Treatment

Maintenance of airway and oxygenation is critical and may be lifesaving in bronchiolitis. Cold vapor produced by bubbling oxygen through water should be administered by means of a croup tent. Hydration—usually by administration of intravenous fluids, since patients handle feedings poorly and may aspirate oral liquids—is essential. Expectorants have been used but seem less satisfactory than moist oxygen. If cardiac failure develops, administer digitalis.

Less well documented therapeutic attempts include administration of epinephrine (0.1 mL of 1:1000 solution subcutaneously) or aminophylline (5 mg/kg intravenously every 6 hours), administration of hydrocortisone (25 mg intravenously every 6 hours), tracheostomy, and intermittent positive pressure breathing. Controlled trials have not shown these methods of therapy to be superior to good nursing care with attention to oxygenation and moist air.

Ribavirin, an antiviral agent approved by the FDA in 1985, is recommended for treatment of moderate to severe RSV infection. Ribavirin is effective in shortening the course of illness and reducing the severity of symptoms and the amount of viral shedding. It is administered by continuous aerosol (6 g in 300 mL of water, delivered by a special aerosol apparatus) for 12–18 hours each day, usually for 3–8 days. Ribavirin is particularly useful in treating children with underlying diseases in whom RSV infection could cause serious morbidity or death.

Antibiotics have also been advocated, but there is no rationale for their use.

Prognosis

Bronchiolitis is rarely fatal, and recovery is usually complete. Respiratory symptoms and signs, cough, and wheezing may persist or may recur with subsequent respiratory infections whether or not they are due to RSV. There is considerable evidence linking RSV bronchiolitis to subsequent asthma.

Hall CB et al: Aerosolized ribavirin treatment of infants with respiratory syncytial virus infection. *N Engl J Med* 1983; **308:**1443.

Hall CB et al: Neonatal respiratory syncytial virus infection. *N Engl J Med* 1979;**300:**393.

Hall CB et al: Possible transmission by fomites of respiratory syncytial virus. *J Infect Dis* 1980;**141:**98.

Henry RL et al: Lung function after bronchiolitis. *Arch Dis Child* 1983;**58:**60.

McConnochie KM: Bronchiolitis: What's in the name? *Am J Dis Child* 1983;**137:**11.

Taber CL et al: Ribavirin aerosol treatment of bronchiolitis associated with respiratory syncytial virus infection in infants. *Pediatrics* 1983;**72:**613.

Twiggs JT et al: Respiratory syncytial virus infection: Ten-year follow-up. *Clin Pediatr* 1981;**20:**187.

MEASLES (Rubeola)

Essentials of Diagnosis

- History of exposure 9–14 days previously.
- Three-day prodrome consisting of fever, conjunctivitis, coryza, and cough.
- Koplik's spots—pathognomonic small whitish specks on a red base on buccal mucous membranes—appear 1–2 days before rash.
- Maculopapular, confluent rash begins at hairline and spreads downward over the face and body in 3 days.
- Leukopenia. Multinucleated giant cells (Warthin-Finkeldey cells) in oral and nasal scrapings.

General Considerations

Measles is an acute, highly contagious disease usually affecting preschool children. Prior to 1957, 95% of children were infected before age 15 years. As of 1984, 95% of school-age children have received vaccine. A residual group of young adults, especially those of college age, remains susceptible to the disease, and epidemics have occurred on college campuses. As many as 40% of measles cases presently occurring in the USA involve refugee children, citizens of the USA traveling abroad, and contacts linked to both groups.

Atypical measles may occur in recipients of killed virus vaccine.

Clinical Findings

A. History: A history of contact can usually be elicited and is particularly important in sporadic episodes. During epidemics, contact may be frequent and usually is with another member of the family.

B. Symptoms and Signs: After an incubation period of 9–14 days, the illness begins with high fever and lassitude, which persist and are accompanied in the next 3 days by increasing cough, coryza, and conjunctivitis. The cough is barking and harsh and is more noticeable at night. Severe conjunctival inflammation may be present, and photophobia is common. Preceding or accompanying the rash, Koplik's spots appear as small white specks on an intensely red base. Koplik's spots may be absent, but when present they are pathognomonic of measles. They may be few in number or may involve the entire buccal mucous membrane and occasionally are seen on the nasal mucous membranes also. The rash begins near the hairline as faint macules and papules and rapidly progresses to involve the face, trunk, and arms. When the rash appears on the lower extremities, it begins to fade on the face and then gradually disappears over an interval of 3–6 days. The lesions begin as discrete macules and papules and rapidly coalesce, involving large areas of skin. Fine desquamation may accompany healing. The coryzal symptoms reach their peak during the first 4–5 days and are accompanied by a harsh "barking" cough that persists throughout the illness, which lasts 9–10 days, and may be manifest after all other symptoms have subsided.

The general appearance (the "measly" look) of a child with florid measles is characteristic. The patient is red-eyed, with puffy eyelids and a swollen bridge of the nose, a distressed look, and copious, thin nasal secretions. The child with measles sits listlessly in bed, roused from apathy by bouts of violent harsh coughing. Combined with a confluent red rash, the clinical picture is one of extreme (though temporary) distress.

A severe form of measles is seen in young adults who received killed measles virus as children prior to 1965. Some cases have occurred despite receipt of live virus vaccine in the intervening period. This illness is characterized by fever, headache, abdominal pain, and pneumonia with or without pleural effusions. Rash occurs in an atypical distribution beginning on the distal extremities and spreading centrally but is usually sparse on the trunk. The rash may be morbilliform, petechial, vesicular, or, rarely, urticarial.

C. Laboratory Findings: Marked leukopenia is present early in the course. White blood cell counts as low as 1500–3000/μL are not uncommon, and lymphocytosis is marked. If bacterial superinfection occurs, abrupt leukocytosis with a shift to the left may be evident.

In the early stages, measles may be identified by fluorescent antibody staining of nasal or pharyngeal cells. However, this is seldom necessary to establish the diagnosis. A 4-fold rise in serum antibody can be demonstrated in paired sera.

D. X-Ray Findings: In typical, uncomplicated measles, chest x-rays may reveal patchy pneumonic infiltrates or the typical "hilar pneumonia" pattern. Overaeration is frequent, and in the presence of bacterial pneumonia the x-ray may reveal lobular or lobar consolidation. With staphylococcal or, less commonly, pneumococcal pneumonia, empyema or pyopneumothorax may be evident.

Differential Diagnosis

Measles must be differentiated from other common exanthematous diseases of childhood. Table 26–1 lists the principal distinguishing features of exanthematous diseases.

Abdominal pain (see below) in measles may be due to appendicitis or may result from gastrointestinal infection without appendicitis.

Acute prodromal measles with central nervous system manifestations must be differentiated from other

Table 26–1. Differential diagnosis of exanthematous diseases.

Disease	Incubation Period	Prodrome	Exanthem	Enanthem	Other Diagnostic Features
Measles	9–14 days	3 days. Cough, coryza, conjunctivitis.	Red, maculopapular, confluent, face to feet, lasts 7–10 days, may desquamate.	Koplik's spots	Cough prominent.
Rubella	14–21 days	Usually none	Pink, maculopapular, discrete, spreads rapidly, lasts 3–5 days.	None or faint	Lymphadenopathy may be prominent.
Roseola infantum	10–14 days	3 days. Fever; "well" child.	Rose, macular, discrete, fleeting.	None	Child remains well. Occasional febrile convulsion with first rise in temperature.
Fifth disease (erythema infectiosum)	About 7–14 days	None	"Slapped cheek," lacelike rash on extremities, may reappear, lasts 7–14 days.	Variable	Rash is characteristic. May appear when extremity is warmed (bathing, clothing, etc).
Scarlet fever	2–5 days	1–2 days. Fever, vomiting, sore throat.	Red, punctate, sandpaper feel, confluent blush, lasts 7 days, desquamation.	Red pharynx, tonsillitis, palatal petechiae, strawberry tongue.	Circumoral pallor, increased rash in skin folds, "toxic" child.
Enteroviral infection	Variable (usually short)	Variable	May resemble any of above. Echo, petechial; coxsackie, vesicular.	Variable	Concurrent familial illness, gastroenteritis, epidemic locally.

causes of fever and convulsions. The presence of conjunctivitis and cough is helpful, as is the finding of giant cells in nasal scrapings or the presence of Koplik's spots.

Complications & Sequelae

A. Upper and Lower Respiratory Tract Complications: Bacterial infection occurs in 5–15% of all cases of measles; otitis media and pneumonia are the most common forms. Sinusitis, mastoiditis, tonsillopharyngitis, and cervical adenitis also occur.

Viral complications include severe bronchial pneumonia and a peculiar viral pneumonia known as Hecht's giant cell pneumonia. The latter occurs frequently without rash and may be fatal.

B. Central Nervous System Complications: Encephalitis occurs in 1:1000 instances of measles. It begins with fever, central nervous system signs (coma, convulsions, bizarre behavior, etc), and vomiting 3–8 days after the onset of rash. Diagnosis can be suspected clinically and confirmed by the finding of cerebrospinal fluid pleocytosis (lymphocytosis) and an elevated cerebrospinal fluid protein, with normal or slightly elevated cerebrospinal fluid glucose content. Sixty percent of patients recover completely; 25% have severe sequelae; and the remainder die.

Rarely, a progressive degenerative central nervous system disease, ending in death, occurs as a late sequel (years after infection) of measles. This disease has had various eponyms attached to it but is currently termed subacute sclerosing panencephalitis. Specimens of brain from affected patients have been cocultured with measles virus-susceptible cells in tissue culture. Whole measles virus has been isolated by this method, providing direct evidence of its role in the disease. It is believed that measles virus remains latent in the neural cells of infected infants and children and produces the slowly progressive panencephalitis at some time in the future.

Some authorities maintain that latent or "slow" measles virus infections are also operative in multiple sclerosis and Jakob-Creutzfeldt disease, both chronic degenerative central nervous system diseases.

C. Hemorrhagic Measles: Rarely, a fulminating form of measles is seen, with hemorrhage into the gastrointestinal tract, mucous membranes, and central nervous system. Fever and toxicity are pronounced, and the rash is purpuric and typically morbilliform. Central nervous system symptoms (coma, convulsions, etc) may be prominent.

D. Thrombocytopenia: Following the onset of the rash, or days later, bleeding may occur into the rash. This is usually associated with a decrease in the platelet count.

E. Gastrointestinal Complications: These are uncommon in the USA but are a leading cause of death elsewhere. True appendicitis, diarrhea, and vomiting may be observed, often with a progressive course and fatal outcome.

F. Ophthalmologic Complications: Secondary bacterial conjunctivitis is common. Corneal ulceration, gangrenous meibomianitis, membranous conjunctivitis, and optic nerve damage are rare complications of measles.

G. Cardiac Complications: Myocarditis and cardiac failure occur occasionally.

H. Effect on Other Diseases and Conditions: Measles during pregnancy may result in stillbirth, abortion, or premature delivery. Tuberculosis is exacerbated by intercurrent measles, and transient anergy to tuberculin is frequent. Nephrosis, asthma, and eczema may temporarily abate during measles virus infection.

Measles can be lethal in immunocompromised individuals; these patients develop severe disease, often associated with pneumonia.

Treatment & Prognosis

Good nursing care is essential, with attention to relief of cough, maintenance of clear nasal passages, reduction of fever, and cleansing of the conjunctivae.

Bacterial complications should be specifically diagnosed and effective antimicrobial therapy employed. Streptococcal infections are common.

Antimicrobial prophylaxis should not be used, since it may result in bacterial infections with resistant organisms.

Measles is usually a self-limited disease lasting 7–10 days. Most often it is without permanent sequelae, although it is a severe infection. The most serious complication, encephalitis, may result in permanent disability or death in 40% of cases.

Amler RW et al: Imported measles in the United States. *JAMA* 1982;**248:**2129.

Bloch AB et al: Measles outbreak in a pediatric practice. *Pediatrics* 1985;**75:**676.

Centers for Disease Control: *Measles Surveillance, Report No. 11*. US Public Health Service, September, 1982.

Hinman AR: Measles and rubella in adolescents and young adults. *Hosp Pract* (Oct) 1982;**17:**137.

Hinman AR: World eradication of measles. *Rev Infect Dis* 1982;**4:**933.

Krause PJ et al: Epidemic measles in young adults. *Ann Intern Med* 1979;**90:**873.

Levy DL: The future of measles in highly immunized populations. *Am J Epidemiol* 1984;**120:**39.

Miller CL: Deaths from measles in England and Wales, 1970–1983. *Br Med J* 1985;**290:**443.

Modlin JF et al: Epidemiologic studies of measles, measles vaccine and subacute sclerosing panencephalitis. *Pediatrics* 1977;**59:**375.

Narain JP et al: Imported measles outbreak in a university. *Am J Public Health* 1985;**75:**397.

Siegel MM, Walter TK, Ablin AR: Measles pneumonia in childhood leukemia. *Pediatrics* 1977;**60:**38.

PICORNAVIRUSES

The picornaviruses include the enteroviruses (poliovirus, echovirus, and coxsackievirus) and the rhinoviruses.

ENTEROVIRAL INFECTIONS

The enteroviruses resemble one another in size, morphology, and biochemical and biophysical characteristics and also in the illnesses they cause. Since a large majority of the types of enteroviral infections can be produced by more than one type of virus, we will present the common clinical categories and then refer to specific syndromes peculiar to each of the groups.

Types of Infection Common to All Enteroviruses

A. Fever Alone: Infection may be accompanied solely by fever of variable height and duration.

B. Respiratory Illness: Undifferentiated upper respiratory infection may occur.

C. Gastrointestinal Illness: Nausea, vomiting, and diarrhea have been associated with enteroviral infection.

D. Exanthematous Illnesses: A variety of rashes have been reported, including scarlatiniform, morbilliform, rubelliform, petechial, and vesicular varieties.

E. Combinations of Above: Illnesses in which all or some of the above symptoms occur together have been recorded. This is particularly true for the echovirus group.

F. Central Nervous System Infections:

1. Aseptic meningitis—Fever, gastrointestinal symptoms associated with nuchal rigidity, headache, lethargy, and cerebrospinal fluid pleocytosis can result from infection with any of the enteroviruses.

2. Encephalitis—Cortical symptoms, including disturbances of sensorium, convulsions, and coma, have been noted.

3. Paralytic illness—Although occasionally due to the echoviruses or coxsackieviruses, this syndrome is almost exclusively produced by polioviruses and will be considered separately below.

G. Isolated Myocarditis: Inflammation of the myocardium with attendant precordial chest pain, dyspnea, cough, tachycardia, cyanosis, and fulminant congestive heart failure has been attributed to poliovirus and coxsackievirus infection.

Krajden S, Middleton PJ: Enterovirus infections in the neonate. *Clin Pediatr* 1983;**22:**87.

Morens DM: Enteroviral disease in early infancy. *J Pediatr* 1978;**92:**374.

Wilfert CM et al: Longitudinal assessment of children with

enteroviral meningitis during the first three months of life. *Pediatrics* 1981;**67:**811.

1. PARALYTIC POLIOMYELITIS

Essentials of Diagnosis

- Muscle weakness, headache, stiff neck, fever, nausea, vomiting, sore throat.
- Lower motor neuron lesion (flaccid paralysis) with decreased deep tendon reflexes and muscle wasting.
- Cerebrospinal fluid shows excess cells. Lymphocytes predominate; rarely more than 500/μL.
- No history of immunization.

Clinical Findings

A. Symptoms and Signs: Following (or blending with) an undifferentiated illness (fever, lassitude, gastrointestinal symptoms), the onset of paralysis is heralded by nuchal rigidity and stiffness of the back. Varying degrees of central nervous system depression or excitability may be observed, followed by pain and tenderness in the affected muscles, a brief period of hypertonicity and spasm with transient hyperactive reflexes, asymmetric flaccid paralysis, and loss of superficial and deep reflexes but maintenance of sensation. Deviations from the above pattern are common, especially in very young infants.

Involvement of the cervical spinal cord segments and the brain stem may lead to respiratory muscle paralysis and cranial nerve involvement with palatal, facial, and laryngeal paralysis. Severe involvement results in loss of function of the respiratory and circulatory centers, with irregular respirations, apnea, and peripheral vascular collapse.

Paralysis generally extends during the first week, reaching its limits as the fever subsides. No change is noted for days or weeks; if spontaneous recovery is to occur, muscle strength and function and reflexes begin to improve at this time. The ultimate extent of paralysis should not be judged until 12–18 months have passed without continuing improvement. In recent years, paralytic poliomyelitis has been observed in the following groups: (1) those infected outside the USA; (2) normal children following oral poliovirus vaccine; (3) contacts of immunized children; and (4) immunodeficient or immunosuppressed individuals.

B. Laboratory Findings: Poliovirus may be isolated from the throat or the stools. Fecal excretion may persist for weeks beyond the acute phase. The specific viral agent can be detected by a serum antibody increase in paired sera.

Cerebrospinal fluid findings are those of aseptic meningitis. There may be mild early pleocytosis with polymorphonuclear leukocytosis rapidly shifting to lymphocytosis. Protein concentration is normal initially, but during the second to third weeks of illness it rises roughly in parallel with the paralysis.

Differential Diagnosis

Most cases of paralytic poliomyelitis occurring in the USA in recent years are (1) due to other enteroviruses, (2) due to infrequent epidemics with wild strains in unimmunized individuals, or (3) secondary to oral poliovirus vaccine. With the dramatic reduction in wild virus, the few cases of nonepidemic paralytic disease are of types (1) and (3). Therefore, the clinician should make every effort both to report paralytic disease and to obtain appropriate viral cultures and paired sera for etiologic identification. Local health departments in liaison with the Centers for Disease Control in Atlanta can provide the necessary consultation and laboratory assistance.

Aseptic meningitis due to any cause may be confused with poliovirus infection. However, paralysis is usually due to poliovirus infection and must be differentiated from Guillain-Barré syndrome or infective polyneuritis (sensory loss frequently present, symmetric paralysis, cerebrospinal fluid shows albuminocytologic dissociation, ie, high protein concentration, little or no increase in leukocytes), other infective polyneuritides (history of preceding illness, mumps, diphtheria, etc), and paralysis or pseudoparalysis due to other causes (signs of scurvy, syphilis, fractures, arthritides, infection of bone, etc).

Complications & Sequelae

Bulbar poliomyelitis may result in respiratory arrest, muscular or central in origin, requiring assisted ventilation and tracheostomy.

Paralysis may remain and result in loss of function, necessitating relearning, bracing, wheelchair ambulation, etc.

Hypertension is usually brief in duration but may persist.

Immobilization in a respirator may result in stasis pneumonia, decubitus ulcers, renal calculi, and disuse atrophy of nonparalyzed muscles. Careful attention to skin care, exercising, and coughing will help to prevent these complications.

Treatment & Prognosis

Complete bed rest is essential. The immediate disability must be accurately assessed so that difficulties can be anticipated and treated promptly rather than as an emergency. Special attention must be given to neurologic evaluation to detect beginning respiratory paralysis.

The Kenny method (heat packs) reduces spasm and tenderness and makes possible early rehabilitation to avoid disease atrophy and reeducate involved muscle groups.

A clear airway should be maintained, preferably without the use of intubation, either endotracheal or transtracheal. If necessary, tracheostomy should be anticipated and performed electively in an operating suite with experts in attendance under optimal conditions. The use of oxygen, assisted ventilation, and humid respirators may be necessary.

The mortality rate in paralytic disease varies from 5 to 10%, and permanent incapacitating paralysis occurs in 15% of cases. Mild paralysis may occur in as many as 30% of cases. In general, pregnant women and other adults are more severely affected than infants and children.

Fulginiti VA: Poliomyelitis. In: *Infectious Diseases,* 3rd ed. Hoeprich P (editor). Harper & Row, 1983.

Fulginiti VA: The problems of poliovirus immunization. *Hosp Pract* (Aug) 1980;**15:**61.

Furesz J et al: Viral and epidemiological links between poliomyelitis outbreaks in unprotected communities in Canada and the Netherlands. *Lancet* 1978;**2:**1248.

Horstmann D: Control of poliomyelitis: A continuing paradox. *J Infect Dis* 1982;**146:**540.

Moore LM et al: Poliomyelitis in the United States, 1969–1981. *J Infect Dis* 1982;**146:**558.

Nathanson N, Martin JR: The epidemiology of poliomyelitis: Enigmas surrounding its appearance, epidemicity and disappearance. *Am J Epidemiol* 1979;**110:**672.

Wyatt HV: Poliomyelitis in the fetus and newborn: Comments on the pathogenesis. *Clin Pediatr* 1979;**18:**33.

2. HERPANGINA (Coxsackie A Virus, Types 2–6, 8, & 10)

There are usually no prodromal symptoms in herpangina. Similar illnesses may be observed in the community, or other forms of coxsackievirus infection may be noted.

Herpangina is characterized by fever, sore throat and painful swallowing, anorexia, and vomiting, which occur with abrupt onset in association with tiny vesicles (which rapidly ulcerate) on the anterior fauces and elsewhere in the posterior pharynx. The ulcers are often arrayed linearly on the anterior fauces, lending a characteristic (diagnostic) appearance to the throat. Fever may be prominent, particularly in the young. Convulsions may occur with the first rise in temperature. Symptoms and signs persist for 2–6 days.

Virus can be isolated from throat swab and stool specimens. Serologic diagnosis is of aid only in epidemics, where the specific virus type has been isolated.

Herpangina in its classic form is seldom confused with other illnesses. Oral ulceration associated with fever is seen in primary herpetic gingivostomatitis (ulcers over most of the oral mucosa, lack of epidemic pattern). Distinguish also from aphthous ulceration (usually no fever; lesions may be anterior), ulcerative pharyngitis associated with leukemia or its treatment (lymphadenopathy, splenomegaly, etc; characteristic peripheral blood and bone marrow changes), and other viral exanthems (history of contact, exanthem, course of disease).

Parotitis or vaginal ulceration may occur, but recovery is complete.

The disease is self-limited, and only symptomatic therapy is required.

3. PLEURODYNIA (Coxsackie B Viruses; Epidemic Myalgia; Bornholm Disease)

Pleurodynia may begin with vague prodromal symptoms of malaise, anorexia, headache, and muscle aches, but the onset is usually unheralded and abrupt. Other coxsackievirus infections may be observed in the community. Pleurodynia may be epidemic.

Pleurodynia characteristically begins with severe, usually unilateral chest pain that frequently is paroxysmal and pleuritic and therefore is aggravated by respiratory movements. The patient is asymptomatic between episodes. The pain is severe and dramatically described by the patient as crushing or viselike (hence the name "devil's grip"). Headache, fever, malaise, apprehension, abdominal pain, hiccups, vomiting, diarrhea, and stiff neck have all been noted. The illness may last as long as a week but is quite variable. Mild forms are also seen. Physical signs include apprehension, fever, limitation of respiratory excursions, muscle tenderness, normal breath sounds, and an ipsilateral pleural friction rub in 25% of cases. Mild to moderate nuchal rigidity may be present.

Virus can be recovered from the stools or from throat swabs. Serologic diagnosis may be possible, since coxsackie B3 and B5 are the most common offenders, but any of the group B coxsackieviruses can produce the disease.

Any cause of sudden pleurisy must be distinguished from pleurodynia. Thus, bacterial pneumonia (leukocytosis, empyema, productive cough, bacteriologic findings), tuberculosis (history of exposure, positive tuberculin test, identification of mycobacteria), and other infectious and noninfectious causes of pleuritis must be differentiated. Abdominal or muscular pain may suggest acute surgical conditions (appendicitis, ulcer, perforation, etc). The superficial nature of the tenderness, the associated fever and pulmonary findings, and epidemiologic evidence may suggest the diagnosis of pleurodynia.

Almost all patients recover completely without complications. A few cases have been reported in association with aseptic meningitis, orchitis, pericarditis, and pneumonia.

Analgesics, splinting of the chest, and other supportive measures are indicated.

Grist NR, Bell EJ, Assaad F: Enteroviruses in human disease. *Prog Med Virol* 1978;**24:**114.

4. GENERALIZED NEONATAL INFECTION (Coxsackie B Viruses)

Sudden onset of fever associated with acute heart failure occurring in more than one infant should arouse the suspicion of generalized neonatal infection. Sick infants are usually in nurseries or recently discharged.

Case finding is important and may lead to the correct diagnosis. A history of mild gastrointestinal symptoms 1–2 days before the major illness is common. The mother may have had an upper respiratory tract infection just prior to delivery. Cyanosis, tachycardia, and increasing size of the liver and heart are all observed. Pneumonic symptoms may predominate early, and cough, dyspnea, and vomiting are prominent manifestations. In more than half of cases, the disease progresses rapidly to death in circulatory collapse. Cardiac murmurs are not heard. Despite the preponderance of cardiac signs and symptoms, the infection is a generalized one, and encephalitis, pancreatitis, focal hepatitis, and myositis are all observed at autopsy. Electrocardiographic changes are those of severe myocardial damage. Chest x-ray reveals a large heart.

In general, the illness is produced by coxsackieviruses B3 and B4. Virus can be recovered from the feces before death and from the myocardium and other tissues postmortem. Serologic confirmation is possible in surviving infants.

Other causes of acute congestive heart failure in neonates must be considered, but the epidemic nature and findings of coxsackievirus infection should be diagnostic.

Intensive supportive measures, including oxygenation, support of ventilation and circulation, and digitalization, are mandatory.

Reported mortality rates are variable but approach or exceed 50%. If the patient survives, recovery is rapid and complete.

Morens DM: Enteroviral disease in early infancy. *J Pediatr* 1978;**92:**374.

5. ISOLATED MYOCARDITIS & PERICARDITIS (Coxsackie B Viruses)

Myocardial or pericardial infection with coxsackieviruses occurs in humans and in several other animal species. The clinical findings are similar to those observed in myocarditis or pericarditis due to other causes. Severity ranges from very mild clinical disease to fulminant fatal infections. The diagnosis is suggested by the clinical findings and substantiated by virus isolation from the stools or pericardial fluid during life, from the myocardium postmortem, or by a rise in serum antibody in paired sera in survivors.

Myocarditis is treated as outlined above for generalized neonatal infection. Pericardial aspiration is indicated for pericarditis.

Barson WJ et al: Survival following myocarditis and myocardial calcification associated with infection by coxsackie virus B-4. *Pediatrics* 1981;**68:**79.

El-Hagrassy MMO et al: Coxsackie B virus-specific IgM responses in patients with cardiac and other diseases. *Lancet* 1980;**2:**1160.

6. ACUTE LYMPHONODULAR PHARYNGITIS (Coxsackie A Virus, Type 10)

Papular whitish-yellow lesions of the uvula, anterior pillars, and pharynx in association with sore throat, fever, and headache have been observed in a single outbreak of coxsackievirus A10 infection. The illness lasted for 1–2 weeks and was uncomplicated. The papules did not vesiculate, which differentiates this disease from herpangina.

Treatment is symptomatic.

7. VESICULAR EXANTHEM (Hand-Foot-Mouth Disease; Coxsackie A Virus, Types 5, 10, & 16)

Several epidemics of a vesicular exanthem, which in its complete form involves the oral mucosa, tongue, and interdigital and digital surfaces of both the upper and lower extremities (hence the term hand-foot-mouth disease), have occurred owing to infection with coxsackievirus A16. Incomplete forms are also seen, and coxsackievirus A16 may cause nonvesicular disease in the community at the same time.

Diagnosis is by virologic isolation and serology. Treatment is symptomatic.

Archibald E, Purdham DR: Coxsackievirus type A-16 infection in a neonate. *Arch Dis Child* 1979;**56:**649.

Ishimaru Y et al: Outbreaks of hand, foot, and mouth disease by enterovirus 71. *Arch Dis Child* 1980;**55:**583.

8. ECHOVIRUS EXANTHEMATOUS DISEASE

Echovirus types 4, 9, and 16 have been definitely associated with epidemics of exanthematous illness; 10 other echovirus types have also been related to such illnesses. Other clinical findings have also been noted, including the aseptic meningitis syndrome.

Echovirus types 4 and 9 cause a usually maculopapular but sometimes petechial rash, and vesicular rashes, even with crusting, have occasionally been noted. Association with aseptic meningitis and lymphadenitis has been observed. The rash is usually present for just a few days but may persist for 10 days.

In echovirus type 16 disease (Boston exanthem), the rash appears during or shortly after defervescence, thus simulating roseola infantum. A punched-out ulcerative exanthem may be seen. Aseptic meningitis due to echovirus 16 usually occurs without rash. The rash lasts 1–5 days and may be associated with pharyngitis and cervical, suboccipital, and postauricular lymphadenopathy, but there are no appreciable respiratory symptoms.

Hall C et al: The return of Boston exanthem. *Am J Dis Child* 1977;**131:**323.

Morens DM, Zweighaft RM, Bryant JM: Non-polio enterovirus disease in the United States, 1971–1975. *Int J Epidemiol* 1979;**8:**49.

RHINOVIRAL INFECTIONS

A large group of viruses with properties similar to those of the enteroviruses have recently been shown to cause the common cold in adults. The role of these rhinoviruses in the production of disease in infants and children is not completely understood at present. They have been isolated from the nose and throat in a wide range of upper respiratory illnesses in children and less frequently in lower tract diseases.

Gwaltney JM, Hendley JO: Rhinovirus transmission. *Am J Epidemiol* 1978;**107:**357.

HERPESVIRUSES

HERPES SIMPLEX

Essentials of Diagnosis

- Recurrent small grouped vesicles on an erythematous base, especially around oral and genital areas.
- May follow minor infections, trauma, stress, or sun exposure.
- Regional lymph nodes may be swollen and tender.

General Considerations

Primary herpesvirus infection is asymptomatic in most individuals. When manifestations occur, they usually take the form of gingivostomatitis in children under 4 or 5 years of age. Secondary (recurrent) infection occurs far more frequently even in the absence of a history of primary infection; thus, the virus is felt to remain hidden or "latent" following first infection. Various excitants (fever, menses, trauma, severe infections, etc) can "uncover" the virus and cause a "fever blister" or "cold sore" type of infection. Thus, immunity is imperfect despite demonstrable levels of circulating antibody.

Two types of herpesvirus have been identified. Type 1 is involved in lesions of the oral cavity, central nervous system, and skin. Type 2 is responsible for genital disease and probably accounts for all cases of congenital herpesvirus infection. Type 2 has also been linked with carcinoma of the cervix. Occasionally, type 1 virus causes infection in sites usually infected by type 2 virus, and vice versa.

Clinical Findings.

A. History: In primary infections, no history of previous disease is elicited. In recurrent disease, a history of severe gingivostomatitis or vulvovaginitis in early childhood can sometimes be elicited, and a history of similar episodes following exposure to the same excitants is usually present.

B. Symptoms and Signs:

1. Herpetic gingivostomatitis—Fever, irritability, pain in the mouth and throat and upon attempted swallowing, and lassitude with disinterest in surroundings are seen in varying degrees. Examination reveals extensive shallow, yellowish ulcers of the buccal, gingival, tonsillar, and pharyngeal mucosae, frequently with crusting of the lips, a half-open mouth with drooling, foul breath odor, and cervical lymphadenopathy. The disease lasts 7–14 days.

2. Herpetic vulvovaginitis or urethritis—Manifestations are similar to those of gingivostomatitis (both may occur) except that they appear on the vulva and vagina. Urination may be painful or withheld, especially in males. Inguinal lymphadenopathy is frequently present.

3. Recurrent herpetic lesions—Sensory symptoms varying from vague discomfort to neuralgic pain may precede or accompany the appearance of erythematous papules on the mucocutaneous junction of the lips. Rapid vesiculation, pustulation, and crusting occur. Fever is usually absent unless it is the inciting factor. Regional lymphadenopathy and lymphadenitis occur infrequently. Lesions appear in groups and tend to involve the same area in recurrences. Severity is variable, and the illness often causes discomfort without being incapacitating.

4. Herpetic keratoconjunctivitis—A variety of forms of herpetic corneal infection have been described according to the depth and extent of the infection. Almost all forms are accompanied by conjunctival inflammation, often purulent in appearance. Cloudiness and ulceration of the cornea may be noted. Ulceration may be diagnosed by application of fluorescein to the eye, whereupon a dendritic (branched) pattern may be seen. Deeper forms include stromal edema and hypopyon with rupture of the globe. Ophthalmologic consultation is indicated for accurate diagnosis and treatment.

5. Herpetic encephalitis—This rare disease may take the form of aseptic meningitis or may begin with cortical symptoms and cranial nerve palsies. Convulsions and coma are frequent, and death occurs in the second to third weeks of illness.

6. Neonatal herpetic infection—This form of infection occurs in infants of nonimmune parents, and a history of recent herpesvirus infection in either parent may be obtained. The illness may be present at birth but usually manifests itself in the first week of life with generalized vesiculation of the skin, high or low temperature, jaundice, progressive hepatosplenomegaly, dyspnea, signs of cardiac failure, hemorrhage, and central nervous system manifestations. Death occurs following a 2- to 4-day course of illness. "Mild" neonatal herpetic infections result in vesicular rash usually unassociated with overt central nervous system disease. The rash may recur repeatedly in the first months of life, and central nervous system function may ultimately be impaired. A congenital anomaly syndrome is associated with early intrauterine infection (microcephaly, mental retardation, intracranial calcifications, microphthalmia, retinal dysplasia, and chorioretinitis).

7. Eczema herpeticum (Kaposi's varicelliform eruption)—The appearance of fever, prostration, and vesicular lesions in a patient with eczema should lead to a diagnosis of intercurrent herpesvirus or vaccinia virus infection. Although varying in severity, eczema herpeticum is frequently fulminant and fatal, especially when large areas of skin are involved.

C. Laboratory Findings: Cerebrospinal fluid pleocytosis (lymphocytosis) is present in aseptic meningitis. Virus can be recovered from vesicular fluid, skin and corneal scrapings, throat swabs, blood, cerebrospinal fluid, and appropriate tissue specimens. Enrichment of the collection medium with protein enhances virus stability if a delay in handling specimens is unavoidable. Brain biopsy is essential in diagnosing encephalitis and in choosing antiviral therapy.

A 4-fold or greater rise in serum antibody is detectable in paired sera from patients with primary infection. This is of little aid in recurrent infection, since titer rises do not occur. A negative titer may help to rule out herpesvirus in vesicular lesions.

Smears taken from the bases of vesicles or ulcers suspected of being herpetic can be stained with hematoxylin and eosin to reveal the typical Cowdry type A intranuclear inclusion bodies. These consist of eosinophilic oval masses within the nucleus, which has marginal chromatin. Fixation produces a distinct halo around the inclusion. Giemsa stains of tissue best visualize the giant cells with their multinucleate or syncytial structure.

Immunofluorescence can rapidly identify herpesvirus in original specimens and in tissue culture; differentiation of types 1 and 2 can also be made.

Electron microscopic examination of vesicular fluid may result in rapid identification of herpes simplex virus, as can fluorescent antibody staining.

Differential Diagnosis

Herpetic gingivostomatitis must be differentiated from herpangina (posterior pharyngeal ulcers only, linear array on anterior pillars, isolation of coxsackie A viruses); aphthous ulceration (one or only a few ulcers, previous history, lack of systemic symptoms); ulcerative pharyngitis of agranulocytic disease (history, other physical findings, blood and bone marrow findings); and Stevens-Johnson syndrome (multiple mucosal involvement, "iris" lesions of skin, history of sulfonamide or other drug ingestion).

Recurrent herpes labialis can easily be differentiated from impetigo by the characteristic history and course of the former and bacterial isolation and response to treatment of the latter.

Herpetic keratoconjunctivitis must be differentiated from vaccinial keratoconjunctivitis (history or presence of recent vaccination or contact, isolation of virus) and from adenovirus keratoconjunctivitis (pain in adenovirus infection of cornea, epidemic nature, isolation of virus).

Meningoencephalitis can only be differentiated from other causes by laboratory studies.

Generalized neonatal infection is differentiated from similar illness due to coxsackie B viruses by lack of skin involvement, epidemic nature in nursery, and isolation of virus.

Eczema vaccinatum can be differentiated from eczema herpeticum by the history of exposure to smallpox vaccination, typical vacciniform lesions, and the fact that eczema vaccinatum lesions tend to be in the same stage. In some cases, differentiation is difficult and laboratory diagnosis is necessary.

Complications, Sequelae, & Prognosis

Primary skin and mucosal infections are usually self-limited, with complete and prompt recovery, although limited recurrences occur.

Herpetic keratoconjunctivitis can lead to blindness or perforation of the cornea with loss of the eye.

Encephalitis or neonatal generalized infection is frequently fatal.

Treatment

A. Specific Measures: A variety of topical agents have proved effective in the treatment of herpetic corneal infection, including 1% trifluridine, 3% acyclovir, 3% vidarabine, and 0.1% and 0.5% idoxuridine. All are about equally effective, but the best results appear to be with trifluridine, approaching 97% cure rates for dendritic and geographic corneal lesions. One drop of the 1% solution of trifluridine is administered every 2 hours during the day until healing has occurred and then every 4 hours while awake during an additional 7 days. Trifluridine should be tried in patients in whom other antiviral solutions or ointments have been ineffective.

Oral acyclovir has been shown to be effective in reducing the amount of viral shedding, the number of new lesions, and the amount of time for crusting to occur in primary and recurrent herpetic lesions of the genital tract. Primary lesions appear to respond better than recurrent lesions. The adult dose is 200 mg 5 times daily for 10 days.

Many topical agents have been advocated for use in either treatment or suppression of recurrent herpetic lesions of the mucosa or skin. Except for topical acyclovir (which has less effect than oral acyclovir), these topical agents are not effective and should be avoided.

Some experience has been gained with the use of systemic antiviral agents in the treatment of herpetic encephalitis and generalized neonatal infection. Idoxuridine and both cytarabine and vidarabine have been utilized, though idoxuridine and cytarabine have been abandoned, and the best results have been obtained with intravenous acyclovir and intravenous vidarabine. Of the 2 drugs, acyclovir appears to be less toxic. Mortality rates are dramatically reduced (3-

fold). Controlled trials are under way comparing both drugs at dosages of 30 mg/kg/d in the treatment of neonatal herpetic infections. At the present time, intravenous acyclovir (30 mg/kg/d for 5–10 days) appears to be the drug of choice of most experts, pending the results of the ongoing trials. It must be administered in a 1-hour infusion 3 times daily (10 mg/kg per dose).

In anecdotal reports, immune globulin has been claimed to be beneficial in neonatal herpetic infections. The doses have been large, and because of the variability of the disease, these reports cannot be validated. This must be regarded as a questionable use of immune globulin (see Chapter 5).

B. General Measures: In gingivostomatitis, considerable discomfort is experienced, with resultant lack of fluid and caloric intake. Since this is a 7- to 14-day illness, maintenance of fluid intake is vital. Dehydration can be avoided by hospitalization and intravenous administration of fluids and electrolytes. In less severe instances, discovering the optimal temperature of fluids tolerated (cool is usually best) can ensure intake. It is rarely necessary to use topical "caine" anesthetics, thus avoiding potential sensitization. Mild antiseptic mouthwashes are occasionally of benefit. Local antibiotics are not useful. Systemic administration of analgesics occasionally is necessary and facilitates intake of food and fluids.

The treatment of encephalitis and neonatal infection is symptomatic and supportive (see above).

Specific measures for treatment of herpetic keratoconjunctivitis are discussed above. The use of topical corticosteroids in the acute ulcerative disease is contraindicated. In instances of stromal edema or of persistent deep lesions, topical corticosteroids may be of aid but should be combined with other topical agents and given only under an ophthalmologist's direction.

Eczema herpeticum is best treated as an extensive "burn" so that appropriate attention is directed to replacement of fluid and electrolytes and to protein nutrition. Prevention of secondary bacterial infection is accomplished by continuous bacteriologic guidance and antibacterial therapy.

In severe complications, the use of systemic corticosteroids is often advocated. There are theoretic objections to the use of such agents, since experimental evidence indicates that they enhance viral spread. Immune globulin has been advocated, but there is no evidence of beneficial effect.

Recurrent herpes labialis has been treated in a variety of ways, including injections of vitamin B_{12}, the use of reticulose (a supposed antiviral substance), and repeat smallpox vaccination. No evidence of a controlled nature is available to indicate that any of these or other forms of therapy are uniformly beneficial. Saline injections and no other treatment can result in "cure" of recurrent infection. Smallpox vaccination has resulted in untoward effects in some patients and should be avoided.

In pregnancies complicated by herpetic cervicitis or infection of the external genitalia, cesarean section has been advocated to prevent contamination of the infant during passage through the birth canal. It is now recommended that all pregnant women be monitored for herpetic cervicitis. If a positive culture is obtained, weekly monitoring in the last trimester is recommended, and vaginal delivery should be allowed only if the last cultures are negative.

American Academy of Pediatrics: Perinatal herpes simplex virus infections. *Pediatrics* 1980;**66:**147.

Bader C et al: The natural history of recurrent facial-oral infection with herpes simplex virus. *J Infect Dis* 1978;**138:**897.

Laskin OL: Acyclovir: Pharmacology and clinical experience. *Arch Intern Med* 1984;**144:**1241.

Light IJ: Postnatal acquisition of herpes simplex virus by the newborn infant: A review of the literature. *Pediatrics* 1979;**63:**480.

Nahmias AJ, Roizman B: Infection with herpes simplex viruses 1 and 2. (3 parts.) *N Engl J Med* 1973;**289:**667, 719, 781.

Nicholson KG: Antiviral therapy: Herpes simplex encephalitis, neonatal herpes infections, and chronic hepatitis B. *Lancet* 1984;**2:**736.

Nicholson KG: Antiviral therapy: Respiratory infections, genital herpes, and herpetic keratitis. *Lancet* 1984;**2:**617.

Parvey LS, Ch'ien LT: Neonatal herpes simplex virus infection introduced by fetal monitor scalp electrodes. *Pediatrics* 1980;**65:**1150.

Schreiner RL et al: Maternal oral herpes: Isolation policy. *Pediatrics* 1979;**63:**247.

Whiteley RJ et al: Herpes simplex encephalitis. *N Engl J Med* 1981;**304:**313.

Whiteley RJ et al: Vidarabine therapy of neonatal herpes simplex virus infection. *Pediatrics* 1980;**66:**495.

VARICELLA (Chickenpox) & HERPES ZOSTER (Shingles)

Essentials of Diagnosis

Varicella:

- History of exposure within 2–3 weeks; appearance of characteristic vesicles over a period of 2–5 days, usually without prodrome.
- Lesions rapidly evolve from macules to papules to "dewdrop" superficial vesicles to encrustation in centripetal distribution. Macules, papules, vesicles, and crusts are all observable at any one time (pleomorphic).

Herpes zoster:

- History of chickenpox.
- Preeruptive pain (infrequent in children) in region of rash.
- Clusters of confluent vesicles in unilateral dermatomal distribution. Successive crops may appear.
- Examination of early vesicular scrapings reveals Tzanck giant cells or characteristic intranuclear inclusions (see Herpes Simplex, above).

General Considerations

Varicella and herpes zoster are caused by the same virus. Varicella is the primary infection, and herpes zoster appears to be a recurrent infection. In the USA, varicella is primarily a disease of childhood; in large areas of the tropics, it is principally a disease of adults. No known animal reservoir exists, and the disease is transmitted from person to person in epidemics with a high degree of contagiousness (80–90% of exposed susceptibles are infected). Herpes zoster is sporadic and considerably less infectious, resulting in varicella in 15% of exposed susceptibles.

Clinical Findings

A. History: A history of contact 10–20 days (average, 12–13 days) prior to onset is typically obtained. There is usually no prodrome, but a mild febrile illness with rhinitis is occasionally noted for 1–3 days before the rash appears. A history of contact may be lacking in zoster, but the disease has occurred (in adults) following exposure to varicella. Severe pain along the nerve root distribution of the rash may precede the rash by several days.

B. Symptoms and Signs:

1. Varicella—In typical varicella, the onset is abrupt with the appearance of the rash. Systemic symptoms, if any, are mild. The rash appears in crops, with faint erythematous macules rapidly developing into papules and vesicles. The vesicles are characteristic; they are thin-walled and superficially located on the skin, with a distinct areola (dewdrop on a red base). They rupture easily, rapidly encrust, and frequently become impetiginized. Successive crops (usually 3) appear in the next 2–5 days, giving rise to the pleomorphic appearance of the rash: lesions in all stages can be seen at one time. The rash is heaviest on the trunk and sparse on the extremities. If there is no bacterial infection, the crust falls off in 1–3 weeks, leaving no scars.

Deviations from the above pattern vary from very mild disease with just a few vesicles to as many as 5 successive crops with involvement of most of the skin. Rarely, hemorrhagic lesions occur and are associated with thrombocytopenia, particularly in children with leukemia receiving antimetabolites. Infrequently, a zosterlike cluster of lesions appears during the course of primary varicella. Bullous and gangrenous forms are recognized.

Systemic symptoms are usually absent or mild but may be severe, and they generally parallel the extent of skin involvement.

An enanthem is recognizable and consists of shallow mucosal ulceration (the vesicle is rarely seen). When it involves the posterior pharynx or esophagus, swallowing may be painful and difficult.

2. Zoster—Herpes zoster is usually unilateral and limited to one or more adjacent dermatomes. Thoracic and lumbar forms are most common, although the ophthalmic division of the trigeminal nerve, cervical roots, and other divisions may be affected. Maculopapules appear in closely arrayed patches, rapidly vesiculate, and frequently coalesce; they follow the dermal distribution of the nerve root and often end abruptly at the midline of the body. Concomitant or preceding pain, often very severe, occurs less frequently in children than in adults.

C. Laboratory Findings: The usual laboratory tests are of little aid. Sepsis may be accompanied by an abrupt increase in the white blood cell count with neutrophilia.

Although virus isolation and serologic tests are available, they are seldom necessary. Etiologic identification may be important in distinguishing varicella from smallpox or in the diagnosis of unusual and atypical forms of the disease.

Giant cells with multinucleate or syncytial structure may be found in vesicular scrapings, as may inclusion bodies of the eosinophilic intranuclear type (Cowdry type A).

D. X-Ray Findings: Chest films may reveal diffuse nodular pneumonia ("viral") and emphysema in varicella pneumonia.

Differential Diagnosis

Typical chickenpox is seldom confused with other illnesses. Severe forms must, in rare cases, be differentiated from smallpox (history of exposure, typical 3-day severe prodrome, lesions all in same stage of development, centrifugal distribution, hard, pearly, nodular, deep-seated lesions, absence of giant cells and intranuclear inclusions, isolation of the virus) and mild forms from the vesicular exanthem due to coxsackievirus infection (sparseness of rash, history of chickenpox, failure to form crusts, isolation of specific virus). Also to be distinguished are impetigo (lack of exposure history, response to therapy), multiple insect bites or papular urticaria (history of bites, papular and excoriated but no vesicles), rickettsialpox (primary eschar, smaller lesions, lack of crusting, serologic diagnosis), and dermatitis herpetiformis (chronic course, symmetry of eruption, urticaria, residual pigmentation).

Complications & Sequelae

Complications are uncommon. Secondary bacterial infection may occur if the lesions are manipulated. Septic sequelae may then ensue, including local abscesses, lymphangitis, septicemia, osteomyelitis, and others.

Varicella pneumonia is rare in children except in severe generalized forms of the disease such as occur in neonatal disease and disseminated forms associated with cancer or immunosuppressive drug therapy. Its onset is in the first week of rash with fulminant pulmonary manifestations (cough, dyspnea and tachypnea, pain, cyanosis, rales, splinting). Chest films show characteristic diffuse pulmonary nodular infiltrates throughout both lung fields. The disease may be fatal, especially in adults and in disseminated forms.

Varicella in the newborn is often mild but may be fulminant, with extensive visceral infection and death.

Varicella occurring in patients with cancer or receiving immunosuppressive therapy can be very severe and often fatal. Hemorrhagic forms of the disease and disseminated visceral lesions, including pneumonia, are common. The role of corticosteroid therapy is controversial, but most authorities feel that the underlying disease is more important in the development of severe infections than is administration of corticosteroids alone.

Patients receiving corticosteroids for illnesses not associated with immunologic suppression (eg, asthma, juvenile rheumatoid arthritis) require no adjustment in dose upon exposure. Those patients whose underlying illness predisposes to disseminated disease should have the dose of corticosteroids reduced as much as possible and varicella-zoster immune globulin (VZIG) administered.

Varicella encephalitis occurs infrequently and is milder than measles encephalitis. Eighty percent of patients fully recover; 15% have sequelae; and 5% die. The onset is insidious, usually in the first week of rash, and is followed by varying central nervous system signs and symptoms.

Fatal hypoglycemia has been reported in infants with varicella and is believed to be associated with decreased carbohydrate intake and concomitant salicylate therapy. Some studies suggest that salicylate administration to children with varicella may be related to subsequent development of Reye's syndrome.

Rare complications include transverse myelitis, optic neuritis, hepatitis, and orchitis.

Treatment

Symptomatic measures include fluids, control of itching (sedative antihistamines, colloidal baths), attention to cleanliness (trimming of nails, hand washing, bathing), and antipyretics where indicated (avoid high or repeated doses of aspirin, especially in young infants). Some experts advocate avoidance of all salicylates in varicella. Antimicrobial agents should not be administered prophylactically, but infections should be treated as they occur. Topical therapy is often sufficient for mild skin infection, but systemic administration may be necessary.

Supportive and symptomatic treatment for the complications of varicella are indicated. In the disseminated forms of infection, massive amounts of passive antibody in the form of varicella-zoster immune globulin (VZIG) may be of aid.

A large-scale controlled study of cytarabine not only failed to demonstrate a favorable effect but reported increased morbidity and mortality rates. However, a recent trial with vidarabine given by intravenous infusion reported findings of accelerated clearing of varicella-zoster virus from vesicles and cessation of new vesicle formation, with no drug toxicity. A placebo-controlled, double-blind study demonstrated that a 1-week course of intravenous acyclovir (1500 $mg/m^2/d$) halted progression of zoster in immunocompromised patients with either skin lesions only or disseminated disease. Most experts will use either vidarabine or acyclovir to treat severe chickenpox, especially in immunocompromised children.

Varicella vaccine, a live attenuated virus vaccine developed in Japan, is undergoing preliminary trials in the USA in patients with leukemia in remission, in healthy children, and in adults.

Prognosis

Varicella is usually benign and self-limited. Complications are infrequent and fatalities rare, except in susceptible immunodeficient persons.

Balfour HH et al: Acyclovir halts progression of herpes zoster in immunocompromised patients. *N Engl J Med* 1983;**308:**1448.

Brawley RL, Wenzel RP: An algorithm for chickenpox exposure. *Pediatr Infect Dis* 1984;**3:**502.

Morgan ER, Smalley LA: Varicella in immunocompromised children. *Am J Dis Child* 1983;**137:**883.

Nicholson KG: Antiviral therapy: Varicella-zoster infections. *Lancet* 1984;**2:**677.

Patel PA et al: Cell-mediated immunity to varicella-zoster virus infection in subjects with lymphoma or leukemia. *J Pediatr* 1979;**94:**223.

Preblud S et al: Varicella: Clinical manifestations, epidemiology and health impact in children. *Pediatr Infect Dis* 1984;**3:**505.

Prober CG et al: Acyclovir therapy of chickenpox in immunosuppressed children: A collaborative study. *J Pediatr* 1982;**101:**622.

Zaia JA et al: Evaluation of varicella-zoster immune globulin: Protection of immunosuppressed children after household exposure to varicella. *J Infect Dis* 1983;**147:**737.

ARBOVIRUSES

Four clinical syndromes of importance in children are associated with arbovirus infection: encephalitis, dengue, yellow fever, and febrile illnesses such as Colorado tick fever. In general, a cycle of infection between an arthropod and nonhuman vertebrates is established in nature, and humans are infected as a secondary host. Dengue and urban yellow fever are exceptions, as the mosquito transmits the viruses directly from human to human.

ENCEPHALITIS SYNDROMES

Essentials of Diagnosis

- High fever, severe headache, nuchal rigidity, stupor, coma, convulsions, and other central nervous system symptoms predominate.
- Cerebrospinal fluid pleocytosis and slight protein elevation (normal in St Louis encephalitis).
- Isolation of virus from blood, cerebrospinal fluid, or postmortem specimens (brain, blood).
- Identification of serum antibody rise in paired specimens obtained 3–4 weeks apart.

General Considerations

The major types of arbovirus encephalitis occurring in the USA are St Louis, California group, and eastern and western equine. In recent years, Venezuelan equine encephalitis has been introduced into the USA from its usual endemic areas in Central and South America. A minor cause of arbovirus encephalitis is Powassan, which occurs in the northern USA and Canada.

Clinical Findings

A. History: A history of encephalitic death in horses may precede human cases of eastern and western equine encephalitis. The epidemic nature of the illness may alert the physician to new cases.

B. Symptoms and Signs: After an incubation period of 5–10 days (as long as 3 weeks in St Louis encephalitis), a sudden onset of high fever and headache heralds the illness. Signs of central nervous system irritability (convulsions, nausea and vomiting) and depression (coma, stupor, lethargy) appear in association with a stiff neck or back, increased deep tendon reflexes, tremors, muscle weakness, and, occasionally, paralysis. Mild or asymptomatic infections are observed in the western equine and St Louis types but are uncommon in the eastern equine type.

The illness may be abortive, with rapid recovery, or may progress to severe illness and even death. In general, eastern equine encephalitis tends to be the most severe.

C. Laboratory Findings: In the eastern and western equine types, cerebrospinal fluid pleocytosis of moderate degree is noted (50–1000 cells/μL), and protein concentration may be slightly elevated. Cerebrospinal fluid glucose concentration remains normal.

Attempts at virus isolation should be made early in the course of an epidemic in order to alert physicians and to inform public health officials. Heparinized blood, cerebrospinal fluid, and central nervous system tissue from fatal cases should be submitted to appropriate diagnostic laboratories. The USPHS maintains diagnostic facilities for this purpose. Serologic diagnosis can be accomplished by demonstration of a 4-fold or greater antibody rise between acute and convalescent sera (21–30 days apart).

Differential Diagnosis

Arbovirus encephalitis must be differentiated from other causes of encephalitis by appropriate laboratory means. Brain tumor, lead and other poisonings, and central nervous system injuries occurring during an epidemic of arbovirus encephalitis must also be differentiated. The history, appropriate neurologic and neurosurgical diagnostic procedures, and negative virologic studies aid in the differentiation.

The abortive forms must be distinguished from aseptic meningitis due to any cause and from enteroviral infections, particularly since the peak incidence of both illnesses often coincides. Only laboratory study can make the distinction, as the clinical syndromes may be identical. For this reason, throat and stool specimens as well as blood and cerebrospinal fluid should be submitted to the viral diagnostic laboratory.

Complications & Sequelae

Infants may develop convulsions, hydrocephalus, mental retardation, and severe central nervous system damage.

Treatment & Prognosis

Control of convulsions by barbiturates is indicated. The unconscious patient requires continuous care, with attention to the airway, oxygenation, and support of the circulation.

Mortality from encephalitis is greatest with the eastern equine type and may exceed 50%, whereas the mortality rate in the western equine and St Louis types is usually less than 25% (often 5–7%).

Chaturvedi UC et al: Transplacental infection with Japanese encephalitis virus. *J Infect Dis* 1980;**141**:712.

Kappus KD et al: Human arboviral infections in the United States in 1980. *J Infect Dis* 1982;**145**:283.

Powell KE, Blakey DL: St Louis encephalitis: The 1975 epidemic in Mississippi. *JAMA* 1977;**237**:2294.

DENGUE (Group B Arboviruses)

Dengue in children usually occurs during the preschool or early school years. It is characterized by a sudden onset of fever, severe headache, and retroocular pain; severe pain in the extremities and back (thus the term breakbone fever); lymphadenopathy; and a maculopapular or petechial (hemorrhagic) rash.

The fever and course are often diphasic, with an "exacerbation" following temporary improvement. Central nervous system and pneumonic symptoms may occur. Shock and peripheral vascular collapse may result in death in the first week of illness.

Leukopenia and thrombocytopenia may be marked. Hemorrhagic disease may be associated with prolonged bleeding time and maturation arrest of megakaryocytes. Virus may be recovered from the blood. Complications include hemorrhage, shock, and postinfectious asthenia.

Treatment consists of supportive measures for shock, blood replacement for severe hemorrhage, and, in severe cases, corticosteroids. Antipyretics and analgesics suffice for uncomplicated cases.

Fatality rates vary from epidemic to epidemic but are usually low. No sequelae have been observed in survivors.

Dengue. (Editorial.) *Lancet* 1976;**2**:239.

Kaplan JE: Epidemiologic investigations of dengue infections in Mexico, 1980. *Am J Epidemiol* 1983;**117**:335.

Ventura AK et al: Placental passage of antibodies to dengue virus in persons living in a region of hyperendemic dengue virus infection. *J Infect Dis* 1975;**131(Suppl)**:62.

YELLOW FEVER

The severity of yellow fever varies, and mild and inapparent infections occur. In the classic illness, 3 phases are seen following an incubation period of 3–7 days. The first is nonspecific, with abrupt onset, fever, headache, lassitude, nausea and vomiting, and vague muscle aching. A short period of remission is followed by the severe "toxic" phase with high fever associated with bradycardia (Faget's sign), severe jaundice, and gastrointestinal hemorrhage often progressing to shock and death. The disease may be fulminant, with no remissive period; or may be abortive, with only mild nonspecific symptoms. The disease is usually less severe in children.

Leukopenia is the rule. Proteinuria, azotemia, hyperbilirubinemia, elevated blood urea nitrogen, and disturbed liver function tests are observed. Virus can be isolated from the blood in the first 3–4 days of illness and irregularly thereafter. Serologic diagnosis is possible by examination of paired sera obtained 2–4 weeks apart. Midzonal hepatic cell necrosis with eosinophilic inclusions (Councilman bodies) and relative absence of inflammation are seen at postmortem examination and can be diagnostic.

Treatment is symptomatic and supportive, including fluid and blood replacement, antipyretics, and support of peripheral circulation.

Despite prolonged convalescence in some severely affected patients, no permanent sequelae are noted in survivors. Mortality rates vary and may be conditioned by age, race, and the status of other arbovirus immunity.

Yellow fever: Cause for concern? *Br Med J* 1981;**282:**1735.

COLORADO TICK FEVER

Three to 6 days after the bite of an infected tick *(Dermacentor andersoni),* a sudden onset of high fever occurs with retro-ocular, back, and muscular pain. This phase lasts 2–3 days, and a remission of 2–3 days may follow, whereupon a second, usually more severe episode of fever, severe headache, and muscular pain occurs. Rarely, several such episodes occur. In 10–15% of patients, a generalized maculopapular or petechial rash may be present. Symptoms subside slowly, and recovery is usually complete within 10–14 days.

Marked leukopenia (often 1500–2000/μL), with a shift to the left occurring on the third to sixth day, is characteristic. In the hemorrhagic forms, thrombocytopenia may be present. Virus may be regularly isolated from the blood during the illness and occasionally from cerebrospinal fluid. Serologic testing reveals an increase in antibody 4–6 weeks after onset.

Any cause of fever must be considered in the early phases, but the typical clinical course, leukopenia, and virus isolation serve to distinguish Colorado tick fever. The appearance of a rash may lead to confusion with other viral exanthems, meningococcemia, and various thrombocytopenic states. Bacteriologic and hematologic studies may be of aid in diagnosis.

Encephalitis and severe hemorrhages have been reported. Nuchal rigidity, stupor, headache, or signs of central nervous system irritability suggest meningoencephalitis and should prompt a lumbar puncture.

Hemorrhage (frequently severe) involving the skin, mucous membranes, gastrointestinal tract, and genitourinary track may occur.

Treatment is symptomatic and supportive. Transfusion of whole blood may be necessary if hemorrhage occurs.

Most cases are uncomplicated and self-limiting.

Spruance SL, Bailey A: Colorado tick fever: A review of 15 laboratory confirmed cases. *Arch Intern Med* 1973;**131:**288.

ADENOVIRUSES

There are more than 24 human types of adenoviruses, but relatively few produce illness in children. A carrier state involving one or more adenoviruses is common in young children. Immunity is type-specific.

Many forms of adenovirus disease are recognized:

(1) Pharyngoconjunctival fever: Fever, exudative pharyngitis, and follicular conjunctivitis.

(2) Follicular conjunctivitis: Sporadic illness with preauricular adenopathy and occasional corneal opacification.

(3) Epidemic keratoconjunctivitis: Epidemics of severe conjunctivitis and corneal infiltration traceable to some common source, eg, ophthalmologic examination.

(4) Others: Adenoviruses have been linked with pertussislike syndrome, with intussusception, and with a form of obliteration pneumonitis in immunodeficient individuals. Enteral adenoviruses have been identified in stools of 5% of children with diarrhea; illness is usually mild and self-limited.

In most of the respiratory infections caused by adenoviruses, the signs and symptoms are not unlike those produced by any of the respiratory viruses. Conjunctivitis and exudative pharyngitis are more commonly due to adenoviral infection than to other viruses and may provide an etiologic clue in local outbreaks. High fever (< 39 °C) may be present.

Specific diagnosis can be made by isolating virus from stools, respiratory secretions, or conjunctival specimens and by testing antibody responses. A 4-fold antibody rise in paired sera is essential to the diagnosis. Since these viruses may be "carried" in the pharynges of normal children, serologic evidence of infection should be sought; lack of evidence of other respiratory viral etiologic agents supports the diagnosis.

Harrison HR et al: A cluster of adenovirus 19 infection with multiple clinical manifestations. *J Pediatr* 1979;**94:**917.

James AG et al: Adenovirus type 21 bronchopneumonia in infants and young children. *J Pediatr* 1979;**95:**530.

Levandowski RA, Rubenis M: Nosocomial conjunctivitis caused by adenovirus type 4. *J Infect Dis* 1981;**143:**28.

Nelson KE et al: The role of adenoviruses in the pertussis syndrome. *J Pediatr* 1975;**86:**335.

Ruuskanen O et al: Adenoviral diseases in children: A study of 105 hospital cases. *Pediatrics* 1985;**76:**79.

Schmitz H et al: Worldwide epidemiology of human adenovirus infections. *Am J Epidemiol* 1983;**117:**455.

Takiff HE, Straus SE, Garon CF: Propagation and in vitro studies of previously non-cultivable enteral adenoviruses in 293 cells. *Lancet* 1981;**2:**832.

POXVIRUSES

VARIOLA (Smallpox) & COMPLICATIONS OF SMALLPOX VACCINATION

Variola has been eradicated from the world; no case has been identified since 1977. Immunization against smallpox has also been eliminated in most of the world, although the military in the USA and elsewhere continues to administer some vaccine to personnel. As a result, rarely, a child may acquire the vaccine virus by contact with an immunized individual and may develop a complication of smallpox immunization, usually limited to lesions on exposed parts of the body. In such instances, the clinician should consult the Centers for Disease Control for advice about management. Those interested in descriptions of variola and discussions about complications of vaccination may wish to refer to Chapter 26 in the 8th edition (1984) of *Current Pediatric Diagnosis and Treatment.*

MOLLUSCUM CONTAGIOSUM

The typical lesions of this uncommon viral infection are white to pink, pearly, hard, rapidly maturing asymptomatic papules that umbilicate and extrude a central core of friable exudate. The most common sites are the face, back, arms, and buttocks. The incubation period is 2–8 weeks.

A history of contact is not usually present in sporadic cases, but outbreaks have been observed in schools or institutions. The histologic picture is diagnostic. Prickle cells of the epithelium undergo degeneration, and round hyaline cytoplasmic masses are seen (molluscum bodies, or Henderson-Paterson inclusions). Virus isolation is possible but not readily available.

Molluscum contagiosum is rarely confused with other lesions. Solitary lesions must be distinguished from malignant tumors.

Surgical excision is rarely necessary. Successful eradication of lesions can be accomplished by incision or cautery (usually chemical) or both. Podophyllum resin, silver nitrate, trichloracetic acid, phenol, and cantharidin 0.9% have all been used with success.

Molluscum contagiosum is usually a self-limited, benign disease. Autoinoculation (rare) results in hundreds of lesions and a chronic course.

Rockoff AS: Molluscum dermatitis. *J Pediatr* 1978;**92:**945.

Rosenberg EW, Yusk JW: Molluscum contagiosum: Eruption following treatment with prednisone and methotrexate. *Arch Dermatol* 1970;**101:**439.

MISCELLANEOUS VIRUSES

RUBELLA

Essentials of Diagnosis

- Variable clinical expression in childhood.

"Typical case":

- Maculopapular, discrete rash with rapid caudal progression (3 days).
- Lymphadenopathy preceding and outlasting rash.
- Minimal respiratory and systemic symptoms.

In congenital rubella (usually in combination):

- Thrombocytopenic purpura.
- Deafness.
- Cataract, glaucoma, retinopathy.
- Congenital heart defect.
- Psychomotor retardation.
- Growth retardation.
- Evidence for specific organ infection (hepatitis, osteomyelitis, etc).

General Considerations

It is now appreciated that rubella may be an asymptomatic illness or one associated solely with lymphadenopathy, although the typical illness in children consists principally of a 3-day exanthem. This virus is of major importance because of its proved teratogenic effects on the unborn fetus of a susceptible woman. Rubella is now occurring in older children, adolescents, and adults in greater proportion than prior to vaccine use.

Clinical Findings

A. History: The incubation period is 14–21 days (usually 17 days), and in children there is no prodrome. (In adults and adolescents, fever, mild respiratory and constitutional symptoms, and lymphadenopathy may precede the eruption by 1–5 days.)

Maternal exposure to rubella, particularly during the first 12 weeks of gestation, may be associated with fetal disease whether or not a history of illness is elicited in the mother.

B. Symptoms and Signs: Lymphadenopathy may be the first sign of the illness and is often present for several days prior to rash. Any nodes may be involved, but the suboccipital and postauricular groups are most frequently enlarged. (Lymph node enlargement is not pathognomonic of rubella.) The rash appears first about the face as a pinkish, discrete, macular eruption and rapidly spreads to the trunk and proximal extremities. Within 2 days, it fades from the face and trunk and involves the distal extremities. Thereafter, it rapidly disappears and only rarely desquamates. In children, the rash may be the first sign of rubella.

Fever and systemic symptoms are usually absent or are very mild. Rarely, in infancy, a severe rash and constitutional symptoms occur. In the epidemic form in 1964, many children were observed with systemic symptoms, some so severe as to suggest rubeola.

Purpura and petechiae may occur in a small percentage of patients during an epidemic. Arthritis is not uncommon, particularly among adolescent girls and young women. The involved joints may be normal in appearance or may simulate acute rheumatoid arthritis.

Rubella infection during pregnancy may result in fetal infection with varied manifestations. Maternal viremia may produce placental infection and may result in infection of fetal tissues. The critical factor is the exact timing of these events in relation to fetal growth and development. Although estimates vary, most data support the concept that teratogenesis is largely confined to rubella infections occurring in the first 16 weeks of pregnancy. There are reports of isolated deafness in association with infections after this time. Chronic infection, persistent for years after birth, also is related to early fetal infection. Depending upon the exact developmental events taking place at the time of infection, the following manifestations may appear in the fetus and newborn:

1. Growth retardation—This is related to inhibition of cellular multiplication by rubella virus and is manifested as low birth weight (''small for gestational age'') and postnatal growth failure.

2. Cardiac anomalies—Among the more common defects are branch stenosis of the pulmonary arteries, patent ductus arteriosus, and ventricular septal defect, although a variety of defects, some very complex, have been described.

3. Eye defects—Congenital glaucoma, cataracts, cloudy corneas, and a distinctive retinopathy (diffuse, sharply demarcated areas of black pigmentation scattered about the retina) are common. Microphthalmia may be noted, particularly in infants with other features of growth retardation.

4. Developmental ear defects—Hearing deficits are usually bilateral and due to maldevelopment of the organ of Corti or the cochlea. The deficit may be so subtle that it is not detected until abnormal speech development calls attention to deafness.

5. Hematologic defects—Thrombocytopenia is the most common defect, ranging from mild to severe, resulting in petechial skin eruption or frank purpura, often at birth or shortly thereafter. The ''blueberry muffin'' skin rash is due to petechial and purpuric bleeding. Lymphocytopenia may occur with an associated immunologic defect. Hemolytic anemia has also been described.

6. Central nervous system defects—Chronic and persistent viral encephalitis begins in the fetus and results in varying degrees of mental retardation. Syndromes noted have included minimal brain dysfunction, behavioral disorders, movement disorders, and a slowly progressive degenerative central nervous system disease resembling subacute sclerosing panencephalitis. The decrease in brain growth may be manifest as microcephaly.

7. Immunologic defects—A variety of immunodeficiencies have been attributed to fetal rubella, including cell-mediated immune disorders, hypoimmunoglobulinemias, and complex deficiencies. The usual immunologic response in congenital rubella uncomplicated by immunodeficiency is high levels of fetal IgM rubella antibody admixed with maternally derived IgG rubella antibody. As maternal antibody wanes, the IgM persists, eventually being replaced with IgG rubella antibody actively synthesized by the child.

8. Gastrointestinal disease—The following have been described, usually in association with chronic rubella: hepatitis, pancreatitis, splenitis, diabetes, and malabsorption syndromes.

9. Bone infection—A characteristic rubella osteomyelitis has been described, with circular metaphyseal radiolucent areas associated with metaphysitis.

10. Miscellaneous—A variety of defects have been described whose association with rubella is less certain than those listed above.

C. Laboratory Findings: Leukopenia or thrombocytopenia is seen in some patients. Virus may be recovered prior to the rash (up to 7 days) and as late as 2 weeks after onset. Throat specimens and urine are good sources, but blood must be examined before the onset of rash. Fecal specimens may also yield the virus.

A rise in rubella antibody titer may be detected between paired sera collected 2 or more weeks apart. Since antibody may be present early in the rash stage of rubella, it is important to collect specimens as early as possible.

In congenital rubella, the following may be detected:

1. Thrombocytopenia, frequently less than 10,000 platelets/μL.

2. Hemolytic anemia, neuroblastemia, reticulocytosis, an erythroid hyperplastic marrow, and eventual decrease in hemoglobin.

3. Increased levels of direct-reacting bilirubin and evidence of hepatocellular dysfunction.

4. Virus may be recovered from peripheral leukocytes, throat, stool, and urine for months or years

after birth. Recovery of virus from the lens has occurred after many years.

5. High and persistent rubella antibody titer in the serum.

6. Abnormalities in immunoglobulin concentration (variable, but includes depression of IgA and IgG levels with increased IgM levels).

7. A defect in cellular immunity.

8. Cerebrospinal fluid pleocytosis and increase in protein.

D. X-Ray Findings: Signs of pneumonia may be present in congenital rubella. Radiographic evidence of rubella osteomyelitis consists of alternating linear densities and translucent streaks in the metaphyses of the long bones.

Differential Diagnosis

Rubella must be differentiated from other acute viral exanthematous diseases (Table 26–1). In general, the 3-day course of the pinkish rash, prior lymphadenopathy, and minimal or absent prodromal symptoms serve as useful clinical criteria for diagnosis. However, in cases where the distinction is important (as in the pregnant woman), virus isolation and serology are essential.

Arthritis or arthralgia raises the possibility of rheumatoid arthritis (fever, splenomegaly, history, multiple joint involvement), and the distinction may be blurred by a positive latex fixation test. The transient nature of rubella arthritis may aid in the differentiation.

Congenital rubella must be differentiated from other infections acquired in utero, including toxoplasmosis (by specific antibody studies), cytomegalovirus infection (by virus recovery and specific antibody studies), and congenital syphilis (by serologic study).

Complications & Sequelae

A. Encephalitis: Encephalitis occurs in no more than one of 6000 cases of rubella. The manifestations are those of postinfectious encephalitis due to any cause, although rubella encephalitis tends to be mild, with less frequent sequelae and few fatalities. A severe encephalitis, much like measles-associated subacute sclerosing panencephalitis, has been described after congenital rubella.

B. Rubella During Pregnancy: Rubella in pregnant women is not unusually severe, but the potential risk to the fetus is great. The following generalizations may be made in the light of currently available evidence:

The risk to infants following maternal rubella is greatest in the first 3–4 months of pregnancy. In one large-scale study, only one of 16 infants born to mothers infected after the fourth month was abnormal, whereas 243 of 291 were abnormal when infection occurred before the end of the fourth month. The risk in this series was greatest in the first 2 months, when 157 of 166 infants were abnormal; next highest in the third month, with 64 of 82 infants affected; and lowest in the fourth month, with 22 of 43 infants involved.

Immune globulin given to an exposed pregnant woman has no effect in preventing fetal infection.

Treatment

A. Specific Measures: Despite the demonstration of antiviral activity of amantadine in vitro, no specific therapy for rubella is available.

B. General Measures: The usual case requires no therapy. Purpura is usually confined to the skin, and no treatment is necessary. It is conceivable that severe hemorrhage might occur, requiring transfusion of whole blood or platelets. Arthritis is controlled with aspirin and limitation of motion.

C. In Pregnancy: Therapeutic abortion is recommended in some pregnancies. This practice is tempered by local standards, religious beliefs, and law.

Prognosis

Rubella is almost always a self-limited, uncomplicated disease with complete recovery. Congenital rubella can result in death or prolonged handicap.

Cherry JD: The "new" epidemiology of measles and rubella. *Hosp Pract* (July) 1980;**15:**49.

Chess S, Fernandez P, Korn S: Behavioral consequences of congenital rubella. *J Pediatr* 1978;**93:**699.

Desmond MM et al: The longitudinal course of congenital rubella encephalitis in non-retarded children. *J Pediatr* 1978;**93:**584.

Lamprecht C et al: An outbreak of congenital rubella in Chicago. *JAMA* 1982;**247:**1129.

Miller E et al: Consequences of confirmed maternal rubella at successive stages of pregnancy. *Lancet* 1982;**2:**781.

Ozsoylu S, Kanra G, Savae G: Thrombocytopenic purpura related to rubella infection. *Pediatrics* 1978;**62:**567.

Preblud SR et al: Current status of rubella in the United States, 1969–1979. *J Infect Dis* 1980;**142:**776.

Sander J et al: Screening for rubella IgG and IgM using an ELISA test applied to dried blood on filter paper. *J Pediatr* 1985;**106:**457.

Stoffman J, Wolfish MG: The susceptibility of adolescent girls to rubella. *Clin Pediatr* 1976;**15:**625.

Weil ML et al: Chronic progressive panencephalitis due to rubella virus simulating subacute sclerosing panencephalitis. *N Engl J Med* 1975;**292:**994.

CYTOMEGALIC INCLUSION DISEASE (Cytomegaloviruses)

Essentials of Diagnosis

- The syndrome of hepatosplenomegaly, microcephaly, and chorioretinitis occurring in a jaundiced infant with a petechial rash is classic.
- Variants occur with only part of the syndrome.
- Periventricular intracranial calcification.
- Inclusion bodies (owl's eye) in cells sedimented from freshly voided urine or in liver biopsy.
- Detection of virus in urine or saliva. (***Note:*** Do not freeze specimens. Keep at 0–4 °C.)

General Considerations

It was originally thought that the cytomegaloviruses produce only a characteristic fulminant, generalized neonatal infection, but it has recently been shown that in older children and adults they may cause pulmonary or gastrointestinal infections also. Patients receiving immunosuppressive therapy may develop clinical disease by unmasking of latent virus infection, usually in the lungs. Each year, 33,000 infected infants are born in the USA; fewer than 1000 of these have the severe form of disease.

Many investigators believe that additional illnesses will be attributable to the cytomegaloviruses, since they are ubiquitous and most individuals are infected (as shown by the finding of serum antibody and, occasionally, asymptomatic virus excretion).

Nurses and other health personnel may acquire cytomegalovirus from patients; the extent of risk and exact source of virus may not be definable.

Cytomegalovirus infection may result from infusion of blood containing the virus. An appreciable risk occurs in a susceptible patient receiving large quantities of whole blood (cardiac surgery, etc). In newborns receiving transfusion, 13–14% will be infected with cytomegalovirus. Breast milk obtained from a breast milk bank may contain cytomegalovirus; storage of milk for 3 days or more at −20 °C will reduce titers by 99%, and pasteurization will eliminate the virus.

Clinical Findings

A. History: Since the maternal disease is asymptomatic, the history is of little value. A history of prior cytomegalovirus infection in an infant virtually ensures that subsequent siblings will be unaffected despite chronic shedding of the virus by the mother.

B. Symptoms and Signs: Jaundice, massive hepatosplenomegaly associated with central nervous system signs (lethargy, convulsions, etc), and a petechial-purpuric rash are present in full-blown neonatal disease. Milder forms of the disease are seen. Fewer infants have chorioretinitis and cerebral calcification, but almost all have some degree of microcephaly, occasionally striking.

Surviving infants are usually severely mentally and physically handicapped, and hepatosplenomegaly and jaundice may persist. Unusual eye abnormalities have been observed in some surviving infants (central corneal defect, anophthalmia). A syndrome resembling infectious mononucleosis may occur without accompanying heterophil antibody rise. Isolated hepatitis has been described. Cytomegalovirus may cause hemophagocytic syndrome (histiocytic proliferation, fever, hepatosplenomegaly, pancytopenia, and erythrophagocytosis), which can be fatal.

Pulmonary disease has been observed in cytomegalovirus-infected children. Interstitial pneumonitis is the most common lesion, but wheezing or tachypnea with positive x-rays is also seen. The illness may be prolonged and intractable and usually occurs in immunodeficient or immunosuppressed individuals. Recently, severe pneumonitis with marked respiratory distress has been noted in very small newborns, possibly acquired from blood used in life support.

C. Laboratory Findings: Anemia, thrombocytopenia, and hyperbilirubinemia are usually present. Cerebrospinal fluid pleocytosis and elevated protein with normal glucose concentration are found. Typical owl's eye intranuclear basophilic inclusions can be found in cells in freshly voided urine. Delay in examination may result in lack of visualization of the inclusions. Tissue from other organs can also be utilized; examination of live biopsy material can establish the diagnosis.

Virus can regularly be isolated from the urine for many months and even years after birth. Salivary and fecal excretion of virus is also detectable, but for shorter periods. Rapid diagnosis is now achievable in many laboratories by electron microscopic identification of cytomegalovirus in clinical specimens. Rheumatoid factor testing, while nonspecific, may identify 35–40% of infected infants.

Diagnosis by antibody determination is clouded by the widespread incidence of infection; more than 70% of all infants have antibody in their cord sera. Therefore, serologic diagnosis is less helpful than isolation of virus and histologic techniques.

Increased levels of total IgM are found in one-third of infected infants and specific IgM cytomegalovirus antibody in three-fourths.

D. X-Ray Findings: Skull films may show typical periventricular calcification.

Differential Diagnosis

Cytomegalic inclusion disease must be differentiated from other causes of jaundice, hepatosplenomegaly, and petechial rash in the newborn, principally toxoplasmosis (diagnosed by elevated Feldman-Sabin dye test antibody titer and suggested by generalized instead of periventricular cerebral calcification); generalized herpetic neonatal infection (presence of vesicular skin lesions, lack of cerebral calcification, specific virologic tests); generalized coxsackievirus infection (myocarditis predominates, epidemic nature, isolation of virus); hemolytic disease of newborn (no microcephaly, positive Coombs tests, demonstration of incompatibility for rhesus or ABO antigens); bacterial sepsis, including syphilis (positive blood culture or serology, osseous changes, lack of microcephaly); and galactosemia (galactosuria, proteinuria, aminoaciduria, and absence of other signs of cytomegalovirus infection).

Pneumonia in older individuals must be differentiated from *Pneumocystis carinii* infection, which is usually accomplished by identification of the parasite.

Complications & Sequelae

Residual cerebral damage frequently results in mental and physical retardation of marked degree. Institutionalization may be necessary for total care.

Treatment

There is no specific treatment. Symptomatic therapy may reduce immediate morbidity but usually does not influence the final outcome.

Floxuridine may be of benefit in severe cytomegalovirus infections in children with leukemia or other diseases associated with immunosuppression. Acyclovir and other forms of therapy and a vaccine are in experimental trials.

Prognosis

The exact mortality rate is difficult to estimate because of a broad base of asymptomatic infections. Fulminant forms of the disease are almost universally fatal in the neonatal period.

Sensorineural hearing loss occurs frequently in both symptomatic and asymptomatic infants with congenital cytomegalovirus infection. Symptomatic cytomegalovirus infection may also result in impaired vision.

Ballard AM et al: Acquired cytomegalovirus infection in preterm infants. *Am J Dis Child* 1979;**133:**482.

Danish EH et al: Cytomegalovirus-associated hemophagocytic syndrome. *Pediatrics* 1985;**75:**280.

Frenkel LD et al: Unusual eye abnormalities associated with congenital cytomegalovirus infection. *Pediatrics* 1980; **66:**763.

Friis H, Andersen HK: Rate of inactivation of cytomegalovirus in raw banked milk during storage at −20 °C and pasteurization. *Br Med J* 1982;**285:**1604.

Hanshaw B: Cytomegalovirus infections. *Pediatr in Rev* 1983;**4:**332.

Lee FK, Nahmias AJ, Stagno S: Rapid diagnosis of cytomegalovirus infection in infants by electron microscopy. *N Engl J Med* 1978;**299:**1266.

Panjvani ZFK, Hanshaw JB: Cytomegalovirus in the perinatal period. *Am J Dis Child* 1981;**135:**56.

Stagno S et al: Comparative study of diagnostic procedures for congenital cytomegalovirus infection. *Pediatrics* 1980; **65:**251.

Yeager A et al: Prevention of transfusion-acquired cytomegalovirus infections in newborn infants. *J Pediatr* 1981;**98:**281.

Yeager A et al: Sequelae of maternally derived cytomegalovirus infections in premature infants. *J Pediatr* 1983;**102:**918.

Yow MD et al: Use of restriction enzymes to investigate the source of a primary cytomegalovirus infection in a pediatric nurse. *Pediatrics* 1982;**70:**713.

ROSEOLA INFANTUM (Exanthem Subitum)

Roseola infantum is a usually benign, self-limited infection that has been transmitted by filtrates of blood. No specific virus has been isolated.

Clinical Findings

A. History: The typical clinical picture is 3 days of sustained high fever, often with a febrile convulsion at onset, in a child who otherwise appears well. Roseola occasionally occurs in epidemics, even in young adults.

B. Symptoms and Signs: A discrete pink rash is the most characteristic finding. It is often evanescent and typically appears as the fever decreases or shortly thereafter. The rash is occasionally generalized and may coalesce. Any sustained fever in an infant or child under age 3 years should therefore alert the physician and parents to look for a rash, which may be mild or transient. The temperature falls to lower than normal after defervescence. Edema of the eyelids has been said to be diagnostic, but this is not regularly observed and may not be specific.

C. Laboratory Findings: Leukocytosis with a shift to the left may be present at onset, but leukopenia is more common and may be marked at the time of rash.

Differential Diagnosis

The presence of high fever and the frequency of initial convulsions may suggest other causes of this combination, including bacterial meningitis and encephalitis. The age of the child, well-being following recovery from the seizure, and the typical course plus a normal spinal fluid are helpful in differentiation.

Complications & Sequelae

Some workers claim that encephalitis is common, but sequelae occur infrequently if at all.

Treatment & Prognosis

Fever can be controlled with supplemental fluids, gentle tepid water sponge baths, and aspirin. Convulsions are usually self-limited and single, requiring no therapy. Barbiturates are rarely required. With a history of prior "febrile" convulsions, administration of elixir of phenobarbital, 15 mg 3 times daily, should be considered. Antimicrobial agents are not indicated and are of no benefit.

Roseola is almost universally benign, and complete recovery is the rule.

ERYTHEMA INFECTIOSUM (Fifth Disease)

A human parvovirus has recently been linked etiologically with erythema infectiosum. This disease is characterized by an intensely erythematous, slightly raised, hot eruption of the cheeks ("slapped face") followed after 1 day by a maculopapular eruption on the extensor surfaces of the proximal extremities. With spread and continued evolution, the rash assumes a striking reticular or lacy pattern. The rash is frequently enhanced by a warm bath or by wrapping the arm in a towel. It lasts for a few days to several weeks, often clearing and reappearing. There are usually no other symptoms, and resolution is eventually complete.

Complications or sequelae are rare. No treatment is necessary.

Anderson MJ et al: Human parvovirus: The cause of erythema infectiosum? *Lancet* 1983;**1:**1378.

Balfour HH: Fifth disease: Full fathom five. *Am J Dis Child* 1976;**130**:239.

Lauer B, MacCormack JN, Wilfert C: Erythema infectiosum: An elementary school outbreak. *Am J Dis Child* 1976; **130**:252.

INFECTIOUS MONONUCLEOSIS

Essentials of Diagnosis

- Fever, pharyngitis, lymphadenopathy, and splenomegaly.
- Lymphocytosis with atypical lymphocytes.
- Positive heterophil test.

General Considerations

Infectious mononucleosis is an acute, self-limiting infectious disease characterized by increased numbers of atypical lymphocytes and monocytes in the peripheral blood. The disease is presumed to be due to a virus (Epstein-Barr [EB] virus). The disorder can occur at any age but is seen most frequently in children and young adults. In the majority of patients, the serum reveals an increased titer of agglutinins for sheep red cells (heterophil antibody test). However, in children under age 5 years, the heterophil test is often negative. Many new disease associations and epidemiologic patterns are being noted with improved serologic diagnosis.

Clinical Findings

A. Symptoms and Signs: Children with infectious mononucleosis often present with fever, sore throat, exudative tonsillitis, malaise, generalized lymphadenopathy, and splenomegaly. Other clinical features may be headache, epistaxis, jaundice, and abdominal pain. A morbilliform or maculopapular exanthem is not unusual. Almost any system may be involved; hepatitis, encephalitis, meningitis, polyradiculoneuritis, pneumonitis, and carditis have all been reported. There is an increased susceptibility to rupture of the spleen. Spatial and visual distortions have been reported in adolescents. In addition, EB virus infection has been noted in newborns, immunocompromised persons, patients with Reye's syndrome, and infants and children with common upper respiratory infections, otitis media, skin rashes, and lymphadenitis. The full spectrum of disease is probably still unknown. Chronic EB virus infection is now known to occur with a highly variable clinical pattern ranging from repetitive episodes of mononucleosislike symptoms to psychiatric syndromes of depression, vague myalgias, and arthralgias to excessive fatigue and malaise.

EB virus infection has recently been associated with increased susceptibility to other infections within a few weeks after onset. Immunologic suppression has been demonstrated and may account for this susceptibility. Acute EB virus infection appears to alter antibody-producing capacity by stimulation of excess numbers of suppressor T cells.

B. Laboratory Findings:

1. Peripheral blood—The leukocyte count varies greatly; although the usual white blood cell count is 10,000–20,000/μL, a normal or low count may be present. A rather constant feature is the appearance of increased numbers of atypical lymphocytes and monocytes in the peripheral blood smear, ranging from 50 to 90% of the total differential count. The hemoglobin, hematocrit, and platelets are usually normal. Thrombocytopenia and autoimmune hemolytic anemia occasionally may be complicating factors.

2. Screening test for mononucleosis—A rapid screening test (Monospot) has been developed for the diagnosis of mononucleosis. This slide test relies upon the differential reactivity of patients' sera with guinea pig kidney and beef red blood cells in the presence of a reactor system, horse erythrocytes. The test is rapid, sensitive, easy to perform, and inexpensive. False-negative reactions are rare; false-positive reactions have been reported in 5–14% of sera containing other heterophil antibodies in such diseases as hepatitis, cytomegalovirus infection, adenovirus infection, leukemia, and rubella. One advantage of this test is its ability to detect patients with low levels of sheep red cell agglutinins (20–40), thus enabling diagnosis to be made where other techniques fail.

3. Serology—The heterophil antibody (Paul-Bunnell) test is often positive in a titer above 1:112.

Precise serologic diagnosis is now possible in many viral laboratories. Antibody to viral capsid antigen (VCA) rises to titers in excess of 1:160 during the acute phase of the disease. Specific IgM antibody to VCA is detectable in 97% of acute infections. In 80% of cases, antibody to "early antigens" is also detectable in the early phase of disease. Antibody to EB nuclear antigen (EBNA) appears only after several weeks of infection.

Thus, in the acute disease, increases in antibody to VCA and "early antigens" can be detected in the absence of antibody to EBNA. During the convalescent phases and for years thereafter, antibody to EBNA predominates, IgG antibody to VCA persists, IgM antibody to VCA disappears, and antibody to "early antigens" also disappears.

Although isolation of the viruses is possible by stimulation of cord blood lymphocytes, it is of no practical value and available in only a few laboratories.

Differential Diagnosis

Differential diagnosis includes leukemia (usually with pancytopenia or circulating "blast" cells), acute infectious lymphocytosis (increase in small mature lymphocytes), viral exanthems (clinical course differs), infectious hepatitis (fewer atypical lymphocytes and absence of lymphadenopathy), and aseptic meningoencephalitis (absence of splenomegaly and lymphadenopathy). In addition, many young infants and children have a few atypical lymphocytes without evidence of illness.

Treatment & Prognosis

Treatment is symptomatic. Emphasis is on supportive care when the major systems (liver, heart, nervous system) are involved. In older children and adolescents, the symptoms may be quite severe, and hospitalization and bed rest are often necessary. In severe disease, some success has been noted in controlled trials with corticosteroids or chloroquine.

The prognosis is good for complete recovery after a period of illness of 3–6 weeks or, with major system involvement, longer. Rupture of the spleen and secondary infection are the major complications.

Bower TJ et al: Transient immunodeficiency during asymptomatic EBV infection. *Pediatrics* 1983;**71:**964.

Fleisher G et al: Intrafamilial transmission of Epstein-Barr virus infections. *J Pediatr* 1981;**98:**16.

Fleisher G et al: Primary EBV infection in association with Reye's syndrome. *J Pediatr* 1980;**97:**935.

Jones JF et al: Evidence for active Epstein-Barr virus infection in patients with persistent, unexplained illnesses: Elevated early antigen antibodies. *Ann Intern Med* 1985;**102:**1.

Krabbe S, Hesse J, Uldall P: Primary Epstein-Barr virus infection in early childhood. *Arch Dis Child* 1981;**56:**49.

Williams LL et al: Sudden hearing loss following infectious mononucleosis: Possible effect of altered immunoregulation. *Pediatrics* 1985;**75:**1020.

RABIES

Essentials of Diagnosis

- History of animal bite (wild, sick, or unidentified).
- Early hypesthesia or paresthesia in area of bite.
- Increasing irritability with clear sensorium.
- Hydrophobia—initially to drinking, later to sight of water.
- Progressive symptoms to death.
- Isolation of rabies virus from animal brain confirming Negri body visualization or fluorescent antibody identification.
- Cerebrospinal fluid may be normal, or there may be pleocytosis and slightly elevated protein.
- Mild to moderate peripheral leukocytosis.

General Considerations

Rabies is an almost unexceptionally fatal disease that is transmitted to humans by the bite of a rabid animal. The variable results following such bites are due to the presence or absence of virus in the animal's saliva, the extent and location of the wound, the promptness with which preventive measures are instituted, and the immune status of the bitten individual. Accurate diagnosis and correct therapy depend upon determination of the presence or absence of rabies. This requires knowledge about the prevalence of rabies in the community, the immunization status of the animal, and observation of the living animal for at least 10 days following the bite.

Clinical Findings

A. History:

1. The animal bite—In most instances, a clear-cut history of animal bite is obtained. The animal is usually a dog, but may be a wild skunk, fox, wolf, etc, or unknown to the patient. Multiple bites may have occurred. If the animal was a pet, unusual behavior and an unprovoked bite should suggest rabies. Death of the animal complicates the history. With prolonged incubation periods, the history of animal bite, particularly in a young child or if the wound was slight, may be lacking.

Rabies may also be transmitted by bats; rarely, the bat's environment, particularly in caves, may serve as a means of transmission where no bite is involved.

2. The animal—Peculiar behavior of an animal during observation is noted. The dog, the usual offender, may become hyperirritable and begin to bite anything in its environment. Conversely, progressive lethargy and paralysis may be seen (''dumb'' rabies). If the animal remains healthy for 10 days or more after the bite, the possibility of rabies is remote.

3. The patient—Following the bite, no symptoms occur for 10 days to many months. The duration of the incubation period is related to the site of the bite in relation to the brain and to the severity of the bite (and therefore to the amount of rabies virus inoculated). Very short incubation periods have been associated with direct intracranial bites and prolonged ones with slight trauma to the distal extremities.

B. Symptoms and Signs: The first symptom in the typical form of the disease relates to the region of the bite. Tingling or loss of sensation is reported. The patient then experiences increasing apprehension, anxiety, and hyperexcitability despite a clear sensorium. Episodes of convulsive movements, irrational behavior, or frank delirium may alternate with lethargy. Progressive aversion to water or the act of swallowing ensues, and drooling and spasmodic contraction of the muscles of deglutition follow.

The course is progressive and culminates in death. Increasing central nervous system depression, cardiovascular and respiratory instability, and fever end in death 5–7 days after onset.

C. Laboratory Findings: Rabies virus may be recovered from saliva during life or from central nervous system tissue or salivary glands after death. Virus identification rarely leads to premortem diagnosis because death occurs before laboratory studies can be completed. A presumptive diagnosis can be made on the basis of examination of the animal's brain, if available, for rabies virus content. Fluorescent antibody or Negri body identification should always be confirmed by virus isolation.

Examination of cerebrospinal fluid is of little aid. Most often it is normal, although elevation of the white blood cell count and protein may occur. The presence of peripheral leukocytosis is of little diagnostic significance.

Differential Diagnosis

Differentiation from other forms of encephalitis is usually not difficult. The history of animal bite, an appropriate incubation period, and the characteristic clinical course should be sufficient. Adequate virologic diagnosis of other forms of encephalitis should be attempted.

Prevention*

Despite adequate support, almost all patients die. Therefore, treatment at the time of the animal bite is directed at preventing the clinical disease.

The World Health Organization has outlined its recommendations for the use of rabies immune globulin and vaccines in the prophylactic treatment of animal bites. However, local conditions should modify these recommendations, particularly because the risk of bites by domestic animals in many areas is almost negligible as a result of absence of a convenient reservoir in the wild animal population or insufficient opportunities for contact between domestic and wild animals. Early and adequate local treatment of the wound, local epidemiologic factors, veterinary consultation, adequate field investigation, and the facts and circumstances associated with the bite may modify the physician's judgment with regard to the systemic treatment indicated in individual cases.

Treatment & Prognosis

Experience with 3 recent cases of rabies suggests that prolonged survival and, in one case, apparent recovery may occur if vigorous early supportive therapy is utilized. Early tracheostomy, careful attention to maintaining oxygenation, circulatory support, and ventilation are suggested.

Although rare instances of survival in suspected rabies have been reported, the disease is almost always fatal.

Berlin BS et al: Rhesus diploid rabies vaccine (adsorbed): A new rabies vaccine. *JAMA* 1983;**249:**2663.

Gode GR et al: Intensive care in rabies. *Lancet* 1976;**2:**6.

Hattwick MAW et al: Recovery from rabies. *Ann Intern Med* 1972;**76:**931.

Mann JM: Systematic decision-making in rabies prophylaxis. *Pediatr Infect Dis* 1983;**2:**162.

Plotkin S: Rabies vaccination in the 1980's. *Hosp Pract* (Nov) 1980;**11:**65.

Shah U, Jaswal GS: Victims of a rabid wolf in India: Effect of severity and location of bites on development of rabies. *J Infect Dis* 1976;**134:**25.

II. RICKETTSIAL INFECTIONS (RICKETTSIOSES)

The rickettsiae are pleomorphic coccobacillary organisms that are intracellular parasites. They are now classified as true bacteria.

Characteristically, human infections occur as a result of arthropod contact. Only those diseases encountered in pediatrics will be considered here.

Common characteristics of rickettsiae and the infections they produce may be listed as follows:

(1) Asymptomatic multiplication in the arthropod host.

(2) Intracellular replication.

(3) Limited geographic and seasonal occurrence related to arthropod ecology.

(4) Local primary lesions (rickettsialpox, scrub typhus, tick typhus).

(5) Fever, rash, and respiratory symptoms predominate.

(6) Nonspecific (Weil-Felix reaction, ≥ 1:320 *Proteus* OX19 or OX2) and specific antibodies develop following human infection.

(7) Infections respond to the tetracyclines and chloramphenicol.

RICKETTSIALPOX

Rickettsialpox is an acute, self-limited disease caused by infection with *Rickettsia akari*. It is transmitted by mites from the common house mouse. Following an incubation period of 10–24 days, fever, chills, myalgia, headache, and photophobia appear abruptly. A primary firm, red papule erupts at the site of the mite bite and then vesiculates and becomes crusted with a black eschar. A generalized papulovesicular eruption appears 2–4 days later and forms crusts within 2 days. The crusts are shed in 1–2 weeks. The differential diagnosis includes varicella, variola, flea typhus, Rocky Mountain spotted fever, and scrub typhus. Leukopenia is frequent early in the illness, and complement-fixing antibodies appear during or after the second week of illness. Treat with tetracycline or chloramphenicol (see Chapter 38).

Wong B et al: Rickettsialpox. *JAMA* 1979;**242:**1998.

TICK TYPHUS (Rocky Mountain Spotted Fever, Boutonneuse Fever, North Queensland Tick Typhus, Spotted Fevers, Etc)

The tick-borne rickettsioses have many features in common and are all produced by rickettsiae that may be considered subspecies of *Rickettsia rickettsii*. They differ in the locale of infection and bear regional names for the illnesses. All are transmitted by the hard ticks, including the genera *Dermacentor, Haemaphysalis, Amblyomma,* and *Rhipicephalus*. Animal hosts vary and include rodents, rabbits, and dogs.

* See also Chapter 5.

1. ROCKY MOUNTAIN SPOTTED FEVER

The name of this disease is a misnomer, since it is seen throughout the USA and is found with greater frequency in some eastern and southeastern states than in the Rocky Mountain region. The ixodid ticks serve as the vector for *Rickettsia rickettsii*. Most cases are seen in the late spring and early summer in children who frequent wooded and rural areas.

There has been a recent increase in the number of cases of Rocky Mountain spotted fever throughout endemic areas in the USA. Most cases occurred in the East (from Massachusetts to Florida), the Southeast, and the Midwest. Very few have been reported in the Rockies or Far West.

Following an incubation period of 3–7 days, chills, fever, and influenzalike symptoms appear suddenly. There may be associated headache, sore throat, retroorbital pain, photophobia, nosebleed, myalgias, arthralgias, gastrointestinal symptoms, and abdominal pain. Severe central nervous system manifestations may occur, ie, coma, delirium, stupor, and profound lethargy. Physical findings initially include conjunctivitis, fever, splenomegaly (in 50% of cases), and, occasionally, cyanosis, hepatomegaly, and jaundice. Within 2–11 days (usually 3–5 days), a tiny red macular eruption appears on the wrists and ankles and spreads to involve the entire extremities and the trunk, usually sparing the face. The macules grow larger and becomes petechial within 2–3 days.

Laboratory findings may include proteinuria, bilirubinuria, and hematuria. The diagnosis may be established by culture or complement fixation tests. *Proteus* OX19 and OX2 agglutinins become detectable during the second week (Weil-Felix reaction). The illness may be complicated by myocarditis, pneumonia, and cerebral infarction.

Before the availability of antimicrobial agents, the mortality rate was 25–75%. Specific therapy includes the tetracyclines or chloramphenicol (see Chapter 38).

Bernard K et al: Surveillance of Rocky Mountain spotted fever in the United States, 1978–1980. *J Infect Dis* 1982;**146:**297.

Donohue JF: Lower respiratory tract involvement in Rocky Mountain spotted fever. *Arch Intern Med* 1980;**140:**223.

Jiminez J et al: Gastrointestinal symptoms in Rocky Mountain spotted fever. *Clin Pediatr* 1982;**21:**581.

Linnemann CC, Janson PJ: The clinical presentations of Rocky Mountain spotted fever. *Clin Pediatr* 1978;**17:**673.

Magnarelli LA, Anderson JF, Burgdorfer W: Rocky Mountain spotted fever in Connecticut: Human cases, spotted-fever group rickettsiae in ticks and antibodies in mammals. *Am J Epidemiol* 1979;**110:**148.

Nieburg PI, D'Angelo LJ, Herrmann KL: Measles in patients suspected of having Rocky Mountain spotted fever. *JAMA* 1980;**244:**808.

Westerman EL: Rocky Mountain spotless fever: A dilemma for the clinician. *Arch Intern Med* 1982;**142:**1106.

2. OTHER FORMS OF TICK TYPHUS

African tick typhus is generally mild, usually terminating by rapid lysis in the second week. An abrupt onset is usual, with severe headache, constipation, insomnia, photophobia, myalgia, and arthralgia. Mental disturbances may occur but are not severe. In a varying proportion of cases, an eschar is already developed at onset, with painful enlargement of regional lymph nodes. The eschar may be anywhere on the body, at the site of the tick bite, but is usually on covered parts. The rash is similar to that of the North American type but is less often petechial and may be transitory or absent, especially outside the Mediterranean region. In the mildest cases, there may be no more than a few days of fever with headache, with or without an eschar and lymphadenopathy.

North Queensland tick typhus has been little studied. Fever lasts less than a week and may be intermittent. The rash is variable in character.

EPIDEMIC TYPHUS (Louse Typhus)

Epidemic typhus is produced by infection with *Rickettsia prowazekii* and is transmitted in the feces of the body louse. Following an incubation period of 8–12 days, during which malaise, cough, nausea, coryza, headache, and chest pain may occur, the disease begins with an abrupt rise in temperature accompanied by chills and severe prostration. Headache, nausea and vomiting, gastrointestinal symptoms, cough, nonpleuritic chest pain, stupor and delirium, and severe muscle aching may occur. Conjunctivitis, flushing, splenomegaly (one-third of cases), rales, low blood pressure, and a rash may be seen. The rash is characteristic, beginning on the third to eighth day of illness with pink maculopapules that appear on the trunk and spread to the extremities. The rash usually spares the face, scalp, palms, and soles and may become hemorrhagic.

Leukopenia may be present during the first week, and leukocytosis during the second. Proteinuria is common, and hematuria may occur. Although rickettsiae can be isolated, the diagnosis is usually made by the appearance of *Proteus* OX19 (and occasionally OX2) agglutinins and specific complement-fixing antibody titers during or after the second week of illness.

The illness usually lasts 2–3 weeks, and convalescence may be prolonged. A recrudescent form of the disease is seen in adults (Brill's disease).

Therapy consists of tetracyclines or chloramphenicol (see Chapter 38).

ENDEMIC TYPHUS (Murine Typhus)

Endemic typhus is caused by *Rickettsia typhi* and is usually transmitted by fleas from a rodent (house rat) reservoir. Body lice may become infected and transmit the agent in their feces.

The illness is gradual in onset. Although the symptoms resemble those of epidemic typhus, they are milder and shorter in duration. The prognosis is also better, and fatalities and complications are rarely seen. *Proteus* OX19 agglutinins and specific complement-fixing antibody titers appear in the second week.

Adams WH et al: The changing ecology of murine (endemic) typhus in Southern California. *Am J Trop Med Hyg* 1970;**19:**311.

SELECTED REFERENCES

Committee on Infectious Diseases: *Report,* 20th ed. American Academy of Pediatrics, 1981.

Feigin RD, Cherry JD: *Textbook of Pediatric Infectious Disease.* Saunders, 1981.

Hoeprich PD: *Infectious Diseases,* 3rd ed. Harper & Row, 1981.

Jawetz E, Melnick JL, Adelberg EA: *Review of Medical Microbiology,* 17th ed. Lange, 1986.

Krugman S, Ward R: *Infectious Diseases of Children,* 7th ed. Mosby, 1981.

Lennette EH, Schmidt NJ: *Diagnostic Procedures for Viral and Rickettsial Diseases,* 5th ed. American Public Health Association, 1974.

Infections: Bacterial & Spirochetal

27

Kenneth McIntosh, MD, & Brian A. Lauer, MD

BACTERIAL INFECTIONS

GROUP A STREPTOCOCCAL INFECTIONS

Essentials of Diagnosis

Streptococcal pharyngitis:

- Clinical diagnosis based entirely on symptoms; signs and physical examination unreliable.
- Throat culture yielding group A streptococci is essential.

Impetigo:

- Rapidly spreading, highly infectious skin rash.
- Erythematous denuded areas and salmon-colored crusts.
- Culture grows group A streptococci in most (not all) cases.

General Considerations

Group A streptococci are common gram-positive bacteria capable of producing a wide variety of clinical illnesses. Prominent among these are acute pharyngitis; impetigo; cellulitis; and scarlet fever, the generalized illness caused by strains that elaborate erythrogenic toxin. Group A streptococci can also cause pneumonia, septic arthritis, osteomyelitis, meningitis, and numerous other syndromes, but these are less common. Group A streptococcal infections have the potential for producing nonsuppurative sequelae (eg, rheumatic fever or acute glomerulonephritis).

The cell walls of streptococci contain both carbohydrate and protein antigens. The C-carbohydrate antigen determines the *group* and the M- or T-protein antigens the specific *type*. In most strains, the M protein appears to confer virulence, and antibodies developed against the M protein are protective against reinfection with that type.

Group A streptococci are almost all β-hemolytic. These organisms are carried asymptomatically on the skin and in the pharynx, rectum, and vagina. Ten to 25% of school children in the USA are asymptomatic pharyngeal carriers.

All group A streptococci are sensitive to penicillin. A small percentage have become resistant to erythromycin, the other mainstay of treatment.

Clinical Findings

A. Symptoms and Signs:

1. Respiratory infections—

a. Infancy and early types (under 3 years of age)—The onset of infection is insidious, with mild symptoms, ie, low-grade fever, serous nasal discharge, and pallor. Otitis media is common. Pharyngitis with exudate and cervical adenitis are rare in this age group.

b. Childhood type—Onset is sudden, with fever and marked malaise and often with repeated vomiting. The pharynx is sore and edematous, and the tonsillar area generally shows exudate. Anterior cervical lymph nodes are tender and enlarged. Small petechiae are frequently seen on the soft palate. Fine discrete petechiae on the upper abdomen and trunk occasionally also appear. In scarlet fever, the skin is diffusely erythematous and appears sunburned. The rash is most intense in the axillas and groin and on the abdomen and trunk. It blanches on pressure except in the skin folds, which do not blanch and are pigmented (Pastia's sign). The rash usually appears 24 hours after the onset of fever and rapidly spreads over the next 1–2 days. Desquamation begins on the face at the end of the first week and becomes generalized by the third week. Early, the surface of the tongue is coated white, with the papillae enlarged and bright red ("white strawberry tongue"). Subsequently, desquamation occurs and the tongue appears beefy red ("red strawberry tongue"). The face generally shows circumoral pallor. Petechiae may be seen on all mucosal surfaces.

c. Adult type—The adult type is characterized by exudative or nonexudative tonsillitis with fewer systemic manifestations, lower fever, and no vomiting. Complications due to sensitization do occur. Scarlet fever is not common in this age group.

2. Impetigo—Streptococcal impetigo begins as a papule that vesiculates and then breaks, leaving a denuded area covered by a honey-colored crust. A mixture of *Staphylococcus aureus* along with streptococci is isolated in about 66% of cases. The lesions spread readily and diffusely. Local lymph nodes often become swollen and inflamed. The affected child may develop high fever and be acutely ill. In some cases of impetigo, the primary lesion is a bulla (''bullous impetigo''). Staphylococci are the major cause in such instances.

3. Cellulitis—The portal of entry is often an insect bite of superficial abrasion on an extremity. There is a diffuse and rapidly spreading cellulitis that involves the subcutaneous tissues and extends along the lymphatic pathways with only minimal local suppuration. Local acute lymphadenitis occurs. The child is usually acutely ill, with fever and malaise. The involved area is swollen, warm, tender, and painful. The infection may extend rapidly from the lymphatics to the bloodstream.

4. Necrotizing fasciitis—Formerly called streptococcal gangrene, this is an uncommon but dangerous entity. Studies have demonstrated that only 20–40% of cases are due to group A streptococci. About 30–40% are due to *S aureus* and the rest to gram-negative organisms. Multiple bacteria are frequently involved. The disease is characterized by extensive necrosis of superficial fasciae, with undermining of surrounding tissue and extreme systemic toxicity. Initially, the skin overlying the infection is pale red without distinct borders, resembling subcutaneous cellulitis. Blisters or bullae may appear. The pale red skin progresses to a distinct purple color. The involved area may develop mild to massive edema.

5. Group A streptococcal infections in newborn nurseries—Group A streptococcal nursery epidemics still occasionally occur. The organism may be introduced into the nursery from the vaginal tract of a mother or from the throat or nose of a mother or a member of the staff. The organism then spreads from infant to infant. The umbilical stump is colonized while the infant is in the nursery. As is true also in staphylococcal infections, there may be no or few clinical manifestations while infants are still in the nursery; most often, a colonized infant develops a chronic, oozing omphalitis days later at home. The organism may spread from the infant to other family members. More serious and even fatal infections may develop, including sepsis, meningitis, empyema, septic arthritis, and peritonitis.

B. Laboratory Findings: Leukocytosis with a marked shift to the left is seen early. Eosinophilia regularly appears during convalescence.

β-Hemolytic streptococci are cultured with ease from the throat. The organism may be cultured from the skin—and by needle aspiration from subcutaneous tissues and other involved sites—and from infected nodes. Occasionally, blood cultures are positive. Group A streptococci may be identified most easily by demonstrable sensitivity to disks containing standardized concentrations of bacitracin. Grouping by immunofluorescence or coagglutination studies is preferred and correlates best with the original precipitin reactions described by Lancefield. Typing is dependent upon the presence of specific M precipitins or T agglutinins in the cell wall and is cumbersome enough to be reserved for epidemiologic surveys.

Rapid antigen detection tests that are now available demonstrate 85% sensitivity and over 95% specificity. They may be useful, particularly when early antibiotic therapy is considered.

Antistreptolysin O (ASO) titers rise about 150 units within 2 weeks after an acute infection. Elevated ASO and anti-DNase B titers are useful in documenting prior throat infections in cases of acute rheumatic fever. On the other hand, elevated anti-DNase B and antihyaluronidase titers are most useful in associating pyoderma and acute glomerulonephritis. The streptozyme test is a useful 2-minute slide test that detects antibodies to streptolysin O, hyaluronidase, streptokinase, DNase B, and NADase. It is somewhat more sensitive than the measurement of ASO titers.

The presence of erythrogenic toxin in scarlet fever may be demonstrated during the first hours of the rash by a blanching reaction following the local intradermal injection of 0.1 mL of human immune globulin. Blanching is best seen 8–14 hours after injection. This is best done on the lateral chest or abdominal wall.

The urine may show proteinuria, cylindruria, and minimal hematuria early. More commonly, true sensitizing poststreptococcal nephritis is seen 2–4 weeks after the respiratory infection.

Differential Diagnosis

Streptococcosis of the early childhood type must be differentiated from pneumococcal fever and from adenovirus and other respiratory virus infections.

Adenoviruses, coxsackieviruses (both A and B), echoviruses, Epstein-Barr virus (infectious mononucleosis), and many other respiratory viruses can produce pharyngitis. The pharyngitis in herpangina (coxsackie A viruses) is vesicular or ulcerative. With other viruses (coxsackie and echoviruses), rashes are common. In infectious mononucleosis, the pharyngitis is often exudative, but generalized lymphadenopathy is also present, and laboratory findings are often diagnostic (atypical lymphocytes, elevated liver enzymes, and a positive heterophil or other serologic test for mononucleosis).

In diphtheria, systemic symptoms, vomiting, and fever are all less marked; the pseudomembrane is confluent and adherent; and the throat is less red.

Pharyngeal tularemia causes white rather than yellow exudate. There is little erythema, and cultures for β-hemolytic streptococci are negative. Response to specific antibiotic therapy is prompt.

Leukemia and agranulocytosis may present with pharyngitis and are diagnosed by bone marrow examination.

Scarlet fever must be differentiated from other exanthematous diseases, principally rubella. Erythema due to sunburn, drug reactions, fever, Kawasaki disease, and staphylococcal scalded skin syndrome must at times be considered.

Complications

The most common suppurative complications of

group A streptococcal infections are purulent or serous rhinitis, sinusitis, otitis, mastoiditis, cervical lymphadenitis (which may be suppurative), pneumonia and empyema, septic arthritis, and meningitis. Spread of streptococcal infection from the throat to other sites, principally the skin (impetigo) and vagina, is common also and should be considered in every instance of chronic vaginal discharge or chronic skin infection such as that complicating childhood eczema.

Both acute rheumatic fever and acute glomerulonephritis are nonsuppurative complications of group A streptococcal infections.

A. Acute Rheumatic Fever: See Chapter 15.

B. Acute Glomerulonephritis: Acute nephritis can follow streptococcal infections of either the pharynx or the skin. This is in contrast to rheumatic fever, which only follows pharyngeal infection. Glomerulonephritis may occur at any age, including infancy. In most reported series of acute glomerulonephritis, males predominate by a ratio of 2:1, whereas acute rheumatic fever occurs with equal frequency in both sexes.

Only certain M types are capable of causing poststreptococcal glomerulonephritis ("nephritogenic types"). Moreover, the serotypes resident on or producing disease on the skin often differ from those found in the pharynx. Pharyngeal infections leading to glomerulonephritis include M types 1, 4, 12, and 18, with limited evidence for 3, 6, and 25. Skin M types leading to nephritis include 2, 31, 49, 52–55, 57, and 60.

The incidence of acute glomerulonephritis after streptococcal infection is variable and has ranged from 0 to 28%. Several outbreaks of acute glomerulonephritis in families have involved 50–75% of siblings of affected patients in 1- to 7-week periods. Second attacks of glomerulonephritis are rare. The median latent period between infection and the development of glomerulonephritis is 10 days. This contrasts with acute rheumatic fever, which has a median latent period of 18 days.

Treatment

A. Specific Measures: Treatment is directed not only toward eradication of acute infection but also at the prevention of rheumatic fever and nephritis. In patients with pharyngitis, antibiotics should be started early to relieve symptoms and should be continued for 10 days to prevent rheumatic fever. On the other hand, glomerulonephritis appears difficult to prevent even when prompt treatment is administered. It seems advisable to treat sibling contacts of patients with pyoderma-associated nephritis as early in the course of skin infection as possible. The use of sulfonamides or trimethoprim-sulfamethoxazole in the treatment of streptococcal disease is to be discouraged because these agents do not prevent the development of sensitizing antibodies and therefore do not lower the incidence of rheumatic fever or nephritis.

1. Penicillin—A single dose of benzathine penicillin G (Bicillin), 0.6–1.2 million units intramuscularly, is preferred for treatment of pharyngitis and impetigo. Oral phenoxymethyl penicillin (penicillin V), 125–250 mg every 6 hours between meals for 10 days, is successful in about 90% of cases. Parenteral therapy is indicated if there is vomiting or sepsis. Mild cellulitis may be similarly treated. Cellulitis requiring hospitalization should be treated with aqueous penicillin G, 150,000 units/kg/d intravenously or intramuscularly in 6 divided doses until there is marked improvement. Oral penicillin V, 125–250 mg every 6 hours, may then be given to complete a 7- to 10-day course. Acute cervical lymphadenitis may require incision and drainage. Treatment of necrotizing fasciitis requires emergency surgical debridement followed by high-dose parenteral antibiotics appropriate to the organisms cultured.

Ampicillin, nafcillin, oxacillin, cloxacillin, and dicloxacillin are also effective in the treatment of streptococcal infections. Penicillinase-producing staphylococci play a controversial role in penicillin treatment failures.

2. Other antibiotics—For pharyngitis or impetigo, give erythromycin, 40 mg/kg/d orally in 4 divided doses for 10 days. Clindamycin and cephalexin are effective oral antibiotics. The dosage of clindamycin is 10–20 mg/kg/d in 4 divided doses; for cephalexin, 25–50 mg/kg/d in 4 divided doses. Each of these drugs should be given for 10 days. Tetracycline-resistant strains have been reported. For serious or life-threatening infections in patients with known penicillin allergy, give cephalothin, 100–200 mg/kg/d intravenously in 6 divided doses, or cefazolin, 100–150 mg/kg/d intravenously or intramuscularly in 4 divided doses.

3. Treatment failure—Reculture after cessation of therapy is only indicated in the patient with pharyngitis who was treated with oral antibiotics and has a personal or family history of rheumatic fever. Even with perfect compliance, organisms will be found at this time in 5–15% of infections. Re-treatment at least once with benzathine penicillin G or a different oral antibiotic is indicated.

4. Control of nursery epidemics—

a. For symptomatic infants with positive cultures, give aqueous penicillin G, 100,000 units/kg/d intramuscularly in 2 divided doses for 10 days. Those with positive cultures but without symptoms or signs may be treated with a single dose of benzathine penicillin G (50,000 units intramuscularly).

b. Apply bacitracin ointment every 8 hours to the umbilical stump of each infant until discharge from the nursery.

c. Treat all other infants prophylactically with a single intramuscular dose of 50,000 units of benzathine penicillin G.

d. Continue prophylactic bacitracin ointment and benzathine penicillin G for 15 days or until the outbreak is controlled.

5. Prevention of recurrences in rheumatic individuals—The preferred prophylaxis for rheumatic individuals is benzathine penicillin G, 1.2 million units intramuscularly once a month. One of the following alternative oral prophylactic regimens may be used: sulfadiazine, 0.5–1 g daily; penicillin G, 200,000 units twice daily; or erythromycin, 250 mg twice daily. Most authorities feel that lifelong prophylaxis is indicated, particularly in the presence of rheumatic heart disease. A similar approach to the prevention of recurrences of glomerulonephritis is debatable but may be indicated during childhood when there is a suspicion that repeated streptococcal infections coincide with flare-ups of acute glomerulonephritis.

B. General Measures: Analgesic lozenges or gargles with 30% glucose or hot saline solution may be used for relief of sore throat. A soft, bland diet that includes noncarbonated high-glucose drinks (such as apple, grape, and pear juice) and iced milk or sherbet is helpful. Acetaminophen may be useful for fever.

With impetigo, local treatment may promote earlier healing. Crusts should first be soaked off; areas beneath the crusts should then be washed with 3% hexachlorophene 3 times daily.

C. Treatment of Complications: Acute complications are best treated with penicillin. Prevention of rheumatic fever is best accomplished by early adequate penicillin treatment of the streptococcal infection (see above).

D. Treatment of Carriers: Spread of disease to contacts is less likely to occur from carriers of group A streptococci than from acutely infected individuals. Carrier states are difficult to abolish, and it is advisable to be certain that a group A strain is involved before it is attempted.

In families with recurrent streptococcal infections or a history of rheumatic fever, contacts should be cultured, and those with positive cultures should be treated. As an alternative plan, all family contacts may be treated. Treatment consists of a single dose of benzathine penicillin G, 1.2 million units intramuscularly, or therapeutic doses of oral penicillin V.

Prognosis

Death is rare except in sepsis or pneumonia in infancy or early childhood. The febrile course is shortened and complications eliminated by early and adequate penicillin treatment.

Bergner-Rabinowitz S et al: The new streptozyme test for streptococcal antibodies. *Clin Pediatr* 1975;**14**:804.

Breese BB, Hall CB: *Beta-hemolytic Streptococcal Infection.* Houghton Mifflin, 1978.

Burech DL, Koranyi KI, Haynes RE: Serious group A streptococcal diseases in children. *J Pediatr* 1976;**88**:972.

Kaplan EL: The group A streptococcal upper respiratory tract carrier state: An enigma. *J Pediatr* 1980;**97**:337.

Krause RM: Prevention of streptococcal sequelae by penicillin prophylaxis: A reassessment. *J Infect Dis* 1975;**131**:592.

Markowitz M, Gordis L: *Rheumatic Fever,* 2nd ed. Saunders, 1972.

Maruyama S et al: Sensitivity of group A streptococci to antibiotics: Prevalence of resistance to erythromycin in Japan. *Am J Dis Child* 1979;**133**:1143.

Peter G, Hazard J: Neonatal group A streptococcal disease. *J Pediatr* 1975;**87**:454.

Randolph MF et al: Effect of antibiotic therapy on the clinical course of streptococcal pharyngitis. *J Pediatr* 1985;**106**:870.

Wannamaker LW: Differences between streptococcal infections of the throat and of the skin. (2 parts.) *N Engl J Med* 1970;**282**:23, 78.

GROUP B STREPTOCOCCAL INFECTIONS

Essentials of Diagnosis:

Early-onset neonatal sepsis or meningitis:

- Newborn infant, age 1 hour to 5 days, with rapidly progressing overwhelming sepsis, with or without meningitis.
- Pneumonia with respiratory failure frequently present. Chest x-ray resembles that seen in hyaline membrane disease.
- Leukopenia with a shift to the left.
- Blood or spinal fluid cultures growing group B streptococci.

Late-onset neonatal sepsis or meningitis:

- Meningitis in a child 1–16 weeks old with spinal fluid or blood cultures growing group B streptococci.

General Considerations

Most patients with group B streptococcal disease are infants under 3 months of age. However, serious or life-threatening infection has been reported occasionally in women with puerperal sepsis, in immunocompromised patients, in patients with cirrhosis and spontaneous peritonitis, and in diabetics with cellulitis. Group B streptococcal infections occur as frequently as gram-negative infections in the newborn period. Two distinct clinical syndromes distinguished by differing perinatal events, age at onset, and serotype of the infecting strain have been described in these infants.

Clinical Findings

The first syndrome, early-onset illness, is observed in the newborn less than 5 days old. The onset of symptoms in the majority of these infants occurs in the first 48 hours of life. Apnea is often the first sign. There is a high incidence of associated maternal obstetric complications, especially premature labor and prolonged rupture of the membranes. Newborns with early-onset disease are severely ill at the time of diagnosis and have a mortality rate of more than 50%. Although the majority of infants with early-onset infections have low birth weights, term infants may also develop fatal infection. Newborns with early-onset infection acquire the group B streptococcal organism from the maternal genital tract in utero or during passage through the birth canal. When early-onset infection is complicated by meningitis, as occurs in approximately 30% of cases, more than 80% of the bacterial isolates belong to serotype III. Postmortem examination of infants with early-onset disease almost always reveals pulmonary inflammatory infiltrates and hyaline membrane formation. These hyaline membranes have been shown by both routine and fluorescent antibody staining to contain large numbers of group B streptococci.

The late-onset infection occurs in infants after the first week of life (between 10 days and 4 months of age); the median age at onset is about 4 weeks. Meningitis is the most common manifestation of serious infection. Maternal obstetric complications are infrequently associated with late-onset infection. These infants are usually not as severely ill at the time of diagnosis as those with early-onset disease, and the mortality rate is significantly lower (approximately 20%). However, up to 50% of infants with late-onset meningitis have neurologic sequelae following recovery. Although the majority of infants with late-onset disease have meningitis, other clinical manifestations have been described. These include septic arthritis and osteomyelitis, asymptomatic bacteremia, otitis media, ethmoiditis, conjunctivitis, cellulitis (particularly of the face or submandibular area), lymphadenitis, breast abscess, pleural empyema, and impetigo. Strains of group B streptococci possessing the capsular type III polysaccharide antigen are isolated from more than 95% of infants with late-onset disease, irrespective of clinical manifestations. The exact mode of transmission of the organisms is not well defined.

Prevention

Many women of childbearing age possess circulating antibody to the neutral buffer polysaccharide antigen of type III group B streptococci. This antibody is transferred to the newborn via the placental circulation. Carriers delivering healthy infants have significant levels of IgG antibody to this antigen in their sera. In contrast, sera obtained from women delivering infants with proved type III group B streptococcal disease of either the early- or late-onset type rarely have detectable antibody in their sera. Similar findings have recently been described for type Ia infections.

Recent studies of use of prophylactic penicillin in newborns to prevent early-onset group B streptococcal disease have produced conflicting results. Many infants with early-onset disease are bacteremic at birth, and use of penicillin in this group fails to control infection. While treatment of parturient mothers with ampicillin probably prevents early-onset disease, widespread use of this treatment cannot be recommended.

Treatment

Penicillin G is usually an effective antibiotic for the treatment of group B streptococcal disease. In vitro and clinical data on susceptibility of group B streptococci to penicillin G with reference to concentration of organisms in cerebrospinal fluid and peak levels of penicillin G in cerebrospinal fluid suggest that doses of penicillin of 250,000 units/kg/d may be necessary to eradicate the organism from the cerebrospinal fluid. The combination of a penicillin with an aminoglycoside may be more effective against group B streptococci than penicillin G alone. For this reason, initial therapy with both drugs may be beneficial. Treatment of group B streptococcal meningitis is with penicillin G for 3 weeks: under 1 week of age, 200,000–250,000 units/kg/d intramuscularly or, preferably, intravenously, divided into 3 doses given every 8 hours; over 1 week of age, 250,000 units/kg/d intravenously or intramuscularly, divided into 6 doses given every 4 hours. Gentamicin in the recommended dosage for the newborn of 5–7.5 mg/kg/d intramuscularly or intravenously may be synergistic with penicillin. For sepsis without meningitis, treatment for 10 days is adequate.

STREPTOCOCCAL INFECTIONS WITH ORGANISMS OTHER THAN GROUP A OR B

Streptococci of groups other than A and B are part of the normal flora of humans and can cause disease. Group C or G organisms occasionally produce pharyngitis (with an ASO rise) but without risk of subsequent rheumatic fever. Group D streptococci (enterococci) are normal inhabitants of the gastrointestinal tract and may produce urinary tract infections, meningitis and sepsis in the newborn, and endocarditis. Alpha (viridans) or nonhemolytic aerobic streptococci are normal flora of the mouth. They are involved in the production of dental plaque and probably dental caries and are the commonest cause of subacute bacterial endocarditis. Finally, there are numerous anaerobic streptococcal species, normal flora of the mouth, skin, and gastrointestinal tract, which alone or in combination with other bacteria may cause sinusitis, dental abscesses, brain abscesses, and intra-abdominal or lung abscesses.

Treatment

A. Group D Streptococcal Infections: Urinary tract infections can be treated with oral ampicillin alone. Sepsis or meningitis in the newborn should be treated intravenously with a combination of ampicillin (100–200 mg/kg/d in 3–4 divided doses) and kanamycin (15–20 mg/kg/d in 2 divided doses). Endocarditis requires 6 weeks of intravenous treatment. Traditionally, this has been with penicillin G, 250,000 units/kg/d in 6–8 divided doses, plus streptomycin, 30 mg/kg/d intramuscularly in 2 divided doses for 2 weeks followed by one-half this dosage for the remaining 4 weeks. Ampicillin plus kanamycin or gentamicin is also adequate treatment, provided the drugs are administered in maximal doses over at least a 6-week period.

Whenever endocarditis, sepsis, or meningitis is being treated, peak and trough serum killing powers should be obtained if possible. A bactericidal level of 1:8 or greater immediately before the next penicillin dose (ie, in the trough) should be maintained.

B. Viridans Streptococcal Infections (Subacute Bacterial Endocarditis): It is important to determine the penicillin sensitivity of the infecting strain as early as possible in the treatment of viridans streptococcal endocarditis. Resistant organisms are most commonly seen in patients receiving chronic penicillin prophylaxis for rheumatic heart disease. Strains sensitive to pencillin G concentrations of less than 0.2 μg/mL (minimum bactericidal concentrations) may be treated for 4 weeks with penicillin, with streptomycin added during the first 2 weeks. Either intramuscular procaine penicillin G, 60,000 units/kg/d in 3 divided doses, or intravenous penicillin G, 150,000 units/kg/d in 6 divided doses, should be used with streptomycin (30 mg/kg/d intramuscularly in 2 divided doses). If a strain requires 0.2 μg/mL or more in vitro to produce killing, longer therapy (at least 4 weeks) and higher doses of parenteral penicillin must be used (200,000–300,000 units/kg/d intravenously or 90,000–100,000 units/kg/d intramuscularly) and a full 4-week course of streptomycin given (the first 2 weeks at 30 mg/kg/d intramuscularly in 2 divided doses and the second 2 weeks at 15 mg/kg/d).

When penicillin sensitivity is suspected, a skin ("scratch") or conjunctival test with 1 unit of penicillin should be performed. If immediate hypersensitivity is seen, desensitization may be carried out. Alternative therapy is vancomycin, 30 mg/kg/d intravenously in 4 divided doses.

Ablow RC et al: A comparison of early-onset group B streptococcal neonatal infection and the respiratory-distress syndrome of the newborn. *N Engl J Med* 1976;**294:**65.

Baker CJ, Kasper DL: Correlation of maternal antibody deficiency with susceptibility to neonatal group B streptococcal infection. *N Engl J Med* 1976;**294:**753.

Edwards MS et al: Long-term sequelae of group B streptococcal meningitis in infants. *J Pediatr* 1985;**106:**717.

Paredes A, Wong P, Yow MD: Failure of penicillin to eradicate the carrier state of group B streptococcus in infants. *J Pediatr* 1976;**89:**191.

Paredes A et al: Nosocomial transmission of group B streptococci in a newborn nursery. *Pediatrics* 1977;**59:**679.

Prevention of early-onset group B streptococcal infection in the newborn. (Editorial.) *Lancet* 1984;**1:**1056.

Pyati SP et al: Penicillin in infants weighing two kilograms or less with early-onset group B streptococcal disease. *N Engl J Med* 1983;**308:**1383.

Sande MA, Scheld WM: Combination antibiotic therapy of bacterial endocarditis. *Ann Intern Med* 1980;**92:**390.

Siegel JD: Single-dose penicillin prophylaxis against neonatal group B streptococcal infection. *N Engl J Med* 1980;**303:**769.

PNEUMOCOCCAL INFECTIONS

Essentials of Diagnosis

Bacteremia:

- High fever (≥ 39.4 °C [102.9 °F]).
- Leukocytosis (≥ 15,000/μL).
- Age 6–24 months.

Pneumonia:

- Fever, leukocytosis, and cough.
- Localized chest pain.
- Localized or diffuse rales. Chest x-ray may show lobar infiltrate (with effusion).

Meningitis:

- Fever, leukocytosis.
- Bulging fontanelle, neck stiffness.
- Irritability and lethargy.

All types:

- Diagnoses confirmed by cultures of blood, spinal fluid, pleural fluid, or other body fluid or by detection of pneumococcal antigen in urine or spinal fluid.

General Considerations

Pneumococcal sepsis, sinusitis, otitis media, pneumonitis, meningitis, osteomyelitis, cellulitis, arthritis, vaginitis, and peritonitis are all part of a spectrum of pneumococcal infection. Clinical findings that correlate with occult bacteremia in ambulatory patients include age (6–24 months), degree of temperature elevation (≥ 39.4 °C [102.9 °F]), and leukocytosis (≥ 15,000/μL). Although each of these findings is in itself nonspecific, a combination of them should arouse suspicion. This constellation of findings in a child who has no focus of infection may be an indication for blood cultures and antibiotic therapy. The cause of two-thirds of such bacteremic episodes is pneumococci. *Haemophilus influenzae* type b is the second most frequent cause.

Streptococcus pneumoniae is the most common cause of acute purulent otitis media. Many physicians suspect that the pneumococcus also causes pharyngitis and purulent rhinitis, but there is no firm evidence to support this belief.

Pneumococci are the organisms responsible for most cases of acute bacterial pneumonia in children. The disease is indistinguishable on clinical grounds from other bacterial pneumonias. Effusions are common, although frank empyema is less common. Abscesses also occasionally occur.

Pneumococcal meningitis is much less common than *H influenzae* type b meningitis in children under age 5, but it is more common in older children. Pneumococcal meningitis, sometimes recurrent, may complicate serious head trauma, particularly if there is persistent leakage of cerebrospinal fluid. This has prompted some physicians to recommend the prophylactic administration of penicillin or other antimicrobials in such cases.

Children with sickle cell disease, other hemoglobinopathies, congenital or acquired asplenia, and some immunoglobulin and complement deficiencies are unusually susceptible to overwhelming pneumococcal sepsis and meningitis. These children often have a catastrophic illness with shock and disseminated intravascular coagulation. Even with excellent supportive care, the mortality rate is 20–50%. The spleen is important in the control of pneumococcal infection by clearing organisms from the blood and producing an opsonin that enhances phagocytosis. Autosplenectomy may explain why children with sickle cell disease are at increased risk for developing serious pneumococcal infections.

For more than 30 years, penicillin has been the agent of choice for pneumococcal infections. The majority of strains are still highly susceptible to penicillin; however, during the last 10 years, there have been increasing reports of pneumococci with moderately increased resistance to penicillin and reports of treatment failure, particularly in meningitis. The prevalence of these relatively penicillin-resistant strains in North America is about 3–15%. An outbreak of infections due to markedly penicillin-resistant pneumococci has been reported from South Africa. Pneumococci from cerebrospinal fluid, blood, and possibly other body fluids should be screened routinely for penicillin susceptibility. Pneumococci may also be resistant to chloramphenicol, erythromycin, and other antimicrobials.

Pneumococci have been classified into 83 serotypes based on capsular polysaccharide antigens. Serotypes 6, 14, 18, 19, and 23 cause most pneumococcal infections in children. The frequency distribution of serotypes varies at different times, in different geographic areas, and with different sites of infection. The most recently developed polyvalent pneumococcal vaccine contains capsular polysaccharides of 23 serotypes and is discussed in Chapter 5. Specific antibody induced by the vaccine protects only against the serotypes included in the vaccine. Children under age 18–24 months generally do not have a good antibody response to this vaccine, and the protective efficacy of the vaccine in older children is controversial. Despite these limitations, the vaccine is recommended for high-risk children over 2 years of age.

Clinical Findings

A. Symptoms and Signs: In pneumococcal sepsis, fever usually appears abruptly, often accompanied by chills. There may be no respiratory symptoms. In pneumococcal sinusitis, mucopurulent nasal discharge may occur. In infants and young children with pneumonia, cough and diffuse rales are found more often than the lobar distribution characteristic of adult forms of pneumococcal pneumonia. Respiratory distress is manifest by flaring of the alae nasi, chest retractions, and tachypnea. Abdominal pain is common. In older children, the adult form of pneumococcal pneumonia with signs of lobar consolidation may be found, but sputum is rarely bloody. Thoracic pain resulting from pleural involvement is sometimes present, but less often in children than in adults. With involvement of the right hemidiaphragm, pain may be referred to the right lower quadrant, suggesting appendicitis. Vomiting is common at onset but seldom persists. Convulsions are relatively common at onset in infants.

Meningitis is characterized by fever, irritability, convulsions, and neck stiffness. The most important sign in very young infants is a tense, bulging anterior fontanelle. In older children, fever, chills, headache, and vomiting are common symptoms. Classic signs are nuchal rigidity associated with positive Brudzinski and Kernig signs. With progression of untreated disease, the child may develop opisthotonos, stupor, and coma.

B. Laboratory Findings: Leukocytosis is often pronounced (20,000–45,000/μL), with 80–90% polymorphonuclear neutrophils. Neutropenia may be seen early in very serious infections. The presence of pneumococci in the nasopharynx is not helpful, because up to 40% of normal children carry pneumococci in the upper respiratory tract. Large numbers of organisms seen on gram-stained smears of endotracheal aspirate are more helpful. Needle aspiration of the lung rarely is indicated. In meningitis, cerebrospinal fluid usually shows an elevated white cell count of several thousand, chiefly polymorphonuclear neutrophils, with decreased glucose and elevated protein levels. Gram-positive diplococci are seen on stained smears of cerebrospinal fluid sediment in 70–90% of cases. Counterimmunoelectrophoresis allows for rapid diagnosis by detection of pneumococcal antigen and is most valuable when a child has been partially treated with antibiotics prior to lumbar puncture and the gram-stained smear and culture of spinal fluid are negative. Counterimmunoelectrophoresis of urine, pleural fluid, or serum may also be useful in selected cases.

Differential Diagnosis

There are many causes of high fever and leukocytosis in young infants; 80–90% of children presenting with these signs have a disease other than pneumococcal bacteremia, such as enteroviral or other viral infection, urinary tract infection, unrecognized focal infection elsewhere in the body, roseola infantum, or early acute shigellosis (diarrhea will appear later).

Infants with upper respiratory tract infection who subsequently develop signs of lower respiratory disease are most likely to be infected with respiratory syncytial virus, parainfluenza virus types 1, 2, or 3, or other respiratory viruses. Hoarseness or wheezing is often present. X-ray of the chest typically shows perihilar infiltrates and increased bronchovascular markings. It must be remembered, however, that viral respiratory infection often precedes pneumococcal pneumonia and that the clinical picture may be mixed.

Staphylococcal pneumonia frequently causes cavity formation and empyema, but it may be indistinguishable early in the course from pneumococcal pneumonia. It is most common in infants.

In primary pulmonary tuberculosis, children are not toxic, and x-rays show a primary focus associated with hilar adenopathy and often with signs of pleurisy. Miliary tuberculosis presents a classic x-ray appearance.

Pneumonia caused by *Mycoplasma pneumoniae* is most common in children 5 years of age and older. Onset is insidious, with infrequent chills, low-grade fever, prominent headache and malaise, cough, and, often, striking x-ray changes. Marked leukocytosis (eg, > 18,000/μL) is unusual.

Pneumococcal meningitis is diagnosed by lumbar puncture. Without a gram-stained smear and culture of spinal fluid, it is not distinguishable from other types of acute bacterial meningitis.

Complications

Complications of sepsis include meningitis and osteomyelitis; complications of pneumonia include empyema, parapneumonic effusion, and, rarely, lung abscess. Mastoiditis and meningitis may follow untreated pneumococcal otitis media. Both pneumococcal meningitis and peritonitis are more likely to occur independently without coexisting pneumonia. Shock, disseminated intravascular coagulation, and Waterhouse-Friderichsen syndrome resembling meningococcemia are occasionally seen in pneumococcal sepsis, particularly in asplenic patients.

Treatment

A. Specific Measures: Penicillin is the drug of choice, but erythromycin and cephalosporins are also effective.

1. Sepsis—All children with blood cultures that grow pneumococci must be reexamined as soon as possible. The child who has a focal infection such as pneumonia or meningitis or who appears septic should be admitted to the hospital and should receive parenteral penicillin G. Only if the child is afebrile and appears well should management on an ambulatory basis be considered. If the physician is assured of close follow-up, a second blood culture is performed (lumbar puncture is not mandatory); oral penicillin V, 50–100 mg/kg/d for 10 days, is prescribed, and the initial dose is given at once. Some children may be intermittently afebrile yet still progress to meningitis.

2. Pneumonia—For infants, severely ill patients, and immunocompromised hosts, give aqueous penicillin G, 150,000–200,000 units/kg/d intravenously in 4–6 divided doses. Aqueous procaine penicillin G, 600,000 units intramuscularly daily for 7–10 days, is recommended for older children. Mild pneumonia may be treated with oral phenoxymethyl penicillin, 50 mg/kg/d in 4 divided doses for 7–10 days. In cases of penicillin allergy, give erythromycin, 40–50 mg/kg/d orally in 4 divided doses. Oral cephalosporins may be used.

3. Otitis media—Treat with oral ampicillin, amoxicillin, trimethoprim-sulfamethoxazole, or erythromycin for 10 days.

4. Meningitis—Until bacteriologic confirmation, give ampicillin plus chloramphenicol intravenously or give cefuroxime or cefotaxime intravenously. After bacteriologic confirmation, give aqueous penicillin G, 300,000 units/kg/d intravenously in 6 divided doses for 10–14 days. Meningitis due to organisms that are resistant or relatively resistant to penicillin should be treated with chloramphenicol or vancomycin.

B. General Measures: Supportive and symptomatic care is required.

Prognosis

In children, case fatality rates of less than 1% should be achieved except in meningitis, in which rates of 5–20% still prevail. The presence of large numbers of organisms without a prominent cerebrospinal fluid inflammatory response or of meningitis due to a penicillin-resistant strain indicates a poor prognosis. Serious neurologic sequelae are more frequent following pneumococcal meningitis than following meningococcal or *H influenzae* type b meningitis.

Alon U, Adler SP, Chan JCM: Hemolytic-uremic syndrome associated with *Streptococcus pneumoniae:* Report of a case and review of the literature. *Am J Dis Child* 1984;**138:**496.

Bortolussi R, Thompson TR, Ferrieri P: Early-onset pneumococcal sepsis in newborn infants. *Pediatrics* 1977;**60:**352.

Bratton L, Teele DW, Klein JO: Outcome of unsuspected pneumococcemia in children not initially admitted to the hospital. *J Pediatr* 1977;**90:**703.

Burman LA, Norrby R, Trollfors B: Invasive pneumococcal infections: Incidence, predisposing factors, and prognosis. *Rev Infect Dis* 1985;**7:**133.

Douglas RM, Miles HB: Vaccination against *Streptococcus pneumoniae* in childhood: Lack of demonstrable benefit in young Australian children. *J Infect Dis* 1984;**149:**861.

Immunizations Practices Advisory Committee, Centers for Disease Control: Update: Pneumococcal polysaccharide vaccine usage—United States. *Ann Intern Med* 1984;**101:**348.

Jackson MA et al: Relatively penicillin-resistant pneumococcal infections in pediatric patients. *Pediatr Infect Dis* 1984; **3:**129.

Jacobs MR et al: Emergence of multiply resistant pneumococci. *N Engl J Med* 1978;**299:**735.

Klein JO: Bacteremia in ambulatory children. *Pediatr Infect Dis* 1984;**3(Suppl):**S5.

Klein JO: The epidemiology of pneumococcal disease in infants and children. *Rev Infect Dis* 1981;**3:**246.

STAPHYLOCOCCAL INFECTIONS

Staphylococcal infections are common and important in childhood. Staphylococcal skin infections range from minor furuncles to the varied syndromes now collected under the encompassing term "scalded skin syndrome." Staphylococci are the major cause of osteomyelitis and, in older children, of septic arthritis. They are an uncommon but important cause of bacterial pneumonia. A toxin produced by certain strains causes staphylococcal food poisoning. Staphylococci are now responsible for most infections of artificial heart valves. They were responsible for outbreaks of skin and systemic diseases in nurseries during the 1950s and early 1960s and remain an important cause of nursery epidemics today. In the 1970s and 1980s, they have been strongly associated with the toxic shock syndrome, a serious multisystem acute illness particularly common in menstruating girls and young women. Finally, they are found in infections at all ages and in multiple sites, particularly when infection is introduced from the skin or upper respiratory tract or when closed compartments become infected (pericarditis, sinusitis, cervical adenitis, surgical wounds, abscesses in the liver or brain, and abscesses elsewhere in the body).

Staphylococcus aureus and *Staphylococcus epidermidis* are normal flora of the skin and respiratory tract. The latter rarely causes disease except in compromised hosts or the newborn or when there is a plastic prosthesis in place.

Many strains of *S aureus* elaborate a β-lactamase that confers penicillin resistance. This can be overcome in clinical practice by the use of a non-penicillin antibiotic, a cephalosporin, or a penicillinase-resistant penicillin such as methicillin, oxacillin, nafcillin, cloxacillin, or dicloxacillin. Methicillin-resistant strains have become a problem in Europe and Britain and are now common in certain hospitals and areas in the USA. Most of these strains retain β-lactamase production, and many are resistant to other antibiotics as well.

S aureus produces a variety of exotoxins, most of which are of uncertain importance. Two toxins are recognized as playing a central role in specific diseases: exfoliatin and staphylococcal enterotoxin. The former is largely responsible for the various clinical presentations of the scalded skin syndrome. Most strains that elaborate exfoliatin are of phage group II. The latter toxin causes staphylococcal food poisoning. Although the toxin causing toxic shock syndrome has not been identified with certainty, it may be what investigators now call "enterotoxin F" or "pyrogenic exotoxin C."

Different strains of *S aureus* vary widely not only in their capacity to produce toxin but also in their virulence. Thus, it is common to observe a colonization rate in nursery infants of 20–40% in the absence of disease; on the other hand, introduction of a virulent strain of *S aureus* in a single infant can lead to a devastating outbreak if proper precautions are not taken.

Clinical Findings

A. Symptoms and Signs:

1. Staphylococcal skin diseases—Dermal infection with *S aureus* is manifested by formation of a furuncle or, occasionally, cellulitis. More superficial infections are often found along with streptococci in impetigo. If the strains produce exfoliatin, localized lesions become bullous (bullous impetigo).

Generalized exfoliative disease (scalded skin syndrome, or toxic epidermal necrolysis) occurs as a result of more generalized involvement with exfoliatin-producing strains. The infection may begin at any site but appears to be introduced through the respiratory tract in most cases. There is a prodromal phase of erythema, often beginning around the mouth, accompanied by fever and irritability. The involved skin becomes tender, and a sick infant will cry when picked up or touched. A day or so later, exfoliation begins, usually around the mouth. The inside of the mouth is red, and a peeling rash is present around the lips, often in a radial pattern resembling rhagades. Generalized, painful peeling may follow, involving the limbs and trunk but often sparing the feet. More commonly, peeling is confined to areas around body orifices. If erythematous but unpeeled skin is rubbed sideways, superficial epidermal layers separate from deeper ones and a blister appears (Nikolsky's sign). In the newborn, the disease is termed **Ritter's disease** and may be fulminating. If there is tender erythema but not exfoliation, the disease is termed nonstreptococcal scarlet fever. The scarlatiniform rash is sandpaperlike, but strawberry tongue is not seen, and cultures grow *S aureus* rather than streptococci.

2. Osteomyelitis and septic arthritis—See Chapter 22.

3. Staphylococcal pneumonia—Staphylococcal pneumonia in infancy is characterized by abdominal distention, high fever, respiratory distress, and toxemia. It often occurs without predisposing factors or after minor skin infections. The organism is necrotizing, producing bronchoalveolar destruction. Pneumatoceles, pyopneumothorax, and empyema are frequently encountered. Rapid progression of disease is characteristic. Frequent chest x-rays to monitor the progress of disease are indicated and may be lifesaving. Presenting symptoms may be typical of paralytic ileus, suggestive of an abdominal catastrophe. When this is suspected, the abdominal films should always be accompanied by a chest film to rule out staphylococcal pneumonitis.

Staphylococcal pneumonia usually is peribronchial and diffuse and begins with a focal infiltrative lesion progressing to patchy consolidation. Most often only one lung is involved (80%), more often the right. Purulent pericarditis occurs by direct extension in about 10% of cases, with or without empyema.

4. Staphylococcal food poisoning—Staphylococcal food poisoning is produced by enterotoxin. The most common source is poorly refrigerated and contaminated food. The disease is characterized by vomiting, prostration, and diarrhea occurring 2–6 hours after ingestion of contaminated foods.

5. Staphylococcal endocarditis—*S aureus* may produce infection of normal heart valves, of valves or endocardium in children with congenital or rheumatic heart disease, or of artificial valves. In large recent series, about 25% of all cases of endocarditis are due to *S aureus*. The great majority of artificial heart valve infections involve either *S aureus* or *S epidermidis*. Infection usually begins in an extracardiac focus, often the skin. Involvement of the endocardium must be suspected in every case of *S aureus* bacteremia regardless of the presence of signs. Suspicion must be highest in the presence of congenital heart disease, particularly ventricular septal defects with aortic insufficiency but also simple ventricular septal defect, patent ductus arteriosus, and tetralogy of Fallot.

Clinical presentation in staphylococcal endocarditis is with fever, weight loss, weakness, muscle pain or diffuse skeletal pain, poor feeding, pallor, and cardiac decompensation. Signs include splenomegaly, cardiomegaly, petechiae, hematuria, and a new or changing murmur. The course of *S aureus* endocarditis is commonly rapid, although subacute disease is occasionally seen. Peripheral septic embolization and uncontrollable cardiac failure are not uncommon, even when optimal antibiotic therapy is administered, and may be indications for surgical intervention (see below).

6. Nursery infections—*S aureus* colonizes the umbilicus and respiratory tract of a highly variable proportion of newborn infants (10–90%) during their nursery stay. The source of colonization is the skin and anterior nares of those handling the infants. Under normal circumstances, such colonization is harmless, since the bacterial strains involved are of low virulence. However, if a virulent strain is introduced (usually from an infected lesion), the proportion of sick to colonized infants can rise from less than 1% to over 50%. Such outbreaks may begin insidiously, since infants usually do not develop symptoms (furuncles, omphalitis, mastitis, impetigo, with occasional more serious disease) until after discharge. Thus, the occurrence of even a single case of staphylococcal disease in a nursery is an indication for epidemiologic surveillance of infants recently resident in that nursery, with possible subsequent institution of control measures.

7. Toxic shock syndrome—In 1978, Todd et al described a new syndrome of fever, blanching erythroderma, diarrhea, vomiting, myalgia, prostration, hypotension, and multiple organ involvement associated with cultures of *S aureus*. In that series, infection occurred equally in male and female children, with apparent heavy mucosal colonization (particularly in the female genital tract) or with clinically evident infection. Bacteremia did not occur.

Subsequently, large numbers of cases have been described almost exclusively in menstruating adolescents and young women using vaginal tampons. The epidemiologic connection with *S aureus* in this group has remained strong. Additional clinical features include sudden onset; conjunctival suffusion; mucosal hyperemia; desquamation of skin on the palms, soles, fingers, and toes during convalescence; disseminated intravascular coagulation in severe cases; renal and hepatic functional abnormalities; and evidence of myolysis. The mortality rate is now about 2%. Recurrences were seen during subsequent menstrual periods in as many as 60% of untreated women who continued to use tampons. Recurrences were reported in up to 15% of those who were treated with antistaphylococcal antibiotics and stopped using tampons. The disease is probably due to a toxin resembling one of the staphylococcal enterotoxins and elaborated by certain strains of *S aureus*.

8. *S epidermidis* infections—Localized and systemic *S epidermidis* infections occur primarily in immunocompromised patients, high-risk newborns, and patients with plastic prostheses or catheters. In one survey, *S epidermidis* was the fourth most common organism isolated from cases of septicemia in children with leukemia; in this group, there was a 10% mortality rate with a high incidence of antibiotic resistance. In low-birth-weight infants, *S epidermidis* has emerged as the commonest nosocomial pathogen in nurseries in the USA. In patients with an artificial heart valve, Dacron patch, ventriculoperitoneal shunt for hydrocephalus, or a Hickman or Broviac vascular catheter, *S epidermidis* is one of the very common causes of sepsis or catheter infection, often necessitating removal of the foreign material and prolonged antibiotic therapy. Because blood cultures are frequently contaminated by this organism, diagnosis of genuine localized or systemic infection is often difficult and sometimes uncertain.

B. Laboratory Findings: Moderate leukocytosis (15,000–20,000/μL) with a shift to the left is occasionally found, although normal counts are common, particularly in infants. The sedimentation rate is elevated. Blood cultures are frequently positive in systemic staphylococcal disease and should always be obtained when it is suspected. Similarly, pus from sites of infection should always be aspirated or obtained surgically, examined with Gram's stain, and cultured both aerobically and anaerobically.

Bacteriophage typing may be useful for epidemiologic studies but is rarely of value in individual cases. There are at present no useful serologic tests for staphylococcal disease.

Differential Diagnosis

Staphylococcal skin disease has many morphologic forms and therefore many differential diagnoses. Bullous impetigo must be differentiated from chemical or thermal burns, from drug reactions, and, in the very young, from the various congenital epidermolytic syndromes or even herpes simplex infections. Staphylococcal scalded skin syndrome resembles scarlet fever in some instances and in others appears similar to mucocutaneous lymph node syndrome, Stevens-Johnson syndrome, erythema multiforme, and other drug reactions. A skin biopsy may be critical in establishing the correct diagnosis. The skin lesions of varicella may become superinfected with exfoliatin-producing staphylococci and produce a combination of the 2 diseases (bullous varicella).

Osteomyelitis of the long bones and septic arthritis must often be differentiated (see Chapter 22).

Severe, rapidly progressing pneumonia, even including ileus, may occasionally be produced by pneumococci. Abscesses and pneumatoceles may be seen in pneumonia due to pneumococci, *Haemophilus influenzae,* and group A streptococci. Empyema formation is common with all bacterial pneumonias.

Staphylococcal food poisoning is often epidemic. It is differentiated from other common-source gastroenteritis syndromes *(Salmonella, Clostridium perfringens, Vibrio parahaemolyticus)* by the short incubation period (2–6 hours), the prominence of vomiting (as opposed to diarrhea), and the general absence of fever.

Endocarditis must be suspected in any instance of *S aureus* bacteremia, particularly when there is a significant heart murmur or preexisting cardiac disease. Multiple blood cultures should be obtained before therapy is instituted. Echocardiography is frequently useful to detect vegetations on valves or the endocardium.

Newborn infections with *S aureus* can resemble infections with streptococci and a variety of gram-negative organisms. Umbilical and respiratory tract colonization occurs with a variety of pathogenic organisms (group B streptococci, *Escherichia coli, Klebsiella*), and both skin and systemic infections occur with virtually all of these. The clinical resemblance of these infections to staphylococcal syndromes can be very close.

Toxic shock syndrome must be differentiated from Rocky Mountain spotted fever, leptospirosis, Kawasaki disease, drug reactions, and measles.

Treatment

A. Specific Measures: Since 85% of *S aureus* strains are penicillin-resistant, it is important to use a β-lactamase-resistant penicillin as the first drug in treatment. In serious systemic disease, in osteomyelitis, and in the treatment of large abscesses, intravenous therapy is indicated, at least at first (oxacillin or nafcillin, 100–200 mg/kg/d in 6 divided doses, or methicillin, 200–300 mg/kg/d in 6 divided doses). When high doses over a long period are required, it is preferable not to use methicillin, because of the frequency with which interstitial nephritis is seen. In life-threatening illness (newborn sepsis, pneumonia, endocarditis), an aminoglycoside antibiotic (kanamycin or gentamicin) may be added to the penicillin for its possible synergistic action.

In those instances where *S aureus* is penicillin-sensitive, penicillin G should be used for treatment.

When children with established penicillin sensitivity are treated, cephalosporins may be used (cephalothin, 100–200 mg/kg/d intravenously in 6 divided doses; cefazolin, 100–150 mg/kg/d intravenously in 4 divided doses; or cephalexin, 50–100 mg/kg/d orally in 4 divided doses). The newer cephalosporins (eg, cefamandole, cefoxitin, moxalactam, cefotaxime) should not generally be used for staphylococcal infections.

For methicillin-resistant infections, vancomycin (40 mg/kg/d in 4 divided doses) should be used, with or without gentamicin. Although such strains are often sensitive to cephalosporins in vitro, resistance emerges rapidly in vivo. Combinations including rifampin may be either synergistic or antagonistic.

1. Skin infections—See Chapter 10.

2. Osteomyelitis and septic arthritis—Treatment should be begun intravenously, with antibiotics selected to cover the most likely organisms (staphylococci in hematogenous osteomyelitis; *H influenzae,* meningococci, pneumococci, staphylococci in arthritic children under the age of 3 years; staphylococci and gonococci in arthritis in older children). Antibiotic levels should be kept high at all times, with monitoring by serum killing powers at least once and at suitable intervals if dosage or route of administration is changed.

In osteomyelitis, clinical studies support the use of intravenous treatment until local symptoms and signs have subsided—at least 1 week—followed by oral therapy (dicloxacillin, 100 mg/kg/d in 4 divided doses, or cephalexin, 100 mg/kg/d in 6 divided doses) for at least 3 additional weeks. Longer treatment may be required, particularly when x-rays show extensive involvement. In arthritis, where drug diffusion into synovial fluid is good, intravenous therapy need be given only for a few days, followed by adequate oral therapy for at least 3 weeks. In all instances, oral therapy should be administered under careful supervision, either in the hospital or, in some instances, at home with frequent support and reinforcement from physicians or visiting nurses.

Surgical drainage of osteomyelitis or septic arthritis is often required (see Chapter 22).

3. Staphylococcal pneumonia—Antibiotic therapy should consist of a parenteral penicillinase-resistant penicillin with or without an aminoglycoside. Empyema or pyopneumothorax should be treated by prompt placement of one or more chest tubes into the pleural space. The tube should be removed as soon as drainage has become clinically insignificant.

If staphylococcal pneumonia is promptly treated and empyema promptly drained, resolution in children is almost always complete—in spite of evidence of widespread parenchymal destruction and the persistence of bullae, blebs, and even pockets of empyema or abscess fluid well into convalescence. Surgical decortication or segmental resection is very rarely required.

4. Staphylococcal food poisoning—Therapy is supportive and usually not required except in severe cases or for small infants with marked dehydration.

5. Staphylococcal endocarditis—As outlined above, high-dose, prolonged, parenteral treatment with oxacillin, nafcillin, or methicillin plus kanamycin or gentamicin is indicated. In penicillin-allergic patients, cefazolin or cephalothin may be used in place of penicillin. With penicillin-sensitive organisms, penicillin G is the drug of choice. Equally effective—though more toxic—is intravenous vancomycin, 40 mg/kg/d in 4 divided doses. Therapy lasts in all instances for at least 6 weeks.

In some patients, medical treatment may fail. Signs of this are (1) recurrent fever without apparent treatable other cause (eg, thrombophlebitis, incidental respiratory or urinary tract infection, drug fever); (2) persistently positive blood cultures; (3) intractable and progressive congestive heart failure; and (4) recurrent (septic) embolization. In such circumstances—

particularly (2), (3), and (4)—operation becomes necessary as part of good management of a difficult situation. The infected valve is removed, and a prosthesis is placed. Antibiotics are continued for at least another 4 weeks. Persistent or recurrent infection may require a second surgical procedure.

6. Nursery infections—(See also Chapter 3.) Methods available to stop a nursery epidemic include the following:

a. Emphasis and reemphasis on the first principle of infection control: thorough washing of hands with soap, an iodophore, or other antiseptic agent between handling of infants.

b. Prompt and adequate management of known infections.

c. Prevention of colonization of newborns with epidemic strains by the following means:

(1) Treatment of the umbilibal cord with triple dye (brilliant green, 2.29 mg; gentian violet, 2.29 mg; and proflavine hemisulfate, 1.14 mg) in 1 mL of distilled water immediately after birth.

(2) Removal and treatment of personnel carrying the epidemic strain.

(3) Segregation of infants according to age, and early discharge (within 3 days after birth).

(4) Cohorting of nursing personnel, ie, division of nurses into multiple units, each of which cares for only a fraction of the infants.

(5) Restriction of visitors to the nursery area.

(6) Complete cleansing and disinfection of nurseries after discharge of colonized and infected infants.

7. Toxic shock syndrome—Treatment is first with colloid solutions and vasopressor drugs to support blood pressure and reduce "shock lung" symptoms and later with oxacillin, nafcillin, or cephalosporins. If a tampon is in place, it should be removed. Antibiotic treatment reduces risk of recurrence.

8. *S epidermidis* infections—*S epidermidis* infections are usually treated with vancomycin (30 mg/kg/d intravenously in divided doses every 12 hours in the first week of life and 40 mg/kg/d intravenously in 4 divided doses after that), often in combination with gentamicin.

B. General Measures: Localized pus should be drained. Oxygen, intravenous fluids, and other supportive care are indicated in staphylococcal pneumonia and other systemic infections. Blood transfusion may be indicated if the patient is severely anemic.

Prognosis

Septicemia, endocarditis, and widespread pneumonitis in infancy all have a serious prognosis. Infants and children who recover from serious staphylococcal pneumonia have a good long-term prognosis without development of chronic respiratory disease. Osteomyelitis is now never fatal if promptly treated.

Baumgart S et al: Sepsis with coagulase-negative staphylococci in critically ill newborns. *Am J Dis Child* 1983;**137**:461.

Friedman LE et al: *Staphylococcus epidermidis* septicemia in children with leukemia and lymphoma. *Am J Dis Child* 1984;**138**:715.

Hieber JP, Nelson AJ, McCracken GH: Acute disseminated staphylococcal disease in childhood. *Am J Dis Child* 1977;**131**:181.

Johnson DH, Rosenthal A, Nadas AS: A forty-year review of bacterial endocarditis in infancy and childhood. *Circulation* 1975;**51**:581.

Johnson JD et al: A sequential study of various modes of skin and umbilical care and the incidence of staphylococcal colonization and infection in the neonate. *Pediatrics* 1976;**58**:354.

Melish ME, Glasgow LA: The staphylococcal scalded skin syndrome: The expanded clinical syndrome. *J Pediatr* 1971;**78**:958.

Shands KN et al: Toxic-shock syndrome in menstruating women. *N Engl J Med* 1980;**303**:1436.

Shulman ST, Ayoub EM: Severe staphylococcal sepsis in adolescents. *Pediatrics* 1976;**58**:59.

Todd J et al: Toxic-shock syndrome associated with phage-group-1 staphylococci. *Lancet* 1978;**2**:1116.

MENINGOCOCCAL INFECTIONS

Essentials of Diagnosis

- Fever, headache, vomiting, convulsions, shock (meningitis).
- Fever, shock, petechial or purpuric skin rash (meningococcemia).
- Diagnosis confirmed by culture or detection of meningococcal antigen in normally sterile body fluids.

General Considerations

Meningococci may be carried asymptomatically for many months in the upper respiratory tract. Fewer than 1% of carriers develop disease. Meningitis and sepsis are the 2 commonest forms of illness, but septic arthritis, pericarditis, pneumonia, chronic meningococcemia, otitis media, conjunctivitis, and vaginitis also occur. The highest attack rate for meningococcal meningitis is in the first year of life. The incidence in the USA is about 1.2 cases per 100,000 people.

Meningococci are classified serologically into groups A, B, C, D, X, Y, Z, 29-E, and W-135. The serologic groups serve as specific markers for studying outbreaks and transmission of disease. Major epidemics of meningococcal disease in the USA prior to 1950 were caused by group A strains. In recent years, however, group A organisms have accounted for only about 2% of meningococcal isolates. Group B, the most common serogroup, accounts for about 40%; group C for 30%; and group Y for 20%. About 25% of all isolates are resistant to sulfadiazine. Resistance is found in 75% of group C strains. In contrast, less than 20% of group B and Y isolates are resistant. Few isolates are resistant to rifampin. Group B is encountered more often in children younger than 9 years of age and in adults over 50 years. Serogroup C predominates in older children and adults. Pathogenic strains differ in their virulence and in their potential for epidemic spread. Serogroup A meningococci have the greatest propensity to cause widespread outbreaks.

Children develop immunity from asymptomatic carriage of meningococci (usually nontypeable, nonpathogenic strains) or other cross-reacting bacteria. Protection correlates positively with the presence of 2 μg or more of bactericidal antibody per microliter of serum. Patients deficient in one of the late components of complement (C6, C7, or C8) are uniquely susceptible to meningococcal infection.

Meningococci are gram-negative organisms containing endotoxin in their cell walls. Endotoxins may damage the walls of blood vessels and may also cause disseminated intravascular coagulation. Myocarditis is a significant factor in the fatal outcome of acute meningococcal infections.

Vaccines prepared from purified meningococcal polysaccharides (Menomune–A/C and Menomune–A/C/Y/W-135) are available for use in control of outbreaks and to prevent spread in special high-risk groups such as household contacts and military recruits. Unfortunately, the vaccines, except for the A component, are ineffective in children under 2 years of age.

Clinical Findings

A. Symptoms and Signs: Many children with clinical meningococcemia also have meningitis, and some may have other foci of infection. All children with suspected meningococcemia should have a lumbar puncture.

1. Meningococcemia—A prodrome of upper respiratory infection is followed within 2 days by high fever, headache, nausea, marked toxicity, and hypotension. A purpuric or petechial rash on the skin and mucous membranes and occasionally bright pink, tender macules or papules over the extremities and trunk are seen and may have hemorrhagic centers.

Fulminant meningococcemia is an extremely virulent and rapidly progressing form of meningococcemia (Waterhouse-Friderichsen syndrome) characterized by disseminated intravascular coagulation, massive skin and mucosal hemorrhages, and shock. This syndrome also may be seen in other generalized bacterial infections, particularly those due to *Haemophilus influenzae* or *Streptococcus pneumoniae,* so the clinical picture is not pathognomonic.

Chronic meningococcemia is characterized by periodic bouts of fever, arthralgia or arthritis, and recurrent petechiae. Splenomegaly is often present. The patient may be free of symptoms between bouts. Chronic meningococcemia occurs primarily in adults and mimics Henoch-Schönlein purpura.

2. Meningitis—In many children, meningococcemia is followed within a few hours by symptoms and signs of acute purulent meningitis, with severe headache, stiff neck, nausea, vomiting, and stupor. Children with meningitis and meningococcemia generally fare better than children with meningococcemia alone.

B. Laboratory Findings: The peripheral white blood cell count may be either low or elevated. Thrombocytopenia may be present with or without disseminated intravascular coagulation. If petechial or hemorrhagic lesions are present, meningococci can sometimes be demonstrated on smear by puncturing the lesions and expressing a drop of tissue fluid. The spinal fluid is generally cloudy and contains more than 1000 white cells per microliter, with many polymorphonuclear cells and gram-negative intracellular diplococci. Meningococci can usually be cultured from the cerebrospinal fluid or other body fluids by the use of chocolate agar incubated in an atmosphere of 5–10% CO_2.

Meningococcal capsular polysaccharide antigen may be detected by counterimmunoelectrophoresis or latex agglutination in the serum, cerebrospinal fluid, synovial fluid, pericardial fluid, and urine. Antigen detection is particularly useful when children have been partially treated with antibiotics.

Severe thrombocytopenia, markedly abnormal prothrombin time and partial thromboplastin time (PTT), an increase in fibrin split products, and significant depletion of prothrombin, factor V, factor VIII, and fibrinogen indicate disseminated intravascular coagulation.

Differential Diagnosis

The lesions of meningococcemia may be mistaken for those seen in sepsis, infections due to *H influenzae* or pneumococci, enterovirus infection, endocarditis, leptospirosis, Rocky Mountain spotted fever, other rickettsial diseases, Henoch-Schönlein purpura, and blood dyscrasias. Other causes of sepsis and meningitis are distinguished by appropriate Gram's stain and cultures.

Complications

Meningitis may lead to permanent central nervous system damage, with deafness, convulsions, paralysis, or impairment of intellectual function. Subdural collections of fluid and hydrocephalus are important complications, but they usually resolve spontaneously. Extensive skin necrosis may complicate fulminant meningococcemia.

Prevention

Household contacts, day-care center contacts, and hospital personnel directly exposed to the respiratory secretions of patients are at increased risk of developing meningococcal infection and should be given chemoprophylaxis with rifampin. The secondary attack rate among household members is 1–5% during epidemics and less than 1% in nonepidemic situations. Children 3 months to 2 years of age are at the greatest risk, presumably because they lack protective antibodies. Secondary cases reported in day-care centers are not uncommon, but school classroom outbreaks are rare. Hospital personnel are not at increased risk unless they have had intimate contact with a patient's oral secretions, eg, mouth-to-mouth resuscitation, intubation, or suctioning. Approximately 50% of secondary cases in households have their onset within 24 hours of identification of the index case. Exposed children should be examined promptly. If they are febrile, they should be fully evaluated and treated with high doses of penicillin pending the results of blood cultures.

All intimate contacts should be given chemoprophylaxis with rifampin in the following dosages twice daily for 2 days: 600 mg for adults, 10 mg/kg for children 1–12 years of age, and 5 mg/kg for infants under 12 months of age. If the organism is sensitive to sulfonamides, sulfadiazine may be used in the following dosages twice daily for 2 days: 1 g for adults, 0.5 g for children, and 0.25 g for infants. Minocycline also is effective but is not recommended, because of its frequent side effects (vertigo, nausea, and vomiting). Penicillin and most other antibiotics are not effective chemoprophylactic agents, probably because they do not enter oropharyngeal secretions sufficiently to eradicate upper respiratory tract carriage of meningococci. In some situations, meningococcal polysaccharide vaccine should be given to contacts in addition to chemoprophylaxis. Throat cultures to identify carriers are not useful, because of the delay in getting culture results and because established carriers usually already possess protective antibody. Children without antibody who will soon acquire the virulent organism are those most needing prophylaxis. A negative throat culture should not be reassuring.

Treatment

Children with meningococcemia or meningococcal meningitis should be managed as though shock were imminent even if their vital signs are stable when they are first seen. If hypotension already is present, supportive measures should be aggressive, because the prognosis is grave in such situations. It is optimal to initiate treatment in an intensive care setting. In addition to the usual supportive measures, corticosteroids in high doses may be useful. Heparin, transfusion of platelets and clotting factors, and exchange transfusion may be indicated for ongoing disseminated intravascular coagulation. To minimize the risk of nosocomial transmission, patients should be placed in respiratory isolation for the first 24 hours of antibiotic treatment.

A. Specific Measures: Give aqueous penicillin G, 250,000–400,000 units/kg/d intravenously in 6 divided doses. Treatment is continued for 7–10 days. Patients allergic to penicillin should be treated with chloramphenicol. Many third-generation cephalosporins are also effective. Antibiotics should be begun promptly.

B. General Measures:

1. Ventilation—The airway and adequate ventilation must be maintained; this may require intubation. Monitor arterial blood gases. Humidified oxygen by nasal catheter is usually required.

2. Fluid management—A central venous pressure catheter should be inserted and the central venous pressure monitored (normal central venous pressure, 3–10 cm water). Hourly urine output should also be monitored (normal, 2–4 mL/kg/h).

Isotonic electrolyte solution, plasma, or blood, 10–20 mL/kg, is infused over a 10-minute period with constant monitoring in order to treat hypovolemic shock. Infusions should be continued until the central venous pressure remains constant in a range of 5–10 cm water and urine output is adequate.

Profound metabolic acidosis occurs in advanced septicemic shock. An infusion of sodium bicarbonate, 1 meq/kg, may be given in an attempt to temporarily correct the acidosis and improve cardiac function, but the primary effort should be directed toward restoring tissue perfusion and aerobic metabolism.

3. Heart failure—There may be decreased cardiac output associated with an increased central venous pressure. Myocarditis is a significant factor in the fatal outcome of acute meningococcal infections. The patient should be treated for heart failure if the central venous pressure exceeds 16 cm water at any time.

a. Isoproterenol—Isoproterenol has the desirable effects of decreasing peripheral vascular resistance and exercising an inotropic effect on the heart. A continuous infusion of 1 mg in 250 mL of isotonic solution given at a rate of about 1 mL/min (0.05–4 μg/min) will often result in increased urine output and a decline in central venous pressure. Cardiac rate and rhythm should be carefully monitored, because of the danger of dysrhythmias. Isoproterenol should not be given until hypovolemia is corrected.

b. Dopamine (Intropin)—Dopamine exercises a direct effect on both beta and alpha receptors. It may be effective in some cases where isoproterenol has failed. Dopamine is administered beginning at a rate of 5 μg/kg/min intravenously. The rate of infusion is gradually increased every 15–20 minutes until blood pressure and urine output are satisfactory.

4. Corticosteroids—Very large doses of hydrocortisone produce an increase in blood pressure and decreased peripheral resistance through arteriolar vasodilation. Nonhemodynamic effects of corticosteroids that may contribute to increased survival include a positive inotropic effect on the heart, stabilization of lysosomes, and binding of endotoxin. Hydrocortisone (Solu-Cortef) is given in a dose of 50 mg/kg as a bolus injection intravenously followed by 100 mg/kg/d. Methylprednisolone also may be used. The efficacy of high doses of corticosteroids in septic shock has not been proved.

Prognosis

Unfavorable prognostic features include shock, disseminated intravascular coagulation, and extensive skin lesions. The case fatality rate in fulminant meningococcemia is very high—over 50%. In uncomplicated meningococcal meningitis, the fatality rate is much lower—generally 10–20%.

Band JD et al: Trends in meningococcal disease in the United States, 1975–1980. *J Infect Dis* 1983;**148:**754.

Dashefsky B, Teele DW, Klein JO: Unsuspected meningococcemia. *J Pediatr* 1983;**102:**69.

Edwards MS, Baker CJ: Complications and sequelae of meningococcal infections in children. *J Pediatr* 1981;**99:**540.

Ellison RT III et al: Prevalence of congenital or acquired complement deficiency in patients with sporadic meningococcal disease. *N Engl J Med* 1983;**308:**913.

Griffiss JM: Epidemic meningococcal disease: Synthesis of a hypothetical immunoepidemiologic model. *Rev Infect Dis* 1982;**4:**159.

Griffiss JM et al: Immune response of infants and children to disseminated infections with *Neisseria meningitidis*. *J Infect Dis* 1984;**150:**71.

Jacobson JA, Filice GA, Holloway JT: Meningococcal disease in day-care centers. *Pediatrics* 1977;**59:**299.

Jacobson JA et al: The risk of meningitis among classroom contacts during an epidemic of meningococcal disease. *Am J Epidemiol* 1976;**104:**552.

Nguyen QV, Nguyen EA, Weiner LB: Incidence of invasive bacterial disease in children with fever and petechiae. *Pediatrics* 1984;**74:**77.

GONOCOCCAL INFECTIONS

Essentials of Diagnosis

- Purulent yellow or green urethral discharge showing intracellular gram-negative diplococci on smear in male patient (usually adolescent).
- Purulent, edematous, sometimes hemorrhagic conjunctivitis showing intracellular gram-negative diplococci on smear in infant 2–4 days of age.
- Fever, arthritis (often polyarticular) or tenosynovitis, and maculopapular peripheral rash that may be vesiculopustular or hemorrhagic.
- Positive culture of blood or pharyngeal or genital secretions.

General Considerations

Gonorrhea is the most commonly reported communicable disease. *Neisseria gonorrhoeae* is a gram-negative diplococcus. Although morphologically similar to other neisseriae, it differs in its ability to grow on selective media and to ferment only glucose. The cell wall of *N gonorrhoeae* contains endotoxin, which is liberated when the organism dies and is responsible for the production of a cellular exudate. The incubation period is short, usually 2–5 days.

Gonococci that elaborate penicillinase and are highly resistant to penicillin are now being encountered. Initially, most isolates of these gonococci in the USA were related to travelers who had returned from the Philippines, but more recent local outbreaks have had no demonstrable epidemiologic connection to travelers returning from the Far East. Nevertheless, since infection with penicillinase-producing gonococci is still uncommon in the USA (fewer than 5% of cases), it has been recommended that the present treatment policies remain unchanged.

Gonococcal disease in children may be transmitted venereally or nonvenereally. Prepubertal girls usually manifest gonococcal vulvovaginitis because of the neutral-alkaline pH of the vagina and thin vaginal mucosa.

Prepubertal gonococcal infection outside the neonatal period should be considered presumptive evidence of sexual play or child abuse. In the adolescent or adult, the workup of every case of gonorrhea should include a careful and accurate inquiry into sexual practices, since pharyngeal infection must be detected if present and may be difficult to eradicate. In addition, efforts should be made to identify and treat all sexual contacts. When prepubertal children are infected, all family members should be cultured, and epidemiologic investigation should be thorough.

Clinical Findings

A. Symptoms and Signs:

1. Asymptomatic gonorrhea—The ratio of asymptomatic to symptomatic gonorrheal infections in adolescents and adults is probably 3–4:1 in women and 0.5–1:1 in men. Asymptomatic infections are considered as infectious as symptomatic ones.

2. Uncomplicated genital gonorrhea—

a. Male with urethritis—Urethral discharge is sometimes painful and bloody and may be white, yellow, or green. There may be associated dysuria. The patient is usually afebrile.

b. Prepubertal female with vaginitis—The only clinical findings initially may be dysuria and polymorphonuclear neutrophils in the urine. Vulvitis characterized by erythema, edema, and excoriation accompanied by a purulent discharge may follow.

c. Postpubertal female with cervicitis—Symptomatic disease is characterized by a purulent discharge, dysuria, and, occasionally, dyspareunia. Lower abdominal pain is absent. Physical examination reveals an afebrile patient with a yellow, foul-smelling discharge. The cervix is frequently hyperemic and tender when touched by the examining finger. This tenderness is not worsened by moving the cervix, nor are the adnexa tender to palpation.

d. Rectal gonorrhea—Rectal gonorrhea is often asymptomatic. There may be purulent discharge, edema, and pain during evacuation.

3. Pharyngeal gonorrhea—Pharyngeal involvement is usually asymptomatic. There may be some sore throat and, rarely, acute exudative tonsillitis with bilateral cervical lymphadenopathy and fever.

4. Conjunctivitis and iridocyclitis—In the adolescent or adult eye, infection probably is spread from infected genital secretions by the fingers.*

5. Pelvic inflammatory disease (salpingitis)—The interval between initiation of genital infection and its ascent to the uterine tubes is variable and may range from days to months, with menses frequently the initiating factor. With the onset of a

* Gonococcal ophthalmia neonatorum is discussed in Chapter 11. Infants may also develop anogenital colonization during birth, with subsequent gonococcal sepsis and arthritis.

menstrual period, gonococci invade the endometrium, causing transient endometritis. Subsequently, salpingitis may occur, resulting in pyosalpinx or hydrosalpinx; rarely, it leads to peritonitis or perihepatitis. Gonococcal salpingitis occurs in an acute, subacute, or chronic form. All 3 forms have in common tenderness on gentle movement of the cervix and bilateral tubal tenderness during pelvic examination.

Not all pelvic inflammatory disease is due to gonococci. In many instances, gonococci may be an initial cause of infection, but the predominant intrapelvic organisms may be enteric bacilli, *Bacteroides fragilis*, or other anaerobes. In other cases, *Chlamydia trachomatis* may be the triggering or sole cause. Nongonococcal salpingitis is sometimes seen in girls or women with intrauterine devices.

6. Gonococcal perihepatitis (Fitz-Hugh-Curtis syndrome)—In the typical clinical pattern, there is right upper quadrant tenderness in association with signs of acute or subacute salpingitis. Pain may be pleuritic and referred to the shoulder. Hepatic friction rub is a valuable but inconstant sign.

7. Disseminated gonorrhea—Dissemination follows asymptomatic more often than symptomatic genital infection and often results from gonococcal pharyngitis or anorectal gonorrhea. The most common form of disseminated gonorrhea is polyarthritis or polytenosynovitis, with or without dermatitis. Monarticular arthritis is less common, and gonococcal endocarditis and meningitis are fortunately rare.

a. Polyarthritis—Disease usually begins with the simultaneous onset of low-grade fever, polyarthralgia, and general malaise. After a day or so, the joint symptoms become acute, and swelling, redness, and acute tenderness occur, frequently over the wrists, ankles, and knees but also in the fingers, feet, and other peripheral joints. Skin lesions may be noted at the same time: individual, tender, evolving 5- to 8-mm maculopapular lesions that may become vesicular, pustular, and then hemorrhagic. They are noted on the fingers, palms, feet, and other distal surfaces and may be single or multiple.

In patients with this form of the disease, blood cultures are often positive, but joint fluids rarely yield organisms. Skin lesions often are positive by Gram's stain but rarely by culture. Genital, rectal, and pharyngeal cultures must always be performed.

b. Monarticular arthritis—In this somewhat less common form of disseminated gonorrhea, fever is often absent. Arthritis evolves in a single joint. Dermatitis usually does not occur. Systemic symptoms are minimal. Blood cultures are negative, but joint aspirates may yield gonococci on smear and culture. Genital, rectal, and pharyngeal cultures must always be performed.

B. Laboratory Findings: Demonstration of gram-negative kidney bean-shaped diplococci on smears of urethral exudate in males is presumptive evidence of gonorrhea. Positive culture confirms the diagnosis. Negative smears do not rule out gonorrhea. Gram-stained smears of cervical or vaginal discharge in girls are more difficult to interpret because of normal gram-negative flora, but they may be useful when technical personnel are experienced. In girls with suspected gonorrhea, both the cervical os and the anus should be cultured. Gonococcal pharyngitis requires culture to substantiate the etiologic diagnosis.

Cultures for *N gonorrhoeae* are plated on Thayer-Martin medium, a chocolate agar containing antibiotics that suppress most normal flora. If bacteriologic diagnosis is critical, suspected material should be cultured on chocolate agar as well. Since gonococci are labile, swabs should be inoculated immediately and agar plates placed without delay in an atmosphere containing CO_2 (candle jar). In circumstances where transportation is necessary, material should be directly inoculated into Transgrow medium prior to shipment to an appropriate laboratory.

All children or adolescents with a suspected or established diagnosis of gonorrhea should have a serologic test for syphilis.

Differential Diagnosis

Urethritis in the male may be gonococcal or "nonspecific." The latter is a syndrome characterized by discharge (rarely painful), mild dysuria, and a subacute course. The discharge is usually scant or moderate in amount but may be profuse. The responsible microorganisms cannot all be identified, but about half of cases are probably due to *C trachomatis*. The remainder are probably due to *Ureaplasma*, trichomonads, or other as yet unknown agents. Most cases respond to tetracycline therapy (2 g daily divided into 4 doses for adolescents) administered orally for 1 week. *C trachomatis* has been shown to cause epididymitis in males and salpingitis in females.

Vulvovaginitis in a prepubertal female may be due to infection caused by miscellaneous bacteria, *Candida*, and herpesvirus; discharges may be caused by trichomonads, *Enterobius vermicularis* (pinworm), or foreign bodies. Symptom-free discharge (leukorrhea) normally accompanies rising estrogen levels.

Cervicitis in a postpubertal female, alone or in association with urethritis and involvement of Skene's and Bartholin's glands, may be due to infection caused by *Candida*, herpesvirus, *Trichomonas*, or discharge resulting from inflammation caused by foreign bodies (usually some form of contraceptive device). Leukorrhea may be associated with birth control pills.

Salpingitis may be due to infection with other organisms. The symptoms must be differentiated from those of appendicitis, urinary tract infection, and ectopic pregnancy.

Disseminated gonorrhea presents a wide differential diagnosis that must include meningococcemia, acute rheumatic fever, Henoch-Schönlein purpura, juvenile rheumatoid arthritis, lupus erythematosus, leptospirosis, secondary syphilis, certain viral infections (particularly rubella, but also enteroviruses), serum sickness, type B hepatitis (in the prodromal phase), infective endocarditis, and even acute leukemia and other types of cancer. The fully evolved skin lesions of disseminated gonorrhea are remarkably specific, and genital, rectal, or pharyngeal cultures, plus cultures of blood and joint fluid, usually yield gonococci from at least one source.

Prevention

Prevention of gonorrhea is principally a problem of sex education and treatment of contacts.

Treatment*

A. Uncomplicated Gonococcal Infections in Adolescents: There are 3 drug regimens of choice: (1) Aqueous procaine penicillin G, 4.8 million units intramuscularly, injected at different sites, with 1 g of probenecid orally just before the injections. (2) Ampicillin, 3.5 g, or amoxicillin, 3 g, orally, together with 1 g probenecid orally administered at the same time. (This regimen is probably somewhat less effective and is not to be used when pharyngeal or anorectal infection is established or suspected.) (3) Tetracycline, 0.5 g orally 4 times daily for 7 days. Spectinomycin, 2 g intramuscularly, should be used only for re-treatment of failures (see below) or primary treatment of those known to be infected with penicillinase-producing *N gonorrhoeae.* Sexual partners should be treated with the same dosages.

Because all of the recommended treatment schedules have a failure rate of about 5%, follow-up cultures must be obtained 3–7 days after completion of treatment. During this time, the patient should abstain from sexual activity. In a small proportion of males, symptoms will persist after bacteriologically sucessful penicillin treatment (postgonococcal urethritis). Such cases are probably due to an original double infection, both gonorrheal and "nonspecific" (ie, chlamydial or mycoplasmal), when penicillin has eradicated *N gonorrhoeae* and left the insensitive organism. Treatment with tetracycline is usually successful.

If cultures obtained after treatment grow *N gonorrhoeae,* the strains should be tested for penicillinase production and penicillin sensitivity. Re-treatment should be with spectinomycin, 2 g intramuscularly, or if this fails, cefoxitin, 2 g intramuscularly, plus probenecid. It is particularly important to report penicillinase-producing organisms.

B. Disseminated Gonorrhea: Strains of *N gonorrhoeae* that disseminate have been uniformly highly sensitive to penicillin. Treatment should therefore be either with penicillin G, 10 million units daily (adult dose) until symptoms subside, followed by ampicillin, 0.5 g orally 4 times a day to complete 7 days; or with tetracycline, 0.5 g orally 4 times a day for 7 days. Oral ampicillin (as above for uncomplicated gonorrhea, followed by 0.5 g 4 times daily for 1 week) or erythromycin, 0.5 g orally 4 times a day for 7 days, may also be used.

C. Prepubertal Gonorrhea: The treatment for uncomplicated gonorrhea in patients under 45 kg is procaine penicillin G, 100,000 units/kg intramuscularly, plus probenecid, 25 mg/kg orally. Alternatively, a single dose of amoxicillin, 50 mg/kg orally, plus probenecid, 25 mg/kg orally, can be given. For penicillin-allergic children, spectinomycin, 40 mg/kg intramuscularly, can be used.

Treat disseminated gonorrhea with penicillin G, 100,000 units/kg/d intravenously for 7 days.

Centers for Disease Control: Sexually transmitted diseases: Treatment guidelines 1982. *MMWR* (Aug 20) 1982;**31:**35S.

Hein K, Marks A, Cohen MI: Asymptomatic gonorrhea: Prevalence in a population of urban adolescents. *J Pediatr* 1977;**90:**634.

Ingram D et al; Sexual contact in children with gonorrhea. *Am J Dis Child* 1982;**136:**994.

Kaufman RE et al: National Gonorrhea Therapy Monitoring Study: Treatment results. *N Engl J Med* 1976;**294:**1.

Litt IF, Edbey SC, Finberg L: Gonorrhea in children and adolescents: A current review. *J Pediatr* 1974;**85:**595.

McCormack WM: Penicillinase-producing *Neisseria gonorrhoeae:* A retrospective. *N Engl J Med* 1982;**307:**438.

Nelson JD et al: Gonorrhea in preschool and school-aged children: Report of the Prepubertal Gonorrhea Cooperative Study Group. *JAMA* 1976;**236:**1359.

BOTULISM

Essentials of Diagnosis

- Dry mucous membranes.
- Nausea and vomiting.
- Diplopia; dilated, unreactive pupils.
- Descending paralysis.
- Difficulty in swallowing and speech occurring within 12–36 hours after ingestion of toxin contaminated home-canned food.
- Multiple cases in a family or group.
- Hypotonia and constipation in infants.
- Diagnosis by clinical findings and identification of toxin in blood, stool, or implicated food.

General Considerations

Botulism is a paralytic disease caused by *Clostridium botulinum,* an anaerobic, gram-positive, spore-forming bacillus normally found in soil. The word botulism is derived from Latin *botulus* "sausage"; the disease derives its name from an outbreak in Germany in 1793 in which contaminated sausage was implicated. The organism produces an extremely potent neurotoxin. Of the 7 types of toxin (A–G), types A, B, and E cause most human disease, and types C and D cause outbreaks of botulism in birds and mammals. The toxin, a polypeptide, is so potent that 0.1 μg is lethal for humans.

Food-borne botulism usually results from ingestion of toxin-containing food. Preformed toxin is absorbed from the gut and produces paralysis by preventing

* These dosages must be modified for use in infants and children. Spectinomycin has not been approved for use in children by the FDA. Tetracycline should not be used for children under 8 years of age. For penicillin-allergic patients, erythromycin or tetracycline may be used.

acetylcholine release from cholinergic fibers at myoneural junctions.

In Japan, a raw fish and vegetable dish that is allowed to ferment for 4 weeks is responsible for most botulism outbreaks. In Germany, smoked sausage is often implicated. In the USA, home-canned vegetables are usually the cause. Commercially canned foods rarely are responsible. Virtually any food will support the growth of *C botulinum* spores into vegetative toxin-producing bacilli if an anaerobic nonacid environment is provided. The food may not appear or taste spoiled. The toxin is heat-labile, but the spores are heat-resistent. Inadequate heating during processing (temperature < 115 °C [239 °F]) allows the spores to survive and later resume toxin production. Boiling of foods for 10 minutes or heating at 80 °C (176 °F) for 30 minutes before eating will destroy the toxin.

Infant botulism is a newly recognized form of the disease seen in infants 2–48 weeks of age. It usually presents as constipation and severe hypotonia. The toxin appears to be produced by *C botulinum* organisms residing in the gastrointestinal tract. In many instances, honey has been the source of spores. Clinical findings include constipation, weak sucking and crying, pooled oral secretions, cranial nerve deficits, generalized weakness, and, on occasion, sudden apnea. A characteristic electromyographic pattern termed "brief, small, abundant motor-unit action potentials" (BSAP) is observed. Infant botulism may be responsible for some cases of sudden infant death syndrome (SIDS). In the USA, 60–80 cases are reported annually. Studies are under way to determine the full clinical spectrum, incidence, and public health importance of this form of botulism.

Wound botulism from contamination with *C botulinum* is uncommon. It should be considered in any patient who develops symmetric cranial nerve paralysis and progressive descending motor weakness. Confirmation of the diagnosis is established by isolating *C botulinum* from the wound or by demonstrating botulinus toxin in the patient's serum.

Clinical Findings

A. Symptoms and Signs: The incubation period is 8–36 hours. Initially, there is lassitude or fatigue, generally with headache. This is followed by double vision, dilated pupils, ptosis, and, within a few hours, difficulty in swallowing and in speech. Pharyngeal paralysis occurs in some cases, and food may be regurgitated. The mucous membranes often are very dry. Descending skeletal muscle paralysis may be seen. The sensorium is clear and the temperature normal. Death usually results from respiratory failure.

B. Laboratory Findings: Feces, vomitus, serum, and suspect food should be examined for the presence of toxin by injection into mice. The organism also may be cultured from feces or the suspect food. Laboratory findings, including cerebrospinal fluid examination, are usually normal. With the use of electrophysiologic techniques, electrical abnormalities can be found. Early in the course, when the patient has marked clinical weakness, the rested muscle shows a depressed response to a single supramaximal stimulus applied to the nerve (normal, 6–12 mV). Later in the course, a marked augmentation of muscle action potential is seen after rapid repetitive stimulation (50/s) of the nerve. This finding is characteristic of neuromuscular block.

Differential Diagnosis

Staphylococcal food poisoning, chemical food poisoning, carbon monoxide poisoning, and Guillain-Barré syndrome are commonly misdiagnosed as botulism. Staphylococcal food poisoning is characterized by nausea, vomiting, and diarrhea; paralysis is not a feature of the illness. Chemical food poisonings generally are characterized by nausea and vomiting beginning minutes after ingestion of contaminated food.

Carbon monoxide poisoning causes unconsciousness without cranial nerve paralysis, and carboxyhemoglobin can be detected in blood. Guillain-Barré syndrome is characterized by ascending paralysis, sensory deficits, and elevated cerebrospinal fluid protein without pleocytosis.

Other illnesses that should be considered include poliomyelitis, postdiphtheritic polyneuritis, certain chemical intoxications, tick paralysis, and myasthenia gravis. The history and elevated cerebrospinal fluid protein characterize postdiphtheritic polyneuritis.

Poisoning with methyl alcohol, organic phosphorus compounds, methyl chloride, sodium fluoride, or atropine may have to be ruled out.

Tick paralysis is characterized by a flaccid ascending motor paralysis that begins in the legs. An attached tick should be sought.

Myasthenia gravis usually occurs in adolescent girls. It is characterized by ocular and bulbar symptoms, with normal pupils, fluctuating weakness, the absence of other neurologic signs, and clinical response to cholinesterase inhibitors such as edrophonium chloride (Tensilon).

Complications

Difficulty in swallowing leads to aspiration pneumonia. Serious respiratory paralysis may be fatal despite assisted ventilation and modern intensive supportive measures.

Prevention

Proper sterilization of foods during canning requires a temperature of 115 °C (239 °F) to destroy the spores of *C botulinum;* this temperature can be reached in a pressure cooker but not by open boiling. Heating food at 80 °C (176 °F) for 30 minutes or allowing it to boil energetically for 10 minutes before eating it will prevent the disease by destroying any toxin produced during storage. Foods that look or smell abnormal and cans with bulging lids or jars with leaking rings should be destroyed.

Prophylactic use of botulism equine antitoxin (available from the Centers for Disease Control) may be given to asymptomatic persons within 72 hours of ingesting an incriminated food, but because of frequent hypersensitivity reactions (20%), this decision should not be made lightly. Vomiting should be induced, and purgatives and high enemas should be administered.

Treatment

A. Specific Measures: Equine botulism antitoxin is of probable value in the treatment of botulism. Trivalent antitoxin (types A, B, and E) should be given intravenously as soon as the diagnosis is made after skin testing for horse serum sensitivity. The antitoxin, 24-hour diagnostic consultation, epidemic assistance, and laboratory testing services are available from the Centers for Disease Control. The trivalent antitoxin contains 7500 IU of type A, 5500 IU of type B, and 8500 IU of type E per vial. Guanidine hydrochloride, 15–35 mg/kg/d orally in 3 doses, may reverse the neuromuscular block, but its efficacy is questionable.

B. General Measures: General and supportive therapy consists of bed rest, tracheostomy or intubation (if necessary), oxygen and assisted respiration for respiratory paralysis, fluid therapy, and administration of purgatives and high enemas. In cases of infant botulism, some authorities recommend penicillin to eliminate organisms continuing to produce toxin within the gastrointestinal tract.

Prognosis

The mortality rate is about 25% and is lower in children than adults. In nonfatal cases, symptoms subside over 2–3 months and recovery is eventually complete. The availability of antitoxin and modern respiratory support affects the prognosis.

Black RE, Gunn RA: Hypersensitivity reactions associated with botulinal antitoxin. *Am J Med* 1980;**69:**567.

Cherington M: Electrophysiologic methods as an aid in diagnosis of botulism: A review. *Muscle Nerve* 1982;**5(Suppl 9):**S28.

Dowell VR Jr.: Botulism and tetanus: Selected epidemiologic and microbiologic aspects. *Rev Infect Dis* 1984;**6(Suppl 1):**S202.

Horwitz MA et al: Food-borne botulism in the United States, 1970–1975. *J Infect Dis* 1977;**136:**153.

Long SS: Botulism in infancy. *Pediatr Infect Dis* 1984;**3:**266.

Merson MH, Dowell VR: Epidemiologic clinical and laboratory aspects of wound botulism. *N Engl J Med* 1973;**289:**1005.

Schmidt-Nowara WW et al: Early and late pulmonary complications of botulism. *Arch Intern Med* 1983;**143:**451.

Smith LDS: *Botulism: The Organism, Its Toxins, the Disease.* Thomas, 1977.

TETANUS

Essentials of Diagnosis

- Unimmunized or partially immunized patient.
- History of skin wound.
- Spasms of jaw muscles (trismus).
- Stiffness of neck, back, and abdominal muscles, with hyperirritability and hyperreflexia.
- Episodic, generalized muscle contractions.
- Diagnosis is based on clinical findings and the immunization history.

General Considerations

Tetanus is caused by *Clostridium tetani,* an anaerobic, gram-positive bacillus that produces a potent neurotoxin, tetanospasmin. Infection depends on immunization status and contamination of a wound by soil containing clostridial spores from animal manure. The toxin reaches the central nervous system by retrograde axon transport, is bound to cerebral gangliosides, and is thought to increase reflex excitability in neurons of the spinal cord by blocking function of inhibitory synapses. Intense muscle spasms result. Two-thirds of cases in the USA follow minor puncture wounds of the hands or feet. In many cases, no history of a wound can be obtained. Narcotic addicts who inject drugs subcutaneously are at special risk of developing tetanus. In the newborn, infection usually results from contamination of the umbilical cord. The incubation period typically is 4–14 days but may be longer.

In the USA, there is an increased incidence of tetanus in the lower Mississippi Valley and in the Southeast. Over the past 25 years, the overall incidence of tetanus in the USA has been declining. In 1982, only 88 cases were reported to the Centers for Disease Control. Tetanus is much more prevalent in developing countries, where immunization is not always available. There are an estimated 500,000 deaths yearly from tetanus worldwide. The World Health Organization estimates that about 1% of newborns in developing countries die of tetanus.

Clinical Findings

A. Symptoms and Signs: In children and adults, the first symptom is often minimal pain at the site of inoculation, followed by hypertonicity and spasm of the regional muscles. Characteristically, difficulty in opening the mouth (trismus) is evident within 48 hours. In newborns, the first signs are irritability and inability to suck at the breast. The disease may then progress to stiffness of the jaw and neck, increasing dysphagia, and generalized hyperreflexia with extreme rigidity and spasms of all muscles of the abdomen and back (opisthotonos). The facial distortion resembles a grimace (risus sardonicus). Difficulty in swallowing and convulsions triggered by minimal stimuli such as sound, light, or movement may occur. Individual spasms may last seconds or minutes. Recurrent spasms are seen several times each hour, or they may be almost continuous. In most cases, the temperature is normal or only mildly elevated. A high or subnormal temperature is a bad prognostic sign. Patients are fully conscious and lucid. A profound circulatory disturbance associated with sympathetic overactivity may occur on the second to fourth day, which may contribute to the mortality. This is characterized by elevated blood pressure, increased cardiac output, tachycardia (> 120 beats/min), and dysrhythmia.

B. Laboratory Findings: The diagnosis is made on clinical grounds. There may be a mild polymorphonuclear leukocytosis. The cerebrospinal fluid is normal with the exception of some elevation of pressure. Severe muscle spasms may produce mild elevations in serum enzyme levels, including AST (SGOT), creatine phosphokinase, and aldolase. Transient electrocardiographic and electroencephalographic abnormalities may occur. Anaerobic culture and microscopic examination of pus from the wound can be helpful, but *C tetani* is difficult to grow, and the drumstick-shaped gram-positive bacilli often cannot be found.

Differential Diagnosis

In areas where tetanus is rarely seen, physicians may not recognize the infection until classic findings are present. Poliomyelitis is characterized by asymmetric paralysis in an incompletely immunized child. The history of an animal bite, absence of trismus, and pleocytosis of the spinal fluid distinguish rabies. Local infections of the throat and jaw should be easily recognized. In strychnine poisoning, spasms of the jaw muscles are not common, and periods of complete relaxation between spasms are more obvious. Bacterial meningitis, phenothiazine reactions, decerebrate posturing, narcotic withdrawal, and spondylitis may be confused with tetanus. Tetany is confirmed by finding hypocalcemia.

Complications

Complications include malnutrition, pneumonitis, asphyxial spasms, nosocomial infections, decubitus ulcers, and fractures of the spine due to intense contractions. They can be prevented in part by skilled supportive care.

Prevention

A. Tetanus Toxoid: Active immunization with tetanus toxoid is the cornerstone of prevention of tetanus. In the USA, primary immunization of infants is completed after 4 injections. A booster is given upon entry into school. A diphtheria and tetanus booster, adult type (Td), is then required every 10 years. A serum antitoxin level of 0.01 unit/mL indicates a protective level and almost always is achieved after the third dose of vaccine. A booster at the time of injury is needed if none has been given in the past 10 years—or within 5 years in case of a heavily contaminated wound. Nearly all cases of tetanus (99%) in the USA are in unimmunized or incompletely immunized individuals. Because an attack of tetanus does not confer immunity, every patient who recovers should be immunized.

B. Tetanus Antitoxin: Horse serum antitoxin was formerly used in nonimmunized individuals with soil-contaminated wounds. Human tetanus immune globulin (TIG) should now be employed instead whenever possible. Much lower doses are required than with horse serum; the child does not require prior sensitivity testing; and, most importantly, there is no danger of serum sickness or sensitization. For children who have had no or one tetanus toxoid immunization, give 250–500 units intramuscularly. Tetanus toxoid and TIG should be administered concurrently at different sites using different syringes; there is no evidence of significant interference with the immune response by concomitantly administered TIG.

C. Treatment of Wounds: Proper surgical cleansing and debridement of contaminated wounds will decrease the risk of tetanus.

D. Prophylactic Antimicrobials: Prophylactic antimicrobials are useful if the child is unimmunized and TIG is not available.

Treatment

A. Specific Measures: Serotherapy lowers the mortality rate from tetanus, but not dramatically. TIG, 500 units intramuscularly for newborns and 3000–6000 units intramuscularly for children and adults, is preferred to horse serum (5000–100,000 units intravenously) because it causes no sensitivity reactions and has a much longer half-life. The 2 are equally efficacious. Surgical debridement of wounds is indicated, but more extensive surgery or amputation to eliminate the site of infection is not necessary. Penicillin G is given in a dosage of 150,000 units/kg/d intravenously for 10–14 days. Cephalosporins may be substituted in penicillin-sensitive children.

B. General Measures: The patient is kept in a quiet room with minimal stimulation. Control of spasms and prevention of hypoxic episodes are crucial. Many sedatives and muscle relaxants have been used for this purpose, but currently diazepam (Valium) is favored by many physicians. It is useful in patients of all ages including newborns. It is usually given in a dosage of 0.6–1.2 mg/kg/d intravenously in 6 divided doses. In the newborn, however, the drug may be given in 2 or 3 divided doses. Large doses (up to 25 mg/kg/d) may be required for older children. Diazepam is given intravenously until muscular spasms become infrequent and the generalized muscular rigidity much less prominent. The drug may then be given orally and the dose weaned as the child improves. Barbiturates, chlorpromazine, and paraldehyde may also be useful.

Tracheostomy or intubation, mechanical ventilation, and muscle paralysis with pancuronium are necessary in severe cases. Hyperbaric oxygen therapy is probably not of value and requires specialized equipment not generally available.

Prognosis

The fatality rate in newborn and heroin addicts is high (70–90%). The overall mortality rate in the USA is 65%. The fatality rate depends primarily on the quality of supportive care. Many deaths are due to pneumonia or respiratory failure. If the patient survives 1 week, recovery is likely.

Mortality rates tend to be high when (1) the incubation time is short, (2) the site of infection is less accessible, (3) there is no immunity, (4) spasms are frequent and severe and are associated with apnea, and (5) the temperature is under 36.7 °C (98 °F) or over 38.9 °C (102 °F).

Bizzini B: Tetanus toxin. *Microbiol Rev* 1979;**43:**224.

Blake PA et al: Serologic therapy of tetanus in the United States, 1965–1971. *JAMA* 1976;**235:**42.

Dowell VR Jr: Botulism and tetanus: Selected epidemiologic and microbiologic aspects. *Rev Infect Dis* 1984;**6(Suppl 1):**S202.

Edmondson RS, Flowers MW: Intensive care in tetanus: Management, complications and mortality in 100 cases. *Br Med J* 1979;**1:**1401.

Stanfield JP, Galazka A: Neonatal tetanus in the world today. *Bull WHO* 1984;**62:**647.

Tetanus. Page 260 in: *Report of the Committee on Infectious Diseases* ("Red Book"), 19th ed. American Academy of Pediatrics, 1982.

GAS GANGRENE

Essentials of Diagnosis

- Contamination of a wound with soil or feces.
- Massive edema, skin discoloration, bleb formation, and pain in an area of trauma.
- Serosanguineous exudate from wound.
- Crepitation of subcutaneous tissue.
- Rapid progression of signs and symptoms.
- Clostridia cultured or seen on stained smears.

General Considerations

Gas gangrene (clostridial myonecrosis) is a necrotizing infection that follows trauma or surgery and is caused by several anaerobic, gram-positive, spore-forming bacilli of the genus *Clostridium.* These are soil, genital tract (female), and fecal organisms. In devitalized tissue, the spores germinate into vegetative bacilli that proliferate and produce toxins causing thrombosis, hemolysis, and tissue necrosis. *Clostridium perfringens,* the species causing approximately 80% of cases of gas gangrene, produces at least 8 such toxins. These toxins, together with tissue distention caused by interference with blood supply and by gas formation, favor the spread of gangrene. The areas involved most often are the extremities, abdomen, and uterus. Nonclostridial infections with gas formation can mimic clostridial infections and are more common.

Clinical Findings

A. Symptoms and Signs: The onset is sudden, usually 1–20 days (mean 3–4 days) after trauma or surgery. The skin around the wound becomes discolored, with hemorrhagic bullae, serosanguineous exudate, and crepitation in the subcutaneous tissues. Pain and swelling are usually intense. Systemic illness appears early and progresses rapidly to intravascular hemolysis, jaundice, shock, toxic delirium, and renal failure. Toxic delirium may precede any obvious signs of wound infection.

B. Laboratory Findings: Isolation of the organism requires anaerobic culture. Gram-stained smears may demonstrate many gram-positive rods and few inflammatory cells.

C. X-Ray Findings: X-ray may demonstrate gas in tissues, but this is a late finding. Gas in tissues is also seen in infections with other gas-forming organisms. Air that is introduced into tissues during trauma or surgery sometimes leads to a false diagnosis of gas gangrene.

D. Surgical Findings: Direct visualization of the muscle at surgery may be necessary to diagnose gas gangrene. Early, the muscle is pale and edematous and does not contract normally; later, the muscle may be frankly gangrenous.

Differential Diagnosis

Gangrene and cellulitis caused by other organisms and clostridial cellulitis (not myonecrosis) must be distinguished. Necrotizing fasciitis may resemble gas gangrene.

Prevention

The prevention of gas gangrene depends upon the adequate cleansing and debridement of all wounds. It is essential that foreign bodies and dead tissue be removed. A clean wound does not provide a suitable anaerobic environment for the growth of clostridial species.

Treatment

A. Specific Measures: Give penicillin G, 300,000–400,000 units/kg/d intravenously in 6 divided doses. The use of polyvalent gas gangrene antitoxin is controversial because of adverse reactions to horse serum and because its effectiveness is questionable.

B. Surgical Measures: Surgery should be prompt and extensive, with removal of all necrotic tissue.

C. Hyperbaric Oxygen: Hyperbaric oxygen therapy has been shown to be effective, but it is not a substitute for surgery. A patient may be exposed to 2–3 atmospheres in pure oxygen for 1- to 2-hour periods for as many sessions as necessary until there is clinical remission.

Prognosis

Clostridial myonecrosis is fatal if untreated. With early diagnosis, antibiotics, and surgery, the mortality rate is about 20–60%. Involvement of the abdominal wall, leukopenia, intravascular hemolysis, renal failure, and shock are ominous prognostic findings.

Bessman AN, Wagner W: Nonclostridial gas gangrene: Report of 48 cases and review of the literature. *JAMA* 1975;**233:**958.

Hart GB et al: Gas gangrene. *J Trauma* 1983;**23:**991.

Unsworth IP, Sharp PA: Gas gangrene: An 11-year review of

73 cases managed with hyperbaric oxygen. *Med J Aust* 1984;**140:**256.

DIPHTHERIA

Essentials of Diagnosis

- A gray, adherent pseudomembrane, most often in the pharynx but also in the nasopharynx or trachea.
- Sore throat, serosanguineous nasal discharge, hoarseness, and fever in a nonimmunized child.
- Peripheral neuritis or myocarditis.
- Positive culture.

General Considerations

Diphtheria is an acute infection of the upper respiratory tract or skin caused by toxin-producing *Corynebacterium diphtheriae*. Corynebacteria are gram-positive rods 0.5–1 μm in diameter and several micrometers long. Characteristically, they possess irregular swellings at one end that give them a club-shaped appearance. Metachromatic granules are irregularly distributed within the rod, often near the poles, and give the rod a beaded appearance.

There are 3 colony types: (1) var *gravis,* (2) var *mitis,* and (3) var *intermedius*. The capacity to produce exotoxin is conferred by a lysogenic bacteriophage and is not present in all strains of *C diphtheriae*. In immunized communities, infection probably occurs through spread of the phage among carriers of susceptible bacteria rather than through spread of phage-containing bacteria themselves.

The toxin is absorbed into the mucous membranes and causes destruction of epithelium and a superficial inflammatory response. The necrotic epithelium becomes embedded in the exuding fibrin and red and white cells so that a grayish "pseudomembrane" is formed, commonly over the tonsils, pharynx, or larynx. Any attempt to remove the membrane exposes and tears the capillaries and results in bleeding. Cervical lymph nodes enlarge, and there may be marked edema of the entire neck. The diphtheria bacilli within the membrane continue to produce toxin actively. This is absorbed and results in distant toxic damage, particularly degeneration and necrosis in heart muscle, liver, kidneys, and adrenals, and is sometimes accompanied by hemorrhage. The toxin also produces nerve damage, resulting in paralysis of the soft palate, eye muscles, or extremities. Death may occur as a result of respiratory obstruction or acute toxemia and circulatory collapse. The patient may succumb after a somewhat longer time as a result of cardiac damage or may recover after perhaps showing evidence of neurotoxic injury. The incubation period is 1–6 days.

Clinical Findings

A. Symptoms and Signs:

1. Pharyngeal diphtheria—Early manifestations of diphtheritic pharyngitis are mild sore throat, moderate fever, and malaise, followed fairly rapidly by severe prostration and circulatory collapse. The pulse is more rapid than the fever would seem to justify. A membrane forms in the throat and may spread into the nasopharynx or the trachea, producing respiratory obstruction. The membrane is tenacious and gray and is surrounded by a narrow zone of erythema and a broader zone of edema. The cervical lymph nodes become swollen, and swelling is associated with brawny edema of the neck ("bull neck").

2. Laryngeal diphtheria—In about 25% of cases, the larynx is invaded. Occasionally, it may be the only manifestation of the disease. Stridor is apparent. Progressive laryngeal obstruction can lead to cyanosis and suffocation.

3. Other forms—Cutaneous or vaginal diphtheria and wound diphtheria comprise fewer than 2% of cases and are characterized by ulcerative lesions with membrane formation.

B. Laboratory Findings: Diagnosis is clinical. Direct smears are unreliable. Material is first obtained from the nose and throat and from skin lesions, if present, for culture on Löffler's blood agar or other media. Sixteen to 48 hours are required before identification of the organism is possible. A toxigenicity test is then performed. Cultures may be negative in individuals who have received antibiotics. The white blood cell count is usually normal, but there may be a slight leukocytosis. The red blood cell count may show evidence of rapid destruction of erythrocytes and hemoglobin. Thrombocytopenia due to peripheral destruction is frequent.

Differential Diagnosis

Pharyngeal diphtheria resembles acute streptococcal pharyngitis, mononucleosis, and, occasionally, other viral pharyngitis. Nasal diphtheria may be mimicked by a foreign body or purulent sinusitis. Other causes of laryngeal obstruction are epiglottitis due to *Haemophilus influenzae* and viral croup. Neuropathy may be a manifestation of Guillain-Barré syndrome, poliomyelitis, or acute poisoning.

Complications

A. Myocarditis: Diphtheritic myocarditis is characterized by a rapid, thready pulse; indistinct heart sounds, dysrhythmias, or cardiac failure; hepatomegaly; and fluid retention. Signs of myocardial dysfunction can occur from 2 to 40 days after the onset of pharyngitis, most commonly during the second week.

B. Toxic Polyneuritis: This complication involves principally the nerves innervating the palate and pharyngeal muscles and occurs during the first or second week. Nasal speech and regurgitation of food through the nose are seen. Diplopia and strabismus occur during the third week or later. Neuritis may also involve peripheral motor nerves supplying the intercostal muscles and diaphragm and other muscle groups. Generalized paralysis usually occurs after the fourth week.

C. Bronchopneumonia: Secondary pneumonia is common in fatal cases.

Prevention

A. Immunization: Immunization with diphtheria toxoid combined with pertussis and tetanus toxoids (DTP) should be used routinely for infants and children (see Chapter 5).

B. Care of Exposed Susceptibles: Children exposed to diphtheria should be examined and nose and throat cultures obtained. If signs and symptoms of early diphtheria are found, treat as for diphtheria. Asymptomatic individuals, regardless of the results of cultures, should receive diphtheria toxoid and either erythromycin orally (20–30 mg/kg/d in 4 divided doses) or benzathine penicillin G intramuscularly (25,000 units/kg) for 10 days and be observed daily.

Treatment

A. Specific Measures:

1. Antitoxin—Every effort must be made to administer diphtheria antitoxin as early as possible. Antitoxin administered beyond 48 hours may have little effect in altering the incidence of severity of complications. A syringe containing epinephrine chloride should always be available when antitoxin is being injected. The dose of epinephrine, 1:1000 aqueous solution, is 0.01 mL/kg (maximum, 0.5 mL). Preliminary sensitivity testing of the patient to horse serum should always be made before antitoxin is administered. Both a skin test and an eye test should be done (see p 134). If either of these tests is positive, desensitization should be accomplished. Diphtheria antitoxin is administered as follows: mild pharyngeal diphtheria, or when the membrane is small or confined to the anterior nares or tonsils, 40,000 units; moderate pharyngeal diphtheria, 80,000 units; severe pharyngeal or laryngeal diphtheria, combined types, or late cases, 120,000 units. These dosages should be given regardless of the child's weight. Diphtheria antitoxin is infused in 200 mL of isotonic saline over a 30-minute period. If this volume of fluid presents problems, up to one-half the dose may be administered intramuscularly as the undiluted preparation.

2. Antibiotics—If the patient can swallow, 250 mg of phenoxymethyl penicillin (penicillin V) is given by mouth 4 times a day. Patients unable to swallow may receive procaine penicillin G, 600,000 units twice daily intramuscularly. The duration of therapy is 10 days. For the patient allergic to penicillin, erythromycin, 25–50 mg/kg/d, is given orally for 10 days.

B. General Measures: Bed rest in the hospital for 10–14 days is usually required. All patients must be strictly isolated from other persons until antibiotic treatment has made respiratory secretions noninfectious (1–7 days). Isolation may be discontinued when 2 successive nose and throat cultures at 24-hour intervals are negative. These cultures should not be taken until at least 48 hours have elapsed since the cessation of antibiotic treatment.

C. Treatment of Carriers: All carriers should be treated. Erythromycin is the drug of choice (20–50 mg/kg/d orally in 3 or 4 divided doses). Treatment is continued for 10 days. All carriers must be confined at home. Before they can be released, carriers must have 2 negative cultures of both the nose and the throat taken 24 hours apart and obtained at least 24 hours after the cessation of antibiotic therapy.

Prognosis

Mortality rates vary from 3 to 25% and are particularly high in the presence of early myocarditis. Neuritis is reversible; it is fatal only if an intact airway and adequate respiration cannot be maintained. Permanent damage due to myocarditis occurs rarely.

Collier RJ: Diphtheria toxin: Mode of action and structure. *Bacteriol Rev* 1975;**39:**54.

McCloskey RV et al: The 1970 epidemic of diphtheria in San Antonio. *Ann Intern Med* 1971;**75:**495.

McCloskey RV et al: Treatment of diphtheria carriers. *Ann Intern Med* 1974;**81:**788.

Nathenson G, Zakzewski B: Current status of passive immunity to diphtheria and tetanus in the newborn. *J Infect Dis* 1976;**133:**199.

Pappenheimer AM, Murphy JR: Studies on the molecular epidemiology of diphtheria. *Lancet* 1983;**2:**923.

INFECTIONS DUE TO *ENTEROBACTERIACEAE*

Essentials of Diagnosis

- Toxigenic or invasive diarrhea *(Escherichia coli).*
- Neonatal sepsis or meningitis.
- Urinary tract infection.
- Opportunistic infections.
- Diagnosis confirmed by culture.

General Considerations

Enterobacteriaceae is a family of gram-negative bacilli that are part of the normal flora of the gastrointestinal tract and are also found in water and soil. They cause gastroenteritis, urinary tract infections, neonatal sepsis and meningitis, opportunistic infections, and, occasionally, other infections. *Escherichia coli* is the organism in this family that most commonly causes infection in children, but *Klebsiella, Morganella, Enterobacter, Serratia, Proteus,* and other genera are also important, particularly in the compromised host. *Shigella* and *Salmonella* will be discussed in separate sections.

E coli causes diarrhea by invasion of the gut mucosa, by production of enterotoxins, and by other ill-defined mechanisms. Toxin production is mediated by plasmids and has little correlation with serotype. Serotyping of "enteropathogenic" *E coli* (EPEC) with commercial reagents is not useful, because it does not distinguish invasive or toxigenic strains from nonpathogenic strains. *E coli* 0157:H7 has recently been identified as a cause of hemorrhagic colitis and hemolytic-uremic syndrome.

Eighty percent of *E coli* strains causing neonatal meningitis possess specific capsular polysaccharide (K1 antigen), which, alone or in association with specific somatic antigens, confers virulence. K1 antigen is also present on approximately 40% of strains causing neonatal septicemia. The *E coli* K1 organisms do not appear to cause gastrointestinal disease.

Approximately 80% of urinary tract infections in children and adults are caused by *E coli*. Five K antigens (1, 2, 3, 12, and 13) account for 70% of isolates from children with acute pyelonephritis. Thus, only a few K polysaccharides are associated with virulent *E coli* infections of the upper urinary tract.

Klebsiella, Enterobacter, Serratia, and *Morganella* are normally found in the gastrointestinal tract and in soil and water. *Klebsiella* may cause a bronchopneumonia with cavity formation. *Klebsiella, Enterobacter,* and *Serratia* are often opportunists associated with antibiotic usage, debilitating states, and chronic respiratory conditions. They frequently cause urinary tract infection or sepsis. Nursery outbreaks have occurred. In many newborn nurseries, nosocomial infection caused by aminoglycoside-resistant *Klebsiella pneumoniae* is a major problem, particularly when associated with necrotizing enterocolitis.

Many of these infections are difficult to treat because of antibiotic resistance. Antibiotic sensitivity tests are desirable. Parenteral third-generation cephalosporins such as cefotaxime are often more useful than ampicillin. Aminoglycoside antibiotics (gentamicin, tobramycin, amikacin) are usually effective.

Clinical Findings

A. Symptoms and Signs:

1. Enteropathogenic *E coli* gastroenteritis—Enteropathogenic *E coli* (EPEC) may cause diarrhea of varying type and severity. Enterotoxin-producing strains usually produce mild self-limiting illness without significant fever or systemic toxicity. However, diarrhea may be severe in newborns and infants, and occasionally an older child or adult will have a choleralike syndrome. Enterotoxigenic *E coli* strains are a major cause of traveler's diarrhea. Invasive strains cause a shigellalike illness characterized by fever, systemic symptoms, blood and mucus in the stool, and leukocytosis. Enteroinvasive strains are uncommon in the USA.

2. Neonatal sepsis—Findings include jaundice, hepatosplenomegaly, fever, temperature lability, apneic spells, irritability, and failure to suck vigorously. Meningitis is associated with sepsis in 25–40% of cases. Other metastatic foci of infection may be present, including pneumonia and pyelonephritis. Sepsis may lead to severe metabolic acidosis, shock, disseminated intravascular coagulation, and death.

3. Neonatal meningitis—Findings include high fever, full fontanelles, vomiting, coma, convulsions, pareses or paralyses, poor or absent Moro reflex, opisthotonos, and, occasionally, hyper- or hypotonia. Sepsis coexists or precedes meningitis in most cases. Thus, signs of sepsis often accompany those of meningitis. Cerebrospinal fluid usually shows a cell count of over 1000/μL, mostly polymorphonuclear neutrophils, and bacteria on Gram's stain. Cerebrospinal fluid glucose concentration is low (usually less than half that of blood), and the protein is elevated above the levels normally seen in newborns and premature infants (> 150 mg/dL).

4. Acute urinary tract infection—Symptoms include dysuria, increased urinary frequency, and fever in the older child. Nonspecific symptoms such as anorexia, vomiting, irritability, failure to thrive, and unexplained fever are seen in children under 2 years of age. Young infants may present with jaundice. As many as 1% of girls of school age and 0.05% of boys have asymptomatic bacteriuria.

B. Laboratory Findings: Serotyping, tests for enterotoxin production or invasiveness, and K antigen typing can be performed in research laboratories, but these diagnostic tests are not available in most laboratories. Blood cultures are positive in neonatal sepsis. Cultures of cerebrospinal fluid and urine should also be obtained. The diagnosis of urinary tract infections is discussed in Chapter 21.

Differential Diagnosis

The clinical picture of enteropathogenic *E coli* infection may resemble salmonellosis, shigellosis, or viral gastroenteritis.

Neonatal sepsis and meningitis caused by *E coli* can be differentiated from other causes of neonatal infection only by blood and cerebrospinal fluid culture.

Treatment

A. Specific Measures:

1. *E coli* gastroenteritis—*E coli* gastroenteritis seldom requires antimicrobial treatment. In nursery outbreaks, infants have been treated with neomycin, 100 mg/kg/d orally in 3 divided doses for 5 days, or colistin, 10–15 mg/kg/d orally in 3 divided doses for 5 days. Clinical efficacy is not established. Trimethoprim-sulfamethoxazole may be used in older children.

2. *E coli* sepsis, pneumonia, or pyelonephritis—Give ampicillin, 150–200 mg/kg/d intravenously or intramuscularly in divided doses every 4–6 hours, and gentamicin, 5–7.5 mg/kg/d intramuscularly or intravenously in divided doses every 8 hours. Treatment is for 10–14 days. Kanamycin, amikacin, or tobramycin may be used instead of gentamicin if the strain is susceptible. Third-generation cephalosporins are often an attractive alternative as single-drug therapy and do not require monitoring for toxicity.

3. *E coli* meningitis—Give ampicillin, 200–300 mg/kg/d intravenously in 4–6 divided doses, and gentamicin, 5–7.5 mg/kg/d intramuscularly or intravenously in 3 divided doses for 3 weeks. Third-generation cephalosporins such as cefotaxime and moxalactam are also effective and are preferred by some when ampicillin resistance occurs. Treatment with intrathecal and intraventricular aminoglycosides is of no value. Newborns treated with chloramphenicol must have serum levels monitored.

4. Acute urinary tract infection—See Chapter 21.

Prognosis

Death due to gastroenteritis can be prevented by early fluid and electrolyte therapy. Neonatal sepsis with meningitis still carries a mortality rate of over 50%. Most children with recurrent urinary tract infections do well if there are no serious underlying anatomic defects. The mortality rate in opportunistic infections usually depends on the severity of infection and the underlying condition.

Cross AS et al: The importance of the K1 capsule in invasive infections caused by *Escherichia coli. J Infect Dis* 1984;**149:**184.

McCracken GH, Mize SG: A controlled study of intrathecal antibiotic therapy in gram-negative enteric meningitis of infancy: Report of the Neonatal Meningitis Cooperative Study Group. *J Pediatr* 1976;**89:**66.

Remis RS et al: Sporadic cases of hemorrhagic colitis associated with *Escherichia coli* 0157:H7. *Ann Intern Med* 184;**101:**624.

Sack RB: Medical perspective: Enterotoxigenic *Escherichia coli:* Identification and characterization. *J Infect Dis* 1980;**142:**279.

Ulshen MH, Rollo JL: Pathogenesis of *Escherichia coli* gastroenteritis in man: Another mechanism. *N Engl J Med* 1980;**302:**99.

PSEUDOMONAS INFECTIONS

Essentials of Diagnosis

- Opportunistic infection.
- Confirmed by cultures.

General Considerations

Pseudomonas aeruginosa is an important cause of infection in children with cystic fibrosis, neoplastic disease, neutropenia, or extensive burns and in those receiving antibiotic therapy. Infections of the urinary and respiratory tracts, ears, mastoids, paranasal sinuses, eyes, skin, meninges, and bones are seen. *Pseudomonas* can be isolated from the respiratory tract of a majority of patients with cystic fibrosis. *Pseudomonas* pneumonia is a common problem in patients receiving assisted ventilation. *P aeruginosa* sepsis may be accompanied by characteristic peripheral lesions called ecthyma gangrenosum. *P aeruginosa* osteomyelitis sometimes complicates puncture wounds of the feet. *P aeruginosa* is the usual cause of malignant external otitis media. Outbreaks of vesiculopustular skin rash have been associated with exposure to contaminated water in whirlpool baths and hot tubs. Nosocomial infections with *P aeruginosa* are spread by means of a variety of hospital equipment and solutions.

Clinical Findings

The clinical findings depend on the site of infection and the patient's underlying disease. Sepsis with these organisms resembles gram-negative sepsis with other organisms. The diagnosis is made by culture. *Pseudomonas* infection should be suspected in neutropenic patients with clinical sepsis.

Prevention

A. Infections in Debilitated Patients: Colonization of extensive second- and third-degree burns by *Pseudomonas* can lead to fatal septicemia. Aggressive debridement and topical treatment with 0.5% silver nitrate solution, 10% mafenide (Sulfamylon) cream, or gentamicin ointment will greatly inhibit *Pseudomonas* contamination of burns. (See Chapter 8 for a discussion of burn wound infections and prevention.)

Experimental *Pseudomonas* vaccines show some potential for preventing infection in high-risk patients.

B. Nosocomial Infections: Faucet aerators, communal soap dispensers, improperly cleaned inhalation therapy equipment, infant incubators, and back rub lotions have all been associated with *Pseudomonas* epidemics. Careful maintenance of equipment and enforcement of infection control procedures are essential to minimize nosocomial transmission.

Treatment

Gentamicin, tobramycin, amikacin, carbenicillin, ticarcillin, piperacillin, and ceftizoxime are active against most *P aeruginosa* strains as well as other enteric gram-negative rods. However, antimicrobial susceptibility patterns vary from area to area, and resistance tends to appear as new drugs become popular. Treatment of infections is best guided by clinical response and susceptibility tests.

The use of gentamicin (5–7.5 mg/kg/d intramuscularly or intravenously in 3 divided doses) in combination with carbenicillin (400–600 mg/kg/d intravenously in 6 divided doses) or with another anti-*Pseudomonas* β-lactam antibiotic is recommended for treatment of serious *Pseudomonas* infections. Treatment should be continued for 10–14 days. Single-dose drug therapy is discouraged. Intravenous immune globulin and neutrophil transfusions may be helpful in selected patients.

Pseudomonas osteomyelitis requires combined surgical and antibiotic treatment. The duration of antimicrobial therapy necessary for cure is unknown; 1–3 weeks is probably sufficient.

Prognosis

Because debilitated patients are most frequently affected, the mortality rate is high. These infections may have a protracted course, and eradication of the organisms may be difficult.

Brown DG, Baublis J: Reservoirs of *Pseudomonas* in an intensive care unit for newborn infants: Mechanisms of control. *J Pediatr* 1977;**90:**453.

Fisher MC, Goldsmith JF, Gilligan PH: Sneakers as a source of *Pseudomonas aeruginosa* in children with osteomyelitis following puncture wounds. *J Pediatr* 1985;**4:**607.

Jackson MA, Wong KY, Lampkin B: *Pseudomonas aeruginosa*

septicemia in childhood cancer patients. *Pediatr Infect Dis* 1982;**1**:239.
Marks MI: The pathogenesis and treatment of pulmonary infections in patients with cystic fibrosis. *J Pediatr* 1981;**98**:173.
Sherman P, Black S, Grossman M: Malignant external otitis due to *Pseudomonas aeruginosa* in childhood. *Pediatrics* 1980;**66**:782.
Wood RE, Pennington JE, Reynolds HY: Intranasal administration of a *Pseudomonas* lipopolysaccharide vaccine in cystic fibrosis patients. *Pediatr Infect Dis* 1983;**2**:367.

SALMONELLA GASTROENTERITIS

Essentials of Diagnosis

- Nausea, vomiting, headache, meningismus.
- Fever, diarrhea, abdominal pain.
- Culture of organism from stool, blood, or other specimens.

General Considerations

Salmonellae are gram-negative rods that frequently cause food-borne gastroenteritis and occasionally bacteremic infection of bone, meninges, and other foci. Three species—*Salmonella typhi, Salmonella choleraesuis,* and *Salmonella enteritidis*—and approximately 1700 serotypes are recognized. The most common serotypes in human disease—exclusive of *S typhi* and *S choleraesuis*—are *S enteritidis* bioserotypes: *Salmonella typhimurium, Salmonella montevideo, Salmonella newport, Salmonella oranienburg, Salmonella paratyphi B, Salmonella bareilly,* and *Salmonella derby. S typhimurium* is the most frequently isolated serotype in most parts of the world. Approximately 50,000 cases of salmonellosis are reported annually in the USA.

Salmonellae are able to penetrate the mucin layer of the small bowel and attach to epithelial cells. Organisms penetrate beneath the epithelial surface and localize there, causing fever, vomiting, watery diarrhea, and, occasionally, mucus with some polymorphonuclear leukocytes in the stool. Although the small intestine is generally regarded as the principal site of infection, colitis also occurs. *S typhimurium* frequently involves the large bowel. Some salmonellae produce a plasmid-mediated enterotoxin that may also be important in the pathogenesis of diarrhea.

Salmonella infections in childhood occur in 2 major forms: (1) gastroenteritis (including food poisoning), which may be complicated by sepsis and focal suppurative complications; and (2) enteric fever (typhoid fever and paratyphoid fever). (See next section.) While the incidence of typhoid fever has decreased in the USA, the incidence of *Salmonella* gastroenteritis has greatly increased in the past 15–20 years. The highest attack rates occur in children under 6 years of age, with a peak in the age group from 6 months to 2 years old.

Salmonellae are widespread in nature, infecting domestic and wild animals. Fowl and reptiles have a particularly high carriage rate. Contaminated egg powder and frozen whole egg preparations used to make ice cream, custards, and mayonnaise are often responsible for outbreaks. Transmission results primarily from ingestion of contaminated food. Transmission from human to human occurs by the fecal-oral route via contaminated food, water, and fomites.

Most cases of *Salmonella* meningitis (80%) and bacteremia occur in infancy. Newborns may acquire the infection from their mothers during delivery and may precipitate outbreaks in nurseries. Newborns are at special risk of developing meningitis.

Clinical Findings

A. Symptoms and Signs: Infants usually develop fever, vomiting, and diarrhea. The older child may also complain of headache, nausea, and abdominal pain. Stools are often watery or may contain mucus and, in some instances, blood, suggesting shigellosis. Drowsiness and disorientation may be associated with meningismus. Convulsions occur less frequently than with shigellosis. Splenomegaly is occasionally noted. In the usual case, diarrhea is moderate and subsides after 4–5 days, but it may be protracted.

B. Laboratory Findings: Diagnosis is made by isolation of the organism from stools, from blood, or, in some cases, from the urine, cerebrospinal fluid, or pus from a suppurative lesion. The white blood cell count usually shows a polymorphonuclear leukocytosis but may show leukopenia. Typing of isolates is done with specific antisera. *Salmonella* isolates should be reported to public health authorities for epidemiologic purposes.

Differential Diagnosis

In staphylococcal food poisoning, the incubation period is shorter (2–4 hours) than in *Salmonella* food poisoning (12–24 hours). Fever is absent, and vomiting rather than diarrhea is the main symptom. In shigellosis, many pus cells are likely to be seen on a stained smear of stool, and there is more likely to be a marked shift to the left in the peripheral white count. *Campylobacter* gastroenteritis resembles shigellosis clinically. *Arizona* organisms are closely related to the salmonellae and cause a similar illness. Culture of the stools will establish the diagnosis.

Complications

Unlike most types of infectious diarrhea, bacteremia is common, especially in newborns and infants. Septicemia with extraintestinal infection is seen most commonly with *S choleraesuis* but also with *S enteritidis, S typhimurium,* and *S paratyphi B* and *C*. The organism may localize in any tissue and may cause arthritis, osteomyelitis, cholecystitis, endocarditis, meningitis, pericarditis, pneumonia, or pyelonephritis. In patients with sickle cell anemia or other hemoglobinopathies, there is an unusual predilection for osteomyelitis to develop. Severe dehydration and shock are more likely to occur with shigellosis but may occur with *Salmonella* gastroenteritis.

Prevention

Measures for the prevention of *Salmonella* infections include thorough cooking of foodstuffs derived from potentially infected sources; proper refrigeration during storage; and recognition and control of infection among domestic animals, combined with proper meat and poultry inspections. Adults with salmonellosis who are food handlers or who have occupations involving care of young children should have 3 negative stool cultures before resuming work.

Treatment

A. Specific Measures: In uncomplicated *Salmonella* gastroenteritis, there is no evidence that antibiotic treatment shortens the course of the clinical illness or the length of time the organism is present in the gastrointestinal tract. In fact, there is evidence that antibiotic treatment prolongs convalescent carriage of the organism.

However, in order to prevent sepsis and focal disease, antibiotic treatment is recommended for newborns, for severely ill young infants, and for children with sickle cell disease, liver disease, recent gastrointestinal surgery, cancer, depressed immunity, and chronic renal or cardiac disease. Ampicillin (150–200 mg/kg/d intravenously in 4 divided doses for 5–10 days), amoxicillin (50 mg/kg/d orally in 3 divided doses), or trimethoprim-sulfamethoxazole is recommended. The efficacy of this prophylactic therapy is not established. Patients developing bacteremia during the course of gastroenteritis should be given parenteral ampicillin for 7–10 days. Longer treatment is indicated for specific complications. If susceptibility tests indicate resistance to ampicillin, chloramphenicol or trimethoprim-sulfamethoxazole should be given.

Salmonella meningitis is best treated with both chloramphenicol (100 mg/kg/d intravenously in 4 divided doses) and ampicillin (200–300 mg/kg/d intravenously in 4–6 divided doses) for 3 weeks. If the child improves rapidly and the cerebrospinal fluid is sterilized, treatment may be completed with a single drug, the choice guided by results of susceptibility tests.

Outbreaks on pediatric wards are difficult to control. Strict hand washing, cohorting of patients and personnel, and ultimate closure of the unit may be necessary.

B. Treatment of the Carrier States: About half of patients are still infectious after 4 weeks. During infancy, there is a tendency to remain a convalescent carrier for up to a year. Antibiotic treatment of carriers is not effective.

C. General Measures: Careful attention must be given to maintaining fluid and electrolyte balance, especially in infants.

Prognosis

In gastroenteritis, the prognosis is good. In sepsis with focal suppurative complications, the prognosis is more guarded.

The case fatality rate for *Salmonella* meningitis is high in infants. There is a strong tendency to relapse if treatment is not prolonged.

Appelbaum PC, Scragg J: *Salmonella* meningitis in infants. *Lancet* 1977;**1:**1052.

Davis RC: *Salmonella* sepsis in infancy. *Am J Dis Child* 1981;**135:**1096.

Nelson JD: Antibiotic therapy for *Salmonella* syndromes. *Am J Dis Child* 1981;**135:**1093.

Rubin RH, Weinstein I: *Salmonellosis: Microbiologic, Pathologic and Clinical Features.* Grune & Stratton, 1977.

TYPHOID FEVER & PARATYPHOID FEVER

Essentials of Diagnosis

- Insidious or acute onset of headache, anorexia, vomiting, constipation or diarrhea, ileus, and high fever.
- Meningismus, splenomegaly, and rose spots.
- Leukopenia; positive blood, stool, bone marrow, and urine cultures.
- Four-fold rise in Widal agglutination titers.

General Considerations

Typhoid fever is caused by the gram-negative bacillus *Salmonella typhi;* paratyphoid fevers, which may be clinically indistinguishable, may be caused by a variety of *Salmonella* species but most frequently by *Salmonella paratyphi A, B,* and *C.* Children have a shorter incubation period than do adults (usually 5–8 days instead of 8–14 days). The organism enters the body through the walls of the intestinal tract and, following a transient bacteremia, multiplies in the reticuloendothelial cells of the liver and spleen. Persistent bacteremia and symptoms then follow. Reinfection of the intestine occurs as organisms are excreted in the bile. Bacterial emboli produce the characteristic skin lesions (rose spots). Symptoms in children may be mild or severe, but in general, except for the very young, the disease is milder than in adults.

Chloramphenicol-resistant typhoid fever has been reported in Southeast Asia, India, and South America, and ampicillin and chloramphenicol-resistant strains are seen in Latin America and elsewhere.

Typhoid fever is transmitted by the fecal-oral route and by contamination of food or water. Unlike other *Salmonella* species, there are no animal reservoirs of *S typhi;* each case is the result of direct or indirect contact with the organism or with an individual who is actively infected or a chronic carrier. Laboratory-acquired infections are common.

About 500 cases per year are reported in the USA, half of which are acquired during foreign travel.

Clinical Findings

A. Symptoms and Signs: In children, the onset is apt to be sudden rather than insidious, with malaise, headache, crampy abdominal pains and distention, and sometimes constipation followed within 48 hours by diarrhea, high fever, and toxemia. An encephalopathy may be seen with irritability, confusion, delirium, and stupor. Vomiting and meningismus may be prominent in the young. The classic prolonged 3-stage disease seen in adult patients is often shortened in children. The prodrome may be only 2–4 days; the toxic stage may last only 2–3 days; and the defervescence stage may last 1–2 weeks.

During the prodromal stage, physical findings may be absent or there may merely be some abdominal distention and tenderness, meningismus, and minimal splenomegaly. The typical typhoidal rash (rose spots) appears during the second week of the disease and may erupt in crops for the succeeding 10–14 days. Rose spots are erythematous maculopapular lesions 2–3 mm in diameter that fade on pressure. They are found principally on the trunk and chest, and they generally disappear within 3–4 days. The lesions usually number less than 20.

B. Laboratory Findings: Typhoid bacilli can be isolated from many sites, including blood, stool, urine, and bone marrow. Blood cultures are positive in 50–80% of cases during the first week and less often later in the illness. Stool cultures are positive in about 50% of cases after the first week. Urine and bone marrow cultures are also valuable. Most patients will have negative cultures (including stool) by the end of a 6-week period. Serologic tests (Widal reaction) are not as useful as cultures. A 4-fold rise in titer of O (somatic) agglutinins is suggestive of infection but not diagnostic.

Leukopenia is common in the second week of the disease, but in the first week, leukocytosis may be seen. Proteinuria, mild elevation of liver enzymes, thrombocytopenia, and disseminated intravascular coagulation are common.

Differential Diagnosis

Typhoid and paratyphoid fevers must be distinguished from other serious prolonged fevers. These include typhus, brucellosis, tularemia, miliary tuberculosis, psittacosis, vasculitis, lymphoma, mononucleosis, and Kawasaki disease.

The diagnosis of typhoid fever is often made clinically in developing countries. In developed countries, where typhoid fever is uncommon and physicians are unfamiliar with the clinical picture, the diagnosis is often not suspected until late. Positive cultures confirm the diagnosis.

Complications

The most important complications of typhoid fever are gastrointestinal hemorrhage (2–10%) and perforation (1–3%). They occur toward the end of the second week or during the third week of the disease.

Intestinal perforation is one of the principal causes of death. The site of perforation generally is the terminal ileum or cecum. The clinical manifestations are indistinguishable from those of acute appendicitis, with pain, tenderness, and rigidity in the right lower quadrant. The x-ray finding of free air in the peritoneal cavity is diagnostic.

Bacterial pneumonia, meningitis, septic arthritis, abscesses, and osteomyelitis are uncommon complications, particularly if specific treatment is given promptly. Shock and electrolyte disturbances may lead to death.

About 1–3% of patients become chronic carriers of *S typhi*. Chronic carriage is defined as excretion of typhoid bacilli for more than 1 year, but carriage is often for life. Adults with underlying biliary or urinary tract disease are much more likely than children to become chronic carriers.

Prevention

Routine typhoid immunization is not recommended in the USA. Selective typhoid fever immunization is indicated in the following circumstances: (1) intimate household exposure to a known typhoid carrier, (2) community or institutional outbreaks of typhoid fever, and (3) foreign travel to areas where typhoid fever is endemic. There are no data to warrant routine typhoid immunization of children attending summer camps.

A. Primary Immunization: For children 6 months to 10 years, give 2 doses of 0.25 mL subcutaneously 3 or more weeks apart. For children over 10 years and adults, give 0.5 mL subcutaneously. Febrile reactions to the vaccine are common.

B. Booster: Under conditions of continued or repeated exposure, a booster dose (0.1 mL intradermally) should be given every 3 years. Even if more than 3 years have elapsed, a single booster injection is sufficient.

Treatment

A. Specific Measures: Chloramphenicol is the drug of choice in typhoid fever. The dosage is 50–100 mg/kg/d orally or intravenously in 4 divided doses. Treatment should be continued for 14–21 days. Temperature usually returns to normal within 3–5 days.

Use of ampicillin, amoxicillin, or trimethoprim-sulfamethoxazole is also effective and is preferred if resistance to chloramphenicol is suspected on the basis of epidemiologic data or demonstrated by susceptibility testing.

B. General Measures: If toxicity is marked, a short course of corticosteroids may be indicated when antibiotics are begun. Prednisone, 1 mg/kg/d orally during the first 4 days of chloramphenicol therapy, often results in marked clinical improvement.

General support of the patient is exceedingly important and includes rest, good nutrition, and careful observation with particular regard to evidence of intestinal bleeding or perforation. Blood transfusions may be needed even in the absence of frank hemorrhage.

Prognosis

A prolonged convalescent carrier stage in children often continues for 3–6 months. This does not require re-treatment with antibiotics or exclusion from school or other activities.

With early antibiotic therapy, the prognosis is excellent. With early treatment, the mortality rate is less than 1%. Relapse occurs 1–3 weeks later in 10–20% of cases despite appropriate antibiotic treatment.

Blaser MJ et al: *Salmonella typhi:* The laboratory as a reservoir of infection. *J Infect Dis* 1980;**142:**934.

Butler T, Mahmoud AA, Warren KS: Algorithms in the diagnosis and management of exotic diseases. 23. Typhoid fever. *J Infect Dis* 1977;**135:**1017.

Colon AR, Gross DR, Tamer MA: Typhoid fever in children. *Pediatrics* 1975;**56:**606.

Hoffman SL et al: Duodenal string-capsule culture compared with bone-marrow, blood, and rectal-swab cultures for diagnosing typhoid and paratyphoid fever. *J Infect Dis* 1984;**149:**157.

Hornick RB: Selective primary health care: Strategies for control of disease in the developing world. 20. Typhoid fever. *Rev Infect Dis* 1985;**7:**537.

Snyder MJ et al: Comparative efficacy of chloramphenicol, ampicillin, and co-trimoxazole in the treatment of typhoid fever. *Lancet* 1976;**2:**1155.

SHIGELLOSIS (Bacillary Dysentery)

Essentials of Diagnosis

- Cramps and bloody diarrhea.
- High fever, malaise, convulsions.
- Pus and blood in diarrheal stools examined microscopically.
- Diagnosis confirmed by stool culture.

General Considerations

Shigellae are nonmotile gram-negative rods of the family *Enterobacteriaceae* and are closely related to *Escherichia coli.* The genus *Shigella* is divided into 4 major groups, A–D: *Shigella dysenteriae, Shigella flexneri, Shigella boydii,* and *Shigella sonnei.* A sharp upswing in isolations of *S sonnei* has occurred in the USA, with a shift to predominance of *S sonnei* over *S flexneri. S dysenteriae* accounts for fewer than 1% of all *Shigella* infections in the USA. It causes the most severe diarrhea of all species and the greatest number of extraintestinal complications. Approximately 20,000 cases of shigellosis are reported each year in the USA.

Shigellosis is often a serious disease, particularly in children under 2 years of age, and without supportive treatment there is an appreciable mortality rate. In older children, the disease tends to be self-limited and milder. For unexplained reasons it is unusual in infants under 3 months of age. However, on rare occasions, shigellae may be transmitted from the mother to the newborn infant during delivery. Shigellosis during the neonatal period often differs from the disease in older children. Diarrhea and refusal to take feedings are the most common symptoms. Bloody diarrhea and fever occur less frequently. Vomiting, convulsions, or high fever is almost never encountered.

Shigella is usually transmitted by the fecal-oral route. The disease is very communicable; as few as 200 bacteria can produce illness in an adult. The secondary attack rate in families is high, and shigellosis is a serious problem in day-care centers and custodial institutions. Food- and waterborne outbreaks occur but are less important overall than person-to-person transmission.

Shigella organisms produce disease by invading the colonic mucosa, causing abscesses and mucosal ulcerations. The Shiga bacillus (*S dysenteriae* type 1) elaborates an enterotoxin and a neurotoxin. Other *Shigella* species may also produce toxins, but invasiveness is thought to be the primary virulence factor.

Clinical Findings

A. Symptoms and Signs: The incubation period usually is 2–4 days. Onset is abrupt, with abdominal cramps, urgency, tenesmus, chills, fever, malaise, and diarrhea. In severe forms, blood and mucus are seen in the watery stool (dysentery), and meningismus and convulsions may occur. In older children, the disease may be mild and the diagnosis therefore missed. In young children, a fever of 39.4–40 °C (103–104 °F) is common. Rarely, there is rectal prolapse. Symptoms generally last 3–7 days.

B. Laboratory Findings: The white blood cell count is high, often with a marked shift to the left. The stool may contain gross blood and mucus, and many neutrophils may be seen if the stool is examined microscopically. Stool cultures usually are positive; however, they may be negative because the organism is somewhat fragile and is present in small numbers late in the disease and because laboratory techniques are suboptimal for the recovery of shigellae.

Differential Diagnosis

Diarrhea due to rotavirus infection is a winter rather than a summer disease. Intestinal infections caused by salmonellae or *Campylobacter* are differentiated by culture. Amebic dysentery is diagnosed by microscopic examination of fresh stools; intussusception by an abdominal mass, currant jelly stools, and absence of fever. Mild shigellosis is not distinguishable clinically from other forms of infectious diarrhea.

Complications

Dehydration, acidosis, shock, and renal failure are the major complications. In some cases, a chronic form of dysentery occurs, characterized by mucoid stools and poor nutrition. Bacteremia and metastatic infections are rare. Febrile seizures are common. Fulminating fatal dysentery (Ikari syndrome) and hemolytic-uremic syndrome are seen rarely.

Treatment

A. Specific Measures: Ampicillin is the antibiotic of choice if the strain is ampicillin-sensitive. It is given intravenously, intramuscularly, or orally in a dosage of 100 mg/kg/d in 4 divided doses for 5 days. Treatment results in a mild reduction in duration of fever and diarrhea and prompt termination of fecal excretion of *Shigella*. Failure of ampicillin correlates closely with in vitro resistance. Sulfonamides are as effective as ampicillin if the organism is susceptible, but most strains are resistant. For ampicillin-resistant strains, give trimethoprim-sulfamethoxazole, 10 mg of the former and 50 mg of the latter per kilogram per day orally in 2 divided doses. Trimethoprim-sulfamethoxazole-resistant strains are beginning to appear in some parts of the world but are very rare in the USA. Antidiarrheal drugs such as diphenoxylate with atropine (Lomotil) and paregoric may worsen the illness.

B. General Measures: In severe cases, immediate rehydration is critical. A mild form of chronic malabsorption syndrome may supervene and require prolonged dietary control.

Prognosis

The prognosis is excellent if vascular collapse is treated promptly by adequate fluid therapy. The mortality rate is high in very young, malnourished infants who do not receive fluid and electrolyte therapy. Convalescent fecal excretion of *Shigella* lasts 1–4 weeks without antimicrobial therapy. Long-term carriers are rare. Experimental vaccines have been developed but are not yet commercially available.

Ashkenazi S et al: Convulsions in shigellosis: Evaluation of possible risk factors. *Am J Dis Child* 1983;**137:**985.

Barrett-Connor E, Connor JD: Extraintestinal manifestations of shigellosis. *Am J Gastroenterol* 1970;**53:**234.

Blaser MJ et al: *Shigella* infections in the United States, 1974–1980. *J Infect Dis* 1983;**147:**771.

Dupont HL, Hornick RB: Adverse effects of Lomotil therapy in shigellosis. *JAMA* 1973;**226:**1525.

Joanes RF et al: Survey of intestinal pathogens in children travelling abroad. *Public Health* 1984;**98:**139.

Keusch GT, Jacewicz M: The pathogenesis of *Shigella* diarrhea. 5. Relationship of shiga enterotoxin, neurotoxin, and cytotoxin. *J Infect Dis* 1975;**131(Suppl):**S33.

Martin T, Habbick BF, Nyssen J: Shigellosis with bacteremia: A report of two cases and a review of the literature. *Pediatr Infect Dis* 1983;**2:**21.

Nelson JD, Kusmiesz H, Jackson LH: Comparison of trimethoprim-sulfamethoxazole and ampicillin therapy for shigellosis in ambulatory patients. *J Pediatr* 1976;**89:**491.

Tacket CO, Cohen ML: Shigellosis in day-care centers: Use of plasmid analysis to assess control measures. *Pediatr Infect Dis* 1983;**2:**127.

CHOLERA

Essentials of Diagnosis

- Sudden onset of severe watery diarrhea.
- Persistent vomiting without nausea or fever.
- Extreme and rapid dehydration and electrolyte loss, with rapid development of vascular collapse.
- Contact with a case of cholera and the presence of cholera in the community.
- Diagnosis confirmed by stool culture and direct microscopy.

General Considerations

Cholera is an acute diarrheal disease caused by *Vibrio cholerae*. It is transmitted by contaminated water or food. The disease is generally so dramatic that in endemic areas the diagnosis is obvious. Individuals with mild illness and young children may play an important role in transmission of the infection.

In endemic areas, rising titers of vibriocidal antibody are seen with increasing age; infection occurs in individuals with low titers. The age-specific attack rate is highest in children under 5 years and declines with age. Cholera is unusual in infancy. Asymptomatic infection is far more common than clinical disease.

A protein enterotoxin produced by *V cholerae* has been shown to be highly active in inducing experimental cholera in animals. The toxin is only active in the small bowel.

Nutritional status is an important factor determining the severity of the diarrhea. Duration of diarrhea is prolonged by 30–70% in those adults and children suffering from severe malnutrition.

Cholera is endemic in India and South and Southeast Asia. Seven major pandemics have occurred since 1817. The most recent pandemic, caused by the El Tor biotype of *Vibrio cholerae* 01, began in 1961 in Indonesia. In 1978, 40 countries were affected and 74,600 cases reported. Outbreaks outside of the area affected by the pandemic occurred in Spain in 1972, in Italy in 1973, and in Guam in 1975. In the USA, there were no cases of cholera between 1911 and 1973; epidemiologic evidence now indicates that a persistent focus of *V cholerae* of a unique phage type exists along the Gulf Coast.

Humans are the only hosts. Chronic carriers are rare. The incubation period is short, usually 1–3 days.

Clinical Findings

A. Symptoms and Signs: There is sudden onset of massive, frequent, watery stools, generally light gray in color ("rice water") and containing some mucus but no pus. Vomiting may be projectile and is not accompanied by nausea. Within 2–3 hours, the tremendous loss of fluids results in severe and life-threatening dehydration, hypochloremia, and hypokalemia, with marked weakness and collapse. *This is a medical emergency.* Renal failure with uremia and irreversible peripheral vascular collapse will occur if fluid therapy is not administered. The illness lasts 1–7 days and is shortened by appropriate therapy.

B. Laboratory Findings: Markedly elevated hemoglobin (20 g/dL), marked acidosis, hypochloremia, and hyponatremia are seen.

A presumptive diagnosis can be made rapidly by fluorescence microscopy or the vibrio-immobilization test (immobilization by specific antisera of the highly motile cholera vibrios). Cultural confirmation using thiosulfate-citrate-bile salt-sucrose (TCBS) agar takes 16–18 hours for a presumptive diagnosis and 36–48 hours for a definitive bacteriologic diagnosis. The 2 major serotypes, Inaba and Ogawa, are distinguished by agglutination tests with specific antisera.

Prevention

Cholera vaccine dosages are discussed in Chapter 5. The vaccine offers only partial protection (60–80%) for 3–6 months and is relatively ineffective in controlling outbreaks. New, experimental vaccines show promise of being more efficacious. In endemic areas, all water and milk must be boiled, food protected from flies, and sanitary precautions observed. All patients with cholera should be isolated.

Chemoprophylaxis is indicated for household and other close contacts of cholera patients. It should be initiated as soon as possible after the onset of the disease in the index patient. Tetracyclines given as a single daily dose of 500 mg for 5 days are effective in preventing infection.

Tourists visiting endemic areas are at little risk if they exercise common sense in what they eat and drink and maintain good personal hygiene.

Treatment

Physiologic saline must be administered in large amounts to restore blood volume and urine output and to prevent irreversible shock. Potassium supplements are required. Sodium bicarbonate, given intravenously, may also be needed initially to overcome profound acidosis. Moderate dehydration and acidosis can be corrected in 3–6 hours by oral therapy alone. The composition of the solution (in meq/L) is as follows: Na^+, 120; HCO_3^-, 48; Cl^-, 37; and K^+, 25—together with glucose, 110 mmol/L. Intravenous fluids should be given initially in severe cases.

Treatment of children with one of the tetracyclines, 40–50 mg/kg/d orally in 4 divided doses for 2–5 days, modifies the clinical course of the disease and prevents clinical relapse but is not as important as fluid and electrolyte therapy.

Prognosis

With early and rapid replacement of fluids and electrolytes, the case fatality rate is 1–2% in children. If significant symptoms appear and no treatment is given, the mortality rate is over 50%.

Berkenbile F, Delaney R: Stimulation of adenylate cyclase by *Vibrio cholerae* toxin and its active subunit. *J Infect Dis* 1976;**133(Suppl):**S82.

Blake PA et al: Cholera: A possible endemic focus in the United States. *N Engl J Med* 1980;**302:**305.

Carpenter CCJ, Mahmoud AAF, Warren KS: Algorithms in the diagnosis and management of exotic diseases. 26. Cholera. *J Infect Dis* 1977;**136:**461.

Glass RI et al: Endemic cholera in rural Bangladesh, 1966–1980. *Am J Epidemiol* 1982;**116:**959.

Kaper JB et al: Recombinant nontoxinogenic *Vibrio cholerae* strains as attenuated cholera vaccine candidates. *Nature* 1984;**308:**655.

Palmer DL et al: Nutritional status: A determinant of severity of diarrhea in patients with cholera. *J Infect Dis* 1976;**134:**8.

Sommer A, Mosley WH: Ineffectiveness of cholera vaccination as an epidemic control measure. *Lancet* 1973;**1:**1232.

CAMPYLOBACTER ENTERITIS

Essentials of Diagnosis

- Fever, vomiting, abdominal pain, diarrhea.
- Blood, mucus, pus in stools (dysentery).
- Presumptive diagnosis by darkfield or phase contrast microscopy of stool wet mount.
- Definitive diagnosis by stool culture.

General Considerations

Campylobacter species (formerly grouped with vibrios and known as *Vibrio fetus*) are small, gram-negative, curved or spiral bacilli that are commensals or pathogens in many animals. *Campylobacter jejuni* frequently causes acute enteritis in humans, and *Campylobacter fetus* causes bacteremia and meningitis in immunocompromised patients.

In the past decade, *C jejuni* has been responsible for 3–11% of cases of acute gastroenteritis in North America and Europe; in many areas, enteritis due to *C jejuni* is more common than that due to *Salmonella* or *Shigella*. *Campylobacter* enteritis often resembles shigellosis clinically.

Like the reservoir for salmonellae, that for *Campylobacter* species is domestic and wild animals, especially poultry. Numerous cases have been associated with sick puppies or other animal contacts. Contaminated food and person-to-person spread by the fecal-oral route are important in transmission. Outbreaks associated with day-care centers, contaminated water supplies, and raw milk have been reported. Newborns may acquire the organism from their mothers at delivery.

Clinical Findings

A. Symptoms and Signs: *C jejuni* enteritis can be mild or severe. In tropical countries, transient asymptomatic stool carriage is common. The disease usually begins with sudden onset of high fever, malaise, myalgia, headache, abdominal cramps, nausea, and vomiting. Diarrhea follows and may be watery or bile-stained, mucoid, and bloody. Passage of up to 20 stools per day is not uncommon. The illness is self-limited, lasting 2–7 days, but relapses occur in 15–25% of cases. Without antimicrobial treatment, the organism remains in the stool for 1–6 weeks.

B. Laboratory Findings: The peripheral white blood cell count generally is elevated, with many band forms. Microscopic examination of stool reveals erythrocytes and pus cells, and darkfield or phase contrast microscopic examination of wet mounts may reveal darting bacilli characteristic of *Campylobacter*. Other bacteria, particularly *Vibrio* species, may exhibit similar motility, but in areas where cholera and

Vibrio parahaemolyticus diarrhea are rare, a positive darkfield examination has a predictive value of about 90%. Isolation of *C jejuni* from stool is not difficult but requires selective agar, incubation at 42 °C, rather than 35 °C, and incubation in an atmosphere of about 5% oxygen and 5% CO_2 (candle jar is satisfactory).

Differential Diagnosis

Campylobacter enteritis cannot be distinguished clinically from viral gastroenteritis, salmonellosis, shigellosis, amebiasis, or other infectious diarrheas. Because it also mimics ulcerative colitis, Crohn's disase, intussusception, and appendicitis, mistaken diagnosis can lead to unnecessary surgery.

Complications

The most important complications are dehydration and inappropriate treatment due to misdiagnosis as inflammatory bowel disease. Other complications include erythema nodosum, convulsions, reactive arthritis, bacteremia, urinary tract infection, and cholecystitis.

Prevention

No vaccine is yet available. Hand washing and adherence to basic food sanitation practices help prevent disease.

Treatment

Treatment of fluid and electrolyte disturbances is most important. Antimicrobial treatment with erythromycin, 30–50 mg/kg/d orally in 4 divided doses for 5 days (or tetracycline in adults), terminates fecal excretion and may prevent relapses, but antimicrobial treatment does not shorten or modify the illness. Supportive therapy is sufficient in most cases. Antidiarrheal drugs may be harmful.

Prognosis

The outlook is excellent if dehydration is corrected and misdiagnosis does not lead to inappropriate diagnostic or surgical procedures.

Anders BJ et al: Double-blind placebo controlled trial of erythromycin for treatment of *Campylobacter* enteritis. *Lancet* 1982;**1:**131.

Blaser MJ, Reller LB: *Campylobacter* enteritis. *N Engl J Med* 1981;**305:**1444.

Blaser MJ, Taylor DN, Feldman RA: Epidemiology of *Campylobacter jejuni* infections. *Epidemiol Rev* 1983;**5:**157.

Blaser MJ et al: *Campylobacter* enteritis in the United States. A multicenter study. *Ann Intern Med* 1983;**98:**360.

Karmali MA, Fleming PC: *Campylobacter* enteritis in children. *J Pediatr* 1979;**94:**527.

Karmali MA et al: *Campylobacter* enterocolitis in a neonatal nursery. *J Infect Dis* 1984;**149:**874.

Nolan CM et al: *Campylobacter jejuni* enteritis: Efficacy of antimicrobial and antimotility drugs. *Am J Gastroenterol* 1983;**78:**621.

Paisley JW et al: Dark-field microscopy of human feces for presumptive diagnosis of *Campylobacter fetus* subsp. *jejuni* enteritis. *J Clin Microbiol* 1982;**15:**61.

BRUCELLOSIS

Essentials of Diagnosis

- Intermittent fevers, primarily in the evenings or at night.
- Easy fatigability, arthralgia, anorexia, sweating, and irritability.
- Relative lymphocytosis, positive blood culture, agglutination titer of 1:160 or greater.

General Considerations

Brucella infections in humans are caused by 4 species: *Brucella abortus* (cattle), *Brucella suis* (hogs), *Brucella melitensis* (goats), and *Brucella canis* (dogs). Infection usually occurs through ingestion of contaminated milk or milk products or by contact with animal tissues through minor skin or mucosal abrasions. The incubation period is 8–30 days but may be as long as 6 months.

Clinical Findings

A. Symptoms and Signs: The onset is insidious, with vague symptoms of weakness, exhaustion, arthralgias, intermittent night fevers, and sweating. The chronic form of the disease, which follows untreated acute or subacute brucellosis, may be characterized by localized abscesses in bone, joints, liver, lung, or spleen. Signs are fever, hepatosplenomegaly, which may be tender, and mild lymphadenopathy.

B. Laboratory Findings: The white blood cell count is normal or reduced, with relative lymphocytosis. The organism can be recovered from the blood or, in chronic forms, from localized areas of infection. There is little difficulty in obtaining positive blood cultures from patients infected with *B melitensis* or *B suis*. However, in *B abortus* infections, there are fewer organisms circulating in the blood. In the case of suspected *B abortus* infection, it is advisable to obtain a larger quantity of venous blood (about 0.5 mL/kg) and distribute it among a series of blood culture bottles. Blood cultures should be subcultured twice a week for at least 3 weeks before a negative result is reported.

Serologic tests are of value in acute cases where cultures are negative or in later or complicated cases. Acutely, the *Brucella* agglutinin titer increases rapidly. A 4-fold rise is diagnostic, and a single titer of 1:160 or more indicates recent infection. False-positive results may occur owing to cross-reactivity with *Francisella tularensis,* cholera vaccine, or even some *Salmonella* infections. Late in infection, agglutinins may fall in titer or may exhibit prozone phenomena, making serial dilution of sera to at least 1:1280 essential.

The agglutinin titer may remain elevated for years, and infections are therefore timed more successfully with other tests, particularly complement fixation or indirect agglutination, which remain positive for shorter periods. Skin tests exist but should not be used if serologic tests are available.

Differential Diagnosis

It is important to distinguish brucellosis from a variety of causes of fever without localization, including bacterial endocarditis; mononucleosis; salmonellosis; tularemia; and neoplastic, collagen vascular, and granulomatous diseases that may cause lymphadenopathy and hepatosplenomegaly.

Complications

Hematogenous spread may lead to endocarditis, pyelonephritis, meningoencephalitis, or osteomyelitis. In older children, infection of the bile ducts results in jaundice. In the malignant form, hepatic necrosis may occur. Neurologic complications may appear at the onset of the illness or at any time during the clinical course, including convalescence, or long after acute symptoms have subsided.

A psychiatric form of the disease is described that is likely to be associated with a mild encephalitis.

Treatment

A. Specific Measures: Tetracycline, 50 mg/kg/d orally in divided doses every 6 hours, is given for 21 days. In case of a relapse, treatment is repeated. In very severe cases of acute brucellosis or in suppurative brucellosis due to *B suis,* simultaneous administration of streptomycin, 20–40 mg/kg intramuscularly as a single daily dose for 1 week, is advised. During the second week, streptomycin is continued at the level of 15 mg/kg while tetracycline is continued orally for the full 21 days.

B. General Measures: Limited physical activity and bed rest are indicated while there is fever. Aspirin will relieve headache and somatic pains.

Prognosis

With antimicrobial therapy, the prognosis is excellent and the chance for prolonged invalidism markedly reduced.

Buchanan TM et al: Brucellosis in the United States, 1960–1972: An abattoir-associated disease. 2. Diagnostic aspects. *Medicine* 1974;**53:**415.

Busch LA, Parker RL: Brucellosis in the United States. *J Infect Dis* 1972;**125:**289.

Feiz J, Sabbaghian H, Miralai M: Brucellosis due to *Brucella melitensis* in children: Clinical and epidemiologic observations on 95 patients studied in central Iran. *Clin Pediatr* 1978;**17:**904.

Street L, Grant WW, Alva JD: Brucellosis in childhood. *Pediatrics* 1975;**55:**416.

TULAREMIA

Essentials of Diagnosis

- A cutaneous or mucous membrane lesion at the site of inoculation and regional lymph node enlargement.
- Sudden onset of fever, chills, and prostration.
- History of contact with infected animals, principally wild rabbits.
- Positive culture or immunofluorescence of mucocutaneous ulcer or regional lymph nodes.
- High serum antibody titer.

General Considerations

Tularemia is caused by *Francisella tularensis,* a gram-negative organism usually acquired from infected animals, principally wild rabbits; by contamination of the skin or mucous membranes with infected blood or tissues; by inhalation of infected material; by bites of ticks, fleas, or deerflies that have been in contact with infected animals; or by ingestion of contaminated meat or water. Strains of high virulence for humans (Jellison type A) are usually associated with tick-borne tularemia of rabbits; those of lowered virulence (Jellison type B) are linked with the waterborne disease of rodents. The incubation period is short, usually 3–7 days, but may vary from 2 to 25 days.

Rabbits are the classic vectors of tularemia. It is important to seek a history of rabbit hunting, skinning, or food preparation in any patient who has a febrile illness with tender lymphadenopathy, often in the region of a draining skin ulcer. However, a history of exposure to other wild game or ticks may also be helpful in diagnosis.

Clinical Findings

A. Symptoms and Signs: Several clinical types are seen in children. Most infections are of the ulceroglandular form and start as a reddened papule that may be pruritic, quickly ulcerates, and is not very painful. Shortly thereafter, the regional lymph nodes become large and tender. Fluctuance quickly follows. At the same time, there may be marked systemic manifestations, including high fever, chills, weakness, and vomiting. Pneumonitis occasionally accompanies the ulceroglandular form or may be seen as the sole manifestation of infection (pneumonic form). A detectable skin lesion is occasionally absent, and localized lymphoid enlargement exists alone (glandular form). Oculoglandular and oropharyngeal forms also occur in children. The latter is characterized by tonsillitis, often with membrane formation, cervical adenopathy, and high fever. In the absence of any primary ulcer or localized lyphadenitis, a prolonged febrile disease reminiscent of typhoid fever can be seen (typhoidal form). Splenomegaly is common in all forms.

B. Laboratory Findings: *F tularensis* can be recovered from ulcers, regional lymph nodes, and sputum of patients with the pneumonic form. However, the organism grows only on an enriched medium (blood-cystine-glucose agar), and laboratory handling is dangerous. Another method of organism detection is immunofluorescence of biopsied material or aspiration of involved lymph nodes. Gram's stain is not useful.

An intradermal skin test is positive early in the disease; it resembles the tuberculin skin tests. The skin test does not result in a significant serologic response and may therefore be used in addition to serologic tests for diagnosis. The white blood cell count is not remarkable. Agglutinins are present after the second week of illness, and in the absence of a positive culture their development confirms the diagnosis. An agglutination titer of 1:160 or higher is considered positive.

Differential Diagnosis

The typhoidal form of tularemia may mimic typhoid, brucellosis, miliary tuberculosis, Rocky Mountain spotted fever, and infectious mononucleosis. Pneumonic tularemia resembles atypical and mycotic pneumonitis. The ulceroglandular type of tularemia resembles pyoderma caused by staphylococci or streptococci, rat-bite fever, plague, anthrax, and cat-scratch fever. The oropharyngeal type must be distinguished from streptococcal or diphtheritic pharyngitis, infectious mononucleosis, herpangina, or other viral pharyngitides.

Prevention

Reasonable attempts should be made to protect children from bites of insects, principally ticks, fleas, and deerflies, by the use of proper clothing and repellents. Since rabbits are the source of most human infections, the dressing and handling of such game should be performed with great care. If contact occurs, thorough washing with soap and water is indicated.

Treatment

A. Specific Measures: Give streptomycin, 30 mg/kg/d intramuscularly in 2 divided doses for 8–10 days. The maximum daily dose is 1 g. Other aminoglycoside antibiotics have been used in individual cases and are probably effective. The tetracyclines and chloramphenicol are also effective, but the organism is not eradicated and relapses occur.

B. General Measures: Antipyretics and analgesics may be given as necessary. Skin lesions are best left open. Glandular lesions occasionally require incision and drainage.

Prognosis

With streptomycin, the prognosis is excellent.

Bloom ME, Shearer WT, Barton LL: Oculoglandular tularemia in an inner city child. *Pediatrics* 1973;**51:**564.

Guerrant RL et al: Tickborne oculoglandular tularemia: Case report and review of seasonal and vectorial associations in 106 cases. *Arch Intern Med* 1976;**136:**811.

Teutsch SM et al: Pneumonic tularemia on Martha's Vineyard. *N Engl J Med* 1979;**301:**826.

Tyson HK: Tularemia: An unappreciated cause of exudative pharyngitis. *Pediatrics* 1976;**58:**864.

PLAGUE

Essentials of Diagnosis

- Sudden onset of fever, chills, and prostration.
- Regional lymph node tender; lymphadenitis with suppuration of nodes (bubonic form).
- Hemorrhages into skin and mucous membranes and shock (septicemia).
- Cough, dyspnea, cyanosis, and hemoptysis (pneumonia).
- History of exposure to infected animals.

General Considerations

Plague is an extremely serious, acute infection caused by a gram-negative bacillus, *Yersinia pestis.* It is a disease of rodents that is transmitted to humans by the bites of fleas. Rodent plague in animals of the field and forest is called sylvatic plague; plague in rodents associated with humans is called murine plague. Plague bacilli have been isolated from rodents in 15 of the western states in the USA. Cases associated with wild rodents occur sporadically. Ten to 20 cases of plague in humans have occurred annually in the USA since 1974. In the western part of the USA, the disease almost always occurs during the period from June through September.

Human plague in the USA appears to occur in cycles that reflect comparable cycles in wild animal reservoirs of infection.

Clinical Findings

A. Symptoms and Signs: The disease assumes several different clinical forms, the 2 most common being bubonic and septicemic. Pneumonic plague, the form that occurs when organisms enter the body through the respiratory tract, is now very uncommon.

1. Bubonic plague—Bubonic plague begins after an incubation period of 2–6 days with a sudden onset of high fever, chills, headache, vomiting, and marked delirium or clouding of consciousness. A less severe form also exists, with a less precipitous onset but with progression over several days to severe symptoms. Although the flea bite is rarely seen, the regional lymph node, usually inguinal and unilateral, is painful and tender, 1–5 cm in diameter, and usually suppurates and drains spontaneously after 1 week. The plague bacillus is known to produce an endotoxin that causes vascular necrosis. Bacilli may overwhelm regional lymph nodes and enter the circulation to produce septicemia. Severe vascular necrosis results in widely disseminated hemorrhages in skin, mucous membranes, liver, and spleen. Myocarditis and circulatory collapse may result from damage by the endotoxin.

A septicemic form of bubonic plague also exists that begins with fever, delirium, and bacteremia, with regional lymphadenopathy and bubo formation occurring after 3–5 days.

Plague meningitis or pneumonia may occur secondarily following bacteremic spread from an infected lymph node.

2. Septicemic plague—The septicemic form is defined as any case of plague without evidence of lymphadenopathy. This form is less common than bubonic plague but carries a worse prognosis, largely because it is less likely to be recognized and treated early. It is frequently complicated by pneumonia.

B. Laboratory Findings: Aspiration of a bubo leads to visualization of bacilli on a stained smear. Pus, sputum, and blood all yield the organism, although laboratory infections are common enough to make isolation dangerous. Blood-agar cultures yield positive results in 48 hours. The white blood cell count is markedly elevated, with a shift to the left.

Sera obtained during disease and convalescence should be collected and stored for use in confirming the diagnosis in cases where the organism may not be recovered.

Differential Diagnosis

The septic phase of the disease may be confused with such illnesses as meningococcemia, sepsis, and rickettsioses. The bubonic form resembles tularemia, anthrax, cat-scratch fever, streptococcal adenitis, and cellulitis. Primary gastroenteritis and appendicitis may have to be distinguished.

Prevention

Proper disposal of household and commercial wastes and chemical control of rats are basic for control of the murine plague reservoir. Flea control is instituted and maintained with the liberal use of insecticides. Children vacationing in remote camping areas should be warned not to handle dead or dying animals. Travelers to wild areas in the enzootic western states are at low risk of infection, and immunization of visitors to these areas is not recommended.

Vaccination is recommended for those traveling or living in areas of high incidence. (See Chapter 5.)

Treatment

A. Specific Measures: Streptomycin and tetracyclines should both be used. The dose of streptomycin is 20–40 mg/kg intramuscularly in 3 divided doses for 5 days, followed by one of the tetracyclines, 50 mg/kg/d intramuscularly or orally in 3 divided doses. Treatment should be continued until the patient has been afebrile for 4 or 5 days. Chloramphenicol, 75–100 mg/kg/d intravenously or orally in 4 divided doses, may be substituted for tetracycline.

In septicemia and pneumonic plague, treatment must be started in the first 15–24 hours of the disease if survival is to be expected. Treatment with streptomycin started 36–48 hours after onset of the disease may result in death due to liberation of plague toxin. The mechanism may be analogous to the Jarisch-Herxheimer reaction, with release of toxin from dead plague bacilli.

Bubonic plague is not highly contagious. Every effort is made to effect resolution of buboes without resorting to surgery. Pus from draining lymph nodes should be handled with rubber gloves.

B. General Measures: Pneumonic plague is highly infectious, and rigid isolation is required. All contacts should receive prophylaxis with sulfadiazine, 100–200 mg/kg/d orally in 4 divided doses for 7 days, or tetracycline, 30 mg/kg/d in 4 divided doses for 7 days.

Prognosis

The mortality rate in untreated bubonic plague is about 50%; it is 90% in the septicemic form and nearly 100% in the pneumonic form. Recent mortality rates in New Mexico were 3% for bubonic plague and 71% for the septicemic form.

Butler T et al: *Yersinia pestis* infection in Vietnam. 1. Clinical and hematologic aspects. *J Infect Dis* 1974;**129(Suppl):**S78.

Isaacson M et al: Unusual cases of human plague in southern Africa. *S Afr Med J* 1973;**47:**2109.

Mann JM, Shandler L, Cushing AH: Pediatric plague. *Pediatrics* 1982;**69:**762.

Meyer KF et al: Plague immunization. 1. Past and present trends. *J Infect Dis* 1974;**129(Suppl):**S13.

Washington RL, Barkin RM, Hillman JR: Septicemic plague that mimics Reye's syndrome. *Am J Dis Child* 1979;**133:**434.

HAEMOPHILUS INFLUENZAE TYPE b INFECTIONS

Essentials of Diagnosis

- Purulent meningitis in children under age 4 years with direct smears of cerebrospinal fluid showing gram-negative pleomorphic rods.
- Acute epiglottitis: High fever, drooling, dysphagia, and croup. White blood cell count over 20,000/μL.
- Septic arthritis: Fever, local redness, swelling, heat, and pain with active or passive motion of the involved joint in a child 4 months to 3 years of age.
- Cellulitis: Sudden onset of fever and distinctive cellulitis in an infant, often involving the cheek or periorbital area, and starting as a mild swelling with central erythema that rapidly progresses to a lesion without a distinct border with central reddish discoloration, surrounded by and merging into purplish areas that fade peripherally.
- In all cases, a positive culture from the blood, cerebrospinal fluid, or aspirated pus confirm the diagnosis.

General Considerations

Haemophilus influenzae type b is perhaps the most important bacterial pathogen in childhood. It causes meningitis, epiglottitis (supraglottic croup), septic arthritis, periorbital and facial cellulitis, pneumonia, and pericarditis. *H influenzae* type b infections occur most frequently in the age group from 4 months to 4 years (epiglottitis: 2–5 years). With the exception of pneumonia and pericarditis, this organism is the leading bacterial cause of all these infections in this age range.

Ninety percent of blood samples from newborns show bactericidal antibody, reflecting passive transfer of antibody from protected mothers. The age distribution of infection is explained by the loss of passive protection by 4–6 months of age, the progressive infection of susceptible individuals, and acquisition of protective antibodies in early childhood. The chief virulence factor for *H influenzae* type b organisms appears to be the polyribose phosphate (PRP) capsule, which is antiphagocytic, and anti-PRP antibody is protective. Many children 4 months to 3 years of age have low or nondetectable levels of anticapsular antibodies. In the period from 3½–8 years of age, anticapsular antibodies appear in the serum and reach adult levels. Although many infants and children are colonized early with *H influenzae* species, most of the strains are nonencapsulated. The very low nasopharyngeal colonization rate of *H influenzae* type b in infants and children suggests that the homologous organism is not the usual stimulus for the development of anticapsular antibodies. The type b capsule is immunologically cross-reactive with the capsules of certain species of bacilli, diphtheroids, lactobacilli, *Staphylococcus aureus, Staphylococcus epidermidis,* streptococci, *Escherichia coli,* and *Pseudomonas.* Thus, it apears that natural immunity is acquired from encapsulated bacteria that share antigenic determinants with *H influenzae* type b PRP.

In the past 3 decades, the incidence of *H influenzae* type b infections serious enough to require hospitalization has been increasing. There is no clear explanation for this increase. Recently, reports of systemic disease in newborns and adults have increased. However, the number of systemic infections has increased in all age groups, and the highest age-specific attack rate still occurs in children from 4 months to 4 years of age.

In 1974, the first 2 cases of illnesses due to ampicillin-resistant *H influenzae* type b were reported. The mechanism of resistance was the elaboration of β-lactamase (penicillinase) by the resistant organisms. At the end of 1980, ampicillin-resistant strains comprised 10–25% of all type b strains isolated in certain regions of the USA. Associated clinical illnesses have included meningitis, pneumonia, epiglottitis, sepsis, and otitis media. *H influenzae* type b resistant to chloramphenicol and rare strains resistant to both drugs have been observed.

Tympanocentesis performed in children with acute otitis media has demonstrated that a pneumococcus can be isolated from about 35% of cases and *H influenzae* from about 25%. However, most of the *H influenzae* strains are nonencapsulated and nontypeable. Type b accounts for about 10% of the *H influenzae* strains. Ampicillin-resistant *H influenzae* should be suspected in situations where ampicillin therapy of otitis media is unsuccessful.

There is epidemiologic evidence that *H influenzae* type b meningitis occurs more frequently in urban and rural areas of low socioeconomic status. Acutely ill children 4–36 months of age, with temperatures higher than 39 °C (102.2 °F) and nonspecific symptoms associated with an elevated white blood cell count, may have *H influenzae* type b bacteremia. This syndrome is associated most frequently with pneumococcal bacteremia and next most frequently with type b bacteremia.

Both ampicillin and chloramphenicol should be used as initial therapy for infants and children over 30 days of age with disease thought to be due to *H influenzae* type b. This includes all bacterial meningitis and epiglottitis, and, in infants under 3 years of age, facial cellulitis and septic arthritis. Ampicillin alone is adequate initial therapy for otitis, sinusitis, and most cases of suspected bacterial pneumonia. If *H influenzae* type b is cultured, sensitivities to ampicillin and chloramphenicol should be determined and therapy continued with the single most appropriate drug. If no organism is cultured and *H influenzae* is a likely cause (as with meningitis or typical cellulitis), chloramphenicol alone should be used.

Clinical Findings

A. Symptoms and Signs:

1. Meningitis—In the USA, *H influenzae* type b is responsible for about 80% of cases of bacterial meningitis in children after the neonatal period. In many other countries, this percentage is lower. Infants usually present with fever, irritability, lethargy, poor feeding with or without vomiting, and a high-pitched cry. Signs of localized disease elsewhere should be looked for carefully, including otitis, cellulitis, arthritis, and pneumonia. (See Chapter 23 for further details.)

2. Acute epiglottitis—The most useful clinical finding in the early diagnosis of *H influenzae* croup is evidence of dysphagia characterized by a refusal to eat or swallow saliva and by drooling. This finding, plus the presence of a high fever in a "toxic" child—even in the absence of cherry-red epiglottis on direct examination of the epiglottis—should strongly suggest the diagnosis and lead to prompt intubation. Stridor is a late sign. (See Chapter 14 for details.)

3. Septic arthritis—*H influenzae* type b is the most common cause of bacterial septic arthritis in children under 3 years of age in the USA. Disease may involve multiple joints and is complicated by osteomyelitis in about 20% of cases. The child is febrile and refuses to move the involved joint and limb because of pain. Examination reveals swelling, warmth, redness, tenderness on palpation, and severe pain on attempted movement of the joint.

4. Cellulitis—Cellulitis due to *H influenzae* type b occurs almost exclusively in the 3-month to 3-year age group. The presentation is typical. The child often gives a history of coryza or otitis media. Fever persists at the same time the cellulitis develops. The cheek or periorbital (preseptal) area is usually involved. There is mild swelling with central erythema, rapidly progressing to a lesion without a distinct border that exhibits central reddish discoloration surrounded by a purplish area. Superficial trauma is characteristically absent. Bacteremia is frequent.

Periorbital cellulitis due to *H influenzae* must be distinguished from 2 other similar entities. The first is periorbital (preseptal) cellulitis caused by other bacteria. This frequently presents with evidence of a primary local infection nearby (conjunctivitis, sinusitis) or trauma to the skin. Staphylococci, streptococci, or a combination of the 2 is usually involved. Bacteremia is rare. The second is true orbital cellulitis. This disease is rare and occurs primarily in older children with ethmoid or splenoid sinusitis. *H influenzae* is usually not involved.

5. Pneumonia—Pneumonia due to *H influenzae* type b usually presents clinically in much the same fashion as pneumonia due to the pneumococcus. Disease is most common in the 3-month to 4-year age group, just as it is with *H influenzae* meningitis. Most cases are segmental or lobar in distribution, but diffuse bronchopneumonia or interstitial involvement is occasionally seen. Both empyema and lung abscesses occur. *H influenzae* involvement of other organs (meningitis, epiglottitis, otitis media) is not uncommon.

The true incidence of *H influenzae* pneumonia is not known. It is likely, however, that it varies according to geographic area. In the USA, *H influenzae* is probably second only to the pneumococcus as a cause of bacterial pneumonia in young children.

B. Laboratory Findings: The white blood cell count in *H influenzae* infections may be high or normal with a shift to the left. Blood culture is frequently positive. Positive culture of aspirated pus or fluid from the involved site or nearby proves the diagnosis.

In meningitis (before treatment), spinal fluid smear may show the characteristic pleomorphic gram-negative rods.

The diagnosis of *H influenzae* pneumonia depends on isolation of the organism from blood, lung tissue, or empyema fluid. A positive culture from the upper respiratory tract is not diagnostic. Detection of antigen in body fluids, including urine, may be helpful. Counterimmunoelectrophoresis or latex agglutination can be used to detect polyribose phosphate (PRP), the capsular antigen of *H influenzae* type b, in cerebrospinal fluid, joint fluid, urine, sputum, and serum. The test is particularly useful in the diagnosis of patients with meningitis or arthritis who have received antibiotic therapy and have negative cultures. Antigenemia may last from days to weeks in certain infants.

C. X-Ray Findings: A lateral view of the neck in suspected acute epiglottitis may be helpful but should not delay intubation. Haziness of maxillary and ethmoid sinuses occurs with orbital cellulitis.

Differential Diagnosis

A. Meningitis: Differentiate from head injury, brain abscess, tumor, lead encephalopathy, and other forms of meningoencephalitis due to viral, fungal, and bacterial agents, including tuberculous meningitis.

B. Acute Epiglottitis: In croup caused by viral agents (parainfluenza 1, 2, and 3, respiratory syncytial virus, influenza A, adenovirus), the child has more definite upper respiratory symptoms, cough, hoarseness, slower progression of obstructive signs, and only low-grade fever. Spasmodic croup occurs typically at night in a child with a history of previous attacks; these attacks may be of allergic origin. A history of sudden onset of choking and paroxysmal coughing suggests aspiration of a foreign body. Occasionally, retropharyngeal abscess or laryngeal diphtheria may have to be differentiated from epiglottitis.

C. Septic Arthritis: Differential diagnosis includes acute osteomyelitis, prepatellar bursitis, cellulitis, rheumatic fever, and fractures and sprains.

D. Cellulitis: Erysipelas, streptococcal cellulitis, insect bites, and trauma may occur. Periorbital cellulitis must be differentiated from paranasal sinus discase without cellulitis, allergic inflammatory disease of the lids, conjunctivitis, and herpes zoster infection.

E. Pneumonia: See Chapter 14.

Complications

A. Meningitis: See Chapter 23.

B. Acute Epiglottitis: Mediastinal emphysema and pneumothorax may occur.

C. Septic Arthritis: Septic arthritis may result in rapid destruction of cartilage and ankylosis if diagnosis and treatment are delayed. Even with early treatment, the incidence of residual damage and disability after septic arthritis in weight-bearing joints may be as high as 25%.

D. Cellulitis: Bacteremia may lead to metastatic meningitis or pyarthrosis.

E. Pneumonia: Complications include empyema and, rarely, pneumatocele and pneumothorax.

Prevention

In Finland, field trials of a purified PRP vaccine for *H influenzae* type b showed greater than 90% protection of infants immunized at 2 years of age and older. This vaccine was licensed in the USA in 1985 and is recommended for routine use in children at 2 years of age (see Chapter 5 for discussion of use in older children). Protein-conjugated PRP vaccines show promise of adequate immunogenicity at younger ages and even during the first 6 months of life; these new vaccines will probably replace the PRP vaccine when efficacy trials have been completed.

Careful epidemiologic studies have demonstrated that families and close contacts of patients with *H influenzae* type b infections are at increased risk of acquiring infection. This has led to the following recommendation: If the infected child has a sibling under 49 months of age, all family members should be given rifampin, 20 mg/kg/d for 4 successive days, in order to avoid illness and further spread to susceptibles. The present recommendation for day-care centers does not indicate prophylaxis unless 2 cases of systemic *H influenzae* infection have occurred within a 60-day period.

Individuals with X-linked antibody synthesis deficiency are susceptible to repeated and severe *H influenzae* type b infections, including meningitis. Passive immunization of these individuals with pooled immune globulin containing anti-type b antibody confers protection.

Treatment

For comments regarding the problem of ampicillin-resistant strains of *H influenzae* type b, see General Considerations (above). With the exception of acute otitis media, all bacteremic or potentially bacteremic *H influenzae* diseases require hospitalization for treatment. The drugs of choice in hospitalized cases are intravenous ampicillin and chloramphenicol, used in combination until the sensitivity of the organism is known, and then singly. Chloramphenicol can also be given by mouth but should never be administered intramuscularly, because of slow and unpredictable absorption. If chloramphenicol is used for more than 3 days, it should be carefully monitored. If serum concentrations can be measured, the dose is adjusted so that peak levels (30 minutes after intravenous infusion or 1 hour after an oral dose) are kept in the range of 15–20 μg/mL. In any case, hemoglobin, white blood cell count and differential, and reticulocyte counts should be measured every second or third day. (See Chapter 38 for further details of dosage at various ages.)

Most second-generation cephalosporins (cefamandole, cefoxitin, and cefaclor) should not be used for any *H influenzae* infection in which meningitis is a possibility, since these drugs do not reach cerebrospinal fluid in concentrations adequate to treat or prevent infection. Cefuroxime and third-generation cephalosporins (moxalactam, cefotaxime, and others) appear to be adequate in treatment of *H influenzae* meningitis, although experience is limited.

Both trimethoprim-sulfamethoxazole and tetracycline have been used successfully in *H influenzae* infections. For otitis, erythromycin-sulfonamide combinations are effective.

A. Meningitis: Therapy is begun as soon as bacterial meningitis has been identified and cerebrospinal fluid, blood, and other appropriate cultures have been obtained. An intravenous push of ampicillin, 100 mg/kg, should be given immediately, followed by 300 mg/kg/d in 6 divided doses. We have not found it necessary to give larger doses. At the same time, chloramphenicol is begun. Infants 3–6 months of age should receive 75 mg/kg/d and those over 6 months 100 mg/kg/d in 4 divided doses. Serum concentrations should be monitored if possible.

Either chloramphenicol or ampicillin should be discontinued when the identity and antibiotic sensitivity of the infecting organism are known, and therapy is continued with one drug. It is preferable to give the entire course of ampicillin intravenously. Administration of chloramphenicol by mouth is permissible as soon as it is tolerated.

Therapy should be employed for at least 10 days. Longer treatment is reserved for those children who respond slowly or in whom septic complications have occurred. Rarely, antibiotics can be discontinued in a febrile child if the clinical response was rapid and satisfactory, but the source of prolonged or recurrent fevers must always be sought with great care. The most common causes for recurrence of fever or persistence of fever beyond 6 days are the following: phlebitis, hospital-acquired viral or bacterial superinfection, metastatic disease requiring drainage (eg, subdural empyema, septic pericarditis, arthritis), drug fever, and subdural effusions.

Repeated lumbar taps are usually not necessary in *H influenzae* meningitis. They should be obtained in the following circumstances: unsatisfactory or questionable clinical response, seizure occurring after several days of therapy, and prolonged (7 days) or recurrent fever. Routine lumbar tap at the end of therapy is not recommended. (See Chapter 23 for additional information.)

Supportive therapy with intravenous fluids, oxygen, and tube feeding should be given as required.

B. Acute Epiglottitis: See Chapter 14.

C. Septic Arthritis: Ampicillin is given in a dosage of 200–300 mg/kg/d intravenously in 6 divided doses until there is marked improvement (usually 4–7 days). This may be followed by oral amoxicillin, 75–100 mg/kg/d in 4 divided doses every 6 hours, administered under careful supervision to complete a 2-week course. Chloramphenicol should be used for ampicillin-resistant organisms. Drainage of infected joint fluid is an essential part of treatment. In joints other than the hip, this can often be accomplished by one or more needle aspirations. In hip infections—and in arthritis of other joints where treatment is delayed or clinical response is slow—open surgical drainage is advised. Local instillation of antibiotics is not necessary and may be injurious.

The joint should be immobilized. Give antipyretics and analgesics as required and maintain adequate hydration.

D. Cellulitis and Orbital Cellulitis: Give ampicillin or chloramphenicol parenterally for about 1 week, followed by oral treatment as for septic arthritis, and supportive and symptomatic treatment as required. There is usually marked improvement after 72 hours of treatment. Antibiotics should be given for 10–14 days.

E. Pneumonia: Give ampicillin (200–300 mg/kg/d intravenously in 6 divided doses) or chloramphenicol as well as oxygen, intravenous fluids, and other supportive care as required. Treat for 3 weeks. Empyema should be treated by placement of one or more chest tubes into the pleural space. When possible, a chest tube should be removed after 4 or 5 days.

Prognosis

The case fatality rate for *H influenzae* meningitis is 5–10%. Young infants have the highest mortality rate. Neurologic sequelae should be watched for but are appreciably reduced with prompt antibiotic treatment.

The case fatality rate in acute epiglottitis is 2–

5%; deaths are associated with bacteremia and the rapid development of airway obstruction.

The prognosis for the other diseases requiring hospitalization is good with the institution of early and adequate antibiotic therapy.

Asman BI et al: *Haemophilus influenzae* type b pneumonia in 43 children. *J Pediatr* 1978;**93:**389.

Committee on Infectious Diseases, American Academy of Pediatrics: Revision of recommendations for use of rifampin prophylaxis of contacts of patients with *Haemophilus influenzae* infection. *Pediatrics* 1984;**74:**301.

Delage G et al: *Haemophilus influenzae* type b infections: Recurrent disease due to ampicillin-resistant strains. *J Pediatr* 1977;**90:**319.

Feigin RD et al: Prospective evaluation of treatment of *Haemophilus influenzae* meningitis. *J Pediatr* 1976;**88:**542.

Gellady AM, Shulman ST: Periorbital and orbital cellulitis in children. *Pediatrics* 1978;**61:**272.

Ginsburg CM et al: *Haemophilus influenzae* type b disease: Incidence in a day-care center. *JAMA* 1977;**238:**604.

Granoff DM: *Haemophilus influenzae* type b and epiglottitis. *J Pediatr* 1976;**88:**1068.

Jacobs NM, Harris VJ: Acute *Haemophilus* pneumonia in childhood. *Am J Dis Child* 1979;**133:**603.

Lindberg J et al: Long-term outcome of *Haemophilus influenzae* meningitis related to antibiotic treatment. *Pediatrics* 1977; **60:**1.

Molteni RA: Epiglottitis. Incidence of extraepiglottic infection: Report of 72 cases and review of the literature. *Pediatrics* 1976;**58:**526.

Peltola H et al: Prevention of *Haemophilus influenzae* type b bacteremic infections with the capsular polysaccharide vaccine. *N Engl J Med* 1984;**310:**1561.

Rotbart HA, Glode MP: *Haemophilus influenzae* type b septic arthritis in children: Report of 23 cases. *Pediatrics* 1985; **75:**254.

Smith AL: Antibiotics and invasive *Haemophilus influenzae:* Current concepts. *N Engl J Med* 1976;**294:**1329.

Todd JK, Bruhn FW: Severe *Haemophilus influenzae* infections: Spectrum of disease. *Am J Dis Child* 1975;**129:**607.

Uchiyame N et al: Meningitis due to *Haemophilus influenzae* type b resistant to ampicillin and chloramphenicol. *J Pediatr* 1980;**97:**421.

Ward J, Smith AL: *Haemophilus influenzae* bacteremia in children with sickle cell disease. *J Pediatr* 1976;**88:**261.

Ward JI et al: *Haemophilus influenzae* meningitis: A national study of secondary spread in household contacts. *N Engl J Med* 1979;**301:**122.

PERTUSSIS (Whooping Cough)

Essentials of Diagnosis

- Prodromal catarrhal stage (1–3 weeks) characterized by mild cough, coryza, and fever.
- Persistent staccato, paroxysmal cough ending with a high-pitched inspiratory "whoop."
- Leukocytosis with absolute lymphocytosis.
- Diagnosis confirmed by fluorescent stain or culture of nasopharyngeal secretions.

General Considerations

Pertussis is an acute, highly communicable infection of the respiratory tract caused by *Bordetella pertussis* and characterized by severe bronchitis. Children usually acquire the disease from symptomatic family contacts. Adults who have mild respiratory illness not recognized as pertussis frequently are the source of infection. Asymptomatic carriage of *B pertussis* occurs rarely. Infectivity is greatest during the catarrhal and early paroxysmal cough stage (for about 4 weeks after onset).

The disease is most common and most severe in early infancy. In the USA, 2400 cases were reported in 1983. Of the affected infants, 73% were hospitalized, and 0.7% died.

Active immunity follows pertussis but is transient. Reinfections occur years to decades later but are apt to be mild.

Bordetella parapertussis causes a similar syndrome and is reported frequently in central Europe.

Clinical Findings

A. Symptoms and Signs: In adults, older children, and partially immunized individuals, symptoms may consist only of low-grade fever and irritating cough lasting 1–2 weeks. In the younger unimmunized child, symptoms of pertussis last about 8 weeks. The onset is insidious, with catarrhal upper respiratory tract symptoms (rhinitis, sneezing, and an irritating cough). Slight fever may be present; high fever suggests complications or another cause of respiratory tract infection. After about 2 weeks, cough becomes paroxysmal, characterized by 10–30 forceful coughs ending with a loud inspiration (the "whoop"). Vomiting commonly follows a paroxysm. Coughing is accompanied by cyanosis, sweating, prostration, and exhaustion. This stage lasts for 2–4 weeks, with gradual improvement. Cough suggestive of chronic bronchitis lasts for another 2–3 weeks. Paroxysmal coughing may continue for some months in the absence of any active infection and may worsen with intercurrent viral respiratory infection.

B. Laboratory Findings: White blood cell counts of 20,000–30,000/μL with 70–80% lymphocytes appear near the end of the catarrhal stage. The blood picture may resemble lymphocytic leukemia or leukemoid reactions. Identification of *B pertussis* by fluorescent antibody technique or culture from nasopharyngeal swabs proves the diagnosis. Cough plates are inferior to nasopharyngeal swabs. The organism may be found in the respiratory tract in diminishing numbers beginning in the catarrhal stage and ending about 2 weeks after the beginning of the paroxysmal stage. After 4–5 weeks of symptoms, cultures and fluorescent antibody tests are almost always negative. Fresh Bordet-Gengou agar or a charcoal agar should be inoculated at the bedside unless the specimen can be transported rapidly to the laboratory. Serum agglutinins appear late in the infection and are of little value in diagnosis. The chest x-ray reveals thickened bronchi and sometimes shows a "shaggy" heart border, indicating bronchopneumonia and patchy atelectasis.

Differential Diagnosis

The differential diagnosis of pertussis includes bacterial pneumonia, tuberculosis, chlamydial pneumonia, and viral pneumonia. Cystic fibrosis and foreign body aspiration may be considerations.

Adenoviruses and respiratory syncytial virus have been reported in association with the pertussis syndrome. Viral infection by itself can probably produce the pertussis syndrome, but more often the presence of a virus in the respiratory tract indicates mixed infection with *B pertussis*.

Complications

Bronchopneumonia due to superinfection is the most common serious complication. It is characterized by abrupt clinical deterioration during the paroxysmal stage, accompanied by high fever and sometimes a striking leukemoid reaction with a shift to predominantly polymorphonuclear leukocytes. Atelectasis is a second common pulmonary complication. Atelectasis may be patchy or extensive and may shift rapidly to involve different areas of lung. Intercurrent viral respiratory infection is also a common complication and may provoke worsening paroxysmal cough. Otitis media is common. Residual chronic bronchiectasis is infrequent despite the severity of the illness. Apnea and sudden death may occur during a particularly severe paroxysm. Convulsions are seen as part of a diffuse encephalopathy of uncertain cause. It is unclear whether anoxic brain damage, cerebral hemorrhage, or pertussis neurotoxins are to blame, but anoxia is most likely the cause. Epistaxis and subconjunctival hemorrhages are common.

Prevention

Active immunization (see Chapter 5) with pertussis vaccine in combination with diphtheria and tetanus toxoids (DTP) should be given in early infancy. Chemoprophylaxis with erythromycin should be given to exposed family and hospital contacts, particularly those under age 2 years, for 10 days. Exposed children under age 4 years also should receive a booster injection of pertussis vaccine. Hospitalized children with pertussis should be isolated because of the great risk of transmission to patients and staff. Several large hospital outbreaks have been reported in the last decade.

Treatment

A. Specific Measures: Antibiotics have no effect on the clinical course of pertussis when administered in the paroxysmal stage of the disease. Erythromycin promptly terminates respiratory tract carriage of *B pertussis* but does not affect the course of the disease. Patients should be treated with erythromycin, 35–50 mg/kg/24 h in 4 divided doses for a period of 10–14 days. Although ampicillin is known to be effective against *B pertussis* in vitro, it is ineffective in vivo. This discrepancy has been explained by its poor penetration of respiratory tract secretions.

In controlled studies, pertussis immune globulin has been shown to be of no benefit in the treatment of pertussis and is therefore no longer recommended.

B. General Measures: Nutritional support during the paroxysmal phase is very important. Frequent small feedings or parenteral fluid supplementation may be needed. Minimizing stimuli that trigger paroxysms is probably the best way of controlling cough. In general, cough suppressants are of little benefit.

C. Treatment of Complications: Respiratory insufficiency due to pneumonia or other pulmonary complications should be treated with oxygen and assisted ventilation if necessary. Control convulsions by means of oxygen and anticonvulsants. Bacterial pneumonia or otitis media may require additional antibiotics.

Prognosis

The prognosis for patients with pertussis has improved in recent years because of adequate nursing care, treatment of complications, nutrition, and modern intensive care. However, the disease is still very serious in infants under 1 year of age; most deaths occur in this age group. Children with encephalopathy have a poor prognosis.

Altemeier WA III, Ayoub EM: Erythromycin prophylaxis for pertussis. *Pediatrics* 1977;**59:**623.

Geller RJ: The pertussis syndrome: A persistent problem. *Pediatr Infect Dis* 1984;**3:**182.

Linnemann CC Jr, Perry EB: *Bordetella parapertussis:* Recent experience and a review of the literature. *Am J Dis Child* 1977;**131:**560.

Linnemann CC Jr et al: Use of pertussis vaccine in an epidemic involving hospital staff. *Lancet* 1975;**2:**540.

Nelson JD: The changing epidemiology of pertussis in young infants. *Am J Dis Child* 1978;**132:**371.

Olson LC: Pertussis. *Medicine* 1975;**54:**427.

Pittman M: The concept of pertussis as a toxin-mediated disease. *Pediatr Infect Dis* 1984;**3:**467.

LISTERIOSIS

Essentials of Diagnosis

Early-onset neonatal disease:

- Signs of sepsis a few hours after birth in an infant born with fetal distress; hepatosplenomegaly. Maternal fever.

Late-onset neonatal disease:

- Meningitis, sometimes with monocytes in the cerebrospinal fluid and peripheral blood. Onset at 9–30 days of age.

General Considerations

Listeria monocytogenes is a gram-positive, nonspore-forming aerobic rod distributed widely in the animal kingdom and in food, dust, and soil. It causes systemic infections in newborn infants and immunosuppressed older children. In pregnant women, infection is relatively mild, with fever, aches, and chills, but it is accompanied by bacteremia and sometimes results in intrauterine or perinatal infection with grave consequences for the fetus or newborn. Disease due to *Listeria* is uncommon even though the organism is widespread and occurs as normal fecal flora in at least 1% of the population. Persons in contact with animals seem to be at particular risk. Several recent food-borne outbreaks have been described, traced in one instance to contaminated cabbage in coleslaw.

As with group B streptococcal infections, *Listeria* infections in the newborn can be divided into early and late forms. Early infections are more common and are frequently severe and generalized, sometimes leading to granulomatosis infantiseptica. Late infections are often characterized by meningitis.

Clinical Findings

A. Symptoms and Signs: In the early neonatal form, symptoms usually appear on the first day of life and always by the third day. Infants are frequently premature and have signs of fetal distress. Respiratory distress, diarrhea, and fever occur. On examination, hepatosplenomegaly and rash are found. A history of maternal fever is common. Meningitis may accompany the septic course.

The late neonatal form usually occurs after 9 days of age and can occur as late as 5 weeks. Meningitis is common, characterized by irritability, fever, and poor feeding.

Listeria infections occur rarely in older children, usually in those with animal contact or those who are immunosuppressed. Signs and symptoms are those of meningitis, usually with insidious onset.

B. Laboratory Findings: In all patients except those receiving white cell depressant drugs, the white blood cell count is elevated, with 10–20% monocytes. When meningitis is found, the characteristic cell count is high (> 500/μL) with a predominance of polymorphonuclear leukocytes in 70%, but monocytes are also present in up to 30%. The chief pathologic feature in severe neonatal sepsis is miliary granulomatosis with microabscesses in liver, spleen, central nervous system, lung, and bowel.

In meningitis, gram-stained smears of cerebrospinal fluid often show short gram-positive rods. In early-onset disease, gram-stained smears of the external ear may show *Listeria.*

Cultures are frequently positive from multiple sites, including blood in the infant and the mother. The organisms form small, weakly hemolytic colonies on blood agar and may be mistaken for streptococci.

Differential Diagnosis

Early-onset neonatal disease resembles hemolytic disease of the newborn, group B streptococcal sepsis or severe cytomegalovirus infection, rubella, or toxoplasmosis. Late-onset disease must be differentiated from meningitis due to echovirus and coxsackievirus, group B streptococci, and gram-negative enteric bacteria.

Treatment

Ampicillin in full antimeningitis doses, 150–300 mg/kg/d every 6 hours intravenously, is the drug of choice in most cases, although gentamicin, 7.5 mg/kg/d every 8 hours intravenously, may be added in severe illnesses, since it has been shown to be synergistic in vitro. If ampicillin cannot be used, erythromycin is also effective (40 mg/kg/d every 6 hours intravenously). Treatment of severe disease should continue for at least 2 weeks.

Prognosis

In a recent outbreak of early-onset neonatal disease, the mortality rate was 27% despite aggressive and appropriate management. Meningitis in older infants has quite a good prognosis. In immunosuppressed children, prognosis depends to a great extent on that of the underlying illness.

Ahlfors CE et al: Neonatal listeriosis. *Am J Dis Child* 1977;**131**:405.

Albritton WL, Wiggins GL, Feeley JC: Neonatal listeriosis: Distribution of serotypes in relation to age at onset of disease. *J Pediatr* 1976;**88**:481.

Perinatal listeriosis. (Editorial.) *Lancet* 1980;**1**:911.

Schlech WF et al: Epidemic listeriosis: Evidence for transmission by food. *N Engl J Med* 1983;**308**:203.

Visintine AM, Oleske JM, Nahmias AJ: *Listeria monocytogenes:* Infection in infants and children. *Am J Dis Child* 1977;**131**:393.

TUBERCULOSIS

Essentials of Diagnosis

- All types: Positive tuberculin test in patient or members of household, suspicious chest x-ray, history of contact, and demonstration of organism by stain and culture.
- Pulmonary: Fatigue, irritability, and undernutrition, with or without fever and cough.
- Glandular: Chronic cervical adenitis.
- Miliary: Classic "snowstorm" appearance of chest x-ray; choroidal tubercles.
- Meningitis: Fever and manifestations of meningeal irritation and increased intracranial pressure. Characteristic cerebrospinal fluid.

General Considerations

Tuberculosis is a granulomatous disease caused by *Mycobacterium tuberculosis.* It remains a leading cause of death throughout the world. Children under 3 years of age are most susceptible, and lymphohematogenous dissemination through the lungs and spread to extrapulmonary sites, including the brain and meninges, eyes, bones and joints, lymph nodes, kidneys, intestines, larynx, and skin, are more likely to occur in infants. Increased susceptibility occurs again in adolescence, particularly in girls within 2 years of menarche. Prolonged household contact with an active adult case usually leads to infection of infants and children. Tuberculosis is a particularly serious problem among crowded urban populations and among refugees from Southeast Asia. The case rate and death rate in nonwhite children are 2–5 times those in white children. The primary complex in infancy and childhood consists of a small parenchymal lesion in any area of the lung with caseation of regional nodes and calcification. Postprimary tuberculosis in adolescents and adults occurs in the apexes of the lungs and is likely to cause chronic, progressive cavitary pulmonary disease with less tendency for hematogenous dissemination.

Clinical Findings

A. Symptoms and Signs:

1. Pulmonary—See Chapter 14.

2. Miliary—Diagnosis is made on the basis of a classic snowstorm appearance of lung fields on x-ray, although early in the course of disseminated tuberculosis, the chest x-ray may show no or only subtle abnormalities. The majority also have a fresh primary complex and pleural effusion. Choroidal tubercles are sometimes seen on funduscopic examination. Other lesions may be present and produce osteomyelitis, arthritis, meningitis, tuberculomas of the brain, enteritis, or infection of the kidneys and liver.

3. Meningitis—Symptoms include fever, vomiting, headache, lethargy, and irritability, with signs of meningeal irritation and increased intracranial pressure, including cranial nerve palsies, convulsions, and coma. Choroidal tubercles are pathognomonic when associated with these signs and symptoms. Otorrhea or acute otitis media may be seen.

4. Glandular—The primary complex may be associated with a skin lesion drained by regional nodes or chronic cervical node enlargement and infection of the tonsils. Involved nodes may become fixed to the overlying skin and suppurative, and they may drain.

B. Laboratory Findings: The Mantoux text (0.1 mL of intermediate strength PPD, 0.0001 mg [5 TU] or 0.0002 mg [10 TU] inoculated intradermally) is read as positive at 48–72 hours if there is over 10 mm of induration. False-negative results are seen in malnourished patients or those with overwhelming disseminated disease. Temporary suppression of tuberculin reactivity may also be seen with viral infections (measles, influenza, varicella, mumps, etc), after live virus immunization, and when corticosteroids or other immunosuppressive drugs are present. For this reason, every Mantoux test should be accompanied by intradermal injection of a control antigen (such as *Candida albicans* or SK-SD) that is uniformly positive in all persons with normal immune response. When tuberculosis is suspected and the child is anergic, family or household members should also be tested immediately.

The erythrocyte sedimentation rate is usually elevated. Cultures of pooled early morning gastric aspirates from 3 successive days are often valuable in children in whom tuberculosis is suspected. The cerebrospinal fluid in tuberculous meningitis shows slight to moderate pleocytosis (50–300 white blood cells), decreased or decreasing glucose, and increased protein. For staining and culture, centrifuged sediment should be used.

The direct detection of mycobacteria in body fluids or discharges is now best done by staining specimens with auramine O and examining them with blue-light fluorescence microscopy; this is superior to the Ziehl-Neelsen method.

C. X-Ray Findings: Chest x-ray should be obtained in all children with suspicion of tuberculosis at any site or with a positive skin test. Positive findings range from a barely detectable primary complex to extensive pneumonia and pleural effusion.

Differential Diagnosis

Pulmonary tuberculosis must be differentiated from sarcoidosis; fungal, parasitic, mycoplasmal, and bacterial pneumonias; lung abscess; foreign body aspiration; lipoid pneumonia; and mediastinal cancer. Cervical lymphadenitis is most apt to be due to streptococcal or staphylococcal infections. Cat-scratch fever and infection with atypical mycobacteria may need to be distinguished from tuberculosis also. Viral meningoencephalitis, head trauma (battered child), lead poisoning, brain abscess, acute bacterial meningitis, brain tumor, and disseminated fungal infections must be excluded in tuberculous meningitis. The skin test in the patient or family contacts is frequently valuable in differentiation of these conditions from tuberculosis.

Prevention

A. BCG Vaccine: BCG vaccination confers definite although not absolute protection. It is used routinely for infants and children in countries with a high prevalence of tuberculosis. In the USA, it is advised for tuberculin-negative children known to be exposed to adults with active or recently arrested disease, particularly those unlikely to take isoniazid on a regular basis or those whose contact with infected adults is difficult to control. It is advisable to give BCG to newborn infants of tuberculous mothers. BCG is administered intracutaneously over the deltoid or triceps muscle. The dosage is 0.05 mL for newborns and 0.1 mL for older infants and children. The child should not remain in contact with the infected member of the family for at least 2 months afterward or until the patient is receiving adequate therapy. A Mantoux test should be done at the end of this time and immunization repeated if it is negative. BCG should never be given to a tuberculin-positive individual; to one with definite or suspected agammaglobulinemia, thymic alymphoplasia, or dysplasia; or to one with skin infection or burns or a recent smallpox vaccination.

B. Isoniazid (INH) Chemoprophylaxis: Daily administration of isoniazid in therapeutic doses is advised for children who cannot avoid intimate household contact with adolescents or adults with active disease. The dose of isoniazid is 10 mg/kg orally, not to exceed 300 mg daily. Isoniazid is continued throughout the period of exposure and for 3 months after the contact has been broken. At the end of this time, a Mantoux test should be done, and therapy should be continued for 1 year if it is positive. BCG is not recommended during the period of isoniazid chemoprophylaxis.

C. Other Measures: The source contact (index case) should be identified, isolated, and treated to prevent other secondary cases. Exposed tuberculin-negative children should be skin tested every 2 months for 6 months after contact has been terminated. Routine tuberculin skin testing is advised at 12 months of age, before live viral vaccines are administered. Routine testing of school children is recommended only in certain populations.

Treatment

A. Specific Measures: Most patients in the USA are hospitalized at the beginning of treatment but receive most of the prolonged drug course as outpatients. Treatment failure is usually due to the inability of patients (and parents) to cooperate in the long program of therapy.

At the present time in the USA, it is recommended that all skin reactors without overt disease in the pediatric age range be treated for 1 year with isoniazid alone (10 mg/kg/d, up to 300 mg, as a single oral dose). In children with overt tuberculosis, there is presently controversy regarding the length and intensity of treatment. While prolonged courses (18–24 months) are of proved efficacy, it is very likely that shorter courses (9 months) will prove equally safe and better tolerated. At present, a 1-year course of isoniazid (10–20 mg/kg/d in a single daily dose) plus rifampin (15–20 mg/kg/d in a single daily dose) is recommended for treatment of uncomplicated infections. Streptomycin should be added for 2–4 months in cases of meningitis or other severe disease. If aminosalicylic acid (PAS) or ethambutol is used instead of either isoniazid or rifampin, consideration should be given to longer therapeutic courses.

1. Isoniazid (INH)—The major toxicity in adults is hepatic. This occasionally occurs in adolescents. It begins 6–12 weeks after onset of therapy. Liver function should be screened before initiation. Pyridoxine, 5–10 mg/100 mg of isoniazid, has been recommended for prevention of peripheral neuropathy, but this is not necessary in patients under 11 years of age.

2. Rifampin—Rifampin should never be used alone for treatment of tuberculosis, because resistance is likely to develop. It is an extremely effective drug as long as bacteria remain sensitive. Hepatic toxicity is rare but occurs without prior hepatic disease. It occurs early (within the first 2 months), if at all, and AST (SGOT) levels should be followed weekly for the first month and then monthly. Rifampin also induces hypersensitivity reactions. Severe hypersensitivity (leukopenia or thrombocytopenia) can be avoided by daily doses. The urine turns red in most patients receiving rifampin.

3. Aminosalicylic acid (PAS)—Since children have a better tolerance for PAS than adults have, there is still a role for PAS as a primary drug in the treatment of tuberculosis in children. The dosage is 200–300 mg/kg/d orally in 2 or 3 divided doses. Toxic reactions are gastrointestinal or allergic. PAS may interfere with the absorption of rifampin.

4. Ethambutol (Myambutol)—Ethambutol is an effective substitute for PAS in older children who can be reliably tested for visual acuity and color vision. The dosage is 15 mg/kg/d orally. Retrobulbar neuritis is dose-related and occurs in about 3% of cases, probably less with the recommended dose. Visual testing should be performed at 2-month intervals during therapy.

5. Streptomycin or kanamycin—In serious or progressive forms, including meningeal, miliary, renal, osseous, cavitary, and chronic pulmonary tuberculosis, give streptomycin, 20–30 mg/kg/d intramuscularly in 1 or 2 doses for 2–4 months in addition to 2 oral drugs. In case of streptomycin resistance, kanamycin, 15 mg/kg/d intramuscularly, is given for 1–3 months. Periodic audiometric tests are advisable when either drug is used.

6. Re-treatment—Re-treating drug-resistant tuberculosis requires 3 drugs which the patient has never had before and to which the organisms are fully susceptible. In vitro determination of drug sensitivities is mandatory.

B. General Measures:

1. Corticosteroids—These drugs may be used for suppressing inflammatory reactions in meningeal, pleural, and pericardial tuberculosis and for the relief of bronchial obstruction due to hilar adenopathy. Prednisone is given orally, 1 mg/kg/d for 6–8 weeks, with gradual withdrawal at the end of that time.

2. Bed rest—Rest in bed is only indicated while the child feels ill. Isolation is necessary only for children with draining lesions or renal disease and those with chronic pulmonary tuberculosis. Most children with tuberculosis are noninfectious and can attend school while being treated.

Prognosis

If bacteria are sensitive and treatment is completed, most patients make lasting recovery. Re-treatment is more difficult and less successful. With antituberculosis chemotherapy (especially isoniazid), there should now be nearly 100% recovery in miliary tuberculosis. Without treatment, the mortality rate in both miliary tuberculosis and tuberculous meningitis is almost 100%. In the latter form, about two-thirds of treated patients survive. There may be a high incidence of neurologic abnormalities among survivors if treatment is started late.

BCG vaccination after the Madras study. (Editorial.) *Lancet* 1981;**1**:309.

Brasfield DM, Goodloe TB, Tiller RE: Isoniazid hepatotoxicity in childhood. *Pediatrics* 1976;**58**:291.

Dutt AK, Stead WW: Present chemotherapy for tuberculosis. *J Inject Dis* 1982;**146:**698.

Greenberg HB, Trachtman L, Thompson DH: Finding recent tuberculous infection in New Orleans: Results of tuberculin skin tests on New Orleans children from the inner city and contact investigation program. *JAMA* 1976;**235:**931.

Idriss ZH, Sinno AA, Kronfol NM: Tuberculous meningitis in childhood: Forty-three cases. *Am J Dis Child* 1976; **130:**364.

Kendig EL: Evolution of short-course antimicrobial treatment of tuberculosis in children, 1951–1984. *Pediatrics* 1985; **75:**684.

Lincoln EM, Sewell EM: Tuberculosis. Chap 34, p 427, in: *Infectious Diseases of Children,* 7th ed. Krugman S, Katz SL (editors), Mosby, 1981.

Smith MHD, Marquis JR: Tuberculosis and other mycobacterial infections. Pages 1016–1060 in: *Textbook of Pediatric Infectious Diseases.* Feigin RD, Cherry JD (editors). Saunders, 1981.

INFECTIONS WITH ATYPICAL MYCOBACTERIA

Essentials of Diagnosis

- Chronic unilateral cervical lymphadenitis.
- Granulomas of the skin.
- Chronic bone lesion with draining sinus (chronic osteomyelitis).
- Reaction to PPD-S (standard) of 5–8 mm, negative chest x-ray, and negative history of contact with tuberculosis.
- Positive skin reaction to a specific atypical antigen.
- Diagnosis by positive acid-fast stain or culture.

General Considerations

Various species of acid-fast mycobacteria other than *Mycobacterium tuberculosis* may cause subclinical infections and, occasionally, clinical disease closely simulating tuberculosis. Strain cross-reactivity with *M tuberculosis* can be demonstrated by simultaneous skin testing (Mantoux) with PPD-S (standard) and PPD prepared from one of the atypical antigens. The larger skin reaction suggests infection with the homologous strain.

The Runyon classification of mycobacteria includes the following:

Group 1—Photochromogens (PPD-Y): Yellow color develops upon exposure to light in previously white colony grown 2–4 weeks in the dark. Group 1 includes *Mycobacterium kansasii* and *Mycobacterium marinum.*

Group II—Scotochromogens (PPD-G): Colonies are definitely yellow-orange after incubation in the dark. Organisms may be found in small numbers in the normal flora of some human saliva and gastric contents. Subclinical infection is widespread in the USA, but clinical disease appears rarely. Group II includes *Mycobacterium scrofulaceum.*

Group III—Nonphotochromogens (PPD-B): "Battey-avian-swine group" grows as small white colonies after incubation in the dark, with no significant development of pigment upon exposure to light. Infection with *Mycobacterium intracellulare* ("Battey bacillus") is prevalent on the east coast of the USA, particularly the Southeast. Infection with avian strains is prevalent in Great Britain.

Group IV—"Rapid growers": *Mycobacterium fortuitum* and *Mycobacterium chelonei* are the recognized pathogens. Within 1 week after inoculation, they form colonies closely resembling *M tuberculosis* morphologically.

Clinical Findings

A. Symptoms and Signs:

1. Lymphadenitis—In children, the commonest form of infection due to mycobacteria other than tuberculosis is cervical lymphadenitis. *M scrofulaceum* or *M intracellulare* is almost always the cause. A submandibular node swells slowly and is firm and usually nontender. Over time, the node suppurates and may drain chronically. Nodes in other areas of the head and neck and elsewhere are sometimes involved.

2. Pulmonary disease—In the western USA, this is usually due to *M kansasii;* in the eastern USA, it may be due to *M intracellulare.* In other countries, disease is usually caused by *M intracellulare* or *Mycobacterium avium.* In adults, there is usually underlying chronic pulmonary disease, but in children, this is often not the case. Immunologic deficiency may be present. Presentation is clinically indistinguishable from that of tuberculosis.

3. Swimming pool granuloma—This is due to *M marinum.* A solitary chronic granulomatous lesion, frequently on the elbow, develops after minor trauma in infected swimming pools.

4. Chronic osteomyelitis—Osteomyelitis is caused by *M kansasii, M scrofulaceum,* or "rapid growers." Findings include swelling and pain over a distal extremity, radiolucent defects in bone, fever, and clinical and x-ray evidence of bronchopneumonia. Such cases are rare.

5. Meningitis—Disease is due to *M kansasii* and may be indistinguishable from tuberculous meningitis.

6. Disseminated infection—Rarely, a clinical syndrome resembling that of acute hematopoietic cancer has been reported in association with isolation of *M kansasii,* scotochromogens, *M fortuitum,* or *M intracellulare* from bone marrow, lymph nodes, or liver. Chest x-rays are usually normal.

B. Laboratory Findings: In most cases, there is a small reaction (< 10 mm) when Mantoux testing is done with PPD-S. The chest x-ray is negative, and there is no history of contact with tuberculosis. Biopsy of the lesion shows a granulomatous reaction with caseation. Acid-fast bacilli are demonstrated in stained biopsy material. Tuberculosis may be suspected and treatment started with antituberculosis drugs. With these findings, including a Mantoux reaction of less than 10 mm, disease due to one of the atypical mycobacteria should be suspected. Simultaneous tuberculin testing with the infecting atypical antigen (PPD-Y, -G, or -B) will usually give a reaction greater than the reaction to PPD-S.

Definitive diagnosis is made by isolating the causative agent from clinical material on media used for the isolation of *M tuberculosis*.

Differential Diagnosis

See section on differential diagnosis in the discussion of tuberculosis above and in Chapter 14.

Treatment

A. Specific Measures: Treatment should be individualized and based on in vitro drug sensitivity studies. The usual treatment of lymphadenitis is complete surgical excision. This may be followed by several months of isoniazid and rifampin. The review by Schaad et al (1979) favors complete excision without chemotherapy whenever possible. Recent data suggest that isoniazid, rifampin, and streptomycin with or without ethambutol (depending on sensitivity to isoniazid) will result in a favorable response in almost all patients with *M kansaii* infection. Chemotherapeutic treatment of *M intracellulare* is much less satisfactory. Most authors favor surgical excision if possible and treatment with at least 3 drugs to which the organism has been shown to be sensitive. Effective drugs may include ethionamide, capreomycin, and pyrazinamide as well as the more familiar antituberculous agents. *M fortuitum* and *M chelonei* are usually susceptible to amikacin plus erythromycin or doxycycline and may be successfully treated with such combinations. Swimming pool granuloma due to *M marinum* is usually self-limited but may be treated either with drugs or by surgical excision, with good results.

B. General Measures: Isolation of the patient is usually not necessary. General supportive care is indicated for the child with disseminated disease.

Prognosis

The prognosis is good for localized disease, though fatalities occur in immunocompromised children with disseminated disease.

Ahn CH et al: Chemotherapy for pulmonary disease due to *Mycobacterium kansasii:* Efficacies of some individual drugs. *Rev infect Dis* 1981;**3:**1028.

Chang MJ, Barton LL: *Mycobacterium fortuitum* osteomyelitis of the calcaneus secondary to a puncture wound. *J Pediatr* 1974;**85:**517.

Dalovisio JR et al: Clinical usefulness of amikacin and doxycycline in the treatment of infection due to *Mycobacterium fortuitum* and *Mycobacterium chelonei. Rev Infect Dis* 1981;**3:**1068.

Davidson PT et al: Treatment of disease due to *Mycobacterium intracellulare. Rev Infect Dis* 1981;**3:**1052.

Kubala E: Some aspects of disease caused by atypical mycobacteria. *Scand J Respir Dis* 1972;**80(Suppl):**11.

Schaad UB et al: Management of atypical mycobacterial lymphadenitis in childhood: A review based on 380 cases. *J Pediatr* 1979;**95:**356.

Schuit KE, Powell DA: Mycobacterial lymphadenitis in childhood. *Am J Dis Child* 1978;**132:**675.

PSITTACOSIS (Ornithosis)

Essentials of Diagnosis

- Fever, cough, malaise, chills, headache.
- Diffuse rales; no consolidation.
- Long-lasting x-ray findings of bronchopneumonia.
- Isolation of the organism or rising titer of complement-fixing antibodies.
- Exposure to infected birds.

General Considerations

Psittacosis is caused by *Chlamydia psittaci*. When the agent is transmitted to humans from psittacine birds (parrots, parakeets, cockatoos, and budgerigars), the disease is often called psittacosis or parrot fever. However, other avian genera (pigeons, turkeys) are common sources of infection in the USA, and the general term ornithosis is often used. The agent is an obligatory intracellular parasite. Human-to-human spread occurs rarely. The incubation period is 7–15 days. The bird from whom the disease was contracted may not be clinically ill.

Clinical Findings

A. Symptoms and Signs: The disease is extremely variable but tends to be mild in children. The onset is rapid or insidious, with fever, chills, headache, backache, malaise, myalgia, and dry cough. Signs include those of pneumonitis, alteration of percussion note and breath sounds, and rales. Pulmonary findings may be absent early. Splenomegaly, epistaxis, prostration, and meningismus are occasionally seen. Delirium, constipation or diarrhea, and abdominal distress may occur. Dyspnea and cyanosis may occur later.

B. Laboratory Findings: The white blood cell count is normal or decreased, often with a shift to the left. Proteinuria is frequently present. The ornithosis agent is present in the blood and sputum during the first 2 weeks of illness and can be isolated by inoculation of clinical specimens into mice or embryonated hens' eggs. Complement-fixing antibodies appear during or after the second week. The rise in titer may be minimized or delayed by early chemotherapy.

C. X-Ray Findings: The x-ray findings in psittacosis are those of central pneumonia, which later becomes widespread or migratory. Psittacosis is indistinguishable from viral pneumonias by x-ray. Signs of pneumonitis may appear by x-ray in the absence of clinical suspicion of pulmonary involvement.

Differential Diagnosis

This disease can be differentiated from acute viral pneumonias only by the history of contact with potentially infected birds. In severe or prolonged cases with extrapulmonary involvement, the differential diagnosis includes a wide spectrum of diseases such as typhoid fever, brucellosis, rheumatic fever, etc.

Complications

Complications include myocarditis, endocarditis, hepatitis, pancreatitis, and secondary bacterial pneumonia.

Treatment

Give tetracyclines in full doses for 14 days. Supportive oxygen may be needed. The patient should be kept in isolation.

Byrom NP, Wells J, Mair IJ: Fulminant psittacosis. *Lancet* 1979;**1**:353.

Durfee PT: Psittacosis in humans in the United States, 1974. *J Infect Dis* 1975;**132**:604.

CAT-SCRATCH DISEASE

Essentials of Diagnosis

- History of a cat scratch or cat contact.
- Primary lesion (papule, pustule, conjunctivitis) at site of inoculation.
- Acute or subacute regional lymphadenopathy.
- Positive cat-scratch skin test.
- Aspiration of sterile pus from a node.
- Laboratory studies excluding other causes.
- Biopsy of node showing histopathologic findings consistent with cat-scratch disease.

General Considerations

Cat-scratch disease is a benign, self-limiting form of lymphadenitis. Patients often report a cat scratch (67%) or contact with a cat or kitten (90%). The cat almost invariably is healthy. Dogs, monkeys, thorns, codfish bones, and wooden splinters also have been implicated. The clinical picture is that of a regional lymphadenitis associated with an erythematous papular skin lesion without intervening lymphangitis. The disease occurs worldwide and is more common in the fall and winter. The most common systemic complication is encephalitis.

An infectious agent has long been presumed to be responsible, but only recently has convincing evidence been found. The agent appears to be a small bacterium.

Clinical Findings

A. Symptoms and Signs: About 50% of patients develop a primary lesion at the site of inoculation. The lesion usually is a papule or pustule and is located most often on the arm or hand (50%), head or leg (30%), or trunk or neck (10%). The lesion may be conjunctival (10%). Regional lymphadenopathy appears 10–30 days later and may be accompanied by mild malaise, lassitude, headache, and fever. Multiple sites are involved in about 10% of cases. Involved nodes may be hard or soft and 1–6 cm in diameter. They are usually tender, and about 25% of them suppurate. The overlying skin may or may not be inflamed. Lymphadenopathy usually resolves in about 2 months, but it may persist for up to 8 months.

Unusual manifestations include nonpruritic maculopapular rash, erythema multiforme or nodosum, purpura, conjunctivitis (Parinaud's oculoglandular fever), parotid swelling, pneumonia, chronic sinus drainage, osteolytic lesions, mesenteric and mediastinal adenitis, peripheral neuritis, hepatosplenomegaly, and encephalitis.

B. Laboratory Findings: For the Hanger-Rose skin test, antigens are prepared from pus aspirated from nodes of infected individuals. Because they are poorly standardized antigens and are not available commercially, we do not encourage their use. The test is performed by the intradermal injection of 0.1 mL of antigen. A positive reaction consists of 5 mm or more of induration or any degree of erythema at the injection site 48–72 hours later. The skin test is positive in about 90% of patients thought to have cat-scratch disease and 5% of normal controls.

Histopathologic examination of involved nodes shows characteristic, but not diagnostic, changes. The lymph node architecture is distorted by multiple areas of central necrosis with acidophilic staining. These areas are surrounded by foci of epithelioid cells and scattered giant cells of the Langhans type. There is usually some elevation in the sedimentation rate. In cases with central nervous system involvement, the cerebrospinal fluid is usually normal but may show a slight pleocytosis and modest elevation of protein. All routine cultures, including anaerobic, fungal, and mycobacterial culture, are negative.

Differential Diagnosis

Cat-scratch disease must be distinguished from pyogenic adenitis, tuberculosis (typical and atypical), tularemia, plague, brucellosis, Hodgkin's disease, lymphoma, rat-bite fever, acquired toxoplasmosis, infectious mononucleosis, lymphogranuloma venereum, and fungal infections.

Treatment

The best therapy is reassurance that the adenopathy is benign and will subside spontaneously within 4–8 weeks in most cases. In cases of suppuration, node aspiration under local anesthesia with an 18- to 19-gauge needle relieves the pain. Excision of the involved node is indicated in cases of chronic adenitis.

Prognosis

The prognosis is good if complications do not occur.

Bradstreet CMP, Dighero MW: Cat-scratch fever skin-test antigen. *Lancet* 1977;**1**:913.

Carithers H: Oculoglandular disease of Parinaud. *Am J Dis Child* 1978;**132**:1195.

Gerber MA et al: The aetiological agent of cat-scratch disease. *Lancet* 1985;**1**:1236.

Margileth AW et al: Cat-scratch disease: Bacteria in skin at the primary inoculation site. *JAMA* 1984;**252:**928.
Wear DJ et al: Cat-scratch disease: A bacterial infection. *Science* 1983;**221:**1403.

SPIROCHETAL INFECTIONS

SYPHILIS

Essentials of Diagnosis

Congenital:

- All types: History of untreated maternal syphilis, a positive serologic test, and a positive darkfield examination.
- Newborn: Hepatosplenomegaly, characteristic x-ray bone changes, anemia, increased nucleated red cells, thrombocytopenia, abnormal spinal fluid, jaundice, edema.
- Young infant (3–12 weeks): Snuffles, maculopapular skin rash, mucocutaneous lesions, pseudoparalysis (in addition to x-ray bone changes).
- Children: Stigmas of early congenital syphilis (saddle nose, Hutchinson's teeth, etc), interstitial keratitis, saber shins, gummas of nose and palate.

Acquired:

- Chancre of genitalia, lip, or anus in child or adolescent. History of sexual contact.

General Considerations

Syphilis is a chronic, generalized infectious disease caused by a slender spirochete, *Treponema pallidum.* In the acquired form, the disease is transmitted by sexual contact. Primary syphilis is characterized by the presence of an indurated chancre. A secondary eruption involving the skin and mucous membranes appears in 4–6 weeks. After a long latency period, late lesions of tertiary syphilis involve the eyes, skin, bones, viscera, central nervous system, and cardiovascular system.

Congenital syphilis results from transplacental infection. Characteristic disease occurs after the fourth month of gestation and may result in stillbirth or manifest illness in the newborn, in early infancy, or later in childhood. First-trimester fetal infection has been found in the products of conception in therapeutic abortions. Syphilis occurring in the newborn and young infant is comparable to secondary disease in the adult but is more severe and life-threatening. Late congenital syphilis (developing in childhood) is comparable to tertiary disease.

Clinical Findings

A. Symptoms and Signs:

1. Congenital syphilis—

a. Newborns—Most newborns with congenital syphilis are well, disease not usually becoming manifest for several weeks. When clinical signs are present, they usually consist of jaundice, anemia with or without thrombocytopenia, increase in nucleated red blood cells, hepatosplenomegaly, and edema. There may be overt signs of meningitis (bulging fontanelle, opisthotonos), but subclinical infection with cerebrospinal fluid abnormalities is more likely. The majority of affected newborns show x-ray changes in the long bones.

b. Young infants (3–12 weeks)—The infant may appear normal for the first few weeks of life only to develop "snuffles," a syphilitic skin eruption, mucocutaneous lesions, and pseudoparalysis of the arms or legs. Shotty lymphadenopathy may sometimes be felt in addition to hepatosplenomegaly. Other signs of disease seen in the newborn may be present. Anemia has been reported as the only presenting manifestation of congenital syphilis in this age group. "Snuffles" (rhinitis) almost always appears and is characterized by a profuse mucopurulent discharge that excoriates the upper lip. A syphilitic rash is common on the palms and soles but may occur anywhere on the body; it consists of bright red, raised maculopapular lesions that gradually fade. Moist lesions occur at mucocutaneous junctions (nose, mouth, anus, genitalia) and lead to fissuring and bleeding.

Syphilis in the young infant may lead to stigmas recognizable in later childhood. Thus, such a child may have rhagades (scars) around the mouth or nose, a "saddle" nose, and a high forehead (secondary to mild hydrocephalus associated with low-grade meningitis and frontal periostitis). The permanent upper central incisors may be peg-shaped with a central notch (Hutchinson's teeth), and the cusps of the sixth-year molars may have a lobulated mulberry appearance.

c. Children—Bilateral interstitial keratitis (at 6–12 years) is characterized by photophobia, increased lacrimation, and vascularization of the cornea associated with exudation. Chorioretinitis and optic atrophy may also be seen. Meningovascular syphilis (at 2–10 years) is usually slowly progressive, with mental retardation, spasticity, abnormal pupil response, speech defects, and abnormal spinal fluid. Deafness sometimes occurs. Thickening of the periosteum of the anterior tibias produces saber shins. A bilateral effusion into the knee joints (Clutton's joints) may occur but is not associated with sequelae. Gummas may develop in the nasal septum, palate, long bones, and subcutaneous tisses.

2. Acquired syphilis—The primary chancre of the genitalia, mouth, or anus may occur as a result of intimate sexual contact. If the chancre is missed, signs of secondary syphilis may be the first manifestation of the disease.

B. Laboratory Findings:

1. Darkfield microscopy—Treponemes can be seen in scrapings from a chancre and from moist lesions.

2. Serologic tests for syphilis (STS)—There are 2 general types of serologic tests for syphilis:

treponemal and nontreponemal. The latter (Venereal Disease Research Laboratory, or VDRL, Hinton, Kolmer, and others) is useful both for screening and for follow-up of known cases. A rapid test (the rapid plasma reagin, or RPR) is useful for screening, but positive sera should be further examined by quantitative nontreponemal and treponemal tests. Treponemal tests, which depended on immobilization of live organisms by antibody (*T pallidum* immobilization, or TPI), have been largely replaced by immunofluorescence tests, the most useful of which is the fluorescent treponemal antibody absorption, or FTA-ABS, test. This test is seldom falsely positive and can be adapted for the measurement of specific IgM antibody as well.

One or 2 weeks after the onset of primary syphilis (chancre), the FTA-ABS test becomes positive. The VDRL or a similar nontreponemal test usually turns positive a few days later. By the time the secondary stage has arrived, virtually all patients show both positive FTA-ABS and positive nontreponemal tests. During latent and tertiary syphilis, the VDRL may become negative, but the FTA-ABS test usually remains positive. The quantitative VDRL or a similar nontreponemal test should be used to follow treated cases (see below).

Positive serologic tests in cord sera may represent passively transferred antibody rather than congenital infection. Such tests must therefore be supplemented by a combination of clinical and laboratory data. Elevated total cord IgM is a helpful but nonspecific finding. A positive IgM-FTA-ABS is considerably more specific: false-positive results may occur in the presence of other infections where rheumatoid factor may be present. Demonstration of characteristic treponemes from a moist lesion (skin, nasal or other mucous membranes) is definitive. Serial measurement of quantitative VDRL is also very useful, since passively transferred antibody in the absence of active infection should decay with a normal half-life of about 18 days.

C. X-Ray Findings: Osteochondritis and periostitis involve the long bones. Occasionally, the phalanges and metatarsals are involved. Periostitis of the skull is seen. Bilateral symmetric osteomyelitis with pathologic fractures of the medial tibial metaphyses (Wimberger's sign) is almost pathognomonic.

Differential Diagnosis

A. Congenital Syphilis:

1. Newborns—Sepsis, congestive heart failure, congenital rubella, toxoplasmosis, disseminated herpes simplex, cytomegalovirus infection, and hemolytic disease of the newborn have to be differentiated. Positive Coombs test and blood group incompatibility distinguish hemolytic disease.

2. Young infants—Pseudoparalysis (a flaccid paralysis) occurs in poliomyelitis, and signs of scurvy do not appear until the latter half of the first year of life. Injury to the brachial plexus, acute osteomyelitis, and septic arthritis must be differentiated from pseudoparalysis. "Snuffles" (coryza due to viral infection) will often respond to symptomatic treatment. Rash (ammoniacal diaper rash) and scabies may be confused with a syphilitic eruption.

3. Children—Interstitial keratitis and bone lesions of tuberculosis are distinguished by positive tuberculin reaction and chest x-ray. Arthritis associated with syphilis is unaccompanied by systemic signs, and joints are not tender. Mental retardation, spasticity, and hyperactivity are shown to be of syphilitic origin by strongly positive serologic tests.

B. Acquired Syphilis: Herpes genitalis, traumatic lesions, and other venereal diseases must be differentiated.

Prevention

A serologic test for syphilis should be performed at the initiation of prenatal care and repeated once during pregnancy. Adequate treatment of mothers with secondary syphilis before the last month of pregnancy will reduce the incidence of congenital syphilis from 90% to less than 2%. The serology of the father and siblings should also be checked.

Treatment

A. Specific Measures: Penicillin is the drug of choice against *T pallidum*. If the patient is allergic to penicillin, erythromycin or one of the tetracyclines may be used.

1. Congenital syphilis—Prompt treatment of the infant with penicillin is indicated if there is clinical or x-ray evidence of disease or the cord blood serology is positive and the mother has not been adequately treated. With equivocal findings, the infant may be given protective treatment or followed at monthly intervals with quantitative serologic tests and physical examinations. Rising titers or clinical signs usually occur within 4 months in infants with infection.

Infants with congenital syphilis should have a cerebrospinal fluid examination before treatment. Infants with abnormal cerebrospinal fluid should receive either of the following: (1) aqueous crystalline penicillin G, 50,000 units/kg/d intramuscularly or intravenously in 2 divided doses for a minimum of 10 days, or (2) aqueous procaine penicillin G, 50,000 units/kg/d intramuscularly for a minimum of 10 days. Infants with normal cerebrospinal fluid should be given benzathine penicillin G, 50,000 units/kg intramuscularly in a single dose. If neurosyphilis cannot be excluded, the aqueous crystalline or procaine penicillin regimen is recommended. Penicillin therapy for congenital syphilis after the neonatal period should use the same dosages recommended for neonatal congenital syphilis. For larger children, the total dose of penicillin need not exceed the dosage used in adult syphilis of more than 1 year's duration.

Follow-up quantitative VDRL tests should be performed at 2, 4, 6, 9, and 12 months. In those infants treated for late infection, follow-up should be longer to demonstrate whether the child, though adequately treated, is "serofast" (ie, seropositive for life).

For interstitial keratitis, a topical corticosteroid

(drops or ointment) should be applied to the affected eye at 2-hour intervals. Herpetic keratitis must be excluded before using topical corticosteroids. The pupil should be kept dilated with a mydriatic.

2. Acquired syphilis—Administration of 1.2 million units of benzathine penicillin G is given intramuscularly in each buttock (total dose of 2.4 million units) to adolescents with primary or secondary disease.

B. General Measures: Care should be given to the maintenance of adequate nutrition.

Penicillin treatment of early congenital or secondary syphilis may result in a febrile Jarisch-Herxheimer reaction. Treatment is symptomatic, with careful follow-up and aspirin or acetaminophen, although transfusion may be necessary in infants with severe hemolytic anemia.

Prognosis

Severe disease, if unexpected, may be fatal in the newborn. Complete cure can be expected if the young infant is treated with penicillin. Serologic reversal will usually occur within 1 year. Treatment of primary syphilis with penicillin is curative. Permanent neurologic sequelae may be seen with meningovascular syphilis.

Fiumara NJ: Syphilis in newborn children. *Clin Obstet Gynecol* 1975;**18:**183.

Harter CA, Benirschke K: Fetal syphilis in the first trimester. *Am J Obstet Gynecol* 1976;**124:**705.

Kaplan JM, McCracken GH: Clinical pharmacology of benzathine penicillin G in neonates with regard to its recommended use in congenital syphilis. *J Pediatr* 1973;**82:**1069.

Primary and secondary syphilis—United States, April 1977. *MMWR* 1977;**26:**207.

Sparling PF: Diagnosis and treatment of syphilis. *N Eng J Med* 1971;**284:**642.

RELAPSING FEVER

Essentials of Diagnosis

- Episodes of fever, chills, malaise.
- Occasional rash, arthritis, cough, hepatosplenomegaly, conjunctivitis.
- Diagnosis confirmed by direct microscopic identification of spirochetes in smears of peripheral blood.

General Considerations

Relapsing fever is a vector-borne disease caused by spirochetes of the genus *Borrelia*. Epidemic relapsing fever is transmitted to humans by body lice *(Pediculus humanus)* and endemic relapsing fever by soft-bodied ticks (genus *Ornithodoros*).

In louse-borne relapsing fever, the vector becomes infected by feeding on an acutely ill individual. Humans become infected when crushed lice are rubbed into the bite wound.

Tick-borne relapsing fever is endemic in the western USA. Transmission usually takes place during the warm months when ticks are active and recreation or work brings people into contact with *Ornithodoros* ticks. Mountain camping areas and cabins are sites where infection often is acquired. The ticks are nocturnal feeders and remain attached for only 5–20 minutes. Consequently, the patient seldom remembers a tick bite.

Rarely, neonatal relapsing fever results from transplacental transmission of *Borrelia*.

Clinical Findings

A. Symptoms and Signs: The disease is characterized by relapses lasting 3–5 days, occurring at intervals of 1–2 weeks with interim asymptomatic periods. The relapses duplicate the initial attack but become progressively less severe. In louse-borne relapsing fever, there is usually a single relapse; in tick-borne infection, there are 2–6 relapses.

The incubation period is 5–11 days. The attack is sudden, with high fever, chills, tachycardia, nausea and vomiting, headache, myalgia, arthralgia, bronchitis, and a dry, nonproductive cough. Hepatomegaly and splenomegaly appear later. An erythematous rash may be seen over the trunk and extremities, and petechiae may be present. After 3–10 days, the fever falls by crisis. Jaundice, iritis, conjunctivitis, cranial nerve palsies, and hemorrhage are more common during relapses.

B. Laboratory Findings: During febrile episodes, the urine contains protein, casts, and, occasionally, erythrocytes; there is a marked polymorphonuclear leukocytosis and, in about one-fourth of cases, a false-positive serologic test for syphilis. Spirochetes can be found in the peripheral blood by direct microscopy in approximately 70% of cases by darkfield examination or by Wright, Giemsa, or acridine orange staining of thick and thin smears. They are not found during afebrile periods. The blood may be injected into young mice and the spirochetes found 1–14 days later in the tail blood. OXK agglutinin titers in serum may be positive.

Differential Diagnosis

Relapsing fever may be confused with malaria, leptospirosis, dengue, yellow fever, typhus, rat-bite fever, Colorado tick fever, Rocky Mountain spotted fever, collagen vascular disease, or any fever of unknown origin.

Complications

Complications include facial paralysis, iridocyclitis, optic atrophy, hypochromic anemia, penumonia, nephritis, myocarditis, endocarditis, and seizures. Central nervous system involvement is seen in 10–30% of cases.

Treatment

For children under 7 years of age with tick-borne relapsing fever, give erythromycin, 40–50 mg/kg/d orally in divided doses every 6 hours for 10 days.

Older children may be given tetracycline instead. Penicillin and chloramphenicol are also efficacious.

In louse-borne relapsing fever, a single dose of tetracycline or erythromycin has been effective.

Severely ill patients should be hospitalized. Antibiotic treatment should be started after the fever has dropped; this will lessen the risk of a severe or even fatal Jarisch-Herxheimer reaction. Isolation precautions are not necessary.

Prognosis

The mortality rate in treated cases is very low, except in debilitated or very young children. With treatment, the initial attack is shortened and relapses prevented. The response to antimicrobial therapy is dramatic.

Boyer KM et al: Tick-borne relapsing fever: An interstate outbreak originating at Grand Canyon National Park. *Am J Epidemiol* 1977;**105:**469.

Edell TA et al: Tick-borne relapsing fever in Colorado: Historical review and report of cases. *JAMA* 1979;**241:**2279.

Johnson RC (editor): *The Biology of Parasitic Spirochetes.* Academic Press, 1976.

Perine PL, Teklu B: Antibiotic treatment of louse-borne relapsing fever in Ethiopia: A report of 377 cases. *Am J Trop Med Hyg* 1983;**32:**1096.

Sciotto CG et al: Detection of *Borrelia* in acridine orange-stained blood smears by fluorescence microscopy. *Arch Pathol Lab Med* 1983;**107:**384.

Warrell DA et al: Pathophysiology and immunology of the Jarisch-Herxheimer-like reaction in louse-borne relapsing fever: Comparison of tetracycline and slow-release penicillin. *J Infect Dis* 1983;**147:**898.

RAT-BITE FEVER

Essentials of Diagnosis

- Agents are *Spirillum minus* (sodoku) or *Streptobacillus moniliformis* (Haverhill fever, streptobacillary fever).
- Rodent bite.
- Fever, chills, nausea, vomiting, rash.
- Myalgia and arthralgia (spirillum fever).
- Migrating polyarthritis (streptobacillary fever).
- Diagnosis is confirmed by culture or serology (streptobacillary fever) or by Giemsa stain or darkfield examination of blood or exudate or by animal inoculation (spirillum fever).

General Considerations

Rat-bite fever is caused by *Streptobacillus moniliformis* (an aerobic, pleomorphic gram-negative rod) or by *Spirillum minus* (a small, noncultivable, gram-negative spiral organism). Infection is transmitted by the bite of a wild or laboratory rat or, less commonly, by mice, cats, squirrels, or weasles. An epidemic of Haverhill fever has been described resulting from ingestion of milk contaminated by rats. In the USA, *S moniliformis* is the usual cause of rat-bite fever. The disease is rarely encountered, or at least rarely recognized, in children.

Clinical Findings

A. Symptoms and Signs: In streptobacillary fever, the healing of the bite is followed in about 3 days by a protracted illness characterized by fever, chills, malaise, and headache. A transient morbilliform or petechial rash then appears, often on the palms and soles. Approximately 50% of cases have migratory polyarthritis. Complications include pneumonia, severe arthritis, and endocarditis.

In spirillum fever, the bite also heals, but 1–6 weeks later the bite site becomes swollen, painful, and dusky and ulcerates. This is followed by lymphadenitis, relapsing fever lasting weeks, chills, myalgia, arthralgia, and a violaceous rash on the palms and soles. Complications include endocarditis and nephritis.

B. Laboratory Findings: Leukocytosis is often present, and in spirillum fever a serologic test for syphilis may be falsely positive. *S minus* may be identified by Giemsa stain or darkfield examination of the ulcer exudate, aspirated lymph node material, or blood. *S minus* cannot be cultured in artificial media; however, blood from patients can be inoculated intraperitoneally into mice or guinea pigs and the organism detected microscopically. *S moniliformis* will grow in enriched media, and a serologic test is available.

Differential Diagnosis

Distinguishing between infection with *S minus* and *S moniliformis* is difficult. *S moniliformis* infection is characterized by a short incubation period (usually < 7 days), lack of flare-up of the primary lesion at the onset of systemic symptoms, a high incidence of migratory polyarthritis (50%), and a low incidence of false-positive serologic tests for syphilis (15%). *S moniliformis* can usually be isolated from blood, joint fluid, or pus. Agglutinins against the organism develop during the second or third week of illness.

S minus infection is suggested by a prolonged incubation period (7–21 days), relapsing instead of sustained fever, arthralgia but not arthritis, and frequent false-positive serologic tests for syphilis (50%).

Rat-bite fever may also need to be distinguished from tularemia, leptospirosis, relapsing fever, malaria, chronic meningococcemia, cat-scratch disease, Kawasaki disease, and rickettsial infections.

Treatment

Treatment of both forms of uncomplicated rat-bite fever is with aqueous penicillin, 100,000 units/kg/d intravenously in divided doses; procaine penicillin G, 25,000 units/kg/d; or tetracycline, 25–50 mg/kg/d orally for 7 days.

Prognosis

The reported mortality rate of untreated streptobacillary fever is about 10%, but this is markedly reduced by prompt diagnosis and treatment. Spirillum fever is more benign; death in treated cases is rare.

Raffin BJ, Freemark M: Streptobacillary fever: A pediatric problem. *Prediatrics* 1979;**64:**214.

Shanson DC et al: *Streptobacillus moniliformis* isolated from blood in four cases of Haverhill fever. *Lancet* 1983;**2:**92.

LEPTOSPIROSIS

Essentials of Diagnosis

- Biphasic course lasting 2 or 3 weeks.
- Initial phase: high fever, headache, myalgia, and conjunctivitis.
- Apparent recovery for 2–3 days.
- Return of fever associated with meningitis.
- Jaundice, hemorrhages, and renal insufficiency (severe cases).
- Culture of organism from blood and cerebrospinal fluid (early) and from urine (later), or direct microscopy of urine or cerebrospinal fluid.
- Positive leptospiral agglutination test.

General Considerations

Leptospirosis is a zoonosis caused by many antigenically distinct but morphologically similar spirochetes. The organism enters through the skin or respiratory tract. Classically, the severe form—Weil's disease, with jaundice and a high mortality rate—was associated with infection with *Leptospira icterohaemorrhagiae* following immersion in water contaminated with rat urine. It is now known that a variety of animals (dogs, rats, cattle, etc) may serve as reservoirs for pathogenic *Leptospira,* that a given serogroup may have multiple animal species as hosts, and that severe disease may be caused by many different serogroups other than *L icterohaemorrhagiae.*

In the USA, leptospirosis occurs more commonly from avocational activities (70% of cases) in children, students, and housewives than from occupational exposure. Urban and suburban cases are more common than rural cases. Cases acquired from contact with dogs are more than twice as frequent as those acquired from cattle, swine, or rodents. Sewer workers, farmers, abattoir workers, animal handlers, and soldiers have occupational exposure. Outbreaks have resulted from swimming in contaminated streams and harvesting field crops.

In the USA, about 100 cases are reported yearly, and about one-third are in children. Approximately 50% of cases occur in the summer or early fall.

Clinical Findings

A. Symptoms and Signs:

1. Initial phase—The incubation period is 4–19 days, with a mean of 10 days. Chills, fever, headache, myalgia, conjunctivitis (episcleral injection), photophobia, cervical lymphadenopathy, and pharyngitis occur commonly. This leptospiremic phase lasts for 3–7 days.

2. Phase of apparent recovery—Symptoms typically (but not always) subside for 2–3 days.

3. Systemic phase—Fever reappears and is associated with headache, muscular pain and tenderness in the abdomen and back, and nausea and vomiting. Lung, heart, and joint involvement occasionally occurs. These manifestations are due to extensive vasculitis.

a. Central nervous system involvement—The central nervous system is involved in 50–90% of cases. Severe headache and mild nuchal rigidity are usual, but delirium, coma, and focal neurologic signs may be seen.

b. Renal and hepatic involvement—In about 50% of cases, the kidney or liver or both are affected. Gross hematuria and oliguria or anuria are sometimes seen. Jaundice may be associated with an enlarged and tender liver.

c. Gallbladder involvement—Leptospirosis may cause acalculous cholecystitis in children. A cholecystogram will reveal a nonfunctioning gallbladder, and cholecystotomy or cholecystectomy may be required. Pancreatitis is unusual.

d. Hemorrhage—Petechiae, ecchymoses, and gastrointestinal bleeding may be severe.

e. Rash—A rash is seen in 10–30% of cases. It may be maculopapular and generalized or may be petechial or purpuric. Occasionally, erythema nodosum is seen. Peripheral desquamation of the rash may occur. Gangrenous areas are sometimes noted over the distal extremities. In such cases, skin biopsy demonstrates the presence of severe vasculitis involving both the arterial and the venous circulations.

B. Laboratory Findings: Leptospires may be seen by direct darkfield or phase contrast microscopy or immunofluorescence techniques, but they do not stain by Gram, Wright, or Giemsa methods. They appear in the blood and cerebrospinal fluid only during the first 10 days of illness. They appear in the urine during the second week, where they may persist for 30 days or longer. The organism can be isolated from blood inoculated into Fletcher's semisolid medium or EMJH semisolid medium, but culture techniques are slow (7–10 days), difficult, and not generally available.

The white blood cell counts often is elevated, especially when there is liver involvement. Serum bilirubin levels usually remain below 20 mg/dL. Other liver function tests may be abnormal, although the AST (SGOT) usually shows only slight elevation. An elevated serum creatinine phosphokinase is frequently found. Cerebrospinal fluid shows moderate pleocytosis ($< 500/\mu L$), increased protein (50–100 mg/dL), and normal glucose. Urine often shows microscopic pyuria, hematuria, and, less often, proteinuria (++ or greater). The erythrocyte sedimentation rate is markedly elevated. Chest x-ray may show pneumonitis.

The most widely used but least specific serologic test for leptospiral disease is the macroscopic slide agglutination test. A microscopic agglutination test using live organisms (performed at the Centers for Disease Control, Atlanta, GA 30333) is superior. Leptospiral agglutinins generally reach peak levels by the third to fourth week. A 1:100 titer is considered suspicious; a 4-fold or greater rise is diagnostic.

Differential Diagnosis

Fever and myalgia associated with the characteristic conjunctival (episcleral) injection should suggest leptospirosis. During the prodrome, malaria, typhoid fever, typhus, rheumatoid arthritis, brucellosis, and influenza may be suspected. Later, depending upon the organ systems involved, a variety of other diseases need to be distinguished, including encephalitis, viral or tuberculous meningitis, viral hepatitis, glomerulonephritis, viral or bacterial pneumonia, rheumatic fever, subacute bacterial endocarditis, acute surgical abdomen, and Kawasaki disease.

Prevention

Preventive measures include the avoidance of contaminated water and soil, the use of rodent control, immunization of dogs and other domestic animals, and good sanitation. Immunization or antimicrobial prophylaxis with doxycycline may be of value to certain high-risk occupational groups.

Treatment

A. Specific Measures: Treatment within the first 4 days of illness may reduce the severity of the disease but has little effect if started later. Give aqueous penicillin G, 150,000 units/kg/d in 4–6 divided doses intravenously for 7–10 days. A Jarisch-Herxheimer reaction may be seen. Tetracycline, 40–50 mg/kg/d, also may be used.

B. General Measures: Symptomatic and supportive care is indicated, particularly for renal and hepatic failure and hemorrhage.

Prognosis

Leptospirosis generally is anicteric and self-limiting. The disease usually last 1–3 weeks but may be more prolonged. Relapse may occur.

There are usually no permanent sequelae associated with central nervous system infection. The mortality rate in reported cases in the USA is 5%, usually from renal failure. The mortality rate may reach 20% or more in elderly patients who have severe kidney and hepatic involvement.

Johnson RC (editor): *The Biology of Parasitic Spirochetes.* Academic Press, 1976.

Martone WJ, Kaufman AF: Leptospirosis in humans in the United States, 1974–1978. *J Infect Dis* 1979;**140:**1020.

Peter G: Leptospirosis: A zoonosis of protean manifestations. *Pediatr Infect Dis* 1982;**1:**282.

Takafuji ET et al: An efficacy trial of doxycycline chemoprophylaxis against leptospirosis. *N Engl J Med* 1984;**310:**497.

Wong ML et al: Leptospirosis: A childhood disease. *J Pediatr* 1977;**90:**532.

LYME DISEASE
(Lyme Arthritis)

Essentials of Diagnosis

- Presence of skin lesion (erythema chronicum migrans) 3–30 days after tick bite.
- Arthritis, usually pauciarticular, occurring about 4 weeks after appearance of skin lesion. Headache, chills, and fever.
- Residence or travel in an endemic area during the late spring, the summer, or early fall.

General Considerations

Lyme disease (see also Chapter 18) is a subacute or chronic spirochetal infection contracted from the bite of an infected deer tick *(Ixodes dammini* or *Ixodes pacificus).* It is usually heralded by a prodromal skin rash (erythema chronicum migrans) characterized by an expanding erythematous papule or sometimes by satellite or generalized smaller maculopapular lesions. This prodrome lasts several days or weeks, and, if untreated, is frequently followed in several weeks by fever and oligoarthritis, usually in the knees. Arthritis may be recurrent, with periods of complete remission between attacks. The syndrome may also involve the nervous system and heart. Episodes recur but are of decreasing intensity in most cases. Circulating immune complexes appear to play a pathogenetic role in the disease. Elevated IgM titers of antibody to the spirochete are found during the acute skin or joint disease.

Because initial cases were seen in the villages of Lyme and Old Lyme, Connecticut, the disease was called Lyme arthritis, or Lyme disease. Most cases now occur in southern New England, eastern Massachusetts, and Long Island. However, distribution of the tick extends to the mid-Atlantic states, the Midwest (Wisconsin and Minnesota), and western states (California, Oregon, Nevada, and Utah), and cases are increasingly recognized in these areas.

Clinical Findings

A. Symptoms and Signs: An expanding erythematous papule as large as 20 cm in diameter appears 3–30 days after a tick bite at the site. Multiple satellite lesions may occur. The center of the lesion may clear completely. There may be headache, fever, chills, and malaise at this stage; in some instances, there are no constitutional symptoms.

Usually several weeks later, arthritis occurs. This is monarticular or oligoarticular, often in the knees, with swelling and pain lasting a few days and remitting but recurring several weeks later. Fewer than 10% of patients develop chronic arthritis.

Ten to 20% develop aseptic meningitis, usually days to weeks after the rash. Facial or other cranial nerve palsy is common, and chorea or cerebellar signs sometimes occur. The neurologic symptoms last several weeks and may recur.

A small number of patients develop cardiac conduction defects or myocardial disease.

B. Laboratory Findings: In those who develop arthritis, the sedimentation rate is elevated, total IgM is high, and cryoprecipitates are found. The joint fluid contains leukocytes (5,000–50,000/μL), with a predominance of neutrophils. Cerebrospinal fluid may show lymphocytosis. Tests for rheumatoid factor, LE cells, and elevated antistreptolysin O are negative.

Differential Diagnosis

Juvenile rheumatoid arthritis, rheumatic fever, viral or septic arthritis, tuberculous or viral meningitis, and infectious mononucleosis must be considered. The benign and recurrent course and the geographic clustering of cases are helpful.

Treatment

Penicillin G (20–30 mg/kg/d orally in 4 divided doses), penicillin V (250 mg orally 4 times a day), or tetracycline (40 mg/kg/d orally in 4 divided doses) given when the skin rash appears and continued for 7–10 days will both shorten the period of the rash and prevent or lessen the chances of subsequent arthritis and meningitis. Tetracycline is probably more effective than penicillin but should not be given to patients under 7 years of age.

Prognosis

All but a few patients have an ultimately benign outcome, even after repeated attacks of arthritis or neurologic symptoms.

Steere AC et al: Antibiotic therapy in Lyme disease. *Ann Intern Med* 1980;**93:**1.

Steere AC et al: Erythema chronicum migrans and Lyme arthritis: The enlarging clinical spectrum. *Ann Intern Med* 1977;**86:**685.

Steere AC et al: The spirochetal etiology of Lyme disease. *N Engl J Med* 1983;**308:**733.

SELECTED REFERENCES

Committee on Infectious Diseases: *Report,* 19th ed. American Academy of Pediatrics, 1982.

Feigin RD, Cherry JD (editors): *Textbook of Pediatric Infectious Disease.* Saunders, 1981.

Jawetz E et al: *Review of Medical Microbiology,* 17th ed. Lange, 1986.

Krugman S, Ward R, Katz S: *Infectious Diseases of Children and Adults,* 6th ed. Mosby, 1977.

28 Infections: Parasitic

L. Barth Reller, MD, DTM&H

Many parasitic diseases of great international importance are not seen in the USA except in immigrants or travelers. Therefore, it is particularly important to obtain a geographic history for all patients, because this history may provide the clue to an otherwise obscure parasitic illness (eg, malaria, schistosomiasis and other fluke infections, trypanosomiasis, and filariasis). Malaria and giardiasis account for most parasitic infections acquired abroad. With rare exceptions, pets are of epidemiologic importance only in the transmission of toxoplasmosis and visceral larva migrans (toxocariasis).

Major clinical syndromes and presenting features of parasitic diseases are listed in Table 28–1. Antiparasitic drugs are shown in Table 28–2.

Table 28–1. Clinical manifestations of parasitic infections.

Clinical Manifestation	Associated Parasitic Diseases
Abdominal pain	Amebiasis, strongyloidiasis, trichinosis, fascioliasis, clonorchiasis, ascariasis
Anemia	Malaria, hookworm disease, diphyllobothriasis, visceral leishmaniasis
Cough	Paragonimiasis, disseminated strongyloidiasis, *Pneumocystis carinii* pneumonia
Diarrhea	Giardiasis, amebiasis, trichinosis, strongyloidiasis, schistosomiasis, cryptosporidiosis, *Dientamoeba fragilis* infection
Dysentery	Amebiasis, acute schistosomiasis, balantidiasis
Dysuria	Schistosomiasis
Encephalopathy	Malaria, African trypanosomiasis, toxoplasmosis
Eosinophilia	Trichinosis, toxocariasis, strongyloidiasis, schistosomiasis, filariasis, fascioliasis, angiostrongyliasis, onchocerciasis
Fever	Malaria, *Pneumocystis carinii* pneumonia, amebic liver abscess, toxoplasmosis, trichinosis, visceral leishmaniasis, African and American trypanosomiasis, toxocariasis
Hematuria	Schistosomiasis
Hemoptysis	Paragonimiasis
Hepatomegaly	Amebic liver abscess, toxocariasis, schistosomiasis, visceral leishmaniasis, echinococcosis
Lymphadenopathy	Toxoplasmosis, trypanosomiasis, filariasis
Malabsorption	Giardiasis, strongyloidiasis, cryptosporidiosis
Pruritus	Onchocerciasis, enterobiasis, cutaneous larva migrans
Rash	Schistosomiasis,strongyloidiasis, onchocerciasis, filariasis
Seizures	Cysticercosis
Splenomegaly	Malaria, schistosomiasis, visceral leishmaniasis

PROTOZOAN INFECTIONS

MALARIA

Essentials of Diagnosis

- Travel to or residence in an endemic area.
- Fever, frequently paroxysmal, with shaking chills and marked diaphoresis.
- Splenomegaly and anemia.
- Severe headache, delirium, coma, and convulsions (in cerebral malaria), vomiting, diarrhea, and jaundice.
- Malarial parasites in blood smears.

General Considerations

Despite all attempts at control or eradication, malaria continues to affect an estimated 200 million people worldwide and kills over a million children annually in Africa alone. In some areas previously controlled (notably the Indian subcontinent, parts of South America, and Turkey), malaria is now resurgent.

Four species of parasites infect humans: *Plasmodium vivax, Plasmodium falciparum, Plasmodium malariae,* and *Plasmodium ovale* (in declining order of frequency). Various species of female anopheline mosquitoes act as vectors. Male and female gametocytes ingested by the mosquito fertilize and develop ultimately into sporozoites that are injected into fresh hosts. They develop in parenchymal cells of the liver (preerythrocytic cycle), resulting in the release of merozoites into the circulation. Those which escape

Table 28–2. Antiparasitic drugs (synonyms and brand names).

Albendazole*	Niridazole (Ambilhar)*
Amodiaquine dihydrochloride (Camoquin)*	Oxamniquine (Vansil)
Amphotericin B (Fungizone)	Paromomycin (Humatin)
Antimony potassium tartrate (tartar emetic)	Pentamidine isethionate (Lomidine, Petam 300)
Antimony sodium gluconate (stibogluconate sodium; Pentostam)†	Piperazine citrate (Antepar)
Bephenium hydroxynaphthoate (Alcopar)*	Praziquantel (Biltricide)
Bithionol (Bitin, Lorothidol)*	Primaquine phosphate
Chloroquine phosphate or sulfate (Aralen and many other trade names)	Proguanil (chloroguanide hydrochloride; Paludrine)*
Dehydroemetine dihydrochloride†	Pyrantel pamoate (Antiminth, Combantrin)
Diethylcarbamazine citrate (Hetrazan [Lederle])	Pyrimethamine (Daraprim)
Difluoromethylornithine (DFMO)*	Pyrimethamine-sulfadoxine (Falcidar, Fansidar)
Diloxanide furoate (Furamide)†	Pyrvinium pamoate (Povan)
Emetine hydrochloride	Quinacrine hydrochloride (mepacrine; Atabrine)
Furazolidone (Furoxone)	Quinidine gluconate (Duraquin)
Iodoquinol (Yodoxin)	Quinine dihydrochloride† and quinine sulfate
Ivermectin*	Spiramycin (Rovamycin)*
Mebendazole (Vermox)	Suramin (Antrypol, Germanin)†
Melarsoprol (Mel B; Arsobal)†	Tetrachloroethylene (perchloroethylene)
Metrifonate (Bilarcil)*	Thiabendazole (Mintezol)
Metronidazole (Flagyl)	Tinidazole (Fasigyn)*
Niclosamide (Niclocide, Yomesan)	Trimethoprim-sulfamethoxazole (co-trimoxazole; Bactrim, Septra)
Nifurtimox (Lampit)†	Tryparsamide*

* Not available in the USA.
† Available in USA only through Parasitic Disease Drug Service, Centers for Disease Control, Atlanta, GA 30333. Telephone: (404) 329-3670.

phagocytosis infect red blood cells, mature, and divide into merozoites that are released when the erythrocytes rupture (erythrocytic cycle, schizogony). Others may continue to develop in liver cells (exoerythrocytic cycle). Merozoites sustain the infection in fresh red cells and repeat the erythrocytic cycle according to a synchronous pattern of 48 or 72 hours, depending on the species of *Plasmodium*. A few merozoites develop into gametocytes. In time, the erythrocytic cycles dwindle and disappear, and the exoerythrocytic cycle forms the source for new erythrocytic cycles, causing relapses, except for falciparum malaria, which has no exoerythrocytic cycle, so that relapses after long intervals do not occur.

Malarial infections constitute an intense form of antigenic stimulation leading to the production of antimalarial antibodies detectable by various techniques. Susceptibility to malarial infection varies in different populations, and some individual genes confer some degree of natural immunity (eg, hemoglobin S, hemoglobin F, G6PD deficiency, thalassemia, and Duffy blood group negativity). Natural immunity appears not to prevent infection by the sporozoites, but the clinical manifestation of the disease is reduced or absent.

Repeated infection confers partial immunity, resulting from both humoral and cellular immunity. IgG is the major protective immunoglobulin; it is species- and strain-specific and prevents reinvasion of erythrocytes by merozoites. Passive immunity appears to be acquired by the newborn via placental antibody transfer. Congenital malaria is relatively common in infants born to nonimmune but infected mothers but is rare in infants of immune mothers despite heavy placental infections with *P falciparum*.

Malaria must be considered even in nonmalarial areas when the clinical syndrome with fever occurs in a patient who has received blood transfusions or shared a syringe or needle during illicit drug use. An exoerythrocytic cycle does not develop in such cases.

Clinical Findings

A. Symptoms and Signs: The clinical manifestations vary to some degree according to the species of parasite. Minor variations also occur between strains of the same species. In children, the initial clinical picture can mimic influenza. In infants, it may be limited at first to fever, vomiting, and diarrhea. On first exposure, the incubation period is 2 weeks for vivax, falciparum, and ovale malaria and about 3–5 weeks for quartan (malariae) malaria. Initially, intermittent or continuous fever occurs and lasts for a variable period. The fever may disappear, only to appear in further episodes. Periodicity characteristic of the species may become established in first or subsequent attacks. In vivax (benign tertian), falciparum (malignant tertian), or ovale malaria, fever occurs on alternate days. In the quartan type, the day of fever is followed by 2 afebrile days. Fever that occurs every day is called quotidian. Considerable variation in the above periodicities can occur as a result of multiple asynchronous cycles of the same species or mixed infection. Each paroxysm consists of chills lasting up to 1 hour accompanied by headache, back and muscle pains, and nausea and vomiting; rapid elevation of temperature lasting for several hours accompanied by prostration; and then remission with intense perspiration. These paroxysms coincide with the periodicity of the erythrocytic cycle of the parasites, which for unknown reasons develops a curious synchrony. Thus, in its classic form, malaria is manifested by remissions and relapses of paroxysmal fever.

Between attacks, the child may feel well or ill. The spleen gradually becomes palpable and continues to enlarge. Rapid splenic enlargement may cause pain. Herpetic lesions may appear on the lips. Anemia and slight jaundice may become manifest. In the absence of reinfections and complications, the relapses die down in less than a year for falciparum malaria and in a few years for vivax malaria. Quartan malaria may remain dormant or cryptic for years or decades and then reappear.

B. Laboratory Findings: The most important part of the investigation is thick and thin blood smears (stained with Giemsa's or Wright's stain), the former for screening and the latter for detailed study. The parasites seen in blood smears are trophozoites, schizonts, and gametocytes—except for falciparum malaria, in which only gametocytes and ring stage trophozoites are ordinarily found in peripheral blood.

Currently available serologic methods of diagnosis include indirect immunofluorescence, passive hemagglutination, and enzyme-linked immunosorbent assay. The latter 2 do not always detect early infection, and the first is the present method of choice. Serologic tests are useful in the detection of carriers among blood donors and also where diagnosis cannot be made by blood smears.

Other laboratory findings include low red and white cell counts, increased unconjugated blood bilirubin, increased serum gamma globulin, and a lowered C3 level. The serologic test for syphilis may be falsely positive.

Differential Diagnosis

Malaria must often be differentiated from tuberculosis, typhoid, and other febrile illnesses, especially recurrent ones such as brucellosis, rat-bite fever, relapsing fever, febrile episodes of lymphoreticular diseases, urinary tract infections, and periodic fevers. Malaria may coexist with other diseases or may be present in unusual circumstances such as undiagnosed postoperative fever. The various complications of *P falciparum* infection are a diagnostic challenge.

Complications & Sequelae

Apart from malignant tertian malaria, the other forms of malaria are relatively free from complications. Chronic malaria may result in anemia and debility. An enlarged spleen may rupture on trivial trauma. Red cells infected with *P falciparum* trophozoites have a tendency to adhere to blood vessels, and in certain viscera, infected red cells and the population of parasites increase in a vicious cycle, causing obstruction and anoxic necrosis that may result in enteritis with gastrointestinal bleeding, interstitial pneumonia, and encephalitis (commonly called cerebral malaria).

Severe intravascular hemolysis resulting in hemoglobinuria and shock (blackwater fever) occurs rarely in falciparum malaria. The mortality rate is very high in cerebral malaria and in blackwater fever. Blackwater fever was very common in the past when quinine was widely used as a therapeutic agent.

The nephrotic syndrome is seen as a complication of chronic *P malariae* infection. Massive splenomegaly may lead to hypersplenism with anemia.

Heavy placental infection with the malarial parasite in the pregnant woman interferes with the growth of the fetus and is a common cause of low birth weight. Though rare, infection across the placenta to the fetus occurs.

Prevention

Widespread prophylaxis may not be justified in malarial areas with immune populations of children, because later withdrawal of prophylaxis leaves the child highly susceptible to severe disease. However, for nonimmune children living in endemic areas and therefore constantly at risk of infection or reinfection, the best procedure is prophylaxis.

Pregnant women from nonendemic areas should be discouraged from traveling to malarial areas. Although chloroquine can be given safely in standard prophylactic doses during pregnancy, other antimicrobials may be fetotoxic.

Since true prophylaxis (prevention of infection by the destruction of sporozoites) is unavailable, a drug is given that suppresses schizogony and clinical symptoms. It should be started 1 week prior to arrival in any endemic area. The most commonly used suppressive drug is chloroquine, given orally each week in a dosage of 5 mg/kg base (8.3 mg/kg salt) up to a maximum adult dose of 300 mg base. Alternatively, amodiaquine may be given, since some studies suggest that it may be effective in areas of low-level chloroquine resistance. Amodiaquine is given orally once a week in a dosage of 7 mg/kg base (9 mg/kg salt) up to a maximum adult dose of 400 mg base. Other suppressive drugs given orally include proguanil, 2–3 mg/kg/d, and pyrimethamine, 0.5 mg/kg/wk. If the suppressive drug is taken for about 6 weeks after a person leaves the endemic area, falciparum malaria usually does not become manifest but the other forms of malaria may because of the uncontrolled exoerythrocytic cycle. To avoid this, a course of primaquine may be given during the final 2 weeks of prophylaxis, as described below.

Falciparum malaria resistant to chloroquine is widespread in Southeast Asia, Indonesia, some islands of the South Pacific (including the Philippines and Papua New Guinea), and South America and has been documented in the Indian subcontinent, East Africa, and parts of Panama. Chemoprophylaxis with chloroquine is not always effective in these areas.

The combination of pyrimethamine (25 mg) and sulfadoxine (500 mg) in a single tablet has been found to be effective against many, but not all, strains of chloroquine-resistant *P falciparum*. In recent years, there have been more deaths from complications of pyrimethamine-sulfadoxine use than from chloroquine-resistant malaria in US travelers. Therefore, rather than receiving routine prophylaxis, travelers with short exposure (3 weeks or less) in high-risk areas for chloroquine-resistant falciparum malaria should carry a therapeutic dose (expressed as portions of a 25-mg/500-mg tablet: ¼ tablet, 2–11 months of age; ½ tablet, 1–3 years; 1 tablet, 4–8 years; 2 tablets, 9–14 years; and 3 tablets, over 14 years as a single dose) to take if fever occurs and there is no access to medical help. For prolonged stays in high-risk areas with substantial nighttime exposure to mosquitoes, the weekly oral dose of pyrimethamine-sulfadoxine is as follows: ⅛ tablet, 2–11 months of age; ¼ tablet, 1–3 years; ½ tablet, 4–8 years; ¾ tablet, 9–14 years; and 1 tablet, over 14 years. ***Caution:*** Pyrimethamine-sulfadoxine is contraindicated in patients with a history of sulfonamide or pyrimethamine intolerance and in infants under 2 months of age. Severe, sometimes fatal, cutaneous reactions (such as Stevens-Johnson syndrome) have occurred; if any mucocutaneous signs or symptoms develop, the drug should be stopped immediately.

Falciparum malaria resistant to pyrimethamine-sulfadoxine has now been documented. Pyrimethamine-sulfadoxine is inadequate for the prevention or treatment of vivax malaria. Consequently, chloroquine chemoprophylaxis should always be given whether or not pyrimethamine-sulfadoxine is indicated as above.

Since most malarial vectors are night biters, mosquito nets to sleep in and mosquito repellants are important preventive measures. While chemoprophylaxis and environmental engineering or chemical control of mosquito populations currently represent the most feasible mass preventive measures, biologic control of mosquitoes and malarial vaccines are under study for future use.

Treatment

Any child with unexplained fever or coma who has a history of travel in a zone of malarial transmission, blood transfusion, or illicit drug injection must be regarded as having malaria until an alternative diagnosis has been established.

A. Specific Measures: In a child with malaria, the first aim of treatment is to terminate the paroxysms with drugs that act on the erythrocytic cycle, ie, chloroquine or quinine. Primaquine may also be used in conjunction with chloroquine to prevent relapses in vivax infections by destroying the exoerythrocytic reservoir of infection.

1. Chloroquine phosphate—Given orally over 3 days, this is the drug of choice for *P vivax* and nonresistant *P falciparum* infections, which it completely eradicates. Toxic symptoms include nausea, vomiting, and diarrhea. The dosage is as follows:

a. Give 10 mg/kg (maximum, 600 mg) as the initial dose. Follow with 5 mg/kg in 6 hours and then 5 mg/kg 18 hours after the second dose and 5 mg/kg 24 hours after the third dose.

b. If oral therapy is impossible, give intravenous quinine or quinidine (see below) initially but switch to oral chloroquine as soon as possible. Parenteral chloroquine is too hazardous to be recommended in children.

2. Quinine or quinidine (alone or in combination with other drugs)—For suspected chloroquine-resistant falciparum infection, treat with quinine or quinidine as follows:

a. Quinine sulfate, 25 mg/kg/d in 3 divided doses for 3 days, plus pyrimethamine according to weight as follows: under 10 kg, 6.25 mg/d; 10–20 kg, 12.5 mg/d; 21–40 kg, 25 mg/d; and over 40 kg, 25 mg twice daily for 3 days; plus sulfadiazine, 100–200 mg/kg/d in 4 divided doses for 5 days (maximum, 2 g/d). Children who are allergic to pyrimethamine or sulfadiazine can be treated with clindamycin in addition to quinine. The dosage of clindamycin is 20–40 mg/kd/d in 3 divided doses for 3 days.

b. Quinine dihydrochloride, 8–10 mg/kg intravenously diluted in 100 mL or more of physiologic saline solution. *(Give very slowly over 2–4 hours.)* The dose may be repeated if necessary in 8 hours and again 8 hours later. Do not exceed 25 mg/kg/d. It is seldom necessary to continue parenteral therapy for more than 24 hours. Switch to oral quinine sulfate, pyrimethamine, and sulfadiazine as soon as oral medication is possible. ***Caution:*** Parenteral quinine is a very dangerous drug; however, it may be lifesaving when required.

c. Quinidine gluconate is more readily available than intravenous quinine, and some experts consider it to be more effective. An intravenous loading dose of 10 mg/kg base (maximum, 600 mg) in physiologic saline solution is given over 4–6 hours and followed by 5 mg/kg (maximum, 300 mg) every 8 hours if oral therapy cannot be started. Electrocardiographic monitoring is imperative to detect dysrhythmias, which require slowing or stopping the influsion.

3. Primaquine phosphate—This drug is used in combination with chloroquine in *P vivax* infections only. It is reported to eradicate the infection and prevent relapses. ***Caution:*** Primaquine is a toxic drug and must be used with careful laboratory follow-up. Never use in blacks without first testing for G6PD deficiency. If anemia, leukopenia, or methemoglobinemia appears, discontinue use of the drug immediately. Never use with quinacrine or within 5 days of quinacrine therapy.

Give orally once daily for 14 days as follows: under 10 kg, 2 mg; 10–20 kg, 4 mg; 21–40 kg, 6 mg; 41–55 kg, 10 mg; and over 55 kg, 20 mg.

Falciparum malaria contracted in an area reporting strains resistant to chloroquine must be treated with other drugs from the beginning to prevent the rapid buildup of a potentially fatal parasitemia.

4. Mefloquine—Although not yet available in the USA, mefloquine is the most promising new drug active against multidrug-resistant strains of *P falciparum*. A single oral dose of 20 mg/kg has been sufficient for treatment of falciparum malaria in partially immune children.

B. General Measures: Fluid therapy is most important. Urge oral intake and, if not satisfactory, give parenteral fluids. Control high fever and treat anemia with iron. Corticosteroids do not improve survival rates for patients with cerebral malaria and should not be given.

Prognosis

In the majority of cases, the prognosis with proper therapy is excellent. In small infants and in the presence of malnutrition or chronic debilitating disease, the prognosis is more guarded.

Bradley-Moore AM et al: A comparison of chloroquine and pyrimethamine as malaria chemoprophylactics in young Nigerian children. *Trans R Soc Trop Med Hyg* 1985;**79:**722.

Centers for Disease Control: Revised recommendations for preventing malaria in travelers to areas with chloroquine-resistant *Plasmodium falciparum*. *MMWR* 1985;**34:**185.

Perrin LH, Mackey LJ, Miescher P: The hematology of malaria in man. *Semin Hematol* 1982;**19:**70.

Phillips RE et al: Intravenous quinidine for the treatment of severe falciparum malaria: Clinical and pharmacokinetic studies. *N Engl J Med* 1985;**312:**1273.

Quinn TC et al: Congenital malaria: A report of four cases and a review. *J Pediatr* 1982;**101:**229.

Randall G, Seidel JS: Malaria. *Pediatr Clin North Am* 1985;**32:**893.

Shann F, Stace J, Edstein M: Pharmacokinetics of quinine in children. *J Pediatr* 1985;**106:**506.

Spencer HC: Drug-resistant malaria: Changing patterns mean difficult decisions. *Trans R Soc Trop Med Hyg* 1985;**79:**748.

Taylor DW, Siddiqui WA: Recent advances in malarial immunity. *Annu Rev Med* 1982;**33:**69.

Tin F, Hlaing N, Lasserre R: Single-dose treatment of falciparum malaria with mefloquine: Field studies with different doses in semi-immune adults and children in Burma. *Bull WHO* 1982;**60:**913.

Warrell DA et al: Dexamethasone proves deleterious in cerebral malaria: A double-blind trial in 100 comatose patients. *N Engl J Med* 1982;**306:**313.

White NJ et al: Quinine pharmacokinetics and toxicity in cerebral and uncomplicated falciparum malaria. *Am J Med* 1982;**73:**564.

Wyler DJ: Malaria: Resurgence, resistance, and research. (2 parts.) *N Engl J Med* 1983;**308:**875, 934.

AMEBIASIS

Essentials of Diagnosis

- Acute dysentery: Evidence of colitis, ie, diarrhea with blood and mucus, pain, and tenderness.
- Chronic dysentery: Recurrent symptoms of diarrhea and abdominal pain.
- Hepatic amebiasis: Enlarged and tender liver.
- Amebic abscess: Reddish-brown pus.
- Amebas or cysts in stools or abscesses.

General Considerations

Amebiasis in children is a common and serious problem in some tropical countries but is rare where sanitation is good. Infants and children of all ages may be infected, and the younger the patient the greater the chance that infection has been acquired within the family.

Only the trophozoites (vegetative forms of *Entamoeba histolytica*) invade tissues, and only the cysts can survive outside the host and infect others. Infection occurs by ingestion of the cysts. The question of pathogenicity of strain variants and other species of amebas is controversial. The so-called small race is now considered a separate nonpathogenic species, *Entamoeba hartmanni*. *Entamoeba coli* is nonpathogenic.

Infection by *E histolytica* causes disease only in a minority (10–25%) of cases. Asymptomatic carriers often pass cysts and, rarely, vegetative forms.

Clinical Findings

A. Symptoms and Signs: The symptoms of amebic dysentery vary greatly in severity. Typically there is diarrhea with several small stools that contain mucus and a variable amount of dark blood. The onset may or may not be sudden. Fever is variable and not usually high. Older children may complain of abdominal pain, either localized over the cecum or sigmoid or generalized. In severe cases, dehydration and prostration may supervene.

Symptoms in chronic intestinal amebiasis also vary greatly in severity. Recurrent complaints of changing bowel habits, abdominal pain, and tenderness over the colon are usual. Chronic dysentery may or may not be preceded by an acute attack. Amebomas are rare in children.

B. Laboratory Findings: The most important investigation is that of satisfactory stool specimens. In acute dysentery, a fresh fecal sample is mounted in warm saline on a warm slide and examined under the microscope. The trophozoites are distinguished by unidirectional movement, size (12–60 μm), a clear ectoplasm, and ingested red cells. If delays in transport are expected, the fecal sample should be preserved in polyvinyl alcohol for later examination after trichrome staining. In acute dysentery in children, sigmoidoscopy is not usually recommended. It may be done, however, for obtaining ulcer scrapings to look for amebas. Characteristically, the mucosa looks inflamed, with shallow ulcers scattered over otherwise intact mucosa.

In suspected chronic amebiasis, a series of stools should be examined for cysts, preferably on alternate days. Cysts are round or oval and measure 10–18 μm in diameter. Immature cysts contain 1–2 nuclei and often 2 chromatoid bodies. More mature cysts contain 4 nuclei and no chromatoid bodies. Staining with Lugol's iodine brings the above features into prominence. If necessary, the stools may be collected after a saline purge. Cysts under 10 μm in diameter are considered to be nonpathogenic *E hartmanni*.

Serologic procedures, such as complement fixation, indirect hemagglutination (IHA), counterelectrophoresis, and latex agglutination tests, are of value in extraintestinal amebiasis. The IHA test for amebiasis is positive at a titer of 1:128 or more in about 90% of patients with invasive amebic colitis and in virtually all patients with amebic liver abscess. Barium enema helps in the differentiation of chronic dysentery from other colonic lesions, but it cannot be used before a search for parasites.

Moderate leukocytosis may be present.

Differential Diagnosis

Acute bacillary dysentery (shigellosis) and campylobacteriosis usually have a more abrupt onset, often with bright red blood and mucus. Fever and leukocytosis are often high. A smear of feces reveals the presence of large numbers of neutrophilic leukocytes and bacteria. The final proof is the cultural demonstration of pathogenic bacteria and the absence of amebas.

Other causes of bloody stools, such as polyps, anaphylactoid purpura, and nonspecific ulcerative colitis, must be differentiated from amebiasis. Schistosomiasis, balantidiasis, regional enteritis, and tuberculous enteritis must be distinguished from acute or chronic amebiasis.

Other causes of chronic and recurrent diarrhea also need to be considered, eg, sprue and malabsorption syndromes.

Complications & Sequelae

Complications may be generally classified as alimentary or extra-alimentary. Acute dysentery may result in perforation of the bowel and peritonitis. Granulomatous proliferations (amebomas) are extremely rare in children.

Amebic hepatitis following amebic colitis consists of hepatic enlargement and tenderness in the absence of demonstrable abscesses. Liver function tests may be only slightly abnormal.

Amebic liver abscess is usually solitary and in the right lobe. Fever, chills, hepatic enlargement, and tenderness are usually present but may be absent in debilitated children. Diagnosis may be readily made with CT scanning, ultrasonography, or radionuclide scanning. Rarely, such abscesses rupture into the peritoneum, pleura, lungs, or pericardium. Metastatic abscesses may occur in the lungs, brain, or spleen. Cutaneous and genital lesions are extremely rare with this disease.

Treatment

A. Specific Measures: Several antiamebic drugs are available, but no drug is consistently effective in eradicating infection in 100% of cases. Moreover, drugs vary in their effect against trophozoites or cysts in the intestinal lumen, in the tissues of the intestinal wall, and in the liver and other organs.

1. Amebic dysentery—Several drugs are available for relief of symptoms and eradication of infection. From among the regimens suggested below, any one may be chosen. Paromomycin is better tolerated than metronidazole and may be preferable in young children unless the disease is severe.

a. Metronidazole is given orally in the following dosage for 10 days: 35–50 mg/kg/d in 3 divided doses, up to a maximum of 2250 mg/d. ***Caution:*** Metronidazole has been shown to be carcinogenic in rodents and mutagenic in bacteria; nevertheless, it is the best single drug currently available for treating invasive amebiasis.

b. Paromomycin, a nonabsorbable antibiotic, given orally in a dosage of 25–30 mg/kg/d in 3 divided doses for 5–10 days, is also usually effective.

c. Emetine hydrochloride or the less toxic dehydroemetine should be used only in life-threatening dysentery. The dosage is 1 mg (emetine) or 1.5 mg (dehydroemetine)/kg/d intramuscularly for up to 5 days. ***Caution:*** Toxicity may result in peripheral neuritis or myocarditis.

d. Diloxanide furoate, 20 mg/kg/d in 3 divided oral doses for 10 days, should also be given to all patients with invasive amebiasis (amebic dysentery, amebic liver abscess, and extragastrointestinal amebiasis). Although metronidazole and dehydroemetine kill *E histolytica* in tissue, diloxanide furoate is the most effective luminal amebicide. Diloxanide furoate is safer and more effective than iodoquinol, which it should replace. Diloxanide furoate should also be given to asymptomatic passers of *E histolytica* cysts. Such treatment prevents recurrences and breaks the cycle of transmission.

2. Amebic liver abscess—Metronidazole or the combination of dehydroemetine (or emetine) and chloroquine phosphate is effective. Most amebic liver abscesses respond to treatment with metronidazole alone with or without needle aspiration. Occasionally, metronidazole therapy seems to fail, and severe illness and a poor response are indications for combined therapy with dehydroemetine (or emetine) and chloroquine phosphate. The dosage of chloroquine is 10 mg/kg once daily for 21 days.

Indications for aspiration of an amebic liver abscess are failure of signs and symptoms to remit with drug therapy alone; persistent localized pain and tenderness (especially when accompanied by referred shoulder pain); a large abscess that results in a markedly elevated diaphragm; and a palpable local mass with impending rupture. A slow response to metronidazole can be accelerated dramatically when a large abscess is drained by needle aspiration.

The most frequent complication of amebic liver abscess is extrahepatic rupture. Rupture into the pericardial sac requires emergency surgical treatment to relieve tamponade. In contrast, neither pleural nor peritoneal ruptures are in themselves indications for surgery unless bacterial superinfection intervenes. If pleural effusion is present, a diagnostic thoracentesis should be performed. Unless the pleural fluid is positive for bacteria on Gram's stain or culture, a thoracostomy tube is unnecessary and metronidazole therapy alone suffices.

3. Chronic amebiasis—Chronic intestinal infection with continued excretion of cysts should be treated to prevent hepatic amebiasis and relapsing amebic colitis. Diloxanide furoate is the most effective drug for asymptomatic infection (cyst passers) with *E histolytica* (see above).

B. General Measures: For follow-up, a diligent examination of 3 fecal specimens collected on alternate days should be done to make sure that infection has been eradicated in all treated cases.

Prognosis

With prompt diagnosis and adequate treatment, if complications can be avoided, the prognosis is good. In ruptured liver abscesses and in brain abscesses, the prognosis is poor. Rupture of an amebic liver abscess into the pericardial sac is frequently fatal.

Adams ED, MacLeod IN: Invasive amebiasis. 1. Amebic dysentery and its complications. 2. Amebic liver abscess and its complications. *Medicine* 1977;**56:**315, 325.

Dykes AC et al: Extraintestinal amebiasis in infancy: Report of three patients and epidemiologic investigations of their families. *Pediatrics* 1980;**65:**799.

Greaney GC, Reynolds TB, Donovan AJ: Ruptured amebic liver abscess. *Arch Surg* 1985;**120:**555.

Harrison HR, Crowe CP, Fulginiti VA: Amebic liver abscess in children: Clinical and epidemiologic features. *Pediatrics* 1979;**64:**923.

Katzenstein D, Rickerson V, Braude A: New concepts of amebic liver abscess derived from hepatic imaging, serodiagnosis, and hepatic enzymes in 67 consecutive cases in San Diego. *Medicine* 1982;**61:**237.

Martinez-Palomo A, Martinez-Baez M: Selective primary health care: Strategies for control of disease in the developing world. 10. Amebiasis. *Rev Infect Dis* 1983;**5:**1093.

Merritt RJ et al: Spectrum of amebiasis in children. *Am J Dis Child* 1982;**136:**785.

Thompson JE Jr, Forlenza S, Verma R: Amebic liver abscess: A therapeutic approach. *Rev Infect Dis* 1985;**7:**171.

Wolfe MS: Treatment of intestinal protozoan infections. *Med Clin North Am* 1982;**66:**707.

DIARRHEA ASSOCIATED WITH *DIENTAMOEBA FRAGILIS*

The pathogenicity of *Dientamoeba fragilis* remains controversial. Most would agree that the diagnosis of diarrhea due to *D fragilis* must be one of exclusion, when other recognized intestinal pathogens cannot be found. Symptoms that have been ascribed to *D fragilis* infection include abdominal pain, diarrhea, flatulence, nausea, anorexia, vomiting, and fatigue. Iodoquinol, 30 mg/kg/d in 3 divided doses for 21 days, has been used with reported success. Given the potential toxicity of therapy and the usual mild nature of the illness, *D fragilis* infection should not be treated routinely.

Spencer MJ, Garcia LS, Chapin MR: *Dientamoeba fragilis:* An intestinal pathogen in children? *Am J Dis Child* 1979;**133:**390.

Turner JA: Giardiasis and infections with *Dientamoeba fragilis. Pediatr Clin North Am* 1985;**32:**865.

PRIMARY AMEBIC MENINGOENCEPHALITIS

Essentials of Diagnosis

Naegleria:

- Upper respiratory syndrome followed by rapidly progressing, usually fatal meningoencephalitis.
- Generally healthy young persons with a history of swimming in soil-contaminated water 3–7 days prior to onset.
- Amebas with large central karyosome in fresh wet mount slide of uncentrifuged cerebrospinal fluid. Can be cultured in Stamm's medium.

Hartmannella-Acanthamoeba (H-A):

- Variable clinical picture, sometimes with multiple organ involvement.
- More insidious onset of severe meningoencephalitis.
- History of preexisting debilitating disease (metabolic, infectious, or malignant), an immunosuppressed state, or trauma to skin, mucous membranes, and eye.

General Considerations

Beginning in 1965, free-living soil- and water-inhabiting amebas of 2 distinct genera were recognized as capable of producing fatal purulent meningoencephalitis. The smaller of the 2, *Naegleria* (8–15 μm), appears to penetrate the posterior nasopharynx, entering the cranium via the cribriform plate. Its higher incidence in children and young adults may reflect their increased exposure through fresh water swimming and possibly an immunity in older persons based on prior undiagnosed infections. The cysts of *Naegleria* are not destroyed even by 10 ppm of residual chlorine in water but are susceptible to a 0.7% concentration of NaCl. *Naegleria* may, under adverse environmental conditions, develop 4–6 flagella transiently.

Acanthamoeba (15–45 μm) does not produce flagella but does possess tapered hyaline projections from its ovoid surface. Both genera are uninucleate, with a large distinguishing central nucleolus. The mechanism by which *Acanthamoeba* enters the central nervous system is unclear. Infection has followed skin or mucous membrane trauma in which initial induration disappeared only to be replaced by multiple organ granulomas and eventual meningoencephalitis. Epidemiologic data for both organisms are far from complete.

Clinical Findings

A. Symptoms and Signs: *Naegleria* infection has been almost invariably fatal within a week from the appearance of central nervous system signs. Presentation is frequently with high fever, severe frontal headache, and nausea and vomiting, although the history may include a prior episode of upper respiratory tract infection. Mental signs include stupor, coma, and convulsions followed by death. Patients with *Acanthamoeba* infections have presented with a variety of clinical pictures, including chronic nodular, granulomatous disease of the skin, kidneys, adrenals, pancreas, and brain. Abscesses and hydrocephalus have also been found in cases of *Acanthamoeba* infection. The amebas themselves produce little exudate in the immediate vicinity but leave behind as they progress a trail of severely lysed and necrotic tissue.

B. Laboratory Findings: Laboratory identification can be made by direct wet mounts of cerebrospinal fluid or nasal smears, antiserum staining of fixed tissue or cerebrospinal fluid, Wright's stain of the sediment from centrifuged cerebrospinal fluid, or cultures on special media.

Differential Diagnosis

Primary amebic meningoencephalitis caused by *Naegleria* has been likened to meningococcal meningitis in its rapid progression and initial upper respiratory symptoms. *Acanthamoeba,* on the other hand, more closely resembles chronic mycotic disease of the brain.

Prevention

Amebic meningoencephalitis appears to be a relatively rare disease, and although it has occurred in time-place clusters of more than one case, its appearance is erratic. Prevention at present would seem to depend upon maintenance of clean swimming pools and education of young people about the danger of swimming anywhere in warm stagnant water. Persons with a history of trauma to the skin, mouth, or eye and those with debilitating disease or who are immunosuppressed for any reason should be suspect if suggestive peripheral lesions or central nervous system signs appear.

Treatment

Animal experiments and the outcome of treated cases suggest that the best chance of success in treatment of *Naegleria* rests in early use of intravenous amphotericin B (1 mg/kg/d), with consideration of intrathecal or intraventricular use (0.1 mg on alternate days)—or both—if improvement does not occur within 48 hours. Some clinicians have used intravenous and intrathecal miconazole and oral rifampin concurrently with amphotericin B. *Acanthamoeba* appears to be sensitive to sulfadiazine given intravenously, although in vitro tests have been less encouraging. There are 3.65 mmol of sodium per gram of sulfadiazine, and this should be borne in mind in planning electrolyte management. Since treatment must be instituted at the earliest possible time, it is best to use both amphotericin B and sulfadiazine pending positive identification of the organism. Attention must be given to supportive care and the prevention of complicating nosocomial infection.

Prognosis

In spite of early successes, the general outlook, especially in infections with *Naegleria,* is grave. The patient must present early, and the diagnosis must be suspected and treatment started before the process becomes irreversible. With *Acanthamoeba* infection of the central nervous system, the time factor may still be critical and the history more difficult to interpret.

Benson RL et al: Cerebrospinal fluid centrifuge analysis in primary amebic meningoencephalitis due to *Naegleria fowleri. Arch Pathol Lab Med* 1985;**109:**668.

John DT: Primary amebic meningoencephalitis and the biology of *Naegleria fowleri. Annu Rev Microbiol* 1982;**36:**101.

Seidel JS: Primary amebic meningoencephalitis. *Pediatr Clin North Am* 1985;**32:**881.

Seidel JS et al: Successful treatment of primary amebic meningoencephalitis. *N Engl J Med* 1982;**306:**346.

Stevens AR et al: Primary amoebic meningoencephalitis: A report of two cases and antibiotic and immunologic studies. *J Infect Dis* 1981;**143:**193.

GIARDIASIS

Giardiasis is the most common protozoan infection of the intestines in people in temperate climates. The number of cases of giardiasis in day-care centers is increasing, with some centers reporting prevalence rates as high as 50% in children 6 months to 3 years of age in comparison with rates of less than 5% in age- and neighborhood-matched controls who do not attend day-care centers. Children with symptomatic or asymptomatic infections may infect family members.

After ingestion of the infective cyst form of *Giardia lamblia,* many people develop few or no symptoms. In others, acute symptoms of diarrhea and abdominal cramps occur 1–3 weeks after exposure. The diarrhea often lasts more than 7 days; it may persist intermittently for months and be accompanied by malabsorption, foul flatulence, bloating, and abdominal discomfort.

The organisms usually reside in the duodenum and jejunum. The diagnostic feature is the presence of the organisms in duodenal aspirate or in fresh stools; vegetative forms in diarrheic stools; and cysts in formed stools. The frequency and the consistency of stools appear to have no relation to the number of organisms seen in the stool specimen. Although examination of several fecal samples obtained on alternate days usually establishes the diagnosis of *G lamblia,* the string test (Entero-Test) for examination of duodenal contents is a simple and useful alternative to collecting and examining multiple stool specimens. A permanent stain such as trichrome is an important tool for the diagnosis of *G lamblia* and should be included in the processing of any diarrheal stool. The most sensitive method of diagnosis is to examine smears and sections of upper small intestinal biopsy for trophozoites that are pear-shaped with 4–5 pairs of notable flagella. There are 2 nuclei with central karyosomes and 2 parabasal bodies, altogether resembling the caricature of a face. They are 12–15 μm in diameter. The cysts are elliptic, with a clear wall and 4 nuclei with karyosomes. Excretion of the cysts is responsible for spread of infection.

Giardiasis must be differentiated from tuberculous enteritis, steatorrhea due to other causes, and chronic amebiasis. Giardiasis may coexist with any of these diseases, and a therapeutic trial may help to clarify the role of *Giardia* in the total clinical picture.

For children 5 years of age and under, furazolidone is the drug of choice. A liquid preparation (50 mg/15 mL) of furazolidone is available; the dosage is 6–8 mg/kg given in 4 divided doses for 7–10 days. Quinacrine is preferred for older children; the dosage is 2 mg/kg orally 3 times daily for 5–10 days. Alternatively, metronidazole,* 5 mg/kg orally 3 times daily for 5–10 days, will usually clear the infection. Outside the USA, tinidazole in a single oral dose of 50 mg/kg (maximum, 2 g) has been shown to be highly effective for treatment of giardiasis.

When an outbreak of giardiasis is suspected in a day-care center, an assessment of infection rates by age, room, and disease status (symptomatic versus asymptomatic) should be performed. Stools from symptomatic family members should also be examined. Although there is agreement that all symptomatic individuals should be treated, the role of therapy for asymptomatic children to prevent spread requires further study.

Black RE et al: Giardiasis in day-care centers: Evidence of person-to-person transmission. *Pediatrics* 1977;**60:**486.

The Child Day-Care Infectious Diseases Study Group: Public health considerations of infectious diseases in child day-care centers. *J Pediatr* 1984;**105:**683.

Craft JC, Murphy T, Nelson JD: Furazolidone and quinacrine: Comparative study of therapy for giardiasis in children. *Am J Dis Child* 1981;**135:**164.

Kavousi S: Giardiasis in infancy and childhood: A prospective study of 160 cases with comparison of quinacrine (Atabrine) and metronidazole (Flagyl). *Am J Trop Med Hyg* 1979;**28:**19.

Murphy TV, Nelson JD: Five versus ten days' therapy with furazolidone for giardiasis. *Am J Dis Child* 1983;**137:**267.

Smith PD: Pathophysiology and immunology of giardiasis. *Annu Rev Med* 1985;**36:**295.

Sokol RJ, Lichtenstein PK, Farrell MK: Quinacrine hydrochloride-induced yellow discoloration of the skin in children. *Pediatrics* 1982;**69:**232.

Speelman P: Single-dose tinidazole for the treatment of giardiasis. *Antimicrob Agents Chemother* 1985;**27:**227.

Thornton SA et al: Comparison of methods for identification of *Giardia lamblia. Am J Clin Pathol* 1983;**80:**858.

CRYPTOSPORIDIOSIS

Cryptosporidium is a protozoan parasite belonging to the same family as *Isospora, Sarcocystis,* and *Toxoplasma.* Primarily an animal pathogen, it also invades the microvilli of epithelial cells and leads to intractable diarrhea in immunocompromised patients, especially those with acquired immunodeficiency syndrome (AIDS). In normal hosts, *Cryptosporidium* can cause a self-limited diarrhea similar to that of giardiasis. It occurs in travelers, in attendees and personnel of day-care centers, and sporadically in household and hospital clusters. Numerous techniques have been used to detect *Cryptosporidium;* the most effective appears to be the modified acid-fast staining method performed directly on a fecal smear or on concentrated 10% formalin-preserved feces. Therapy with spiramycin can be tried, but proof of efficacy is lacking. Fluid and electrolyte therapy should suffice in immunocompetent children.

Navin TR, Juranek DD: Cryptosporidiosis: Clinical, epidemiologic, and parasitologic review. *Rev Infect Dis* 1984;**6:**313.

Taylor JP et al: Cryptosporidiosis outbreak in a day-care center. *Am J Dis Child* 1985;**139:**1023.

Wolfson JS et al: Cryptosporidiosis in immunocompetent patients. *N Engl J Med* 1985;**312:**1278.

BALANTIDIASIS

Dysentery due to *Balantidium coli* infection is far less common than amebiasis. The clinical picture may mimic that of amebic dysentery. It is believed that pigs are the main source of infection. Ingested cysts result in colonic infection by trophozoites. *B coli* usually will live free in the lumen of the intestine; rarely, it may cause ulceration in the colon. In severe infection, the entire lower bowel may be affected.

Patients may be asymptomatic or may have symptoms that mimic those of acute amebic colitis, eg, diarrhea with or without blood and mucus. Slight leukocytosis may be present, and mild eosinophilia may be present.

Examination of fresh feces discloses motile trophozoites, ciliated ovoid bodies approximately 100 × 50 μm with a kidney-shaped macronucleus, a micronucleus, and several vacuoles. The cysts are about 40 × 60 μm and contain most of the internal features of the trophozoite.

Intestinal perforation is the major complication. Liver lesions do not occur.

Traditionally, tetracycline, 10 mg/kg orally 4 times daily for 10 days, has been used to treat balantidiasis. An alternative is iodoquinol, 30–40 mg/kg/d orally in 3 divided doses for 20 days. Metronidazole, 5 mg/kg orally 3 times daily for 10 days, has also been successful.

TOXOPLASMOSIS

Essentials of Diagnosis

- Congenital toxoplasmosis: Fever, rash, hepatosplenomegaly, chorioretinitis, hydrocephalus or microcephalus, and mental retardation (in various combinations).

* For ***Caution,*** see p 901 under amebiasis.

- Acquired toxoplasmosis: Fever, rash, lymphadenopathy, chorioretinitis, encephalitis, and myocarditis (in various combinations). Chronic infection may be afebrile and associated only with lymphocytosis.
- In both cases, the demonstration of *Toxoplasma gondii* or serologic evidence of infection is required for confirmation.

General Considerations

Toxoplasma gondii is a protozoan parasite of various animals and humans and has a life cycle similar to that of the coccidian parasite *Isospora*. The tachyzoite is crescentic, 4–7 μm long, and has a single nucleus. In tissues, the parasites appear intracellularly, often in small clusters. True cysts with large numbers of bradyzoites form in various tissues but are particularly common in the brain. Ingestion of tissue cysts (eg, cats eating mice with infected brains; humans eating infected meat) is a form of transmission.

Toxoplasmosis may be congenital or acquired. Congenital toxoplasmosis is acquired in utero from the mother. Most acquired infections, including those of pregnant women, remain clinically unrecognized.

The main modes of transmission to humans are handling and eating raw or undercooked meat (especially lamb, pork, and beef) and contact with oocyst-containing feces (in litter pans and soil) from cats infected with *T gondii*. Recent work has established that the cat and other felines are probably the normal final hosts and the only ones in which an intestinal *Isospora*-like stage is found, with infective oocysts being passed in the feces.

Clinical Findings

A. Congenital Toxoplasmosis: The infected newborn may manifest skin rash (hemorrhagic or otherwise), hepatosplenomegaly, and jaundice. Thrombocytopenia is common. Some infants exhibit central nervous system disease during the first several weeks of life. Hydrocephalus, microcephalus, cerebrospinal fluid pleocytosis and elevated protein, intracranial calcifications, and mental retardation occur in various combinations. Chorioretinitis is common. The systemic manifestations may occur alone or be accompanied or followed by encephalitic features depending upon the stage in utero when the transplacental infection took place.

The organisms may be visualized in or isolated (usually in mice) from infected tissues or cerebrospinal fluid. The indirect fluorescent antibody (IFA) test has largely replaced the Sabin-Feldman dye test for the serologic diagnosis of toxoplasmosis, because it is relatively easy to perform. Mothers with high IFA test titers (1:512 or more) and a positive IgM-IFA test should be highly suspect for recently acquired infection. In the absence of a placental leak, a positive (1:2 or more) IgM-IFA test in the newborn is firm evidence for congenital toxoplasmosis.

B. Acquired Toxoplasmosis: Symptomatic acquired infection, though rare, may occur at any age. The clinical manifestations include fever and the following features in varying combinations: generalized lymphadenopathy, muscular pain, maculopapular rash, hepatosplenomegaly, encephalitis, chorioretinitis (usually unilateral), pneumonia, and myocarditis. The course may be short or may extend over several weeks. The diagnosis may be confirmed by the demonstration of the organisms or by serology. Titers of greater than 1:1000 in the indirect fluorescent antibody test suggest acute infection. Biopsy material rarely shows or yields trophozoites.

C. Toxoplasmosis in the Immunocompromised Host: *T gondii* is an important treatable cause of illness and death in immunocompromised patients, especially those with malignant lymphomas, leukemia, and acquired immunodeficiency syndrome (AIDS). Acute necrotizing encephalitis, myocarditis, and pneumonitis are the most frequent findings at necropsy. In over 50% of cases, there are manifestations of central nervous system disorders, including seizures, impaired consciousness, and motor abnormalities.

Differential Diagnosis

Congenital toxoplasmosis may be mistaken for hepatitis due to other causes, septicemia, cytomegalovirus infection, and maternal rubella syndrome. The acquired form must be differentiated from viral encephalitis, viral myocarditis, infectious mononucleosis, and lymphoreticular and lymphoproliferative diseases. Because of the lymphoid proliferation, it may be difficult to differentiate lymphoid toxoplasmosis from lymphosarcoma even on biopsy.

Demonstration of the trophozoites of *T gondii* in tissue or body fluids establishes the diagnosis of acute toxoplasmosis. In the absence of a histologic diagnosis, a 4-fold change in titer is required for serologic confirmation, owing to the prevalence of antibodies to *T gondii* in the general population.

Complications

Nephritis and nephrotic syndrome have recently been recognized as complications of both acquired and congenital toxoplasmosis.

Prevention

Toxoplasma infection acquired during pregnancy in previously seronegative women can result in congenital infection of the fetus or in spontaneous abortion. To prevent primary infection during pregnancy, pregnant women should be instructed to avoid touching mucous membranes of the mouth and eye after handling raw meat, to wash hands thoroughly after handling raw meat, to cook meat to 66 °C or greater, to wash fruits and vegetables before consumption, and to avoid contact with cat feces (eg, wear gloves when handling litter boxes or when gardening).

Treatment

A combination of pyrimethamine and a sulfonamide (sulfadiazine or trisulfapyrimidines) is recommended for 3–4 weeks in suspected or proved cases. Pyrimethamine is given orally in doses of 0.5 mg/kg twice daily in infants and 1 mg/kg/d in older children. Sulfadiazine or trisulfapyrimidines are given orally in a dosage of 100 mg/kg/d in 4 divided doses. Both of these drugs may cause gastrointestinal upsets that may necessitate interruption of treatment.

Pyrimethamine may cause leukopenia, thrombocytopenia, and, very rarely, agranulocytosis; frequent blood counts should be performed and the drug stopped if the counts fall very low. Folinic acid, 1–3 mg intramuscularly once a week, may be given to combat the drug's toxicity.

The neurologic damage that occurs in congenital toxoplasmosis does not subside after treatment. In acquired toxoplasmosis, in the absence of encephalitis and myocarditis, one must use discretion in instituting potentially dangerous therapy. The infection is usually self-limited.

In chorioretinitis, especially in the acquired form, a course of corticosteroids should be given along with antitoxoplasmosis drugs, eg, prednisone, 1 mg/kg orally initially and then reduced gradually. The corticosteroid may be stopped in 3–4 weeks and anti-infective therapy continued until activity of the eye lesion abates. For recurrence of eye lesions, corticosteroids may be given alone.

Anderson SE, Remington JS: The diagnosis of toxoplasmosis. *South Med J* 1975;**68:**1433.

Desmonts G, Couvreur J: Congenital toxoplasmosis: A prospective study of 378 pregnancies. *N Engl J Med* 1974;**290:**1110.

Frenkel JK: Toxoplasmosis. *Pediatr Clin North Am* 1985; **32:**917.

Mahmoud AAF, Warren KS: Algorithms in the diagnosis and management of exotic diseases. 20. Toxoplasmosis. *J Infect Dis* 1977;**135:**493.

Masur H et al: Outbreak of toxoplasmosis and documentation of acquired retinochoroiditis. *Am J Med* 1978;**64:**396.

Stagno S et al: An outbreak of toxoplasmosis linked to cats. *Pediatrics* 1980;**65:**706.

Swartzberg JE, Remington JS: Transmission of *Toxoplasma*. *Am J Dis Child* 1975;**129:**777.

Teutsch SM et al: Epidemic toxoplasmosis associated with infected cats. *N Engl J Med* 1979;**300:**695.

Townsend JJ et al: Acquired toxoplasmosis: A neglected cause of treatable nervous system disease. *Arch Neurol* 1975; **32:**335.

Wilson CB, Remington JS: What can be done to prevent congenital toxoplasmosis? *Am J Obstet Gynecol* 1980;**138:**357.

PNEUMOCYSTIS CARINII PNEUMONIA

Acute pulmonary disease caused by *Pneumocystis carinii* is characterized by fever, tachypnea, cough, dyspnea, and cyanosis. It occurs in immunocompromised patients, including those with acquired immunodeficiency syndrome (AIDS), and malnourished or premature infants. Chest radiograph discloses a bilateral diffuse pneumonitis. Arterial blood gases show hypoxemia and normal or low P_{CO_2} and a pH that is increased to the alkaline range.

Specific diagnosis requires demonstration of *P carinii* in secretions or tissue from the infected lungs. An open lung biopsy by a standard surgical procedure gives the best specimen for diagnostic studies. The characteristic round or ovoid cysts, 6–8 μm in diameter, may also be found in pulmonary secretions obtained by tracheobronchial aspiration or percutaneous transthoracic needle aspiration. Methenamine silver nitrate and toluidine blue O stains both provide marked contrast between the organisms and host cells, thus permitting easy recognition. The developmental stages and internal structure of *P carinii* can best be delineated with a polychrome methylene blue, Giemsa, or Wright stain.

Because the rate of adverse reactions to therapy with trimethoprim-sulfamethoxazole is high in patients with AIDS, they may require therapy with pentamidine, 4 mg/kg/d intravenously slowly over 60 minutes for 14–21 days. In other patients, trimethoprim-sulfamethoxazole has now replaced pentamidine as the drug of choice. The therapeutic dosage schedule for established or suspected acute pneumonitis is 20 mg of trimethoprim and 100 mg of sulfamethoxazole per kilogram orally daily in 4 divided doses for 14–21 days. Trimethoprim-sulfamethoxazole has also been shown to be highly effective in preventing *P carinii* pneumonia in high-risk patients undergoing immunosuppressive and cytoxic therapy for acute leukemias and other forms of cancer. The dosages for chemoprophylaxis are 5 mg of trimethoprim and 25 mg of sulfamethoxazole per kilogram daily, given by mouth in 2 divided doses. The drug combination must be administered throughout the period of markedly increased susceptibility to be fully effective.

Recently, there has been further suggestive evidence that *P carinii* is communicable among immunosuppressed patients. Respiratory isolation has been recommended for patients with acute *P carinii* pneumonia until the end of therapy with trimethoprim-sulfamethoxazole.

Giebink GS et al: *Pneumocystis carinii* pneumonia in two Vietnamese refugee infants. *Pediatrics* 1976;**58:**115.

Hughes WT: *Pneumocystis carinii* pneumonia. *N Engl J Med* 1977;**297:**1381.

Hughes WT et al: Comparison of pentamidine isethionate and trimethoprim-sulfamethoxazole in the treatment of *Pneumocystis carinii* pneumonia. *J Pediatr* 1978;**92:**285.

Hughes WT et al: Successful chemoprophylaxis for *Pneumocystis carinii* pneumonitis. *N Engl J Med* 1977;**297:**1419.

Lau WK, Young LS, Remington JS: *Pneumocystis carinii* pneumonia: Diagnosis by examination of pulmonary secretions. *JAMA* 1976;**236:**2399.

Pifer LL et al: *Pneumocystis carinii* infection: Evidence for high prevalence in normal and immunosuppressed children. *Pediatrics* 1978;**61:**35.

Sands M, Kron MA, Brown RB: Pentamidine: A review. *Rev Infect Dis* 1985;**7:**625.

Singer C et al: *Pneumocystis carinii* pneumonia: A cluster of eleven cases. *Ann Intern Med* 1975;**82:**772.

LEISHMANIASIS

1. VISCERAL LEISHMANIASIS (Kala-Azar)

Essentials of Diagnosis

- High fever, remittent or intermittent—occasionally hectic.
- Splenomegaly and hepatomegaly; often lymphadenitis.
- Progressive anemia, leukopenia, and wasting.
- Demonstration of *Leishmania donovani* in smears of bone marrow or in splenic, hepatic, or lymph node aspirate.
- Positive formol-gel test, complement fixation test, or immunofluorescence test.

General Considerations

Leishmania donovani is a protozoan parasite transmitted by the sandfly (species of *Phlebotomus*) from human to human (India), from dogs to humans (Mediterranean region), or from various carnivores or rodents to humans (Sudan). Infantile kala-azar is common in the Mediterranean area; in India, older children are more susceptible; and in other parts of the world, leishmaniasis is primarily an adult disease, probably varying with the timing and intensity of exposure.

The parasites infect and multiply in the reticuloendothelial cells of the spleen, liver, bone marrow, and lymph nodes. In the human body, they exist as ovoid bodies 2–4 μm in diameter. With Leishman's or Giemsa's stain, they exhibit a round nucleus and a rod-shaped kinetoplast enclosed in faintly bluish cytoplasm. Appropriate touch-preparation smears show these organisms intracellularly or extracellularly, though the normal site of infection is the macrophage. In the sandfly as well as in artificial (NNN) medium, the parasites exist in a flagellated form, the promastigote.

Clinical Findings

A. Symptoms and Signs: In infants and children, the onset is usually acute, with high fever and gastrointestinal upsets. The spleen enlarges rapidly. There may also be enlargement of the liver (though to a lesser degree) and lymphadenopathy.

In older children, the illness is usually less severe and more prolonged. Patients remain febrile over long periods, develop hyperpigmentation, lose weight, and become progressively anemic and wasted.

Hypopigmented patches and nodular lesions of varying severity may occur on the face, forearms, and thighs in patients a year or longer after treatment for visceral leishmaniasis. This condition, called dermal leishmanoid or post-kal-azar dermal leishmaniasis, has been reported in India and Africa. The nodular lesions harbor numerous parasites.

B. Laboratory Findings: The diagnosis is confirmed by the presence of *L donovani* in smears of bone marrow or splenic or lymph node aspirate. Rarely, blood smears may reveal the organisms. Blood or bone marrow may be cultured on NNN medium to prove the diagnosis. In chronic cases, a drop of commercial formalin coagulates about 1 mL of serum at room temperature (aldehyde or formol-gel test). Although not species-specific, a direct agglutination test can provide serologic evidence of leishmanial infection. The test is available through the Centers for Disease Control, Atlanta, GA 30333.

Leukopenia is common and often quite marked. Thrombocytopenia (with skin hemorrhages) also is common. Anemia and markedly elevated serum gamma globulins are also characteristic.

Differential Diagnosis

Febrile illnesses associated with splenomegaly, such as infective endocarditis, typhoid fever, brucellosis, lymphoproliferative and lymphoreticular diseases, trypanosomiasis, schistosomiasis, and malaria, must be differentiated from kala-azar. Dermal leishmanoid simulates leprosy, yaws, or lupus vulgaris.

Treatment

Correction of nutritional deficiencies (including anemia) and treatment of complicating infections should be done along with specific therapy.

The drugs used in kala-azar are a pentavalent antimony compound (stibogluconate, or antimony sodium gluconate) and pentamidine isethionate.

Indian leishmaniasis is easily controlled by treatment, but in Africa the response to specific treatment has been less satisfactory.

The antimony compound may be given intramuscularly or by slow intravenous injection. Antimony sodium gluconate is given in doses of 10 mg/kg/d for 6 daily injections. It may cause vomiting, diarrhea, and muscle cramps; temporary interruption of therapy may be necessary.

Pentamidine may be given intramuscularly in doses of 3 mg/kg daily for 10 days. This drug is useful where the disease is resistant to antimony compounds.

For the nodular type of dermal leishmanoid, a course of a pentavalent antimony compound must be given.

Prognosis

In untreated cases, death usually occurs as a result of bacterial complications such as pneumonia.

Chance ML: Leishmaniasis. *Br Med J* 1981;**283:**1245.

Evans T et al: American visceral leishmaniasis (kala-azar). *West J Med* 1985;**142:**777.

Naik SR et al: Kala-azar in north-western India: A study of 24 patients. *Trans R Soc Trop Med Hyg* 1979;**73:**61.

2. CUTANEOUS LEISHMANIASIS (Oriental Sore)

Leishmania tropica is morphologically identical to *Leishmania donovani*. The vector is also the sandfly, but of a different species from the vectors of kala-azar. Cutaneous leishmaniasis has been reported from all inhabited continents. Endemic foci are mostly in India, the Asian countries west of India, and North Africa. Russian investigators recognize 2 forms: the dry type, in urban areas, spread from human to human; and the moist type, in rural areas, transmitted from rodents to humans. An area of autochthonous transmission has been identified in south central Texas.

The lesions develop at the sites of sandfly bites after an incubation period of weeks to months. They begin as itchy papules and develop into granulomatous ulcers with scabs. The ulcers gradually extend, and satellite lesions occasionally appear. These lesions occur mostly on the face and limbs, especially in children. The lesions occasionally remain atypical with no ulceration. The onset may or may not be accompanied by fever. After several months, the lesions heal slowly, leaving behind depressed and deforming scars.

In endemic areas, the diagnosis is suspected on clinical grounds and confirmed by demonstration of the causative organisms in smears or fluid aspirated from the margins of the lesions. Such specimens may also be cultured on NNN medium.

The leishmanin skin test is positive in all cases except in anergic individuals.

Discrete ulcers may be cleaned and treated with systemic antibacterial therapy for secondary infections and allowed to heal, ensuring immunity and avoiding potentially toxic drugs. In cases of multiple or extensive ulceration and lesions on the face, provide antibacterial therapy plus specific therapy with a pentavalent antimony compound as for visceral leishmaniasis except that 10 days of daily injections are required to treat cutaneous leishmaniasis of the Old World.

The prognosis is good except for deforming scars, which can be minimized by early treatment.

Al-Taqi M, Behbehani K: Cutaneous leishmaniasis in Kuwait. *Ann Trop Med Parasitol* 1980;**74:**495.

Ridley DS: The pathogenesis of cutaneous leishmaniasis. *Trans R Soc Trop Med Hyg* 1979;**73:**150.

3. MUCOCUTANEOUS LEISHMANIASIS

Except for a few reports, most cases of mucocutaneous *Leishmania* infection are reported from South America. Several different species are now recognized and cause widely varying clinical manifestations. *Leishmania braziliensis* causes espundia, the most destructive form of the disease; *Leishmania mexicana* causes chiclero ulcer in Mexico, Guatemala, and Honduras; *Leishmania peruviana* causes uta in Guyana, French Guiana, and Peru; and several other forms have recently been described. *L braziliensis* is morphologically identical with *Leishmania donovani* and is also transmitted by sandflies. The chronic ulcerative lesions may be indistinguishable from those of oriental sore, or they may develop into destructive mucocutaneous lesions over the naso-oral regions. Healing is slow, and in untreated cases heavy scarring occurs. Lesions similar to oriental sore or punched-out ulcers may occur on the face or limbs.

The diagnosis is confirmed by demonstration of *L braziliensis* at the margins of the ulcer. The leishmanin test is usually positive.

Treatment is similar to that of oriental sore and visceral leishmaniasis, with a pentavalent antimony compound; however, as many as 30 injections are required for refractory cases of cutaneous leishmaniasis of the New World.

Lainson R, Shaw JJ: Epidemiology and ecology of leishmaniasis in Latin-America. *Nature* 1978;**273:**595.

Oster CN et al: American cutaneous leishmaniasis: A comparison of three sodium stibogluconate treatment schedules. *Am J Trop Med Hyg* 1985;**34:**856.

Shaw PK et al: Autochthonous dermal leishmaniasis in Texas. *Am J Trop Med Hyg* 1976;**25:**788.

AFRICAN TRYPANOSOMIASIS (Sleeping Sickness)

Essentials of Diagnosis

- Trypanosome chancre and erythematous nodule at the site of fly bite.
- Fever, progressive anemia and debility, splenomegaly, lymphadenitis, skin rash.
- Changes in personality, disturbances of speech and gait, progressive apathy and somnolence, involuntary movements, and coma.
- Detection of trypanosomes in a wet blood film in rhodesiense infections and by lymph node puncture in gambiense infections.

General Considerations

Trypanosomiasis occurs in parts of tropical Africa. The more virulent Rhodesian form, caused by *Trypanosoma brucei rhodesiense,* occurs chiefly in East Africa, but the Gambian form, caused by *T brucei gambiense,* is more widespread. Both species are transmitted by the bites of tsetse flies (various species of *Glossina*). In human blood, the 2 are morphologically similar—actively motile, slender, wavy, spindlelike bodies with a central nucleus and a prominent flagellum, the trypomastigote stage. Variation in size and body form occurs, with both elongated and "stumpy" forms. This is apparently related to antigenic variation by the parasite and infectivity for the vector.

Gambian trypanosomiasis occurs more commonly in children than the Rhodesian form, except in epidemics of the latter.

Clinical Findings

A. Symptoms and Signs:

1. Rhodesian trypanosomiasis—During the first week, an erythematous, pruritic, and occasionally painful nodule appears at the site of the fly bite, which subsides in a few days. Some patients do not develop this reaction. Fever appears by the second week. It varies in intensity but occurs intermittently or continuously, accompanied by headache, muscular pain, tenderness, and transient skin rashes. Progressive splenomegaly and, to a lesser degree, hepatomegaly are common. Cervical, femoral, or axillary lymph nodes may become palpable. In a few months, weakness, lassitude, emaciation, personality changes, disturbances of speech and gait, and involuntary movements appear. Death may occur before the onset of the classic somnolence.

2. Gambian trypanosomiasis—The early and intermediate stages are similar to those of the Rhodesian form, but the progression is slower. Lymphadenitis is more prominent, especially of the posterior cervical glands (Winterbottom's sign). Central nervous system involvement sets in after several months to years. The child becomes very lethargic and sleeps most of the time. Severe emaciation and edema are common. Terminally, coma is followed by death.

B. Laboratory Findings: A wet or stained thick blood smear should be examined for trypanosomes. Repeated examinations are sometimes necessary. Bone marrow aspirate or, preferably, a lymph node aspirate is more likely to be positive in the early and intermediate stages. In the late stages, cerebrospinal fluid, especially after centrifugation, may exhibit the organisms. Cerebrospinal fluid pleocytosis and elevated protein are usually found. Even in the absence of gross central nervous system symptoms and signs, pleocytosis and elevated protein are evidences of central nervous system invasion.

Anemia, elevated erythrocyte sedimentation rate and serum gamma globulins, and hypoproteinemia are some of the accompanying nonspecific features.

Differential Diagnosis

Malaria is not usually difficult to distinguish, but kala-azar may at times be mistaken for trypanosomiasis. Fever, splenomegaly, and lymphadenitis may occur also in lymphoreticular and lymphoproliferative diseases and should be differentiated from trypanosomiasis in endemic areas. Meningitis, especially tuberculous and cryptococcal, and intracranial neoplasms may mimic the central nervous system manifestations of this disease.

Treatment

A. Specific Measures:

1. Suramin—Suramin is the drug of choice in the early and intermediate hemolymphatic stages without central nervous system involvement in both the Rhodesian and Gambian forms. It should be given as fresh 10% aqueous solution intravenously in the following dosage: Give a test dose of 20–50 mg with facilities for resuscitation in the event of severe reaction. Continue with 5 doses of 20 mg/kg on days 1, 3, 7, 14, and 21. The appearance of heavy and persistent proteinuria or dermatitis is an indication for discontinuing therapy.

2. Pentamidine isethionate—This is an alternative drug that may be given in doses of 4 mg/kg intramuscularly daily for 10 days. It may induce hypotension or hypoglycemia. It is less effective in the Rhodesian form than the Gambian form.

Suramin and pentamidine do not penetrate the central nervous system, so that treatment with arsenicals is necessary when the brain is involved.

3. Melarsoprol—Melarsoprol, an arsenical, is the drug of choice in stages with central nervous system involvement, especially in patients with average nutrition and little renal or hepatic damage. It is given intravenously as 3.6% solution in propylene glycol, 3.6 mg/kg on alternate days for 3 injections. In severe central nervous system disease, the course may be repeated after 3 weeks. Any evidence of arsenical toxicity such as mental confusion, encephalopathy, or peripheral neuritis should immediately be treated with dimercaprol (BAL). Headache, vomiting, and proteinuria are indications for discontinuing therapy.

4. Tryparsamide—Tryparsamide, another arsenical, is less toxic than melarsoprol but may cause optic atrophy. It is more effective against *T b gambiense* in the central nervous system than against *T b rhodesiense*. The dose is 20–40 mg/kg intravenously given at weekly intervals for 10 injections. Treatment should be stopped at the appearance of the slightest symptom related to the eyes. In severe and late cases, the course may be repeated after a month.

During the treatment of central nervous system disease, suramin or pentamidine also should be given to eradicate parasites from the blood and reticuloendothelial system.

5. Difluoromethylornithine (DFMO)—DFMO has been used successfully in the treatment of late-stage *T b gambiense* disease. Therapy with doses of about 400 mg/kg/d for 5–6 weeks was associated with disappearance of parasites from cerebrospinal fluid, a decrease in cerebrospinal fluid leukocyte counts and protein concentrations, and reversal of clinical signs. Side effects included diarrhea, abdominal discomfort, and anemia. In early-stage disease, a dosage of about 200 mg/kg/d for 6 weeks appeared adequate and was tolerated well.

B. General Measures: When facilities are available, patients should be hospitalized for therapy. Concurrent infections and nutritional deficiencies should be adequately treated.

Prognosis

Spontaneous recovery occurs occasionally in early cases, and patients with early and intermediate disease do well with treatment. After the central nervous system has been invaded, the prognosis is less favorable. Untreated patients have an extremely high mortality rate; ie, death occurs within 1 year in Rhodesian and within 10 years in Gambian forms.

Greenwood BM, Whittle AC: The pathogenesis of sleeping sickness. *Trans R Soc Trop Med Hyg* 1980;**74:**716.

Haller L et al: Clinical and pathological aspects of human African trypanosomiasis *(Trypanosoma brucei gambiense)* with particular reference to reactive arsenical encephalopathy. *Am J Trop Med Hyg* 1986;**35:**94.

Molyneux DH: Selective primary health care: Strategies for control of disease in the developing world. 8. African trypanosomiasis. *Rev Infect Dis* 1983;**5:**945.

Olowe SA: A case of congenital trypanosomiasis in Lagos. *Trans R Soc Trop Med Hyg* 1975;**69:**57.

Robins-Browne RM, Schneider J, Metz J: Thrombocytopenia in trypanosomiasis. *Am J Trop Med Hyg* 1975;**24:**226.

Spencer HC Jr et al: Imported African trypanosomiasis in the United States. *Ann Intern Med* 1975;**82:**633.

Van Nieuwenhove S et al: Treatment of gambiense sleeping sickness in the Sudan with oral DFMO (DL-α-difluoromethylornithine), an inhibitor of ornithine decarboxylase: First field trial. *Trans R Soc Trop Med Hyg* 1985;**79:**692.

AMERICAN TRYPANOSOMIASIS (Chagas' Disease)

Essentials of Diagnosis

- Chagoma—an erythematous, painful nodule at the site of primary cutaneous infection.
- Unilateral conjunctivitis and palpebral and facial edema—"Romaña's sign."
- Fever, lymphadenitis, myocarditis, occasionally meningoencephalitis.
- Megaesophagus, megacolon.
- *Trypanosoma cruzi* in blood, bone marrow, or aspirates of lymph nodes or spleen.

General Considerations

Chagas' disease is confined to South and Central America, with the highest incidence in Brazil and Argentina. The causative agent, *Trypanosoma cruzi,* infects humans and various animals. It is transmitted through the feces of reduviid bugs—by rubbing feces in skin abrasions or the eye. The organisms multiply locally and invade blood and other tissues. Chagas' disease can also be transmitted by blood transfusions from donors with inapparent parasitemia. An estimated 25,000 cases of transfusion-induced disease occur annually in Brazil alone. Congenital Chagas' disease with pneumonitis has also been described.

Clinical Findings

A. Symptoms and Signs: Infants and children are frequently infected in endemic areas. In most cases, a transient lesion (chagoma) develops at the site of primary infection, characterized by an erythematous painful nodule. It is soon followed by local lymphadenitis, unilateral palpebral and facial edema, conjunctivitis, intermittent or continuous fever, generalized lymphadenitis, hepatosplenomegaly, and myocarditis (tachycardia, cardiomegaly, dysrhythmias, and cardiac failure). Occasionally, meningoencephalitis may occur.

In chronic cases, especially in older children and young children who survive the early stages, the main abnormality is myocardial damage. Damage to the myenteric nerve plexuses may result in megaesophagus and megacolon.

B. Laboratory Findings: In acute Chagas' disease, wet and Giemsa-stained blood smears should be examined for *T cruzi.* If they are negative, bone marrow and lymph node or splenic aspirate should be examined. Blood or other specimens may be inoculated into mice, rats, or guinea pigs or cultured in NNN medium. Another method, suitable only during the early, blood-borne phase of the disease, is to feed clean laboratory-grown bugs on patients and to look for the organisms in the bugs' feces after 3–8 weeks. A complement fixation test is also available.

In the acute phase, there is often severe leukocytosis, mostly due to mononuclear cells. Patients with myocarditis have radiographic and electrocardiographic abnormalities.

Differential Diagnosis

Trichinosis, kala-azar, and bacterial sepsis should be differentiated. In endemic areas, nonpathogenic trypanosomes *(Trypanosoma rangeli)* may be found in blood.

Treatment

Unfortunately, there is no safe and specific drug active against *T cruzi.* Nifurtimox, a nitrofuran derivative, has been used with some success in acute Chagas' disease in a dosage of 5–15 mg/kg/d for 120 days. Rapid arrest of the chagoma, negative blood smears and cultures for 2 years, and a decreasing titer of antibody to *T cruzi* in the complement fixation test have been achieved with the regimen despite some relapses. Nifurtimox, however, is a highly toxic drug; it has no place in the treatment of chronic Chagas' disease. Within 48 hours, amphotericin B can eliminate the trypomastigote from of *T cruzi* from blood stored at 4 °C.

Prognosis

Acute infection may prove fatal to infants and children. The mortality rate is particularly high in meningoencephalitis. Chronic disease with myocardial damage carries a poor prognosis.

Bittencourt AL et al: Pneumonitis in congenital Chagas' disease: A study of ten cases. *Am J Trop Med Hyg* 1981;**30:**38.

Cruz FS, Marr JJ, Berens RL: Prevention of transfusion-induced Chagas' disease by amphotericin B. *Am J Trop Med Hyg* 1980;**29:**761.

Hoff R et al: *Trypanosoma cruzi* in the cerebrospinal fluid during the acute stage of Chagas' disease. *N Engl J Med* 1978;**298:**604.

Mahmoud AAF, Warren KS: Algorithms in the diagnosis and management of exotic diseases. 4. American trypanosomiasis. *J Infect Dis* 1975;**132:**121.

Schipper H et al: Tropical diseases encountered in Canada. 1. Chagas' disease. *Can Med Assoc J* 1980;**122:**165.

METAZOAN INFECTIONS

NEMATODE INFECTIONS

1. ENTEROBIASIS (Oxyuriasis; Pinworm or Seatworm Infection)

Essentials of Diagnosis

- Pruritus ani, especially at night.
- Worms in stool; ova on perianal skin.

General Considerations

Enterobiasis occurs all over the world. Infection is caused by *Enterobius vermicularis*, a pinworm or seatworm. The adult worms reside in the cecum and colon. The gravid females crawl out and deposit thousands of eggs in the skin folds of the anus, especially at night, causing intense itching. When the child scratches, the ova stick to the fingertips and under the nails and eventually get to the mouth and are swallowed, resulting in autoinfection. Contamination of clothes and the environment leads to the infection of fresh hosts; it is not unusual for several members of the same household to harbor pinworms.

Clinical Findings

A. Symptoms and Signs: Pinworms have been blamed for a multitude of minor ills for which proof is difficult to find (eg, bruxism, insomnia, short attention span). A cause and effect relationship can be observed, however, for pruritus ani and pruritus vulvae. Pinworms can induce tiny mucosal ulcers and have been identified in the submucosa and the deeper layers of the bowel wall. They are rarely a cause of appendiceal inflammation. The ability of parasites to penetrate the intact mucosa is controversial, but there seems to be little doubt that they can exploit any breach that is already present. The female worm may become disoriented in her normal migration to deposit eggs, reaching instead the peritoneal cavity via the human female genital tract. Migration into the female urethra may be one cause of urinary tract infection. In any of these ectopic sites, the parasites may produce a granuloma. They often produce no symptoms.

B. Laboratory Findings: The diagnosis is confirmed by the detection of ova on the perianal skin. A transparent adhesive tape held tight over the bottom of a test tube with the sticky surface outward is applied to the anus and perianal skin; this is preferably done in the morning, before defecation or washing. The tape is then mounted over a drop of toluene on a glass slide and examined under the microscope. Occasionally, ova and even adult worms may be seen in stools.

The ova measure about 50–60 × 20–30 μm and are oval with one flat surface. The coiled larva is usually visible through the translucent shell.

Differential Diagnosis

All instances of pruritus ani or vulvae are not caused by enterobiasis, though in the absence of other demonstrable causes a therapeutic trial is justifiable.

Treatment

A. Specific Measures: To prevent intrafamilial cross-infection, it is worthwhile treating all individuals in a household simultaneously. Treatment should be repeated after 2 weeks to eradicate infection.

1. Pyrantel pamoate—This drug is highly effective against *Ascaris* and hookworm and pinworm. It is given in a single dose (11 mg/kg up to a maximum of 1 g), is tasteless, and has minimal side effects.

2. Mebendazole—Mebendazole is a highly effective drug active against pinworm as well as whipworm, *Ascaris*, and hookworm. It is given in a single dose of 100 mg irrespective of age. ***Caution:*** Avoid in pregnant women. Experience is scanty in children under 2 years of age.

3. Pyrvinium pamoate—The syrup form is given in a single dose of 5 mg/kg (maximum, 0.25 g). It may cause nausea and vomiting, and it turns the stools red.

4. Piperazine compounds—Piperazine compounds (citrate, adipate, hydrate, or phosphate) are relatively nontoxic in therapeutic dosage and are widely used in syrup form. The dosage is 50 mg/kg/d (maximum, 2 g/d) in the evenings for 7 days.

B. General Measures: Strict personal hygiene helps prevent autoinfection. Infected children should wear undergarments even while sleeping so that direct contact of fingers with perianal skin can be avoided. The nails should be kept short and clean. Bedclothes and undergarments of infected children should be removed without shaking (to prevent dispersal of ova) and laundered frequently. Since treatment is satisfactory and clinical complications minor, it is often necessary to reassure concerned parents and to prevent their undertaking extreme measures at household sanitation ("pinworm psychosis").

Brugmans JP et al: Mebendazole in enterobiasis: Radiochemical and pilot clinical study in 1,278 subjects. *JAMA* 1971; **217:**313.

Chandrasoma PT, Mendis KN: *Enterobius vermicularis* in ectopic sites. *Am J Trop Med Hyg* 1977;**26:**644.

Mayers CP, Purvis RJ: Manifestations of pinworms. *Can Med Assoc J* 1970;**103:**489.

Simon RD: Pinworm infestation and urinary tract infection in young girls. *Am J Dis Child* 1974;**128:**21.

Warren KS, Mahmoud AAF: Algorithms in the diagnosis and management of exotic diseases. 5. Enterobiasis. *J Infect Dis* 1975;**132:**229.

2. ASCARIASIS

Essentials of Diagnosis

- Abdominal discomfort and colic.
- The passage of roundworms in feces or the demonstration of *Ascaris* ova.

General Considerations

The roundworm *Ascaris lumbricoides* is a cosmopolitan human parasite. Where indiscriminate defecation by children is allowed, the ova are spread widely in the soil, where they remain viable for long periods. The ova contaminate food, fingers, toys, etc, and are swallowed and then hatch in the upper small intestine. The escaping larvae penetrate the gut wall and, through the portal circulation and the right side of the heart, reach the pulmonary capillaries. They penetrate into the alveoli, are coughed up and swallowed, and mature in the small intestine. Males and females mate, and the female lays thousands of eggs each day.

Clinical Findings

A. Symptoms and Signs: In the great majority of instances, the infection remains silent. However, abdominal pain, anorexia, gastrointestinal upsets, loss of weight, irritability, and short febrile episodes have been attributed to the presence of these worms. Occasionally, the worms are excreted in feces or ascend to the stomach and are vomited out.

Large numbers of the larvae migrating through the lungs may cause an acute and often transient "pneumonia" accompanied by eosinophilia (Löffler's syndrome). This syndrome, however, seems to be rare. In pediatric patients, large numbers of worms in the gut lumen can cause symptoms of intestinal obstruction.

B. Laboratory Findings: Except when a history of passing roundworms is obtained, the diagnosis is made by the detection of ova in fecal smears. They are approximately 45 × 60 μm with a brown (bile-stained), heavily mamillated outer coat, a thick middle, and a delicate inner coat covering a densely granular egg cell.

Complications

Large numbers of worms occasionally cause intestinal obstruction, which may be precipitated by treatment in cases of massive infection.

Worms may penetrate the gut wall and cause peritonitis; block the appendiceal lumen, causing acute appendicitis; or block the common bile duct and cause actue obstructive jaundice.

Treatment

In asymptomatic infections, especially in older children, there is no urgency for treatment. The infection is self-limited within a year unless reinfection occurs.

Pyrantel pamoate and mebendazole are the currently recommended drugs of choice. The dosage of pyrantel pamoate is 11 mg/kg (maximum, 1 g) as a single oral dose. The dosage of mebendazole is 100 mg twice daily for 3 days. If follow-up stool examination is positive for ova, treatment should be repeated. Mebendazole is contraindicated in pregnancy and not recommended for children under 2 years old.

Piperazine compounds (citrate, adipate, hydrate, or phosphate) are also highly effective and are available as tablets or syrup. Dosage is usually calculated in terms of the hydrous base, piperazine hexahydrate. Piperazine citrate is widely used as a single dose of 75–100 mg/kg (maximum, 3 g) taken orally after breakfast, either once, or, preferably, on 2 consecutive days. No purge is required, and treatment can be repeated after a week in heavy infections. Little or no toxicity is encountered.

In massive infection, treatment may result in intestinal obstruction by masses of paralyzed worms.

In the presence of surgical complications, enterotomy with evacuation is perhaps the safest procedure. The administration of a piperazine drug is recommended after about 2 weeks.

Prognosis

The prognosis is good except when massive infection results in bowel gangrene or perforation and peritonitis; in these instances, death may result.

Cremin BJ, Fisher RM: Biliary ascariasis in children. *Am J Roentgenol* 1976;**126:**352.

Ihekwaba FN: *Ascaris lumbricoides* and perforation of the ileum: A critical review. *Br J Surg* 1979;**66:**132.

Katz Y et al: Intestinal obstruction due to *Ascaris lumbricoides* mimicking intussusception. *Dis Colon Rectum* 1985;**28:**267.

Stephenson LS: The contribution of *Ascaris lumbricoides* to malnutrition in children. *Parasitology* 1980;**81:**221.

Warren KS, Mahmoud AAF: Algorithms in the diagnosis and management of exotic diseases. 22. Ascariasis and toxocariasis. *J Infect Dis* 1977;**135:**868.

Williams D, Burke G, Hendley JO: Ascariasis: A family disease. *J Pediatr* 1979;**84:**853.

Wolfe MS, Wershing JM: Mebendazole: Treatment of trichuriasis and ascariasis in Bahamian children. *JAMA* 1974; **230:**1408.

3. TRICHURIASIS (Trichocephaliasis, Whipworm)

The whipworm *Trichuris trichiura* is a worldwide human and animal parasite. It is still found with regularity in the southern USA and is common among impoverished children living in warm, humid tropical areas. The adult worms reside in the cecum and colon, and ova are passed in feces, where they develop to the infective stage in 3–4 weeks. Infective (larvated) eggs then reach the human alimentary canal in contaminated soil, vegetables, toys, etc, and hatch in the upper small intestine. There are usually no symptoms except when infection is heavy, causing abdominal pain (especially in the right iliac fossa), abdominal distention, and diarrhea. Massive colonic infection commonly causes rectal prolapse and may cause dysentery clinically similar to amebic dysentery. The diagnosis is based on demonstrations of ova in fecal smears. They are about 50 × 20 μm, brown, and oval, with 2 polar plugs in the shell. Proctoscopy may disclose grayish-white worms with narrow anterior and broad posterior portions attached to hyperemic mucosa. The whole worm measures 3–5 cm. Mild to moderate eosinophilia may occasionally be present.

The treatment of choice is mebendazole, which has been shown to be highly effective against trichuriasis as well as roundworm, pinworm, and hookworm. The drug is contraindicated in pregnancy and not recommended for children under 2 years old. The dosage of mebendazole is 100 mg twice daily for 3 days for children older than 2 years. Alternatively, a single oral dose of 600 mg can be given to children 6 years of age and older when compliance with the standard 3-day regimen would be difficult. Albendazole can also be used in a single oral dose of 400 mg.

Bundy DAP et al: Rate of expulsion of *Trichuris trichiura* with multiple and single dose regimens of albendazole. *Trans R Soc Trop Med Hyg* 1985;**79:**641.

Gilman RH et al: The adverse consequences of heavy *Trichuris* infection. *Trans R Soc Trop Med Hyg* 1983;**77:**432.

Kan SP: Efficacy of single doses of mebendazole in the treatment of *Trichuris trichiura* infection. *Am J Trop Med Hyg* 1983;**32:**118.

Scragg JN, Proctor EM: Mebendazole in the treatment of severe symptomatic trichuriasis in children. *Am J Trop Med Hyg* 1977;**26:**198.

4. HOOKWORM DISEASE

Essentials of Diagnosis

- Weakness and pallor, with a hypochromic microcytic anemia.
- Abdominal discomfort, weight loss.
- Occult blood in stool.
- Ova in fecal smears.

General Considerations

The hookworms that commonly infect humans are *Ancylostoma duodenale* and *Necator americanus*. Their life cycles are identical, and both occur widely in the tropical and subtropical regions of the world, with *Necator* the predominant form in the Americas and elsewhere in tropical areas. The larger *Ancylostoma* is the predominant form in temperate regions, especially North Africa, Europe, Asia, and Japan. It is considerably more pathogenic, since it can withdraw substantially more blood per worm.

The adult worms reside mostly in the jejunum. They feed on blood; blood loss from on *Ancylostoma* worm may be 0.1–0.5 mL/d, and that from *Necator* somewhat less. Ova are deposited in the bowel and expelled in feces. In suitable damp, shaded soil, the eggs hatch and develop after about 2 weeks into infective larvae. On contact with human skin (walking barefoot or handling soil), they penetrate and enter the bloodstream, reach the lungs, exit into the alveoli, migrate toward the pharynx, and are swallowed. In the upper intestine, they develop into adults.

In some communities where no organized drainage and sanitation are available, over 90% of individuals may be infected.

Another species, *Ancylostoma braziliense*, a dog or cat hookworm, is a rare human parasite. The infective larvae cause cutaneous larva migrans. This condition occurs mainly on the American continents.

Clinical Findings

A. Symptoms and Signs: At the skin sites where large numbers of larvae penetrate, especially on and between the toes, intense itching ("ground itch") may occur, particularly in rainy seasons. In cutaneous larva migrans, the larvae penetrate the skin and wander under it, causing irritation, redness, and a slowly creeping eruption.

Small numbers of worms cause no symptoms, and symptoms directly related to the presence of these parasites are never notable. Abdominal pain, discomfort, and distention and changes in bowel habits occasionally occur with heavy infection.

B. Laboratory Findings: Diagnosis is made by identification of ova in fecal smears. They are oval, about 60 × 40 μm, with a segmented egg of 4–16 cells visible through the thin eggshell. Eggs of *N americanus* and *A duodenale* are identical, but identification by means of geographic distribution usually is possible. Moderate to severe anemia of the microcytic hypochromic type is usually present in patients who are chronically ill with hookworm disease. Hypoalbuminemia is an integral part of the disease in these patients and is related to the worm load.

Tests for occult blood in feces are usually positive if there are a sufficient number of worms. Mild to moderate eosinophilia is common.

Complications & Sequelae

By causing a continuous loss of blood, hookworm aggravates nutritional deficiencies. Thus, a progressive iron deficiency anemia is produced in people who are on a low iron intake. Supplemental iron usually prevents hookworm anemia. In patients with borderline folic acid intake, megaloblastic anemia may be produced. The anemia is so insidious that patients may seek medical attention only after cardiac decompensation has occurred. In addition to cardiac failure, hypoalbuminemia may also exist and contribute to anasarca.

Prevention

Prevention of hookworm infection is achieved by avoiding fecal contamination of soil and skin contact with contaminated soil.

Treatment

A. Specific Measures:

1. Mebendazole—This is now the drug of choice for both kinds of hookworm infection in humans; the dosage is 100 mg twice daily by mouth for 3 days for children older than 2 years. Mebendazole is also effective for the treatment of ascariasis, enterobiasis, and trichuriasis; it is particularly convenient and helpful for mixed infections with susceptible intestinal nematodes. Mebendazole is contraindicated in pregnancy and not recommended for children under 2 years old.

2. Pyrantel pamoate—In a single oral dose of 11 mg/kg, pyrantel pamoate is an effective alternative to mebendazole for both kinds of human hookworm infections.

3. Bephenium hydroxynaphthoate—This is a useful alternative, particularly for *A duodenale* infection. It is also effective against roundworms *(Ascaris)* and can be administered in mixed infections. It is given in a single dose, on an empty stomach, 2.5 g for children under 20 kg and 5 g for those over 20 kg. Food should be withheld for 2 hours after administration, but no purgation is necessary. Because of its bitter taste, bephenium hydroxynaphthoate is best mixed with fruit juice, flavored liquid, or milk. It may provoke nausea and vomiting, but other side effects are few. Treatment may be repeated after an interval of 3–4 weeks.

4. Tetrachloroethylene—Tetrachloroethylene is also effective and widely used, especially for *N americanus.* It is given orally in a single dose of 0.1–0.12 mL/kg (maximum, 5 mL) on an empty stomach. No purgation is necessary, but a light supper with no fat on the previous night is recommended to prevent absorption of the fat-soluble drug. In severely anemic or debilitated children, treatment for anemia should precede the above therapy. Since it may stimulate roundworms into activity and migration, tetrachloroethylene is better avoided in mixed infection or only given after the roundworms have been eliminated. The drug may cause abdominal discomfort and nausea and vomiting. It deteriorates unless kept in a cool place in dark airtight containers.

5. Thiabendazole—Thiabendazole is used to treat cutaneous larva migrans. The condition may be arrested by a topical preparation of 15% thiabendazole powder in a water-soluble base. Oral thiabendazole is the drug of choice; the dose is 25 mg/kg twice daily for 2 days.

B. General Measures: In many anemic children, oral iron therapy is of greater value than anthelmintics. Exchange blood transfusions may be lifesaving in severely anemic children in cardiac failure. In less severe cases, parenteral iron therapy is of value.

Prognosis

Except in severely anemic children, the prognosis is good.

Botero D, Castano A: Comparative study of pyrantel pamoate, bephenium hydroxynaphthoate, and tetrachloroethylene in the treatment of *Necator americanus* infections. *Am J Trop Med Hyg* 1973;**22:**45.

Hutchison JGP et al: Clinical trial of mebendazole, a broad-spectrum anthelminthic. *Br Med J* 1975;**2:**309.

Lozoff B, Warren KS, Mahmoud AAF: Algorithms in the diagnosis and management of exotic diseases. 8. Hookworm. *J Infect Dis* 1975;**132:**606.

Mebendazole: A new anthelmintic. *Med Lett Drugs Ther* 1975;**17:**37.

5. STRONGYLOIDIASIS

Essentials of Diagnosis

- Productive cough, blood-streaked sputum.
- Abdominal pain, distention, diarrhea.
- Progressive nutritional deficiencies, eosinophilia.
- Larvae in stool, duodenal aspirate, or sputum.

General Considerations

Unlike the other helminths considered in this chapter, *Strongyloides stercoralis* has parasitic and free-living forms, which can survive and multiply for a few generations as free-living soil dwellers. As a human parasite, it has been found in most tropical and subtropical regions of the world. The adult worms live in the submucosal tissue and the mucosal folds of the duodenum and occasionally occupy the entire length of the intestines. Eggs are deposited in the intestinal mucosa and hatch rapidly. Therefore, both in feces and in duodenal aspirates, the rhabditiform larvae are found commonly but the eggs rarely. However, rhabditiform larvae can occasionally change to the infective stage (filariform larvae) before leaving the anus, penetrate the bowel wall, enter the bloodstream, and initiate an internal autoinfection.

In suitable soil and moisture, the larvae develop rapidly into the skin-penetrating, infective filariform larvae. Under less suitable conditions, free-living adult worms may develop and reproduce for several nonparasitic generations. Contact with human skin (walking barefoot or handling soil) facilitates the penetration of skin by the infective larvae, which follow a course much like that of the hookworms and reach the pulmonary capillaries through the bloodstream. They escape into alveoli, travel up the bronchial tree, and enter the alimentary canal. In the duodenum, they mature into adults.

Older children and adults are more often affected than young children. Even in areas where the general incidence of strongyloidiasis is low, an occasional patient presents with massive parasitization, chiefly due to internal autoinfection. Immunosuppressed patients may develop fatal disseminated strongyloidiasis.

Clinical Findings

A. Symptoms and Signs: The site of skin penetration may go unnoticed, or a transient pruritic papular eruption may occur. After heavy exposure, respiratory signs and symptoms may be caused by the migrating larvae. Cough, often productive, with streaks of blood in the sputum, may occur. Abdominal pain, distention, vomiting, and diarrhea with large and pale stools, often with mucus, are the common features.

B. Laboratory Findings: The diagnosis is confirmed by the presence of larvae in feces and duodenal aspirates. They are about 225 μm long, with a double-bulb esophagus that is almost half the length of the larva.

Larvae can sometimes be seen in sputum. A mild to moderate eosinophilia may be present.

C. Radiographic Findings: There may be patchy areas of infiltration on chest radiograph. A barium meal may reveal evidence of duodenitis, including coarse mucosal folds, a widened lumen, and clumping of barium. In severe cases, a pipelike appearance may occur in the duodenum and elsewhere. These findings simulate those of sprue, regional enteritis, and, occasionally, ulcerative colitis.

Differential Diagnosis

Symptomatic strongyloidiasis must be differentiated from sprue, other causes of malabsorption, regional enteritis, tuberculous enteritis, and hookworm disease.

Complications & Sequelae

In heavy infection with *Strongyloides,* chronic diarrhea and malabsorption eventually lead to severe nutritional deficiencies and debility. Several workers have reported fatal strongyloidiasis, nearly all of which were cases of internal hyperinfection, with massive numbers of larval worms found throughout the viscera.

Overwhelming strongyloidiasis is a recently recognized opportunistic infection in patients from endemic areas who undergo intensive cytotoxic and immunosuppressive therapy (especially high-dose corticosteroids) for a variety of conditions. In these patients, diffuse bilateral pulmonary infiltrates and paralytic ileus on chest and abdominal radiographs are clues to the diagnosis, which can be established readily by finding larvae of *S stercoralis* on microscopic examination of upper small bowel fluid, feces, or sputum.

Treatment

A. Specific Measures: The treatment of choice is with thiabendazole, 25 mg/kg orally twice daily for 2 days. Patients with severe, disseminated strongyloidiasis should be treated with thiabendazole for at least 5–7 days. Close follow-up of treated patients is recommended, as relapses are common. In such instances, specific therapy should be repeated.

B. General Measures: In serious infections, attention to the nutritional and fluid and electrolyte needs is urgent. In many fatal cases, death appears to be due to the severe nutritional defects or to paralytic ileus.

Prognosis

The prognosis is good in mild infection but poor in symptomatic heavy infections with complications.

Burke JA: Strongyloidiasis in childhood. *Am J Dis Child* 1978;**132:**1130.

Grove DI, Warren KS, Mahmoud AAF: Algorithms in diagnosis and management of exotic diseases. 3. Strongyloidiasis. *J Infect Dis* 1975;**131:**755.

Harris RA Jr et al: Disseminated strongyloidiasis: Diagnosis made by sputum examination. *JAMA* 1980;**244:**65.

Milder JE et al: Clinical features of *Strongyloides stercoralis* infection in an endemic area of the United States. *Gastroenterology* 1981;**80:**1481.

Purtillo DT, Meyers WM, Connor DH: Fatal strongyloidiasis in immunosuppressed patients. *Am J Med* 1974;**56:**488.

Rivera E et al: Hyperinfection syndrome with *Strongyloides stercoralis. Ann Intern Med* 1970;**72:**199.

Scowden EB, Schaffner W, Stone WJ: Overwhelming strongyloidiasis: An unappreciated opportunistic infection. *Medicine* 1978;**57:**527.

Smith SB et al: Fatal disseminated strongyloidiasis presenting as acute abdominal distress in an urban child. *J Pediatr* 1977;**91:**607.

6. VISCERAL LARVA MIGRANS (Toxocariasis)

Essentials of Diagnosis

- Marked eosinophilia and hepatomegaly in children with pica.
- The demonstration of larvae in liver biopsy.

General Considerations

Visceral larva migrans occurs in young children infected with the larvae of *Toxocara canis* or *Toxocara cati* (dog or cat roundworm). Most of the reported cases are from North America and the British Isles. A history of pica is helpful in diagnosis. The presence of worm-infested dogs in the environment leads to the ingestion of eggs.

The life cycle and transmission of dog and cat roundworms are quite similar to those of *Ascaris* in humans. When the eggs are ingested in large numbers by children via feces-contaminated soil, the larvae hatch in the intestines, migrate through the bloodstream, and are caught up in granulomatous inflammatory lesions in the liver, occasionally in the lungs, and rarely in other tissues, where they may remain or migrate for months to several years.

A similar syndrome can also be caused by *Capillaria hepatica,* a rodent whipworm.

Clinical Findings

A. Symptoms and Signs: The common presenting symptoms are anorexia, fever, and pallor. Abdominal distention and cough occur occasionally. Hepatomegaly is common, and splenomegaly is not unusual. Cutaneous hemorrhagic lesions have been reported in a few instances. Blindness and epileptiform convulsions may be atypical forms of presentation.

B. Laboratory Findings: Anemia is usually present and may be the reason for the pica. Severe leukocytosis, mainly due to eosinophilia (30–90%), is almost a constant feature. Hypergammaglobulinemia and high titers of blood group isoagglutinins are commonly found. The diagnosis may be confirmed by finding nematode larvae in a liver biopsy specimen, preferably performed by the open method. The larvae may be seen in secretions in granulomatous lesions or in crushed or papain-digested specimens. In fatal cases, larvae have been found in muscle and brain also.

C. Radiographic Findings: Infiltrations can often be seen on chest radiograph.

Differential Diagnosis

Pallor and pica in children with other symptoms may be associated with lead poisoning. These 2 conditions have been reported to occur simultaneously. Transient eosinophilia (< 3 weeks) may occur during the migration of *Ascaris* larvae. More prolonged eosinophilia may occur in strongyloidiasis and trichinosis. Other helminths do not usually cause eosinophilia to a comparable degree.

Tropical eosinophilia, probably due to filariasis, may occur in infants and toddlers, especially in India. Pulmonary signs and symptoms are common, and hepatomegaly and fever may occur. Pica is not a feature.

Eosinophilia may be prominent in schistosomiasis and hydatid disease in association with hepatomegaly. Collagen diseases with eosinophilia and eosinophilic leukemia also should be differentiated.

Complications & Sequelae

Myocarditis, convulsive disorders, encephalitis, and ocular involvement such as retinal mass and endophthalmitis may occur owing to the presence of larvae in these tissues. The ocular complications may be mistaken for retinoblastoma.

Treatment

A. Specific Measures: Thiabendazole is considered the best available drug for visceral larva migrans (25 mg/kg orally twice a day for 5–7 days). Diethylcarbamazine is also active against the larvae. The dosage is 2–4 mg/kg orally 3 times a day for 3 weeks. Medical treatment is especially indicated when pulmonary symptoms are prominent.

B. General Measures: In most cases, the prevention of reinfection is all that is required, since the condition disappears without treatment. Removal of the source of *Toxocara* ova is important. The treatment of anemia with iron may be of value in stopping pica.

For endophthalmitis or for severe cases, especially with massive pulmonary infiltrates, corticosteroids may be lifesaving. These appear to reduce hepatocyte necrosis and cellular infiltration without changing the fibrous lesions.

Prognosis

Some severe cases have been fatal. Endophthalmitis leads to blindness. The majority of patients recover if continued infection is avoided.

Attah EB et al: Hepatic capillariasis. *Am J Clin Pathol* 1983;**79:**127.

Beshear JR, Hendley JO: Severe pulmonary involvement in visceral larva migrans. *Am J Dis Child* 1973;**125:**599.

Glickman LT, Schantz PM, Cypess RH: Epidemiological characteristics and clinical findings in patients with serologically proven toxocariasis. *Trans R Soc Trop Med Hyg* 1979; **73:**254.

Schantz PM, Glickman LT: Toxocaral visceral larva migrans. *N Engl J Med* 1978;**298:**436.

Woodruff AW: Toxocariasis. *Br Med J* 1970;**3:**663.

Zinkham WH: Visceral larva migrans: A review and reassessment indicating two forms of clinical expression: Visceral and ocular. *Am J Dis Child* 1978;**132:**627.

7. TRICHINOSIS

Essentials of Diagnosis

- Vomiting, diarrhea, and abdominal pain within 48 hours of ingesting infected meat.
- Fever, periorbital edema (80–85% of patients), myalgia, and eosinophilia (90–95% of patients) about 1 week later.
- Encysted *Trichinella spiralis* larvae in muscle (biopsy).

General Considerations

Trichinella spiralis is a small roundworm (1.5 mm male, 4 mm female) that inhabits the intestines of hogs and several other flesh-eating animals. The larvae are ingested in the muscle meats of pork, bear, walrus, etc. They are liberated by digestion of their capsule and immediately enter the mucosa of the upper small intestine, where they develop into adult worms before emerging. The fertilized female burrows again into the mucosa, where she may release more than 1000 larvae within the next few weeks to months. The larvae enter the bloodstream and reach the striated musculature before becoming encysted. They may cause significant damage to many tissues as they migrate. Humans are thereby a dead end for the parasite. Trichinosis is largely a disease of North America, parts of Europe, and the Soviet Union. Humans usually become infected by eating undercooked pork. Smoking, salting, and drying do not kill infective larvae. Ground beef may be contaminated with pork left in the grinding machine.

Clinical Findings

Illness begins when excysted larvae from infected meat penetrate the small bowel mucosa, producing nausea, vomiting, diarrhea (occasionally with some bleeding), and abdominal cramps. This occurs 1–2 days after ingestion. Most patients are without symptoms or experience only the gastrointestinal phase in a mild form. In some cases, the migration of larvae is heralded by fever, edema (especially face and eyelids), and moderate to severe myalgia. Muscles with a low glycogen content (eg, diaphragm) are more apt to be heavily invaded. Larval migrations are extensive, however, and symptoms may indicate involvement of the heart, lungs, kidneys, and brain. The patient may become progressively more neurotoxic and die at 4–6 weeks. Although recuperation may begin about the fifth week, the continued release of larvae can result in symptoms for several months. A rash can occur, as can splenomegaly.

Differential Diagnosis

At times, a typhoidal picture may be seen in trichinosis. The triad of periorbital edema, eosinophilia, and myalgia is so characteristic that it is only necessary to be aware of its meaning (ie, trichinosis) to make the presumptive diagnosis.

Complications & Sequelae

Marked inflammation of virtually any tissue can occur. If the mass of larvae is sufficiently large, the toxicity can threaten life.

Prevention

The United States Department of Agriculture does not inspect meat in the USA for trichinosis. There are, however, laws in all 50 states requiring the cooking of swill fed to hogs. Since hog-to-hog or hog-to-rat cycles of transmission are still possible, it is necessary to educate the public about personal prevention. All pork should be heated to at least 65 °C (149 °F) at the center of the cut. The same applies to all sylvatic meats (bear, walrus, etc). It is thought that freezing meat at −15 °C (5 °F) for 3 weeks prevents transmission, but there is some recent question about this.

No animal that is used for food should be allowed access to carrion. Hog farms in particular should be cleared of rats.

Treatment

Although thiabendazole (25 mg/kg twice daily by mouth for 5 days) has been successful in some cases in treating the larval phase of trichinosis, its use is sometimes limited by side effects. Mebendazole has recently shown promise in its larvicidal effects (including the encysted form) as well as some effect against the mature worm. Insufficient data exist to justify a recommendation for the use of thiabendazole in pregnant women or children under 2 years of age. Corticosteroids have proved useful in decreasing the severity of symptoms, but their use may aid survival of the mature female worm and thus the total numbers of larvae liberated. General supportive measures are indicated. Where exposure has been recognized before the onset of initial gastrointestinal symptoms, saline purgatives may help eliminate some developing larvae. No therapy to date is considered truly specific.

Prognosis

The vast majority of symptomatic cases can be managed without significant threat to life or fear of residual disability. Death, when it occurs, generally occurs at about the fifth week. Survivors of this critical period usually recover.

Grove DI, Warren KS, Mahmoud AAF: Algorithms in the diagnosis and management of exotic disease. 7. Trichinosis. *J Infect Dis* 1975;**132:**485.

Margolis HS, Middaugh JP, Burgess RD: Arctic trichinosis: Two Alaskan outbreaks from walrus meat. *J Infect Dis* 1979;**139:**102.

Most H: Trichinosis—preventable but still with us. *N Engl J Med* 1978;**298:**1178.

Wand M, Lyman D: Trichinosis from bear meat: Clinical and laboratory features. *JAMA* 1972;**220:**245.

8. DRACUNCULIASIS (Dracontiasis, Guinea Worm Infection)

Dracunculus medinensis (guinea worm) is a common parasite of humans in some parts of India, southwest Asia, and Africa. Infection results from drinking water containing small copepod crustaceans *(Cyclops)* harboring mature larvae. The larvae penetrate the intestinal mucosa, develop in the abdominal cavity for about a year, and then the mated female worms migrate to the subcutaneous tissues of the lower extremities or back. They may also reach various other tissues and die, causing few or no symptoms. The female lies under the skin, from which larvae are discharged through a skin blister near the head of the female adult worm, when the skin is in contact with water. Thus, farm workers and water carriers who wade into step-in wells both suffer from and perpetuate dracunculiasis.

There have been few reports on the infection in children, though pediatric infection is known to occur in India.

The symptoms mostly refer to the blister or ulcer caused by the worm. The lesion is usually on the lower limb and discharges a milky fluid that shows the white worm. Fever and urticaria may occur prior to or during the blister formation. In cryptic infection, eosinophilia may be the sole evidence, although intense pruritus occasionally occurs. Calcified worms can be seen on radiographs and may be palpable. The ulcer may become bacterially infected. Premature death of worms in the subcutaneous tissues may result in inflammatory lesions and sometimes in a sterile abscess. A filarial skin test is available but is seldom needed for diagnosis.

In ulcerated dracunculiasis, a moist antiseptic dressing (eg, acriflavine) accelerates the discharge of larvae and the death of the worm. Afterward, the worm can be pulled out gradually, about 2–3 cm a day, using a suitable instrument such as a clean match stick, on which it can be wound. If more rapid withdrawal is attempted, the worm might rupture and cause a severe cellulitis.

Niridazole, 25 mg/kg/d orally in 2 divided doses for 15 days, appears to be effective in the treatment of dracunculiasis. In one study, patients reported rapid relief of pain, tenderness, and swelling; the adult guinea worms were extracted more easily; and there was less tendency for fresh worms to emerge. Alternatively, metronidazole, 25 mg/kg orally in 3 divided doses for 10 days, can be used. Its therapeutic effects resemble those of niridazole except that it has no preventive or vermicidal action. With either drug, the adult guinea worms should be extracted carefully once they begin to emerge.

Patients with secondary bacterial infections at the site of the ulcer must be given local care and, occasionally, appropriate systemic antimicrobial therapy.

Hopkins DR: Dracunculiasis: An eradicable scourge. *Epidemiol Rev* 1983;**5**:208.

Muller R: Guinea worm disease: Epidemiology, control, and treatment. *Bull WHO* 1979;**57**:683.

Sharma VP, Rathore HS, Sharma MM: Efficacy of metronidazole in dracunculiasis: A clinical trial. *Am J Trop Med Hyg* 1979;**28**:658.

9. ONCHOCERCIASIS

Essentials of Diagnosis

- Localized or generalized pruritus.
- Subcutaneous nodules (adult worms).
- Superficial punctate keratitis.
- Late iridocyclitis.
- Eosinophilia.
- Biopsy evidence of *Onchocerca volvulus.*

General Considerations

Onchocerca volvulus is a filarial nematode found across central Africa and in Central America and southern Mexico. It is transmitted by species of *Simulium* (black flies). The infective larvae deposited after the bite of an infected *Simulium* will slowly develop in the subcutaneous tissues, which form an enclosing tumor, encapsulating the large female and possibly several smaller male worms. Microfilariae are developed in the female and shed in large numbers. These minute prelarvae wander in subcutaneous tissue fluids and the eyes but do not enter the bloodstream, as do the other pathogenic filariae of humans.

Clinical Findings

A. Symptoms and Signs: About half of infected patients develop localized areas of nodularity or skin tumors associated with itching and resulting in excoriation and chronic pigmentary and morphologic skin changes. Common sites include the bony prominences of the trunk, extremities, and head.

Ocular infestation results in an early superficial punctate keratitis. Iridocyclitis may ultimately occur and is a serious complication that may lead to glaucoma, cataracts, and blindness.

B. Laboratory Findings: Eosinophilia of 15–50% is common. Aspiration of nodules will usually reveal microfilariae, and adult worms may be demonstrated in excised nodules. Microfilariae are not found in the blood but can be identified in skin or conjunctival snips or in skin shavings. The snip is performed by tenting the skin with a needle and cutting off a bit of skin above the needle tip. A blood-free shaving may be cut with a razor blade from the top of a ridge of skin firmly pressed between thumb and forefinger. The snip or shaving is examined in a drop of saline under a coverslip on a slide. Shavings or snips should be taken from several sites over bony prominences of the scapular region, hips, and thighs. In ocular onchocerciasis, slit lamp examination will usually reveal many microfilariae in the anterior chamber. Complement fixation and skin tests are of doubtful value because of high false-positive reaction rates.

Treatment

A. Specific Measures:

1. Diethylcarbamazine citrate—This drug is almost nontoxic and fairly effective. Give 2–3 mg/kg orally 3 times daily for 14–21 days. To prevent severe allergic symptoms, which may be provoked early in therapy as microfilariae are rapidly killed, start treatment with small doses and increase the dosage over 3–4 days. When the eyes are involved, particular caution is necessary, starting with a single daily dose of 0.25 mg/kg. Use antihistamines to control allergic symptoms.

One course of diethylcarbamazine will eradicate the infection in about 40% of patients and halt progression in the remainder. Two or 3 courses will cure almost all cases.

2. Suramin sodium—Suramin sodium is more effective than diethylcarbamazine in eradicating infection in a single course, but it has the disadvantage of potential renal toxicity (proteinuria, casts, red cells). Renal disease is a contraindication. Give 20 mg/kg as a 10% solution in distilled water intravenously weekly for a total of 5 weeks. Start treatment with a test dose of 10–20 mg.

3. Ivermectin—This drug, which is already widely used for helminthic infections in veterinary medicine, now appears to be a better-tolerated, safer, and more effective microfilaricidal agent than diethylcarbamazine for the treatment of onchocerciasis. Ivermectin is given as a single oral dose of 0.2 mg/kg. Counts of microfilariae in skin remain reduced for at least 6 months after ivermectin treatment.

B. Surgical Measures: Surgical removal of nodules is not curative but removes many adult worms and is particularly justifiable when nodules are located close to the eyes. Nodulectomy may also be indicated for cosmetic reasons.

Prognosis

With chemotherapy, progression of all forms of the disease usually can be checked. The prognosis is unfavorable only for patients seen for the first time with already far-advanced ocular onchocerciasis.

Connor DH, George GH, Gibson DW: Pathologic changes in human onchocerciasis: Implications for future research. *Rev Infect Dis* 1985;**7**:809.

Greene BM et al: Comparison of ivermectin and diethylcarbamazine in the treatment of onchocerciasis. *N Engl J Med* 1985;**313:**133.

Ottesen EA: Efficacy of diethylcarbamazine in eradicating infection with lymphatic-dwelling filariae in humans. *Rev Infect Dis* 1985;7:341.

10. FILARIASIS

Essentials of Diagnosis

- Lymphangitis of the legs and genitalia; obstructive lymphatic disease.
- Recurrent episodes lacking in periodicity.
- Characteristic microfilariae in blood.
- Leukocytosis with marked eosinophilia.
- Positive indirect hemagglutination and bentonite flocculation tests.

General Considerations

Filariasis is caused by infection with filarial worms that produce microfilariae and parasitize the blood and lymphatic systems and involve muscles, serous cavities, and connective tissues. The 2 principal human pathogens are *Wuchereria bancrofti* and *Brugia malayi.* Both are transmitted by mosquitoes *(W bancrofti* by *Culex* and *Aedes* and *B malayi* by *Anopheles* and *Mansonia). W bancrofti* infection is widely prevalent in the tropics and subtropics throughout the world; *B malayi* is found mostly in India, Ceylon, and Southeast Asia. Microfilariae are ingested by the mosquito vector and migrate to the thoracic muscles; larvae are deposited on the skin of humans close to the bite of the mosquito. The larvae migrate into the puncture wound and pass to the lymphatics, where they reside for approximately 1 year, reaching maturity in the interval. Adult worms reside in the lymphatics of the extremities and genitalia, where they give rise to microfilariae that reach the circulation. Microfilariae of *W bancrofti* are in the peripheral blood at night (an exception is a nonnocturnal variety in the South Pacific). *B malayi* may show nocturnal periodicity but can be subperiodic (present at all times but more plentiful at night).

Humans are the only definitive hosts for both filariae, except for a zoonotic strain of *B malayi* found infecting wild cats in northern Malaya. *B malayi* tends to occur in regions along coastlines dotted with multiple ponds bearing water plants of the genus *Pistia,* in which *Mansonia* mosquitoes breed.

Other species of filarial worms infect humans but are of little consequence clinically. These include *Dipetalonema perstans* (African and South American tropics), *Mansonella ozzardi* (West Indies and Central and South America), and worms of the genus *Dirofilaria* (southern USA, especially Florida), including the common heartworm of dogs, *Dirofilaria immitis.*

Clinical Findings

A. Symptoms and Signs: Three clinical forms are apparent in children: the asymptomatic, the inflammatory, and the obstructive stages.

Asymptomatic infection is observed with both *W bancrofti* and *B malayi.* Children are exposed early in life and may exhibit microfilariasis in the blood without symptoms. By age 6, most children will be affected in endemic regions. Physical examination may show moderate lymphadenopathy, commonly of the inguinal nodes but not limited to this group. With death of the adult worms, the disease is "cured" and microfilariae disappear.

Inflammatory disease is probably related to hypersensitivity to antigens or products of the living and dead adult worms. Localized areas of lymphangitis involving the lower extremities and episodes of epididymitis, orchitis, and funiculitis are common. Systemic manifestations include fever, chills, vomiting, and malaise lasting for days or weeks. Abscesses occasionally occur in areas where adult worms have died. A chronic proliferative fibroblastic reaction eventually results in obstructive lymphatic disease.

The obstructive stage develops in only a portion of those infected with filariae. Obstructive filariasis is a slow, chronic, progressive state resulting in edema of the affected parts. Elephantiasis results from multiple channel obstruction and can terminate in gross distortion of the extremities and genitalia. Recurrent inflammatory episodes may punctuate the progressive obstructive signs. Lymphatic rupture can result in the extrusion of lymph into serous cavities or organs (chyluria, chylous ascites, hydrocele).

B. Laboratory Findings: Eosinophilia may occur in 5–25% of pediatric patients early in the disease. With progression and reduction of inflammatory episodes, the eosinophil count falls.

Microfilariae may be found in night blood specimens in the asymptomatic form as well as in the inflammatory form, but they decrease in number as the obstructive phase progresses. A microfilariae filtering technique with a clear plastic membrane (Nucleopore) is more sensitive than older methods; moreover, it can eliminate the need for night blood in looking for microfilariae with nocturnal periodicity. Differentiation of *W bancrofti* and *B malayi* from nonpathogenic microfilariae requires an experienced observer. Adult worms can be identified in biopsy specimens, but biopsies should be performed judiciously to avoid damage to lymphatic channels.

Antibody determinations may be useful when microfilariae cannot be identified. Indirect hemagglutination and bentonite flocculation tests are available.

Differential Diagnosis

During the inflammatory stage, diagnosis may be difficult, and many common childhood infections must be considered. In endemic areas or with a history of a stay in such areas, the presence of fever, lymphangitis, and lymphadenitis associated with eosinophilia should suggest filariasis. Various inflammatory lesions of the genitalia (gonorrhea, mumps orchitis, epididymitis) must be differentiated. Elephantiasis is strongly suggestive of filariasis but must be differentiated from hernia or hydrocele, Milroy's disease, venous thrombosis, or lesions resulting in anasarca or dependent edema (congestive heart failure, nephrosis, hepatic disease).

Prevention

Control of mosquitoes and human sources is necessary. Insecticide control of mosquitoes and attempts to reduce breeding areas are useful. Diethylcarbamazine therapy in humans results in a diminishing reservoir for mosquito transmission.

Treatment

A. Specific Measures: Diethylcarbamazine citrate is the drug of choice. The dose is 2 mg/kg orally 3 times daily for 14–21 days. Allergic reactions are minimized by reducing each dose in relation to the occurrence and severity of prior reactions. The drug kills microfilariae but has little effect on the adult worms. Relapses can occur 3–12 months after a course of therapy, and re-treatment over a period of 1–2 years is often necessary. Obstructive filariasis is not benefited by drug therapy.

B. General Measures: Rest and relocation in a cooler climate appear to aid in alleviation of inflammatory episodes. All secondary infections—particularly those affecting the lymphatics, such as streptococcal infections—should be diagnosed promptly and treated vigorously. Inflammatory genital lesions in the male are relieved by suspension of the affected part.

C. Surgical Measures: Plastic surgical correction of the involved genitalia may be accomplished with good results. Surgical treatment of limbs is unsatisfactory. Drainage of chyle, when it results in discomfort or reduced function, may be useful on a temporary basis.

Prognosis

In asymptomatic disease, the prognosis is excellent in young children. With progression, relocation can result in improvement provided the disease is in its early stages and is mild. Severe elephantiasis requires surgical correction, which may have a satisfactory result in the genital region but a poor result if extremities are involved.

Dennis DT, McConnell E, White GB: Bancroftian filariasis and membrane filters: Are night surveys necessary? *Am J Trop Med Hyg* 1976;**25:**257.

Grove DI: Selective primary health care: Strategies for the control of disease in the developing world. 7. Filariasis. *Rev Infect Dis* 1983;**5:**933.

Weller PF et al: Endemic filariasis on a Pacific island. 1. Clinical, epidemiologic, and parasitologic aspects. *Am J Trop Med Hyg* 1982;**31:**942.

11. TROPICAL EOSINOPHILIA

Tropical eosinophilia is characterized by chronic or recurrent cough, exertional dyspnea, and wheezing, especially nocturnal. Generalized lymphadenitis and splenomegaly may occur. Fever is uncommon. Chest x-ray usually shows miliary mottling or other forms of interstitial infiltration. Marked leukocytosis, predominantly eosinophilic, is a diagnostic feature. Since mild to moderate eosinophilia is common in children where tropical eosinophilia is prevalent, an absolute eosinophil count of 4000/μL or more is generally considered an essential diagnostic criterion. Counts of 2000–4000/μL are equivocal, and lower counts speak against this diagnosis.

This disease is prevalent in the southwestern Pacific islands, southeastern and southern Asia, central and northwestern Africa, and some parts of South America. It may occur at any age but is uncommon in infants and very young children. It is believed to be due to infection with an unknown species of filaria. Microfilariae have been demonstrated in biopsies of lymph nodes, liver, and lung but not in the peripheral blood.

Treatment with the antifilarial drug diethylcarbamazine is usually effective. The recommended dosage is 2 mg/kg orally 3 times daily for 7–10 days. In case of recurrence or treatment failure, the course may be repeated for 10–20 days.

Neva FA, Ottesen EA: Tropical (filarial) eosinophilia. *N Engl J Med* 1978;**298:**1129.

Spry CJF, Kumaraswami V: Tropical eosinophilia. *Semin Hematol* 1982;**19:**107.

12. ANGIOSTRONGYLIASIS (Eosinophilic Meningitis, Intestinal Eosinophilic Granuloma)

The rat lungworm *Angiostrongylus cantonensis* has an intermediate host in mollusks. Most important among them are the amphibious snails of the genus *Pila,* found in gardens and fresh waters on the Pacific islands and in southeastern Asia, and the giant land snails of the genus *Achatina.* Larvae in these snails, when ingested raw, infect humans, and the developing parasites migrate through the liver and lungs to reach the central nervous system. After an incubation period of about 1–4 weeks, signs and symptoms of meningitis develop as well as eosinophilic pleocytosis of cerebrospinal fluid. The parasite may occasionally be seen in cerebrospinal fluid. The disease is usually self-limited but may be prolonged or fatal. This infection has been reported from Taiwan, Hawaii, several other Pacific islands, Thailand, and Australia. It may occur at any age. Avoidance of raw mollusks in the diet is the best preventive measure. In addition to the meningitic form, an ocular form of disease also has been reported.

Intestinal eosinophilic granuloma is a newly recognized disease caused by infection with *Morerastrongylus (Angiostrongylus) costaricensis.* The most extensive clinical experience has been reported from Costa Rica. Humans are accidental hosts; the usual life cycle of *M costaricensis* involves rodents (principal hosts) that feed on infected snails or slugs. The main clinical findings are abdominal pain, fever, leukocytosis with eosinophilia, and inflammatory mass lesions in the ascending colon, cecum, appendix, or small intestine. Many cases are recognized only after surgery for acute appendicitis. There is no known medical therapy.

Kuberski T, Wallace GD: Clinical manifestations of eosinophilic meningitis due to *Angiostrongylus cantonensis*. *Neurology* 1979;**29:**1566.

Loria-Cortés R, Lobo-Sanahuja JF: Clinical abdominal angiostrongylosis: A study of 116 children with intestinal eosinophilic granuloma caused by *Angiostrongylus costaricensis*. *Am J Trop Med Hyg* 1980;**29:**538.

Punyagupta S, Juttijudata P, Bunnag T: Eosinophilic meningitis in Thailand: Clinical studies of 484 typical cases probably caused by *Angiostrongylus cantonensis*. *Am J Trop Med Hyg* 1975;**24:**921.

Yii C-Y et al: Epidemiologic studies of eosinophilic meningitis in Southern Taiwan. *Am J Trop Med Hyg* 1975;**24:**447.

13. CAPILLARIASIS

Intestinal capillariasis in humans was first recognized in the northern Philippines but has also been reported in Thailand. It is caused by the roundworm *Capillaria philippinensis*. The adult worms are about 4–5 mm long, and the characteristic ova are peanut-shaped (45 × 21 μm) with pitted shells and nonprotuberant bipolar plugs. Capillariasis is thought to be acquired from eating raw fish or shellfish and is characterized by protracted diarrhea. Many patients develop a severe protein-losing enteropathy and malabsorption syndrome that leads to debility and death within 2–4 months if treatment is not given. The drug of choice is mebendazole, given in an oral dose of 200 mg twice daily for 20 days to children over 2 years of age.

Singson CN, Banzon TC, Cross JH: Mebendazole in the treatment of capillariasis. *Am J Trop Med Hyg* 1975;**24:**932.

CESTODE INFECTIONS

1. TAENIASIS & CYSTICERCOSIS

Essentials of Diagnosis

- Abdominal discomfort, pain, or diarrhea (taeniasis).
- Passage of segments (proglottids) or ova of tapeworm per rectum (taeniasis).
- Demonstration of cysticerci in tissue biopsy specimens or on radiograph (cysticercosis).

General Considerations

Taeniasis may be caused by beef tapeworm *(Taenia saginata)* or pork tapeworm *(Taenia solium)*. The adult worms reside in the alimentary canal of humans. The mature segments passed per rectum discharge ova in feces and soil, which are then ingested by cattle and pigs. The hatched larvae develop into encysted forms mainly in the skeletal muscles (cysticercosis). When humans consume raw or undercooked meat, the larvae are liberated and develop into adults in the small intestine. The worm attaches itself to the mucosa by its scolex, with suckers and (in *T solium)* a double ring of eversible hooks.

Human cysticercosis is caused by the larvae of *T solium*. It occurs as a result of ingestion of eggs, which hatch in the intestines, or from internal autoinfection following reverse peristalsis and release of eggs from a broken segment of gravid *T solium* in the duodenal area. The swallowed or released eggs hatch, and the hexacanth larvae then penetrate the gastric or intestinal wall, enter the bloodstream, and migrate into muscle and other tissues.

Both of these disorders are worldwide in distribution. They are more prevalent in areas where control over the quality of meat is inadequate.

Clinical Findings

A. Symptoms and Signs: In the majority of tapeworm infections, there are no symptoms other than the passage of segments in feces—sometimes up to several dozen a day per worm—seen as white motile bodies about 1–2 cm long and 5 mm thick. Occasionally, the proglottid moves out of the rectum and crawls on the skin of the thigh—especially *T saginata*, whose segments are more muscular than the flaccid *T solium* segments.

Infants are not infected, since they are not exposed. Toddlers and older children may harbor the infection for years. Abdominal pain, diarrhea, excessive appetite, failure to gain weight, abdominal distention, and anorexia may occur. Symptoms may be related to the number of worms present.

Most cases of cysticercosis go undiagnosed, since there are few or no symptoms. The development of subcutaneous or muscle nodules is often the sole manifestation. After several years, the cysticerci calcify and appear as opacities on radiograph. Cysticerci in the brain may remain silent or may cause symptoms and signs of epilepsy, brain tumor, hydrocephalus, and basal meningitis. In the eye, they may cause uveitis, retinal detachment, and hemorrhage. The diagnosis is difficult to confirm except when nodules are available for biopsy or are visible in radiographs. CT scanning of the head is a sensitive method for demonstrating cysticerci in the brain. The presence of *T solium* in the gut is of diagnostic significance.

B. Laboratory Findings: The diagnosis is confirmed by the demonstration of the proglottids or eggs. Eggs may be seen in fecal smears or may be detected on the perianal skin by the method used in the diagnosis of enterobiasis (see above). They are globular, 30–60 μm in diameter, with a double wall showing radial striations and an embryo with 6 hooklets (hexacanth).

If a proglottid is compressed between 2 glass slides, the main lateral branches of the uterus may be examined. *T saginata* has 18 or more and *T solium* fewer than 12 such branches to each side.

Eosinophilia is mild or absent in most cases.

Treatment

A. Taeniasis: Niclosamide is the best available drug for all tapeworm infections. Toxicity is slight or absent in therapeutic doses. The vanilla-flavored niclosamide tablets should be chewed or crushed thoroughly before swallowing; they are best taken on an empty stomach the morning after a light nonresidue supper. Niclosamide is given as a single dose of 1 g (2 tablets) for children weighing 11–34 kg and 1.5 g for those weighing over 34 kg. Teenagers should take the adult dose of 2 g (4 tablets).

Paromomycin is an alternative drug that also works, but niclosamide is definitely preferred. The dosage of paromomycin is 11 mg/kg every 15 minutes for a total of 4 doses.

If segments are not passed per rectum for at least 3 months, that is sufficient evidence of complete expulsion of the worms.

B. Cysticercosis: Previously, there was no specific treatment for cerebral cysticercosis apart from surgical removal of accessible cysticerci. CT scanning now allows for recognition of infection before calcification takes place, and medical therapy may be successful. The drug of choice is praziquantel, 50 mg/kg/d orally in 3 divided doses for 14 days. A concurrent short, tapering course of oral dexamethasone may be required to control transient cerebral edema associated with killing of cysticerci by praziquantel. Neurosurgical consultation must be available. Follow-up CT scans at 3, 6, and 12 months are recommended to assess the response to therapy.

Prognosis

The prognosis is good in taeniasis. In cerebral cysticercosis, the prognosis is less favorable: Symptoms may disappear after a variable interval, or heavy infections may result in death.

Botero D, Castaño S: Treatment of cysticercosis with praziquantel in Colombia. *Am J Trop Med Hyg* 1982;**31:**811.

Brown WJ, Voge M: Cysticercosis: A modern plague. *Pediatr Clin North Am* 1985;**32:**953.

Loo L, Braude A: Cerebral cysticercosis in San Diego. *Medicine* 1982;**61:**341.

Nash TE, Neva FA: Recent advances in the diagnosis and treatment of cerebral cysticercosis. *N Engl J Med* 1984;**311:**1492.

Percy AK, Byrd SE, Locke GE: Cerebral cysticercosis. *Pediatrics* 1980;**66:**967.

Perera DR, Western KA, Schultz MG: Niclosamide treatment of cestodiasis: Clinical trials in the United States. *Am J Trop Med Hyg* 1970;**19:**610.

Sotelo J et al: Therapy of parenchymal brain cysticercosis with praziquantel. *N Engl J Med* 1984;**310:**1001.

2. HYMENOLEPIASIS

Hymenolepis nana commonly infects children; *Hymenolepis diminuta* does so rarely. *H diminuta* is a rat tapeworm with cysticercoid stages in fleas and insects. Children acquire the infection by eating insect-contaminated grains. *H nana* occurs in South and Southeast Asia, North Africa, southern Europe, South America, and the southern USA. *H nana* is primarily a parasite of humans. Occasionally, humans are infected via an intermediate flea or beetle with *H nana* var *fraterna,* which is common in mice and rats. *H nana* may be passed to humans by infected grain beetles and other insects, but it also has the unique ability to infect directly by its eggs without passing through a developmental (cysticercoid) stage in an intermediate host. The eggs hatch in the intestinal lumen and the larvae penetrate the villi, where they form the larval stage, then return to the gut lumen, attach, and mature to become adult tapeworms. Fecal-oral contamination is necessary for infection of fresh human hosts.

Unlike other tapeworms, *H nana* is very small (2–5 cm), and numerous worms may be present in the intestine. Infection is usually asymptomatic, but diarrhea and abdominal pain may occur. The diagnosis is confirmed by detecting eggs in feces. They appear oval, rarely globular, 30–50 μm, and double-walled without radial striations; as with other tapeworms of humans, the embryo has 6 hooklets. The eggs of *H nana* have 4–8 polar filaments at each end; this characteristic feature serves to distinguish eggs of *H nana* from those of *H diminuta*.

The drug of choice for treatment of hymenolepiasis is niclosamide (for dosage, see Taeniasis). Alternatively, paromomycin may be used (see Taeniasis). The duration of treatment, however, for *H nana* infection is 5–7 days. This is important because both niclosamide and paromomycin are active only against adult tapeworms. The longer therapy for *H nana* enables killing of newly emerging adults from the intestinal villi, where the larvae develop uniquely in humans in contrast to the larvae of all other tapeworms.

Jones WE: Niclosamide as a treatment for *Hymenolepsis diminuta* and *Dipylidium caninum* infection in man. *Am J Trop Med Hyg* 1979;**28:**300.

Most H et al: Yomesan (niclosamide) therapy of *Hymenolepis nana* infections. *Am J Trop Med Hyg* 1971;**20:**206.

Wittner M, Tanowitz H: Paromomycin therapy of human cestodiasis with special reference to hymenolepiasis. *Am J Trop Med Hyg* 1971;**20:**433.

3. DIPHYLLOBOTHRIASIS

Human infection with *Diphyllobothrium latum,* a broad fish tapeworm, occurs in the Scandinavian, Baltic, and Mediterranean regions; in Japan, Chile, and Argentina; and in Alaska and around the Great Lakes region of the USA and Canada. One or more adult worms live inside the human intestine, attached to the mucosa by a scolex with twin sucking grooves. Adults and children are infected.

The ova develop in copepod crustaceans *(Diaptomus),* which are eaten by fish. The larvae develop further in the muscle and connective tissues of the fish. Pike, salmon, trout, whitefish, and turbot may become infected. The cycle is maintained in nature by many species of fish-eating mammals that can serve as definitive hosts, including the bear, fox, seal, sea lion, walrus, dog, and cat. Humans acquire the infection by consuming raw or undercooked fish. Smoking or ordinary kippering does not destroy the larvae.

In many cases, the infection remains silent. No segments (proglottids) are passed per rectum. Abdominal pain, vomiting, diarrhea, and nutritional deficiency occur occasionally.

The diagnosis is made by the detection of ova in stools. They are oval, operculated, 45 × 70 μm, with a brownish operculated shell enclosing several granulated, tightly packed yolk cells.

In fewer than 1% of cases—but a higher percentage in Finland—progressive macrocytic, megaloblastic anemia occurs as a result of vitamin B_{12} (cobalamin) deficiency. The megaloblastic anemia may be complicated by spinal cord lesions.

Niclosamide is the drug of choice for treatment of fish tapeworm; a single dose is highly effective (for dosage, see Taeniasis). Alternatively, paromomycin can be used as with other tapeworm infections.

In the majority of instances of megaloblastic anemia, the explusion of the worms results in a hematologic remission. In severe cases, cobalamin (vitamin B_{12}) may be given parenterally in a single dose of 15–30 μg by deep subcutaneous or intramuscular injection. Oral cobalamin is of little value until after the expulsion of the worms.

Anemia and the fish tapeworm. (Editorial.) *Lancet* 1977;**1**:292.

4. ECHINOCOCCOSIS

Essentials of Diagnosis

- Cystic tumor of liver or lung; rarely, of kidney, bone, brain, and other organs.
- Urticaria and pruritus secondary to rupture of cyst.
- Eosinophilia.
- Protoscoleces, brood capsules, or daughter cysts in lesion.
- Elevated titers on indirect hemagglutination (≥ 1:128) or bentonite flocculation (≥ 1:5) tests.

General Considerations

Echinococcus granulosus is a tapeworm that infects dogs and some cats and other carnivores. The adult worm lives in the intestines, and eggs are excreted in the feces. Humans serve as intermediate (never final) hosts. When eggs from dog feces are ingested by a child, the embryo hatches and passes into intestinal lymphatics, reaching various parts of the body via the circulation. A cyst develops in the organ where the embryo settles. There is a predilection for the liver (60–70%) and the lungs (20–25%). A unilocular spherical cyst is the most common expression of the infection. It grows over a period of years and may reach 25 cm in diameter, although most are between 1 and 8 cm. A well-defined structure exists in the cyst. Infection with *Echinococcus multilocularis* results in cysts that are multilocular or alveolar, without the heavy enclosing capsule that typifies the unilocular cyst of *E granulosus* and prevents rapid, uncontrolled growth as is seen in *E multilocularis*.

Clinical Findings

A. Symptoms and Signs: Clinical findings are dependent upon several phenomena: pressure by the enlarging cysts, erosion of blood vessels, and circulation of sensitizing parts of the cyst or worm. Cysts in the liver present as slowly growing tumors. Jaundice may be present if biliary obstruction occurs. Most cysts are in the right lobe, extending downward into the abdomen; one-fourth are on the upper surface and may go undetected for many years.

Hemorrhage may result from erosion. Omental torsion is also observed.

Pulmonary cysts rarely produce pressure symptoms but may erode into a bronchus, resulting in cough and atelectasis.

Rupture of a cyst and discharge of its contents may result in sudden episodes of coughing if in the lung. Asthma, urticaria, and pruritus may be observed. The sputum is blood-tinged and frothy and contains bits of the cyst and worm. Common signs in pulmonary cyst rupture are coughing, dyspnea, hemoptysis, chest pain, and increase in pulse and respiratory rates.

Cysts of the brain may produce focal neurologic signs and convulsions; of the kidney, hematuria and pain; of bone, pain.

B. Laboratory Findings: In suspected cases of echinococcosis with allergic manifestations, a search for protoscoleces, brood capsules, or daughter cysts should be made. Specimens for examination will depend on the site of the cyst but include sputum or bronchoscopic aspirates, urine, ascitic fluid or pleural fluid, and cerebrospinal fluid.

Eosinophilia occurs irregularly and to a variable extent.

Serologic tests can assist both in the diagnosis of hydatid cyst and in evaluation of the success of cystectomy. It is best to use more than one type of immunodiagnostic test and to bear in mind that the diagnostic titer varies in different laboratories. The bentonite flocculation test is considered positive at a titer of 1:5 or higher, whereas a significant titer in the indirect hemagglutination test is 1:128 or higher at the Centers for Disease Control, Atlanta, GA 30333. When secondary echinococcosis is present, the titers are usually 10- to 1000-fold higher. Titers in all of these immunodiagnostic tests remain high for at least 1 year after surgery, even when it is successful. They drop significantly by 3–4 years postoperatively and are usually negative by the tenth year. If the parasite has not been completely removed at operation, the titers remain higher. Continued presence of the parasite should be suspected when titers remain markedly elevated. The indirect hemagglutination titer takes longer to drop under all circumstances.

The intradermal (Casoni) skin test for echinococcosis is no longer recommended. The antigen, hydatid fluid from humans or animals, is not readily available. Moreover, the Casoni skin test is not reliable, since it has never been standardized and false-positive results are obtained in up to 40% of patients. Radiographs, CT scans, and serologic studies should establish the diagnosis in patients with an appropriate history.

C. Radiographic Findings: Radiography of the chest may reveal the cyst. Special studies of the central nervous system may reveal evidence of an intracranial mass and increased pressure. Calcified cysts in any organ may be noted; destruction of bony structure is visible in osseous lesions. CT scanning or ultrasonography can delineate the location and size of echinococcal cysts.

Differential Diagnosis

Hydatid cysts in any site may be mistaken for a variety of malignant and nonmalignant tumors or for abscesses, both bacterial and amebic. In the lung, a cyst may be confused with an advanced tubercular lesion. Syphilis may also be confused with echinococcosis. Allergic symptoms arising from cyst leakage may resemble those associated with many other diseases.

Complications

Sudden rupture of a cyst leading to anaphylaxis and sometimes death is the most important complication of echinococcosis. If the patient survives the rupture, there is still the danger of multiple secondary cyst infections arising from seeding of daughter cysts. Segmental lung collapse, secondary infections of cysts, secondary effects of increased intracranial pressure, and severe renal damage due to kidney cysts are other potential complications.

Treatment

The only definitive treatment is surgical removal of the intact cysts, preferably preceded by inoculation into the cyst of a 1% aqueous iodine solution or formalin. A recent advance in surgical technique is the freezing of the cyst wall and instillation of silver nitrate immediately prior to removal.

Often, however, the presence of a cyst is only recognized when it begins to leak or when it ruptures. Such an event calls for vigorous treatment of allergic symptoms or emergency management of anaphylactic shock. In cases where spillage of hydatid cyst fluid at surgery is recognized or inevitable and in the inoperable case, drug therapy may be tried. Oral treatment with mebendazole (50 mg/kg/d) or albendazole (10 mg/kg/d) has resulted in a clinical response. Albendazole therapy for 1 month has recently been shown to be effective in patients who failed to respond to earlier therapy with mebendazole for 6 months. The precise role of medical therapy for echinococcosis remains to be defined.

Prognosis

Patients may live for years with relatively large hydatid cysts before their condition is diagnosed. Liver and lung cysts often can be removed surgically without great difficulty, but for cysts in sites less accessible to surgery, the prognosis is less favorable. The prognosis is always grave in secondary echinococcosis and with alveolar cysts. About 15% of patients with echinococcosis eventually die because of the disease or its complications.

Bryceson ADM et al: Experience with mebendazole in the treatment of inoperable hydatid disease in England. *Trans R Soc Trop Med Hyg* 1982;**76:**510.

Grove DI, Warren KS, Mahmoud AAF: Algorithms in the diagnosis and management of exotic diseases. 10. Echinococcosis. *J Infect Dis* 1976;**133:**354.

Katz R, Murphy S, Kosloske A: Pulmonary echinococcosis: A pediatric disease of the Southwestern United States. *Pediatrics* 1980;**65:**1003.

McCorkle SJ, Lewall DB: Computed tomography of intracerebral echinococcal cysts in children. *J Comput Assist Tomogr* 1985;**9:**514.

Morris DL et al: Albendazole: Objective evidence of response in human hydatid disease. *JAMA* 1985;**253:**2053.

Nourmand A: Hydatid cysts in children and youths. *Am J Trop Med Hyg* 1976;**25:**845.

Pearl M et al: Cerebral echinococcosis, a pediatric disease: Report of two cases with one successful five-year follow-up. *Pediatrics* 1978;**61:**915.

Schantz PM: Effective medical treatment for hydatid disease? (Editoral.) *JAMA* 1985;**253:**2095.

Wilson JF, Rausch RL: Alveolar hydatid disease: A review of clinical features of 33 indigenous cases of *Echinococcus multilocularis* infection in Alaskan Eskimos. *Am J Trop Med Hyg* 1980;**29:**1340.

Wilson JF, Rausch RL: Mebendazole and alveolar hydatid disease. *Ann Trop Med Parasitol* 1982;**76:**165.

TREMATODE INFECTIONS

1. PARAGONIMIASIS, CLONORCHIASIS, FASCIOLIASIS, & FASCIOLOPSIASIS

Paragonimiasis, caused by the lung fluke *Paragonimus westermani,* occurs in East and Southeast Asia, parts of Africa, and in South America. Humans and carnivorous animals acquire the infection by consuming uncooked crabs and other crustacea, the intermediate hosts carrying encysted larvae.

Clonorchiasis and fascioliasis are caused by the Oriental liver fluke *Clonorchis sinensis* and the sheep liver fluke *Fasciola hepatica.* The former occurs in East and Southeast Asia, and the latter is worldwide. Ingestion of raw fish containing encysted *Clonorchis* larvae or fresh aquatic plants with attached encysted *Fasciola* larvae results in infections.

Fasciolopsis buski, the giant intestinal fluke of humans, causes fasciolopsiasis, found in East and Southeast Asia. The encysted larvae remain attached to water plants, as in the case of *Fasciola.*

Clinical Findings

A. Paragonimiasis: The young lung flukes digested free of their cysts migrate from the intestines to the lungs, where they mature and form cystic lesions with fibrous walls, often 2 worms to a cyst. Fibrous nodules also appear around masses of eggs. The usual symptoms are cough with copious brownish sputum and frequent hemoptysis. In heavy infections, the worms are also found in various abdominal viscera and even in the brain. In such instances, abdominal pain, dysentery, and convulsive and paralytic disease may occur. Radiographic changes in the lungs and clubbing of the fingers are common. The diagnosis depends on the demonstration of ova in sputum or feces.

B. Clonorchiasis and Fascioliasis: The hatched worms of these liver flukes migrate from the intestine to mature in the bile ducts of the liver. Most infections remain asymptomatic. Fever, upper abdominal pain, hepatomegaly, jaundice, urticaria, and eosinophilia in various combinations are the early features in heavy and continued infections, especially in older children. Cholangitis, cholecystitis, and cholelithiasis may occur in episodes. Cirrhosis of the liver is a late complication, as is cholangiocarcinoma. Confirm the diagnosis by demonstrating ova in feces or duodenal aspirate.

C. Fasciolopsiasis: The flukes inhabit the duodenum and the jejunum. The usual symptoms are abdominal pain and diarrhea. Gradually, progressive malnutrition, ascites, and generalized edema appear. Severe and untreated infections may cause death. The diagnosis is confirmed by the presence of ova in feces.

Treatment

Praziquantel is now the drug of choice for treatment of all lung, liver, and intestinal flukes. The drug's effectiveness against fluke infections has rendered past regimens obsolete; its major drawback at present is cost. Praziquantel is given orally, 75 mg/kg on a single day in 3 divided doses. Bithionol, 30–50 mg/kg/d divided evenly into a morning and evening dose on alternate days for 10–15 doses, is a less effective, more troublesome alternative drug for paragonimiasis and fascioliasis. There is no alternative drug for clonorchiasis. Fasciolopsiasis may also be treated with tetrachloroethylene in the same dosage as for hookworm disease (see p 914).

Burton K et al: Pulmonary paragonimiasis in Laotian refugee children. *Pediatrics* 1982;**70:**246.

Flavell DJ: Liver-fluke infection as an aetiological factor in bile-duct carcinoma of man. *Trans R Soc Trop Med Hyg* 1981;**75:**814.

Horstmann RD et al: High efficacy of praziquantel in the treatment of 22 patients with *Clonorchis/Opisthorchis* infections. *Tropenmed Parasitol* 1981;**32:**157.

Johnson JR et al: Paragonimiasis in the United States: A report of nine cases in Hmong immigrants. *Chest* 1982;**82:**168.

Jong EC et al: Praziquantel for the treatment of *Clonorchis/Opisthorchis* infections: Report of a double-blind, placebo-controlled trial. *J Infect Dis* 1985;**152:**637.

Pearson RD, Guerrant RL: Praziquantel: A major advance in anthelminthic therapy. *Ann Intern Med* 1983;**99:**195.

Schiappacasse RH, Mohammadi D, Christie AJ: Successful treatment of severe infection with *Fasciola hepatica* with praziquantel. *J Infect Dis* 1985;**152:**1339.

Spitalny KC et al: Treatment of pulmonary paragonimiasis with a new broad-spectrum antihelmintic, praziquantel. *J Pediatr* 1982;**101:**144.

2. SCHISTOSOMIASIS (Bilharziasis)

Essentials of Diagnosis

- A transient itchy papular rash following exposure to fresh water.
- Fever, urticaria, joint pain, cough, lymphadenitis, eosinophilia.
- Anorexia, loss of weight, diarrhea or dysentery.
- Hematuria (usually terminal), painful micturition.
- Demonstration of ova in stools, urine, or rectal biopsy specimen.

General Considerations

Schistosomiasis is caused by the blood flukes *Schistosoma haematobium, Schistosoma japonicum, Schistosoma mekongi,* and *Schistosoma mansoni.* Worldwide, more than 200 million people harbor these blood flukes; schistosomiasis is one of the world's most common serious diseases. *S haematobium* is prevalent in tropical and subtropical Africa, Yemen, and some parts of Saudi Arabia. *S japonicum* and *S mekongi* occur in East and Southeast Asia. *S mansoni* is common in tropical Africa, South America, and parts of the Caribbean.

The infective swimming larvae (cercariae) are found in fresh water. When in contact with human skin, they penetrate, invade the blood vessels, migrate to the liver, and finally move up the mesenteric vessels to specific final preferred sites. Respectively, the preferential sites of *S haematobium, S japonicum* and *S mekongi,* and *S mansoni* are the vesical venous plexus, the draining veins of the small intestine, and those of the large bowel. They mature in the liver, mate, and migrate to these sites where the females lay eggs. The eggs escape into the perivascular tissues, cause inflammatory lesions, and enter into the lumens of the bladder and bowel. This is accompanied by extravasation of blood.

The eggs that escape in urine and feces hatch in fresh water, and the ciliated larvae (miracidia) enter and develop in the appropriate freshwater intermediate snail host. The parasite multiplies in the snail, and after 3–4 weeks large numbers of cercariae emerge and seek the skin of new final hosts—human for *S haematobium* and *S mansoni;* human and dog for *S mekongi;* and human, cattle, dog, and many others for *S japonicum*.

Clinical Findings

In highly endemic areas, large proportions of the population may be infected, with many showing no symptoms but discharging eggs. Symptoms follow heavy and continued exposure. The diagnosis is readily suspected in endemic areas. Otherwise, a history of residence in endemic areas is of great value in alerting the pediatrician.

A. Symptoms and Signs: Irritation of the skin may occur at sites of cercarial entry with a transient itchy papular rash. During the ensuing migration of the larvae, fever and urticaria may occur. The larvae may escape into the alveoli, causing cough and hemoptysis. Liver and spleen gradually enlarge and become tender. After lodgment of the flukes in their favorite venous plexuses, fever and toxemia occur and last for several days to weeks. In bladder infection, painful and frequent micturition and hematuria are common. Bladder stones and incontinence of urine may follow. Secondary pyelonephritis, vesicoureteral reflux, and anatomic changes in the ureters demonstrable by excretory urography are common. In the intestinal types, abdominal pain, diarrhea (often bloody), and progressive abdominal enlargement due to increasing splenomegaly and ascites occur.

B. Laboratory Findings: The diagnosis should be confirmed by the demonstration of schistosome eggs in feces or urine. *S japonicum* and *S mekongi* eggs are seen only in feces. *S mansoni* eggs are frequently seen in feces and occasionally in urine. If there are no eggs in the feces and urine, a rectal biopsy specimen may reveal *S mansoni* eggs. *S haematobium* eggs are frequently seen in urine and occasionally in feces.

The eggs of *S mansoni* and *S haematobium* measure about 140 × 60 μm and those of *S japonicum* about 90 × 70 μm. *S haematobium* eggs have a terminal spine, whereas the eggs of *S mansoni* and *S japonicum* have a lateral hook or spine, though it is often hidden or hard to see clearly in the smaller eggs of *S japonicum*. *S mekongi* eggs are almost spherical, lack a spine, and measure about 60 × 65 μm.

Complications & Sequelae

The complications and sequelae of *S haematobium* infection are anemia, renal calculi, ascending bacterial infection of the urinary tract, strictures and fistulas, lymphedema of the genitalia, uremia, hypertension, and cancer of the bladder. Schistosomal granulomas in the female genital tract or in the spinal cord (with paraplegia) have been described.

Anemia, cirrhosis of the liver, portal hypertension, and bleeding from esophageal varices may occur in alimentary forms of schistosomiasis. Pulmonary hypertension and cor pulmonale may occur late in *S mansoni* infections.

Severe nutritional deficiencies and death are not uncommon in unchecked and heavy infections.

Prevention

In edemic areas, prevention of infection by avoiding skin contact with contaminated fresh water (bathing, wading) is of paramount public health importance.

Treatment

A. Specific Measures: There have been important improvements in the chemotherapy of schistosomiasis in recent years, the most important of which has been the introduction of praziquantel. As a result, hycanthone and stibophen should no longer be used owing to excessive toxicity. Oxamniquine is now considered to be an alternative drug to praziquantel.

1. Praziquantel—Praziquantel is the drug of choice for all types of schistosomiasis. In clinical trials, praziquantel has been effective in a single oral dose of 40 mg/kg for infections caused by *S mansoni* or *S haematobium* and in a dosage of 30 mg/kg twice in 1 day for infections caused by *S japonicum* or *S mekongi*. Alternatively, all types of schistosomiasis can be treated with praziquantel, 60 mg/kg given in 1 day in 3 divided doses to minimize the occasional abdominal discomfort experienced with a single oral dose. No major toxic reactions have been observed with praziquantel.

2. Oxamniquine—Oxamniquine is an alternative drug for *S mansoni* infection. For western hemisphere strains of *S mansoni*, the recommended oral dosage in children under 30 kg is 20 mg/kg in 2 divided doses 2–8 hours apart on the same day. For children over 30 kg, as in adults, a single dose of 15 mg/kg should be given. African strains of *S mansoni* seem to require a higher dosage of 15 mg/kg twice daily for 2 days. Toleration is improved if capsules are given after food. Transitory dizziness or drowsiness occurs in about one-third of patients. Nausea, vomiting, and abdominal pain are less common. Rarely, epileptiform convulsions have occurred within a few hours following ingestion of oxamniquine. Patients with known seizure disorders should remain under medical observation for at least 6 hours after receiving the drug.

3. Metrifonate—This organophosphorus insecticide is used only as an alternative drug for *S haematobium* infections. Metrifonate is given orally in a dosage of 10 mg/kg every other week for a total of 3 doses. Side effects to date have been negligible (mainly gastrointestinal), and results have been excellent. Metrifonate temporarily reduces cholinesterase levels in blood and should be used with care where exposure to organophosphorus insecticides is a possibility.

4. Niridazole—Niridazole is an alternative drug for *S japonicum* and is a second alternative to oxamniquine for *S mansoni* infection and to metrifonate for *S haematobium* infection. The dosage of niridazole is 25 mg/kg/d in 3 divided doses taken by mouth for 5–7 days. Niridazole should not be given to patients with impaired liver function or portacaval shunts or to those with a history of psychosis. The main toxic reactions of depression, insomnia, mania, confusion, convulsions, and coma result from unmetabolized drug reaching the brain. These effects usually abate promptly when the drug is stopped. Patients and parents should be forewarned that the urine turns dark brown during treatment.

5. Antimony compounds—Antimony potassium or sodium tartrate is recommended only for *S japonicum* and *S mekongi* infections when praziquantel is unavailable. It is given intravenously as a freshly prepared 0.5% solution as follows: For children under 15 kg, give doses of 0.5, 1, 2, 3, 4, 5, and 6 mL on alternate days, then 7 mL on alternate days to a total of 90 mL. For those weighing 15–30 kg, give doses of 1, 2, 4, 6, 8, 10, and 12 mL on alternate days, then 14 mL on alternate days to a total of 180 mL. The solution must be given very slowly, avoiding leakage into perivascular tissue. The patient must rest in bed during the injection and for several hours afterward.

Another alternative drug for *S japonicum* infection is antimony sodium dimercaptosuccinate, 8 mg/kg intramuscularly once or twice a week for a total of 5 doses. Antimony sodium dimercaptosuccinate is also used for patients with *S mansoni* infection when neither praziquantel nor niridazole can be given.

B. General Measures: It is important to look for and treat intercurrent bacterial or parasitic infections and nutritional deficiencies. For fibrotic and calcified lesions in the older child, especially of the urinary tract, corrective surgery should be done to relieve symptoms or arrest the progression of renal damage. Splenectomy and portacaval shunt are palliative measures in advanced alimentary schistosomiasis.

Prognosis

The prognosis is good in mild infections and in heavy symptomatic infections treated early. Otherwise, the prognosis is poor, especially with involvement of the lungs, liver, spleen, and urinary tract.

Doehring E et al: Reduction of pathological findings in urine and bladder lesions in infection with *Schistosoma haematobium* after treatment with praziquantel. *J Infect Dis* 1985;**152:**807.

Feldmeier H et al: Efficacy of metrifonate in urinary schistosomiasis: Comparison of reduction of *Schistosoma haematobium* and *S mansoni* eggs. *Am J Trop Med Hyg* 1982; **31:**1188.

Hofstetter M et al: Infection with *Schistosoma mekongi* in Southeast Asian refugees. *J Infect Dis* 1981;**144:**420.

Keittivuti B et al: Treatment of *Schistosoma mekongi* with praziquantel in Cambodian refugees in holding centers in Prachinburi Province, Thailand. *Trans R Soc Trop Med Hyg* 1984;**78:**477.

Kilpatrick ME et al: Oxamniquine versus niridazole for treatment of uncomplicated *Schistosoma mansoni* infection. *Am J Trop Med Hyg* 1982;**31:**1164.

Lambertucci JR et al: A double blind trial with oxamniquine in chronic schistosomiasis mansoni. *Trans R Soc Trop Med Hyg* 1982;**76:**751.

Mott KE et al: Effect of praziquantel on hematuria and proteinuria in urinary schistosomiasis. *Am J Trop Med Hyg* 1985;**34:**1119.

Pearson RD, Guerrant RL: Praziquantel: A major advance in anthelminthic therapy. *Ann Intern Med* 1983;**99:**195.

Pugh RNH, Teesdale CH: Single dose oral treatment in urinary schistosomiasis: A double blind trial. *Br Med J* 1983; **286:**429.

Warren KS: Selective primary health care: Strategies for control of disease in the developing world. 1. Schistosomiasis. *Rev Infect Dis* 1982;**4:**715.

SELECTED REFERENCES

Beaver PC, Jung RC, Cupp EW: *Clinical Parasitology,* 9th ed. Lea & Febiger, 1984.

Binford CH, Connor DH (editors): *Pathology of Tropical and Extraordinary Diseases.* Vols 1 and 2. Armed Forces Institute of Pathology, 1976.

Brown HW, Neva FN: *Basic Clinical Parasitology,* 5th ed. Appleton-Century-Crofts, 1983.

Drugs for Parasitic Infections: *Handbook of Antimicrobial Therapy.* The Medical Letter, Inc., 1984.

James DM, Gilles HM (editors): *Human Antiparasitic Drugs: Pharmacology and Usage.* Wiley, 1985.

Jawetz E et al: *Review of Medical Microbiology,* 17th ed. Lange, 1986.

Katz M, Despommier DD, Gwadz RW: *Parasitic Diseases.* Springer-Verlag, 1982.

Maegraith BG, Gilles HM (editors): *Management and Treatment of Tropical Diseases.* Blackwell, 1971.

Manson-Bahr PEC, Apted FIC: *Manson's Tropical Diseases,* 18th ed. Bailliere Tindall, 1982.

Marcial-Rojas RA (editor): *Pathology of Protozoal and Helminthic Diseases With Clinical Correlation.* Williams & Wilkins, 1971.

Markell ED, Voge M: *Medical Parasitology,* 5th ed. Saunders, 1981.

Peters W, Gilles HM: *A Colour Atlas of Tropical Medicine and Parasitology.* Wolfe, 1977.

Strickland G: *Hunter's Tropical Medicine,* 6th ed. Saunders, 1984.

Warren KS, Mahmoud AAF (editors): *Tropical and Geographic Medicine.* McGraw-Hill, 1984.

29 Infections: Mycotic

Vincent A. Fulginiti, MD

ACTINOMYCOSIS

Essentials of Diagnosis

- Chronic suppurative lesions of the skin, with sinus tract formation.
- "Sulfur granules"—*Actinomyces* colonies 1–2 mm in diameter—found in pus from lesion.
- Gram-positive hyphae.
- Association with gram-negative bacteria.
- Isolation of organism from sulfur granule or pus.

General Considerations

Human actinomycosis is almost always caused by *Actinomyces israelii*. Although traditionally classified as a fungus, *A israelii* is actually a bacterium.* The symptoms and course of the diseases produced resemble those of the chronic mycoses, but successful therapy with antibacterial antibiotics is more in keeping with the true nature of these organisms.

The organism is a frequent oral and dental saprophyte, and infection is endogenous. Actinomycosis is characteristically a chronic, slowly progressive disease.

Clinical Findings

A. Symptoms and Signs: Three primary forms of the disease are recognized: cervicofacial, thoracic, and abdominal.

1. Cervicofacial actinomycosis (lumpy jaw)—Granulomas appear in the mandible or maxilla and are of dental or oral origin. These break down and suppurate and may seal over but do not heal. Sinus tracts form and re-form, and without treatment the disease has a chronic unremitting course.

2. Thoracic actinomycosis—This form is heralded by fever (often of septic nature), pleural pain, cough, and weight loss. There may be mucopurulent or sanguineous sputum or sinus tract drainage. Dullness to percussion and signs of consolidation may be present, and sinus tracts may communicate with the skin.

3. Abdominal actinomycosis—This usually begins with inflammation of the appendix and weight loss. Fever, chills, and vomiting over a protracted course are associated with painful, palpable masses.

4. Infections in other sites—*A israelii* can also infect the brain, liver, kidney, genitourinary tract, and bone. Bacteremia can occur, particularly in immunocompromised individuals, and may last for months, with symptoms and signs of low-grade chronic infection.

B. Laboratory Findings: Identification of typical sulfur granules and gram-positive hyphae in secretions should lead to culture of *A israelii*.

C. X-Ray Findings: With bony involvement, periostitis and osteomyelitis are visible on x-ray examination. Heavy hilar and basilar infiltration is characteristic of pulmonary actinomycosis.

Differential Diagnosis

Actinomycosis must be distinguished from fungal diseases causing similar manifestations (culture); pulmonary, intestinal, or lymphatic tuberculosis (PPD, isolation of mycobacteria, response to therapy); and lymphomas (biopsy, absence of sinuses, blood or bone marrow changes). Bacterial infection of the cervical lymph nodes, bones, chest, or abdomen can usually be differentiated on the basis of culture, acuteness, and response to therapy.

Complications

Extension of the infection from the primary site to contiguous structures (irrespective of anatomic limits) results in osteomyelitis, brain abscess, hepatic or renal involvement, abscesses, and sinus tracts.

Treatment

A. Specific Measures: Penicillin is the drug of choice. Daily doses range up to 2 million units in infants and up to 20 million units in older children. Initial intravenous therapy for 2–4 weeks is followed by intramuscular and then by oral administration and must usually be continued for as long as 6 months to 1 year or more. Broad-spectrum antibiotics and sulfadiazine are useful adjuncts but should not be used alone.

B. General Measures: Surgical excision is frequently necessary, particularly with chronic, multiple sinus tracts. Preoperative therapy with penicillin is always indicated.

Prognosis

Penicillin therapy has greatly improved the prognosis. Unless the course has been prolonged and complications such as brain abscess or meningitis have appeared, recovery is the rule. A defective cell-mediated immune response has been noted in patients with

* Discussed in this chapter by convention. See also Nocardiosis, p 936.

deep actinomycosis. Convalescence may be prolonged.

Larsen J et al: Cervicofacial *Actinomyces* infections. *J Pediatr* 1978;**93:**797.

Rose HD, Varkey B, Kutty CP: Thoracic actinomycosis caused by *Actinomyces meyeri. Am Rev Respir Dis* 1982;**125:**251.

Spinola SM, Bell RA, Henderson FW: Actinomycosis. *Am J Dis Child* 1981;**135:**336.

Stanley TV: Deep actinomycosis in childhood. *Acta Paediatr Scand* 1980;**69:**173.

ASPERGILLOSIS

Opportunistic infection due to *Aspergillus fumigatus* and other species of this genus is rare in childhood. These organisms are found commonly in nature, particularly in decaying vegetation. A number of cases have occurred in children receiving corticosteroids or immunosuppressive drugs; other predisposing causes include chronic bronchopulmonary disease, tuberculosis, and morphologic abnormalities of the respiratory tract. Recently, marihuana contaminated with *Aspergillus* has been found.

A chronic course is characteristic, and a history of long-standing symptoms may be elicited. Fever, productive cough, and increasing lassitude often precede cavitary pulmonary changes. Pulmonary infection may become disseminated to other viscera, often with a fatal outcome. Mucopurulent sputum or hemoptysis is frequently present. Chronic otomycosis is manifested by obstruction of the auditory canal with a plug composed of fungus, wax, and epithelial debris. In the absence of bacterial infection, the canal is dry. There are no laboratory aids to the diagnosis save for culture of the fungus or identification of hyphae in sodium hydroxide preparations from specimens of sputum, pus, or ear curettage.

In recent years, a variety of syndromes have been recognized in association with this organism, particularly allergic pulmonary disease, endophthalmitis following eye surgery, and disseminated disease.

Pulmonary symptoms resemble those of allergic asthma. Patients with true asthma may also have clinical exacerbation upon exposure to *Aspergillus*. The diagnosis is suggested by positive immediate-type skin tests and by the presence and increase in titer of serum precipitins and other antibodies. Transient infiltrates may be seen on x-ray examination of the lungs and may be due to bronchial plugging with the organisms in association with bronchospasm. Therapy is symptomatic; a few patients seem to benefit from desensitization.

Early systemic administration of amphotericin B (Fungizone) in high doses may cure invasive aspergillosis. Surgical resection of pulmonary fungal masses may be coupled with local instillation of amphotericin B. Disseminated disease and endophthalmitis may be treated with amphotericin B; however, many of the organisms are resistant to the serum levels of this antibiotic usually achieved, and the fulminant nature of the disease process may preclude successful therapy. Some experts argue for aggressive early diagnosis and application of surgical therapy and amphotericin B or flucytosine in attempts to decrease morbidity and mortality rates. Imidazoles may be useful if organ failure precludes use of the usual antifungal agents.

Brueton MJ et al: Allergic bronchopulmonary aspergillosis complicating cystic fibrosis in childhood. *Arch Dis Child* 1980;**55:**348.

D'Silva H et al: Disseminated aspergillosis in a presumably immunoincompetent host. *JAMA* 1982;**248:**1495.

Imbeau SA, Cohen M, Reed CE: Allergic bronchopulmonary aspergillosis in infants. *Am J Dis Child* 1977;**131:**1127.

Park GR: Disseminated aspergillosis occurring in patients with respiratory, renal and hepatic failure. *Lancet* 1982;**2:**179.

Rinaldi MG: Invasive aspergillosis. *Rev Infect Dis* 1983;**5:**1061.

NORTH AMERICAN BLASTOMYCOSIS

Blastomyces dermatitidis, a budding yeast form in human infection, is present in soil, but its exact mode of transmission is not known. Blastomycosis is widely distributed in North and Central America, with a high prevalence in the Mississippi Valley. Childhood illness is uncommon.

There are 2 basic forms—pulmonary and cutaneous—and a disseminated form that may arise from either. The disseminated form is characterized by chronic suppurative bronchopulmonary disease with insidious and often prolonged (months) early symptoms of cough, fever, weight loss, increasing chest pain, and hoarseness. Purulent or bloody sputum may be present. With dissemination, cutaneous lesions, bone pain, chills, and sweats become apparent. Central nervous system symptoms are heralded by severe headache, and focal neurologic signs, particularly paralysis, are common.

Cutaneous lesions are usually single, beginning as a nodular papule on an exposed surface and gradually ulcerating and failing to heal. Multiple sites may be present and are all associated with pulmonary disease. Spread is believed to be via the bloodstream. The individual lesion has a raised border with a multiply abscessed crater. Purplish discoloration is frequent, and small abscesses can be found in the border.

Dissemination results in involvement of the brain, kidneys, bones, skin, and subcutaneous tissues. Symptoms referable to these tissues in a patient with chronic pulmonary infection should lead the clinician to suspect blastomycosis.

Skin tests and serologic tests are of little value in the diagnosis of blastomycosis. Cytologic examination of sputum often reveals the organism.

Hydroxystilbamidine isethionate appears to be effective in a dosage of 5–8 mg/kg/d intravenously for a total dose of 8 g. It is recommended that it be used only for nonprogressive cutaneous infections. Amphotericin B (Fungizone) by intravenous infusion may be helpful (see Chapter 38). Surgical drainage and excisional therapy are of limited benefit but may be useful in selected cases and as an adjunct to antifungal therapy.

Mild forms of the pulmonary disease may exist, but the usual clinically apparent case, if untreated, usually disseminates, leading to death.

Eberle DE, Evans RB, Johnson RH: Disseminated North American blastomycosis. *JAMA* 1977;**238:**2629.

Laskey WK, Serosi GA: Blastomycosis in children. *Pediatrics* 1980;**65:**111.

Miller D et al: Erythema nodosum and blastomycosis. *Arch Intern Med* 1982;**142:**1839.

Trumbull ML, Chesney TM: The cytological diagnosis of pulmonary blastomycosis. *JAMA* 1981;**245:**836.

CANDIDIASIS

Essentials of Diagnosis

- Plaquelike and ulcerative lesions of the oral mucosa.
- Vulvovaginitis, skin fold infections, paronychia; pulmonary, central nervous system, and disseminated disease.
- A compatible clinical picture, a susceptible host, and the repeated finding of oval, budding yeasts in clinical specimens should establish the diagnosis.

General Considerations

Candida albicans is the major human pathogen of the genus. It is a ubiquitous, dimorphic fungus that usually reproduces by budding. The yeast forms are vegetative; in most human tissue infections, the mycelial form is observed. Although many host defense factors have been described, no consistent relationship to infection or disease has been established. Delayed hypersensitivity to *Candida* appears to be important in that clinically significant disease states are almost always associated with a lack of skin test reactivity.

C albicans exists as a normal inhabitant of the gastrointestinal flora, and its growth is held in check by the presence of other members of the flora. With the expections of thrush in newborns and vaginitis in pregnant women, it seldom produces disease in healthy individuals. Reduction in host defenses or a significant change in the indigenous flora results in overgrowth of *Candida* and can lead to local and systemic disease. Thus, lymphopenic immunologic deficiencies, the use of corticosteroids or other immunosuppressive therapy, and the administration of antibiotics all may result in systemic candidiasis. Candidiasis is also commonly associated with diabetes mellitus. Topical candidiasis may occur in areas of the skin macerated or exposed to excessive moisture (eg, the diaper area).

Clinical Findings

A. Symptoms and Signs:

1. Oral candidiasis—White patches with superficial mucosal ulceration appear on the entire oral and pharyngeal mucosa and frequently result in loss of appetite, difficulty in swallowing, and even respiratory distress. Individual lesions are surrounded by intensely red areolas; occasionally, in severe forms, coalescence occurs. The illness may be seen in newborns or even 1–2 weeks later.

A new form of oropharyngeal candidiasis has been associated with the use of beclomethasone dipropionate inhalations in the treatment of asthma. Clinical signs may be seen in 5–10% of patients; as many as 4–8 times this number are colonized. This incidence is higher than that associated with oral corticosteroid use and may reflect the higher local concentrations or the increased potency of this agent.

2. Skin infection—Diaper dermatitis is common, with an intensely red, "scorched" appearance extending to the perianal and anterior abdominal areas. Sharp demarcation is sometimes evident. Scaling, weeping lesions, vesicles, pustules, and papules are occasionally present. Satellite lesions are frequent.

Vulvovaginitis may present with the above changes plus a thick, often yellowish exudate associated with itching (often intense).

3. Mucocutaneous infection—This chronic disease is characterized by mucous membrane and skin infection associated with T cell-deficient immunity.

4. Pulmonary infection—*C albicans* pneumonia (uncommon) tends to occur only in diseases associated with deficiency or abnormalities of lymphocyte function. On the other hand, *Candida* is commonly isolated from sputum or on autopsy, and it is sometimes difficult to determine what etiologic role *Candida* played in the pneumonia. This is especially true if antibiotics or corticosteroids have been administered. Symptoms include low-grade fever, chronic cough, and mucoid or mucosanguineous sputum. Rales, signs of pleuritis, and effusion may be present.

5. Other forms—Meningitis, endocarditis, pyelonephritis, and candidemia are seen. All of these forms are limited to patients who are rendered susceptible by therapy with antibiotics, corticosteroids or other immunosuppressive agents, or underlying disease.

A relatively new phenomenon has emerged as a major problem in the care of premature and ill newborn infants. Antibiotic therapy combined with the use of life support systems (respirators, central venous lines, and hyperalimentation) has increased the risk of systemically introduced or seeded candidal infections. Systemic candidiasis may produce signs of generalized sepsis, changes in the homeostasis of glucose, and localization of infection in critical organs. Diagnosis is made difficult by the ubiquitous nature of the organism, which is frequently present among the normal flora but may also be found in sites that are normally sterile (eg, the trachea). The presence of organisms in these sites does not necessarily imply causation of the illness observed in the infant.

A chronic progressive granulomatous skin lesion,

occasionally associated with oral candidiasis, is characterized by horny excrescences.

Paronychia and onychia due to *Candida* are observed in children as part of the clinical illness characterized by hypoadrenalism, hypoparathyroidism, pernicious anemia, and steatorrhea. Candidiasis usually precedes the other manifestations, but all combinations are seen.

Candidiasis has also been implicated in diarrheal illness associated with watery stools and abdominal cramping pain but no blood or mucus in the stools. This isolated form of the disease responds to minimal (3–4 days) oral therapy with nystatin.

B. Laboratory Findings: Direct examination of scrapings, pus, or sputum will reveal ovoid, budding yeast cells in large numbers. With tissue invasion, typical mycelial elements may be found. In the newborn, the best diagnostic indicator of systemic infection, apart from isolation of *Candida* in blood or cerebrospinal fluid, is the identification of budding yeasts or pseudomycelial or mycelial elements in the urine. For many physicians, this finding is considered diagnostic and is sufficient to institute appropriate therapy.

The organism is readily cultured on the usual laboratory media or on Sabouraud's medium.

A skin test is available, but the ubiquity of the fungus and the large number of positive reactions preclude its clinical usefulness. Furthermore, lymphopenic states associated with a high incidence of candidiasis are frequently characterized by anergy to *Candida* extract injected intradermally.

Serologic tests are of little use in diagnosis. Precipitins may be found in most patients with disseminated disease and in only a few asymptomatic individuals.

Differential Diagnosis

Characteristic mucosal or skin lesions, isolation of the fungus, and response to therapy establish the diagnosis in most cases. To be differentiated are agranulocytic mucosal lesions, herpes simplex, herpangina, contact or allergic dermatitis, avitaminosis, bacterial infections, and toxic or drug eruptions of the skin.

Complications

Dissemination from oral and skin infection is the most serious complication. The severity of candidal infection is directly related to the type of underlying disease and the amount of therapy with antibiotics, corticosteroids, or immunosuppressive agents.

In cases of systemic disease, meningitis and osteoarthritis occur more frequently in neonates than in older infants and children.

Treatment

Oral candidiasis in normal infants is best treated by local instillation of nystatin (Mycostatin) (see Chapter 38). Resistant and persistent oral candidiasis, such as is seen in immunodeficient individuals, may be treated with large doses of nystatin (over 3–4 million units/d; as much as 10–15 million units/d is often necessary). The imidazoles (miconazole, clotrimazole, and ketoconazole) have been used successfully both orally (clotrimazole as a buccal troche) and parenterally.

Skin and mucosal infections have been treated successfully with creams containing nystatin or one of the imidazoles.

If oral, skin, or mucosal infection is secondary to local irritative factors, antibiotics, or corticosteroids, adjustment of these factors, when possible, often hastens clinical improvement or cure.

The visceral, systemic, and chronic forms of candidiasis are more difficult to treat because of the underlying disease process or because it is necessary to continue antibiotic, corticosteroid, or immunosuppressive therapy for other reasons. In these forms of candidiasis, amphotericin B (Fungizone) may have to be employed adjunctively (see Chapter 38). Whenever possible, modification or elimination of predisposing causes should be attempted.

The introduction of flucytosine (Ancobon) has improved the outlook for some patients with severe candidiasis. Used alone or in conjunction with amphotericin B, flucytosine has produced cures or improvement in patients with disseminated disease, urinary tract infections, and other forms of candidiasis. In several series, neonatal infants with disseminated disease improved with administration of amphotericin B (0.1–0.25 mg/kg/d given initially and slowly increased to a maximum of 0.5–1 mg/kg/d) with the concomitant administration of flucytosine in doses ranging from 50 to 200 mg/kg/d (precise adequate dosage is unknown). The duration of treatment was individualized; in one series, therapy ranged from 30 to 120 days. Unfortunately, flucytosine is a toxic drug; leukopenia, thrombocytopenia, nausea, diarrhea, and disturbances in liver function are among the more common adverse effects.

Miconazole has been employed successfully in the treatment of severe candidiasis. Miconazole is a synthetic imidazole derivative with a broad spectrum of antifungal and antibacterial activity. Intravenous administration may be associated with phlebitis.

Ketoconazole has been used successfully in some patients.

Some investigators have been successful in treating the underlying immunodeficiency and secondarily benefiting the patient with candidiasis. Immunotherapy, usually directed at correcting disorders of cell-mediated immunity, has included bone marrow transplantation and administration of transfer factor.

Prognosis

Most superficial forms are self-limited and, with topical therapy, curable. In some cases, only suppression is achieved, and the disease recurs upon discontinuing antifungal therapy.

The prognosis is usually grave in systemic or visceral forms of the disease.

Baley JE, Annable WL, Kliegman RM: *Candida* endophthalmitis in the premature infant. *J Pediatr* 1981;**98**:458.
Carpentieri U et al: Clinical experience in prevention of candidiasis by nystatin in children with acute lymphatic leukemia. *J Pediatr* 1978;**92**:593.
Hughes WT et al: Ketoconazole and candidiasis: A controlled study. *J Infect Dis* 1983;**147**:1060.
Jacobs RF et al: Laryngeal candidiasis presenting as inspiratory stridor. *Pediatrics* 1982;**69**:234.
Johnson DE et al: Systemic candidiasis in very low birth weight infants (< 1500 grams). *Pediatrics* 1984;**73**:138.
Katz ME, Cassileth PA: Disseminated candidiasis in a patient with acute leukemia: Successful treatment with miconazole. *JAMA* 1977;**237**:1124.
Kobayashi RH et al: *Candida* esophagitis and laryngitis. *Pediatrics* 1980;**66**:380.
Kressel B et al: Early clinical recognition of disseminated candidiasis by muscle and skin biopsy. *Arch Intern Med* 1978;**138**:429.
Mansour A et al: A new approach to the use of antifungal agents in infants with persistent oral candidiasis. *J Pediatr* 1981;**98**:161.
Montes LF, Wilborn WH: Fungus-host relationship in candidiasis. *Arch Dermatol* 1985;**121**:119.
Pazin GJ et al: Topical clotrimazole treatment of chronic mucocutaneous candidiasis. *J Pediatr* 1979;**94**:322.
Rosenblatt HM et al: Successful treatment of chronic mucocutaneous candidiasis with ketoconazole. *J Pediatr* 1980;**97**:657.
Smith H, Congdon P: Neonatal systemic candidiasis. *Arch Dis Child* 1985;**60**:365.
Whyte RK et al: Antenatal infections with *Candida* species. *Arch Dis Child* 1982;**57**:528.

COCCIDIOIDOMYCOSIS

Essentials of Diagnosis

- History of residence in or travel to an endemic area.
- Primary pulmonary form: Fever, pleuritis, productive cough, anorexia, weight loss, and (in 10%) generalized macular skin rash.
- Erythema nodosum or multiforme with arthralgia ("desert rheumatism").
- Extrapulmonary form: Traumatic site, indurated ulcer 1–3 weeks later, regional adenopathy.
- Disseminated lesions in skin, bones, viscera, and meninges.
- Sporangia (30–60 μm) in pus, sputum, cerebrospinal fluid, etc.
- Gray, cottony growth on Sabouraud's medium.
- Delayed-type skin test reaction (induration > 5 mm) to coccidioidin.
- Precipitin (early, 1–4 weeks) and complement-fixing (late, 6–12 weeks) antibodies develop.

General Considerations

Coccidioidomycosis is caused by the dimorphic fungus *Coccidioides immitis*. The infective forms (arthrospores) are found in soil in the lower Sonoran life zone, and the disease is endemic in parts of California, Arizona, New Mexico, Texas, Mexico, and South America; however, because of extensive air travel, the disease is now seen generally in the USA. Infection is acquired by inhalation or skin inoculation. Many rodents are naturally infected. The human disease is not contagious, but laboratory infections can occur from cultured *Coccidioides*.

Almost two-thirds of infections are asymptomatic; of the remainder, less than 0.5% will disseminate.

Clinical Findings

A. History: The diagnosis may be suspected on the basis of the patient's residence in or travel to an endemic area. Even brief exposure, such as during an automobile trip through an infective area, given the right environmental circumstances, may result in acquisition of arthrospores. The incubation period is usually 7–28 days, and a history of appropriate exposure in that interval, combined with a compatible clinical illness, should strongly suggest coccidioidomycosis. A dry climate, windy conditions, and large areas of open soil such as those found in the Sonoran life zone in the southwestern USA allow for airborne dissemination of the fungus.

B. Symptoms and Signs:

1. Primary disease—The child may be asymptomatic or may have mild, nonspecific upper respiratory tract symptoms with cough. Fever may be prominent and prolonged, and chest pain on breathing varies from mild to severe. Myalgia, arthralgia ("desert rheumatism"), headache, lassitude, malaise, anorexia, weight loss, and skin rash may occur in varying combinations. Physical findings other than fever and skin rash are often few. Rales may be present, and in the more severe forms of disease, signs of lobar consolidation can be elicited. Pleural friction rubs are occasionally heard.

2. Dermal disease—Skin rash (erythema multiforme or erythema nodosum) occurs in up to 10% of children. If traumatized skin is inoculated with arthrospores, an indolent, indurated ulcer may occur in association with regional lymphadenopathy. Infected skin lesions may also occur in association with breakdown of underlying bone or with lymph node infections.

3. Chronic pulmonary disease—Several forms of chronic lung disease are found, especially in patients with diabetes mellitus and in immunosuppressed patients. Chronic pneumonia with associated symptoms and signs of consolidation may be seen. There may be parenchymal signs of cavitary disease or, if the cavity empties into the pleura, signs of pleural effusion or pneumothorax. Chronic disease may be asymptomatic, suspected only because of radiologic findings, or may be associated with chronic cough. Sputum production is uncommon; when present, sputum is sometimes bloody.

4. Disseminated disease—In children, limited dissemination from a symptomatic or asymptomatic primary pulmonary focus may occur. If dissemination is limited to a single bone, signs of osteomyelitis may be present, with fever and localized pain, induration, and erythema. If limited to a lymph node or group of nodes, signs of node enlargement, induration, tenderness, and overlying erythema may be apparent.

With systemic, multiorgan dissemination (rare in children), severe debility, fever, and signs related to the organs involved may be seen.

Renal coccidioidomycosis may present with urinary symptoms or with pain referable to the urinary tract.

Coccidioidal meningitis in children commonly presents with vomiting and disturbances in equilibrium (ataxia, changes in gait). In older children, severe, persistent headache occurs. Physical signs are those typical of meningeal irritation, eg, stiff neck, positive Kernig and Brudzinski signs, and focal neurologic signs, including ataxia.

C. Laboratory Findings: Direct examination of pus, cerebrospinal fluid, sputum, or other clinical specimens treated with sodium hydroxide may reveal the characteristic sporangia (30–60 μm). India ink may be useful for contrast, but staining is of no value. The fungus can be cultured on Sabouraud's agar, but to avoid laboratory infections, the slants should be sealed and never opened. *C immitis* grows rapidly, and gray, cottony colonies appear in a few days. Occasionally, mouse inoculation will aid in diagnosis.

Precipitating antibodies appear in the first to third weeks of infection and disappear by 4–6 weeks. Complement-fixing antibodies develop much later, if at all. Mild and asymptomatic illness is associated with no complement-fixing antibodies; moderate to severe illness is associated with a complement-fixing antibody rise that disappears in 6–8 months; and disseminated illness is associated with a persistent and high titer of complement-fixing antibodies. The presence of complement-fixing antibody in cerebrospinal fluid is diagnostic of meningitis.

Immunodiffusion is as sensitive as the complement fixation test and is specific. It is often used in screening sera initially and is especially useful in anticomplementary serum. Some laboratories are utilizing counterimmunoelectrophoresis (CIE) for detection of low levels of antibody.

A skin test with coccidioidin results in an area of induration more than 5 mm in diameter within 2–21 days after onset. In patients with allergic manifestations (erythema nodosum), extreme skin sensitivity is present, and the coccidioidin should be diluted 10–100 times before testing. Reactivity may persist for years in convalescence but may decrease or disappear with dissemination. Spherulin can also be used in usual or high test concentrations; 5 mm of induration within 24–48 hours is a positive test.

The sedimentation rate is elevated during the acute phase. An intense eosinophilia has been described just prior to dissemination.

D. X-Ray Findings: Roentgenologic evidence of pneumonia, pleural effusion, granuloma, or cavitation may be present at various stages of the pulmonary disease. Osteomyelitis may be noted. Contrast-enhanced CT scanning will diagnose ventriculitis, hydrocephalus, and basal meningitis.

Differential Diagnosis

Coccidioidomycosis must be distinguished from acute viral and bacterial pneumonias and acute tuberculosis. The chronic pulmonary lesion must be distinguished from chronic tuberculosis and cancer. The disseminated forms will resemble diseases of the organs involved (osteomyelitis, meningitis, etc).

Complications

These are primarily pulmonary, with pleural effusion, empyema, pneumothorax, or combinations occurring in association with a subpleural cavity.

Treatment

A. Specific measures: In mild forms of coccidioidomycosis, no specific therapy is warranted.

In severe disease, especially with dissemination and localization in vital organs or tissues, amphotericin B has been the drug of choice. In some centers today, amphotericin B is still given both systemically and intraventricularly (see Chapter 38 for dosage) for all forms of disseminated disease, including meningitis. In recent years, ketoconazole has proved to be of benefit in children with disseminated disease, especially meningitis; this has not been true for many adult patients. Currently, in our unit in Arizona, we initiate therapy for meningitis with oral ketoconazole (see Chapter 38 for dosage) and instill miconazole (3–5 mg) daily into the ventricles by means of a device that connects directly to the ventricle or to the shunt placed for management of hydrocephalus. Duration of therapy is indeterminant; we have several children who are still being maintained on this form of therapy after receiving it for many years. Adjustment of the frequency of intraventricular miconazole is based on the response as judged by symptom relief, reduction in white cell count and protein concentration in the cerebrospinal fluid, lack of positive cultures, and the course of complement-fixing antibody titers in the serum and cerebrospinal fluid.

Mandibular infection, an indolent form of osteomyelitis, may require systemic administration of amphotericin B and local irrigation following adequate surgical debridement.

Experimental regimens have focused on attempts to improve the immunologic status of patients who are immunodeficient. Transfer factor has been administered orally and intravenously in an effort to render lymphocytes competent to fight *C immitis*. Reports are sporadic, and results show varying efficacy of transfer factor.

B. General Measures: Most children with pulmonary coccidioidomycosis require little therapy. They may feel ill for a day or 2 and limit their own activities. Cough and chest pain rarely require treatment. Bed rest is required only for children with severe symptoms or excessive fatigue. It is surprising how active children with this disease can be despite severity of symptoms and chest findings.

C. Surgical Measures: Surgery may be indicated in cavitary lesions or with chronic draining sinuses. Neurosurgical intervention is often required in central nervous system disease to ameliorate hydrocephalus and to place reservoirs for drug therapy. Amphotericin B should be administered prior to and for 4 weeks following excisional surgery.

Osteomyelitis may require surgical curettage for optimal management. Single lesions respond well to this form of treatment combined with systemic administration of amphotericin B.

Prognosis

Complete recovery is the rule for all but a very few patients. Those with disseminated disease are at greatest risk, and as many as 50% died prior to the availability of amphotericin B. Blacks and Filipinos appear to be at greater risk of dissemination (10 times the rate for whites) and, therefore, a fatal outcome. Meningitis and diffuse disseminated disease carry the worst prognosis. An increasing complement-fixing antibody titer and a decrease or reversion of a positive skin test are unfavorable prognostic signs.

Doto IL et al: Coccidioidin, histoplasmin, and tuberculin sensitivity among school children in Maricopa County, Arizona. *Am J Epidemiol* 1972;**95:**464.

Drutz DJ, Huppert M: Coccidioidomycosis: Factors affecting the host-parasite relationship. *J Infect Dis* 1983;**147:**372.

Fulginiti V: Coccidioidomycosis for all of us. *J Pediatr* 1981;**98:**411.

Harrison ER et al: Amphotericin B and imidazole therapy for coccidioidal meningitis. *Pediatr Infect Dis* 1983;**2:**216.

Kafka JA, Catanzaro A: Disseminated coccidioidomycosis in children. *J Pediatr* 1981;**98:**355.

Sieber O, Larter W, Fulginiti V: Limited extrapulmonary coccidioidomycosis as a form of disseminated disease in children. In: *Coccidioidomycosis: Current Clinical & Diagnostic Status.* Ajello L (editor). Symposia Specialists, Florida, 1977.

Stadalnik RC et al: Use of radiologic modalities in coccidioidal meningitis. *Arch Intern Med* 1981;**141:**75.

Warlick MA et al: Rapid diagnosis of pulmonary coccidioidomycosis. *Arch Intern Med* 1983;**143:**723.

CRYPTOCOCCOSIS

Cryptococcus neoformans is a spherical fungus found worldwide in soil and in the old excreta of pigeons. It is an opportunistic organism that is frequently associated with seriously altered host mechanisms, eg, leukemia. It is commonly found at autopsy. Humans are probably infected by inhalation.

Systemic cryptococcosis may result in widespread infection. Particular sites of localization include the central nervous system, eyes, skin, and bone. Skin lesions vary from papules to ulcerative abscesses. Bony lesions are indurated and painful and result in extensive local destruction, although periosteal proliferation is minimal or absent.

Several forms of the disease exist. Most commonly observed is the insidious cryptococcal meningitis. Recurrent or progressive headache, changes in personality and ambition, dizziness, and vomiting herald the onset of meningeal infection. The patient may have mild fever, slight nuchal rigidity, and alteration in lower extremity reflexes. Signs of progressive increase in intracranial pressure follow, with papilledema, cranial nerve paresis, and optic atrophy. The symptoms usually progress slowly over a period of several months, but chronic forms may last for years.

Sporadic cases of acute pulmonary cryptococcosis are seen, and asymptomatic granulomas are frequently detected at necropsy. Thus, it is likely that the lungs are the portal of entry for the fungus.

Clinical laboratory specimens are usually very mucoid owing to the capsule of the fungus. Direct visualization of the 5- to 20-μm fungi is enhanced by India ink contrast. Any specimen containing cellular debris should be digested with 10% sodium hydroxide. Culture from pus, sputum, bone marrow, or cerebrospinal fluid is possible. When cerebrospinal fluid is inoculated, care must be taken to use sufficient volume. As much as 2–20 mL should be inoculated into a single culture, as the fungus cell content may be quite low.

Latex agglutination can detect small amounts of cryptococcal antigen in body fluids (cerebrospinal fluid, urine, serum). False-negative results can occur.

Chest x-rays may reveal solitary or multiple lesions; bone films may show areas of osteolysis.

Amphotericin B (Fungizone) (see Chapter 38) is of proved value, and its use (intravenously or intrathecally) may result in complete cure. Surgical excision may be of adjunctive value.

Flucytosine (Ancobon) offers additional therapy. Patients have received both amphotericin B and flucytosine. Flucytosine is toxic, and leukopenia, thrombocytopenia, nausea, diarrhea, and disturbances in liver function have been reported.

Miconazole may be useful in cryptococcal disease. A newer imidazole, ketoconazole, may prove to be superior to other drugs.

The disease process may be relatively acute or may progress slowly over a period of several years. In the chronic forms, remissions and exacerbations are frequent. The disseminated and meningeal forms are frequently fatal.

Bennett JE et al: A comparison of amphotericin B alone and combined with flucytosine in the treatment of cryptococcal meningitis. *N Engl J Med* 1979;**301:**126.

Friedman GD: The rarity of cryptococcosis in northern California: The 10 year experience of a large, defined population. *Am J Epidemiol* 1983;**117:**230.

Gauder JP: Cryptococcal cellulitis. *JAMA* 1977;**237:**672.

Graybill JR, Levine HB: Successful treatment of cryptococcal meningitis with intraventricular miconazole. *Arch Intern Med* 1978;**138:**814.

Hammerschlag MR et al: Cryptococcal osteomyelitis. *Clin Pediatr* 1982;**21:**109.

Robert F, Durant JR, Gams RA: Demonstration of *Cryptococcus neoformans* in a stained bone marrow specimen. *Arch Intern Med* 1977;**137:**688.

Stamm AM, Polt SS: False-negative cryptococcal antigen test. *JAMA* 1980;**244:**1359.

HISTOPLASMOSIS

Essentials of Diagnosis

- History of residence in or travel to endemic areas.
- Pulmonary calcification.
- Hepatosplenomegaly, anemia, leukopenia.
- Positive skin test.
- Isolation of organism or identification in smears (2- to 4-μm oval budding yeasts with narrow neck).

General Considerations

Histoplasmosis is caused by the dimorphic fungus *Histoplasma capsulatum.* Its tissue form is a budding oval yeast, 2–4 μm in diameter. Benign histoplasmosis was first noted in tuberculin-negative individuals with pulmonary calcifications. Such individuals were histoplasmin-reactive (positive). The endemic areas include the central and eastern USA. The fungus is found in soil, especially when enriched by bat feces. It is believed that infection is acquired by inhalation, and over 65% of children acquire asymptomatic infections in the endemic areas.

Clinical Findings

A history of residence or travel to the endemic areas is essential. Heavy contact with potentially infected soil or excreta (bat feces) may provide an etiologic clue.

A. Symptoms and Signs: Three forms of infection are recognized: asymptomatic benign infection, pneumonia, and disseminated disease.

1. Asymptomatic infection—The diagnosis is made by observation of pulmonary calcifications in the absence of delayed hypersensitivity to other antigens and a positive histoplasmin skin test.

2. Histoplasmal pneumonia—This form of the disease is manifested by nonproductive cough, chest pain, hemoptysis, and dyspnea. Cyanosis and hoarseness may also be noted. Influenzalike symptoms sometimes occur, with fever, muscle and joint pains, and malaise. Night sweats and weight loss may simulate tuberculosis. Physical signs may be absent, or typical findings of pneumonia (rales, bronchial breathing, etc) may be observed. A chronic pulmonary disease may be seen in adults but almost never in children.

3. Disseminated histoplasmosis—The disseminated form of the disease has all of the pulmonary features plus signs and symptoms referable to the lymphatic system. Thus, hepatosplenomegaly, severe wasting, and generalized lymphadenopathy occur. Ulceration of the gastrointestinal and respiratory tracts occurs occasionally. Pallor may be a prominent finding. Multifocal choroiditis with visual loss may occur.

B. Laboratory Findings: Anemia and leukopenia, often profound, occur in the disseminated form. Isolation of the fungus provides a specific diagnosis. This usually is unrewarding in the benign infection, although rarely the organism may be found in the urine. Examination of sputum, urine, biopsy material, bone marrow, or blood may yield the organism in the disseminated form. Morphologically, *H capsulatum* appears as 2- to 4-μm oval cells on a smear stained with Giemsa's or Wright's stain. A large vacuole and crescent-shaped eosinophilic masses of cytoplasm may be visible in the larger end of the ovoid. If budding is observed, the neck is seen to be narrow and may appear as a separate ovoid. Such cells are identified within monocytes or macrophages but often are found free. Upon culture (with agar at 20–30 °C), the organism may be isolated and specifically identified. Mouse inoculation is an extremely sensitive method for isolation of *Histoplasma.* Complement fixation and precipitin antibody tests are available. Both are positive in the first few weeks after infection and remain elevated only with dissemination.

C. X-Ray Findings: Pulmonary calcifications, solitary or multiple, may be noted in an asymptomatic child. In acute pulmonic disease, bilateral bronchial pneumonia is the rule. Miliary distribution occasionally occurs.

Differential Diagnosis

Pulmonary histoplasmosis with or without symptoms must be differentiated from tuberculosis. The use of skin tests and serologic and isolation techniques permits differentiation. The disseminated form of the disease mimics miliary tuberculosis and leukemia. Differentiation is based upon isolation of the organism. Serology may be helpful if the disease is not fulminant.

Complications

Benign and mild symptomatic infections require no specific therapy, and recovery is the rule. With concomitant disease (lymphatic cancer, tuberculosis) or with immunosuppressive therapy, dissemination may occur.

Treatment

Benign or mild forms require no treatment. Selective extirpative surgical therapy may be of benefit in localized pulmonary disease. Amphotericin B (Fungizone) appears to be effective. (See Chapter 38.)

Prognosis

In benign or mild forms, the prognosis is excellent for recovery and complete healing. Chronic infection may result from more marked pulmonary disease. Disseminated histoplasmosis has a variable course and severity. Fulminant histoplasmosis, histoplasmosis associated with concomitant tuberculosis or cancer, or histoplasmosis occurring in a patient receiving immunosuppressive therapy has a very poor prognosis.

Feman SS, Tilford RH: Ocular findings in patients with histoplasmosis. *JAMA* 1985;**253:**2534.

Henochowicz S et al: Histoplasmosis diagnosed on peripheral

blood smear from a patient with AIDS. *JAMA* 1985; **253:**3148.

Hughes WT: Hematogenous histoplasmosis in the immunocompromised child. *J Pediatr* 1984;**105:**569.

Shore RN et al: African histoplasmosis in the United States. *JAMA* 1981:**245:**734.

Waldman RJ et al: A winter outbreak of acute histoplasmosis in northern Michigan. *Am J Epidemiol* 1983;**117:**68.

Wheat LJ et al: Histoplasmosis in renal allograft recipients. *Arch Intern Med* 1983;**143:**703.

NOCARDIOSIS

Nocardiosis is infrequent in childhood. It is caused by *Nocardia asteroides,* an aerobic, gram-positive, partially acid-fast actinomycete.* Pulmonary infection is common and may lead to chronic pneumonia or dissemination to the meninges or brain. Typical gram-positive, short-branching rods or coccal forms are seen, and these are acid-fast. Culture establishes the diagnosis.

The sulfonamides are the drugs of choice (see Chapter 38). Gentamicin and amikacin are also active but should only be used as an adjunct and in difficult therapeutic circumstances. Trimethoprim-sulfamethoxazole appears to offer no advantage over sulfonamides alone.

Curry WA: Human nocardiosis. *Arch Intern Med* 1980;**140:**818.

Law BJ, Marks MI: Pediatric nocardiosis. *Pediatrics* 1982; **70:**560.

Mills V et al: Central nervous system *Nocardia* infection. *Clin Pediatr* 1982;**21:**248.

Yogev R et al: Successful treatment of *Nocardia asteroides* infection with amikacin. *J Pediatr* 1980;**96:**771.

* A bacterium, not a fungus. Discussed in this chapter by convention, since *Nocardia asteroides* (like *Actinomyces israelii*) was thought for many years to be a fungus.

SPOROTRICHOSIS

Sporotrichosis is caused by *Sporothrix schenckii.* Localized lymphatic sporotrichosis may follow a prick with a thorn or splinter that results in an ulcer or nodule followed by others along the route of lymphatic return from the injured part. Dissemination to the skin and mucosa can occur, but the viscera are usually spared. Diagnosis is best accomplished by culture of aspirates or drainage from local lesions or nodes.

Potassium iodide is said to be effective, although some cases may require amphotericin B (Fungizone) (see Chapter 38). Potassium iodide can be administered orally as the saturated solution. The dose is variable. Initially, give 3–5 drops 3 times daily after meals. Increase the dose to 40 drops 3 times daily by adding 1 drop per dose. Continue therapy for 2 weeks or until signs of disease activity have disappeared. Then reduce the dose by 1 drop per dose until 5 drops is reached, at which time therapy is discontinued. ***Note:*** If signs of iodism appear, the dosage must be reduced. Potassium iodide is indicated only in sporotrichosis and not in other fungal diseases.

Lynch PJ, Botero F: Sporotrichosis in children. *Am J Dis Child* 1971;**122:**325.

Orr ER, Riley HD: Sporotrichosis in children: Report of 10 cases. *J Pediatr* 1971;**78:**951.

Pepper MC, Rippon JW: Sporotrichosis presenting as facial cellulitis. *JAMA* 1980;**243:**2327.

SELECTED REFERENCES

Bennett JE: Chemotherapy of systemic mycoses. (2 parts.) *N Engl J Med* 1974;**290:**30, 320.

Campbell MC, Stewart JL: *The Medical Mycology Handbook.* Wiley, 1980.

Cohen J: Antifungal chemotherapy. *Lancet* 1982;**2:**532.

Conant NF et al: *Manual of Clinical Mycology,* 3rd ed. Saunders, 1971.

Ehrlich GE: Fungal arthritis. *JAMA* 1978;**240:**563.

Emmons CW et al: *Medical Mycology,* 3rd ed. Lea & Febiger, 1977.

Halde C: Infectious diseases: Mycotic. Chapter 27 in: *Current Medical Diagnosis & Treatment 1986.* Krupp MA, Chatton MJ, Tierney LM Jr (editors). Lange, 1986.

Medoff G, Kobayashi GS: Strategies in the treatment of systemic fungal infections. *N Engl J Med* 1980;**302:**145.

Rockoff AS: Fungus cultures in a pediatric outpatient clinic. *Pediatrics* 1979;**63:**276.

Thienpont D et al: Ketoconazole: A new broad-spectrum, orally active antimycotic. *Experientia* 1979;**35:**606.

Treating fungal infections. *Br Med J* 1980;**1:**698.

Van den Bossche H et al: In vitro and in vivo effects of the antimycotic drug ketoconazole on sterol synthesis. *Antimicrob Agents Chemother* 1980;**17:**922.

Wade TR, Jones HE, Chanda JJ: Intravenous miconazole therapy of mycotic infections. *Arch Intern Med* 1979;**139:**784.

Poisoning

30

Barry H. Rumack, MD

Poisonings, the fourth most common cause of death in children, result from the complex interaction of the agent, the child, and the family environment. The peak incidence is at age 2 years, and most of these episodes are not actual poisonings but ingestions that do not produce toxicity. Accidents occur most often in children under 5 years of age as a result of insecure storage of drugs, household chemicals, etc. Repeated poisonings may be a sign of a family problem requiring intervention on the child's behalf, although 25% of children will have a second episode of ingestion of a toxic substance within a year following the first one. Accidental poisonings are unusual after age 5 years. "Poisonings" in older children and adolescents usually represent manipulative or genuine suicide attempts. Toxicity may also result in this group following the use of drugs or chemicals for their mind-altering effects.

PHARMACOLOGIC PRINCIPLES OF TOXIOCOLOGY

In the evaluation of the poisoned patient, it is important to compare the anticipated pharmacologic or toxic effects with the clinical presentation of the patient. If the history, for example, is that the patient ingested phenobarbital 30 minutes ago but the clinical examination reveals dilated pupils, tachycardia, dry mouth, absent bowel sounds, and active hallucinations, then clearly the major toxicity is anticholinergic and therapy should be given accordingly.

Knowledge of the pharmacokinetics of the toxic agent will help the physician to plan a rational approach to definitive care after necessary life-supporting measures have been instituted.

LD50, MLD

Many health professionals, when confronted with an episode of ingestion of a potentially poisonous agent, are eager to look up the LD50 or the MLD (minimum lethal dose) because they think this information will help them decide whether or not the child is going to be ill. Unfortunately, such information is seldom of value, since it is usually impossible to tell how much the child has ingested, how much has been absorbed, the metabolic status of the patient, or where the patient's response to the agent will fall in the normal distribution curve. Furthermore, these values are often not valid in humans even if the history is accurate.

Half-Life ($t_{1/2}$)

Knowledge of the $t_{1/2}$ of an agent can be confusing in the overdose situation. For example, one cannot rely upon the published $t_{1/2}$ for salicylate (2 hours) to assume rapid elimination of the drug with a concomitant short toxic course. In salicylate overdose (> 100 mg/kg), the $t_{1/2}$ is prolonged to 24–30 hours. Most published $t_{1/2}$ values are for therapeutic dosages. The $t_{1/2}$ may increase as the quantity of the ingested

Table 30–1. Some examples of pK_a and V_d.*

Drug	pK_a	Diuresis	Dialysis	Apparent V_d
Amobarbital	7.9	No	No	200–300% body weight
Amphetamine	9.8	No	Yes	60% body weight
Aspirin	3.5	Alkaline	Yes	15–40% body weight
Chlorpromazine	9.3	No	No	40–50 L/kg (2800–3500% body weight)
Codeine	8.2	No	No	5–10 L/kg (350–700% body weight)
Desipramine	10.2	No	No	30–40 L/kg (2100–2800% body weight)
Ethchlorvynol	8.7	No	No	5–10 L/kg (350–700% body weight)
Glutethimide	4.5	No	No	10–20 L/kg (700–1400% body weight)
Isoniazid	3.5	Alkaline	Yes	61% body weight
Methadone	8.3	No	No	5–10 L /kg (350–700% body weight)
Methicillin	2.8	No	Yes	60% body weight
Phenobarbital	7.4	Alkaline	Yes	75% body weight
Phenytoin	8.3	No	No	60–80% body weight
Tetracycline	7.7	No	No	200–300% body weight

* See Table 37–2 for additional V_d values.

substance increases for many common intoxicants such as barbiturates, salicylates, and phenytoin.

Volume of Distribution (V_d)

The volume of distribution (V_d) of a drug represents the percentage of the body mass in which a drug is distributed. It is obtained by dividing the amount of drug absorbed by the blood level. With theophylline, for example, this is roughly equivalent to the body water volume and can be expressed as 0.46 L/kg body weight, or 32 L in an adult. Ethchlorvynol, a lipophilic drug, on the other hand, distributes well beyond total body water. Since the calculation produces a volume above body weight (300 L in an adult, 500% of body weight in children), this figure is frequently referred to as an **apparent** volume of distribution, a designation shared by many drugs (Table 30–1).

When a drug is differentially concentrated in body lipids or is heavily tissue- or protein-bound and has a high volume of distribution, only a small proportion of the ingested drug will be in the blood and thereby accessible to diuresis, dialysis, or exchange transfusion. On the other hand, a drug that is water-soluble and has a low volume of distribution may cross the dialysis membrane well and also respond to diuresis. The V_d can be useful in predicting which drugs will be removed by dialysis or exchange transfusion. In general, agents with a V_d greater than 1 L/kg are not significantly removable by these maneuvers.

Metabolism & Excretion

The route of detoxification of an agent—correlated with other information—will help in making therapeutic decisions. Methanol, for example, is metabolized to a toxic product. This metabolic step may be blocked by the administration of ethanol. Long-acting barbiturates are primarily metabolized in the liver but are also partially excreted in the urine, which means that forced diuresis will be an effective therapeutic measure. Secobarbital, a short-acting barbiturate, is poorly excreted in the urine and has a larger V_d, and forced diuresis is therefore ineffective.

Blood Levels

Care of the poisoned patient should never be guided solely by the results of laboratory measurements. Treatment should be directed first against the clinical signs and symptoms, followed by more specific therapy based on laboratory determinations. The laboratory pathologist should be given whatever information is needed regarding the history and the class of the suspected toxic agent (sedative-hypnotic, opiate, amphetamine, etc), so that the specific agent can be identified as rapidly as possible. The laboratory should know its own normal levels of therapeutic ranges so that interpretation can be rational.

Handling of Specimens

A. Vomitus and Gastric Lavage Fluid: Collect and send to the laboratory initial material produced in separate containers plus an aliquot of the remainder. Include any material that appears to be pill fragments.

B. Blood: Ask the laboratory pathologist specifically what type of container and anticoagulant are desired before drawing the sample.

C. Urine: Collect an initial sample—if possible, 100 mL—for analysis and then begin a timed 6- to 12-hour collection, which may be useful in determining the rate of excretion of the agent.

GENERAL TREATMENT OF POISONING

The first contact in the case of possible poisoning by ingestion involving a child under age 5 will usually be over the telephone. Proper handling of the situation by phone can significantly reduce morbidity and prevent unwarranted or excessive treatment.

After initial telephone advice has been given, a decision is made about whether or not the child should be seen. The decision as to which child should be seen will depend upon the ingested agent, the age of the child, the time of day, the reliability of the parent, and whether or not child neglect is suspected.

Initial Telephone Contact

Evaluate the urgency of the situation and decide whether immediate emergency transportation to a health facility is indicated. Transportation of seriously poisoned patients should be by competent emergency rescue personnel who have suction, oxygen, and other equipment available to provide or continue emergency procedures. Determine whether the patient is in immediate danger, potential danger, or no danger.

Basic information that should be *written down* at the first telephone contact includes the patient's name, age, weight, address and telephone number, and the time elapsed since ingestion or other exposure.

Type of Ingestion

This information is usually given by the parent in the first few words of the call. (***Example:*** "My little boy just swallowed the vitamin pills!") After a decision is made about whether the ingestion is a dangerous one and basic information has been obtained, the physician should develop more details about the suspected toxic agent. It may be difficult to obtain an accurate history. For example, an empty bottle of iron tablets may have rolled out of sight under the couch, and the parent may then assume that the empty vitamin bottle means that only the vitamin capsules have been swallowed. Obtain names of drugs or ingredients, manufacturers, prescription numbers, names and phone numbers of prescribing physician and pharmacy, etc. Find out whether the substance was shared among several children, whether it had been recently purchased, who had last used it, how full it was, and how much was spilled if any.

PREVENTING CHILDHOOD POISONINGS

Each year, thousands of children are accidentally poisoned by medicines, polishes, insecticides, drain cleaners, bleaches, household chemicals, and garage products. It is the responsibility of adults to make sure that children are not exposed to potentially toxic substances.

Here are some suggestions:

(1) Insist on safety closures and learn how to use them properly.
(2) Keep household cleaning supplies, medicines, garage products, and insecticides out of the reach and sight of your child. Lock them up whenever possible.
(3) Never store food and cleaning products together. Store medicine and chemicals in original containers and never in food or beverage containers.
(4) Avoid taking medicine in your child's presence. Children love to imitate. Always call medicine by its proper name. Never suggest that medicine is "candy"—especially aspirin and children's vitamins.
(5) Read the label on all products and heed warnings and cautions. Never use medicine from an unlabeled or unreadable container. Never pour medicine in a darkened area where the label cannot be clearly seen.
(6) If you are interrupted while using a product, take it with you. It only takes a few seconds for your child to get into it.
(7) Know what your child can do. For example, if you have a crawling infant, keep household products stored above floor level, not beneath the kitchen sink.
(8) Keep the phone number of your doctor, poison center, hospital, police department, and fire department or paramedic emergency rescue squad near the phone.

FIRST AID FOR POISONING

Always keep syrup of ipecac and Epsom salt (magnesium sulfate) in your home. The former is used to induce vomiting, and the latter may be used as a laxative. These drugs are used sometimes when poisons are swallowed. Only use them as instructed by your poison center or doctor, and *follow their directions for use.*

Inhaled Poisons

If smoke, gas, or fumes have been inhaled, immediately drag or carry the patient to fresh air. Then call the poison center or your doctor.

Poisons on the Skin

If the poison has been spilled on the skin or clothing, remove the clothing and flood the involved parts with water. Then wash with soapy water and rinse thoroughly. Then call the poison center or your doctor.

Swallowed Poisons

If the substance swallowed is a medicine, give nothing. If the substance is a household product or other chemical, give one glass of water or milk. Then call the poison center or your doctor. ***CAUTION:*** antidote labels on products may be incorrect. Do not give salt, vinegar, or lemon juice. Call before doing anything else.

Poisons in the Eye

Flush the eye with lukewarm water poured from a pitcher held 3–4 inches from the eye for 15 minutes. Call the poison center or your doctor.

DOCTOR ____________________ POISON CENTER ______________ AMBULANCE ______________

POLICE ____________________ FIRE DEPARTMENT ______________ HOSPITAL ______________

Bring the Poison to the Hospital

If the patient is to be seen in the emergency department, everything in the vicinity of the patient that may be a cause of poisoning should be brought along.

Initial Therapy Over the Phone

Treatment at home should include external and internal decontamination if appropriate.

A. External:

1. Skin—If the patient has been exposed to an insecticide or has spilled a caustic agent on the skin, the area should be immediately flooded with water and washed well with soap and a soft washcloth or sponge.

2. Eye—Irrigation of the eye with plain water should begin *before* the patient arrives at the emergency room. Use plain tap water—do not try to neutralize acids or alkalies. Have the head held back over the sink and direct a gentle stream of water into the eye from the tap, or pour water into the eye from a drinking glass or pitcher. Irrigation should be continued for 15–20 minutes. Then transport the patient to the hospital for ophthalmologic examination.

B. Internal: Milk or water should be immediately administered to any patient who has ingested a strongly acid or alkaline agent. Do not induce vomiting in patients who are comatose or convulsing or who have lost the gag reflex. If vomiting occurs, the vomitus should be retained for further analysis. If emesis is induced on the way to the hospital, syrup of ipecac should be administered as described in the section on prevention of absorption (see p 941).

Poison Information

Up-to-date data on ingredients of commercial products and medications can usually be obtained from the regional poison information center. *POISINDEX* is a quarterly publication that offers current data about toxic ingredients based on computer contact with over 8000 manufacturers. It is important to have the actual container at hand when calling the manufacturer so that information about serial numbers, label colors, etc, can be conveyed. In some cases, the experience of the company physician may be of value in management. ***Caution:*** Antidote information on labels of commercial products is frequently incorrect and may contain bad advice such as administration of an acidic agent like vinegar to a child who has ingested a caustic substance.

Follow-Up

In over 95% of cases of ingestion of potentially toxic substances by children, a trip to the hospital is not required. If it is decided that an ingestion is not toxic or that vomiting induced at home is the only treatment required, it is important to call the parent at 1 and 4 hours after an ingestion. If the child has actually ingested an additional unknown agent and is gradually becoming comatose, a change in management may be instituted, including transportation to the hospital. An additional call should be made 24 hours after the ingestion to begin the process of poison prevention.

Poison Prevention Over the Telephone

This may be instituted with a few simple questions about storage of hazardous substances in unsafe locations. The following is a partial list of potentially poisonous substances that must be stored safely if there are small children in the home: drain-cleaning crystals or liquid, dishwasher soap and cleaning supplies, paints and paint thinners, medicines, garden spray and other insecticide materials, automobile products.

If it seems that there are problems that may lead to further episodes of hazardous exposure of small children to potential poisons, it will be useful to arrange an appointment with the parent to discuss the matter or to send a public health nurse to the home to examine storage practices and make suitable arrangements to improve the situation.

PREVENTION OF POISONING

A major goal of pediatricians is to reduce the number of accidental ingestions in the high-risk age group under 5 years of age. A systematic poison education effort should be part of the routine care of every patient. Parents of very young children should be encouraged to search the house and identify all hazardous substances that should be removed from the home or locked up.

The chart entitled "Preventing Childhood Poisonings," reproduced on p 939, may be copied from this book and given to parents along with a bottle of syrup of ipecac at the 6-month checkup.* Reinforcement should occur at the 1-year checkup to make certain that adequate poison-proofing measures have been instituted and maintained.

INITIAL EMERGENCY ROOM CONTACT

If the decision has been made to see the child in the hospital, or if the patient has bypassed the initial phone call and is brought to the hospital emergency room—as in the case of many severe ingestions or adolescent overdoses—the following steps should be followed:

Make Certain the Patient Is Breathing

This is sometimes overlooked in the emergency room frenzy of getting intravenous lines started and searching for treatment protocols. The adequacy of

* No request for permission to reproduce the chart is necessary provided it is done without modification.

tidal volume should be checked, normal being 10–15 mL/kg.

Treat Shock

Initial therapy of the hypotensive patient should consist of laying the patient flat and administering colloids, blood, or isotonic solutions. Because of potential interaction and toxicity, vasopressors should be reserved for poisoned patients in shock who do not respond to these standard measures.

Treat Burns

Burns may occur following exposure to strong acid or strong alkaline agents or petroleum distillates. Burned areas should be cleaned and debrided (if extensive) and fully decontaminated by flooding with sterile saline solution or water. Skin decontamination should be performed in a patient with cutaneous exposure. Emergency department personnel in contact with a critically ill patient who has been contaminated with (for example) an organophosphate insecticide should themselves be decontaminated if their skin or clothing has been exposed to the agent. So-called barbiturate burns require treatment as for any other kind of burn. These bullous lesions, usually on the fingers, may occur following exposure to one of a wide variety of sedating agents.

Take a Pertinent History

The history should be taken from family or friends or from the patient if he or she is old enough and sufficiently alert to give useful answers to questions. It may be crucial to determine all of the kinds of toxicants in the home (eg, toxic drugs used by ill family members, chemicals associated with hobbies, occupations of family members, or purity of the water supply), unusual eating or medication habits, or other clues to the possible cause of poisoning.

Coma, Hyperactivity, & Withdrawal

It is useful to determine the level of coma, degree of hyperactivity, or severity of withdrawal symptoms as a means of assessing the efficacy of treatment.

A. Determine the Level of Coma: Coma is graded on a scale of 0–4:

0 Asleep but can be aroused and can answer questions.
1 Comatose; withdraws from painful stimuli; reflexes intact.
2 Comatose; does *not* withdraw from painful stimuli; most reflexes intact; no respiratory or circulatory depression.
3 Comatose; most or all reflexes absent; no depression of respiration or circulation.
4 Comatose; reflexes absent; respiratory depression with cyanosis, circulatory failure, or shock.

B. Determine the Degree of Hyperactivity:

1 + Restlessness, irritability, insomnia, tremor, hyperreflexia, sweating, mydriasis, flushing.
2 + Confusion, hyperactivity, hypertension, tachypnea, tachycardia, extrasystoles, sweating, mydriasis, flushing, mild hyperpyrexia.
3 + Delirium, mania, self-injury, marked hypertension, tachycardia, dysrhythmias, hyperpyrexia.
4 + The above symptoms and signs plus convulsions, coma, circulatory collapse.

C. Determine the Severity of Narcotic Withdrawal Symptoms: Score the following findings on a scale of 0–2:

Diarrhea	Insomnia
Dilated pupils	Lacrimation
Gooseflesh	Muscle cramps
Hyperactive bowel sounds	Restlessness
	Tachycardia
Hypertension	Yawning

A score of 1–5 represents mild, 6–10 moderate, and 11–15 severe withdrawal symptoms.

Seizures, which are unusual in narcotic withdrawal, indicate severe withdrawal problems.

DEFINITIVE THERAPY OF POISONING

Antidotes

There are few specific antidotes. Many of these agents are discussed in the section on treatment of specific agents. A few poisons that may require immediate antidotal therapy are listed here:

Poison	Antidote
Carbon monoxide	Oxygen
Cyanide	Sodium nitrite (pediatric dosage), sodium thiosulfate
Nitrites and nitrates	Treat methemoglobinemia with methylene blue
Organophosphate insecticides	Atropine, pralidoxime (2-PAM)
Anticholinergics	Physostigmine
Narcotics	Naloxone (Narcan)
Methanol, ethylene glycol	Ethanol

Prevention of Absorption

A. Emesis: Induced vomiting is *contraindicated* in patients who are comatose or convulsing, who have lost the gag reflex, or who have ingested strong acids, strong bases, or 50 mL of hydrocarbons. However, in the case of hydrocarbons, vomiting should be induced if more than 1 mL/kg has been ingested, if they contain heavy metals, or if the solvent is a central nervous system depressant.

1. Ipecac method—Adult dose, 30 mL; pediatric dose, 15 mL. Give orally and repeat once only in 20 minutes if necessary. The procedure is as follows:

a. Give ipecac orally.

b. Follow with large amounts of water or whatever fluid the child will drink (ipecac on an empty stomach is "like squeezing an empty balloon").

c. Keep the patient ambulatory.

d. After 15 minutes, stimulate the patient's throat, if necessary, to induce vomiting.

2. Other emetics—The only approved oral emetic agent is syrup of ipecac. Use of sodium chloride may lead to lethal hypernatremia. Apomorphine should not be used, as its depressant effect outlasts the duration of reversal by naloxone. Other emetic agents are not as effective as syrup of ipecac and should be avoided.

B. Lavage: If the patient is or is becoming unconscious, is convulsing, or has lost the gag reflex, gastric lavage (see p 1046) following endotracheal or nasotracheal intubation should be performed rather than induction of vomiting. Lavage is less effective than emesis if a small (8–16F) tube is utilized but not if the recommended 28–36F Ewald tube is used. The tube should be inserted orally, and lavage should be with warm saline solution in a small child to avoid hyponatremia or hypothermia. Save the initial aspirate for laboratory determination and lavage until the returns have been clear for 1 L.

Emesis and lavage recover an average of about 30% of the stomach contents. While this may be helpful in reducing the amount of toxin available for absorption, it means that approximately 70% of an ingested dose will remain. Additional measures such as charcoal and cathartics should be instituted to prevent further absorption.

C. Charcoal: Thirty grams of charcoal should be made into a slurry with water. The mixture will keep without affecting the activity of the charcoal. A few drops of anise may be added. The patient may regurgitate some of the charcoal, but 70% is usually retained. Charcoal has been shown to reduce the $t_{1/2}$ even following intravenous administration of phenobarbital or theophylline.

D. Catharsis: *Caution:* Do not give cathartics containing magnesium to patients in renal failure. Pneumonitis and "mineral oil pneumonia" may occur following aspiration of oil-based cathartics.

Give either magnesium sulfate (Epsom salt), 30 g orally for an adolescent or 250 mg/kg orally for a child, or sodium sulfate (Glauber's salt) in a similar dosage. A convenient alternative is Fleet's Phospho-Soda, 15–30 mL diluted 1:4, with the entire amount administered to an adolescent and one-fourth the amount administered to a child.

Enhancement of Urinary Excretion

Urinary excretion of certain toxins can be hastened by forced alkaline diuresis or by dialysis (hemodialysis or peritoneal dialysis).

A. Diuresis: Forced diuresis is often useful in serious poisonings if the drug is excreted in the urine in active form. The technique should not be used unless it is specifically indicated, as it may increase the likelihood of cerebral edema, a common cause of death in poisonings.

Excretion of any of the following can be hastened by forced alkaline diuresis: jequirity beans, phenobarbital, and salicylates.

Hypertonic or pharmacologic diuretics should be given along with adequate fluids. The usual urine flow is 0.5–2 mL/kg/h; with forced diuresis, urine flow should increase to 3–6 mL/kg/h. Alkaline diuresis should be chosen on the basis of the toxin's pK_a, so that ionized drug will be trapped in the tubular lumen and not reabsorbed. (See Table 30–1.) Thus, if the pK_a is less than 7.5, alkaline diuresis is appropriate; if it is over 8.0, this technique will not usually be beneficial. Osmotic load is also important, and the diuretic should be given at intervals. Proximal reabsorption will occur if adequate osmotic load is not maintained in the tubule. The pK_a is usually supplied with general drug information.

1. Alkaline diuresis—Alkaline diuresis can usually be accomplished with bicarbonate. It is well to observe for potassium depletion, in which case administration of potassium citrate, which has both potassium and considerable alkalinizing ability, may be used. Potassium citrate is also available orally as K-Lyte "fizzies," which are a quite palatable form. Follow serum K^+ and observe for electrocardiographic evidence of K^+ deficiency.

2. Acid diuresis—Acid diuresis has been abandoned owing to renal complications in the face of rhabdomyolysis or myoglobinuria associated with some poisons.

B. Dialysis: Hemodialysis (or peritoneal dialysis if hemodialysis is unavailable) is useful in the poisonings listed below. Dialysis should be considered part of supportive care if the patient satisfies any of the following criteria:

1. Clinical criteria—

a. Stage 3 or 4 coma or hyperactivity that is caused by a dialyzable drug and cannot be treated by conservative means.

b. Hypotension threatening renal or hepatic function that cannot be corrected by adjusting circulating volume.

c. Apnea in a patient who cannot be ventilated.

d. Marked hyperosmolality that is not due to easily corrected fluid problems.

e. Severe acid-base disturbance not responding to therapy.

f. Severe electrolyte disturbance not responding to therapy.

g. Marked hypothermia or hyperthermia.

2. Immediate dialysis—Immediate dialysis may be considered in ethylene glycol and methanol poisoning only if acidosis is refractory and blood levels of methanol of 100 mg/dL are consistently maintained.

3. Dialysis indicated on basis of condition of patient—(In general, dialyze if patient is in coma deeper than level 3.)

Alcohols	Bromides	Paraldehyde
Ammonia	Calcium	Potassium
Amphetamines	Chloral hydrate	Quinidine
Anilines	Fluorides	Quinine
Antibiotics	Iodides	Salicylates
Barbiturates (long-acting)	Isoniazid	Strychnine
	Meprobamate	Thiocyanates
Boric acid		

(Other drugs may be dialyzable, but the information should be verified prior to institution of dialysis therapy.)

4. Dialysis not indicated except for support—Therapy consists of intensive care.

Antidepressants (cyclics and MAO inhibitors also)	Heroin and other opiates
Antihistamines	Methaqualone (Quaalude)
Barbiturates (short-acting)	Methyprylon (Noludar)
Chlordiazepoxide (Librium)	Oxazepam (Serax)
Diazepam (Valium)	Phenothiazines
Digitalis and related drugs	Phenytoin (Dilantin)
Diphenoxylate with atropine (Lomotil)	Synthetic anticholinergics and belladonna compounds

While the long-acting barbiturates (cleared by the kidneys) are more readily dialyzable than the short-acting ones (cleared by the liver), dialysis may be helpful if the patient satisfies the criteria for supportive dialysis needs as outlined above.

Salicylates generally respond very well to intensive alkaline diuretic therapy, but if complications such as renal failure or pulmonary edema develop, hemodialysis alone or with hemoperfusion may be helpful.

Peritoneal dialysis and **exchange transfusion** may be more useful in small children than hemodialysis, as much for fluid and electrolyte homeostasis as for poison removal.

Dialysis should *not* be performed as initial therapy but only when the criteria listed above are met.

Hemoperfusion

Perfusion of blood through charcoal- or resin-filled devices is gradually becoming more widely available in many centers. These techniques will probably allow rapid removal of many substances previously considered dialyzable but will not be likely to remove large quantities of agents with large V_ds.

MANAGEMENT OF SPECIFIC COMMON POISONS

Unless otherwise directed, syrup of ipecac should be given to all conscious patients poisoned by the substances listed in the following section. Gastric lavage is usually indicated for comatose patients after an endotracheal tube is inserted. Apomorphine should not be used, because of the high incidence of complications.

ACETAMINOPHEN

Acetaminophen is an analgesic antipyretic contained in numerous preparations often accessible to children. In prescribed doses, the drug is a safe and effective agent for relief of fever and pain. In overdosage, acetaminophen can cause severe hepatotoxicity. The incidence of hepatotoxicity in adults and adolescents has been reported to be 10 times higher than in young children; in the latter group, only 3 of 417 patients under the age of 5 years developed transient hepatotoxicity.

Acetaminophen is normally metabolized in the liver. A small percentage of the drug goes through a pathway leading to a toxic metabolite. Normally, this nucleophilic reactant is removed harmlessly by conjugation with glutathione. In overdosage, the supply of gluthathione becomes exhausted, and the metabolite may bind covalently to hepatic macromolecules to produce necrosis.

Treatment

Treatment is to supply a surrogate glutathione by giving acetylcysteine (Mucomyst). In the USA, it may only be given orally. Consultation may be obtained from the Rocky Mountain Poison Center (telephone number: [800] 525–6115). Blood levels should be obtained as soon as possible after 4 hours and plotted on Fig 30–1. Acetylcysteine is the drug of choice if given within 16 hours after ingestion. It is administered to patients whose acetaminophen levels plot in the toxic range on the nomogram (Fig 30–1).

The dose is 140 mg/kg orally, diluted to a 5% solution in sweet fruit juice or carbonated soft drink. After this loading dose, 70 mg/kg should be administered orally every 4 hours for 3 days. AST (SGOT), ALT (SGPT), serum bilirubin, and plasma prothrombin time should be followed closely; if the patient develops hepatic encephalopathy, supportive measures should be provided and acetylcysteine withdrawn.

Peterson RG, Rumack BH: Pharmacokinetics of acetaminophen in children. *Pediatrics* 1978;**62:**877.

Rumack BH: Acetaminophen overdose in young children. *Am J Dis Child* 1984;**138:**428.

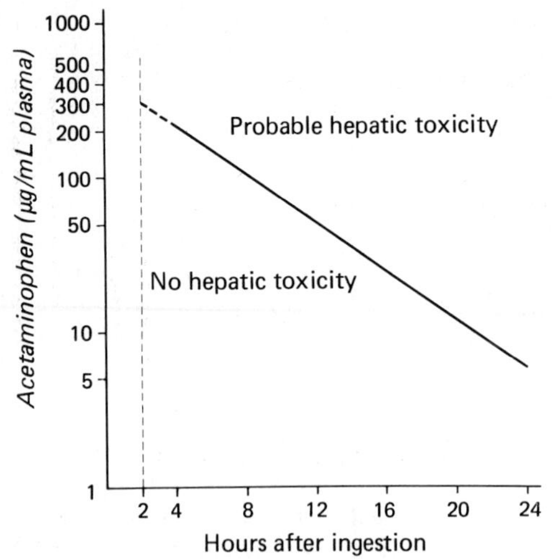

Figure 30–1. Semilogarithmic plot of plasma acetaminophen levels versus time. (Reprinted, with permission, from Rumack BH, Matthew H: Acetaminophen poisoning and toxicity. *Pediatrics* 1975;**55**:871.)

Rumack BH et al: Acetaminophen overdose. *Arch Intern Med* 1981;**141**:380.

ALCOHOL, ETHYL (Ethanol)

Alcoholic beverages, tinctures, cosmetics, and rubbing alcohol are common sources of poisoning in children. Concomitant exposure to other depressant drugs increases the seriousness of the intoxication. (Blood levels cited are for adults; comparable figures for children are not available. In most states, alcohol levels of 50–80 mg/dL are considered compatible with impaired faculties, and levels of 80–150 mg/dL are considered evidence of intoxication.)

50–150 mg/dL: Incoordination, slow reaction time, and blurred vision.

150–300 mg/dL: Visual impairment, staggering, and slurred speech. Marked hypoglycemia may be present.

300–500 mg/dL: Marked incoordination, stupor, hypoglycemia, and convulsions.

> **500 mg/dL:** Coma and death except in individuals who have developed tolerance.

Complete absorption of alcohol by the stomach and small bowel requires 30 minutes to 6 hours depending upon the volume, the presence of food, the time spent in consuming the alcohol, etc. The rate of metabolic degradation is constant (about 10 mL of 50% alcohol per hour in an adult). Less than 10% is excreted in the urine. Absolute ethanol, 1 mL/kg, results in a peak blood level of about 100 mg/dL in 1 hour after ingestion. Acute and chronic alcoholism increases the risk of subarachnoid hemorrhage.

Treatment

Supportive treatment, including aggressive management of hypoglycemia and acidosis, is usually the only measure required. Glucagon does not correct the hypoglycemia, because hepatic glycogen stores are reduced. If the patient is conscious, vomiting may be induced with syrup of ipecac. Monitoring of blood gases and oxygen administration are indicated in serious overdoses, since death is usually caused by respiratory failure. In severe cases, cerebral edema should be treated with dexamethasone, 0.1 mg/kg intravenously every 4–6 hours. Peritoneal dialysis and hemodialysis are indicated in life-threatening intoxication.

Hammond K, Rumack B, Rodgerson D: Blood ethanol. *JAMA* 1973;**226**:63.

Sellers EM, Kalant H: Alcohol intoxication and withdrawal. *N Engl J Med* 1976;**294**:757.

Seppälä M et al: Ethanol elimination in a mother and her premature twins. *Lancet* 1971;**1**:1188.

AMPHETAMINES & RELATED DRUGS (Methamphetamine, Phenmetrazine [Preludin])

Acute poisoning. Amphetamine poisoning is common because of the widespread availability of "diet pills" and the use of "speed" by adolescents. Symptoms include central nervous system stimulation, anxiety, hyperactivity, hyperpyrexia, hypertension, abdominal cramps, nausea and vomiting, and inability to void urine. A toxic psychosis indistinguishable from paranoid schizophrenia may occur.

Chronic toxicity. Amphetamines are common causes of dependency and addiction. Chronic users develop such a high tolerance that more than 1500 mg of intravenous methamphetamine can be used daily. Hyperactivity, disorganization, and euphoria are followed by exhaustion, depression, and coma lasting 2–3 days. Upon awakening, the patient is ravenously hungry. Heavy users, taking more than 100 mg/d, have restlessness, incoordination of thought, insomnia, nervousness, irritability, and visual hallucinations. Psychosis may be precipitated by the chronic administration of high doses. Depression, weakness, tremors, gastrointestinal complaints, and suicidal thoughts occur frequently.

Treatment

Because chlorpromazine (Thorazine) (0.5–1 mg/kg every 30 minutes as needed) brings about dramatic decreases in hyperactivity, it is used in the management of intoxication. However, if ingestion of 2,5-dimethoxy-4-methylamphetamine (STP), methylenedioxyamphetamine (MDA), or dimethyltryptamine (DMT) is suspected, diazepam (Valium) should be used instead of chlorpromazine because of the risk of hypotension with the latter drug. When combinations of amphetamines and barbiturates (diet pills) are used, the action of the amphetamines begins first, followed by a rebound depression caused by the barbiturates. In these cases, treatment with additional barbiturates is contraindicated because of the risk of respiratory failure. Emesis or lavage, charcoal, and cathartics should be used.

Chronic users may be withdrawn rapidly from amphetamines. On the other hand, if amphetamine-barbiturate combination tablets have been used, the barbiturates must be withdrawn gradually to prevent withdrawal seizures. Psychiatric treatment should be considered.

Cohen S: Amphetamine abuse. *JAMA* 1975;**231:**414.

Espelin DE, Done AK: Amphetamine poisoning: Effectiveness of chlorpromazine. *N Engl J Med* 1968;**278:**1361.

ANESTHETICS, LOCAL

Intoxication from local anesthetics may be associated with central nervous system stimulation, acidosis, delirium, shock, convulsions, and death. Methemoglobinuria has been reported following local dental analgesia.

Local anesthetics used in obstetrics cross the placental barrier and are not efficiently metabolized by the fetal liver. Mepivacaine, lidocaine, and bupivacaine can cause fetal bradycardia, neonatal depression, and death. Prilocaine causes methemoglobinemia, which should be treated if levels in the blood exceed 40% or if the patient is symptomatic.

Accidental injection of mepivacaine (Carbocaine) into the unborn infant's head during paracervical anesthesia has caused neonatal asphyxia, cyanosis, acidosis, bradycardia, convulsions, and death.

Treatment

If the anesthetic has been ingested, induced vomiting should be followed by activated charcoal. Any contaminated mucous membranes should be carefully cleansed. Oxygen administration, with assisted ventilation if necessary, is indicated. Methemoglobinemia is treated with methylene blue, 1%, 0.2 mL/kg intravenously over 5–10 minutes; this should dramatically relieve the cyanosis. Therapeutic levels of mepivacaine, lidocaine, and procaine are less than 5 μg/mL.

Rothstein P, Dornbusch J, Shaywitz BA: Prolonged seizures associated with the use of viscous lidocaine. *J Pediatr* 1982;**101:**461.

ANTIHISTAMINES

Although antihistamines typically cause central nervous system depression, children often react paradoxically with excitement, hallucinations, delirium, tremors, and convulsions followed by central nervous system depression, respiratory failure, or cardiovascular collapse. Anticholinergic effects such as dry mouth, fixed dilated pupils, flushed face, and fever may be prominent.

Antihistamines are widely available in allergy, cold, and antiemetic preparations, and many are supplied in sustained-release forms, which increases the likelihood of dangerous overdoses. They are absorbed rapidly and metabolized by the liver, lungs, and kidneys. A potentially toxic dose of most antihistamines is 25–50 mg/kg, or 20–30 tablets of the most commonly used antihistamines.

Treatment

Activated charcoal should be used to delay drug absorption. Emetics may be ineffective if the antihistamine is structurally related to phenothiazines. A saline cathartic is indicated for sustained-release preparations. Physostigmine, 0.5–2 mg intravenously, dramatically reverses the central and peripheral anticholinergic effects of antihistamines. Diazepam (Valium), 1–2 mg/kg intravenously, can be used to control seizures. Forced diuresis is not helpful. Exchange transfusion should be considered in very severe intoxications, since most antihistamines are highly protein-bound and are concentrated in the serum.

Nigro SA: Toxic psychosis due to diphenhydramine hydrochloride. *JAMA* 1968;**203:**301.

Rumack BH et al: Ornade and anticholinergic toxicity, hypertension, hallucinations and arrhythmia. *Clin Toxicol* 1974; **7:**573.

Wallace AR, Allen E: Recovery after massive overdose of diphenhydramine and methaqualone. *Lancet* 1968;**2:**1241.

ARSENIC

Acute poisoning. Abdominal pain, vomiting, watery and bloody diarrhea, cardiovascular collapse, paresthesias, neck pain, garlic odor on breath, difficulty in walking, and exfoliative dermatitis occur. Convulsions, coma, and anuria are later signs. Inhalation may cause pulmonary edema. Death is the result of cardiovascular collapse.

Chronic toxicity. Anorexia, generalized weakness, giddiness, colic, abdominal pain, polyneuritis, dermatitis, nail changes, alopecia, and anemia often develop.

Arsenic is commonly used in insecticides (fruit tree or tobacco sprays), rodenticides, weed killers, and wallpaper. It is well absorbed primarily through the gastrointestinal and respiratory tracts, but skin absorption may occur. Arsenic can be found in the urine, hair, and nails by laboratory testing.

Poisoning with arsenic trioxide, an insoluble precursor of most arsenicals, is associated with a 12% mortality rate. Highly toxic soluble derivatives of this compound, such as sodium arsenite, are frequently found in liquid preparations and can cause death in as many as 65% of victims. The alkyl methanearsonates found in "persistent" or "preemergence" type weed killers (eg, Ortho Crabgrass Killer) are relatively less soluble and do not cause deaths. Poisonings with a liquid arsenical preparation that does not contain alkyl methanearsonate compounds should be considered potentially lethal. Patients with any clinical signs other than minor gastrointestinal irritation should be treated until laboratory tests indicate it is no longer necessary.

Treatment

In acute poisoning, induce vomiting and put activated charcoal into the stomach. Then immediately give dimercaprol (BAL), 2.5 mg/kg intramuscularly, and follow with 2 mg/kg intramuscularly every 4 hours. The dimercaprol-arsenic complex is dialyzable. Penicillamine (Cuprimine), 100 mg/kg orally to a maximum of 1 g/d in 4 divided doses, should be used instead of BAL after the first day or even immediately if the patient is not acutely ill.

Dimercaprol is not effective in the treatment of arsine gas intoxication, which should be treated by exchange transfusion when the plasma hemoglobin is 1.5 g/dL or more and then by hemodialysis if there is renal damage. Vomiting should always be induced.

Chronic arsenic intoxication should be treated with penicillamine. Collect a 24-hour baseline urine specimen and then begin chelation. If the 24-hour urine arsenic level is greater than 50 μg, continue chelation for 5 days. After 10 days, repeat the 5-day cycle once or twice depending on how soon the urine arsenic level falls below 50 μg/24 h.

Done AK: . . . and old lace. *Emergency Med* 1973;**5:**246.
Peterson RG, Rumack BH: Arsenic poisoning treated with D-penicillamine. *J Pediatr* 1977;**91:**661.

BARBITURATES

A patient who has ingested barbiturates in toxic amounts can present with a variety of findings, including confusion, poor coordination, coma, miotic or fixed dilated pupils, and increased or (more commonly) decreased respiratory effort. Respiratory acidosis is commonly associated with pulmonary atelectasis, and hypotension frequently occurs in severely poisoned patients. Ingestion of more than 6 mg of long-acting or 3 mg of short-acting barbiturates per kilogram is usually toxic; however, chronic users of barbiturates can tolerate blood levels up to 25 mg/dL.

Treatment

If the patient is awake, vomiting should be induced and activated charcoal, 50–100 g every 4 hours, should be given. Careful, conservative management with emphasis on maintaining a clear airway, adequate ventilation, and control of hypotension is critical. Forced alkaline diuresis is useful and often eliminates the need for dialysis. If the patient develops increasing respiratory acidosis after initial improvement during forced alkaline diuresis, pulmonary edema ("shock lung") is suggested and may require dialysis or hemoperfusion if the blood level is high. Forced alkaline diuresis or hemodialysis is not of significant help in the treatment of poisoning with short-acting barbiturates.

Analeptics are contraindicated.

Berg MJ et al: Acceleration of the body clearance of phenobarbital by oral activated charcoal. *N Engl J Med* 1982;**307:**642.
Gröschel D, Gerstein A, Rosenbaum J: Skin lesions as a diagnostic aid in barbiturate poisoning. *N Engl J Med* 1970;**283:**409.
Matthew H: Barbiturates. *Clin Toxicol* 1975;**8:**495.

BELLADONNA ALKALOIDS (Atropine, Jimsonweed, Potato Leaves, Scopolamine, Stramonium)

Patients with atropinism have been characterized as "red as a beet, dry as a bone, and mad as a hatter." Common complaints include dry mouth; thirst; decreased sweating with hot, dry, red skin; high fever; and tachycardia that may be preceded by bradycardia. The pupils are dilated, and vision is blurred. Speech and swallowing may be impaired. Hallucinations, delirium, and coma are common. Leukocytosis may occur, confusing the diagnosis.

The onset of symptoms is quite rapid, but symptoms usually last only 3–4 hours unless large overdoses have been taken. Atropinism has been caused by normal doses of atropine or homatropine eye drops, especially in children with Down's syndrome. Many common plants and over-the-counter sleeping medications contain belladonna alkaloids.

Treatment

Emesis or lavage should be followed by activated charcoal and cathartics. Physostigmine, 0.5–2 mg intravenously (can be repeated every 30 minutes as needed), dramatically reverses the central and peripheral signs of atropinism. Neostigmine is ineffective because it does not enter the central nervous system. High fever must be controlled. Catheterization may be needed if the patient cannot void.

Gowdy JM: Stramonium intoxication: Review of symptomatology in 212 cases. *JAMA* 1972;**221:**585.
Mikolich JR, Paulson GW, Cross CJ: Acute anticholinergic syndrome due to Jimson seed ingestion. *Ann Intern Med* 1975;**83:**321.
Rumack BH: Anticholinergic poisoning: Treatment with physostigmine. *Pediatrics* 1973:**52:**449.

BORIC ACID

Boric acid is a worthless antiseptic that has been commonly used to treat diaper rash and burns. It is rapidly absorbed through broken skin and is potentially toxic to all organs, especially the central nervous system, kidneys, and pancreas. About half of the ingested dose will be excreted in the first 24 hours. The estimated lethal dose in children is 5–6 g. The amount of boric acid present in a baby powder is relatively safe, but other boric acid preparations should be discarded.

Anorexia, weight loss, and mild diarrhea are the most common initial findings. Later, the "boiled lobster" skin, a characteristic erythematous exfoliating rash that desquamates in 1–2 days, is seen. Fever, vomiting, dehydration, anuria, and convulsions are commonly associated with the rash. Central nervous system signs (irritability, high-pitched cry, exaggerated startle reflex, and opisthotonos) are common in children.

Treatment

Unless contraindicated, induced vomiting followed by catharsis should be used to remove ingested boric acid. If boric acid is being absorbed through the skin or mucous membranes, it should be removed with water and its use discontinued. Ten percent glucose in water given intravenously will induce diuresis. Anticonvulsants may be needed. Peritoneal dialysis and hemodialysis are more effective than exchange transfusion in severe boric acid poisoning.

Baliah T. McLeish HP, Drummond KN: Acute boric acid poisoning. *Can Med Assoc J* 1969;**101:**166.
Levin S: Diapers. *S Afr Med J* 1970;**44:**256.

CARBON MONOXIDE

The degree of toxicity correlates well with the carboxyhemoglobin level. Symptoms are more severe if the patient has exercised or taken alcohol or lives at a high altitude. Normal blood may contain up to 5% carboxyhemoglobin.

The most prominent early clinical effect is headache. Other symptoms occur in relation to levels as shown in Table 30–2.

Proteinuria, glycosuria, elevated serum transaminase levels, or electrocardiographic changes (including ST segment and T wave abnormalities, atrial fibrillation, and interventricular block) may be present in the acute phase. Myocardial infarction most commonly occurs about a week after an acute serious exposure. Permanent cardiac, liver, renal, or central nervous system damage occasionally occurs. Even in extremely severe poisoning, central nervous system damage may be completely reversible, although months may be required for total recovery.

Treatment

The half-life of carbon monoxide in room air is approximately 200 minutes; in 100% oxygen, it is 40 minutes. After the level has been reduced to near zero, therapy is aimed at the nonspecific sequelae of anoxia. The addition of CO_2 is more hazardous than beneficial. A hyperbaric chamber (if readily

Table 30–2. Clinical symptoms of carbon monoxide poisoning.

Saturation of Blood	Symptoms
0–10%	None.
10–20%	Tightness across forehead; slight headache; dilatation of cutaneous vessels.
20–30%	Headache; throbbing in temples.
30–40%	Severe headache; weakness and dizziness; dimness of vision; nausea and vomiting; collapse and syncope; increased pulse and respiratory rate.
40–50%	As above, plus increased tendency to collapse and syncope; increased pulse and respiratory rate.
50–60%	Increased pulse and respiratory rate; syncope; Cheyne-Stokes respiration; coma with intermittent convulsions.
60–70%	Coma with intermittent convulsions; depressed heart action and respiration; death possible.
70–80%	Weak pulse; depressed respiration; respiratory failure and death.

available) at 2–2.5 atmospheres of oxygen is the ideal treatment. Hypothermia appears to be a useful adjunct to therapy. Dexamethasone, 0.1 mg/kg intravenously or intramuscularly every 4–6 hours, should be started to combat cerebral edema.

The patient should be closely observed for at least a week following severe acute poisoning, because myocardial infarction, pulmonary edema, and myoglobinuria may occur during convalescence.

Clark CJ, Campbell D, Reid WH: Blood carboxyhaemoglobin and cyanide levels in fire survivors. *Lancet* 1982;**1:**1332.
Gore I: Treatment of carbon-monoxide poisoning. *Lancet* 1970;**1:**468.
Myers RA et al: Value of hyperbaric oxygen in suspected carbon monoxide poisoning. *JAMA* 1981;**246:**2478.
Smith JS, Brandon S: Morbidity from acute carbon monoxide poisoning at three-year follow-up. *Br Med J* 1973;**1:**318.

CAUSTICS

1. ACIDS (Hydrochloric, Nitric, & Sulfuric Acids; Sodium Bisulfate)

Strong acids are commonly found in metal and toilet bowl cleaners, batteries, etc. Sulfuric acid is the most toxic and hydrochloric acid the least toxic of these 3 substances. However, even a few drops can be fatal if aspirated into the trachea.

Painful swallowing, mucous membrane burns, bloody emesis, abdominal pain, respiratory distress due to edema of the epiglottis, thirst, shock, and renal failure can occur. Coma and convulsions sometimes are seen terminally. Residual lesions include esophageal, gastric, and pyloric strictures as well as scars of the cornea, skin, and oropharnyx.

Treatment

Emetics and lavage are contraindicated. Water or milk is the ideal substance to dilute the ingestant, because a heat-producing chemical reaction does not occur. Alkalies should not be used. The use of gas-forming carbonates is contraindicated, since they increase the likelihood of perforating an already weakened stomach wall. Burned areas of the skin, mucous membranes, or eyes should be washed with copious amounts of warm water. Olive oil should not be applied to denuded areas unless the surgeon concurs. Opiates for pain and antibiotics may be needed. Treatment of shock is often necessary. An endotracheal tube may be required to alleviate laryngeal edema. Esophagoscopy should be performed if the patient has significant burns or difficulty in swallowing. Acids are more likely to produce gastric burns than esophageal burns. Corticosteroids may be of use.

2. BASES (Clinitest Tablets, Clorox, Drano, Liquid-Plumr, Purex, Sani-Clor)

Alkalies produce more severe injuries than acids do. Some substances, such as Clinitest Tablets or Drano, are quite toxic, while the chlorinated bleaches (3–6% solutions of sodium hypochlorite) are not as toxic as formerly thought. When sodium hypochlorite comes in contact with the acid pH of the stomach, hypochlorous acid, which is very irritating to the mucous membrane and skin, is formed. However, the rapid inactivation of this substance prevents systemic toxicity from developing. If a chlorinated bleach is mixed with a strong acid such as a toilet bowl cleaner, chloramine, which is extremely irritating to the eyes and respiratory tract, is produced.

Alkalies can cause burns of the skin, mucous membranes, and eyes. Respiratory distress may be due to edema of the epiglottis, pulmonary edema resulting from inhalation of fumes, or pneumonia. Mediastinitis or other intercurrent infections or shock can occur. Perforation of the esophagus or stomach is rare.

Treatment

The skin and mucous membranes should be cleansed with copious amounts of water. A local anesthetic can be instilled in the eye if necessary to alleviate blepharospasm. The eye should be irrigated for at least 20–30 minutes. Ingestions should be treated with water or milk as a diluent. Routine esophagoscopy is no longer indicated to rule out burns of the esophagus due to chlorinated bleaches unless an unusually large amount has been ingested or the patient is symptomatic. The absence of oral lesions does not rule out the possibility of laryngeal or esophageal burns following granular alkali ingestion. A 3-week course of corticosteroids in high doses (dexamethasone, 10 mg initially, then 1 mg every 4 hours) is indicated for the treatment of esophageal burns. Bougienage may be helpful in selected cases. Antibiotics may be needed if mediastinitis is likely, but they should not be used prophylactically.

Cello JP, Fogel RP, Boland CR: Liquid caustic ingestion: Spectrum of injury. *Arch Intern Med* 1980;**140:**501.

Haller JA Jr et al: Pathophysiology and management of acute corrosive burns of the esophagus. *J Pediatr Surg* 1971;**6:**578.

Muhletaler CA et al: Acid corrosive esophagitis: Radiographic findings. *Am J Radiol* 1980;**134:**1137.

Rumack BH, Burrington JP: Antidotal therapy of caustic reactions. *Clin Toxicol* 1977;**11:**27.

CONTRACEPTIVE PILLS

The only known toxic effects following acute ingestion of oral contraceptive agents are nausea, vomiting, and vaginal bleeding in girls.

COSMETICS & RELATED PRODUCTS

The relative toxicities of commonly ingested products in this group are listed in Table 30–3.

Permanent wave neutralizers may contain bromates, peroxides, or perborates. Bromates have been removed from most products because they can cause nausea, vomiting, abdominal pain, methemoglobinemia, shock, hemolysis, renal failure, and convulsions. Four grams of bromate salts is potentially lethal. Poisoning is treated by induced emesis or gastric lavage with 1% sodium thiosulfate followed by demulcents to relieve gastric irritation. Sodium thiosulfate, 1%, 100–500 mL, can be given intravenously, but methylene blue should not be used to treat methemoglobinemia in this situation, because it increases the toxicity of bromates. Dialysis is indicated in severe

Table 30–3. Relative toxicities of cosmetics and similar products.

High toxicity	**Low toxicity**
Permanent wave neutralizers	Perfume
Fingernail polish remover	Hair removers
	Deodorants
	Bath salts
Moderate toxicity	**No toxicity**
Fingernail polish	Liquid makeup
Metallic hair dyes	Vegetable hair dye
Home permanent wave lotion	Cleansing cream
Bath oil	Hair dressing (nonalcoholic)
Shaving lotion	Hand lotion or cream
Hair tonic (alcoholic)	Lipstick
Cologne, toilet water	

bromate poisoning. Perborate can cause boric acid poisoning.

Fingernail polish removers used to contain toluene or aliphatic acetates, which produce central nervous system irritation and depression. They now usually have an acetone base, which does not require treatment.

Cobalt, copper, cadmium, iron, lead, nickel, silver, bismuth, and tin are sometimes found in metallic hair dyes. In large amounts, they can cause skin sensitization, urticaria, dermatitis, eye damage, vertigo, hypertension, asthma, methemoglobinemia, tremors, convulsions, and coma. Treatment for ingestions is to administer demulcents and the appropriate antidote for the heavy metal involved.

Home permanent wave lotions, hair straighteners, and hair removers usually contain thioglycolic acid salts, which cause irritation and perhaps hypoglycemia.

Shaving lotion, hair tonic, hair straighteners, cologne, and toilet water contain denatured alcohol, which can cause central nervous system depression and hypoglycemia.

Deodorants usually consist of an antibacterial agent in a cream base. Antiperspirants are aluminum salts, which frequently cause skin sensitization. Zirconium oxide can cause granulomas in the axilla.

Chronic inhalation of hair sprays containing synthetic and natural resins has reportedly caused thesaurosis (hilar lymphadenopathy and diffuse pulmonary infiltration) as well as ocular irritation and keratitis.

Arena JM: *Poisoning: Toxicology, Symptoms, Treatments,* 3rd ed. Thomas, 1974.

CYANIDE

Cyanide poisoning may cause a bitter, burning taste with an odor of bitter almonds on the breath, salivation, nausea (usually without vomiting), anxiety, confusion, vertigo, giddiness, stiffness of the lower jaw, coma, convulsions, opisthotonos, paralysis, dilated pupils, cardiac irregularities, and transient respiratory stimulation followed by respiratory failure. A prolonged expiratory phase is characteristic.

Cyanide is commonly used in rodenticides, metal polishes (especially silver), electroplating, and photographic solutions as well as in fumigation products. Aqueous solutions are readily absorbed through the skin, mucous membranes, and lungs, but alkali salts are toxic only when ingested. Lethal doses vary greatly with the individual, but death has usually been associated with ingestion of 200–300 mg of the sodium or potassium salt, or blood cyanide levels of 0.26–3 mg/dL. Death usually occurs within minutes following inhalation but may be delayed several hours following ingestion.

Treatment

If the patient is apneic or has gasping respirations, artificial respiration must be started immediately. The patient should inhale amyl nitrite for 15–30 seconds of every minute while a sodium nitrite solution is being prepared for intravenous injection. Amyl nitrite alone is not adequate treatment, because the maximum methemoglobin level obtainable in this way is about 5%. Cyanide kits (Cyanide Antidote Package [Lilly]) that contain instructions *(for use in adults)* should be carried in all emergency vehicles. Intravenous sodium nitrite is given first and followed immediately by sodium thiosulfate. Doses for children are listed in Table 30–4. Oxygen increases the effects of nitrites and thiosulfates but is not adequate treatment by itself. It should be continued after the thiosulfate is given, because methemoglobinemia decreases the ability of blood to carry oxygen. Exchange transfusion or infusion of whole blood is indicated if methemoglobin levels rise over 50%.

Table 30–4. Pediatric dosages of sodium nitrite and sodium thiosulfate.

Hemoglobin	Initial Dose 3% Sodium Nitrite (mL/kg)	Initial Dose 25% Sodium Thiosulfate (mL/kg)
8 g/dL	0.22 mL (6.6 mg)	1.1 mL
10 g/dL	0.27 mL (8.7 mg)	1.35 mL
12 g/dL*	0.33 mL (10 mg)	1.65 mL
14 g/dL	0.39 mL (11.6 mg)	1.95 mL

* Normal child.

The patient should be observed for 24–48 hours, since toxicity may reappear. If a relapse occurs, the patient should be treated again, using one-half of the above doses of sodium nitrite and sodium thiosulfate.

Berlin CM Jr: The treatment of cyanide poisoning in children. *Pediatrics* 1970;**46:**793.

Lasch EE, Elshawa R: Multiple cases of cyanide poisoning by apricot kernels in children from Gaza. *Pediatrics* 1981;**68:**5.

CYCLIC ANTIDEPRESSANTS

Cyclic antidepressants (amitriptyline [Elavil], imipramine [Tofranil], etc) are utilized in adolescents and adults as antidepressants. Unfortunately, these drugs have a very low toxic:therapeutic ratio, and in a young child even a moderate overdose can have a disastrous effect. The 5 features of cyclic antidepressant overdosage that make it more of a problem than other drugs with anticholinergic properties are dysrhythmias, coma, convulsions, hypertension (and, later, hypotension), and hallucinations. These may be life-threatening and require rapid intervention. A newer agent, amoxapine, differs significantly in that it has a much lower incidence of cardiovascular complications, and seizures may be associated with normal QRS complexes.

If the patient has symptoms—dry mouth, tachycardia, etc—an ECG should be taken. If there is any dysrhythmia, the patient should be admitted and monitored until free of irregularity for 24 hours. Another indication for monitoring is tachycardia of more than 110/min plus additional findings of anticholinergic toxicity. The onset of dysrhythmias is rare beyond 24 hours after ingestion.

Treatment

Physostigmine is a dangerous drug that must be given slowly to avoid iatrogenic convulsions. It is contraindicated in asthma, vascular gangrene, or urinary tract obstruction. The dosage is as follows: (1) For children under 12 years of age, give 0.5 mg intravenously over 60 seconds. If there is no effect, the dose may be repeated at 5-minute intervals to a maximum of 2 mg. Repeat as necessary only for life-threatening situations. (2) For adolescents and adults, give 2 mg intravenously over 60 seconds. If there is no effect, repeat in 10 minutes to a maximum dose of 4 mg. Repeat for life-threatening situations.

Phenytoin or lidocaine may be used primarily for treatment of dysrhythmia, and physostigmine for tachyarrhythmia. Alkalinization with sodium bicarbonate, 0.5 meq/kg intravenously, may dramatically reverse *ventricular* dysrhythmias. Sodium bicarbonate should be administered to all patients with significant dysrhythmias to achieve a plasma pH of 7.5–7.6. Forced diuresis is contraindicated. A QRS interval greater than 100 ms specifically identifies patients with major cyclic antidepressant overdosage. Diazepam should be given for convulsions.

Hypotension is a major problem, since cyclic antidepressants block the reuptake of catecholamines. This may produce a rebound hypotension following initial hypertension. Treatment with physostigmine is not effective. Infusion of sodium bicarbonate, 0.5 meq/kg, to produce a plasma pH of 7.5 or 7.6, will help avert hypotension. Vasopressors are generally ineffective, and the mortality rate is 60% in patients with hypotension who prove unresponsive to initial fluids. Orogastric charcoal, 0.5 g/kg every 4–6 hours during the first 24 hours following ingestion, appears to interrupt an enterohepatic recirculation of cyclic antidepressants and shorten the plasma $t_{1/2}$.

Burks JS et al: Tricyclic antidepressant poisoning: Reversal of coma, choreoathetosis, and myoclonus by physostigmine. *JAMA* 1974;**230:**1405.

Callahan M et al: Epidemiology of fatal tricyclic antidepressant ingestion. *Ann Emerg Med* 1985;**14:**1.

Kulig K et al: Amoxapine overdose: Coma and seizures without cardiotoxic effects. *JAMA* 1982;**248:**1092.

Swartz CM et al: The treatment of tricyclic antidepressant overdose with repeated charcoal. *J Clin Psychopharmacol* 1984;**4:**336.

DIGITALIS & OTHER CARDIAC GLYCOSIDES

Manifestations include nausea, vomiting, diarrhea, headache, delirium, confusion, and, occasionally, coma. Cardiac irregularities such as atrial fibrillation, paroxysmal atrial tachycardia, and atrial flutter often occur. Death usually is the result of ventricular fibrillation.

Toxic reactions occur with doses of digoxin greater than 0.07 mg/kg.

Transplacental intoxication by digitalis has been reported. An accurate radioimmunoassay for digitalis is now available.

Treatment

If vomiting has not occurred, induce emesis or provide lavage followed by charcoal cathartics. Potassium should not be given in acute overdosage unless there is laboratory evidence of hypokalemia. In acute overdosage, hyperkalemia is more common.

The patient must be monitored carefully for electrocardiographic changes. The correction of acidosis will better demonstrate the degree of potassium deficiency present. In some cases, phenytoin (Dilantin), a β-adrenergic blocking agent such as propranolol (Inderal), or procainamide (Pronestyl) is necessary to correct dysrhythmias. A pacemaker may be needed.

Clinical investigations using digoxin antibody fragments (Fab), supplied by Burroughs Wellcome Company, are currently under way. Preliminary results indicate that this is the most effective agent for treatment of cardiac glycoside poisoning.

Hobson JD, Zettner A: Digoxin serum half-life following suicidal digoxin poisoning. *JAMA* 1973;**223:**147.

Rumack BH et al: Phenytoin (diphenylhydantoin) treatment of massive digoxin overdose. *Br Heart J* 1974;**36:**405.

Smith TW et al: Treatment of life-threatening digitalis intoxication with digoxin-specific Fab antibody fragments: Experience in 26 cases. *N Engl J Med* 1982;**307:**1357.

DIPHENOXYLATE HYDROCHLORIDE (Lomotil)

Lomotil is a combination of diphenoxylate hydrochloride, a synthetic narcotic, and atropine sulfate. Early signs of Lomotil intoxication are due to its anticholinergic effect and consist of fever, facial flush, tachypnea, and lethargy. However, the miotic effect of the narcotic predominates. Later, hypothermia, increasing central nervous system depression, and loss of the facial flush occur. Seizures are probably secondary to hypoxia. Small amounts of Lomotil are potentially lethal when ingested by children; it is contraindicated as a drug under age 2 years.

Treatment

After an adequate airway has been established with an endotracheal tube, gastric lavage may be useful because of the prolonged delay in gastric emptying time. Narcotics are not adsorbed by activated charcoal, but atropine is. Naloxone (Narcan), 0.02 mg/kg intravenously, should be given. A transient improvement in respiratory status may be followed by respiratory depression, since the duration of action of diphenoxylate is considerably longer than that of the antagonists. The anticholinergic effects do not usually require treatment but can be reversed temporarily by the use of physostigmine, 0.5–2 mg intravenously.

Rumack BH, Temple AR: Lomotil poisoning. *Pediatrics* 1974;**53:**495.

DISINFECTANTS & DEODORIZERS

1. NAPHTHALENE

Naphthalene is commonly found in mothballs as well as in disinfectants and deodorizers commonly used in bathrooms, toilets, and garbage cans.

Naphthalene's toxicity is often not fully appreciated. It is absorbed not only when ingested but also through the skin and lungs. Naphthalene is very soluble in oil and relatively insoluble in water. It is potentially hazardous to store baby clothes in naphthalene because baby oil is an excellent solvent that increases absorption of the drug through the skin.

Metabolic products of naphthalene cause a severe hemolytic anemia similar to that due to primaquine toxicity 3–7 days after ingestion. Other physical findings include nausea, vomiting, diarrhea, jaundice, oliguria, anuria, coma, and convulsions. The urine may contain hemoglobin, protein, and casts.

Treatment

Induced vomiting should be followed by a saline cathartic. Forced alkaline diuresis prevents blocking of the renal tubules by acid hematin crystals. Repeated small blood transfusions may be necessary to bring the hemoglobin level up to 60–80% of normal. Corticosteroids are said to be useful in minimizing naphthalene hemolysis. Anuria may persist for 1–2 weeks and still be completely reversible.

2. *p*-DICHLOROBENZENE & PHENOLIC ACIDS

Disinfectants and deodorizers containing *p*-dichlorobenzene or sodium bisulfate are much less toxic than those containing naphthalene. Disinfectants containing phenolic acids are highly toxic, especially if they contain a borate ion. Phenol precipitates proteins and causes respiratory alkalosis followed by metabolic acidosis. Some phenols cause methemoglobinemia.

Local gangrene occurs after prolonged contact with tissue. Phenol is readily adsorbed from the gastrointestinal tract, causing diffuse capillary damage and, in some cases, methemoglobinemia. Pentachlorophenol, which has been used in terminal rinsing of diapers, has caused infant fatalities.

The toxicity of alkalies, quaternary ammonium compounds, pine oil, and halogenated disinfectants varies with the concentration of active ingredients. Wick deodorizers are usually of moderate toxicity. Iodophor disinfectants are the safest. Spray deodorizers are not usually toxic, because a child is not likely to swallow a very large dose.

Manifestations of acute ingestion include diaphoresis, thirst, nausea, vomiting, diarrhea, cyanosis, hyperactivity, coma, convulsions, hypotension, abdominal pain, and pulmonary edema. Acute liver or renal failure may develop later.

Treatment

Activated charcoal should be used prior to emesis or gastric lavage. Castor oil dissolves phenol and retards its absorption. Mineral oil and alcohol are contraindicated because they increase the gastric absorption of phenol. A saline cathartic should follow the castor oil. The metabolic acidosis must be carefully managed. Anticonvulsants or measures to treat shock may be needed.

Because phenols are absorbed through the skin, exposed areas should be irrigated copiously with water.

Arena JM: *Poisoning: Toxicology, Symptoms, Treatments,* 5th ed. Thomas, 1985.

George JN, Miller DR, Weed RI: Heinz body hemolytic anemias. *NY State J Med* 1970;**70:**2574.

DISK BATTERY

Small, flat, smooth disk-shaped batteries are used in watches, calculators, hearing aids, games, etc. They measure between 10 and 25 mm in diameter. In the past, treatment for disk battery ingestion was the same as for other smooth foreign bodies such as coins. It is now known that batteries are associated with different hazards and may represent a major emergency.

Batteries impacted in the esophagus may, like any other foreign body, cause presenting symptoms of refusal to take food, increased salivation, vomiting with or without blood, and pain or discomfort. Aspiration into the trachea may also occur. Fatalities have been reported in association with esophageal perforation.

When a history of disk battery ingestion is obtained, x-rays of the entire respiratory tract and gastrointestinal tract should be taken to locate the battery, since this will help determine therapy.

Treatment

If the disk battery is located in the esophagus, it must be removed immediately. If ingestion occurred within the previous 24-hour period, the battery may be removed by the balloon catheter technique. The patient is placed in the steep head-down, prone-oblique position. The catheter is placed beyond the object; the balloon is inflated with barium; and the catheter is withdrawn. If the battery has been in the esophagus for more than 24 hours, the risk of caustic burn is greater, and removal by endoscopic means may be necessary.

Location of the disk battery below the esophagus has been associated with erosion, tissue damage, and colored residue in the stomach and bowel, but the course has been benign in most cases. Perforated Meckel's diverticulum has been the major complication. It may take as long as 7 days for spontaneous passage to occur, and lack of movement in the gastrointestinal tract may not be a reason for removal. Some have suggested x-rays every 4–6 hours and surgical intervention if passage of the battery pauses, but this approach may be excessive. Batteries that have opened in the gastrointestinal tract have been associated with some toxicity due to mercury, but the patients have recovered.

Emesis is ineffective in removal of the battery from the stomach. Asymptomatic patients may simply be observed, and stools may be examined for passage of the battery. If the battery has not passed within 7 days or if the patient becomes symptomatic, x-rays should be repeated. If the battery has come apart or appears not to be moving, a purgative or enema should be administered. If these methods are not successful, surgical intervention may be required. Levels of heavy metals (mainly of mercury) should be measured in patients in whom the battery has opened or symptoms have developed.

Kulig K et al: Elevated mercury levels after ingestion of a disk battery. *JAMA* 1983;**249:**2502.

Litovitz TL: Button battery ingestions. *JAMA* 1983;**249:**2495.

Rumack BH, Rumack CM: Disk battery ingestion. *JAMA* 1983;**249:**2509.

Votteler TP, Nash JC, Rutledge JC: The hazard of ingested alkaline disk batteries in children. *JAMA* 1983;**249:**2504.

GLUTETHIMIDE (Doriden)

Patients may have nystagmus, mydriasis, dry mouth, ileus, and central nervous system depression manifested by absent deep tendon reflexes, coma, and either hypothermia or hyperpyrexia. Respiratory depression with normal respiratory rates, sudden apnea, and alternating levels of consciousness occur. The anticholinergic effects of glutethimide often predominate in children.

There is a narrow range between therapeutic and toxic blood levels. Doses exceeding 25–50 mg/kg are toxic in children. Blood levels greater than 3 mg/dL are generally associated with coma and serious illness. Glutethimide levels usually fall at a rate of 1.5–2 mg/dL/d. As in any other sedative poisoning, coma often is prolonged and varies in depths from moment to moment, but patients usually awake when blood levels decline to 1.5 mg/dL, although in some cases the patient awakens at levels higher than at the beginning of coma.

Treatment

Meticulous conservative management is the most successful approach and consists of adequate lavage and administration of activated charcoal and magnesium sulfate. Forced diuresis, peritoneal dialysis, and hemodialysis (including lipid dialysis) have not been helpful in reducing the duration of coma or the morbidity or mortality rate, although enhanced excretion of inert metabolites of the drug has been demonstrated. Fluids should be used cautiously because there is an increased likelihood of pulmonary or cerebral edema.

Chazan JA, Garella S: Glutethimide intoxication: A prospective study of 70 patients treated conservatively without hemodialysis. *Arch Intern Med* 1971;**128:**215.

Comstock EG: Glutethimide intoxication. *JAMA* 1971; **215:**1668.

Hansen AR et al: Glutethimide poisoning: A metabolite contributes to morbidity and mortality. *N Engl J Med* 1975;**292:**250.

Vestal RE, Rumack BH: Glutethimide dependence: Phenobarbital treatment. (Correspondence.) *Ann Intern Med* 1974; **80:**670.

Wright N, Roscoe P: Acute glutethimide poisoning: Conservative management of 31 patients. *JAMA* 1970;**214:**1704.

HYDROCARBONS (Benzene, Charcoal Lighter Fluid, Gasoline, Kerosene, Petroleum Distillates, Turpentine)

Ingestion causes irritation of mucous membranes, vomiting, blood-tinged diarrhea, respiratory distress, cyanosis, tachycardia, and fever. Although 10 mL is potentially fatal, patients have survived ingestion of several ounces of petroleum distillates. The more aromatic and the lower the viscosity rating of a hydrocarbon, the more toxic it is. Benzene, gasoline, kerosene, and red seal oil furniture polish are the most dangerous. A dose exceeding 1 mL/kg is likely to cause central nervous system depression. A history of coughing or choking, as well as vomiting, suggests aspiration with resulting hydrocarbon pneumonia, an acute hemorrhagic necrotizing disease that usually develops within 24 hours of the ingestion and resolves without sequelae in 3–5 days. However, several weeks may be required for resolution of a hydrocarbon pneumonia. Pneumonia may be caused by a few drops of petroleum distillate being aspirated into the lung or by absorption from the circulatory system. Pulmonary edema and hemorrhage, cardiac dilatation and dysrhythmias, hepatosplenomegaly, proteinuria, and hematuria can occur following large overdoses. Hypoglycemia is occasionally present. A chest film may reveal pneumonia shortly after the ingestion. An abnormal urinalysis in a child with a previously normal urinary tract suggests a large overdose.

Treatment

Both emetics and lavage should be avoided if only a small amount has been ingested. It is impossible to do a "cautious gastric lavage" unless a cuffed endotracheal tube is inserted. Under these circumstances, gastric lavage may be done using saline or 3% sodium bicarbonate solution. Following lavage, magnesium or sodium sulfate should be left in the stomach. (Mineral oil should not be given, because it is capable of causing a low-grade lipoid pneumonia.)

Emetics are probably preferable to gastric lavage if massive ingestion has occurred. Epinephrine should not be used, since it may affect an already sensitized myocardium. Analeptic drugs are contraindicated. The usefulness of corticosteriods is debated, and antibiotics should be reserved for patients with infections. Oxygen and mist are helpful.

Brown J et al: Experimental kerosene pneumonia. *J Pediatr* 1984;**84:**396.

Kulig K, Rumack BH: Hydrocarbon ingestion. *Curr Top Emerg Med* 1981;**3:**1.

INSECT STINGS (Bee, Wasp, & Hornet)

Insect stings are painful but not usually dangerous; however, these insects cause more deaths in the USA than snakes do. Deaths from insect stings are usually due to severe allergic reactions. Bee venom, for example, has hemolytic, neurotoxic, and histaminelike activities that can on rare occasions cause hemoglobinuria and severe anaphylactoid reactions.

Treatment

If possible, a tourniquet should be applied above the bite and the stinger removed, care being taken not to squeeze the venom sac. Epinephrine 1:1000 solution, 0.01 mL/kg, should be administered intravenously or subcutaneously above the site of the sting. Three to 4 whiffs from an isoproterenol (Isuprel) aerosol inhaler may be given at 3- to 4-minute intervals as needed. Corticosteroids (hydrocortisone), 100 mg intravenously, and diphenhydramine (Benadryl), 1.5 mg/kg intravenously, are useful ancillary drugs but have no immediate effect. Ephedrine or antihistamines may be used for 2 or 3 days to prevent recurrence of symptoms.

A patient who has had a potentially life-threatening insect sting should be desensitized against the Hymenoptera group, since the honey bee, wasp, hornet, and yellow jacket have common antigens in their venom.

For the more usual stings, cold compresses, aspirin, and diphenhydramine (Benadryl), 1 mg/kg orally, are useful.

Russell F et al: Insect and scorpion bites and stings. *JAMA* 1973;**224:**131.

Yunginger JW: Advances in the diagnosis and treatment of stinging insect allergy. *Pediatrics* 1981;**67:**325.

INSECTICIDES

The petroleum distillates or other organic solvents used in these products are often as toxic as the pesticide. Unless otherwise indicated, induced vomiting or gastric lavage is warranted after insertion of an endotracheal tube.

DePalma AE, Kwalich DS, Zukerberg N: Pesticide poisoning in children. *JAMA* 1970;**211:**1979.

Rumack BH (editor): *POISINDEX: An Emergency Poison Management System:* Micromedex, Denver, Colorado. [Published quarterly.]

1. CHLORINATED HYDROCARBONS (Aldrin, Carbinol, Chlordane, DDT, Dieldrin, Endrin, Heptachlor, Lindane, Toxaphene, Etc)

Signs of intoxication include salivation, gastrointestinal irritability, abdominal pain, nausea, vomiting, diarrhea, central nervous system depression, and convulsions. Inhalation exposure causes irritation of the eyes, nose, and throat; blurred vision; cough; and pulmonary edema.

Chlorinated hydrocarbons are absorbed through the skin, respiratory tract, and gastrointestinal tract. These compounds or their metabolic products are chronically stored in fat. Decontamination of skin (tincture of green soap) and evacuation of the stomach contents are critical. All contaminated clothing should be removed. Castor oil, milk, and other substances containing fats or oils should not be left in the stomach, since they increase absorption of the chlorinated hydrocarbons. Convulsions should be treated with diazepam (Valium), 0.1–0.3 mg/kg intravenously. Epinephrine should not be used, as it may cause cardiac dysrhythmias.

2. ORGANOPHOSPHATE (CHOLINESTERASE-INHIBITING) INSECTICIDES (Chlorthion, Co-Ral, DFP, Diazinon, Malathion, Paraoxon, Parathion, Phosdrin, TEPP, Thio-TEPP, Etc)

Dizziness, headache, blurred vision, miosis, tearing, salivation, nausea, vomiting, diarrhea, hypoglycemia, cyanosis, sense of constriction of the chest, dyspnea, sweating, weakness, muscular twitching, convulsions, loss of reflexes and sphincter control, and coma can occur.

The clinical findings are the result of cholinesterase inhibition, which causes an accumulation of large amounts of acetylcholine. The onset of symptoms is within 12 hours of the exposure. Red cell cholinesterase levels should be measured as soon as possible. (Some normal individuals have a low serum cholinesterase level.) Normal values vary in different laboratories. A screening test apparatus for cholinesterase levels should be available in every hospital emergency room. In general, a decrease of red cell cholinesterase to below 25% of normal indicates significant exposure to organophosphate insecticides and is an indication for treatment with pralidoxime.

Repeated low-grade exposure may result in sudden, acute toxic reactions. This syndrome usually occurs after repeated household spraying rather than agricultural exposure.

Although all organophosphates act by inhibiting cholinesterase activity, they vary greatly in their toxicity. Parathion, for example, is 100 times more toxic than malathion. The toxicity is influenced by the specific compound, the type of formulation (liquid or solid), the vehicle, and the route of absorption (lungs, skin, or gastrointestinal tract).

Treatment

Atropine plus a cholinesterase reactivator, pralidoxime (Protopam), is a chemical antidote for organophosphate insecticide poisoning. After establishing a clear airway and eliminating any cyanosis, large doses of atropine should be given and repeated every few minutes until signs of atropinism are present. An appropriate starting dose of atropine is 2–4 mg intravenously in an adult and 0.05 mg/kg in a child. The patient should receive enough atropine to stop secretions (approximately 10 times the normal dose). As much as 1 g of atropine per 24 hours may be needed in an adult.

Because atropine antagonizes the parasympathetic effects of the organophosphates but does not alter the muscular weakness, pralidoxime should also be given immediately in more severe cases and repeated every 8–12 hours as needed (1 g intravenously for older children and 250 mg intravenously for infants at a rate of no more than 500 mg/min). Pralidoxime should be used in addition to—not in place of—atropine if red cell cholinesterase is less than 25% of normal. Pralidoxime is probably not useful later than 36 hours after the exposure. Morphine, theophylline, aminophylline, succinylcholine, and tranquilizers of the reserpine and phenothiazine types are contraindicated. Hyperglycemia is common.

Decontamination of the skin (including nails and hair) and clothing with soapy water is extremely important. Decontamination of the skin must be done carefully to avoid abrasions, which increase organophosphate absorption significantly.

Melby TH: Prevention and management of organophosphate poisoning. *JAMA* 1971;**216:**2131.

Nelson DL, Crawford CR: Organophosphorus compounds: The past and the future. *Clin Toxicol* 1972;**5:**223.

3. CARBAMATES (Carbaryl, Sevin, Zectran, Etc)

Carbamate insecticides are reversible inhibitors of cholinesterase. The usual laboratory procedures used to determine red cell cholinesterase will not show a depression after carbamate exposure. The reversal is often so rapid that measurements of blood cholinesterases are near normal, whereas β-naphthol, a metabolite, is present in significant amounts. The signs and symptoms of intoxication are similar to those associated with organophosphate poisoning but are generally less severe. Atropine in large doses is sufficient treatment. Pralidoxime should not be used with carbaryl (Sevin) poisoning but is of value with other carbamates. In combined exposures to organophosphates, give atropine but reserve pralidoxime for cases in which the red cell cholinesterase is depressed below 25% of normal.

4. BOTANICAL INSECTICIDES (Black Flag Bug Killer, Black Leaf CPR Insect Killer, Flit Aerosol House & Garden Insect Killer, French's Flea Powder, Raid, Etc)

Pyrethrins, allethrin, ryania, and rotenone do not commonly cause signs of toxicity. Antihistamines, short-acting barbiturates, and atropine are helpful when needed.

IRON

Five stages of intoxication occur following iron intoxication: (1) Hemorrhagic gastroenteritis, which occurs 30–60 minutes after ingestion and may be associated with shock, acidosis, coagulation defects, and coma. This phase usually lasts 4–6 hours and is commonly followed by a 6- to 24-hour asymptomatic period. (2) Phase of improvement during which patient looks better. Lasts 2–12 hours. (3) Delayed shock, which may occur 12–48 hours after ingestion and is usually associated with a serum iron level greater than 500 mg/dL. Metabolic acidosis, fever, leukocytosis, and coma may also be present. (4) Liver damage with hepatic failure. (5) Residual pyloric stenosis, which usually develops at least 4 weeks after the ingestion.

Diarrhea, vomiting, leukocytosis ($> 15,000/\mu L$), hyperglycemia, and a positive abdominal x-ray have been shown to correlate positively with serum iron levels exceeding 300 μg/dL. If any of these signs are present, chelation with deferoxamine should be initiated and further serum iron levels obtained.

Once iron is absorbed from the gastrointestinal tract, it is not normally eliminated in feces but may be partially excreted in the urine, giving it a red color prior to chelation. A reddish discoloration of the urine suggests a serum iron level greater than 350 μg/dL.

Treatment

Shock must be treated in the usual manner. After inducing vomiting, leave sodium bicarbonate or Fleet's Phospho-Soda (15–30 mL diluted 1:2 with water) in the stomach to form the insoluble phosphate or carbonate. Deferoxamine (Desferal), a specific chelating agent for iron, is a useful adjunct in the treatment of severe iron poisoning. When given parenterally, it forms a soluble complex that is excreted in the urine. It is contraindicated in patients with renal failure unless dialysis can be used.

Deferoxamine should not be delayed in serious cases of poisoning until serum iron levels are available. Intravenous administration is indicated if the patient is in shock, in which case it should be given at a rate not to exceed 15 mg/kg/h for 8 hours. Rapid intravenous administration causes hypotension, facial flushing, urticaria, tachycardia, and shock. The dose may be repeated every 8 hours if clinically indicated. Deferoxamine, 90 mg/kg intramuscularly every 8 hours, may be given if clinically indicated. Blood levels of deferoxamine given intramuscularly and intravenously are about equal in 15 minutes if the patient is not in shock. The drug should not be given orally.

Hemodialysis, peritoneal dialysis, or exchange transfusion can be used to increase the excretion of the dialyzable complex, if necessary. Urine output should be monitored and urine sediment examined for evidence of renal tubular damage. Initial laboratory studies should include blood typing and crossmatching; total protein; total iron-binding capacity; serum iron, sodium, potassium, and chloride; CO_2; pH; and liver function tests. Serum iron levels fall rapidly even if deferoxamine is not given.

After the acute episode, liver function studies and an upper gastrointestinal series are indicated to rule out residual damage.

Lacouture PG et al: Emergency assessment of severity in iron overdose by clinical and laboratory methods. *J Pediatr* 1981;**99:**89.

Propper RD, Shurin SB, Nathan DG: Reassessment of the use of desferrioxamine B in iron overload. *N Engl J Med* 1976;**294:**1421.

Westlin WF: Deferoxamine as a chelating agent. *Clin Toxicol* 1971;**4:**597.

LEAD

Lead poisoning causes weakness, irritability, weight loss, vomiting, personality changes, ataxia, constipation, headache, transient abdominal pain, opaque flakes in the gastrointestinal tract, and a "lead line" on the gums and in many bones at the metaphyseal area. Late manifestations consist of retarded development, convulsions, and coma associated with increased intracranial pressure. The latter is a medical emergency.

Plumbism usually occurs insidiously in children under 5 years of age. The most likely sources of lead include flaking leaded paint, artist's paints, fruit tree sprays, solder, brass alloys, home-glazed pottery, and fumes from burning batteries. Only paint containing less than 1% lead is safe for interior use (furniture, toys, etc). Tetraethyl lead poisoning from gasoline sniffing is manifested by pyramidal and cerebellar dysfunction and encephalopathy. Repetitive ingestions of small amounts of lead are far more serious than a single massive exposure.

Toxic reactions are likely to occur if more than 0.5 mg of lead per day is absorbed. Only uncombined lead is removed by deleading agents. Children under 2 years of age have a poor prognosis, whereas children who develop peripheral neuritis without evidence of mental retardation or encephalitis usually recover completely.

Laboratory tests are necessary to establish a diagnosis of plumbism. Urinary coproporphyrins or, preferably, red cell δ-aminolevulinic acid dehydratase or free erythrocyte protoporphyrin (FEP) levels are satisfactory screening tests. Urine lead levels are the definitive test. The 24-hour urinary lead level exceeds 80 μg/d without treatment and should increase to greater than 1.5 mg/d on any one of the first 3 days on calcium disodium edetate (EDTA) or penicillamine therapy (or both). Dehydration and acidosis may falsely lower urinary lead levels. Glycosuria, proteinuria, hematuria, and aminoaciduria occur frequently. Blood lead levels usually exceed 80 μg/dL in symptomatic patients. Blood lead levels exceeding 40 μg/dL on 2 occasions warrant further investigation. Abnormal blood and urinary lead levels should be repeated in asymptomatic patients to rule out laboratory error. Specimens must be meticulously obtained in acid-washed containers. A normocytic, slightly hypochromic anemia with basophilic stippling of the red cells and reticulocytosis is usually present in plumbism. Stippling of red blood cells is absent in cases of sudden massive ingestion.

The cerebrospinal fluid protein is elevated, and the white cell count is usually less than 100 cells per milliliter. Cerebrospinal fluid pressure is usually elevated. Lumbar punctures must be performed cautiously to prevent herniation of the brain stem in patients with encephalopathy.

Treatment

Induced vomiting followed by a saline cathartic is indicated. Combination therapy with dimercaprol (BAL), 4 mg/kg per dose every 4 hours intramuscularly, and calcium disodium edetate, 12.5 mg/kg per dose (maximum dose, 75 mg/kg/d) intravenously or intramuscularly starting with the second dose of dimercaprol, should reduce the mortality rate of acute lead encephalopathy to less than 5%. Penicillamine (Cuprimine), 100 mg/kg/d (maximum, 1 g), should be added as soon as the patient can take oral medication. This treatment is indicated for a symptomatic patient or one with a blood lead level of 100 μg/

dL. It should be started as soon as urine flow is initiated. If urine flow is delayed over 4 hours, simultaneous hemodialysis must be started. Unless the patient is severely affected, a lower dose (50 mg/kg/d) of calcium disodium edetate is adequate and is less likely to damage the kidneys or cause hypercalcemia. Elevated lead levels will usually return to normal in 3–5 days when the combination method is used; this is rarely true when calcium disodium edetate is used alone. After a 2-day pause, another course of treatment can be given if desired, again including oral penicillamine. Dimercaprol can be used with complete renal shutdown but not in patients with severe hepatic insufficiency. Dimercaprol (but not calcium disodium edetate) increases the fecal excretion of lead. The development of lacrimation, blepharospasm, paresthesias, nausea, tachycardia, and hypertension suggests a toxic reaction to dimercaprol. Iron should not be given to patients being treated for plumbism, since it forms a toxic substance with dimercaprol.

If the blood lead level is 80–100 μg/dL, one of the following regimens can be used: calcium disodium edetate and dimercaprol given for 2 days and then replaced with penicillamine orally for 5 days if there is no lead in the gut; calcium disodium edetate given alone for 5 days; or dimercaprol and calcium disodium edetate given concomitantly for 3 days.

A brief course of calcium disodium edetate or a longer course of penicillamine is indicated for lead levels of 60–80 μg/dL. Chelation therapy is not indicated for lead levels below 60 μg/dL unless there is additional evidence of toxicity.

Anticonvulsants may be needed. Mannitol or corticosteroids are indicated in patients with encephalopathy. Fluid intake should be restricted. One expert investigator feels that surgical decompression is contraindicated, but others disagree. Hypothermia and corticosteroid therapy have not altered mortality rates significantly. A high-calcium, high-phosphorus diet and large doses of vitamin D remove lead from the blood by depositing it in the bones.

Urinalysis should be done daily; serum calcium and phosphorus and blood urea nitrogen every 2 days. Calcium gluconate given intravenously as a 10% solution is helpful in controlling the colic that sometimes occurs.

A public health team should evaluate the source of the lead. Necessary corrections should be completed before the child is returned home.

Boeckx RL, Postl B, Coodin FJ: Gasoline sniffing and tetraethyl lead poisoning in children. *Pediatrics* 1977;**60:**140.

Chisholm J et al: Recognition and management of children with increased lead absorption. *Arch Dis Child* 1979;**54:**249.

Houk VN: Preventing lead poisoning in young children: A statement by the Center for Disease Control. *J Pediatr* 1978;**93:**709.

Lin-Fu J: Lead exposure among children: A reassessment. *N Engl J Med* 1979;**300:**731.

MERCURY

Mercury poisoning is manifested by a metallic taste, thirst, severe vomiting, bloody diarrhea, cough, pharyngeal and abdominal pain, dyspnea, pulmonary embolization, dermatitis, corneal ulcers, nephrosis, renal failure, hepatic damage, ulcerative colitis, and shock. Acrodynia occurs in children after chronic exposure to small amounts of mercury in diaper rash ointments and teething lotions.

Chronic inorganic mercury poisoning causes salivation, loosening of teeth, bad oral odor, gingivitis, mouth ulcerations, dermatitis, fatigue, loss of memory, irritability, apprehension, tremors, decreased visual acuity and night vision, and staggering and slurred speech ("mad hatter syndrome"). Both organic and inorganic mercury poisoning can cause similar physical signs, although organic mercury intoxication characteristically causes dysarthria, ataxia, and constricted visual fields.

Elevated mercury levels have recently been noted in tuna and swordfish, and human mercury poisoning has been attributed to eating large amounts of contaminated swordfish. Mercury is a possible constituent of antiseptics, cathartics, diuretics, fumigants, and fungicides. All forms of mercury are potentially poisonous, but organic mercurials are generally less toxic than inorganic mercurials because they are poorly absorbed. The small amount of metallic mercury from a thermometer is nontoxic, as it is not well absorbed.

Treatment

Activated charcoal should be followed by induced vomiting and a saline cathartic. Dimercaprol (BAL) as for lead poisoning (see above) is often used. (Calcium disodium edetate is contraindicated.) Penicillamine (Cuprimine), 100 mg/kg/d orally (maximum, 1 g), is as effective as dimercaprol. Demulcents and analgesics are indicated, as well as correction of fluid and electrolyte imbalances. Hemodialysis may be indicated for renal failure but not for removal of mercury.

Eyl TB: Alkylmercury contamination of foods. *JAMA* 1971;**215:**287.

Javett SN, Kaplan B: Acrodynia treated with D-penicillamine. *Am J Dis Child* 1968;**115:**71.

Kark RAP et al: Mercury poisoning and its treatment with N-acetyl-D,L-penicillamine. *N Engl J Med* 1971;**285:**1.

Teitelbaum DT, Ott JE: Elemental mercury self-poisoning. *Clin Toxicol* 1969;**2:**243.

MUSHROOMS

Many toxic species of mushrooms are difficult to separate from edible varieties. Symptoms vary with the species ingested, the time of year, the stage of maturity, the quantity eaten, the method of preparation, and the interval since ingestion. A mushroom that is toxic to one individual may not be toxic for another. Drinking alcohol and eating certain mushrooms may cause a reaction similar to that seen with disulfiram (Antabuse) and alcohol. Cooking destroys some toxins but not the deadly one produced by *Amanita phalloides,* which is responsible for 90% of deaths due to mushroom poisoning. Mushrooms toxins are absorbed relatively slowly. Onset of symptoms within 2 hours of ingestion suggests muscarinic toxin, whereas a delay of symptoms for 6–48 hours after ingestion strongly suggests *Amanita* poisoning. Patients who have ingested *A phalloides* may relapse and die of hepatic or renal failure following initial improvement.

Mushroom poisoning may be manifested by muscarinic symptoms (salivation, vomiting, diarrhea, cramping abdominal pain, tenesmus, miosis, and dyspnea), coma, convulsions, hallucinations, hemolysis, and hepatic and renal failure.

Treatment

Induce vomiting and follow with activated charcoal and a saline cathartic. If the patient has muscarinic signs, give atropine, 0.05 mg/kg intramuscularly (0.02 mg/kg in toddlers), and repeat as needed (usually every 30 minutes) to keep the patient atropinized. Atropine, however, is only used when there are cholinergic effects and not for all mushrooms. Hypoglycemia is most likely to occur in patients with delayed onset of symptoms. It is important, if at all possible, to specifically identify the mushroom if the patient is symptomatic. Local botanical gardens, university departments of botany, and societies of mycologists may be able to help. Supportive care is usually all that is needed except in the case of *A phalloides,* where thioctic acid or hemodialysis may be indicated.

Litton W: The most poisonous mushrooms. *Sci Am* (March) 1975;**232:**90.

Rumack BH, Salzman E: *Mushroom Poisoning, Diagnosis and Treatment.* CRC Press, 1978.

NARCOTICS & SYNTHETIC CONGENERS* (Codeine, Heroin, Methadone, Morphine, Propoxyphene)

Physicians may be called upon to treat various narcotic problems, including drug addiction, withdrawal in a newborn infant, and accidental overdoses. Accidental ingestions of propoxyphene (Darvon) and diphenoxylate (in Lomotil) are frequent.

Unlike other narcotics, methadone is readily absorbed from the gastrointestinal tract. Drug abusers often use the intravenous route of administration. Most narcotics, including heroin, methadone, meperidine, morphine, and codeine, are excreted in the urine within 24 hours and can be readily detected.

Narcotic addicts often have other medical problems, including cellulitis, abscesses, thrombophlebitis, tetanus, infective endocarditis, tuberculosis, hepatitis, malaria, foreign body emboli, thrombosis of pulmonary arterioles, diabetes mellitus, obstetric complications, nephropathy, and peptic ulcer.

Treatment of Overdosage

Children receiving an overdose of opiates can develop respiratory depression, stridor, coma, increased oropharyngeal secretions, sinus bradycardia, and urinary retention. Pulmonary edema rarely occurs in children; deaths usually result from respiratory arrest and cerebral edema. Convulsions may occur with propoxyphene overdosage.

While suggested doses for naloxone (Narcan) range from 0.01 to 0.1 mg/kg, it is generally unnecessary to calculate the dosage on this basis. This extremely safe antidote should be given in sufficient quantity to reverse opiate binding sites. For children under 1 year of age, 1 ampule (0.4 mg) should be given initially; if there is no response, give 5 more ampules (2 mg) rapidly. Older children should be given 1–2 ampules, followed by 5–10 more ampules if there is no response. An improvement in respiratory status may be followed by respiratory depression, since the depressant action of narcotics may last 24–48 hours but the antagonist's duration of action is only 2–3 hours.

Withdrawal in the Addict

The severity of withdrawal signs should be evaluated as explained on p 941.

Diazepam (Valium), 10 mg every 6 hours orally, has been recommended for the treatment of mild narcotic withdrawal in ambulatory adolescents. Ambulatory or hospitalized patients with moderate or severe withdrawal signs can be given the same dose of diazepam intramuscularly. Diazepam is recommended because it is nonhepatotoxic and nonmutagenic, does not affect the fetus when given to pregnant women, and is a good anticonvulsant. Diazepam therapy can be discontinued when the withdrawal score falls below 2. Diphenoxylate with atropine (Lomotil) is used to treat severe diarrhea and abdominal cramps. Chloral hydrate is the drug of choice for insomnia.

Methadone maintenance is not usually recommended for adolescents, although it may be used for withdrawal purposes. One method of administration is to give methadone orally every 12 hours, starting with a 25-mg dose and decreasing the amount by 5 mg every 12 hours. When the dose of methadone is 10 mg, add 3 tablets of diphenoxylate with atropine (Lomotil) 3 times daily for 1 day followed by 2 tablets 3 times daily for 2 days. If signs of withdrawal recur, give 10 mg of methadone orally or diazepam orally or intramuscularly.

The abrupt discontinuation of narcotics (cold turkey method) is not recommended and may cause severe physical withdrawal signs.

Withdrawal in the Newborn

A newborn infant in narcotic withdrawal is small

* See p 950 for diphenoxylate (Lomotil) poisoning.

for gestational age and demonstrates yawning, sneezing, decreased Moro reflex, hunger but uncoordinated sucking action, jitteriness, tremor, constant movement, a shrill protracted cry, increased tendon reflexes, convulsions, vomiting, fever, watery diarrhea, cyanosis, dehydration, vasomotor instability, and collapse. The onset of symptoms commonly begins in the first 48 hours but may be delayed as long as 8 days depending upon the timing of the mother's last fix and her predelivery medication. The diagnosis can be easily confirmed by identifying the narcotic in the urine of the mother and baby.

Several methods of treatment have been suggested for narcotic withdrawal in the newborn. Phenobarbital, 8 mg/kg/d intramuscularly or orally in 4 doses for 4 days and then reduced by one-third every 2 days as signs decrease, may be continued for as long as 3 weeks. Methadone may be necessary in those infants with congenital methadone addiction who are not controlled in their withdrawal by large doses of phenobarbital. Dosage should be 0.5 mg/kg/d in 2 divided doses but can be gradually increased as needed. Slow tapering off may be necessary over 4 weeks for methadone addiction.

It is not clear whether prophylactic treatment with these drugs decreases the complication rate. The mortality rate of untreated narcotic withdrawal in the newborn may be as high as 45%.

Bradberry JC, Raebel MA: Continuous infusion of naloxone in the treatment of narcotic overdose. *Drug Intell Clin Pharm* 1981;**15**:945.

Cunningham EE et al: Heroin nephropathy: A clinicopathologic and epidemiologic study. *Am J Med* 1980;**68**:47.

Litt I, Colli A, Cohen M: Diazepam in the management of heroin withdrawal in adolescents: Preliminary report. *J Pediatr* 1971;**78**:692.

Lovejoy FH Jr, Mitchell AA, Goldman P: The management of propoxyphene poisoning. *J Pediatr* 1974;**85**:98.

Martin WR: Naloxone. *Ann Intern Med* 1978;**85**:765.

Reddy AM, Harper RG, Stern G: Observations on heroin and methadone withdrawal in newborn. *Pediatrics* 1971;**48**:353.

NITRITES, NITRATES, ANILINE, PENTACHLOROPHENOL, & DINITROPHENOL

Nausea, vertigo, vomiting, cyanosis (methemoglobinemia), cramping abdominal pain, tachycardia, cardiovascular collapse, tachypnea, coma, shock, convulsions, and death are possible manifestations of nitrite or nitrate poisoning.

Nitrite and nitrate compounds found in the home include amyl nitrite, nitroglycerin, pentaerythritol tetranitrate (Peritrate), sodium nitrite, nitrobenzene, and pyridium. Pentachlorophenol and dinitrophenol, which are found in wood preservatives, produce methemoglobinemia and high fever because of uncoupling of oxidative phosphorylation. High concentrations of nitrites in water or spinach have been the most common cause of nitrite-induced methemoglobinemia. Symptoms do not usually occur until 40–50% of the hemoglobin has been converted to methemoglobin. A rapid test is to compare a drop of normal blood with the patient's blood on a dry filter paper. Brown discoloration of the patient's blood indicates a methemoglobin level of more than 15%.

Treatment

After administering activated charcoal, induce vomiting and follow with a saline cathartic. Decontaminate any affected skin with soap and water. Oxygen and artificial respiration may be needed. If the blood methemoglobin level exceeds 40% or if levels cannot be obtained, give a 1% solution of methylene blue, 0.2 mL/kg intravenously over 5–10 minutes. Avoid perivascular infiltration, since it causes necrosis of the skin and subcutaneous tissues. A dramatic change in the degree of cyanosis should occur. Transfusion is occasionally necessary. Epinephrine and other vasoconstrictors are contraindicated. If reflex bradycardia occurs, atropine can be used to block it.

Bakshi SP, Fahey JL, Pierce LE: Sausage cyanosis: Acquired methemoglobinemic nitrite poisoning. *N Engl J Med* 1967; **277**:1072.

McDermott JH: Health aspects of toxic materials in drinking water. *Am J Public Health* 1971;**61**:2269.

PHENOTHIAZINES (Chlorpromazine [Thorazine], Prochlorperazine [Compazine], Trifluoperazine [Stelazine], Etc)

Extrapyramidal crisis. Episodes characterized by torticollis, stiffening of the body, spasticity, poor speech, catatonia, and inability to communicate although conscious are typical manifestations. These episodes usually last a few seconds to a few minutes but have rarely caused death. Extrapyramidal crises may represent idiosyncratic reactions and are aggravated by dehydration. The signs and symptoms occur most often in children who have received prochlorperazine (Compazine). They are commonly mistaken for psychotic episodes.

Overdose. Lethargy and deep prolonged coma commonly occur. Promazine, chlorpromazine, and prochlorperazine are the drugs most likely to cause respiratory depression and precipitous drops in blood pressure. Occasionally, paradoxic hyperactivity and extrapyramidal signs as well as hyperglycemia and acetonemia are present. Seizures are uncommon.

Phenothiazines are rapidly absorbed from the gastrointestinal tract and bound to tissue. They are principally conjugated with glucuronic acid and excreted in the urine.

Treatment

Extrapyramidal signs are alleviated within minutes by the slow intravenous administration of diphenhydramine (Benadryl), 1–5 mg/kg. No other treatment is usually indicated. Dialysis is contraindicated.

Patients with overdoses should be treated conservatively. An attempt should be made to induce vomiting with ipecac after administration of activated charcoal. Charcoal adsorbs chlorpromazine and probably other phenothiazines very well. Emetics are often unsuccessful in this situation because phenothiazines are potent antiemetics; gastric lavage, therefore, may be the only practical way to remove gastric contents. A large amount of intravenous fluid without vasopressor agents is the preferred method of treating tranquilizer-induced neurogenic hypotension. If a pressor agent is required, norepinephrine (levarterenol) should be used. Epinephrine should *not* be used, because phenothiazines reverse epinephrine's effects.

Barry D, Meyskens FL Jr, Becker CE: Phenothiazine poisoning: A review of 48 cases. *Calif Med* (Jan) 1973;**118:**1.

Davies DM: Treatment of drug-induced dyskinesias. *Lancet* 1970;**1:**567.

Thomas J: Fatal case of agranulocytosis due to chlorpromazine. *Lancet* 1970;**1:**44.

PLANTS

Many common ornamental, garden, and wild plants are potentially toxic. Small amounts of a plant may cause severe illness or death. These effects usually involve the cardiovascular, gastrointestinal, and central nervous systems and the skin. Table 30–5 lists the most toxic plants, symptoms and signs of poisoning, and treatment.

Hardin JW, Arena JM: *Human Poisoning From Native and Cultivated Plants,* 2nd ed. Duke Univ Press, 1974.

Kozma JJ: *Killer Plants: A Poisonous Plant Guide.* Milestone Publishing Co., 1969.

PSYCHOTROPIC DRUGS

Psychotropic drugs consist of 4 general classes: stimulants (amphetamines, cocaine), depressants (narcotics, barbiturates, etc), antidepressants and tranquilizers, and hallucinogens (LSD, PCP, etc).

The following clinical findings are commonly seen in patients abusing drugs:

Stimulants. Agitation, euphoria, grandiose feelings, tachycardia, fever, abdominal cramps, visual and auditory hallucinations, mydriasis, coma, convulsions, and respiratory depression.

Depressants. Emotional lability, ataxia, diplopia, nystagmus, vertigo, poor accommodation, respiratory depression, coma, apnea, and convulsions. Dilatation of conjunctival blood vessels suggests marihuana ingestion. Narcotics cause miotic pupils and, occasionally, pulmonary edema.

Antidepressants and tranquilizers. Hypotension, lethargy, respiratory depression, coma, and extrapyramidal reactions.

Hallucinogens and psychoactive drugs. Belladonna alkaloids cause mydriasis, dry mouth, nausea, vomiting, urinary retention, confusion, disorientation, paranoid delusions, hallucinations, fever, hypotension, aggressive behavior, convulsions, and coma. **Psychoactive drugs** such as LSD cause mydriasis, unexplained bizarre behavior, hallucinations, and generalized undifferentiated psychotic behavior.

See also other entries discussed in alphabetic sequence in this chapter.

Management of the Patient Who Abuses Drugs

Only a small percentage of the persons using drugs come to the attention of physicians; those who do are usually suffering from adverse reactions such as panic states, drug psychoses, homicidal or suicidal thoughts, and respiratory depression that could not be satisfactorily managed by friends.

Even with cooperative patients, an accurate history is difficult to obtain. The user often does not really know what drug has been taken or how much. "Street drugs" are almost always adulterated with one or more other compounds. Multiple drugs are often taken together, making it impossible to clinically define the type of drug. Friends may be a useful source of information. A drug history is most easily obtained in a quiet spot by a gentle, nonthreatening, honest examiner.

The general appearance, skin, lymphatics, cardiorespiratory status, gastrointestinal tract, and central nervous system should be stressed during the physical examination, since they often provide clues suggesting drug abuse. A drug history should not be taken from an adolescent in the parents' presence.

Although it is desirable to know the specific drug taken, it is often impossible to obtain this information. Hallucinogens are not life-threatening unless the patient is frankly homicidal or suicidal. A specific diagnosis is usually not necessary for management; instead, the presenting signs and symptoms are treated. Does the patient appear intoxicated? In withdrawal? "Flashing back?" Is some illness or injury (eg, head trauma) being masked by a drug effect? (Remember that a known drug user may still have hallucinations from meningoencephalitis.)

The signs and symptoms in a given patient are a function of not only the drug and the dose but also the level of acquired tolerance, the "setting," the patient's physical condition and personality traits, the potentiating effects of other drugs, and many other factors.

A common drug problem in hospital emergency rooms is the "bad trip," which is usually a panic reaction. This is best managed by "talking the patient down" and minimizing auditory and visual stimuli. It is sometimes helpful to communicate a light mood and "join the party" while looking for opportunities to restore reality orientation. If the response is adverse, the attempt should be abandoned. The physician should not use "street language" if not fluent

Table 30–5. Poisoning due to plants.*

	Symptoms and Signs	Treatment
Arum family: *Caladium, Dieffenbachia,* calla lily, dumb cane (oxalic acid)	Burning of mucous membranes and airway obstruction secondary to edema caused by calcium oxalate crystals.	Accessible areas should be thoroughly washed. Corticosteroids relieve airway obstruction. Apply cold packs to affected mucous membranes.
Autumn crocus (colchicine)	Abdominal cramps, severe diarrhea, CNS depression, and circulatory collapse. Occasionally, oliguria and renal shutdown. Delirium or convulsions occur terminally.	Fluid and electrolyte monitoring. Abdominal cramps may be relieved with meperidine or atropine.
Castor bean plant (ricin—a toxalbumin)	Mucous membrane irritation, nausea, vomiting, bloody diarrhea, blurred vision, circulatory collapse, acute hemolytic anemia, convulsions, uremia.	Fluid and electrolyte monitoring. Saline cathartic. Forced alkaline diuresis will prevent complications due to hemagglutination and hemolysis.
Foxglove and cardiac glycosides	Nausea, diarrhea, visual disturbances, and cardiac irregularities (eg, heart block).	See treatment for digitalis drugs in text (p 950).
Jequirity bean (abrin—a toxalbumin)	Nausea, vomiting, abdominal and muscle cramps, hemolysis and hemagglutination, circulatory failure, respiratory failure, and renal and liver failure.	Symptomatic. Renal failure can be prevented by alkalinizing the urine. Gastric lavage or emetics are contraindicated because the toxin is necrotizing. Saline cathartics are indicated.
Jimsonweed: See Belladonna Alkaloids, p 946		
Larkspur (ajacine, *Delphinium,* delphinoidine)	Nausea and vomiting, irritability, muscular paralysis, and CNS depression.	Symptomatic. Atropine may be helpful.
Monkshood (aconite)	Numbness of mucous membranes, visual disturbances, tingling, dizziness, tinnitus, hypotension, bradycardia, and convulsions.	Activated charcoal, oxygen. Atropine is probably helpful.
Oleander (dogbane family)† (oleandrin)	Nausea, bloody diarrhea, respiratory depression, tachycardia, and muscle paralysis.	Symptomatic. See treatment for poisoning with digitalis drugs in text (p 950).
Poison hemlock (coniine)	Mydriasis, trembling, dizziness, bradycardia, CNS depression, muscular paralysis, and convulsions. Death is due to respiratory paralysis.	Symptomatic. Oxygen and cardiac monitoring equipment are desirable. Assisted respiration is often necessary. Give anticonvulsants if needed.
Rhododendron (andromedotoxin)	Abdominal cramps, vomiting, severe diarrhea, muscular paralysis, CNS and circulatory depression. Hypertension with very large doses.	Atropine can prevent bradycardia. Epinephrine is contraindicated. Antihypertensives may be needed.
Yellow jessamine (active ingredient, gelsemine, is related to strychnine)	Restlessness, convulsions, muscular paralysis, and respiratory depression.	Symptomatic. Because of the relation to strychnine, activated charcoal and diazepam (Valium) for seizures would be worth trying.

* Many other plants cause minor irritation but are not likely to cause serious problems unless large amounts are ingested. See Hardin JW: Poisonous plants. In: *POISINDEX: An Emergency Poison Management System.* Rumack BH (editor). Micromedex, Denver, Colorado, 1975.

† Done AK: Ornamental and deadly. *Emergency Med* (April) 1973;**5:**255.

in it. Sitting with a friend while the drug effect dissipates may be the best treatment that can be offered. This may take 8 hours or more. The physician's job is not to terminate the drug effect but to help the patient over the bad experience.

Drugs are often unnecessary and may complicate the clinical course of a patient with a panic reaction. Although phenothiazines have been commonly used to treat "bad trips," they should be avoided if the specific drug is not known, since they may cause a precipitous drop in blood pressure if STP has been taken or paradoxic hyperactivity that makes management difficult. Diazepam (Valium), 20 mg orally every 30 minutes as necessary, is the drug of choice if a sedative effect is required. Physical restraints are rarely if ever indicated and usually increase the patient's panic reaction.

For treatment of life-threatening drug abuse, consult the section on the specific drug elsewhere in this chapter and the section on general management at the beginning of the chapter.

After the acute episode, the physician must decide whether psychiatric referral is indicated; in general, patients who have made suicidal gestures or attempts and adolescents who are not communicating with their families should be referred. On the other hand, adolescents who are "experimenting" with drugs often do not need psychiatric referral.

Cohen S: The "angel dust" states: Phencyclidine. *Pediatr in Rev* 1979;**1:**17.
Consroe PF: Treatment of acute hallucinogenic drug toxicity: Specific pharmacological intervention. *Am J Hosp Pharm* 1973;**30:**80.
Gabel M: Treatment for ingestion of LSD. *J Pediatr* 1972; **81:**634.
Hollister LE: Marihuana in man: Three years later. *Science* 1971;**172:**21.
Marijuana. *Med Lett Drugs Ther* (Aug 13) 1976;**18:**69.
Smith D et al: PCP problems and prevention. *J Psychedelic Drugs* 1980;**12:**181.
Teitelbaum DT: Poisoning with psychoactive drugs. *Pediatr Clin North Am* 1970;**17:**557.

SALICYLATES

The use of childproof containers and publicity regarding accidental poisoning have reduced the incidence of acute salicylate poisoning. Serious intoxication still occurs and must be regarded as an emergency.

Salicylates uncouple oxidative phosphorylation, leading to increased heat production, excessive sweating, and dehydration. They also interfere with glucose metabolism and may cause hypo- or hyperglycemia. Respiratory center stimulation occurs early.

Patients usually have signs of hyperventilation, sweating, dehydration, and fever. Vomiting and diarrhea sometimes occur. In severe cases, disorientation, convulsions, and coma are often present.

The severity of acute intoxication can in some measure be judged by serum salicylate levels (Fig 30–2). High levels are always dangerous irrespective of clinical signs, and low levels may be misleading in chronic cases. Other laboratory values usually indicate metabolic acidosis despite hyperventilation; low serum K^+ values; and, often, abnormal serum glucose levels.

Salicylate poisoning is classified as mild when plasma pH is greater than 7.4 and urine pH is greater than 6.0; as moderate when plasma pH is greater than 7.4 and urine pH is less than 6.0; and as severe when plasma pH is less than 7.4 and urine pH is less than 6.0.

In mild poisoning, stimulation of the respiratory center produces respiratory alkalosis. The kidney responds by producing alkali.

In moderate poisoning, the respiratory center is still stimulated and produces respiratory alkalosis. The kidney becomes less able to excrete alkali owing to depletion of K^+. Consequently, the kidney exchanges K^+ for H^+, and a relatively acidic urine is seen.

In severe intoxication (seen in severe acute ingestion with high salicylate levels and in chronic toxicity with lower levels), respiratory response is unable to overcome the metabolic overdose.

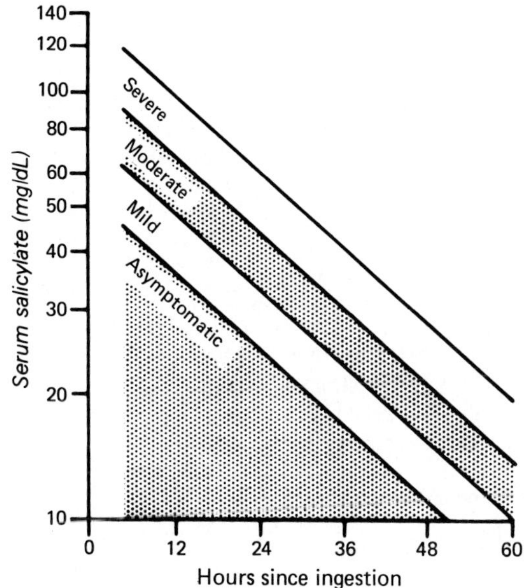

Figure 30–2. Nomogram relating serum salicylate concentration and expected severity of intoxication at varying intervals following ingestion of a single dose of salicylate. (Redrawn and reproduced, with permission, from Done AK: Salicylate intoxication. *Pediatrics* 1960;**26:**800.)

Once the urine becomes acidic, progressively smaller amounts of salicylate are excreted. Until this is reversed, the half-life will remain extended, since metabolism contributes little to the removal of these substances.

Chronic severe poisoning may be seen as early as 3 days after a regimen of salicylate is begun. Findings usually include vomiting, diarrhea, and dehydration due to accumulation of salicylates in the body.

Treatment

Salicylates can be recovered from the body in substantial amounts for as long as 20 hours following accidental or intentional ingestion. Charcoal binds salicylates well and, after emesis or lavage, should be given on a cyclic basis every 4 hours until charcoal appears in stool.

Mild poisoning may require only the administration of oral fluids and confirmation that the salicylate level is falling.

Moderate ingestion is reflected by moderate dehydration and depletion of renal potassium. Fluids must be administered at a rate sufficient to correct dehydration and produce urine with a pH of greater than 7.0 at a rate of flow of 3–6 mL/mg/min. Initial hydrating solutions should be isotonic, with sodium bicarbonate constituting half the electrolyte content. Once the patient is rehydrated, the solution can contain more free water and approximately 40 meq of potassium per liter.

Severe ingestion is marked by major dehydration in cases of chronic poisoning with a delay in diagnosis.

Symptoms may be confused with those of Reye's syndrome, encephalopathy, and metabolic acidosis. Salicylate levels may even be in the "therapeutic range." Major fluid correction of dehydration is required. Once this has been accomplished, hypokalemia must be corrected and sodium bicarbonate given. Urine pH will not become alkaline until adequate potassium has been provided. Usual requirements are sodium bicarbonate, 0.5–2 meq/L over the first 6–8 hours, and K^+, 40–80 meq/L. A urine flow of 3–6 mL/kg/h should be established.

Vitamin K should be administered, although hemorrhaging is rare except in severely poisoned patients. Renal failure or pulmonary edema is an indication for dialysis. Hemodialysis is most effective and peritoneal dialysis relatively ineffective. Acetazolamide should not be used unless large quantities of sodium bicarbonate are also administered. Failure to do this results in high levels of salicylate in cerebrospinal fluid.

Hill JB: Salicylate intoxication. *N Engl J Med* 1973;**288:**1110.

Snodgrass W et al: Salicylate toxicity following therapeutic doses in young children. *Clin Toxicol* 1981;**18:**247.

SCORPION BITES

Scorpion bites are common in arid areas of the southwestern USA. Scorpion venom is more toxic than most snake venoms, but only minute amounts are injected. Although neurologic manifestations of the bite may last a week, most clinical signs subside within 24–48 hours.

Bites by less toxic scorpion species cause local pain, redness, and swelling. Bites by more toxic species cause tingling or burning paresthesias that begin at the site of the bite and tend to progress up the extremity; other findings include throat spasm, a feeling of a thickening of the tongue, restlessness, muscular fibrillation, abdominal cramps, convulsions, urinary incontinence, and respiratory failure.

Treatment

A specific antiserum for scorpion bites is available from laboratories "MYN," S.A., Av. Coyoacan 1707, Mexico 12, D.F. In addition, calcium gluconate, 10% solution, 5–20 mL intravenously, relieves muscular cramps. Hot compresses of sodium bicarbonate will soothe the bitten area. Sedation and corticosteroids may be indicated.

The prognosis for life is good except in infants and young children.

Bartholomew C: Acute scorpion pancreatitis in Trinidad. *Br Med J* 1970;**1:**666.

Gueron M et al: Cardiovascular manifestations of severe scorpion sting: Clinicopathologic correlations. *Chest* 1970;**57:**156.

Zlotkin E et al: Recent studies on the mode of action of scorpion neurotoxins: A review. *Toxicon* 1969;**7:**217.

SNAKEBITE

Despite the lethal potential of venomous snakes, human morbidity and mortality rates are surprisingly low. The outcome depends on the size of the child, the site of the bite, the degree of envenomation, and the effectiveness of treatment.

Poisonous snakebites are most common and most severe in the early spring. Children in snake-infested areas should wear boots and long trousers, should not walk barefoot, and should be cautioned not to explore under ledges or in holes where a snake might be hiding.

Ninety-eight percent of poisonous snakebites in the USA are caused by pit vipers (rattlesnakes, water moccasins, and copperheads). A few are caused by elapids (coral snakes), and occasional bites occur from cobras and other nonindigenous exotic snakes kept as pets. Snake venom is a complex mixture of enzymes, peptides, and proteins that may have predominantly cytotoxic, neurotoxic, hemotoxic, or cardiotoxic effects but other effects as well. The snake seldom uses all its venom in a single bite. Up to 70% of bites by pit vipers do not result in venom injection.

Pit viper venom is predominantly cytotoxic and hemotoxic, causing a severe local reaction with pain, discoloration, and edema, as well as hemorrhagic effects. Peripheral and central neurologic abnormalities can also occur. Convulsions are common in children.

Swelling and pain occur soon after rattlesnake bite and are a certain indication that envenomation has occurred. During the first few hours, swelling and ecchymosis extend proximally from the bite. The bite is often obvious as a double puncture mark surrounded by ecchymosis. Hematemesis, melena, hemoptysis, and other manifestations of coagulopathy develop in severe cases. Respiratory difficulty and shock are the ultimate causes of death. Even in fatal rattlesnake bite, there is usually a period of 6–8 hours between the bite and death; there is, therefore, usually enough time to start effective treatment.

Coral snake envenomation causes little local pain, swelling, or necrosis, and systemic reactions are often delayed for 10 hours, although children may convulse within 1 hour after being bitten. The early signs of coral snake envenomation include bulbar paralysis, dysphagia, and dysphoria; these may appear in 5–10 hours and may be followed by total peripheral paralysis and death in 24 hours.

Snakebites are an important hazard in many parts of the world; in India there are thought to be over 30,000 deaths per year from cobra bites. The general principles outlined here apply to any bite, but specific therapy will naturally vary between species.

Treatment

The treatment of snakebite envenomation is controversial, but the following approach seems most useful.

A. Emergency (First Aid) Treatment: The most

important first aid measure is reassurance. If possible, clean the wound with a germicidal preparation. Splint the affected extremity and minimize the patient's motion. Tourniquets are of questionable value, and ice packs are contraindicated.

Incision and suction are useful only if done soon after envenomation. Because most bites are into the deep subcutaneous layer or muscle, small skin incisions are not effective. In making an incision, consideration must be given to the danger of damaging underlying tendons, nerves, or vessels. Incision is not effective for coral snake bites.

B. Definitive Medical Management: Blood should be drawn for typing and cross-matching, hematocrit, clotting time and platelet function, and serum electrolyte determinations. Close monitoring of the hematocrit and electrolytes is indicated. The massive destruction of red cells may be associated with hyperkalemia. Establish 2 secure intravenous sites for the administration of antivenin, blood, and other medications.

Specific antivenin is indicated only when signs of severe envenomation are present. Polyvalent pit viper antivenin and coral snake antivenin (Wyeth Laboratories) are widely available from drugstores. Coral snake antivenin can also be obtained on an emergency basis from state epidemiologists and is stockpiled (mainly in the southeastern USA) at over 75 locations, including the Centers for Disease Control, Atlanta, GA 30333 (central telephone number: [404] 329–3311).

After horse serum sensitivity tests (see Chapter 5) are negative, antivenin should be given intravenously and can be given at any desired concentration or rate. Ten to 100 mL may be required. (Antivenin should not be given intramuscularly or subcutaneously, because it is slow-acting, inefficient, and impossible to control if adverse reactions occur. Antivenin injected into the bite site has little effect.) If anaphylaxis occurs despite negative skin tests, it will occur at the onset of treatment. Epinephrine, 0.3 mL of 1:1000 solution, should be drawn up in a syringe before antivenin is administered. Horse serum sensitivity must be reevaluated if another course of antivenin is required over 36 hours after the first. The hemorrhagic tendency, pain, and shock are rapidly diminished by adequate amounts of antivenin.

Codeine, 1–1.5 mg/kg per dose orally, or meperidine (Demerol), 0.6–1.5 mg/kg per dose orally or intramuscularly, is occasionally necessary to control pain during the first 24 hours. Cryotherapy is contraindicated, since it commonly causes tissue damage severe enough to necessitate amputation. Early physiotherapy minimizes contractions. In rare cases, fasciotomy to relieve pressure within muscular compartments is required to save the function of a hand or foot. The evaluation of function as well as of pulses will better predict the need for fasciotomy. Corticosteroids (hydrocortisone, 1–2 g intravenously every 4–6 hours) are useful in the treatment of serum sickness or anaphylactic shock and may be useful treatment by themselves, especially if the patient is already sensitive to antivenin. Ampicillin (200 mg/kg/d orally) is given to treat gram-negative infections that are often associated with snakebite.

A fluid tetanus toxoid booster is adequate if the patient was previously immunized against tetanus. If the patient has not completed the primary series of immunizations, 250 units of tetanus immune globulin (human) should be given intramuscularly. Tetanus antitoxin is not given if tetanus immune globulin is available.

Russell FE: *Snake Venom Poisoning*. Lippincott, 1980.

Russell FE et al: Snake venom poisoning in the United States: Experience with 550 cases. *JAMA* 1975;**233**:841.

SOAPS, HEXACHLOROPHENE, & DETERGENTS

1. SOAPS

Soap is made from salts of fatty acids. Some toilet soap bars contain both soap and detergent. Ingestion of soap bars may cause vomiting and diarrhea, but they have a low toxicity.

Dilute with milk or water. Induced emesis is unnecessary.

2. HEXACHLOROPHENE

Hexachlorophene is an antibacterial agent found in soaps, detergents, creams, etc. It is also dispensed as a solution (pHisoHex). Cleansing of extensive areas of burned or abraded skin with pHisoHex and the application of pHisoHex wet dressings have resulted in a significant degree of absorption, central nervous system irritation, and convulsions. Concentrations in products have been reduced, however, and toxicity is now infrequent. pHisoHex should be thoroughly cleaned off with water or saline to minimize its absorption.

pHisoHex placed in a cup or glass has also been confused with milk of magnesia and formula, resulting in ingestion, absorption of large amounts of the agent, and death. Nausea, vomiting, diarrhea, abdominal cramps, convulsions, dehydration, and shock have occurred following ingestion of pHisoHex.

Induce vomiting and carefully monitor fluid and electrolyte balance. Anticonvulsants, vasoconstrictors, and sedatives may be needed.

Hexachlorophene: Its use in the nursery. *Pediatrics* 1973; **51(Suppl)**:329.

Lockhart JD: How toxic is hexachlorophene? *Pediatrics* 1972; **50**:229.

3. DETERGENTS

Detergents are nonsoap synthetic products used for cleaning purposes because of their surfactant properties. Commercial products include granules, powders, and liquids. Electric dishwasher detergent granules are very alkaline and can cause caustic burns. Low concentrations of bleaching and antibacterial agents as well as enzymes are found in many preparations. These pure compounds are moderately toxic, but the concentration used is too small to significantly alter the product's toxicity, although occasional primary or allergic irritative phenomena have been noted in housewives and in employees manufacturing these products.

There are 3 general types of detergents: cationic, anionic, and nonionic.

Cationic Detergents (Ceepryn, Diaperene, Phemerol, Zephiran)

Nausea, vomiting, collapse, coma, and convulsions may occur. The estimated fatal dose is approximately 1 g of pure product per square meter of body area. Death is most likely in the first 4 hours, as cationic detergents are rapidly inactivated by tissues and ordinary soap.

Induce vomiting and follow with a saline cathartic. Ordinary soap is an effective antidote for unabsorbed cationic detergents. Anticonvulsants may be needed. Analeptics are likely to aggravate seizures and should not be used.

Anionic Detergents

Most common household detergents are anionic—Tide, Cheer, etc. Laundry compounds (All, etc) have water softener (sodium phosphate) added, which acts as a corrosive and may reduce ionized calcium. Anionic detergents irritate the skin by removing natural oils. Although ingestion causes diarrhea, intestinal distention, and vomiting, no fatalities have been reported. The LD50 in animals ranges from 1 to 5 g/kg.

The only treatment usually required is to discontinue use if skin irritation occurs. Induced vomiting is not indicated following ingestion of electric dishwasher detergent, because of its strong alkalinity. Dilute with water or milk. Give 5 mL of 10% calcium gluconate intravenously if the patient has hypocalcemia.

Nonionic Detergents (Brij Products; Tritons X-45, X-100, X-102, & X-144)

These compounds include lauryl, stearyl, and oleyl alcohols and octyl phenol. They have a minimal irritating effect on the skin and are nontoxic when swallowed.

Deichmann WB, Gerarde HW: Hazards of alkaline laundry detergents. *JAMA* 1972;**220:**1014.

Enzyme detergents. (Editorial.) *Br Med J* 1970;**1:**518.

Jeven JE: Severe dermatitis and "biological" detergents. *Br Med J* 1970;**1:**299.

Newhouse ML et al: An epidemiological study of workers producing enzyme washing powders. *Lancet* 1970;**1:**689.

SPIDER BITES

At least 50 species of spiders have been implicated in human spider bites, but most toxic reactions in the USA are caused by the black widow spider *(Latrodectus mactans)* and the North American brown recluse (violin) spider *(Loxosceles reclusus)*. Many spider venoms have common chemical and pharmacologic properties. It is helpful if positive identification of the spider can be made, since many spider bites may mimic those of the brown recluse spider.

Black Widow Spider

The black widow spider, which is endemic to nearly all areas of the USA, causes most of the deaths due to spider bites. The initial bite may be hemorrhagic and associated with a sharp fleeting pain. Local and systemic muscular cramping, abdominal pain, nausea and vomiting, and shock can occur. Convulsions are more commonly seen in small children. Systemic signs of black widow spider bite are often confused with other causes of acute abdomen. Although paresthesias, nervousness, and transient muscle spasms may persist for months in survivors, recovery from the acute phase is generally complete within 3 days.

Antivenin is no longer in general use, because of the self-limiting nature of the injury and the danger of serum sickness with its use. Give 5–20 mL of 10% calcium gluconate intravenously to relieve muscle cramps. Hydrocortisone, 25–100 mg intravenously, or diazepam may be useful. Morphine or barbiturates may occasionally be needed for control of pain or restlessness, but they increase the possibility of respiratory depression.

Local treatment of the bite is not helpful.

Brown Recluse Spider (Violin Spider)

The North American brown recluse spider is most commonly seen in the central and midwestern areas of the USA. Its bite characteristically produces a localized reaction with progressively severe pain within 8 hours. The initial bleb on an erythematous ischemic base is replaced by a black eschar within a week. This eschar separates in 2–5 weeks, leaving a poorly healing ulcer that may result in keloid formation. Systemic signs include cyanosis, morbilliform rash, fever, chills, malaise, weakness, nausea and vomiting, joint pains, hemolytic reactions with hemoglobinuria, jaundice, and delirium. Fatalities are rare. Fatal disseminated intravascular coagulation due to the brown recluse spider has recently been reported.

Hydrocortisone sodium succinate (Solu-Cortef),

1 g/24 h intravenously, is indicated for systemic complications. Hydroxyzine (Atarax, Vistaril), 1 mg/kg/d intramuscularly, is reportedly useful because of its muscle relaxant, antihistaminic, and tranquilizing effects. The advisability of total excision of the lesion at the fascial level to minimize necrosis is debatable.

Arena JM: *Poisoning: Toxicology, Symptoms, Treatments,* 5th ed. Thomas, 1985.

Bolton M: The brown spider bite. *J Kans Med Soc* 1970;**71:**197.

Frazier CA: *Insect Allergy: Allergic and Toxic Reactions to Insects and Other Arthropods.* Warren Green, 1969.

Russell FE, Waldron WG: Spider bites, tick bites. *Calif Med* 1967;**106:**247.

Vorse H: Disseminated intravascular coagulopathy following fatal brown spider bite. *J Pediatr* 1971;**80:**1035.

STRYCHNINE

Strychnine poisoning is characterized by restlessness, apprehension, perceptual difficulties, and simultaneous contraction of all muscles, resulting in opisthotonos, respiratory depression, cyanosis, and a characteristic tetanic contraction of the face (risus sardonicus). The patient is conscious throughout the convulsion and is in great pain. Complete muscle relaxation frequently occurs between convulsions. The onset of symptoms is 10–20 minutes after exposure.

Strychnine can be found in household products such as rodenticides, tonics, and cathartics. It is also occasionally added to hallucinogenic drugs. Deaths have been reported after ingestion of as little as 15 mg.

Treatment

If the patient is seen before the onset of symptoms, activated charcoal should be administered, since it is a very efficient adsorber of strychnine. Vomiting should not be induced, owing to risk of convulsions. Convulsions can be controlled with diazepam (Valium), 0.1–0.3 mg/kg to a maximum of 10 mg. External stimulation should be minimized. Forced acid diuresis has been abandoned because it carries the risk of renal complications. The hyperacute nature of strychnine intoxication makes hemodialysis impractical.

Maron BJ, Krupp JR, Tane B: Strychnine poisoning successfully treated with diazepam. *J Pediatr* 1971;**78:**697.

Teitelbaum DT, Ott JE: Management of strychnine intoxication. *Clin Toxicol* 1970;**3:**267.

THYROID PREPARATIONS (Desiccated Thyroid, Sodium Levothyroxine [Synthroid])

Ingestion of the equivalent of 50–150 g of desiccated thyroid can cause signs of hyperthyroidism, including irritability, mydriasis, hyperpyrexia, tachycardia, and diarrhea. Maximal clinical effect occurs about 9 days after ingestion—several days after the protein-bound iodine level has fallen dramatically.

Induce vomiting. If the patient develops clinical signs of toxicity, chlorpromazine (Thorazine) is useful because of its adrenergic and anticholinergic activity.

Funderburk SJ, Spaulding JS: Sodium levothyroxine (Synthroid) intoxication in a child. *Pediatrics* 1970;**45:**298.

VITAMINS

Accidental ingestion of excessive amounts of vitamins rarely causes significant problems. Occasional cases of hypervitaminosis A and D do occur, however, particularly in patients with poor hepatic or renal function. The fluoride contained in many multivitamin preparations is not a realistic hazard, since a 2- or 3-year-old child could eat 100 tablets, containing 1 mg of sodium fluoride per tablet, without producing serious symptoms. Iron poisoning has been reported with multiple vitamin tablets containing iron.

Armstrong GD: Vitamin ingestions. *National Clearinghouse Poison Control Center Bull 1–6,* April–June, 1972.

Morrice G: Papilledema and hypervitaminosis A. *JAMA* 1970;**213:**1344.

Seelig MS: Vitamin D and cardiovascular, renal, and brain damage in infancy and childhood. *Ann NY Acad Sci* 1969;**147:**539.

WARFARIN

Warfarin is used as a pesticide. It causes hypoprothrombinemia and capillary injury. It is readily absorbed from the gastrointestinal tract but is absorbed poorly through the skin. One to 2 mg/kg/d (or 0.5 kg of rat bait at one ingestion) is required to cause severe toxic effects in humans. Warfarin is more toxic to dogs. A prothrombin time is helpful in establishing the severity of the poisoning. Chloral hydrate potentiates the hypoprothrombinemic effect of warfarin.

Treatment consists of induced vomiting followed by a saline cathartic. If bleeding occurs or the prothrombin is prolonged, give 10–50 mg of vitamin K intravenously.

Filmore SJ, McDevitt M: Effect of coumarin compounds on the fetus. *Ann Intern Med* 1970;**73:**731.

Monro P: Iatrogenic encephalopathy. *Postgrad Med J* 1970;**46:**327.

Sellers EM: Potentiation of warfarin-induced hypoprothrombinemia by chloral hydrate. *N Engl J Med* 1970;**283:**827.

SELECTED REFERENCES

AMA Drug Evaluations, 5th ed. American Medical Association, 1983.

Arena JM, Drew RH: *Poisoning: Toxicology, Symptoms, Treatments,* 5th ed. Thomas, 1985.

Bayer MJ, Rumack BH (editors): *Poisonings and Overdose.* Aspen Systems, 1982.

Bayer MJ, Rumack BH, Wanke L: *Toxicologic Emergencies: A Manual of Diagnosis and Management.* Brady-Prentice Hall, 1983.

Billups NF: *American Drug Index,* 29th ed. Lippincott, 1985.

Browning E: *Toxicity of Industrial Metals,* 2nd ed. Butterworth, 1969.

Browning E: *Toxicity and Metabolism of Industrial Solvents.* Elsevier, 1965.

Childhood poisoning: Prevention and first-aid management. *Br Med J* 1975;**4:**483.

Doull J, Klaassen C, Amdur M (editors): *Cassarett and Doull's Toxicology: The Basic Science of Poisons,* 3rd ed. Macmillan, 1985.

Dreisbach RH: *Handbook of Poisoning: Prevention, Diagnosis, & Treatment,* 12th ed. Lange, 1986.

Gilman AG et al (editors): *Goodman and Gilman's The Pharmacological Basis of Therapeutics,* 7th ed. Macmillan, 1985.

Gosselin RE, Smith RP, Hodge HC: *Clinical Toxicology of Commercial Products,* 5th ed. Williams & Wilkins, 1984.

Hamilton A, Hardy HL: *Industrial Toxicology,* 4th ed. Publishing Sciences Group, Inc., 1982.

Handbook of Nonprescription Drugs, 7th ed. The American Pharmaceutical Association, 1982.

Hayes WJ: *Clinical Handbook on Economic Poisons.* US Department of Health, Education, & Welfare, 1963. [Available through most state health departments.]

Kozma JJ: *Killer Plants: A Poisonous Plant Guide.* Milestone Publishing Co., 1969. [Available from the author: Director, Poison Control Center, Passavant Memorial Area Hospital, Jacksonville, IL 62650.]

Lampe KF, McCann MA: *AMA Handbook of Poisonous and Injurious Plants.* American Medical Association, 1985.

Matthew H, Lawson AA: *Treatment of Common Acute Poisonings,* 3rd ed. Churchill Livingstone, 1975.

Meyler L, Herxheimer A: *Side Effects of Drugs.* Vol. 7. Excerpta Medica, 1972.

Rumack BH (editor): *POISINDEX: An Emergency Poison Management System.* [Published quarterly.] Micromedex, Denver, Colorado.

Rumack BH, Salzman E: *Mushroom Poisoning: Diagnosis and Treatment.* CRC Press, 1978.

Rumack BH, Temple AR: *Management of the Poisoned Patient.* Science Press, 1977.

Samter M, Parker CW: *Hypersensitivity to Drugs.* Vol 1. Pergamon Press, 1972.

Neoplastic Diseases

31

David G. Tubergen, MD

Cancer is the most common cause of death due to disease in children over the age of 1 year. Malignant diseases occur in about 10 per 100,000 children per year and account for about 4000 deaths annually. Leukemias and lymphomas constitute about 40% of pediatric malignant diseases, with the solid tumors, chiefly sarcomas, making up the remaining 60%. The signs and symptoms of pediatric cancer may be subtle. Any mass—solid, cystic, or mixed—should be considered malignant until a definitive histologic diagnosis is established or until specific therapy directed at another cause has resulted in its disappearance within the expected period.

The causes of cancer in children remain elusive. Genetic disorders play an important role in some cases, eg, retinoblastoma and the tumors associated with neurofibromatosis. Chromosomal excess, as in trisomy 21, or chromosomal instability, as in Fanconi's hypoplastic anemia, is associated with an increased incidence of cancer. Somatic growth disturbances, as seen in hemihypertrophy, may be associated with liver, kidney, or adrenal tumors.

A wide variety of immunologic deficiencies have been associated with an increased incidence of many types of cancer. This may reflect a decrease in the host's surveillance mechanism against transformed cells or may result from prolonged exposure to oncogenic agents as a consequence of failure to mount an adequate immune response. Our lack of information regarding the causes of cancer makes prevention virtually impossible and emphasizes the importance of early detection and specific diagnosis followed by aggressive treatment.

Once cancer is suspected or diagnosed, there are several considerations that affect the ultimate outcome. The initial evaluation requires determination of the nature of the malignant tumor and the precise extent of disease. Since many pediatric tumors fit the broad description of "small cell neoplasm," the pathologic material should be examined by pediatric pathologists using special stains, histochemical techniques, and electron microscopy when necessary. Determination of the extent of disease requires a knowledge of potential metastatic sites and selected utilization of many radiographic, isotopic scanning, and ultrasonic techniques as well as biochemical and biopsy procedures. The surgeon must not only have sound judgment and expert technical skills but must also include with the operative notes an accurate description of the extent of tumor involvement and the location and extent of local metastases or extensions. These observations are critical to further therapeutic planning.

Therapy is multidisciplinary and ideally involves a surgeon, a radiation therapist, and a pediatric oncologist before therapy is started. Certainly once the diagnosis has been made, a comprehensive treatment plan must incorporate all 3 major modalities. The significant progress that has been made in the management of several pediatric cancers as a result of aggressive multimodal therapy emphasizes the importance of this approach and the advantage of beginning treatment in a medical center where personnel and facilities are available to implement this concept. The primary physician serves several roles as a member of this team: as the diagnostician best situated to facilitate early detection; as the person administering therapy in the home community; as the physician most likely to observe early complications or toxic reactions; and as counselor to the patients and their families.

The current goal of cancer chemotherapy is to cure the patient. This implies an aggressive approach, as will be evident in the following pages. Chemotherapeutic agents fall into several general classes based on mode of action, and almost all programs utilize combinations of agents of differing actions in an attempt to increase tumor kill. This can only happen, of course, if each agent has some activity against the tumor in question. Ideally, the agents used together should have nonadditive toxicities. In other words, one attempts to use combinations with additive or synergistic antitumor effects and nonadditive toxic effects. In the treatment of solid tumors, the concept of adjunctive chemotherapy is important to achieve better results. In the case of many tumors, microscopic metastases are already present at the time of initial therapy, and local treatment alone will not be curative. Owing to the growth characteristics of small tumor implants and probably because of their relatively better blood supply, these microscopic tumors appear more susceptible to drugs than are clinically obvious metastases. Thus, in beginning chemotherapy, one should reason that metastasis has already occurred, because the potential for cure is greater at this time than if one waits for clinical metastases to appear. In the management of some tumor types, the efficacy of drug therapy against microscopic residual disease lessens the need for extensive local tumor bed irradiation.

Table 31–6 lists the commonly used chemotherapeutic agents, the tumors for which they are used, and the most common toxicities.

LEUKEMIA

1. ACUTE LYMPHOBLASTIC LEUKEMIA

Essentials of Diagnosis

- Pallor, petechiae, purpura, fatigue, fever, bone pain.
- Hepatosplenomegaly, lymphadenopathy.
- Thrombocytopenia, normal or low hemoglobin.
- Diagnosis confirmed by bone marrow examination.

General Considerations

Acute lymphoblastic leukemia (ALL) comprises about 85% of leukemias in childhood. About 12% of cases are acute myeloblastic or monoblastic, and 3% are chronic granulocytic leukemia. Acute stem cell leukemia and acute undifferentiated leukemia are terms used to denote leukemia cells with slightly different morphologic characteristics, but clinically these leukemias behave as acute lymphoblastic leukemia.

The peak incidence of onset of acute lymphoblastic leukemia is at 4 years of age, but the disease may occur at any time during childhood. Before the advent of chemotherapy, this disease was usually fatal within 3–4 months, with virtually no survivors 1 year after diagnosis. Current estimates are that over half of children receiving aggressive combination chemotherapy and early central nervous system treatment may be expected to survive free of disease for 5 years or longer. Not all patients have the same likelihood of achieving long-term remission. Those with the best prognosis are 3–7 years of age with white counts at presentation of less than 10,000/μL. Patients who present with a white blood cell count over 50,000/μL or who are less than 1 year of age have the poorest prognosis. The leukemic cells of approximately 15% of patients have surface characteristics of thymus-dependent lymphocytes. These patients tend to have higher white counts; many of them are adolescents; and mediastinal masses may be present on chest x-ray. This group of patients is less likely to achieve prolonged remission.

Clinical Findings

A. Symptoms and Signs: The variable presenting complaints of children with acute leukemia are referable to organ infiltration and marrow replacement with malignant cells that crowd out normal elements of the marrow. The absence of red cell precursors leads to anemia, which may make the child pale, listless, irritable, and chronically tired. The lack of mature granulocytes makes the child more susceptible to infection, and a history of repeated infections prior to a definitive diagnosis of leukemia is not unusual. The thrombocytopenia predisposes to bleeding episodes: epistaxis, petechiae, hematomas, or life-threatening hemorrhage. Organs may be infiltrated by disease and not function properly; may cause discomfort because of their large size; or may cause symptoms due to pressure on other structures.

Organ infiltration, especially of the kidney, may cause significant dysfunction. This may result in serious uric acid toxicity when therapy is initiated and must be assessed prior to treatment.

B. Laboratory Findings: The white count at presentation is below normal in one-third of patients, normal in another third, and elevated in the remainder. Thrombocytopenia is present in about 85% of patients, and varying degrees of anemia are reported in almost that many. The peripheral blood smear may or may not demonstrate the malignant cells. The diagnosis is established by bone marrow examination, which shows a homogeneous infiltration of blast cells replacing the normal elements. Special stains may be useful in classification of the various types of leukemia, and T and B lymphocyte markers should be sought on the lymphoblasts. Elevated serum lactate dehydrogenase and an elevated sedimentation rate are nonspecific findings. An elevated serum uric acid level requires careful monitoring and treatment (see below).

Diagnostic Workup

A. Complete History and Physical Examination: Important features of the history are a family history of cancer, drugs used, radiation exposure, immunizations, and infectious diseases.

B. Laboratory Studies:

1. Complete blood count, platelet count, reticulocyte count, prothrombin time, and bone marrow aspiration or biopsy (or both). (Bone marrow aspiration is discussed in Chapter 35.)

2. Lumbar puncture with study of a special Wright-stained smear of the sediment for blast cells; sugar and protein determinations.

3. Blood urea nitrogen and serum levels of creatinine, uric acid, bilirubin, AST (SGOT), alkaline phosphatase, proteins, sodium, potassium, lactate dehydrogenase, and immunoglobulins.

4. Urinalysis.

5. Cultures and smears of mouth, throat, blood, bone marrow, skin lesions, urine, cerebrospinal fluid, and stool should be taken immediately if infection is suspected (see also Chapter 35). Fungal and viral cultures and serologic tests should also be done when needed.

6. PPD intermediate-strength skin test and endemic fungal skin tests.

C. X-Ray Studies: A chest x-ray should be obtained to look for mediastinal enlargement.

D. Psychosocial Evaluation: An inventory of the patient's and family's strengths, coping abilities, and economic status helps in anticipating problems.

Differential Diagnosis

Early in the course of the disease, leukemia may produce signs and symptoms similar to those of rheumatic fever, rheumatoid arthritis, viral diseases such as infectious mononucleosis or hepatitis, or other neoplastic diseases such as neuroblastoma or histiocytosis X. The peripheral blood picture may be indistinguishable from that of aplastic anemia.

Specific Treatment

The goal of therapy is to eradicate disease or, at a minimum, to produce a prolonged period free of disease. Therapy can be divided into (1) sytemic therapy, consisting of induction and maintenance phases, and (2) treatment of the central nervous system.

A. Systemic Therapy: The theoretic objective of antileukemic therapy is elimination of lymphoblasts from the body. A child weighing 20–30 kg may present with a tumor weighing approximately 1 kg, which represents about 10^{12} cells. Current techniques do not permit detection of disease when cell numbers are 10^9 or fewer, so it is impossible to determine whether the objective is being approached.

Induction therapy is designed to achieve a complete remission, ie, absence of detectable tumor tissue and presence of normal bone marrow and peripheral blood counts. This generally requires 3–6 weeks of therapy and can be achieved in 95% of patients. The drugs most commonly used are vincristine, 1.5 mg/m^2 intravenously once a week, and a corticosteroid given daily, usually prednisone, 40 mg/m^2 orally in 3 divided doses, or, less commonly, dexamethasone, 6 mg/m^2 orally in 3 divided doses. Asparaginase in doses of 6000 units/m^2 intramuscularly given 3 days a week for 9 doses has been included in several large studies. Once remission has been achieved, some programs call for 2–3 weeks of more intensive chemotherapy with other agents in an attempt to further reduce the tumor burden. This has been called the consolidation phase.

Maintenance therapy is designed to prevent reappearance of the disease while further reducing the number of leukemic cells. Current information indicates that therapy should be continued for at least 2½ years, but the optimal duration has not yet been established. The most common maintenance programs are with mercaptopurine, 75 mg/m^2 orally daily, plus methotrexate, 20 mg/m^2 orally once a week. Other agents may be added at periodic intervals. Some programs add periodic (1–3 months) "mini-inductions" with vincristine and 5–14 days of a corticosteroid to attempt to eliminate cells that develop resistance to the other agents.

Alternative maintenance programs using agents such as doxorubicin (Adriamycin) or intravenous methotrexate (Mexate) on an intermittent, intensive basis have had about the same effect as other agents given on a continuous basis.

In any treatment program, the dosages of drugs must be carefully adjusted to the patient's tolerance. The goals are to give the maximum tolerated amounts of drugs while preventing unacceptable toxicities or the hazards of severe marrow depression, particularly infections associated with profound neutropenia. This generally means maintaining the white count between 2000 and 3000/μL and the absolute neutrophil count above 1000/μL.

B. Therapy for Central Nervous System Leukemia: In the absence of specific therapy directed at leukemic cells within the central nervous system, as many as 50% of children with acute lymphoblastic leukemia may develop clinical central nervous system involvement. The symptoms are most commonly headache, stiff neck, vomiting, and lethargy and may include cranial nerve palsies, hyperphagia and rapid weight gain, polydipsia, and polyuria. Physical examination may show papilledema; in younger children, a skull x-ray may reveal spread cranial sutures. The diagnosis is established by Wright-stained cytocentrifuge preparations of spinal fluid, which demonstrate the presence of lymphoblasts. Occasional patients will have definite symptoms of central nervous system leukemia without detectable lymphoblasts in the cerebrospinal fluid; in others, unequivocal lymphoblasts will be present in the absence of any associated symptoms.

Central nervous system leukemia appears to originate from leukemia cells that gain access to the central nervous system early in the course of the disease. Many of the antileukemic drugs do not penetrate the blood-brain barrier in adequate concentrations, and the cells can proliferate in the central nervous system while the disease is being controlled systemically.

Overt central nervous system leukemia can be prevented by "prophylactic" treatment. This can be accomplished by the use of cranial irradiation, 1800 rads, with cobalt or the linear accelerator, plus intrathecal methotrexate, 12 mg/m^2 dissolved in 3–5 mL of preservative-free saline solution or sterile water and given 3–6 times concomitantly with the irradiation (maximum single dose of intrathecal methotrexate is 12 mg). The amount of spinal fluid withdrawn should equal the volume injected. Such treatment will reduce the incidence of overt central nervous system symptoms from as high as 50% to 5–10%. It does, of course, expose a significant number of children who would not develop central nervous system disease to irradiation. In children with a relatively low risk for developing central nervous system leukemia, current data show that disease can be prevented by use of intrathecal methotrexate alone.

If overt central nervous system disease develops, the use of intrathecal methotrexate given twice weekly for 4–6 doses will usually relieve the symptoms and clear the spinal fluid of lymphoblasts. However, the disease tends to recur within a few months, and total eradication is rarely achieved. Cytarabine may also be used intrathecally, and a repeated course of irradiation may be used to control the debilitating symptoms. Oral corticosteroids may also offer some temporary relief. If central nervous system disease develops, a bone marrow examination is needed because systemic relapse may also be present.

The best means of achieving long-term survival is by prolongation of the first remission. If bone marrow relapse occurs, second and third remissions are obtainable in 40–70% of children using vincristine and corticosteroids. Maintenance programs may then employ combinations of drugs such as cytarabine, cyclophosphamide, daunorubicin, doxorubicin, asparaginase, or newer experimental agents.

Supportive & Adjunctive Treatment

A. Massive Tumor Tissue: Uric acid nephropathy, which can be fatal, can occur during initial therapy in the presence of leukemic leukocytosis, massive hepatosplenomegaly, mediastinal mass, or compromised renal function due to infiltrates. In some patients, hyperuricemia is present prior to therapy. Prevention of uric acid nephropathy depends upon decreasing uric acid production by the use of a xanthine oxidase inhibitor, increasing uric acid solubility in urine by keeping the urine pH above 6.5, and ensuring a large urine volume. These measures are important for the first 3–7 days of therapy.

Hyperphosphatemia and hypocalcemia may occur with rapid tumor destruction. On occasion, the patient will be symptomatic and require temporary calcium supplementation. Specific measures of treatment are as follows:

1. Give allopurinol, 100 mg/m^2 orally 3 times a day. This should be started 24 hours before beginning specific antileukemic therapy.
2. Provide fluids, 2–3 L/m^2 daily orally or intravenously. Avoid potassium-containing parenteral solutions during the stage of tumor catabolism.
3. Maintain a careful record of fluid intake and urinary output.
4. Alkalinize the urine with intravenous sodium bicarbonate, 50–75 meq/L intravenously. Measure urine pH of each voiding to ensure adequate alkalinization. Increase the dose, if necessary, to maintain the urine pH at 7.0–7.4.
5. Perform a daily urinalysis and measure blood urea nitrogen and serum uric acid, potassium, calcium, and phosphorus daily for 3 days or until normal levels are reported.
6. Give a regular diet for age, with no added salt.

B. Hepatic Dysfunction: When there is evidence of hepatic dysfunction as manifested by elevated enzymes or bilirubin or prolonged prothrombin time, vincristine toxicity is likely, since vincristine is excreted by the liver. Subsequent doses of vincristine may need to be reduced if toxicity is moderate to severe.

C. Infection: Cultures of blood and bone marrow and smears and cultures of pharyngeal, nasopharyngeal (if no bleeding), rectal, and urine specimens should be taken on admission and repeated as necessary. Gram-stained smears of infected lesions and body orifices should be examined immediately. Full doses of appropriate bactericidal antibiotics should be used as soon as infection is suspected. If paronychia or other skin infections occur, 0.3 mL of saline solution should be injected and aspirated for smear and culture. Do not wait for "pointing." Urinary tract infections may exist without pyuria in the granulocytopenic child. Do not delay antibiotic chemotherapy. Suspect *Escherichia coli, Klebsiella-Enterobacter,* or staphylococcal infection if the child has been receiving penicillin. Therapy should be initiated with broad-spectrum combinations such as carbenicillin plus gentamicin or carbenicillin plus cephalothin. Tobramycin may also be useful. Therapy should be given intravenously. Prolonged antibiotic therapy should be avoided.

The organisms responsible for infections in leukemic children are almost always their own skin or enteric organisms. This has 2 important implications: "Reverse" precautions are unlikely to reduce the incidence of infections beyond that obtained by good hand washing (and this tends to make good medical and nursing care more difficult to provide), and prolonged use of antibiotics may modify the gut flora and select for increasingly resistant organisms.

In the severely neutropenic child with sepsis, transfusions of granulocytes may be extremely useful. Once started, they should be used for at least 4–6 days or until the patient's own neutrophils appear in the blood in adequate numbers.

Pneumocystis carinii pneumonia may be treated with trimethoprim-sulfamethoxazole (Bactrim, Septra) orally. Recent evidence indicates that *Pneumocystis* infection may be prevented in susceptible patients by daily low-dosage trimethoprim therapy. Fungal infections require prolonged treatment with amphotericin B given intravenously.

The classic symptoms of infection may be masked by immunosuppressive chemotherapy. Children may have life-threatening infections with rubeola and varicella. Parents, teachers, and school nurses need to be educated regarding notification of the physician when the child shows symptoms of infection or has been exposed to contagious diseases. Varicella-zoster immune globulin or convalescent plasma given within 48 hours of exposure may prevent or modify varicella. No live virus vaccines should be given to leukemic children or those receiving immunosuppressive therapy.

D. Thrombocytopenia and Anemia: The patient with thrombocytopenia is at risk of bleeding. Platelet transfusions should be given for episodes involving difficult to control epistaxis, gastrointestinal bleeding, or signs and symptoms of central nervous system hemorrhage (retinal hemorrhage is an important finding). Prophylactic platelet transfusion is usually not indicated in thrombocytopenic patients who are not bleeding, although some clinicians give platelets prior to lumbar puncture. Because patients with fever and infection tend to have more frequent serious bleeding episodes, prophylactic platelet transfusions may be indicated.

Anemia is present in more than two-thirds of patients at the time of diagnosis. Even with successful induction therapy, it takes 2–3 weeks before adequate numbers of erythrocytes can be produced, and red cell transfusion is often needed. An attempt is made to maintain the hemoglobin concentration at greater than 10 g/dL by the use of packed red blood cell transfusions. Each transfusion is limited to 8–10 mL/kg, and in thrombocytopenic patients the transfusions are given over 3–4 hours to prevent rapid expansion of the vascular space that might precipitate hemorrhage.

E. Additional Precautions:

1. A "no salt added" diet is prescribed when the patient is taking corticosteroids.

2. Avoid deep venipunctures, intramuscular injections, and instrumentation with catheters, laryngoscopes, etc, in children with bleeding tendencies. Avoid tight clothing.

3. Avoid administration of barium sulfate during vincristine therapy, and give the child fruit, fruit juice, and plenty of liquids to help prevent constipation due to vincristine. Stool softeners may be indicated.

4. For nausea and vomiting, give antiemetics orally (or as suppositories) and fluids if needed.

5. Good nutrition and well-balanced meals are essential. Providing extra fluids on the day before and the day of cyclophosphamide therapy helps decrease bladder toxicity.

F. Psychologic Support of Patient and Family: The emotional impact of the diagnosis of leukemia is usually overwhelming and affects the entire family. A thorough discussion with the parents regarding diagnosis, prognosis, therapy, toxic reactions to drugs, and their own role in the care of the child is mandatory initially and throughout the course of the disease. Psychologic problems are common in the patient's siblings, and anticipatory guidance is needed.

What to tell the patient depends upon the maturity of the child and the judgment of physicians and family about the problems at hand. The author recommends frank discussion of the disease with the adolescent patient. The discussion should be factual and honest, emphasizing the hopeful aspects and offering reassurance that progress is being made.

Psychologic guidance may be needed for siblings, parents, and patient, and appropriate professional consultation should be obtained.

Prognosis

Centers are now reporting greater than 50% projected 5-year survival rates with various programs that have in common aggressive combination chemotherapy, treatment for occult central nervous system disease, and the use of intensive supportive therapy as needed. It is likely that we will now begin to see significant numbers of long-term survivors. The word "cure" as applied to leukemia is difficult to define but is undoubtedly a reality for some patients.

See references below.

2. ACUTE NONLYMPHOCYTIC LEUKEMIA

The acute nonlymphocytic leukemias include acute myeloblastic leukemia, acute monoblastic leukemia, and leukemias whose morphologic features suggest both cell lines, the myelomonocytic leukemias.

The clinical features are similar to those of acute lymphoblastic leukemia, and the supportive care is basically the same. Therapy is more difficult, with different drugs, and produces remission rates of about 70% and a median duration of remission of about 12 months. Bone marrow transplantation done after the patient is in remission offers a 40–50% opportunity for long-term remission and is the best treatment currently available.

See references below.

3. CHRONIC MYELOCYTIC LEUKEMIA

Chronic myelocytic leukemia (CML) of the adult form that demonstrates the Philadelphia (Ph) chromosome is treated with busulfan (Myleran), beginning with 5–8 mg/m^2/d orally and reducing the dosage to 2–4 mg/d when the white count reaches 15,000/μL. The white count should remain between 5000 and 10,000/μL, and the dosage is adjusted as necessary to achieve this response.

The juvenile non-Philadelphia chromosome (Ph-negative) form of chronic myelocytic leukemia is seen in younger children. Bleeding secondary to thrombocytopenia, organomegaly, and repeated infections makes this form of disease difficult to control clinically. Attempts at various forms of chemotherapy have not been successful. Transient relief of pressure symptoms has been accomplished by splenic irradiation with ^{60}Co. Splenectomy has resulted in longer survival times in a few patients.

Bleyer WA et al: Reduction in central nervous system leukemia with a pharmacokinetically derived intrathecal methotrexate dosage regimen. *J Clin Oncol* 1983;**1:**317.

Grier HE, Weinstein HJ: Acute nonlymphocytic leukemia. *Pediatr Clin North Am* 1985:**32:**653.

Lampkin BC et al: Current status of the biology and treatment of acute non-lymphocytic leukemia in children. *Blood* 1983;**61:**215.

Miller DR et al: Prognostic factors and therapy in acute lymphoblastic leukemia of childhood. *Cancer* 1983;**51:**1041.

Pizzo PA: Infectious complications in the child with cancer. (2 parts.) *J Pediatr* 1981;**98:**341, 513.

Poplack D: Acute lymphoblastic leukemia in childhood. *Pediatr Clin North Am* 1985;**32:**669.

Sallan SE, Weinstein HJ, Nathan DG: The childhood leukemias. *J Pediatr* 1981;**99:**676.

Smithson WA et al: Childhood acute lymphocytic leukemia. *CA* 1980;**80:**158.

Thomas DE et al: Marrow transplantation for malignant diseases. *J Clin Oncol* 1983;**1:**517.

LYMPHOMAS

1. HODGKIN'S DISEASE

Essentials of Diagnosis

- Lymphadenopathy.
- Hepatomegaly with or without splenomegaly.
- Fever, night sweats, fatigue, weight loss, generalized pruritus.

General Considerations

The clinical course of Hodgkin's disease has been favorably altered by advances in diagnostic techniques that have improved our understanding of the disease and by the application of combined modality therapy. Optimal results depend on precise definition of the extent of disease and selection of therapy based on these results.

The histologic classification currently used is shown in Table 31–1. Nodular sclerosing Hodgkin's disease is the type most commonly seen in the second decade. Hodgkin's disease is less frequent in the first decade but has occurred in children as young as 3 years. The mixed cellularity type is more common in younger children. The response to therapy is nearly equal in these 2 types. Lymphocyte-depleted Hodgkin's disease is less common and is much less responsive to therapy.

Table 31–1. Histologic classification of Hodgkin's disease.

Designation	Distinctive Features	Relative Frequency
Lymphocyte predominance	Abundant stroma of mature lymphocytes, histiocytes, or both; no necrosis; Reed-Sternberg cells may be sparse.	10–15%
Nodular sclerosis	Nodules of lymphoid tissue partially or completely separated by bands of doubly refractile collagen of variable width; atypical Reed-Sternberg cells in clear spaces ("lacunae") in the lymphoid nodules.	20–50%
Mixed cellularity	Usually numerous Reed-Sternberg and atypical mononuclear cells with a pleomorphic admixture of plasma cells, eosinophils, lymphocytes, and fibroblasts; foci of necrosis commonly seen.	20–40%
Lymphocyte depletion	Reed-Sternberg and malignant mononuclear cells usually, though not always, numerous; marked paucity of lymphocytes; diffuse fibrosis and necrosis may be present.	5–15%

Clinical and pathologic staging of the disease is carried out according to the Ann Arbor classification (Table 31–2). The subclassification of (A) absence or (B) presence of systemic symptoms (fever, night sweats, or loss of over 10% of body weight) is also of prognostic value. For a given stage, treatment may be more aggressive in the presence of systemic symptoms.

Clinical Findings

A. Symptoms and Signs: The most common presentation of Hodgkin's disease is painless enlargement of lymph nodes. The most common sites of involvement are the cervical node areas. The involved nodes are firm or rubbery, often matted together and nontender to palpation. They may cause symptoms by compressing other structures, such as a chronic cough due to tracheal compression from a large mediastinal mass. Extranodal disease may occur in any organ. Symptoms may be absent but may include anorexia, fatigue, weight loss, night sweats, and pain upon ingesting alcohol. Generalized pruritus may occur.

B. Laboratory Findings: Hematologic findings are often normal but may include anemia, elevated or depressed leukocytes and platelets, and, sometimes, modest eosinophilia. The sedimentation rate and the serum copper level may be elevated. With hepatic involvement, the serum alkaline phosphatase, AST (SGOT), and ALT (SGPT) may be elevated. Many patients have tumors that take up gallium, and in these patients the gallium scan may help identify areas of involvement. Gallium scanning does not differentiate between Hodgkin's disease and inflammatory tissue, and its usefulness is limited in the subdiaphragmatic area.

Immunologic abnormalities may occur, primarily in the cell-mediated system, with anergy to the common delayed hypersensitivity antigens. Coombs-posi-

Table 31–2. Staging classification for Hodgkin's disease. (Ann Arbor classification.)

Stage I	Involvement of a single lymph node region (I) or a single extralymphatic organ or site (I_E).
Stage II	Involvement of 2 or more lymph node regions on the same side of the diaphragm (II) or localized involvement of an extralymphatic organ or site (II_E).
Stage III	Involvement of lymph node regions on both sides of the diaphragm (III) or localized involvement of an extralymphatic organ or site (III_E) or spleen (III_{SE}).
Stage IV	Diffuse or disseminated involvement of one or more extralymphatic organs with or without associated lymph node involvement. The organs involved should be identified by a symbol.
	A = Asymptomatic. B = Fever, sweats, weight loss > 10% of body weight.

tive hemolytic anemia and abnormal immunoglobulin levels have also been described.

The diagnosis is established by histologic examination of an excised lymph node or other involved tissue. After the diagnosis is made, bone marrow biopsy and radiologic examinations, including lymphangiography, are done. This is followed in almost all cases by pathologic staging, involving laparotomy with multiple abdominal lymph node biopsies, liver biopsy, wedge bone marrow biopsy, and splenectomy and may include moving the ovaries laterally to remove them from the contemplated radiation field.

C. X-Ray Findings: Chest x-ray may show parenchymal or mediastinal nodal disease. Skeletal survey may show bone involvement. CT scanning and ultrasonography may help identify abdominal and pelvic disease. Lymphangiography may reveal "foamy" filling defects in an enlarged node, which implies tumor involving the node. Allergy to iodides and severe pulmonary disease are contraindications to lymphangiography.

Complications

Patients with Hodgkin's disease have an increased susceptibility to herpes zoster and fungal infections. Therapy may induce acute toxicities that include nausea, vomiting, anorexia, alopecia, bone marrow suppression, and radiation pneumonitis. The patient must be carefully monitored so that necessary adjustments can be made in treatment. Chronic toxic effects of therapy include retardation of bone growth and an increased incidence of second malignant tumors. The splenectomy that is done as part of pathologic staging is associated with an increased incidence of sepsis, most commonly pneumococcal, which can occur days to years after the splenectomy. These septic episodes have a high mortality rate. All such splenectomized patients should be given prophylactic antibiotics to prevent sepsis and should receive pneumococcal vaccine.

A fatal complication that may develop in up to 4% of Hodgkin's disease patients is acute myelogenous leukemia. It appears to be treatment-related in that it occurs with greater frequency in patients treated with both intensive radiation therapy and chemotherapy. This occurrence emphasizes the need to refine therapy to the minimum consistent with disease eradication, so as to minimize exposure to treatment that is itself carcinogenic.

The psychologic effects of this disease and its treatment in the adolescent age group require good rapport between the patient, the family, the school, and the physician.

Treatment

Following establishment of the patient's stage of disease, therapy is planned by the chemotherapist and radiation therapist. Optimum results will be obtained by a radiation therapist skilled in the treatment of growing children by means of megavoltage irradiation. Combination chemotherapy is vastly superior to single agent therapy. Several combinations have been used effectively, including mechlorethamine, vincristine (Oncovin), procarbazine, and prednisone (MOPP); cyclophosphamide, vincristine (Oncovin), procarbazine, and prednisone (COPP); and lomustine (CCNU), vinblastine, procarbazine, and prednisone. Programs using doxorubicin (Adriamycin), bleomycin, vinblastine, and dacarbazine (ABVD) also are effective. The dosage, frequency of administration, and duration of therapy depend upon the patient's tolerance to therapy and the stage of disease.

In general, for stage IA or IIA disease, treatment may consist of extended field irradiation alone or may employ irradiation only of clinically involved areas, with or without chemotherapy. When chemotherapy is used, doses of radiation therapy can be reduced. In stage IB or IIB, extended field irradiation is followed by 6 months of chemotherapy. In stage IIIA disease, therapy is initiated with 3 cycles of chemotherapy and the patient then receives total nodal irradiation. Following hematologic recovery, chemotherapy is resumed for a total of 9 courses.

Stage IIIB or stage IV disease is treated with chemotherapy plus irradiation to areas of bulky disease. If the liver or lungs are involved, these organs are also irradiated as tolerated.

The goal of therapy is to eradicate malignant tissue. Recurrences in nonirradiated areas may require further irradiation. The various chemotherapy programs are not cross-resistant, and second prolonged remissions often can be obtained.

Prognosis

The 5-year survival rate of pathologically staged and aggressively treated patients with stage IA and IIA disease is about 90%. Most of these will be without relapse, and a high proportion are curable. In more advanced stage IIIA disease, the 5-year survival rate is about 70%, and even in stage IV disease, survival of more than 2 years with no evidence of disease can be achieved in a majority of cases.

Gilchrist GS, Evans RG: Contemporary issues in pediatric Hodgkin's disease. *Pediatr Clin North Am* 1985;**32:**721.

Kaplan H: *Hodgkin's Disease*, 2nd ed. Harvard Univ Press, 1980.

Lacher MJ: Hodgkin's disease: Historical perspective, current status, and future directions. *CA* 1985;**35:**88.

Lange B, Littman P: Management of Hodgkin's disease in children and adolescents. *Cancer* 1983;**51:**1371.

Tan C et al: Hodgkin's disease in children: Results of management between 1970–1981. *Cancer* 1983;**51:**1720.

2. NON-HODGKIN'S LYMPHOMA

The non-Hodgkin's lymphomas form a relatively diverse group of cancers of the lymphoid organs. Recent advances in our understanding of normal lymphocyte subpopulations have enabled investigators to clarify the origin of these cancers. Lymphoma cells may carry the membrane markers of T (thymus-dependent) lymphocytes, the surface markers of immunoglobulin-producing B lymphocytes, or no distinctive markers (null cells). Many classification systems have been used for the lymphomas, resulting in confusing terminology. For pediatric lymphomas, it appears sufficient to consider 2 major histologic categories: lymphoblastic lymphoma and nonlymphoblastic lymphoma. The latter category includes Burkitt's lymphoma and pleomorphic lymphoma. This simple classification system as applied by expert pathologists has been found to be very useful in planning therapy.

The lymphoblastic histologic type of lymphoma is often associated with T cell surface markers. Patients with this disease often have a mediastinal mass, and the disease tends to involve bone marrow and the central nervous system early. This disease appears very closely related to, if not identical with, T cell leukemia.

Burkitt's lymphoma is a lymphoma involving the B lymphocyte line. It is responsible for over half the pediatric cancer deaths in Uganda and Central Africa, and in that area the Epstein-Barr virus appears to play an important role in tumor development. Its prevalence is much lower in the USA, where it tends to present with primary abdominal involvement and an extremely aggressive pattern of spread to viscera, marrow, and bones.

Clinical Findings

A. Symptoms and Signs: The non-Hodgkin's lymphomas in general are more common in boys than in girls, and the single most common site of origin is in the lymphoid structures of the intestinal tract, usually in the ileocecal area. The most common presentation in these children is with symptoms of an acute surgical abdomen. Disease originating elsewhere generally presents as nontender lymph node involvement, which may produce symptoms due to compression. Central nervous system involvement consists of symptoms due to cord compression or increased intracranial pressure.

B. Laboratory Findings: The evaluation is similar to that used in patients with Hodgkin's disease except that routine laparotomy and splenectomy are not done. Owing to the frequency of central nervous system involvement, lumbar puncture with careful cytologic examination of the fluid needs to be done on all patients. Clinical staging permits determination of whether disease is localized, involving a single or 2 contiguous nodal areas, or nonlocalized, with either widespread nodal involvement or extranodal involvement (eg, in bone marrow or the central nervous system).

Treatment

The lymphomas are sensitive to both chemotherapy and irradiation. A number of combination chemotherapy programs are effective in producing clinical remissions. The most commonly used agents are vincristine, prednisone, cyclophosphamide, asparaginase, methotrexate, and doxorubicin in varying doses, combinations, and sequences. Radiation therapy has generally been recommended for areas of bulky disease, although recent studies suggest that with the more effective chemotherapy programs, irradiation may not be necessary. Burkitt's lymphoma and lymphomas with a mediastinal primary site have a high incidence of involvement of the central nervous system, and presymptomatic treatment of the central nervous system with irradiation or intrathecal methotrexate (or both) is therefore recommended. Maintenance chemotherapy with multiple agents is continued for 6 months to 2 years depending on the stage of disease and the particular program being followed. Relapses in early-stage disease are very uncommon after 1 year from diagnosis; in all stages, relapses are rare after 2 years of complete remission.

Prognosis

The prognosis for children with non-Hodgkin's lymphoma has improved dramatically in the past decade. Early-stage disease (isolated intestinal involvement or single lymph node involvement other than in the mediastinum) is curable in about 90% of patients. For all patients with non-Hodgkin's lymphoma, the 2-year survival rate is about 70%. Treatment failures are often related to relapses in the bone marrow or central nervous system. Because of rapid developments in treatment for children and the importance of careful histologic evaluation in determining optimum therapy, these patients must be treated at a major pediatric cancer center.

Anderson JR et al: Childhood non-Hodgkin's lymphoma: The results of a randomized therapeutic trial comparing a 4-drug regimen (COMP) with a 10-drug regimen (LSA_2–L_2). *N Engl J Med* 1983;**308**:559.

Graham-Pole J: *Non-Hodgkin's Lymphomas in Children.* Masson, 1980.

Link MP: Non-Hodgkin's lymphoma in children. *Pediatr Clin North Am* 1985;**32**:699.

Sullivan MP et al: Pediatric oncology group experience with modified LSA_2–L_2 therapy in 107 children with non-Hodgkin's lymphoma (Burkitt's lymphoma excluded). *Cancer* 1985;**55**:323.

Wilson JF et al: Studies on the pathology of non-Hodgkin's lymphoma of childhood: 1. The role of routine histopathology as a prognostic factor: A report from the Children's Cancer Study Group. *Cancer* 1984;**53**:1695.

NEUROBLASTOMA

Essentials of Diagnosis

- Asymptomatic abdominal mass, subcutaneous nodules, posterior mediastinal mass, and organomegaly.
- Fever, anemia, weakness, "black eyes," proptosis, opsoclonus, diarrhea, and hypertension.
- Bone pain, paraplegia, and ataxia.

General Considerations

Neuroblastoma is a tumor arising from cells in the sympathetic ganglia and adrenal medulla. It is the third most frequent pediatric neoplasm. Clinically, the survival rates are much better in children under 2 years of age, in children with extra-adrenal tumor, and in those with localized disease. These tumors may spontaneously regress in 5–10% of cases. In routine autopsies of infants under 3 months of age dying of other causes, neuroblastoma in situ in the adrenal is seen 40 times more frequently than expected, suggesting a high rate of spontaneous regression or differentiation.

Immunologic factors may be very significant in understanding the biology of neuroblastoma. Many tumors show infiltration with lymphocytes and plasma cells. The colony inhibition test (Hellström) has shown the lymphocytes of neuroblastoma patients, and in some cases of their mothers as well, to react against neuroblastoma cells in tissue culture.

Clinical staging of extent of disease is the basis of therapeutic planning. The system developed by Evans is shown in Table 31–3.

Clinical Findings

A. Symptoms and Signs: The child most commonly presents at about age 2 with a palpable abdominal mass, although the tumor may present at any time from neonatal life to adolescence. Symptoms depend upon the extent of disease at the time of diagnosis. Bone pain, weight loss, and fever may be the presenting complaints. Newborn infants may present with subcutaneous nodules and adrenal masses with marrow involvement. Early diagnosis depends on keeping the disease in mind so that obscure presentations will not be missed.

B. Laboratory Findings: Anemia and thrombocytopenia may be present secondary to marrow replacement by neuroblasts that may mimic leukemia.

Table 31–3. Clinical staging of neuroblastoma (Evans).

Stage I	Tumors confined to the organ or structure of origin.
Stage II	Tumors extending in continuity beyond the organ or structure of origin but not crossing the midline. Regional lymph nodes on the ipsilateral side may be involved.
Stage III	Tumor extending in continuity beyond the midline. Regional lymph nodes bilaterally may be involved.
Stage IV	Remote disease involving skeleton, parenchymatous organs, soft tissues, or distant lymph node groups. (See IV-S.)
Stage IV-S	Tumors which would be stage I or II except for the presence of remote disease confined to one or more of the following sites: liver, skin, and bone marrow (without radiographic evidence of bone metastases on complete skeletal survey).

The urinary excretion of catecholamines is elevated in the majority of patients. A 24-hour urine collection for vanilmandelic acid (VMA) and homovanillic acid (HVA) should be done preoperatively. This test is useful in following the patient if levels are elevated initially. If the vanilmandelic acid levels increase during follow-up, recurrence may be suspected and re-evaluation is advised. Urinary cystathionine is increased in 50% of children with neuroblastoma; it is independent of vanilmandelic acid excretion and may offer additional diagnostic help if vanilmandelic acid levels are normal.

Measurement of other urinary catecholamines is sometimes useful.

C. X-Ray Findings: Chest x-ray, skeletal survey, and intravenous urography aid in preoperative staging of the disease. Angiography may aid the surgeon in identifying the extent of the tumor and its blood supply; the tumor may be extremely vascular. Bone scanning may detect skeletal metastases before gross lesions on x-rays can be observed.

Treatment & Prognosis

Therapy involves the combined use of surgery, irradiation, and chemotherapy. Initial surgical efforts are directed at removal of as much of the primary tumor as possible. The massive size of some tumors precludes a vigorous surgical approach, and only a biopsy may be advisable. Following irradiation and chemotherapy, a second surgical procedure may permit more definitive removal. Chemotherapy with drugs such as vincristine, cyclophosphamide, doxorubicin, and dacarbazine produces remissions in about 80% of patients.

Infants under 1 year of age with stage IV-S disease have a generally good prognosis, with 80% or more 2-year disease-free survival. These infants may need little if any therapy of any kind to effect a cure.

Approximately two-thirds of children with neuroblastoma after age 2 years have widely disseminated disease at the time of diagnosis. Death due to the tumor occurs in over 80%, although chemotherapy may provide remissions. In children under age 2, the prognosis is significantly better.

Evans AE (editor): *Advances in Neuroblastoma Research.* Vol 12 in: *Progress in Cancer Research and Therapy.* Raven Press, 1980.

Lopez-Ibor B, Schwartz AD: Neuroblastoma. *Pediatr Clin North Am* 1985;**32:**755.

Pochedly C (editor): *Neuroblastoma: Clinical and Biological Manifestations.* Elsevier, 1982.

Rosen EM et al: Neuroblastoma: The Joint Center for Radiation Therapy/Dana-Farber Cancer Institute/Children's Hospital experience. *J Clin Oncol* 1984:**2:**719.

WILMS' TUMOR

Essentials of Diagnosis

- Asymptomatic abdominal mass or abdominal pain.

- Hematuria, genitourinary anomalies, aniridia.
- Hypertension, fever.

General Considerations

Wilms' tumor follows neuroblastoma in frequency of occurrence of pediatric solid tumors. It is believed to be embryonal in origin, develops within the kidney parenchyma, and enlarges with distortion and invasion of the adjacent renal tissue. This tumor may be associated with congenital anomalies, and patients should be evaluated for Wilms' tumor if the following entities occur: hemihypertrophy, aniridia, ambiguous genitalia, hypospadias, undescended testes, duplications of the ureters or kidneys, horseshoe kidney, or Beckwith's syndrome.

Wilms' tumor more commonly presents as an abdominal mass—in contrast to renal tumors in adults, which usually present with hematuria. The incidence of bilateral Wilms' tumor is 5–10%. Metastatic disease in liver, lungs, bone, or (rarely) brain is present in about 11% of patients at the time of diagnosis.

The prognosis in Wilms' tumor is dependent upon 2 major criteria: the clinical grouping, which is a reflection of the extent of disease at the time of diagnosis; and the histologic features of the lesion. The clinical grouping as defined by the National Wilms' Tumor Studies extends from those lesions entirely confined to the kidney and totally resected through varying degrees of extension and finally hematogenous dissemination to such organs as lung, liver, bone, and brain. Beckwith and Palmer have identified 2 histologic variants of Wilms' tumor—the anaplastic and sarcomatous varieties—which in a large series comprised only 11.5% of the cases but accounted for over 50% of the deaths due to Wilms' tumor.

Clinical Findings

A. Symptoms and Signs: Children with Wilms' tumor may be asymptomatic, and a mass may be felt by the parent while dressing or washing the child, or less commonly, by a physician on a routine well baby examination. Occasionally, a tumor may be ruptured by a fall or trauma to the abdomen, with symptoms of an acute surgical abdomen.

B. Laboratory Findings: Complete blood count, reticulocyte count, platelet count, and bone marrow examination are needed as baselines for staging and for following therapy. Wilms' tumor rarely metastasizes to bone marrow, whereas neuroblastoma does so frequently. Urinalysis and urine culture may reveal hematuria or infection. Blood urea nitrogen and serum creatinine, uric acid, bilirubin, alkaline phosphatase, lactate dehydrogenase, and AST (SGOT) are other baseline studies of importance for following treatment. Erythropoietin levels are followed in some centers and may aid in detecting tumor activity.

C. X-Ray Findings: Posteroanterior, lateral, and oblique views of the chest should be taken to search for pulmonary metastases. Ultrasonography, CT scans, or intravenous urograms to define the tumor mass and an inferior venacavogram to rule out vascular invasion are useful. A liver scan is helpful to rule out hepatic metastases.

Treatment & Prognosis

In 1956, a 47% cure rate with total excision of Wilms' tumor was reported. It is now proper to use a transabdominal approach to allow early ligation of the renal vessels, to avoid manipulation of the tumor, and to examine the abdominal viscera, nodes, and opposite kidney for staging.

Radiation therapy to the renal fossa postoperatively increased the survival rate in some series to 60%. Therapy with megavoltage equipment is begun following surgery. Dosages of 2000–3500 rads are given, depending on the age of the patient and the stage of the tumor. If the tumor is ruptured, the entire abdomen should be treated using lead shields to protect the remaining kidney. The entire vertebral body is treated to prevent scoliosis if the spine is included in the radiation field. Radiation hepatitis may occur in the treatment of right-sided Wilms' tumor, and the early chemotherapy doses may need to be adjusted downward.

In 1966, survival rates of 89% were reported when chemotherapy with dactinomycin was added to surgery and radiation therapy in 53 patients with operable tumors; 53% survival rates were reported in 15 children presenting with metastases. Chemotherapy with vincristine and dactinomycin in courses of 6–12 weeks has been effective, with tolerable toxicity. Radiation therapy and chemotherapy are given concurrently; wound healing and adequate nutrition are important factors in following patients postoperatively. Chest films, complete blood counts, and renal function studies should be monitored during therapy. The duration of therapy depends on the patient's age and the extent of the disease.

In patients with early-stage disease and favorable histologic features, there is now a tendency to decrease the amount and duration of therapy. Thus, in patients under 2 years of age who have grossly resectable tumors, no irradiation is given, and chemotherapy consists of several months of vincristine and dactinomycin. In the presence of more extensive local disease or metastases, irradiation is added, and chemotherapy is given for longer periods, with doxorubicin added.

Currently, the 2-year disease-free survival rate is about 80% in patients with tumor extending beyond the kidney by contiguity but without apparent hematogenous spread. It is about 90% in patients with tumor confined to the kidney, and in this group patients under 2 years of age do better than older patients. Even in patients with metastatic disease, an aggressive approach is rewarded with a significant number of cures.

Beckwith JB, Palmer NF: Histopathology and prognosis of Wilms' tumor: Results from the first National Wilms' Tumor Study. *Cancer* 1978;**41:**1937.

Breslow N et al: Prognosis for Wilms' tumor patients with

nonmetastatic disease at diagnosis: Results of the second National Wilms' Tumor Study. *J Clin Oncol* 1985;**3:**521.
Green DM: The diagnosis and management of Wilms' tumor. *Pediatr Clin North Am* 1985;**32:**735.
Machin GA: Persistent renal blastoma as a frequent percursor of Wilms' tumor. *Am J Pediatr Hematol Oncol* 1980;**2:**253.

HEPATIC TUMORS

Essentials of Diagnosis

- Abdominal mass.
- Weight loss, malaise, fever.
- Nausea, vomiting, diarrhea, rarely jaundice.
- Liver function studies usually normal; mild to moderate anorexia, hyperlipemia, osteoporosis, elevated alpha-fetoprotein, masculinization.

General Considerations

Hepatic carcinoma is the most commonly seen cancer in the newborn period, although hepatic cancer in general is a rare tumor. A survey of the Surgical Section of the American Academy of Pediatrics revealed data on 375 children with liver tumors over a period of 10 years: 252 (67%) were malignant; of these, 129 (51%) were hepatoblastoma and 98 (39%) hepatocellular carcinoma. The leading benign tumors were hemangioma (38 cases), hamartoma (37 cases), and hemangioendothelioma (16 cases).

Hepatic tumors decline in incidence after a peak in the first year of life, although hepatocellular carcinoma shows a substantial increase in incidence during adolescence. Children with tyrosinemia are particularly susceptible to these tumors.

Norethandrolone and other androgenic hormones used in the treatment of aplastic anemias have recently been associated with benign and malignant tumors.

Clinical Findings

A. Symptoms and Signs: A painless, firm right upper quadrant mass is the most common finding; anorexia, weight loss, fever, or (rarely) jaundice may be the initial complaint.

B. Laboratory Findings: The workup should include specific inquiries about chemical or drug exposure or hepatitis in addition to bone marrow examination, reticulocyte count, and renal and liver function studies, including serum bilirubin, protein electrophoresis, serum alkaline phosphatase, serum lactate dehydrogenase, and tests for hepatitis-associated antigen titer and alpha-fetoprotein.

C. X-Ray Findings: Radiologic examination includes posteroanterior, lateral, and oblique chest films, an intravenous urogram, skeletal and liver scans, and angiography in some cases.

D. Staging: The staging of primary hepatic tumors is based on resectability of the hepatic tumor and the extent of extrahepatic spread (Table 31–4). The value of differentiating stages II, III, and IV is questionable, since the outcome is virtually the same in these stages.

Table 31–4. Staging of hepatic tumors.

Stage I	Tumor confined to liver and completely resected.
Stage II	Tumor confined to liver with microscopic residual tumor at the surgical margins.
Stage III	Tumor confined to liver but unresectable or with gross residual disease.
Stage IV	Extrahepatic tumor: A. Regional spread by contiguity. B. Hematogenous metastases.

Treatment & Prognosis

The prognosis for children with primary hepatic tumors is grave. In the past, only 20–50% of patients with completely resectable lesions survived and very few with unresectable lesions. Recent data suggest improved survival with stage I tumors when multiagent chemotherapy is given. Chemotherapy often reduces or may completely destroy the tumor. A tumor that is initially unresectable may be reduced by chemotherapy so that resection is possible at a later time. When the liver is already compromised, multimodal therapy is difficult and is associated with significant toxicity.

Evans AE et al: Combination chemotherapy (vincristine, Adriamycin, cyclophosphamide, and 5-fluorouracil) in the treatment of children with malignant hepatoma. *Cancer* 1982;**50:**821.
Randolph JG et al: Liver resection in children with hepatic neoplasms. *Ann Surg* 1978;**187:**599.

SOFT TISSUE TUMORS

Tumors arising in tissues of mesodermal origin may be malignant or benign. Histologically, they are of connective, fatty, or muscle tissue origin. The most common clinical complaint is of a painless lump that may arise at any site. These lumps should not be "watched" for long periods of time; surgical consultation with excisional biopsy is warranted. These tumors are too often diagnosed by means of incisional biopsy, which may disseminate the tumor and make a potentially curable lesion a widespread disease.

The malignant soft tissue tumors are rhabdomyosarcoma, malignant mesenchymoma, and fibrosarcoma.

1. RHABDOMYOSARCOMA

Rhabdomyosarcoma is the most common type of sarcoma among the somatic soft tissues of children. It is most commonly found in the first 2 decades of life and is an embryonal tumor. The 4 histologic types (with definite overlapping) are embryonal, alveolar, botryoid, and pleomorphic. Common sites of occurrence are the head and neck, extremities, orbits, and pelvic regions. The histologic pattern is variable and may be related to the site—ie, if arising in a luminal structure such as the bladder or nasopharynx where there is poor support, the tumor may assume a gelatinous or botryoid ("grapelike") appearance, in contrast to the fleshy sarcomatous tumor within the body of a muscle bundle in an extremity, where a more alveolar pattern with cross-striations may be noted. This tumor is often misdiagnosed as neuroblastoma; special electron microscopic studies may be needed for clarification and show primitive Z bands in the myofibrils.

Chest x-ray, intravenous urograms, and bone marrow examination should be done. Rhabdomyoblasts may appear in the marrow as primitive "tadpole" cells. Creatine phosphokinase and lactate dehydrogenase may be elevated. Renal and liver function studies should be obtained as baselines.

Staging is based on a scheme developed for a nationwide cooperative therapy trial (Table 31–5).

When single therapeutic modalities are used, cures are rare because of the tumor's microscopic local extensions and early infiltration of blood and lymphatic vessels. Surgical procedures should be designed to produce wide margins of normal tissue, but amputations or mutilating procedures need not be employed. Megavoltage therapy in the range of 4000–6000 rads is used locally for any residual disease or, in initially inoperable lesions, may precede surgical extirpation. Chemotherapeutic agents with demonstrated effectiveness include dactinomycin, cyclophosphamide, vincristine, doxorubicin, and dacarbazine (Table 31–6).

Group I patients (Table 31–5) have a greater than 90% chance of long-term survival. With only microscopic residual disease and no regional spread, about 70% of children will survive for 3 years. With regional or distant metastases at the time of diagnosis, the long-term survival rate drops to about 30%. On a stage-for-stage basis, extremity lesions tend to do less well than more central ones. This reflects in part a poorer prognosis for alveolar as compared to embryonal histologic types and reflects in part the early spread of extremity tumors to regional nodes where microscopic disease may not be initially appreciated.

Table 31–5. Staging of rhabdomyosarcoma.

Group I	Localized disease, completely resected: (a) Confined to muscle or organ of origin. (b) Infiltration outside the muscle or organ of origin, but regional nodes not involved.
Group II	(a) Grossly resected tumor with microscopic residual disease. (b) Regional disease completely resected. (c) Regional disease grossly resected but with evidence of microscopic residual.
Group III	Incomplete resection or biopsy with gross residual disease.
Group IV	Distant metastases present at diagnosis.

Miser JS, Pizzo PA: Soft tissue sarcomas in childhood. *Pediatr Clin North Am* 1985;**32:**779.

2. MALIGNANT MESENCHYMOMA

Malignant mesenchymoma consists of 2 or more anaplastic mesenchymal elements. It is the second most frequent soft tissue cancer. It may be found in any superficial soft tissue as well as viscera.

Since the most common differentiated element is the rhabdomyosarcoma, treatment is as above.

3. FIBROSARCOMA

Fibrosarcoma may be found as a nodule of varying size that invades locally and may metastasize to the lung. It may be present at birth but more commonly is noted in the first year of life. A variant called neurilemoma, arising in the nerve sheath, may be seen in Recklinghausen's disease.

Surgical excision is the treatment of choice. The prognosis is good for the completely resected infantile variety of fibrosarcoma. In patients with incomplete resection, local recurrence is more common than metastases. Radiation therapy and drugs such as are used for rhabdomyosarcoma may be used to treat recurrences or metastases, although the responses are often poor.

BRAIN TUMORS

Brain tumors comprise about 20% of malignant disease in pediatrics. Two-thirds of these tumors arise in the infratentorial region. The most common histologic types are cerebellar **astrocytoma, medulloblastoma,** and **brain stem glioma.** Symptoms may be generalized as a result of increased intracranial pressure secondary to obstruction of normal cerebrospinal fluid flow or may be localized to the involved area of brain. In young children, the sutures may spread in response to increased pressure, and rapid head enlargement may occur. Headaches and vomiting—especially soon after rising in the morning—and lethargy are the most common symptoms of increased pressure. Papilledema is found in older children with increased pressure but may be absent in infants when the sutures spread to provide decompression.

In addition to a careful neurologic examination, skull x-rays, brain scanning, and CT scanning are important noninvasive diagnostic procedures. Cerebral angiography and pneumoencephalography contribute to precise tumor localization.

Therapy depends upon the tumor type. Cerebellar astrocytomas can often be totally excised, and no other therapy is indicated. With incomplete removal of more aggressive lesions, radiotherapy may be added. The 10-year survival rate is about 65%. Che-

Table 31–6. Antineoplastic agents commercially available in common use.

Agent	Dosage and Route	Indications	Toxicity
Asparaginase (Elspar)	6000 IU/m^2 IM 3 times a week for 3 weeks.	Acute lymphoblastic leukemia.	Allergic reactions, anaphylaxis, hyperglycemia, coagulopathy, pancreatitis.
Cisplatin (Platinol)	50 mg/m^2 IV every 3 weeks.	Ovarian and testicular tumors.	Nausea, vomiting, nephrotoxicity, ototoxicity, bone marrow suppression.
Cyclophosphamide (Cytoxan)	75–100 mg/m^2/d orally or 300 mg/m^2/wk IV.	Leukemia, Hodgkin's lymphoma, neuroblastoma, sarcomas, retinoblastoma, hepatoma, rhabdomyosarcoma, Ewing's sarcoma.	Nausea, vomiting, anorexia, alopecia, bone marrow depression, hemorrhagic cystitis.
Cytarabine (cytosine arabinoside; Cytosar-U)	100–300 mg/m^2/wk IV or IM; 5–50 mg/m^2 once or twice weekly intrathecally for CNS leukemia until CSF clears.	Acute myeloblastic and acute lymphocytic leukemia.	Nausea, vomiting, anorexia, bone marrow depression, hepatotoxicity.
Dactinomycin (Cosmegen)	0.4 mg/m^2/wk IV in 6 doses in phases with varying rest periods.	Wilms' tumor, sarcomas, rhabdomyosarcoma.	Nausea, vomiting, anorexia, bone marrow depression, alopecia, chemical dermatitis if leakage at intravenous site, tanning of skin if used with radiation therapy.
Doxorubicin (Adriamycin)	40–75 mg/m^2 IV every 21 days, not to exceed 550 mg/m^2 total dose.	Acute lymphoblastic and myelocytic leukemia, lymphoma, Hodgkin's disease, Wilms' tumor, neuroblastoma, ovarian or thyroid carcinoma, Ewing's sarcoma, osteogenic sarcoma, rhabdomyosarcoma, other soft tissue sarcomas.	Alopecia, stomatitis, esophagitis, nausea, vomiting, severe chemical cellulitis and necrosis if extravasated; bone marrow suppression, myocardial damage if dose exceeds 550 mg/m^2; monitor ECG.
Fluorouracil (Adrucil)	300–360 mg/m^2 IV. Dosage should be scheduled based upon the specific disease stage. Maximum dose: 800 mg/d.	Hepatoma, gastrointestinal carcinoma.	Nausea, vomiting, oral ulceration, bone marrow depression, gastroenteritis, alopecia, anorexia.
Lomustine (CCNU; CeeNu)	100–130 mg/m^2 orally every 6 weeks.	Brain tumors, Hodgkin's disease.	Nausea and vomiting, alopecia, stomatitis, hepatotoxicity. Bone marrow suppression with 4- to 6-week delay in onset.
Mercaptopurine (Purinethol)	50–100 mg/m^2/d orally.	Acute myeloblastic and acute lymphocytic leukemia.	Nausea, vomiting, rare oral ulcerations, bone marrow depression.
Methotrexate (Mexate)	15–20 mg/m^2 orally twice a week until relapse. Give 12 mg/m^2/wk intrathecally for CNS leukemia until CSF clears.	Acute lymphocytic leukemia, CNS leukemia, lymphomas, choriocarcinoma, brain tumors, Hodgkin's disease.	Oral ulcers, gastrointestinal irritation, bone marrow depression, hepatotoxicity. Do not use in presence of impaired renal function.
Prednisone (Deltasone)	40 mg/m^2/d orally in 3 divided doses for 4–6 weeks.	Acute myeloblastic and lymphocytic leukemia, lymphoma, Hodgkin's disease, bone pain from metastatic disease, CNS tumors.	Increased appetite, sodium retention, hypertension, provocation of latent diabetes or tuberculosis, osteoporosis.
Procarbazine (Matulane)	100–125 mg/m^2/d orally for 4–6 weeks depending on schedule.	Hodgkin's disease, lymphomas.	Nausea, vomiting, anorexia, bone marrow depression (3-week delay). Do not give with narcotics or sedatives; has "disulfiram effect." Monitor liver and renal function.
Vincristine (Oncovin)	1.5 mg/m^2/wk IV for 4–6 weeks, then every 2 weeks. Maximum dose: 2 mg.	Acute lymphocytic and myeloblastic leukemia, lymphoma (Hodgkin's), rhabdomyosarcoma, Wilms' tumor, neuroblastoma, Ewing's sarcoma, retinoblastoma, hepatoma, sarcomas, osteosarcoma, brain tumors.	Alopecia, constipation, abdominal cramps, jaw pain, paresthesia, myalgia and muscle weakness, neurotoxicity, decrease in deep tendon reflexes, chemical dermatitis. Do not use in presence of severe liver impairment.

motherapy is not of proved effectiveness in primary management but may play a role in tumor recurrence.

Medulloblastoma is radiosensitive. Following surgery to reduce the tumor burden, radiation therapy is given to the primary and to the entire neuraxis because of the predilection of the tumor to metastasize to other areas of the brain and spinal cord via the cerebrospinal fluid. This therapy may produce 25% 10-year survival rates. Trials of various chemotherapeutic agents that may improve survival are under way.

Brain stem gliomas are usually not amenable to operation, and biopsy may not be feasible. Radiation therapy may produce survivals ranging from a few months in high-grade tumors to 3–5 years in low-grade ones. Chemotherapy with nitrosoureas and methotrexate, either intrathecally or in high doses by the intravenous route, has caused tumor regression, but the role of drugs is not established.

Allen JC: Childhood brain tumors: Current status of clinical trials in newly diagnosed and recurrent disease. *Pediatr Clin North Am* 1985;**32:**633.

Allen JC, Epstein F: Medulloblastoma and other primary malignant neuroectodermal tumors of the central nervous system: The effect of age and extent of disease on prognosis. *J Neurosurg* 1982;**57:**446.

Bleyer WA et al: Eight drugs in 1-day chemotherapy for brain tumors: A new approach and rationale for preradiation chemotherapy. *Med Pediatr Oncol* 1983;**11:**213.

Danoff BF et al: Assessment of the long-term effects of primary radiation therapy for brain tumors in children. *Cancer* 1982;**49:**1580.

Sung DI: Suprasellar tumors in children: A review of clinical manifestations and managements. *Cancer* 1982;**50:**1420.

BONE TUMORS

A variety of benign and malignant tumors may originate in bone. Bones are also common sites of metastatic disease. The principal symptoms of bone tumors, whether primary or metastatic, are pain and swelling. A fracture may first call attention to an area of cortical destruction due to cancer. The diagnosis must be based on careful and complete clinical evaluation and examination of an adequate biopsy specimen.

Ewing's sarcoma occurs most commonly in the long bones of the lower extremities and in the pelvis. Radiographically, it shows cortical bone destruction, often with periosteal elevation and an "onion skin" appearance beneath the periosteum. It must be differentiated from neuroblastoma, rhabdomyosarcoma, and non-Hodgkin's lymphoma. Metastasis occurs to other bones and to the lungs and may be present at diagnosis in one-third of patients. Ewing's sarcoma is treated with radiation doses of 6000–8000 rads over a 6- to 8-week period and with combination chemotherapy for 2 years employing vincristine, cyclophosphamide, and doxorubicin, with dactinomycin substituting for doxorubicin after a dose of 300–400 mg/m^2 of the latter has been given. If metastatic lesions are present, these are also irradiated. In patients without overt metastasis, 75% or more should live 3 years with no evidence of recurrent disease.

Surgical resection rather than irradiation should be considered for treatment of Ewing's sarcoma. The high doses of radiation required may predispose adjacent normal tissues to the development of radiation-induced osteogenic sarcoma.

Osteogenic sarcoma is the most common malignant bone tumor in the pediatric age group. It is most frequently seen during adolescence and usually occurs in long bones, with the distal femur, proximal tibia, and proximal humerus being the most common sites. The diagnosis is made by biopsy, and the therapeutic approach is jointly planned after a careful review of the x-ray and histologic findings and the bone scan results.

Therapy for this tumor is undergoing rapid change. The traditional and still most widely used surgical approach is amputation above the joint proximal to the involved bone or, in the case of femoral lesions, amputation across the femur as high as possible to avoid the tumor while retaining enough femoral shaft to fit well into a prosthesis. This is followed by intensive chemotherapy with vincristine, high doses of methotrexate with folinic acid rescue, and doxorubicin. Chemotherapy extends over a period of 2 years. In some centers, carefully selected patients are being treated either with 10,000 rads of electron beam therapy to the entire bone containing the primary or by en bloc resection of the tumor followed by prosthetic replacement in an attempt to avoid the problems of amputation. Current results indicate that aggressive chemotherapy and surgery with or without irradiation may permit a 2-year disease-free survival of 60%.

Jaffe N: Advances in the management of malignant bone tumors in children and adolescents. *Pediatr Clin North Am* 1985;**32:**801.

Meadows AT et al: Bone sarcoma as a second malignant neoplasm in children. *Cancer* 1980;**46:**2603.

Rosen G et al: Ewing's sarcoma: Ten-year experience with adjuvant chemotherapy. *Cancer* 1981;**47:**2207.

Rosen G et al: Preoperative chemotherapy for osteogenic sarcoma: Selection of postoperative adjuvant chemotherapy based on the response of the primary tumor to preoperative chemotherapy. *Cancer* 1982;**49:**1221.

Thomas PR et al: Controversies in the management of Ewing's sarcoma: Role of radiotherapy in local tumor control. *Cancer Treat Rep* 1984;**68:**703.

Winkler K et al: Neoadjuvant chemotherapy for osteogenic sarcoma: Results of a cooperative German/Austrian study. *J Clin Oncol* 1984;**2:**617.

RETICULOENDOTHELIOSES

The diseases to be discussed under this heading comprise a heterogeneous group of proliferative disorders that involve the reticuloendothelial system and are of unknown cause. Eosinophilic granuloma of bone, Hand-Schüller-Christian disease, and Letterer-Siwe disease constitute a complex of diseases of unknown cause, of histiocytic proliferation, and of unpredictable prognosis. They are sometimes grouped under the term histiocytosis X. These disorders, frequently showing Langerhans' cells on ultrastructural study, should be differentiated from reactive histiocytosis seen in diseases caused by infection and immunodeficiency.

Certain patients present primarily with signs and symptoms of lytic lesions limited to the bones—especially the skull, ribs, clavicles, and vertebrae. These lesions are well demarcated and occasionally painful. Biopsy reveals eosinophilic granuloma, which may be the only lesion the patient will develop, although further bone and even visceral lesions may occur.

Another group of patients often present with otitis media, seborrheic skin rash, and evidence of bone lesions, usually in the mastoid or skull area. They frequently also have visceral involvement, which may be indicated by lymphadenopathy and hepatosplenomegaly. This chronic disseminated form is usually known as Hand-Schüller-Christian disease and is associated with "foamy histiocytes" on biopsy. The classic triad of Hand-Schüller-Christian disease (bony involvement, exophthalmos, and diabetes insipidus) is rarely seen; however, diabetes insipidus is a common complication.

A third group of patients present early in life primarily with visceral involvement. They often have a petechial or macular skin rash, generalized lymphadenopathy, enlarged liver and spleen, pulmonary involvement, and hematologic abnormalities such as anemia and thrombocytopenia. Bone lesions can occur. This acute visceral form—Letterer-Siwe disease—is often fatal.

The principal diseases to be differentiated from histiocytosis X are bone tumors (primary or metastatic), lymphomas or leukemias, granulomatous infections, storage diseases, reactive histiocytosis, sinus histiocytosis, and lymphohistiocytosis reticulosis. The diagnosis is established by biopsy of bone marrow, lymph node, liver, or mastoid or other bone. Tissue should be preserved for electron microscopy.

Almost any system or area can become involved during the course of the disease. Rarely, these will include the heart (subendocardial infiltrates), bowel, eye, mucous membranes such as vagina or vulva, and dura mater.

Isolated bony lesions are best treated by curettage and local radiotherapy. Multiple bony involvement and visceral involvement often respond well to prednisone, vinblastine (Velban), mechlorethamine (Mustargen), or methotrexate. The current treatment of choice at the author's institution is prednisone and vinblastine or etoposide, given in repeated courses or continuously until healing of lesions occurs.

If diabetes insipidus occurs, treatment with vasopressin (Pitressin) gives good control (see Chapter 25).

In idiopathic histiocytosis, the prognosis is often unpredictable. Many patients with considerable bony and visceral involvement have shown apparent complete recovery. In general, however, the younger the patient and the more extensive the visceral involvement, the worse the prognosis.

Greenberger JS et al: Results of treatment of 127 patients with systemic histiocytosis (Letterer-Siwe syndrome, Schüller-Christian syndrome, and multifocal eosinophilic granuloma). *Medicine* 1981;**60**:311.

Matus-Ridley M et al: Histiocytosis X in children: Patterns of disease and results of treatment. *Med Pediatr Oncol* 1983;**11**:99.

SELECTED REFERENCES

Ablin AR: Supportive care for children with cancer: Guidelines of the Children's Cancer Study Group. *Am J Pediatr Hematol/Oncol* 1984;**6**:245.

Altman AJ, Schwartz AD: *Malignant Diseases of Infancy, Childhood and Adolescence,* 2nd ed. Saunders, 1983.

Lanzkowsky P: *Pediatric Oncology.* McGraw-Hill, 1983.

Levine AS: *Cancer in the Young.* Masson, 1982.

Sutow WW, Fernbach DJ, Vietti TJ (editors): *Clinical Pediatric Oncology.* Mosby, 1984.

32 Allergic Disorders

David S. Pearlman, MD

Allergic disorders include a variety of local and systemic manifestations that commonly are ultimate expressions of the union between antigen and antibody. Although this union triggers the chain of events that culminates in the clinical allergic reaction, nonimmunologic factors are important in modifying this chain of events. In some instances, nonimmunologic factors can be completely responsible for clinical reactions indistinguishable from immunologically induced reactions (eg, urticaria caused by histamine-releasing drugs such as codeine and polymyxin B).

Allergic reactivity is normal. The reaction that results from the transfusion of mismatched blood is an allergic reaction; the repeated injection of antitoxin in the form of foreign serum often leads to serum sickness; and contact with poison ivy frequently causes an allergic dermatitis. Some forms of allergic reactivity, however, occur only in certain members of the population. These disorders (which include allergic rhinitis, asthma, and atopic dermatitis) are called **atopic disorders,** signifying an unusual form of reactivity for which there is some unknown predisposition.

GENERAL PRINCIPLES OF DIAGNOSIS

By definition, allergic reactions stem from an antigen-antibody interaction; identification of these participants is of prime importance both in the diagnosis and in the therapy of allergic disorders. It is often difficult to identify the antigens (allergens) responsible for a particular clinical disorder, but the most helpful procedure by far is a thorough and detailed history. Tests for the presence of a specific antibody that will implicate specific allergens are helpful but are never a substitute for a thorough history.

Antibodies differ in their biologic activities. Since certain types of antibodies are involved in some disorders and others in different disorders, it is essential to select the appropriate immunologic tests for the disorder being investigated. In atopic disorders, reaginic or skin-sensitizing (IgE) antibody is important. The usual immunologic test for this type of antibody is the scratch, prick, or intradermal skin test. In this test, the union of skin-sensitizing antibody with antigen is responsible for the liberation of histamine, which in turn induces local vasodilatation and edema with consequent wheal and erythema ("hive") formation. As with all immunologic tests, the presence of antibody does not itself signify its clinical importance, since antibody can often be identified in the absence of any clinical symptoms. When correlated with the history, however, the results of skin tests for this type of antibody can be highly informative.

IgE antibody plays no significant role in contact dermatitis. In this type of disorder, cellular immunity (delayed hypersensitivity), which also characterizes the tuberculin reaction, is responsible. Delayed hypersensitivity reactions are characterized by infiltration around the allergen of a variety of cells, including sensitized lymphoid cells, which cause tissue destruction by mechanisms different from those operative in IgE-mediated reactions. In contact dermatitis, "patch testing" (placing the suspected allergen in direct contact with the skin for 24–48 hours under cover of a "patch") is used to detect the presence of specific sensitivity to the allergen.

The presence of a particular antibody does not always identify the cause of a given allergic disorder; ie, the presence of antibody is necessary but not in itself sufficient to produce allergic symptoms. The suspicion of the clinical importance of an allergen, however, may be confirmed by the use of a "provocative test," ie, challenging a given individual with the suspected allergen and observing the response. In a sense, "patch testing" in contact dermatitis is a provocative test, since this is both the route of sensitization and the point of reaction. Inhalation of pollens and molds by patients with asthma or hay fever and the feeding of milk to patients with suspected milk allergy are other examples of provocative tests. However, since allergic sensitivity can be inordinately great, provocative testing is potentially dangerous and should not be used routinely. Provocative tests may prove a relationship between the provoking substance and a clinical reaction, but they do not necessarily establish that the reaction is allergic. For example, in children with lactase deficiency, milk may elicit gastrointestinal symptoms similar to those of milk allergy.

GENERAL PRINCIPLES OF TREATMENT

Environmental Control of Exposure

Since the clinical allergic reaction stems from the union of antigen with antibody, avoidance of the offending antigen is the most effective means of therapy of all allergic disorders. In many instances, complete avoidance of identified allergens is impossible, but it is frequently feasible to reduce the incidence and severity of reactions by minimizing the contact. Many nonimmunologic factors can precipitate or aggravate atopic disorders (eg, irritating smoke; cold air in asthma), and avoidance of such known or suspected irritants is also of prime importance in the therapy of allergic disorders.

The following are sample directions for environmental control of common allergens. They refer mainly to the patient's bedroom, but the principles are applicable to the rest of the house as well.

(1) House dust is a common offender. The accumulation of dust may be minimized by the avoidance of dust catchers and dust producers such as wool (in rugs, blankets), flannel (in bedding, pajamas), upholstered furniture, toys stuffed with plant or animal products, chenille (bedspreads, drapes, and rugs), cotton quilts, stuffed cotton pads, and venetian blinds.

(2) Rooms should be dusted daily with a damp or oiled cloth. The room should be cleaned thoroughly at least once a week—never with the patient present.

(3) All forced air ducts, which frequently contain dust and molds and tend to stir up room dust, should be sealed off. An electric radiator may be substituted as a source of heat, if necessary. If pollenosis is a problem, windows should be kept closed during the pollen seasons. Air cleaners (central or room) and refrigerated air conditioners may be useful. Automatic humidifiers with provision for humidity not to exceed 40% can be helpful in dry climates and with heating systems. Humidifiers should be kept as mold-free as possible.

(4) Plant products (kapok, cotton) and animal products sometimes used for pillows, stuffing of furniture, toys, bedding, and hair pads for rugs should be eliminated. Alternatively, all mattresses, box springs, and pillows in the bedroom should be completely enclosed in impermeable plastic or rubber casings. Inexpensive casings may be obtained from department stores; better quality encasings may be obtained from Allergen-Proof Encasings, Inc, 1450 E 363rd Street, Eastlake, OH 44094. Especially if plastic casings are used, they should be checked periodically for tears or punctures. Furniture and bedding stuffed solely with synthetic products or rubber are permissible; rubber pillows, however, may harbor molds. Toys stuffed with old nylon stockings or synthetic foam and covered with plain nonfuzzy cotton or synthetic materials are satisfactory.

(5) Cleaning equipment, wool, and fur coats should not be kept in or near the child's room or closet.

(6) Sensitization to animals develops so frequently in atopic individuals that close contact with animals of any sort should be avoided. Danders, saliva, and urine are the important sources of allergen. With existing sensitivity, it is important to rid the environment of animals.

Hyposensitization (Immunotherapy)

If avoidance of offensive allergens is not possible, specific hyposensitization is sometimes attempted. The value of hyposensitization is limited mainly to atopic disorders and to severe insect allergy. There are a variety of hyposensitization procedures, but the same general principle applies to all: Extremely small amounts of allergen are injected subcutaneously at frequent intervals and in increasing amounts until a "top dose" is reached; this is usually the highest tolerated dose of a given allergen extract, or that amount which induces a state of clinical hyporeactivity to the allergen as demonstrated after natural contact. When perennial therapy is adopted, the top tolerated dose is used as a maintenance dose, with carefully regulated lengthening of intervals (by not more than an additional week at a time) up to 6 weeks, as tolerated.

Most allergists agree that the majority of well-selected patients with pollen asthma or hay fever are significantly improved after 1–2 years of therapy on a "perennial" injection regimen of aqueous antigens, and there is evidence to substantiate the beneficial effects of hyposensitization even in perennial asthma. The effectiveness of therapy is dose-related. Repository therapy using alum-precipitated extracts (Allpyral, Center-Al) is useful mainly in increasing the antigen dosage in individuals who are extremely sensitive to small amounts of aqueous antigen. Theoretically, fewer injections of alum-precipitated material are required to reach a maintenance dose of antigen, and maintenance injections need to be given less frequently. However, information on the efficacy of this form of therapy is not as complete as that relating to aqueous therapy. Mold hyposensitization therapy is believed to offer significant protection, but adequate documentation of this is lacking. The value of hyposensitization against house dust mites is substantiated; it appears beneficial but is no substitute for good environmental control. Venom therapy for stinging insect sensitivity is efficacious. The use of bacterial extracts appears to be of little value and has been largely abandoned.

Drug Therapy

A variety of drugs are effective in the treatment of allergic disorders (Table 32–1). The principal groups include adrenergic agents, antihistamines, methylxanthines, cromolyn sodium, expectorants, oxygen, and adrenocorticosteroids. The selection of drugs depends upon the pathologic processes involved.

A. Adrenergic Agents: As a group, adrenergic agents exhibit many different pharmacologic effects. Their usefulness in allergic disorders depends mainly on their ability to constrict blood vessels and relax other smooth muscle. The manifestations of many allergic reactions are due, at least in part, to chemical mediators, such as histamine and leukotrienes, that produce varying degrees of vasodilatation, edema,

Table 32–1. Preparations and dosages of drugs commonly used in allergic disorders.

Agent	Dosage
Adrenergic agents	
Epinephrine aqueous, 1:1000 (Adrenalin)	0.01 mL/kg SC or IM up to 0.25 mL. (May repeat at 20-minute intervals—total of 3 doses.)
Terbutaline* (Bricanyl), 1 mg/mL	0.01 mL/kg SC or IM up to 0.25 mL. (May repeat at 20-minute intervals—total of 2 doses.)
Epinephrine suspension, long-acting, 1:200 (Sus-Phrine)	0.1–0.2 mL SC every 8–12 hours. (Shake well before administering.)
Pseudoephedrine hydrochloride (Sudafed)	1 mg/kg/dose orally, 4–6 times a day.
Metaproterenol (Alupent, Metaprel)	10–20 mg orally, every 6–8 hours.
Terbutaline* (Brethine, Bricanyl)	2.5 mg orally, every 8 hours.
Albuterol* (salbutamol; Proventil, Ventolin), 2- to 4-mg tablets	2–4 mg orally, 3 times a day.
Adrenergic aerosols	
Albuterol* (salbutamol; Proventil, Ventolin) Bitolterol* (Tornalate) Isoetharine mesylate (Bronkometer) Metaproterenol* (Alupent, Metaprel) Terbutaline* (Brethaire)	1–2 inhalations from pressurized aerosol. May use as often as every 4 hours. *Avoid excessive use.*
Isoetharine (Bronkosol) 1% solution	0.15–0.5 mL diluted with 1 mL water or saline and administered by hand or compressor-driven nebulizer.
Metaproterenol* (Alupent, Metaprel) 5% inhalant solution	0.1–0.3 mL diluted with 1 mL water or saline and administered by hand or compressor-driven nebulizer.
Drugs with antihistaminic activity	
Diphenhydramine hydrochloride (Benadryl) Injectable	1 mg/kg/dose (up to 50 kg) orally, 4 times a day. 25–50 mg IV (slowly) or IM (ampules, 50 mg/mL; vials, 10 mg/mL).
Chlorpheniramine maleate (Chlor-Trimeton, Chlor-Trimeton Repetabs, Teldrin) Injectable	0.1 mg/kg/dose (up to 50 kg) orally, 4 times a day. 0.1–0.2 mg/kg/dose (up to 50 kg) orally, 2 times a day. 4–8 mg IV (slowly) or IM (10 mg/mL in 1-mL vials; 100 mg/mL in 2-mL vials).
Brompheniramine maleate (Dimetane)	0.1 mg/kg/dose (up to 50 kg) orally, 4 times a day.
Tripelennamine hydrochloride (PBZ)	0.5–1 mg/kg/dose (up to 50 kg) orally, 4 times a day.
Hydroxyzine (Atarax, Vistaril)	0.2–0.5 mg/kg/dose (up to 50 kg) orally, 3 times a day.
Cyproheptadine (Periactin)	0.05 mg/kg/dose (up to 50 kg) orally, 3–4 times a day.
Combination drugs for allergic rhinitis and conjunctivitis	
Pseudoephedrine and triprolidine (Actifed)	Syrup: ½–2 tsp 3 times a day depending on age. Tablets: ½–1 tablet 3 times a day depending on age.
Pseudoephedrine and dexbrompheniramine* (Drixoral)	Tablets: 1 tablet 2 times a day (older children).
Pseudoephedrine and carbinoxamine (Rondec)	Drops: ¼–1 dropperful 4 times a day (infants). Syrup: ½–1 tsp 4 times a day (older children). Tablets: ½–1 tablet 4 times a day (older children).
Phenylpropanolamine, pyrilamine, and pheniramine (Triaminic)	Drops: 5–10 drops 3 times a day (infants). Syrup: ½–2 tsp 4 times a day depending on age. Juvulets: 1–2 tablets 4 times a day (older children).
Expectorants	
Guaifenesin (glyceryl guaiacolate; Robitussin)	1 tsp every 4–6 hours.
Methylxanthines	
Aminophylline, theophylline (Choledyl, Elixophyllin, Quibron, Respbid, Slo-Bid, Slo-Phyllin, Somophyllin, Sustaire, Theo-24, Theo-Dur, Theolair, Theophyl, Theospan, Theostat, Uniphyl)	IV: 4–6 mg†/kg every 4–6 hours (infuse over 10- to 20-minute period or as 0.6–1 mg/kg/h at constant drip). Oral: 4–6 mg†/kg every 6 hours. Longer-acting preparations can be used every 8–12 hours (eg, Slo-Bid, Theo-Dur) or every 24 hours (Theo-24, Uniphyl) in children over 12 years of age. Rectal: Enema (Somophyllin), 4–6 mg†/kg every 6 hours.

* Not recommended by manufacturer for children under 12 years of age.
† Refers to theophylline dose. See text for further discussion of dosage.
‡ Not recommended by manufacturer for children under 6 years of age.
§ Not recommended by manufacturer for children under 4 years of age.

Table 32–1 (cont'd). Preparations and dosages of drugs commonly used in allergic disorders.

Agent	Dosage
Adrenal glucocorticoids	
Most rapid therapeutic effect follows intravenous or oral administration, but there may be no perceptible effect for hours. In acute situations, high doses of corticosteroids (eg, 100–200 mg hydrocortisone or 40–80 mg methylprednisolone [Solu-Medrol] every 4–6 hours) are generally employed the first day and the dose tapered as rapidly as possible to maintenance levels or withdrawn completely.	
Approximate equivalents of activity: 100 mg hydrocortisone = 4 mg dexamethasone = 25 mg prednisolone = 20 mg methylprednisolone.	
Intravenous preparations	
Hydrocortisone sodium succinate (Solu-Cortef)	100 mg in 2-mL vials.
Methylprednisolone (Solu-Medrol)	40 mg in 1-mL vials.
Dermatologic preparations	
Fluocinolone acetonide (Synalar)	0.025% cream or ointment and 0.01% cream.
Flurandrenolide (Cordran)	0.05% and 0.025% cream or ointment.
Hydrocortisone (Cort-Dome)	0.125% up to 2% hydrocortisone in acid mantle base.
Hydrocortisone (Hytone)	0.5% and 1% hydrocortisone cream or ointment.
Topical corticosteroid preparations for severe asthma	
Beclomethasone dipropionate‡ (Beclovent, Vanceril)	Not to exceed 3 inhalations 4 times a day.
Flunisolide‡ (AeroBid)	2 inhalations 2 times a day.
Triamcinolone acetonide‡ (Azmacort)	1–2 inhalations 3 times a day.
Topical inhalant preparations for prophylaxis	
Cromolyn sodium (Intal), 20-mg capsules or vials	1 capsule or vial is diluted (20 mg in 2 mL) and the preparation inhaled 3–4 times a day or just prior to exercise or contact with asthma-precipitating agents.
Topical inhalant preparations for rhinitis	
Beclomethasone dipropionate* (Beconase, Vancenase)	1 inhalation in each nostril up to 3 times a day. Discontinue if there is any nasal bleeding.
Dexamethasone sodium phosphate‡ (Turbinaire Decadron Phosphate)	1–2 sprays in each nostril 2 times a day. (Should be used for short periods only.) Discontinue if there is any nasal bleeding.
Flunisolide 0.025% nasal solution‡ (Nasalide)	1 inhalation in each nostril 3 times a day, or 2 inhalations in each nostril 2 times a day. Discontinue if there is any nasal bleeding.
Cromolyn sodium‡ (Nasalcrom)	1 inhalation in each nostril every 3–4 hours.
Topical preparations for allergic conjunctivitis	
Decongestant-antihistamines	
Naphazoline 0.025% and pheniramine 0.3% solution (Muro's Opcon-A), 15-mL bottles	1–2 drops in each eye 3–4 times a day as needed.
Naphazoline 0.05% and antazoline 0.5% solution (Albalon-A Liquifilm), 15-mL bottles	1–2 drops in each eye 3–4 times a day as needed.
Phenylephrine 0.12%, pyrilamine 0.1%, and antipyrine 0.1% solution (Prefrin-A), 15-mL bottles	1–2 drops in each eye 3–4 times a day as needed.
Corticosteroid preparations	
Dexamethasone phosphate 0.1% solution (Decadron Phosphate), 2.5- and 5-mL bottles	1–2 drops up to every 1–2 hours initially until relief, then up to every 4 hours as needed.
Hydrocortisone acetate 2.5% suspension (Hydrocortisone Acetate), 5-mL bottles	1–2 drops up to every 1–2 hours initially until relief, then up to every 4 hours as needed.
Prednisolone phosphate 0.5% solution (Hydeltrasol, Metreton), 5-mL bottles	1–2 drops up to every 1–2 hours initially until relief, then up to every 4 hours as needed.
Medrysone 1% suspension (HMS Liquifilm), 5- and 10-mL bottles	1–2 drops every 4 hours as needed.
Preparations for prophylaxis	
Cromolyn sodium 4% solution§ (Opticrom 4%), 10-mL bottles	1–2 drops in each eye 4–6 times a day.

* Not recommended by manufacturer for children under 12 years of age.

† Refers to theophylline dose. See text for further discussion of dosage.

and smooth muscle spasm. Adrenergic agents are the principal pharmacologic antagonists of these chemical mediators and at times may even reverse their effects completely. However, the pharmacologic properties of adrenergic drugs as a group are not shared uniformly by all members of the group, and these drugs cannot be used interchangeably to produce a given effect. In rhinitis, for example, phenylephrine, an effective vasoconstrictor but a poor smooth muscle dilator, would be especially useful. Albuterol, on the other hand, although devoid of vasoconstrictor action, is an effective bronchodilator and is useful in asthma. In asthma and in anaphylaxis—in which vasodilatation, edema, and asthma may all be a problem—epinephrine, which is a potent antagonist of all of these effects, is the drug of choice.

Adrenergic drugs are not always effective in a given disorder and are not without undesirable effects. Epinephrine resistance may occur in severe asthma, for example, and its use in such cases may actually aggravate the disorder by increasing the patient's anxiety and contributing to venous congestion and mucus plugging. The injection of epinephrine when severe hypoxemia and acidosis are present may produce cardiac dysrhythmia or arrest. Adrenergic aerosols can be extremely effective in acute asthma, but some (eg, isoproterenol) have been shown to severely aggravate asthma if used excessively. Aerosols containing newer B_2-adrenergic drugs appear to be safer.

B. Antihistamines: The antihistamines act through competition with histamine for receptor sites, thereby preventing histamine from exerting its activity. There are 2 classes of antihistamines: H_1 receptor inhibitors, the classic antihistamines used for many years in allergic disorders, and H_2 receptor inhibitors, a newer class of drugs useful in inhibiting gastric acid secretion. H_1 antihistamines are particularly useful in urticaria, anaphylaxis, and allergic rhinitis; they may not be effective in certain other syndromes such as asthma, in which other mediators besides histamine also appear to be involved. This may relate in part to the presence of H_2 as well as H_1 receptors in some tissues. In certain curcumstances, the combination of H_1 and H_2 antihistamines is therapeutic when either alone is not. In addition, numerous mediators unrelated to histamine are important in allergic conditions.

Although antihistamines may be useful in severe allergic disorders, they are not the drug of first choice in medical emergencies due to allergic reactions but may be administered after epinephrine has been given. Antihistamines have antipruritic properties and are useful in atopic dermatitis and in contact dermatitis, in which histamine may play a major role. The sedation that occurs as a side effect, although undesirable in many instances, may be an advantage in others. Some antihistamines possess atropinelike drying actions.

C. Methylxanthines: Theophylline and its ethylenediamine derivative, aminophylline, are effective bronchodilators that appear to act at a different point but in the same pathway through which epinephrine exerts its smooth muscle dilating effect. The improper use of these agents has been associated with severe toxic reactions, in some cases resulting in death. Overdosage frequently occurs as a result of failure to appreciate the variability of rate and extent of absorption with different routes of administration. Toxic reactions include headache, palpitations, dizziness, stomach ache, nausea and vomiting, excessive thirst, and hypotension. *Nausea and stomach ache may be related to local irritation but can also represent a central nervous system-mediated toxic effect of the drug when administered by any route.* When used properly, theophylline and aminophylline are valuable drugs with a potent bronchodilating effect. There is great individual variation in the metabolism of methylxanthines, and dosage must be highly individualized. Optimal therapeutic blood levels of theophylline are considered to be 10–20 μg/mL serum or plasma, with levels over 20 μg/mL more likely to be associated with drug toxicity. However, side effects such as behavioral changes and effects on attention span and learning can occur at significantly lower levels. Average dosages likely to achieve therapeutic blood levels of 10–20 μg/mL are 25 ± 5 mg/kg/d between ages 1 and 8, then 20 ± 5 mg/kg/d until about age 16; thereafter, average daily dosage is closer to 12 ± 3 mg. A single daily dose can be given, or the daily dosage can be divided into 2–4 doses (every 6–24 hours), depending on the preparation used. Safe peak blood levels appear to be those below 15 μg/mL. *In early to mid infancy, metabolism is markedly diminished, and theophylline should be employed with particular caution.*

Rectal administration of theophylline in fluid form usually results in prompt and efficient absorption of the drug that may be almost as efficient as intravenous administration. Absorption from rectal suppositories is unpredictable, and these preparations should not be used. Long-acting preparations given orally are preferred for chronic administration of methylxanthines.

D. Expectorants: Expectorants such as guaifenesin (glyceryl guaiacolate) are used mainly in bronchial asthma to liquefy thick, tenacious mucus, but it is not clear whether any therapeutic effectiveness of those agents is in fact due to their expectorant action. Iodides seem more effective than guaifenesin, but—especially with prolonged use—goiter, salivary gland inflammation, gastric irritation, skin eruptions, and acne may occur. ***Note:*** It is important to keep in mind that adequate hydration is essential to effective expectoration. In general, expectorant preparations containing narcotics should not be used in asthma.

E. Corticosteroids: Adrenal glucocorticoids have been used in the treatment of all of the allergic disorders. Their effectiveness is apparently due to their "anti-inflammatory" actions. The untoward side effects of prolonged corticosteroid administration (eg, growth suppression, myopathy, Cushing's syndrome, hypertension, peptic ulcer [controversial], diabetes, and electrolyte imbalance) limit their use mainly to those conditions which are refractory to other measures or are life-threatening. Even then, however, their slow onset of action (even when given intravenously) precludes first-choice administration of these drugs in acute allergic emergencies. Most allergic syndromes are amenable to other forms of therapy, and the systemic use of the corticosteroids usually is unnecessary. When chronic use is necessary, alternate-day corticosteroid therapy with a short-acting preparation (eg, prednisone) in the early morning every other day should be attempted. Alternatively, for asthma or rhinitis, use by inhalation can be considered. There are virtually no advantages to the use of corticotropin over the glucocorticoids themselves when glucocorticoid action is deemed necessary.

The main indications for the use of systemic corticosteroids are acute life-threatening asthma and control of chronic severe disorders, such as asthma, that are refractory to other appropriate therapy. In some instances, administration of a short course of corticosteroids for self-limiting allergic disorders (eg, serum sickness) may be warranted.

Topical corticosteroids are extremely effective anti-inflammatory agents in the control of allergic dermatitis—mainly contact dermatitis and atopic dermatitis. Topical application is the preferred route of administration in such disorders, keeping long-term use of the more potent preparations to a minimum.

F. Sedatives: Sedatives have been grossly misused in asthma and have been responsible for some deaths. Although the psyche undoubtedly exerts a significant influence on asthma and other allergic disorders, the anxiety associated with extreme asthma is more often a reflection of the severity of the respiratory distress than the main cause of it. Sedatives that suppress the respiratory center (as the barbiturates do) should not be used in the therapy of severe asthma. If sedatives are necessary, chloral hydrate may be used.

G. Oxygen: Oxygen is extremely important in the treatment of severe asthma. Hypoxemia usually occurs early in the course of moderately severe or severe asthma, much in advance of any detectable cyanosis. Oxygen is potentially very drying and should be humidified when administered. Excessively high concentrations of oxygen should be avoided, since they can lead to atelectasis or possibly lessening of respiratory drive.

H. Antibiotics: There are no special indications for the use of antibiotics in allergic disorders. Antibiotics should of course be used when evidence of bacterial infection exists. However, their excessive use in children with allergic disorders should be avoided to reduce the risk of sensitization to these drugs.

Erythromycin seems to be one of the least sensitizing antibiotics and offers good coverage against many respiratory pathogens.

I. Cromolyn Sodium (Intal): This drug is used in the management of asthma and noninfectious rhinitis and conjunctivitis. It blocks release of pharmacologic mediators such as histamine resulting from antigen-antibody interaction, and it is useful in the prevention of chronic symptomatic asthma. In many children, it is interchangeable with theophylline as a first-line drug for chronic asthma therapy. However, it does not reverse tissue changes induced by chemical mediators and is therefore of no value in the treatment of acute asthmatic paroxysms. It is useful in blocking exercise-induced asthma and irritant- and allergen-provoked asthma if used just prior to anticipated exposure to irritating agents.

Buckley J, Pearlman DS: Controlling the environment. Chap 22, p 300, in: *Allergic Diseases of Infancy, Childhood, and Adolescence*. Bierman CW, Pearlman DS (editors). Saunders, 1980.

Morris HG: Mechanisms of action and therapeutic role of corticosteroids in asthma. *J Allergy Clin Immunol* 1985;**75**:1.

Pearlman DS: Allergic disorders. Chap 17, p 229, in: *Medical Care of the Pregnant Patient*. Abrams R, Wexler P (editors). Little, Brown, 1983.

Pearlman DS: Antihistamines: Pharmacology and clinical use. *Drugs* 1976;**12**:258.

MEDICAL EMERGENCIES DUE TO ALLERGIC REACTIONS

The most common causes of severe allergic reactions are skin testing; hyposensitization with allergen extracts; drugs, vaccines, toxoids, sera, blood transfusions, and insect stings; and food sensitivity. Recently, anaphylaxis related to strenuous exercise has been described. Anaphylactic shock, angioedema, and bronchial obstruction, alone or in combination, are the principal life-threatening manifestations of severe allergic reactions. Light-headedness, paresthesias, sweating, flushing, palpitations, and urticaria may precede or accompany severe reactions.

Prevention

Prevention consists mainly of avoiding allergens known or believed to be responsible for allergic reactions. A history suggestive of a reaction to a given drug is an indication for the selection of an alternative and unrelated drug for therapeutic use. Perform skin tests *cautiously* before foreign serum is administered.

Treatment

A. Emergency Measures: Immediate treatment is essential for management of these reactions.

1. Epinephrine—Epinephrine, 1:1000, 0.2–0.4 mL, should be injected intramuscularly without delay. This may be repeated at intervals of 15–20 minutes as necessary. If the reaction is due to the recent injection of a drug, serum, or other substance, a tourniquet should be applied proximal to the injection. If the offending substance has been injected intradermally or subcutaneously, absorption of the material may be delayed further by injecting epinephrine, 0.1 mL subcutaneously, near the site of injection. Subsequent therapy depends partly upon the response.

2. Antihistamines—Antihistamines (Table 32–1) should be given intramuscularly or intravenously. When intravenous infusions are used, they should be given over a period of 5–10 minutes, since untoward reactions, particularly hypotension, have been induced by too rapid administration.

3. Theophylline—Theophylline is useful when bronchospasm occurs. (See also p 994.)

4. Tracheostomy—Tracheostomy may be lifesaving in cases of profound laryngeal edema.

5. Fluids—Since anaphylactic shock is in part produced by hypovolemia secondary to massive exudation of intravascular fluid, maintenance of a proper volume by intravenous fluids (isotonic saline, 5% dextrose in water, or 5% dextrose in saline) is particularly important.

B. Follow-Up Measures: Adrenocorticosteroids should be given only after epinephrine and antihistamines have been administered. The onset of action of these drugs is slow (hours, even by intravenous administration). A combination of H_1 antihistamines (eg, chlorpheniramine) and H_2 antihistamines (eg, cimetidine) is recommended.

Mild sedation may also be indicated.

C. Hyposensitization for Insect Stings: Children who have experienced life-threatening reactions following an insect sting should by hyposensitized. A large local reaction or generalized urticaria *without* respiratory or cardiovascular compromise is probably *not* an indication for hyposensitization. The main allergens responsible for severe allergic reactions are found in the venoms of Hymenoptera (bees, wasps, hornets, and fire ants). Venom antigens for diagnosis and treatment of anaphylactic sensitivity to stinging insects have become available only recently. These are much more efficacious than whole body extracts, and the latter should no longer be employed. Hyposensitization with venom antigens, however, is associated with a high incidence of significant reactions in the course of treatment, and testing and therapy are best left to physicians experienced in dealing with insect allergy. Treatment kits for anaphylactic reactions should be available for immediate use in individuals with insect hypersensitivity and should be kept in the home or taken along by a responsible person when the sensitive person travels in an area likely to be infested with the offensive insects. The single most important item in such a kit is epinephrine. The patient and parents should be instructed in proper use of the kit and in ways to avoid insects. (The kits should also be available for patients with severe recurrent allergic reactions from any cause.)

Gershwin ME, Keslin MH (editors): Allergic emergencies. *Clin Rev Allergy* 1985;**3**:1. [Entire issue.]

Schuberth KC et al: Epidemiologic study of insect allergy in children. 2. Effect of accidental stings in allergic children. *J Pediatr* 1983;**102**:361.

Yunginger JW: Advances in the diagnosis and treatment of stinging insect allergy. *Pediatrics* 1981;**670**:325.

ATOPIC DISORDERS

Certain individuals are predisposed to asthma, allergic rhinitis, or atopic dermatitis. The incidence tends to be familial, but little is known about the constitutional basis. Sensitization is usually to substances considered to be innocuous for other people. Animal danders, feathers, spores from indoor molds, and house dust mites are the most common perennial allergens. Animal danders and emanations of house dust mites (high in mattress flock) and of cockroaches (abundant in poor housing situations) are important factors contributing to the allergenicity of house dust. Many varieties of trees, grass and weed pollens, and molds cause atopic disorders in a more or less seasonal incidence. Foods and a number of other substances may contribute to perennial or seasonal problems. Atopic individuals commonly become sensitized to one or more of these sensitizing substances, and "environmental control" (see above) is therefore recommended for any child with an atopic syndrome.

It is important to remember that many atopic disorders, including many cases of asthma and atopic dermatitis, are due to or are influenced by causes other than allergic sensitization.

Diagnosis

The diagnosis of atopic disease is based primarily on the clinical findings. Laboratory procedures (including allergy testing) can be very helpful, but results should be interpreted in the light of the history and physical findings. To arrive at a diagnosis of any or all atopic diseases, a detailed history and complete physical examination are essential. More than one atopic disease may be present, and a history of familial atopic disorders or of other past or present atopic symptoms is especially useful. The following is a guideline for the overall history and physical examination. Indicated laboratory procedures will be included under individual atopic diseases.

A. History:

1. Chief complaint of patient.

2. Family history—Past or present specific allergen sensitivity or any atopic disease in other family members (asthma, allergic rhinitis, atopic dermatitis).

3. First episode—Details of development of first episode (eg, infection), change in environment (family move, acquisition of pets or toys, different household furnishings), season of year, ingestion of "new" food, special occasions, emotional and social upheavals.

4. Circumstances of subsequent and most recent episodes—See above details.

5. Other allergic diseases—Associated atopic or other allergic diseases (past or present), especially allergic rhinitis, bronchial asthma, "allergic cough," atopic dermatitis, food intolerance, "allergic rashes," angioedema.

6. Infections; tonsils and adenoids—History of pneumonia, "bronchitis," bronchiolitis, "croup," recurrent ear infections, sinusitis, removal of tonsils and adenoids.

7. Food-related symptoms—Vomiting, colic, diarrhea, abnormal stools, abdominal pain, skin rashes, headache, etc.

8. Presence of "continuity symptoms"—Itchy or stuffy nose; fatigue; irritability; diminished exercise tolerance; night cough; prolonged cough; breathlessness, cough, or wheezing when exercising, laughing, crying, or experiencing frustration.

9. Wheezing, cough, rashes, or nose, ear, or eye symptoms following contact with the following:

a. Animals—Especially house pets of the child or of friends or relatives; direct or indirect contact with horses or other animals.

b. Seasonal agents—In winter, predominantly house dust and viral respiratory infections; in spring, trees; in late spring to early summer, grasses; in late summer to early fall, weeds. (Most sporulation [see below] also is seasonal.)

c. Seasonal sources of pollen—Grass mowing, harvesting, play or work in weed patches, etc.

d. Mold—Outside seasonal molds (wet, warm periods), moldy foods, mildew, old storage areas (attics, damp basements), grass mowing, thatching, etc.

e. Cosmetics—Bubble bath, hair spray, facial cosmetics, shampoos, soaps, enzyme detergents, etc.

10. Emotional and social factors and habits—Family structure; general attitudes and behavior; family, school, and social adjustments.

11. Past therapy and response to it.

B. Physical Examination: A complete physical examination is essential. The following signs deserve special emphasis:

1. General appearance of patient—State of nourishment and physical development, including weight and height; degree of activity; signs of fatigue; sneezing; cough and its character; dyspnea.

2. Attitudes, responses, and relationships of patient to parents, physician, nurses, etc.

3. Vital signs—Blood pressure, temperature, pulse rate, and character of respirations.

4. Skin—Rashes, pallor, cyanosis, temperature changes, sweating, degree of dryness.

5. Eyes—"Allergic shiners" (lower lid edema, eyeshadowing), conjunctival injection, blebs, itching, cataracts (in severe, long-standing atopic dermatitis), blepharitis (from chronic rubbing), tearing.

6. Nose—Itching ("allergic salute," "bunny nose," nasal crease), excoriation of nares, hyperemia, mucosal edema, polypoid changes, purplish pallor, excessive serous or mucoid discharge.

7. Ears—With auditory tube dysfunction, retraction of drums and decreased drum mobility; with recurrent serous otitis media, hearing loss, changes in drum (immobility, distortion, retraction, fullness, opacity, narrow and "chalky" malleus), evidence of fluid in middle ear.

8. Mouth—For palatal malformations, character of speech, "canker sores," changes in tongue (geographism, grooving).

9. Throat—Presence and appearance of tonsils and pharyngeal lymphoid tissue, appearance of mucosal epithelium (anterior pillars, soft palate, pharyngeal wall), character of secretions.

10. Chest—Configuration ("barrel chest," "pigeon breast," prominent Harrison's grooves—all may be present in long-standing asthma), evidence of hyperinflation, pattern of breathing, development and use of accessory muscles for respiration (eg, hypertrophy of pectorals, trapezii, sternocleidomastoids), retractions.

11. Lungs—Relationship to inspiratory-expiratory cycle of gross or auscultatory wheezes (including after exercise and forced expiration), rhonchi, or rales; degree and equality of air exchange; level and movement of diaphragm.

12. Heart—Tachycardia, size, accentuation of pulmonic second sound (for evidence of pulmonary hypertension in asthma), murmurs.

13. External genitalia—Vulvitis (girls in pollen season), meatal ulcer (boys with contact dermatitis).

14. Signs of associated infections—Pyoderma, purulent nasal or ear discharge, purulent bronchial secretions, significant adenopathy.

C. Supplementary Diagnostic Procedures:

1. Allergy tests—In all atopic disorders, testing for the presence of IgE antibody is potentially useful in identifying allergens that may play a role in the disorder. Atopic individuals often have IgE antibody to many antigens.

a. Skin tests—Scratch or prick testing should be done first, since it is less likely than intradermal testing to cause severe reactions in sensitive individuals. Intradermal testing is about 100 times more sensitive than scratch testing. The tests are read at the peak of the urticarial reaction, usually within 15–20 minutes. If scratch tests are negative, intradermal tests (on an extremity) may be used. Skin testing is potentially dangerous in highly sensitive individuals, and epinephrine and a tourniquet should always be at hand.

A positive test reaction consists of erythema, wheal, and flare (triple response). In interpreting the skin tests and assessing their clinical significance, the following should be kept in mind: (1) A diluent ("negative") control and a histamine ("positive") control should always be used for comparison. (2) Infants may react predominantly with flaring; older children, with wheal and flare reactions. (3) Mild reactions (1−2+) are less likely to be clinically significant than more strongly positive (pseudopodic wheal) reactions. Also, a positive reaction elicited by scratch or puncture testing is more likely to be clinically significant than a positive reaction that can be elicited only by intradermal testing. (4) When a skin test does correlate with clinical sensitivity, the size of the reaction cannot be taken as an index of the severity of the clinical syndrome. (5) Large (3−4+) reactions to foods are likely to be of clinical significance (in contrast to mild reactions), but negative reactions do not rule out allergic or nonallergic clinical sensitivity. (6) A positive skin test suggests only that antibody is present in the skin. It may reflect past, present, or potential clinical hypersensitivity, but it is not necessarily clinically significant. The patient may never develop an atopic disease due to the specific allergen. (7) A positive skin test may be clinically relevant to one but not necessarily to all the allergic disorders present. (8) Up to 10% of nonatopic individuals may have positive skin reactions to a few allergens, especially house dust.

b. Serologic tests—Immunoassays to measure serum IgE antibody are being used increasingly. The best known is the radioallergosorbent test (RAST), a radioimmunoassay, but enzyme-linked immunoassays that eliminate the need for radioactive material are also available.

Results of RAST and similar tests correlate well with those of skin tests, although the former are somewhat less sensitive. They are advantageous because they allow for testing of individuals in whom skin testing would be difficult (eg, patients with extensive dermatitis) and there is no risk of provoking a hypersensitivity reaction. These tests should be especially useful in testing for severe drug and stinging insect hypersensitivity when the appropriate problematic antigens can be identified. The number of antigens available for testing is limited, and considering the greater expense of these tests and the delay in obtaining results, skin testing is much preferable at this time.

2. Measurement of IgE immunoglobulin levels—The radioimmunosorbent test (RIST) measures the concentration of IgE immunoglobulin in the blood. Elevated IgE levels as measured by RIST or PRIST (paper RIST) suggest an atopic disorder, but the correlation is so imperfect that this is not a generally useful screening procedure. Greatly elevated IgE levels in infancy (> 2 SD above the mean) are highly predictive of an atopic diathesis, and elevated IgE levels in ''bronchiolitis'' suggest the diagnosis of asthma. However, a normal or low IgE level does not rule out an atopic disorder or allergic sensitization.

3. The Prausnitz-Küstner reaction—Passive transfer of antibody by injecting serum from a sensitized individual into the skin of a nonsensitized individual, followed by local challenge of the transfer site with the suspected allergen, was occasionally employed when skin testing was not feasible. This has been supplanted by serologic tests.

4. Provocative testing—Provocative testing may be employed but is not recommended as a routine procedure for any potentially severe disorder such as asthma. Provocative tests are most valuable in determining clinical sensitivity to foods. Elimination and subsequent challenge with the following may be especially revealing: (1) Foods eaten more or less daily (unless there is a history of vomiting or angioedema involving the mouth and throat immediately following ingestion), eg, cow's milk, legumes, cereal grains, potatoes, chocolate, eggs. (2) Foods eaten less often, eg, nuts, peanuts, fish or seafood, sunflower seeds, and melons—if vomiting and angioedema have not occurred. Usually, the parent or patient is already aware of the relationship between allergen and reaction if symptoms have immediately followed ingestion.

Procedure for provocative testing. After environmental factors are stabilized, withhold all suspected foods for at least 1 week; then challenge with a single food. Repeated offerings for a few days may be necessary to establish a hypersensitivity reaction.

Direct provocative inhalant testing is potentially hazardous and is best performed in a hospital setting.

5. Eosinophilia—Increased numbers of eosinophils in the blood or bodily secretions (nasal, gastrointestinal) are frequently present in a variety of allergic conditions, especially in atopic disorders, and the presence of eosinophilia may strengthen a suspicion of allergic diathesis. Nasal eosinophilia (> 15%) is highly suggestive of allergic rhinitis, but eosinophilia can occur in the absence of clinical allergies. Conversely, the absence of eosinophilia does not rule out allergy, particularly since a variety of factors (eg, concurrent infection) may suppress eosinophilia. The degree of eosinophilia correlates inversely with the degree of control of allergic and nonallergic asthma. Nasal eosinophilia in infants up to 3 months of age is considered normal.

Controversial Techniques for Diagnosis & Treatment

Intracutaneous end point titration, sublingual and serial intracutaneous provocative titration tests, cytotoxic tests, and sublingual desensitization all have been claimed by some to be of value in diagnosing and treating allergic disorders. Their merit is yet to be validated scientifically, and they remain techniques of unproved value that are not recommended.

Prophylaxis of Atopic Disorders

There is suggestive evidence that avoidance of cow products, eggs, wheat, and chicken during the first 9 months of life significantly lessens the likelihood of development of allergic rhinitis and asthma. Recently, evidence has been presented also that a diet excluding cow products, fish, and eggs for the first 6 months of life coupled with general environmental precautions minimizing house dust and animal dander contact is associated with a diminished likelihood of developing atopic dermatitis, at least in the first year. It seems prudent, therefore, to institute dietary and environmental restrictions mentioned above in the first few months of life in children with a strong family history of atopy.

Grieco MH: Controversial practices in allergy. *JAMA* 1982; **247:**3106.

Johnstone DE, Dutton AM: Dietary prophylaxis of allergic disease in children. *N Engl J Med* 1976;**274:**715.

Kniker WT, Hales SW, Lee LK: Diagnostic methods to demon-

strate IgE antibodies: Skin testing techniques. *Bull NY Acad Med* 1981;**57**:524.
Matthew DJ et al: Prevention of eczema. *Lancet* 1977;**1**:321.
Nelson H: Diagnostic procedures in allergy. 1. Allergy skin testing. *Ann Allergy* 1983;**4**:411.
Zieger RS: Atopy in infancy and early childhood: Natural history and role of skin testing. (Editorial.) *J Allergy Clin Immunol* 1985;**75**:633.
Zieger RS, Schatz M: Immunotherapy of atopic disorders: Present state of the art and future perspectives. *Med Clin North Am* 1981;**65**:987.

BRONCHIAL ASTHMA ("Reactive Airways Disorder")

Essentials of Diagnosis

- Paroxysmal or chronically exacerbating dyspnea characterized by bilateral wheezing, prolongation of expiration, hyperinflation of the lungs, and cough (overt wheezing may *not* occur).
- Reversal of abnormal pulmonary function to (or significantly toward) normal by injection of epinephrine, inhalation of adrenergic aerosols, or other therapeutic measures (can also reverse spontaneously).
- Eosinophilia of sputum and blood (common).
- Positive immediate skin test reactions to provoking allergens (common but not necessary).

General Considerations

Bronchial asthma is a largely reversible obstructive process of the tracheobronchial tree caused by mucosal edema, increased and unusually viscid secretions, and smooth muscle constriction. Especially in protracted asthmatic episodes, the obstructive pathologic changes may cause not only hypoxemia but retention of CO_2 and respiratory acidosis.

The incidence of asthma is reportedly less than 3% of the total population, but in the author's opinion, this is a gross underestimation. Before adolescence, boys are affected twice as frequently as girls. Onset is common in early childhood (but asthma frequently begins in adulthood). In the majority of cases in childhood, the onset is by the seventh year.

Evidence of sensitization to inhalant allergens is found in the majority of children with asthma. However, in many patients, offensive allergens cannot be identified by history or suggested by allergy testing, and IgE-mediated allergy, at least, does not appear to be related to the pathogenesis of the disorder. One does *not* have to be allergic to have asthma. Nevertheless, allergic sensitization probably plays a major role in the pathogenesis of asthma in many children and adults. When allergens contribute to or are major precipitants of asthma, "allergy" rarely is the sole significant factor involved (see below). The most common allergens causing asthma in children are inhalants: house dust mites, indoor molds, epidermals (especially the saliva and danders of cats and dogs), airborne pollens (trees, grasses, weeds), and out-of-doors seasonal molds. Foods occasionally provoke asthma, especially in infants, but this is less common in later childhood. The same allergens that cause asthma frequently cause allergic rhinitis in the same patient; many children with initial hay fever develop asthma.

An important pathogenic feature of asthma is an extraordinary "nonspecific" hyperreactivity of the tracheobronchial tree to various chemical mediators (eg, acetylcholine, histamine, leukotrienes) and, in turn, various insulting agents or events that cause their activation or liberation. Because of this feature, asthma is sometimes called "reactive airways disorder." (However, airway hyperreactivity is not always present in asthma.) In addition to allergic reactions, numerous factors trigger or aggravate asthma, principally upper and lower respiratory tract infections of *viral* origin. The role of bacterial organisms in the precipitation of asthma is a disputed question. Other triggering factors are rapid changes in temperature or barometric pressure, the common air pollutants in cities, cooking, odors, smoke, paint fumes, and exercise. Psychologic factors appear to be important in some cases but are seldom the sole cause. Aspirin idiosyncrasy can be a cause of asthma in childhood as well as in adult life.

Clinical Findings

A. History: Onset may be as early as the first few weeks of life. In infancy in particular, the first attack usually is associated with an upper respiratory tract infection or "bronchiolitis." As age increases, there is a progressively greater tendency for initial and subsequent episodes to be associated with inhalant allergens or irritants. The initial inciting event appears to render the tracheobronchial tree more susceptible to reactions to both similar and unrelated precipitants.

A history of atopic dermatitis or allergic rhinitis is often obtainable. A family history of atopic diseases (especially allergic rhinitis and bronchial asthma) is often present and is helpful in arousing suspicion of the diagnosis. Asthma can (and all too frequently does) occur in the absence of overt wheezing, and complaints may range from frequent "chest congestion" to recurrent cough. A careful physical examination, including chest auscultation on a forced expiratory maneuver rather than on simple tidal volume, or pulmonary function tests, can be revealing, especially when the patient is experiencing clinical discomfort.

B. Progressive Symptoms and Signs: The following may occur during an acute severe attack or if an attack is prolonged.

1. Distressing cough, dyspnea, increasing prolongation of expirations, high-pitched rhonchi and wheezes throughout the chest (diminishing in intensity as the obstruction becomes more severe), secretions (variable), hyperinflation, retractions, use of accessory respiratory muscles, poor air exchange.

2. Restlessness, apprehension, fatigue, drowsiness, coma.

3. Increasing tachycardia; initially, there may be

mild hypertension; ultimately, hypotension; rarely, signs of cardiac failure; pulsus paradoxicus.

4. Flushed, moist skin; pallid cyanosis; dry mucous membranes.

5. Initially good response to epinephrine or other adrenergic drugs or methylxanthines. If the attack is prolonged, the response to the above drugs may be poor.

C. Special Clinical Findings:

1. Episodes of asthma in association with infections are frequently insidious in onset and prolonged; those due to specific identifiable allergens tend to be acute in onset and relatively brief if the causative agent is removed.

2. Bronchial asthma in infants (under 2 years of age) deserves special comment. The first attack usually follows by a few days the onset of a respiratory infection; some degree of cough or wheezing may persist for prolonged periods and becomes worse with subsequent "colds."

3. In infants, the predominant symptoms may be dyspnea, excessive secretions, noisy and rattly breathing, cough, and, in many cases, some intercostal and suprasternal retractions—rather than the typical pronounced expiratory wheezes that occur in older children. Initial and repeated diagnoses of these episodes are apt to be "croup," "bronchiolitis," and "pneumonia." Infection (viral) is often present.

4. Cough frequently is a presenting symptom, with or without wheezing. Asthma can exist *without overt wheezing,* and "subclinical" wheezing may be detected only by careful physical examination including auscultation on a forced vital capacity maneuver, examination during an episode of "chest congestion," or pulmonary function testing.

5. A syndrome of paroxysmal cough, presumably tracheal in origin ("irritable trachea," "allergic cough"), occurs and may be difficult to differentiate from true asthma, particularly since bronchodilator drugs are sometimes effective in this condition. In this condition, wheezing generally does not occur and signs of lower respiratory tract obstruction are lacking. The condition frequently is provoked by a (viral) respiratory infection, and allergic factors may or may not play a role. This also may presage later asthma.

Chronic recurrent bronchial asthma may lead to invalidism (both organic and psychologic), barrel chest, and distensive emphysema; atelectasis and massive pulmonary collapse; mediastinal emphysema and pneumothorax; and death due to respiratory insufficiency, improper medication (sedatives, tranquilizers, narcotics), drug overdose (eg, with theophylline), or delayed or inadequate therapy. Sudden death may occur as a result of causes unknown and unrelated to respiratory insufficiency. Although asthma often is defined as a "reversible" obstructive airway disorder, chronic moderately severe to severe asthma may, in time, have a significant irreversible element, especially with prolonged exposure to cigarette smoke.

D. Laboratory Findings: Eosinophil accumulations (eg, clumps of eosinophils on sputum smear) and blood eosinophilia are commonly found but are often absent in infection or when corticosteroids are given. Their presence tends to reflect disease activity and does *not* necessarily mean that allergic factors are involved.

Hematocrit can be elevated with dehydration, as in prolonged attacks, or in severe chronic disease. In severe asthma, the first sign is hypoxemia without CO_2 retention. Respiratory acidosis and increased CO_2 tension may ensue. (Moderately severe hypoxemia may occur with low CO_2 tension due to a combination of hyperventilation and ventilation-perfusion disturbances.)

E. X-Ray Findings: Bilateral hyperinflation, bronchial thickening and peribronchial infiltration, and areas of densities (patchy atelectasis or associated bronchopneumonia) may be present. (Patchy atelectasis is common and often misread as pneumonitis.) The pulmonary arteries may also appear prominent.

F. Pulmonary Function Studies: (See Chapter 14.) Increased airway resistance occurs with a decrease in flow rates, decreased vital capacity (VC), and increased functional residual capacity (FRC) and residual volume (RV). The first 3 may be normal in asymptomatic intervals, but frequently there is residual hyperinflation chronically.

G. Allergy Tests: IgE antibodies to allergens may be present.

H. Provocative Tests:

1. Food and drugs—Clinical reactions occur within minutes to hours after ingestion.

2. Inhalants—A clinical reaction usually occurs immediately after inhalation and may occur again a few hours after challenge ("late" reaction). Asthma may occasionally be provoked by skin testing in unusually sensitive children.

Differential Diagnosis*

Bronchial asthma may be confused with middle and lower respiratory tract infections (eg, laryngotracheobronchitis, acute bronchiolitis, bronchopneumonia, and pertussis), especially in the very young.

Nasal "wheezes" may be transmitted to the chest (especially in infants) from upper airway edema, increased secretions, or other obstructing factors such as allergic rhinitis, upper respiratory tract infections, adenoidal hypertrophy, foreign body, choanal stenosis, and nasal polyps (eg, in cystic fibrosis).

Congenital laryngeal stridor is usually associated with other anomalies.

In tracheal or bronchial foreign body, dyspnea or wheezing is usually of sudden onset; on auscultation, the wheezes are usually but not always unilateral. Characteristic x-ray findings are not always present.

The differentiation between bronchial asthma and cystic fibrosis is made on the basis of high sweat sodium and chloride, a history (often present) in cystic

* See also Other Allergic Pulmonary Disorders, p 1005.

fibrosis of serious pulmonary infections since birth, a personal and family history of associated intestinal disturbances with profuse, bulky stools, and pancreatic enzyme deficiency. Chronic inflammatory changes seen on chest x-ray in cystic fibrosis also can be a helpful differential point. There is evidence, however, for a significant reactive airway (asthmatic) component with or without allergic precipitants in many children with cystic fibrosis, and it is clear that cystic fibrosis and asthma can coexist.

Tracheal or bronchial compression by extramural forces may resemble asthma and may be due to foreign body in the esophagus, aortic ring, anomalous vessels, or inflammatory or neoplastic lymphadenopathy.

Treatment of Mild & Moderate Asthma

A. Specific Measures: Insofar as possible, the patient should avoid contact with proved or suspected irritants and allergens. (See Environmental Control of Exposure, above.) Hyposensitization therapy is for allergens that cannot be avoided (eg, pollens, seasonal molds, and house dust mites) when such allergens play a substantial role in the disorder.

B. General Measures: Depending upon the frequency and severity of asthma, some or all of the measures listed below may be used, either with the onset of an asthmatic attack or as a constant regimen—especially during the times of year when asthma is most severe.

1. Education—The parents (and patient, if old enough) must understand the asthmatic process. Complete understanding of all recommendations is essential.

2. Liquefaction and expectoration of mucus—Maintain adequate hydration by encouraging oral fluid intake, or give intravenous fluids if necessary. The value of expectorants is dubious. Postural drainage, preceded by use of an adrenergic aerosol, up to every 4 hours *if tolerated* may be useful.

3. Bronchodilatation—The major bronchodilating drugs are theophylline (aminophylline) and adrenergic drugs used alone or in combination. Adrenergic aerosols are extremely useful but must not be abused. They can be as effective as injected drugs in reversing acute severe asthma and have fewer side effects.

4. Correction of metabolic acidosis—Correct metabolic acidosis, if present, by providing an adequate energy source to diminish ketosis (eg, 5% dextrose intravenously), food if tolerated, and bicarbonate (see below).

5. Corticosteroids—In severe acute asthma or in chronic asthma unresponsive to other measures, adrenal glucocorticoids may be indicated (see below). If chronic use of corticosteroids is necessary for adequate control of asthma, prednisone or other short-acting equivalent given before 8:00 AM on alternate days should be attempted. Topical aerosolized corticosteroids are a useful alternative. Before resorting to chronic corticosteroid therapy, cromolyn sodium, 20 mg by inhalation 3–4 times daily, should be given a therapeutic trial for at least 1 month.

6. Antibiotics—If there is evidence of bacterial infection, give antibiotics. Leukocytosis up to 15,000/μL is common in severe asthma without any evidence of bacterial infection (even higher counts can be seen after epinephrine administration). Patchy atelectasis can be confused with pneumonitis on x-ray.

7. Breathing and fitness exercises—In children with chronic or recurrent asthma, breathing and fitness exercises under the guidance of a properly trained physical therapist may assist the patient in aborting some attacks of asthma and improving muscular functions of the thoracic cage.

Exercise should be encouraged rather than restricted. Exercise-induced bronchospasm can be ameliorated, if necessary, by theophylline given 1–2 hours before exercise; by cromolyn sodium or adrenergic aerosol (albuterol is recommended), or both, just prior to exercise; or by a combination of these.

8. Airflow assessment—In instances when perception of the degree of airflow limitation may be poorly appreciated by the parents or patient, have the patient use a peak flow meter at home to assist in assessment of airflow.

9. Daily regimen for control of asthma—Children with frequent overt asthma attacks (eg, 1 or 2 per week) and evidence of more or less constant pulmonary obstruction should be on constant pharmacologic therapy. A daily regimen stimulating coughing and encouraging expectoration (eg, postural drainage at least twice a day) may be useful. Theophylline (taken orally) and cromolyn sodium (20 mg 3–4 times daily by inhalation) may be considered first-line drugs for chronic symptomatic asthma. Adrenergic drugs (and, if necessary, corticosteroids) may be added to the regimen.

Treatment of Acute Severe Asthma (Status Asthmaticus, Intractable Asthma)

This is a medical emergency!

A. Emergency Care: Epinephrine (1:200 solution; Sus-Phrine) or, if the child is cooperative, aerosolized adrenergic drugs given by a compressed air device, preferably with oxygen, are the drugs of first choice. Aerosolized adrenergic drugs have been found to be as effective as epinephrine, as least in older children, and have the advantage of minimizing systemic side effects. These drugs can be used every ½–1 hour. The shorter-acting β_2 agonist isoetharine is recommended initially rather than longer-acting β_2 drugs or isoproterenol. Dosages that do not induce jitteriness or tachycardia are used. The lack of therapeutic response to adrenergic drugs is sometimes used as the criterion for "status asthmaticus." Relative or apparent complete lack of responsiveness to these drugs may be due to hypoxemia and acidosis, bronchial obstruction with thick mucus plugs, pneumothorax, or simply severe asthma. Sensitivity to adrenergic drugs may improve after initiation of other therapy.

B. Hospital Care: If signs are relatively early, an overnight stay may suffice.

1. Give 5% dextrose solution with 0.2% saline intravenously at the first sign of resistance to epinephrine or with poor fluid intake, vomiting, or dehydration. (Use maintenance requirements; *do not overhydrate.*) Particularly if corticosteroids are used, remember to add potassium (10–20 meq/L of intravenous fluid) after urination is established.

2. Give moisturized oxygen (by mask or nasal prongs—not by tent) at a flow rate of approximately 4 L/min. All patients with acute severe asthma will be hypoxemic, largely as a result of the ventilation-perfusion imbalance that is integral to asthma.

3. Give aminophylline, 4–6 mg/kg, in intravenous tubing over a 10- to 20-minute period (if not used in previous 4 hours) and repeat every 4–6 hours, or give as a constant infusion beginning with a loading dose of 4–6 mg/kg over 15 minutes and then 0.6–1 mg/kg/h.*

4. Take an arterial or venous blood sample for pH and an arterial sample for P_{CO_2} and P_{O_2} determinations. Early in the course of an asthmatic paroxysm, the patient usually hyperventilates and blows off CO_2, with a resultant low P_{aCO2}. As the severity of the episode increases, the patient may become fatigued and may be unable to perform the necessary work, contributing to an increasing P_{aCO2}. (A "normal" as well as increased P_{aCO2} in acute severe asthma, in other words, is an indication of respiratory failure.) Continued close monitoring of blood gases and pH is essential to proper management of severe asthma. (Determination of gases or pH on capillary blood generally is unreliable.) An ear oximeter can be used to measure oxygen saturation of the blood; this is a useful substitute for measurement of arterial blood gases.

5. Correction of acidosis (pH 7.3 or below) with sodium bicarbonate should be attempted. With the increased work of breathing and hypoxemia, there may be metabolic acidosis due to lactic acid production. This may be compensated by a respiratory alkalosis due to hyperventilation. The appropriate bicarbonate dose may be calculated with the following formula:

$$\text{meq Bicarbonate needed} = \text{Negative base excess} \times 0.3 \times \text{Body weight in kg}$$

The bicarbonate can be given rapidly by the intravenous route.† Arterial or venous pH should be redetermined 5–10 minutes later, and further correction of acidosis, using bicarbonate, should be considered at that time if necessary. In respiratory failure, in the absence of a pH determination, 2 meq/kg may be infused initially.

6. Give isoetharine, 1% by inhalation (or other adrenergic aerosols) every 2–4 hours followed by postural drainage *as tolerated.* (The proper use of aerosolized adrenergic agents early in the course of acute severe asthma may obviate the need for injected epinephrine.)

7. If the patient is already receiving corticosteroids, do not withdraw but increase the dose temporarily. Corticosteroids may be withheld in attacks of mild to moderate severity responding satisfactorily to the other treatment measures. However, they should be used at once when the asthmatic attack is of sufficient severity to be life-threatening or when the patient has been on prolonged daily corticosteroid therapy (at least 2 weeks) in the past year. If it is decided that corticosteroids are to be used, one of the following should be given intravenously in the following initial doses every 4 hours around the clock: hydrocortisone sodium succinate (Solu-Cortef), 100 mg, or methylprednisolone (Solu-Medrol), 20 mg. (Add at least usual daily potassium requirements to intravenous fluids.) With amelioration of symptoms, the dose should be decreased as rapidly as possible. (If the patient has not been on prolonged corticosteroid therapy within the past year, the corticosteroids can be discontinued abruptly rather than tapered. It is frequently feasible to use high doses of corticosteroids for 48 hours or less.)

8. Give antibiotics as indicated.

9. In respiratory failure unresponsive to the above therapy, intravenous isoproterenol therapy or assisted ventilation by a mechanical respirator may be required. Failure to respond to the above measures can be defined as 2 arterial P_{CO_2} determinations above 45 mm Hg over a 15- to 30-minute period. This is the indication for insertion of an indwelling arterial catheter if that has not been done. If the steady-state arterial P_{CO_2} remains above 45 mm Hg in the blood drawn from the indwelling line, continuous isoproterenol infusions should be considered. This is *not* generally recommended for older adolescents or adults, however, because of the increased risk of inducing cardiac dysrhythmias. *Such an infusion should be undertaken only in an intensive care unit where continuous cardiac and blood pressure monitoring facilities are available.* An additional intravenous line should be started for the isoproterenol so that it is not infused into the only existing line. The infusion

* In patients receiving chronic theophylline therapy, use their usual total daily maintenance dose infused over a 24-hour period. Theophylline blood levels of 10–20 μg/mL serum are considered "optimally therapeutic" for hospitalized patients, but levels should be on the low side of this range when theophylline is used on a long-term basis. Average total daily dosages of theophylline to achieve therapeutic levels are listed below, but there is much individual variation in requirements. ***Caution:*** In the first few months of life, theophylline (aminophylline) is metabolized very slowly, and this drug should be used with extreme caution in patients at this age.

Age	Average Total Daily Dose ± SD
12 months to 8 years	25 ± 5 mg/kg
8–16 years	20 ± 5 mg/kg
Over 16 years	12 ± 3 mg/kg

† Sodium bicarbonate for injection may be obtained in ampules or multidose vials that contain approximately 1 meq/mL.

should be started at a rate of 0.1 μg/kg/min and increased by this amount every 10–15 minutes until there is clinical improvement or until the heart rate approaches 200 beats/min. The development of significant dysrhythmias is an indication for decreasing the rate of isoproterenol infusion. If a favorable response occurs, it is necessary to very slowly wean the patient from the isoproterenol, decreasing the rate of infusion over a period of 30–36 hours. Rebound bronchospasm may occur if the rate is decreased too rapidly.

If the arterial P_{CO_2} remains high or continues to increase despite the continuous isoproterenol infusion, endotracheal intubation should be performed and assisted ventilation initiated. A volume respirator capable of producing high inspiratory pressures should be used. Since these patients have prolonged expiratory times as a result of the marked airway resistance, it is necessary to set an adequate expiratory time on the ventilator to avoid further air trapping within the lung. The need for assisted ventilation for status asthmaticus in children has been reduced since the introduction of the continuous isoproterenol infusion. *Intubation and assisted ventilation should be performed only by medical personnel trained in such techniques.*

C. Precautions in Therapy: Note the following "don'ts":

1. Don't use narcotics or barbiturates. (They depress the respiratory center. Tranquilizers may do the same in the presence of severe hypoxemia.)

2. Don't use epinephrine excessively. (It tends to thicken secretions, depletes glycogen stores, and increases apprehension.)

3. Don't use adrenergic aerosols excessively. (Discontinue temporarily if responsiveness to aerosol therapy is not apparent. Reduce dosage if systemic side effects occur.)

D. Follow-Up Therapy:

1. Fluids—When the patient is improved and is able to take fluids and oral medications, give oral fluids in the form of fruit juices but not fluids containing caffeine and chocolate. Give no milk or iced drinks.

2. Drugs—The following medications are of value at this stage:

a. Adrenergic aerosol every 4–6 hours, followed by postural drainage for 20 minutes as tolerated.

b. Theophylline orally (dosage according to weight).

c. If corticosteroids have been started, withdraw after 72 hours or taper gradually and discontinue as soon as possible.

Prognosis

There is no evidence that bronchial asthma can be cured, and the old adage still holds: "Once an asthmatic, always an asthmatic." However, the prognosis for symptom-free control in childhood asthma is fairly good. The majority of asthmatic children have less symptomatic asthma in their teens, and some appear to lose any asthmatic symptomatology for life. Unfortunately, however, only a minority (probably < 30%) fall into this category, and it is usually the pediatrician rather than the disorder that the child outgrows. Many have persistent, significant (though often unrecognized) chronic pulmonary obstruction, and others later redevelop symptomatic obstruction.

Reports indicate that in the past 25–30 years the morbidity and mortality rates in asthma may have increased, but it is not clear whether this increase is due to the diagnosis of more cases of "infectious" or "intrinsic" asthma, increased air pollution, the use of isoproterenol aerosols, or corticosteroid therapy. Mortality statistics indicate that a high percentage of deaths have been due to indiscriminate use of sedatives, narcotics, and aminophylline, but many also are from undertreatment, particularly in labile asthmatics and asthmatics whose perception of pulmonary obstruction is poor.

"Continuity" symptoms of night cough, breathlessness, and provocation of wheezing with exercise or stress are usually indicative of more serious disease than occasional, spontaneous, and brief attacks due to recognizable allergens, with symptom-free periods in between. "Mild" asthma is more likely to be "outgrown" than moderate or severe asthma. Prolonged exposure of asthmatic children to cigarette smoke ("passive smoking") is associated with increased risk of irreversible small airway obstruction in adulthood.

Bierman CW, Pearlman DS: Asthma. Chap 41, p 496, in: *Disorders of the Respiratory Tract in Children,* 4th ed. Kendig EL Jr, Chernick V (editors). Saunders, 1983.

Lichtenstein LM, Valentine MD, Norman PS: A reevaluation of immunotherapy for asthma. *Am Rev Respir Dis* 1984;**129:**657.

Mansmann HC Jr: The evaluation, control, and modification of continuing asthma. *Clin Chest Med* 1980;**1:**339.

Mellis CM, Phelan PD: Asthma death in children: A continuing problem. *Thorax* 1977;**32:**29.

Pearlman DS. Bronchial asthma: A perspective from childhood to adulthood. *Am J Dis Child* 1984;**138:**459.

Welliver RC: Pediatric asthma: The role of infection. *J Respir Dis* 1983;**4:**46.

Zeiger RS: Special considerations in the approach to asthma in infancy and early childhood. *J Asthma* 1983;**20:**341.

ALLERGIC RHINITIS

Essentials of Diagnosis

- Chronic or recurrent nasal obstruction; itching and sneezing (frequently paroxysmal) with seromucoid discharge. There may be accompanying conjunctival injection and itching, with or without tearing.
- Mucosal hyperemia to purplish pallor and edema of nasal mucous membranes.
- Eosinophilia of nasal secretions when symptomatic. (May be absent with infections or possibly with corticosteroid therapy.)
- Presence of IgE antibody to provoking allergens (supportive evidence only).

General Considerations

Allergic rhinitis is the most common atopic disease, perhaps because the nose is anatomically and physiologically vulnerable to inhalant allergens. The pathologic changes are chiefly hyperemia, edema, and increased serous and mucoid secretions due to mediator release, all of which lead to variable degrees of nasal obstruction, rhinorrhea, and pruritus. Inhalant allergens are principally responsible for causation of symptoms, but food allergens on occasion may provoke rhinitis.

Classification

Allergic rhinitis may be classified as perennial, seasonal (hay fever), or episodic, but these entities frequently occur concomitantly. Children with allergic rhinitis seem to be more susceptible to upper respiratory infections, which in turn intensify the symptoms of existing allergic rhinitis.

A. Perennial Allergic Rhinitis: Perennial allergic rhinitis occurs to some degree all year long but may be more severe in winter. Frequently, it "blows up" when forced air heating systems are turned on in the fall, causing increased exposure to house dusts. Nasal stuffiness, frequent sniffing, and constant rhinorrhea with evidence of mild to moderate itching (frequent nose rubbing) are often the dominant symptoms, although more severe symptoms, including paroxysmal sneezing, may occur. Sneezing is often most pronounced in the morning shortly after waking. Poor appetite, fatigue, and pharyngeal irritation from nasopharyngeal mucus drainage are not unusual accompanying symptoms. Greater exposure to house dust during the winter months is due to increased indoor activities and heating systems that raise, disperse, and circulate dust. The increased dryness of heated air and greater exposure to pets housed indoors may also add to the problem.

This disease frequently begins before the second year of life. It often accompanies bronchial asthma and may be provoked by the same allergens. Dental abnormalitites, including disturbances in dental arch growth and malocclusion, have been attributed to long-standing perennial allergic rhinitis with nasal obstruction.

B. Seasonal Allergic Rhinitis (Hay Fever): Hay fever occurs seasonally as a result of exposure to specific wind-borne pollens. The major important pollen groups in the temperate zones are trees (late winter, early spring), grasses (spring to early summer), and weeds (late summer to early fall). Seasons may vary significantly in different parts of the country. Mold spores also cause seasonal allergic rhinitis, principally in the summer and fall.

The age at onset is generally later than for perennial allergic rhinitis, usually after 2 years of age. Worsening or extension of pollen sensitivities over a period of several years after onset can be expected.

C. Vasomotor (Nonallergic, Noninfectious) Rhinitis: This form of perennial rhinitis, which occurs in children and adults, masquerades as allergic rhinitis. Manifestations of the condition include variable degrees of serous or mucoid rhinorrhea and nasal stuffiness, often with pharyngeal drainage and with or without significant nasal itching. Diagnosis depends upon ruling out an allergic or infectious cause. Rarely, there may be nasal eosinophilia.

Clinical Findings

A. Symptoms and Signs: Nasal obstruction is manifested by mouth breathing, snoring, difficulty in nursing or eating, nasal speech, and inability to clear the nose with blowing. Nasal seromucoid secretions are increased, with anterior drainage, sniffling, "nasal stuffiness," postnasal drip, and loose cough. Nasal itching leads to nose rubbing ("allergic salute," "bunny nose"), nose picking, epistaxis, and sneezing. Eye manifestations consist of itching, tearing, conjunctival injection, lid and periobital edema, and circumorbital cyanosis ("allergic shiners"). Palatal and pharyngeal itching may occur, as well as pharyngeal soreness, irritation, and hoarseness. Headache, head "fullness," lassitude, or frank fatigue often occurs. In perennial rhinitis, nasal obstruction tends to be a predominant symptom; in seasonal rhinitis, there tends to be more intense itching, coryza, and sneezing.

Examination shows decreased patency of nasal airways and increased seromucoid discharge (usually more serous in seasonal rhinitis). The mucous membranes range from reddened with little edema to pale blue, swollen, and boggy, with dimpling in the turbinates. Increased pharyngeal lymphoid tissue from chronic pharyngeal drainage or enlarged tonsillar and adenoid tissue may be present. Bleeding points or ulceration may be seen on the anterior nasal septum. There may be a horizontal crease extending across the lower third of the nose, owing to frequent upward rubbing of the nose. Malocclusion (overbite), presumably due to excess pressure of digit sucking to relieve palatal itching, may be seen in long-standing cases.

The florid conjunctival injection, coryza, intense itching of the eyes and nose, and violent sneezing experienced by older children and adults are not so commonly seen in young children. Paroxysmal sneezing, however, is frequent even in young children.

B. Laboratory Findings: Eosinophilia frequently can be demonstrated on smears of nasal secretions or blood (usually higher in seasonal than perennial rhinitis). The technique of examination of nasal secretions is as follows:

1. Obtain nasal secretions by having the patient blow onto a piece of wax paper or by nasal swab; spread on a microscope slide and allow to dry.
2. Cover the slide with Hansel's stain for 1–2 minutes.
3. Add enough distilled water to take up staining solution and allow to stand 1 minute.
4. Wash with distilled water.
5. Flood with 95% ethanol and drain off immediately; allow to dry.
6. Examine under the oil immersion objective.

Look for consistently greater than 15% eosinophils or accumulation (clumps) of eosinophils.

C. Allergy Testing: Skin or serologic tests may reveal IgE antibody to offending allergens.

D. Associated Conditions: Sinusitis may accompany allergic rhinitis and is frequently demonstrable on x-ray (mucosal thickening, fluid levels, or complete opacification of sinuses). Vigorous treatment is indicated until there is complete resolution of x-ray as well as clinical findings. Auditory (eustachian) tube dysfunction and chronic or recurrent serous or secretory otitis media can also be a complication of allergic rhinitis.

Some cases of secretory or serous otitis media are thought to be an extension of the pathologic changes of allergic rhinitis (edema and increased secretory activity of the mucosa) involving the auditory tubes and the epithelial lining of the middle ear. The results are episodic obstruction of the auditory tubes, metaplastic mucosal changes, accumulation of viscid secretions within the middle ear, and decreased mobility (with or without fullness or retraction) of the tympanic membrane. The membrane sometimes ruptures. Hearing loss, earache and ear plugging, and frequent "colds" are common complaints. This entity is most common in small children and is seldom seen after 8 years of age.

The atopic young child seems to be particularly prone to the development of serous otitis media. The middle ear probably is not a "shock organ" for allergy per se; there is little evidence that allergy-associated serous otitis media exists in the absence of allergic rhinitis. Etiologic allergens are those responsible for the rhinitis. Intercurrent ear infections are common in this disorder and tend to complicate the underlying problem. Although allergic factors appear to be important in many cases of serous otitis media, most cases do not appear to be associated with "allergy."

Differential Diagnosis

These disorders must be differentiated from the common cold, other infectious diseases (eg, purulent rhinitis and sinusitis), adenoidal hypertrophy, foreign bodies (usually unilateral), nasal polyposis with cystic fibrosis or aspirin idiosyncrasy (nasal polyposis is rarely due to allergy), choanal stenois or atresia, nasopharyngeal neoplasms, palatal malformations (eg, congenitally high arch, cleft palate), and "vasomotor" rhinitis.

Treatment

A. Specific Measures:

1. Avoid exposure to proved allergens insofar as is reasonably possible. (See Environmental Control of Exposure, above.)

2. Hyposensitization should be considered when symptoms are severe and other symptomatic measures have failed and when the disease is associated with complications such as chronic or recurrent sinusitis, recurrent serous otitis media, and hearing loss. There is controversial evidence that hyposensitization for hay fever may prevent the onset of asthma; some allergists (but not this author) therefore favor hyposensitization therapy in all children with hay fever in whom an inciting allergen can be identified.

B. General Measures:

1. Give antihistamines with or without vasoconstricting adrenergic drugs by mouth. (See Table 32–1.)

2. Treat associated infections.

3. Topical decongestants (eg, phenylephrine) can be used for *no more than 5 days* for severe episodes. Corticosteroids (topical or systemic) can be used for short periods in polypoid states or up to a few weeks for severe nasal symptoms not controllable by other means.

4. Surgical procedures (removal of nasal polyps, creation of antral windows for maxillary sinusitis, insertion of ventilating tubes for chronic otitis media) should be considered only when medical therapy fails.

Prognosis

A. Perennial Allergic Rhinitis: Unless specific allergens can be identified and eliminated from the environment or diet (unusual cases), this atopic disease tends to be very protracted. If polypoid growths do not appear, nasal obstruction may become less troublesome as the child grows and the nasal airway increases in caliber.

B. Seasonal Allergic Rhinitis: Hay fever patients tend to repeat their seasonal symptoms if exposure to offending allergens is high. On moving to a region devoid of problem allergens, they may be free of seasonal allergic rhinitis for 1–3 years but frequently acquire new pollen hypersensitivities from airborne pollens in the areas to which they move. (*Example:* On moving to the Rocky Mountain region from mideastern USA, patients usually become less symptomatic to ragweed because of low exposure but acquire hypersensitivity to tumbleweeds and sages.)

Bierman CW (editor): ENT allergy. *Clin Rev Allergy* 1984;**2:**169.

Bluestone CD: Eustachian tube function: Physiology, pathophysiology, and role of allergy in the pathogenesis of otitis media. *J Allergy Clin Immunol* 1983;**72:**242.

Forstot L: Diseases of the eye. In: *Allergic Disease of Infancy, Childhood, and Adolescence.* Bierman CW, Pearlman DS (editors). Saunders, 1980.

Kraemer MJ et al: Risk factors for persistent middle-ear effusions: Otitis media, catarrh, cigarette smoke exposure, and atopy. *JAMA* 1983;**249:**1022.

Norman PS: Allergic rhinitis. *J Allergy Clin Immunol* 1985;**75:**531.

Pearlman DS: Chronic rhinitis in children. *Clin Rev Allergy* 1984;**2:**197.

Zeiger RS, Schatz M: Chronic rhinitis: A practical approach to diagnosis and treatment. (2 parts.) *Immunol Allergy Pract* 1982;**4:**63, 108.

ATOPIC DERMATITIS*
(Infantile Eczema)

Essentials of Diagnosis

- Lesions varying from erythematous and papular to scaling, vesicular, and oozing; lichenification in more chronic forms.
- Predilection in infants for cheeks and extensor areas and in older children and adolescents for flexural creases.
- Pruritus, frequently intense.

General Considerations

Atopic dermatitis is considered by many to be an atopic disorder because of its frequent association with allergic rhinitis and asthma and because of the high incidence of IgE antibodies in children with this disorder. However, the role of IgE antibody (particularly antibody to inhalant allergens) in its pathogenesis is controversial. Children with atopic dermatitis have many immune aberrations, but the role of these immune defects is unclear. The common denominator in all individuals with atopic dermatitis appears to be a lowered threshold for itching; atopic dermatitis has been called "an itch that rashes."

In some infants, certain foods precipitate or aggravate eczema, and IgE antibody to these foods may be demonstrated. When eczema persists beyond age 2 years in such children, food-induced aggravation may disappear. Eczema may be made worse by exposure to environmental substances considered to be allergens (eg, animal danders), but this aggravation may be based upon nonallergic mechanisms in some cases. In some older children and adolescents, a striking seasonal worsening of eczema correlates with other evidence of sensitivity to inhalant allergens, and there are frequent claims that hyposensitization to unavoidable allergens leads to amelioration of dermatitis. Allergic reactions to foods or other substances may precipitate or aggravate eczema but are rarely the only or even the predominant causative factor. Certain foods, especially citrus fruits and tomatoes, will not uncommonly induce facial erythema in children with atopic dermatitis, but it is not clear whether they induce more extensive dermatitis. Other foods implicated with some frequency in atopic dermatitis include egg white, milk, legumes (including peanut butter), wheat, and corn.

Scratching plays a major role in the occurrence and progression of dermatitis, predisposing the skin to infection. Factors that aggravate itching include dryness, sweating, and contact with rough materials and detergents. Psychologic factors may intensify itching and complicate management at home and at school.

Clinical Findings

A. Symptoms and Signs: Although infantile eczema ordinarily begins in infancy, it can begin at almost any time in childhood. In infants, lesions typically appear after 2 months of age, beginning on the cheeks and forehead and spreading in a patchy or generalized distribution over the extremities and trunk. Initially, involvement of extremities is primarily on extensor surfaces, but after infancy, involvement of flexural creases (antecubital, popliteal, neck) predominates; frequently, the wrists, hands, feet, face, and eyelids are also involved. The lesions may vary from facial erythema and minimal scaling to frank oozing and "weeping." As the child grows older, the eczema tends to wax and wane, sometimes disappearing completely for months, and in many children abating altogether by age 3 years. The skin may be thickened and somewhat plaquelike (lichenified) because of long-standing irritation from scratching. Although scarring is unusual, hyper- and hypopigmentation may occur. Excessive skin dryness is a frequent concomitant finding in eczema, and a form of congenital ichthyosis often accompanies atopic dermatitis. Infection sometimes occurs, although it is not usual, even though the concentration of staphylococci in and on the skin of children with atopic dermatitis tends to be much higher than normal.

B. Laboratory Findings: There are no practical tests for atopic dermatitis. IgE immunoglobulin levels are frequently elevated, and there may be specific IgE antibodies to various inhalant and food allergens. Eosinophilia may occur but is not necessarily evidence of allergy.

Differential Diagnosis

Seborrheic dermatitis may be distinguished by lack of significant pruritus, its predilection for the scalp ("cradle cap"), and its coarse yellowish "potato chip" scales. Seborrheic dermatitis may occur in association with atopic dermatitis. Candidiasis occurs predominantly in the diaper region and is characteristically intensely red, with satellite lesions. Contact dermatitis is distinguished chiefly by the distribution of lesions (usually on extensors and exposed areas), generally with a greater demarcation of dermatitis than in atopic dermatitis. Nummular eczema is characterized by coin-shaped plaques, with minimal to sometimes intense eczema. Scabies is more papulovesicular and relatively nonerythematous, occurring chiefly in the interdigital and waistline areas, with itching that may be intense particularly at night; because of scratching, an eczematous dermatitis may develop.

Various other disorders have associated skin eruptions that may resemble atopic dermatitis. These include Wiskott-Aldrich syndrome, X-linked agammaglobulinemia, ataxia-telangiectasia, severe combined immunodeficiency disease, phenylketonuria, Hurler's syndrome, Hartnup syndrome, and ahistidinemia.

In Buckley's syndrome, there is marked elevation of IgE, with a dermatitis associated with increased susceptibility to infectious agents, especially staphylococci. The skin eruption is easily distinguishable from atopic dermatitis.

* From the perspective of a pediatric allergist (see also Dermatitis, Chapter 10).

Complications & Sequelae

Bacterial skin infections, particularly those produced by staphylococcal and streptococcal organisms, occur with some frequency. Viral infections, mainly with herpesvirus (Kaposi's varicelliform eruption), can occur from exposure to individuals with herpetic lesions, and varicella can be unusually severe in children with atopic dermatitis, although this generally is not a problem.

Nutritional disturbances may result from unwarranted and unnecessarily vigorous dietary restrictions imposed by physicians and parents. Cataracts in late childhood or adulthood occur in a small percentage of cases, even when corticosteroids are not used in treatment. Temporary or chronic emotional disturbances may occur as a result of feelings of disfigurement, imposed restrictions, and unhealthy attitudes of parents toward a child with this disease. Poor academic performance and behavioral disturbances may be a result of uncontrolled intense or frequent itching.

Treatment

Good general skin care and vigorous specific dermatologic treatment are the most important aspects of treatment of atopic dermatitis. Any foods that have been shown to aggravate eczema should be eliminated, as long as the diet remains nutritionally adequate. Minimizing direct contact with irritants (wool and other rough materials, irritating soaps and detergents), avoiding excessive sweating, and maintaining good skin hydration are important. Hyposensitization is rarely of value.

A. General Skin Care: Provide good skin hydration and have the patient bathe at least daily, using a bath oil (Alpha Keri or Lubath) added halfway through the bath; superfatted and nonirritating soaps (Basis, Dove, Lowila, or Neutrogena) should be used, and soap should be thoroughly rinsed off the skin. The skin may be patted partly dry, and areas that are ordinarily excessively dry can then be coated with a small amount of bland cream (eg, Eucerin) to help trap water in the skin.

B. Acute Weeping Stage: Apply Burow's solution (aluminum subacetate) soaks made up to 1:20 solution (Domeboro tablets or packets) for 20 minutes, using 3 layers of gauze or linen thoroughly moistened with solution 4 times a day. Do not use for more than 3 days. Treat infection with a systemic antibiotic (eg, cephalexin, erythromycin). Antihistamines can be used as antipruritic agents but are of secondary importance to topical treatment in controlling pruritus. Hydroxyzine (Atarax) is of value.

C. Subacute and Chronic Stages: The liberal use of emollients along with the *cautious* use of corticosteroid topical agents to control inflammation is the mainstay of therapy. Encourage daily bathing followed by application of corticosteroid cream to allow for penetration of the corticosteroid through the skin barrier and to aid in trapping water in the skin. Although creams are generally preferred to ointments, ointments may be more effective in some situations. Corticosteroids should be applied 2–3 times a day until inflammation is controlled. With subsidence of active inflammation, bland creams should be substituted. The choice of a corticosteroid preparation depends upon the degree of inflammation and, to some extent, the location of the lesions. Potent (fluorinated) topical agents are used for short periods of time to bring inflammation under control; with more chronic use, the weakest preparations compatible with control are used. (Hydrocortisone cream, 0.5–1%, is recommended.) Corticosteroid absorption from a potent agent used for a prolonged period and over large areas of inflamed skin (especially if used under occlusive dressing) can produce adrenal suppression and other complications of systemic corticosteroid therapy. Prolonged use of topical corticosteroids may also produce skin thinning. Potent topical corticosteroids should not be used with any frequency or duration on the face or periorbital areas.

An alternative approach to therapy (the Scholtz regimen) avoids bathing with water completely. A moist washcloth can be used to clean the groin and axillary areas; otherwise, Cetaphil lotion, which consists primarily of propylene glycol, sodium lauryl sulfate, and acetyl alcohol in water, is applied liberally until it foams and is then gently wiped from the skin, leaving a thin film of lotion on the skin. In the author's experience, this regimen is of limited value in a dry climate. Topical ointments of any kind, except for topical corticosteroid preparations in the form of creams or solutions, are avoided.

Systemic corticosteroids may in rare instances be necessary to aid in controlling severe eczema. They should be used for the shortest period of time possible (no more than 3–5 days).

Prognosis

Most cases of atopic dermatitis resolve spontaneously by 3 years of age, but atopic dermatitis may persist through childhood and even into adult life. With severe dermatitis, emotional problems may require special consideration. There is a high likelihood (up to 80% of children in some series) that a child with atopic dermatitis will develop allergic rhinitis, asthma, or both. Consequently, it seems wise to institute simple environmental control procedures in the homes of children with atopic dermatitis and to follow these children particularly closely for the development of these disorders.

Clark SD, Wolf JE Jr: Current management of atopic dermatitis. *Immunol Allergy Pract* 1984;**6:**457.

Pearlman DS: Management of atopic dermatitis: An allergist's point of view. *Cutis* 1974;**13:**1029.

Rajka G: *Atopic Dermatitis.* Saunders, 1975.

Sampson H: Increased plasma histamine concentrations after food challenges in children with atopic dermatitis. *N Engl J Med* 1984;**311:**372.

ADVERSE REACTIONS TO FOODS

Adverse reactions to foods occur quite frequently. Although these reactions are often diagnosed as "allergic," they can be caused by many other factors that are nonimmune in origin, such as pharmacologic or biochemical mechanisms, or by food toxins. Reactions can occur in all body tissues. A wide variety of signs and symptoms can be encountered, many of which may appear extremely vague. Serious allergic reactions include anaphylaxis, acute angioedema of the upper airway, and severe bronchial asthma provoked especially by eggs, shellfish, fish, cow's milk (see Chapter 19), walnuts, peanuts, pork, melons, and certain seeds (sesame, sunflower). Such reactions usually occur from within minutes to 2 hours. Other symptom complexes of lesser consequence, both allergic and nonallergic, can also occur in response to a variety of common foods. These are more likely to appear after several hours.

Syndromes Sometimes Associated With Food Sensitivity

A. Angioedema: Angioedema is often accompanied by urticaria. In mild cases, findings include periorbital and lip edema, a few hives, mild arthralgia, and malaise. In severe cases, there may be tongue, pharyngeal, and laryngotracheal edema and joint swelling. Death may occur from asphyxia. (See Medical Emergencies Due to Allergic Reactions.)

B. Anaphylaxis: Immediate reaction is characterized by light-headedness to syncope, flushing to pallor, paresthesias, generalized itching, palpitations, and tachycardia. There may be symptoms and signs of pulmonary edema, bronchial asthma, and vascular collapse. (See Medical Emergencies Due to Allergic Reactions.)

C. Gastrointestinal Intolerance: In mild cases, findings may include nausea, diarrhea, flatulence, bloating, and abdominal discomfort. In severe cases, there may be forceful vomiting, severe colic, bloody and mucoid diarrhea, and dehydration. Prolonged episodes of gastrointestinal intolerance can result in malnutrition and growth retardation. In many instances, food-associated symptoms are attributed to "allergy" but the mechanism upon which the reaction is based is unclear.

D. Perennial Allergic Rhinitis, Bronchial Asthma, Atopic Dermatitis, Urticaria: See elsewhere in this chapter.

E. Tension-Fatigue Syndrome: A combination of fatigue, lassitude, irritability, sleeplessness, disturbed behavior, disinterest, pallor, "shadowy" eyes with "allergic pleats," "run-down feeling," and sometimes a generalized headache with vague abdominal complaints has been reported. This syndrome may or may not be associated with atopic disorders. It may be related to inhalant allergens but frequently seems to be provoked by foods commonly and abundantly eaten, eg, cow's milk, cereal grains, chocolate, eggs, pork. The diagnosis of this syndrome is frequently difficult and is one of exclusion of many other mild and chronic disease states, particularly in a patient who has no other evidence of allergic disease. It is not clear that these food-associated symptoms are mediated by an allergic mechanism. Claims that salicylates, dyes, sugar, and other food ingredients may add to hyperactivity in children with minimal brain dysfunction are controversial, and in the occasional child who appears to be benefited by restricted diets (eg, the "Feingold diet") there is no evidence of an allergic reaction to the foodstuffs involved.

F. Migraine: In addition to other causes, foods may precipitate a migrainous episode. Certain foods such as chocolate, cheeses, liver, and some wines and beers in which significant amounts of vasoactive amines have been found have been demonstrated to precipitate migraine.

Clinical Findings

A. History; Symptoms and Signs: See above in the section on history in the discussion of atopic disorders and see individual disorders.

B. Laboratory Findings:

1. Eosinophilia of stool mucus may be present in cases of gastrointestinal allergy but may be a normal finding in the first 3 months of life; blood eosinophilia may occur.

2. Large positive reactions in skin tests (use scratch or prick tests only) are likely to be clinically relevant; mild (1–2+) reactions correlate poorly with clinical sensitivity. Negative reactions do not rule out a nonimmune clinical reaction or even an allergic reaction to some elements of food (eg, partially hydrolyzed product).

3. Serologic tests are in principle the same as skin tests. RAST scores of less than 3 are usually not associated with clinical sensitivity.

4. Provocative food tests are important in the less serious entities. Elimination, challenge, and rechallenge must be relied upon for definitive diagnosis. In very serious reactions such as angioedema, anaphylaxis, and bronchial asthma, the causative food is usually known by the patient or parents or can be identified by the physician with the aid of a history. Food challenges and food skin testing would be hazardous in these situations. In the less serious and more obscure symptom entities, the likely food is a common one (eg, milk); the suspected food should be withdrawn for 1 week before challenge.

Differential Diagnosis of Important Symptoms

A. Gastrointestinal Intolerance: Differentiate from cystic fibrosis, pyloric stenosis, celiac disease, acute or chronic intestinal infections, gastrointestinal malformations, carbohydrate enzyme deficiencies (eg, lactase), and irritable bowel syndrome.

B. Angioedema of the Upper Airway: Differentiate from acute epiglottitis and foreign body in the upper airway.

Treatment & Prognosis

Treatment consists of eliminating the offending food, but with specific advice for ensuring the nutritional adequacy of the diet. If milk or a milk substitute is withdrawn from the diet for over 1 month, the daily maintenance requirement of calcium should be administered (see Chapter 4). ***Note:*** To be condemned—especially in the growing child—is the unnecessary and unjustified restriction of many foods over an indefinite period merely because they *might* be involved or happened to give a positive skin test reaction.

Treat specific signs or symptoms as indicated.

The prognosis is good if the offending food can be identified. In some of the vague chronic syndromes, this may not be possible, in which case the patient will remain symptomatic. In the severe syndromes, the responsible food is usually known and can be avoided.

Anderson JA, Sogn DD (editors): *Adverse Reactions to Foods: AAAI and NIAID Report.* US Department of Health and Human Services Publication No. (NIH) 84–2442, 1984.

Bahna SL, Heiner DC: *Allergies to Milk.* Grune & Stratton, 1980.

Bock SA: Food sensitivity: A critical review and practical approach. *Am J Dis Child* 1980;**134:**973.

Defined diets and childhood hyperactivity: Consensus Development Conference (NIH). *JAMA* 1982;**248:**290.

Heiner DC (editor): Food allergy. *Clin Rev Allergy* 1984;**2:**1. [Entire issue.]

CONTACT DERMATITIS

Essentials of Diagnosis

- Erythematous, papular eruption that may progress to include vesiculation, bulla formation, and denudation.
- Pruritus, often intense.
- Eruption confined more or less to areas of direct skin contact with allergen.

General Considerations

Contact dermatitis is a delayed hypersensitivity reaction in the skin. The allergen is believed to conjugate locally with skin tissue elements. Sensitization after initial contact requires at least a few days, but an already sensitized individual may react to allergen contact in as little as 24 hours. Fur, leather and fabric dyes, formalin, dichromates (used in leather), nickel, rubber compounds, ethylenediamine (used in topical medications), neomycin, poison ivy, poison oak, and poison sumac are the most common offenders in contact dermatitis. Although most contact is local, dermatitis can be induced systemically in an already sensitized individual by ingestion of the antigen.

Clinical Findings

A. History: A history of contact with possible allergens appropriate to the distribution of the lesions, in conjunction with the appearance of the lesions, may be sufficient for the diagnosis or may serve only as a starting point for further investigation. Itching is the rule, is frequently intense, and may precede the onset of observable lesions.

B. Physical Examination: The appearance and distribution of the lesions are the main criteria for diagnosis. Eruptions may be confined to areas of contact with the offending allergen, and inflammations may be sharply demarcated from normal skin. With more severe and chronic eruptions, however, dissemination may occur as a result of scratching and repeated contact with the allergen. If the eruption is mild, only erythema with some papulation may be present; more intense reactions include vesiculation with denudation of skin and frank weeping. Exfoliative dermatitis and secondary infection can also occur. There may be evidence of excoriation reflecting the pruritic nature of these lesions. With chronic dermatitis, skin thickening may be present.

C. Patch Testing: Patch testing with suspected allergens can be used to identify the contactants involved. In general, patch testing should not be performed when the dermatitis is active, since this procedure may exacerbate the dermatitis. Patch testing kits of common contact allergens can be obtained from a variety of firms dealing with allergenic materials.

Differential Diagnosis

Seborrheic dermatitis, atopic dermatitis, scabies, papular urticaria, nummular eczema, dermatophytoses, and candidiasis may at times be confused with contact dermatitis.

Prevention

Sensitizing substances should be avoided. Inflamed skin is more susceptible to sensitization than normal skin, and virtually any substance applied to the skin is potentially sensitizing; use only those topical agents considered necessary for treatment.

Parenteral or oral hyposensitization is not generally successful and can induce serious reactions. Moreover, the striking beneficial effects of a brief course of local or systemic corticosteroid treatment virtually nullify justification for hyposensitization at the present time.

Treatment

A. Early Treatment:

1. Terminate exposure to the contactant.

2. Soaks with Burow's solution (Domeboro powder or tablet, 1 package or tablet to 1–2 pints of water) or with a 1:6000 solution of potassium permanganate (0.3-g tablet plus 2 quarts of water) may be used in the early stage of treatment, especially if oozing is present, to diminish itching.

B. Mild Dermatitis: A short period of treatment with a mild adrenocorticosteroid cream or ointment is recommended.

C. Severe Dermatitis: Creams or ointments containing potent corticosteroids are helpful. These should be applied liberally and frequently so as to keep the inflamed areas covered at all times. In unusual circumstances, when the dermatitis is extremely severe and extensive, systemic corticosteroids should be considered. A short course of systemic corticosteroids followed by topical corticosteroid administration is frequently helpful in controlling acute severe contact dermatitis (eg, poison ivy dermatitis). Pastes, ointments, and creams should not be applied to weeping skin.

D. General Measures:

1. Avoid all secondary irritants to the skin, eg, wool, detergents.

2. Treat infection, if present. Early, potassium permanganate solution may be employed instead of Burow's solution. This topical treatment may be sufficient; however, with extensive lesions, systemic antibiotic therapy must be used. Topical antibiotics should not be used, because they have potential for sensitization.

3. Give antihistamines orally for pruritus (hydroxyzine is recommended). Colloidal soaks, such as starch baths, may be employed with extensive dermatitis.

DeWeck AL: Contact eczematous dermatitis. Pages 669–680 in: *Dermatology in General Medicine*. Fitzpatrick TB et al (editors). McGraw-Hill, 1971.

Fisher AA: *Contact Dermatitis*, 2nd ed. Lea & Febiger, 1973.

Parker F: Contact dermatitis. Chap 32, pp 431–439, in: *Allergic Diseases of Infancy, Childhood and Adolescence*. Bierman CW, Pearlman DS (editors). Saunders, 1980.

SERUM SICKNESS

Essentials of Diagnosis

- Fever, malaise.
- Skin rash (usually urticarial).
- Local or generalized lymphadenopathy, polyarthralgia, or polyarthritis is frequent.
- History of recent administration of foreign serum or drug.

General Considerations

Antibiotics—particularly penicillin—have largely replaced foreign serum as the principal cause of serum sickness. Vaccines, toxoids, and virtually any injectable foreign substance also may cause this disorder. It may occur after the first encounter with a substance, usually requiring 7–10 days for sufficient sensitization to occur. Reexposure to the antigen in an already sensitized individual may result in symptoms as early as 1–4 days later. In unusually sensitive individuals, exposure to antigen may result in anaphylactic shock. Administration of antigen or, in atopic individuals, natural exposure (eg, to horse allergens) may sensitize an individual to the antigen without inducing clinically apparent symptoms.

Clinical Findings

A. Symptoms and Signs: This disorder usually begins with a low-grade fever and malaise, which are followed to a variable extent by skin rash, lymphadenopathy, polyarthritis, and neurologic symptoms. Skin rashes occur in over 90% of cases. Most commonly, the skin rash is urticarial with an accompanying severe pruritus (which may precede the urticaria), but other erythematous eruptions may occur. Development of a localized erythematous or frankly urticarial reaction may first occur at the injection site. Lymphadenopathy may be localized to an area that drains the injection site, or it may be generalized. Neurologic lesions, when they occur, are most commonly those of peripheral neuritis, but there may be central nervous system involvement as well. Gastrointestinal symptoms sometimes occur.

B. Laboratory Findings: Leukopenia may occur early, followed later by leukocytosis. Eosinophilia is not common but does occur. Proteinuria and microscopic hematuria may be seen. Complement (CH_{50}, C3) may be decreased.

Prevention

The patient should always be questioned about a history of previous reactions before the administration of drugs, sera, or other injectable foreign substances. (In atopic individuals, a history of respiratory allergy induced by contact with an animal from which the serum to be administered has been derived is strongly suggestive that the patient may react adversely.)

Since foreign sera are highly sensitizing, skin tests with the serum should be performed if a history of previous contact or suspected allergy is obtained. Caution is required, since anaphylactic reactions after skin tests have been known to occur. Scratch testing should be done first, followed by intradermal testing with a 1:20 dilution of the scratch test material. Unfortunately, the reliability of the skin test in predicting clinical sensitivity is much less than desired; both false-positive and false-negative reactions occur. Conjunctival tests are also unreliable.

Treatment & Prognosis

Treatment consists mainly of the discontinuance of the drug or other offending agent, the use of antihistamines with or without adrenergic drugs, and, in more severe and prolonged cases, administration of adrenocorticosteroids. When angioneurotic edema, bronchial constriction, and vascular collapse occur, epinephrine and theophylline may be lifesaving. (See Medical Emergencies Due to Allergic Reactions, above.)

In most cases, serum sickness subsides in less than a week, but on occasion it may be more prolonged. The symptoms usually abate with the clearance of offending antigen from the circulation; persistence, therefore, suggests continued exposure.

Frick OL: Serum sickness. Chap 33, p 574, in: *Allergy: Principles and Practice*, 2nd ed. Middleton E Jr, Reed CE, Ellis EF (editors). Mosby, 1983.

DRUG ALLERGY

Drugs are so widely used that drug reactions of one type or another are commonplace. **Toxic drug reactions** are due to the inherent pharmacologic properties of the drug and are most frequently encountered after drug overdosage. Some individuals exhibit inordinate sensitivity to the recognized pharmacologic effects of a drug, however, and may therefore develop toxicity after administration of amounts that are usually nontoxic. **Drug idiosyncrasy** is an unusual response to the pharmacologic action of the drug (eg, hyperactivity rather than sedation following the administration of phenobarbital). **Allergic reactions to drugs** are independent of the drug's pharmacologic action and are the result of antigen-antibody interaction. The allergen may not be the drug administered but a metabolic derivative of it produced in the body. Although the immune reaction is highly specific, cross-reactions with chemically related drugs are not infrequent, for example, among the various kinds of penicillins. **Anaphylactoid (pseudoallergic) reactions** mimic true allergic reactions but are caused by release of histamine or other vasoactive mediators from most cells following an antigen-IgE reaction (eg, some reactions to iodinated radiocontrast dyes).

The manifestations of drug allergy are extremely varied, and virtually all allergic syndromes can be produced by drugs. The most common manifestations are skin eruptions (see Chapter 10) and fever.

In recent years, various syndromes related to reactivity to aspirin have been recognized, predominantly in adults but also in children. The reactions appear to be nonallergic, based rather on some peculiar biochemical idiosyncrasy. Production of nasal polyposis, severe aspirin-induced bronchospasm, and rhinitis with sinusitis have been well publicized, but a more subtle bronchospastic influence also has been documented in many children with asthma. Urticaria or angioedema also occurs in association with rhinitis and nasal polyposis, generally without bronchospasm in the urticarial forms.

Although any drug is a potential sensitizer, some (particularly penicillin and the sulfonamides) are more often associated with allergic reactions than others. The likelihood of sensitization is increased by repeated exposure. It is also probable that parenteral administration is more sensitizing than oral administration. Topical administration of drugs, especially over inflamed skin, is particularly sensitizing.

Exposure to sunlight may activate skin reactions to photosensitizing drugs such as sulfonamides, tetracycline antibiotics, and topically applied coal tar products.

In questioning a patient about drug reactions, it should be remembered that certain drugs such as benzathine penicillin G remain in the body for a long time. Reactions to a single depot injection of penicillin have been known to last for months.

With the exception of patch testing in contact dermatitis, allergy testing has usually been a disappointing procedure in identifying or predicting drug allergy. The reasons are many, and in some cases at least, the allergic reaction is due to a metabolically altered form of the drug. In the case of penicillin, some of the offensive metabolic derivatives have been identified. When these substances are used in testing, prediction of allergic reactions on the basis of a test reaction is more successful. However, these reagents are not readily available, and until the exact allergens in other drugs are identified and preparations containing the appropriate allergens become widely available, skin and serologic testing for drug allergy cannot be considered a reliable procedure. The basis for "hypersensitivity" reactions to urographic or other radiocontrast material is unknown, and skin testing and other tests, including use of a smaller "test dose" of the material, to predict reactivity to these agents are unreliable.

The history of previous reactions to drugs remains the best means of diagnosing drug sensitivity. This is often difficult, however, and in any instance in which a reaction to a drug is questionable, an alternative drug should be used (if possible) and the patient advised to avoid the drug even though a definite drug allergy has not been established.

Treatment & Prognosis

Regardless of the manifestation, the treatment of drug allergy includes discontinuance of the offending drug at the first sign of an adverse reaction and making certain that further contact with the drug is avoided. Small amounts of drugs to which a patient may be sensitive may be found in vaccines, foods, and other substances. Individuals with extreme hypersensitivity to a given drug should be warned, therefore, of other hidden sources of contact with the drug. Although desensitization has been used successfully, it is not recommended, and it is better to substitute a chemically unrelated drug for the offending drug.

Symptomatic treatment is usually effective. Patients suspected of being reactive to a radiocontrast dye should be pretreated with corticosteroids and antihistamines if the use of the dye is considered necessary.

The prognosis is good, especially with early identification of drug allergies.

Anderson JA: Drug allergies. Chap 54, pp 690–708, in: *Allergic Disorders of Infancy, Childhood and Adolescence*. Bierman CW, Pearlman DS (editors). Saunders, 1980.

Goldstein RA, Patterson R (editors): Symposium proceedings on drug allergy: Prevention, diagnosis, and treatment. *J Allergy Clin Immunol* 1984;**74(Suppl)**:549. [Entire issue.]

Mathews KP: Clinical spectrum of allergic and pseudoallergic drug reactions. *J Allergy Clin Immunol* 1984;**84**:558.

Settipane GA, Pudupakkam RK: Aspirin intolerance. 3. Subtypes, familial occurrence, and cross-reactivity with tartrazine. *J Allergy Clin Immunol* 1975;**56**:215.

Van Arsdel PP Jr: Allergy and adverse drug reactions. *J Am Acad Dermatol* 1982;**6**:833.

URTICARIA

Essentials of Diagnosis

- Multiple (occasionally single) macular lesions, consisting of localized edema (wheal) with surrounding erythema.
- Pruritus, frequently intense.

General Considerations

Urticaria is a vascular reaction of the upper dermis consisting mainly of vasodilatation and perivascular transudation, resulting in the classic "hive" or wheal and flare. Lesions are characteristically pruritic. Ordinarily, this vascular reaction is due to the liberation of histamine, but other mediators may be involved.

Urticarial reactions are usually transient (hours) but can persist for months or more. They may be the sole allergic manifestation or may represent only a part of the clinical picture, as in serum sickness and erythema multiforme. Emotional tension may be an aggravating factor. **Angioedema** is essentially an urticarial reaction of the lower parts of the dermis, resulting in the production of a more diffuse edema.

Hereditary angioneurotic edema is a rare syndrome characterized by periodic bouts of angioedema usually involving one or more extremities but sometimes affecting other anatomic areas as well. It is inherited as an autosomal dominant trait and appears to be related to a deficiency of C1 esterase and kinin inhibitor. There is no evidence that an allergic mechanism is involved. Characteristically, pruritus is absent.

Cholinergic urticaria, which is uncommon, seems to occur in some individuals during and following exercise, increased environmental heat, and emotional stress. Characteristically, the lesions appear as extremely small wheals accompanied by a large bright-red flare. Abdominal cramps, diarrhea, increased sweating, and headache may also occur.

Papular urticaria is a term given to a syndrome characterized by multiple papules resembling insect bites, found especially on the extremities. It is thought to be due to hypersensitivity to the bites of fleas, mites, mosquitoes, lice, or bedbugs.

Dermatographism (the ability to "write" on the skin by stroking it with a fingernail, for example, and producing a wheal and erythema) can occur in allergic and nonallergic individuals. It generally is of no pathologic significance but may accompany chronic urticaria or urticaria pigmentosa (mastocytosis).

Clinical Findings

A. History: The history is of prime importance in ascertaining the possible cause. The most common causes of urticaria include the following:

1. Drugs, hyposensitization extracts, vaccines, toxoids, and hormone preparations.
2. Infections, including bacterial (especially staphylococcal and group A β-hemolytic streptococcal), parasitic, fungal, and viral, including viral hepatitis and herpesvirus.
3. Foods (especially eggs, milk, wheat, corn, pork, shellfish, fish, berries, cheese, and nuts) and food dyes and other food additives.
4. Inhalants, pollens, and molds.
5. Psychologic factors (probably overrated).
6. Physical factors (cold, heat), exercise, histamine liberators, and dermatographism.

B. Symptoms and Signs: Urticarial lesions characteristically appear as erythematous areas with a pale center and usually occur in large numbers. Pruritus is the rule and is frequently intense; it may precede the appearance of the lesions. Pruritus is not characteristic of angioneurotic edema, however, which occurs most often as a solitary lesion or together with multiple urticaria. When angioedema involves the laryngeal area, it may be a threat to life.

Dermatographism may be symptomatic and occurs in a small percentage of allergic and nonallergic patients.

C. Laboratory Findings: Diagnostic procedures may include drug elimination, dietary elimination and challenge of suspected foods, and a thorough search for infection elsewhere in the body. Allergy testing is occasionally of value.

Differential Diagnosis

Urticaria is a prominent feature of mastocytosis (urticaria pigmentosa) and may occur in systemic diseases such as lupus erythematosus, various liver diseases, lymphoma, leukemia, and carcinoma.

Treatment & Prognosis

Treatment consists mainly of the detection and elimination of the appropriate allergens, when possible. Aspirin should be avoided, as it may secondarily aggravate the urticaria. Antihistamines are usually the most useful therapeutic agents in urticarial disorders, but adrenergic agents with vasoconstrictor properties can be a useful adjunct. Epinephrine is especially effective when rapid relief is needed. Hydroxyzine (Atarax, Vistaril) is among the most effective antihistamines, especially in treatment of chronic urticaria and dermatographism. In most resistant cases, combining an H_1 antihistamine (eg, hydroxyzine) with an H_2 antihistamine (eg, cimetidine) may be helpful. Cyproheptadine (Periactin) is most effective in some patients with cold urticaria. Mild sedation may also be indicated.

Adrenocorticosteroids are sometimes used in the more chronic form of urticaria but are reserved for more refractory cases. Topical medications generally are not effective.

Except for life-threatening laryngeal edema, the prognosis is good. Identification of the offending agent is most important.

Epstein JH: Photoallergy. *Arch Dermatol* 1972;**106:**741.

Guin JD: Treatment of urticaria. *Med Clin North Am* 1982; **66:**831.

Kaplan AP: Urticaria and angioedema. Chap 60, pp 1341–1360, in: *Allergy: Principles and Practice,* 2nd ed. Middleton E Jr, Reed CE, Ellis EF (editors). Mosby, 1983.

Sheffer A: Urticaria and angioedema. *Pediatr Clin North Am* 1975;**22:**193.

OTHER ALLERGIC PULMONARY DISORDERS

Various pulmonary disorders either known or thought to stem from an allergic reaction to inhaled or ingested antigens have been described. In some cases, evidence implicating an allergic mechanism in the development of the disease is substantial; in others, the role of allergic mechanisms is mainly conjectural.

A syndrome thought to be related to **cow's milk hypersensitivity** has been described and consists of recurrent pulmonary infiltrates, wheezing, chronic cough, chronic or frequent otitis media and rhinorrhea, and iron deficiency anemia related to excessive gastrointestinal blood loss. Gastrointestinal symptoms (diarrhea, vomiting) and poor weight gain are also features of this disorder, which is seen in children chiefly in the first 2 years of life. Some of these children have evidence of pulmonary hemosiderosis, and blood eosinophilia is sometimes seen. Multiple precipitins to cow's milk can be demonstrated, but the significance of this finding is controversial. Dietary elimination of cow's milk antigens is followed by improvement of the disorder, although symptoms also have been reported to subside spontaneously.

Hypersensitivity pneumonitis is an inflammatory reaction involving principally the alveoli and bronchioles and characterized clinically by malaise, fever, chills, cough, and dyspnea. Tissue damage stems from a hypersensitivity reaction to any of a variety of inhaled organic dusts or of fungi that may or may not also be infective. The disease is seen predominantly in adults as a result of occupational exposure to large concentrations of certain antigens (eg, proteinaceous material from bird droppings in bird fancier's lung; thermophilic actinomycetes from hay in farmer's lung or from contaminated air conditioners), but it can occur at any age. The onset may be insidious or acute. Symptoms of these disorders—particularly in the acute onset form—typically occur 4–8 hours after exposure to the offending antigen. In asthmatic individuals, wheezing also may be present, with involvement of IgE-mediated mechanisms. Rales may be heard, but physical findings referable to the lungs may be minimal. Chest x-ray reveals a variable pattern, with mottled densities or infiltrates early in the disease and a picture of interstitial fibrosis in more chronic cases. Pulmonary function studies show a restrictive defect with diminished diffusing capacity. Treatment consists mainly of avoiding the offensive inhalants. Glucocorticoids may be very helpful in minimizing the hypersensitivity reaction early in the disease. If recognized early, lesions are largely reversible and the prognosis is excellent. With chronic severe disease, pulmonary fibrosis may result, leading to severe respiratory insufficiency and death.

Allergic bronchopulmonary aspergillosis, with or without tissue invasion by the organism, is seen with some frequency in Great Britain but is rare in the USA (especially in children). The syndrome occurs in allergic asthmatics and includes symptoms of asthma and pneumonitis. High tissue and blood esoinophil levels, high IgE levels, and the presence of IgE and precipitating antibody to *Aspergillus* are characteristic laboratory findings. *Aspergillus* also may be found on sputum smear or culture. Treatment includes use of corticosteroids and antifungal agents.

An association between **tissue and blood eosinophilia** and **pulmonary infiltrates** has been observed in various disorders (eg, asthma, allergic bronchopulmonary aspergillosis, connective tissue diseases) and is thought to reflect an allergic mechanism in these disorders. Pulmonary infiltrates with eosinophilia sometimes occur as an apparently distinct clinical entity characterized by mild (mainly cough) to absent clinical symptoms and fleeting pulmonary infiltrates that, on x-ray, appear to migrate from one area of the lungs to another over a few days (often called Löffler's syndrome). A number of drugs (especially sulfonamides and nitrofurantoin), parasites (eg, *Ascaris*), and other antigens have been implicated at times in the production of this syndrome, but frequently no cause can be found. The disorder is generally self-limited, lasting less than a month; however, more severe forms may be seen (eg, in many cases of so-called tropical eosinophilia associated with filariasis), and the tissue reaction may proceed to pulmonary fibrosis. Corticosteroids may be extremely beneficial, particularly early in the reaction, and should be used when the severity of the disorder warrants.

Bierman CW, Pierson WE, Massie FS: Nonasthmatic allergic pulmonary disease. Chap 42, p 543, in: *Disorders of the Respiratory Tract in Children,* 4th ed. Kendig EL Jr, Cherniak V (editors). Saunders, 1983.

Lee SK et al: Cow's milk-induced pulmonary disease in children. *Adv Pediatr* 1978;**25:**39.

Schatz M, Patterson R: Hypersensitivity pneumonitis. *Clin Rev Allergy* 1983;**1:**451.

Stankus RP, Salvaggio JE (editors): Immunologically mediated lung disease. *Clin Rev Allergy* 1985;**3:**143. [Entire issue.]

SELECTED REFERENCES

References for Physicians

Berman BA, MacDonnell KF: *Differential Diagnosis and Treatment of Pediatric Allergy.* Little, Brown, 1981.

Bierman CW, Pearlman DS (editors): *Allergic Diseases of Infancy, Childhood, and Adolescence.* Saunders, 1980.

Friedlaender MH: *Allergy and Immunology of the Eye*. Harper & Row, 1979.

Gershwin ME (editor): *Bronchial Asthma: Principles of Diagnosis and Treatment*. Grune & Stratton, 1981.

Lockey RF (editor): *Allergy and Clinical Immunology*. Medical Examination Publishing Co., 1979.

Middleton E Jr, Reed CE, Ellis EF (editors): *Allergy: Principles and Practice,* 2nd ed. Mosby, 1983.

Mygind N: *Nasal Allergy,* 2nd ed. Blackwell, 1979.

Patterson R (editor): *Allergic Diseases: Diagnosis and Management,* 2nd ed. Lippincott, 1980.

Salvaggio JE (editor): Primer in allergic and immunologic diseases. *JAMA* 1982;**248:**2579.

Sly M: *Pediatric Allergy,* 2nd ed. Medical Examination Publishing Co., 1981.

References for Parents & Patients

Plaut TF: *Children With Asthma.* PediPress, 1983.

Slavin RG, Norback CT: *The Allergy Encyclopedia.* New American Library, 1981.

Young SH, Shulman SA, Shulman MD: *The Asthma Handbook: A Complete Guide for Patients and Their Families.* Bantam Books, 1985.

Genetic & Chromosomal Disorders, Including Inborn Errors of Metabolism

33

Arthur Robinson, MD, Stephen I. Goodman, MD, & Edward R. B. McCabe, MD, PhD

I. GENETIC & CHROMOSOMAL DISORDERS

Recent developments in the science of genetics have greatly increased our understanding of the basic processes of heredity. Genetics is an essential discipline for an understanding of human biology; it helps to unify the physician's concept of disease and has increasing relevance to clinical experience.

THE CELL

The central structure of any living cell is its complement of genes (located on the chromosomes) within the cell nucleus and consisting of a molecule whose 3-dimensional structure is that of a double helix. This molecule, deoxyribonucleic acid (DNA), is the chief constituent of the gene, which has a dual function: (1) to replicate itself (the central act of biologic reproduction); and (2) to be responsible, through the enzymes, for specific aspects of the cell's metabolism.

The information residing within a specific gene is necessary to permit synthesis of the polypeptide, a linear array of amino acids, which forms a segment of a protein. The enzymes, which are proteins, are necessary as catalysts for chemical reactions in the cell.

A series of consecutive triplet pyrimidine and purine base pairs in the linear DNA chain code for the series of consecutive amino acids in the polypeptide chain, although strict colinearity between the DNA base pairs and the amino acid sequences in the related protein is no longer believed always to be present in eukaryotes. Many of the details of how this information is transcribed and translated have been worked out, and protein synthesis has been observed in vitro in a cell-free system.

The majority of the genes are probably not "structural" (ie, not responsible for the production of specific proteins) but are regulatory. These latter genes permit the cell to respond sensitively to its environment and to differentiate into the various kinds of cells within the organism. It has recently been demonstrated that genetic regulation is much more complex in humans than in bacteria. The gene, for example, has coding regions (**exons**) and, interspersed among them, noncoding regions (**introns**). The latter may be involved in regulation and are one cause of the absence of strict colinearity mentioned above. In addition, the degree of methylation of DNA relates directly to the inability of at least some genes to be expressed.

CELL DIVISION

The cell cycle can be divided into 4 periods (Fig 33–1): S, the period of DNA replication; M, the period of cell division; and G1 and G2, the periods separating S and M, in which protein synthesis may occur.

Cell division is of 2 types: meiosis, a form of cell division limited to those cells (germ cells or gam-

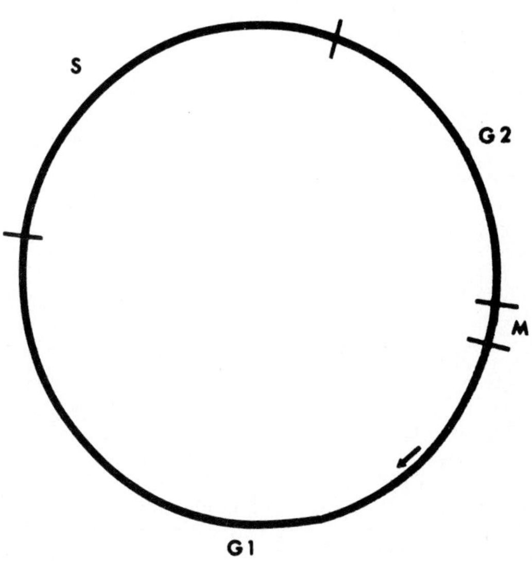

Figure 33–1. Diagram of the life cycle of a mammalian cell.

etes) which participate in sexual reproduction; and mitosis, a form of asexual division occurring in somatic cells.

Meiosis occurs during gametogenesis (Fig 33–2). During the first meiotic division, homologous chromosomes are arranged in pairs (synapsis) along the equatorial plate, permitting genetic recombination, a process essential to human variability and evolution. The 2 homologs then separate and move to opposite poles (disjunction). Unlike the situation that exists in mitosis, described below, division occurs between (not through) the centromeres. As a result, the daughter cells have one member of each chromosome pair (haploid). Following the first meiotic (reduction) division, a second division, mitotic in character, occurs. Hence the mature germ cells, both sperm and ova, have the haploid number of 23 chromosomes. After fertilization, the fertilized egg (zygote) has the full diploid chromosome complement of somatic cells, 46.

It is worth stressing that during the first meiotic division, chance alone determines which member of a chromosome pair, the maternally or paternally derived one, will migrate to a given pole. This permits 2^{23} different combinations of chromosomes in the gametes and, in addition to the process of recombination, is responsible for the major part of human genetic variability. No 2 humans, with the exception of monozygotic twins, have ever been genetically identical.

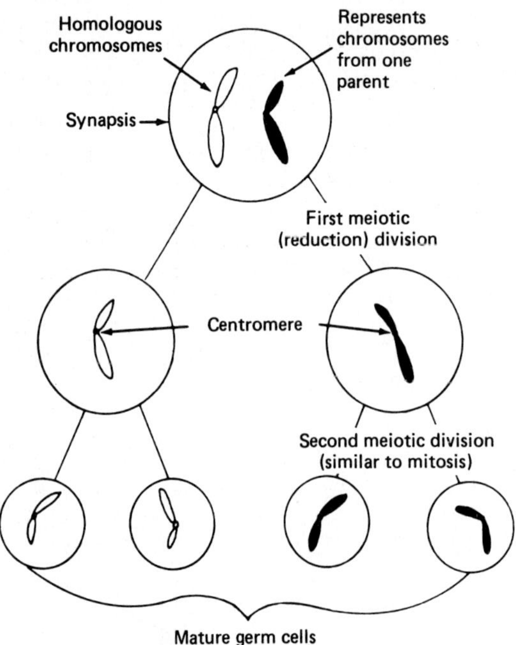

Figure 33–2. Diagrammatic representation of meiosis, demonstrating the conversion from the diploid somatic cell to the haploid gamete.

During **mitosis,** the DNA coils up tightly so that the chromosomes become short and thick, which explains why they are only visible during this relatively brief segment of the cell cycle. During metaphase (Fig 33–3), the shortened chromosomes arrange themselves on the spindle; the centromere undergoes longitudinal division; and the separated chromosomal halves disjoin to opposite poles before the cell divides into 2 daughter cells. This permits the 2 daughter cells to have the identical genetic material that was present in the parent cell.

THE HUMAN CHROMOSOMES

A new era in cytogenetics began in 1956 with the discovery, by Tjio and Levan, that the human chromosomal number was 46. Since then, this field has advanced with explosive rapidity. Its importance to medicine may be judged by the fact that grossly abnormal karyotypes occur in about 1% of human live births.

Since the chromosomes can only be delineated during mitosis, it is important to examine human material containing many cells in a dividing state. The only tissue in the body where this condition exists to any degree is the bone marrow. Because bone marrow is not readily available for routine biopsy, it becomes necessary to utilize tissue culture techniques to stimulate rapid in vitro growth, so that many cells in mitosis may be examined. The period of culture varies with the tissues sampled. The lymphocytes of the blood, being most readily available, are most commonly cultured, requiring 3 days of growth in the presence of phytohemagglutinin (PHA), a mitogenic agent.

Chromosomes prepared from cultures consist of 2 arms separated by a light-staining centromere by

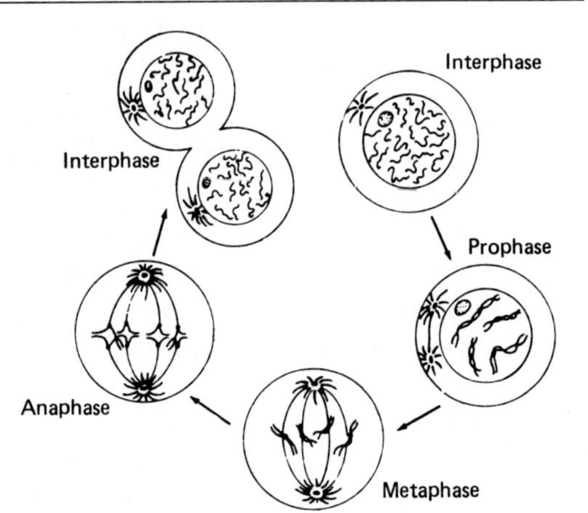

Figure 33–3. Diagram demonstrating the various stages of the mitotic cycle.

which they are normally attached to the spindle. Because the DNA has already replicated (in the S period), each arm consists of 2 identical chromatids. Chromosomes may be designated, according to the position of the centromere, as metacentric, submetacentric, and acrocentric (nearly terminal centromere). The 10 acrocentrics are satellited and are responsible for the synthesis of ribosomal RNA.

The human somatic cell has 22 pairs of autosomes and 2 sex chromosomes. The female, being the homogametic sex, has two X chromosomes; the heterogametic male has one X and one Y (Fig 33–4).

New staining techniques have now made it possible to identify all of the chromosomes in the karyotype and to arrange them in homologous pairs. The first of these utilizes the differential affinity of the various chromosomes and parts of chromosomes for the fluorescent dye quinacrine mustard. Segments of chromosomes that take up the dye fluoresce brightly under ultraviolet microscopy, whereas the other segments do not. This gives the individual pairs of chromosomes unique and characteristic banding patterns. The long arm of the Y chromosome fluoresces particularly intensely. The other staining methods produce a very similar banding pattern on the chromosomes when they are stained with an alkaline Giemsa stain. Many variants are being described.

Dutrillaux B, Lejeune J: New techniques in the study of human chromosomes: Methods and applications. *Adv Hum Genet* 1975;**56:**119.

Puck TT, Kao FT: Somatic cell genetics and its application to medicine. *Annu Rev Genet* 1982;**16:**225.

Yunis JJ: Mid-prophase human chromosomes: The attainment of 2000 bands. *Hum Genet* 1981;**56:**293.

CHROMOSOMAL ABERRATIONS

With current techniques, the cytogeneticist is able to recognize 2 classes of abnormality: numerical and morphologic. **Numerical abnormalities** are due to nondisjunction, ie, the failure of the chromosomes to divide equally between the 2 daughter cells. This may occur during either meiosis or mitosis, ie, during gametogenesis or as a postzygotic phenomenon. In the former eventuality, 2 types of gametes will be formed: those which lack a chromosome and those with an extra chromosome. If either of these gametes unites with a normal germ cell, the resulting conceptus will be either monosomic or trisomic for the involved chromosome rather than having the normal pair.

When the nondisjunction is postzygotic, the resulting individual may be a mosaic, ie, may have 2 or more cell populations that differ in their chromosomal number. Mosaicism may also be due to chromosome lag, the failure of a chromosome to migrate to one pole of the dividing cell and its subsequent loss from one of the daughter cells. The phenotype of the mosaic individual will then depend upon when in develop-

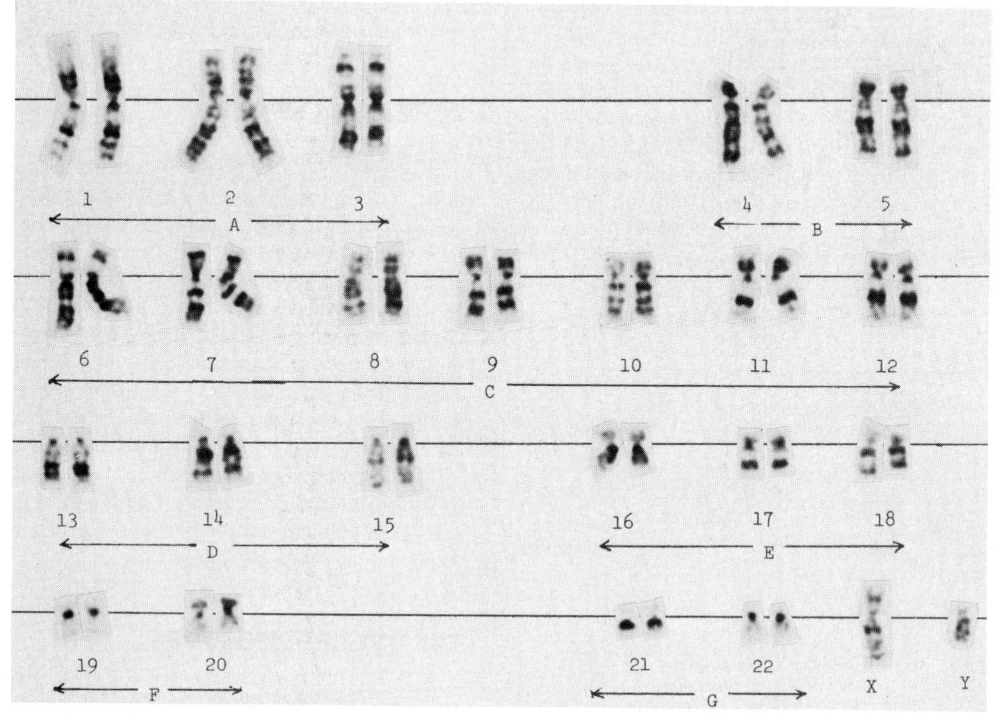

Figure 33–4. Male human chromosomes (Giemsa banding).

ment the nondisjunction occurred and which anlage had the aneuploid cells.

Morphologic aberration is the result of the breakage of chromosomes and the rejoining of the damaged ends in new ways. When such a rearrangement occurs between 2 nonhomologous chromosomes (reciprocal translocation) without significant loss of chromatin material (Fig 33–5), this is a balanced translocation and the individual is phenotypically normal. However, if duplication or loss of chromatin material (deletion) occurs, the somatic effects are frequently severe—even lethal. A break may occur at the centromere, with rehealing to form a metacentric structure known as an isochromosome, both arms of which originate from the chromatids of a single arm of the original chromosome. Thus, the isochromosome will lack the genes on the other arm.

CAUSE OF CHROMOSOMAL ABERRATIONS

As many as 0.5% of human live births and 25–50% of spontaneous abortions are aneuploid, a fact that marks nondisjunction as one of the major causes of human disease.

Nondisjunction has been observed to increase with maternal age. An explanation of this "maternal age effect" may be that the ovary contains a full complement of oocytes at birth, at which time meiotic prophase has already begun. These oocytes remain in prophase until ovulation, which may occur 40 years later. It may well be that the completion of oogenesis in these older cells is attended by an increased risk of nondisjunction.

Another possible cause of nondisjunction is ionizing radiation. At least 3 retrospective studies suggest that the mothers of children with Down's syndrome (which results from nondisjunction involving chromosome 21) have a history of significantly higher exposure to ionizing radiation than do control groups.

Viral infections, both in vivo and in vitro, have been shown to cause chromosomal breaks with or without abnormal rehealing. In 3 diseases—congenital aplastic anemia (Fanconi), Bloom's dwarfism, and ataxia-telangiectasia—an increased incidence of chromosomal breakage has been found. Whether viral infections are involved in the etiology of these breaks is unknown. All 3 of these diseases are associated with an increased risk of cancer.

Finally, a variety of chemical agents, especially drugs, have been implicated as causes of chromosomal breakage. In many cases, the data are conflicting and a final conclusion has not yet been reached. If these drugs do, in fact, break chromosomes, their influence on the production of congenital malformations is also not yet known.

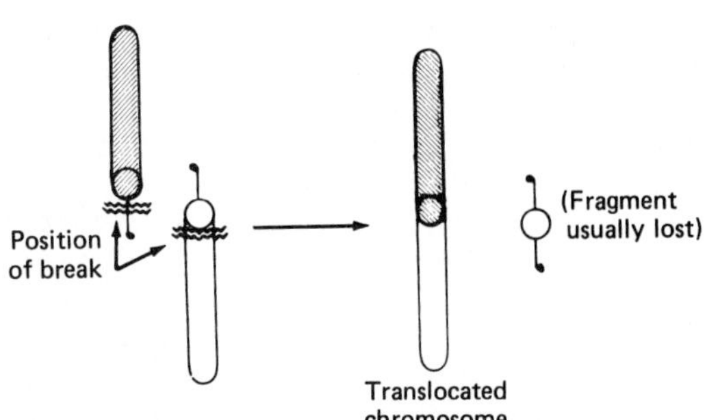

Figure 33–5. Reciprocal translocation (Robertsonian) between 2 nonhomologous satellited chromosomes.

Arlett CF, Lehmann AR: Human disorders showing increased sensitivity to the induction of genetic damage. *Annu Rev Genet* 1978;**12:**95.

Carr DH, Gedeon M: Population cytogenetics of human abortions. In: *Population Cytogenetics.* Hook EB, Porter IH (editors). Academic Press, 1977.

Denniston C: Low-level radiation and genetic risk estimation in man. *Annu Rev Genet* 1982;**16:**329.

Sandberg AA: *The Chromosomes in Human Cancer and Leukemia.* Elsevier, 1980.

CHROMOSOMAL DISEASES

Numerical abnormalities may involve either the sex chromosomes or the autosomes, predominantly the former in live births. Gross autosomal imbalances produce severe phenotypic disturbances and, particularly when they involve loss of chromosomal material, are usually incompatible with life.

DERMATOGLYPHICS

In persons with a variety of congenital malformations, and especially in those with chromosomal disease, the dermatoglyphic patterns, ie, the fingerprints, palm prints, and footprints, deviate from the normal.

Since the fine dermal ridges on the hands and feet begin to develop in their characteristic patterns between the second and fourth months of embryogenesis, deviations from normal embryonic development during this period may be reflected in abnormalities of the dermatoglyphic pattern. As a result, the presence of abnormal dermatoglyphics in a patient suggests some developmental trauma during the second to fourth months of pregnancy and should prompt a careful examination of the patient for associated, less obvious, congenital malformations.

THE SEX CHROMOSOMES

Unlike *Drosophila,* in which the fly with the XO pattern is the male, in the human the Y chromosome is necessary (but not sufficient) for maleness. The

Y chromosome presumably contains few genes other than those necessary to produce "maleness." It has recently been demonstrated that a gene for the so-called H-Y antigen exists on the Y chromosome (close to the centromere). The evidence suggests that this gene may be concerned with the primary determination of sex through the development of the undifferentiated gonad in the direction of a testicle. Other genes on the autosomes and the X chromosome interact with the Y chromosomal gene to control expression of the antigen. The X chromosome, on the other hand, carries many X-linked ("sex-linked") genes, most of which are not involved with either sex determination or sex development.

The X chromosome has some unique characteristics that have thrown light on some fundamental properties of mammalian cells and have been of great importance to medicine. The first indication of this was the demonstration by Moore and Barr of a sexual dimorphism in the somatic cells of humans that consisted of a deeply staining chromatin body in some cells of the normal female and its absence in the male (Fig 33–6). Subsequent studies revealed that humans may have 0–4 chromatin (Barr) bodies and that the number of such bodies is one less than the number of X chromosomes in the individual's karyotype (the "nuclear sex rule").

A hypothesis was proposed by Lyon and Russell (independently) to account both for the above phenomenon and for the "dosage compensation" effect—the fact that the amount of protein produced by a given X-linked gene such as the one for antihemophilic globulin is independent of the number of X chromosomes the individual has (eg, the female with two X chromosomes does not produce twice as much antihemophilic globulin as the male with only one). They suggested that only one X chromosome in any cell is fully active and that all others are genetically inactive during the major part of the cell's life cycle. Moreover, the hypothesis suggests that, early in embryogenesis (about the tenth to 12th day in humans), a random choice is made by each somatic cell about which X will remain active. Thereafter, the same X will remain active for all future progeny of a given cell. The normal female would then constitute a mosaic of clones with respect to the identity of the active X chromosome.

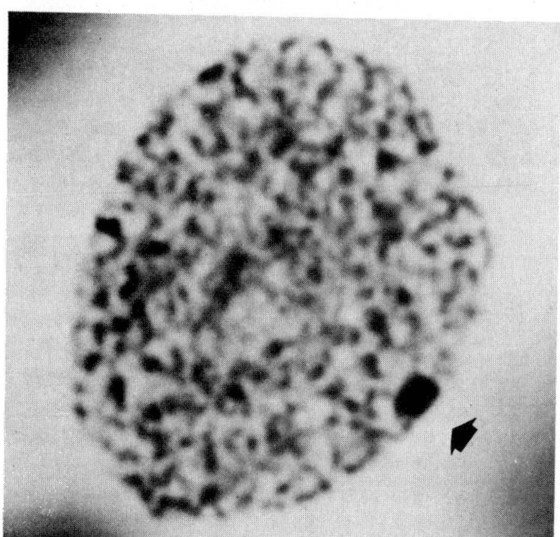

Figure 33–6. Nucleus of cell obtained from the buccal mucosa, demonstrating the densely staining chromatin body. Arrow points to chromatin body.

Much evidence has been accumulated to support the basic validity of the Lyon-Russell hypothesis. At present, it is thought that the Barr body represents the X chromosome, most of which is genetically inactive. Recent evidence suggests that some loci on the short arm of the inactive X are not inactive, namely, the genes for the Xga blood group and the enzyme steroid sulfatase (which is deficient in X-linked ichthyosis). It has also recently been demonstrated that X-chromosomal inactivation is related to methylation of DNA, since inhibition of methylation at least partially prevents this inactivation. Autoradiography has demonstrated that the various chromosome pairs have specific patterns of replication. The X chromosomes are remarkable for the degree of asynchrony they show in their patterns of replication, one of them being the last chromosome to replicate its DNA during the S period of the cell cycle. Whenever X polysomy (an increased number of X chromosomes) exists, all but one of the X chromosomes replicate late; and when one of the two X chromosomes has a morphologic abnormality, it too (with rare exceptions) is late in replicating. The Barr body, then, is thought to represent the genetically inactive, late-replicating X chromosome.

The Lyon-Russell hypothesis provides an explanation for the observation that abnormalities of X chromosomal constitution are more likely to be compatible with life and to be associated with less severe phenotypic defects than those of autosomes.

The Barr test has become an effective means of screening patients for sex chromosomal abnormalities. The test may be performed rapidly by means of a buccal smear. Normal males have less than 3% positive cells in their buccal smears, whereas normal females have 25–50% positive cells. Intermediate counts suggest mosaicism. The amniotic membrane stripped from the placenta has been utilized to great advantage in screening populations of newborns for abnormalities of the X chromosomes.

The affinity of the long arm of the Y chromosome for fluorescent dyes is also being used in screening newborns for abnormalities of the Y chromosome by looking for the "Y body" in interphase cells.

Naftolin F, Butz E: Sexual dimorphism. *Science* 1981; **211:**1263.

Shapiro LJ: X-chromosome and X-chromosome-linked disorders. Chap 7, pp 91–106, in: *Genetic Issues in Pediatric and Obstetric Practice.* Kaback M (editor). Year Book, 1981.

Smith DW: *Recognizable Patterns of Human Malformation,* 3rd ed. Saunders, 1982.

DISEASES OF THE SEX CHROMOSOMES

The characteristics of diseases involving sex differentiation are shown in Table 33–1.

About 0.25% of all live infants born at term and about 1% of the inmates of institutions for the retarded have sex chromosomal anomalies. Since most affected newborns have a normal phenotype, little is known about the developmental course of those identified at birth. This is increasingly important because of the frequency with which these conditions are diagnosed in utero and the associated need of parents to know the prognosis. Several longitudinal studies of these infants are currently being conducted to define their prognosis.

Indications for Examining the Sex Chromatin

An incidence of sex chromosomal anomalies of 0.35% has been found in a survey of 40,000 newborns born in 2 Denver hospitals. Since most of the abnormal cases would not have been diagnosed by physical examination alone, it may eventually be desirable for obstetric services to establish the chromatin status of all newborns at birth by routine examination of the amniotic membranes.

Robinson A et al: Sex chromosomal abnormalities (SCA): A prospective and longitudinal study of newborns identified in an unbiased manner. *Birth Defects* 1982;**18(4)**:7.

TURNER'S SYNDROME (Gonadal Dysgenesis)

Essentials of Diagnosis

- Short stature, primary amenorrhea, and sexual infantilism in adults.
- "Streak" gonads and partial or complete X-chromosomal monosomy (Fig 33–7) are found at all ages.

General Considerations

Turner's syndrome has an incidence of about one in 3000 live births, but the "45,X anomaly" is 40 times as common in spontaneous abortions. The occurrence of some of the somatic stigmas of the disease varies greatly from case to case. Most cases are chromatin-negative.

Clinical Findings

The family history is noncontributory except that an increased incidence of twinning has been reported in families with gonadal dysgenesis. Birth weight tends to be low (especially for those with webbed neck and coarctation of the aorta). Newborns often display lymphedema, especially of the lower parts of the legs and the distal arms. This may last for several years.

Table 33–1. Diseases involving sex differentiation.

Lesion and Disease	Chromosome Number	Symptoms
XX male. Sex chromatin–positive.	46	Like Klinefelter's or partial feminization, as in true hermaphrodite. Usually does not have a eunuchoid build, usually H-Y antigen–positive.
45,X/46,XY male pseudohermaphrodite, "mixed gonadal dysgenesis." Sex chromatin–negative.	45/46	A variable degree of Turner's phenotype with infantile female secondary sex characteristics and a variable amount of masculinization of the genitalia. Tendency to develop gonadoblastomas.
"Pure" gonadal dysgenesis, 46,XY male pseudohermaphroditism. Sex chromatin–negative.	46	Tall female with underdeveloped secondary sex characteristics, streak gonads, primary amenorrhea, and sterility. Tendency to develop gonadal tumors. May be familial.
Testicular feminizing syndrome, male pseudohermaphroditism, 46,XY. Sex chromatin–negative.	46	Tall, well-feminized, sterile female with testes. An "end-organ" insensitivity to androgens. May be suspected in sterile women with primary amenorrhea and in girls with bilateral inguinal hernias. Inherited as an X-linked recessive disease. Tendency to develop gonadal tumors.
True hermaphrodite, 46,XX; 46,XY or 46,XX/46,XY (the latter possibly due to an ovum being fertilized by 2 sperm).	46	Varying degrees of abnormal phenotypic sexual indeterminacy. May have ovum on one side, testis on the other (lateral hermaphrodite) or ovotestis on one (unilateral) or both sides (bilateral hermaphrodite). In lateral hermaphrodites, internal genitalia usually conform to gonad on that side. External genitalia may vary widely.

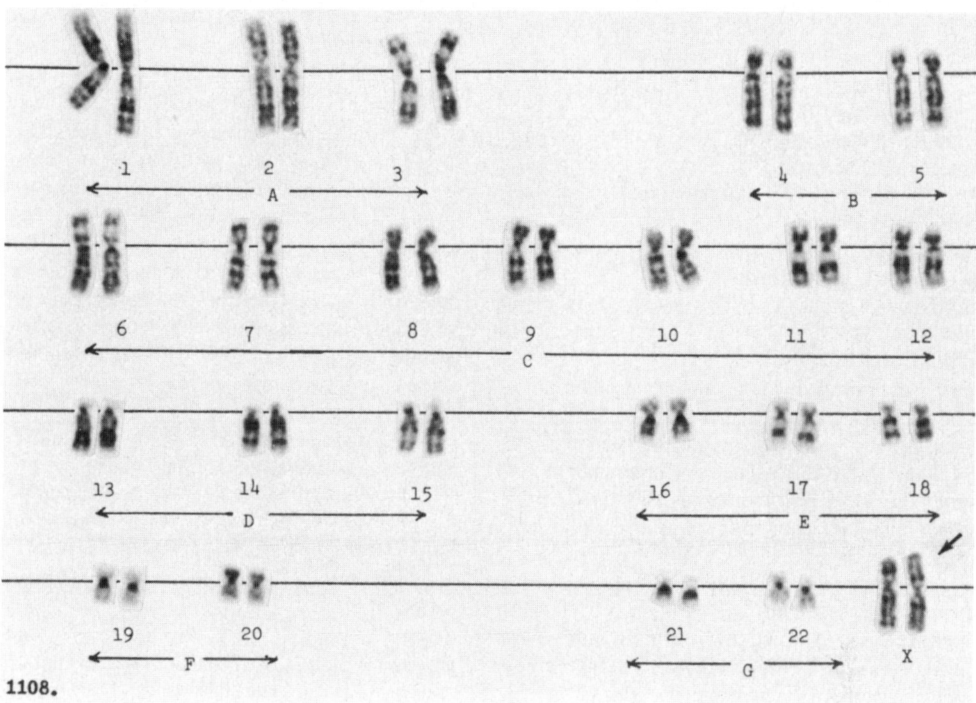

Figure 33–7. 46,X,i(Xq) karyotype of girl with Turner's syndrome. Arrow points to isochromosome of the long arm of the X.

A. Symptoms and Signs: The characteristic findings are sexual infantilism and primary amenorrhea in a postpubertal female, shortness of stature, congenital lymphedema, cubitus valgus, a small "turned down" mouth, low hairline, retrognathia or micrognathia, webbing of the neck, and short neck. Other abnormalities may include coarctation of the aorta, pigmented nevi, deep-set nail beds, and hypoplastic nails. The IQ is usually normal, although many patients have perceptual difficulties and space blindness or have trouble with numbers (dyscalculia). Congenital malformations of the urinary tract are common, especially horseshoe kidneys and double ureter and pelvis. In addition, there may be "shield chest" combined with widely spaced nipples, abnormalities of the spine (epiphysitis), retardation of bone age, and osteoporosis. The growth rate throughout childhood is slow, and the ultimate height is usually 130–150 cm. Occasional patients have been reported who menstruate and have normal height; these are probably chromosomal mosaics. Several reportedly 45,X females have borne normal children.

B. Laboratory Findings: Sex chromatin is usually negative. 45,X/46,XX mosaicism is not uncommon; in these cases, there may be some chromatin-positive cells but a lower percentage ($< 20\%$) than one would normally expect to find. Occasionally, the buccal smear is chromatin-positive but the bodies look particularly large; this suggests that the patient has an X-isochromosome of the long arm 46,X,i(Xq).*

In the typical case, the karyotype reveals a 45,X condition. Mosaicism (45,X/46,XX or 45,X/46,XX/47,XXX)* is not rare. In these cases, the phenotype may be modified so that many of the characteristic clinical findings are absent. Even mosaics, however, may have "streak" gonads and primary amenorrhea.

Patients with 46,X,i(Xq) usually have the typical Turner phenotype. In addition, they have an increased incidence of Hashimoto's thyroiditis. When a deletion of part or all of the long arm of one X chromosome occurs, many of the characteristic signs and symptoms, including shortness of stature, are absent, but amenorrhea and the sterility that results from dysgenetic gonads persist.

Urinary FSH excretion is elevated by the 13th to 14th year. Prior to this, FSH may be higher than normal for the age.

The gonads appear as long, slender white "streaks" in the broad ligaments. They are composed of wavy connective tissue without any germinal epithelium.

C. X-Ray Findings: X-ray studies often reveal rarefaction of the bones, especially in the hands, feet, and spine, where epiphysitis may also be present.

* Terminology adopted by Paris Conference on the Human Chromosomes (1971).

Bone age is only slightly retarded. Intravenous urography will often reveal urinary tract anomalies.

Differential Diagnosis

Turner's syndrome must be ruled out in all cases of females with shortness of stature, amenorrhea, webbing of the neck, or coarctation of the aorta. The diagnosis depends on the buccal smear and the chromosomal analysis. Patients with pseudohypoparathyroidism may have many of the stigmas of gonadal dysgenesis.

Complications & Sequelae

These relate primarily to the dangers of coarctation of the aorta when that is present. Rarely, the dysgenetic gonads may become neoplastic (gonadoblastoma). Sexual infantilism and the perceptual motor difficulties to which these patients are prone may have concomitant psychologic hazards. Essential hypertension often develops.

Treatment & Prognosis

Treatment consists of identifying and treating perceptual problems before they become established. Replacement hormone therapy should be started at 12–14 years of age to develop secondary sex characteristics and permit normal menstrual periods. This is psychologically most important. Teenage patients need careful counseling so that they will have no doubt about their femininity and to help them to cope with the stigmas of their condition. The need for hormone therapy should be carefully explained. Some pediatricians initiate therapy at about 10 years of age with an anabolic agent (eg, oxandrolone, 0.1 mg/kg/d) in order to stimulate growth. It is important to monitor bone growth to avoid too rapid advance. The hormone is usually given for a 4-month period, then stopped for 4 months, and then restarted for another 4 months. It should be stressed, however, that there is currently no unanimity of opinion about the usefulness or desirability of oxandrolone therapy for this purpose.

Replacement therapy consists of a daily oral dose (1.25 mg) of conjugated estrogens. Vaginal bleeding usually begins after 3–6 months. At that time, cyclic therapy is started, with the medication being administered during the first 3 weeks of each month. Because of the possible risk of endometrial carcinoma related to unopposed estrogen therapy, it is desirable to use a combination oral contraceptive (estrogen and progesterone) for long-term replacement therapy.

The prognosis for life is good, limited only by complications such as coarctation of the aorta. Sterility is permanent.

Simpson JL: Gonadal dysgenesis and sex chromosome abnormalities: Phenotypic-karyotypic correlations. Pages 365–405 in: *Genetic Mechanisms of Sexual Development*. Vallet H, Porter I (editors). Academic Press, 1979.

POLYSOMY X SYNDROME (XXX & XXXX)

The incidence of polysomy X in newborns is about 0.1% (significantly higher among retardates). Affected patients are phenotypic females with 2 or more sex chromatin bodies (Table 33–2). In an as yet undetermined proportion of adult cases, mild mental retardation and emotional disturbance occur. Tall stature, low IQ, learning difficulties, and delayed language development are common in prepubescent girls.

Treatment is supportive. Cyclic hormone therapy is indicated for older girls with underdeveloped secondary sex characteristics and amenorrhea.

When the condition is diagnosed in the newborn, the prognosis for mental development and language development must be guarded.

The offspring of women with polysomy X have for the most part had normal sex chromosomal constitutions, although there have been several children with Down's syndrome and some XXY and XXYY males.

Robinson A et al: Sex chromosomal abnormalities (SCA): A prospective and longitudinal study of newborns identified in an unbiased manner. *Birth Defects* 1982;**18(4):**7.

KLINEFELTER'S SYNDROME

Essentials of Diagnosis

- Micro-orchidism due to prepubertal testicular atrophy, azoospermia, and sterility in the adult (about 4 patients with this syndrome are said to have been fertile).
- Elevated urinary gonadotropins in puberty. 47,XXY chromosomal constitution.
- Chromosomal variants are occasionally seen.

General Considerations

The incidence in the newborn population is roughly one in 500, but it is about 1% in groups of male retardates and 3% in males seen at infertility clinics. The maternal age at birth is often advanced. The diagnosis is rarely made before puberty except as a result of screening tests for sex chromatin. Unlike gonadal dysgenesis, this lesion is rarely found in spontaneous abortions.

Clinical Findings

A. Symptoms and Signs: The characteristic findings do not usually appear until after puberty.

Table 33–2. Sex chromatin in polysomy X.

Sex Chromatin	Karyotype
Two bodies	47,XXX
Three bodies	48,XXXX
Four bodies	49,XXXXX
Few double bodies	46,XX/47,XXX;45,X/47,XXX
Few triple bodies	45,X/48,XXXX

Therefore, it is improper to stigmatize a child with a 47,XXY karyotype with a diagnosis of Klinefelter's syndrome. The most that can be said is that such a child is at an unmeasurable increased risk of developing the syndrome during adolescence. Micro-orchidism associated with otherwise normal external genitalia, azoospermia, and sterility is almost invariable in diagnosed cases. Gynecomastia, normal to borderline IQ, diminished facial hair, lack of libido and potency, and a tall, eunuchoid build are frequent. In chromosomal variants with 3 and 4 X chromosomes, mental retardation may be severe, and radioulnar synostosis may be present as well as anomalies of the external genitalia and cryptorchidism. In the XXXXY cases, these findings are especially prominent, as well as microcephaly, hypertelorism, epicanthus, prognathism, short stature, and incurved fifth fingers.

The adult XXYY patient tends to be taller and more retarded than the average XXY patient.

In general, the physical and mental abnormalities in Klinefelter's syndrome increase with the number of sex chromosomes.

B. Laboratory Findings: Sex chromatin is positive. Twenty to 40% of the cells of the buccal mucous membrane usually have one Barr body, although 2 and 3 Barr bodies may be found in individuals having one of the rare variants of Klinefelter's syndrome with more than two X chromosomes.

The majority of cases have a 47,XXY constitution. However, rare variants may have 48,XXXY, 49,XXXXY, 49,XXXYY, or 48,XXYY. A variety of mosaics containing combinations of the above and including 46,XY/47,XXY mosaicism have been reported. Some of these latter have been fertile.

Urinary excretion of gonadotropins is high in adults, the levels being comparable to those found in postmenopausal women.

Histology of the testis in the adult is characterized by hyalinization and atrophy of the majority of seminiferous tubules, with large clumps of abnormal Leydig cells in between. A marked deficiency of germ cells (spermatogonia) has been found also in prepubertal patients (even in a 10-month-old child).

Differential Diagnosis

Chromatin-positive Klinefelter's syndrome must be differentiated from 2 chromatin-negative varieties: postpubertal testicular atrophy and germ cell aplasia. In both cases, the diagnosis can be made by buccal smear for sex chromatin and testicular biopsy.

Adolescent obesity with delayed puberty and Prader-Willi syndrome may be confused with Klinefelter's syndrome. In both cases, the sex chromatin determination, absence of a eunuchoid build, and absence of true testicular atrophy should rule out Klinefelter's syndrome.

Complications & Sequelae

Affected patients may be more prone to a variety of conditions, including antisocial personality (especially sex crimes), schizophrenia, male breast cancer, and thyroid disease.

Treatment & Prognosis

Treatment consists of supportive care for the psychologic stresses of the disease and, occasionally, plastic surgery for gynecomastia. Therapy with androgens has been claimed to be helpful as patients reach adolescence.

The prognosis is good for life but poor for fertility. It is not known what percentage of patients will have normal intelligence, but undoubtedly many do.

XYY SYNDROME

The incidence of the 47,XYY karyotype in the newborn population is as yet unknown, although current estimates are that it occurs in about one in 1000 male births. It is worth stressing that affected newborns in general are perfectly normal and do *not* have the "XYY syndrome," which may be present in 10% of tall men (> 180 cm [> 6 ft]) who come into conflict with the law because of their grossly defective, aggressive personalities.

Affected individuals may on occasion exhibit an abnormal behavior pattern from early childhood and may be slightly retarded. Fertility may be normal. They are chromatin-negative except for an occasional chromatin-positive individual with a 48,XXYY karyotype. Hence, these patients are not identified by examination of the X chromatin. However, they can be identified by a buccal smear stained for the fluorescent "Y body."

There is no treatment. Many males with an XYY karyotype are normal. Long-term problems may relate to IQ and environmental stress.

FRAGILE X SYNDROME

X-linked (sex-linked) mental retardation is a common form of mental retardation, possibly as common as Down's syndrome, and may account for 25% of cases of mental retardation in males. A frequent form of this syndrome is associated with a fragile site on the end of the X chromosome, giving an appearance similar to that of the satellites which normally occur on chromosomes 13–15, 21, and 22. Demonstration of this heritable fragile site (46,XY,fra[X]q28) requires exacting tissue culture methods (eg, low folic acid in the medium).

Phenotypically normal males may be positive for fragile X and pass the fragile site on to their daughters, who may be mildly retarded. All people with undiagnosed "nonspecific" mental retardation should probably be karyotyped for fragile X.

Carrier females have a similar but less severe lesion; about one-third have a mild mental retardation. Males with the fragile X syndrome frequently have a characteristic phenotype, most typically with macroorchidism.

Rhoads FA: X-linked mental retardation and fragile-X or marker-X syndrome. *Pediatrics* 1982;**69:**668.
Stewart DA (editor): Children with sex chromosome aneuploidy: Follow-up studies. *Birth Defects* 1982;**18(4).** [Entire issue.]
Summitt RL: Abnormalities of the sex chromosomes. Chap 6, pp 63–89, in: *Genetic Issues in Pediatric and Obstetric Practice.* Kaback M (editor). Year Book, 1981.

AUTOSOMAL DISEASES

Humans are even more susceptible to autosomal disorders (Table 33–3) than to abnormalities of the sex chromosomes. Uniform autosomal monosomy is not compatible with life and has been observed only in spontaneously aborted fetuses. Similarly, only complete trisomy of the small autosomes (13, 18, 21, and 22) occurs in living individuals and then only in the presence of serious disease. The newer banding techniques have made us aware that there are many patients with minor morphologic changes of the autosomes (partial trisomies and monosomies) who have varying pathologic features, often associated with mental retardation. The belief that many abnormalities of the chromosomes do not permit the birth of a viable infant is strengthened by the finding of gross chromosomal aberrations in 30–50% of cases of spontaneous abortion.

Indications for Chromosomal Analysis

The following conditions or circumstances are in-

Table 33–3. Other diseases of the autosomes.

Lesion and Disease	Symptoms
Deletion of long arm of chromosome 22–the Ph[1] chromosome. The deleted segment is translocated onto the terminal portion of the long arm of a "C-group" chromosome, usually No. 9.	Chronic granulocytic leukemia. The chromosomal abnormality is present in the bone marrow in 90% of cases. Less often, it is also present in cells cultured from the peripheral blood unstimulated by PHA.
Bloom's dwarfism: multple chromosome breaks, quadriradial figures, occasionally "pulverization" of chromosomes, increased sister chromatid exchange.	Dwarfism, chronic erythematous rash, tendency to develop cancer, especially leukemia. Inherited as a single gene autosomal recessive. Increased chromosomal breaks may be seen in close relatives.
Congenital aplastic (Fanconi's) anemia: increased number of chromosomal breaks; chromosomes probably more susceptible to breakage by virus (especially SV40).	Skeletal (especially upper extremities) and hematopoietic abnormalities, increased hemoglobin F. Anemia often does not appear until 6–10 years of age. Hyperpigmentation, sexual and mental retardation, and microcephaly may also be present. Autosomal recessive inheritance.
Trisomy 8 mosaicism (46/47+8).	Mild to moderate mental retardation, strabismus, large ears, upturned nose, thick everted lower lip, high-arched palate, micrognathia, vertebral anomalies, genitourinary anomalies, thick bulging skin with deep furrows (especially on hands and feet), restricted movement of some small and large joints. Absence of patellas is very characterisitc.
9p– trisomy (47,XY[XX]+9p–)	A relatively frequent syndrome with craniofacial dysmorphia, microcephaly, brachycephaly, bulbous nose, downturned mouth, single palmar crease, and mental retardation.
46,XY(XX),18q– Partial deletion of long arm of No. 18.	Mental retardation, microcephaly, midfacial dysmorphia, prominent antihelix, atretic ear canals, "carp-shaped" mouth, cryptorchidism, long, tapering fingers. IgA often absent.
46,XY(XX),13q– Partial deletion of long arm of No. 13.	Mental retardation, failure to thrive, microcephaly, hypertelorism, ptosis, microphthalmia and colobomas, hypoplastic or absent thumbs, occasional retinoblastoma, congenital heart disease, genitourinary abnormalities.
46,XY(XX),4p– Partial deletion of short arm of No. 4.	Severe mental retardation, microcephaly, epicanthi, coloboma, beaked nose, cleft palate, micrognathia, inguinal hernia, hypospadias, growth deficiency of prenatal onset.
46,XY(XX), 18p– Partial deletion of short arm of No. 18.	Variable mental retardation, micrognathia, flat nasal bridge, low-set and large ears, short hands.
46,XY(XX)del(15q11)	An interstitial deletion involving the proximal part of the long arm of chromosome 15 has been found in many persons with Prader-Willi syndrome, using recently developed techniques for high-resolution study of chromosomes.

dications for chromosomal analysis: (1) the phenotypic and chromatin sex do not agree; (2) the chromatin examination suggests sex chromosome mosaicism; (3) the Barr body is morphologically abnormal; (4) the clinical condition suggests one of the autosomal syndromes, eg, the patient has gross structural anomalies involving a variety of systems and is retarded; (5) there is an abnormal number of "Y bodies"; (6) nonspecific mental retardation is seen in a patient with 2 or more somatic abnormalities, even minor ones; (7) a familial disorder, especially X-linked mental retardation, is present (look for fragile X); or (8) the couple has a history of recurrent spontaneous abortions.

Bergsma D (editor): New chromosomal and malformation syndromes. *Birth Defects* 1975;**11(5).** [Entire issue.]

De Grouchy J, Turleau C: *Clinical Atlas of Human Chromosomes,* 2nd ed. Wiley, 1984.

Schinzel A: *Catalogue of Unbalanced Chromosome Aberrations in Man.* De Gruyter, 1984.

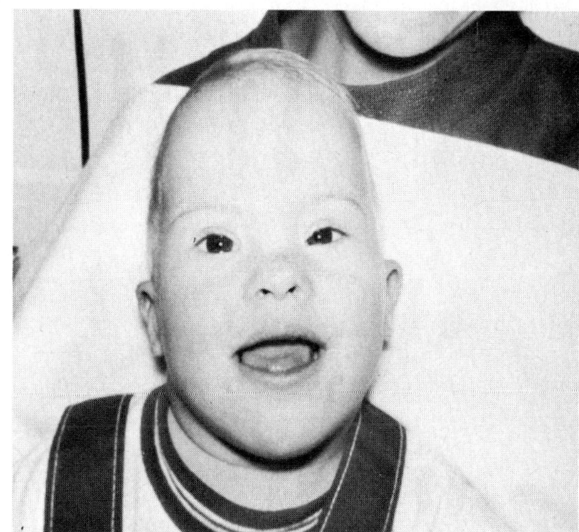

Figure 33–8. Facies of a child with Down's syndrome.

DOWN'S SYNDROME

Essentials of Diagnosis

- Slow development, characteristic facies, short stature, abnormal dermatoglyphics.
- Trisomy 21 or chromosomal translocation.

General Considerations

The term Down's syndrome is preferred to mongolism, since the latter term is descriptively inaccurate and is offensive to some. The most constant characteristic of the disease is mental retardation. IQs may vary between 20 and 80, with the great majority being between 45 and 55. The incidence of Down's syndrome has been dropping with the lowering of the average maternal age. In the author's series, Down's syndrome currently occurs in about one in 900 newborns, whereas the less recent literature states its incidence to be about one in 600 newborns. The patient's mother's age at the time of conception and the nature of the chromosomal malformation are important in genetic counseling.

Clinical Findings

A. Symptoms and Signs: The principal findings are a small, brachycephalic head, flat nasal bridge, ruddy cheeks, dry lips, large protruding "scrotal" tongue, small ears, oblique palpebral fissures that narrow laterally, epicanthic folds, occasional Brushfield spots, and a short fleshy neck (Fig 33–8). Irregular development of teeth is common; in about one-third of cases, the upper lateral permanent incisors are missing or defective. About one-third have congenital heart disease, most often an endocardial cushion defect or other septal defect. Patients tend to have short, stubby, spadelike hands with transverse palmar ("simian") lines and abnormal dermatoglyphics (see below). Generalized hypotonia is often present, as well as umbilical hernia. There is often a cleft between the big toe and second toe. Sexual development is retarded, especially in males. The affected newborn is prone to have a third fontanelle, prolonged physiologic jaundice, polycythemia, and a transient leukemoid reaction. Cutis marmorata is often present.

Patients with Down's syndrome display an increased sensitivity to the mydriatic effects of atropine instilled into the conjunctiva.

Dermatoglyphic patterns are characteristic. In general, the dermal ridges are poorly formed, and the frequencies of arches, radial and ulnar loops on the fingers, the distal location of the axial triradius on the palm, and the hallucal pattern on the sole of the foot differ from normals. Ford-Walker has combined frequency data on dermatoglyphic patterns on the fingers, palms, and soles into a "dermal index" that delineates 3 ranges—"mongol," "normal," and "overlap." A single flexion crease on the fifth finger is often found.

B. Laboratory Findings: The chromosomal abnormalities are pathognomonic. The great majority of cases (95%) have 47 chromosomes with trisomy of 21. However, about 4% of sporadic cases have 46 chromosomes, including an abnormal translocated chromosome formed as a result of centric fusion between 2 acrocentric chromosomes,* one of which is chromosome 21 (Fig 33–9). On the other hand, about one third of the familial cases have a translocation. Ten percent of patients whose mothers are younger will have these "interchange" lesions, whereas this is true in only 3% of those with older mothers.

Mosaicism of the 46/47 type can also occur in persons with Down's syndrome. This may result in

* Fusion between 2 centromere regions—a robertsonian translocation.

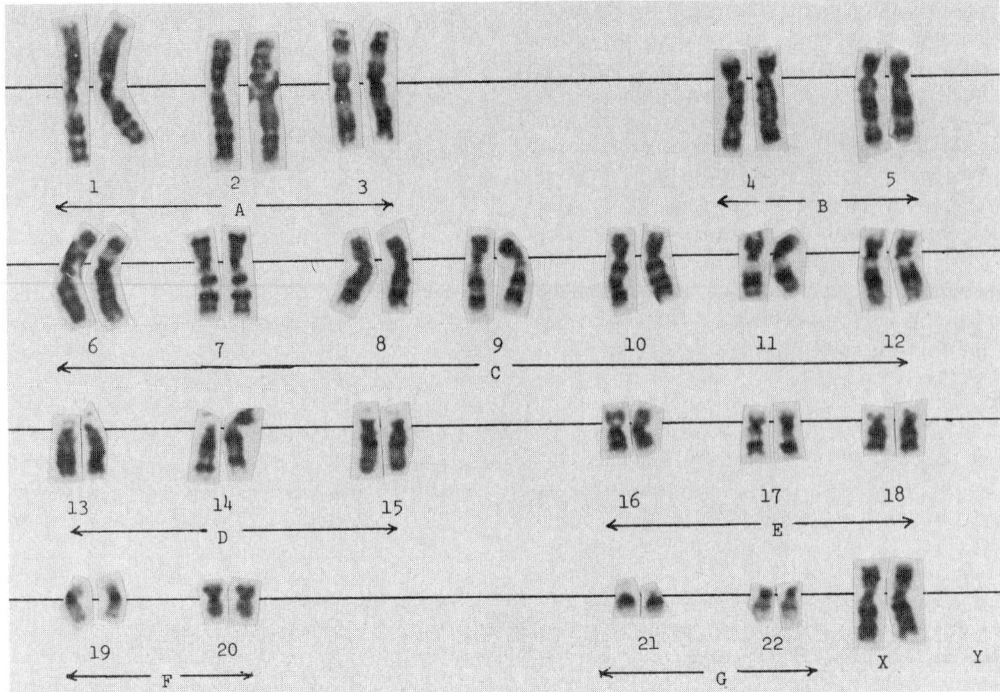

Figure 33–9. Karyotype demonstrating an unbalanced translocation resulting in chromosome 21 being present in the trisomic state. 46,XX,−4,+t(14;21)(p11;q11).

milder symptoms, especially in higher than expected IQ. Apparently normal mothers of affected children have occasionally been mosaics.

Band q22 on the long arm of chromosome 21 is the only part of the long arm that needs to be trisomic to produce Down's syndrome. Some genes such as those for superoxide dismutase, the interferon receptor, and several enzymes involved in the pathway of de novo purine biosynthesis are located near this band but do not seem to be the cause of Down's syndrome.

C. X-Ray Findings: X-rays of the pelvic bones of affected infants reveal flattening of the inner edges of the ileum and widening of the iliac wings. The "iliac index" is one-half the sum of both acetabular and iliac angles. This index is low (< 65) in about 80–90% of infants under 9 months of age with Down's syndrome (index is > 80 in the controls).

Skull x-rays often reveal brachycephaly, with flattening of the occiput. The sinuses may be absent or poorly developed. X-rays of the hand show shortening of the metacarpal bones and phalanges. The second phalanx of the little finger, in particular, is often abnormally small.

Differential Diagnosis

Most of the individual signs and symptoms of Down's syndrome also occur in the normal population, and the diagnosis is based on the presence of a *combination* of symptoms. Patients with other autosomal trisomies, and occasionally girls with a triple X karyotype, may have similar findings. The dermatoglyphics, sex chromatin status, and chromosomal analysis will differentiate the latter from Down's syndrome.

Complications

Leukemia (not the transient leukemoid reaction of the newborn) is 20 times more common than normal in individuals with Down's syndrome. These patients are very susceptible to intercurrent infections and are subject to the complications of congenital heart disease, when they have it, and to hypothyroidism.

Prevention

In general, Down's syndrome is not familial, and the risk of having an affected child in a sibship varies with maternal age (1:2000 for mothers under 25; 1:50 for mothers 35–39 years of age; 1:20 over 40 years of age). These figures are fairly accurate for families with trisomy 21 but much too low when one of the parents is a balanced translocation carrier.

In counseling parents who have produced one child with Down's syndrome about the risk of having a second affected child, the prognostic accuracy can be improved by studying the karyotypes of the affected child and the parents. Several situations may occur:

A. Child Has Trisomy 21, Parents Have Normal Karyotypes: The risk is only slightly greater than for parents in the general population (1–2%).

B. Trisomic Child, One Parent Mosaic: The risk will depend upon the degree of gonadal mosaicism of the affected parent. A rough estimate will be half of the proportion of abnormal cells in fibroblast cultures of the cells obtained from the parent.

C. Child Has 14/21 (D/G) Translocation, Parents Have Normal Karyotypes: The risks are unknown but should be considered slightly increased.

D. Child Has 14/21 Translocation, One Parent Is a Balanced Translocation Carrier:

1. When the mother is the carrier, 10–15% of the children will be affected, one-third will be carriers, and the remainder will be completely normal.
2. When the father is the carrier, there is a 3–5% chance of having another affected child, and half of the apparently unaffected children may be carriers.

E. Child Has a 21/22 (G/G) Translocation:

1. If both parents have normal karyotypes, the prognosis is roughly the same as under (A), although there is some evidence that advancing paternal age may increase this risk slightly.
2. If one parent carries the translocation and it is an isochromosome of 21 (21/21), the risk is 100%. If it is a 21/22 translocation, the risk is as in (D).

Treatment

No form of medical treatment has been shown to have much merit. Therapy is directed toward specific problems, eg, cardiac surgery or digitalis for heart problems, antibiotics for infections, checking thyroid function, special education and occupational training, etc. Affected children should be helped to make the most of their limited abilities. Early institutionalization is not recommended. Infant stimulation programs are helpful, and support of the parents is important.

Bungio G et al (editors): *Trisomy 21.* Springer-Verlag, 1981.
Pueschel SM (editor): *Down Syndrome: Growing and Learning.* Andrews, McMeel, 1978.

TRISOMY 18 SYNDROME (E$_1$ Trisomy)

Essentials of Diagnosis

- Mental retardation, failure to thrive, hypertonicity.
- Abnormal dermatoglyphics.
- Trisomy of chromosome 18 or, occasionally, an unbalanced translocation involving chromosome 18.

General Considerations

Trisomy 18 has an incidence of about one in 4500 live births, and there is an approximately 1:3 sex ratio (male:female). The mean maternal age is advanced. Affected individuals usually die in early infancy, although patients occasionally survive into childhood.

Clinical Findings

A. Symptoms and Signs: Trisomy 18 is characterized by failure to thrive, low birth weight, mental retardation, hypertonicity, prominent occiput, low-set and malformed ears, micrognathia, abnormal flexion of the fingers (index over third), equinovarus or "rocker bottom" feet, short sternum and narrow pelvis, congenital heart disease (often ventricular septal defect or patent ductus arteriosus), and inguinal or umbilical hernias. There is an increased occurrence of single umbilical arteries.

Dermatoglyphics show simple arches on fingers, a single flexion crease on the fifth finger, and transverse palmar lines.

B. Laboratory Findings: In place of uniform trisomy 18, chromosomal analysis occasionally reveals mosaicism for trisomy 18 or an unbalanced translocation involving a third number 18 and a chromosome of the 13–15 group. Rarely, double trisomies have been found in which trisomy X or trisomy 21 is present in addition to trisomy 18.

C. X-Ray Findings: X-ray often reveals gross retardation of osseous maturation, eventration of the diaphragm, and kidney abnormalities.

Differential Diagnosis

Trisomy 18 is differentiated from trisomy 13, in which failure to thrive, congenital heart disease, and retardation are also present. In the latter condition, the following findings differ from those of trisomy 18: shape of the head; eye, ear, and palatal anomalies; dermatoglyphics; and the occurrence of apneic spells. Other causes of failure to thrive must be considered.

Complications

Complications are related to associated lesions. Death is often due to heart failure or pneumonia.

Treatment & Prognosis

There is no treatment other than general supportive care. Death usually occurs in infancy, although patients have sometimes reached early childhood.

De Grouchy J, Turleau C: *Clinical Atlas of Human Chromosomes,* 2nd ed. Wiley, 1984.

TRISOMY 13 SYNDROME (D Trisomy)

The incidence of trisomy 13 is about one in 5000 live births, and 60% of the patients are female. The mean maternal age is high. Death usually (but not always) occurs by the second year of life, commonly as a result of heart failure or infection.

The symptoms and signs consist of failure to thrive, mental retardation, arhinencephaly, sloping forehead, eye deformities (anophthalmia, colobomas), low-set ears, cleft lip and palate, capillary hemangiomas, deafness, apneic spells, seizures, polydactyly or syndactyly, and congenital heart disease (usually ventricular septal defect). The facies of an infant with trisomy 13 is shown in Fig 33–10. Other abnormal findings may include hyperconvex, narrow fingernails, flexed and overlapping fingers, "rocker bottom" feet, retroflexible thumbs, urinary tract anomalies, umbilical hernia, and cryptorchidism or bicornuate uterus.

Although most patients have trisomy 13 (D trisomy), occasional patients are mosaic, and there are rare cases of an unbalanced (D/D) translocation with one of the parents carrying a similar translocation in the balanced state. Multiple projections and abnormal lobulation of the neutrophils are often present. Grossly elevated fetal hemoglobin and the presence of embryonic Gower's hemoglobin often occur.

Trisomy 18 patients are more hypertonic than these infants, and the head shape is different. The diagnosis of trisomy 13 should be considered in all cases of failure to thrive associated with retardation and palatal anomalies.

Other forms of the first arch syndrome are differentiated by the absence of a sloping forehead and the usual absence of other generalized malformations.

Treatment is supportive. Since on occasion it is necessary to decide immediately after birth how extensive and definitive therapy should be for a severely malformed infant, an immediate confirmation of this diagnosis (as well as one of trisomy 18) can be arrived at by direct examination of mitotic figures obtained from bone marrow. Prevention in the form of genetic counseling is indicated when one of the parents carries a balanced translocation, in which case the risks for future affected children are high (as in the analogous situation in Down's syndrome).

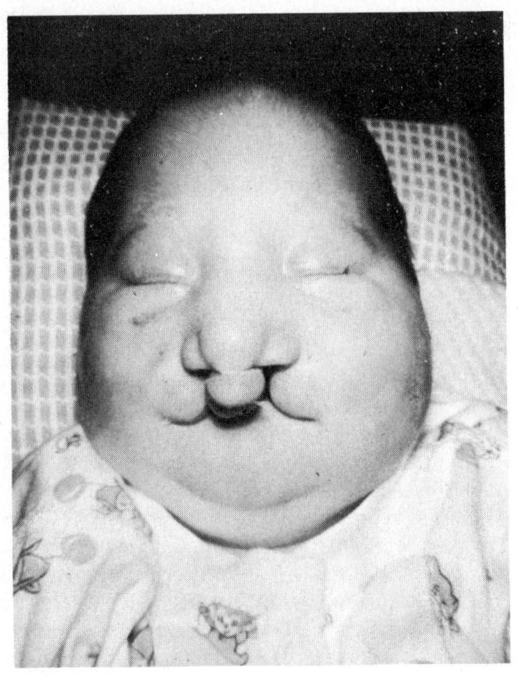

Figure 33–10. Facies of an infant with trisomy 13.

De Grouchy J, Turleau C: *Clinical Atlas of Human Chromosomes,* 2nd ed. Wiley, 1984.

CRI DU CHAT ("CAT CRY") SYNDROME

The incidence of cri du chat syndrome is not known. It occurs more commonly among females. Life expectancy is not seriously curtailed. The dimensions of the deleted chromosomal fragment are variable, which explains the variations observed in the phenotype.

Symptoms and signs consist of severe mental retardation, low birth weight, failure to thrive, microcephaly, hypertelorism, obliquity of palpebral fissures, epicanthic folds, low-set ears, a broad, flattened nasal bridge, "moonlike" facies, and micrognathia. The cry has a unique mewling quality like that of a kitten. It has a sharp timbre and plaintive tonality when emitted on expiration. It is due to small, flaccid, and somewhat rudimentary laryngeal structures and becomes less typical as the child gets older.

Patients often have repeated respiratory infections and persistent feeding problems. Breathing may be difficult. Hypospadias, cryptorchidism, and curved little fingers have been reported.

Chromosomal analysis shows deletion of part of the short arm of chromosome 5. This is occasionally replaced by a "ring" chromosome 5 or by a translocation.

Dermatoglyphics are often abnormal, with distal axial triradii. Transverse palmar lines may be present.

Because of the lack of specificity of many of the symptoms associated with abnormalities of the autosomes, all children with severe mental retardation, microcephaly, and failure to thrive enter into the differential diagnosis.

Newborn infants with various kinds of weak cry and laryngeal stridor may be differentiated by the fact that the "cat cry" is an expiratory sound and that an affected infant has the associated malformations.

Few cases have been familial. However, when one parent carries a balanced translocation involving chromosome 5 with deletion of the short arm, the risks are increased as in Down's syndrome.

Supportive care is all that can be given.

"NEW" CHROMOSOMAL SYNDROMES

A variety of new syndromes have recently been described, primarily because of the greater diagnostic accuracy resulting from the chromosomal banding techniques. Many of these syndromes are seen in a group of patients with more subtle chromosomal defects in whom one of the parents often has a balanced translocation. Prenatal diagnosis makes possible the prevention of future children with the same phenotype. New techniques that provide greatly extended chromosomes for study permit the visualization of many more bands and promise the elucidation of more chromosomal diseases resulting from interstitial deletions (see Prader-Willi syndrome, Table 33–3).

De Grouchy J, Turleau C: *Clinical Atlas of Human Chromosomes,* 2nd ed. Wiley, 1984.

Yunis JJ, Chandler MR: High resolution chromosome analysis in clinical medicine. Pages 267–287 in: *Progress in Clinical Pathology,* Vol. 8. Stefanini M et al (editors). Grune & Stratton, 1977.

THE GENE

The genes, which occur in pairs in somatic cells, occur at similar sites on the homologous chromosomes. The members of a pair, although they encode for the same function, are not always the same but may constitute alternate forms (alleles). When the homologs are the same, the individual is said to be "homozygous" for the gene; if they are different, the individual is "heterozygous." Since the male has only one X chromosome, he is said to be "hemizygous" for X-linked genes. If both alleles have different mutations, the individual is said to be a compound heterozygote.

GENE EXPRESSION

Most of what is currently known about a gene stems from how it expresses itself—its phenotype.

The phenotypic expression of a gene is the result of an interaction between the gene and its environment. The latter, in addition to the surrounding nucleoplasm and cytoplasm, includes the rest of the genome (genetic complement), which may have a modifying effect on the expression of a particular gene. It is this interaction that results in the variable severity of genetic diseases (expressivity) and occasionally completely prevents the expression of a defective gene (penetrance). The primary gene product, a protein, is least affected by environmental conditions. Hence, one of the criteria for determining that a gene product is primary is complete penetrance and little variation in expressivity. This would be true, for example, of hemoglobin S, a protein that is the direct result of a single mutation in the gene which produces the beta polypeptide chain of hemoglobin. An important point in clinical genetics is that the defective gene which is not expressed at all (nonpenetrant) can still be passed on to offspring, where it may be expressed.

It appears that with new techniques involving somatic cell hybridization, DNA probes, molecular hybridization, and restriction endonucleases, the study of defective genes can be performed without examination of the gene product, and many genes can be localized to specific areas on the chromosome. In short, the gene is no longer a symbol to explain the observable facts of mendelian segregation but is now a physically recognizable unit whose detailed structure and function are known. Of importance is the fact that many genes are discontinuous and may be characterized as mosaics of coding regions (exons) and noncoding regions (introns), and this gives the genome much more flexibility in gene expression and regulation.

Riggs AD, Itakura K: Synthetic DNA and medicine. *Am J Hum Genet* 1979;**31**:531.

RECOMBINANT DNA

A revolutionary advance in biology in recent years has been the development of recombinant DNA technology, which has major implications for medicine in general and medical genetics in particular. Fragments of DNA containing specific genes of interest are produced by a variety of bacterial enzymes called **restriction endonucleases,** which have the property of cleaving the DNA at sequence-specific sites. These specific DNA fragments are incorporated into the DNA of a vector (plasmid) by recombination, and the vector is then reintroduced into its host (eg, *Escherichia coli*), which is cultured. This produces multiple copies of the human DNA fragments, and clones of the fragment of interest can be selected and harvested in large quantities to be studied. The fragment may contain, for example, a complementary DNA copy (cDNA) produced from a specific messenger RNA (mRNA) by **reverse transcriptase,** an RNA-dependent polymerase. In this way, so-called libraries of specific DNA fragments can be produced. These specific DNA fragments are being utilized to manufacture human proteins, such as insulin, growth hormone, interferon, and blood clotting factors for pharmacologic applications, and also are being used as probes, which may be thought of as gene-specific, radioactively labeled reagents for mapping and diagnosis.

The diagnostic applications of molecular genetics are most commonly targeted to changes in genomic DNA using southern blot analysis, but the similar technique of northern blot analysis is being used increasingly to look at mRNA abnormalities. Southern blot analysis relies on the use of restriction endonucleases to cleave human genomic DNA at specific nucleotide sequences and produce DNA fragments of different lengths. When these DNA fragments are separated by agarose gel electrophoresis and overlaid with a probe, the probe will hybridize only with a fragment to which its DNA is complementary. This fragment, representing the gene of interest, is identified by autoradiography and its size determined.

There are 3 basic recombinant DNA techniques that are being used diagnostically. The first involves detection of **restriction fragment length polymorphisms** (RFLPs). Restriction enzymes cleave DNA at specific sequences 4–6 nucleotide base pairs in length, known as restriction recognition sequences. There is a normal variation in DNA sequences between individuals, and this variation may change the recognition sequence for a particular restriction enzyme, making the site unrecognizable to that endonuclease. When this occurs, the enzyme will not cut there, and a longer fragment spanning the interval between 2 unchanged recognition sequences (ie, the RFLP) will be detected by the specific cDNA probe. If closely linked to a point mutation under investigation, an RFLP may be used as a marker for that mutation. RFLPs have been extremely useful in the diagnosis of globin gene abnormalities (Fig 33–11), phenylketonuria, hemophilia A, and Huntington's chorea. In other heritable disorders in which specific mutations are not known, RFLP studies can be performed in the affected family member and the results compared with those in other family members. Since an RFLP is only a linked marker, it does not provide direct information about the mutation. However, restriction enzyme haplotyping with several different nucleases increases the probability that a given pedigree will be informative. This same approach may also be used to detect gene deletions and duplications.

The second diagnostic technique depends on the point mutation of interest altering a specific restriction sequence and making it unrecognizable to a particular endonuclease. This is known as a **restriction recognition site mutation** and provides a direct means for diagnosis of a disorder without the necessity of determining mutations in a previously affected individual in the family. Such is the case with sickle cell anemia and the use of the restriction enzyme *Mst*II, where a recognition site is lost as a consequence of the point mutation, leading to a longer fragment in the presence of the sickle cell gene.

The third diagnostic technique utilizes **synthetic oligonucleotide probes.** This approach is possible when the base change at a point mutation is known, as well as the nucleotide sequence surrounding the mutation. Synthetic probes may be constructed so that they are complementary to either the normal sequence or the mutant sequence. Under appropriate conditions, the single base pair mismatch will prevent hybridization, eg, between the normal genomic sequence and the probe complementary to the mutant sequence. Among the disorders for which synthetic oligonucleotide probes are being used diagnostically are sickle cell anemia and α_1-antitrypsin deficiency.

The knowledge gained using recombinant DNA technology is dramatically improving our understanding of gene structure and regulation. This not only will increase the diagnostic applications of these techniques but also will provide the basis for gene therapy in the future. Models utilizing experimental animals and human cells in culture show the feasibility of gene therapy for genetic disease.

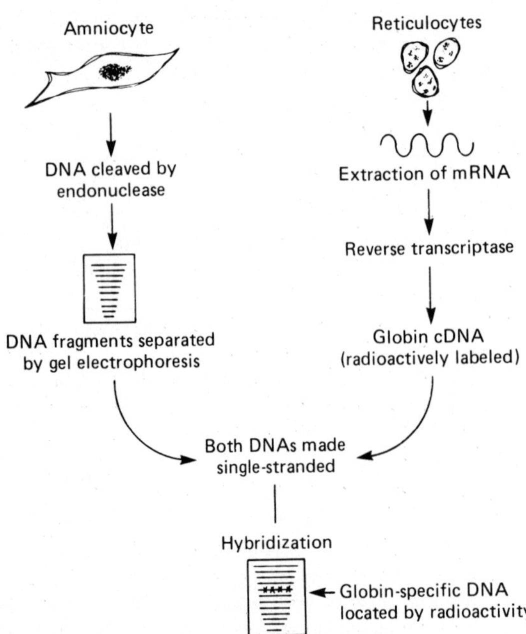

Figure 33–11. Recombinant DNA.

Antonarakis SE et al: Genetic disease: Diagnosis by restriction endonuclease analysis. *J Pediatr* 1982;**100:**845.

Cederbaum SD et al: Symposium on genetic engineering and phenylketonuria. (4 parts.) *Pediatrics* 1984;**74:**406, 408, 412, 424.

Kidd VJ et al: Prenatal diagnosis of α_1-antitrypsin deficiency by direct analysis of the mutation site in the gene. *N Engl J Med* 1984;**310:**639.

Miller AD et al: Expression of a retrovirus encoding human HPRT in mice. *Science* 1984;**225:**630.

Molecular genetics for the clinician. (Editorial.) *Lancet* 1984;**1:**257.

Oberle I et al: Genetic screening for hemophilia A (classic hemophilia) with a polymorphic DNA probe. *N Engl J Med* 1985;**312:**682.

Orkin S: Prenatal diagnosis of hemoglobin disorders by DNA analysis. *Blood* 1984;**63:**249.

Palmiter RD et al: Metallothionein-human growth hormone fusion genes stimulate growth of mice. *Science* 1983; **222:**809.

Prowchownik EV at al: Molecular heterogeneity of inherited antithrombin III deficiency. *N Engl J Med* 1983;**308:**1550.

White R at al: Construction of linkage maps with DNA markers for human chromosomes. *Nature* 1985;**313:**101.

SINGLE GENE DEFECTS

Diseases that are due to defects in a single gene are said to be "autosomal" or "X-linked" depending on whether the defective gene is located on an auto-some or X chromosome. If the disease is present when the defective gene is present either in the heterozygous or in the homozygous state, it is a dominantly inherited disease. If, however, it is present only when the gene involved is in the homozygous state, it is a recessively inherited disease.

AUTOSOMAL DOMINANT INHERITANCE

Some characteristics of dominantly inherited diseases (Table 33–4) are as follows:

(1) One of the parents of the propositus will have the disease. An exception to this is a mutation occurring in the parent's germ cell (see below) or when the disease in the parent was either not penetrant or of a greatly diminished expressivity.

(2) There is a 50% risk of involvement in each sibling of an affected individual if the parent is affected.

(3) The disease is usually not as serious as a recessively inherited disease.

(4) Either sex may be affected.

(5) The pedigree tends to be "vertical"—ie, there are affected individuals in several generations.

AUTOSOMAL RECESSIVE INHERITANCE

Some characteristics of recessively inherited diseases (Table 33–5) are as follows:

The disease tends to be rare and more severe than many dominantly inherited conditions.

Table 33–4. Some dominantly inherited diseases (autosomal).

Achondroplasia	Marfan's syndrome
Ehlers-Danlos-syndrome	Neurofibromatosis
Epidermolysis dystrophica hereditaria	Osteogenesis imperfecta
Gardner's syndrome	Polycystic kidneys (adult type)
Hereditary spherocytosis	Porphyria, hepatic form
Huntington's chorea	Retinoblastoma
	Tuberous sclerosis

Table 33–5. Some recessively inherited diseases (autosomal).

Albinism	Morquio's syndrome
Cystic fibrosis of the pancreas	Niemann-Pick disease
Familial nonhemolytic jaundice with kernicterus	Phenylketonuria
Galactosemia	Sickle cell anemia
Glycogen storage disease	Thalassemia
Hurler's syndrome	Virilizing adrenal hyperplasia
Microcephaly	Wilson's disease

(2) Affected individuals tend to be in the same generation. Pedigree is horizontal.

(3) Normal parents are carriers.

(4) The rarer the trait, the greater the incidence of consanguinity in the parents.

(5) There is a 25% risk of involvement of the sibs of an affected individual.

(6) Either sex may be affected.

X-LINKED (SEX-LINKED) DISEASE

When a gene is located on the X chromosome, it is said to be X-linked (sex-linked). A disease due to a single gene defect, which is inherited in an X-linked fashion, may be inherited either as an X-linked dominant or X-linked recessive.

X-linked dominant traits are rare (Table 33–6). They have the following characteristics:

(1) The hemizygous male will exhibit the full disease. None of his sons will be involved. All of his daughters will be involved, but they will show a milder form of the disease. There will be a 50% risk of involvement in each of his daughter's children.

(2) The homozygous female will have severe disease, and all of her children will be involved.

(3) The heterozygous female will have a milder form of disease, and there will be a 50% chance in all of her children, regardless of sex, of their being involved.

The X-linked recessive form of disease (Table 33–7) will have the following characteristics:

(1) Affected individuals are nearly always males.

(2) The mother is usually a carrier. She transmits the disease to half of her sons; ie, there is a 50% chance that each of her sons will be involved. She may on occasion show mild symptoms of the disease.

(3) One-half of a carrier mother's daughters will be carriers. All of an affected father's daughters will be carriers.

Table 33–6. X-linked dominant inheritance.

Hereditary hematuria: some types
Vitamin D-resistant rickets: some types
Xg(a) blood group

Table 33–7. X-linked recessively inherited diseases.

Agammaglobulinemia
Color blindness
Glucose 6-phosphate dehydrogenase deficiency
Glycerol kinase deficiency
Hemophilia A and B
Hereditary anhidrotic ectodermal dysplasia
Lesch-Nyhan syndrome
Ornithine transcarbamoylase deficiency
Pseudohypertrophic muscular dystrophy (Duchenne)
Steroid sulfatase deficiency (X-linked ichthyosis)
X-linked mental retardation

(4) The uninvolved sons do not transmit the disease.

(5) There is no father-son transmission.

MUTATION

The word mutation means a sudden change in genotype. In the case of a gene, this is a point mutation to distinguish it from more gross de novo changes in chromosomal structure. A mutation occurring in a germ cell will result in a child who differs at the given genetic locus from the parents. This mutant gene, however, will be passed on to the descendants of the individual having the mutation in the same manner as any other gene. It is obvious that mutations can only be recognized when the trait exhibits itself in the heterozygous condition—in other words, is dominantly inherited.

The causes of mutation are not completely known, although some factors, particularly high-energy radiation, that increase the rate of mutation are recognized.

SPORADIC OCCURRENCE OF DISEASE

It is especially important to investigate sporadic cases of disease occurring in a family when it is known that the disease is usually due to a single gene defect. The following causes should be considered.

(1) The mutation occurred in one of the parents. If this is true, then the disease should be dominantly inherited in the offspring of the affected individual. Since the mutant event was a point mutation occurring in one germ cell, the parents of the affected individual are not at an increased risk that further affected children will result from conceptions involving other, nonmutated germ cells.

(2) The disease is a rare recessive. Both parents are healthy carriers, and any future children that the parents have will run the usual 25% risk of being involved.

(3) The disease is a phenocopy, ie, a predominantly environmentally determined disease that mimics a genetic disease. An example of this would be the microcephaly occurring as part of the rubella syndrome versus genetically determined microcephaly.

(4) The disease is dominantly inherited but has low penetrance and has for this reason skipped the previous generation. It is possible that if one were to examine the parents by very sensitive techniques, some abnormal manifestation might be found to show that they were, in fact, involved.

(5) One must always consider the possibility in sporadic cases of genetic diseases that there may be illegitimacy and that one of the supposed parents is not really the parent.

SEX-LIMITED DISEASE

A sex-limited disease is one which is actually autosomally inherited but which, because of factors in the environment such as the presence of certain sex hormones, is expressed only in one sex. An example of this is baldness, which is inherited as an autosomal dominant but occurs predominantly in the male.

POLYGENIC DISEASE (Multifactorial Inheritance)

In addition to those traits which are due to the inheritance of a single gene, there are many traits and genetically determined diseases that are multifactorial in origin. Many of these traits occurring in the general population do not sharply divide the population into those who have and those who do not have the trait but exhibit a continuous variability representing a varying interaction between a genotype of a certain composition and an environment. The inheritance of certain quantitative characteristics such as blood pressure, intelligence, and height is multifactorial.

A number of relatively common defects and diseases that are clearly familial cannot be made to fit *all* the expectations for single gene (autosomal) inheritance. These discontinuous manifestations (Table 33–8) have been recognized during the last 4 decades to be examples of the multifactorial inheritance of a continuously distributed variable (liability or susceptibility). When the combination of genetic susceptibility and toxic environmental factors exceeds a developmental threshold, the defect or disease becomes manifest.

Cleft of the secondary palate is an example of such a threshold having been exceeded. In order for the palate to close, the palatal shelves must move from a vertical position alongside the tongue to a horizontal one above the tongue so that their medial edges may fuse. A variety of factors are involved in the timing of these embryologic events. Any delay will prevent meeting of the edges at the critical time (the threshold), and a cleft palate will result.

Some of the characteristics of this type of inheritance may be listed as follows:

(1) The risk of recurrence in relatives of the index case is increased.

(2) Recurrence risks for all first-degree relatives (those with 50% of their genes in common) are the

Table 33–8. Some common polygenically determined diseases.

Cleft lip and palate
Anencephaly/meningomyelocele
Pyloric stenosis
Congenital dislocated hips
Asthma

same. However, risks for second-degree relatives (grandchildren, nieces and nephews, aunts and uncles) and still more distant relatives drop off greatly in a nonlinear fashion.

(3) There is an increased risk of recurrence after 2 affected children. This is in marked contrast to single gene inheritance.

(4) There is an increased recurrence risk with increased severity of the defect. The risk of recurrence is greater in future siblings of a child with cleft lip or palate when the index case has bilateral cleft lip and palate (5.6%) as opposed to unilateral cleft lip (2.6%).

(5) The sex of the index case (proband) may affect the recurrence risk. In defects that occur more frequently in one sex than the other, when the index case is of the less frequently affected sex, it must be assumed that susceptibility is greater and thus the risk for recurrence is greater. Pyloric stenosis occurs more commonly in males. If a female has it, the risk for recurrence increases significantly.

Unfortunately for the practical application of genetics to medicine, the more common diseases tend to be etiologically heterogeneous and due to many genetic and environmental factors. As a result, genetic counseling about these conditions is not as simple as it is when discussing the aforementioned diseases in which simple types of inheritance occur.

EMPIRIC RISK FIGURES

Where the pattern of inheritance is obscure, as in diseases in which a number of genes interacting with the environment seem to be responsible, it becomes difficult to provide accurate risk rates. In this case, so-called empiric risk figures must be used. These are obtained from the literature and pooled data on a large number of families with the disease. These figures represent averages that may have little meaning in a specific case. However, they are the best available. Where the pattern of inheritance is not clear, a risk of a repeat is generally about one in 30, a figure much lower than the risks that must be quoted when single gene defects are involved (Table 33–9).

II. INBORN ERRORS OF METABOLISM

In his Croonian Lecture to the Royal College of Physicians of London in 1908, Sir Archibald Garrod described 4 diseases—alkaptonuria, cystinuria, albinism, and pentosuria—at the same time coining the term "inborn errors of metabolism." Since that time, the field has expanded greatly in fundamental under-

Table 33–9. Empiric risks for some congenital diseases.

Mental deficiency of unknown cause: Incidence 3:100
- Risks among siblings
  - Both parents normal, 15% defective
  - One parent defective, 35% defective
  - Both parents defective, 85% defective

Anencephaly and spina bifida: Incidence 1:1000
- Male:female = 1:3. Incidence increases with maternal age and parity, and also in firstborn of very young mothers.
- Risk of repeat = about 3%. Risk of abnormal child or abortion = 25%.

Hydrocephalus: Incidence 1:2000 newborns
- Occasional X-linked recessive
- Often associated with meningocele or spina bifida
- May be nongenetic (toxoplasmosis, aminopterin, x-ray)
- Chance of repeat of some central nervous system anomaly = 3%
- Chance of repeat of hydrocephalus = 1%

Central nervous system malformations in general: Incidence 29:10,000
- Siblings 6 times more likely to have central nervous system malformation
- Stillborn and abortion rates increased

	Cleft lip ± cleft palate (% of risk of repeat)	Cleft palate (% of risk of repeat)
Incidence	0.1	0.04
Negative family history	4	2
Normal parents; relative involved	4	4
2 affected children	9	7
1 affected parent; no affected children	4	6
1 affected parent; 1 affected child	17	15

Congenital heart disease: Incidence 2:1000
- Neither parent involved, 1.4–1.8% risk of repeat*
- One parent involved, 5% risk of repeat*

Diabetes: Incidence 5:100
- One parent involved, 15% risk of repeat*
- Both parents involved, 25–75% risk of repeat*

Pyloric stenosis

Male index patients:		
Brothers	3.2%	10 times greater than normal risk
Sons	6.8%	
Sisters	3.0%	20 times greater than normal risk
Daughters	1.2%	
Female index patients:		
Brothers	13.2%	35 times greater than normal risk
Sons	20.5%	
Sisters	2.5%	70 times greater than normal risk
Daughters	11.1%	

Clubfoot: Incidence 1:1000 (male:female = 2:1)
- Sibling risk = 3–8%

Congenital dislocated hip: Incidence 1:1000
- Siblings of index case, 40 times greater than normal risk
- Aunts, uncles, nephews, nieces (of index case), 4 times greater than normal risk

* Many exceptions.

standing, in the identification of new conditions, and in possibilities for treatment and prevention.

Most inborn errors of metabolism are caused by mutations of structural genes that code for enzymes. These mutations lead to the production of proteins (enzymes) that are inactive. The enzyme deficiency causes changes in the local concentrations of the enzyme substrate and products, causing the clinical manifestations or phenotypes.

Treatment is usually directed at correcting the alterations in the substrate or product concentrations (or both), or it may be aimed at increasing the activity of the mutant apoenzyme by providing large quantities of coenzyme. Treatment with enzyme itself is more difficult because the enzyme must be obtained in large quantities and directed to the appropriate tissues and organelles and also because enzyme inactivation by antibodies or rapid hydrolysis by intracellular proteases must be prevented. Current examples of enzyme replacement therapy involve organ transplantation and include the treatment of nephropathic cystinosis by renal transplantation and treatment of Wilson's disease by liver transplantation.

Treatment with genetic material that could itself code for active enzyme has not been successfully performed in humans but could proceed in the following manner: The appropriate gene could be cloned or synthesized and then amplified. The gene could then be given to the patient, with or without prior insertion into host cells in culture. This has been accomplished in tissue culture and in experimental animals, but regulation of insertion and expression remain the key issues (see Recombinant DNA, above).

Prevention for most inborn errors is by genetic counseling on risks for the particular pattern of inheritance, which is usually autosomal recessive but occasionally X-linked. Carrier detection for many of the conditions is possible but is usually complex and relatively expensive and is thus restricted to close relatives of known patients. Occasionally, however, as in Tay-Sachs disease, carrier detection is simple enough to justify screening programs in high-risk populations. Most of the conditions can be diagnosed in utero, and testing should be done with all at-risk couples who desire this service. Some of the better known and more common syndromes are described below. Others are described elsewhere in this book—eg, the hyperbilirubinemias in Chapter 20, glucose 6-phosphate dehydrogenase deficiency and the hemoglobinopathies in Chapter 16, and the immune globulin disorders in Chapter 17.

Burton BK, Nadler HL: Clinical diagnosis of inborn errors of metabolism in the neonatal period. *Pediatrics* 1978;**61:**398.

McCabe ERB: Principles of newborn screening for metabolic disease. *Perinatol Neonatol* 1982;**6:**63.

DISORDERS OF CARBOHYDRATE METABOLISM*

GALACTOSEMIA

The term galactosemia now denotes 2 conditions of galactose intolerance, one due to galactose-1-phosphate uridyl transferase deficiency and the other due to galactokinase deficiency.

1. GALACTOSE-1-PHOSPHATE URIDYL TRANSFERASE DEFICIENCIES

Although many variants and mixed heterozygotes are now known (such as the Indiana, Hammarsen, Negro, Kelly, Rennes, unstable, and the much more common Duarte variants), classic galactosemia occurs only when there is virtual absence of either galactose-1-phosphate uridyl transferase or galactose-4-epimerase activity. The resulting accumulations of galactose 1-phosphate in the liver, brain, and proximal convoluted tubules of the kidney cause hepatic parenchymal failure, mental retardation, and the renal Fanconi syndrome. The accumulation in the lens of galactitol, a reduction product of galactose, produces cataracts.

The disorder is inherited as an autosomal recessive trait with an incidence of approximately one in 40,000 live births; the carrier frequency is thus 1:100. Neonatal screening can be carried out using the Beutler fluorescence or the Paigen bacterial inhibition assay: the former test can also pick up carriers. These tests are in increasingly wide use because of the unreliability of early clinical diagnosis. In utero diagnosis of the deficiency in an affected fetus can be made by demonstrating enzyme deficiency in cultured amniotic cells.

Clinical Findings

A. Symptoms and Signs: In the severe form of the disease, the onset is with vomiting and diarrhea in the newborn period after a milk feeding. The infant becomes jaundiced and develops hepatomegaly. Without treatment, death frequently occurs in the first month of life, frequently from *Escherichia coli* sepsis. Cataracts usually develop within 2 months in untreated cases, and hepatic cirrhosis is progressive.

Not all cases are severe, as shown by the occasional identification of a patient with galactosemia in mental institution surveys. Mental retardation occurs unless treatment is given, and it seems to be irreversible. Even with early dietary restriction, there appears to be an increased risk for speech and language deficits

* A good general reference is Cornblath M, Schwartz R: *Disorders of Carbohydrate Metabolism in Infancy,* 2nd ed. Saunders, 1976.

and ovarian failure, and some patients develop progressive delay, tremor, and ataxia. Clinical and laboratory evidence of the disease abates gradually with effective treatment.

B. Laboratory Findings: In infancy, these include galactosuria and hypergalactosemia in patients receiving galactose-containing feedings, as well as proteinuria and aminoaciduria. Specific confirmation of defective red cell galactose-1-phosphate uridyl transferase activity must always be carried out. Normal levels are above 300 international milliunits (mIU)/g hemoglobin; in galactosemia, they are below 8 mIU/g hemoglobin.

Treatment & Prognosis

A galactose-free diet should be instituted as soon as the diagnosis is made. In the USA, regimens based on hydrolysates (eg, Nutramigen) or soy protein isolates (eg, Isomil, Prosobee) have proved satisfactory. For the detailed implementation of such a regimen, the reader should consult the references given below.

The efficacy of the diet should be monitored by measuring red cell galactose 1-phosphate concentration, which should not exceed 3 mg/dL packed red cell lysate. However, results must be corroborated with dietary history, since in certain conditions galactose 1-phosphate can be produced endogenously from UDP-galactose. Avoidance of galactose should be lifelong in severe cases, although there is some increased tolerance with age. Galactose is a component of stachyose and raffinose in soy products: as such, it is not absorbed, however, unless there is digestion in the colon. Heterozygous and homozygous mothers are advised to take a galactose-free diet during pregnancies.

With prompt institution of a galactose-free diet, the prognosis for life is excellent. Long-term follow-up suggests, however, that most severely affected individuals suffer some intellectual impairment. Infertility may be a late complication.

Garibaldi LR et al: Galactosemia caused by generalized uridine diphosphate galactose-4-epimerase deficiency. *J Pediatr* 1985;**103:**927.

Kaufman FR et al: Hypogonadotropic hypogonadism in female patients with galactosemia. *N Egl J Med* 1981;**304:**994.

Levy HL, Hammarsen G: Newborn screening for galactosemia and other galactose metabolic defects. *J Pediatr* 1978; **92:**871.

Levy HL et al: Sepsis due to *Escherichia coli* in neonates with galactosemia. *N Engl J Med* 1977;**297:**823.

Lo W et al: Curious neurological sequelae in galactosemia. *Pediatrics* 1984;**73:**309.

Segal S: Disorders of galactose metabolism. Chap 7, pp 167–191, in: *The Metabolic Basis of Inherited Disease,* 5th ed. Stanbury JB et al (editors). McGraw-Hill, 1983.

2. GALACTOKINASE DEFICIENCY

Increasing numbers of patients with galactosemia and galactosuria due to galactokinase deficiency are being described. These individuals show no renal or hepatic disease but do develop cataracts, often within the first few months of life, and the condition should thus be suspected in any child with cataracts. It is now recognized that many of these patients also have central nervous system disease, including developmental and neurologic abnormalities and seizures. Confirmation is made by identifying the presence of galactosuria and by demonstrating galactokinase deficiency in erythrocytes or cultured skin fibroblasts. The cataracts may regress upon institution of a galactose-free diet. The disorder is transmitted as an autosomal recessive trait and may be as common as galactosemia due to galactose-1-phosphate uridyl transferase deficiency. Heterozygotes have mild galactose intolerance and may have an increased incidence of cataracts.

Beutler E et al: Galactokinase deficiency as a cause of cataracts. *N Engl J Med* 1973;**288:**1203.

Gitzelman R: Additional findings in galactokinase deficiency. *J Pediatr* 1975;**87:**1007.

Segal S et al: Galactokinase deficiency and mental retardation. *J Pediatr* 1979;**95:**750.

HEREDITARY FRUCTOSE INTOLERANCE

Hereditary fructose intolerace is an autosomal recessive disorder in which there is deficient cleavage of fructose 1-phosphate into glyceraldehyde and dihydroxyacetone phosphate by fructose 1-phosphate aldolase. Affected individuals are symptom-free except after the ingestion of fructose, when hypoglycemia appears as well as failure to thrive, vomiting, jaundice, hepatomegaly, proteinuria, generalized aminoaciduria, and tyrosyluria. While the untreated condition can progress to death in liver failure, treatment is simple and consists of removal of fructose-containing foods from the diet. In fact, as less severely affected individuals grow up, they may recognize the association of nausea and vomiting with fructose-containing foods and selectively avoid them.

The diagnosis is supported by the demonstration of fructosuria following an oral fructose load. The presence of hypoglycemia and hypophosphatemia following fructose loading (24 g/m^2) is diagnostic, as is reduced activity of fructose 1-phosphate aldolase in liver.

Treatment consists of eliminating cane sugar from the diet. If the diet is subsequently relaxed, there may be retardation of physical growth, but growth will resume when more stringent dietary restrictions are instituted. If the disorder is recognized early enough, the prospects for normal development are good.

Fructose 1,6-diphosphatase deficiency, another form of fructose intolerance, usually presents as neonatal hypoglycemia.

Melancon SB et al: Metabolic and biochemical studies in fructose 1,6-diphosphatase deficiency. *J Pediatr* 1973;**82:**650.

Mock DM et al: Chronic fructose intoxication after infancy in children with hereditary fructose intolerance: A cause of growth failure. *N Engl J Med* 1983;**309:**764.

Odierre M et al: Hereditary fructose intolerance in childhood: Diagnosis, management and course in 55 patients. *Am J Dis Child* 1978;**132:**605.

GLYCOGEN STORAGE DISEASES

Glycogen is a branched-chain polysaccharide that is stored in liver and muscle. The usual end-to-end linkage in the molecule, which may contain about 10,000 glucosyl residues, is between carbon atoms 1 and 4. The branching links, however, are formed by α1,6-glucosidic bonds. About half of the bulk of the molecule is made up of free-end chains that are 7–10 glucosyl units long.

In the synthesis of glycogen, glucose is phosphorylated first in the 6 and then in the 1 position. Uridine diphosphoglucose is then formed by the enzyme UDPG pyrophosphorylase. In the next step, activated by glycogen synthetase, a glucosyl unit is added to the growing chain in a 1:4 bond. At the same time, the branching enzyme amylo-1,4:1,6-transglucosidase dislodges appropriate terminal chain segments and reattaches them in the 1,6 position. In the breakdown of glycogen, a small amount of glucose is liberated by the action of the debranching enzyme amylo-1,6-glucosidase; however, the bulk of the molecule is broken down to glucose 1-phosphate by phosphorylase. The activity of the latter enzyme is subject to a complex control mechanism initiated by glucagon and epinephrine and dependent on cyclic AMP.

About 10 different disorders of glycogen synthesis and breakdown have been described and the specific enzymic defects identified. In the hepatic forms, the diagnosis is suggested by growth failure and hepatomegaly with a tendency to fasting hypoglycemia. Other types predominantly affect muscle glycogen. These include acid maltase deficiency with cardiomegaly and macroglossia and muscle phosphorylase and phosphofructokinase deficiency, where the most striking features are easy fatigability and muscle weakness and stiffness.

Precise diagnosis is dependent on liver or muscle biopsy and appropriate biochemical tests. Treatment is for the most part symptomatic. In the more severe hepatic forms, some good results have been reported following continuous nighttime high-carbohydrate feeding.

Ambruso DR et al: Infectious and bleeding complications in patients with glycogenosis Ib. *Am J Dis Child* 1985;**139:**691.

Angelini C, Engel AG, Titus JL: Adult acid maltase deficiency: Abnormalities in fibroblasts cultured from patients. *N Engl J Med* 1972;**287:**498.

Fernandes J et al: Hepatic phosphorylase deficiency. *Arch Dis Child* 1974;**49:**186.

Greene HL et al: Type I glycogen storage disease: A metabolic basis for advances in treatment. *Adv Pediatr* 1979;**26:**63.

THE HYPOGLYCEMIAS

Impaired ability to sustain normal serum glucose levels is a common metabolic problem in infancy and childhood. Since precise definitions are difficult, diagnosis and treatment are designed to detect and treat either hyperinsulinism or disorders of glycolysis, gluconeogenesis, and absorption.

Table 33–10 sets out many of the recognized forms of infantile hypoglycemia and summarizes the differential diagnosis. The special importance of this group of disorders is worth repeated emphasis—namely, that failure to diagnose and treat correctly can lead to significant permanent cerebral damage.

Clinical Findings

A. Symptoms and Signs: Symptoms of hypoglycemia are quite variable. In the newborn, especially, there may be none, or the infant may show difficulty in feeding, apathy, hypothermia, pallor, cyanosis, a weak cry, and, later, episodes of tremors, eye rolling, or actual convulsions. The fontanelle is sometimes distended, and there may be cardiomegaly in severe cases. In older children, the usual symptoms are those of faintness, headache, sweating, and feeling hungry. Patients may look pale and complain of muscle pains and paresthesia; they may become irritable and drowsy and ultimately develop convulsions. Clinical response to restoration of normal serum glucose levels is usually rapid at all ages unless neurologic involvement is marked.

B. Laboratory Findings:* Hypoglycemia is usually defined as a serum glucose level of less than 20 mg/dL in premature infants, less than 30 mg/dL in full-term newborns, and less than 40 mg/dL in older infants and children. The possibility of this diagnosis always warrants complete laboratory evaluation, which can usually be done as an elective procedure. Where toxic or other specific cause is indicated, the diagnosis is that of the supposed underlying condition. In other cases, the following procedure is suggested:

1. Initial tests—After 3 days of a high-carbohydrate diet, the child is admitted to the hospital and, after an overnight fast, is given a standard glucose test lasting 4 hours. This is followed immediately after the last sample by a glucagon tolerance test. An abrupt fall in blood glucose between 30 and 60 minutes is indicative of hyperinsulinism, including leucine sensitivity. Late hypoglycemia at 3–4 hours suggests the delayed hyperinsulinemia of prediabetes. A flat curve may suggest malabsorption. A normal glucagon tolerance test indicates adequate hepatic glycogen and serves also as a screening test for normal

* See Chapter 39 for details of the tests discussed in this section.

glycolytic mechanisms. Simultaneous insulin levels are often helpful.

Since prediabetic hypoglycemia is very unusual in younger children, the initial glucose tolerance test can be restricted to samples taken during fasting and at 20, 40, and 60 minutes. Specimens for insulin levels can be taken at the same time, although a fasting and 20-minute sample are sufficient. Specimens for serum glucagon and cortisol levels should be drawn with the fasting sample.

2. Subsequent tests—Preliminary tests described above may indicate whether the problem is one of malabsorption, hyperinsulinism, or defective glycolysis or gluconeogenesis. Depending on the test results and on the severity of the hypoglycemia, it may be appropriate to carry out further tests for disorders such as galactosemia, fructose intolerance, propionic acidemia, isolated growth hormone insufficiency, panhypopituitarism, etc.

In infants and toddlers, the investigator may have to take refuge in a diagnosis of "ketotic hypoglycemia," an imprecise term that covers many metabolic aberrations in which the fasting child is unable to mobilize homeostatic amounts of glucose. Some of these children have low alanine levels. In these cases, it is usually of little value either to try a ketogenic diet or to seek a precise enzymatic diagnosis. Instead, treatment should be started, since many will improve with time.

Complications

Uncontrolled hypoglycemic episodes may lead to progressive cerebral damage, with epilepsy and developmental retardation. In cases in which a pancreatectomy has been performed, diabetes is an occasional complication.

Treatment

Treatment is directed at counteracting the imbalance in glucose homeostasis; it is not necessarily specific to the nature of the imbalance. The following program can be used as a guide:

A. Hypoglycemia in the Newborn: Treat initially with 5 or 10% dextrose infusion. This sometimes does not prevent hypoglycemia and may occasionally provoke hypoglycemia if suddenly discontinued. One of the following is sometimes required for a few days in addition to a glucose infusion: prednisone, 5 mg/d orally; glucagon, 15 μg/kg every 4 hours intramuscularly; or epinephrine, 1:200 (Sus-Phrine), 0.005 mL/kg intramuscularly. Fructose can be used instead of glucose in equimolar amounts. It is less likely to cause reactive hypoglycemia if temporarily discontinued.

B. Specific Hypoglycemias: When the specific cause of hypoglycemia is understood, treatment should be directed at relieving that primary cause, eg, nocturnal feeding in glycogen storage disease type I.

C. Hyperinsulinism: Patients with hyperinsulinism are often difficult to treat, especially since frequent feedings may precipitate hyperinsulinism. Diazoxide, 6–12 mg/kg/d in 2 divided doses, may be helpful and may be continued for a number of years, although hypertrichosis is a problem. Many affected children ultimately come to surgery either for the removal of an adenoma or for partial (85%) pancreatectomy for islet cell hyperplasia.

D. Undifferentiated Hypoglycemia: Acute episodes can be managed by giving glucagon, 20 μg/kg intramuscularly, followed by 10% dextrose in an appropriate electrolyte solution intravenously at a rate of 100 mL/kg/24 h. A combination of frequent feedings high in protein and carbohydrate and a high-protein feeding just before bedtime may help. Prednisone, 1–2 mg/kg/d in 2–3 divided doses, may be effective, but if a child requires prednisone for control, every effort should be made to define the cause of the hypoglycemia. Diazoxide may control hypoglycemia even when the cause is not hyperinsulinism. Uncontrolled hypoglycemia carries a grave risk of cerebral damage, epilepsy, and diminished cerebral function.

Prognosis

Treatment may be complex but is usually successful. Symptoms may persist into adult life.

Cornblath M, Schwartz R: Page 82 in: *Disorders of Carbohydrate Metabolism in Infancy,* 2nd ed. Saunders, 1976.

Greenberg RE, Christiansen RD: The critically ill child: Hypoglycemia. *Pediatrics* 1970;**46:**915.

Pagliara A: Hypoglycemia in infancy and childhood. (2 parts.) *J Pediatr* 1973;**82:**365, 559.

DISORDERS OF AMINO ACID METABOLISM

The widespread introduction of newborn screening programs and the use of increasingly sophisticated laboratory technology to study the components of physiologic fluids has led to the almost routine discovery of previously unrecognized inherited disorders of amino acid metabolism. The list of these disorders is now long, and only a few of special interest or importance are described in the following paragraphs.

PHENYLKETONURIA & THE HYPERPHENYLALANINEMIAS

Essentials of Diagnosis

- Serum phenylalanine levels persistently in excess of 20 mg/dL after the first few days of life, with low serum tyrosine levels.
- Phenylalanine levels can only be lowered by a special low-phenylalanine formula.

Table 33–10. Guide to the diagnosis of hypoglycemic states.

Causes and Types	Diagnosis
Newborn period	
Infants of diabetic mothers, prematurity, placental insufficiency, intracranial injury, sepsis, erythroblastosis fetalis, neonatal cold injury, cessation of intravenous glucose	Clinical history and serum glucose determination. Increased K_t following intravenous glucose may predict severe cases.
Cardiomegaly and neonatal hypoglycemia	
Metabolic disorders in older infants and children (disorders of glycolysis) Glycogen storage diseases Glucagon deficiency	Ideally, specific enzyme assay on liver biopsy.
Glucagon-resistant and hypoalaninemic ketotic hypoglycemia	Hypoglycemia with ketonuria. Hypoglycemia induced by ketosis. Small-for-gestational-age infants. Some respond to diazoxide.
Hypopituitarism with or without hyperinsulinism	Clinical history and supportive laboratory evidence. hGH levels unresponsive to arginine.
Hypoadrenocorticism	Clinical history and supportive laboratory evidence.
Primary liver disease	Poor response to glucagon and epinephrine.
Malnutrition	Rarely < 20 mg/dL, but serious if associated with hypothermia, coma, and bacterial or parasitic infection.
Catechol insufficiency (Zetterström type)	Defective catechol response to hypoglycemia.
Systemic carnitine deficiency	Associated myopathy and marked hepatic dysfunction.
Other disorders of hexose metabolism	
Galactosemia	Screen for red cell UDPgal transferase deficiency.
Fructose intolerance	Hypoglycemia after fructose load. Test for specific aldolase deficiency.
Fructose 1,6-diphosphatase deficiency	Acidosis and hypoglycemia on fasting; glycerol and fructose provoke hypoglycemia.
Hypoglycemia induced by lactose and other monosaccharides	Flat oral glucose tolerance test. Hypoglycemic response to lactose.
Hypoglycemia induced by glycerol	Poor response to glycogen. Sustained hypoglycemia produced by glycerol, 1 g/kg.
Phosphoenolpyruvate carboxykinase deficiency	Severe infantile hypoglycemia. Fatty changes in liver and kidney.
Pyruvate carboxylase deficiency	Thiamine-responsive.
Disorders of glyconeogenesis	
Idiopathic spontaneous hypoglycemia	Increased insulin sensitivity as shown by insulin/glucose tolerance test.
Hyperinsulinism	Often but not always an excessive insulin response to a glucagon, tolbutamide, or epinephrine tolerance test. Prompt and exaggerated hypoglycemic response to glucose loading.
Islet cell hyperplasia, nesidioblastosis	Increased K_t on intravenous glucose tolerance test.
Islet cell adenoma or adenocarcinoma	Irregular hyperinsulinemia after a glucose load. May have paradoxic response to diazoxide. May only be diagnosed at exploratory laparotomy.
Some extrapancreatic tumors	
Beckwith's syndrome	Associated with macroglossia, microcephaly, hepatomegaly, somatic gigantism, omphalocele.
Prediabetes	Delayed hypoglycemia following oral glucose tolerance test; later, glucose intolerance.
Leucine sensitivity	Positive leucine sensitivity test.
Maple syrup urine disease	Presence of typical smell, neurologic symptoms, acidosis, branched-chain ketoaciduria.
Miscellaneous disorders	
Hypothyroidism	Clinical history; serum glucose levels.
Primary neurologic disorders	Clinical history; serum glucose levels.
Reye's syndrome	Clinical picture of encephalopathy, hepatomegaly, and acidosis.
Chronic diarrhea	Especially with enteric infection.
Familial glucocorticoid deficiency	Body pigmentation, normal growth.
L-Asparaginase	In therapy for leukemia.

Table 33–10 (cont'd). Guide to the diagnosis of hypoglycemic states.

Causes and Types	Diagnosis
Miscellaneous disorders (cont'd)	
Methylmalonic aciduria	Specific organic aciduria.
Toxic	
Salicylates	Positive ferric chloride test; elevated blood salicylates.
EDTA	
Sulfonylureas	History of diabetes in the mother.
Manganese	Has been used in treatment of diabetes.
Propranolol	Tachycardia and sweating may be absent.
Biotin deficiency	Vomiting, glossitis, and scaly dermatitis.

- Tolerance to phenylalanine is very poor, and serum levels rise rapidly with any increase in intake. Tolerance is unchanged with increasing age.
- Untreated cases excrete phenylpyruvic and *o*-hydroxyphenylacetic acid in the urine and show a positive ferric chloride test.

General Considerations

Probably the most studied and best known disorder of amino acid metabolism, phenylketonuria was first recognized in 1934 by Folling in 10 severely retarded children who excreted phenylpyruvic acid in the urine. The disorder is due to diminished activity of phenylalanine hydroxylase, a complex enzyme system that converts phenylalanine to tyrosine and is transmitted as an autosomal recessive trait with a frequency of approximately one in 10,000 live births. The biochemical block leads to hyperphenylalaninemia and to the formation and excretion of such alternative phenylalanine metabolites as phenylacetylglutamine and phenylpyruvic, phenyllactic, phenylacetic, and *o*-hydroxyphenylacetic acids. The clinical picture includes severe mental retardation, a "mouselike" odor of the urine, light complexion and eczema, hyperactivity, and seizures. While decreased pigmentation is thought to be due to inhibition of melanin synthesis by hyperphenylalaninemia, the biochemical basis of the central nervous system dysfunction remains unclear. Postulated mechanisms have included inhibition of cerebroside, sulfatide, dopamine, serotonin, and protein synthesis by phenylalanine and inhibition of brain pyruvate kinase by phenylpyruvic acid.

Early favorable results in phenylketonuric children treated from early infancy with a diet low in phenylalanine led to the development of programs that were designed to detect hyperphenylalaninemia early in life, the notion being that phenylalanine restriction would then prevent the severe neurologic consequences. In general terms, this expectation has been fulfilled.

Present data suggest that diagnosis should be established and diet therapy begun in the first month of life—hence the necessity for newborn screening, which is usually performed in the first few days of life. When this is carried out in the first 24 hours of life, a repeat test should be done before the third week of life. Routine second tests are not recommended.

A. The Enzyme Defect: The 3 cosubstrates of phenylalanine hydroxylase are L-phenylalanine, atmospheric oxygen, and tetrahydrobiopterin; the products of the reaction are L-tyrosine, water, and the quininoid form of dihydrobiopterin. The latter is then reconverted to tetrahydrobiopterin by dihydropteridine reductase. In classic phenylketonuria, the mutant enzyme is phenylalanine hydroxylase, and little or no residual activity is demonstrable; in the less severe hyperphenylalaninemias, significant residual activity (10–20%) is present. There are 2 rare variants, one due to dihydropteridine reductase deficiency and the other due to a defect in biopterin synthesis.

B. Genetic Considerations: All of the hyperphenylalaninemias and phenylketonurias are inherited as autosomal recessives; some are true homozygous traits, while others probably represent heterozygosity for 2 different mutant alleles at the same locus.

Because phenylalanine hydroxylase is not normally present in fibroblasts or cultured amniotic cells, in utero diagnosis relies on the use of recombinant DNA techniques (see earlier section). However, dihydropteridine reductase activity is normally present in these cells, allowing the enzymatic diagnosis of this deficiency disorder.

Tests for the phenylketonuria carrier state have relied in the past on analysis of serum phenylalanine and tyrosine concentrations after natural protein or phenylalanine loading. These are now being replaced by recombinatant DNA techniques.

Clinical Findings

In infants, one of the earliest manifestations of phenylketonuria is vomiting. Another is a "mouselike" odor of the urine and sweat, which contain excessive amounts of phenylacetic, phenyllactic, and phenylpyruvic acids. By 1 year of age, the untreated phenylketonuric infant is often quite obese. The excessive accumulation of phenylalanine also impairs melanin production; thus, the untreated phenylketonuric individual often has a lighter complexion than unaffected relatives. For example, blacks, Orientals, and Hispanics have been noted to have brown hair; eczema is also common. Neurologic impairment is usual but not universal. Most patients are mentally retarded and hypertonic and have hyperactive reflexes. Seizures and tremors may be noted. Some have autistic or psychotic manifestations.

Differential Diagnosis

The diagnosis of phenylketonuria in a severely retarded older child with typical biochemical and physical characteristics is straightforward, but in the newborn period, especially when there is no family history, the condition must be differentiated from other forms of hyperphenylalaninemia as summarized below. A liver biopsy to determine the hydroxylase level may be helpful occasionally.

A. Classic Phenylketonuria: Findings include persistently elevated serum levels of phenylalanine (> 20 mg/dL on a regular diet), normal or low serum levels of tyrosine, and urinary excretion of phenylpyruvic and *o*-hydroxyphenylacetic acids. There is poor tolerance to oral phenylalanine throughout life, and serum tyrosine levels do not rise after a phenylalanine load. Phenylalanine restriction, which lowers the serum phenylalanine level, is indicated.

B. Persistent Hyperphenylalaninemia: Serum phenylalanine levels may exceed 20 mg/dL early but eventually range from 4 to 20 mg/dL on a normal protein intake. The serum tyrosine level rises after a phenylalanine load, and phenylketones are not excreted in urine or are only transiently excreted. Dietary treatment may or may not be required, depending on phenylalanine tolerance.

C. Transient Hyperphenylalaninemia: Serum phenylalanine levels are elevated early but progressively decline toward normal. If required at all, dietary restriction is only temporary.

D. Dihydropteridine Reductase Deficiency: Serum phenylalanine levels are variable but may be in the range of classic phenylketonuria. Serum tyrosine levels are normal. The activity of dihydropteridine reductase can be measured in fibroblasts, and the disorder may be suspected on screening of urinary biopterin metabolites. Seizures and psychomotor regression are seen, even if diet therapy is instituted. Neurotransmitter deficiencies require treatment with levodopa, carbidopa, and 5-hydroxytryptophan.* Treatment with tetrahydrobiopterin* is still debated.

E. Defects in Biopterin Biosynthesis: Serum phenylalanine levels are variable but may be in the range of classic phenylketonuria. Serum tyrosine levels are normal. The disorder is diagnosed by evaluation of urinary biopterin metabolites. Clinical findings include myoclonus, tetraplegia, and other movement disorders. Treatment is the same as that for dihydropteridine reductase deficiency.

F. Persistent Hyperphenylalaninemia and Tyrosinemia: Findings include elevated serum levels of phenylalanine and tyrosine; increased urinary levels of phenylethylamine, mandelic acid, and *p*-hydroxymandelic acid; and progressive clinical deterioration, with ataxia and seizures appearing at 12–18 months of age. Treatment consists of dietary restriction of phenylalanine.

G. Tyrosinemia of the Newborn: Hyperphenylalaninemia is accompanied by even greater transient hypertyrosinemia. Patients respond to vitamin C administration (see Tyrosinemia, below).

H. Maternal Phenylketonuria: The heterozygous (for phenylketonuria) offspring of phenylketonuric mothers have transient hyperphenylalaninemia after birth. Dietary treatment of the neonate is not indicated, since serum phenylalanine levels fall rapidly. Nearly all offspring are mentally retarded; the majority are microcephalic; and there is a significantly increased risk for low birth weight and congenital heart disease. The risk for the maternal PKU syndrome appears to be diminished if the mother's disorder is treated with phenylalanine restriction prior to conception and throughout pregnancy; this requires extremely close nutritional monitoring.

Treatment & Prognosis

Treatment is aimed at limiting the intake of phenylalanine to amounts that allow normal growth and development without excessive hyperphenylalaninemia, an approach made possible by the availability of several low-phenylalanine milk substitutes. Since excessive restriction of phenylalanine may produce bone changes, anemia, and retardation of growth and development, it is essential to monitor the treatment closely through serial serum phenylalanine determinations as well as by ascertaining general health, growth, development, and nutritional intake. Such coordination of care is frequently best done at clinics where specialists in each of these areas are in attendance. Although dietary treatment is most effective when initiated during the first few months of life, it is sometimes beneficial in reversing maladaptive behavior such as hyperactivity and excessive lethargy when started later in life.

It is now generally accepted that phenylalanine restriction should continue throughout life. As noted above, females with phenylketonia merit special attention during the childbearing years, with counseling during adolescence and closely monitored diet therapy prior to conception and throughout pregnancy.

Children treated promptly after birth and properly managed in terms of phenylalanine and tyrosine homeostasis will develop well physically and can be expected to have normal or nearly normal intellectual development.

Acosta PB et al: *Dietary Management of Inherited Metabolic Diseases*. Department of Pediatrics, Emory University School of Medicine, 1976.

Committee on Genetics, American Academy of Pediatrics: New issues in newborn screening for phenylketonuria and congenital hypothyroidism. *Pediatrics* 1982;**69:**104.

Committee on Nutrition, American Academy of Pediatrics: Special diets for infants with inborn errors of metabolism. *Pediatrics* 1976;**57:**783.

* Available only at authorized centers. For information, consult FDA sources.

Danks DM et al: Malignant hyperphenylalaninemia: Current status (June 1977). *J Inherited Metab Dis* 1978;**2**:49.

Lenke RR, Levy HL: Maternal phenylketonuria: Results of dietary therapy. *Am J Obstet Gynecol* 1982;**142**:548.

McCabe ERB et al: Newborn screening for phenylketonuria: Predictive validity as a function of age. *Pediatrics* 1983; **72**:390.

Scriver CR, Clow CL: Phenylketonuria: Epitome of human biochemical genetics. (2 parts.) *N Engl J Med* 1980; **303**:1336, 1394.

Tourian A, Sidbury JB: Phenylketonuria and hyperphenylalaninemia. In: *The Metabolic Basis of Inherited Disease,* 5th ed. Stanbury JB et al (editors). McGraw-Hill, 1983.

Williamson ML et al: Correlates of intelligence test results in treated phenylketonuric children. *Pediatrics* 1981;**68**:161.

TYROSINEMIA

The normal metabolism of tyrosine is by transamination to *p*-hydroxyphenylpyruvic acid (*p*HPPA) followed by oxidation to homogentisic acid by *p*-hydroxyphenylpyruvic acid oxidase; homogentisic acid is then oxidized to fumaric and acetoacetic acids. The tyrosinemias are disorders in which defects in this pathway result in high serum concentrations of tyrosine (tyrosinemia) and urinary excretion of various tyrosine metabolites like *p*-hydroxyphenylpyruvic and *p*-hydroxyphenyllactic acids (tyrosyluria). The most important forms of tyrosinemia are summarized below.

Classification

A. Tyrosinemia of the Newborn: Tyrosinemia of the newborn (serum tyrosine levels of ⩾ 6 mg/dL) is due to immaturity of *p*-hydroxyphenylpyruvic acid oxidase and is thus especially common in premature infants; it is accentuated by vitamin C deficiency and high protein intake. Recovery of enzyme activity is usually quite sudden and may occur at any time between a few days and 3 months of age.

Tyrosinemia in this condition may be reduced by lowering protein intake to 2 g/kg/d or by giving ascorbic acid, 100 mg intramuscularly. The response to these measures may help differentiate the condition from other causes of tyrosinemia described below. Prolonged tyrosinemia (> 6 weeks) may be associated with central nervous system damage (the relation is unclear), and thus lowering tyrosine levels may be important in preventing neurologic sequelae.

B. Hereditary Tyrosinemia: Hereditary tyrosinemia is an inherited syndrome of progressive hepatic parenchymal damage, renal tubular dystrophy with generalized aminoaciduria and hypophosphatemic rickets, hypermethioninemia, mild tyrosinemia, and tyrosyluria. The course may be rapidly fatal in infancy or somewhat more chronic. It has become apparent that this clinical picture is nonspecific and may occur with a number of disorders, including those caused by deficiencies in fumarylacetoacetase, fructose 1-phosphate aldolase (hereditary fructose intolerance), galactose-1-phosphate uridyl transferase (galactosemia), and fructose 1,6-diphosphatase.

C. Hypertyrosinemia (Oregon Type): This disorder is probably due to inherited deficiency of hepatic cytosol tyrosine aminotransferase and is characterized by profound tyrosinemia (35–50 mg/dL), a syndrome of palmar and plantar keratoses and corneal dystrophy (Richner-Hanhart syndrome) whose severity fluctuates with the elevation of serum tyrosine, and mental retardation.

Treatment

There is only tentative evidence that transient *p*HPPA deficiency in the newborn leads to any neurologic impairment. However, some animal studies show an effect of tyrosinosis on myelination. It seems reasonable, therefore, to use a low-protein formula until enzyme activity is restored to normal and to ensure an adequate vitamin C supplement.

In the groups with liver damage, control with a low-phenylalanine and low-tyrosine diet (50 mg of each per kilogram in 24 hours) now seems mandatory, but these patients may still develop hepatic disease despite diet therapy.

Hostetter MK et al: Evidence for liver disease preceding amino acid abnormalities in hereditary tyrosinemia. *N Engl J Med* 1983;**308**:1265.

Mamunes P et al: Intellectual deficits after tyrosinemia in term neonates. *Pediatr Res* 1974;**8**:344.

Rizzardini M, Abeliuk P: Tyrosinemia and tyrosinuria in low birth weight infants. *Am J Dis Child* 1971;**121**:182.

MAPLE SYRUP URINE DISEASE (Branched-Chain Ketoaciduria)

Maple syrup urine disease is due to generalized deficiency of the enzymes that catalyze oxidative decarboxylation of the keto acid derivatives of the branched-chain amino acids leucine, isoleucine, and valine. The keto acids of leucine and isoleucine contribute to the characteristic odor, while only the keto acid of leucine has been implicated in central nervous system dysfunction. Many variants of this disorder have been described, including mild, intermittent, and thiamine-dependent forms.

In the classic form, patients are normal at birth but soon develop the characteristic odor, lethargy, feeding difficulties, coma, and seizures. If the diagnosis is not made and diet therapy begun, most will die in the first month of life. Peritoneal dialysis may be necessary in initial therapy, but long-term treatment is dietary and directed toward restriction of branched-chain amino acids to amounts necessary for normal growth and development. If such treatment is begun prior to about 10 days of age, normal growth and development can be achieved. Problems include (1) maintenance of dietary restriction throughout life, (2) necessity for and cost of biochemical monitoring, and (3) hyperleucinemia and central nervous system symptoms accompanying catabolic episodes during infections.

This rare disorder is transmitted as an autosomal recessive trait. It can be diagnosed during fetal life on the basis of absent branched-chain keto acid decarboxylase activity in cultured amniotic cells.

Acosta PB et al: *Dietary Management of Inherited Metabolic Diseases.* Department of Pediatrics, Emory University School of Medicine, 1976.

Clow CL et al: Outcome of early and long-term management of classical maple syrup urine disease. *Pediatrics* 1981; **68:**856.

Hammersen G et al: Maple syrup urine disease: Treatment of the acutely ill newborn. *Eur J Pediatr* 1978;**129:**157.

Scriver CR et al: Thiamine responsive maple syrup urine disease. *Lancet* 1971;**1:**310.

DISORDERS OF THE UREA CYCLE

The urea cycle is a series of 5 enzymes that convert ammonia to one of the amino groups in urea. Inherited deficiency of one of the first enzymes in the sequence (carbamoyl phosphate synthetase and ornithine transcarbamoylase) usually presents in infancy with a syndrome of episodic vomiting, hyperammonemia, and neurologic signs (coma, seizures, etc) that can lead to early death. Similar symptoms may occur in citrullinemia (argininosuccinic acid synthetase deficiency) and argininosuccinic acidemia (argininosuccinic acid lyase deficiency), but a more chronic course with mental retardation is more usual in these conditions and in argininemia (arginase deficiency).

Diagnosis is based on the presence of hyperammonemia, specific aminoacidemia or aminoaciduria (in citrullinemia, argininosuccinic aciduria, and argininemia), and specific enzyme assay. Treatment, which is variably effective, is by lowering blood ammonia acutely with peritoneal dialysis or exchange transfusion and, in citrullinemia and arginosuccinic acidemia, by providing arginine to augment waste nitrogen excretion. Useful long-term treatment is with a low-protein diet, sodium benzoate, and, possibly, the keto analogs of essential amino acids.

With the exception of ornithine transcarbamoylase deficiency, which is inherited in X-linked fashion, all of these disorders are inherited as autosomal recessive traits. Citrullinemia and argininosuccinic aciduria can be diagnosed in utero; carbamoyl phosphate synthetase deficiency and ornithine transcarbamoylase deficiency cannot.

Batshaw ML et al: Arginine-responsive asymptomatic hyperammonemia in the premature infant. *J Pediatr* 1984;**105:**86.

Brusilow SW et al: Treatment of episodic hyperammonemia in children with inborn errors of urea synthesis. *N Engl J Med* 1984;**310:**1630.

Hokanson JT et al: Carrier detection in ornithine transcarbamylase deficiency. *J Pediatr* 1978;**93:**75.

Lindgren V et al: Human ornithine transcarbamylase locus mapped to band Xp21.1 near the Duchenne muscular dystrophy locus. *Science* 1984;**226:**698.

Msall M et al: Neurologic outcome in children with inborn errors of urea synthesis: Outcome of urea cycle enzymopathies. *N Engl J Med* 1984;**310:**1500.

Qureshi IA et al: Treatment of hyperargininemia with sodium benzoate and arginine-restricted diet. *J Pediatr* 1984; **104:**473.

CONGENITAL METHYLMALONIC ACIDEMIA

Four essential amino acids (L-threonine, L-valine, L-isoleucine, and L-methionine) are metabolized through D-methylmalonyl-CoA. Under normal conditions, this compound is converted to L-methylmalonyl-CoA by methylmalonyl-CoA racemase and then to succinyl-CoA by methylmalonyl-CoA mutase, an enzyme that requires adenosyl-B_{12} as coenzyme. Congenital methylmalonic aciduria can thus be caused by deficiencies of methylmalonyl-CoA racemase, methylmalonyl-CoA mutase, or enzymes that function in the synthesis of adenosyl-B_{12}.

There are several diseases in the latter category, including 2 that affect the synthesis of adenosyl-B_{12} and 2 that affect the synthesis of both adenosyl-B_{12} and methyl-B_{12}. The latter is the coenzyme for N^5-methyltetrahydrofolate methyltransferase, an enzyme necessary for the conversion of homocysteine to methionine.

Clinical symptoms in methylmalonic aciduria depend on the location and severity of the enzyme block. Those with severe blocks present with acute, life-threatening metabolic acidemia and hyperammonemia early in infancy or with metabolic acidemia, vomiting, and failure to thrive during the first few months of life. Children with less severe blocks may show only moderate mental retardation. Laboratory findings include hyperglycinemia and hyperglycinuria, a positive methylmalonic aciduria screening test, the presence of methylmalonic acid in the urine on organic acid chromatography, and, in the case of an appropriate block in B_{12} metabolism, hypomethioninemic homocystinuria.

Patients with enzyme blocks in B_{12} metabolism usually respond to massive (1 mg/d) doses of vitamin B_{12}, while nonresponders require protein restriction and correction of their rather constant metabolic acidemia.

All types of methylmalonic aciduria described to date are transmitted as autosomal recessive traits. The disorder can be diagnosed in utero by demonstrating defective metabolism of propionate in cultured amniotic fluid cells.

Matsui SM et al: The natural history of the inherited methylmalonic acidemias. *N Engl J Med* 1983;**308:**857.

Packman S et al: Severe hyperammonemia in a newborn infant with methylmalonyl-CoA-mutase deficiency. *J Pediatr* 1978; **92:**769.

Shinnar S, Singer HS: Cobalamin C mutation (methylmalonic aciduria and homocystinuria) in adolescence: A treatable cause of dementia and myelopathy. *N Engl J Med* 1984;**311:**451.

DISORDERS OF PURINE & PYRIMIDINE METABOLISM

Hereditary Orotic Aciduria

Orotate phosphoribosyltransferase and orotidylate decarboxylase are sequential and physically complexified enzymes in the biosynthesis of uridine monophosphate, and a defect in the activity of one or both enzymes leads to an autosomal recessive condition characterized by failure to thrive, hypochromic anemia with megaloblastic changes in the marrow, and increased urine excretion of orotic acid. The enzyme defect may be demonstrated in tissue biopsy, erythrocytes, and cultured skin fibroblasts.

Two types have been described: one in which both enzyme activities are deficient (type I) and one in which only decarboxylase activity is deficient (type II). Although the former situation was once thought to be due to mutation of a regulator gene, both types are in fact due to decarboxylase mutations. The type I mutation does not allow proper aggregation of phosphoribosyltransferase and decarboxylase subunits, so that both activities appear to be deficient, whereas the type II mutation affects only its active site and not aggregation.

Brown GK, O'Sullivan WJ: The subunit structure of the orotate phosphoribosyltransferase-orotidylate decarboxylase complex from human erythrocytes. *Biochemistry* 1977;**16:**3235.

Kelley WN, Smith LH Jr: Hereditary orotic aciduria. Chap 56, pp 1202–1226, in: *The Metabolic Basis of Inherited Disease*, 5th ed. Stanbury JB et al (editors). McGraw-Hill, 1983.

Adenosine Deaminase Deficiency

Adenosine deaminase is the enzyme responsible for the conversion of adenosine to inosine in the purine salvage system. The autosomal recessive disorder due to its deficiency chiefly affects the immune system, causing the most common form of combined immunodeficiency disease, a syndrome characterized by the onset of severe infections early in life, lymphopenia, and deficiency of both B and T cell-mediated immunity. Without treatment, patients die at age 2 years or after.

The combined immunodeficiency disease caused by this enzymopathy may be distinguished from adenosine deaminase-positive forms by (1) enzyme assay of lymphocytes, erythrocytes, or cultured fibroblasts; (2) the presence of various radiologic abnormalities of pelvis, spine, and ribs; and (3) the presence in the thymus of Hassall's corpuscles and differentiated thymic epithelium.

Unlike the adenosine deaminase-positive forms of combined immunodeficiency disease, which respond only to bone marrow or fetal liver transfusions, enzyme replacement by repeated transfusions of normal irradiated erthyrocytes rapidly restores and maintains immunocompetence in the adenosine deaminase-negative patient.

Meuwissen HJ et al: Combined immunodeficiency disease associated with adenosine deaminase deficiency. *J Pediatr* 1975;**86:**169.

Polmar SH et al: Enzyme replacement therapy for adenosine deaminase deficiency and severe combined immunodeficiency. *N Engl J Med* 1976;**295:**1337.

Purine Nucleoside Phosphorylase Deficiency

Purine nucleoside phosphorylase is the enzyme responsible for the respective conversions of inosine, guanosine, and xanthosine to hypoxanthine, guanine, and xanthine in the purine salvage system, and the autosomal recessive disease caused by its deficiency is, like adenosine deaminase deficiency (see above), primarily one of the immune system. In this situation, however, only T cell-mediated immunity is severely deficient, and the clinical condition is characterized by recurrent infections, hypochromic anemia with megaloblastic changes in the bone marrow, lymphopenia, hypouricemia, and hypouricosuria. Erythrocytes and cultured fibroblasts are completely deficient in purine nucleoside phosphorylase activity.

Cohen A et al: Abnormal purine metabolism and purine overproduction in a patient deficient in purine nucleoside phosphorylase. *N Engl J Med* 1976;**295:**1449.

Giblett ER et al: Nucleoside-phosphorylase deficiency in a child with severely defective T-cell immunity and normal B-cell immunity. *Lancet* 1975;**1:**1010.

Hypoxanthine-Guanine Phosphoribosyltransferase Deficiency (Lesch-Nyhan Syndrome)

Hypoxanthine-guanine phosphoribosyltransferase (HPRT) is the enzyme that converts the purine bases hypoxanthine and guanine to inosine monophosphate (IMP) and guanosine monophosphate (GMP), respectively, and the X-linked recessive disorder due to its complete deficiency is characterized by central nervous system dysfunction and purine overproduction with hyperuricemia and hyperuricosuria. Depending on the residual activity of the mutant enzyme, male hemizygotes may be severely retarded and show choreoathetosis, spasticity, and compulsive, mutilating lip and finger biting, or they may present with only gouty arthritis and urate ureterolithiasis. The enzyme deficiency can be demonstrated in erythrocytes, fibroblasts, and cultured amniotic cells; this disorder can thus be diagnosed with certainty in utero.

Although the cause of the central nervous system dysfunction in Lesch-Nyhan syndrome remains obscure, the absent or less severe central nervous system manifestations of purine nucleoside phosphorylase deficiency (in which HPRT is functionally inactive because of lack of substrate) suggest that the problem relates to accumulation of substrate behind the block.

Allopurinol and probenecid may be given to reduce hyperuricemia, but they do not affect neurologic status. Insertions of the HPRT gene into cultured cells from affected patients and into experimental animals have been effective and offer promise as models for human gene therapy in the future.

Cohen A et al: Abnormal purine metabolism and purine overproduction in a patient deficient in purine nucleoside phosphorylase. *N Engl J Med* 1976;**295:**1449.

Kelley WN, Wyngaarden JB: The Lesch-Nyhan syndrome. Chap 51, pp 1115–1143, in: *The Metabolic Basis of Inherited Disease,* 5th ed. Stanbury JB et al (editors). McGraw-Hill, 1983.

DISORDERS OF MUCOPOLYSACCHARIDE & LIPID METABOLISM

The lysosome is the cellular organelle responsible for the degradation of complex macromolecules. When one of its specific hydrolases is genetically altered so as to become inactive, the substrate of the enzyme accumulates in the lysosomes of tissues degrading it, thus causing the characteristic clinical picture. Depending on the nature of the stored material, disorders of this type fall into 2 main groups: mucopolysaccharidoses and lipidoses.

MUCOPOLYSACCHARIDOSES

Mucopolysaccharidoses are characterized by mucopolysacchariduria and by the storage of products of partial mucopolysaccharide digestion in lysosomes throughout the body. Features of these conditions and closely related diseases are given in Table 33–11.

Diagnosis of these conditions, usually suspected on clinical grounds, can be confirmed by a number of tests that screen for mucopolysacchariduria. The specific mucopolysaccharides excreted can then be determined by chromatography. Especially when parents are considering having additional children, enzyme diagnosis is mandatory and can be made on tissue biopsy (eg, liver), cultured skin fibroblasts, or peripheral leukocytes. Most of these disorders can be diagnosed in utero by enzyme assays of cultured amniotic cells. Bone marrow transplantation may affect the course of some of these diseases.

Hobbs JR et al: Reversal of clinical features of Hurler's disease and biochemical improvement after treatment by bone marrow transplantation. *Lancet* 1981;**2:**709.

McKusick VA: *Heritable Disorders of Connective Tissue,* 4th ed. Mosby, 1972.

LIPIDOSES

Lipidoses are characterized by lysosomal accumulation of lipids that usually contain sphingosine. Features of these conditions are given in Table 33–12.

When suspected, diagnosis may be confirmed by appropriate enzyme assays of biopsy specimens, cultured skin fibroblasts, and peripheral leukocytes. Most can be diagnosed in utero by appropriate enzyme assays of cultured anmiotic cells.

Hers HG, Van Hoff F (editors): *Lysosomes and Storage Diseases.* Academic Press, 1973.

Malone MJ: The cerebral lipidoses. *Pediatr Clin North Am* 1976;**23:**303.

O'Brien JS: Ganglioside storage diseases. In: *Advances in Human Genetics.* Vol 3. Harris H, Hirschhorn K (editors). Plenum Press, 1972.

Stanbury JB et al (editors): Disorders of lysosomal enzymes. Chaps 36–46, pp 751–972, in: *The Metabolic Basis of Inherited Disease,* 5th ed. McGraw-Hill, 1983.

DISORDERS OF THE PLASMA LIPOPROTEINS

The intravascular transport of lipids is mediated via 2 protein-binding systems: one for free fatty acids and one involving lipoproteins. Free (unesterified) fatty acids are the main currency of energy in the body during the postabsorptive state. They circulate as an albumin-fatty acid complex and are derived in part from enteric absorption of fatty acids with fewer than 12 carbons, but they are mainly derived from the triglyceride stores from which they are released by a series of complex homeostatic mechanisms. Primary disorders of this system are very rare and are not further discussed in this section.

Other lipids—primarily glycerides but also phospholipids, cholesterol, and the fat-soluble vitamins—are transported in the plasma in lipoprotein complexes. There are 4 main subdivisions of these lipoproteins characterized by their basic apoprotein, electrophoretic mobility, density, molecular size, and lipid composition as shown in Table 33–13.

Exogenous glycerides are derived from the intestine. Ingested triglyceride is broken down by pancreatic lipase to micelles of monoglyceride and fatty acid. The short-chain fatty acids move directly across the mucosal cell to the portal vein. The longer-chain fatty acids and monoglycerides also enter the mucosal cell, where hydrolysis is completed and where triglycerides are resynthesized. The latter pass into the bloodstream via the thoracic duct and are carried as chylomicrons to adipose tissue, liver, heart, and other organs, where they are immediately hydrolyzed as they enter the cells. In fasting plasma, the glyceride content is derived primarily from the liver.

Table 33–11. Disorders of lysosomal hydrolases. (See also Table 23–9.)*

Disorder	Enzyme Defect	Mucopolysaccharides in Urine	Clinical Features
Hurler's syndrome	α-Iduronidase	Heparan sulfate and dermatan sulfate	Autosomal recessive. Mental retardation, hepatosplenomegaly, umbilical hernia, coarse facies, corneal clouding, skeletal changes with gibbus, severe heart disease.
Scheie's syndrome	α-Iduronidase (allele to Hurler mutant but probably more residual activity to natural substrate)	Dermatan sulfate and lesser amounts of heparan sulfate	Autosomal recessive. Corneal clouding, stiff joints, normal intellect. Clinical types intermediate between Hurler and Scheie are quite common; aortic valves may be involved.
Hunter's syndrome	Sulfoiduronate sulfatase	Heparan sulfate and dermatan sulfate	X-linked recessive. Variable mental retardation, coarse facies, hepatosplenomegaly, severe heart disease. Corneal clouding and gibbus not present. Mild forms are seen.
Sanfilippo's syndrome			
Type A	Sulfamidase	Heparan sulfate	Autosomal recessive. Severe mental retardation with comparatively mild skeletal changes, visceromegaly, and facial coarseness. Types *cannot* be differentiated clinically.
Type B	α-N-Acetylglucosaminidase	Heparan sulfate	
Type C	Acetyl-CoA: α-glucosaminide N-acetyltransferase	Heparan sulfate	
Type D	N-Acetylglucosamine-6-sulfate sulfatase	Heparan sulfate	
Morquio's syndrome	N-Acetylhexosamine-6-sulfatase	Keratosulfate	Autosomal recessive. Severe skeletal changes, platyspondylisis, corneal clouding.
Maroteaux-Lamy syndrome			
Type A	N-Acetylgalactosamine-4-sulfatase	Dermatan sulfate	Autosomal recessive. Coarse facies, growth retardation, severe skeletal deformities with gibbus, corneal clouding, hepatosplenomegaly, normal intellect.
β-Glucuronidase deficiency[1]	β-Glucuronidase	Chondroitin sulfates A and C	Autosomal recessive. Varies from mental retardation, skeletal changes with gibbus, corneal clouding, and hepatosplenomegaly to mild facial coarseness, retardation, and loose joints. Hearing loss common.
Mannosidosis[2]	α-Mannosidase	Oligosaccharides in urine	Autosomal recessive. Varies from severe mental retardation, coarse facies, short stature and skeletal changes, and hepatosplenomegaly to mild facial coarseness, retardation, and loose joints. Hearing loss common.
Fucosidosis[3]	α-Fucosidase	Oligosaccharides in urine	Autosomal recessive. Variable: coarse facies, skeletal changes, hepatosplenomegaly, occasional angiokeratoma corporis diffusum.
I-cell disease[4]	Multiple lysosomal hydrolases	Sialyl oligosaccharides in urine	Autosomal recessive; milder forms are known. Very short stature, mental retardation, early facial coarsening, clear cornea, stiffness of joints, normal head circumference.
Sialidosis[5]	N-Acetylneuraminidase (sialidase)	Sialyl oligosaccharides in urine	Autosomal recessive. Mental retardation, coarse facies, skeletal dysplasia, myoclonic seizures, cherry-red macular spot.

* For further details, see McKusick VA: *Heritable Disorders of Connective Tissue,* 4th ed. Mosby, 1972. See also specific references:

[1] *J Pediatr* 1973;**82:**249.

[2] *Acta Paediatr Scand* 1973;**62:**555.

[3] *J Pediatr* 1974;**84:**727.

[4] *J Pediatr* 1971;**79:**360.

[5] *Am J Med Genet* 1977;**1:**21.

Table 33–12. Clinical features of lipidoses.

Disorder	Enzyme Defect	Clinical Features
Niemann-Pick disease	Sphingomyelinase	Autosomal recessive. Acute neuronopathic form most common and especially frequent in eastern European Jews. Accumulation of sphingomyelin in lysosomes of cells of reticuloendothelial system and CNS. Onset at age 3–6 months, with hepatosplenomegaly, mental retardation, and cherry-red spot on retina. Death by 1–4 years.
Metachromatic leukodystrophy	Arylsulfatase A	Autosomal recessive; late infantile form most common. Accumulation of sulfatide in white matter. Onset at age 1–4 years, with disturbances of gait (ataxia), motor incoordination, and dementia. Death usually in first decade.
Krabbe's disease (globoid cell leukodystrophy)	Galactocerebroside β-galactosidase	Autosomal recessive. Globoid cells in white matter and myelin deficiency. Onset at age 3–6 months, with seizures, irritability, and retardation. Death by 1–2 years.
Fabry's disease, angiokeratoma corporis diffusum	α-Galactosidase A	X-linked recessive. Storage of trihexosylceramide in blood vessels, renal tubules, and glomeruli. Pain in extremities, lack of sweating, proteinuria, fever, and skin lesions. In later stages, fatigability, poor vision, high blood pressure, and renal failure.
Farber's disease, lipogranulomatosis	Ceramidase	Autosomal recessive. Storage of ceramide in various organs. Subcutaneous nodules and plaques. Arthropathy, hoarseness, irritability, and poor growth and development. Deformed and painful joints. Death within first year due to respiratory infections and malnutrition.
Gaucher's disease	Glucocerebroside β-glucosidase	Autosomal recessive. Acute neuronopathic form: Accumulation of glucocerebroside in lysosomes of cells of reticuloendothelial system and CNS. Onset at age 6 months, with hepatosplenomegaly, mental retardation, cherry-red spot on retina, and Gaucher's cells on biopsy. Death by 1–2 years. Chronic form: Especially frequent in eastern European Jews. Accumulation of glucocerebroside in lysosomes of reticuloendothelial system. Hepatosplenomegaly and flask-shaped osteolytic bone lesions. Often compatible with normal life expectancy.
G_{M1} gangliosidosis	G_{M1} ganglioside β-galactosidase	Autosomal recessive. Accumulation of G_{M1} ganglioside in lysosomes of reticuloendothelial system and CNS. Infantile form: Patient abnormal at birth, with dysostosis multiplex, hepatosplenomegaly, mental retardation, and cherry-red spot on retina. Death by 2 years. Juvenile form: Normal development to 1 year of age, then ataxia, weakness, dementia, and occasional inferior beaking of the vertebral bodies of L1 and L2. Death by 4–5 years.
G_{M2} gangliosidosis, Tay-Sachs disease, Sandhoff's disease	G_{M2} ganglioside β-N-acetylhexosaminidase	Autosomal recessive. Tay-Sachs disease 100 times more common in eastern European Jews than in other groups; Sandhoff's disease is panethnic. The A isoenzyme is deficient in Tay-Sachs disease; the A and B isoenzymes are deficient in Sandhoff's disease. Phenotypes identical, and accumulation of G_{M2} ganglioside in lysosomes of CNS. Onset at age 3–6 months, with hypotonia, hyperacusia, retardation, and cherry-red spot on retina. Death by 2–3 years.
Wolman's disease	Acid lipase	Autosomal recessive. Accumulation of cholesterol esters and triglycerides in lysosomes of reticuloendothelial system. Onset in first weeks of life, with gastrointestinal symptoms and hepatosplenomegaly. Death by 3–6 months. Enlargement and calcification of the adrenals is usual. (Young EP: *Arch Dis Child* 1970;**45:**664.)

Modified and reproduced, with permission, from Wenger DA: Defects in metabolism of lipids. Page 556 in: Vaughan VC, McKay RJ, Behrman RE: *Textbook of Pediatrics.* Saunders, 1975.

Transport of cholesterol within the body is quantitatively much less than that of free fatty acids or glycerol. Exogenous cholesterol moves to the liver in the chylomicrons. From then on, transport of endogenous and exogenous cholesterol is on the various lipoproteins.

The protein components of lipoproteins are called apoproteins A, B, C, D, and E. They are important in relation to conditions in which there is an inborn abnormality of these proteins.

Patton JS, Carey MC: Watching fat digestion. *Science* 1979;**204:**145.

Table 33–13. Percentage composition of plasma lipoproteins.*

	Apoprotein	Protein	Cholesterol†	Phospho-lipid	Glyceride	Electrophoresis
Chylomicrons (exogenous glyceride)	Major A-I, A-II, A-IV, B, C-I, C-II, C-III Minor E	1–2	1–2 (C) 1–2 (EC)	4–6	85–95	chylo
Low-density lipoproteins (LDL)	Major A-IV Minor E	18–22	5–8 (C) 45–50 (EC)	16–25	3–9	β
Very low density, or pre-β, lipoproteins (VLDL)	Major B, C-I, C-II, C-III, E Minor A-I, A-II, D	6–10	4–7 (C) 15–22 (EC)	15–22	45–65	pre-β
High-density, or α, lipoproteins (HDL)	Major A-I, A-II Minor A-IV, B, C-I, C-II, C-III, D, E	45–55	3–5 (C) 15–20 (EC)	26–32	2–7	α

* For normal values, see Chapter 39.
† C = Unesterified cholesterol. EC = Esterified cholesterol.

LIPOPROTEIN DEFICIENCY SYNDROMES

Familial High-Density Lipoprotein (HDL) Deficiency (Tangier Disease)

This rare autosomal recessive condition was first identified in a kindred from Tangier Island in Chesapeake Bay. Abnormal storage of cholesterol esters in many organs accounts for the large lobulated tonsils with red, orange, or yellowish banding; hepatosplenomegaly; lymphadenopathy; and neurologic complications, including loss of pain and temperature sensation and peripheral neuropathy.

Plasma cholesterol levels are abnormally low owing to a deficiency of apoprotein A, and high-density lipoprotein (HDL) and very low density lipoproteins (VLDL) band are about 8% of normal on electrophoresis. Serum triglycerides are normal or modestly elevated. The diagnosis can be confirmed by finding typical foam cells in the bone marrow or rectal mucosa. The appearance of the tonsils, together with hypoalphaproteinemia, is unique except for LCAT deficiency (see below).

Tonsillectomy may be required for enlarged tonsils.

Clifton-Bligh P et al: Tangier disease. *N Engl J Med* 1972;**286:**567.

Herbert PN et al: Tangier disease. *N Engl J Med* 1978;**299:**519.

Lecithin:Cholesterol Acyltransferase (LCAT) Deficiency

LCAT deficiency is a rare inborn error of metabolism characterized by hypertriglyceridemia and hypercholesterolemia with lipid deposits in the corneas, proteinuria, renal failure, and normochromic anemias.

This is also a disorder of HDL that may be inherited or secondary to liver disease. The lipoprotein classes are involved. Plasma and tissue phosphatidylcholine and unesterified cholesterol are increased, and there is a corresponding cholesterol ester deficit in plasma. A low-fat diet may help.

Norum KR et al: Familial plasma lecithin:cholesterol acyltransferase deficiency. *Acta Med Scand* 1970;**188:**323.

Abetalipoproteinemia

This rare autosomal recessive condition is manifested in early infancy with failure to thrive and steatorrhea. Later in life, neurologic deficits include weakness, nystagmus, and posterior column, pyramidal tract, and cerebellar signs. Retinitis pigmentosa is also described.

Cholesterol and phospholipid levels are all extremely low owing to low levels of apoprotein B, and chylomicrons are not formed after fat ingestion. Fasting glyceride levels are also abnormally low. Lipoprotein electrophoresis shows no chylomicron band and no VLDL or LDL bands. The red blood cells demonstrate acanthocytosis.

Low cholesterol levels with steatorrhea are also found in celiac disease but without acanthocytosis, neurologic findings, or the typical lipoprotein pattern. In cystic fibrosis, there are respiratory symptoms and an elevated sweat chloride. In IgA deficiency, the immunoglobulin change can be measured.

Prescribe a low-fat diet. Medium-chain triglycerides are helpful as an additional source of calories. Supplements of water-soluble vitamin A (5000 IU/d) and vitamin D (500 IU/d) should be given.

Neurologic complications shorten life expectancy. A variant with normal triglyceride levels has been described.

Gotto AM et al: On the protein defect in abetalipoproteinemia. *N Engl J Med* 1971;**284:**813.

Herbert PN, Gotto AM, Fredrickson DS: Familial lipoprotein deficiency (abetalipoproteinemia, hypobetalipoproteinemia, and Tangier disease). Chap 29, pp 589–621, in: *The Meta-*

bolic Basis of Inherited Disease, 5th ed. Stanbury JB et al (editors). McGraw-Hill, 1983.

Hypobetalipoproteinemia

There have been reports of a small number of patients with reduction of serum β-lipoprotein concentrations to 10–50% of normal and with decreased serum levels of cholesterol, phospholipids, and glycerides. Acanthocytosis and neurologic symptoms may be seen. The condition must be differentiated from hypobetalipoproteinemias secondary to the celiac syndrome or the thalassemia trait and from abetalipoproteinemia. Heterozygotes in the former state have low plasma cholesterol and LDL. These levels are normal in the latter state.

A syndrome has also been described with low α- and β-lipoprotein, raised cholesterol and triglycerides, retardation, and hepatomegaly.

THE FAMILIAL HYPERLIPOPROTEINEMIAS

There have been many classifications of hyperlipoproteinemias based on clinical, biochemical, and inheritance characteristics. No one approach is completely satisfactory.

The primary lipoproteinemias are a group of heritable disorders of serum lipoprotein components; the secondary hyperlipoproteinemias are a reflection of a number of disorders such as nephrosis, hypothyroidism, diabetes, systemic lupus erythematosus, and obstructive liver disease.

Glueck CJ et al: Risk factor for coronary artery disease in children: Recognition, evaluation and therapy. *Pediatr in Rev* 1980;**2:**131.

Motulsky AG: The genetic hyperlipidemias. *N Engl J Med* 1976;**294:**823.

Stanbury JB et al: Disorders of lipoprotein and lipid metabolism. Chaps 29–35, pp 589–747, in: *The Metabolic Basis of Genetic Disease,* 5th ed. McGraw-Hill, 1983.

Type I: Familial Hyperchylomicronemia (Lipoprotein Lipase Deficiency)

The onset is usually early in life, with bouts of abdominal pain. Later, moderate hepatosplenomegaly is noted, and the retinal vessels are seen to be especially pale. Small cutaneous xanthomas are common.

The serum is characteristically lactescent, and on standing, the chylomicrons rise to the top as a creamy layer on the plasma. Serum HDL and LDL levels are decreased. Postheparin lipoprotein lipase activity is reduced. Hyperglycemia and glycosuria have been reported but are not common (as in type IV; see below).

Hyperchylomicronemia usually decreases on a low-fat diet (< 0.2 g/kg/d). The α- and β-lipoprotein bands will increase somewhat, and the pre-β-band that carries endogenous triglyceride will increase further. Caloric intake can be supplemented on a low-triglyceride diet (< 0.5 g/kg/d) by giving medium-chain triglycerides, either as a milk formula (Portagen) or as a special diet using MCT oil. Episodes of abdominal pain (which may be accompanied by pancreatitis) and hepatosplenomegaly can be controlled on this regimen. There is no increased risk of artherosclerosis. The diagnosis is consistent with a normal life.

Apoprotein C-II deficiency causes a similar disorder.

Ford S et al: Familial hyperchylomicronemia. *Am J Med* 1971;**50:**536.

Type IIA: Familial Hyperbetalipoproteinemia; Essential Familial Hypercholesterolemia

Familial hyperbetalipoproteinemia is the commonest lipoprotein disorder of childhood and is inherited as an autosomal dominant. The basic defect is the lack of the normal LDL receptor on the cell membrane, which results in a failure of the feedback inhibition of cholesterol synthesis. Evidence of hypercholesterolemia in at least one parent is essential to the diagnosis. The most striking clinical manifestations in homozygotes are the xanthomatous deposits in tendons (particularly the Achilles tendon), over extensor surfaces of knees, hands, and elbows and in pressure or trauma areas such as the buttocks. Xanthomas of the eyelids (xanthelasma) and corneal arcus are also common. Coronary atherosclerosis may be an early and life-threatening complication. Heterozygotes usually have no abnormal physical findings prior to the onset of early atherosclerosis.

Elevated levels of cholesterol have been reported in cord blood, and levels over 500 mg/dL have been seen at 3 months of age. As with the appearance of xanthomas, the age at which hypercholesterolemia develops varies considerably, and the expression of the disease is more marked in the homozygote. Total cholesterol levels in childhood vary with age and methodology, but any level exceeding 240 mg/dL should be considered abnormal. Homozygotes usually have levels in excess of 600 mg/dL, and levels are elevated in the parents. Serum phospholipid is moderately elevated but not to the same extent as cholesterol, and in some cases there may be a modest elevation of VLDL. Lipoprotein electrophoresis shows a characteristic intense increase in the LDL, with lipoprotein cholesterol exceeding 210 mg/dL. Hypercarotenemia is also seen because of the increased β-lipoprotein.

Hyperbetalipoproteinemia is reported in hypothyroidism, obstructive liver disease, nephrosis, and disseminated systemic lupus erythematosus. Florid xanthomatosis is, however, rare in children with these conditions.

A history of coronary infarction before age 50 in either parent is the best screening test for this disease.

Nenonatal cholesterol values do not seem to be helpful.

Treatment possibilities are as follows:

A. Dietary Management: With the overall proviso that the diet should be palatable and contain adequate protein and calories, it is justifiable to limit the fat intake to 20% of calories, primarily polyunsaturated. Increasing dietary polyunsaturates is more important than reducing dietary cholesterol. Obesity, if present, should be controlled.

Whether to treat moderate elevations of cholesterol in the heterozygote is still a difficult decision. The evidence that treating the child will diminish the risk of later myocardial infarction is still inferential, besides which treatment itself is not always effective, nor is compliance easy, especially in older children. In the future, improved cholesterol-reducing agents and a better understanding of the protective action of plasma HDL on elevated LDL levels may make this decision easier.

B. Drug Therapy:

1. Cholestyramine is a resin that bonds bile acids, prevents their reabsorption, and, in turn, enhances the hepatic conversion of cholesterol to more bile acids. The dose is 0.3 g/kg/d orally, but the drug is unpleasant to take and may cause steatorrhea. In some cases, the effect is to remove feedback inhibition of endogenous cholesterol synthesis, and levels rise. Sucrose polyester is not yet available but may soon replace the resin.

2. Nicotinic acid, 0.15 mg/kg/d orally, may lower cholesterol levels. The mechanism is not understood but may relate to liver damage. Liver function tests should be followed closely. The drug may be more effective when used with cholestyramine; it is of little value in the homozygote.

3. Compactin, a new penicillin derivative, has been found to be a potent inhibitor of HMG-CoA reductase in vitro. It may become a highly effective therapeutic agent.

4. There is evidence that a portacaval shunt will substantially lower serum cholesterol levels and that plasmapheresis may be an even better mode of therapy for homozygous type II hyperlipidemia.

5. Plasmapheresis at 2- and 3-week intervals plus drug and diet therapy will lower serum LDL levels; the impact on cardiovascular disease is not known.

Ahrens AH: Homozygous hypercholesterolemia and the portacaval shunt. *Lancet* 1974;**2:**449.

Brown MS et al: Familial hypercholesterolemia: A genetic defect in the low density lipoprotein receptor. *N Engl J Med* 1976;**294:**1386.

West RJ et al: Long-term follow-up of children with familial hypercholesterolemia treated with cholestyramine. *Lancet* 1980;2:873.

Witztum JL et al: Successful plasmapheresis in a 4-year-old child with homozygous familial hypercholesterolemia. *J Pediatr* 1980;**97:**615.

Yeshurun D et al: Drug treatment of hyperlipidemia. *Am J Med* 1976;**60:**379.

Type IIB: Familial Combined Hyperlipoproteinemia

Some hypercholesterolemic patients have elevations of endogenous triglyceride (VLDL) as well as LDL. Many of these conditions have come to be regarded as a separate autosomal dominant clinical entity with variable expression of the phenotype. Therefore, relatives may show elevations of cholesterol, triglyceride, or both. In childhood, the diagnosis may be confusing because the hypertriglyceridemia is expressed before the hypercholesterolemia. Some type IIA patients will have environmentally elevated triglycerides (as found with inadequate exercise or obesity). Some type IV patients will have secondary hypercholesterolemia as VLDL is normally converted in part to LDL, which then results in elevated cholesterol levels. It is wise to look at the height of elevation of the 2 lipids and the life-style of the patient in attempting to separate contaminating phenotypes from true "familial combined hyperlipoproteinemia." Parent phenotypes may also be helpful. Subjects with combined hyperlipoproteinemia usually manifest characteristics of the type IV disorder—impaired glucose tolerance, obesity, and hyperuricemia—and not characteristics of the type IIA disorder such as skin xanthomas. Patients should be treated as for the type IV disorder.

Glueck CJ et al: Familial combined hyperlipoproteinemia. *Metabolism* 1973;**22:**1403.

Tall AR, Small DM: Current concepts: Plasma high density lipoprotein. *N Engl J Med* 1978;**299:**1232.

Type III: Hyperbetalipoproteinemia

Type III hyperbetalipoproteinemia is an autosomal recessive condition that has not been described in childhood; in late adolescence, it would be distinguished by the small papular xanthomas on palm creases and fingertips, by the "tubero-eruptive" lesions at the elbows, and, in the laboratory, by the opalescent serum with increased cholesterol and glyceride. Lipoprotein electrophoresis shows an intense conjoined broad β- and pre-β-band. The disorder is due to an abnormality of apoprotein E and to the consequent accumulation in plasma of VLDL remnants. Estrogen treatment may be of value, as are diet and drugs.

Chait A et al: Type III hyperlipoproteinemia. *Lancet* 1977; **1:**1176.

Type IV: Familial Hypertriglyceridemia

This is a common form of hyperlipoproteinemia in adults and is also seen in childhood. It is characterized by turbid plasma and an increase in endogenous glyceride with a marked increase in VLDL and a decrease in HDL and LDL. There are no chylomicrons on a low-fat diet. Hyperuricemia is common, and in most cases the lipemia is carbohydrate-induced.

The condition may be secondary to uncontrolled diabetes, type I glycogen storage disease, idiopathic hypercalcemia, hypoparathyroidism, nephrosis, and obesity. If a patient does not fast for 12 hours before testing, a false diagnosis may be made.

Treatment consists of providing 40% of calories as fat, primarily polyunsaturated, and restricting carbohydrate sufficiently to reduce endogenous hyperlipemia. Nicotinic acid and clofibrate (Atromid-S) may also be helpful.

Glueck CJ et al: Familial hypertriglyceridemia in children: Dietary management. *Pediatr Res* 1977;**11**:953.

Type V: Familial Hyperprebetalipoproteinemia With Hyperchylomicronemia

This condition is usually not seen until adult life, but it has been reported in childhood. Clinically, patients tend to be obese and to have a family history of diabetes. There are widespread xanthomas with lipemia retinalis, hepatosplenomegaly, and foam cells in the bone marrow. There is an increase in both endogenous and exogenous glyceride (chylomicrons), and cholesterol levels may also be elevated. Lipoprotein lipase activity is normal. Cases of type IV hyperlipoproteinemia and familial combined hyperlipidemia may occur in the kindred.

Treatment consists of reducing weight by caloric and fat restriction. Clofibrate (Atromid-S) and nicotinic acid may also be helpful.

Kwiterovich PO et al: Type V hyperlipoproteinemia in childhood. *Pediatrics* 1977;**59**:513.

GENETIC COUNSELING

The most direct application of the advances in our understanding of basic genetic mechanisms is in the provision of genetic advice or genetic counseling. The advice usually stems from an inquiry about whether a given disease is likely to recur in the family, and its primary purpose is thus to help people make responsible decisions about reproduction. Other questions may relate to the desirability of cousin marriage, the reasons for multiple miscarriages, the risk of having malformed children when the parents are at advanced ages, the effects of hallucinatory drugs, or the possible hazards of ionizing radiation.

Genetic counseling is expensive but is an effective way of diminishing society's burden of chronic disease, which is far more expensive.

The prime requisite for giving advice is the possession of all available facts about the patient and the disease. In order to give genetic advice, the physician must ponder the following questions:

(1) What is the disease in the propositus? This requires the most accurate diagnosis available.

(2) Is the disease hereditary or is it a phenocopy? For example, is the cleft palate due to abortifacients? Is the mental deficiency due to a birth injury? Is the pseudohermaphroditism due to the use of oral progestins?

FAMILY HISTORY

History taking is a fundamental tool in every physician's armamentarium. In genetic counseling, however, there are points in the family history that should be stressed in order to pinpoint the genetic factors involved.

(1) Parental age: Mention has already been made of the maternal age effect, ie, the increasing risk of nondisjunction and the increasing risk of other congenital malformations with increasing parental age. Elevated paternal age has recently been associated with an increased incidence of dominant mutations.

(2) Siblings: Their age, sex, and state of health are important. The larger the number of unaffected sibs, the less likely the condition is to be due to a single segregating gene.

(3) Consanguinity: The chance of both parents carrying the same rare recessive gene is greater if they are related. The likelihood of the patient's disease being recessively inherited is thus increased in the presence of consanguinity. Consanguinity rates in the general population have been decreasing throughout the world. In the USA, the overall rate is about 0.05%. Among the parents of children with albinism, however, there is a consanguinity rate of about 20%. This fact should be borne in mind when one is asked, "Should I marry my cousin?"

(4) Radiation history: The deleterious effect of x-irradiation on the embryo has been well documented, although it should be stressed that there is little if any evidence that diagnostic irradiation produces birth defects. In addition, there occur genetic effects of irradiation such as point mutations, chromosomal breaks with abnormal healing, and an increased incidence of nondisjunction. These effects are likely to occur prior to conception during gametogenesis. For this reason, a history of radiation exposure to the gonads of either parent prior to conception is important. Because of the nature of gametogenesis in the female, inquiries should be made concerning exposure of the mother to x-ray at a time when she herself was an embryo.

(5) History of exposure to drugs and virus infections early in pregnancy: A positive history of exposure to a known teratogen may help in determining whether genetic or environmental factors were etiologically important in the child's disease.

(6) History of previous pregnancies in the family: Many abortions in the family may suggest the carrier state of a translocation chromosome, which should then be looked for in the patient. Similarly, diabetes or "prediabetes" should be ruled out.

(7) Construction of a pedigree: The diagrammatic representation of the family history helps one decide whether a disease is familial and, if so, whether it follows one of the single gene patterns of inheritance, ie, the vertical patterns of dominant inheritance, the horizontal pattern of recessive inheritance, or the oblique pattern of X-linked recessive inheritance. The larger the pedigree, the more typical the pattern (Fig 33–12). A pedigree also helps identify other family members who may be at risk and be unaware of it.

PHYSICAL EXAMINATION

In addition to the physical examination that is performed on the affected patient for diagnostic purposes, it is frequently desirable to examine the parents and the unaffected siblings of the patient in order to pick up cases where expressivity is diminished. This is important in determining whether a gene mutation has occurred in a parental germ cell, a fact that changes risk figures greatly. Sometimes a laboratory test on the parents, such as a blood phosphorus level when the patient has vitamin D-resistant rickets, will bring to light an expression of a previously unrecognized defective gene in a seemingly normal parent.

Finally, the literature on a specific disease should be carefully reviewed in order to determine the usual type of transmission and, if this is not clear, to estimate the empiric risks. This is particularly helpful if the patient's pedigree data are not too complete.

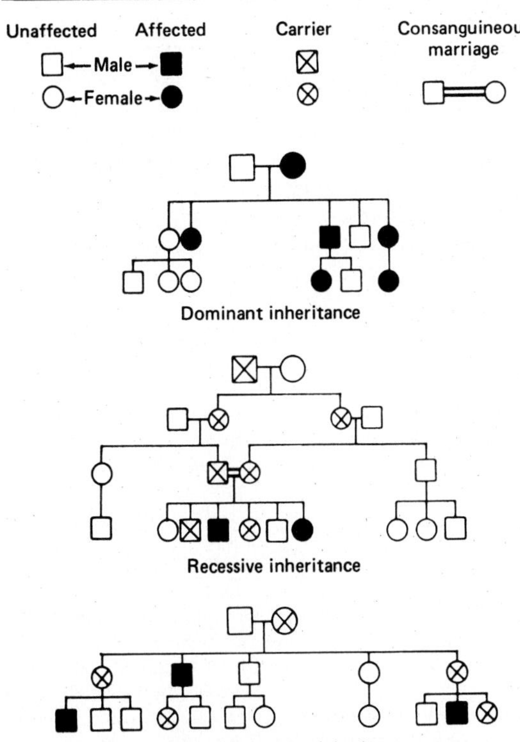

Figure 33–12. Pedigrees demonstrating various types of single gene inheritance.

NATURE OF ADVICE

Counseling should be given with both parties present. Knowledge of the cultural, religious, and educational background of the family is helpful. Advantage should be taken of the opportunity for a thorough discussion of the nature of the disease in order to dispel the store of misinformation, anxiety, and guilt that is often present.

It is often helpful to remind the patient of the 2–4% chance in every pregnancy of a congenital abnormality. The defect in question will frequently not add significantly to this risk.

When the patients are fully informed about the nature of the disease and the risks they will incur in future pregnancies, the actual decision about their future action is left up to them. This decision is based on an understanding of both the odds (a statistic) and the stakes (the seriousness and the long-term prognosis of the disease). The latter part of the counseling should attempt to be supportive. The counselor should be aware of possible feelings of guilt, anger, and fear and attempt to deal with them. This supportive side of genetic counseling is essentially no different from other kinds of medical counseling. The difficulty in communication between patient and physician is a continuing challenge, especially as the patient's understanding of a probability estimate is often confused.

The physician should be ready, however, to offer information on alternatives to normal reproduction, such as sterilization, artificial insemination, contraception, and adoption. For young couples, it may be desirable to delay reproduction for 5 years in the hope of further developments in treatment or intrauterine diagnosis. Other family members at risk should be identified and, if possible, counseled (an important form of family medicine). The counselor in general attempts to be nondirective in counseling, even though this is often misunderstood and resented by the patient, who is accustomed to being told what to do by the physician. An earnest attempt is made by the counselor to help the patient arrive at what the patient determines is an appropriate decision.

The above type of preconceptional counseling, which is generally **retrospective** in the sense that the question usually relates to the risk of a couple having a second affected child, may often lead to **prospective** counseling, ie, in the identification of other individuals in the kindred who may be at risk of a genetic disease but are unaware of their risk because they have not yet borne affected children. It is an important responsibility of the counselor and the primary care physician to communicate with these individuals after the necessary permission is obtained from the patient.

Another type of prospective counseling is related

to genetic screening of 2 types: (1) screening of the general population of newborns (as for phenylketonuria or hypothyroidism) in order to diagnose and treat disease early enough to prevent serious and irreversible symptomatology and (2) screening of a defined population (as for Tay-Sachs disease) in order to identify those at risk of having an affected child before tragedy occurs. Essential features of these procedures are that people be fully informed prior to being tested; that rights to privacy be carefully guarded; and that those who are at risk have adequate counseling. Occasionally, those *not* at risk also need counseling, since many are made needlessly anxious by virtue of having been screened. The psychologic implications of being "branded" as a carrier must be considered in counseling carriers. It has been helpful to remind these individuals that we all carry several potentially harmful genes. In any form of population screening, the benefits to be derived should outweigh the cost of the screening. The frequency of the disease in the population tested, the simplicity and accuracy of the test, the ease of follow-up, and the availability of treatment should all be considered.

Genetic counseling may be postconceptional as well as preconceptional. In most cases, the investigative procedure is similar to what has been discussed above, and the patient is told the probability of the unborn child being affected, which may vary from 1% to 50%. On the basis of this figure, one must decide whether there is a valid genetic indication for interrupting pregnancy. It is hoped that better diagnostic and treatment procedures for intrauterine disease will become available, so that abortion will not be the only alternative to having a defective child in these cases.

INTRAUTERINE DIAGNOSIS

Intrauterine diagnosis constitutes the greatest single advance in medical genetics of the last decade. It usually converts an estimate of probable fetal disease to a certainty, giving the couple scientifically reliable information on which to base a decision about whether or not to proceed to delivery.

Methods of Intrauterine Diagnosis

Several methods of intrauterine diagnosis are currently being used or are becoming available as follows:

A. X-Ray: X-ray is used only if there is a significant risk for gross skeletal lesions.

B. Ultrasonography: This method is used for diagnosis of anencephaly, hydrocephaly, polycystic kidneys, twins, fetal death, and gross skeletal disease.

C. Fetoscopy: Fetoscopy permits direct visualization of the fetus by insertion of an appropriate endoscopic tube into the uterus. This procedure, still in an experimental stage, will identify gross structural malformations and will make possible the sampling of fetal blood for the intrauterine diagnosis of hemoglobinopathies.

D. Amniography: A radiopaque substance is introduced into the uterus and attaches to fetal skin. An x-ray may then outline the fetus and demonstrate structural abnormalities such as meningomyelocele. The efficacy of this procedure has been questioned.

E. Chorionic Villus Sampling: This recently developed technique permits much earlier (eighth to tenth weeks) prenatal diagnosis than the usual genetic amniocentesis (17th to 20th weeks). Although still somewhat experimental, this method is less physically and emotionally traumatic because it allows for earlier interruption of a pregnancy.

F. Amniocentesis: This is currently the most widely used form of antenatal diagnosis. The procedure has made possible intrauterine diagnosis for some diseases—in particular, the cytogenetic diseases and those biochemical diseases that can be diagnosed (1) by assaying for a specific enzyme in cultured fetal cells obtained from amniotic fluid, (2) by recombinant DNA analysis of amniocytes, or (3) by direct assay of metabolites in the amniotic fluid (Table 33–14).

1. Procedure—The procedure consists of the suprapubic insertion of a needle into the uterine cavity at about 15 weeks of pregnancy and the aspiration of 20–25 mL of sterile amniotic fluid. Thus far, the complications have been few. For this reason, it seems reasonable to perform the procedure when the risk of diagnosable fetal disease exceeds 1%.

An important preliminary to the actual procedure of amniocentesis is genetic counseling. During this session, a pedigree is obtained and examined for other conditions that might be of importance. This session is utilized to describe in detail the procedure, potential complications, and what can and what cannot be learned from it. The patient must be made aware that there is no guarantee of a normal child.

Ultrasonography is usually employed prior to the procedure in order to rule out a missed abortion or

Table 33–14. Some biochemical disorders that can be diagnosed antenatally.

Argininosuccinic aciduria	Juvenile G_{M1} gangliosidosis
Branched-chain ketoaciduria	Krabbe's syndrome
Cystathionine synthase deficiency	Lesch-Nyhan syndrome and variants
Cystinosis	Mannosidosis
Fabry's disease	Metachromatic leukodystrophy
Fucosidosis	Methylmalonic aciduria
Galactokinase deficiency	Niemann-Pick disease
Galactosemia	Orotic aciduria
Gaucher's disease (infantile)	Phenylketonuria
Generalized gangliosidosis	Pompe's disease
Hunter's and Hurler's syndromes	Refsum's disease
I-cell disease	Sandhoff's disease
	Sanfilippo's syndrome
	Tay-Sachs disease

twinning and to locate the placenta, which one hopes not to puncture, although this is not always possible.

The extracted amniotic fluid contains fetal cells that are cultured in vitro so that karyotyping and enzyme assays can be performed. The noncellular part of the fluid is assayed for alpha-fetoprotein (AFP). The procedure usually takes 1½–2 weeks to complete.

By extracting DNA from amniocytes and using appropriate restriction endonucleases, it is now possible to diagnose thalassemia, sickle cell anemia, and phenylketonuria without time-consuming cell culture or examination of the gene product. The ability to diagnose specific gene mutations without the requirement of looking for the enzyme produced by the gene should eventually greatly expand the diagnostic capabilities of intrauterine diagnosis (see Recombinant DNA, above).

2. Indications—The indications for amniocentesis are as follows:

a. Either parent is a carrier of a balanced translocation. The risk of an affected child is about 3–15% depending upon which parent is the carrier.

b. A previous child was born with trisomy 21. The risk of a repeat may be as high as 2%, especially for mothers under 30 years of age.

c. The parents are carriers of an autosomal recessively inherited disease that can be diagnosed in utero (Table 33–14).

d. The mother is a carrier of an X-linked recessively inherited disease that cannot be diagnosed in utero (eg, muscular dystrophy, hemophilia A). However, the risk of being affected is 50% if the fetus is a male and close to zero if a female.

e. The mother is over 35 years of age.

f. The mother is at increased risk of having a child with a neural tube defect (anencephaly, meningomyelocele). The amniotic fluid level of AFP (the predominant protein in fetal serum) is significantly higher than normal in 90% of affected fetuses. However, the level will frequently not be elevated in the presence of closed neural tube defects, which may represent 5–10% of the total number.

Amniotic fluid AFP can also be elevated in the absence of a neural tube defect, in the presence of intrauterine death, Turner's syndrome, congenital nephrosis, and exomphalos. When anencephaly is suspected, examination of the uterine contents by ultrasonography will often reveal an absent or disturbed fetal head. It has recently been shown that by measuring amniotic fluid acetylcholinesterase and AFP, diagnostic accuracy is improved.

Unfortunately, more than 90% of infants with neural tube defects are born to mothers without a previous history suggesting risk. It has recently been reported that the maternal serum AFP is elevated in a pregnancy with a neural tube defect. This makes it possible to screen *all* pregnant women by a simple blood test (radioimmunoassay) for neural tube defect and identify most of the 90% that cannot be identified today. This is being done in some communities in Great Britain, where the incidence of neural tube defect is roughly 10 times that in the USA. However, because of the relative rareness in the USA and the number of false-positive results, which would mean that many more patients would require both ultrasonography and amniocentesis, screening of *all* pregnancies for neural tube defect is not currently being attempted in the USA except in a few pilot studies but will probably soon be used generally.

CONCLUSION

Who should give genetic counseling? The primary care physician who knows the family, its attitudes, and its social and financial stresses may be the best person to provide counseling. Ideally, genetic counseling—an important form of preventive medicine—should be part of primary care. The primary care physician may not have the training in medical genetics, the facilities for sophisticated laboratory tests, the acquaintance with rare syndromes, or the considerable amount of time necessary to do the complete job but nevertheless should be in a position to reinforce the counseling that is provided by the genetics clinic, which may be a satellite clinic of the main clinic at the university medical center staffed by a medical geneticist, genetic associate, and public health nurse.

It is clear that the general public is largely unaware of the existence of genetic counseling and its benefits. A greater public education effort is required to make these services available to those who need them.

Brock DJH: Neural tube defects and α-fetoprotein: An international perspective. Chap 24, pp 471–488, in: *Genetic Issues in Pediatric and Obstetric Practice*. Kaback M (editor). Year Book, 1981.

Kaback MM: Screening for recessive gene carriers in clinical practice. Chap 25, pp 489–500, in: *Genetic Issues in Pediatric and Obstetric Practice*. Kaback MM (editor). Year Book, 1981.

Riccardi VM, Robinson A: Preventive medicine through genetic counseling: A regional program. *Prev Med* 1975;**4**:126.

GLOSSARY OF GENETIC TERMS

Alleles: Genes that occupy homologous loci on homologous chromosomes. An individual can never have more than 2 allelic genes at a given locus.

Aneuploid: This refers to the chromosomal number of a cell population which is not an integral multiple of the haploid number.

Autosomes: All of the chromosomes other than the 2 sex chromosomes.

Colinearity: The relationship between DNA and protein in which the sequence of components of the former (bases) specifies the sequence of components of the latter (amino acids).

Consanguinity: The blood relationship of 2 individuals. It usually refers to a married couple.

Crossing-over: The physical process of exchange between chromatids in synapsis, which permits the process of recombination. This has the result that genes lying in one chromosome are not always passed on together to the descendants.

Diploid: The double set of chromosomes in the somatic cells of the organism. The diploid number in humans is 46.

Exons: Portions of the DNA of a gene that are transcribed into mRNA and then translated into protein.

Genotype: The genetic constitution of an organism.

Haploid: One-half of the diploid complement of chromosomes, in which only one chromosome of each homologous pair is present. The haploid number in humans is 23.

Introns: Intervening sequences or portions of the DNA of genes that do not contribute to functional mRNA and protein. These regions are excised after producing precursor RNA.

Isochromosome: A morphologically abnormal chromosome that results from an abnormal ("horizontal") division of the centromere, instead of its normally vertical division, during mitosis. The result is that the chromosome is metacentric, with the centromere in the center. Such a chromosome would possess a double set of genes from the arm of the parent chromosome that supplied the chromatids and would be lacking the genes normally provided by the other arm of the parent chromosome.

Karyotype: The chromosomal constitution of an individual, as typified by the systematized array of the chromosomes of a single cell prepared by photography.

Meiosis: A form of cell division in which the haploid gametes are produced from diploid cells.

Messenger RNA (mRNA): RNA that serves as a template for protein synthesis: an intermediate in the transcription of DNA to protein.

Monosomy: Having only one chromosome of a particular homologous pair, instead of 2.

Mosaic: An individual whose tissues are of 2 or more genetically different kinds, usually of different chromosomal constitution.

Phenocopy: A nongenetic condition which mimics that produced by a certain genotype.

Phenotype: The manifest constitution of an individual as determined by careful examination. This is the result of an interaction between genetic makeup and environment.

Proband or propositus: The index case, or starting case, from which a genetic investigation is undertaken.

Restriction endonuclease: An enzyme, usually of bacterial origin, that cleaves DNA at sequence-specific sites. About 200 are known.

Restriction fragment length polymorphisms (RFLPs): Variations in nucleotide sequences distributed at random throughout the genome, without phenotypic effect, producing fragments of DNA of different lengths in different people with the same restriction enzyme.

Reverse transcriptase: An enzyme that produces a DNA copy of mRNA.

Satellites: These are small deeply staining bodies situated at the end of the short arm of an acrocentric chromosome and separated from it by a short distance.

Sister chromatic exchange: Exchange of segments of DNA between chromatids of a chromosome. The frequency is greatly increased in Bloom's syndrome.

Trisomy: The presence of a single chromosome in 3 homologous forms, rather than the usual 2.

SELECTED REFERENCES

Ampola MG: *Metabolic Diseases in Pediatric Practice.* Little, Brown, 1982.

Emery AEH, Rimoin DL: *Principles and Practice of Medical Genetics.* Churchill Livingstone, 1983.

Kaback MM (editor): *Genetic Issues in Pediatric and Obstetric Practice.* Year Book, 1981.

McKusick VA: *Mendelian Inheritance in Man,* 6th ed. Johns Hopkins Univ Press, 1983.

Nyhan WL (editor): *Heritable Disorders of Amino Acid Metabolism: Patterns of Clinical Expression and Genetic Variation.* Wiley, 1974.

O'Brien D, Goodman SI: The critically ill child: Life-threatening metabolic disease in infancy. *Pediatrics* 1970;**45:**620.

Puck TT, Kao FT: Somatic cell genetics and its application to medicine. *Annu Rev Genet* 1982;**16:**225.

Riccardi VM: *The Genetic Approach to Human Disease.* Oxford, 1977.

Scriver CR, Rosenberg LE: *Amino Acid Metabolism and Its Disorders.* Saunders, 1973.

Smith DW: *Recognizable Patterns of Human Development,* 3rd ed. Saunders, 1982.

Stanbury JB et al (editors): *The Metabolic Basis of Inherited Disease,* 5th ed. McGraw-Hill, 1983.

Symposium on treatment of amino acid disorders. *Am J Dis Child* 1967;**113:**1. [Entire issue.]

The Dysmorphic Infant

34

David K. Manchester, MD

The term "birth defect" is conventionally used to describe dysmorphologies visible at birth; these may occur in 2–3% of infants. Various structural abnormalities can be found in up to 7% of the population at autopsy. The infant mortality rate in the presence of congenital anomalies is high. Each year in the USA, about one-half million pregnancies end in miscarriage or in fetal or neonatal death as a direct result of congenital malformations. Survivors may have substantial defects, including incapacitating handicaps and severe impairment of organ function. Twenty to 30% of pediatric hospital admissions are for genetic conditions and birth defects.

Proper treatment of dysmorphic infants depends on an understanding of pathophysiology and an organized approach to diagnosis. This chapter will describe mechanisms of teratogenesis and outline a general and practical approach to the management of newborn infants with birth defects. Congenital abnormalities of specific organs are discussed also in other chapters.

INTERACTING SYSTEMS IN TERATOGENESIS

Human congenital malformations can be caused by chromosomal aberrations, single gene defects, mechanical stresses, and certain environmental agents (teratogens). Most birth defects are multifactorial—ie, they are the product of genetic, developmental, and environmental interactions. Single etiologic factors are recognized in only about 30% of cases.

GENETIC FACTORS

About 25% of birth defects can be directly attributed to single gene defects and chromosomal aberrations. Genetic contributions to multifactorial disorders are more difficult to identify, but their presence is evident from studies in twins and from empirical data documenting increased risk of recurrence in families of affected individuals. Although there is a strong association between genotype and phenotype, the mechanisms by which extra or missing chromosomes produce birth defects are not understood. It appears that many biologic responses to environmental exposures are genetically regulated. A closer link between genetic abnormalities and morphology can be seen in mendelian disorders where abnormal structures of proteins or enzymes have been identified. Some of these biochemical disorders are recognizable by the morphologic abnormalities they produce. The recently established fields of pharmacogenetics and genetic epidemiology attempt to deal with clinical aspects of genetic and environmental interactions.

ENVIRONMENTAL FACTORS

Clustering of birth defects has resulted in identification of a few specific human teratogens, but epidemiologic evidence consistently indicates that other factors (eg, ethnic background, maternal age and health, socioeconomic status, exposure to other environmental agents) also interact to cause birth defects. Since it is impossible to control the human environment, animal models have been used to systematically determine the relationship of birth defects to exposure to environmental agents. Clear dose-related responses to chemicals can be seen in animals, and important mechanisms of cytotoxicity have been identified.

Chemical exposures during pregnancy can be divided into 3 general categories: exposures to abused substances and prescribed drugs (high-dose), exposures to food and environmental contaminants (moderate- to low-dose), and exposures to poisons (low-dose).

Prescription drugs are generally taken in high doses in order to be pharmacologically active. Most drugs readily traverse the placenta and achieve significant concentrations in the conceptus. However, extensive preclinical testing and studies of long-term use have shown that most drugs have a low potential for toxicity, and few drugs are potent teratogens at therapeutic doses. On the other hand, all drugs have a potential for adverse effects from dose-related toxicity or idiosyncrasy. The psychoactive drug ethanol, for instance—relatively safe at low doses in adults but clearly toxic at higher levels—produces a similar spectrum of effects in fetuses. Many apparently drug-related embryopathies may fall into the category of idiosyncratic reactions. Idiosyncratic drug reactions in adults often appear to be due to genetically controlled differences in drug disposition or receptor interactions. Drugs that are frequently linked with idiosyncratic reactions in adults (eg, phenytoin) are suspected of causing problems in fetuses during development.

Chemical contamination of the environment and the presence of natural toxins also cause concern during pregnancy. Environmentally related cancer in adults warns of a potential for significant cytotoxicity in fetuses during development. Although most chemical carcinogens are also teratogens, the relationship of dose to response is important. Concentrations of chemicals in the food and environment are generally low but may be increased through improper handling of food or inadequate ventilation. An increase in exposure increases the risk for toxicity. Monitoring reproductive outcome may, unfortunately, be a good way of identifying adverse effects of environmental contamination in humans.

Poisons cause damage even at low levels. Methyl mercury is a good example. Relatively small amounts of this compound present in foods produced significant neurotoxicity in infants in Japan and Iran. This agent is particularly dangerous, since it tends to concentrate in fetal tissues.

Not all teratogens are chemicals. Mechanical stresses, extremes of temperature, radiation exceeding usual diagnostic exposures, and infectious agents are also potential teratogens. The effects of congenital infections are discussed in Chapters 26–29.

DEVELOPMENTAL FACTORS

Each organ passes through a number of critical periods during its development (Fig 34–1). Abnormal development or interruption of normal development at any one of these stages for whatever reason is likely to produce a structural defect. The anlage for a single structure may be affected, but since critical periods overlap and there are important functional interactions between tissues, less specific processes may interfere with the development of several organs. At the cellular level, processes leading to cell death or to abnormal migration appear to contribute most significantly to structural defects.

Familiarity with human embryology is essential to dysmorphology. It is useful to divide human gestation into 5 stages. The first (preconception) stage includes the processes of gametogenesis and fertilization. Our understanding of the role of these processes in human congenital problems is limited, but studies in animals indicate that the role is significant.

The second stage, implantation, begins with fertilization and is complete by 13–14 days. During this time, the blastocyst invades the endometrium, and the placenta differentiates and begins to function. (Note that, in humans, placentation precedes organogenesis.) Perfusion of the fetal placenta by maternal blood at this early stage puts the developing embryo in close contact with the maternal environment. Although the trophoblastic tissues that separate maternal and embryonic circulation are readily permeable by most xenobiotics (compounds foreign to the biologic system), environmental exposures during this stage of development are not often associated with birth defects. The reason for this is unknown but could be explained by spontaneous abortion during implantation. It is known that the genetically abnormal conceptus frequently aborts during this period.

The third stage of embryonic development is organogenesis, extending from the second to the eighth week after conception. Most critical periods of organ formation occur during this stage; thus, most structural abnormalities can be traced to these or preceding weeks. While considerations of teratogenic mechanisms necessarily concentrate on this stage of development, it should not be assumed that adverse effects of environmental agents or genetic disorders are limited to this period.

The fourth stage, fetal development (weeks 9–38), is the longest phase of human gestation. During this stage, cytotoxicity is less likely to be expressed as a structural defect but is not necessarily less likely to occur. Although organs are formed by this time, functional differentiation and growth occur during these weeks. This is an especially important period for the brain. Investigators in the field of behavioral teratology, which concentrates on this period, are just beginning to study relationships between events in fetal life and later brain function.

The final phase of intrauterine development is the intrapartum period. Fetal presentation at the time of delivery as well as route of delivery and any trauma sustained can affect morphologic features in the neonate. Many abnormal findings are related to molding of the head or the position of the extremities and are transient in nature.

CLASSIFICATION OF DYSMORPHIC FEATURES

Accurate diagnosis is the key to prognosis and management. Great efforts have been spent, therefore, in describing recognizable patterns of dysmorphism. Recognition of specific syndromes and patterns can be extremely valuable but is often difficult in the neonatal period. A dysmorphologist should be consulted, if possible, but classification of defects on the basis of suspected origin can also be useful and requires less first-hand experience than does recognition of specific patterns. This approach to classification begins with an attempt to distinguish intrinsic from extrinsic causes on the basis of history and physical examination. Each anomaly found is then assigned to one of the etiologic categories listed in Fig 34–2.

Malformations are the result of intrinsically abnormal processes of development. The conceptus is abnormal from the outset of gestation, and malforma-

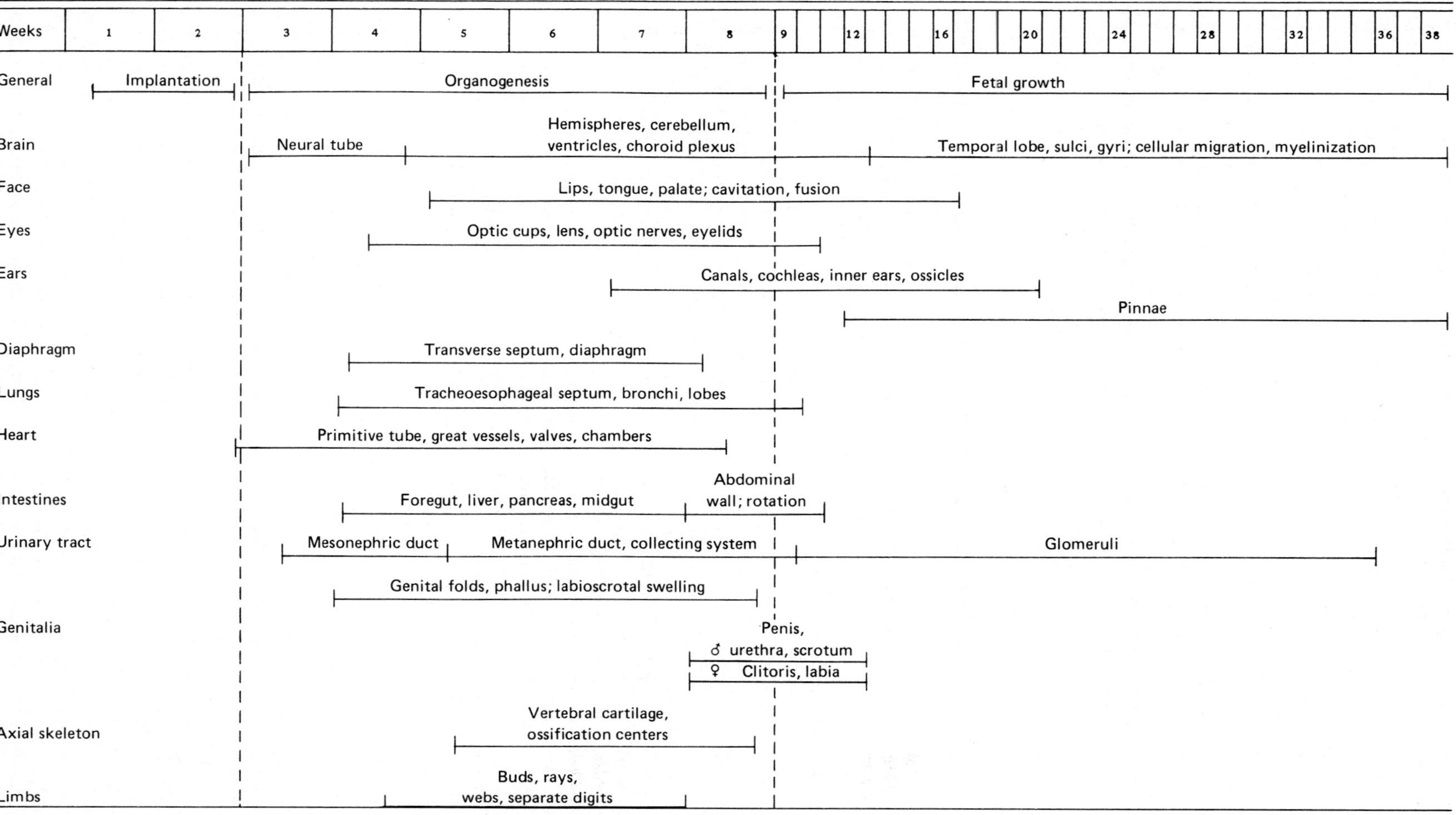

Figure 34–1. Critical periods in human gestation.

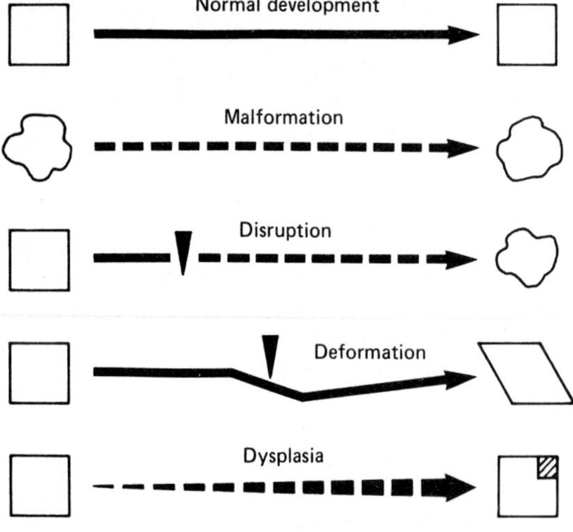

Figure 34–2. Etiologic classification of congenital anomalies. (Modified and reproduced, with permission, from Spranger J et al: Errors of morphogenesis: Concepts and terms. Recommendations of an international working group. *J Pediatr* 1982;**100**:161.)

tions are generally attributed to genetic pathology. The characteristic morphologic features of Down's syndrome and the hypoplastic thumbs and pancytopenia associated with Fanconi's syndrome are classified as malformations.

Disruptions are the result of extrinsic processes. Development is perceived as proceeding normally when factors external to the conceptus interfere at a cellular level. Note that external factors need not be distributed in the general environment; they also include maternal factors. Drug-related embryopathies such as those associated with use of thalidomide are prototypic disruptions, but multifactorial processes such as neural tube defects are currently classified as disruptions despite their considerable genetic influence. The distinction between a disruption and a malformation may be difficult to discern on the basis of form alone. Careful histories—especially family histories and cytogenic studies—are useful in this case. It is easier to establish the classification of malformation on the basis of a positive family history or abnormal karyotype than it is to rule out a disruption. Disruptions, however, are more common by far.

Deformations are the result of extrinsic mechanical forces. Deformations rarely involve internal organs but may range from minor malpositioning of limbs to major disturbances of the head and trunk. Intrauterine problems resulting in deformations include multiple pregnancies, abnormal uterine shape, fetal positioning, rupture of the amnion, and oligohydramnios caused by loss of or failure to produce fluid or by failure of the fetus to urinate. Deformations are characteristically asymmetric. Deforming processes may bend, cut, or fuse tissues.

Dysplasias occur as a result of abnormal tissue differentiation. In theory, extrinsic processes may be involved, but intrinsic, genetically determined factors are most often responsible. Dysplasias emphasize the link between cell function and morphogenesis. Examples include osteogenesis imperfecta (a disorder in which poorly ossified bone is easily fractured) and mucopolysaccharidoses (inborn errors of metabolism that result in growth deficiency, skeletal abnormalities, and unusual facies). Most dysplasias are the result of single gene disorders.

Assignment to an etiologic category may also involve a statement about prognosis. The presence of deformations, for instance, often means that the development and function of unaffected organs will be normal. Specific therapy can be applied to deformations, and, not uncommonly, significant improvement occurs. When deformations are the result of neurologic abnormalities, however, the prognosis is poorer. Many dysplasias are not recognizable in the neonatal period. Those presenting at birth (eg, thanatophoric dwarfism) frequently have poor prognoses. Disruptions are probably the most common cause of birth defects and demonstrate the vulnerability of the developing human to extrinsic factors. Isolated disruptions, such as congenital heart defects, have excellent prognoses if repair is possible. Malformations are often multiple and, like dysplasias, often have poor prognoses.

Etiologic categorization also provides information about risks for recurrence. The highest risks are associated with single gene disorders, producing dysplasias and malformations. Most chromosomally mediated malformations occur sporadically, but careful cytogenetic analysis is required. Risks for recurrence are higher if parents carry balanced translocations. Disruptions also tend to occur sporadically, but many are the result of multifactorial processes with substantial genetic input. Empirical data indicate higher than normal risks for recurrence in relatives of infants affected with disruptions. Isolated deformations that do not occur as a result of uterine abnormalities have a low risk for recurrence.

MULTIPLE MALFORMATIONS

Many dysmorphic infants will have more than one abnormality. Relationships between multiple malformations also provide important clues to etiology and prognosis.

A **developmental field** is a region or part of an embryo that responds as a coordinated unit to intrinsic or extrinsic stimuli. The pathogenesis of developmental field defects may involve functional disturbances in primordial cells, interacting tissues, or processes common to multiple tissues. Disturbances in the rostral mesoderm, for instance, may lead to multiple anomalies of the head and face. Genital and cardiac abnormalities may be related to disturbances in other tissues or organs such as the hypothalamus and vascular structures.

A **sequence** is a pattern of anomalies that are all caused by a single abnormality. Renal agenesis, for instance, results in decrease of amniotic fluid, fetal compression, pulmonary hypoplasia, and limb deformations. This same sequence may occur as a result of loss of amniotic fluid or urethral obstruction. The sequence of micrognathia, glossoptosis, and cleft soft palate (Pierre Robin syndrome) may begin with mandibular hypoplasia, which pushes the developing tongue posteriorly so that it interferes with movements of the posterior palatal shelves.

The term **association,** when used to describe multiple anomalies, refers to their nonrandom occurrence outside any known developmental field. It denotes statistical but not necessarily causal relationships. The pathogenesis may involve both developmental field defects and sequences. Knowledge of associations is useful because it alerts the clinician to investigate other specific organs further if a defect is recognized in one.

The term **syndrome** is applied to patterns of multiple anomalies that recur with such regularity that they are considered to be pathogenetically related. Down's syndrome and Turner's syndrome are disorders with morphologic features found in individuals with specific chromosomal abnormalities: trisomy 21 and 45,X karyotype, respectively.

DYSMORPHIC PATTERNS IN NEONATES

The following are examples of patterns of abnormalities in the neonate. Numerous other patterns have been described in newborns (see references by Smith and Jones [1982] and by Warkany [1971] at end of chapter).

Chromosomal Abnormalities

Common chromosomal abnormalities are reviewed in Chapter 33. These include trisomy 13, 18, and 21, Turner's and Klinefelter's syndromes, and the XYY and fragile X syndromes, among others.

Cornelia de Lange's Syndrome

Cornelia de Lange's syndrome, a sporadically occurring constellation of congenital anomalies, has typical features that can be recognized in the newborn. Intrauterine growth retardation and characteristic facial features, including prominent eyebrows with a tendency toward central fusion (synophrys) and thin, downturned lips with a midline peak on the upper lip, are invariable. These infants are hirsute, and limb abnormalities occur in over 50%. Hypoplastic hands and feet are most common, but major limb reductions occur in 30%. One infant in 4 has congenital heart disease. No specific chromosomal abnormalities have been found. The immediate prognosis depends largely upon the presence of congenital heart disease or respiratory failure. Subsequent failure to thrive and severe mental deficiency are the rule.

Meckel's Syndrome (Meckel-Gruber Syndrome)

Meckel's syndrome is rare and is inherited as an autosomal recessive trait. Infants with this syndrome have encephaloceles, polydactyly, and renal cysts. The prognosis is generally poor, owing to central nervous system and renal dysfunction. Central nervous system anomalies are variably expressed and range from anencephaly and holoprosencephaly to small posterior or dorsal encephaloceles. Oligohydramnios due to renal hypoplasia may lead to a sequence including pulmonary hypoplasia and clubfeet. The renal cysts are bilateral and typically small and uniform. They must be distinguished from the more commonly occurring multicystic renal dysplasia, which may be associated with other anomalies. Meckel's syndrome is often recognized only at autopsy—an unfortunate fact that emphasizes the importance of early diagnosis in dysmorphic infants.

VATER (VACTERL) Association

Vertebral anomalies and abnormalities of the heart, trachea, esophagus, kidneys, and limbs are found in association with each other and in association with anal atresia more often than would be expected (ie, the association is nonrandom). The acronym VATER (*v*ertebral defects, imperforate *a*nus, *t*racheo*e*sophageal fistula, and *r*adial and *r*enal dysplasia) is sometimes written as VACTERL to include *c*ardiac and *l*imb anomalies. The limb defects seen are usually preaxial (radial or fibular). The association occurs sporadically, but some authors have suggested that exposures to progestational agents may be involved. While the anomalies themselves may be immediately or ultimately life-threatening, primary neurologic abnormalities are characteristically absent; the prognosis for intellectual development is good if the VATER association is recognized early enough for proper treatment to be instituted.

Amnion Rupture Sequence

The amniotic membrane is separated from the chorion early in gestation. Partial or complete rupture of the amniotic membrane may occur and cause loss of fluid and entrapment of the developing conceptus. Early rupture is often associated with major structural abnormalities that are incompatible with life. Later rupture may lead to complex deformations of the head and limbs or to amputation of structures by constricting amniotic bands. It may be difficult to distinguish these deformations from malformations unless the placenta is also carefully examined for the presence of amniotic bands that may have been removed during delivery. If the head has escaped significant deformation, neurologic development proceeds normally. The amniotic rupture sequence occurs sporadically. Its recognition, especially in cases where fetal death occurs, allows encouraging information about the unlikelihood of recurrence of the disorder in future pregnancies to be passed on to parents.

Twins

Multiple pregnancies are at high risk for abnormal development. Crowding may result in deformations in both identical and nonidentical twins. In one sense, monozygosity itself is a "birth defect," since it occurs after conception. Depending upon the timing of division, placental circulations and amniotic sacs may or may not be shared. Division after day 13 of gestation results in conjoined twins. Despite genetic concordance, congenital abnormalities in monozygotes are frequently discordant. This observation demonstrates the role of environmental factors in multifactorial birth defects. Monochorionic twins are particularly at risk for abnormalities resulting from vascular accidents, since emboli are more likely to form in shared circulations.

Short-Limbed Dwarfism

Several distinct dysplasias of bone and cartilage produce a phenotype with short, curved, or malformed limbs. The head and trunk may appear normal in a few of these disorders, but more frequently there is a protuberant abdomen with or without ascites. Many of these dysplasias result in death due to pulmonary hypoplasia associated with small or poorly compliant chest walls. The differential diagnosis includes achondroplasia, achondrogenesis, osteogenesis imperfecta, several types of skeletal dysplasia, camptomelic syndrome, asphyxiating thoracic dystrophy, and thanatophoric dwarfism. These dysplasias may be due to single gene disorders or may be sporadic occurrences. Accurate diagnosis is extremely important, especially in the case of stillbirth or neonatal death. Specific diagnoses are made radiographically. Films should be taken of all extremities and should include a lateral view of the spine, which may be critical to the diagnosis. The immediate prognosis depends largely on the extent of pulmonary hypoplasia. The long-term prognosis is variable.

DRUG-RELATED DISORDERS

Very few human teratogens have been described. Thalidomide is the classic example of a human teratogen producing a relatively specific syndrome. Although the compounds discussed below appear to be significantly less potent teratogens than thalidomide, they are associated with specific abnormalities.

Warfarin

The use of warfarin derivatives as anticoagulants during pregnancy was initially felt to be safe, but closer examination of exposed fetuses has shown untoward effects including nasal hypoplasia, significant visual problems, stippling of uncalcified areas of bone, and abnormalities of brain development and function. Central nervous system abnormalities in the fetus can occur with exposure to warfarin during the second or third trimester of pregnancy, demonstrating the potential susceptibility of the brain to drug-related disorders during this period. Not all exposed infants are affected, however. The reason for this is not clear but may relate to differences in dose, metabolism, or drug action in different individuals. A rough estimate of risks indicates that untoward effects occur in as many as one-third of exposed fetuses.

Anticonvulsants

The relationship between anticonvulsant drugs and congenital abnormalities seen in offspring of women with seizure disorders is controversial and complex. There appears to be an interaction between genetic and pharmacologic factors, and the seizures themselves may be important. Significant abnormalities may occur as frequently as once in every 10 pregnancies in this population. A broad gamut of structural abnormalities have been reported with most anticonvulsants, but specific anomalies have also been reported with certain drugs. Maternal use of phenytoin (a hydantoin) is associated with fetal growth retardation; midface hypoplasia; hypertelorism; a broad, depressed nasal bridge; and, occasionally, cleft lip and palate and hypoplasia of distal phalanges and nails. This group of abnormalities has been termed the fetal hydantoin syndrome. Maternal use of trimethadione has also been associated with growth retardation, decreased mentation, and unusual facies (fetal trimethadione syndrome). An increased risk for neural tube defects has recently been linked to maternal use of valproic acid.

Ethyl Alcohol

Admonitions against heavy use of alcohol during pregnancy have existed since ancient times. More recently, a specific syndrome has been recognized in the offspring of heavy drinkers. The fetal alcohol syndrome consists of intrauterine and postnatal growth retardation, microcephaly, significant mental dysfunction, and a group of craniofacial changes including short palpebral fissures, short nose, and a long, smooth philtrum. A variety of other structural abnormalities have also been reported.

While it is clear that high concentrations of alcohol are cytotoxic, the mechanisms of alcohol toxicity are poorly understood. The dose-response relationship is not entirely clear, but maternal alcohol intake exceeding 2–3 oz daily is considered toxic. The timing of fetal exposure to alcohol is important. Structural abnormalities occur with increased frequency in offspring of chronic alcohol abusers, but neurologic abnormalities can be decreased if women stop drinking by 16–20 weeks of gestation. Approximately two-thirds of pregnancies in active alcoholics will have significant complications, including prematurity, growth retardation, and perinatal asphyxia. Fetal alcohol syndrome is seen in about one-third of offspring of active alcoholics. The relationship of episodic maternal use of alcohol or paternal alcoholism to congenital problems is less well defined.

CLINICAL APPROACH TO THE DYSMORPHIC INFANT

The physician caring for an abnormal neonate has 2 immediate concerns: first, to provide care, and second, to make an accurate diagnosis. Often these must be done under conditions of great stress. The extent of the neonate's abnormalities may not be immediately apparent, and parents who feel grief and guilt are often desperate for information. As with any medical problem, however, the history and physical examination provide most of the clues to diagnosis. Special aspects of these procedures are outlined below.

HISTORY

Environmental, family, and pregnancy histories may contain important clues to the diagnosis. In the postpartum period, when frightened parents are attempting to cope with their grief and fears, the guilt they feel is likely to be heightened by suggestions made when the history was being taken. Nonetheless, parents are eager to discuss the history and will often bring up a variety of issues as they attempt to explain the problem. Thus, the interviewer must be prepared to answer as well as ask questions. Studies of parental responses indicate that recall after delivering an abnormal infant is better than recall after a normal birth.

Use of a wheel that relates calendar dates to gestational age may be helpful in documenting many of the following details: the last menstrual period, the onset of symptoms of pregnancy, the date of diagnosis of the pregnancy, the date of the first prenatal visit, and the physician's impressions of fetal growth at that time. This line of questioning establishes gestational age. Many parents will be able to indicate when they believe conception occurred, and this information can also be useful.

Next, it is important to establish the patterns of fetal growth and development. Prenatal visits should be noted and, using the gestational wheel, a record made of the patterns of fetal growth, the onset of fetal movement (usually at 16 weeks), and the mother's perceptions of fetal movements. Although the degree of movement is variable, normal fetal movement is usually strong enough at some point to hurt the mother and be visible to the father. Abnormal fetal movement or no perceived change in fetal position may indicate neuromuscular dysfunction or fetal constraint. These inquiries are particularly important when asphyxia accompanies the birth of a dysmorphic infant. A history of decreased fetal movement will distinguish neuromuscular abnormalities (which result in a low Apgar score) from intrapartum events (which depress the infant).

Abnormal patterns of uterine growth may also provide clues to fetal function. Increased uterine size may indicate accumulation of amniotic fluid (hydramnios). Fluid may accumulate if the fetus fails to swallow (eg, owing to neuromuscular disorder, obstruction of the fetal esophagus or proximal small bowel, or fetal heart failure) or if fetal urine output is increased. Hydramnios also can occur without apparent explanation and is associated with certain maternal complications, especially diabetes. Lack or delay of uterine growth may reflect fetal growth directly or may indicate too little amniotic fluid (oligohydramnios). Amniotic fluid may be lost through premature rupture of membranes with or without formation of amniotic bands, or it may be the result of compromised function of fetal kidneys. The mother should be questioned about loss or leakage of amniotic fluid, which is often mistakenly perceived as a vaginal discharge. Information from prenatal ultrasound examination is often very helpful in distinguishing different entities associated with altered uterine growth.

The history should also include details about the onset and progression of labor.

A family history should be taken next. It is not appropriate to ask simply whether there are other similarly affected family members. This question may be perceived as an accusation by the parents and may increase anxiety and guilt in the immediate as well as the extended family. A better approach is to outline the pedigree of first- and second-degree relatives, documenting the health of each member of both sides of the family. This approach is more likely to uncover relevant pathologic features than is focusing solely on dysmorphism. It is less threatening but may still lead to anxiety. The interviewer should be prepared to respond to specific questions from parents.

Finally, an environmental history that documents parental habits and their work and home environments should be obtained. Maternal and paternal health, use of medications, and environmental exposures during the embryonic period should be reviewed. Questions should be considered carefully because of their emotional impact. Society is currently preoccupied with the roles of drugs, radiation, and chemical exposures in birth defects. While these may be important, immediate focus on these issues greatly increases parental anxiety and may lead to erroneous perceptions. For example, exposure to diagnostic radiation is seldom high enough to cause birth defects, but immediate questioning about x-ray exposures during pregnancy gives parents the message that they may have hurt their infant by submitting to such procedures. This approach can lead to incapacitating anxiety in parents at precisely the time when their informed input into decision making is vital. History taking under these circumstances should therefore be approached with careful planning.

PHYSICAL EXAMINATION

Meticulous physical examination is crucial to accurate diagnosis in dysmorphic infants. Delivery of an affected infant may necessitate immediate attention to potentially life-threatening problems, but it is precisely because intensive support may be required that a complete examination becomes urgent. The examination should be performed as soon as possible.

In addition to the routine procedures described in Chapter 3, special attention should be paid to the neonate's physical measurements (Fig 34–3). Photographs are very helpful and should include a scale of measurements for reference. The placenta should also be examined.

Since most syndromes occur infrequently in the general population and patterns of abnormalities are therefore difficult to recognize, a dysmorphologist should be consulted if possible.

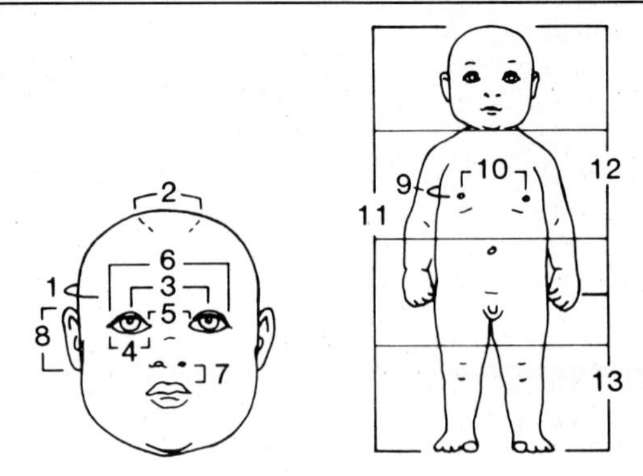

Measurement	Range (cm) Term (38–40 weeks)	Preterm (32–33 weeks)
1 Head circumference	32–37	27–32
2 Anterior fontanelle $\left(\frac{L-W}{2}\right)$	0.7–3.7	. . .
3 Interpupillary distance	3.3–4.5	3.1–3.9
4 Palpebral fissure	1.5–2.1	1.3–1.6
5 Inner canthal distance	1.5–2.5	1.4–2.1
6 Outer canthal distance	5.3–7.3	3.9–5.1
7 Philtrum	0.6–1.2	0.5–0.9
8 Ear length	3–4.3	2.4–3.5
9 Chest circumference	28–38	23–29
10 Internipple distance*	6.5–10	5–6.5
11 Height	47–55	39–47
12 13 Ratio Upper body segment / Lower body segment	1.7	. . .
14 Hand (palm to middle finger)	5.3–7.8	4.1–5.5
15 Ratio of middle finger to hand	0.38–0.48	0.38–0.5
16 Penis (pubic bone to tip of glans)	2.7–4.3	1.8–3.2

*Internipple distance should not exceed 25% of chest circumference.

Figure 34–3. Neonatal measurements.

LABORATORY STUDIES

Radiologic and ultrasonographic examinations can be extremely helpful in the evaluation of dysmorphic infants. In general, films of infants with apparent limb or skeletal anomalies should include the skull and all of the long bones in addition to frontal and lateral views of the axial skeleton. Chest and abdominal films should be obtained when indicated. The pediatrician should consult a radiologist for further workup. Nuclear scanning, CT scanning, ultrasonographic imaging, and contrast studies are all useful diagnostic tools, but their performance and interpretation require specialized skills.

Cytogenetic analysis (see Chapter 33) can provide specific diagnoses in approximately 5% of dysmorphic infants who survive and in perhaps as many as 10–15% who die during the newborn period. The most accurate tests require banding of chromosomes grown from several lines of circulating lymphocytes or fibroblasts. These procedures take several days. Speeding up the process may limit the interpretation, but rapid results can be obtained in certain cases. Analysis of cells in bone marrow, for example, can be performed rapidly but should always be accompanied by complete analysis of cultured cells. Any case requiring rapid diagnosis should be thoroughly discussed with an experienced cytogeneticist. The clinician should not base decisions about further workup and management on the results of only one test. The finding of normal karyotypes does not rule out significant genetic disease, nor does the sole finding of abnormal karyotypes indicate the prognosis.

When death of a dysmorphic infant occurs, autopsy examination can provide important diagnostic information and should include sampling of tissue for cytogenetic analysis. To avoid overlooking important areas of investigation, the pediatrician should discuss the case thoroughly with the pathologist before tissue samples are obtained. Photographs should always be taken.

IMMEDIATE MANAGEMENT OF THE DYSMORPHIC INFANT

Birth defects in the newborn may be life-threatening. One physician should assume responsibility for overall care as soon as possible. The skills of several other health professionals will usually be required, and their efforts should be coordinated by the primary physician.

Vital functions should be supported until a firm diagnosis is made. Occasionally, lethal or inoperable anomalies will be immediately recognized, and humane, compassionate treatment and support directed at ensuring comfort should be provided. All neonates should be dried, kept warm, and provided with an opportunity to interact with their families.

PROTOCOL FOR DECISION MAKING

The birth of a dysmorphic infant is a highly emotional event and may raise profound ethical and medical dilemmas. In some cultures at one time, such infants were simply discarded, since families lacked the means to care for affected individuals and severe handicaps would jeopardize the economic survival of others. Modern medicine and technology now offer life support systems that have the potential to sustain life under most extraordinary circumstances. Very often, the appropriate use of this capability is not immediately apparent. Our society is currently agonizing over the dilemmas presented by such cases, and it is clear that agreement on general principles does not always lead to agreement on what to do in specific cases. The following protocol is based on the premise that decisions are best made in a supportive atmosphere by parents who are well informed and aware of the options open to them and who have been given clear medical recommendations.

After historical, physical, and laboratory data are obtained, it is useful to review the clinical situation from 3 different perspectives. The first review with the parents involves describing each abnormality in detail and discussing what is known and not known about why it occurs and what can be done about it. At this point, the purpose of the review is to make the parents aware of all the findings, and no effort is made to correlate findings.

The second review follows immediately, and its purpose is to correlate the findings. The parents are informed about the immediate importance of specific abnormalities, their relationship to one another, and their combined effect on overall prognosis. If a definitive diagnosis can be made, it is introduced at this point.

Implementation of the plan does not go forward until the parents have had an opportunity to ask specific questions about the information communicated in the first and second reviews. It may not be necessary to move to the next review immediately.

A third review takes into account the immediate priorities and outlines all possible options for care to the parents. Parents contribute as much as health professionals to the formulation of these options. After all options have been described and their implications discussed, a medical recommendation should be made to the parents. This is not the final decision; rather, it is a medical opinion expressed by the infant's physician. Parents should not be required to weigh the merits of various treatment options. They have a right to the physician's best opinion, and the physician has an obligation to apply his or her judgment and experience.

The above protocol is designed to clearly separate the process of informing parents and making recommendations from the process of making decisions. The latter may be obvious and straightforward or complex and painful. Most parents need both time and support from within their own community. A sense of the time available before a decision must be made should be given to the parents, and they should have an opportunity to discuss their problem with supportive individuals. Other health professionals may also be able to provide additional support. The infant's physician has an important role in this process but should not be the sole individual involved.

SELECTED REFERENCES

Juchau M: *The Biochemical Basis of Chemical Teratogenesis.* Elsevier, 1981.

Kalter H, Warkany J: Congenital malformations. (2 parts.) *N Engl J Med* 1983;**308:**424, 491.

Kushner H: *When Bad Things Happen to Good People.* Schocken, 1982.

Merlob P, Sivan Y, Reisner SH: Anthropomorphic measurements of the newborn infant. *Birth Defects* 1984;**20(7):**1. [Entire issue.]

Smith DW: Fetal drug syndromes: Effects of ethanol and hydantoins. *Pediatr in Rev* 1979;**1:**165.

Smith DW, Jones KL: *Recognizable Patterns of Human Malformation.* Saunders, 1982.

Spranger J et al: Errors of morphogenesis: Concepts and terms: Recommendations of an international working group. *J Pediatr* 1982;**100:**160.

Thompson JS, Thompson MW: *Genetics in Medicine.* Saunders, 1981.

Warkany J: *Congenital Malformations.* Year Book, 1971.

Wilson JG, Fraser FC (editors): *Handbook of Teratology.* Vols 1–4. Plenum Press, 1977.

35 Diagnostic & Therapeutic Procedures

*Ronald W. Gotlin, MD, & Henry K. Silver, MD**

The care of children optimally does not end with a diagnostic and treatment plan but includes an understanding of the specific procedures referable to this age group.

This chapter records those methods which have proved to be useful and effective. No claim is made of originality, and all possible pediatric procedures have not been included.

We recognize what may appear to be a lack of sufficient emphasis regarding the comfort and feelings of our pediatric patients and their parents. Were it not for limited space, we would continually reiterate the importance of patience and understanding when conducting procedures in children.

PREPARATION OF THE PATIENT & ORIENTATION OF THE PROCEDURE TEAM

With any diagnostic or treatment procedure, proper positioning and restraint are of greatest importance.

In the majority of cases, failure to complete a procedure is directly related to undue haste in preparing the patient. Young patients often have levels of apprehension and fear that do not lend themselves to ''classic'' adult physician-patient understanding; competence needs to be developed to balance reassurance and determination to carry out a procedure. This should be done by individualizing the approach for each patient.

Patience and adequate preparation are also necessary when dealing with understandably anxious parents. A few words of explanation to concerned family members will be most reassuring. In general, procedures go more smoothly when parents are not in the procedure room. However, in the event that a parent wants to be present, forcible ejection from the scene may be associated with harmful effects both to the patient and to the procedure team, and it is usually advisable to allow the parent to remain under these circumstances. If parents are allowed to remain in the room, they should not be asked to become part of the procedure team or to play an active part in restraining the patient.

Most procedures should have consent from parents. As full an explanation as possible, even to children as young as 3 years, should be given to the patient.

In all procedures, either diagnostic or therapeutic, the need for the particular procedure should be weighed against the possible complications.

RESTRAINT & POSITIONING

The physician should be acquainted with various methods of properly restraining and positioning a patient. It is usually very difficult and sometimes dangerous to attempt any procedure on an unrestrained young patient. Before actually starting a procedure, the physician should be certain that all necessary items of equipment are available and arranged for immediate use.

Specially designed restraint devices (eg, ''papoose boards'') are commercially available. Following immobilization of any extremity, the fingers or toes should be examined for adequate circulation by noting the color and capillary filling of the nail bed.

When total body restraint is necessary, the physician must be certain before and during the procedure that cardiorespiratory function has not been impaired. To assist in doing this, a stethoscope may be taped to the anterior chest of the patient to permit frequent evaluation.

Local subcutaneous infiltration with procaine or lidocaine (Xylocaine) before performing a lumbar puncture, bone marrow aspiration, or thoracic, pericardial, or peritoneal aspiration is frequently necessary and advisable. Whenever drugs are employed, a history of previous reactions to the drugs should be ascertained, and equipment (suction apparatus, oral airway or endotracheal tube, laryngoscope, tourniquet, and epinephrine, 1:1000 solution) should be readily available to manage the rare but dangerous untoward reaction that may occur.

After any procedure is performed, the physician should personally observe the child long enough to be certain that no adverse reactions have developed.

* With contributions by Craig Schramm, MD.

DIAGNOSTIC PROCEDURES

COLLECTION & PROCESSING OF BLOOD SAMPLES

1. VENIPUNCTURE

The antecubital superficial veins of the hand and external jugular veins are used most frequently for venipuncture and withdrawal of blood (Fig 35–9). Venipuncture of the femoral and internal jugular veins may be associated with serious complications (see below), particularly in the newborn, and should be avoided if possible. In some instances, blood may be withdrawn from other peripheral veins. Large, accessible veins are best for purposes of injection.

The skin should be cleansed thoroughly with an iodinated solution and alcohol. Iodinated solutions should not be used when blood is to be tested for various iodinated compounds, and alcohol should be avoided when blood is drawn for alcohol levels. When blood is obtained for culture and for various tests, it should be put into media-containing tubes or bottles before being placed in vacutainer tubes, since the latter may not be sterile.

Antecubital Vein Puncture

If available, the antecubital vein should be used for venipuncture in children, infants, and newborns.

A soft elastic tourniquet is applied proximal (cephalad) to the vein and the venous pattern observed. Dilation of a vein may be facilitated by local warming in a wash basin or with warm, moist towels. Frequently, light palpation of the antecubital fossa will reveal a distended vein not visible on the surface.

A short, sharp-beveled, 20- or 22-gauge needle (disposable syringes and needles are recommended) applied firmly to an appropriate-sized syringe is used.

The skin is entered with the needle at an approximately 10- to 30-degree angle with the bevel up. If gentle suction is applied to the syringe barrel, blood will be aspirated as the vessel is entered. Blood should be withdrawn gently and rapidly to avoid clotting and hemolysis. In a struggling patient, the use of a needle and catheter (eg, butterfly assembly) attached to the syringe will lessen leverage between the vein and needle. When the required quantity of blood has been obtained, the tourniquet is released and the needle withdrawn quickly. After the needle is removed, a dry sterile cotton ball is applied with pressure over the puncture site and held for approximately 3 minutes or until any evidence of bleeding has subsided. To avoid excessive hemolysis, the needle should be removed from the syringe and the stopper taken out of vacuum tubes prior to expelling the blood from the syringe into the specimen tube.

Puncture of Superficial Dorsal Veins of the Hand & Wrist

The superficial dorsal veins of the hand and wrist are particularly readily accessible for diagnostic venipuncture in the newborn infant. After thorough preparation of the skin, a 22-gauge needle, preferably with a clear hub, can be inserted into the vein. Blood will be seen to flow into the hub and can be easily collected into capillary or specimen tubes.

External Jugular Vein Puncture (Fig 35–1)

Wrap the child firmly so that arms and legs are adequately restrained. The wraps should not extend higher than the shoulder girdle. Place the child on a flat, firm table so that both shoulders are touching the table; the head is rotated fully to one side and extended partly over the end of the table so as to stretch the vein. Adequate immobilization is essential.

Use a very sharp 20- or 22-gauge needle or a 21-gauge scalp vein needle with attached catheter (Fig 35–4) for withdrawing blood. The child should be crying and the vein distended when entered. First thrust the needle just under the skin; then enter the vein. Pull constantly on the barrel of the syringe and be certain that air is not drawn into the vein during aspiration.

After removing the needle, exert firm pressure over the vein for 3–5 minutes while the child is in a sitting position.

The next 2 procedures can result in significant complications, particularly in the newborn infant, and should be performed by someone skilled in their techniques.

Femoral Vein Puncture (Fig 35–2)

This is a hazardous procedure, particularly in the newborn, and should be employed only in emergencies.

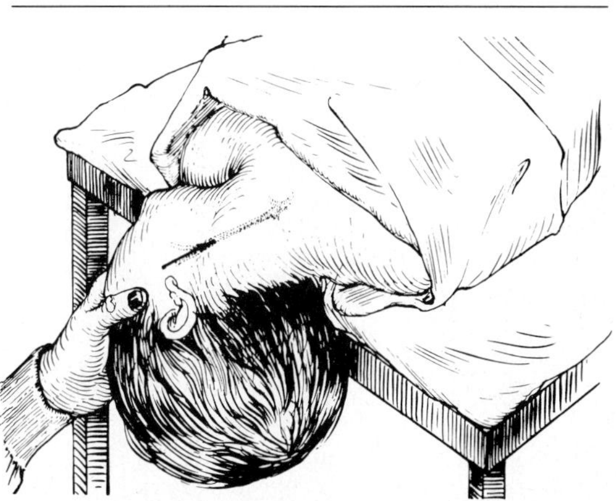

Figure 35–1. External jugular vein puncture.

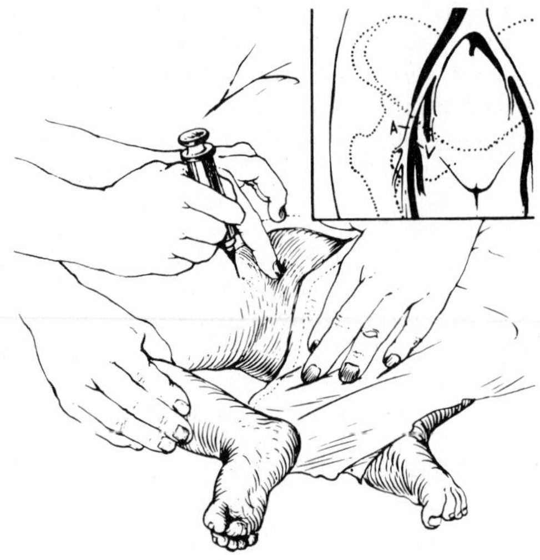

Figure 35–2. Femoral vein puncture.

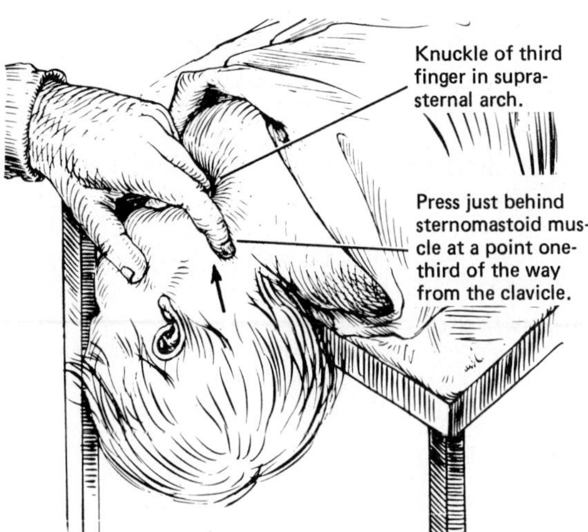

Figure 35–3. Direction of needle for internal jugular vein puncture.

Place the child on a flat, firm table. Abduct the leg so as to expose the inguinal region. Locate the femoral artery by its pulsation. The vein lies immediately medial to it. Be certain of the position of the femoral pulse at the time of puncture. Prepare the skin carefully with an antiseptic solution and carry out the procedure using strict sterile precautions. Insert a short-beveled, 21- or 22-gauge needle into the vein (perpendicularly to the skin) about 3 cm below the inguinal ligament; use the artery as a guide. If blood does not enter the syringe immediately, withdraw the needle slowly, gently drawing on the barrel of the syringe; the needle sometimes passes through both walls of the vein, and blood is obtained only when the needle is being withdrawn. Use a large enough syringe to produce adequate suction to assist in withdrawing the blood.

After removing the needle, exert firm, steady pressure over the vein for 3–5 minutes. If the artery has been entered, check the limb periodically for several hours.

Dangers: Septic arthritis of the hip may complicate femoral vein puncture secondary to accidental penetration of the joint capsule. Arteriospasm that has resulted in serious vascular compromise of the extremity, particularly in the debilitated and dehydrated infant, has been reported secondary to arterial puncture or venipuncture.

Internal Jugular Vein Puncture (Figure 35–3)

Prepare the child as for an external jugular vein puncture. Insert the needle beneath the sternocleidomastoid muscle at a point marking the junction of its lower and middle thirds. Aim at the suprasternal notch and advance the needle until the vein is entered. Avoid the trachea and the upper pleural space. Alternatively, the needle may be inserted at the apex of a triangle formed by the clavicle and the sternal and clavicular segments of the sternocleidomastoid muscle and advanced toward the ipsilateral nipple.

If no blood is obtained on inserting the needle, withdraw slowly and continue to pull gently on the barrel of the syringe. Not infrequently, the needle passes through both walls of the vein, and blood is obtained only when the needle is being withdrawn.

After completing the procedure, remove the needle and exert firm pressure over the area for 3–5 minutes with the child in a sitting position so as to reduce pressure in the vein.

Dangers: When properly performed, complications are rare. However, careless deep probing of the internal carotid vessel may result in injury to the trachea, vagus nerve, and pleura; the pleural cavity may be entered, and a hemothorax or a pneumothorax may be induced.

Cote CJ et al: Two approaches to cannulation of a child's internal jugular vein. *Anesthesiology* 1979;**50:**371.

2. COLLECTION OF CAPILLARY BLOOD

The majority of determinations may be made on blood obtained from a finger or heelstick. An expertly performed heelstick is much less traumatic for a small infant than is a femoral puncture and has the additional advantage that it may be repeated frequently and does not have the same risk of complications. The earlobe is not a satisfactory site, since puncture here may be associated with excessive bleeding that may be relatively difficult to control.

After the skin is cleaned with alcohol, a stab is made with either a No. 11 Bard-Parker blade or a lancet. Free-flowing blood is collected in capillary tubes.

Frequent wiping of the puncture site with a dry swab may be necessary to prevent clotting and to ensure good blood flow. Collection of capillary blood may be difficult, and proficiency may be gained only after prolonged practice. Hemostasis can be obtained by applying pressure with a sterile cotton ball. The site of puncture should be examined several times during the next 1–2 hours for evidence of oozing or ecchymoses. A rare complication of this procedure is the development of osteomyelitis of the calcaneus as a result of puncture by the lancet. Because of the shallow depth of the calcaneus in small infants, premature newborns are at particular risk for this complication.

3. COLLECTION OF MULTIPLE SPECIMENS OF BLOOD

When a number of blood samples must be obtained over a short period of time (eg, when glucose and electrolyte determinations are needed for a diabetic patient with ketoacidosis), multiple venipunctures may be avoided by employing a pediatric scalp vein catheter (butterfly needle) or an indwelling 22-gauge or larger Teflon intravenous catheter. The catheter and stylet are inserted in an arm or hand vein in the usual manner. When the stylet is removed, the catheter hub is attached by means of a male Luer adapter to a buffalo cap filled with heparinized saline (10 units/mL) or, alternatively, to a 3-way stopcock. Blood may be withdrawn at intervals by applying a tourniquet to the extremity and inserting a needle attached to a syringe through the sterilely prepared rubber port or by opening the stopcock and drawing off and discarding the saline solution. A second needle and syringe are then used to collect the blood specimen. The tourniquet is removed, and the buffalo cap and catheter are subsequently cleared by injecting heparinized saline through the rubber port.

4. ARTERIOPUNCTURE

Arteriopuncture is routinely employed in obtaining blood for blood gas determinations essential in monitoring many patients with cardiopulmonary disease. The radial, brachial, temporal, dorsalis pedis, and posterior tibial arteries are punctured most readily; the umbilical artery may be used in the newborn period. The femoral artery should be employed only in extreme emergencies.

Procedure

A. Radial and Brachial Arteries: The radial artery is the site of choice for obtaining arterial blood. It is relatively immobile in its position at the wrist, and since it does not course with an accompanying vein, erroneous sampling of venous blood will not easily occur. The right radial artery in the newborn has the advantage of providing preductal arterial blood samples. If the brachial artery is selected, it is entered either in the antecubital fossa or just proximal to the antecubital fossa along the anteromedial aspect of the arm. An effort should be made to maintain constant inspired oxygen delivery for the child or newborn receiving supplemental oxygen. A syringe fitted with a suitable needle (25-gauge for newborns and younger children to 22-gauge for adolescents) is flushed with heparin (200 units/mL), allowing a small amount to remain in the "dead space" of the syringe. A butterfly needle may be more useful in a struggling child. The wrist is supported slightly dorsiflexed and supine. The radial artery is located by palpation, and the overlying skin is cleaned first with an iodine-containing solution and then with alcohol.

The needle is inserted into the artery at a 30- to 45-degree angle, and blood is withdrawn into the syringe. When a butterfly needle is used, pulsatile flow of blood can be observed in the tubing. After the pulsatile flow of bright red blood has cleared the tubing of solution, the syringe is connected and the sample collected. To avoid hematoma formation, firm pressure is applied for at least 5 minutes after specimen withdrawal.

B. Posterior Tibial Artery: The posterior tibial artery is relatively constant in its position between the medial malleolus and the Achilles tendon. Careful palpation will identify its course. Care should be taken to avoid the Achilles tendon.

C. Dorsalis Pedis Artery: The dorsalis pedis artery can be palpated along the dorsum of the foot and can be safely entered for sampling.

D. Branches of the Superficial Temporal Artery: These branches are safe and suitable for arterial sampling. Either the frontal or parietal branch of the temporal artery is located by palpation. Overlying hair is shaved and the skin suitably cleansed. The palpating fingers partially immobilize the artery while the heparin-filled scalp vein needle is inserted with the bevel up (Fig 35–4). The needle is advanced until the artery is entered.

Dangers: Arterial punctures may be hazardous because of the risks of laceration, spasm, hematoma formation, and damage to adjacent structures. Septic arthritis may complicate inadvertent hip joint penetration deep in a femoral artery puncture. Damage to the median nerve may occur with repeated brachial artery blood sampling. Firm pressure should be applied for at least 10–15 minutes after withdrawal of the blood specimen to avoid hematoma formation. Temporary or persistent arteriospasm with serious vascular compromise may occur, leading to sloughing of the skin. Distal obstruction of an artery due to the inadvertent injection of clots into the vessel during arteriopuncture has been reported. Arteriospasm may be relieved by the application of heat or by the subcutaneous administration of 2% procaine proximal to the site of puncture.

Schlueter MA et al: Blood sampling from scalp arteries in infants. *Pediatrics* 1973;**51**:120.

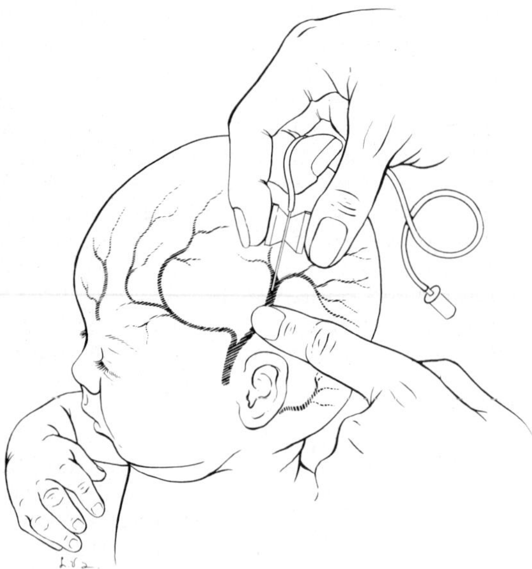

Figure 35–4. Scalp arteries suitable for blood sampling in infants. Note that the artery is palpated during cannulation. This helps immobilize the artery.

UMBILICAL VESSEL CATHETERIZATION

The use of an indwelling catheter in an umbilical artery or vein has become a common procedure in hospital nurseries. Catheterization of the artery generally provides a more useful source of diagnostic information and is safer than catheterization of the umbilical vein. The umbilical vessels are employed to obtain reliable arterial access for sampling and pressure monitoring, to administer fluids and electrolytes, and to perform exchange transfusions. The risks of umbilical vessel catheterization are significant. Transcutaneous blood gas measurements, Doppler ultrasound blood pressure measurements, and other noninvasive procedures should be substituted whenever possible.

Procedure

The catheter should be made of flexible, nontoxic radiopaque material that will not kink when advanced through a vessel and will not collapse during blood withdrawal. Nonwettable material and a single, smooth-surfaced end hole reduce clot formation. A 3.5-gauge catheter is used for infants weighing less than 1500 g and a 5-gauge for larger infants. Dead space of the catheter system should be determined prior to catheterization.

The infant is warmed (preferably under an overhead radiant heater) and loosely restrained. The procedure is carried out under sterile conditions.

A standard cut-down tray is opened, and the wide end of the umbilical artery catheter is cut off so that the blunt needle adapter fits snugly into the catheter. Discarding the wide end and utilizing the needle adapter reduces the catheter capacity. A sterile syringe is filled with flushing fluid (eg, heparinized saline) and attached to a 3-way stopcock and, in turn, to the umbilical catheter. The entire system is filled with flushing fluid.

An assistant may elevate the umbilical cord by the cord clamp while the operator prepares the cord and adjacent skin with 1% iodine solution, which should then be removed with alcohol to prevent an iodine burn of the skin. All areas of the skin should be inspected for the presence of iodine solution. The area is then draped. A loop of umbilical tape is placed at the base of the umbilical cord and tied loosely in order to control bleeding if necessary. The cord is then cut 1–1.5 cm above the skin with scissors or a scalpel blade.

The 2 thick-walled, round arteries and the single, thin-walled vein are identified. The rim of the cut vessel is grasped with a pointed forceps. The lumen of the vessel is then dilated with the tips of the forceps. Initially, the lumen may allow only one tip to enter. Both tips may then be inserted and allowed to spread, further dilating the vessel. The fluid-filled catheter is inserted into the lumen of the artery or vein and advanced. Any obstruction to advancement usually can be overcome by steady, gentle pressure. Forceful probing may lead to increased arteriospasm in the artery or perforation of the vein or artery. If the obstruction in one of the arteries cannot be overcome, the catheter should be removed and an attempt made to catheterize the other umbilical artery. If a similar obstruction occurs, 0.1–0.2 mL of 1% or 2% lidocaine without epinephrine is instilled into the artery, and after 2–3 minutes the catheter can usually be advanced.

Frequent aspiration will demonstrate blood return. In arterial catheterization, the tip may be left at the level of the third to fifth lumbar vertebrae as determined by anteroposterior abdominal x-ray. The catheter is tied in place by a pursestring suture at the base of the umbilical cord, with the ends of the suture secured to the catheter and the catheter taped to the abdomen.

Complications

The principal complications of umbilical artery catheterization are thrombosis, embolism, and vasospasm. Portal vein thrombosis with subsequent development of presinusoidal portal hypertension may complicate umbilical vein catheterization. Infection and accidental disconnection of the catheter system may complicate either umbilical artery or vein catheterization. Thrombogenic complications of umbilical artery catheterization may result in paraplegia, infarction of the kidneys or bowel, gangrene of the buttocks or lower extremities, and renal hypertension in later childhood.

Adelman RD: Neonatal hypertension. *Pediatr Clin North Am* 1978;**25:**99.

Mokrohisky ST et al: Low positioning of umbilical-artery catheters increases associated complications in newborn infants. *N Engl J Med* 1978;**299**:561.

Moore TD (editor): *Iatrogenic Problems in Neonatal Care: Sixty-Ninth Ross Conference on Pediatric Research.* Ross Laboratories, 1976.

Wesström G: Umbilical artery catheterization in newborns: Clinical follow-up study. *Acta Paediatr Scand* 1980;**69**:371.

URINE COLLECTION

Attached Receptacle Method

A pediatric urine collector (a Sterilon product)—a plastic bag with a round opening surrounded by an adhesive surface that adheres to the skin—may be used. If a specimen is to be used for culture, the genitalia should be scrupulously cleansed with soap and water and benzalkonium chloride solution. In the male, the penis is placed in the plastic bag and the adhesive surface is applied to the surrounding skin. In the female, the opening of the bag is placed around the external genitalia. After voiding occurs, the bag is removed and emptied of urine. For collection of a 24-hour specimen, bags with a catheter outlet from which urine may be periodically removed are commercially available.

Clean Catch Method

The "clean catch" technique is a useful method for urine collection in toilet-trained children. The male prepuce and glans of the penis or the opening of the female urethra and external vaginal vestibule are cleansed with benzalkonium chloride-soaked cotton balls. (In uncircumcised males, the foreskin should first be retracted.) The disinfectant should be removed with sterile water. An uninterrupted midstream clean catch specimen can then be obtained and sent to the laboratory.

Metabolic Bed Method

The metabolic bed is a crib in which the mattress has been replaced by a taut synthetic cloth mesh. The infant or young child is maintained without a diaper in the crib, and any urine that is passed flows through the mesh and onto a sloping surface beneath the crib. Children can usually tolerate the mesh for periods up to 24–48 hours without difficulty.

Catheterization of the Urinary Bladder

Catheterization is necessary to obtain a sterile urine specimen from a child who cannot produce a clean catch sample or when continuous measurement of urine output is needed. When it is used, sterile technique, including the use of sterile gloves and towels and adequate antiseptic preparation with hexachlorophene (pHisoHex) and benzalkonium chloride (Zephiran), should be employed.

If catheterization is necessary, catheters measuring 3–6 mm in diameter are usually satisfactory for most patients. A No. 5 feeding tube may be used for all age groups beyond the newborn period. Catheters made of inert Silastic- or Teflon-coated materials are preferred. They may be either straight or indwelling. The latter are double lumen tubes with an inflatable balloon near the distal opening. When inflated, removal is prevented until the bulb is deflated. This type of catheter is employed when continuous urine collection is necessary. If a retention catheter is employed, a closed drainage system should be used to reduce the risk of infection.

The patient is placed supine on a bed or table and immobilized and restrained when necessary. The skin is cleansed, and the catheter is inserted into the external urethra. In the male, the penis is held initially at a right angle to the body. In the female, the labia majora and minora are widely separated. The female urethra is somewhat C-shaped and is more easily traversed than the relatively acute-angled male urethra. Continue to thread the catheter gently until urine flow is obtained. Allow the first aliquot of urine to drain out of the catheter. Collect subsequent urine for culture. If a Foley catheter is used, inflate the balloon with the appropriate volume of normal saline solution (the volume is written on the catheter); inflation is through a one-way valve in the sidearm tubing. Pull back on the catheter to test that the balloon is in the bladder and that the catheter is secured. Tape the tubing to the thigh and attach the sterile collection unit and tubing. Trauma to the urethra or bladder can be minimized by using a catheter of the proper size and by gentle technique.

To prevent phimosis in male patients, remember to return the foreskin to its normal position after catheter insertion. Some authorities recommend use of a single dose of a urinary tract antibiotic (eg, nitrofurantoin [Macrodantin], 2 mg/kg) following in-and-out catheterization in an attempt to prevent infection resulting from the possible introduction of bacteria into the bladder during the procedure.

Suprapubic Percutaneous Bladder Aspiration

This method is useful when a sterile urine sample is necessary—particularly in the newborn infant, in whom the bladder is high and easily accessible. It is indicated in selected cases but does not lend itself to routine use.

The bladder *must* be full before the procedure is attempted and should be enlarged to palpation or percussion above the os pubis before an attempt is made to aspirate urine. Local anesthesia may be used but is generally not necessary.

A. Procedure:

1. Prepare the skin carefully with an antiseptic solution, using strict sterile precautions, while an assistant holds the child either in the frog-leg position or with thighs and hips together.

2. Firmly insert a sterile 22- or 25-gauge (for newborns) needle attached to a syringe through the skin and abdominal muscle in the midline 1–2 cm

above the symphysis pubis, with the needle perpendicular to the skin. Slight negative pressure should be exerted as the needle is advanced into the bladder. The appearance of urine in the syringe will therefore indicate a successful tap. After the skin and anterior wall have been penetrated, the tip of the needle will be lying against the bladder.

3. After urine has been obtained, withdraw the needle with a single, swift motion and cover the area with a small dressing. Failure to obtain urine usually indicates either that the bladder was not full or that the needle did not enter the bladder but passed to one side. The procedure may be repeated.

B. Dangers: When the procedure is performed as outlined above, complications are uncommon but include transient hematuria, abdominal wall abscess, and penetration of the bowel. Rarely, prolonged hemorrhage may occur.

COLLECTION OF NASOPHARYNGEAL FLUID

Nasopharyngeal secretions are frequently collected for culture in upper respiratory infections. In the newborn period, removal of fluid from the pharynx is frequently necessary after birth; passage of a nasopharyngeal tube and DeLee suction apparatus is helpful in excluding choanal atresia.

Fluid is easily obtained with the use of an ordinary polyvinyl feeding tube to which a syringe has been attached for suction. The tube is introduced into either nostril or into the oral cavity and directed downward as necessary, applying gentle suction with the syringe.

GASTRIC ASPIRATION

Gastric aspiration may be indicated to remove ingested drugs or toxins, to relieve intestinal distention, or to diagnose esophageal atresia in the newborn.

Infants and children unable to cooperate are restrained in the supine position. A cooperative older child is best intubated in the sitting position, with neck and chin held forward without flexion or extension of the neck. When restraint is necessary, the patient is placed on the left side after insertion of the nasogastric tube, allowing the stomach to assume a dependent position. When the danger of pulmonary aspiration is present (ie, toxic ingestions), the patient should be placed with the head in a dependent position while gastric aspiration is being carried out. In ingestions, use a large-bore orogastric tube (Ewald). If there is danger of aspiration, the patient should be intubated with an inflated cuffed orotracheal or endotracheal tube in place.

The desired tube length is determined by measuring the distance from the patient's nose to the xiphoid process and adding 10 cm. This point is marked on the tube, and another mark is made approximately 15 cm distal to that point for reference. The tube is lubricated and introduced into one nasal passage and directed posteriorly while the tip of the nose is held up (Fig 35–5). The tube is then advanced for a distance of 5–7.5 cm as the patient swallows water. If the tube coils, it is best to remove it entirely and start over. To minimize coiling, the tube may be made stiff by prior cooling in ice. After passage of the tube, aspiration with a syringe is attempted. If gastric fluid is not obtained, a bolus of air is introduced while an assistant auscultates over the area of the stomach. A characteristic "gurgling" noise heard by the second observer will indicate that the stomach has been intubated properly; coughing indicates that the patient's respiratory tract has been intubated inadvertently.

The tube may have to be relocated by passing it farther or by withdrawing it 2.5–5 cm.

When prolonged intubation is necessary, the tube is secured to the cheekbone or forehead with nonirritating tape.

As an alternative, the oral route may be used and is preferable in the newborn.

COLLECTION OF DUODENAL FLUID

Bile, duodenal, or pancreatic fluid may be needed for diagnostic analysis. The Miller-Abbott tube with weighted metal tip and double lumen is introduced as described above for gastric aspiration, and the gastric contents are aspirated with the patient placed on the right side. The tube is advanced approximately 15 cm and the patient asked to remain in that position for 30–60 minutes. In this position, the normal stomach will pass the tube beyond the gastric pylorus and into the duodenum. Alternatively, a standard feeding tube may be placed in the stomach and advanced 1–2 cm/h while the patient lies on the right side. The appearance of bile and change in pH of the aspirated duodenal fluid or roentgenographic visualiza-

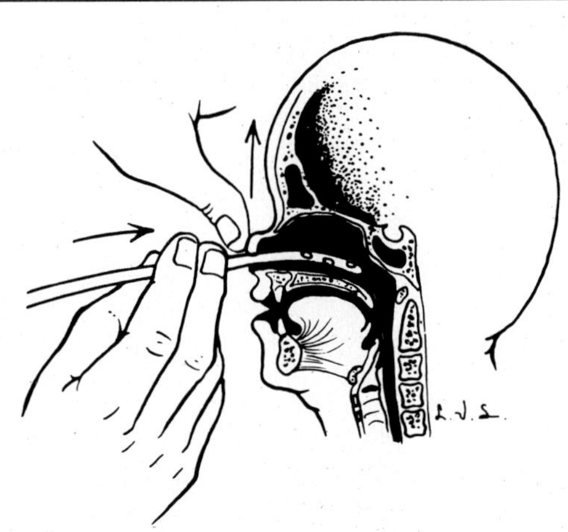

Figure 35–5. Inserting the nasogastric tube.

tion of the metal tip verifies proper positioning of the tube.

OBTAINING SPINAL FLUID

The 4 procedures for the collection of cerebrospinal fluid are lumbar, subdural, cisternal, and ventricular punctures. Lumbar puncture is most frequently used for obtaining cerebrospinal fluid for diagnostic purposes.

Lumbar Puncture

The patient should be restrained in either the sitting or lateral recumbent position according to the preference of the operator (Fig 35–6).

The needle should be inserted through the L4–5 interspace into the subarachnoid space. This point is marked by the intersection of an imaginary line drawn between the iliac crests and the spine. The interspace above and below this may also be used. The skin around this area is cleansed with iodine and alcohol solutions and the area suitably draped. Local anesthetic may be used.

With the operator comfortably seated, the 22-gauge lumbar puncture needle with stylet in place is inserted into the chosen intervertebral space in the midline and perpendicular to the plane of the body. The needle is directed toward the umbilicus, with the bevel of the needle parallel to the spine. In older children, a distinct "give" is usually felt when the dura is pierced. However, this may not be appreciated in newborns or in young infants. If in doubt, remove the stylet and examine the needle hub for the appearance of fluid.

When fluid is obtained and with the child quiet, the 3-way stopcock and manometer are attached and the stopcock opened. Pressure measurements are made before collection (opening pressure) and at the completion of collection (closing pressure). In addition, the presence of pressure changes with compression of the neck veins (Queckenstedt's test) is indicative of patency between the intracranial system and cerebrospinal canal.

After the closing pressure is obtained, the needle is removed with a quick deliberate movement and pressure applied for several minutes with a sterile sponge over the puncture site. Pressure measurements are meaningless in the struggling, crying patient.

Note: When fluid is obtained in the infant or child for glucose determination, a concomitant blood sugar should be obtained for comparison. Without such a comparison, a low cerebrospinal fluid glucose may be difficult to interpret.

A "bloody tap" may occur without obvious cause and is most likely the result of penetration of the needle into the anterior venous plexus of the vertebral body. The counting of red blood cells in the first and third tubes of bloody spinal fluid will help distinguish a traumatic from a nontraumatic tap.

Dangers: Herniations of the cerebellar tonsils may occur when increased intracranial pressure is present in the posterior fossa at the time of lumbar puncture; preoperative ophthalmoscopic examination of the retina may be helpful in indicating increased pressure. Increased intracranial pressure is not necessarily an absolute contraindication to the procedure if provision is made for neurosurgical management of possible complications. Introduction of chemical irritants and infectious agents should be avoided by the use of proper technique. Postspinal headache is common when large amounts of cerebrospinal fluid are removed rapidly or when leakage from the spinal canal into the subarachnoid space occurs. An analgesic may be required. The use of needles without stylets for lumbar puncture has been associated with the development of intraspinal dermoids resulting from the introduction of islets of epidermis into the subarachnoid space.

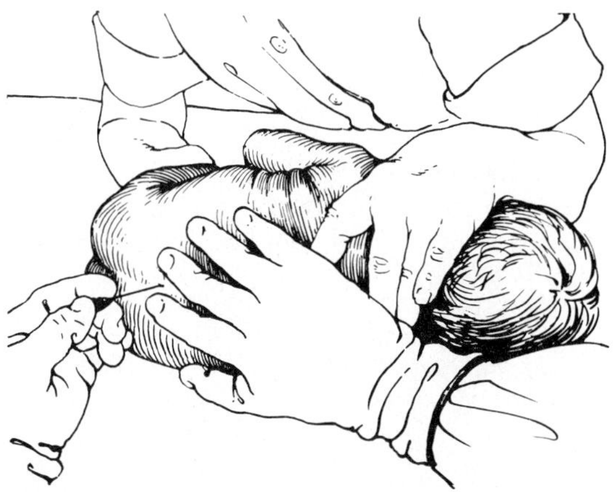

Figure 35–6. Restraining the infant for lumbar puncture with assistance of nurse. (Drapes omitted to show positioning.)

Subdural Puncture (Fig 35–7)

Subdural taps are performed to confirm the presence of and remove a postinfectious or posttraumatic subdural effusion. The anterior two-thirds of the scalp are shaved and cleaned with iodine and alcohol solutions. The patient is restrained as shown. Draw the scalp taut to one side and insert a short 19- or 20-gauge lumbar puncture needle with a very short bevel through the skin at the extreme lateral corner of the fontanelle or farther out through the suture line, depending on the size of the fontanelle. Release the tension and advance the needle for a distance of 0.2–0.5 cm. A hemostat clamped on the needle will prevent the operator from going too deep. Piercing the tough dura is easily recognized by a sudden "popping through" feeling. Normally, not more than a few drops (up to 1 mL) of clear fluid are obtained. If a subdural hematoma is present, the fluid will be grossly

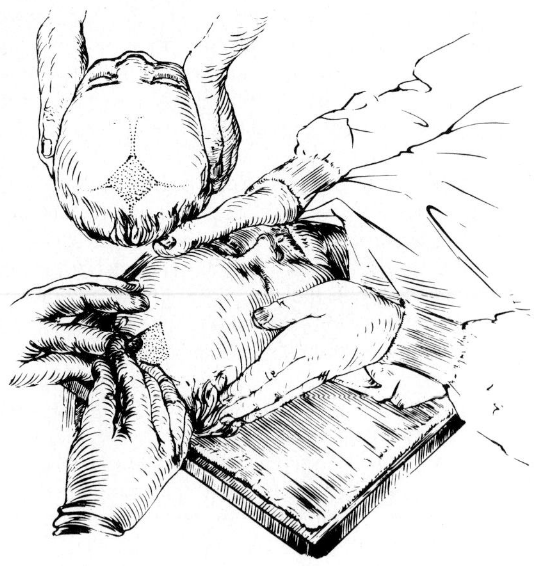

Figure 35–7. Subdural puncture.

xanthochromic or bloody and more abundant. Repeat the procedure on the other side. Do not remove more than 15–20 mL of fluid at any one time and allow the fluid to drip from the needle without aspiration. Remove the needle, exert firm pressure for a few minutes, and apply a sterile collodion dressing.

If the fontanelle and sutures are closed, neurosurgical assistance should be sought.

Note: Hemorrhage may occur if the needle causes a laceration of a tiny vein communicating with the sagittal sinus. This may result in subsequent taps yielding xanthochromic fluid from the blood introduced during the preceding procedures. Fistulous drainage is prevented by covering the orifice with a sterile collodion dressing.

BONE MARROW ASPIRATION

Bone marrow puncture is indicated in the diagnosis of neuroblastomas, blood dyscrasias, metastatic disease, reticuloendothelioses, and "storage diseases" and is occasionally used for marrow culture.

Sites for Punctures

The sites that may be used at different ages are listed in Table 35–1.

Table 35–1. Sites for bone marrow puncture.*

Site	Age to Which Adaptable
Anterior iliac crest	Any age
Posterior iliac crest	Any age
Femur	Birth to 2 years
Spinous vertebral process	2 years and older
Sternum	6 years and older
Tibia	Birth to 2 years

* Reproduced, with permission, from Hughes WT: *Pediatric Procedures.* Saunders, 1964.

The site of choice for children is the posterior iliac crest, because it is easy to locate and the child can easily be restrained in this position.

Procedure

For the performance of a posterior iliac crest aspiration, restrain the child on the abdomen with a rolled sheet placed under the hips. Sedation is often necessary for children. Prepare the skin surrounding the area as for a surgical procedure. Scrub and wear sterile gloves. Infiltrate with 1% procaine or lidocaine solution through the skin and subcutaneous tissues to the periosteum at a point 1 cm below the lip of the posterior crest.

Use an 18- or 19-gauge bone marrow needle in children and a 21-gauge needle in infants. Insert the needle with obturator in place perpendicular to the skin, through the skin and tissues, down to the periosteum. Push the needle through the cortex, using a screwing motion with firm, steady, well-controlled pressure. Some "give" is usually felt as the needle enters the marrow; the needle will then be firmly in place.

Fit a dry 20-mL syringe onto the needle and apply strong suction for a few seconds. A small amount of marrow will come up into the syringe. To prevent dilution of the marrow specimen by peripheral blood, no more than 0.5–1 mL of marrow should be aspirated. Marrow spicules should be smeared on glass coverslips or slides for subsequent staining and counting.

Remove the needle after replacing the obturator, and exert local pressure for 3–5 minutes or until all evidence of bleeding has ceased. Apply a dry dressing.

Bone marrow aspiration is a relatively safe procedure. Possible complications include infection and bleeding, the latter especially in hemophiliacs.

COLLECTION OF FLUID FROM BODY CAVITIES

Thoracentesis

Thoracentesis is used in the removal of pleural fluid for diagnosis or treatment or in the emergency relief of a pneumothorax.

A. Site: Locate the fluid or air by physical examination and by x-ray if necessary.

B. Equipment: Use an 18- to 19-gauge needle with a very short bevel and a sharp point. The needle and a 10- or 20-mL syringe are attached to a 3-way stopcock (10-mL syringe is easier). If much fluid is to be removed, it can be pumped through a rubber tube attached to the sidearm of the stopcock, thereby avoiding leakage of air into the pleural space. A catheter with an external needle can also be inserted;

after the catheter has entered the pleural space, the needle is removed. This will lessen damage to the lung parenchyma.

C. Procedure: When possible, the patient should be in a flexed position and leaning forward against a chair back or bed stand. If too ill to sit, the patient can lie on the involved side on a firm, flat surface with an area of lateral chest wall extending over the edge of the procedure table.

Use strict sterile precautions, scrub, and wear sterile gloves. Prepare the skin surgically and use suitable drapes, preferably a large drape with a hole in the center. Infiltrate through the skin and down to the pleura with 1% procaine or lidocaine. A 3-way stopcock is attached to the aspiration needle, a section of rubber tubing is applied to the sidearm, and a 10-mL syringe is applied to the hub.

Insert the needle through an interspace, passing just above the edge of the rib. The intercostal vessels lie immediately below each rib. With gentle aspiration of the syringe, the needle is advanced a few millimeters at a time until the pleural space is reached. It is usually not difficult to know when the pleura is pierced: suction on the needle at any stage will show whether or not fluid has been reached. In long-standing infection, the pleura may be thick and the fluid may be loculated, necessitating more than one puncture site. To prevent accidental penetration of the lung after the needle is in place, apply a surgical hemostat to the needle adjacent to the skin. Pleural fluid is apt to coagulate unless it is frankly purulent, and an anticoagulant should be added after removal to facilitate examination. If a large amount of fluid is present, it should be removed slowly at intervals, 100–500 mL each time, depending on the size of the patient.

D. Dangers: Complications of this procedure include introduction of a new infection, pneumothorax or hemothorax from tearing of the lung, and hemoptysis. Careful sterile technique will decrease the risk of introducing infection. Insertion of the needle into a blood vessel, heart, liver, and spleen can be prevented by proper selection and positioning of the puncture site. Pneumothorax should not occur if care is taken to avoid advancing the needle beyond the point where fluid should be present.

If the patient starts to cough, the needle should be removed.

Pericardiocentesis (Fig 35–8)

Pericardiocentesis should be performed only by a skilled practitioner. The procedure is indicated for the diagnosis of purulent pericarditis or to relieve cardiac tamponade due to collection of large amounts of blood or other fluid.

A. Site: Several points for needle insertion are illustrated in Fig 35–8. The most common site used is at the chondroxiphoid angle. Echocardiography, fluoroscopy, and ultrasonography may aid in pericardial fluid location.

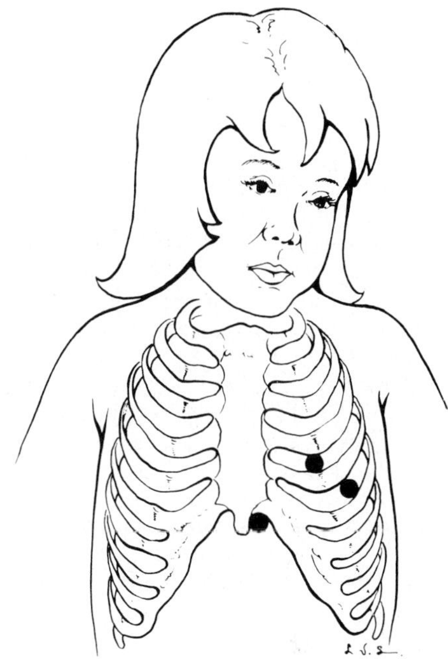

Figure 35–8. Sites of needle insertion for pericardiocentesis.

B. Procedure: The patient leans backward, restrained, at a 60-degree angle supported by bed or pillows. Using sterile technique, infiltrate the skin and subcutaneous tissues with 1% procaine. Connect a 50-mL syringe, 3-way stopcock, and 18-gauge needle. The V lead of an electrocardiograph machine attached with an alligator clip to the needle may be used to detect a current of injury tracing, should the myocardium be inadvertently entered. Insert the needle slowly at the lower border of the interspace just above the edge of the rib, directing it posteriorly and toward the spine. The needle is aimed posteriorly and upward when the chondroxiphoid approach is used. Aspirate slowly, and then turn the stopcock to discharge fluid via the rubber tubing. When fluid is being aspirated with ease, attach a surgical clamp to the needle next to the skin to prevent the needle from slipping farther.

The ECG should be continuously recorded and the needle pulled back if a current of injury pattern is observed. The blood pressure and pulse rate should be frequently recorded. The needle is removed in one quick movement at the completion of the procedure, and a dressing is applied.

C. Dangers: Cardiac dysrhythmias and penetration of the heart or coronary vessels have been reported.

Peritoneal Paracentesis

Peritoneal paracentesis can be used as a therapeutic measure to remove excessive fluid in cases of nephrotic syndrome or hepatic cirrhosis or diagnostically for evidence of blood or intestinal contents. In cases of known or suspected trauma, a puncture in each of the 4 quadrants of the abdomen may be made ("4-quadrant tap") in search of blood or intestinal contents. Infrequently, peritoneal paracentesis may be used as a diagnostic measure to obtain bacteriologic specimens in peritonitis, but this involves the danger of puncturing the distended bowel, which frequently is adherent to the abdominal wall. Electrolyte solutions, albumin, blood, and antibiotics may be administered by the peritoneal route. Peritoneal dialysis may be of value for renal insufficiency and in the treatment of certain poisonings.

A. Procedure: Use an 18- or 19-gauge needle with a short bevel and a sharp point. The skin is cleansed and surgical safeguards employed to avoid peritoneal infection. A local anesthetic is injected and a needle advanced along a zigzag course to prevent leakage. Enter at a level about halfway between the symphysis and the umbilicus in the lower quadrant or in the midline. The needle should enter obliquely to avoid leakage afterward. Ascitic fluid will flow out readily. Pus may require aspiration.

B. Dangers: Perforation of the intestine has resulted when the intestines are distended or adhesions are present. Perforation of the bladder has resulted when the bladder is not empty. The removal of excessive amounts or excessively rapid removal of fluid may result in circulatory embarrassment. Peritonitis from the introduction of infectious agents has been observed; "prophylactic" antibiotics are no substitute for proper surgical technique and are usually not indicated.

THERAPEUTIC PROCEDURES

ADMINISTRATION OF FLUIDS

The administration of fluids may be necessary in a number of clinical situations. The available routes of administration are as follows: (1) alimentary—oral, gastric (gavage or gastrostomy), duodenal, or rectal; (2) intravascular—intravenous or intra-arterial; (3) hypodermoclysis; (4) intraosseous; (5) intraperitoneal; and (6) intramuscular.

1. ALIMENTARY ROUTE

Oral, Gastric, or Duodenal

When available, the alimentary tract is the route of choice for the administration of all nutrients and fluids with the exception of blood. When the oral-gastric avenue is not competent, intubation of the stomach and duodenum is safe and easily accomplished.

Rectal

The rectal route may be used for diagnosis (culture or roentgenologic examination with barium), for cleansing (fecal impaction), or for therapy (administration of fluids, electrolytes, or drugs).

Because the vascular drainage of the rectum does not enter the portal system, the liver is bypassed and administered fluids and drugs that are absorbed can enter the systemic circulation directly without hepatic conjugation or detoxification. The portal bypass may be avoided by administering fluids into the colon by high enema or colonic flush.

A. Procedure: The older patient is placed in either the left lateral recumbent or the knee-chest position. The small infant may be placed supine with legs flexed and elevated. A rectal examination should be performed initially to rule out the presence of a foreign body. A rectal catheter of appropriate size is lubricated and introduced beyond the anal sphincter. Fluid (preferably warmed) is administered by the gravity method, holding or taping the buttocks together if necessary to prevent the loss of fluid.

B. Dangers: Rectal perforation, particularly in the small infant, is not rare but can be avoided with the use of a soft rubber catheter.

2. INTRAVENOUS ROUTE

Intravenous fluid may be administered to infants and children by either a standard gravity apparatus or by a constant infusion pump. Fluids are best administered through a 21- or 23-gauge needle. *The rate of flow should be checked frequently.* An accurate record must be kept of the amount of fluid added. For small infants (particularly those who were prematurely born), never permit more than one-third of the daily fluid requirements to be in the container at any one time. It is advisable to remove the needle and change location each 48–72 hours to avoid phlebitis. If possible, avoid hypertonic solutions.

A. Site: (Fig 35–9.) For small infants, a scalp vein or one on the wrist, hand, foot, or arm will usually be most convenient. The superficial veins of the scalp do not have valves, and fluids may therefore be infused in either direction. In infants under the age of 2 years, these veins are easily visualized and can be distinguished from the superficial arteries of the scalp by palpation. Any accessible vein may be used in an older child.

B. Procedure: The child should be positioned and the site for infusion immobilized. If an extremity is to be used, this should be taped to an adequately padded board. The skin is cleaned with iodine-containing solution and alcohol. When scalp veins are used, special care in cleansing the skin is mandatory, since they communicate with the dural sinuses. The dead space of a 21- to 25-gauge butterfly needle or

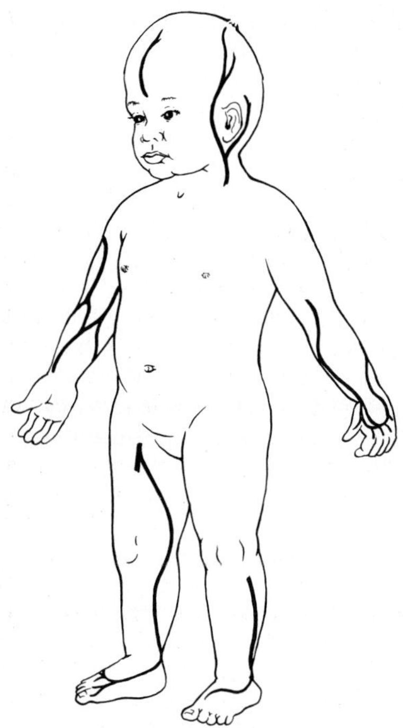

Figure 35–9. Superficial veins used most frequently for intravenous infusion.

similar gauge intravenous catheter needle (Medicut, Angiocath) should be filled with saline. A tourniquet is placed proximal to the site to enhance the distention of the vein. Warming in water or gentle percussion over the vein will increase its filling. The needle is introduced bevel up and parallel to the long axis of the vein at a point just beneath the skin. A characteristic "give" is perceptible, and blood usually flows back into the catheter. In the infant, venous pressure may be low and blood return not appreciated until negative pressure is applied with the syringe. The tourniquet is released and the flow tested by opening the intravenous clamp or by slowly injecting some saline. If there is no extravasation, the wing of the butterfly may be taped securely. Final restraints are applied when necessary and the flow rate adjusted. If a percutaneous needle catheter is used, the needle is inserted as described above. When blood is observed in the hub of the needle, the outer plastic catheter sleeve is gently advanced into the vein and the intravenous tubing connected. The plastic catheter is then securely taped in position.

Filston HC, Johnson DG: Percutaneous venous cannulation in neonates and infants: A method for catheter insertion without "cutdown." *Pediatrics* 1971;**48:**896.

Intravenous Cutdown

If fluids or intravenous medications are urgently needed by a seriously ill child and difficulty is encountered in entering a vein percutaneously, expose a vein surgically and tie a piece of polyethylene tubing in place or enter the vein subcutaneously with a plastic catheter equipped with an inner needle stylet.

A. Site: The internal saphenous vein has been found to be the most satisfactory site. Its position is constant, running anterior to the medial malleolus of the tibia to the groove between the upper medial end of the tibia and the calf muscle. It can be entered at any point along its course. The novice can easily identify it on his or her own leg first.

Other veins (external jugular, median, basilic, and cephalic) may also be used for cutdowns, but their courses are more variable and difficult to define.

B. Equipment:

1. Sterile solution, container, tubing, drip bulb, and clamp are prepared as for continuous venoclysis.

2. Thin polyethylene tubing with the end cut on the slant is easiest to use and least irritating. A 19-gauge tubing is preferred, but tubing as small as 22-gauge may be used. A 20- to 22-gauge intravenous catheter needle (Medicut, Angiocath) may also be used.

C. Procedure:

1. Preparation—Apply a tourniquet, cleanse the skin, and drape the leg as for a surgical procedure, using sterile precautions. The foot can be securely taped to a sandbag or board splint. Make a large wheal with 1% or 2% procaine solution in the skin over the vein.

2. Incision—With a scalpel, make an incision about 1 cm long just through the skin. The incision should be at a right angle to the direction of the vein. Using small, curved, sharp-pointed scissors or fine forceps, spread the incision widely.

3. Identifying the vein—The vein is usually seen lying on the fascia. Some dissection of subcutaneous fat may be necessary. Insert a curved clamp to the periosteum and bring the vein to the surface (Fig 35–10). Be certain it is a vein, not a nerve or tendon, by observing for the passage of blood. Using a small hook (eg, strabismus hook), dissect the vein

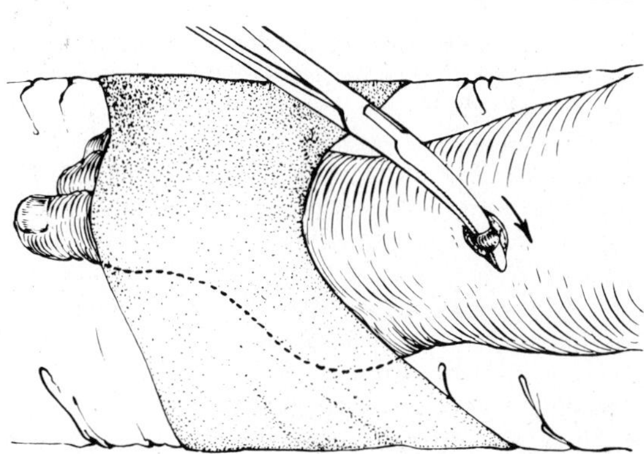

Figure 35–10. Isolation of vein for intravenous cutdown. (Drapes not shown.)

free for a length of 1–2 cm. In small infants, the vein is small and fragile, and great care must be taken in handling it.

4. Placing ties—Using No. 00 black silk, tie the vein off at the extreme distal (lower) end of the exposed portion. Leave the ends of the suture long so that they may be used later for traction. At the proximal end of the vein, loop a piece of suture loosely around the vein.

5. Insertion and fixation of the catheter—Introduce the catheter with the stylet needle bevel up. When the needle is in vessel lumen, hold the stylet stationary and gently advance the catheter. Withdraw the stylet and release tension on the proximal tie so that the catheter may be threaded and blood return ascertained. If there is no blood flow, remove the tourniquet and attempt to inject a small amount of intravenous solution into the vein. Watch for a wheal or extravasation of fluid, indicating that the catheter is not in the vessel. If the catheter flushes easily, remove the proximal ligatures and suture the plastic wings of the catheter hub to the skin. This can most easily be accomplished by placing a skin closure suture on either side of the catheter hub. Tie the suture, and then pass the free ends through holes provided in the wings of the plastic hub. Tie the suture again. This should hold the catheter securely in the vessel. Apply tape across the hub and tubing for further security.

When a needle or cannula is used, a pad of gauze under the hub will keep it in alignment with the vein. Cover the wound with gauze and roller bandage. Avoid restraint, which interferes with adequate circulation or causes pressure lesions.

3. INTRAOSSEOUS, INTRAPERITONEAL, & INTRAMUSCULAR THERAPY

Intraosseous (into the bone marrow) administration of fluids is a form of intravenous therapy. The effluent vessels of bone marrow provide a rapid and relatively complete drainage into the systemic circulation. However, the obvious consequences of infection preclude its general use.

Isotonic fluids and blood may be administered by the intraperitoneal route, but the intravenous route is generally preferred.

Intramuscular injections may be given into the upper outer quadrant of the gluteal area. With the child prone on a flat surface, locate the head of the greater trochanter of the femur and the posterior superior iliac spine. Direct the needle perpendicular to the table or bed in this space cephalad to the head of the trochanter. Other satisfactory sites include (1) the anterolateral aspect of the thigh (use a 2.5-cm needle), with the needle directed downward at an oblique angle toward the bone; and (2) the ventral gluteal muscles, to the center of an area outlined by locating the anterior iliac tubercle, placing the index finger on the tubercle, and extending the middle fingertip along the crest of the ileum as far as possible, forming a triangle. The needle is directed slightly toward the iliac crest.

EXCHANGE TRANSFUSION FOR NEONATAL JAUNDICE

After an adequate preparation of the infant (respirations and temperature stabilized and maintained, gastric contents removed, proper restraint), drape the umbilical area, employing sterile technique. Cut off the cord about 1.5 cm or less from the skin. Control any bleeding with umbilical tape. Identify the vein (the 2 arteries are white and cordlike; the single vein is larger and thin-walled). If the vein cannot be visualized in the cord stump, make a small transverse incision above the umbilicus, and cannulate the vein.

Selection & Amount of Blood

Employ sterile packaged equipment specifically prepared for this procedure (eg, Pharmaseal Laboratories).

Use freshly collected heparinized blood or blood preserved with anticoagulant acid-citrate-dextrose (ACD) or citrate-phosphate-dextrose (CPD). Blood should always be less than 3 days old and should be warmed before use. Give twice the blood volume (BV = 85 mL/kg) for a complete 2-volume exchange.

Remove blood in 5- to 20-mL amounts and save the first aliquot for laboratory studies. Replace with an equivalent amount of blood. The hydropic infant requires slow, carefully packed red cell exchanges with careful observation of signs of heart failure.The blood pressure and central venous pressure should also be frequently monitored in these patients. An assistant should accurately record each volume exchange as well as the total exchange volume.

The administration of calcium gluconate has been suggested by some when ACD blood is employed. If signs of hypocalcemia develop, administer calcium gluconate, 1 mL of 10% solution, slowly through the polyethylene tubing (rinsing tubing with saline solution before and after the drug is introduced). Do not give any further calcium if there is slowing of the pulse.

Give protamine sulfate, 0.5 mg intramuscularly, to terminate the heparin effect at the end of an exchange employing heparinized blood.

VENOUS & ARTERIAL ACCESS & MONITORING OF THE CRITICALLY ILL CHILD

With the current use of more complex monitoring devices and more aggressive forms of therapy, central venous and arterial access is frequently necessary to monitor the critically ill child's progress. Most of these procedures should be performed only by someone familiar with techniques of pediatric intensive care.

VENOUS ACCESS & MONITORING

Peripheral Venous Catheters

One or more functional indwelling venous catheters are essential to ensure optimal delivery of fluids and medications. If necessary, a cutdown should be performed (see above).

Central Venous Pressure Lines

Intermittent or continuous monitoring of central venous pressure is often essential to the management of an unstable patient. A central venous pressure line is indicated when (1) a secure and large-gauge venous catheter is needed to administer fluids or blood products; (2) vasoactive medications must be reliably administered; (3) an additional line is needed to monitor intravascular volume status; or (4) hypertonic parenteral nutrition must be administered.

When the central venous pressure monitoring line is used, the pressure transducer or water manometer should be carefully adjusted so the zero will be at the level of the right atrium. When the line is properly positioned within the thoracic cavity, the pressure should be an indication of right ventricular filling pressures and, in the absence of heart disease, an index of the intravascular volume.

A cutdown on the right basilic or cephalic vein will provide access if the vein cannot be entered percutaneously (see cutdown procedure, above). A long 18- or 20-gauge catheter can usually be threaded to a central site within the thoracic cavity. Respiratory variation of the subsequent pressure tracing will confirm the position of the catheter tip within the thoracic cavity. A Valsalva maneuver or extension of the arm at a 90-degree angle from the body may facilitate passage of the catheter through the axilla.

The internal jugular vein is also a good site for the central venous pressure line placement, and the right side provides the most direct access. Prepare the child as for internal jugular vein puncture (see earlier section of this chapter), locate the vein with a 22-gauge needle, and note the angle and depth of the needle. Insert a catheter with the external needle along the same tract until the vessel is entered. The catheter is then advanced until pressure measurements indicate placement in the thoracic cavity. The needle is withdrawn and the catheter secured to the skin by sutures. An intravenous solution of normal saline with 1 unit of heparin per milliliter should be infused to maintain patency of the catheter.

The external jugular vein can be used, but the route is less direct. Placement of a central venous pressure line should always be followed by a chest x-ray to confirm its position. The line should be carefully watched to prevent infusion of air.

Central Venous Catheters

The recent development of pediatric wire-guided catheters (Seldinger type) has facilitated central venous catheterization in young children. These catheters are equipped with steel guide wires that have either a straight flexible tip or a J-shaped flexible tip; the latter is useful when sharp turns must be followed in the venous system (eg, at the entrance of the external jugular into the subclavian vein). The wires are available in 3 diameters that can pass through 21-, 19-, and 18-gauge needles. Any suitable vein may be cannulated in the following manner: The site is prepared in the usual fashion and is surrounded by a sterile drape. The needle on a syringe is inserted into the vein. Once steady blood flow is obtained, the syringe is removed and the wire threaded through the needle into the vein. The wire should meet with no resistance in its path. Enough wire must remain outside the vein so that its opposite end will extend beyond the catheter when the catheter is placed over the wire. When the wire is in place in the vein, the needle is removed and is replaced on the wire by the catheter. A tiny incision made in the skin near the wire will ease the subsequent passage of the wire through the skin. The catheter is then threaded over the wire into the vein. Some force may initially be required to advance the catheter through the subcutaneous tissues to the vein, but the catheter should pass very freely once the vein is entered. After the catheter is inserted to the desired position, the wire is removed, and blood should flow readily from the catheter. Some catheter sheaths have an end access port for passage of a long, more narrow catheter for central venous monitoring and a side port for simultaneous fluid administration.

Complications

Infection, thrombosis, phlebitis, or hemorrhage can occur when any vein is cannulated. Femoral vein catheterization often compromises venous drainage from the leg and can cause reversible edematous enlargement of the extremity. Intracardiac placement of central venous catheters has been associated with perforations of the right atrium, endocarditis, and premature ventricular contractions and other dysrhythmias when intra-atrial catheters slip into the right ventricle.

Dailey RH: Use of wire-guided (Seldinger-type) catheters in the emergency department. *Ann Emerg Med* 1983;**12:**489.

ARTERIAL ACCESS & MONITORING

Arterial access allows for accurate repeated blood gas determination, continuous pressure monitoring, and withdrawal of reliable blood specimens. An arterial line can eliminate the pain of repeated needle punctures for frequent tests. However, this should not be its sole indication. Arterial access may be provided by percutaneous catheterization or by a cutdown procedure. The radial and posterior tibial arteries are most commonly used, because each normally has an alternative arterial supply to distal tissue (eg, ulnar or dorsalis pedis arteries). This prevents vascular compromise to the foot or hand in the event of occlusion of the catheterized artery. In the newborn, the umbilical artery is usually used as described previously.

Percutaneous Arterial Catheterization

Secure the forearm or leg to an armboard with the wrist in 30-degree extension or the foot dorsiflexed. After locating the artery by palpation, prepare the area with an iodine-containing solution followed by alcohol. Determine patency of alternative arterial supply to distal parts of the extremity by Doppler probe or palpation of the pulse. In the newborn, a bright light carefully placed under or to the side of the area will, when pressed against the skin, allow visible pulsations to be seen. (***Caution:*** Heat generated by the light can cause burns.) A 20- to 22-gauge catheter with a central needle is inserted into the skin at a 45-degree angle; either the artery is entered directly or both walls are pierced. If both walls have been pierced, remove the needle and very slowly withdraw the catheter until a gush of blood signifies that the catheter tip is in the artery. The catheter can then be advanced easily until only the hub is seen externally. Connect the catheter to the intravenous line containing heparinized normal saline (0.5–2 units/mL) and run under pressure at a rate of 2–3 mL/h. Connect to a pressure transducer and evaluate the wave form.

Although arterial punctures may be performed safely in the temporal artery, this artery should not be cannulated, because there is a risk of developing ipsilateral cerebral infarcts and neurologic deficits following its catheterization.

Arterial catheterization can be complicated by bleeding, which is usually brief and can be controlled by direct pressure. More seriously, arteriospasm or thromboembolic events may severely impair distal blood flow and cause necrosis of areas of the extremity.

Cutdown Arterial Access

Secure the arm or leg to a board. After determining that alternative arterial supply is adequate, locate the artery by palpation and prepare the area with an iodine-containing solution. Drape the area with sterile towels. Make a 1-cm incision over the artery and perpendicular to its course. Isolate the artery by blunt dissection. Pass one length of No. 000 silk suture around the artery at the distal end and a second length at the proximal end of the isolated vessel. Apply a hemostat to the ends of each suture to better control the artery. Pierce the artery with a catheter with an interior needle and advance the catheter proximally while withdrawing the needle. A prompt flow of blood indicates correct placement. Attach the catheter to a pressure intravenous solution with transducer and observe the wave form. Remove the 2 sutures that were used to control the artery. No ligatures should be left around the artery. Close the skin wound and suture the catheter hub to the skin.

Complications include bleeding, which is generally brief and can be controlled by direct pressure, and loss of patency of the artery after discontinuation of the line. The latter is more common with this technique than with the percutaneous technique.

Pulmonary Artery Catheters & Pulmonary "Wedge" Pressure Lines

With the introduction of smaller (eg, No. 3F) catheters, the pulmonary artery and "wedge" pressures as well as cardiac output by thermodilution can be measured in all but the smallest newborns. Indications are (1) congenital heart disease with pulmonary hypertension in a perioperative period; (2) shock states with myocardial dysfunction; (3) severe congestive heart failure; and (4) instances of respiratory failure secondary to noncardiogenic pulmonary edema. This procedure requires a skillful practitioner and should be done at centers with facilities for monitoring and maintaining such lines. The pressures obtained and the measurement of cardiac output by thermodilution can give much useful information, but the risks include dysrhythmias, endocarditis, air embolization, pulmonary infarction, and rupture of a peripheral pulmonary vessel.

Pollack MM et al: Bedside pulmonary artery catheterization in pediatrics. *J Pediatr* 1980;**96:**274.

Todres ID et al: Swan-Ganz catheterization in the critically ill newborn. *Crit Care Med* 1979;**7:**330.

SELECTED REFERENCES

Avery GB: *Neonatology*, 2nd ed. Lippincott, 1981.

Gellis SS, Kagan BM: *Current Pediatric Therapy*, 10th ed. Saunders, 1982.

Hughes WT, Buescher ES: *Pediatric Procedures*, 2nd ed. Saunders, 1980.

Lewis DL, Morriss FC, Moore GC: *A Practical Guide to Pedi-*

atric Intensive Care. Mosby, 1979.
Rudolph AM, Hoffman JE: *Pediatrics,* 17th ed. Appleton-Century-Crofts, 1982.
Shirkey HC (editor): *Pediatric Therapy,* 6th ed. Mosby, 1980.
Silver HK et al: *Handbook of Pediatrics,* 15th ed. Lange, 1986.
Vaughan VC III et al (editors): *Nelson Textbook of Pediatrics,* 11th ed. Saunders, 1979.

36 Fluid & Electrolyte Therapy

Donough O'Brien, MD, FRCP

I. PHYSIOLOGY OF THE FLUID SPACES IN CHILDHOOD

BODY FLUIDS, MEMBRANES, & OSMOLALITY

After early infancy, the total water in the body (TBW) consists of roughly two-thirds intracellular water (ICW) and one-third extracellular water (ECW). Between the ECW and ICW lie all the cell membranes of the body, which may be considered as one large (aggregate) membrane. This so-called cell membrane possesses 2 qualities of importance to clinicians: (1) It is water-permeable, and (2) it permits passage of Na^+ into the ECW and K^+ into the ICW by means of a membrane-associated Na^+-K^+ "pump."

Water molecules cross the cell membrane constantly and equally in both directions; hence, the volumes of the ECW and ICW do not change. Particles dissolved in the water interfere with the movement of water molecules and thus lower the number that find "pores" in the membrane and cross to the opposite side. The number of dissolved particles per number of water molecules must therefore be equal on both sides of the cell membrane, or a net transfer of water or particles (or both) would result. If the membrane is impermeable to certain solute particles, addition of such particles to one side will lower the number of water molecules leaving that side and the number of water molecules entering from the opposite side will then be greater. A net transfer of water will occur until the ratio of particles to water molecules has again been equalized on both sides. The number of dissolved particles per number of water molecules is seldom computed as such, but a closely related value, osmolality, is employed. Osmolality is customarily expressed as mosm/L* of water.

The forces generated by separating solutions of differing osmolalities by a semipermeable membrane may be substantial and will cause the transfer of water or particles or both. Much evidence exists that osmolality is the same throughout the TBW. Osmolality is often referred to as tonicity, and solutions that contain approximately 285 mosm/kg are referred to as isosmolal, as isotonic, or, occasionally, as normal. ("Normal" in this sense does not imply equivalents per liter.) Solutions containing less than or more than 285 mosm/kg are spoken of as hypo- or hyperosmolal or hypo- or hypertonic, respectively. Osmolality can be changed by selectively adding or taking away water or by selectively adding or taking away solute particles. It is generally true that isosmolality (ie, 285 mosm/kg) of the body fluids is a desirable therapeutic end point.

* mosm/L = mmol/L × number of particles formed when 1 molecule dissolves, eg, 1 for glucose, 2 for NaCl, 3 for $MgCl_2$.

EXTRACELLULAR FLUID (ECF)

1. COMPONENTS

The components of the ECF are (1) plasma, (2) interstitial fluid, (3) connective tissue, cartilage, and bone fluids, and (4) transcellular fluids.

Plasma

After early infancy, the plasma constitutes about one-sixth of the ECF volume, about one-twelfth of the TBW, and about one-twentieth of the weight of the patient (Table 36–1). It is separated from the interstitial fluid by the endothelial membranes lining the blood vessels. Endothelium allows the immediate passage of water and very rapid passage of ions but confines most of the albumin and globulin molecules to the intravascular compartment proper. This is presumably due to the large size of the protein molecules. The plasma proteins consist mostly of albumin of

Table 36–1. Blood and plasma volume formulas.*

Boys

Blood volume in mL/kg = 75.7 − (0.114 × wt in kg)
Blood volume in mL/m² = 697 × surface area (in m²) + 1312

Girls

Blood volume in mL/kg = 82.4 − (0.374 × wt in kg)
Blood volume in mL/m² = 360 × surface area (in m²) + 1575

$$\text{Plasma volume} = \text{Blood volume} \times 1 - \left(\frac{0.95 \times \text{Hct}}{100}\right)$$

* From Cropp JA: Changes in blood and plasma volumes during growth. *J Pediatr* 1971;**78:**220.

approximately 60,000 MW and globulins ranging in molecular weight from 180,000 to 1,000,000. The albumin molecules, though smaller, are much more numerous and contribute roughly three-fourths of the osmotic pressure attributable to the plasma proteins. This is frequently called colloid osmotic pressure. Compared to the osmotic pressure due to the more numerous low-molecular-weight electrolyte molecules of the plasma (eg, Na^+, K^+, Cl^-, HCO_3^-), the colloid osmotic pressure is negligible and constitutes only about 1 mosm out of 285. Nevertheless, this difference plays a critical role in the maintenance of plasma volume.

Plasma is delivered to capillary beds under hydrostatic pressure. This pressure forces fluid out of the intravascular compartment into the interstitial fluid, concentrating the plasma proteins and raising the colloid osmotic pressure in the capillaries. As hydrostatic pressure falls and colloid osmotic pressure rises with further passage down the capillaries, a point is reached where the fluid, initially exuded, is reabsorbed into the capillaries.

Interstitial Fluid (ISF)

The ISF may be regarded as an ultrafiltrate of plasma. Thus, the concentrations of Na^+, K^+, HCO_3^-, and Cl^- in ISF closely resemble those of plasma, and for all practical purposes plasma electrolyte analyses reflect interstitial fluid composition.

The ISF is the perfusate of the cells. Its composition is regulated chiefly by renal and pulmonary action on plasma. It represents a fluid "space" or "compartment" of considerable volume and therefore acts as a buffer against changes occurring in the much smaller plasma compartment. Excessive volume of ISF is manifested as edema. When ISF volume is diminished, the clinical signs include poor skin turgor, sunken eyes, depressed fontanelles, and small tongue size. The ISF is thus an integral component of soft tissue structure.

Connective Tissue, Cartilage, & Bone Water

No particular symptoms are known to derive specifically from alterations in these fluid spaces.

Transcellular Fluids

Transcellular fluids are body fluids that have been directly elaborated by cells. The fluids involved are spinal and ventricular fluid, bile, the humors of the eye, synovial fluid, and gastrointestinal fluids. Ordinarily, these fluids comprise less than 2% of TBW. The volume of gastrointestinal fluids, however, can expand enormously, creating a fluid pool of considerable size and importance.

2. CONTROL OF THE ECF

A wide variety of mechanisms play a role in the control of the composition and volume of the ECF. The most important ones are discussed below.

Thirst

Thirst is the perception of the need to drink, and control mechanisms operate with astonishing precision. ECF volume deficits evoke thirst, and the organism will use water to control volume at the expense of osmolality. Many fluid balance problems arise when thirst cannot be perceived, communicated, or satisfied.

Aldosterone

This potent adrenocortical hormone acts to enhance the tubular resorption of Na^+. Aldosterone secretion plays an important role in the control of ECF volume, which depends mainly on the amount of Na^+ that it contains.

Antidiuretic Hormone (Vasopressin, ADH)

ADH acts to enhance renal resorption of water and thus allows formation of a concentrated urine of small volume. Inhibition of secretion or absence of ADH results in free excretion of water and diuresis. ADH is secreted from the posterior pituitary after synthesis in the anterior hypothalamus. ADH secretion is dominated by a decrease in plasma (or ECF) volume but is also affected by an increase in osmolality, emotional stress (pain, fear, rage), exercise, and a number of drugs, including morphine, ether, barbiturates, nicotine, histamine, acetylcholine, and epinephrine. ADH secretion is inhibited by dilution of body fluids, distention of the left atrial wall, and ingestion of alcohol. Inappropriate ADH excretion is discussed in a subsequent section of this chapter.

INTRACELLULAR WATER

The bulk of the body water is intracellular, and for technical reasons quantitative assays are difficult.

It is clearly inappropriate to conceive of intracellular water as a simple homogeneous solution. As yet there is no useful information about regional differences in the volume and composition of intracellular water as between cytoplasm and organelles.

DISTRIBUTION OF BODY WATER WITH AGE

An understanding of fluid and electrolyte problems requires some concept of the differences in ionic composition between extracellular and intracellular water (Fig 36–1) and a knowledge that the proportions of TBW in the various compartments vary with age (Table 36–2).

ACID-BASE PHYSIOLOGY

Definitions

An acid is a substance that, when in solution, dissociates into hydrogen ions (H^+) and anions (A^-).

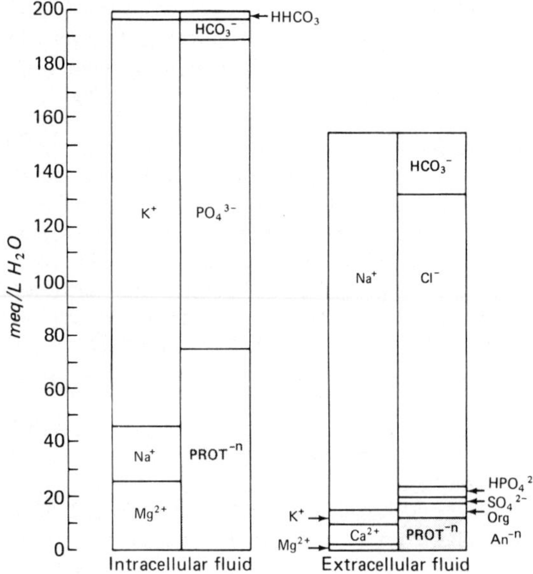

Figure 36–1. Electrolyte composition of intracellular and extracellular water.

Acids are, therefore, hydrogen ion donors, and a strong acid dissociates more completely than a weak acid. Acidity is thus directly proportionate to the concentration of hydrogen ions in solution. In contrast, a base dissolved in water yields anions that react with hydrogen ions to remove them from solution. A base is consequently a hydrogen ion acceptor, and the strength of a base is proportionate to its affinity for H^+.

Acidity and alkalinity are not independent of one another; the product of $[H^+] \times [OH^-]$ is constant. Thus, a rise in $[H^+]$ (or acidity) is accompanied by an equivalent fall in $[OH^-]$ (or alkalinity) and vice versa.

The acidity of body fluids has come to be described not in terms of $[H^+]$ but by another term, pH, which is equal to $-\log [H^+]$. This relationship may be rewritten as follows:

$$\text{pH} = \log \frac{1}{[H^+]}$$

Hence, it can be seen that as acidity or $[H^+]$ rises, pH falls, and vice versa.

The pH of arterial blood is normally 7.40 ± 0.02. When the pH of blood is 7.40, the $[H^+]$ is only 0.04 μeq/L. At that pH, the buffer acids and buffer bases are present in milliequivalents per liter, making buffer acid and buffer base molecules many times more numerous than hydrogen ions.

Table 36–2. Distribution of body water with age (in percentage of total body weight).

Age	Total (TBW)	Extra-cellular (ECW)	Intra-cellular (ICW)
0–11 days	77.8 (69–84)	42 (34–53)	34.5 (28–40)
11 days–6 months	72.4 (63–83)	34.6 (28–57)	38.8 (20–47)
6 months–2 years	59.8 (52–72)	26.6 (20–30)	34.8 (28–38)
2–7 years	63.4 (55–73)	25 (21–30)	40.4 (31–53)
7–16 years	58.2 (50–64)	20.5 (18–26)	46.7

Normal Control

Normal fine control of pH is achieved by 3 mechanisms. The first is the normal buffering capacity of the body fluid (except gastric fluid). A buffer is a mixture of a weak acid and its conjugate base. In the equilibrium $H_2CO_3 \rightleftharpoons HCO_3^- + H^+$, carbonic acid ($H_2CO_3$) is a weak acid and bicarbonate ion (HCO_3^-) is the conjugate base. In a buffer, or buffered solution, the weak acid is called a buffer acid and the weak base is called a buffer base. When hydrion is added to the bicarbonate system, the above reaction is shifted to the left, and carbonic acid is in turn lost via the lungs as CO_2.

The second mechanism is the respiratory control of carbonic acid as the most important buffer acid.

The third homeostatic mechanism is the kidneys' ability to conserve bicarbonate, the principal buffer base, and to excrete H^+ into the urine against a gradient and in exchange for Na^+ as well as to form NH_4^+. The action of the last 2 mechanisms is slower than buffering.

Relationships Between pH, P_{CO_2}, Serum $[HCO_3^-]$, & Other Buffers

Acid-base relationships are governed by the following equation:

$$\text{pH} = \text{pK} + \log \frac{[\text{Buffer base}]}{[\text{Buffer acid}]}$$

Because 53% of all blood buffering is in the bicarbonate system and because it is this system that is predominantly altered in acid-base disorders, this equation can be conveniently rewritten as follows:

$$\text{pH} = 6.1 + \log \frac{[HCO_3^-]}{0.03\ P_{CO_2}}$$

A complete evaluation of acid-base status thus requires a knowledge of 2 of its 3 variables: pH, serum bicarbonate, and P_{CO_2}.

Some understanding is still required of the interchangeability between bicarbonate and nonbicarbonate buffers in the blood. The latter are primarily erythrocyte hemoglobin and, to a lesser extent, anionic groups on plasma proteins, and phosphates.

Consider the second equation:

$$H_2CO_3 + Hb^- = HCO_3^- + HProt$$

An increase in H_2CO_3 or P_{CO_2} will shift the reaction to the right. This will reduce $[Hb^-]$ and increase the $[HCO_3^-]$. The sum of $[Hb^-] + [HCO_3^-]$ or "total buffer base" is not changed, however. The same is also true in reverse—ie, total buffer base is independent of P_{CO_2}. Normal values for total buffer base are about 46–50 meq/L; it has, however, become popular instead to use the term "base excess" for deviations from normal values. The interrelationship of all these buffer systems, however, cannot be expressed in one simple equation, and a nomogram (Fig 36–2) is therefore used. Again, this requires knowing 2 of the 3 variables (pH, P_{CO_2}, and $[HCO_3^-]_s$) as well as knowing hemoglobin concentration.

In "metabolic" acidosis or alkalosis, where the changes are due to loss or excess of buffer base, therapy can be based on changes in serum bicarbonate concentration ($[HCO_3^-]_s$). The Siggaard-Andersen nomogram (Fig 36–3) is useful in determining the metabolic component in mixed respiratory and metabolic situations such as may be seen in salicylate intoxication. Other nomograms also help to separate the respiratory and metabolic components.

Total body buffering capacity is only about 20% in the blood, about 30% in extracellular water, and 50% in intracellular water. However, therapy can be successfully based on an estimate of total body water multiplied by the base excess in plasma.

Anion Gap

Most up-to-date and well-automated clinical laboratories report the anion gap when electrolyte measurements are requested. The anion gap is the difference between ($Na^+ + K^+$) and ($Cl^- + HCO_3^-$), which is an approximation of the sum of unmeasured anions (eg, sulfate, lactate, phosphate, protein, and 3-hydroxybutyrate). Normal values must be set for each laboratory, and the usefulness of the measurement is dependent on the precision with which each component is assayed. An elevated anion gap value is of use clinically primarily as an index of metabolic acidosis, including ketoacidosis and salicylism. In diabetic acidosis, this measurement is of special value because in severely dehydrated patients, lack of tissue oxygenation favors 3-hydroxybutyrate levels over acetoacetate levels, and measurement of the anion gap rather than urinary ketones may give a truer picture of the degree of acidosis. Abnormally low anion gap measurements, if not artifactual, may indicate hypoalbuminemia.

The anion gap. *Lancet* 1977;**1:**785.

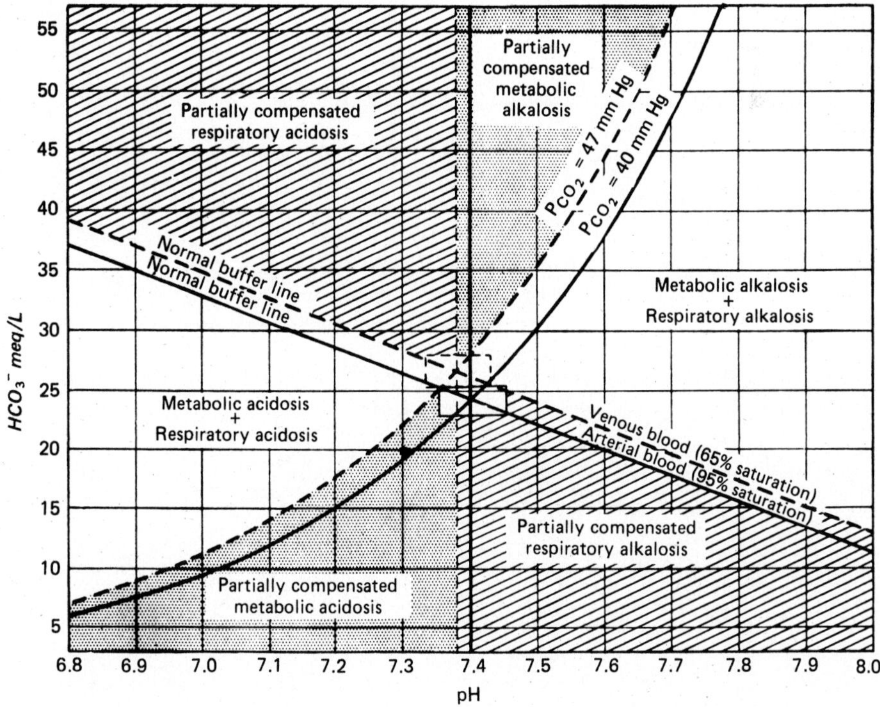

Figure 36–2. The relation of blood pH to plasma bicarbonate in acidosis and alkalosis. (Reproduced, with permission, from Pickering DE, Fisher DA. *Fluid and Electrolyte Therapy.* Medical Research Foundation of Oregon, 1959.)

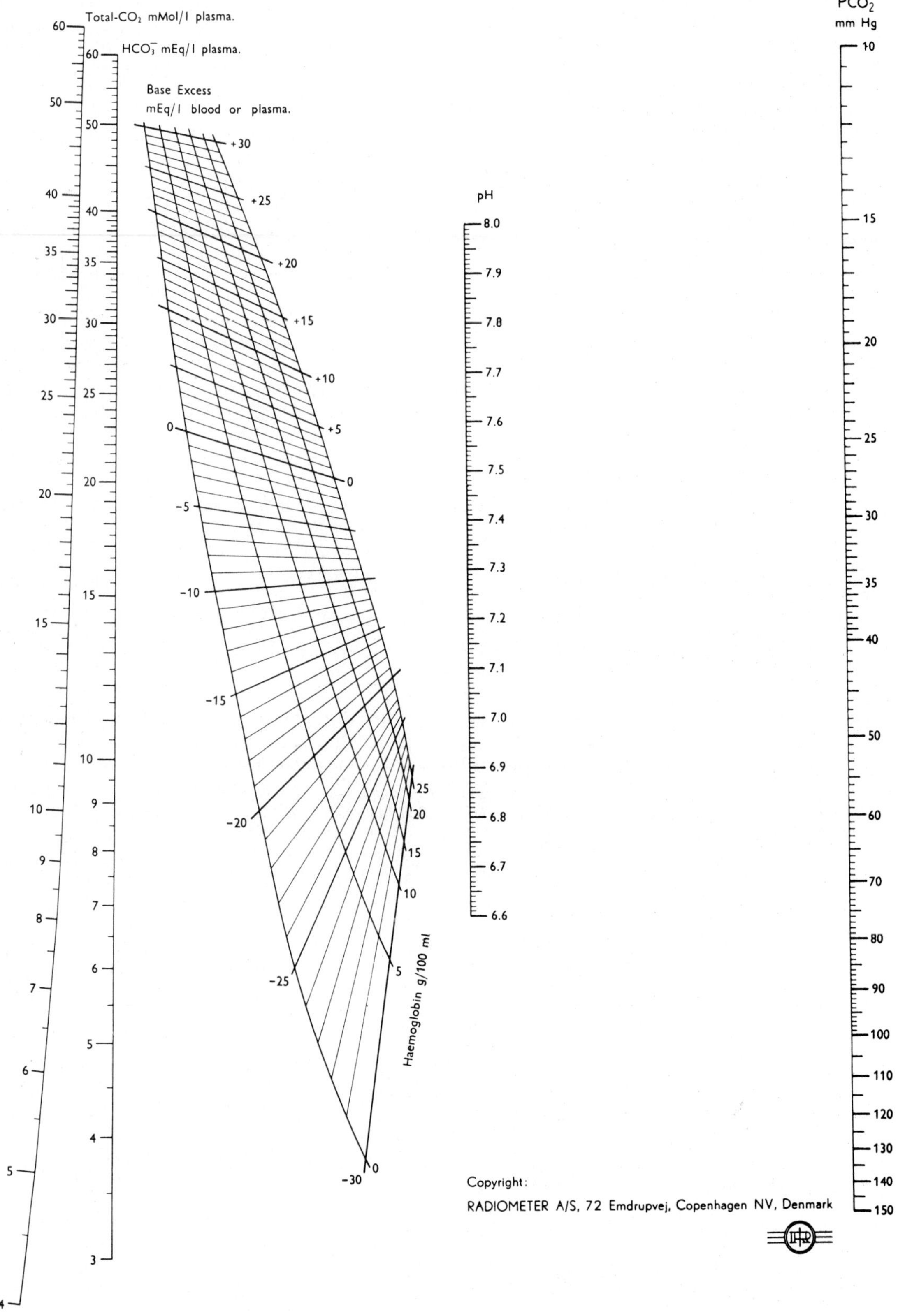

Figure 36–3. Siggaard-Andersen alignment nomogram.
(Reproduced by permission of the copyright holder, Radiometer A/S, Copenhagen.)

II. GENERAL PRINCIPLES OF FLUID & ELECTROLYTE MANAGEMENT

All plans for the repair of fluid and electrolyte distortions are based on calculations first of maintenance requirements and then of volume and qualitative changes (correctional requirements).

MAINTENANCE REQUIREMENTS

Maintenance requirements are the fluids and electrolytes that must be given to maintain homeostasis for the next balance period (usually 24 hours). Predictions must be made for (1) sensible and insensible losses, (2) urinary output, (3) gastrointestinal (or other) losses, and (4) sufficient calories to prevent undue expenditure of the patient's own energy stores.

A number of years ago, these components were measured separately, and this is still useful in patients with anuria or oliguria, severe burns, or unusual loss of fluids from the intestine, as may occur with a stoma. In these circumstances, the information in Tables 36–3 and 36–4 and Fig 36–4 may be helpful. Now, when short-term administration of fluids and electrolytes is required, it is usually done according to Table 36–3.

Table 36–3. Maintenance requirements for water and electrolytes.

Water	100 mL/kg for the first 10 kg 50 mL/kg for the second 10 kg 20 mL/kg after 20 kg
Na^+	3 meq/dL water
K^+	2 meq/dL water

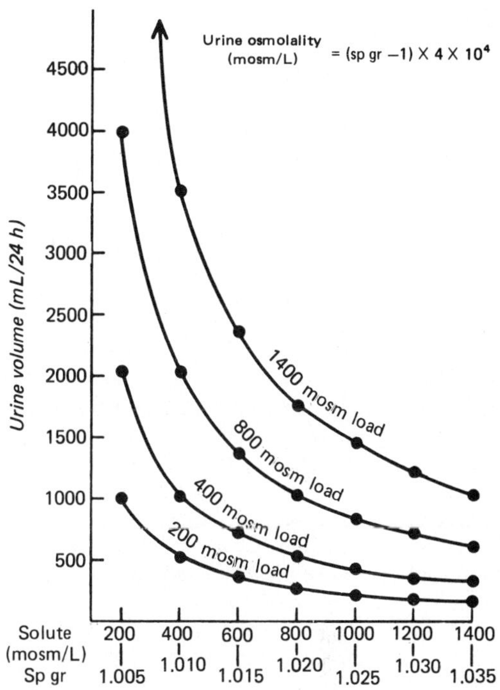

Figure 36–4. Total solute excretion and urine volume per given sp gr. (Redrawn and reproduced, with permission, from Bland JH: *Clinical Recognition and Management of Disturbances of Body Fluids.* Saunders, 1956.)

Modifications of this regimen may be needed when there is fever, hyperventilation, or special losses of body fluids or when changes in environmental humidity occur. Correction of imbalances is most readily made when the patient is weighed daily and plasma electrolyte measurements are taken frequently. Measurement of urine osmolality is particularly helpful in judging the need for water when renal function is normal. If these values are between 200 and 600 mosm/L, no major changes in water intake are required. A special situation exists in diabetic ketoacidosis, where it is crucial to replace water and salt lost in the urine as a result of osmotic diuresis of glucose.

Table 36–4. Estimated 24-hour requirements for infants and children on an intravenous regimen.

	Sensible and Insensible Losses (mL/kg)	Urinary Losses		
		Water (mL/kg)	Na^+ (meq/kg)	K^+ (meq/kg)
Prematures	20 (in mist) 30 (dry air)	40	1.5–2	1–2
Birth–2 months	25 (in mist) 35 (normal) 45 (hypermetabolic)	65	1.5–2	1–2
2–12 months (10 kg)	20	80	1.5–2	1–2
15 kg 30 kg 45 kg	400 mL/m²/24 h	1000 mL/24 h 1300 mL/24 h 1500 mL/24 h	25 meq/24 h 37 meq/24 h 50 meq/24 h	20 meq/24 h 30 meq/24 h 40 meq/24 h

CALORIES

If maintenance requirements are given as 5% glucose solutions, no additional source of calories need be added provided that such a regimen is not continued for longer than 2–3 days and the patient's caloric needs are not markedly increased, as in salicylate intoxication or the respiratory distress syndrome of prematurity. In these instances, 10% glucose in water may be substituted. Maintenance fluids given as 5% glucose solutions contain few calories, but they provide enough to prevent the patient from being hungry; they exert a protein-sparing effect; and they prevent ketosis. Ordinarily, all intravenous fluids should contain at least 5% glucose. If water restriction is in force, however, insufficient protein-sparing calories will be administered if only 5% glucose is given. Fifteen to 20% glucose may then be used—if need be, with ethyl alcohol. Such solutions rapidly inflame veins and shorten the life of an intravenous site. If oral intake is allowed, cookies and candy may provide an alternative source of calories.

A special section of Chapter 4 is devoted to the problem of prolonged intravenous alimentation.

REPAIR OF EXISTING DEFICITS OR SURPLUSES

Calculations must be designed to correct both volume and qualitative distortions. In theory, adjustments should apply to all the body water compartments; however, knowledge of changes in the intracellular water in disease is limited because of the technical difficulties of measurement. From a practical viewpoint, therefore, correctional changes are applied as extracellular water, and there is experimental evidence that sodium may temporarily substitute for potassium as the main intracellular cation. Clinical response certainly justifies this approach. In making calculations, appraisals are made for (1) ECF volume changes and (2) qualitative changes in osmolality, acid-base balance, and electrolyte potassium balance.

CHANGES IN THE VOLUME OF BODY FLUIDS

DEHYDRATION

Clinical Features

Dehydration, usually due to gastroenteritis, is one of the most common clinical problems in pediatrics. The symptoms and signs vary with the severity of fluid depletion. Skin turgor begins to be lost after 3–5% of the body weight is lost as isotonic ECF. The patient is thirsty, and urinary output is reduced. With a 10% loss of body weight, skin turgor becomes strikingly depressed, the eyes become sunken and soft, the fontanelle (if present) is sunken, and the sutures in the skull may become prominent. Pulse rate is increased and pulse volume diminished, and central venous pressure is diminished. Orthostatic hypotension may occur in older children. Fever, oliguria, a dry mouth, diminished tearing, and lethargy are present. The skin, however, is pink, and the capillary refill time is prompt. The hematocrit is elevated. When 15% of the body weight is lost as ECF, the above signs become more prominent, but the hallmark of this end stage of acute ECF depletion is progressive cardiovascular collapse. Tachycardia increases, pulse volume decreases further, the skin becomes cool and pale, and renal function diminishes.

In hyponatremic dehydration, there is a relatively greater loss of fluid from the extracellular and intravascular spaces along with a correspondingly greater need for sodium as opposed to potassium in the replacement fluid (Table 36–5). Conversely, in hypernatremic dehydration, proportionately more water is lost from the intracellular compartment, which may result in a clinical underestimation of dehydration and potassium needs (Table 36–6).

Table 36–5. The approximate concentration of electrolytes (meq/L) in fluids obtained from the gastrointestinal tract.*

Fluid Type	Sodium	Potassium	Chloride	Total HCO_3^-
Stomach	20–120	5–25	90–160	0–5
Duodenal drainage	20–140	3–30	30–120	10–50
Biliary tract	120–160	3–12	70–130	30–50
Small intestine				
Initial drainage	100–140	4–40	60–100	30–100
Established	4–20	4–10	10–100	40–120
Pancreatic	110–160	4–15	30–80	70–130
Diarrheal stool	10–25	10–30	30–120	10–50

* Because of the wide range of normal values, specific analyses are suggested in individual cases.

Table 36–6. Assessment of water loss in relation to Na^+ levels.

Serum Sodium	Degree of Dehydration as Percent of Body Weight		
	Mild	Moderate	Severe
Isotonic	5%	10%	15%
$Na^+ \leq 130$ meq/L	4%	6%	8%
$Na^+ \geq 150$ meq/L	7%	12%	17%

Treatment

The treatment of dehydration, which involves replacement of both intracellular and extracellular fluid, may be achieved by oral or intravenous administration of fluids.

A. Oral Rehydration: The need for an inexpensive, effective remedy for infantile gastroenteritis, which has an appallingly high death rate worldwide, led to the development of oral electrolyte replacement solutions (Table 36–7). Extensive, global experience has confirmed the effectiveness of these solutions, the use of which has now been extended to developed countries.

Initially, the World Health Organization advocated a solution containing Na^+, 90 meq/L. This was suitable for the rehydration of patients with cholera, but the Na^+ content was sufficiently high to cause hypernatremia in patients with diseases associated with smaller losses of stool sodium or in those living in cooler climates. When used after the initial rehydration period, this solution had to be diluted with water or breast milk or supplemented by juices, especially potassium-containing ones.

In other parts of the world, such as the USA, needs are different. The solution that seems least likely to cause salt or water overloading is one containing approximately 2% glucose; Na^+, 50–60 meq/L; K^+, 20–30 meq/L; HCO_3^- or citrate, 30 meq/L; and the balance of anion as Cl^-. This solution has a lower osmolality than some commercial solutions but sufficient glucose to facilitate Na^+ absorption. Usually, 150 mL/kg/24 h is given and supplemented as necessary with breast milk, water, or fruit juice.

Adding glycine to the oral solution may further enhance absorption of electrolyte and water; such a solution is not available commercially.

B. Intravenous Rehydration: In the USA, oral solutions can be given with a modest amount of laboratory monitoring in most cases of dehydration, especially those associated with gastroenteritis. In emergency situations in less technologically developed countries, isotonic saline solution injected intraperitoneally may be lifesaving and can be given with minimal equipment and at low risk. In most instances of severe dehydration, however, intravenous fluid restoration and adequate laboratory measurements are essential.

General principles of parenteral rehydration therapy are as follows: (1) Restore peripheral circulatory volume if necessary; (2) restore combined intracellular and extracellular deficits of water and electrolytes within 24 hours; (3) maintain adequate water and electrolytes; and (4) resolve homeostatic distortions (eg, acidosis, potassium or magnesium deficiency).

To restore peripheral circulatory volume, give isotonic fluid, 20 mL/kg intravenously as rapidly as possible. Saline solution, plasma or other colloid, or whole blood may be used, depending on amount of volume lost and availability of fluids. If necessary, an additional 20 mL/kg can be given immediately following the first quantity. (For treatment of shock, see Chapter 8.)

Restoration of intracellular and extracellular water and electrolytes is made according to the amount and composition of fluids lost. Table 36–4 gives a clinical approximation of volume deficits. An alternative approach is to assume that the volume deficit is equivalent to any known recent weight loss. In most instances, the electrolyte composition of the rehydration fluid can be determined according to the figures given in Table 36–8 prorated for percent of dehydration. In rare circumstances involving unusual types of losses (eg, stomal losses), it may be necessary to analyze the specific fluids lost in order to ensure adequate replacement. Treatment of qualitative changes in body fluids is discussed in a subsequent section of this chapter.

Sample calculations for isotonic and hypertonic dehydration are given in Tables 36–9 and 36–10. The figures do not reflect calculation for homeostatic distortions. Usually, approximately 20% of the anion is given as a buffered base, specifically potassium acetate, because the sodium bicarbonate space is approximately equal to the total volume of body water. In the presence of metabolic acidosis, additional base is needed, and this is usually given by substituting appropriate amounts of $NaHCO_3$ for NaCl in the final calculations.

The rehydration regimen should be reevaluated at least once every 24 hours according to amount of weight gain, output of urine and other fluids, and serum electrolyte levels.

Finberg L et al: Oral rehydration for diarrhea. *J Pediatr* 1982;**101:**497.

Santosham M et al: Oral rehydration therapy of infantile diarrhea. *N Engl J Med* 1982;**306:**1070.

Snyder JD: From Pedialyte to popsicles: A look at oral rehydration therapy used in the United States and Canada. *Am J Clin Nutr* 1982;**35:**157.

EXTRACELLULAR FLUID EXCESS

The accumulation of excess extracellular water, whether due to retention of water or salt and water or to a proportion shift between ECF and ICF, constitutes edema. The various forms are described below.

Table 36–7. Composition of frequently used oral electrolyte replacement solutions.

Solutions	Percent CHO	Na^+ (meq/L)	K^+ (meq/L)	Cl^- (meq/L)	HCO_3^- or Other Base (meq/L)	mosm/L
Normal saline		154		154		308
Ringer's lactate		130	4	109	28	271
Dextrose 5% in 0.25% NaCl	5% glucose	38		38		320
WHO solution	2% glucose or 4% sucrose	90	20	30	80	330
WHO solution, modified	2% glucose	55	25	30	50	271
Rice water	2.5% carbohydrate	90	20	30	80	
Pedialyte (Ross)	2.5% glucose	45	20	35	30 citrate	269
Lytren (Mead Johnson)	1.6% glucose, 6.4% corn syrup	30	25	25	36 citrate	290
Infalyte (Pennwalt)	2% glucose	50	20	40	30	290
Gatorade	2.6% glucose, 2% fructose	20	3	20	3	330
Apple juice	3.2% glucose, 1.3% sucrose, 7.5% fructose	0.4–3.5	24–40			650–700
Orange juice 1:3	1% glucose, 1.2% fructose	0.1–0.6	12–16		12	135–180
Grape juice	1.6% glucose, 2.1% fructose	0.2–0.7	8–11		8	290–300
One package cherry gelatin dissolved in 4 cups water		24	Needs added K^+			290
Coca-Cola		1.8	4.1			600
Pepsi-Cola		6.5	0.8			590
Beef broth		120	10			350
Chicken broth		250	10			500

Table 36–8. Approximate electrolyte deficits in infants with 10–12% dehydration.

Serum Osmolality	Na^+ (meq/kg)	K^+ (meq/kg)
Isotonic	8–10	8–10
Hypotonic ($Na^+ \leqslant$ 130 meq/L)	10–12	8–10
Hypertonic ($Na^+ \geqslant$ 150 meq/L)	2–4	2–4

Systemic Edema

By the time edema is evident, significant ECF excess is already present. Rapid weight gain with no change in [Na^+] indicates accumulation of ECF and may be the only sign available until edema appears. Edema fluid is an ultrafiltrate of plasma, and its presence implies sodium excess.

Edema fluid is mobile and is distributed to the most dependent portions of the body. Children may have periorbital edema that is seen upon arising in the morning and disappears in a short time as the edema fluid is redistributed. Paroxysmal nocturnal dyspnea may occur when edema fluid within the legs is added to the circulation upon lying down, giving rise to acute episodes of pulmonary edema. Pulmonary edema is generally the most serious complication of systemic edema.

Edema of Hypoproteinemia

Significant hypoproteinemia (albumin concentration less than about 2 g/dL) is usually accompanied by edema. This comes about in 2 ways. First, inadequate albumin concentrations cause the colloid osmotic pressure of plasma to fall below that necessary to reabsorb fluid filtered from capillaries under hydrostatic pressure. Second, the resulting decrease in plasma volume activates the renin-angiotensin-aldosterone system and increases the renal tubular reabsorption of sodium.

The "Third Space" Phenomenon

A special situation exists when edema fluid is sequestered in a particular location and can no longer readily exchange with the plasma. Such an accumulation of fluid is called a "third space." Examples include ascites, lymphedema, dermal sequestration in burns, and bowel edema in enterocolitis.

In all these instances, the third space must be allowed to form and sufficient isotonic saline or other

Table 36–9. Calculation of 24-hour fluid replacement in a 10-kg infant with 10% isotonic dehydration.*

	H_2O (mL)	Na^+ (meq/L)	K^+ (meq/L)	Total Anion (meq/L)
Maintenance	1000	30	20	50
Deficit (see also Tables 36–6 and 36–8)	1000	80	80	160
Total	2000	110	100	210
Composition per liter	1000	55	50	105

* Give fluids intravenously as follows: 5% dextrose in water, 85 mL/h, with NaCl, 65 meq/L; KCl, 20 meq/L; and potassium acetate, 20 meq/L. Note that K^+ should not exceed 40 meq/L except in carefully monitored circumstances and that 50% of replacement fluids should be given in the first 4–6 hours and 50% in the remainder of the first 24-hour period.

Table 36–10. Calculation of 24-hour fluid replacement in a 10-kg infant with 10% hypertonic dehydration.*

	H_2O (mL)	Na^+ (meq/L)	K^+ (meq/L)	Total Anion (meq/L)
Maintenance	1000	30	20	50
Deficit (see also Tables 36–6 and 36–8)	1200	40	40	80
Total	2200	70	60	130
Composition per liter	1000	33	27	60

* Give fluids intravenously as follows: 10% dextrose in water, 90 mL/h, with NaCl, 33 meq/L; KCl, 17 meq/L; and potassium acetate, 10 meq/L. Serum osmolality should be monitored and, in order to avoid cerebral edema, should not be allowed to fall at a rate exceeding 2 mosm/h or 1 meq of Na^+ per liter per hour. The initial fluid should not be less than a one-third isotonic solution, because of the danger of inducing cerebral edema in hypernatremia. As an additional precaution, it may be wise to use 10% dextrose in water as a base solution.

ECF substitute made available. However, any third space may rapidly return its borrowed sodium to the circulation, as is frequently seen 3–4 days after a severe burn. The resulting volume distortion may be sufficient to cause pulmonary edema.

ICF to ECF Shifts

Occasionally in renal failure, a shift occurs in the distribution of water between extracellular and intracellular fluid, and children will become edematous without any change in total body water.

Treatment

The treatment of ECF excess depends upon whether the edema fluid is generalized or localized (third space) and whether or not serious hypoproteinemia exists (causing "obligate" edema).

Treatment involves the restriction of both dietary and parenteral Na^+ and water, and dialysis is sometimes necessary. If rapid correction of edema is desired, the following diuretics (alone or in combination) may be employed: furosemide (Lasix), 1–2 mg/kg/d; hydrochlorothiazide (HydroDiuril), 2 mg/kg/d; and spironolactone (Aldactone), 2 mg/kg/d.

Neither sodium restriction nor diuretic therapy should be used to alleviate a third space in a patient in otherwise satisfactory fluid balance.

The treatment of edema due to hypoproteinemia consists of treatment of the primary disease. Administration of parenteral albumin is rational, but the rate of administration should be slow enough to avoid plasma volume overload. Combinations of intravenous protein administration, diuretics (particularly furosemide), and sodium restriction are usually effective but seldom provide more than transient benefit unless protein can ultimately be retained in the plasma.

CHANGES IN THE COMPOSITION OF BODY FLUIDS

DISORDERS OF OSMOLALITY

1. HYPONATREMIA

Hyponatremia Due to Water Overload

Patients with normal renal function can ordinarily excrete a sudden water load with relative ease. However, many patients with impaired renal function and virtually all patients with acute renal failure or total obstructive uropathy are unable to tolerate water loading. Such patients are prone to develop hyponatremia with great rapidity and often make this fact known with an unexpected seizure. Treatment consists of water restriction, relief of urinary tract obstruction, and hypertonic glucose to control convulsions.

Inappropriate ADH Secretion

If a patient receives vasopressin (ADH) either iatrogenically or from inappropriate endogenous secretion, the urine output falls and the urine concentration increases. Thirst is unaffected, and the patient, if allowed access to water, will drink. As water is retained, the serum osmolality and serum sodium concentrations begin to fall. After 1–3 days, sufficient ECF volume expansion has occurred to inhibit aldosterone secretion, and a saline diuresis occurs and normalizes the ECF volume but leaves the osmolality and serum sodium concentration low. Administration of isotonic or hypertonic saline may result in transient rises of $[Na^+]_s$ but is quickly followed by brisk saline diuresis. Restriction of water can prevent this and will rectify the situation once it has developed.

The most common cause of this disorder is inappropriate secretion of vasopressin in the face of a normal ECF volume. Vasopressin is secreted in a variety of intracranial diseases, including tumors, head injuries, hydrocephalus, and meningitis. It also occurs with a variety of intrathoracic disorders varying from pneumonia to cystic fibrosis. Drugs such as barbiturates, ether, morphine, and histamine may have this effect, and strong emotional stress, rage, fear, and pain, as well as surgery, occasionally initiate this inappropriate chain of events.

Hyponatremia is seldom associated with significant signs or symptoms until Na^+ concentrations fall below 120 meq/L. If hyponatremia develops gradually, anorexia, apathy, and mild nausea and vomiting may be the only symptoms. If it develops rapidly, headache, mental confusion, muscular twitching, eventual delirium, and, finally, convulsions occur. The signs and symptoms are related almost as much to the rate at which the hyponatremia developed as to the severity achieved. Extremely low Na^+ concentrations (90–110 meq/L) invariably cause central nervous system dysfunction but are not incompatible with either survival or recovery. Central nervous system dysfunction due to rapid onset hypo-osmolality is sometimes called water intoxication.

Treatment consists of water restriction. Administration of isotonic or hypertonic saline solution results in overexpansion of the ECF. Three-percent saline solutions should be reserved for severe water intoxication with frank central nervous system disturbance. An occasional patient is helped by administration of ethanol, 7% solution, 20 mL/kg/24 h, to inhibit ADH secretion.

Hyponatremia With Diminished ECF Volume

Depletion of the ECF in gastroenteritis, vomiting, adrenal insufficiency, renal salt-losing states, diabetic ketoacidosis, etc, calls into play a number of mechanisms that act to protect plasma volume. Aldosterone conserves Na^+, thirst prompts the patient to drink, renin and catecholamines help to maintain blood pressure, and decreased glomerular filtration rate enhances both Na^+ and water resorption. In addition to the above, vasopressin is secreted, and as a result the organism will conserve water alone to maintain an adequate plasma volume at a lower than normal osmolality, if necessary. In the presence of a lowered ECF volume, renal clearance of free water (C_{H_2O}) is strikingly impaired. Thus, even though the organism is hypo-osmolal, excess water is now conserved. Rigid restriction of water will cause severe oliguria and will tend to normalize the osmolality, but it is poor treatment for the patient. If water alone is made available, the patient will drink water when sodium is needed.

The signs and symptoms are those typical of ECF depletion, ie, thirst, tenting skin, dehydrated appearance, dry mucous membranes, tachycardia, and oliguria.

Therapy is directed toward restoring a normal ECF volume by the administration of normal ECF-like fluids. This is usually associated with a water diuresis from the ICF compartment and rapid resolution of the hyponatremic state. If the hyponatremia is severe, correction of ECF depletion by saline may be combined with free water restriction.

Hyponatremia With Expanded ECF Volume

This type of hyponatremia is by far the most serious and most difficult to treat. The presence of hyponatremia in combination with edema implies that the osmoregulatory mechanisms have been reset at a lower level. It occurs with severe heart failure, liver disease, renal failure, or, occasionally, central nervous system disease. If the underlying circulatory disturbance can be corrected, hyponatremia with edema usually resolves spontaneously. These patients may have gross edema and therefore a high total body Na^+ content.

The signs and symptoms are overshadowed by those of the underlying disease. Edema is obvious, and both the $[Na^+]$ and osmolality are low.

Vigorous water restriction should be instituted despite complaints of thirst.

The Dysequilibrium Syndrome

Any sudden reduction in serum osmolality—as in acute intravenous water overloading, in too rapid dialysis, or with overly prompt reduction of glucose levels in diabetic acidosis—will produce an osmotic gradient between the intracalvarial and other extracellular fluid spaces. Water will move into the brain quicker than sodium moves out, leading to acute nausea, vomiting, headaches, and convulsions.

Artifactual Hyponatremia

Plasma ordinarily contains about 93% water and 7% solids. The serum sodium concentration may be affected by the amount of solid present. Marked hyperproteinemia or hyperlipidemia may thus cause falsely low serum sodium concentrations. Osmolality, as determined by vapor pressure depression, is not significantly affected by this phenomenon. In children, this is most common in diabetes and nephrotic syndrome.

Laboratory Findings

Certain indices of sodium and water excretion may be helpful in deciding whether hyponatremia is renal or prerenal in origin. In prerenal hyponatremia, urine osmolality usually exceeds 800 mosm/L and urine sodium is maximally conserved (ie, usually < 10 meq/L). Fractional sodium excretion (FE_{Na}) or

$$\frac{U_{Na}}{P_{Na}} \div \frac{U_{Cr}}{P_{Cr}} \times 100$$

is less than 1, plasma urea is elevated, and the urine/plasma urea ratio is greater than 5.

Keisch RC, Oliver WJ: Hyponatremia in children. *Pediatr in Rev* 1980;**2:**187.

2. HYPERNATREMIA

Hypernatremia always implies a deficit of water with respect to solute throughout the entire body. Therefore, it always indicates hyperosmolality. It may arise primarily from too little water or too much solute but is usually due to a combination of both. Hypernatremia is said to exist whenever the $[Na^+]_s$ exceeds 150 meq/L. Values over 160 meq/L are serious, yet patients have survived $[Na^+]_s$ in excess of 190 meq/L. Serious hypernatremia frequently causes intracerebral bleeding, brain damage, and subsequent mental retardation, convulsions, and death.

Hypernatremia Due to Primary Inability to Maintain Normal Body Water Content

A. Inadequate Water Intake: Patients who are denied access to water (or are unable to retain water, as in diabetes insipidus) are at risk of developing hypernatremia. Renal water conservation becomes extreme, but sensible and insensible water losses through the skin and lungs are unavoidable and, if continued, may cause hypernatremia. Unconscious or mentally retarded patients are unable to communicate thirst and may develop water deficiency hypernatremia in spite of normal osmoregulatory capability.

B. Defective Osmoregulation: Tumors in or near the anterior hypothalamus, the third ventricle, or the cerebral aqueduct and certain other lesions associated with noncommunicating hydrocephalus may destroy the perception of thirst.

Patients with hypothalamic or hypophyseal diabetes insipidus, although generally thirst-perceptive, are at risk of developing hypernatremia if denied access to water or overloaded with solute.

Also at risk are patients with nephrogenic (vasopressin-resistant) diabetes insipidus and those with chronic hypercalciuria or chronic hypokalemia, both of which cause a vasopressin-resistant clinical picture similar to diabetes insipidus. In recovery from acute tubular necrosis, a water-losing state may exist.

C. Extrarenal Water Loss: Large sensible and insensible water losses occurring through the skin and lungs may predispose to hypernatremia. Patients with burns over large areas, prolonged high fevers, heat exhaustion (occasionally), tracheostomies, or hyperpnea due to diabetic ketoacidosis or salicylism are all at risk.

Hypernatremia Due to Primary Salt Overloading

Salt overloading occurs as a form of child abuse and when salt is used accidentally instead of sugar in making up formula. In severe cases, the symptoms, signs, and treatment are the same as in hypertonic dehydration. If the mistake is detected early in an otherwise healthy infant, serum sodium levels may be restored by giving hydrochlorothiazide, 2 mg/kg/24 h for 1 or 2 days. Peritoneal dialysis has also been used.

Hypernatremia Due to Water Loss in the Presence of Solute Gain

A. Hypernatremia Due to Infantile Diarrhea: This type of hypernatremia begins by lowering the ECF volume. The usual mechanisms of sodium and water conservation (thirst, vasopressin secretion, and aldosterone secretion) are called into play. If the patient is fed a high sodium load, hypernatremia may develop.

B. Hypernatremia Due to Large Solute Loads: The solute load required to produce hypernatremia need not be particularly rich in NaCl. Tube feeding of protein-rich foods to an unconscious patient or an infant creates a heavy solute load for renal excretion and results in an osmotic diuresis with the loss of much more water than salt. Hypernatremia may quickly follow if additional water is not provided. Chronic glycosuria in uncontrolled diabetes mellitus occasionally leads to hypernatremia in this fashion, as does overzealous therapy with mannitol or the absorption of the breakdown products of a gastrointestinal hemorrhage.

The signs and symptoms are referable to central nervous system dysfunction. Irritability, twitching, mental confusion, stupor, irregular respirations, frank convulsions, and, eventually, coma may occur. Thirst is severe, but the patient may be unable to swallow solid foods owing to dryness of the mucosa. Weight loss may amount to 20–25% of body weight. There may be moderate fever due to lack of substrate with which to sweat.

Skin turgor may be normal, but the skin often feels "doughy" and inelastic. Subcutaneous fat may feel stiff or unusually firm. Pulse and blood pressure are usually normal. The hemoglobin tends to rise, mean corpuscular volume decreases, and the hematocrit changes little. Blood urea nitrogen may be greatly elevated (> 100 mg/dL). Red cells, hyaline and granular casts, and protein appear in the urine.

Treatment consists of restoring deficits in ECW with isotonic solutions followed by slow, careful reduction of the $[Na^+]_s$ at a rate that should not exceed 15 meq/24 h. This is best accomplished by administering solutions that contain sodium concentrations about 60 meq less than the patient's $[Na^+]_s$, with the rate of administration being governed by frequent laboratory determinations of $[Na^+]_s$. The $[Na^+]_s$ should never be lowered rapidly, because doing so may precipitate convulsions. The administration of hypertonic saline solution may be helpful if convulsions do occur.

Patients with hypernatremia frequently have metabolic acidosis. Rapid alkalinization with sodium bicarbonate should not be attempted unless the acidemia is severe, since alkalinization enhances central nervous system irritability. Hypocalcemia commonly accompanies hypernatremia, although the reason for it is not clear. Therapy with calcium is, however, seldom necessary.

Lastly, not all patients with hyperosmolality have hypernatremia. The presence of large quantities of glucose may osmotically draw water into the plasma from the cells. A blood glucose level of 100 mg/dL is approximately equivalent to 3 meq/L added to the $[Na^+]_s$. A patient with a blood glucose level of 800 mg/dL and a $[Na^+]_s$ of 140 meq/L thus has about the same osmolality as a patient with a $[Na^+]_s$ of 156 meq/L. These changes are also a complication of intravenous alimentation. Urea also contributes to osmolality, and uremia is frequently associated with a hyperosmolal state. However, because urea readily crosses cell membranes, shrinkage of the ICF volume does not occur.

Finberg L: Hypernatremia (hypertonic) dehydration in infants. *N Engl J Med* 1973;**289:**196.

POTASSIUM DISORDERS

Physiology

The total body potassium (TBK^+) of a 20-kg child is normally about 900 meq. Roughly 20 meq of this is in extracellular fluid; the remainder is intracellular. The $[TBK^+]$ has been measured by whole body analysis and by counting the naturally occurring $^{40}K^+$ in whole body counters in "background-free" rooms. Ninety to 95% of the total body K^+ is more or less freely exchangeable, and this quantity, the "exchangeable K^+," may be assessed by following the 24- to 48-hour dilutional distribution of an injection of $^{40}K^+$ or $^{42}K^+$. Tissue $[K^+]$ may be investigated in muscle biopsy specimens, but such studies require rather broad inferences in their interpretation. $[K^+]_s$ is the only simple potassium determination available in most laboratories and is usually the only direct assessment of $[K^+]$ available to the physician. Red blood cell $[K^+]$ does not reflect total body or intracellular $[K^+]$.

The preponderance of K^+ lies within cells—about 60% of it specifically within skeletal muscle cells. Expressed as $[K^+]$/kg body weight, $[TBK^+]$ correlates well with total body water and lean body mass. The correlation of $[TBK^+]$ with weight falls off in obese patients and in those with malnutrition due to starvation or wasting illness. Newborns contain roughly 35–40 meq/kg, a value that increases gradually to 50–55 meq/kg in adult males and changes little throughout life in females.

Maintenance of normal $[K^+]_s$ is primarily dependent upon the Na^+-K^+ pump at the cell membrane. The normal skeletal muscle $[K^+]$ approximates 150–160 meq/L cell water. For comparison, in extracellular fluid the $[K^+]$ is normally only 4.5–5 meq/L.

The second most important regulator of $[K^+]$ is the kidney. The normal kidney is able to excrete a large load of K^+ in exchange for Na^+ but is poorly equipped to conserve K^+ on short notice.

The distribution of K^+ between ICF and ECF is dependent upon ECF pH. Alkalemia promotes entry of K^+ into cells and lowers $[K^+]_s$. Acidemia, on the other hand, promotes exit of K^+ from cells and may raise $[K^+]_s$ if renal K^+ excretion lags behind. A normal $[K^+]_s$ in the presence of acidemia therefore suggests that K^+ depletion exists and that rapid correction of pH may be followed by a sharp fall in $[K^+]_s$.

When glycogen deposition occurs, K^+ enters cells and the serum level tends to fall. This is one of the factors explaining the low $[K^+]_s$ seen in diabetics following institution of insulin therapy.

$[K^+]_s$ may be raised artifactually in a number of ways. Hemolysis of red cells occurring between the time of sampling and centrifuging is well known and requires that blood drawn for $[K^+]_s$ determination be handled gently. Elevations of $[K^+]_s$ in patients with acute intravenous hemolysis are more difficult to evaluate. Storing of blood samples on ice (without freezing) is followed by rises in $[K^+]_s$. Blood with a grossly elevated leukocyte count (as in leukemia) may show artifactual elevations in $[K^+]_s$ due to damage of the leukocytes during clotting. Platelets are also rich in K^+, and thrombocythemic blood samples may show hyperkalemia if clotting is allowed to occur. The simple alternative is to do $[K^+]$ determinations on fresh plasma rather than serum.

Renal Aspects of $[K^+]$ Control

Under normal circumstances, the K^+ filtered by the glomerular membrane is mostly reabsorbed in the proximal tubule. Most of the potassium excreted is the product of distal tubular secretion. The quantity secreted by the distal tubular cells appears to result from an exchange with Na^+ from the distal tubular urine.

The amount of K^+ secreted also depends on there being an adequate amount of Cl^- (or other directly reabsorbable anion) in the glomerular filtrate. Put another way, the Na^+ in the proximal tubule is absorbed in proportion to the sum of the amounts of chloride and bicarbonate in the tubular fluid. Any remaining Na^+ will be excreted with nonreabsorbable anion.To a limited extent, it may still be exchanged for H^+, but in the distal tubule it will also be exchanged for K^+, depending on the amount of Na^+ in the tubule fluid and the amount of intracellular K^+. Tubular potassium loss is thus proportionate to the tubular content of nonreabsorbable anion. Potassium losses should therefore be replaced with potassium chloride and not with a salt such as gluconate, which is a nonreabsorbable anion.

If dietary K^+ intake is totally curtailed, K^+ excretion will continue, decreasing only gradually for 2–3 weeks, by which time a significant negative K^+ balance will exist. The finding of a lowered urinary $[K^+]$ strongly implies that a K^+-depleted state exists and virtually excludes a renal K^+-wasting condition as the cause.

A number of factors enhance the renal secretion of K^+. Hypochloremia (eg, due to vomiting, prolonged nasogastric suction, $AgNO_3$ treatment of burns, chloriduria, or diuretic therapy) has been mentioned. Adrenal corticosteroids, by causing renal retention of Na^+, increase the quantity of Na^+ exchanging for K^+ ions in the distal tubule. If dietary Na^+ intake is minimized, corticosteroid-induced K^+ loss ceases. Diuretics of many types—in particular, thiazides, mercurials, and acetazolamide—effectively enhance the secretion of K^+.

1. POTASSIUM DEPLETION

When 10–20% of the TBK^+ of the patient has been lost, symptoms of apathy and muscular weakness ensue. Paresthesias and tetany are occasionally seen. If the depletion worsens, the muscular weakness extends to a flaccid paralysis, eventually interfering with respiration. Extracellular replacement of K^+ may bring about dramatic relief.

During serious K^+ depletion, typical electrocardiographic changes occur. These include T wave depression, the appearance of a U wave, and, eventually, ST segment depression. The QT interval may appear prolonged if a QU interval is mistakenly measured instead. A number of dysrhythmias occur (Fig 36–5).

In the kidney, concentrating ability is impaired, and a clinical picture similar to that of diabetes insipidus is produced and gives rise, occasionally, to hypernatremia. Tubular degeneration is seen on renal biopsy. Of the effects of hypokalemia, this is the slowest to resolve after proper therapy, and 2–3 weeks may be required for restoration of normal renal function. K^+ depletion also predisposes to digitalis intoxication, and a $[K^+]_s$ determination is always indicated when digitalis toxicity exists.

Treatment

The treatment of K^+ depletion is to restore a $[K^+]_s$ sufficient to dispel any signs of muscular weakness

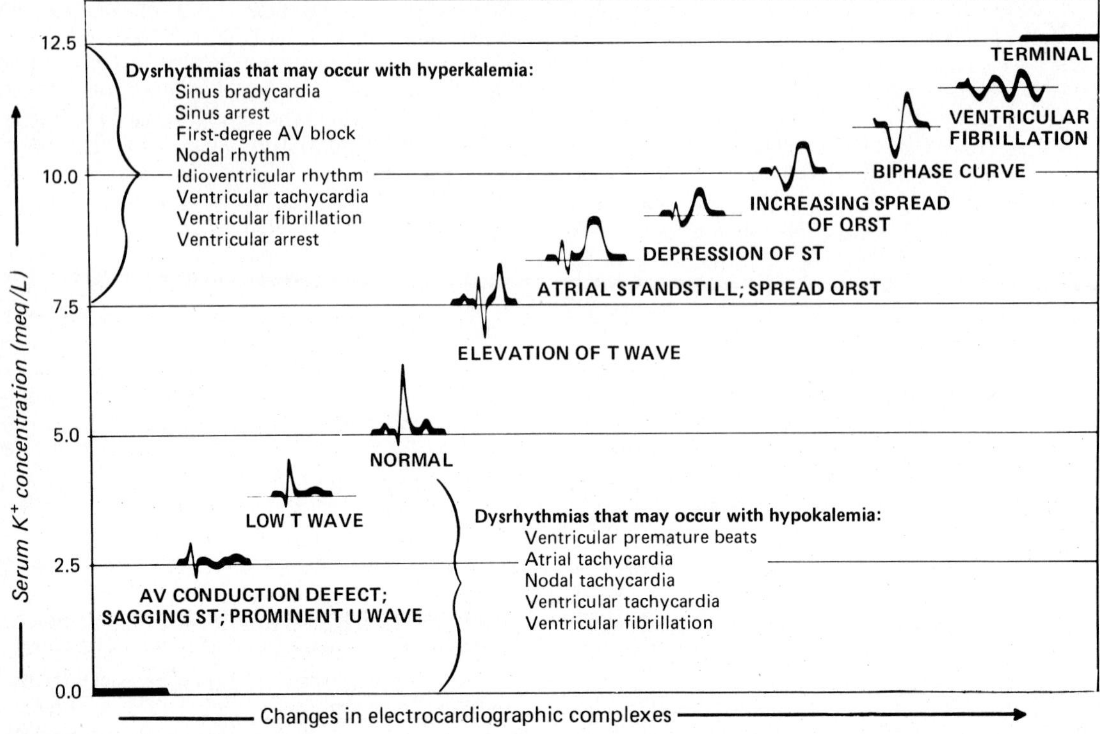

Figure 36–5. Rough correlation between $[K^+]_S$ and the ECG. In hyperkalemia, the cardiotoxicity at a given $[K^+]_S$ becomes more marked by a decrease of $[Na^+]_S$. Thus, with severe hyponatremia, far-advanced cardiotoxicity may be seen with a $[K^+]_S$ of 7.5 mg/L. (Reproduced, with permission, from Krupp MA, Chatton MJ [editors]: *Current Medical Diagnosis & Treatment 1974.* Lange, 1974.)

or electrocardiographic abnormalities and to return the $[TBK^+]$ to normal. Such replacement may require several days.

Chronic K^+ depletion frequently complicates hypochloremic metabolic alkalosis. Until the Cl^- deficiency is corrected, administered K^+ continues to be wasted. Thc administration of KCl, therefore, corrects both the metabolic alkalosis and the K^+ depletion at the same time. The administration of K^+ with virtually any other anion (see above) effectively corrects neither. A variety of K^+-containing foods and juices provide excellent oral medication for this purpose (Table 36–11).

Table 36–11. Juices high in potassium.

	Approximate Content*	
	meq	mg
Apple juice	2.5	100
Apricot juice	2.4	94
Pineapple juice	3.5	140
Grape juice	3	120
Grapefruit juice	4	150
Orange juice	5	190
Prune juice	6.5	260
Tomato juice	6	230

* ½-cup quantities (120 mL)

Additional KCl, up to 5 meq/kg/24 h, may be given to infants and small children as a correctional measure (in addition to maintenance K^+). As K^+ depletion is corrected, the amount and especially the rate of administration should be lowered lest hyperkalemia occur. Actually, intravenous K^+ therapy in excess of that required for maintenance is not necessary to relieve symptoms of K^+ depletion; therefore, K^+ depletion should be treated without haste.

All intravenous K^+ should be evenly infused throughout the 24-hour balance period. If concentrations of K^+ greater than 40 meq/L are present in any bottle of intravenous solution, there should be a maximum rate and laboratory control. Concentrated K^+ solution must never be given by intravenous "push."

2. HYPERKALEMIA

The symptoms and signs of hyperkalemia are few. They include muscle weakness and, occasionally, tetany or paresthesias with ascending central paralysis. The major toxic symptoms and signs are cardiac in origin. Electrocardiographic changes include tenting and then elevation of T waves, spreading of the QRS complex, atrial arrest, and, finally, a sine wave followed by ventricular fibrillation and death. These changes, with their attendant dysrhythmias, are shown in Fig 36–5.

Treatment

The extent of treatment required depends upon the severity of the hyperkalemia, the electrocardiographic findings, the electrolyte profile of the serum, and the predicted behavior of the underlying disorder.

Ordinarily, $[K^+]_s$ values less than 6.5 meq/L require little more than curtailment of all K^+ intake. Such levels might cause serious concern if, for example, QRS complex widening were noted, if the $[Na^+]_s$ were low, if alkalemia existed, if a previous value indicated a sharp rate of rise of $[K^+]_s$, if acute renal failure had occurred, or if digitalis toxicity were evident.

Serious hyperkalemia (levels > 8 meq/L) or serious electrocardiographic changes (widened QRS complexes, heart block, ventricular dysrhythmias, etc) warrant vigorous measures. These are aimed at accomplishing 4 objectives: (1) counteracting the depolarization of cardiac muscle, (2) shifting K^+ from serum into cells, (3) ridding the body of excess K^+, and (4) preventing tissue catabolism.

Depolarization of cardiac muscle may be effectively counteracted for several minutes by administration of Ca^{2+}. A slow intravenous infusion of 10% calcium gluconate, 0.2–0.5 mL/kg, is given over a period of 2–10 minutes. The infusion should be stopped at the first sign of bradycardia. It should be stressed that although Ca^{2+} infusion may be lifesaving, it has no effect on $[K^+]_s$ and its cardiac effects are of brief duration.

K^+ may be shifted into cells by administration of sodium in high amounts, by raising the pH with HCO_3^-, and by promoting the deposition of intracellular glycogen with insulin. $NaHCO_3$ is usually marketed in hypertonic form in ampules that contain 44.6 meq/50 mL. One to 3 mL/kg (at ampule strength) is given over a 5- to 20-minute time span by intravenous infusion. Ten to 20% glucose solutions may also be infused over 30–60 minutes at a dose of 1 g/kg body weight. The effects of these measures may persist for several hours.

K^+ may be removed from the body by oral or rectal administration of ion exchange resins in their Na^+ or Ca^{2+} cycles. For example, sodium polystyrene sulfonate (Kayexalate), 0.2 g/kg, is mixed with 3–4 mL of water or syrup per gram of resin and given orally or by intragastric tube; or resin, 1 g/kg, is mixed into a loose slurry with water and administered as a well-mixed retention enema into the sigmoid or descending colon, where it is held for 4–8 hours and then flushed out with isotonic saline solution. In an emergency, $[K^+]_s$ may be rapidly lowered by the administration of insulin, 0.25 unit/kg subcutaneously or 0.1 unit/kg intravenously. Each unit of insulin should be covered by 3 g of glucose given orally or intravenously.

Peritoneal dialysis—or, preferably, hemodialysis—may be used to reduce $[K^+]_s$ but only at some increased risk and a significant cost in time.

The administration of maximal calories is of great value in minimizing tissue catabolism.

Lastly, whenever hyperkalemia occurs, stop the administration of all oral and parenteral K^+.

MAGNESIUM DISORDERS

Magnesium is the fourth most abundant cation in the body and is second only to potassium in the intracellular water and soft tissues. Approximately half of the total body magnesium is contained in bone; the remainder exists primarily in the intracellular water of the soft tissues, where it acts as a cofactor in a wide spectrum of enzymic reactions.

Clinically, hypomagnesemia can present with muscular weakness and wasting, irritability, a positive Chvostek sign with a negative Trousseau sign, vertigo, tremors, and, in the newborn especially, convulsions. Hypomagnesemia (serum levels < 1 meq/L) is seen in the newborn as a familial condition or with hypoparathyroidism; in older infants and children with malabsorption syndromes, protein-calorie malnutrition, chronic renal disease, and renal tubular dystrophies; and in diabetic acidosis and hyperparathyroidism. Hypomagnesemia may lead to rickets.

Hypermagnesemia may be seen in the newborn if the mother has been given magnesium sulfate and in older children in renal failure. It is usually asymptomatic, but levels of over 6 meq/L may produce drowsiness, and levels of over 10 meq/L may cause respiratory failure and heart block.

Treatment

Hypomagnesemia can be treated with magnesium (0.5 mL $MgSO_4$, 50% w/v aqueous solution USP), 2 meq/kg twice daily intramuscularly. Oral therapy can be sustained initially by 3 meq/kg/d. Magnesium gluconate, 42 g/L w/v, will give 1 meq/5 mL.

Hypermagnesemia only requires treatment in renal failure, in which case levels greater than 7 meq/L would justify dialysis.

Niklasson E: Familial early hypoparathyroidism associated with hypomagnesemia. *Acta Paediatr Scand* 1970;**59:**715.

O'Brien D: Treatment of magnesium deficiency in childhood. In: Gellis SS, Kagan BM (editors): *Current Pediatric Therapy 7.* Saunders, 1976.

ACID-BASE DISORDERS

1. CHRONIC RESPIRATORY ACIDOSIS

Chronic respiratory acidosis involves a gradual impairment of the rate of CO_2 removal by the lungs, with a consequent trend to low blood pH. It can arise with normal lungs as a result of central nervous system damage or when skeletal or chest wall deformities prevent normal lung volume changes during the respiratory cycle. More typically, chronic respiratory acidosis results from primary pulmonary disease.

Disease entities in which chronic respiratory acidosis is seen include bulbar poliomyelitis, advanced muscular dystrophy, polymyositis, osteogenesis imperfecta, rickets, chronic severe asthma, and cystic fibrosis.

Clinically, the patient is dyspneic, shows peripheral cyanosis with clubbing of the fingernails, and may be uncooperative, disagreeable, depressed, and occasionally confused. Laboratory data typically show pH values only slightly below normal (7.27–7.35). The P_{CO_2} is, by definition, abnormally high, and base excess values are significantly elevated above normal (+3 to +15 meq/L). The elevated base excess values derive from augmented renal conservation of HCO_3^-, a so-called compensatory mechanism that acts to prevent dangerous depressions in pH.

Treatment

Treatment consists of correcting the ventilatory problem to the fullest possible degree, making sure that adequate oxygenation is achieved. Na^+ administration should be carefully controlled in the presence of cardiovascular complications.

2. ACUTE RESPIRATORY ACIDOSIS

Acute respiratory acidosis involves an abruptly developing retention of CO_2 and consequent H_2CO_3 elevation, as a result of which blood pH may fall abruptly. Acute respiratory acidosis can result from a variety of causes: perfusion failure (due to cardiac arrest, ventricular fibrillation), respiratory failure (due to central nervous system damage, poliomyelitis), upper airway obstruction (due to croup, epiglottitis, aspiration of foreign body), lower airway obstruction (due to asthma, aspiration of vomitus), and ventilation/perfusion disturbances (due to hyaline membrane disease).

Clinically, the patient is acutely "air hungry"; chest wall retraction may be evident; accessory muscles of respiration may be in use; and the patient is commonly dusky or frankly cyanotic.

Laboratory data include an elevated P_{CO_2}; a lowered arterial blood pH, occasionally to levels below 7.0; and a variable depression in base excess that usually ranges from −5 to −15 meq/L. The acidemia results directly from acute hypercapnia.

A greater hypobasemia is observed in premature and newborn infants with the respiratory distress syndrome. This is because prematures have larger ISF volumes (on a percentage basis) than older children and adults.

Treatment

The management of acute respiratory acidosis depends upon the underlying cause. In cases due to acute upper airway obstruction, relief of the obstruction may be the only measure required. If it is impossible to correct the lesion, adequate ventilation should be provided by mechanical ventilation. Bicarbonate is of limited value in respiratory acidosis because, with CO_2 retention, the equation $H^+ + HCO_3^- \rightleftharpoons H_2CO_3$ cannot move to the right. Thus, addition of bicarbonate only raises the P_{CO_2} without increasing the pH.

Eidelman AI, Hobbs JF: Bicarbonate therapy revisited. *Am J Dis Child* 1979;**132:**846.

3. RESPIRATORY ALKALOSIS

Respiratory alkalosis is characterized by hyperventilation that lowers the P_{CO_2} below normal and thereby tends to raise the pH of blood above normal. The hyperventilation is nearly always the result of abnormal central nervous system stimulation and thus is usually seen in one of 3 clinical settings: hysterical hyperventilation, salicylate or salicylamide poisoning, or irritative central nervous system disorders such as meningitis and encephalitis.

Clinically, the patient may experience paresthesias about the fingers, toes, and lips and may complain of dizziness, faintness, palpitations, heart pain, and even a bandlike feeling about the chest. Hypocalcemic tetany is occasionally observed, and susceptible patients may have convulsions. Hyperventilation is usually apparent, and in salicylate intoxication this may mimic the Kussmaul respirations seen in diabetic ketoacidosis.

Laboratory data are helpful. The P_{CO_2} is depressed, occasionally to levels as low as 10 or 15 mm Hg. Arterial pH values above 7.65 are sometimes reported. Acutely, the base excess tends to be normal or slightly low. With greater chronicity (several days), base excess values as low as −15 meq/L may be observed. Whether such depressions in base excess derive from a compensatory process is not known, although hypocapnia stimulates red cells to produce abnormally large quantities of lactic acid.

Treatment

The management of respiratory alkalosis depends upon the disorder. If hysterical hyperventilation is the cause, simple rebreathing into a paper bag followed by administration of tranquilizers or psychotherapy (or both) usually suffices. If the disorder is caused by salicylate intoxication, give suitable fluids and electrolytes to enhance excretion of the drug. In patients younger than about age 5 years, metabolic acidosis with significant acidemia may soon supervene. Acccordingly, zealous treatment of respiratory alkalosis due to salicylate intoxication is seldom practiced. Prolonged irritative central nervous system lesions may require administration of 2–4% CO_2. Apparatus designed to increase dead space or to allow partial rebreathing may be helpful. Careful laboratory monitoring of acid-base values is essential. The most effective therapy is usually directed at the underlying lesion.

4. METABOLIC ACIDOSIS

Metabolic acidosis is the primary pathophysiologic process that tends to lower the pH of blood by causing abnormal production or retention of strong nonvolatile acid or by enhancing the loss of buffer base.

A wide variety of illnesses are associated with metabolic acidosis—eg, diabetic or starvational ketoacidosis, lactic acidosis due to tissue hypoxia or metabolic poisoning, and ingestion of one of a large number of acidic or acidogenic products such as NH_4Cl and ethylene glycol. Diminished acid excretion is seen in renal failure, in primary renal tubular dystrophies of several kinds, and in renal hypoperfusion due to dehydration, shock, and other causes. Abnormal base loss occasionally causes metabolic acidosis in diarrheal states (especially cholera) in which the stools are strongly alkaline. Biliary fistulas and certain HCO_3^--wasting nephropathies also produce metabolic acidosis through loss of base. Late metabolic acidosis of prematurity is a recognizable entity.

Regardless of the cause, the clinical and laboratory pictures are similar. There is significant hypobasemia. Base excess values as low as −23 meq/L are occasionally encountered. There is usually a brisk compensatory hyperventilation, but compensation is seldom, if ever, complete. Arterial blood pH values lower than 7.0 are sometimes found.

Treatment

Management consists of the administration of $NaHCO_3$ and appropriate treatment of the underlying disorder. There is no advantage to using lactate, phosphate, or citrate instead of $NaHCO_3$. Once the pH approaches 7.25 or 7.30, then the rate of correction may be tapered. The compensatory hyperventilation that usually attends serious metabolic acidosis ordinarily requires 1–2 days to abate once hypobasemia has been resolved. If full correction of hypobasemia is undertaken in the first few hours of treatment, a transient (though seldom severe) respiratory alkalosis may occur. As usual, acid-base therapy is directed toward achieving a blood pH of 7.40 and then keeping the pH at that level.

In most cases, the objective is to correct the base excess in extracellular fluid within 48 hours. The dose of $NaHCO_3$ is calculated according to the following formula:

Dose of $NaHCO_3$ (meq) = 0.3 × body weight (kg) × base excess. This formula usually provides a dose of bicarbonate that fully corrects the negative base excess if given on 2 successive days.

When calculating the total daily requirement, equivalent amounts of sodium and chloride must be deducted from maintenance or replacement solutions.

Alberti KGMM, Nattrass M: Lactic acidosis. *Lancet* 1977;**2:**25.

5. METABOLIC ALKALOSIS

Metabolic alkalosis is caused by losses of excessive quantities of strong, nonvolatile acid or excessive gains of buffer base. The most frequent cause of metabolic alkalosis is loss of gastric fluid (HCl) via nasogastric tube or vomiting. Vomiting due to pyloric obstruction (eg, pyloric stenosis) is especially prone to cause metabolic alkalosis, since the acidic emesis fluid is not contaminated with pancreatic (alkaline) fluid.

Any condition that selectively depletes the patient of Cl^- or provides insufficient Cl^- in the diet or formula may cause a metabolic alkalosis in which hypokalemia, hypochloremia, hyperkaluria, and paradoxic aciduria are prominent features. Besides vomiting and nasogastric suction, diuretics, silver nitrate treatment of burns, and certain chronic diarrheas ("chloridorrheas") are well-known causes.

Likewise, any condition that selectively conserves Na^+ without selectively conserving Cl^- results in the same syndrome, the only difference being a normal $[Cl^-]_s$. Examples include Calcagno's syndrome, adrenal 11β-hydroxylase deficiency, and Bartter's syndrome.

The laboratory picture is classic and consists of elevated blood pH, elevated base excess, and normal to very slightly elevated P_{CO_2}. Respiratory compensation appears to be limited, however, by oxygen need. A common denominator underlies most cases of metabolic alkalosis, ie, a widened gap between $[Na^+]_s$ and $[Cl^-]_s$ (see Potassium Depletion, above).

Treatment

The mainstay of management is the administration of Cl^-. A common misconception exists that K^+ is essential to treat the alkalosis. This is now known not to be so. Cl^+, as NaCl, KCl, or NH_4Cl, will correct the alkalosis. K^+ plus Cl^- is required to repair the K^+ depletion. Potassium gluconate, acetate, citrate, and bicarbonate have all been ineffective in treating either the K^+ depletion or the metabolic alkalosis.

PLANNING & ADMINISTRATION OF INTRAVENOUS FLUIDS

WRITING INTRAVENOUS FLUID ORDERS

Once maintenance and correctional requirements have been calculated and combined into 24-hour totals, intravenous fluid orders may be written. Some rounding-off of numbers is permissible. Unless emergency considerations dictate otherwise, the 24-hour totals are evenly administered over a 24-hour balance period. The necessity for regular review of fluid orders in the light of clinical changes and ongoing laboratory data cannot be overestimated.

The sequence number and composition of each bottle should be stated in the orders and on the bottles themselves.

It is preferable that intravenous infusions for small children be constituted in a number of small bottles rather than a single large one. If 24-hour totals are mixed in a single bottle and then delivered to the patient by way of a smaller increment chamber (eg, Pedatrol or Buratrol), then a hemostat should be placed between the large reservoir bottle and the increment chamber. As a general rule, quantities exceeding 150 mL should not be connected to children under 2 years of age, nor should quantities greater than 250 mL be connected to children under 5, nor quantities greater than 500 mL to children under 10.

All orders for intravenous fluids should contain specific instructions regarding the rate of infusion for each bottle, and one of a number of calibrated intravenous pumps should be used. Bottles containing K^+ should contain instructions regarding the maximum rate of infusion lest a nurse fall behind schedule and try to catch up.

All orders for intravenous fluid therapy should be accompanied by orders to carefully record daily weights and intake and output.

All output, whether gastric fluid or urine, should be saved and measured at the end of each therapy period. All empty or partly emptied intravenous fluid bottles should also be saved for the duration of each period.

ROUTES OF PARENTERAL FLUID ADMINISTRATION

A variety of routes other than the intravenous one are available for administration of parenteral fluids. These include hypodermoclysis, proctoclysis, and the intraperitoneal route. These are poor substitutes for intravenous infusion. Scalp vein needles have been perfected to such a degree that the above routes are seldom if ever indicated. If a vein cannot be found and it is important to use intravenous fluids, a venous cutdown (see Chapter 35) should be attempted on a saphenous vein at the ankle.

HAZARDS IN THE ADMINISTRATION OF INTRAVENOUS FLUIDS

Infection is usually preventable with proper hygiene and rotation of sites. If an intravenous or cutdown site becomes infected, the site should be changed and appropriate therapy begun.

Sloughing can occur owing to extravasation of hypertonic fluids, inadvertent administration into an artery, or pressure necreosis. Adequate padding is essential, especially beneath the heel when veins in the dorsum of the foot are used.

Rapid injection of certain substances may be fatal. K^+-induced ventricular fibrillation is a well-known hazard. Rapid Ca^{2+} infusion may cause cardiac arrest that is preceded by bradycardia. Ca^{2+} infusions should never be given without monitoring the pulse. Ca^{2+} should never be infused through umbilical artery catheters, because of the risk of gastrointestinal bleeding and skin necrosis over the buttocks, thighs, anus, and scrotum. NH_4Cl or any $NH_4{}^+$-containing salt should never be given to patients with liver disease and should never be injected rapidly. They are in any case only rarely used in the evaluation of renal tubular acidosis.

KEEPING AN INTRAVENOUS INFUSION RUNNING

A variety of means may be employed to prolong the usable life of an intravenous site. Adequate immobilization of the site is extremely important, and so is nontraumatic insertion of the needle. This may sometimes be facilitated by warming the extremity around the vein and by the infiltration of small amounts of 1% lidocaine (Xylocaine).

Metal needles last longer than plastic catheters. Whichever is used, constant vigilance must be maintained for signs of phlebitis or infection. Teflon catheters with a removable introducing needle (Intracath) are useful for long-duration infusions.

Hypertonic solutions should be avoided.

The addition of 100 units of heparin and 1 mg of prednisolone to each liter of intravenous solution lengthens the life of a vein without causing significant systemic effects.

SOLUTIONS COMMERCIALLY AVAILABLE FOR PEDIATRIC INTRAVENOUS USE

Carrier Solutions

Dextrose, 2.5%, 250 mL
Dextrose, 5%, 250, 500, and 1000 mL
Dextrose, 10%, 500 mL
Dextrose, 20%, 500 mL
Dextrose, 50%, 50 and 500 mL
Water, 20, 250, and 500 mL

Straight Solutions

Lactated Ringer's injection, 500 mL (contains sodium, 130 meq/L; potassium, 4 meq/L; calcium, 3 meq/L; chloride, 109 meq/L; and lactate, 28 meq/L)
Dextrose, 2.5%, and sodium chloride, 0.45% (0.5 N), 250 and 500 mL

Dextrose, 5%, and sodium chloride, 0.2% or 0.45%, 250 and 500 mL
Dextrose, 5%, and sodium chloride, 0.9% (N), 250 and 500 mL
Dextrose, 10%, and sodium chloride, 0.9%, 500 mL
Sodium lactate, 1/6 M, 500 mL
Dextrose, 5%, and ethanol, 5% or 10%

Concentrated Electrolytes

(for use in carrier solutions)
Sodium bicarbonate, 44.6 meq in 50 mL
Ammonium chloride, 3 meq/mL in 30 mL
Potassium chloride, 2 meq/mL in 10 or 20 mL
Sodium chloride, 3 meq/mL in 30 mL
Potassium phosphate, 3 meq/mL in 10 mL
Potassium acetate, 4 meq/mL in 10 mL

Special Solutions

Volume Expander: Dextran, 10% in 0.9% sodium chloride solution

Osmotic Diuretic: Mannitol, 15%, 150 and 500 mL

Amino Acids: FreAmine HBC contains 34 g of protein equivalent in 500 mL. L-Amino acid concentrations (in g/dL) are isoleucine, 0.76; leucine, 1.37; lysine, 0.41; methionine, 0.25; phenylalanine, 0.32; threonine, 0.2; tryptophan, 0.09; valine, 0.88; alanine, 0.4; arginine, 0.58; histidine, 0.16; proline, 0.63; serine, 0.33; glycine, 0.33; and cysteine hydrochloride, < 0.02.

The electrolyte content is sodium, 10 meq/L; chloride, < 3 meq/L; and acetate, 57 meq/L.

For Peritoneal Dialysis: In meq/L: Na^+, 131 or 141; K^+, 0 or 4; Ca^{2+}, 3.5; Mg^{2+}, 1.5; Cl^-, 101; lactate, 35; dextrose, 1.5% or 4.25%.

SPECIAL CLINICAL SITUATIONS

BURNS

Burns (see also Chapter 8) are the third commonest cause of accidental death in childhood (after automobile accidents and drownings). Many thousands of burned children who do not die have to endure prolonged and painful hospitalization, with complications and aftereffects that may go on for many years. These tragedies are the worse because so many are preventable.

The management of severe burns, ie, burns involving more than 15% of body surface (see Fig 8–5), is primarily a surgical responsibility and ideally carried out in a special burn center. Details of care are given in Chapter 8, and this section is concerned only with the fluid and electrolyte problems.

Fluid and electrolyte abnormalities in burned patients can present a major challenge for a number of reasons. Capillary leakage into the burned areas in the first 48 hours may substantially diminish blood volume. Myoglobinuria from electrical burns and hemoglobinuria from initial hemolysis may also contribute to poor renal perfusion and oliguria or anuria. Acute tubular necrosis or renal cortical necrosis can also occur if there is hypotension.

For the first 24 hours, an isotonic ECF-like fluid should be given at the rate of 100 mL/kg/24 h. Transfusions of whole blood, albumin, or other intravascular volume expanders are not indicated at this stage.

The subsequent fluid and electrolyte plan focuses on maintenance needs and should take into account the loss of plasma volume and also the need for a urine flow of at least 1 mL/kg/h with an osmolality close to 300 mosm/L. It is usually necessary to catheterize the patient, to install a central venous pressure line, and to have a separate catheter access for fluids into a large vein. A convenient routine is to give isotonic lactated Ringer's injection or equivalent solution (3 mL per percentage of area burned per kilogram of body weight per 24 hours) plus additional fluid containing calories and maintenance sodium and potassium (at least 1500 mL/m^2/24 h). Serum protein concentration should still be maintained at 3.5 g/dL or greater. The appropriateness of the plan is checked by repeatedly monitoring serum electrolytes and proteins, body weight, urine flow, and osmolality.

If the plasma hematocrit rises above 50%, if central venous pressure falls, or if urine flow drops below 0.5 mL/kg/h, then the rate of infusion of isotonic lactated Ringer's injection should be increased to as much as 300 mL/m^2/h. If this fails, plasma volume must be sustained by colloid, initially giving 1 g/kg of albumin.

Half of the first 24-hour allocation should be given in the first 8 hours. Subsequent therapy must be planned on the basis of clinical and laboratory progress.

ANURIA & OLIGURIA

The principles of conserving extracellular water homeostasis are the same in renal failure irrespective of its cause or duration. Careful attention to detail may sustain life for several weeks or until peritoneal dialysis or hemodialysis is begun. Treatment of the primary condition, when possible, is implicit.

The first rule is to keep meticulous input and output records that are clear both to physicians and to nursing staff. Reconciliation of these records must be made at regular intervals, never exceeding 24 hours. In difficult problems, calculations should be made on an 8-hour basis. Apart from reports of clinical changes, it is necessary to chart urine volume, patient's weight, and, if possible, plasma pH and levels of Na^+, K^+, Cl^-, and HCO_3^-. It may also be helpful to know the ionic composition of any urine, gastric fluid, etc.

The most difficult problem is to provide calories and to manipulate electrolyte distortions within a limited water intake. A suitable water allowance is 400 $mL/m^2/24$ h; to this may be added the volume of passed urine in the previous calculation period plus the volume of any other extraneous losses. Water should be given as 20% dextrose. Electrolyte losses are replaced. Correction problems are dealt with as indicated elsewhere in this chapter. Hypersomolality or hypernatremia is a considerable problem, since it restricts alkali administration unless extracellular water is present in increased amounts. This is of no concern in the short term but may require dialysis if sustained. Hypo-osmolality requires treatment, but at the same time it affords an opportunity to counteract acidosis with parenteral bicarbonate administration. Hyperkalemia is usually satisfactorily managed by potassium restriction. Resins by enema will remove 1 meq/g. If necessary, dialysis may be used, and insulin, 0.1 unit/kg intravenously, may be given in an emergency. Low potassium levels are particularly likely to occur in the period immediately following recovery from acute tubular necrosis. Acidosis is treated with bicarbonate in the usual manner; it is more important to correct acidosis than to correct extracellular water volume unless cardiac failure is present.

Peritoneal dialysis and sometimes hemodialysis are now used early in the course of renal failure, as it is no longer acceptable to wait for clinical deterioration and intractable acidosis and hyperkalemia to use these procedures.

Finally, it is essential not to neglect caloric intake. Where anuria is complete and due to acute tubular damage that promises to be relatively short-lived (ie, < 2 weeks), it is advisable to depend entirely on the intravenous route for the first week. Thereafter, if good electrolyte control has been achieved or if some urine flow exists, hard candy and renal cookies can be allowed with some oral water intake—also products such as Polycose or Ensure Plus.

SALICYLATE POISONING

See Chapter 30.

PREOPERATIVE & POSTOPERATIVE FLUID & ELECTROLYTE MANAGEMENT

Surgery in a child should, if possible, be deferred until fluid and electrolyte balance has been achieved and the general nutritional status is optimal.

Special problems can be corrected according to instructions given elsewhere in this chapter. The following points should be considered.

(1) Complete volume replacements in plasma and ECF prior to surgery. Correct all electrolyte distortions.

(2) Arrange a planned review of fluid, electrolyte, and caloric balance for the operative and postoperative period.

(3) Except for minor procedures, use an intravenous infusion for at least 24 hours postoperatively.

(4) Maintenance fluid and electrolytes should be given evenly over the period of the operation. Whole blood is replaced in proportion to operative losses.

(5) The carrier vehicle for water and electrolytes should be 5% dextrose to provide minimum calories until normal alimentation is restored. Prolonged parenteral feeding is discussed in Chapter 4.

PYLORIC STENOSIS

The main problem in pyloric stenosis is that repeated vomiting of gastric contents without diarrhea leads to extracellular water depletion complicated by excessive potassium and chloride losses and metabolic alkalosis. Calculations of replacement and maintenance volumes follow the usual guidelines. The alkalosis per se is not treated except by administration of Cl^- and indirectly by giving maximum permissible K^+ concentrations in the solutions employed.

In both pyloric and lower intestinal obstruction, surgery should be delayed if possible until fluid and electrolyte homeostasis has been achieved.

SELECTED REFERENCES

Gamble JL: Early history of fluid replacement therapy. *Pediatrics* 1953;**11:**554.

Winters RW: *The Body Fluids in Pediatrics.* Little, Brown, 1973.

Drug Therapy

37

Henry K. Silver, MD, Robert G. Peterson, MD, PhD, & Barry H. Rumack, MD

INTRODUCTION

Precautions

Older children should never be given a dose greater than the adult dose. Adult dosages are given below to show limitation of dosage in older children when calculated on a weight basis. All drugs should be used with caution in children, and dosage should be individualized. In general, the smaller the child, the greater the metabolic rate; this may increase the dose needed. Dosage may also have to be adjusted for body temperature (metabolic rate is increased about 10% for each degree celsius); for obesity (adipose tissue is relatively inert metabolically); for edema (depending on whether the drug is distributed primarily in extracellular fluid); for the type of illness (kidney and liver disease may impair metabolism of certain substances); and for individual metabolic rates. The dosage recommendations on the following pages should be regarded only as estimates; careful clinical observations and the use of pertinent laboratory aids are necessary. Established drugs should be used in preference to newer and less familiar drugs.

Drugs should be used in early infancy only for significant disorders. In both full-term and premature infants, detoxifying enzymes may be deficient or absent; renal function relatively inefficient; and the blood-brain barrier and protein binding altered.

Dosages have not been determined as accurately for newborn infants as for older children.

At any age, oliguria requires a reduction of dosage of drugs excreted via the urine.

Whenever possible, reference should also be made to the printed literature supplied by the manufacturer or other recent authoritative sources, particularly for drugs that are used infrequently.

Determination of Drug Dosage

Dosage rules based on proportions of the adult dose are not entirely satisfactory but have been widely used in the past and may serve as a rough guide. Dosage based on surface area is probably the most accurate method of estimating the dose for a child if extrapolated adult doses are to be used. Converting kilogram weights of children to surface area can be done using Fig 37–1.

Administration of Drugs

A. Route of Administration:

1. Oral—Tablets may be crushed between spoons and given with chocolate, honey, jam, or maple or corn syrup. Many regularly prescribed drugs are commercially available in special pediatric preparations. The parent should be warned that the attractively flavored drug must be kept out of reach of children in the home. Avoid administering drugs with food. Attempt to administer the entire dose in one spoonful.

2. Parenteral—Parenteral administration of certain drugs may be necessary, especially in the hospital. Its use as a matter of convenience should be evaluated in the light of the psychic trauma that may result.

3. Rectal—Rectal administration is often very useful, especially for home use. The physician must make certain, however, that rectal absorption is predictable before depending upon this route for a specific drug. Many drugs are prepared in suppository form, but pediatric dose forms are mandatory. It is not good practice to cut an adult suppository.

B. Flavoring Agents for Drugs: Drugs for children should not be so flavorful that they are sought out as "candy." Syrups are more useful as flavoring agents than alcoholic elixirs, since the ethanol content of the latter may produce toxicity.

Refusal of Medications

The administration of a drug to a child requires tact and skill. The parent or nurse should proceed as if protest is not anticipated. Persuasion before it is necessary sets the stage for struggle. The child must understand that the drug will be given despite protest, but great care should be exercised to avoid aspiration in a struggling child.

SPECIAL CONSIDERATIONS IN PEDIATRIC DRUG DOSAGE

When treating children by means of drugs, the pediatrician must not only be aware of the correct dosage and indications but must also take into account optimal frequency of administration as well as rates of absorption, metabolism, and elimination, which may vary widely at different ages and under different conditions. The following approach to rational drug administration in the pediatric age group takes into account various states of renal function, liver metabolism, and body size that affect drug dosage in children.

Therapeutic Range

Determination of plasma levels of drugs can be

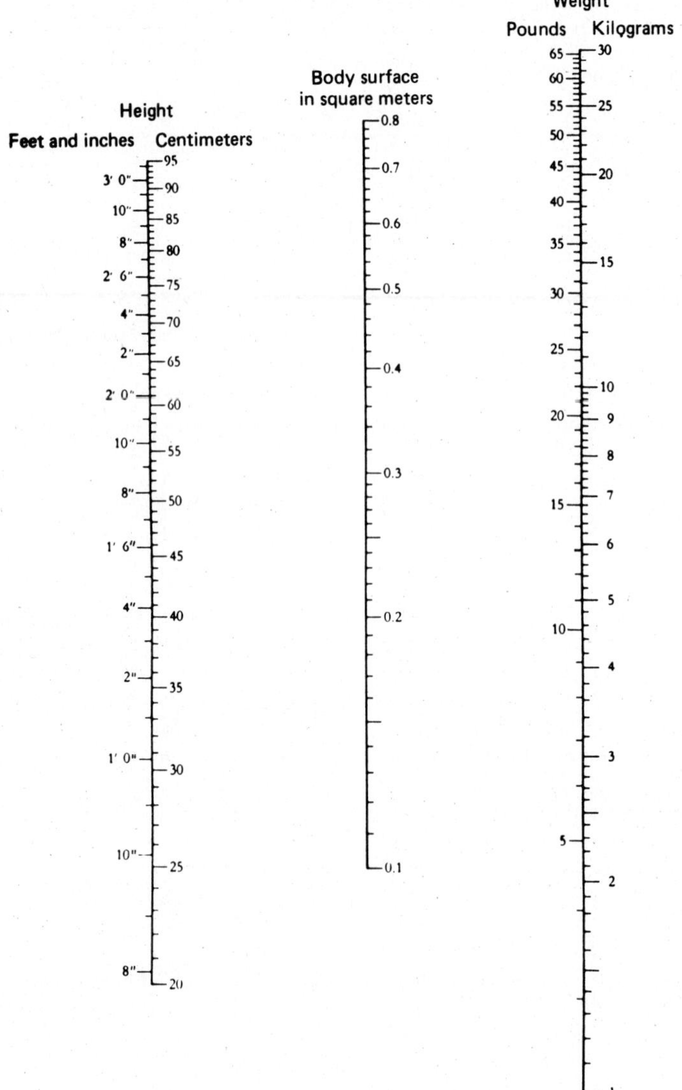

Figure 37–1. Nomogram for the determination of body surface area of children. (Reproduced, with permission, from DuBois EF: *Basal Metabolism in Health and Disease.* Lea & Febiger, 1936.)

extremely useful in monitoring therapy. For some drugs (eg, digoxin, theophylline, phenobarbital), the plasma level is well correlated with the drug's physiologic effect and is easier to determine than the physiologic effect itself. For other classes of drugs (eg, antibiotics, anticoagulants, insulin), it is more important to measure the physiologic effect: serum bactericidal level, prothrombin time, blood glucose, etc.

The therapeutic range is defined as the range of plasma levels for any given drug at which the majority of a treated population will receive the drug's intended therapeutic benefit without experiencing serious toxic side effects. Table 37–1 lists the therapeutic ranges for some drugs commonly used in pediatric practice. Drug toxicity can be expected when plasma levels exceed the therapeutic range.

To obtain a therapeutic level for a particular drug, one must take into account the distribution of the drug throughout the body, whereas maintenance of a therapeutic level requires consideration of elimination processes.

Volume of Distribution

Following the intravenous administration of a drug, plasma levels will fall rapidly as the drug is distributed from the vascular compartment to the extracellular, cellular, central nervous system, and other "compartments" of the body. Its final concentration

Table 37–1. Therapeutic blood levels.*

Drug	Blood Levels: Expressed as Fraction of g/mL	Blood Levels: Expressed as Fraction of mol/L (SI Units)
Acetaminophen (Tylenol)	10–20 μg/mL†	65–130 μmol/L
Amikacin	15–30 μg/mL (peak) < 5 μg/mL (trough)	. . . . . .
Amobarbital (Amytal, Tuinal)	< 5 μg/mL	< 20 μmol/L
Aprobarbital (Alurate)	< 5 μg/mL	< 20 μmol/L
Bromide	< 500 μg/mL	< 6 mmol/L
Bupivacaine (Marcaine)	< 100 ng/mL	< 0.3 μmol/L
Butalbital (Fiorinal)	≤ 5 μg/mL	≤ 20 μmol/L
Carbamazepine (Tegretol)	4–12 μg/mL	16–48 μmol/L
Chloramphenicol	15–30 μg/mL	45–90 μmol/L
Digoxin (Lanoxin)	0.9–2.4 ng/mL	1–2 nmol/L
Ethanol	1000 μg/mL ("under the influence")	20 mmol/L
Ethchlorvynol (Placidyl)	10–20 μg/mL	70–140 μmol/L
Ethosuximide (Zarontin)	40–100 μg/mL	280–700 μmol/L
Gentamicin	8–10 μg/mL (peak)	. . .
Glutethimide (Doriden)	< 4 μg/mL	< 20 μmol/L
Hexobarbital	< 5 μg/mL	< 20 μmol/L
Lidocaine (Xylocaine)	< 100 ng/mL (newborn) 1.5–2.5 μg/mL (adult)	< 0.4 μmol/L (newborn) 6–9 μmol/L (adult)
Meprobamate (Equanil, Miltown)	5–20 μg/mL	20–80 μmol/L
Methsuximide (Celontin) as the metabolite N-des methsuximide	10–40 μg/mL	50–200 μmol/L
Methyprylon (Noludar)	< 5 μg/mL	< 25 μmol/L
Pentobarbital (Nembutal)	< 5 μg/mL	< 20 μmol/L
Phenobarbital	15–40 μg/mL	60–160 μmol/L
Phensuximide (Milontin)	10–20 μg/mL	50–100 μmol/L
Phenytoin (diphenylhydantoin, Dilantin)	10–20 μg/mL	40–80 μmol/L
Primidone (Mysoline)	4–12 μg/mL	20–55 μmol/L
Procainamide (Pronestyl)	4–6 μg/mL	15–20 μmol/L
Quinidine	3–5 μg/mL	10–15 μmol/L
Salicylate	< 350 μg/mL	< 2.5 mmol/L
Secobarbital (Seconal, Tuinal)	< 5 μg/mL	< 20 μmol/L
Sulfisoxazole (Gantrisin)	100 μg/mL	375 μmol/L
Theophylline	10–20 μg/mL	55–110 μmol/L
Tobramycin	8–10 μg/mL (peak)	17–21 μmol/L (peak)
Valproic acid	50–120 μg/mL	350–800 μmol/L

* Therapeutic level or range for drugs that can be routinely analyzed.
† Conversions: 1 μg/mL = 1 mg/L. 1 μg/mL = 0.1 mg/dL.

in the plasma will be dependent upon the dilution of the drug in the various body spaces. Mathematically, this is expressed as

$$\text{Plasma level} = \frac{\text{Dose}}{\text{Volume of distribution}}$$

Since different drugs have differing solubilities in the body fluids or bind to tissues to varying degrees, the volume of distribution (V_d) will vary from drug to drug. Table 37–2 gives the V_d values for a number of commonly used drugs. With the therapeutic level (from Table 37–1) and the volume of distribution (from Table 37–2), one can calculate the appropriate loading dose for a number of drugs as follows:

$$\text{Dose (mg/kg)} = \text{Plasma level (mg/L)} \times V_d \text{ (L/kg)}$$

It should be emphasized that this calculation is appropriate for initial or loading doses only. Maintenance doses are discussed below.

Although the V_d is determined from data gathered after intravenous use, it is also a valuable constant for use with oral or intramuscular preparations. Pro-

Table 37–2. Approximate volumes of distribution (V_d) in L/kg.

Acetaminophen	1.0
Amobarbital	1.1
Secobarbital	1.5
Phenobarbital	0.75 (1.0)*
Pentobarbital	1.0
Phenytoin	0.75 (1.0)
Amphetamine	0.6
Caffeine	0.9
Salicylate†	0.2 (therapeutic doses) 0.6 (toxic doses)
Furosemide	0.2
Phenothiazines	> 30
Theophylline	0.46 (0.69)
Narcotics	> 5
Penicillins	0.2–0.3
Digoxin	7.5
Local anesthetics	1.0–1.5
Aminoglycosides	0.3–0.5
Benzodiazepines	> 10

* Values in parentheses are for newborns.
† The V_d of salicylate increases with increasing dose owing to saturation of plasma protein binding.

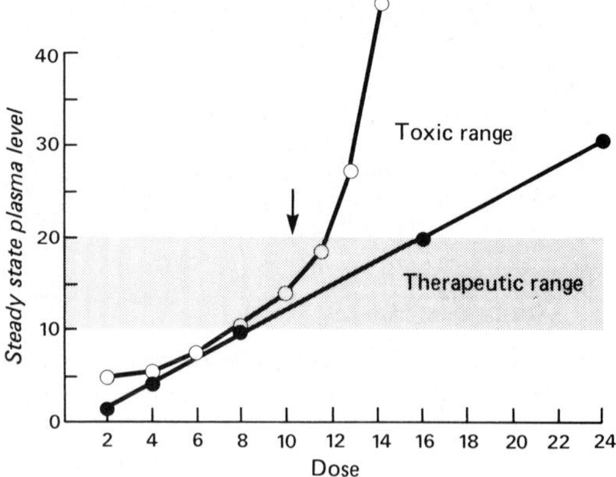

Figure 37–2. Plot (○—○) represents plasma level as a function of increasing dosage of any drug eliminated by hepatic metabolism. Arrow indicates dose at which rapid accumulation of drug occurs. This quantity of administered drug equals capacity of liver metabolism. Dosages above this level cause further rapid increase in plasma level. Plot (●—●) shows data observed with drugs eliminated directly by the kidney without metabolism; observe the difference.

vided the drug's absorption is complete, there is little difference between a slow intravenous infusion and an intramuscular injection. In an instance where an immediate effect is desired but intramuscular absorption is poor (eg, digoxin, phenytoin, diazepam), the slow intravenous route is preferred.

Renal Elimination

Maintenance of a therapeutic level requires that drugs be administered in amounts equivalent to their elimination. Charged or polar drugs (eg, penicillins, aminoglycosides) are directly excreted by the kidneys, and there is little danger of drug accumulation unless the drug is given more frequently than every half-life. Thus, the recommendation for dosage interval for this type of drug is approximately every 1–2 half-lives. When drugs are eliminated by renal processes alone, a steady state will be reached after approximately 5 half-lives, and the plasma level will depend upon the dose and volume of distribution of the drug (see above).

Recommendations for dose and frequency of administration of a large number of medications are given in Average Drug Dosages for Children (below).

Hepatic Elimination

Nonpolar drugs are first metabolized in the liver to make them polar and are then excreted by the kidneys. A steady-state plasma level will be achieved only when the dose given is equivalent to the amount of drug metabolized in the interval between doses.

In deciding on dosages of drugs metabolized in the liver, care must be exercised to make certain that an amount of drug given at a particular frequency does not overwhelm the liver's capacity to metabolize it during the prescribed interval. Fig 37–2 demonstrates the effect of increasing dosage for a drug such as phenytoin upon the plasma level of the drug. As can be observed, one can determine a safe maximum dose (indicated by arrow) above which drug accumulation rapidly occurs. This dose approximates the maximum capacity of the liver for metabolism of this drug.

Drug toxicity can occur rapidly with drugs requiring hepatic elimination. When plasma levels in the upper portion of the therapeutic range are required, frequent plasma determinations should be utilized to avoid drug accumulation.

An example is as follows: A 20-kg child receiving phenytoin (V_d = 0.75 L/kg; see Table 37–2) has a plasma level of 18 μg/mL 4 hours following a daily oral dose. Just prior to the next dose (given at 24-hour intervals), a plasma level is 10 μg/mL. One can estimate the amount metabolized by this child and, therefore, the appropriate maintenance dose by means of the following equations:

$$\text{Fall in plasma level} = 8 \text{ mg/L}$$
$$V_d = 20 \text{ kg} \times 0.75 \text{ L/kg} = 15 \text{ L}$$
$$\text{Dose} = 15 \text{ L} \times 8 \text{ mg/L} = 120 \text{ mg}$$

In 20 hours, 120 mg was eliminated, or 144 mg would be eliminated in 24 hours. The appropriate dose of phenytoin for this child is 144 mg, or 7.2 mg/kg, given every 24 hours.

Table 37–3 outlines examples of drugs that are eliminated by the 2 routes discussed above.

Continuous intravenous infusions. Recently, several drugs have been administered by continuous intravenous infusion. Examples are theophylline, in-

Table 37–3. Principal routes of drug elimination.

Renal	Liver
Aminoglycosides	Acetaminophen*
Digoxin	Alcohol
Furosemide	Caffeine
Penicillins	Digitoxin (75%)
Phenobarbital (25%)	Phenobarbital (75%)
	Phenytoin
	Salicylates
	Theophylline*

* Liver metabolism is rapid, and kinetics appear to be similar to those of drugs excreted by primary renal elimination.

sulin, tolazoline, nitroprusside, lidocaine, and dopamine. Continuous intravenous infusion provides a constant amount of drug in the plasma and avoids the "peaks" and "troughs" in plasma levels. For several of the shorter-acting drugs such as dopamine or nitroprusside, it has not been important to measure an actual plasma level, since the effect of the drug is readily apparent to the clinician and toxicity can be rapidly terminated by stopping the infusion. For other drugs such as theophylline or lidocaine, however, measurement of plasma levels during continuous infusion is essential, particularly if the drugs are used aggressively. For example, in the case of aminophylline (theophylline ethylenediamine), an infusion rate of 0.9 mg/kg/h is widely used, but this infusion rate is correct only in adults and will result in an average steady-state theophylline level of 10 μg/mL. Since this level is near the lower end of the therapeutic range (Table 37–1), many asthmatics in status asthmaticus will not be adequately treated with this infusion rate. A useful calculation in estimating the infusion rate required to obtain a higher steady-state continuous plasma level is as follows:

$$\text{Infusion rate (mg/kg/h)} = \text{Plasma level (mg/L)} \times \text{Plasma clearance (L/kg/h)}$$

The utility of this formula is that the clinician who has decided on the therapeutic plasma level that is appropriate for an asthmatic patient (low [10 μg/mL], middle [15 μg/mL], or high [20 μg/mL]) can then estimate an appropriate infusion rate. The plasma level in the formula is in mg/L for the sake of equality in the units, but 1 mg/L = 1 μg/mL. The additional value necessary for this estimation, the plasma clearance, is given in Table 37–4. Note that there are distinct differences in plasma clearance in different age groups; the greater theophylline clearance in younger children requires a larger rate of infusion than used in adults.

Table 37–4. Plasma theophylline clearance.

Age	Clearance (L/kg/h)
Newborn	0.018
Children (1–10 years)	0.10
Adults	0.07

If one wishes to estimate the theophylline infusion rate necessary to maintain a plasma level of 15 μg/mL in a 5-year-old child, the calculation would be:

$$\begin{aligned}\text{Rate (mg/kg/h)} &= 15\ \text{(mg/L)} \times 0.1\ \text{(L/kg/h)} \\ &= 1.5\ \text{(mg/kg/h)}\end{aligned}$$

A continuous infusion should be initiated following a loading dose of theophylline based upon the V_d calculation to give an initial plasma level of 15 μg/mL.

These calculations do not take the place of laboratory monitoring of theophylline levels but provide a reference point to aid in dosage recommendations. In the case of theophylline, the use of a higher molecular weight dosage form, ie, aminophylline, will require an increment to be made in the dose administered.

DRUGS & BREAST FEEDING

Most drugs are excreted to some degree in breast milk, but this is not a pharmacologically important route for maternal drug elimination, since toxic quantities are rarely delivered to the infant by this route. Levels of drugs in breast milk rarely exceed levels in maternal plasma. In those cases where levels in milk have been reported to exceed the plasma level, the ratio is seldom beyond 1.5:1; ratios above 10:1 have not been reported for therapeutic agents. Quantitative drug overdose of the infant via breast milk is virtually never a problem.

Before administering a drug to a lactating woman, the following questions should be answered:

(1) Is the maternal drug therapy really necessary?

(2) Is this the least toxic drug that is effective?

(3) Can the dosing schedule be arranged to minimize delivery of the drug to the infant?

(4) Would this drug be given directly to the infant if the infant had an appropriate pediatric illness?

(5) In those instances where parenteral medications are given to the mother, is the drug absorbed by the oral route as it is delivered to the infant?

(6) Are idiosyncratic or allergic reactions a particular concern for this infant?

(7) Are there side effects? Will they be easily recognized (eg, drowsiness, rash, etc)?

(8) Does the infant have a known medical problem (eg, hepatic disease or renal disease) that would diminish the drug's excretion and thereby allow it to accumulate in the infant?

(9) Does the infant have a suspected medical problem (eg, suspected infection masked by low-dose antibiotic delivery via milk) whose eventual diagnosis might be delayed by subtherapeutic doses of the maternal drug?

(10) Will the amount of drug delivered via breast

milk come close to approaching a therapeutic dose in the infant?

The answers to these questions usually will give the health care provider the information needed to know whether a drug should be given to the mother.

Quantitative drug overdose of the infant via breast milk is virtually never an issue, but idiosyncratic or allergic reactions to drugs are often not dose-related, and this aspect of drug administration should be kept in mind.

Some drugs are relatively safe in the adult (eg, radioactive iodine) but are associated with higher toxicity rates in children. These drugs, as well as other radiolabeled compounds, many cancer chemotherapeutic agents, and organ-selective toxic substances, should not be given to the mother if breast feeding is to be continued.

SUMMARY

The therapeutic ranges for a number of drugs are presented in Table 37–1. The measurement of plasma levels during therapy will facilitate the regulation of dosage to produce therapeutic effects without toxicity. Drugs whose elimination is dependent chiefly upon hepatic metabolism require special surveillance. Average Drug Dosages for Children (below) lists a number of drugs used in pediatric patients along with the appropriate dose and frequency for each.

AVERAGE DRUG DOSAGES FOR CHILDREN*

Acetaminophen (Tempra, Tylenol): Dose based on weight is 10–15 mg/kg orally. Dose based on age is generally as follows: 12–24 months, 120 mg; 2–3 years, 160 mg; 4–5 years, 180 mg; 6–8 years, 320 mg; 9–10 years, 400 mg; and 11–12 years, 480 mg. May be repeated up to 5 times in 24 hours.

Acetazolamide (Diamox): 5–30 mg/kg/d orally every 6–8 hours. (Adult = 5 mg/kg/d.) For hydrocephalus, 20–55 mg/kg/d orally in 2 or 3 divided doses. For anticonvulsant use, see Table 23–3.

Acetylcysteine (Mucomyst): For acetaminophen antidote, use 20% solution diluted 1:4 with juice or carbonated beverage, 140 mg/kg orally (loading dose) followed by 70 mg/kg orally every 4 hours either until plasma acetaminophen levels are not detectable or until the drug has been used for 72 hours (whichever comes first).

ACTH (adrenocorticotropic hormone, corticotropin): Aqueous solution, 1.6 units/kg/d intravenously, intramuscularly, or subcutaneously in 3 or 4 divided doses. Gel, 0.8 unit/kg/d intramuscularly or subcutaneously as a single dose or in 2 divided doses; for infantile spasms, usually 5–8 units/kg/d intramuscularly in 2 divided doses for 14–21 days. For anticonvulsant use, see Seizure Disorders, Chapter 23.

Albumin, salt-poor: 0.5–1 g/kg intravenously as 25 g/dL solution. Maximum, up to 25 g per dose, as required.

Aluminum hydroxide gel: 15–30 mL orally with meals.

Aminocaproic acid: 100 mg/kg orally or intravenously by slow infusion and then 30 mg/kg/h intravenously until bleeding is controlled. Maximum, 600 mg/kg/24 h. (Adult maximum = 30 g/24 h.)

Aminophylline: Orally, 4–6 mg/kg every 6 hours. (Adult = 0.25 g every 6 hours.) Intravenously, 4–6 mg/kg every 6 hours or by continuous infusion of 0.9 mg/kg/h. High infusion rates may be necessary in children (see Special Considerations in Pediatric Drug Dosage, above). Intramuscular or rectal administration not recommended.

Ammonium chloride: 75 mg/kg/d orally in 4 divided doses. Single expectorant dose, 0.06–0.3 g orally. (Adult = 0.3 g.) For urine acidification, 60–75 mg/kg every 6 hours. (Adult = 4 g/d.)

Amobarbital sodium (Amytal): Intravenously or intramuscularly, 5 mg/kg every 6 hours. (Adult = 0.125–0.5 g 2 or 3 times daily.) Use freshly prepared 10% solution and give slowly. Try smaller dose first. Orally, 1–2 mg/kg every 6–8 hours.

Amphetamine sulfate: 0.5 mg/kg/d orally in 3 divided doses. Maximum, 15 mg/d. (Adult = 5–15 mg/d.)

Apomorphine: Not indicated in pediatric practice.

Asparaginase: 5000–10,000 IU/m^2 intravenously daily to weekly. See also Table 31–6.

Aspirin: As analgesic, 10 mg/kg orally every 4 hours. (Adult = 0.3–0.65 g every 4 hours.) For rheumatic fever, 65–100 mg/kg/d to maintain a blood level of 20–30 mg/dL. (Adult maximum = 6–8 g/d.) As antipyretic, 30–65 mg/kg/d. Obtain blood levels for higher doses.

Atropine sulfate: 0.005–0.02 mg/kg subcutaneously or orally. Maximum, 0.4 mg. (Adult = 0.3–1 mg.) For cardiac arrest, use intravenous or endotra-

*For drugs discussed in other chapters, consult the Index.

cheal route. For breath-holding spells, see Seizure Disorders, Chapter 23. ***Caution.***

Azathioprine (Imuran): 3–5 mg/kg/d orally.

Beclomethasone: For reactive airway disease, 1–2 puffs every 6–8 hours. Metered aerosol delivers 50 μg per puff.

Benzoyl peroxide: Apply once daily after washing face. Begin with 2.5% gel, and increase gel concentration (5%, 10%, 20%) as tolerated and required.

Bethanechol chloride (Duvoid, Urecholine): Orally, 0.6 mg/kg/d in 3 divided doses. (Adult = 10–30 mg 3 or 4 times daily.) Subcutaneously, 0.15–0.2 mg/kg/d. (Adult = 2.5–5 mg/d.)

Bisacodyl (Dulcolax): 0.3 mg/kg orally or rectally.

Brompheniramine (Dimetane): For children under 6 years, 0.1 mg/kg/d orally. For children over 6 years, 4 mg 3 or 4 times daily. (Adult = 4–8 mg 3 or 4 times daily.)

Busulfan (Myleran): 0.06 mg/kg/d orally. (Adult = 2 mg 1–3 times daily.)

Calcium chloride (27% calcium): For newborns, 0.3 g/kg/d orally as a 2–5% solution. For infants, 1–2 g/d as dilute solution. For children, 2–4 g/d. (Adult = 2–4 g 3 times daily.) ***Caution.***

Calcium gluconate (9% calcium): Orally, for infants, 3–6 g/d; for children, 6–10 g/d in divided doses as a 5–10% solution. (Adult = 8 g 3 times daily.) Intravenously, for cardiac arrest in children, give 10% solution, 0.3–1 mL/kg. Inject slowly and stop if bradycardia occurs. (Adult = 5–10 mL.) ***Caution.***

Calcium lactate (13% calcium): 0.5 g/kg/d orally in divided doses as dilute solution. (Adult = 4–8 g 3 times daily.)

Calcium mandelate: 2–8 g/d orally, depending on age. (Adult = 3 g 4 times daily.)

Charcoal, activated: 0.5 g/kg mixed in water and given orally or by orogastric tube.

Chloral hydrate (Noctec): As hypnotic, 12.5–50 mg/kg (up to 1 g) orally or rectally. (Adult = 0.5–2 g.) As sedative, 4–20 mg/kg (up to 1 g) orally or rectally. (Adult = 0.25–1 g.) May be repeated in 1 hour to obtain desired effect, and then may be repeated every 6–8 hours.

Chlorambucil (Leukeran): 0.1–0.2 mg/kg/d orally. (Adult = 0.2 mg/kg/d.)

Chlordiazepoxide (Librium): For children over 6 years, 0.5 mg/kg/d orally in 3 or 4 divided doses.

Chlorothiazide (Diuril): For children under 6 months, 30 mg/kg/d orally in 2 divided doses. For older children, 20 mg/kg/d. (Adult = 0.5–1 g once or twice daily.)

Chlorpheniramine (Chlor-Trimeton, Teldrin): 0.35 mg/kg/d orally in 4 divided doses or subcutaneously. (Adult = 2–4 mg 3 or 4 times daily; long-acting, 8–12 mg 2 or 3 times daily.)

Chlorpromazine (Thorazine): Orally, 0.5 mg/kg every 4–6 hours. (Adult maximum = 1–2 g/d.) Intramuscularly, for children up to 5 years, 0.5 mg/kg every 6–8 hours as necessary but not over 40 mg/d; for children 5–12 years, not over 75 mg/d. (Adult = 25–100 mg per dose.) Rectally, 2 mg/kg per dose. (Adult = 10–50 mg per dose.)

Cholestyramine (Questran): For children under 6 years, dose not yet established. For children over 6 years, 240 mg/kg/d orally in 3 divided doses. (Adult = 4 g 3 or 4 times daily.)

Cimetidine (Tagamet): 20–40 mg/kg/d orally or intravenously in 4 divided doses. (Adult = 300 mg 4 times daily.)

Citrovorum factor (leucovorin calcium): 1–6 mg/d orally. (Adult = 3–10 mg/d.)

Clonazepam (Clonopin): 0.01 mg/kg/d orally in divided doses every 8 hours to start. Increase slowly to 0.1–0.2 mg/kg/d. See also Table 23–3.

Codeine phosphate: Orally, 0.8–1.5 mg/kg as a single sedative or analgesic dose. (Adult = 8–60 mg every 4–6 hours.) Subcutaneously, 0.8 mg/kg. (Adult = 30 mg.) For cough, 0.2 mg/kg every 4–6 hours.

Cromolyn sodium (Intal): One 20-mg capsule inhaled with a Spinhaler 4 times daily. ***Caution:*** Should not be used during asthmatic attack.

Cyclizine (Marezine): For children, 3 mg/kg/d orally in 3 divided doses. For adolescents, 50 mg every 4–6 hours as necessary (same as adult dose).

Cyclophosphamide (Cytoxan): 2–8 mg/kg/d orally or intravenously for 7 or more days or 20–50 mg/kg once a week. See also Table 31–6.

Cyproheptadine (Periactin): 0.25 mg/kg/d orally in 3 or 4 divided doses. (Adult = 12–16 mg/d.)

Cytarabine (cytosine arabinoside; Cytosar-U): 2 mg/kg/d by direct injection or 0.5–1 mg/kg/d by infusion. See also Table 31–6.

Dactinomycin (actinomycin D; Cosmegen): 0.015 mg/kg/d intravenously for 5 days (same as adult dose). See also Table 31–6.

Dantrolene: For malignant hyperthermia prophylaxis, 1 mg/kg orally every 8 hours, starting 24 hours prior to anesthesia. For malignant hyperthermia treatment, 1 mg/kg intravenously as initial dose and then increase by 0.5–1 mg/kg as required. Maximum dose, 10 mg/kg.

Deferoxamine mesylate (Desferal): Intramuscularly,

*For drugs discussed in other chapters, consult the Index.

90 mg/kg (up to 1 g) every 8 hours. Intravenously, 15 mg/kg/h by continuous infusion. ***Caution:*** Hypotension.

Dextroamphetamine (Dexedrine): 2–15 mg/d orally in 3 divided doses. (Adult = 5–15 mg/d.) For anticonvulsant use, see Table 23–3. For attention deficit disorder, see Chapter 23.

Dextromethorphan (Romilar): 1 mg/kg/d orally.

Diazepam (Valium): Orally, 0.12–0.8 mg/kg/d in 4 divided doses. (Adult = 5–10 mg per dose.) Intravenously, 0.04–0.2 mg/kg slowly as a single dose. (Adult = 5–10 mg per dose.) See also Table 23–3.

Diazoxide: For hypertensive crisis, 3–5 mg/kg intravenously as bolus into peripheral vein within 30 seconds. May repeat in 30 minutes and then every 2–5 hours. ***Caution:*** Monitor for sodium retention and hyperglycemia.

Dicyclomine (Bentyl): For infants, 5 mg orally (as syrup) 3 or 4 times daily. For children, 10 mg 3 or 4 times daily. (Adult = 10–20 mg 3 or 4 times daily.)

Dihydrotachysterol (Hytakerol): Initially, 1–4 mL (1.25 mg/mL) orally daily. As maintenance, 0.5–1 mL 3–5 times a week. (Adult = 4–10 mL initially and then 1–2 mL 3–5 times a week.)

Dimenhydrinate (Dramamine): 1–1.5 mg/kg orally every 6 hours as needed. (Adult = 50–100 mg every 6 hours as needed.)

Dimercaprol (BAL): 2.5 mg/kg intramuscularly every 4 hours. For lead poisoning, see Chapter 30.

Diphenhydramine (Benadryl): Orally, 4–6 mg/kg/d in 3 or 4 divided doses. (Adult = 100–200 mg/d.) Intravenously, 1 mg/kg over 5 minutes as an antidote for phenothiazine toxicity.

Diphenoxylate (in Lomotil): Contraindicated for children under 2 years; not recommended for those under 6 years. For older children, 2.5 mg orally 2 or 3 times daily and decrease dose as symptoms are relieved. (Adult = 5 mg 3 or 4 times daily and then decrease dose.) ***Caution:*** Overdose produces narcotic poisoning.

Docusate sodium (dioctyl sodium sulfosuccinate; Colace, Doxinate): 3–5 mg/kg/d orally in 3 divided doses. (Adult = 60–480 mg/d.)

Dopamine (Intropin): 5–20 μg/kg/min by continuous intravenous infusion.

Doxylamine succinate: 2 mg/kg/d orally.

Edrophonium chloride (Tensilon): As test dose for infant, 0.2 mg/kg intravenously. Give only one-fifth of dose slowly initially; if tolerated, give remainder. (Adult = 5–10 mg.) For myasthenia gravis, see Chapter 23. ***Caution:*** Atropine should be available as antidote.

EDTA (calcium disodium salt, calcium EDTA, edetate calcium disodium; Versenate): 12.5 mg/kg intramuscularly in solution containing procaine, 0.5–1.5%.

Ephedrine sulfate: Orally, 0.5–1 mg/kg. May repeat every 4–6 hours. (Adult = 25 mg per dose.) Intravenously, 50 mg/L, adjusting drip rate to patient's response (same as adult dose).

Epinephrine solution, 1:1000 aqueous: Subcutaneously, 0.01–0.025 mL/kg. Maximum, 0.5 mL. (Adult = 0.5–1 mL.) For cardiac arrest, 0.01 mL/kg intravenously or via endotracheal tube.

Epinephrine solution, 1:200 aqueous (Sus-Phrine): 0.05–0.1 mL subcutaneously, one dose only. Use smallest effective dose.

Ergocalciferol (vitamin D_2; Calciferol): For renal osteodystrophy, 25,000–200,000 units/d orally. For hypoparathyroidism, 2000 IU/d (50 μg/kg/d) orally.

Estradiol valerate (Delestrogen): For teenage girls, 10 mg/month intramuscularly. (Adult = 10–20 mg every 2–3 weeks.)

Ethinyl estradiol (Estinyl): For teenage girls, 0.02–0.05 mg orally 1–3 times daily. (Adult = 0.05 mg 1–3 times daily.)

Ethosuximide (Zarontin): For children under 6 years, 250 mg/d orally as starting dose. For children over 6 years, 250 mg twice daily as starting dose. See also Table 23–3.

Ferrous salts (medicinal iron): Elemental iron, 4.5–6 mg/kg/d orally in 3 divided doses. See also Table 4–1. For iron deficiency anemia, see Chapter 16.

Fluorescein: 2 mL of 5% solution intravenously. (Adult = 3–4 mL of 20% solution.)

Fluorouracil (Adrucil): 12 mg/kg intravenously (up to 800 mg/d) for 4 successive days. If no toxicity is observed, give 6 mg/kg on the sixth, eighth, tenth, and 12th days. If toxicity has not been a problem, the course of therapy may be repeated beginning 30 days after the last day of the previous course. See also Table 31–6.

Fluoxymesterone (Halotestin): For prepubertal children, up to 0.15 mg/kg/d orally in 2 divided doses. For pubertal children, up to 0.1 mg/kg/d. (Adult = 2–10 mg/d.)

Flurazepam: Not recommended for children under 15 years. For adolescents and adults, 15–30 mg orally at bedtime for sleep.

Folic acid: 0.2–1 mg/d orally. (Adult = 10–15 mg/d.)

Furosemide (Lasix): 1 mg/kg intravenously, intra-

*For drugs discussed in other chapters, consult the Index.

muscularly, or orally. (Adult = 40–80 mg intravenously, intramuscularly, or orally in the morning for diuresis or 40 mg orally twice daily for hypertension.) For altered states of consciousness, see Chapter 23.

Gallamine (Flaxedil): 1–2 mg/kg intravenously.

Glucagon: For newborns, 0.025–0.1 mg/kg intravenously as a single dose. Try smaller dose first. May repeat in 30 minutes. For older children, 0.25–1 mg subcutaneously, intramuscularly, or intravenously as a single dose. Maximum, 1 mg.

Gold sodium thiomalate: 1 mg/kg/wk intramuscularly.

Gonadotropin, chorionic: 500–1000 units intramuscularly 2 or 3 times a week for 5–8 weeks.

Guanethidine (Ismelin): 0.2 mg/kg/d orally as a single dose. Increase dose at weekly intervals by same amount. (Adult = 10 mg/d; larger doses possible for hospitalized adults.) ***Caution.***

Haloperidol (Haldol): Contraindicated in children under 12 years; safety is not yet established. (Adult = 1–2 mg orally 2 or 3 times daily initially and then 1–2 mg 3 or 4 times daily for maintenance; maximum, 15 mg/d.)

Heparin: 50–100 units/kg intravenously as loading dose. May be followed by continuous infusion of 10–25 units/kg/h or by 40–100 units/kg subcutaneously every 4 hours. Control dosage with clotting times, and follow partial thromboplastin time. May prolong clotting for 24 hours.

Hexylresorcinol: 0.1 g per year of age orally. Maximum, 1 g. (Adult = 1 g.)

Histamine: For provocative test, 0.02 mg/m^2 intravenously. ***Caution:*** Phentolamine should be available.

Hydralazine (Apresoline): Orally, 0.15 mg/kg 4 times daily. Increase to tolerance. (Adult = 100 mg as single oral dose.) Intravenously or intramuscularly, 1.5–3.5 mg/kg/d in 4–6 divided doses. (Adult = 20–40 mg as initial parenteral dose.)

Hydrochlorothiazide (Esidrix, HydroDiuril): For children under 6 months, 2–3 mg/kg/d in 2 divided doses. For older children, 2 mg/kg/d as a single dose or in 2 divided doses. (Adult = 25–200 mg/d.)

Hydrocodone (Hycodan): 0.6 mg/kg/d orally in 3 or 4 divided doses. (Adult = 5–10 mg/d.)

Hydroxyprogesterone caproate (Delalutin): For teenage girls, 125 mg intramuscularly.

Hydroxyzine (Atarax): Orally, 1–2 mg/kg/d in 3 divided doses. (Adult = 25–50 mg 3 times daily.) Intramuscularly for preoperative use, 1 mg/kg/d.

*For drugs discussed in other chapters, consult the Index.

Idoxuridine (Herplex, Stoxil): For newborns, 50 mg/kg/d by continuous intravenous drip over 4 days. (Adult = 600 mg/kg maximum total dose.)

Imipramine (Tofranil): Not generally recommended for children under 6 years. For older children, 25 mg/d orally as initial dose; may increase according to response and tolerance. For adolescents, generally not more than 75 mg/d. (Adult = 75 mg initially, increased to up to 150 mg/d.) ***Caution.***

Indomethacin: For closure of patent ductus arteriosus, 0.1–0.25 mg/kg every 12–24 hours until 3 doses have been given. ***Caution:*** Monitor vital signs and urinary output.

Iodine solution, strong (Lugol's solution): 1–10 drops orally daily for 10–21 days.

Iodochlorhydroxyquin (Vioform): 0.25 g orally 3 times daily for 14 days.

Iodopyracet (Diodrast): 35% for intravenous urography and retrograde aortography. 70% for intravenous angiocardiography. 7% in saline with hyaluronidase for subcutaneous injection.

Iodoquinol (Yodoxin): 40 mg/kg/d orally in 2 or 3 divided doses.

Ipecac syrup: 15–20 mL orally initially. (Adult = 30 mL.) Give water. Ambulate. Repeat in 20 minutes if necessary. ***Caution:*** Never use fluid extract of ipecac as emetic.

Isoproterenol hydrochloride: For asthma in older children, 2–5 mg sublingually 4 times daily (never more often than every 3–4 hours) or 5–15 breaths of 1:200 solution by oral inhalation (not more than 0.5 mL). (Adult = 5 mg sublingually 4 times daily.) For hypotension, 0.1–1 μg/kg/min by continuous intravenous infusion.

Isoproterenol sulfate (Norisodrine): 1–2 inhalations of a 1:200 or 1:400 solution.

Kaolin with pectin (Kaopectate): For children 3–6 years, 1–2 tbsp. For children 6–12 years, 2–4 tbsp.

Levothyroxine sodium (L-thyroxine sodium; Synthroid): 0.1 mg of levothyroxine sodium = 65 mg of thyroid USP = 25–30 μg of triiodothyronine. For hypothyroidism, see Chapter 25.

Lidocaine (Xylocaine): For ventricular ectopy, 1 mg/kg intravenously slowly. May repeat after 5–10 minutes for additional control. Give continuous intravenous infusion of 20–50 mg/kg/min following loading dose. Measure plasma levels during infusions. For seizures, 0.2–0.5 mg/kg as loading dose, followed by 5–15 mg/kg/min by continuous intravenous infusion. (Adult = 50–100 mg.) See also Table 23–3.

Lorazepam: For seizures, 0.05 mg/kg slowly intravenously. (Adult maximum = 2 mg.) Repeat once in 15 minutes if required.

Lypressin (8-lysine vasopressin): 30–55 units/d as a nasal spray.

Magnesium hydroxide (milk of magnesia): 0.5–1 mL/kg orally. (Adult = 30–60 mL.)

Magnesium sulfate: As cathartic, 250 mg/kg orally. As anticonvulsant for hypertension, use 50% solution, 0.1–0.4 mL/kg intramuscularly every 4–6 hours, if renal function is adequate; otherwise, use 1% solution, 10 mL/kg (100 mg/kg) intravenously slowly. ***Caution:*** Check blood pressure carefully, and have calcium gluconate available.

Mannitol (Osmitrol): As test dose for oliguria, 0.2 g/kg intravenously. For cerebral edema, 1–3 g/kg over a period of 30 minutes to 6 hours. For altered states of consciousness, see Chapter 23.

Mebendazole: 100–200 mg/d as a single oral dose.

Mechlorethamine (nitrogen mustard; Mustargen): 0.1 mg/kg/d intravenously for 4 days (same as adult dose). Dilute and inject slowly.

Meclizine (Bonine): 2 mg/kg orally every 6–12 hours. (Adult = 25–50 mg every 6–12 hours.)

Medroxyprogesterone acetate (Depo-Provera): For children under 4 years, 100–150 mg per intramuscular injection every 2 weeks. For children over 4 years, 150–200 mg per intramuscular injection every 2 weeks.

Menadiol sodium diphosphate (vitamin K analog; Synkayvite): For newborns, see Phytonadione. For older infants and children, 1 mg intramuscularly. (Adult = 3–6 mg.)

Menadione sodium bisulfite: Contraindicated for infants. For children, 1 mg intramuscularly. (Adult = 0.5–2 mg.)

Meperidine (pethidine hydrochloride; Demerol): 0.6–1.5 mg/kg intramuscularly, intravenously, or orally as a single analgesic dose. Maximum, 6 mg/kg/d. (Adult = 50–100 mg intramuscularly, intravenously, or orally every 4–6 hours.)

Mephentermine (Wyamine): 0.4 mg/kg orally, intramuscularly, or slowly intravenously as a single dose. (Adult = 15–20 mg intramuscularly.)

Mephenytoin (Mesantoin): 3–10 mg/kg/d orally. Start with smaller dose and gradually increase. (Adult = 0.1–0.3 g 3 times daily.) See also Table 23–3.

Meprobamate (Equanil, Miltown): For children over 3 years, 7–30 mg/kg/d orally in 2 or 3 divided doses. (Adult = 400–800 mg 3 times daily.)

Mercaptopurine (6-MP; Purinethol): 2.5–4 mg/kg/d orally in 3 divided doses (same as adult dose). See also Table 31–6. ***Caution.***

Metaraminol (Aramine): Subcutaneously or intramuscularly, 0.04–0.2 mg/kg. Intravenously, 0.3–2 mg/kg in 500 mL of solution. Titrate by effect or by blood pressure readings. (Adult = 2–10 mg intramuscularly or 0.5–5 mg intravenously.)

Methacholine: For dysrhythmia in young children, 0.1–0.4 mg/kg subcutaneously or intramuscularly. May be increased by 25% every 30 minutes. Oral starting dose is about 18 times greater.

Methadone: For analgesia, 0.7 mg/kg/d orally in 4–6 divided doses.

Methandrostenolone: 0.04 mg/kg/d orally. (Adult = 2.5–5 mg/d.)

Methantheline (Banthine): 4–8 mg/kg/d orally or intramuscularly in 4 divided doses. (Adult = 50–100 mg orally 3 times daily.)

Methimazole (Tapazole): Initially, 0.4 mg/kg/d orally in 3 divided doses. Maximum, 30 mg/d. For maintenance, half of initial dose. (Adult = 15–60 mg/d.)

Methionine: 250 mg/kg/d orally in 3 or 4 divided doses. (Adult dose to acidify urine = 12–15 g/d orally.)

Methocarbamol (Robaxin): 40–65 mg/kg/d orally in 4–6 divided doses. (Adult = 1.5–2 g 3 or 4 times daily.)

Methotrexate (amethopterin; Mexate): Orally or intramuscularly, 0.12 mg/d. (Adult = 5–10 mg/d.) Intrathecally, 0.25–0.5 mg/kg/wk. Intravenously, 3–5 mg/kg as a single dose every other week. See also Table 31–6. ***Caution.***

Methoxamine (Vasoxyl): 0.25 mg/kg intramuscularly as a single dose. (Adult = 15 mg.)

Methsuximide (Celontin): 20 mg/kg/d orally in divided doses. (Adult = 300 mg 1–3 times daily.) See also Table 23–3.

Methylatropine nitrate: 1:10,000 alcoholic solution, 0.05 mg subcutaneously initially. Increase to 0.3 mg as necessary. (Adult = 1–3 mg.)

Methylcellulose: 0.5 g orally at bedtime.

Methyldopa (Aldomet): Intravenously, 2–4 mg/kg initially. Double the dose in 4 hours if no effect. Dilute in 50–100 mL of fluid and infuse over 30–60 minutes. Orally, 10 mg/kg/d in divided doses every 6 hours, increasing at 2-day or greater intervals to 65 mg/kg/d. For moderate to severe hypertension, 20–40 mg/kg/d orally in divided doses every 6 hours, continuing with regular oral doses when controlled. (Adult = 250 mg orally 3 times daily initially, adjusted at 2- to 7-day intervals.) ***Caution.***

Methylene blue: 1% solution, 0.1–0.2 mL/kg (1–2

*For drugs discussed in other chapters, consult the Index.

mg/kg) slowly intravenously. (Adult = 100–150 mg per dose.)

Methylphenidate (Ritalin): Not recommended for children under 6 years. For children over 6 years, 5 mg given orally with breakfast and lunch. (Adult = 10 mg 3 times daily.) For attention deficit disorder, see Chapter 23. ***Caution.***

Methyltestosterone (Metandren, Oreton Methyl): 0.08–0.15 mg/kg/d sublingually. (Adult = 5–10 mg/d.)

Metoclopramide: To speed gastric emptying in children 5–14 years, 2.5–5 mg orally 3 times daily before meals. As antiemetic during chemotherapy, 0.5–2 mg/kg intravenously.

Mineral oil (liquid paraffin, liquid petrolatum): 0.5 mL/kg orally. (Adult = 15–30 mL.)

Morphine sulfate: 0.1–0.2 mg/kg subcutaneously, intramuscularly, or intravenously every 4 hours as necessary. Single dose maximum, 10 mg. (Adult = 10–15 mg.)

Naloxone (Narcan): Usual dose is 0.01 mg/kg intravenously. In patients who are significantly depressed, the first dose should be 0.4 mg for those under 5 years and 0.8 mg for those over 5 years. If still unresponsive, 2–4 mg may be given once intravenously to rule out opiate overdose.

Nandrolone (Durabolin): For infants, 12.5 mg intramuscularly every 2–4 weeks. For children, 25 mg intramuscularly every 2–4 weeks.

Neostigmine (Prostigmin): Orally, 0.25 mg/kg. (Adult = 15 mg.) Intramuscularly, 0.025–0.045 mg/kg. (Adult = 0.25–1 mg.) For myasthenia test, 0.04 mg/kg intramuscularly (see also Chapter 23). ***Caution:*** Atropine should be available.

Nitroprusside (Nipride): For hypertensive emergencies, 0.5–8 μg/kg/min as a continuous intravenous infusion. Start with lowest dose, and titrate blood pressure by increasing infusion by 0.3 μg/kg/min every 5 minutes.

Norepinephrine (levarterenol; Levophed): Start at 0.05 μg/kg/min intravenously and titrate rate by blood pressure. For adrenal crisis, see Chapter 25.

Oxandrolone: 0.05–0.1 mg/kg/d orally.

Oxtriphylline (Choledyl): 7 mg/kg orally every 6 hours. Equivalent to 65% theophylline base (ie, 100 mg of oxtriphylline = 65 mg of theophylline).

Oxymetholone (Androl-50): 1–3 mg/kg/d orally or 2.5 mg for children weighing less than 20 kg and 3.75 mg for those over 20 kg.

Pancreatin (pancreatic enzymes): 0.3–0.6 g orally with each feeding. Increase as necessary. (Adult = 2.5 g/d.)

Pancrelipase (pancreatic replacement; Cotazym, Viokase): For Cotazym, 0.3–0.6 mg orally with each feeding. For Viokase, 0.3–0.6 g orally with each feeding.

Papaverine: 1–6 mg/kg/d orally, intravenously, or intramuscularly in 4 divided doses. (Adult = 0.1 g/d.)

Paraldehyde: Orally, 0.1–0.15 mL/kg. (Adult = 4–16 mL.) Rectally, 0.3–0.6 mL/kg in 1 or 2 parts of vegetable oil. (Adult = 16–32 mL.) Intramuscularly, 0.1 mL/kg as a single anticonvulsant dose. Maximum, 10 mL. (Adult = 4–10 mL.) Intravenously, 0.02 mL/kg very slowly. (Adult = 1–2 mL.) See also Table 23–3. ***Caution:*** Intramuscular administration may cause fat necrosis. Intravenous administration may cause respiratory distress or pulmonary edema. Do not use plastic equipment.

Paregoric (opium tincture, camphorated): Morphine content is 0.4 mg/mL. For newborns, 0.2–0.5 mL (0.08–0.2 mg morphine equivalents) every 3–4 hours until symptoms of withdrawal are controlled. For children, 0.25–0.5 mL/kg (not to exceed 10 mL) up to 4 times daily.

Penicillamine (D-isomer penicillamine; Cuprimine): For infants over 6 months, 100 mg/kg/d orally in 4 divided doses. Maximum, 1 g/d.

Pentobarbital (Nembutal): 1–1.5 mg/kg orally. Up to 3–5 mg/kg as a single sedative dose. (Adult = 100 mg.)

Phenobarbital: As sedative, 0.5–2 mg/kg orally every 4–6 hours. As anticonvulsant loading dose, 5–10 mg/kg intramuscularly (to receive 20 mg/kg in 24 hours). For maintenance, 5 mg/kg/d in 2 or 3 divided doses. See also Table 23–3.

Phentolamine (Regitine): For hypertensive crisis, 0.05–0.1 mg/kg intravenously every 5 minutes until blood pressure is controlled. ***Caution:*** Avoid hypotension.

Phenytoin: For loading dose, 10–20 mg/kg intravenously slowly, not to exceed 1 mg/kg/min. (Adult = 500–1000 mg per dose.) For maintenance, 5–10 mg/kg/d orally as a single dose or in 2 divided doses. (Adult = 0.3–0.5 g/d.) See also Table 23–3.

Phytonadione (vitamin K_1; AquaMephyton, Konakion, Mephyton): For prophylactic dose, 0.5–5 mg intramuscularly. For therapeutic dose, 5–10 mg intramuscularly, intravenously, or orally. (Mephyton for oral use; others for parenteral use.)

Pilocarpine: 0.5%, 1%, and 2% as eye drops; 0.1 mg/kg as a single intramuscular or subcutaneous dose.

Piperoxan: For test dose, 0.25 mg/kg intravenously slowly (same as adult dose).

*For drugs discussed in other chapters, consult the Index.

Pituitary, posterior, powder: Small pinch of powder (approximately 40–50 mg) nasally 4 times daily as necessary. (Adult = 30–60 mg 2 or 3 times daily.)

Potassium iodide: Saturated solution, 0.1–0.3 mL orally in cold milk or fruit juice. (Adult = 0.3 mL.)

Pralidoxime (Protopam): 5% solution, 25–50 mg/kg intravenously.

Primidone (Mysoline): 10–25 mg/kg/d orally. For children under 8 years, start with 125 mg twice daily; for those over 8 years, start with 250 mg twice daily. Increase dose slowly as necessary. (Adult = 250 mg as initial dose.) See also Table 23–3.

Probenecid (Benemid): 25 mg/kg orally as initial dose and then 10 mg/kg every 6 hours. (Adult = 1–2 g as initial dose and then 0.5 g every 6 hours.)

Procainamide (Pronestyl): Orally, 8–15 mg/kg every 4–6 hours. Intramuscularly, 6 mg/kg every 4–6 hours. Intravenously, for emergency use only, 2 mg/kg slowly over a 4- to 20-minute period. ***Caution:*** Monitor by continuous electrocardiography and blood pressure recording every minute.

Procarbazine (Matulane): 8 mg/kg orally as initial dose. See also Table 31–6. ***Caution.***

Prochlorperazine (Compazine): Orally or rectally, 0.25–0.375 mg/kg/d in 2 or 3 divided doses. (Adult = 25 mg rectally twice daily or 5 mg orally 3 or 4 times daily.) Intramuscularly, 0.25 mg/kg/d. ***Caution:*** Avoid overdosage; irritating to tissue.

Promethazine (Phenergan): As antihistaminic, 0.5 mg/kg orally at bedtime; 0.1 mg/kg orally 3 times daily. For nausea and vomiting, 0.25–0.5 mg/kg rectally or intramuscularly. For sedation, 0.5–1 mg/kg intramuscularly.

Propantheline (Pro-Banthine): 1–2 mg/kg/d orally in 4 divided doses after meals. (Adult = 15–30 mg 3 or 4 times daily.)

Propoxyphene (dextropropoxyphene; Darvon): 3 mg/kg/d orally. (Adult = 32–65 mg 3 or 4 times daily.)

Propranolol (Inderal): Intravenously, 0.01–0.15 mg/kg as slow push; tetralogy spells may require up to 0.25 mg/kg intravenously. Orally, 0.5–1 mg/kg every 6–8 hours. For headaches, see Chapter 23.

Propylthiouracil: 6–7 mg/kg/d in 3 divided doses at intervals of 8 hours. For maintenance, one-third to one-half the initial dose. For hyperthyroidism, see Chapter 25.

Prostaglandin E_1: To maintain patency of ductus arteriosus in patients with congenital heart lesions, 0.05–0.1 μg/kg/min by continuous infusion.

Protamine sulfate: 1 mg per 100 units of administered heparin.

Pseudoephedrine hydrochloride (Sudafed): 4 mg/kg/d orally in 4 divided doses. (Adult = 30–60 mg every 6–8 hours.)

Pyridostigmine (Mestinon): 7 mg/kg/d orally in 4–6 divided doses. Increase as necessary. (Adult = 600 mg/d as average dose.) For myasthenia gravis, see Chapter 23.

Pyrimethamine (Daraprim): 12.5 mg orally (in syrup) weekly.

Pyrvinium pamoate (Povan): 5 mg/kg/d orally.

Quinidine: For test dose, 2 mg/kg orally. If tolerated, give 3–6 mg/kg every 2–3 hours. For therapeutic dose, 30 mg/kg/d orally in 4 or 5 divided doses.

Reserpine: Orally, 0.005–0.03 mg/kg/d in 4 divided doses. (Adult = 0.1–0.5 mg/d.) Intramuscularly, 0.02–0.07 mg/kg every 12–24 hours. Initially, try smaller dose (except in life-threatening situations) and double in 4–6 hours if response is inadequate. May give with hydralazine.

Scopolamine (Hyoscine): 0.006 mg/kg as a single dose orally or subcutaneously.

Secobarbital sodium (Seconal): Orally, 2–6 mg/kg as a single sedative or light hypnotic dose. (Adult = 100 mg.) Rectally, 6 mg/kg as a minimal hypnotic dose. (Adult = 200 mg.)

Sodium phosphate: 150–200 mg/kg orally. (Adult = 4–8 g.)

Sodium polystyrene sulfonate (Kayexalate): 1 meq of potassium per gram of resin. Calculate dose on basis of desired exchange. Instill rectally in 10% glucose. May be administered every 6 hours. (Adult = 15 g orally 1–4 times daily in small amount of water or syrup; 3–4 mL per gram of resin.)

Sodium sulfate: 150–200 mg/kg orally. Give as 50% solution. (Adult = 8–12 g.)

Spironolactone (Aldactone): For diagnostic testing, 0.5–1.5 $g/m^2/d$ orally in divided doses. For edema and ascites, 1.7–3.3 mg/kg/d orally in divided doses. Start with smaller dose. (Adult = 25 mg 3–6 times daily.) ***Caution.***

Sulfasalazine (Azulfidine): 50–100 mg/kg/d orally in 4–6 divided doses. (Adult = 1 g 4–6 times daily.)

Tetraethylammonium chloride: For test dose, 250 mg/m^2 intravenously. (Adult = 10–15 mg/kg intravenously or intramuscularly.) ***Caution:*** Phentolamine should be available.

Theophylline: 10–20 mg/kg/d orally in 4 divided

*For drugs discussed in other chapters, consult the Index.

doses. See discussion on aminophylline for intravenous use.

Thiopental (Pentothal): For basal anesthesia, 10–20 mg/kg rectally slowly.

Thioridazine (Mellaril): For children under 2 years, do not use. For behavior disorder in children 2–12 years, 0.5–3 mg/kg/d (maximum) orally; for older children, 20–40 mg/d. (Adult = 200–800 mg/d for psychosis.)

Tobramycin (Nebcin): 5 mg/kg/d intravenously or intramuscularly in 3 or 4 divided doses.

Tolazoline (Priscoline): For newborns, 1 mg/kg intravenously, followed by 1 mg/kg/h by continuous intravenous infusion. For children up to 5 years, 2–10 mg orally. For children over 5 years, 5–15 mg orally or intramuscularly. ***Caution:*** Potent vasodilator.

Trichlormethiazide: 0.03–0.1 mg/kg/d orally. (Adult = 2–8 mg/d.)

Triiodothyronine (liothyronine; Cytomel): 25–30 μg of triiodythyronine = 65 mg of thyroid USP = 0.1 mg of levothyroxine sodium.

Trimethaphan (Arfonad): 50–100 μg/kg/min intravenously. (Adult = begin at 0.5–1 mg/min and titrate rate by blood pressure.) ***Caution:*** Hypotension, including orthostatic hypotension.

Tripelennamine (PBZ): 3–5 mg/kg/d orally in 3–6 divided doses. Maximum, 300 mg/d. (Adult = 50 mg 3 or 4 times daily.)

Tubocurarine (curare): Initially, 0.2–0.4 mg/kg intravenously. Subsequently, 0.04–0.2 mg/kg as needed to maintain paralysis. ***Caution.***

Urea: Orally, 0.8 g/kg/d in 3 divided doses. Intravenously, 0.5–1 g/kg over a period of 30–60 minutes. (Adult = 1–1.5 g/kg/d intravenously.)

Valproic acid (Depakene): 15 mg/kg/d as a single dose or in 2 or 3 divided doses. May increase by 5 mg/kg/d every 1–2 weeks. Maximum, 60 mg/kg/d. See also Table 23–3.

Vasopressin injection (Pitressin): 0.125–0.5 mL (20 units/mL) intramuscularly. Short duration. (Adult = 0.25–0.5 mL.)

Vasopressin tannate injection (Pitressin): 0.2 1 mL (5 units/mL in oil) intramuscularly every 2–4 days as necessary. Start with smaller dose and increase. Effective 1–3 days. (Adult = 0.3–1 mL per dose.)

Verapamil: For supraventricular tachycardia, 0.1 mg/kg intravenously over 30 seconds (repeat once if required) or 4–10 mg/kg/d orally in divided doses every 12 hours. ***Caution:*** Transient hypotension.

Vinblastine (Velban): 0.1–0.2 mg/kg/wk intravenously as a single dose. (Adult = 0.1–0.15 mg/kg/wk.)

*For drugs discussed in other chapters, consult the Index.

SELECTED REFERENCES

Connor CS, Rumack BH: *Drugdex, Drug Information,* 24th ed. Micromedex, 1984.

Gellis SS, Kagan BM: *Current Pediatric Therapy 11.* Saunders, 1984.

Gilman AG et al (editors): *Goodman and Gilman's The Pharmacological Basis of Therapeutics,* 7th ed. Macmillan, 1985.

Peterson RG, Bowes WA Jr: Drugs, toxins, and environmental agents in breast milk. Chap 13, pp 367–403, in: *Lactation: Physiology, Nutrition, and Breast-Feeding.* Neville M, Neifert M (editors). Plenum Press, 1983.

Physicians' Desk Reference, 39th ed. Medical Economics Co., 1985.

Roberts RJ: *Drug Therapy in Infants.* Saunders, 1984.

Shirkey HC (editor): *Pediatric Therapy,* 6th ed. Mosby, 1980.

Silver HK et al: *Handbook of Pediatrics,* 15th ed. Lange, 1986.

Wood BSL (editor): *A Paediatric Vade-Mecum,* 9th ed. Lloyd-Luke, 1977.

38 Anti-infective Chemotherapeutic Agents & Antibiotic Drugs

Ziad M. Shehab, MD, C. George Ray, MD, Anne S. Yeager, MD, & C. Henry Kempe,* MD*

Success in the use of antibiotics depends upon (1) identification of the pathogens to be eliminated, (2) selection of the therapeutic agent or agents most active against the pathogen (Table 38–1), and (3) selection of the best route of administration so that the drug can effectively reach and destroy the pathogen.

Resistance may develop (1) if strains in the bacterial population that are genetically resistant to the agent being used become dominant by selection, (2) if "spontaneous" mutation to a state of resistance occurs, or (3) if genetic material or plasmids transfer resistance from one organism to another.

This chapter will discuss the major agents that are currently available for treatment of pediatric patients. Some newer agents that may be in use more commonly in the future are listed in the references. These include the monobactams (eg, aztreonam) and recently described cephalosporin and cephalosporin-like drugs.

Problems in Prescribing Aminoglycosides

Tobramycin and gentamicin are aminoglycosides useful in the therapy of *Pseudomonas* and other gram-negative infections. These 2 drugs are very similar in dosage rate, route of excretion, and toxicity. They have a narrow therapeutic:toxic ratio. Amikacin is also effective against some strains of *Pseudomonas* as well as many other gram-negative organisms. The ability to achieve higher blood levels with amikacin may widen the therapeutic:toxic ratio and make the drug easier to use. Whether amikacin will be more clinically efficacious than the other aminoglycosides remains to be shown.

Blood levels of aminoglycosides show more scatter at a standard dose than is desirable, and any dose recommendations should be regarded as "best guesses." Dosages are listed in the text as mg/kg amounts and as mg/m^2 amounts when the latter information is available.

* Deceased.

Dosages in Newborn & Premature Infants (Table 38–2)

The term "newborn" usually refers to an infant in the first 7 days of life. In premature and full-term newborn infants, caution is necessary to prevent overdosage and avoid causing serious and permanent damage. However, undertreatment is a definite risk if doses are not adjusted as the infant's renal function matures. Failure to recognize that there is a marked increase in excretion of drugs such as penicillin G, methicillin, ampicillin, gentamicin, and kanamycin by the second week of life—and failure to increase drug dosages at this time—will result in unsatisfactory blood levels as well as clinical failure. The need for higher drug dosages in infants 8 or more days of age is especially important if therapy of gram-negative infections, including meningitis, is to be successful. Whatever the age of the child, about 30 times as much ampicillin is required in blood or cerebrospinal fluid to kill a sensitive *Escherichia coli* strain as is required to kill a sensitive *Haemophilus influenzae* strain. Some strains of group B streptococci are 50 times more resistant to penicillin G than are group A strains. Marginal penicillin levels in the cerebrospinal fluid will result if the infant's increasing ability to excrete penicillin is not taken into account.

Indications for the use of cephalothin in the neonatal period are rare because the drug does not penetrate the cerebrospinal fluid and therefore does not protect bacteremic patients from meningitis.

The small, sick, premature infant who is neither "just born" nor old enough in conceptual age to be considered "term" remains in no-man's-land, and drug dosages should be intermediate between those used for premature infants who are less than 3 days of age and those used for term infants who are more than 7 days of age.

Therapeutic Monitoring of Antibiotics With Potential for Toxicity

Drug concentrations of aminoglycosides, chloramphenicol, vancomycin, and other antibiotics that are

Table 38–1. Choice of anti-infective agents.

Organism (and Gram Reaction)	Drug(s) of First Choice	Drug(s) of Second Choice
Actinomyces (+)	Penicillin	Tetracyclines or sulfonamides
Bacillus anthracis (+)	Penicillin	Tetracyclines or erythromycin
Bacteroides (−)*	Chloramphenicol or clindamycin	Metronidazole or penicillin
Bordetella pertussis (−)	Erythromycin	Ampicillin
Brucella (−)	Tetracycline + streptomycin	Kanamycin
Candida albicans	Nystatin or amphotericin B	Flucytosine or ketoconazole
Chlamydiae	Erythromycin or tetracyclines	Chloramphenicol or sulfonamides
Clostridia (+)	Antitoxin + penicillin	Erythromycin, kanamycin, or vancomycin
Corynebacterium diphtheriae (+)	Antitoxin + penicillin	Erythromycin
Erysipelothrix (+)	Penicillin	Tetracyclines or erythromycin
Francisella tularensis (−)	Streptomycin + tetracycline	
Haemophilus influenzae (−)*	Chloramphenicol or ampicillin	Trimethoprim-sulfamethoxazole or third-generation cephalosporins
Leptospira	Tetracyclines	Penicillin
Listeria monocytogenes (+)	Ampicillin or tetracyclines	Penicillin
Mycobacterium leprae (+)	Sulfones	Sulfonamides, sulfoxone, or rifampin
Mycobacterium tuberculosis (+)*	Isoniazid + rifampin **or** Isoniazid + PAS + streptomycin **or** Isoniazid + ethambutol† **or** In meningitis: isoniazid + rifampin	Ethionamide, pyrazinamide, cycloserine, or viomycin
Mycoplasma pneumoniae	Erythromycin	Tetracyclines
Neisseria gonorrhoeae (−)	Penicillin + probenecid	Ampicillin + probenecid **or** Spectinomycin or third-generation cephalosporins
Neisseria meningitidis (−)	Penicillin	Ampicillin or chloramphenicol
Nocardia (+)*	Sulfonamides	Sulfonamides + agent chosen by sensitivity tests
Proteus mirabilis (−)*	Ampicillin or penicillin	Cephalothin, kanamycin, or gentamicin
Pseudomonas aeruginosa (−)*	Tobramycin + either carbenicillin, ticarcillin, or piperacillin	Gentamicin or ceftazidime
Rickettsiae (−)	Chloramphenicol	Tetracyclines
Spirillum minor (−)	Penicillin	Tetracyclines
Staphylococcus (+)* if sensitive to penicillin	Penicillin	Erythromycin, cephalothin, or cephalexin
Staphylococcus (+)* if resistant to penicillin	Methicillin, nafcillin, oxacillin, dicloxacillin, or cloxacillin	Cephalothin, cefazolin, clindamycin, erythromycin, or vancomycin
Streptococcus (+) (group A, group B, and nonenterococcal group D)	Penicillin	Erythromycin, cephalothin, ampicillin, or clindamycin
Streptococcus faecalis (+)* (group D enterococci)	Penicillin + gentamicin **or** Ampicillin	Vancomycin
Streptococcus pneumoniae	Penicillin	Cephalothin, erythromycin, or clindamycin
Treponema pallidum	Penicillin	Cephalothin or erythromycin
Yersinia pestis (−)	Streptomycin + tetracycline	

* Sensitivity test usually indicated.

† Ethambutol should be used with caution in children too young to complain of or be tested for changes in visual acuity.

potentially toxic should be carefully monitored. Through proper timing and interpretation of drug concentrations in the blood, the doses and intervals between doses can be adjusted to ensure safe and therapeutic drug levels.

A. Guidelines: The following are guidelines for monitoring patients receiving intravenous infusions of these drugs: (1) The schedule for drawing blood samples for evaluation will depend on the drug (see below). "Steady-state" concentrations are the most useful measurements, and the steady state is reached at 5 half-lives after initiation of drug therapy. (2) For interpretation of drug concentration reports, it is of primary importance to know when the blood specimens were actually drawn and when and how the infusions were actually given—not just when and

Table 38–2. Suggested doses for newborn and premature infants.

Antibiotic	Preferred Route	Dosage and Frequency*	
		0–7 Days	8–30 Days
Amikacin	IV, IM	7.5 mg/kg every 12 h	10 mg/kg every 8–12 h
Ampicillin	IV	25–50 mg/kg every 12 h	25–75 mg/kg every 6–8 h
Carbenicillin	IV	LBW: 75 mg/kg every 8 h NBW: 100 mg/kg every 6 h	100 mg/kg every 6 h
Cefotaxime	IV, IM	50 mg/kg every 12 h	50 mg/kg every 8 h
Ceftriaxone	IV	50 mg/kg every 12 h	50 mg/kg every 12 h
Chloramphenicol	IV	12.5 mg/kg every 12 h†	LBW: 12.5 mg/kg every 12 h† NBW: 25 mg/kg every 12 h†
Clindamycin	IV, IM, oral	LBW: 5 mg/kg every 12 h NBW: 5 mg/kg every 8 h	5 mg/kg every 6 h
Erythromycin estolate	Oral	10 mg/kg every 12 h	10 mg/kg every 8 h
Gentamicin	IM, IV	LBW: 2.5 mg/kg every 24 h NBW: 2.5 mg/kg every 12 h	2.5 mg/kg every 8 h
Kanamycin	IM	LBW: 7.5 mg/kg every 12 h NBW: 7.5–10 mg/kg every 12 h	LBW: 7.5–10 mg/kg every 12 h NBW: 7.5–10 mg/kg every 8 h
Methicillin (or nafcillin or oxacillin)	IV, IM	25–50 mg/kg every 12 h	25–50 mg/kg every 6–8 h
Mezlocillin	IV, IM	75 mg/kg every 12 h	75 mg/kg every 8 h
Moxalactam	IV	50 mg/kg every 12 h	50 mg/kg every 8 h
Penicillin G	IV, IM	25,000–50,000 units/kg every 12 h	25,000–50,000 units/kg every 6–8 h
Ticarcillin	IV, IM	LBW: 75 mg/kg every 12 h NBW: 75 mg/kg every 8 h	75 mg/kg every 6–8 h
Tobramycin	IV, IM	2 mg/kg every 12 h	2 mg/kg every 8 h
Vancomycin	IV	15 mg/kg every 12 h	15 mg/kg every 8 h

* LBW = infant of low birth weight (< 2000 g). NBW = infant of normal birth weight (> 2000 g).
† Chloramphenicol must be used with extreme caution. Start with a loading dose of 20 mg/kg, and then follow schedule in table. Serum levels should be carefully monitored to adjust dosage (therapeutic serum levels are 5–10 μg/mL for troughs and 10–25 μg/mL for peaks; toxic level is probably > 40 μg/mL).

how they were supposed to be done. Stress this in working with nurses and other members of the health care team. Check the medical records and make the appropriate inquiries. (3) If the drug is likely to be discontinued within 24 hours, further drug concentration measurements are usually not needed, and the costs of unnecessary measurements should be avoided.

B. Specific Recommendations:

1. Aminoglycosides—Erratic administration of the dose can cause confusion in interpreting results. Therefore, it is recommended that blood specimens be drawn approximately 2 hours and 4 hours after the start of the intravenous infusion. Plot the drug levels on semilog graph paper to extrapolate the peak (concentration at 1 hour after the start of a 30-minute intravenous infusion) and the trough (concentration just prior to giving the next dose). For gentamicin and tobramycin, peaks are normally 5–8 μg/mL (in some patients, peaks of 8–12 μg/mL may be needed), and troughs are 0.5–2 μg/mL. For amikacin, peaks of 15–25 μg/mL and troughs of less than 5 μg/mL are preferred. If extrapolated levels lie outside of this range, if drug administration difficulties may have confused interpretation of results, or if large dosage changes are contemplated, consultation should be obtained.

2. Chloramphenicol—Measurement of peak levels may be complicated by erratic infusion rates; therefore, trough levels are generally recommended. Blood specimens should be drawn just prior to the fourth or fifth dose. Trough levels should be 5–10 μg/mL.

3. Vancomycin—Multicompartment distribution and difficulties with accurately delivering 1-hour infusions may make levels of vancomycin more variable. Peak levels with blood drawn immediately at the end of the infusion should be in a range of 25–40 μg/mL. Trough levels with blood drawn just prior to the next dose should be 5–10 μg/mL.

Precautions in Oliguric Children (Table 38–3)

Regular drug dosages and intervals may result in drug levels that are too high in children with reduced renal function. Dosage and time schedules must be adjusted to renal output in the case of the more toxic agents (amikacin, gentamicin, kanamycin, tobramycin, and vancomycin), and serum half-lives should

Table 38–3. Use of anti-infective agents in patients with renal failure.*

Adjustment Needed	Drug	Approximate Half-Life in Serum (Hours)		Usual Initial Dose	Significant Removal by:	
		Normal	Renal Failure		Hemo-dialysis	Peritoneal Dialysis
Major	Amikacin	2	44–86	7.5 mg/kg	Yes	Small amount
	Flucytosine	3–6	70	30 mg/kg	Yes	Yes
	Gentamicin	2.5	72–96	2 mg/kg	Yes	Small amount
	Kanamycin	3	72–97	7.5–10 mg/kg	Yes	Small amount
	Streptomycin	2.5	72–96	10 mg/kg	Yes	Small amount
	Tobramycin	2.5	48–72	2 mg/kg	Yes	Small amount
	Vancomycin	6	> 96	10 mg/kg	No	No
Moderate	Azlocillin	1	5	50 mg/kg	Yes	No
	Carbenicillin	0.5–1	12	75 mg/kg	Yes	No
	Cefazolin	2	32	35 mg/kg	Yes	No
	Cephalothin	0.5	15	35 mg/kg	Yes	Variable
	Moxalactam	2	19	25–50 mg/kg	Yes	No
	Penicillin G	0.5	10	70,000 units/kg	No	No
	Sulfamethoxazole	9	27	20–40 mg/kg	Yes	Small amount
	Ticarcillin	1	13	50 mg/kg	Yes	No
	Trimethoprim	11	25	5–10 mg/kg	Yes	Small amount
Minor or none	Amoxicillin	1	16	25 mg/kg	Yes	No
	Ampicillin	0.5–1	8–20	50 mg/kg	Yes	No
	Cefotaxime	1.5	3	50 mg/kg	Yes	No
	Ceftriaxone	4–7	12–15	50 mg/kg	?	?
	Chloramphenicol	3	4	30 mg/kg	No	No
	Clindamycin	4	8	5 mg/kg	No	No
	Cloxacillin	0.5	0.8	25–50 mg/kg	No	No
	Erythromycin	1.5	5	20 mg/kg	No	No
	Isoniazid	2	4	5 mg/kg	Yes	Yes
	Rifampin	2–3	2–5	10 mg/kg	No	No

* This table should be used only as a guide. Renal failure is considered here to be marked by a creatinine clearance of 10 mL/min or less. Sources of data include the following: Bennett WM et al: *Ann Intern Med* 1980;**93:**62. Moellering RC: *Ann Intern Med* 1981;**94:**343. Nelson JD: *1985 Pocketbook of Pediatric Antimicrobial Therapy.* Williams & Wilkins, 1985.

be carefully estimated as a basis for individual dosing. The usual dosing interval is every 3 half-lives for patients with significant renal failure. Subsequent doses are one-half to two-thirds of the initial loading dose. Patients on dialysis will need an additional dose at the end of each procedure if a significant amount of drug is removed (Table 38–3). In patients being treated with aminoglycosides during continuous peritoneal dialysis, it may be convenient to merely adjust antibiotic doses in the dialysate.

AMINOCYCLITOLS

Amikacin (Amikin)

Use: Active against most gram-negative organisms, including most strains of *Serratia* and some strains of *Pseudomonas.*

Dosage:

Intramuscular: For children, 7.5 mg/kg every 8 hours or 300–425 mg/m^2 every 8 hours. For adolescents, 7.5 mg/kg every 8 hours.

Intravenous: The dose should be given over a 30-minute period and is the same as the intramuscular dose.

Toxicity: Renal toxicity and damage to eighth nerve (similar to adverse effects of gentamicin).

Comment: Peak blood levels should fall between 15 and 30 μg/mL. Trough level should be less than 5 μg/mL.

Gentamicin (Garamycin)

Use: Active against gram-negative organisms, including *Pseudomonas, Proteus,* and *Serratia.* Some activity against coagulase-positive staphylococci. Relatively inactive against pneumococci, streptococci, and anaerobic organisms.

Dosage:

Intramuscular: For children, 2.5–3 mg/kg every 8 hours or 60 mg/m^2 every 8 hours. For adolescents, 1.75 mg/kg every 8 hours.

Intravenous: The dose should be given over a 30-minute period and is the same as the intramuscular dose.

Intraventricular: For children and adolescents, 1–2 mg/d (gives cerebrospinal fluid levels of 3–20 μg/mL or more 24 hours after injection).

Toxicity: Irreversible vestibular damage has occurred, most often in uremic patients, and is related to excessive plasma levels. Transient proteinuria, elevated blood urea nitrogen, oliguria, azotemia, macular skin eruption, and elevated serum hepatic enzymes.

Comment: Dosage schedule for uremic patients should be modified. Should be used with caution in patients receiving other ototoxic drugs. Overall toxicity is probably the same as or less than that of kanamycin. ***Caution:*** Parenteral therapy should be reserved for serious *Pseudomonas* infections, hospital-acquired infections, and life-threatening infections of unknown but suspected gram-negative origin. If cultures later are positive for an organism sensitive to penicillin, methicillin, cephalothin, or ampicillin, therapy should be changed to one of these drugs. Every effort should be made to use gentamicin as little as possible in order to discourage the development of drug resistance. Serum levels should be measured in any patient requiring long-term therapy, since blood levels are variable despite standard dose in mg/kg. Peak blood levels of 8–10 μg/mL are usually necessary to control serious infections. Levels exceeding 10–12 μg/mL may be toxic to the eighth nerve. In young children, peak serum levels of less than 5 μg/mL are common on currently recommended doses. After measurement of serum levels, dose increases may be necessary in serious gram-negative infections. Oral therapy is recommended only for nursery outbreaks of diarrhea due to enteropathogenic *Escherichia coli*.

Kanamycin (Kantrex)

Use: Bactericidal for coliforms, *Proteus*, staphylococci, mycobacteria, and some strains of *Pseudomonas*. Of use in special circumstances for treatment of some *Vibrio*, *Salmonella*, and *Shigella* infections.

Dosage:

Oral: Not absorbed. Used for sterilization of bowel. For children and adolescents, 50–100 mg/kg/d in divided doses every 6 hours.

Intramuscular or intravenous: For children, 10 mg/kg every 8 hours. For adolescents, 1 g/d in divided doses every 12 hours (for serious infection, give 2 g/d for a short time).

Toxicity: Limit use to 10 days. Irreversible deafness occurs after prolonged administration of high doses. There is cumulative ototoxicity with other ototoxic drugs. Nephrotoxicity is transient unless there has been prior renal impairment.

Comment: Modify dosage and use with caution in oliguric patients. Measurement of blood levels is desirable. Peak blood levels should fall between 15 and 30 μg/mL.

Neomycin (Mycifradin, Neobiotic)

Use: Parenteral uses superseded by penicillinase-resistant penicillins. Some role remains for use of neomycin in reducing bowel flora in surgery and hepatic coma.

Comment: Because neomycin therapy can result in the development of disaccharidase deficiency, it is no longer recommended for treatment of enteropathogenic *Escherichia coli* infection.

Spectinomycin (Trobicin)

Use: Active against *Neisseria gonorrhoeae*.

Dosage (intramuscular): For children, 40 mg/kg as a single dose. For adolescents, 2 g as a single dose.

Toxicity: Toxicity reported after a single dose includes urticaria, dizziness, nausea, chills, fever, and insomnia.

Comment: This drug is in the same class of drugs as streptomycin and kanamycin.

Streptomycin Sulfate

Use: Active against *Mycobacterium tuberculosis*, *Haemophilus influenzae*, and some gram-negative organisms. Synergistic with penicillin against enterococci. Resistance develops quickly.

Dosage (intramuscular): For children, 20 mg/kg every 12–24 hours. For adolescents, 1 g every 12–24 hours.

Toxicity: Damage to vestibular apparatus. Fatal central nervous system and respiratory depression. Bone marrow depression, renal toxicity, hypersensitivity, and superinfection.

Comment: Should never be used as a single drug.

Tobramycin (Nebcin)

Use: Active against most *Escherichia coli*, *Enterobacter*, *Klebsiella*, *Proteus*, and *Pseudomonas* strains.

Dosage (intramuscular or intravenous): For children, 2–2.5 mg/kg every 6 hours. For adolescents, 1–1.7 mg/kg every 8 hours.

Toxicity: Renal and eighth nerve toxicity (similar to gentamicin).

Comment: Some *Pseudomonas* strains are more sensitive to tobramycin than to gentamicin;

hence, tobramycin may be clinically more effective than gentamicin at the same concentration in μg/mL. With this possible exception, these 2 drugs are very similar in dosage and excretion. Gram-negative strains that are resistant to gentamicin but sensitive to tobramycin occur but are relatively rare. More commonly, gentamicin-resistant strains are also resistant to tobramycin.

CEPHALOSPORINS & RELATED ANTIBIOTICS

Cephalosporins are active against pneumococci; *Staphylococcus aureus,* including penicillinase producers; streptococci (except enterococci); and many gram-negative organisms, including *Escherichia coli, Klebsiella, Proteus mirabilis,* and *Bacteroides* (except *Bacteroides fragilis*). They are *not* active against *Listeria monocytogenes.* Despite their widespread use (in part due to intense promotion), the indications for cephalosporins in pediatric patients are currently rather limited. These include (1) treatment of infections due to susceptible organisms when the patient is allergic to the drug of choice (eg, penicillin) and (2) initial treatment (usually in combination with an aminoglycoside) of life-threatening sepsis in which the etiologic agent is not initially known. However, it must be kept in mind that the cephalosporins all share similar problems with regard to toxicity as well as possible cross-sensitivity in penicillin-allergic individuals (estimated to be 5–16%). In addition, transport of active drug into the cerebrospinal fluid is variable, and the majority of cephalosporins (first- and second-generation) should *not* be used for the treatment of patients with meningitis or those in whom the diagnosis of meningitis is being considered.

The major therapeutic advantages and disadvantages of each class of cephalosporin are briefly outlined below.

FIRST- & SECOND-GENERATION CEPHALOSPORINS

Use

The first-generation cephalosporins are generally highly active against gram-positive cocci (pneumococci, staphylococci, and most streptococci except enterococci) and some gram-negative organisms (eg, *Klebsiella, Escherichia coli,* and *Proteus mirabilis*). Because of long-term experience with cephalothin, it is still a good choice for susceptible gram-positive organisms.

The so-called expanded-spectrum (second-generation) cephalosporins sometimes appear to be *less* reliable than the first group for the treatment of infections caused by gram-positive cocci, and they are also ineffective against enterococci. On the other hand, they are quite resistant to many β-lactamases produced by *Enterobacteriaceae* and by *Proteus, Bacteroides,* and *Haemophilus* species.

Cefamandole appears slightly more effective against gram-positive cocci and *Haemophilus influenzae,* while cefoxitin seems to be better for the treatment of some *Bacteroides fragilis* infections. Both have good activity against many strains of *E coli, Clostridium* species (except *Clostridium difficile*), *Proteus* species, *H influenzae, Neisseria gonorrhoeae,* and *Neisseria meningitidis.* They have variable effects on *Serratia* and are ineffective for the treatment of infections due to *Pseudomonas aeruginosa.*

Cefuroxime, a new second-generation parenteral agent, may be useful for infections due to streptococci, staphylococci, or *H influenzae.* It is ineffective against most strains of *B fragilis.*

Cefaclor, an oral cephalosporin, has good gram-positive activity and appears to be reasonably effective against ampicillin-resistant *H influenzae* strains. It has enjoyed some recent popularity in the treatment of otitis media and some respiratory infections.

Dosage & Toxicity

Cefaclor (Ceclor): For children, 15 mg/kg orally every 6–8 hours. For adolescents, 750–1500 mg orally every 8 hours. Toxicity includes rash and arthritis.

Cefamandole (Mandol): For children, 17–25 mg/kg intramuscularly or intravenously every 4–6 hours. For adolescents, 6–8 g/d intramuscularly or intravenously in divided doses every 4–8 hours (up to 12 g/d in very serious infections). Toxicity includes skin rash, drug fever, and eosinophilia. Cross-allergy with penicillin is reported in up to 15% of cases.

Cefazolin (Ancef, Kefzol): For children, 25 mg/kg intramuscularly or intravenously every 6 hours. For adolescents, 2–6 g/d intramuscularly or intravenously. Renal toxicity has been proved in experimental animals at doses of 300 mg/kg or more.

Cefoxitin (Mefoxin): For children, 32.5 mg/kg intramuscularly or intravenously every 4 hours. For adolescents, 6–8 g/d intramuscularly or intravenously in divided doses every 4–6 hours (up to 12 g/d in very serious infections). Cefoxitin causes false-positive increases in the serum creatinine level. Intramuscular administration is painful. Intravenous injection can result in thrombophlebitis. Allergic reactions, gastrointestinal disturbances, eosinophilia, transient leukopenia, neutropenia, and hemolytic anemia have been described.

Cefuroxime (Zinacef): For children, 50 mg/kg intramuscularly or intravenously every 6–8 hours. For adolescents, 0.75–1.5 g intramuscularly or intravenously every 8 hours. Cefuroxime may produce a false-positive Clinitest response for glucose (but not glucose oxidase) in the urine. Toxicity includes transient eosinophilia and elevated hepatic enzyme levels.

Cephalexin (Keflex): For children, 25 mg/kg orally every 6–8 hours. For adolescents, 1–2 g/d orally in divided doses every 6–8 hours. Toxicity includes nausea, vomiting, diarrhea, elevated serum hepatic enzymes, rash, and pruritus.

Cephalothin (Keflin): For children, 50 mg/kg intramuscularly or intravenously every 4–6 hours. For adolescents, up to 12 g/d intramuscularly or intravenously. Oral form is not absorbed. Toxicity includes pain on injection, drug fever, sterile abscesses, positive results in the direct Coombs test, thrombocytopenic purpura, and a brown-black Clinitest response (normal glucose oxidase).

THIRD-GENERATION CEPHALOSPORINS & RELATED ANTIBIOTICS

Use

The third-generation cephalosporins are reputed to possess almost all of the effective attributes of the second-generation cephalosporins. The exceptions are that the third-generation drugs have decreased activity against staphylococci and, in the case of moxalactam, against group B streptococci and pneumococci. In addition, they are active against some strains of *Pseudomonas aeruginosa, Serratia,* and *Citrobacter* species. While many strains of *Salmonella typhi* are also susceptible, cefotaxime has not been effective in a few cases of typhoid fever where it was tried. Unlike most of the other cephalosporins, the third-generation agents enter the cerebrospinal fluid reasonably well. They currently appear to be potentially useful agents, but it seems advisable to restrict their use to serious gram-negative infections, including *Haemophilus influenzae* infections, when susceptibility studies clearly indicate that they may be effective *and* other agents cannot be used—for example, in cases of gram-negative meningitis in which other antibiotics are shown to be ineffective or are not tolerated well by the patient. The third-generation drugs appear to be significantly less effective against staphylococci than the first-generation cephalosporins. They should not be trusted for treatment of group B streptococcal infections. As with other cephalosporins, they are not active against enterococci or *Listeria monocytogenes.*

Dosage

Cefoperazone (Cefobid): For children, not available for use at present. For adolescents, 1–2 g intramuscularly or intravenously every 12 hours.

Cefotaxime (Claforan): For children, 50 mg/kg intramuscularly or intravenously every 6 hours. For adolescents, 1–2 g intramuscularly or intravenously every 4–6 hours.

Ceftazidime (Fortaz): For children, 50–75 mg/kg intravenously every 6 hours. For adolescents, 1–2 g intravenously every 8–12 hours.

Ceftriaxone (Rocephin): For children, 25–50 mg/kg intravenously every 12 hours. For adolescents, 0.5–1 g intravenously every 12–24 hours.

Moxalactam (Moxam): For children, 50 mg/kg intramuscularly or intravenously every 6 hours. For adolescents, 1–2 g intramuscularly or intravenously every 8 hours (for serious infections, 12 g/d in divided doses every 8 hours).

Toxicity

In general, the toxicity of third-generation cephalosporins is the same as that of other cephalosporins. Fungal overgrowth is common because of extreme sensitivity of normal flora (aerobes and anaerobes) to these agents. Bleeding diathesis can be seen with all 5 drugs listed above. All cause prolongation of the prothrombin time; routine administration of vitamin K is recommended. In addition, moxalactam and cefoperazone cause decreased platelet aggregation. Neutropenia may occur. The third-generation cephalosporins can produce disulfiramlike effects if combined with alcohol. Moxalactam displaces bilirubin from protein-binding sites in vitro, and this may be a clinical consideration in neonatal usage.

Comment

In renal failure, there is little accumulation of cefoperazone, ceftriaxone, or cefotaxime until the creatinine level falls to less than 20 mL/m^2 because of biliary excretion or acetylation. Moxalactam has a longer half-life, and about 90% is excreted by the kidneys; therefore, accumulation is greater. Probenecid will elevate serum levels of cefotaxime but not cefoperazone or moxalactam. The minimal inhibitory concentration for group B streptococci is 4–8 μg/mL for moxalactam and 0.06 μg/mL for cefotaxime. Ceftazidime is most active against many strains of *Pseudomonas.*

THE PENICILLINS

All penicillins are cross-allergenic. The mechanism of action of the tetracyclines and chloramphenicol is often antagonistic to that of the penicillins.

In serious infections, all penicillins should be given in divided doses at least every 4 hours.

PENICILLINASE-SENSITIVE PENICILLINS

Amoxicillin (Amoxil, Larotid, Polymox)

Use: Active against gram-positive cocci, except for penicillinase-producing staphylococci, *Neisseria meningitidis, Neisseria gonorrhoeae,* and *Listeria.* Most *Haemophilus influenzae* strains are sensitive, but 10–30% are resistant. Fifty to 80% of strains of *Escherichia coli,* most *Salmonella* and *Shigella* strains, and 90% of *Proteus mirabilis* strains are sensitive. *Enterobacter* and *Klebsiella* strains are usually resistant.

Dosage (oral): For children, 25 mg/kg every 6–8 hours. For adolescents, 250–500 mg every 8 hours.

Toxicity: Generally of low toxicity. Diarrhea, skin rash (especially in mononucleosis), drug fever, and superinfection occur.

Comment: Amoxicillin is slightly less active than ampicillin against shigellae and *H influenzae* and slightly more active against enterococci and *Salmonella typhi.* Amoxicillin achieves a blood level about double that of the same dose of ampicillin (see Ampicillin, below). Less diarrhea may occur with amoxicillin than with ampicillin.

Amoxicillin With Potassium Clavulanate (Augmentin)

Use: Amoxicillin is combined with a β-lactamase inhibitor for presumed expanded-spectrum coverage of otitis media, sinusitis, and respiratory, skin, and urinary tract infections. Further experience is necessary to confirm the usefulness of this combination.

Dosage (oral): For children, give amoxicillin component dosage of 40–60 mg/kg/d in 3 divided doses. For adolescents, give 250–500 mg of amoxicillin component every 8 hours.

Toxicity: Diarrhea, nausea, and skin rashes.

Comment: Can cause false-positive results in the direct serum antiglobulin test.

Ampicillin (Omnipen, Polycillin, Totacillin)

Use: Same as amoxicillin (see above).

Dosage:

Oral: For children and adolescents, 50–150 mg/kg/d in divided doses.

Intramuscular or intravenous: For children, 50–65 mg/kg every 4–6 hours. For adolescents, 12–18 g/d in divided doses every 4 hours.

Toxicity: Same as amoxicillin (see above). See also comments for amoxicillin.

Comment: An ampicillin loading dose of 50–100 mg/kg is desirable in serious infections. Five hundred milligrams of ampicillin contain about 1.7 meq of Na^+. Ampicillin levels in the cerebrospinal fluid decrease after the third day in meningitis as the pleocytosis resolves; the drug should be given parenterally for the entire course. Higher blood levels are achieved on oral administration if the drug is given in the fasting state. Peak blood levels following oral administration are in the range of 1 μg/mL, which is sufficient for sensitive gram-positive organisms but inadequate for systemic infections with gram-negative organisms. Higher levels are achieved in urine. In intravenous solutions, ampicillin is not stable; it should be reconstituted immediately prior to use.

Carbenicillin (Geocillin, Geopen)

Use: Generally covers the same organisms as ampicillin but is active also against *Pseudomonas, Proteus,* and some strains of *Serratia.*

Dosage:

Oral (carbenicillin indanyl sodium): For children, 15–25 mg/kg every 6 hours. For adolescents, 0.5–1 g every 6 hours.

Intramuscular: Do not use.

Intravenous (carbenicillin disodium): For children, 100 mg/kg every 4 hours. For adolescents, up to 30 g/d in divided doses every 4 hours.

Toxicity: Bleeding diathesis secondary to platelet dysfunction. Rises in AST (SGOT) levels have been reported and may be due to anicteric hepatitis as well as muscle necrosis after intramuscular injection. Hypokalemia also occurs.

Comment: High doses are required. The oral form is useful only in urinary tract infections. Of value in *Pseudomonas* infections in patients with compromised renal function (toxicity low). Probably synergistic with gentamicin, tobramycin, and amikacin. Because of the rapid development of resistance and the difficulty of treating systemic infections, intravenous carbenicillin should be used only in combination with an aminoglycoside. Contains 4.7 meq of Na^+ per gram.

Mezlocillin (Mezlin)

Use: Same as for carbenicillin except is also active against many strains of *Bacteroides fragilis, Klebsiella,* and enterococci.

Dosage (intravenous): For children, 50 mg/kg in divided doses every 4 hours. For adolescents, 3 g every 4 hours (up to 24 g/d).

Toxicity: Same as carbenicillin.

Comment: Least likely of anti-*Pseudomonas* penicillins to alter bleeding time. Contains 1.9 meq of Na^+ per gram.

Penicillin G, Potassium or Sodium Salt

Use: Active against gram-positive cocci, gram-negative cocci, and gram-positive bacilli. In high doses, active against some gram-negative bacilli.

Dosage:

Oral: For children and adolescents, 100,000–400,000 units ½ hour before meals every 4–6 hours.

Intramuscular: For children and adolescents, 20,000–50,000 units/kg/d in divided doses every 4–6 hours.

Intravenous: For children, 100,000–400,000 units/kg/d in divided doses every 4 hours. For adolescents, 5–20 million units/d.

Toxicity: Hypersensitivity (anaphylaxis, urticaria, rash, and drug fever). Change in bowel flora, candidiasis, diarrhea, hemolytic anemia, hematuria, and interstitial nephritis. Neurotoxic in very large doses.

Comment: Some group B streptococci require penicillin G levels of 0.5 unit/mL for inhibition. This compares to the amount (< 0.009 unit/mL) required to inhibit group A streptococci. These higher penicillin G doses are unlikely to cause seizures in the newborn if the dose is administered over a 20-minute period. Not all group B streptococcal infections will respond to these increased doses in newborns. High concentration in the urine makes this agent useful in treatment of some urinary tract infections with gram-negative rods. One million units of potassium penicillin G contain 1.7 meq of K^+. Avoid pushing large doses of potassium salt, as in initiating therapy for meningitis; use sodium salt instead. Note that 1.7 units equal 1 μg of penicillin G.

Penicillin G, Procaine

Use: Same as penicillin G.

Dosage (intramuscular): For children and adolescents, 100,000–600,000 units every 12–24 hours.

Toxicity: Agitation, hallucinations, and bizarre behavior (Hoigné's syndrome).

Penicillin G, Benzathine (Bicillin L-A, Permapen)

Use: The preferred drug for rheumatic fever prophylaxis.

Dosage (intramuscular): For children and adolescents, 50,000 units/kg (up to 1.2 million units/d) for acute illness; 1.2 million units every 25–27 days for rheumatic fever prophylaxis.

Toxicity: Same as penicillin G.

Comment: Increasing the dose gives a more sustained rather than a higher blood level. Penicillin cannot be detected in cerebrospinal fluid. In acute illness, the procaine penicillin in Bicillin C-R (see below) may be desirable.

Penicillin G, Benzathine & Procaine Combined (Bicillin C-R, Bicillin C-R 900/300)

Use: For treatment of acute streptococcal infections. Do not use for rheumatic fever prophylaxis.

Dosage (intramuscular): Bicillin C-R contains 600,000 units of benzathine penicillin and 600,000 units of procaine penicillin. Bicillin C-R 900/300 contains 900,000 and 300,000 units of benzathine and procaine penicillin, respectively. For children and adolescents, give 1.2 million units.

Toxicity: Same as penicillin G.

Penicillin V (Phenoxymethyl Penicillin; Pen-Vee K, V-Cillin K)

Use: Same as penicillin G.

Dosage (oral): For children, 30–60 mg/kg/d in 4 divided doses (for serious infection, 100 mg/kg/d in divided doses every 4–6 hours). For adolescents, 1–4 g/d in divided doses every 6 hours (for serious infections, 4–6 g/d in divided doses every 4–6 hours).

Comment: Note that 200,000 units equal 125 mg of penicillin V. Penicillin V is better absorbed than penicillin G.

Piperacillin (Pipracil)

Use: Same as for carbenicillin except is also active against enterococci, *Klebsiella, Enterobacter,* and *Citrobacter* strains and against many strains of *Bacteroides fragilis* and peptostreptococci.

Dosage (intravenous): For children, 50–75 mg/kg every 4 hours or 1.5 g/m^2 every 4 hours. For adolescents, 3–4 g every 4 hours.

Toxicity: Eosinophilia, drug fever, and rash. Reversible platelet dysfunction and neutropenia.

Comment: Piperacillin is more active on a weight basis (mg/kg) against most enteric gram-negative organisms than carbenicillin or ticarcillin. It is 4–16 times more active against *Pseudomonas* than carbenicillin, ticarcillin, or mezlocillin. Because of emergence of resistant strains, piperacillin should be used with another antibiotic in serious infections. Contains 1.98 meq of Na^+ per gram, in comparison to 4.7 meq/g for carbenicillin and 5.2 meq/g for ticarcillin.

Ticarcillin (Ticar)

Use: Same as for carbenicillin.

Dosage (intravenous): For children, 50 mg/kg every 4 hours. For adolescents, 3 g every 4–6 hours (up to 24 g).

Toxicity: As with carbenicillin, side effects include platelet dysfunction and hypokalemia.

Comment: Ticarcillin is 2–4 times more active in vitro than carbenicillin against isolates of *Pseudomonas, Escherichia coli,* and *Proteus.* Improved clinical efficacy not yet documented. May have better therapeutic:toxic ratio than carbenicillin. Contains 5.2 meq of Na^+ per gram.

PENICILLINASE-RESISTANT PENICILLINS

Cloxacillin (Tegopen), Dicloxacillin (Dynapen, Veracillin), Methicillin (Staphcillin), Nafcillin (Unipen), & Oxacillin (Prostaphlin)

Use: Active against penicillinase-producing and non-penicillinase-producing staphylococci. These penicillins are probably somewhat less effective than penicillin G against pneumococci and streptococci. Enterococci are insensitive.

Dosage:

Oral:

Cloxacillin or dicloxacillin: For children and adolescents, 12.5–25 mg/kg every 6 hours.

Methicillin or nafcillin: Do not use oral form.

Oxacillin: For children and adolescents, 50–100 mg/kg/d in divided doses every 6 hours.

Intravenous:

Oxacillin, methicillin, or nafcillin: For children, 50 mg/kg in divided doses every 4 hours. For adolescents, 12 g/d.

Toxicity: Hypersensitivity, kidney damage, and hematuria (the latter is thought to be a hypersensitivity phenomenon) in all age groups with methicillin and in infants with oxacillin. Reversible bone marrow depression occurs. When neutropenia develops with this class of drugs, it sometimes recurs about 10 days after beginning cephalothin (Keflin) therapy. Peak serum drug levels after oral administration vary from patient to patient. With dicloxacillin, 32% of children have peak serum drug levels 2 hours or more after ingestion.

Comment: Deterioration of methicillin in dextrose in water or normal saline solution is rapid and lessened by adding 3 meq of $NaHCO_3$ per liter. If therapy is initiated with a drug in this class because of suspected penicillin resistance, therapy should be changed to penicillin G when sensitivity to this agent is shown. One gram of methicillin contains 2.5 meq of Na^+. Nafcillin causes a false-positive sulfosalicylic acid reaction for urinary protein.

OTHER ANTIBACTERIAL AGENTS (In Alphabetical Order)

Aminosalicylic Acid (PAS)

Use: For treatment of tuberculosis.

Dosage (oral): For children, 250–300 mg/kg/d in divided doses every 6 hours; for salts of PAS, increase dose by 25%. For adolescents, 12 g/d.

Toxicity: Gastrointestinal symptoms, hypersensitivity (skin, fever, general), and renal irritation. Goitrogenic, hematologic, and hepatic effects.

Comment: Avoid or reduce dosage by half when renal function is impaired. Stop drug at first sign of skin rash.

Chloramphenicol (Chloromycetin)

Use: Bacteriostatic for a wide range of gram-positive and gram-negative organisms, rickettsiae, and chlamydiae. Active against most species of *Bacteroides* and anaerobic streptococci. Bactericidal for *Haemophilus influenzae.* For treatment of *Haemophilus* meningitis (including cases due to ampicillin-resistant strains), meningococcal meningitis in penicillin-sensitive persons, *Bacteroides* infections, typhoid fever, brain abscess, and peritonitis.

Dosage:

Oral (crystalline or palmitate): For children, 50–75 mg/kg/d in divided doses every 6 hours. For adolescents, 35–50 mg/kg/d in divided doses every 6 hours.

Intramuscular: Intramuscular injection should not be used, since absorption is poor.

Intravenous (succinate): For children, 15–20 mg/kg every 6 hours. For adolescents, 50–75 mg/kg/d.

Toxicity: In newborns up to 4 months of age, vasomotor collapse (gray syndrome); myocardial depression can also occur at high serum levels at any age. Irreversible aplastic anemia (one in 60,000 cases estimated) and reversible suppression of granulocyte production (associated with peak levels > 35 μg/mL). Gastrointestinal symptoms, stomatitis, and candidal infections. Allergy, hepatitis, optic neuritis, and neurologic abnormalities occur rarely.

Comment: Adjust dose to attain a trough level of 5–10 μg/mL or a peak level of 20–25 μg/mL 60–90 minutes after dose. Dose increases may be necessary if the patient is receiving phenobarbital or rifampin, and dose decreases may be necessary if the patient is receiving phenytoin (Dilantin). Should not be used when an equally effective drug is available. Diffuses better than most penicillins (eyes, cerebrospinal fluid).

Clindamycin (Cleocin)

Use: Active against common anaerobic organisms, including various species of *Bacteroides* and anaerobic streptococci. Most aerobic gram-positive cocci are sensitive, but clindamycin is relatively ineffective against *Streptococcus faecalis, Neisseria gonorrhoeae, Neisseria meningitidis,* and *Haemophilus influenzae.*

Dosage:

Oral: For children, 8–20 mg/kg/d in divided doses every 6–8 hours. For adolescents, 0.6–1.8 g/d in divided doses every 6 hours.

Intravenous: For children, 25–40 mg/kg/d in divided doses every 6–8 hours. For adolescents, 1.8 g/d in divided doses every 6–8 hours.

Toxicity: Gastrointestinal disturbances, pseudomembranous colitis, rash (10% of cases), thrombophlebitis, and sterile abscess.

Comment: If diarrhea develops, the drug should be discontinued, the patient should be examined by sigmoidoscopy to rule out pseudomembranous colitis, or the stool should be assayed for *Clostridium difficile* toxin. Pseudomembranous colitis appears to be an uncommon complication of therapy in children.

Colistin (Coly-Mycin S) & Colistimethate (Coly-Mycin M)

Use: Active against *Pseudomonas aeruginosa* and some strains of *Escherichia coli, Enterobacter,* and *Klebsiella. Proteus* and gram-positive organisms are resistant.

Dosage:

Oral (colistin sulfate): Not absorbed. For children, 15 mg/kg/d in divided doses every 8 hours.

Intramuscular (colistimethate sodium): This agent has little (if any) use. For children, 2.5–5 mg/kg/d in divided doses every 8 hours given deep into a muscle. For adolescents, 2.5–5 mg/kg/d in divided doses every 8 hours.

Toxicity: Proteinuria, cylindruria, hematuria, and increased blood urea nitrogen levels (reversible). Paresthesias, ataxia, drowsiness, and confusion. Fever, rash, and pain at injection site.

Comment: May be used orally for enteropathogenic *E coli* infections. Use with care if renal function is abnormal. Do not use colistimethate intrathecally, because the preparation contains dibucaine.

Erythromycin (Erythrocin, Ilosone, Ilotycin, Pediamycin)

Use: Active against *Legionella, Chlamydia, Bordetella pertussis, Corynebacterium diphtheriae,* rickettsiae, clostridia, *Brucella,* some *Bacteroides,* and some gram-positive cocci. Resistance of some group A streptococci and some pneumococci has been reported, although this is rare at present. Probably as effective as tetracycline for symptomatic relief of *Mycoplasma pneumoniae* infection, although the organisms continue to be shed.

Dosage:

Oral: For children, 30–50 mg/kg/d in divided doses every 6 hours. For adolescents, 2–4 g/d in 4 divided doses.

Intravenous: For children, 10–20 mg/kg/d in divided doses every 6 hours (over a 20- to 60-minute period). For adolescents, 2–8 g/d.

Toxicity: Pain at injection site, gastrointestinal symptoms, candidiasis, and drug fever. Erythromycin estolate (Ilosone) is rarely associated with intrahepatic cholestatic jaundice when treatment is for more than 10 days.

Ethambutol (Myambutol)

Use: For treatment of tuberculosis.

Dosage (oral): Experience in the pediatric age range is limited. For adolescents, 15 mg/kg/d; retreatment, 25 mg/kg/d for 60 days, then 15 mg/kg/d.

Toxicity: Retrobulbar neuritis (3% of cases). Patients should be routinely followed with monthly examination of visual acuity and color discrimination. Anaphylactoid reaction, peripheral neuritis, and hyperuricemia.

Isoniazid (INH; Nydrazid)

Use: For treatment of tuberculosis.

Dosage:

Oral: For children, 10–15 mg/kg as a single dose every 24 hours. For adolescents, 300–500 mg/d.

Intramuscular: For children, 10–15 mg/kg as a single dose every 24 hours. For adolescents, 2.5–5 mg/kg every 24 hours (up to 600 mg/d).

Toxicity: Hepatitis; neurotoxic as a result of pyridoxine deficiency. Gastrointestinal symptoms, seizures, and hypersensitivity.

Comment: Avoid use in patients with preexisting liver disease. Although it is generally stated that addition of pyridoxine is unnecessary in children, exceptions to this rule occur; therefore, routine supplementation with pyridoxine is recommended. Always use with other drugs, such as rifampin, for the treatment of active tuberculosis. Dose should not exceed 10 mg/kg when used with rifampin.

Methenamine Mandelate (Mandelamine)

Use: For treatment of genitourinary infections. Not effective against *Proteus.*

Dosage (oral): For children, 100 mg/kg immediately and then 50 mg/kg/d given in divided doses every 6–8 hours. For adolescents, 4 g/d in divided doses every 6–8 hours.

Toxicity: Gastrointestinal disturbances, rash, and hematuria.

Comment: Urine should be kept acid.

Nalidixic Acid (NegGram)

Use: Useful in uncomplicated gram-negative urinary tract infections with *Escherichia coli, Enterobacter, Klebsiella,* or *Proteus. Pseudomonas* strains are generally resistant.

Dosage (oral): For children, 40–50 mg/kg/d in divided doses every 6 hours; may be reduced to 20–25 mg/kg/d for maintenance therapy. For adolescents, 4 g/d in divided doses every 6 hours; may be reduced to 2 g/d for maintenance therapy.

Toxicity: Gastrointestinal symptoms, hypersensitivity (pruritus, rash, urticaria, and eosinophilia), seizures, pseudotumor cerebri, and pneumonitis.

Comment: Toxicity is low, and the drug may be used for months. Resistance may develop. Use cautiously in patients with liver disease or those with impaired renal function. Do not use in children under 1 month of age or for infections other than those of the urinary tract.

Nitrofurantoin (Furadantin)

Use: Many gram-negative organisms are susceptible to concentrations achieved in urine.

Dosage (oral): For children, 5–7 mg/kg/d; reduce dosage to 2.5–5 mg/kg/d after 10–14 days. For adolescents, 400 mg/d in divided doses every 6 hours.

Toxicity: Primaquine-sensitive hemolytic anemia, peripheral neuropathy, rash, chills, fever, myalgialike syndrome, and cholestatic jaundice.

Comment: Used only for urinary tract infections.

Rifampin (Rifadin, Rimactane)

Use: Active against *Neisseria, Mycobacterium, Staphylococcus aureus,* and some enteric bacteria.

Dosage (oral): Not available in solution; suspensions in Supalta solution made by the pharmacist are stable for 6 weeks if kept in an amber bottle at 4 °C.

For treatment of tuberculosis: For children, place contents of 300-mg capsule in 1 tablespoon of applesauce or pudding (each teaspoonful equals 100 mg) and administer 15 mg/kg once daily; mix freshly each time. For adolescents, 600 mg/d.

For treatment of carriers of *Neisseria meningitidis*: For children, 20 mg/kg/d in divided doses every 12 hours for 2 days (10 mg/kg/d for children 1 year of age). For adults, 1200 mg/d in divided doses every 12 hours for 2 days.

For treatment of carriers of *Haemophilus influenzae*: For children, 20 mg/kg once daily for 4 days (10 mg/kg/d for children under 1 year of age). For adults, 600 mg/d once daily for 4 days.

Toxicity: Hepatotoxicity has been reported, especially when used with isoniazid. AST (SGOT) levels should be followed when used with isoniazid.

Comment: The most striking contribution of rifampin has been in the care of patients infected with resistant strains of *Mycobacterium tuberculosis.* The main indications for its use in children are (1) contact with an adult with a drug-resistant strain, (2) isoniazid intolerance, (3) isoniazid resistance, and (4) meningitis due to *M tuberculosis.* Although the results have been good, when used alone the development of resistance is rapid; therefore, the drug should always be used in combination with one or 2 drugs to which the organisms are sensitive. In addition, rifampin is effective in reducing the carrier state due to *N meningitidis* and *H influenzae,* but the development of rifampin resistance is relatively common.

Sulfonamides: Sulfadiazine, Sulfamethoxazole (Gantanol), Sulfisoxazole (Gantrisin), & Trisulfapyrimidines

Use: Bacteriostatic for gram-positive and gram-negative organisms. Active against *Nocardia.* Approximately 80% of shigellae are resistant. Useful in urinary tract infections and rheumatic fever prophylaxis. (Should not be used for treatment of active group A streptococcal infection.)

Dosage:

Sulfadiazine, sulfisoxazole, or trisulfapyrimidines: For children, 120–150 mg/kg/d orally in divided doses every 6 hours or 120 mg/kg/d intravenously in divided doses every 6–12 hours (alkalinize urine). For adolescents, 2–4 g/d orally in divided doses every 6 hours or 2–6 g/d intravenously in divided doses every 6–12 hours.

Sulfamethoxazole: For children, 50 mg/kg/d orally in divided doses every 12 hours. For adolescents, 1–3 g/d orally in divided doses every 8–12 hours.

Toxicity: To prevent crystalluria (mechanical urinary obstruction), *keep fluid intake high.* Hypersensitivity (fever, rash, hepatitis, lupuslike state, and vasculitis). Neutropenia, agranulocytosis, aplastic anemia, and thrombocytopenia. Hemolytic anemia in individuals deficient in glucose 6-phosphate dehydrogenase (G6PD deficiency is seen in association with sickle cell anemia).

Comment: Sulfadiazine is preferred for central nervous system infections, since diffusion into cerebrospinal fluid is better. Sulfamethoxazole is intermediate-acting and has a slightly greater propensity than sulfisoxazole for causing urinary sediment abnormalities.

Tetracyclines: Chlortetracycline, Doxycycline, Minocycline, Oxytetracycline, & Tetracycline (many trade names)

Use: Active against gram-positive bacteria, rickettsiae, chlamydiae, *Mycoplasma pneumoniae, Brucella, Bacteroides,* and some gram-negative bacteria. Many gram-negative bacteria are resistant.

Dosage:

Tetracycline, chlortetracycline, or oxytetracycline: For children, 20–40 mg/kg/d orally in divided doses every 6 hours (do not give with milk) or 15–25 mg/kg/d intramuscularly in divided doses every 12 hours (achieves poor levels; painful). For adolescents, 1–2 g/d orally in divided doses every 6 hours or 250–300 mg/d intramuscularly in divided doses every 8–24 hours. Intravenous therapy is used only in rare circumstances.

Doxycycline or minocycline: For children, 4 mg/kg orally once; then 2–2.5 mg/kg orally every 12 hours. For adolescents, 200 mg orally once; then 100 mg orally every 12 hours.

Toxicity: In children under 8 years of age, tetracyclines cause damage to teeth and bones. Deposition in teeth and bones of premature and newborn infants can result in enamel dysplasia and growth retardation. Outdated tetracyclines can produce Fanconi's syndrome. Other adverse effects include pseudotumor cerebri, bulging fontanelles, nausea, vomiting, diarrhea, stomatitis, glossitis, proctitis, candidiasis, overgrowth of staphylococci in bowel, disturbed hepatic and renal function, drug fever, rash, and photosensitivity.

Comment: Cross-resistance among the tetracyclines is complete. Minocycline, however, offers an advantage at this time over other tetracyclines in the therapy of carriers of *Neisseria meningitidis,* but it has been reported to cause vestibular dysfunction with high frequency.

Trimethoprim-Sulfamethoxazole (Co-trimoxazole; Bactrim, Septra)

Use: A combination agent with a wide range of activity against gram-positive and gram-negative organisms. Most promising therapeutic applications are in chronic or recurrent urinary tract infections with sensitive organisms. Beneficial in certain *Salmonella* and *Shigella* infections and in *Pneumocystis carinii* infections.

Dosage (oral or intravenous): Combination tablets contain 80 mg of trimethoprim and 400 mg of sulfamethoxazole; 5 mL of suspension contains 40 mg of trimethoprim and 200 mg of sulfamethoxazole. The intravenous route is used in rare instances. For children, give trimethoprim, 8–10 mg/kg/d, and sulfamethoxazole, 40–50 mg/kg/d, orally in divided doses every 12 hours; for serious gram-negative infections and for therapy of *P carinii* infections, give trimethoprim, 20 mg/kg/d, and sulfamethoxazole, 100 mg/kg/d, in divided doses orally or intravenously every 6–8 hours; and for *Pneumocystis* prophylaxis, give trimethoprim, 4 mg/kg/d, and sulfamethoxazole, 20 mg/kg/d, in divided doses orally every 12 hours. For adolescents, give trimethoprim, 160 mg, and sulfamethoxazole, 800 mg, orally every 12 hours.

Toxicity: Kernicterus in newborns. Gastrointestinal irritation, bone marrow depression, and allergic reactions. Should not be used in patients with renal or liver disease or blood dyscrasias, patients with a history of hypersensitivity to sulfonamides, or those with G6PD deficiency. Use in pregnancy is not recommended, since large doses are teratogenic in animals.

Vancomycin (Vancocin)

Use: Active against staphylococci, other gram-positive cocci, clostridia, and corynebacteria. Main use is in treatment of pseudomembranous enterocolitis, severe disseminated staphylococcal disease, and methicillin-resistant staphylococcal infection. Has been used successfully in the treatment of subacute bacterial endocarditis, osteomyelitis, shunt infections, and serious soft tissue infections. Oral doses are effective in pseudomembranous enterocolitis associated with *Clostridium difficile.*

Dosage:

Oral: Not absorbed. For children and adolescents, 20–40 mg/kg/d in divided doses every 6 hours.

Intravenous: For children, 40 mg/kg/d in divided doses every 6 hours. For adolescents, 2 g/d in divided doses every 12 hours. Infusion should be over a minimum of 1 hour. Concomitant administration of corticosteroids may be necessary.

Intramuscular: Painful when given intramuscularly; do not use.

Toxicity: Troublesome symptoms during intravenous administration include hypotension, rash, chills, thrombophlebitis, and fever. Nephrotoxicity and ototoxicity have occurred, most commonly when an aminoglycoside has been administered concurrently.

ANTIFUNGAL AGENTS

Amphotericin B (Fungizone)

Use: Active against *Candida, Cryptococcus, Blastomyces, Sporotrichum, Coccidioides,* and *Histoplasma.*

Dosage:

Intravenous: For children and adolescents, 0.6 mg/kg/d or 1 mg/kg every other day, given over 1–4 hours; begin as 0.2 mg/kg/d and increase by 0.2 mg/kg per dose.

Intrathecal, intraventricular, or cisternal: For children and adolescents, 0.5–1 mg in 10 mL spinal fluid every other day; begin with 0.1 mg and increase.

Toxicity: Chills, fever, and malaise. Significant renal, hepatic, and bone marrow damage. Thrombophlebitis and calcifications.

Comment: Indicated only in severe systemic fungal infections. Administration of corticosteroids, diphenhydramine, and acetaminophen before the daily dose of amphotericin is given may ameliorate side effects.

Flucytosine (Ancobon)

Use: Active against some strains of *Candida, Cryptococcus neoformans,* and *Torulopsis glabrata.*

Dosage (oral): For children and adolescents, 50–150 mg/kg/d in divided doses every 6 hours.

Toxicity: Rash, diarrhea, and hepatic dysfunction. Serious toxicity (leukopenia, thrombocytopenia, and enterocolitis) can develop when flucytosine is used in patients with impaired renal function or when it is administered concomitantly with amphotericin B.

Comment: Ninety percent of the drug is excreted in urine. Drug resistance has been reported during therapy. Sensitivity studies are indicated. Currently, it is suggested that patients on therapy be followed with measurements of creatinine or blood urea nitrogen, AST (SGOT), and alkaline phosphatase levels; hemoglobin concentrations; and white blood cell counts.

Griseofulvin (Fulvicin U/F or P/G, Grifulvin V, Grisactin)

Use: Active against *Microsporum* and *Trichophyton.* Ineffective against *Candida, Cryptococcus, Blastomyces, Histoplasma,* and *Coccidioides.*

Dosage (oral):

Griseofulvin microsize: For children, 10 mg/kg once daily; for difficult infections, twice daily. For adolescents, 500 mg once daily; for difficult infections, twice daily.

Griseofulvin ultramicrosize: For children, 5 mg/kg once daily; for difficult infections, twice daily. For adolescents, 250 mg once daily; for difficult infections, twice daily.

Toxicity: Leukopenia and other blood dyscrasias, headache, incoordination and confusion, gastrointestinal disturbances, rash (allergic and photosensitivity), renal damage, and lupuslike syndrome.

Comment: Do not use in patients with hepatocellular failure or porphyria.

Ketoconazole (Nizoral)

Use: Active against *Candida, Coccidioides, Histoplasma,* and dermatophytes.

Dosage (oral): For patients weighing less than 20 kg, 50 mg once daily; 20–40 kg, 100 mg once daily; and more than 40 kg, 200–400 mg once daily (up to 8 mg/kg/d). For treatment of coccidioidal meningitis, 20 mg/kg once daily.

Toxicity: Hepatocellular dysfunction, gynecomastia, depressed testosterone levels with prolonged use, and depressed cortisol levels while drug is in bloodstream. Nausea, vomiting, abdominal pain, pruritus, headache, somnolence, and dizziness.

Comment: Useful in chronic mucocutaneous candidiasis and probably of benefit in *Candida* esophagitis. Indicated as adjunctive therapy for some forms of systemic mycosis. (Doses of up to 30 mg/kg/d are being studied for efficacy in treating systemic mycoses and for toxicity.) Patients receiving long-term therapy should have liver function tests performed monthly. Antacids decrease ketoconazole absorption; administer the dose at least 2 hours after ingestion of antacids. Gastrointestinal side effects are decreased by administration with meals or at bedtime.

Miconazole (Monistat)

Use: For treatment of coccidioidomycosis, candidiasis, cryptococcosis, and paracoccidioidomycosis.

Dosage:

Intravenous: For children, 15 mg/kg every 8 hours, given over 30–60 minutes. For adolescents, 200–1200 mg every 8 hours, given over 30–60 minutes.

Intraventricular: For children and adolescents with coccidioidal meningitis, 3–5 mg per dose.

Toxicity: Phlebitis, pruritus, rash, anorexia, nausea, vomiting, fever, drowsiness, flushes, and peripheral neuritis. Anemia, hyponatremia, and thrombocytopenia. Enhances action of coumarin drugs.

Nystatin (Mycostatin)

Use: Active against *Candida albicans* and other yeasts.

Dosage:

Oral: Not absorbed. For children under 2 years of age, 400,000–800,000 units/d; for children over 2 years of age and for adolescents, 1–2 million units/d in divided doses every 6–8 hours.

Topical: For all patients, 100,000 units/d to treat eye or skin infection.

Toxicity: None.

ANTIPARASITIC AGENTS

Chloroquine (Aralen)

Use: Active against *Plasmodium vivax, Plasmodium malariae, Plasmodium ovale,* and chloroquine-sensitive strains of *Plasmodium falciparum.*

Dosage (oral):

Chloroquine phosphate (for treatment): For children, 10 mg/kg base (16.6 mg salt) once; then 5 mg/kg base at 6, 24, and 48 hours. For adolescents, 600 mg base (1 g salt) once; then 300 mg base at 6, 24, and 48 hours.

Chloroquine phosphate (for prophylaxis): For children, 5 mg/kg base (8.3 mg salt) once a week beginning 1–2 weeks before entry to endemic area and continuing until 6 weeks after leaving area. For adolescents, 300 mg base (500 mg salt) once a week beginning 1–2 weeks before entry to endemic area and continuing until 6 weeks after leaving area.

Chloroquine sulfate (for prophylaxis): For children, 5 mg/kg base (6.8 mg salt) once a week during exposure and for 6 weeks after leaving endemic area. For adolescents, 300 mg base (410 mg salt) once a week during exposure and for 6 weeks after leaving endemic area.

Toxicity: Headaches, visual disturbances, gastrointestinal upset, pruritus, confusion, and agitation.

Furazolidone (Furoxone)

Use: Active against *Giardia* and *Vibrio cholerae* (also has antibacterial activity).

Dosage (oral): For children, 8 mg/kg/d in 3–4 divided doses for 10 days. For adolescents, 100 mg every 6 hours for 10 days.

Toxicity: Nausea, vomiting, abdominal pain, diarrhea, and brownish discoloration of urine.

Comment: Tolerated well by children but is expensive and requires a large volume of medication, since concentration of the suspension is 50 mg/15 mL.

Mebendazole (Vermox)

Use: Active against *Trichuris, Enterobius, Ascaris, Ancylostoma,* and *Necator.*

Dosage:

Oral: For anyone over 2 years of age with *Enterobius* infection, one 100-mg tablet once. For those with *Ascaris, Trichuris, Ancylostoma,* or *Necator* infection, one 100-mg tablet twice a day for 3 days and repeat dosage in 3 weeks if infection persists.

Intravenous: For children and adolescents, 15 mg/kg loading dose; then 7.5 mg/kg every 6–8 hours (up to 4 g/d).

Toxicity: Neutropenia, thrombophlebitis (with intravenous administration), seizures, and peripheral neuropathy. Increases serum warfarin levels. Use with alcohol or disulfiram may produce psychotic state or confusion.

Comment: Contraindicated in pregnancy.

Metronidazole (Flagyl, Metryl)

Use: For treatment of trichomoniasis, giardiasis, and amebiasis (also has activity in anaerobic infections).

Dosage:

Oral: For children, 15–50 mg/kg/d in divided doses every 8 hours. For adolescents, 250 mg every 8 hours.

Intravenous: For children and adolescents, 30–50 mg/kg/d in divided doses.

Toxicity: Nausea, anorexia, and other gastrointestinal effects. Glossitis, stomatitis, leukopenia, dizziness, vertigo, ataxia, urticaria, and pruritus.

Comment: Has been used for treatment of giardiasis or amebic dysentery in children in doses up to 50 mg/kg/d.

Niclosamide (Niclocide)

Use: Active against *Taenia saginata, Diphyllobothrium latum,* and *Hymenolepis nana.*

Dosage (oral):

For treatment of *T saginata* or *D latum* infection: For children weighing 11–34 kg, 2 tablets (1 g) chewed thoroughly as a single dose. For children over 34 kg, 3 tablets (1.5 g) chewed thoroughly as a single dose. For adolescents, 4 tablets (2 g) chewed thoroughly as a single dose.

For treatment of *H nana* infection: For children weighing 11–34 kg, 2 tablets (1 g) chewed thoroughly on day 1 and 1 tablet (0.5 g) chewed thoroughly on days 2–7. For children over 34 kg, 3 tablets (1.5 g) chewed thoroughly on day 1 and 2 tablets (1 g) chewed thoroughly on days 2–7. For adolescents, 4 tablets (2 g) chewed thoroughly as a single dose on days 1–7.

Toxicity: Nausea, loose stools, and abdominal pain.

Comment: To ensure ingestion by young children, crush tablet and mix with water to form paste. Treat again if segments or ova of *T saginata* or *D latum* are present after day 7. Not effective in extraintestinal infections (cysticercosis).

Praziquantel (Biltricide)

Use: For treatment of schistosomiasis, clonorchiasis, paragonimiasis, and cysticercosis; perhaps also useful in treatment of echinococcosis.

Dosage (oral): For children and adolescents, 75 mg/kg/d in 3 divided doses for 1 day; for cysticercosis, give 50–60 mg/kg/d in 3 divided doses for 15 days.

Toxicity: Gastrointestinal upset most common. May need to treat simultaneously with dexamethasone in cerebral cysticercosis when intracranial pressure is elevated.

Primaquine

Use: For eradication of *Plasmodium vivax* or *Plasmodium ovale* from exoerythrocytic sites.

Dosage (oral): For children, 0.3 mg/kg/d base (0.5 mg salt) for 14 days. For adolescents, 15 mg/d base (26.3 mg salt) for 14 days.

Toxicity: Can cause hemolytic anemia in persons with G6PD deficiency.

Quinacrine (Atabrine)

Use: Active against *Giardia*.

Dosage (oral): For children and adolescents, 6 mg/kg/d in 3 divided doses (up to 300 mg/d).

Toxicity: Nausea, vomiting, diarrhea, toxic hepatic necrosis, acute psychosis, aplastic anemia, and hemolysis in G6PD deficiency. Diffuse yellow skin pigmentation.

Sulfadoxine-Pyrimethamine (Fansidar)

Use: Active against chloroquine-resistant *Plasmodium falciparum*.

Dosage (oral): Each Fansidar tablet contains 500 mg of sulfadoxine plus 25 mg of pyrimethamine.

Sulfadoxine-pyrimethamine (for treatment, single dose): For patients 2–11 months of age, ¼ tablet; 1–3 years of age, ½ tablet; 4–8 years, 1 tablet; and 9–14 years, 2 tablets. For adolescents, 2–3 tablets.

Sulfadoxine-pyrimethamine plus chloroquine (for prophylaxis): Administer weekly from 1–2 days before departure through 4–6 weeks after return. For patients 2–11 months of age, ⅛ tablet; 1–3 years of age, ¼ tablet; 4–8 years, ½ tablet; and 9–14 years, ¾ tablet of sulfadoxine-pyrimethamine. For adolescents, 1 tablet of sulfadoxine-pyrimethamine. For chloroquine treatment, see above.

Toxicity: Same as trimethoprim-sulfamethoxazole (see above). Crystalluria (keep fluid intake high). Hemolysis in presence of G6PD deficiency. Folate deficiency. Severe cutaneous reactions, including Stevens-Johnson syndrome.

Comment: Contraindications are age less than 2 months, breast feeding, pregnancy, and hypersensitivity to either drug. Chloroquine must be used along with sulfadoxine-pyrimethamine in areas in which any of the other types of malaria coexist with chloroquine-resistant *P falciparum*. Folinic acid can be given if signs of folinic acid deficiency occur. Strains of *P falciparum* resistant to this drug combination now occur and must be treated with quinine and tetracycline or with quinine, pyrimethamine, and sulfadiazine.

Thiabendazole (Mintezol)

Use: For treatment of cutaneous larva migrans and infections due to *Ascaris, Trichuris, Enterobius, Ancylostoma, Necator americanus,* or *Strongyloides*.

Dosage (oral): For children and adolescents, 25 mg/kg twice a day up to a total daily dose of 3 g/d: for 4 days for *Trichuris* infection; for 2 days for *Ascaris, Ancylostoma, N americanus,* or *Strongyloides* infection or cutaneous larva migrans; and for 1 day for *Enterobius* infection and repeat once 7 days later.

Toxicity: Anorexia, nausea, vomiting, dizziness, angioneurotic edema, and pruritus.

ANTIVIRAL AGENTS

Few therapeutic agents are available for viral infections. The following drugs have some usefulness.

OPHTHALMIC ANTIVIRAL AGENTS

Trifluridine (Viroptic) & Vidarabine (Adenine Arabinoside; Vira-A)

Use: At present, limited to treatment of acute superficial herpes simplex or vaccinia virus keratitis.

Dosage (ophthalmic):

Trifluridine: For any patient, solution (1%) should be used initially; place 1 drop in each infected eye every hour while awake and every 2 hours at night; with definite improvement, decrease to every 2 hours around the clock and continue treatment for 7 days after healing appears to be complete.

Vidarabine: For any patient, ointment (3%) is administered 5 times a day (every 3 hours).

Toxicity: Too frequent administration may lead to small punctate defects in the cornea.

Comment: Should be administered under an ophthalmologist's supervision. Some prefer concomitant local corticosteroid administration.

TOPICAL ANTIVIRAL AGENTS

Acyclovir (Zovirax)

Use: For treatment of initial genital infections due to herpes simplex virus and severe local infections in the immunocompromised host.

Dosage (topical): For adolescents, apply sufficient 5% ointment (by use of a finger sheath) to adequately cover all lesions.

Toxicity: Possible discomfort and burning on application.

Comment: Should not be used for prevention of recurrent genital lesions.

SYSTEMIC ANTIVIRAL AGENTS

Acyclovir (Zovirax)

Use: For treatment of disseminated varicella-zoster virus infections in the immunocompromised host, severe herpes simplex infections in the immunocompromised host, and severe initial attacks of genital herpes. Treatment of other infections due to herpes simplex is still under investigation.

Dosage (intravenous): For infants, children, and adolescents, 10 mg/kg administered over 1 hour and repeated every 8 hours.

Toxicity: Can precipitate in kidneys and cause acute renal failure if given as bolus or if urine flow is not adequate. Adjust dose downward in patients with renal dysfunction. Phlebitis and rash. Rarely, encephalopathic changes (jitters, lethargy, tremors, and confusion).

Amantadine (Symmetrel)

Use: Prophylactic administration during identified influenza A virus epidemics.

Dosage (oral): For children 1–9 years of age, 4.4–8.8 mg/kg/d (do not exceed 150 mg/d) in 1 or 2 doses. For children 9–12 years of age, 200 mg/d in 1 or 2 doses. For adolescents, 200 mg/d in 1 or 2 doses.

Toxicity: Central nervous system irritability (nervousness, insomnia, dizziness, light-headedness, feelings of drunkenness, slurred speech, ataxia, and inability to concentrate). Occasional depression and feelings of detachment; blurred vision (heightened with higher dosage, 300–400 mg/d, in elderly); less commonly, dry mouth, gastrointestinal upset, and skin rash. Rarely, tremors, anorexia, pollakiuria, and nocturia. Use with care and consider reduced dosage in patients with seizure disorders or renal insufficiency.

Comment: Amantadine can ameliorate influenza A illness if started within 24–48 hours of onset and continued for 5–7 days. Does not appear to interfere with immunity induced by vaccination.

Ribavirin (Virazole)

Use: Investigational drug. Major pediatric use is for treatment of severe lower respiratory tract infections caused by respiratory syncytial, influenza A or B, and parainfluenza viruses.

Dosage (aerosol): For infants, administered as a continuous small-particle aerosol, 18 hours per day for 3–8 days or longer, until clinical improvement is clearly apparent.

Toxicity: Occasional mild decrease in white blood cell count or rise in liver enzyme levels.

Vidarabine (Adenine Arabinoside; Vira-A)

Use: For treatment of disseminated varicella-zoster infections, herpes simplex encephalitis, and neonatal herpes simplex infections. Not indicated for treatment of genital infections due to herpes simplex virus.

Dosage (intravenous): For neonates, children, and adolescents, 15 mg/kg/d as continuous infusion over 12 hours.

Toxicity: Water intoxication due to necessity of administering drug in a relatively dilute form owing to its insolubility. Anorexia, nausea, neutropenia, thrombocytopenia, and elevated AST (SGOT) levels. Rarely, tremors, aphasia, dizziness, and confusion. Rash. Use with care in patients with impaired renal or hepatic function.

SELECTED REFERENCES

Adler SP, Markowitz SM: Failure of moxalactam in the treatment of neonatal sepsis and meningitis from *Salmonella typhimurium*. *J Pediatr* 1983;**103:**913.

Alpert G et al: Vancomycin dosage in pediatrics reconsidered. *Am J Dis Child* 1984;**138:**20.

Axelrod JL et al: Ceftazidime concentrations in human aqueous humor. *Arch Ophthalmol* 1984;**102:**923.

Barson WJ, Miller MA: Relapse of *Haemophilus influenzae* type b meningitis following therapy with ceftriaxone. *Pediatr Infect Dis* 1984;**3:**241.

Brown CH et al: The hemostatic defect produced by carbenicillin. *N Engl J Med* 1984;**291:**265.

Bryson YJ: The use of amantadine in children for prophylaxis and treatment of influenza A infections. *Pediatr Infect Dis* 1982;**1:**44.

Bryson YJ et al: Treatment of first episodes of genital herpes simplex virus infection with oral acyclovir: A randomized double-blind controlled trial in normal subjects. *N Engl J Med* 1983;**308:**916.

Conlon CP, Ellis CJ: Praziquantel. *J Antimicrob Chemother* 1985;**15:**1.

Cox F et al: Rifampin prophylaxis for contacts of *Haemophilus influenzae* type B disease. *JAMA* 1981;**245:**103.

Craft JC, Murphy T, Nelson JD: Furazolidone and quinacrine: Comparative study of therapy for giardiasis in children. *Am J Dis Child* 1981;**135:**164.

Dolin R: Antiviral chemotherapy and chemoprophylaxis. *Science* 1985;**227:**1296.

Drusano GL et al: The acyclampicillins: Mezlocillin, piperacillin and azlocillin. *Rev Infect Dis* 1984;**6:**13.

Faden H et al: Renal and auditory toxic effects of amikacin in children with cancer. *Am J Dis Child* 1982;**136:**223.

Finitzo-Hieber T et al: Prospective controlled evaluation of auditory function in neonates given netilmicin or amikacin. *J Pediatr* 1985;**106:**129.

George WL et al: Intravenous metronidazole for treatment of infections involving anaerobic bacteria. *Antimicrob Agents Chemother* 1982;**21:**441.

Ginsburg CM, McCracken GH Jr, Olsen K: Pharmacology of ketoconazole suspension in infants and children. *Antimicrob Agents Chemother* 1983;**23:**787.

Granati B et al: Clinical pharmacology of netilmicin in preterm and term newborn infants. *J Pediatr* 1985;**106:**664.

Greenberg RN et al: Treatment of serious gram-negative infections with aztreonam. *J Infect Dis* 1984;**150:**623.

Gutman LT: The use of trimethoprim-sulfamethoxazole in children: A review of adverse reactions and indications. *Pediatr Infect Dis* 1984;**3:**349.

Higlam M et al: Ceftriaxone administered once or twice a day for treatment of bacterial infections of childhood. *Pediatr Infect Dis* 1985;**4:**22.

Hintz M et al: Neonatal acyclovir pharmacokinetics in patients with herpes virus infections. *Am J Med* 1982;**73:**210.

Hoecker JL: Clinical pharmacology of tobramycin in children. *J Infect Dis* 1978;**137:**593.

Kafetzis DA et al: Treatment of severe neonatal infections with cefotaxime: Efficacy and pharmacokinetics. *J Pediatr* 1982;**100:**483.

Kaplan SL et al: Prospective comparative trial of moxalactam versus ampicillin or chloramphenicol for treatment of *Haemophilus influenzae* type b meningitis in children. *J Pediatr* 1984;**104:**447.

Kasik JW et al: Postconceptional age and gentamicin elimination half-life. *J Pediatr* 1985;**106:**502.

Krasinski K, Kusmiesz H, Nelson JD: Pharmacologic interactions among chloramphenicol, phenytoin and phenobarbital. *Pediatr Infect Dis* 1982;**1:**232.

Laskin OL et al: Effects of probenecid on the pharmacokinetics and elimination of acyclovir in humans. *Antimicrob Agents Chemother* 1982;**21:**804.

Leff RD et al: Simplified gentamicin dosing in neonates: A time- and cost-efficient approach. *Pediatr Infect Dis* 1984;**3:**208.

Markowitz SM: Nafcillin-induced agranulocytosis. *JAMA* 1975;**232:**1150.

Martin E et al: Pharmacokinetics of ceftriaxone in neonates and infants with meningitis. *J Pediatr* 1984;**105:**475.

Marx CM, Alpert SE: Ticarcillin-induced cystitis. *Am J Dis Child* 1984;**138:**670.

Matzke GR et al: Pharmacokinetics of vancomycin in patients with various degrees of renal functions. *Antimicrob Agents Chemother* 1984;**25:**433.

McCracken GH Jr, Threlkeld NE, Thomas ML: Pharmacokinetics of cefotaxime in newborn infants. *Antimicrob Agents Chemother* 1982;**21:**683.

McCracken GH Jr et al: Moxalactam therapy for neonatal meningitis due to gram-negative enteric bacilli. *JAMA* 1984;**252:**1427.

Mulhall A, de Louvois J: The pharmacokinetics and safety of ceftazidime in the neonate. *J Antimicrob Chemother* 1985;**15:**97.

Nelson JD: Cefuroxime: A cephalosporin with unique applicability to pediatric practice. *Pediatr Infect Dis* 1983;**2:**394.

Nelson JD, McCracken GH Jr: Mezlocillin and related antibiotics. *Pediatr Infect Dis* 1982;**1:**42.

Nelson JD et al: Cefuroxime therapy for pneumonia in infants and children. *Pediatr Infect Dis* 1982;**1:**159.

Odio C et al: Nephrotoxicity associated with vancomycin-aminoglycoside therapy in four children. *J Pediatr* 1984;**105:**491.

Padoan R et al: Ceftazidime in treatment of acute pulmonary exacerbations in patients with cystic fibrosis. *J Pediatr* 1983;**103:**320.

Salzer W, Pegram PS Jr, McCall CE: Clinical evaluation of moxalactam: Evidence of decreased efficacy in gram-positive aerobic infections. *Antimicrob Agents Chemother* 1983;**23:**565.

Saxon A et al: Lack of cross-reactivity between aztreonam, a monobactam antibiotic, and penicillin in penicillin-allergic subjects. *J Infect Dis* 1984;**149:**16.

Schaad UB et al: An extended experience with cefuroxime therapy of childhood bacterial meningitis. *Pediatr Infect Dis* 1984;**3:**410.

Scully BE, New HX: Clinical efficacy of ceftazidime. *Arch Intern Med* 1984;**144:**57.

Shankaran S, Kauffman RE: Use of chloramphenicol palmitate in neonates. *J Pediatr* 1984;**105:**113.

Siber GR: Pedictability of peak serum gentamicin concentration with dosage based on body surface area. *J Pediatr* 1979;**94:**135.

Steele RW: Ceftriaxone: Decreasing the half-life and activity of third-generation cephalosporins. *Pediatr Infect Dis* 1985;**4:**188.

Steele RW, Bradsher RW: Comparison of ceftriaxone with standard therapy for bacterial meningitis. *J Pediatr* 1983;**103:**138.

Stutman HR et al: Potential of moxalactam and other new antimicrobial agents for bilirubin-albumin displacement in neonates. *Pediatrics* 1985;**75:**294.

Tuckman AJ et al: Cerebrospinal fluid penetration of anti-infective agents. *South Med J* 1984;**77:**1443.

Tuomanen EI et al: Oral chloramphenicol in the treatment of *Haemophilus influenzae* meningitis. *J Pediatr* 1981;**99:**968.

Vogelstein B, Kowarski A, Lietman PS: The pharmacokinetics of amikacin in children. *J Pediatr* 1977;**91:**333.

Weitekamp MR, Aber RC: Prolonged bleeding times and bleeding diathesis associated with moxalactam administration. *JAMA* 1983;**249:**69.

Whitley RJ et al: Vidarabine therapy of neonatal herpes simplex virus infection. *Pediatrics* 1980;**66:**495.

Wilkinson JD et al: Chloramphenicol toxicity: Hemodynamic and oxygen utilization effects. *Pediatr Infect Dis* 1985;**4:**69.

Wilson CB et al: Piperacillin pharmacokinetics in pediatric patients. *Antimicrob Agents Chemother* 1982;**22:**442.

Wilson R, Feldman S: Toxicity of amphotericin B in children with cancer. *Am J Dis Child* 1979;**133:**731.

Yaeger AS: Use of acyclovir in premature and term neonates. *Am J Med* 1982;**73:**205.

Zarfin Y et al: Possible indomethacin-aminoglycoside interaction in preterm infants. *J Pediatr* 1985;**106:**511.

39 Normal & Therapeutic Biochemical & Hematologic Values

Donough O'Brien, MD, FRCP, & Keith B. Hammond, MS, FIMLS

Pediatricians and other health professionals caring for children have the responsibility to insist on accurate, rapid, and comprehensive laboratory testing. Collecting large blood samples for biochemical assay is not suitable for the proper care of children—especially for premature infants or older children in intensive care, where repetitive sampling may be essential. Technology for performing biochemical assays on blood samples of 100 μL or less has been available for 30 years or more. Most of the earlier automated systems for assay were better adapted to larger samples, and thus many central laboratories continued to request these. However, the newest automated systems have the capacity to work with small volumes.

In infants and young children, blood samples attained by heel-prick are better collected by laboratory personnel than by physicians or nurses.

INTERPRETATION OF LABORATORY VALUES

Accreditation by the American College of Pathologists and by state or federal agencies has done much to ensure standardized laboratory working conditions. Methods employed in various laboratories differ, as do normal values for the methods. Normal range is, of course, a combination of biologic variation and of intrinsic laboratory variation; thus, an acceptable range of normal values should be composed of data developed within the laboratory for the population it serves. Any laboratory should be able to provide information on the coefficient of variation and standard deviation applicable to each test performed in that laboratory. Each laboratory should maintain a rigorous procedure of checks with daily standards and control specimens. Errors may still occur but can usually be detected by retesting before a questionable result is reported. Fortunately, errors occur much less commonly today than in the past.

The range of normal values may be narrow or wide, depending upon the test. Serum sodium or bilirubin levels should be accurate within narrow limits, whereas a wider range is clinically acceptable with serum cholesterol or insulin levels, for example.

The clinical value of a test—especially a screening test—is related to its sensitivity and specificity. Sensitivity is an expression of the incidence of positive test results in those who have the disease. Specificity is an expression of the incidence of negative test results in those free of the disease. Sensitivity and specificity are calculated as follows:

$$\text{Sensitivity \%} = \frac{\text{TP}}{\text{TP} + \text{FN}} \times 100 \text{ (ie, how many TP are missed)}$$

$$\text{Specificity \%} = \frac{\text{TN}}{\text{TN} + \text{FP}} \times 100 \text{ (ie, how many TN are missed)}$$

where TP = true-positive result; FP = false-positive result; TN = true-negative result; and FN = false-negative result.

Screening tests must be interpreted with appreciation of sensitivity and specificity. These expressions are illustrated in Fig 39–1 in terms of a screening test for phenylketonuria in newborns. The figures are not strictly correct but serve the purpose of illustration. According to Fig 39–1, a blood phenylalanine level of 4 mg/dL is the discriminating point above which all infants are presumed to have the disease and below which they are presumed to be normal. However, no test is ever quite that exact. Some normal infants will have levels above 4 mg/dL; the test results in these will be false positive. Some abnormal infants will have levels below 4 mg/dL; the test results in these will be false negative. The discriminating point is a compromise between sensitivity and specificity. Moving the point to 2 mg/dL would effect 100% sensitivity, but there would be a large increase in the number of false-positive results. Moving it to 6 mg/dL would make it very specific, but this would increase the number of false-negative responses, which would result in failure to detect phenylketonuria in a much larger proportion of affected children.

These concepts can be viewed in yet another way. Suppose this test were set at a specificity of 99.9%. This would mean that in a sample of 10,000 tests, there would be 10 false-positive results. In a rare condition like phenylketonuria, however, the true incidence of the disease may be only 1 in 12,000. The ratio of true- to false-positive results is thus 1:12;

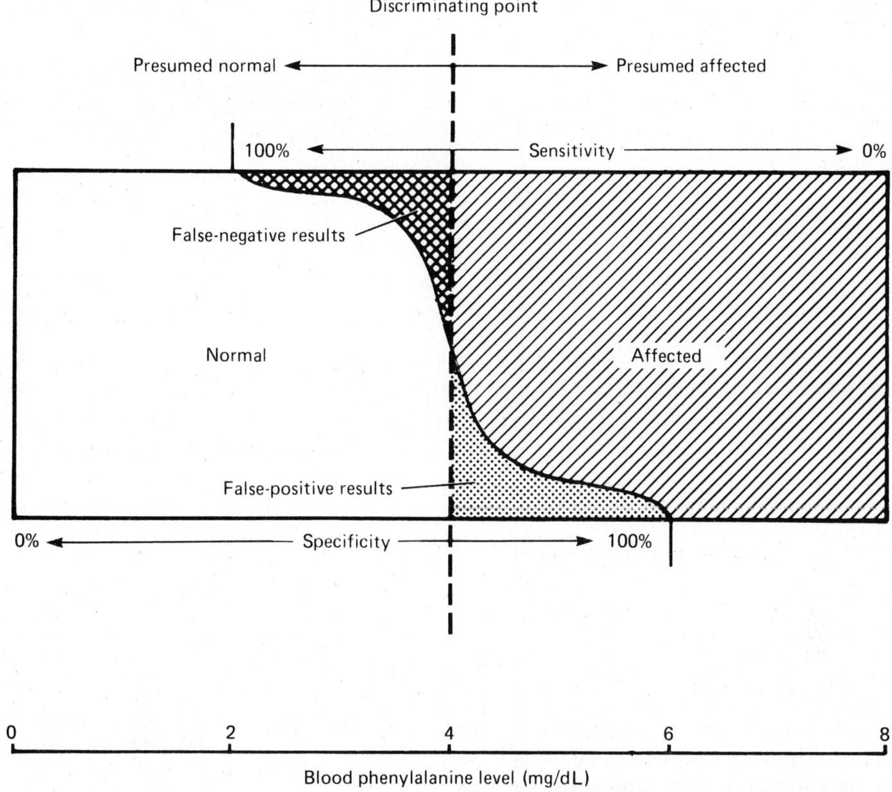

Figure 39–1. Screening test for phenylketonuria in newborns. Data have been simplified to illustrate the concepts of sensitivity and specificity (see text).

this is a reflection of the low incidence of the disease and the relatively high incidence of false-positive results due to the nature of the assay. These considerations, of course, apply to the interpretation of all laboratory tests.

LABORATORY VALUES

Normal blood chemistry values and miscellaneous other laboratory values are shown in Tables 39–1 through 39–3.

Table 39–1. Normal values of amino acids and other Ninhydrin-positive substances in plasma* and urine.†

	Newborn	Premature		Full Term		Years 2–12		Adult		% Tubular Reabsorption		
	Plasma (Week 1)	Plasma (Week 6)	Urine (Week 6)	Plasma (Week 6)	Urine (Week 6)	Plasma	Urine	Plasma	Urine	Infancy	Childhood	Adult
Phosphoethanol-amine	tr	. . .	. . .	. . .	. . .	. . .	0.08–0.28	. . .	. . .	. . .	. . .	. . .
Taurine	0.01–0.20	0.05–0.08	0.03–0.08	0.02–0.11	0.01–0.18	0.06–0.11	0.76–1.9	0.05–0.08	0.4–1.3	96–98	93–95	72–95
Hydroxyproline	0–tr	tr–0.08	1.1–2.1	0–tr	0.7–2.6	0–tr	0	0–tr	0	‡	. . .	. . .
Aspartic acid	tr–0.02	0.01–0.02	tr–0.04	0.008–0.02	tr–0.32	0.004–0.02	tr–0.07	0.004–0.01	0.03–0.09	§	92–99	85–98
Threonine	0.04–0.05	0.15–0.33	0.9–1.9	0.17–0.23	0.67–1.4	0.04–0.10	0.04–0.17	0.09–0.14	0.09–0.14	71–91	92–99.5	97–99
Serine	0.04–0.30	0.10–0.16	0.8–1.3	0.16–0.20	1.1–2.3	0.08–0.11	0.09–0.34	0.08–0.11	0.09–0.31	54–86	92–99	97–99
Asparagine Glutamine	0.3–2.1	0.40–0.44	0.5–1.5	0.36–0.57	1.1–2.0	0.06–0.47	0.04–0.75	0.4–0.5	0.17–0.48	90–96	98–9.99	99+
Proline	0.02–0.43	0.10–0.31	0.6–1.7	0.40–0.48	0.7–5.4	0.07–0.15	tr–0.04	0.15–0.25	0	53–94	99.5–100	99+
Glutamate	tr–0.26	0.08–0.14	0.02–0.13	0.06–0.21	0.04–0.62	0.02–0.25	0.01–0.13	0.05–0.20	0.008–0.16	95–99	98.5–99.8	99+
Citrulline	. . .	0.04–0.07	0.02–0.17	tr–0.04	tr–0.04	. . .	tr–0.03	tr–0.03	0–tr	92–98	. . .	99+
Glycine	0.05–0.44	0.12–0.21	2.5–4.2	0.18–0.24	3.7–8.4	0.12–0.22	0.33–1.5	0.15–0.24	0.40–0.90	15–63	93–99	94–99
Alanine	0.04–0.44	0.20–0.39	0.5–0.7	0.46–0.52	1.2–2.1	0.14–0.30	0.04–0.35	0.35–0.37	0.09–0.27	87–92	99–99.9	99+
α-Amino adipic	. . .	0	0.1–0.23	0	0.17–0.23	. . .	. . .	0	0–0.02	‡	. . .	‡
α-Amino butyric	tr–0.07	0–tr	tr	tr–0.02	0	. . .	tr–0.06	0.01–0.03	0.01–0.04	‡	. . .	99
Valine	0.03–0.32	0.12–0.22	tr–0.2	0.32–0.35	0.10–0.16	0.13–0.28	tr–0.08	0.05–0.08	tr–0.05	98–99+	99.6–99.9	99+
Homocitrulline	. . .	tr	0.13–0.37	0	0.12–0.24	. . .	. . .	0	0.02–0.04	‡	‡	‡
1/2 Cystine	0.02–0.07	tr–0.07	0.04–0.25	0	0.14–0.34	. . .	. . .	0	0.02–0.08	60–90	. . .	99+
Cystathionine	. . .	0.005–0.01	0.09–0.12	0–tr	0.11–0.17	. . .	. . .	0	0.01–0.02	35–65	. . .	‡
Methionine	tr–0.08	0.02–0.04	0.08–0.14	0.03–0.05	0.12–0.14	0.01–0.02	0.01–0.04	0.01–0.04	0.02–0.04	85–97	98.3–99.7	98–99+

Isoleucine	0.01–0.09	0.04–0.08	0.03–0.07	0.08–0.12	0.10–0.16	0.03–0.08	0.01–0.07	0.05–0.08	0.01–0.04	96–99+	99.2–99.9	99+
Leucine	0.01–0.18	0.1–0.5	0.04–0.08	0.14–0.22	0.15–0.18	0.06–0.18	0.02–0.11	0.10–0.14	0.02–0.05	97–99+	99.6–99.9	99+
Tyrosine	0.05–0.30	0.1–0.4	0.17–0.60	0.11–0.21	0.22–0.38	0.03–0.07	0.03–0.12	0.04–0.07	0.06–0.10	93–99	98.2–99.3	98–99+
Phenylalanine	0.02–0.12	0.05–0.07	0.08–0.13	0.06–0.12	0.11–0.14	0.03–0.06	0.01–0.11	0.04–0.07	0.04–0.07	94–99	98.8–99.7	99+
β-Alanine	...	0	0	0	0	0.02–0.05	tr	0	0	...	...	...
BAIB	...	0	0.09–0.16	0	0.17–0.42	...	0–0.19	0	0.01–0.09	...	...	...
Methylglycine	...	...	...	...	...	< 0.01	< 0.05	...	...	...	...	...
Hydroxylysine	...	0	0.13–0.27	0	0.05–0.11	...	...	0	0–0.02	‡	...	...
GABA	tr–0.1	0	0–tr	0	0–tr	...	...	0	tr	...	...	‡
Ornithine	0.01–0.22	0.08–0.11	0–0.08	0.07–0.10	0.05–0.08	0.03–0.09	0.01–0.03	0.58–0.90	tr	96–99+	99.5–99.8	99+
Lysine	0.05–0.35	0.08–0.15	0.2–0.6	0.21–0.34	0.7–1.4	0.07–0.15	0.04–0.21	0.16–0.18	0.02–0.20	81–96	98.5–99.8	99+
1-Methylhistidine	...	0	0	0	0–0.03	...	...	0	0.58–0.90	...	...	...
Histidine	tr–0.13	0.05–0.13	0.34–0.83	0.05–0.08	0.8–1.8	0.02–0.08	0.11–1.0	0.06–0.07	0.15–0.53	30–80	90.3–98.4	92–98
3-Methylhistidine	...	0	0	0	0–0.07	...	...	0	0.08–0.28	...	...	...
Arginine	tr–0.12	tr–0.07	0	0.04–0.10	tr–0.1	0.02–0.09	0.01–0.04	0.03–0.06	0.02–0.20	99+	99–99.9	99+

* Measured in μmol/mL (fasting).
† Measured in μmol/min/1.73 m^2.
‡ 0—trace in plasma but significant amounts in urine.
§ Detectable in plasma but not in urine except in traces.

Table 39–2. Normal blood chemistry values and miscellaneous other hematologic values.*
(Values may vary with the procedure employed.)

Determinations for:	
(S) = Serum	(P) = Plasma
(B) = Whole blood	(RBC) = Red blood cells

Acid-Base Measurements (B)
pH: 7.38–7.42 from 14 minutes of age and older.
P_{aO_2}: 65–76 mm Hg (8.66–10.13 kPa).
P_{aCO_2}: 36–38 mm Hg (4.8–5.07 kPa).
Base excess: −2 to +2 meq/L, except in newborns (range, −4 to −0).

Acid Phosphatase (S, P)
Values using *p*-nitrophenyl phosphate buffered with citrate (end-point determination).
Newborns: 7.4–19.4 IU/L at 37 °C.
2–13 years: 6.4–15.2 IU/L at 37 °C.
Adult males: 0.5–11 IU/L at 37 °C.
Adult females: 0.2–9.5 IU/L at 37 °C.

ACTH: See Corticotropin.

Adenosine Triphosphate (RBC)
Premature infants: 5.66 μmol/g of hemoglobin.
Adults: 3.86 μmol/g of hemoglobin.

Alanine Aminotransferase (ALT, SGPT) (S)
Newborns (1–3 days): 1–25 IU/L at 37 °C.
Adult males: 7–46 IU/L at 37 °C.
Adult females: 4–35 IU/L at 37 °C.

Aldolase (S)
Newborns: 17.5–47.8 IU/L at 37 °C.
Children: 8.8–23.9 IU/L at 37 °C.
Adults: 4.4–12 IU/L at 37 °C.

Aldosterone (P)
First year: 25–140 ng/dL.
Second year: 9–25 ng/dL.

Alkaline Phosphatase (S)
Values in IU/L at 37 °C using *p*-nitrophenol phosphate buffered with AMP (kinetic).

Group	Males	Females
Newborns (1–3 days)	95–368	95–368
2–24 months	115–460	115–460
2–5 years	115–391	115–391
6–7 years	115–460	115–460
8–9 years	115–345	115–345
10–11 years	115–336	115–437
12–13 years	127–403	92–336
14–15 years	79–446	78–212
16–18 years	58–331	35–124
Adults	41–137	39–118

Amino Acids (P)
(See Table 39–1.)

Ammonia (P)
Newborns: 90–150 μg/dL (53–88 μmol/L); higher in premature and jaundiced infants.
Thereafter: 0–60 μg/dL (0–35 μmol/L) when blood is drawn with proper precautions.

Amylase (S)
Values using maltotetrose substrate (kinetic).
Neonates: Undetectable.
2–12 months: Levels increase slowly to adult levels.
Adults: 28–108 IU/L at 37 °C.

Androstenedione (P)
Values in ng/dL (nmol/L).

Group	Males	Females
Cord blood	31–139 (1.1–4.9)	17–186 (0.6–6.5)
1–3 months	12–56 (0.1–2.0)	11–27 (0.4–0.9)
3–5 months	3–54 (0.1–1.9)	3–31 (0.1–1.1)
5–7 months	3–31 (0.1–1.1)	4–24 (0.1–0.8)
7–12 months	3–22 (0.1–0.8)	. . .
Adults	57–157 (2.0–5.5)	75–227 (2.6–7.9)

Antihemophilic Globulin (Factor VIII) (P)
Children: 82–157 units/dL.

α_1-Antitrypsin (S)
1–3 months: 127–404 mg/dL.
3–12 months: 145–362 mg/dL.
1–2 years: 160–382 mg/dL.
2–15 years: 148–394 mg/dL.

Ascorbic Acid: See Vitamin C.

Aspartate Aminotransferase (AST, SGOT) (S)
Newborns (1–3 days): 16–74 IU/L at 37 °C.
Adult males: 8–46 IU/L at 37 °C.
Adult females: 7–34 IU/L at 37 °C.

Base Excess: See Acid-Base Measurements.

Bicarbonate, Actual (P)
Calculated from pH and P_{aCO_2}.
Newborns: 17.2–23.6 mmol/L.
2 months–2 years: 19–24 mmol/L.
Children: 18–25 mmol/L.
Adult males: 20.1–28.9 mmol/L.
Adult females: 18.4–28.8 mmol/L.

* Adapted from Meites S (editor): *Pediatric Clinical Chemistry,* 2nd ed. American Association for Clinical Chemistry, 1982, and many other sources.

Table 39–2 (cont'd). Normal blood chemistry values and miscellaneous other hematologic values. (Values may vary with the procedure employed.)

Bilirubin (S)
Values in mg/dL (μmol/L).
Levels after 1 month are as follows:
Conjugated: 0–0.3 mg/dL (0–5 μmol/L).
Unconjugated: 0.1–0.7 mg/dL (2–12 μmol/L).

Peak Newborn Level	Percentage of Newborns (Birth Weight) Exceeding Peak Level		
	< 2001 g	2001–2500 g	> 2500 g
20 (342)	8.2%	2.6%	0.8%
18 (308)	13.5%	4.6%	1.5%
16 (274)	20.3%	7.6%	2.6%
14 (239)	33.0%	12.0%	4.4%
11 (188)	53.8%	23.0%	9.3%
8 (137)	77.0%	45.4%	26.1%

Bleeding Time
1–3 minutes.

Blood Volume
Premature infants: 98 mL/kg.
At 1 year: 86 mL/kg (range, 69–112 mL/kg).
Older children: 70 mL/kg (range, 51–86 mL/kg).

BUN: See Urea Nitrogen.

C Peptide (S)
5–15 years (8:00 AM fasting): 1–4 ng/mL.
Adults (8:00 AM fasting): < 4 ng/mL.
Adults (nonfasting): < 8 ng/mL.

Calcium (S)
Premature infants (first week): 3.5–4.5 meq/L (1.7–2.3 mmol/L).
Full-term infants (first week): 4–5 meq/L (2–2.5 mmol/L).
Thereafter: 4.4–5.3 meq/L (2.2–2.7 mmol/L).

Carbon Dioxide, Total (S, P)
Cord blood: 15–20.2 mmol/L.
Children: 18–27 mmol/L.
Adults: 24–35 mmol/L.

Carboxyhemoglobin (B)
5% of total hemoglobin (0.05 mol/mol).

Carnitine (S)
Fasting levels: 20–45 μmol/L.

Carotene (S, P)
0–6 months: 0–40 μg/dL (0–0.75 μmol/L).
Children: 50–100 μg/dL (0.93–1.9 μmol/L).
Adults: 100–150 μg/dL (1.9–2.8 μmol/L).

Cation-Anion Gap (S, P)
5–15 mmol/L.

Ceruloplasmin (Copper Oxidase) (S, P)
21–43 mg/dL (1.3–2.7 μmol/L).

Chloride (S, P)
Premature infants: 95–110 mmol/L.
Full-term infants: 96–116 mmol/L.
Children: 98–105 mmol/L.
Adults: 98–108 mmol/L.

Cholesterol (S, P)
Premature cord blood: 47–98 mg/dL (1.2–2.5 mmol/L).
Full-term cord blood: 45–98 mg/dL (1.1–2.5 mmol/L).
Full-term newborns: 45–167 mg/dL (1.2–4.3 mmol/L).
3 days–1 year: 69–174 mg/dL (1.8–4.5 mmol/L).
2–14 years: 120–205 mg/dL (3.1–5.3 mmol/L).
14–19 years: 120–210 mg/dL (3.1–5.4 mmol/L).
20–29 years: 120–240 mg/dL (3.1–6.2 mmol/L).
30–39 years: 140–270 mg/dL (3.6–7 mmol/L).
40–49 years: 150–310 mg/dL (3.9–8 mmol/L).
50–59 years: 160–330 mg/dL (4.1–8.5 mmol/L).

Cholinesterase (S, RBC)
2.5–5 μmol/min/mL of serum (pseudocholinesterase).
2.3–4 μmol/min/mL of red cells.

Christmas Factor (Factor IX) (P)
Children: 100 ± 22 units/dL.

Circulation Time, Decholin
3–6 years: 8–12 seconds.
6–12 years: 7.5–15 seconds.
12–15 years: 10–16 seconds.

Circulation Time, Fluorescein
Upper limit of normal, based on weight.
10 kg: 8 seconds
20 kg: 8.4 seconds.
40 kg: 11.3 seconds.

Coagulation Time (Test Tube Method)
3–9 minutes.

Complement (S)
C3: 96–195 mg/dL.
C4: 15–20 mg/dL.

Copper (S)
Cord blood: 26–32 μg/dL (4.1–5.2 μmol/L).
Newborns: 26–32 μg/dL (4.1–5.2 μmol/L).
1 month: 73–93 μg/dL (11.5–14.6 μmol/L).
2 months: 59–69 μg/dL (9.3–10.9 μmol/L).
6 months–5 years: 27–153 μg/dL (4.2–24.1 μmol/L).
5–17 years: 94–234 μg/dL (14.8–36.8 μmol/L).
Adults: 70–118 μg/dL (11–18.6 μmol/L).

Copper Oxidase: See Ceruloplasmin.

Corticotropin (ACTH) (P)
Morning (8:00 AM): 20–100 pg/mL (4.4–22 pmol/L).

Table 39–2 (cont'd). Normal blood chemistry values and miscellaneous other hematologic values. (Values may vary with the procedure employed.)

Cortisol (S, P)
Morning (8:00 AM): 5–25 μg/dL (0.14–0.68 μmol/L).
Evening: 5–15 μg/dL (0.14–0.41 μmol/L).

Creatine (S, P)
0.2–0.8 mg/dL (15.2–61 μmol/L).

Creatine Kinase (S, P)
Newborns (1–3 days): 40–474 IU/L at 37 °C.
Adult males: 30–210 IU/L at 37 °C.
Adult females: 20–128 IU/L at 37 °C.

Creatinine (S, P)
Values in mg/dL (μmol/L).

Group	Males	Females
Newborns (1–3 days)*	0.2–1.0 (17.7–88.4)	0.2–1.0 (17.7–88.4)
1 year	0.2–0.6 (17.7–53.0)	0.2–0.5 (17.7–44.2)
2–3 years	0.2–0.7 (17.7–61.9)	0.3–0.6 (26.5–53.0)
4–7 years	0.2–0.8 (17.7–70.7)	0.2–0.7 (17.7–61.9)
8–10 years	0.3–0.9 (26.5–79.6)	0.3–0.8 (26.5–70.7)
11–12 years	0.3–1.0 (26.5–88.4)	0.3–0.9 (26.5–79.6)
13–17 years	0.3–1.2 (26.5–106.1)	0.3–1.1 (26.5–97.2)
18–20 years	0.5–1.3 (44.2–115.0)	0.3–1.1 (26.5–97.2)

* Values may be higher in premature newborns.

Creatinine Clearance
Values show great variability and depend on specificity of analytical methods used.
Newborns (1 day): 5–50 mL/min/1.73 m^2 (mean, 18 mL/min/1.73 m^2).
Newborns (6 days): 15–90 mL/min/1.73 m^2 (mean, 36 mL/min/1.73 m^2).
Adult males: 85–125 mL/min/1.73 m^2.
Adult females: 75–115 mL/min/1.73 m^2.

Dehydroepiandrosterone Sulfate (S)
Values in μg/dL (μmol/L).

Group	Males	Females
Premature infants	223–303 (5.8–7.9)	223–303 (5.8–7.9)
Full-term infants	54–64 (1.4–1.7)	54–64 (1.4–1.7)
1–8 years	12–23 (0.3–0.6)	18–36 (0.5–0.9)
8–10 years	49–69 (1.3–1.8)	. . .
8–12 years	. . .	75–155 (2.0–4.1)
10–14 years	105–155 (2.7–4.1)	. . .
12–14 years	. . .	150–188 (3.9–4.9)
14–20 years	203–325 (5.3–8.5)	198–288 (5.2–7.5)

2,3-Diphosphoglycerate (B)
Values vary with method employed and with altitude.
4.5–6 mmol/L.

17β-Estradiol (P)
Values in pg/mL.
(See Table, top of next column.)

Estrone (P)
Values in pg/mL.

Group	17β-Estradiol		Estrone	
	Males	Females	Males	Females
0–8 years	2–4	1–10	7–20	11–20
Tanner I	2–6	7–14	10–20	16–20
Tanner II and III	2–16	24–126	15–51	23–91
Tanner IV and V	11–29	41–270	23–50	41–177
Adults				
Follicular	. . .	40–150	. . .	. . .
Luteal	. . .	100–400	. . .	. . .

Factor: See Antihemophilic Globulin, Christmas Factor, Proaccelerin, and Prothrombin.

Fatty Acids, "Free" (P)
Newborns: 435–1375 μeq/L.
4 months–10 years (14-hour fast): 500–900 μeq/L.
4 months–10 years (19-hour fast): 730–1200 μeq/L.
Adults (14-hour fast): 310–590 μeq/L.
Adults (19-hour fast): 405–720 μeq/L.

Fatty Acids, Total Esterified (P, RBC)
Values in mg/dL.

Fatty Acid*	Plasma		Erythrocytes	
	mg/dL	% of Total	mg/dL	% of Total
16:0	29.4–55.8	20.7–28.3	24.8–49.0	18.5–28.3
16:1	1.4–6.8	1.1–2.5	0.0–9.4	0.0–4.9
18:0	11.2–28.6	6.9–16.1	13.7–47.3	13.1–26.5
18:1	21.9–51.1	16.9–24.5	11.6–46.8	12.7–23.3
18:2	24.5–78.5	19.5–39.1	0.7–47.9	6.1–22.1
20:3	0.0–8.0	0.0–4.9	0.8–7.6	0.8–4.4
20:4	5.5–26.9	3.2–15.6	14.2–46.2	12.5–26.3

* Ratio of number of carbons to number of unsaturated bonds.

Ferritin (S)
Newborns: 20–200 ng/mL (mean, 117 ng/mL).
1 month: 60–550 ng/mL (mean, 350 ng/mL).
1–15 years: 7–140 ng/mL (mean, 31 ng/mL).
Adult males: 50–225 ng/mL (mean, 140 ng/mL).
Adult females: 10–150 ng/mL (mean, 40 ng/mL).

Fibrinogen (P)
200–500 mg/dL (5.9–14.7 μmol/L).

Folate (S)
Prepubertal children: Mean folic acid values are reported to be slightly higher than mean adult values but remain within the normal range.
Adults: 3–21 ng/mL.

Table 39–2 (cont'd). Normal blood chemistry values and miscellaneous other hematologic values. (Values may vary with the procedure employed.)

Follicle-Stimulating Hormone (FSH) (S)
Values in mIU/mL. Based on World Health Organization Human Pituitary Standard 69/104.

Group	Males	Females
Newborns (1–7 days)	< 1–2.4	< 1–2.4
2 weeks–1 year	< 1–20	< 1–31
Prepubertal children	< 1–3.2	< 1–5
Tanner II	2–7	< 1–6
Tanner III	2–8	1.5–9
Tanner IV	2–8	2–9
Tanner V	2–8	1–9
Adults	1–8	...
Follicular	...	1–9
Midcycle	...	4–30
Luteal	...	< 1–7
Postmenopausal	...	20–160

FSH: See Follicle-Stimulating Hormone.

Galactose (S, P)
1.1–2.1 mg/dL (0.06–0.12 mmol/L).

Galactose 1-Phosphate (RBC)
Normal: 1 mg/dL of packed erythrocyte lysate; slightly higher in cord blood.
Infants with congenital galactosemia on a milk-free diet: < 2 mg/dL.
Infants with congenital galactosemia taking milk: 9–20 mg/dL.

Galactose-1-Phosphate Uridyl Transferase (RBC)
Normal: 308–475 mIU/g of hemoglobin.
Heterozygous for Duarte variant: 225–308 mIU/g of hemoglobin.
Homozygous for Duarte variant: 142–225 mIU/g of hemoglobin.
Heterozygous for congenital galactosemia: 142–225 mIU/g of hemoglobin.
Homozygous for congenital galactosemia: < 8 mIU/g of hemoglobin.

Gastrin (S)
Newborns (1–7 days): 20–300 pg/mL.
Children (8- to 12-hour overnight fast): < 10–125 pg/mL.
Adults (8- to 12-hour overnight fast): < 10–100 pg/mL.

GHL See Growth Hormone.

Glomerular Filtration Rate
Newborns: About 50% of values for older children and adults.
Older children and adults: 75–165 mL/min/1.73 m^2 (levels reached by about 6 months).

Glucose (S, P)
Premature infants: 20–80 mg/dL (1.11–4.44 mmol/L).
Full-term infants: 30–100 mg/dL (1.67–5.56 mmol/L).
Children and adults (fasting): 60–105 mg/dL (3.33–5.88 mmol/L).

Glucose 6-Phosphate Dehydrogenase (RBC)
150–215 units/dL.

Glucose Tolerance Test (S)
(See Table, bottom of page.)

λ-Glutamyl Transpeptidase (S)
0–1 month: 12–271 IU/L at 37 °C (kinetic).
1–2 months: 9–159 IU/L at 37 °C (kinetic).
2–4 months: 7–98 IU/L at 37 °C (kinetic).
4–7 months: 5–45 IU/L at 37 °C (kinetic).
7–12 months: 4–27 IU/L at 37 °C (kinetic).
1–15 years: 3–30 IU/L at 37 °C (kinetic).
Adult males: 9–69 IU/L at 37 °C (kinetic).
Adult females: 3–33 IU/L at 37 °C (kinetic).

Glycogen (RBC)
Cord blood: 10–338 μg/g of hemoglobin.
4½–19 hours: 48–361 μg/g of hemoglobin.
2–12 months: 32–134 μg/g of hemoglobin.
1–12 years: 22–109 μg/g of hemoglobin.
Adults: 20–105 μg/g of hemoglobin.

Glucose tolerance test results in serum.

Normal levels based on results in 13 normal children given glucose, 1.75 g/kg orally in one dose, after 2 weeks on a high-carbohydrate diet.

	Glucose		Insulin		Phosphorus	
Time	mg/dL	mmol/L	μU/mL	pmol/L	mg/dL	mmol/L
Fasting	59–96	3.11–5.33	5–40	36–287	3.2–4.9	1.03–1.58
30 minutes	91–185	5.05–10.27	36–110	258–789	2.0–4.4	0.64–1.42
60 minutes	66–164	3.66–9.10	22–124	158–890	1.8–3.6	0.58–1.16
90 minutes	68–148	3.77–8.22	17–105	122–753	1.8–3.6	0.58–1.16
2 hours	66–122	3.66–6.77	6–84	43–603	1.8–4.2	0.58–1.36
3 hours	47–99	2.61–5.49	2–46	14–330	2.0–4.6	0.64–1.48
4 hours	61–93	3.39–5.16	3–32	21–230	2.7–4.3	0.87–1.39
5 hours	63–86	3.50–4.77	5–37	36–265	2.9–4.4	0.94–1.42

Table 39–2 (cont'd). Normal blood chemistry values and miscellaneous other hematologic values. (Values may vary with the procedure employed.)

Glycohemoglobin (hemoglobin A_{1c}) (B)
Normal: 6.3–8.2% of total hemoglobin.
Diabetic patients in good control of their condition ordinarily have levels < 10%.
Values tend to be lower during pregnancy; they also vary with technique.

Growth Hormone (GH) (S)
After infancy (fasting specimen): 0–5 ng/mL.
In response to natural and artificial provocation (eg, sleep, arginine, insulin, hypoglycemia): > 8 ng/mL.
During the newborn period (fasting specimen); GH levels are high (15–40 ng/mL) and responses to provocation variable.

Haptoglobin (S)
50–150 mg/dL as hemoglobin-binding capacity.

Hematocrit (B)
At birth: 44–64%.
14–90 days: 35–49%.
6 months–1 year: 30–40%.
4–10 years: 31–43%.

Hemoglobin (P)
No more than 0.5 mg/dL (0.3 μmol/L).

Hemoglobin A_{1C}: See Glycohemoglobin.

Hemoglobin Electrophoresis (B)
A_1 hemoglobin: 96–98.5% of total hemoglobin.
A_2 hemoglobin: 1.5–4% of total hemoglobin.

Hemoglobin, Fetal (B)
At birth: 50–85% of total hemoglobin.
At 1 year: < 15% of total hemoglobin.
Up to 2 years: Up to 5% of total hemoglobin.
Thereafter: < 2% of total hemoglobin.

17-Hydroxyprogesterone: See Progesterone.

Immunoglobulins (S)
Values in mg/dL.

Group	IgG	IgA	IgM
Cord blood	766–1693	0.04–9	4–26
2 weeks–3 months	299–852	3–66	15–149
3–6 months	142–988	4–90	18–118
6–12 months	418–1142	14–95	43–223
1–2 years	356–1204	13–118	37–239
2–3 years	492–1269	23–137	49–204
3–6 years	564–1381	35–209	51–214
6–9 years	658–1535	29–384	50–228
9–12 years	625–1598	60–294	64–278
12–16 years	660–1548	81–252	45–256

Insulin: See Glucose Tolerance Test and Table (bottom of previous page).

Inulin Clearance
< 1 month: 29–88 mL/min/1.73 m^2.
1–6 months: 40–112 mL/min/1.73 m^2.
6–12 months: 62–121 mL/min/1.73 m^2.
> 1 year: 78–164 mL/min/1.73 m^2.

Iron (S, P)
Newborns: 20–157 μg/dL (3.6–28.1 μmol/L).
6 weeks–3 years: 20–115 μg/dL (3.6–20.6 μmol/L).
3–9 years: 20–141 μg/dL (3.6–25.2 μmol/L).
9–14 years: 21–151 μg/dL (3.8–27 μmol/L).
14–16 years: 20–181 μg/dL (3.6–32.4 μmol/L).
Adults: 44–196 μg/dL (7.2–31.3 μmol/L).

Iron-Binding Capacity (S, P)
Newborns: 59–175 μg/dL (10.6–31.3 μmol/L).
Children and adults: 275–458 μg/dL (45–72 μmol/L).

Lactate (B)
Venous blood: 5–18 mg/dL (0.5–2 mmol/L).
Arterial blood: 3–7 mg/dL (0.3–0.8 mmol/L).

Lactate Dehydrogenase (LDH) (S, P)
Values using lactate substrate (kinetic).
Newborns (1–3 days): 40–348 IU/L at 37 °C.
1 month–5 years: 150–360 IU/L at 37 °C.
5–8 years: 150–300 IU/L at 37 °C.
8–12 years: 130–300 IU/L at 37 °C.
12–14 years: 130–280 IU/L at 37 °C.
14–16 years: 130–230 IU/L at 37 °C.
Adult males: 70–178 IU/L at 37 °C.
Adult females: 42–166 IU/L at 37 °C.

Lactate Dehydrogenase Isoenzymes (S)
LDH_1 (heart): 24–34%.
LDH_2 (heart, red cells): 35–45%.
LDH_3 (muscle): 15–25%.
LDH_4 (liver [trace], muscle): 4–10%.
LDH_5 (liver, muscle): 1–9%.

LATS: See Long-Acting Thyroid Stimulator.

LDH: See Lactate Dehydrogenase.

Lead (B)
< 30 μg/dL (< 1.4 μmol/L).

Leucine Aminopeptidase (S, P)
Up to 1 month: 29–59 IU/L.
Thereafter: 15–50 IU/L.

LH: See Luteinizing Hormone.

Lipase (S, P)
20–136 IU/L based on 4-hour incubation.

Table 39–2 (cont'd). Normal blood chemistry values and miscellaneous other hematologic values. (Values may vary with the procedure employed.)

Lipoprotein Cholesterol (P)
Fasting levels for lipoprotein cholesterol in children 4–17 years:
High-density lipoprotein (HDL) cholesterol: 37–73 mg/dL.
Low-density lipoprotein (LDL) cholesterol: 66–145 mg/dL.
Very low density lipoprotein (VLDL) cholesterol: 6–15 mg/dL.

Lipoprotein Cholesterol, High-Density (HDL) (S)
Values in mg/dL (mmol/L).

Group	Males	Females
6–7 years	24–78 (0.62–2.02)	31–67 (0.80–1.73)
8–9 years	36–76 (0.93–1.97)	31–75 (0.80–1.94)
10–11 years	36–76 (0.93–1.97)	31–71 (0.80–1.94)
12–13 years	25–85 (0.65–2.20)	38–78 (0.98–2.09)
14–15 years	28–68 (0.72–1.76)	30–70 (0.78–1.81)
16–17 years	28–68 (0.72–1.76)	31–79 (0.80–2.04)

Long-Acting Thyroid Stimulator (LATS) (S)
None detectable.

Luteinizing Hormone (LH) (S)
Values in mIU/mL. Based on World Health Organization Human Pituitary Standard 68/40.

Group	Males	Females
Newborns (1–7 days)	1.5–3	1.5–3
2 weeks–1 year	3.5–25	2.1–14
Prepubertal children	< 1–4	< 1–4
Tanner II	< 1–5	< 1–5
Tanner III	2–10	< 1–10
Tanner IV	2–10	3–11
Tanner V	4.5–11	2–12
Adults	3–10	...
Follicular	...	3–11
Midcycle	...	18–70
Luteal	...	2–11
Postmenopausal	...	25–70

Magnesium (RBC)
3.92–5.28 meq/L (1.96–2.64 mmol/L).

Magnesium (S, P)
Newborns: 1.5–2.3 meq/L (0.75–1.15 mmol/L).
Adults: 1.4–2 meq/L (0.7–1 mmol/L).

Manganese (S)
Newborns: 2.4–9.6 μg/dL (0.44–1.75 μmol/L).
2–18 years: 0.8–1.2 μg/dL (0.15–0.38 μmol/L).

Methemoglobin (B)
0–0.3 g/dL (0–186 μmol/L).

Mucoprotein, Tyrosine (S)
2.5–3.5 mg/dL.

Osmolality (S, P)
270–290 mosm/kg.

Oxygen Capacity (B)
1.34 mL/g of hemoglobin.

Oxygen Saturation (B)
Newborns: 30–80% (0.3–0.8 mol/mol of venous blood).
Thereafter: 65–85% (0.65–0.85 mol/mol of venous blood).

P_{aCO_2}: See Acid-Base Measurements.

P_{aO_2}: See Acid-Base Measurements.

Partial Thromboplastin Time (P)
Children: 42–54 seconds.

pH: See Acid-Base Measurements.

Phenylalanine (S, P)
0.7–3.5 mg/dL (0.04–0.21 mmol/L).

Phosphatase: See Acid Phosphatase and Alkaline Phosphatase.

Phospholipid (S)
Cord blood: 48–160 mg/dL (0.62–2.07 mmol/L).
2–13 years: 166–247 mg/dL (2.14–3.19 mmol/L).
13–20 years: 193–338 mg/dL (2.49–4.37 mmol/L).

Phosphorus, Inorganic (S, P)
Premature infants:
- At birth: 5.6–8 mg/dL (1.81–2.58 mmol/L).
- 6–10 days: 6.1–11.7 mg/dL (1.97–3.78 mmol/L).
- 20–25 days: 6.6–9.4 mg/dL (2.13–3.04 mmol/L).

Full-term infants:
- At birth: 5–7.8 mg/dL (1.61–2.52 mmol/L).
- 3 days: 5.8–9 mg/dL (1.87–2.91 mmol/L).
- 6–12 days: 4.9–8.9 mg/dL (1.58–2.87 mmol/L).

Children:
- 1 year: 3.8–6.2 mg/dL (1.23–2 mmol/L).
- 10 years: 3.6–5.6 mg/dL (1.16–1.81 mmol/L).

Adults: 3.1–5.1 mg/dL (1–1.65 mmol/L).
(See also Glucose Tolerance Test.)

Potassium (RBC)
87.2–97.6 mmol/L.

Potassium (S, P)
Premature infants: 4.5–7.2 mmol/L.
Full-term infants: 3.7–5.2 mmol/L.
Children: 3.5–5.8 mmol/L.
Adults: 3.5–5.5 mmol/L.

Table 39–2 (cont'd). Normal blood chemistry values and miscellaneous other hematologic values. (Values may vary with the procedure employed.)

Progesterone and 17-hydroxyprogesterone in serum.

Group	Progesterone		17-Hydroxyprogesterone	
	Males	Females	Males	Females
Prepubertal children (1–10 years)	7–33	7–33	3–90	3–82
Tanner II	< 10–33	< 10–55	5–115	11–98
Tanner III	< 10–48	10–450	10–138	11–155
Tanner IV	10–108	< 10–1300	29–180	18–230
Tanner V	21–82	< 10–950	24–175	20–265
Adults	13–97	. . .	27–199	. . .
Follicular	. . .	15–70	. . .	15–70
Luteal	. . .	200–2500	. . .	35–290

Proaccelerin (Factor V) (P)
Children: 61–127 units/dL.

Progesterone (S)
Values in ng/dL.
Cord blood: 8000–56,000 ng/dL.
Newborns (1–7 days): Levels are markedly elevated in the neonate but fall rapidly to reach prepubertal levels by 7 days, where they remain until puberty.
For levels in children over 1 year of age and levels in adults, see Table (top of page).

Progesterone (17-Hydroxyprogesterone) (S)
Values in ng/dL.
Cord blood: 900–5000 ng/dL.
Newborns (1–7 days): Levels decrease rapidly during the first week to reach 60–150 ng/dL by 7 days.
Males (1–12 months): Levels increase after the first week to peak values (120–200 ng/dL) between 30 and 60 days. Values then decline gradually to reach prepubertal levels by 1 year.
Females (1–12 months): Levels gradually decrease during the first 12 months to reach prepubertal levels.
For levels in children over 1 year of age and levels in adults, see Table (top of page).

Prolactin (S)
Cord blood: 61–590 ng/mL.
Newborns (1–7 days): 30–495 ng/mL.
1–8 weeks: Levels decline during the first 2 months of life to levels observed in prepubertal and pubertal children and adults.
Male children and adults: 3–18 ng/mL.
Female children and adults: 3–24 ng/mL.

Prostaglandin E (P)
Newborns: 1000–1730 pg/mL.
2–3 days: 60–150 pg/mL.
1–6 years: 125–200 pg/mL.
6–14 years: 160–340 pg/mL.
Adults: 450–550 pg/mL.

Proteins (S)
(See Table, bottom of page.)

Prothrombin (Factor II) (P)
Children: 81–123 units/dL.

Prothrombin Time (P)
Children: 11–15 seconds.

Protoporphyrin, "Free" (FEP, ZPP) (B)
Values for free erythrocyte protoporphyrin (FEP) and zinc protoporphyrin (ZPP) are 1.2–2.7 μg/g of hemoglobin.

Pseudocholinesterase (S)
2.5–5 μmol/mL/min.

Pyruvate (B)
Resting adult males (arterial blood); 50.5–60.1 μmol/L.
Adults (venous blood): 34–102 μmol/L.

Pyruvate Kinase (RBC)
7.4–15.7 units/g of hemoglobin.

Proteins in serum.

Values are for cellulose acetate electrophoresis and are in g/dL. SI conversion factor: g/dL × 10 = g/L.

Group	Total Protein	Albumin	α_1-Globulin	α_2-Globulin	β-Globulin	γ-Globulin
At birth	4.6–7.0	3.2–4.8	0.1–0.3	0.2–0.3	0.3–0.6	0.6–1.2
3 months	4.5–6.5	3.2–4.8	0.1–0.3	0.3–0.7	0.3–0.7	0.2–0.7
1 year	5.4–7.5	3.7–5.7	0.1–0.3	0.5–1.1	0.4–1.0	0.2–0.9
> 4 years	5.9–8.0	3.8–5.4	0.1–0.3	0.4–0.8	0.5–1.0	0.4–1.3

Table 39–2 (cont'd). Normal blood chemistry values and miscellaneous other hematologic values. (Values may vary with the procedure employed.)

Renin Activity (P)
3–6 days: 8–14 ng/mL/h.
0–3 years: 3–6 ng/mL/h.
Children: 1.3–2.6 ng/mL/h.

Sedimentation Rate (Micro) (B)
< 2 years: 1–5 mm/h.
> 2 years: 1–8 mm/h.

Serotonin S,P)
Children: 127–187 ng/mL.
Adults: 119–171 ng/mL.

SGOT: See Aspartate Aminotransferase.

SGPT: See Alanine Aminotransferase.

Sodium (S, P)
Children and adults: 135–148 mmol/L.

Somatomedin C (S)
Newborns: 0.17–0.62 units/mL.
1–5 years: 0.14–0.94 units/mL.
6–12 years: 0.87–2.06 units/mL.
13–17 years: 1.35–3 units/mL.
Adults: 0.61–2.04 units/mL.

Sugar: See Glucose.

T_3: See Triiodothyronine.

T_4: See Thyroxine.

TBG: See Thyroxine-Binding Globulin.

Testosterone (S)
Values in ng/dL.
Males:
Newborns: 75–400 ng/dL.
1–7 months: Levels decrease rapidly the first week to 20–50 ng/dL and then increase to 60–400 ng/dL between 60 and 80 days. Levels then decline gradually to the prepubertal range by 7 months.
Females:
Newborns: 20–64 ng/dL.
1–7 months: Levels decrease during the first month to < 10 ng/dL and remain there until puberty.
Levels in children over 1 year of age and levels in adults are as follows:

Group	Males	Females
Prepubertal children	< 3–10	3–10
Tanner II	18–150	7–28
Tanner III	100–320	15–35
Tanner IV	200–620	13–32
Tanner V	350–970	20–38
Adults	350–1030	10–55

Thrombin Time (P)
Children: 12–16 seconds.

Thyroid-Stimulating Hormone (TSH) (S)
Levels increase shortly after birth to levels as high as 30–40 μIU/mL. Levels return to the adult normal range (1.6–10.9 μIU/mL) by about 10–14 days.

Thyroxine (T_4) (S)
1–2 days: 11.4–25.5 μg/dL (147–328 nmol/L).
3–4 days: 9.8–25.2 μg/dL (126–324 nmol/L).
1–6 years: 5–15.2 μg/dL (64–196 nmol/L).
11–13 years: 4–13 μg/dL (51–167 nmol/L).
> 18 years: 4.7–11 μg/dL (60–142 nmol/L).

Thyroxine, "Free" (Free T_4) (S)
1–2.3 ng/dL.

Thyroxine-Binding Globulin (TBG) (S)
1–7 months: 2.9–6 mg/dL.
7–12 months: 2.1–5.9 mg/dL.
Prepubertal children: 2–5.3 mg/dL.
Pubertal children and adults: 1.8–4.2 mg/dL.

α-Tocopherol: See Vitamin E.

Transaminase: See Alanine Aminotransferase and Aspartate Aminotransferase.

Triglycerides (S, P)
< 19 years (12- to 14-hour fast): < 10–130 mg/dL (0.11–1.47 mmol/L).
20–29 years (12- to 14-hour fast): < 10–140 mg/dL (0.11–1.58 mmol/L).
30–39 years (12- to 14-hour fast): < 10–150 mg/dL (0.11–1.69 mmol/L).
40–49 years (12- to 14-hour fast): < 10–160 mg/dL (0.11–1.81 mmol/L).
50–59 years (12- to 14-hour fast): < 10–190 mg/dL (0.11–2.14 mmol/L).

Triiodothyronine (T_3) (S)
1–3 days: 89–405 ng/dL.
1 week: 91–300 ng/dL.
1–12 months: 85–250 ng/dL.
Prepubertal children: 119–218 ng/dL.
Pubertal children and adults: 55–170 ng/dL.

Trypsinogen, Immunoreactive (S, P)
Newborns: 5–97 ng/mL.
99.5th percentile: 136 ng/mL.
99.8th percentile: 162 ng/mL.

TSH: See Thyroid-Stimulating Hormone.

Tyrosine (S, P)
Premature infants: 3–30.2 mg/dL (0.17–1.67 mmol/L).

Table 39–2 (cont'd). Normal blood chemistry values and miscellaneous other hematologic values. (Values may vary with the procedure employed.)

Full-term infants: 1.7–4.7 mg/dL (0.09–0.26 mmol/L).
1–12 years: 1.4–3.4 mg/dL (0.08–0.19 mmol/L).
Adults: 0.6–1.6 mg/dL (0.03–0.09 mmol/L).

Tyrosine Mucoprotein: See Mucoprotein.

Urea Clearance
Premature infants: 3.5–17.3 mL/min/1.73 m^2.
Newborns: 8.7–33 mL/min/1.73 m^2.
2–12 months: 40–95 mL/min/1.73 m^2.
$\geqslant$ 2 years: $>$ 52 mL/min/1.73 m^2.

Urea Nitrogen (S, P)
1–2 years: 5–15 mg/dL (1.8–5.4 mmol/L).
Thereafter: 10–20 mg/dL (3.5–7.1 mmol/L).

Uric Acid (S, P)
Males:
0–14 years: 2–7 mg/dL (119–416 μmol/L).
$>$ 14 years: 3–8 mg/dL (178–476 μmol/L).
Females:
0–14 years: 2–7 mg/dL (119–416 μmol/L).
$>$ 14 years: 2–7 mg/dL (119–416 μmol/L).

Vitamin A (S, P)
Values of $<$ 20 μg/dL (0.7 μmol/L) should be considered abnormally low.

Vitamin B_{12} (S, P)
330–1025 pg/mL (243–756 pmol/L).

Vitamin C (Ascorbic Acid) (S, P)
0.2–2 mg/dL (11–114 μmol/L).

Vitamin D (S)
1,25-Dihydroxycholecalciferol:
Normal: 37 $\pm$ 12 pg/mL.
X-linked vitamin D-resistant disease: 16 $\pm$ 8 pg/mL.
Vitamin D dependency: 9.5 $\pm$ 3 pg/mL in type I. Normal in type II.
Hypophosphatemic bone disease: 30 $\pm$ 6 pg/mL.
Lead poisoning: 20 $\pm$ 1 pg/mL.
25-Hydroxycholecalciferol:
Normal: 26–31 ng/mL.

Vitamin E (α-Tocopherol) (S, P)
Premature infants: 0.05–0.35 mg/dL (1.2–8.4 μmol/L).
Full-term infants: 0.10–0.35 mg/dL (2.4–8.4 μmol/L).
2–5 months: 0.2–0.6 mg/dL (4.8–14.4 μmol/L).
6–24 months: 0.35–0.8 mg/dL (8.4–19.2 μmol/L).
2–12 years: 0.55–0.9 mg/dL (13.2–21.6 μmol/L).
Breast-fed infants: 0.6–1.1 mg/dL (14.4–26.4 μmol/L).

Volume (B)
Premature infants: 98 mL/kg (mean).
Full-term infants: 75–100 mL/kg.
1 year: 69–112 mL/kg (mean, 86 mL/kg).
Older children: 51–86 mL/kg (mean, 70 mL/kg).

Volume (P)
Full-term neonates: 39–77 mL/kg.
Infants: 40–50 mL/kg.
Older children: 30–54 mL/kg.

Water (B, S, RBC)
Whole blood: 79–81 g/dL.
Serum: 91–92 g/dL.
Red blood cells: 64–65 g/dL.

Xylose Absorption Test (B)
Following a 5-g loading dose, the laboratory will report the D-xylose concentration of the baseline and 60-minute samples in mg/dL. The difference between these 2 values should be corrected to a constant surface area of 1.73 m^2 according to the formula shown below.
The actual surface area can be derived from a number of available nomograms using the patient's weight and height.
Normal corrected blood values:* 9.8–20 mg/dL.
Effect of age and sex: No significant differences between males and females. No significant differences in ages 14–92.

Zinc (S)
Males: 83–88 μg/dL (12.7–13.5 μmol/L).
Females: 85–91 μg/dL (13–13.9 μmol/L).
Females taking oral contraceptives: 86–93 μg/dL (13.2–14.2 μmol/L).
At 16 weeks of gestation: 66–70 μg/dL (10.1–10.7 μmol/L).
At 38 weeks of gestation: 54–58 μg/dL (8.3–8.9 μmol/L).

$$\text{* Corrected blood value} = \frac{(\text{Value}_{60\ min} - \text{Value}_{baseline}) \times \text{Actual surface area}}{1.73}$$

Table 39–3. Normal values: Urine, bone marrow, duodenal fluid, feces, sweat, and miscellaneous.*

Urine

Acidity, Titratable
20–50 meq/d.

Addis Count
Red cells (12-hour specimen): < 1 million.
White cells (12-hour specimen): < 2 million.
Casts (12-hour specimen): < 10,000.
Protein (12-hour specimen): < 55 mg.

Albumin
First month: 1–100 mg/L.
Second month: 0.2–34 mg/L.
2–12 months: 0.5–19 mg/L.

Aldosterone
Newborns: 0.5–5 μg/24 h (20–140 μg/g of creatinine).
Prepubertal children: 1–8 μg/24 h (4–22 μg/g of creatinine).
Adults: 3–19 μg/24 h (1.5–20 μg/g of creatinine).

Amino Acids
(See Table 39–1.)

δ-Aminolevulinic Acid: See Porphyrins.

Ammonia
2–12 months: 4–20 μeq/min/m^2.
1–16 years: 6–16 μeq/min/m^2.

Calcium
4–12 years: 4–8 meq/L (2–4 mmol/L).

Catecholamines (Norepinephrine, Epinephrine)
Values in μg/24 h (nmol/24 h).
(See Table, bottom of page.)

Chloride
Infants: 1.7–8.5 mmol/24 h.
Children: 17–34 mmol/24 h.
Adults: 140–240 mmol/24 h.

Copper
0–30 μg/24 h.

Coproporphyrin: See Porphyrins.

Corticosteroids (17-Hydroxycorticosteroids)
0–2 years: 2–4 mg/24 h (5.5–11 μmol).
2–6 years: 3–6 mg/24 h (8.3–16.6 μmol).
6–10 years: 6–8 mg/24 h (16.6–22.1 μmol).
10–14 years: 8–10 mg/24 h (22.1–27.6 μmol).

Creatine
18–58 mg/L (1.37–4.42 mmol/L).

Creatinine
Newborns: 7–10 mg/kg/24 h.
Children: 20–30 mg/kg/24 h.
Adult males: 21–26 mg/kg/24 h.
Adult females: 16–22 mg/kg/24 h.

Epinephrine: See Catecholamines.

Follicle-Stimulating Hormone (FSH)
Values in IU/24 h.

Group	Males	Females
Prepubertal children	< 1–3.3	< 1–3.4
Tanner II	1–7	2–6
Tanner III	2–9	3–8
Tanner IV	2–10	3–9
Tanner V	3–12	2–11
Adults	3–11	2–15

FSH: See Follicle-Stimulating Hormone.

Homovanillic Acid
Children: 3–16 μg/mg of creatinine.
Adults: 2–4 μg/mg of creatinine.

17-Hydroxycorticosteroids: See Corticosteroids.

5-Hydroxyindoleacetic Acid
0.11–0.61 μmol/kg/7 h, based on results in 15 well-nourished, apparently healthy, mentally defective children on a tryptophan load.

Hydroxyproline, Total
5–14 years: 38–126 mg/24 h (290–961 μmol/24 h).

17-Ketosteroids
Values in mg/24 h (μmol/24 h)
(See Table, top of next page.)

Catecholamines in urine.

Group	Total Catecholamines	Norepinephrine	Epinephrine
< 1 year	20	5.4–15.9 (32–94)	0.1–4.3 (0.5–23.5)
1–5 years	40	8.1–30.8 (48–182)	0.8–9.1 (4.4–49.7)
6–15 years	80	19.0–71.1 (112–421)	1.3–10.5 (7.1–57.3)
> 15 years	100	34.4–87.0 (203–514)	3.5–13.2 (19.1–72.1)

* Adapted from Meites S (editor): *Pediatric Clinical Chemistry,* 2nd ed. American Association for Clinical Chemistry, 1982, and many other sources.

Table 39–3. (cont'd). Normal values: Urine, bone marrow, duodenal fluid, feces, sweat, and miscellaneous.

Group	Males	Females
0–14 years	0.5–2.5 (1.7–8.7)	0.5–2.5 (1.7–8.7)
2 weeks–2 years	0.0–0.5 (0.0–1.7)	0.0–0.5 (0.0–1.7)
2–6 years	0.0–2.0 (0.0–6.9)	0.0–2.0 (0.0–6.9)
6–8 years	0.0–2.5 (0.0–8.7)	0.0–2.5 (0.0–8.7)
8–10 years	0.7–4.0 (2.4–13.9)	0.7–4.0 (2.4–13.9)
10–12 years	0.7–6.0 (2.4–20.8)	0.7–5.0 (2.4–17.3)
12–14 years	1.3–10.0 (4.5–34.7)	1.3–8.5 (4.5–29.5)
14–16 years	2.5–13.0 (8.7–45.1)	2.5–11.0 (8.7–38.1)

Luteinizing Hormone (LH)
Values in IU/24 h.

Group	Males	Females
Prepubertal children	< 1–5.6	1.4–4.9
Tanner II	1.5–11	3–10
Tanner III	2.5–13	5–18
Tanner IV	5–16	6–21
Tanner V	4–28	5–24
Adults	9–23	4–30

Mercury
< 50 μg/24 h (249 nmol/24 h).

Metanephrine and Normetanephrine
< 2 years: < 4.6 μg/mg of creatinine (23.3 nmol).
2–10 years: < 3 μg/mg of creatinine (15.2 nmol).
10–15 years: < 2 μg/mg of creatinine (10.3 nmol).
> 15 years: < 1 μg/mg of creatinine (5.1 nmol).

Mucopolysaccharides
Acid mucopolysaccharide screen should yield negative results. Positive results after dialysis of the urine should be followed up with a thin-layer chromatogram for evaluation of the acid mucopolysaccharide excretion pattern.

Norepinephrine: See Catecholamines.

Normetanephrine: See Metanephrine and Normetanephrine.

Osmolality
Infants: 50–600 mosm/L.
Older children: 50–1400 mosm/L.

Phosphorus, Tubular Reabsorption
78–97%.

Porphobilinogen: See Porphyrins.

Porphyrins
δ-Aminolevulinic acid: 0–7 mg/24 h (0–53.4 μmol/24 h).
Porphobilinogen: 0–2 mg/24 h (0–8.8 μmol/24 h).
Coproporphyrin: 0–160 μg/24 h (0–244 nmol/24 h).
Uroporphyrin: 0–26 μg/24 h (0–31 nmol/24 h).

Potassium
26–123 mmol/L.

Pregnanetriol
2 weeks–2 years: 0–0.2 mg/24 h (0–0.59 μmol/24 h).
2–16 years: 0.3–1.1 mg/24 h (0.89–3.27 μmol/24 h).

Sodium
Infants: 0.3–3.5 mmol/24 h (6–10 mmol/m^2).
Children and adults: 5.6–17 mmol/24 h.

Testosterone
Prepubertal children: 0.2–2.3 μg/24 h (0.3–5 μg/g of creatinine).
Adult males: 40–130 μg/24 h.
Adult females: 2–11 μg/24 h.

Urobilinogen
< 3 mg/24 h (< 5.1 μmol/24 h).

Uroporphyrin: See Porphyrins.

Vanilmandelic Acid (VMA)
Because of the difficulty in obtaining an accurately timed 24-hour collection, values based on microgram per milligram of creatinine are the most reliable indications of VMA excretion in young children.
1–12 months: 1–35 μg/mg of creatinine (31–135 μg/kg/24 h).
1–2 years: 1–30 μg/mg of creatinine.
2–5 years: 1–15 μg/mg of creatinine.
5–10 years: 1–14 μg/mg of creatinine.
10–15 years: 1–10 μg/mg of creatinine.
Adults: 1–7 μg/mg of creatinine (1–7 mg/24 h; 5–35 μmol/24 h).

VMA: See Vanilmandelic Acid.

Xylose Absorption Test
Mean 5-hour excretion expressed as percentage of ingested load.
< 6 months: 11–30%.
6–12 months: 20–32%.

Xylose Absorption (cont'd)
1–3 years: 20–42%.
3–10 years: 25–45%.
> 10 years: 25–50%.
Or: % excretion > (0.2 × age in months) + 12.

Bone Marrow Cytology

Eosinophils (all stages): 1–10%.
Lymphocytes: 5–45%.
Metamyelocytes: 7–30%.
Monocytes: 0–7%.
Myeloblasts: 0–4%.
Myelocytes: 7–25%.

Table 39–3. (cont'd). Normal values: Urine, bone marrow, duodenal fluid, feces, sweat, and miscellaneous.

Normoblasts: 4–35%.
Polymorphonuclear leukocytes (PMNs): 5–30%.
Promyelocytes: 0–6%.
Pronormoblasts: 0–8%.
Other cells: Occasionally seen.

Duodenal Fluid Values

Enzymes
Amylase: (Anderson).
0–2 months: 0–10 units/mL.
2–6 months: 10–20 units/mL.
6–12 months: 40–150 units/mL.
1–2 years: 100–225 units/mL.
2–5 years: 125–275 units/mL.
Carboxypeptidase:
0.4–1 unit (Ravin).
Chymotrypsin:
11–65 units (Ravin).
Protease:
18–70 units (Free-Meyers).
Trypsin: (Anderson or as noted).
0–2 months: 110–160 units/mL.
2–6 months: 115–160 units/mL.
6–12 months: 120–290 units/mL; 3–10 units (Nothman et al).
1–2 years: 200–300 units/mL.
2–5 years: 200–275 units/mL.

pH
6–8.4.

Viscosity
< 3 minutes (Shwachman).

Feces

Chymotrypsin
3–14 mg/kg 72 h.

Fat, Percentage of Dry Weight
2–6 months: 5–43%.
6 months–6 years: 6–26%.

Fat, Total
2–6 months: 0.3–1.3 g/d.
6 months–1 year: < 4 g/d.
Children: < 3 g/d.
Adolescents: < 5 g/d.
Adults: < 7 g/d.

Lipids, Split Fat
Adults: > 40% of total lipids.

Lipids, Total
Adults: Up to 7 g/d on normal diet, 10–27% of dry weight.

Nitrogen
Infants: < 1 g/d.
Children: < 1.2 g/d.
Adults: < 3 g/d.

Urobilinogen
2–12 months: 0.03–14 mg/d.
5–10 years: 2.7–39 mg/d.
10–14 years: 7.3–99 mg/d.

Sweat

Electrolytes
Values for sodium or chloride or both. Elevated values in the presence of a family history or clinical findings of cystic fibrosis are diagnostic of cystic fibrosis.
Normal: < 55 mmol/L.
Borderline: 55–70 mmol/L.
Elevated: > 70 mmol/L.

Miscellaneous

Amylo-1,6-Glucosidase Debrancher (Liver)
> 1 μmol/min/g of wet tissue.

Chloride
Breast milk: 2.5–30 mmol/L.
Cow's milk: 20–80 mmol/L.
Muscle: 20–26 mmol/kg of wet fat-free tissue.
Spinal fluid: 120–128 mmol/L.

Copper (Liver)
< 20 μg/g of wet tissue.

Glucose 6-Phosphatase (Liver)
> 5 μmol/min/g of wet tissue.

Lactate Dehydrogenase (LDH) (CSF)
17–59 IU/L at 37 °C.

Potassium
Breast milk: 12–17 mmol/L.
Cow's milk: 20–45 mmol/L.
Muscle: 160–180 mmol/kg of wet fat-free tissue.

Proteins (CSF)
Total proteins:
Newborn: 40–120 mg/dL (0.4–1.2 g/L).
1 month: 20–70 mg/dL (0.2–0.7 g/L).
Thereafter: 15–40 mg/dL (0.15–0.4 g/L).
Gamma globulin:
Children: Up to 9% of total.
Adults: Up to 14% of total.

Sodium
Breast milk: 4.7–8.3 mmol/L.
Cow's milk: 22–26 mmol/L.
Muscle: 33–43 mmol/kg of wet fat-free tissue.

Index

Lange Medical Books are available at medical bookstores within the United States. To order directly from the publisher, complete and mail the postage-paid card below.

BASIC SCIENCE TEXTBOOKS

1. **Correlative Neuroanatomy & Functional Neurology, 19th Ed.**, *Chusid*, A0001-6, $21.50
2. **Biochemistry: A Synopsis**, *Colby*, A0033-9, $14.00
3. **Review of Medical Physiology, 13th Ed.**, *Ganong*, A8435-8, $24.00
4. **Physiology: A Study Guide**, *Ganong*, 2nd Ed., A7864-0, $16.50
5. **Review of Medical Microbiology, 17th Ed.**, *Jawetz et al.*, A8432-5, $22.00
6. **Basic Histology, 5th Ed.**, *Junquiera et al.*, A0570-0, $24.00
7. **Basic & Clinical Pharmacology, 3rd Ed.**, *Katzung*, A0553-6, $29.50
8. **Pharmacology: A Review**, *Katzung and Trevor*, A0031-3, $14.00
9. **Harper's Review of Biochemistry, 21st Ed.**, *Murray et al.*, A3648-1, $29.00
10. **Basic & Clinical Immunology, 6th Ed.**, *Stites et al.*, A0548-6, $29.00

CLINICAL SCIENCE TEXTBOOKS

11. **Principles of Clinical Electrocardiography, 12th Ed.**, *Goldman*, A0008-1, $22.00
12. **Review of General Psychiatry**, *Goldman*, A0030-5, $27.50
13. **Electrocardiography: Essentials of Interpretation**, *Goldschlager and Goldman*, A0029-7, $16.50
14. **Basic & Clinical Endocrinology, 2nd Ed.**, *Greenspan and Forsham*, A0547-8, $27.00
15. **General Urology, 11th Ed.**, *Smith*, A0009-9, $28.00
16. **Clinical Cardiology, 4th Ed.**, *Sokolow and McIlroy*, A0023-0, $26.50
17. **General Ophthalmology, 11th Ed.**, *Vaughan and Asbury*, A3108-6, $23.50

CURRENT CLINICAL REFERENCES

18. **Current Obstetric & Gynecologic Diagnosis & Treatment, 6th Ed.**, *Pernoll and Benson*, A1412-4, $34.50
19. **Current Pediatric Diagnosis & Treatment, 9th Ed.**, *Kempe et al.*, A1414-0, $31.50
20. **Current Medical Diagnosis & Treatment 1988, 27th Ed.**, *Schroeder et al.*, A1344-9, $32.50 (approx.)
21. **Current Emergency Diagnosis & Treatment, 2nd Ed.**, *Mills et al.*, A0027-1, $29.50
22. **Current Surgical Diagnosis & Treatment, 8th Ed.**, *Way*, A1415-7, $34.50

HANDBOOKS

23. **Handbook of Obstetrics & Gynecology, 8th Ed.**, *Benson*, A0014-9, $13.00
24. **Handbook of Poisoning, 12th Ed.**, *Dreisbach and Robertson*, A3643-2 $16.50
25. **Physician's Handbook, 21st Ed.**, *Krupp et al.*, A0002-4, $16.50
26. **Handbook of Pediatrics, 15th Ed.**, *Silver et al.*, A3635-8, $16.50

ORDER CARD

Please send the books I've circled below on 30-day approval:

1. Chusid, A0001-6, $21.50
2. Colby, A0033-9, $14.00
3. Ganong, A8435-8, $24.00
4. Ganong, A7864-0, $16.50
5. Jawetz, A8432-5, $22.00
6. Junquiera, A0570-0, $24.00
7. Katzung, A0553-6, $29.50
8. Katzung, A0031-3, $14.00
9. Murray, A3648-1, $29.00
10. Stites, A0548-6, $29.00
11. Goldman, A0008-1, $22.00
12. Goldman, A0030-5, $27.50
13. Goldschlager, A0029-7, $16.50
14. Greenspan, A0547-8, $27.00
15. Smith, A0009-9, $28.00
16. Sokolow, A0023-0, $26.50
17. Vaughan, A3108-6, $23.50
18. Pernoll, A1412-4, $34.50
19. Kempe, A1414-0, $31.50
20. Schroeder, A1344-9, $32.50
21. Mills, A0027-1, $29.50
22. Way, A1415-7, $34.50
23. Benson, A0014-9, $13.00
24. Dreisbach, A3643-2, $16.50
25. Krupp, A0002-4, $16.50
26. Silver, A3635-8, $16.50

☐ Payment enclosed. (Publisher pays postage & handling.) Please include your state sales tax.
☐ Bill me later.
Charge to: ☐ VISA ☐ Mastercard

Card #__________ Exp. Date______

Signature__________

NAME__________

ADDRESS__________

CITY/STATE/ZIP__________

Prices advertised are in U.S. dollars and applicable in the U.S. only. All prices are subject to change without notice.

In Canada, contact Prentice-Hall Canada, 1870 Birchmount Rd., Scarborough, Ontario M1P 2J7.

Outside the U.S. and Canada, contact Simon & Schuster Intl., Englewood Cliffs, NJ 07632.

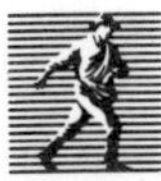

APPLETON & LANGE
25 Van Zant St.
E. Norwalk, CT 06855
Simon & Schuster Higher Education Group

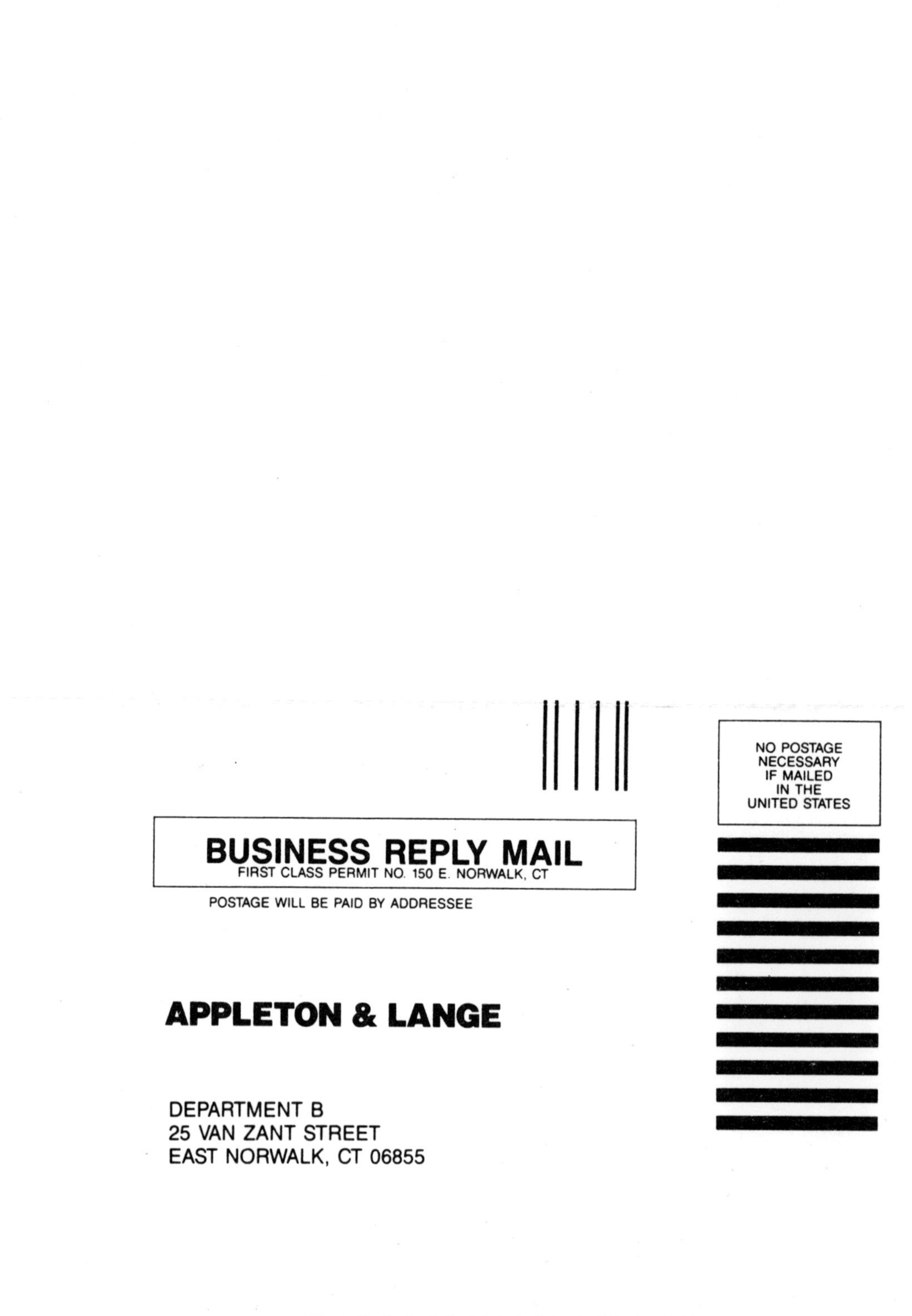
NO POSTAGE
NECESSARY
IF MAILED
IN THE
UNITED STATES
BUSINESS REPLY MAIL
FIRST CLASS PERMIT NO. 150 E. NORWALK, CT
POSTAGE WILL BE PAID BY ADDRESSEE
APPLETON & LANGE
DEPARTMENT B
25 VAN ZANT STREET
EAST NORWALK, CT 06855